MUSCULOSKELETAL IMAGING CASES

Editor: Jamshid Tehranzadeh, MD

The McGraw-Hill Radiology Series

Series Editor: Robert J. Ward, MD

This innovative series offers indispensable workstation reference material for the practicing radiologist. Within this series is a full range of practical, clinically relevant works divided into three categories:

- **Patterns:** Organized by modality, these books provide a pattern-based approach to constructing practical differential diagnoses.
- **Variants:** Structured by modality as well as anatomy, these graphic volumes aid the radiologist in reducing false positive rates.
- **Cases:** Classic case presentations with an emphasis on differential diagnoses and clinical context.

MUSCULOSKELETAL IMAGING CASES

Editor: Jamshid Tehranzadeh, MD
Director of Musculoskeletal Imaging
Chief of Radiology and Nuclear Medicine Imaging at Long Beach, VA
Emeritus Professor & Vice Chair of Radiology at
University of California (Irvine)

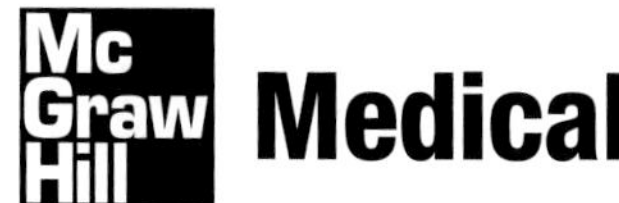

New York Chicago San Francisco Lisbon London Madrid Mexico City
Milan New Delhi San Juan Seoul Singapore Sydney Toronto

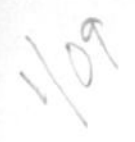

The McGraw-Hill Companies

Musculokseletal Imaging Cases

1 2 3 4 5 6 7 8 9 0 CTP/CTP 12 11 10 9 8

ISBN 978-0-07-146542-7
MHID 0-07-146542-1

Notice

Medicine is an ever-changing science. As new research and clinical experience broaden our knowledge, changes in treatment and drug therapy are required. The authors and the publisher of this work have checked with sources believed to be reliable in their efforts to provide information that is complete and generally in accord with the standards accepted at the time of publication. However, in view of the possibility of human error or changes in medical sciences, neither the authors nor the publisher nor any other party who has been involved in the preparation or publication of this work warrants that the information contained herein is in every respect accurate or complete, and they disclaim all responsibility for any errors or omissions or for the results obtained from use of the information contained in this work. Readers are encouraged to confirm the information contained herein with other sources. For example and in particular, readers are advised to check the product information sheet included in the package of each drug they plan to administer to be certain that changes have not been made in the recommended dose or in the contraindications for administration. This recommendation is of particular importance in connection with new or infrequently used drugs.

This book was set in TradeGothic Light by Aptara®, Inc.
The editors were Ruth W. Weinberg and Kim J. Davis
Project Management was provided by Sandhya Joshi, Aptara®, Inc.
The production supervisor was Phil Galea.
The designer was Eve Siegel; the cover designer was the Gazillion Group.
The index was prepared by Aptara®, Inc.
China Translation & Printing Service, Ltd., was the printer and binder.

This book is printed on acid-free paper.

Library of Congress Cataloging-in-Publication Data

Musculoskeletal imaging cases / editor, Jamshid Tehranzadeh.
p. ; cm. — (The McGraw-Hill radiology series)
Includes index.
ISBN-13: 978-0-07-146542-7 (hardcover : alk. paper)
ISBN-10: 0-07-146542-1 (hardcover : alk. paper) 1. Musculoskeletal system—Imaging—Case studies. I. Tehranzadeh, Jamshid, 1947- II. Series.
[DNLM: 1. Musculoskeletal Diseases—radiography—Case Reports. 2. Musculoskeletal System—radiography—Case Reports. 3. Diagnosis, Differential—Case Reports. 4. Diagnostic Imaging--Case Reports. WE 141 M9856 2009]
RC925.7.M8716 2009
616.7'07572—dc22

2008000307

To my wife, Shahla, to my children, Arash, Ashkan, and Anna,
and to the memory of my parents, Abraham and Rosy

CONTENTS

CONTRIBUTORS

Ibrahim F. Abdelwahab, MD
Forest Hills, New York

Tod G. Abrahams, MD
Clinical Professor, Department of Radiology, University of Vermont School of Medicine, Burlington, Vermont; Attending Radiologist and Chief, Musculoskeltal Section, Maine Medical Center, Portland, Maine

Alipasha Adrangui, MD
Department of Internal Medicine, University of Southern California, Los Angeles, California

Ashkan Afshin, MD
Department of Radiology, University of California, Irvine Medical Center, Orange, California

Atul Agarwal, MD
Resident, Department of Radiology, University of Southern California Medical Center, University of Southern California, Los Angeles, California

Piran Aliabadi, MD
Associate Professor of Radiology, Harvard Medical School, Brigham and Women's Hospital, Boston, Massachusetts

Maria Pia Altavilla, MD
Resident, Harbor UCLA Medical Center, Torrance, California

Arash Anavim, MD
Assistant Clinical Professor, Department of Radiological Sciences, University of California, Irvine, Orange, California

Janice C. Ancheta, MD
Resident, Department of Radiology, Harbor-UCLA Medical Center, Torrance, California

Derek R. Armfield, MD, MS
Diagnostic Radiologist, Department of Radiology, Jefferson Regional Medical Center, Pittsburgh, Pennsylvania

Oganes Ashikyan, MD
Chief Resident, Department of Radiological Sciences, University of California Irvine, Orange, California

Timothy Auran, MD
Department of Radiology, Harbor-UCLA Medical Center, Torrance, California

Eli J. Bendavid, MD
Director, Musculoskeletal Imaging, Department of Radiology, Good Samaritan Hospital, Los Angeles, California

Stefano Bianchi, MD
Consultant Radiologist, Institut de Radiologie, Clinique des Grangettes, Founding Member, Fondation des Grangettes, Geneva, Switzerland

Marcia F. Blacksin, MD
Professor, Department of Radiology, University of Medicine and Dentistry of New Jersey, Newark, New Jersey

Peyman Borghei, MD
Research Fellow, Department of Diagnostic Radiology, Division of Musculoskeletal Imaging, University of California Irvine Medical Center, Orange, California

Nathalie Boutry, MD
Doctor, Department of Musculoskeletal Radiology, Hospital Roger Salengro, Lille, France

Michael A. Bruno, MS, MD
Associate Professor of Radiology and Medicine, Penn State College of Medicine, Hershey, Pennsylvania

Charles H. Bush, MD
Clinical Assistant Professor, Department of Radiology, University of Florida College of Medicine, Gainesville, Florida

Michelle Chandler, MD
Health Sciences Assistant Clinical Professor, Radiology and Pediatrics, Children Hospital, Imaging Department, Oakland, California

Eric Chen, MD
Tustin, California

Kira Chow, MD
Assistant Professor, Musculoskeletal Imaging, Department of Radiology, David Geffen School of Medicine, University of California Los Angeles, Los Angeles, California

Anne Cotten, MD
Professor and Head of the Department of Musculoskeletal Radiology, Hospital Roger Salengro, Lille, France

James Coumas, MD
Musculoskeletal Radiologist, Charlotte Radiology; Carolina Healthcare System Charlotte, North Carolina

Neerjana Doda, MD
Clincial Associate, Department of Radiology, Changi General Hospital, Singapore

Joshua Farber, MD
Cincinnati, Ohio

Amilcare Gentili, MD
Department of Radiology, University of California, San Diego Thornton Hospital, La Jolla, California

Joseph C. Giaconi, MD
Radiology Resident, Keck School of Medicine, University of Southern California, Los Angeles, California

Melitus Maryam Golshan, MD
Tustin, California

Mohammad Reza Hayeri, MD
Research Fellow, Department of Radiology Science, University of California, Irvine, Orange, California

George Hermann, MD, FACR
Professor, Department of Radiology, Mount Sinai School of Medicine, New York, New York

Thomas L. Huang, MD, MS
Musculoskeletal Radiologist, BMC Diagnostics, Inc., Saint Mary's Medical Center, San Francisco, California

John C. Hunter, MD
Professor, Department of Radiology, UC Davis Medical Center, Sacramento, California

Hakan Ilaslan, MD
Assistant Professor of Radiology, Cleveland Clinic Lerner Medical College, Cleveland, Ohio

Joon Kim, MD
Musculoskeletal Fellow, Department of Radiology, University of California, David Geffen School of Medicine, Los Angeles, California

Scott Kingston, MD
Medical Director, Health South Diagnostic Center of Los Angeles, Consultant, Kerlan-Jobe Orthopedic Medical Group, Los Angeles, California

Ingrid B. Kjellin, MD
Musculoskeletal Radiologist,
Radsource
Brentwood, Tennessee

Rosemary J. Klecker, MD
Department of eRadiology, Cleveland Clinic, Independence, Ohio

Rajendra Kumar, MD, FACR
Professor of Radiology, Department of Diagnostic Radiology, The University of Texas M.D. Anderson Cancer Center, Houston, Texas

Raymond Kuo, MD
Staff Radiologist, Radnet Management, Inc., Orange, California

Roy C. Kwak, MD
Harbor-UCLA Medical Center, Torrance, California

Thomas Learch, MD
Department of Radiology, Musculoskeletal Radiology Section, Cedars-Sinai Medical Center, Los Angeles, California

Christopher Lee, MD
Department of Radiological Sciences, University of California Medical Center, Orange, California

Gregory T. Lee, MD
Department of Radiology, Harbor-UCLA Medical Center, Torrance, California

Stephen E. Ling, MD
Assistant Professor of Radiology, Temple University School of Medicine, Attending Radiologist, Temple University Health System, Philadelphia, Pennsylvania

Jeffrey N. Masi, MD
Resident, Department of Radiology, University of Southern California, Los Angeles, California

Sulabha Masih, MD
Clinical Professor of Radiology, University of California, Los Angeles Staff Radiologist, West Los Angeles Veteran's Administration, Los Angeles, California

Shahla Modarresi, MD
Clinical Assistant Professor, Department of Radiology, Veteran Administration Hospital/UCLA Medical Center, Los Angeles, California

Carlos Molina, MD
Resident, Department of Radiology, Harbor-UCLA Medical Center, Torrance, California

Sandra Leigh Moore, MD
NYU Medical Center and Medical School, Department of Radiology, Musculoskeletal Division, New York, New York

Mélanie Morel, MD
Doctor, Department of Musculoskeletal Radiolgy, Hospital Roger Salengro, Lille, France

Edward Mossop, MD
Resident Internal Medicine, Cedars-Sinai Medical Center, Los Angeles, California

Daria Motamedi, MD
Resident, Department of Radiology, Cedar-Sinai Medical Center, Los Angeles, California

Kambiz Motamedi, MD
Assistant Professor, Musculoskeletal Imaging, Department of Radiology, David Geffen School of Medicine at UCLA, Los Angeles, California

Ayodale S. Odulate, MD
Clinical Fellow in Radiology, Harvard Medical School, Brigham and Women's Hospital, Boston, Massachusetts

Janis Owen, MD
Department of Radiology, King-Drew Medical Center, Los Angeles, California

Nuttya Pattamapasong, MD
Instructor, Department of Radiology, Faculty of Medicine, Chiang Mai University, Chiang Mai, Thailand

Wilfred CG Peh, MD
Senior Consultant Radiologist, Alexandra Hospital, Singapore; Clinical Professor of Diagnostic Radiology, National University of Singapore, Singapore; Visiting Consulting Radioloist, Changi General Hospital, Singapore; Visiting Consultant Radiologist, KK Women's and Children's Hospital, Singapore

Albert Quan, MD
Department of Radiological Sciences, University of California Medical Center, Orange, California

William R. Reinus, MD
Vice Chairman and Professor of Radiology and Chief, Musculoskeletal and Trauma Radiology, Temple University Medical School, Philadelphia, Pennsylvania

Zehava Sadka Rosenberg, MD
Professor of Radiology and Orthopedic Surgery, New York University School of Medicine, New York, New York

Amita Sapra, MD
Department of Radiology, Section of Musculoskeletal Radiology, LA County/USC Medical Center, Los Angeles, California

Alya Sheikh, MD
Chief Cardiothoracic Imaging Harbor-UCLA Medical Center, Assistant Professor of Radiological Sciences, David Geffen School of Medicine at UCLA, Los Angeles, California

John Shin, MD
Department of Radiology, University of California, Irvine Medical Center, Orange, California

Robert D. Simon, MD
Department of Radiology, Harbor-UCLA Medical Center, Torrance, California

Lynne Steinbach, MD
Professor of Clinical Radiology and Orthopaedic Surgery, Department of Radiology, University of California San Francisco, San Francisco, California

Gideon Strich, MD
Associate Clinical Professor, Department of Radiology, University of California, Irvine, Orange, California

Cliff Tao, DC, DACBR
Chiropractic Radiologist, Private Practice of Chiropractic Radiology, Orange County, California; Assistant Professor of Radiology, Southern California University of Health Sciences, Whitier, California

Arash Tehranzadeh, MD
Musculoskeletal Radiology Division, Centinela Radiology Medical Group, Kerlan-Jobe Orthopaedic Clinic, Anaheim, California

Jamshid Tehranzadeh, MD
Director of Musculoskeletal Imaging
Chief of Radiology and Nuclear Medicine Imaging at VALBHS
Emeritus Professor & Vice Chair of Radiology at University of California (Irvine)

Stephen Thomas, MD
University of Pittsburgh, Pittsburgh, Pennsylvania

Jimmy Ton, MD
Diagnostic Radiology Resident, Morristown Memorial Hospital, Morristown, New Jersey

Hamidreza R. Torshizy, MD
Department of Radiology, University of California, Irvine Medical Center, Orange, California

Binh-To Tran, MD
Harbor-UCLA Medical Center, Torrance, California

Rajeev K. Varma, MD
Chief, Musculoskeletal Radiology, Assistant Clinical Professor of Radiological Sciences,
David Geffen School of Medicine at UCLA, Los Angeles, California

Tatiana Voci, MD
Tatiana Voci, MD, Inc., Los Angeles, California

Minh-Chau Vu, MD
Harbor-UCLA, Los Angeles, California

Robert J. Ward, MD
Chief, Division of Musculoskeletal Imaging,
Department of Radiology, Tufts Medical Center, Boston, Massachusetts

Sailaja Yadavalli, MD, PhD
Staff Radiologist, Musculoskeletal Division,
Department of Radiology, William Beaumont Hospital, Royal Oak, Michigan

Adam C. Zoga, MD
Assistant Professor of Radiology,
Director of Ambulatory Imaging Services and Musculoskeletal MRI,
Thomas Jefferson University Hospital,
Philadelphia, Pennsylvania

FOREWORD

I am deeply honored to be able to write a foreword for this first-rate educational endeavor, *Musculoskeletal Imaging Cases*, and I do so for a number of reasons. First, I have known the author and editor of this text, Dr. Jamshid Tehranzadeh, for over 20 years, and I recognize his credentials as a world-class educator. Jim is dedicated and enthusiastic, and his approach to teaching is effective and based on considerable experience at the podium, viewbox, and computer console. Second, I am a true fan of a case-based approach as a uniquely personal way of getting teaching points across and, in many ways, far better than the traditional method of presenting material in textbook format. Third, the success of any educational tool is based on thoughtful organization, and this book, among many other fine attributes, is highly organized.

The material for this text has been contributed by over 50 authors who come from the United States and abroad. Each brings to the table his/her own set of teaching credentials. Although the style of one contributor may vary somewhat from that of another, the fabric of this book is tightly woven into an easy and uniform read. This is critical, ensuring that the reader can move effortlessly from one case to a second, and so forth. The subject material includes all of the musculoskeletal conditions that might be encountered in a busy private practice, although cases related to sports medicine and trauma are presented initially and most extensively. This makes perfect sense because of the prominent role played by MR imaging in the assessment of such cases. But congenital, metabolic, systemic, articular, neoplastic, and infectious disorders are not forgotten, each covered in turn. The text that accompanies each case is carefully and succinctly written, containing all the pearls and hints that could be asked for. Differential diagnostic considerations are included, and the illustrations are carefully chosen for their clarity and appropriateness. A regional approach is employed, with individual chapters dealing with all of the major anatomical skeletal locations.

Based on personal experience, I know full well the considerable time and energy that are required to bring a project like this to fruition. I know also that the process of writing and editing has its "great moments" that are occasionally separated by periods of doubt and frustration. It takes a qualified and dedicated person who takes prime responsibility for the whole process in order to ensure that the final product is worth the wait. Clearly, Jamshid Tehranzadeh was the right person for this job, and he should be proud of what he has accomplished. We, the readers, will benefit greatly from Jim's efforts. With this in mind, I am honored to be able to offer this foreword to mark the publication of a terrific educational tool.

Donald Resnick, MD
Professor of Radiology
University of California, San Diego

PREFACE

Case-based and problem-based learning are rapidly being adopted in professional programs in medicine, business, law, engineering, and technology. As a student and a teacher for more than 50 years I know case studies are the most effective way of learning. A case will allow the reader to address more than one goal at a time. I have always been more intrigued and stimulated by studying and analyzing an interesting case than by reading a general topic about a subject. Studying a case is like reading a true story; it stimulates your curiosity and makes you think. In choosing a good case one should consider the importance of the potential learning issue. Is it central to the diagnosis, or is the case too difficult or too mundane or just right? Is it relevant for everyday practice or so bizarre that no one really cares about it? Is the case open-ended enough to stimulate the reader to go beyond fact finding? Is the text relevant to the case; is it too short or too long? Does it provide pertinent differential diagnosis? Does it tell you how to distinguish this condition from other conditions that may present similarly or masquerade the same appearance? Does the text provide you with pearls or the highlight of current literature about this condition? And finally are the findings in the main case and differential diagnosis well illustrated and present superb image quality?

The objective of this book is to provide the above points and present a comprehensive collection of cases that are relevant and constitute the core of knowledge that a musculoskeletal radiologist must know. The thrust of this book is to present interesting and relevant cases using advance imaging modalities such MRI, CT, US, and scintigraphy. What makes this book unique is that over 70 contributors from the United States and different corners of the globe have contributed to the pool of the cases presented here.

Coverage begins with conditions of the shoulder and ends with ankle and foot and finally spine and miscellaneous cases. In each joint section, sport medicine and trauma cases are discussed first then congenital, systemic and metabolic diseases followed by arthritis and connective tissue and crystal deposition disorders, then infection and tumor and tumor-like lesions and miscellaneous conditions.

I am highly indebted to all of the contributors to this book for their great support and priceless contributions. I would also like to thank my research fellows, Dr. Ashkan Afshin, Dr. Peyman Borghei, and Dr. Maryam Golshan, for their assistance in writing their cases and helping me coordinate materials for the publisher. I am also indebted to McGraw-Hill's Senior Editor, Ruth Weinberg, for her support and constructive guidance. Thanks to Dr. Robert J. Ward for his contribution and helpful critiques. And last but not least thanks to Kim Davis, the Project Development Editor of McGraw-Hill, who turned my submission into a wonderful book.

Jamshid Tehranzadeh, MD

SECTION I

SHOULDER

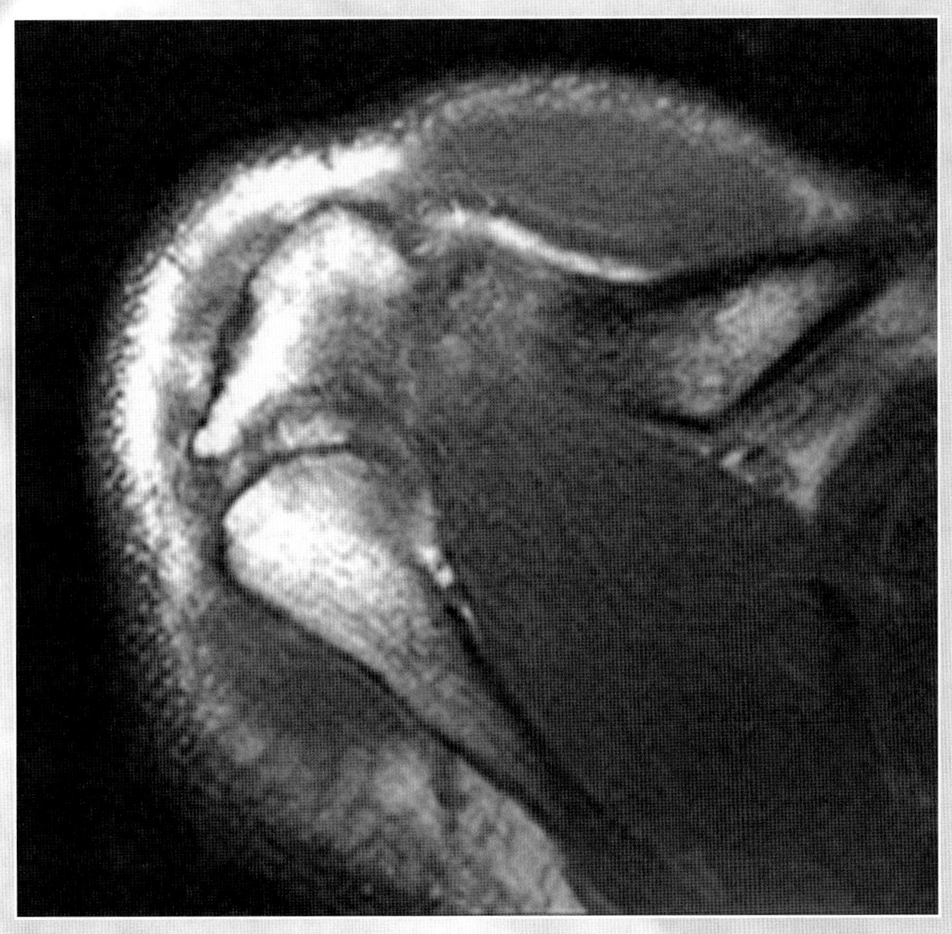

Chapter 1

Sport Medicine and Trauma

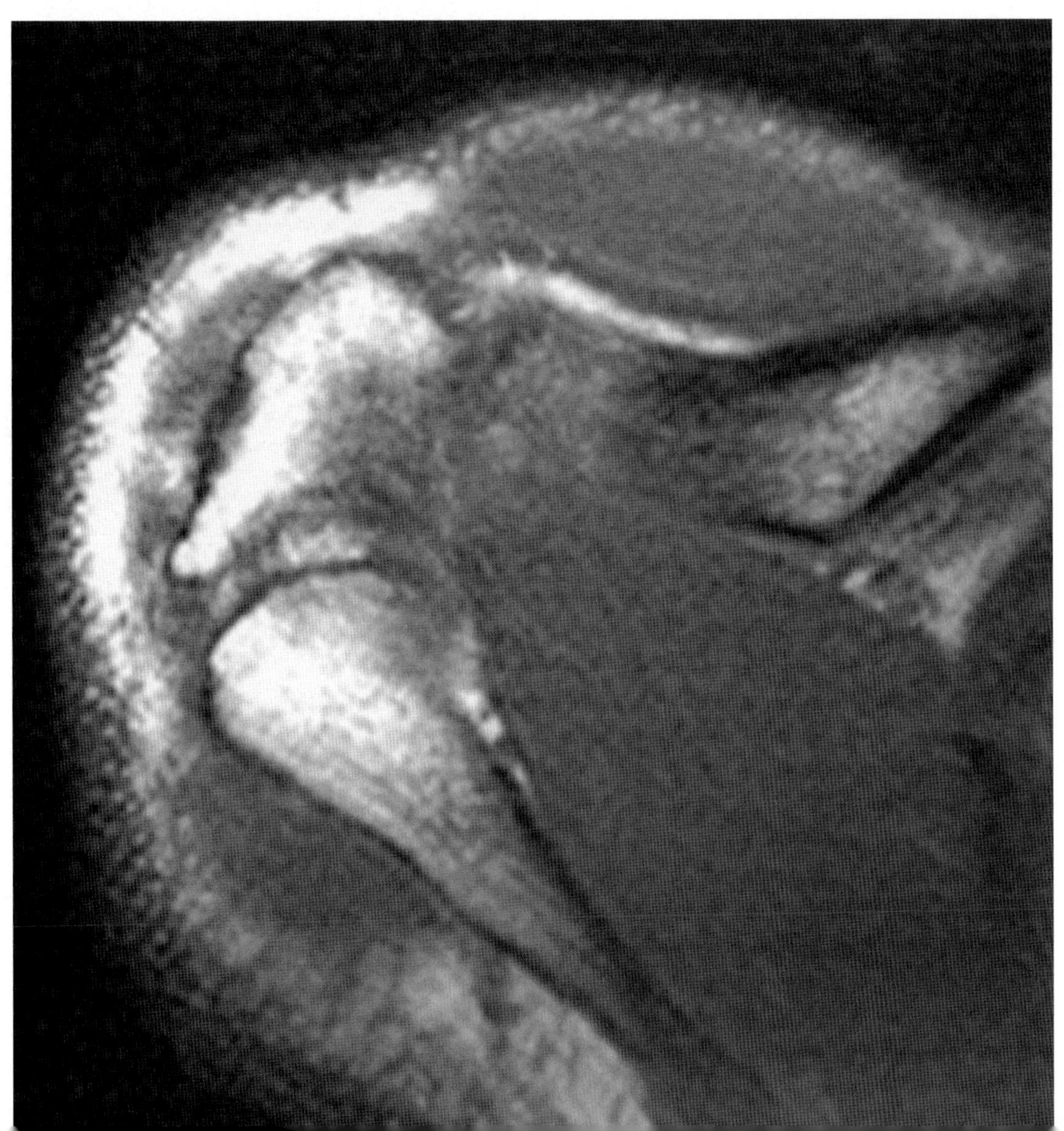

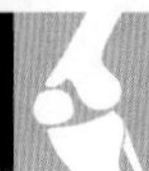

1–1 Os Acromiale

Ashkan Afshin and Jamshid Tehranzadeh

PRESENTATION

Pain with overhead activities

FINDINGS

MR images demonstrate an extra ossicle known as os acromiale between acromial process and the clavicle.

DIFFERENTIAL DIAGNOSES

- *Calcific tendinosis of supraspinatus tendon:* Calcium hydroxyapatite deposition in the tendon and or the bursa of supraspinatus is associated with severe pain and tendinosis.
- *Curved acromion (type II):* This curve-shaped acromion process (43% of shoulders) is associated with higher incidence of impingement of the rotator cuff tendon.
- *Hooked acromion (type III):* This hook-shaped acromion (40% of shoulders) has the highest association with impingement of the rotator cuff tendon.

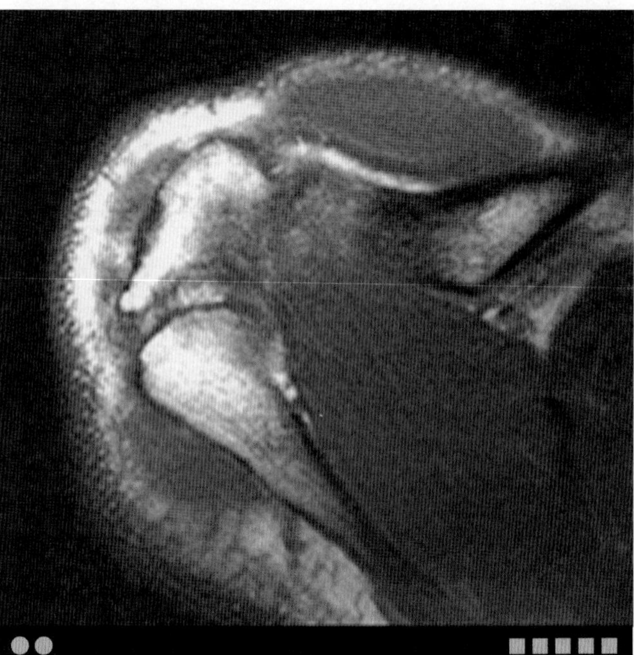

A. Os acromiale: Axial T1WI shows os acromiale located in the corner between acromion process posteriorly and clavicle anteriorly.

COMMENTS

Os acromiale is an anatomical condition resulting from the failure of an anterior acromial ossification center to fuse to the acromial process. At age 15, three separate ossification centers appear in the acromion: preacromion, mesacromion, and metacromion. These centers should fuse by age 22 to 25. Failure of one of these three ossification centers causes one of four subtypes of os acromiale: preacromion, mesacromion, metacromion, and basiacromion types. The most common sites of fusion failure are at the mesacromion and metacromion.

Os acromiale is a relatively rare condition. Its frequency has been documented in radiographic and anatomical studies to be between 1% and 15%, of which 62% are bilateral. Patients may show impingement-like symptoms including chronic pain, stiffness, and weakness of the shoulder with limited range of motion. They will also experience localized tenderness. Os acromiale has strong association with rotator cuff tear. The double-density sign on a standard anteroposterior radiograph of the shoulder and a cortical irregularity on the supraspinatus outlet view are highly suggestive of an os acromiale. MR images of the shoulder of patient with os acromiale demonstrate that the anterior portion of the acromion is ununited with the remainder of the acromion. Os acromiale is often mistaken for a fracture on the axial view.

PEARLS

- **Caused by failure of one of three ossification centers**
- **Unfused acromial apophysis**
- **Mesacromion is the most common subtype**
- **Associated with impingement-like symptoms and localized tenderness**
- **Highly associated with rotator cuff tears**

ADDITIONAL IMAGES

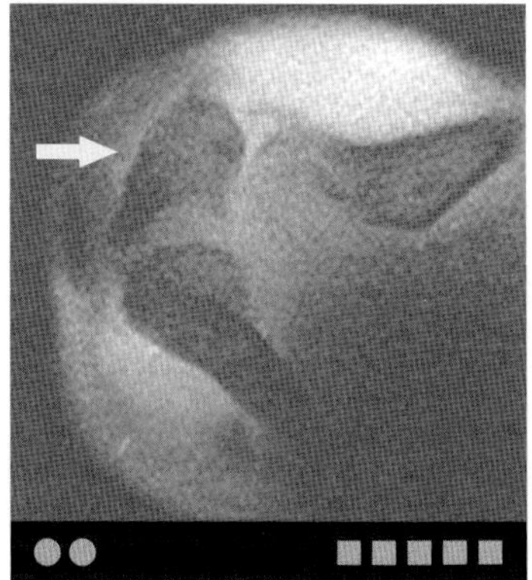

B. Os acromiale: Axial gradient echo image of the shoulder shows os acromiale (arrow).

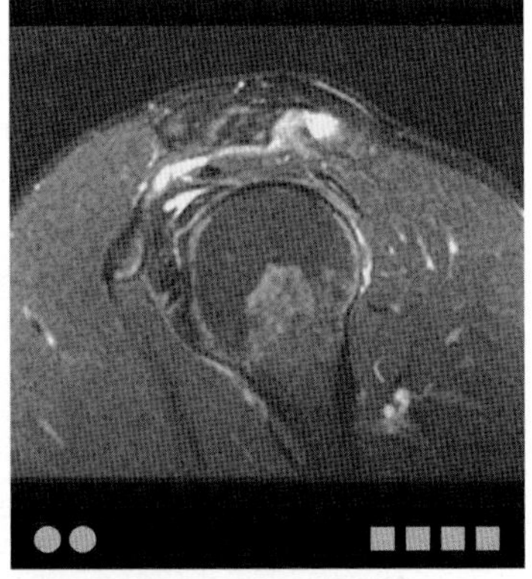

C. Os acromiale: Sagittal fat-saturated T2-weighted image shows os acromiale posterior to distal tip of clavicle.

DIFFERENTIAL DIAGNOSES IMAGES

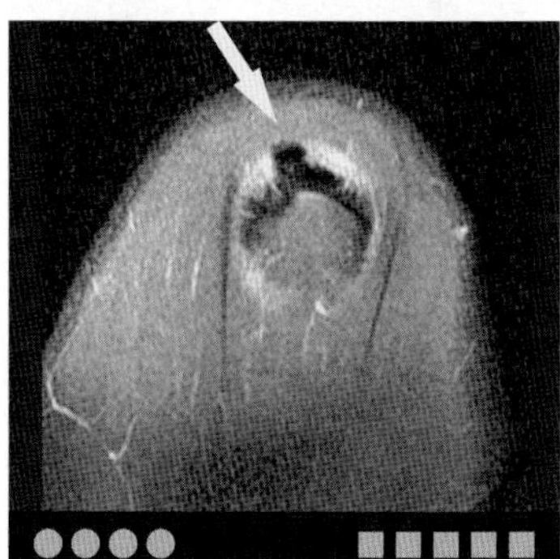

D. Calcific tendinosis of supraspinatus tendon: Sagittal fat-saturated T2-weighted image shows focal dark signal (arrow) at the supraspinatus tendon near subdeltoid bursa consistent with calcific tendinosis and bursitis.

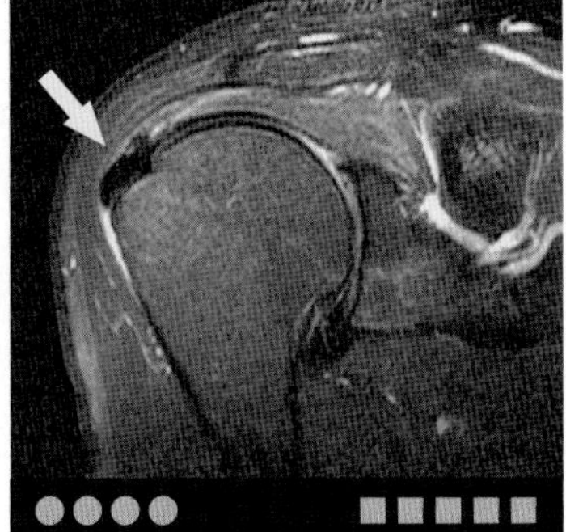

E. Calcific tendinosis of supraspinatus tendon: Coronal fat-saturated T2-weighted image shows calcification in the form of dark signal at the supraspinatus tendon at the insertion site to the greater tuberosity consistent with calcific tendinosis.

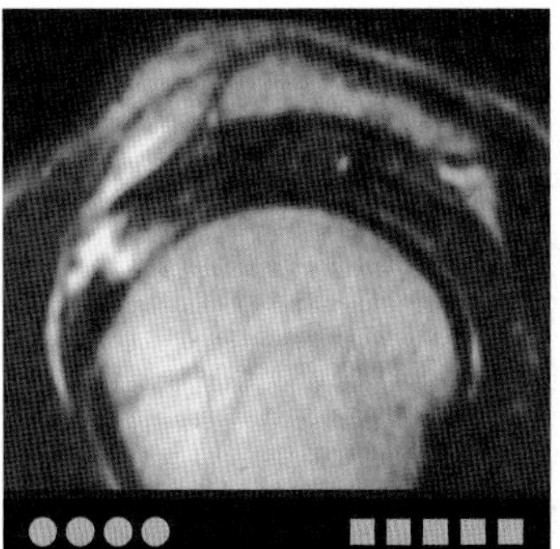

F. Curved acromion (type II): Sagittal T2-weighted image shows curved acromion (type II) associated with full-thickness tear of supraspinatus tendon.

IMAGE KEY

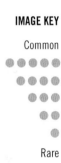

Typical

Unusual

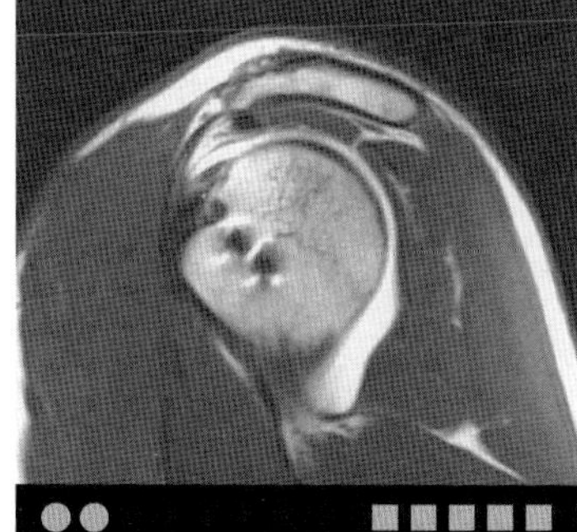

G. Hooked acromion (type III): Sagittal T1 MR arthrogram shows hooked acromion (type III) in a patient who has been previously operated for rotator cuff repair with metallic anchors artifact.

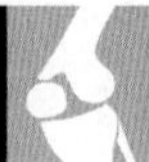

1–2 Calcific Tendinosis of Supraspinatus Tendon

Amilcare Gentili

PRESENTATION

Shoulder pain

FINDINGS

A focal area of low signal intensity, corresponding to large focus of calcification, is present in the supraspinatus tendon.

DIFFERENTIAL DIAGNOSES

- *Rotator cuff tear:* On MR imaging fluid signal is seen in the tear.
- *Greater tuberosity fracture:* Usually a history of direct trauma can be elicited.
- *Impingement:* Symptoms of impingement and calcific tendinosis may overlap since calcium deposit in the tendon may cause impingement.

COMMENTS

Calcific tendinosis is caused by the deposition of hydroxyapatite crystals in the tendons. Calcific tendinosis usually affects middle-aged persons, with a slightly male predilection. Patients with calcific tendinosis around the shoulder may be completely asymptomatic or may present with acute severe pain or chronic or recurrent symptoms of pain of varying severity. The pain my cause limitation in range of motion, which is similar to symptoms of rotator cuff tears. The supraspinatus tendon is the most commonly involved tendon of the rotator cuff, but any tendon can be involved. Different phases of the disease have been described. In the first phase, or the silent phase, calcium is contained within the tendon. There are minimal, if any, clinical signs and symptoms. MR imaging shows calcification within an otherwise normal tendon. In the second phase, or the mechanical phase, calcium deposit increases in size and produces an elevation of the floor of the subacromial bursa. At this stage, elevated tension within the tendon produces pain and an accompanying bursitis may be present because of mass effect on the bursa. MR imaging may demonstrate fluid in the subacromial bursa. In the third phase, adhesive periarthritis is seen. In this stage, calcium deposits of variable size are present in the tendon and an adhesive bursitis is also seen. MR imaging shows fluid and calcification in the bursa and inflammation in the surrounding tissues. In the fourth phase, intraosseous extension of calcium deposits is present. This phase is rarely seen and can be confused with the presence of intraosseous neoplasms.

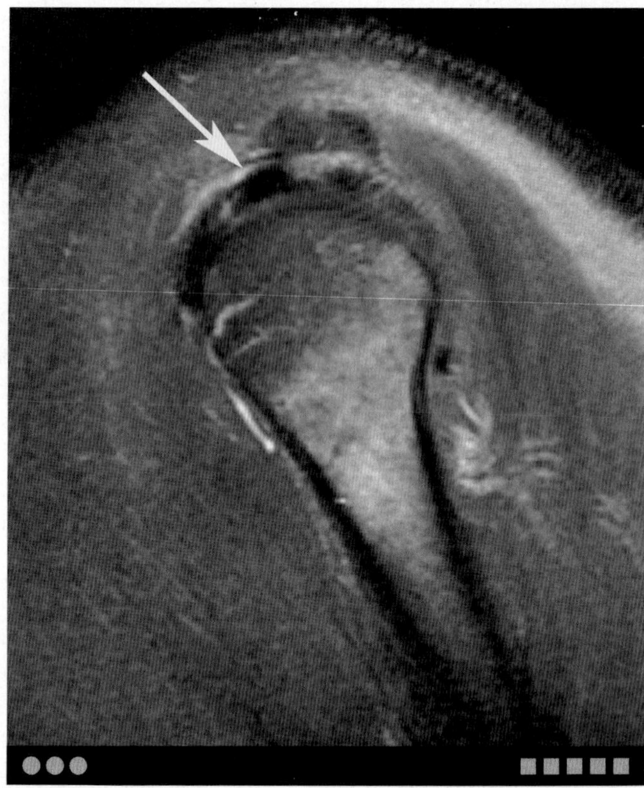

A. Calcific tendonitis of supraspinatus tendon: Sagittal T2-weighted fat-suppressed MR image shows a focal area (arrow) of low signal intensity within the supraspinatus tendon.

PEARLS

- **Radiographs are useful in confirming the diagnosis**
- **Inflammatory changes may be present surrounding the calcification and may simulate a rotator cuff tear**

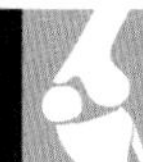

ADDITIONAL IMAGES

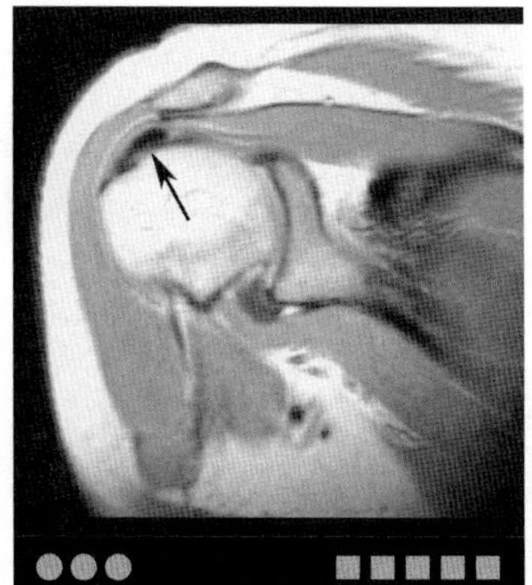

B. Calcific tendonitis of supraspinatus tendon: Coronal T1-weighted MR image shows a focal area (arrow) of low signal intensity within the supraspinatus tendon.

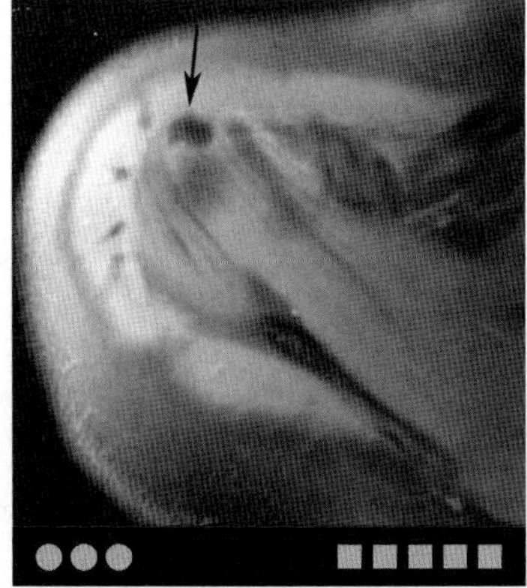

C. Calcific tendonitis of supraspinatus tendon: Axial gradient echo MR image shows a focal area (arrow) of low signal intensity within the supraspinatus tendon.

DIFFERENTIAL DIAGNOSES IMAGES

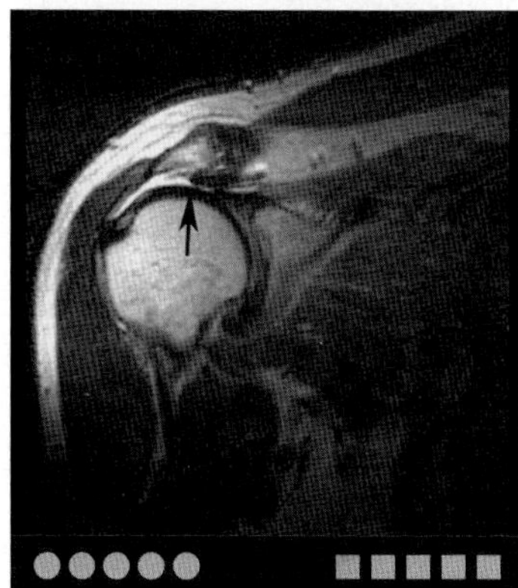

D. Rotator cuff tear: Coronal T2-weighted MR image shows a large tear of the supraspinatus tendon with retraction of the torn tendon (arrow).

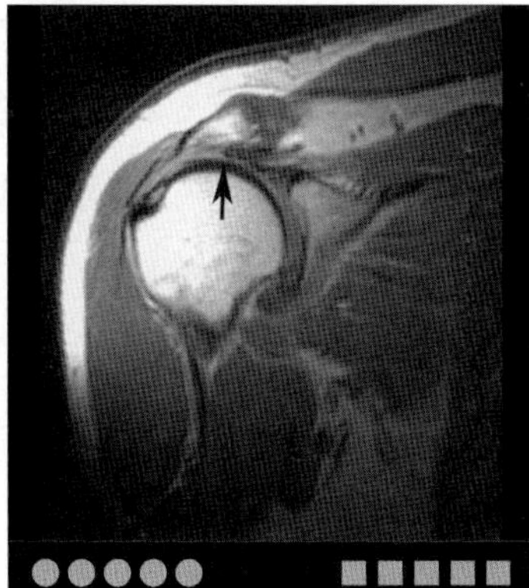

E. Rotator cuff tear: Coronal T1-weighted MR image shows a large tear of the supraspinatus tendon with retraction of the torn tendon (arrow).

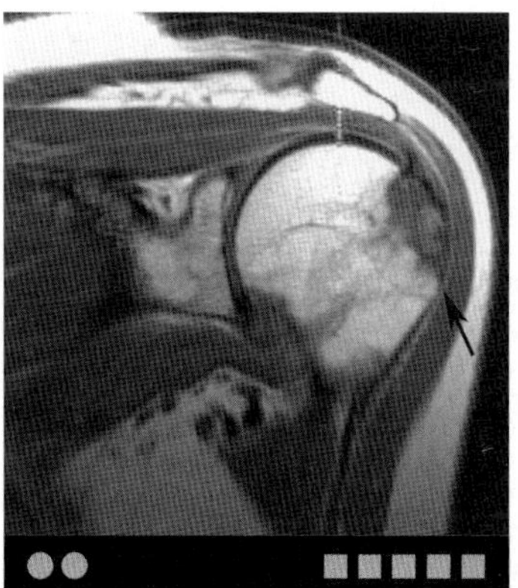

F. Greater tuberosity fracture: Coronal T1-weighted MR image shows an undisplaced fracture (arrow) of the greater tuberosity of the humerus.

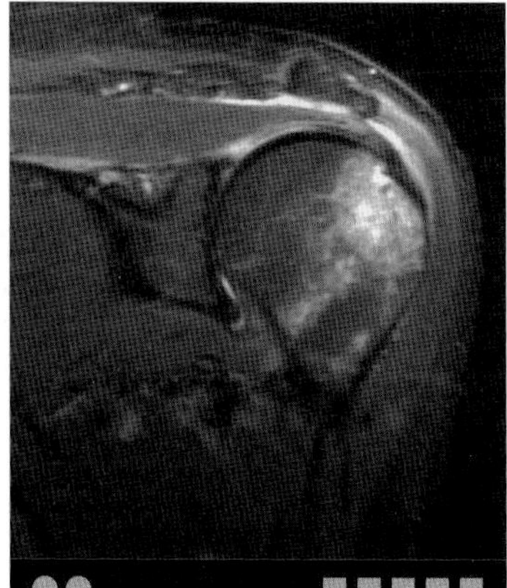

G. Greater tuberosity fracture: Coronal T2-weighted fat suppressed MR image shows extensive bone marrow edema in the greater tuberosity of the humerus (arrow).

IMAGE KEY

Common

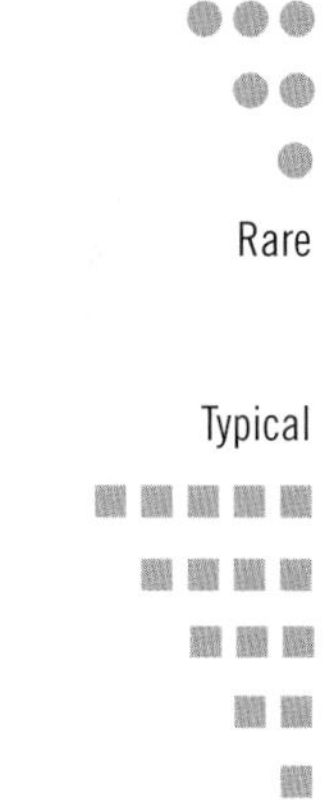

Rare

Typical

Unusual

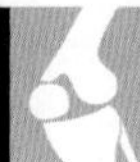

1–3 Geyser Phenomenon After Full-Thickness Rotator Cuff Tear

Marcia F. Blacksin

PRESENTATION

Supraclavicular mass

FINDINGS

Supraspinatus tendon tear, allowing fluid in the acromial–clavicular (AC) joint to form a supraclavicular bursa.

DIFFERENTIAL DIAGNOSES

- *Lymphadenopathy:* Lymph node chains occupy the supraclavicular region. Lymph node enlargement can be seen with infectious etiologies like tuberculosis.
- *Neurofibroma:* The brachial plexus can rise to pathologic processes. Neurofibromatosis will predispose patients for development of peripheral nerve sheath tumors like schwannoma and neurofibromas.

COMMENTS

Chronic rotator cuff tears are often seen with effusions, and may be massive, with more than one tendon torn. When the torn cuff retracts, there is no soft tissue occupying the space between the glenohumeral joint and the AC joint. This allows joint fluid to enter the AC joint, and as the volume increases, an adventitial bursa may form proximal to the AC joint. The "geyser" is the extravasation of fluid from the joint, into the cuff tear, and erupting through the AC joint. Extravasation of fluid from the bursa will cause increased pain and soft tissue edema. Patients with massive rotator cuff tears can be sent for examination of the supraclavicular masses or because of pain in this region, which is actually caused by these bursae. Evaluation of bursae in this region must always include an assessment of the rotator cuff. Other soft tissue masses in this region include masses related to peripheral nerve sheath tumors and lymphadenopathy. Peripheral nerve sheath tumors are sharply marginated and usually oval or round in shape. Neurofibromas can demonstrate a low signal intensity center or "target sign" on T2-weighted images. Peripheral nerve sheath tumors of the extremities show variable enhancement with gadolinium, and can be best seen on T2-weighted images. A conglomerate of enlarged lymph nodes can also present as a supraclavicular mass. These findings can be seen with head and neck tumors, lymphoma, and infectious etiologies like tuberculosis or cat scratch disease.

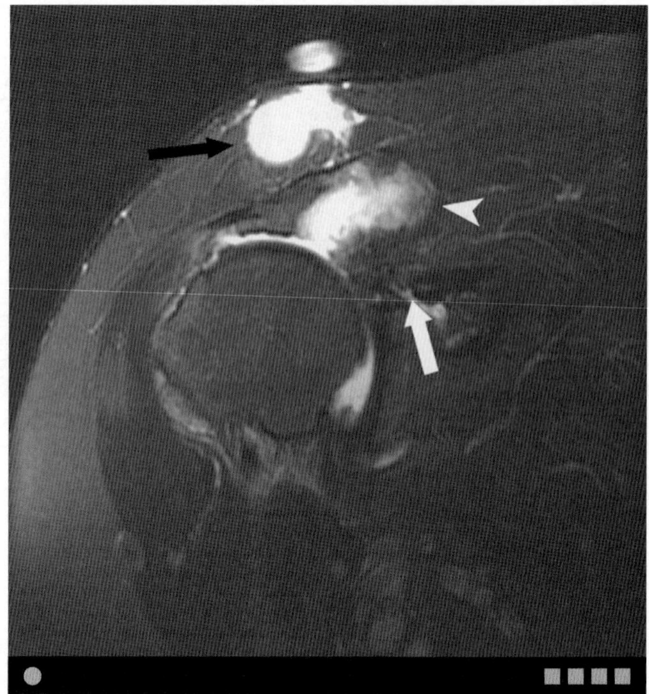

A. Geyser phenomenon: Coronal fat-saturated T2-weighted MR shows fluid-filled bursa proximal to the AC joint (black arrow). Full thickness retracted supraspinatus tear (white arrow) and fluid extravasating from joint, through cuff into AC joint (arrowhead).

PEARLS

- **Massive rotator cuff tears can show supraclavicular bursitis masquerading as soft tissue masses.**
- **Evaluation of soft tissue masses around the shoulder should, if possible, always include some assessment of the joint and relationship of the mass to the capsule.**
- **Other common soft tissue masses in the supraclavicular region include lymphadenopathy and neurofibromata.**

ADDITIONAL IMAGES

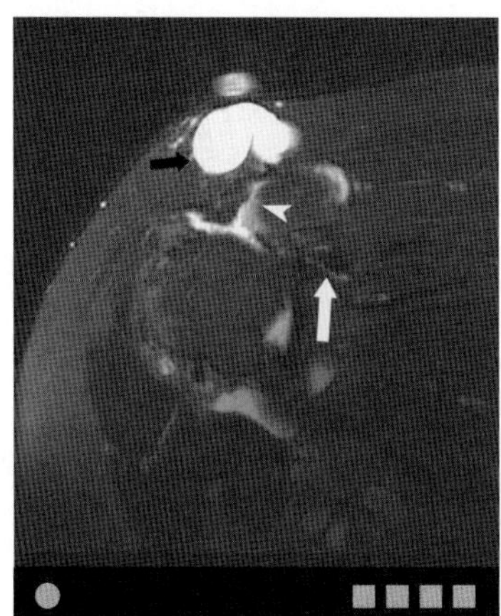

B. Geyser phenomenon: Sagittal fat-saturated T2-weighted MR shows fluid-filled bursa proximal to the AC joint (black arrow). Full thickness retracted supraspinatus tear (white arrow) and fluid extravasating from joint, through cuff into AC joint (arrowhead).

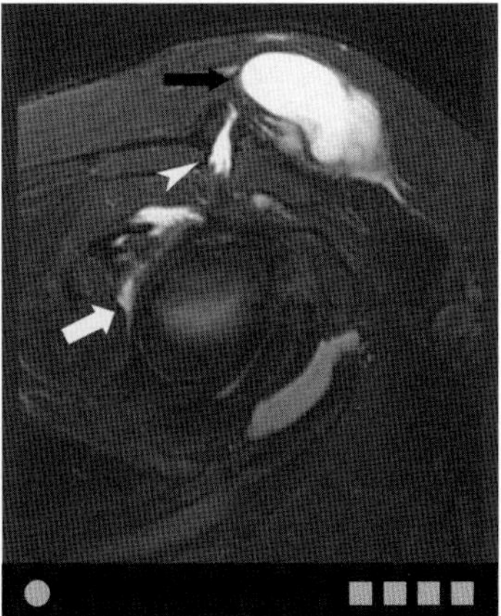

C. Geyser phenomenon: Sagittal fat-saturated T2-weighted image shows bursa (black arrow), fluid entering AC joint (arrowhead), and tear of infraspinatus tendon, partial (white arrow).

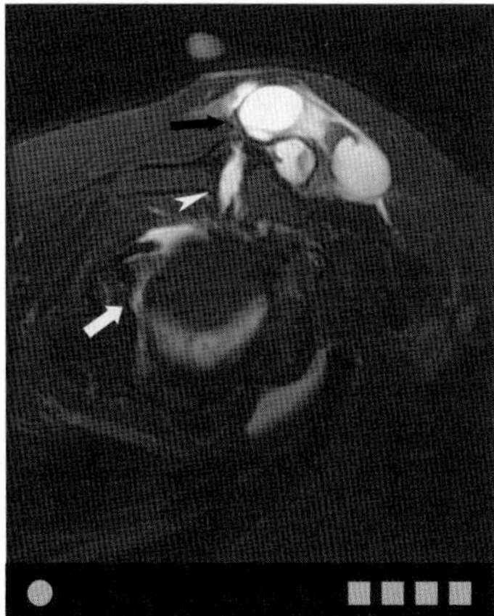

D. Geyser phenomenon: Sagittal fat-saturated T2-weighted image shows bursa (black arrow), fluid entering AC joint (arrowhead), and tear of infraspinatus tendon, partial (white arrow).

DIFFERENTIAL DIAGNOSES IMAGES

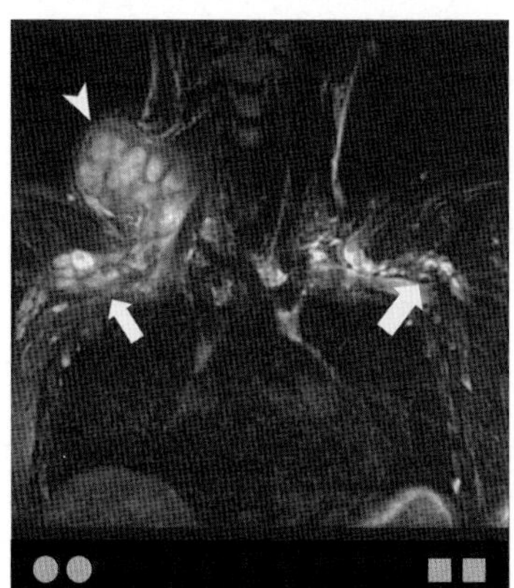

E. Neurofibroma: Coronal fat-saturated T2-weighted image in patient with neurofibromatosis shows extensive involvement of bilateral brachial plexus with neurofibromata (white arrows). Enlarging brachial conglomerate in right neck is noted (arrowhead).

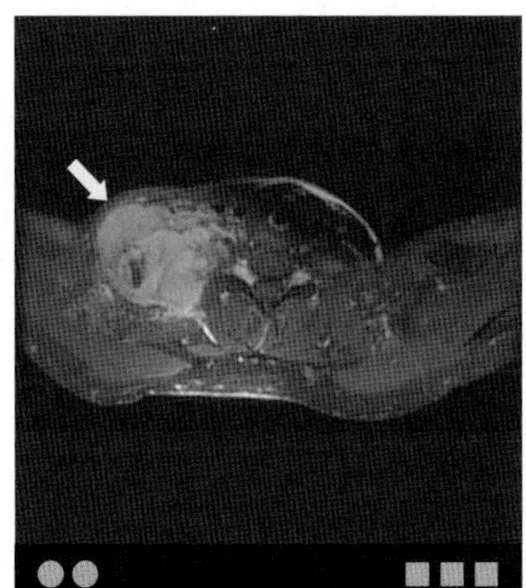

F. Neurofibroma: Axial fat-saturated T1-weighted image after contrast shows significant enhancement of mass (arrow) with low signal central target sign. This mass was not malignant.

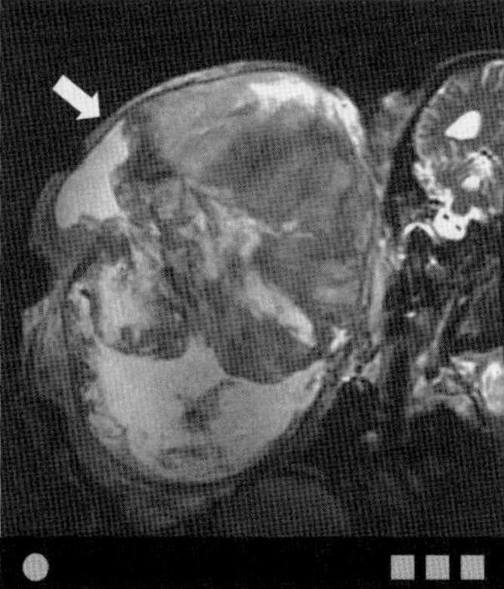

G. Neurofibrosarcoma: Coronal fat-saturated T2-weighted image shows large necrotic neurofibrosarcoma of brachial plexus (arrow) in a patient with neurofibromatosis. Head deviated by mass.

IMAGE KEY

Common

Rare

Typical

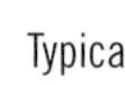

Unusual

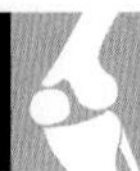

1–4 Full-Thickness Partial-Width Supraspinatus Tear Using Multidetector CT

Joshua Farber

PRESENTATION

Shoulder pain

FINDINGS

Multidetector computed tomography (MDCT) reformatted image (MPR) of the right shoulder after arthrography demonstrates contrast extending through the supraspinatus tendon, infiltrating from anterior to the midportion. The posterior portion of the supraspinatus is intact.

DIFFERENTIAL DIAGNOSES

- *Full-thickness full-width (complete) tear of the supraspinatus tendon:* Full-thickness full-width tears involve the entire tendon and the tendon is often retracted.
- *Full-thickness partial-width pinhole tear of the supraspinatus tendon:* Pinhole tears involve a small, discrete portion of the tendon.
- *Partial-thickness supraspinatus tear:* No contrast from the arthrogram should extend from the shoulder joint through the tendon and into the subacromial bursa in the absence of a full-thickness tear.

COMMENTS

This 73-year-old female patient presented with right shoulder pain and was suspected to have rotator cuff pathology; since she had a cardiac pacemaker, MRI exam was contraindicated. Therefore, an MDCT arthrogram was performed. The arthrographic technique involves injecting 10cc to 15 cc of full strength contrast by using a 22 gauge 3.5 inch spinal needle under fluoroscopic guidance. The patient is then scanned with an MDCT with the shoulder in external rotation. Axial slices, 2 mm, are obtained at 1-mm intervals with a pitch of less than one. The thin, overlapping slices create an essentially isotropic data set that allows for robust MPR images. The low pitch allows high mAs (300–400) to scan through the chest wall. This combination of factors produces high-resolution images with excellent detail. The MPR images are 2-mm thick. Rotator cuff tears are common in elderly people, many of whom have contraindications for MRI. MDCT arthrography is an excellent alternative in this patient population and is useful in postoperative patients as well, who may have a large amount of metal in the joint. In addition to diagnosing the rotator cuff tears, MDCT arthrography offers information about the health of the "nontorn" cuff as well. In the current case, for example, contrast is seen extending into the anterior tendon. This process is called "imbibition" and indicates the presence of a diseased, friable cuff that may respond poorly to surgery. This information, obviously, is useful to a surgeon who may attempt a repair. MDCT arthrography also allows evaluation of the labrum, biceps anchors, ligaments, and bony structures about the joint.

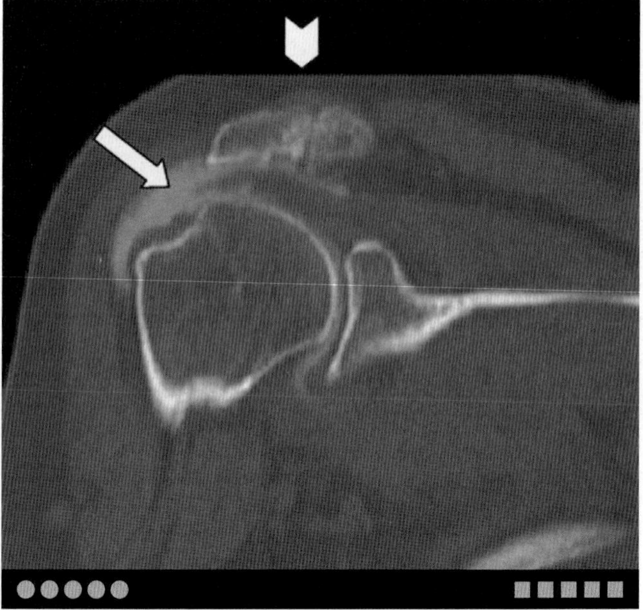

A. Full-thickness partial-width supraspinatus tear: Coronal MPR image from a right shoulder MDCT arthrogram demonstrates contrast extension through the supraspinatus tendon, indicating a full-thickness tear (arrow). Note also the degenerative disease involving the acromio-clavicular joint (arrow head).

PEARLS

- **Rotator cuff tears have width as well as thickness, and the sagittal images in MDCT arthrography or MRI often best demonstrate the extent of the width.**
- **Imbibition of contrast by a tendon is a sign of disease and often indicates a poor surgical outcome.**
- **MDCT arthrography is an excellent imaging modality for patients who have a contraindication to MRI or who have significant amounts of metal in the joint.**
- **Proper scanning technique is essential to produce diagnostic images.**

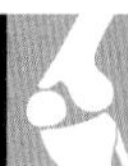

ADDITIONAL IMAGES

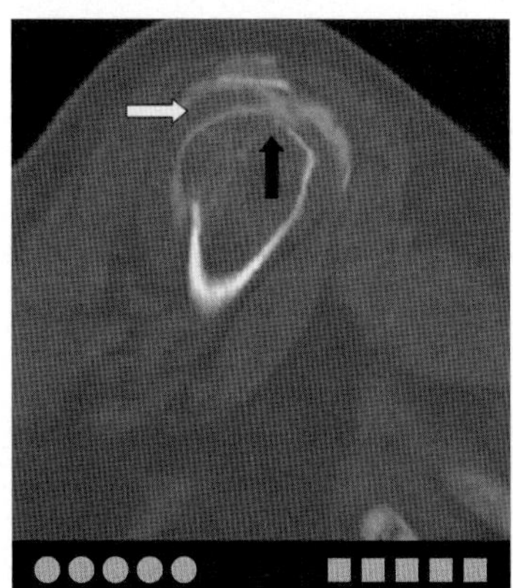

B. Full-thickness partial-width supraspinatus tear: Sagittal MPR image from a right shoulder MDCT arthrogram demonstrates contrast extension through the midportion of the supraspinatus tendon (black arrow). The posterior portion of the tendon is intact (white arrow).

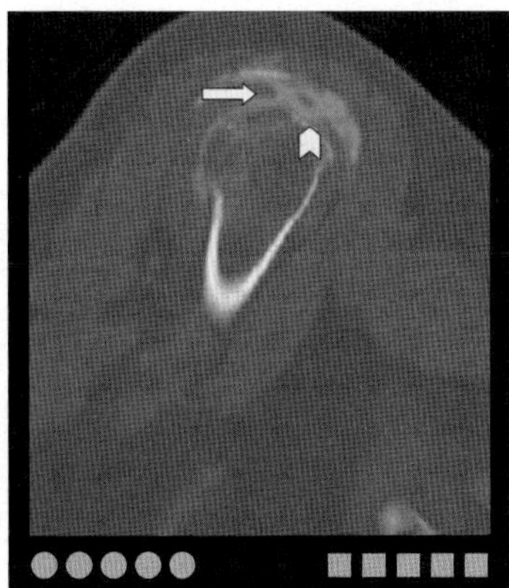

C. Full-thickness partial-width supraspinatus tear: Sagittal MPR image from a right shoulder MDCT arthrogram demonstrates contrast extension through the midportion of the supraspinatus tendon (arrow). The anterior portion of the tendon is diseased and has imbibition of contrast (arrow head), which indicates a badly diseased, friable tendon.

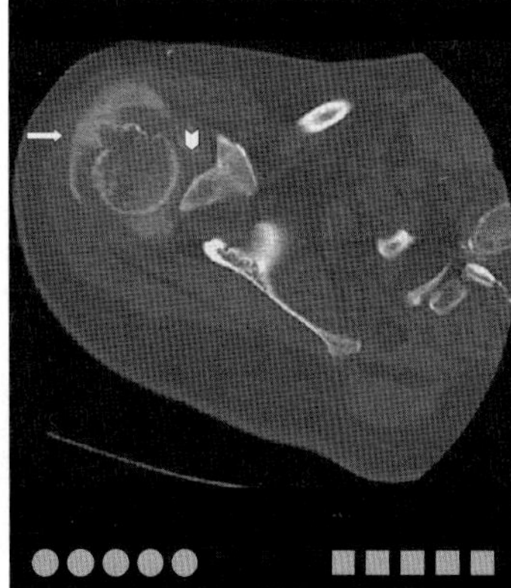

D. Full-thickness partial-width supraspinatus tear: Axial source image from a right shoulder MDCT arthrogram at the top of the humeral head demonstrates contrast extending through the midportion of the supraspinatus tendon (arrow). Note that the long head of the biceps attachment on the superior labrum is intact (arrow head).

IMAGE KEY

Common

Rare

Typical

Unusual

DIFFERENTIAL DIAGNOSES IMAGES

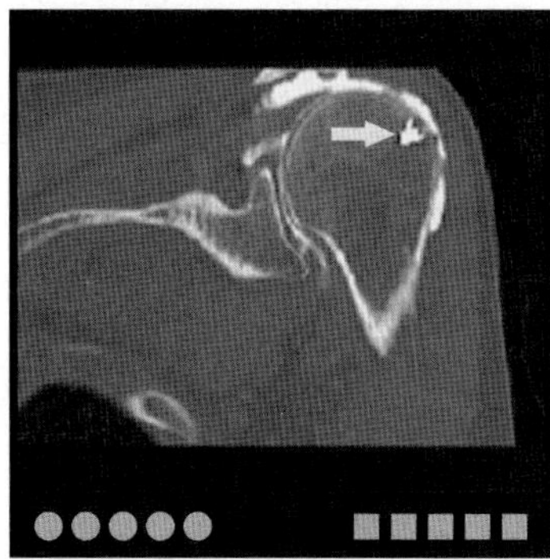

E. Full-thickness full-width supraspinatus tear: Coronal MPR image from a left shoulder MDCT arthrogram demonstrates contrast extending through the supraspinatus tendon, which is retracted. This patient had a supraspinatus repair that has failed. Note the tendon anchor in the humeral head (arrow).

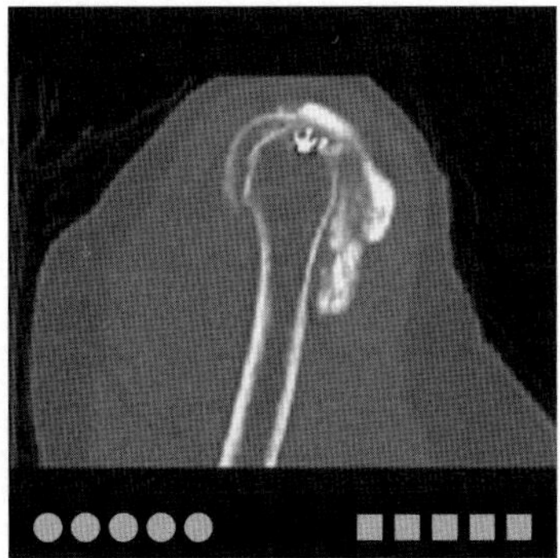

F. Full-thickness full-width supraspinatus tear: Sagittal MPR image from a left shoulder MDCT arthrogram demonstrates contrast extending through the entire width of the supraspinatus tendon. The sagittal orientation demonstrates the width of tendon tears nicely. Again noted is a tendon anchor from prior surgery in the humeral head.

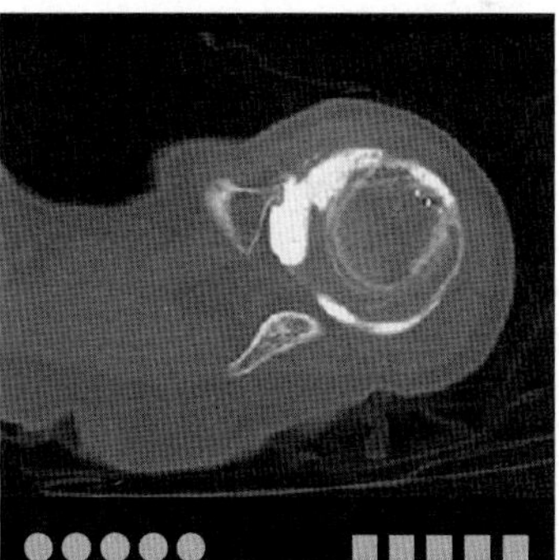

G. Full-thickness full-width supraspinatus tear: Axial source image from a left shoulder MDCT arthrogram demonstrates contrast extending through the entire insertion site of the supraspinatus tendon, which indicates a full-thickness full-width tear.

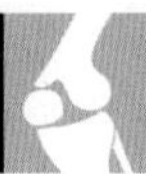

1–5 Chronic Supraspinatus Rotator Cuff Tear

Michael A. Bruno

PRESENTATION

Pain and limited range of motion

FINDINGS

MRI of the shoulder reveals fluid signal and retraction of the supraspinatus with superior migration of humeral head and loss of subacromial space.

DIFFERENTIAL DIAGNOSES

- *Infraspinatus tear:* The principal differential is an infraspinatus tear, which is a much less common lesion. The infraspinatus is seen in more posterior slices and more obliquely oriented.
- *Teres minor tear:* This is even more infrequent. Teres minor is located below infraspinatus.

COMMENTS

Supraspinatus is the major muscle of the rotator cuff. It originates above the spine of the scapula and inserts on the greater tuberosity. Impingement syndrome plays an important role in chronic tendinosis of supraspinatus tendon, which leads initially to partial tear and then full thickness and ultimately complete tear of this tendon. The supraspinatus tendon is torn in more than 95% of rotator cuff injuries. Chronic tear of supraspinatus creates a void in the subacromial space that allows superior migration of humeral head and finally loss of normal space between acromion and humeral head. Conventional radiograph in a normal patient shows the subacromial space measuring 15 mm or more. Patients with chronic atrophy or tear of the supraspinatus have a subacromial space, which measures less than 7 mm on conventional radiograph. Coronal or sagittal T2-weighted MR images show fluid has replaced this space, which should be normally filled with supraspinatus tendon. The main differential diagnosis is with a less common condition, namely, tear of infraspinatus tendon. Isolated tear of infraspinatus is an unusual injury pattern because the infraspinatus only rarely tears in isolation. An isolated infraspinatus tear, without an accompanying supraspinatus tear, is a relatively rare finding, with an estimated incidence of fewer than 5%, and perhaps is as low as 1%. It can be diagnosed on either MRI or ultrasound, with approximately equal sensitivity, specificity, and accuracy.

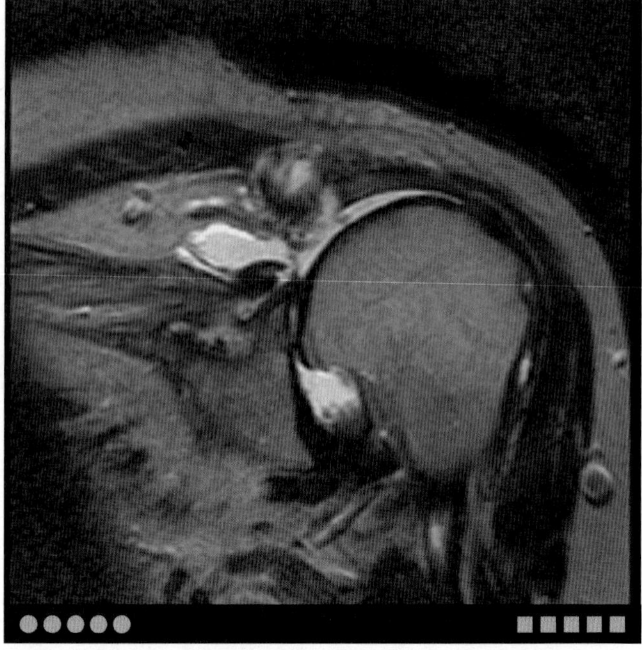

A. Chronic complete supraspinatus tear: Coronal oblique T2-weighted image shows complete tear and retraction of the supraspinatus tendon. Note loss of subacromial space.

PEARLS

- **Rotator cuff tears may be asymptomatic.**
- **The supraspinatus is involved in RCT in more than 95% of cases.**
- **The infraspinatus tendon's contribution to the conjoined tendon of the rotator cuff lies posterior and inferior to the supraspinatus tendon.**
- **Isolated infraspinatus tears are extremely rare, perhaps as few as 1% of cases.**

ADDITIONAL IMAGES

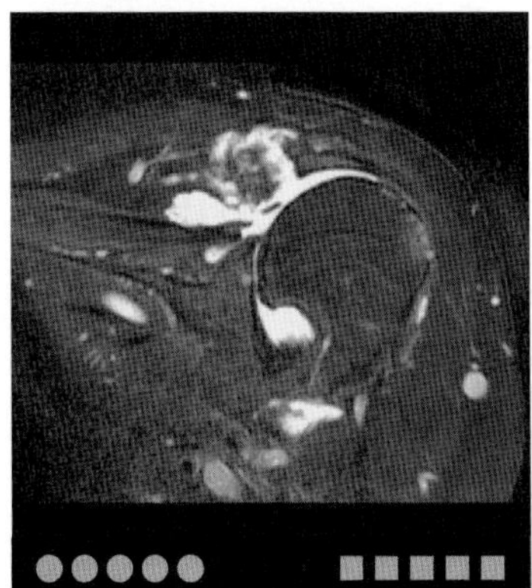

B. Chronic complete supraspinatus tear: Coronal oblique T2-weighted FS image shows complete tear and retraction of the supraspinatus tendon. Note loss of subacromial space and severe arthritis of acromioclavicular joint.

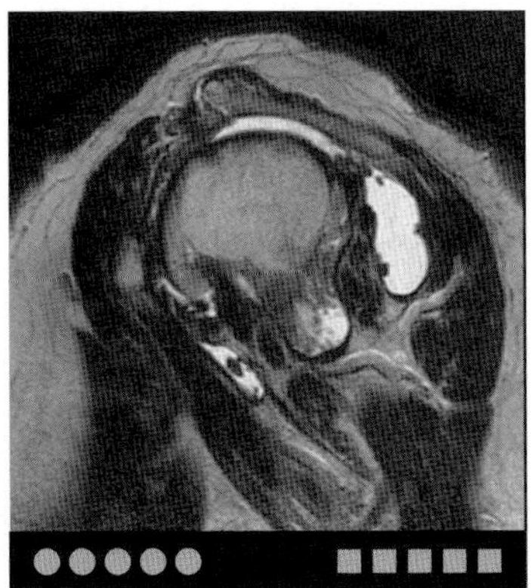

C. Chronic complete supraspinatus tear: Sagittal T2-weighted image shows loss of subacromial space. The supraspinatus site is replaced by fluid.

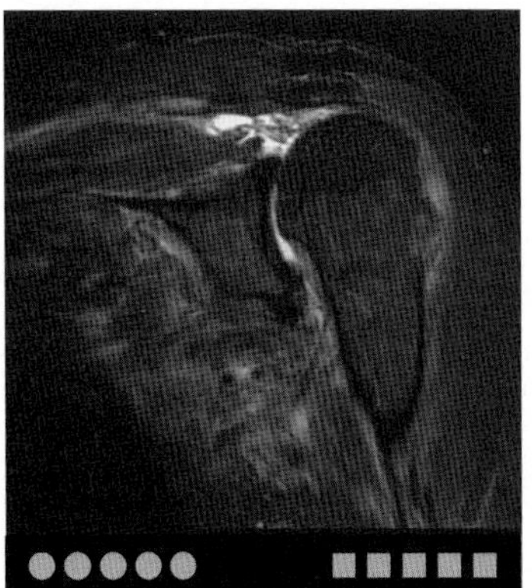

D. Chronic complete supraspinatus tear: Oblique coronal fat-suppressed T2-weighted MRI in another patient showing full-thickness supraspinatus tear with retraction. Note the fairly anterior slice location and cephalad migration of the humeral head. Recognition of anatomic landmarks allows this to be distinguished from an infraspinatus tear.

IMAGE KEY

Common

Rare

Typical

Unusual

DIFFERENTIAL DIAGNOSES IMAGES

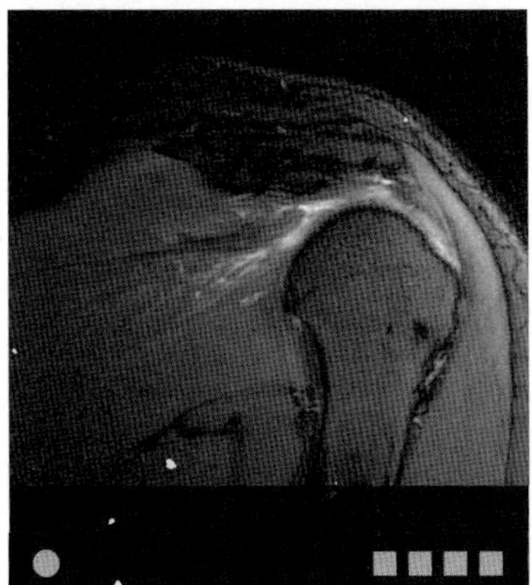

E. Infraspinatus tear: Oblique coronal T2-weighted FS MR image shows a full-thickness tear of the infraspinatus with retraction. High fluid signal is present in the gap of the tear.

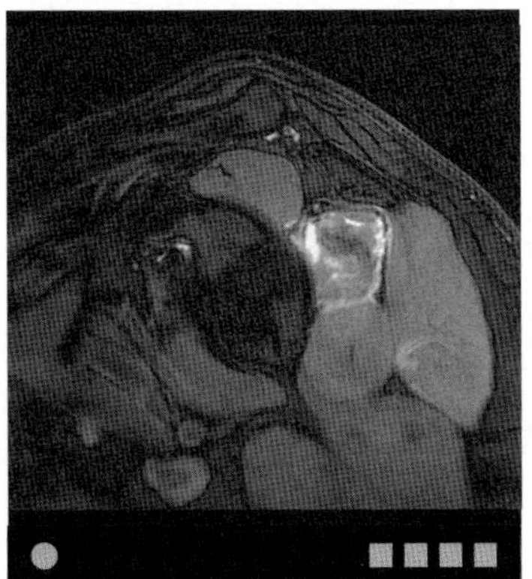

F. Infraspinatus tear: Image from an oblique sagittal sequence shows the intact supraspinatus and torn infraspinatus with fluid signal outlining the margins of the muscle belly. This section is near the plane of the glenohumeral joint and does not include the scapular spine.

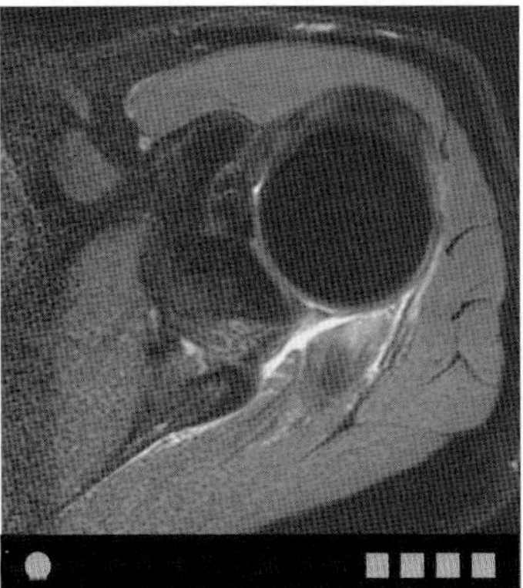

G. Infraspinatus tear: Axial T2-weighted MR sequence shows infraspinatus tear. Note the more anteriorly located subscapularis tendon is intact.

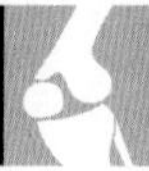

1–6 Tendinosis of Supra and Infraspinatus Tendon

Ashkan Afshin and Jamshid Tehranzadeh

PRESENTATION

Shoulder pain

FINDINGS

MR images show intermediate to increased signal on proton density, T1- and T2-weighted images (however these signals are not as bright as fluid signal) in supra and infraspinatus tendon.

DIFFERENTIAL DIAGNOSES

- *Calcific tendinosis:* This condition results from deposition of calcium hydroxyapatite most commonly near the insertion of the supraspinatus tendon. MR images of these patients show a focal decreased signal lesion of the tendon.
- *Partial tear of supraspinatus:* The signal intensity is brighter (fluid signal) on T2-weighted images than tendinosis; however, only partial thickness of the tendon is affected.
- *Full-thickness tear of supraspinatus:* This condition results from full-thickness disruption of the supraspinatus tendon, which extends to both articular and bursal surfaces. Imaging studies demonstrate focal bright (fluid) signal in supraspinatus tendon.
- *Complete tendon tear of supraspinatus:* In this condition there is full-thickness and full-width tear of the tendon and the tendon is ruptured and retracted.

COMMENTS

Tendinosis refers to intratendinous degeneration that results from atrophy (aging, microtrauma, vascular compromise). Clinically, there is often a palpable tendon nodule that can be asymptomatic or possibly have point tenderness. There is no swelling of a tendon sheath. Supraspinatus tendinosis is a relatively common condition that is more prevalent in athletes who are involved in sports requiring repetitive overhead arm movements such as baseball, swimming, and lifting heavy weights over the shoulder. These patients experience pain at the shoulder, eliciting with active abduction, in a small arc of movement between 60 and 120 degrees (painful arc syndrome). MR images show intermediate to increased signal on T1-weighted images within the tendon, which persists or is slightly decreased on T2-weighted spin echo sequences. In partial- or full-thickness tears, the signal would further increase (focal fluid signal) on T2-weighted sequences. In complete tear, the tendon is disrupted and is associated with retraction of proximal part. One of the major pitfalls in the diagnosis of tendinosis is the magic angle phenomenon. Infraspinatus tendinosis is a rare condition and presents with pain exacerbated by external rotation and tenderness around the point of insertion on the lateral aspect of greater tuberosity of humerus. Infraspinatus is posteriorly located and similar pattern of MR findings is expected.

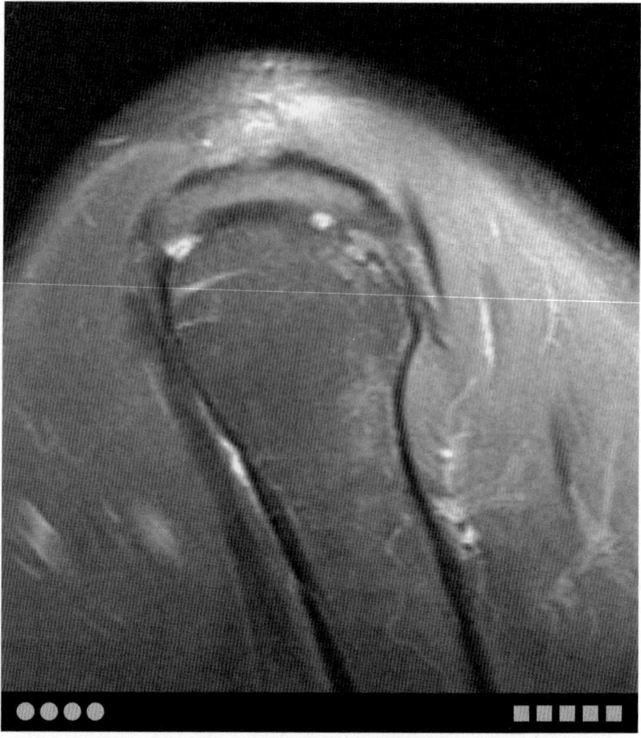

A. Tendinosis of supra and infraspinatus tendon: Sagittal fat-saturated T1-weighted image shows intermediate to increased signal noted in the supra and infraspinatus tendon.

PEARLS

- **Supraspinatus tendinosis is a common cause of shoulder pain associated with repetitive overhead arm movements.**
- **Shoulder pain is aggravated with active abduction.**
- **Intermediate to increased signal on T1-weighted images with similar or slightly lower signal on T2-weighted images.**
- **Magic angle phenomenon is a major pitfall in diagnosis.**
- **Infraspinatus tendinosis is uncommon and associated with pain exacerbated by external rotation with MR signal findings similar to that of supraspinatus tendinosis.**

ADDITIONAL IMAGES

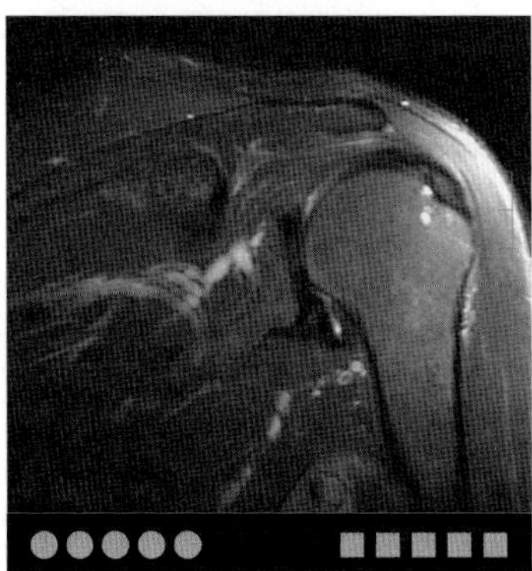

B. Tendinosis of supraspinatus tendon: Coronal oblique fat-saturated T2-weighted image shows intermediate signal in supraspinatus tendon.

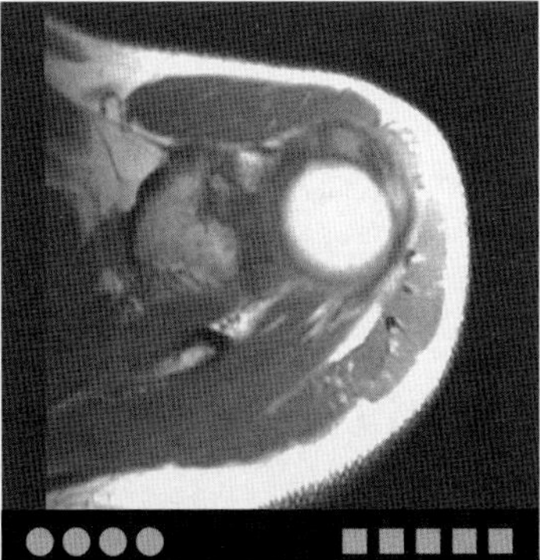

C. Tendinosis of supra and infraspinatus tendon: Axial T1-weighted image shows intermediate to increased signal in supra and infraspinatus tendon.

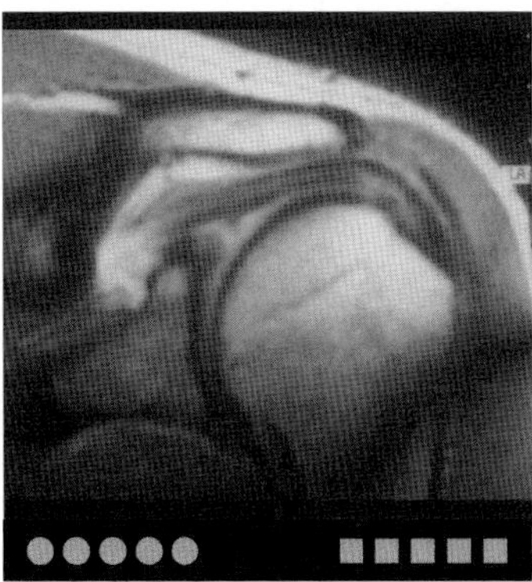

D. Tendinosis of supraspinatus tendon: Coronal oblique Proton density image in another patient shows intermediate to increased signal in the supraspinatus tendon.

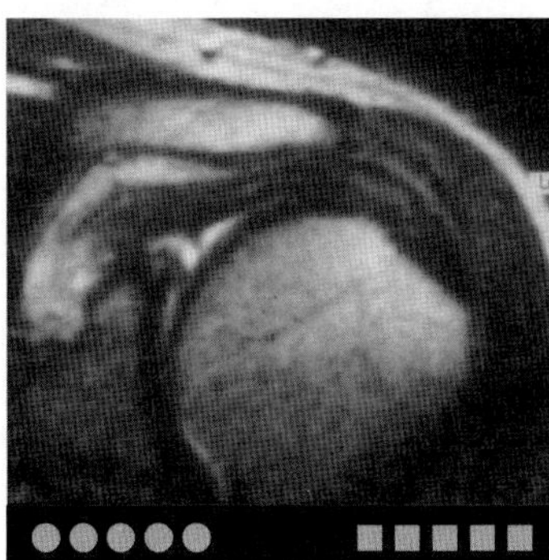

E. Tendinosis of supraspinatus tendon: Coronal oblique T2-weighted image (same patient as in image D) shows intermediate signal in the supraspinatus tendon.

DIFFERENTIAL DIAGNOSES IMAGES

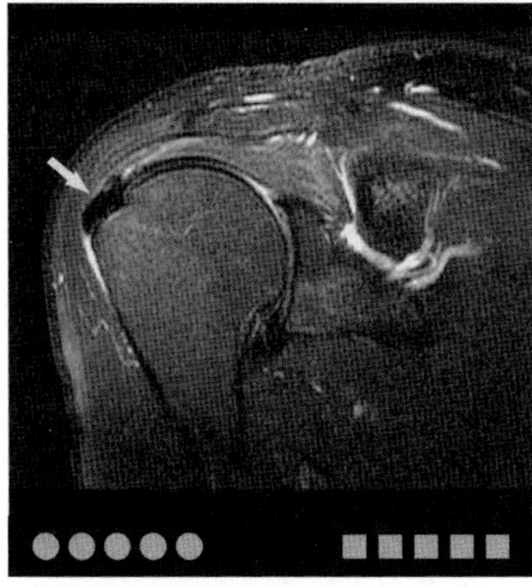

F. Calcific tendinosis: Coronal oblique fat-saturated T2-weighted image shows focal area of low signal lesion in the supraspinatus tendon (arrow) because of calcific tendinosis.

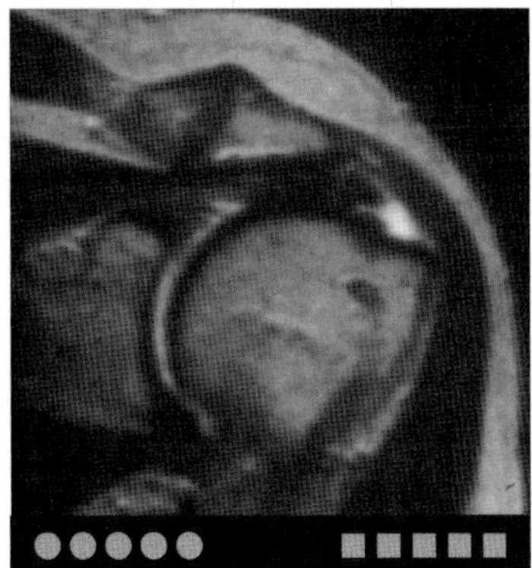

G. Full-thickness tear of supraspinatus: Coronal oblique T2-weighted image shows focal bright (fluid) signal in the supraspinatus tendon because of full-thickness supraspinatus tear at the insertion site.

IMAGE KEY

Common
●●●●●
●●●●
●●●
●●
●
Rare

Typical
■■■■■
■■■■
■■■
■■
■
Unusual

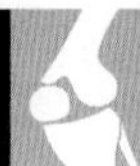

1–7 Partial-Thickness Tear of Supraspinatus

Ashkan Afshin and Jamshid Tehranzadeh

PRESENTATION

Shoulder pain

FINDINGS

MR image shows intrasubstance intermediate signal of supraspinatus tendon on proton density image. T2-weighted images show intrasubstance bright (fluid) signal within the tendon without full thickness involvement.

DIFFERENTIAL DIAGNOSES

- *Supraspinatus tendinosis:* MR images show intermediate to increased signal on T1 and similar or slightly lower signal on T2-weighted images (however, these signals are not as bright as fluid signal) of supraspinatus tendon.
- *Calcific tendinosis:* This condition results from deposition of calcium hydroxyapatite most commonly near the insertion of the supraspinatus tendon. MR images of these patients show a focal decreased signal lesion of the tendon.
- *Full-thickness tear of supraspinatus:* This condition results from full-thickness disruption of the supraspinatus tendon. Bright signal (fluid) extends to both articular and bursal surfaces.
- *Complete tear:* The tendon is completely torn and disrupted; the proximal segment of the tendon is pulled and retracted.

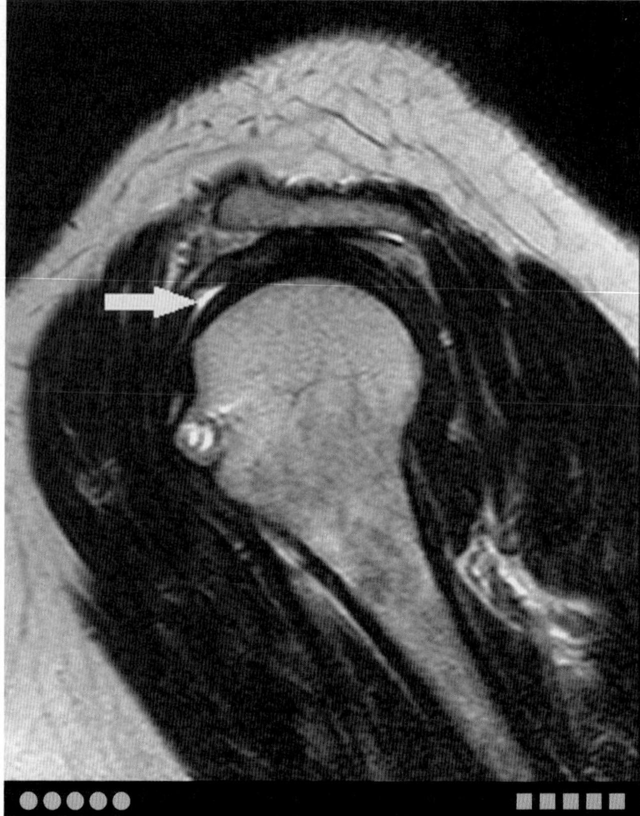

A. Partial-thickness tear of supraspinatus: Sagittal T2-weighted image shows partial intrasubstance tear of the anterior supraspinatus musculotendinous junction (arrow). This intrasubstance tear extends to articular surface but not bursal surface.

COMMENTS

Partial tear usually occurs near the anterior insertion of the tendon and, depending on the involved surface of the tendon, can be classified as articular, bursal, and intrasubstance. Partial tear of the articular surface is the most common form of this lesion. Patients with partial tear of the supraspinatus tendon usually complain of shoulder pain with overhead activities, which is more severing than pain in full-thickness tear. They may also experience pain in the shoulder at night, which causes discomfort during sleep. Muscle weakness, especially when trying to lift the arm, is another clinical finding in these patients. Ultrasonographic findings in partial tear of supraspinatus consists of focal areas of decreased echogenicity (hypo echoic cleft) within the tendon (hyper echoic). The most important MR finding in partial tear is a focal intermediate signal on PD images, which changes to bright signal on T2-weighted sequences and disrupts the normal low-signal surface of the supraspinatus tendon. Particular conditions such as degenerative changes of acromioclavicular (AC) joint and hooked acromion (type III acromion) have been associated with a higher incidence of partial tear of supraspinatus. Therefore, these should prompt a careful evaluation of the supraspinatus muscle. The MRI findings include intermediate to increased signal in T1-weighted and proton density images, which changes to bright (fluid) signal in T2-weighted or STIR sequences.

PEARLS

- **Incomplete tendon tear that does not qualify for full thickness**
- **Classified as articular, bursal, and intrasubstance**
- **Pain in the shoulder, with overhead activities, at night or while sleeping is a common clinical finding**
- **Ultrasound shows focal areas of decreased echogenicity within the tendon**
- **MRI shows intermediate to increased signal on T1-weighted or proton density images, which changes to bright signal on T2-weighted images**

ADDITIONAL IMAGES

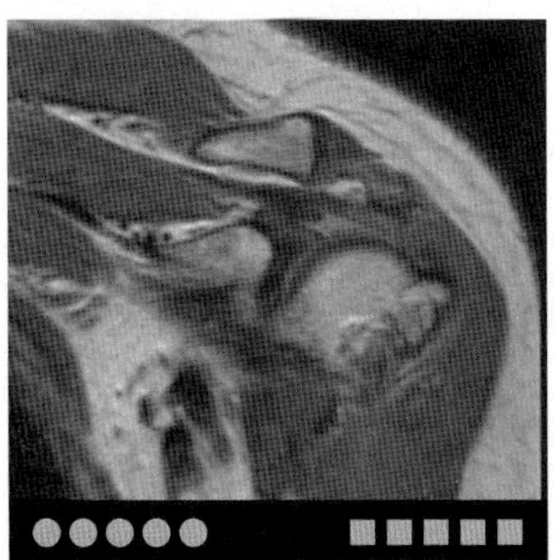

B. Partial-thickness tear of supraspinatus: Coronal proton density image shows intermediate signal in the anterior supraspinatus musculotendinous junction.

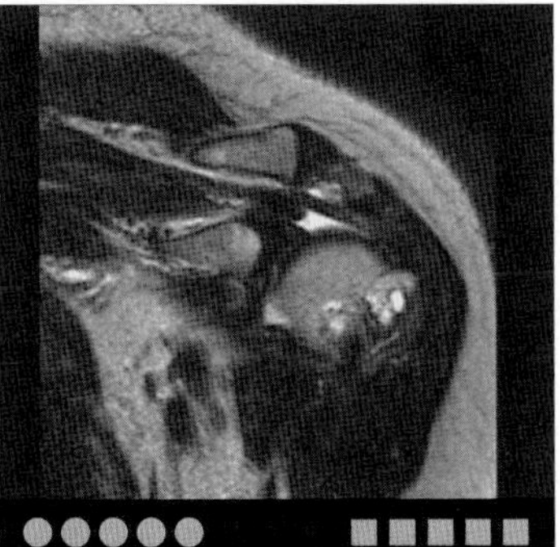

C. Partial-thickness tear of supraspinatus: Coronal T2-weighted image shows bright (fluid) signal in the intrasubstance of supraspinatus tendon and musculotendinous junction consistent with partial-thickness tear.

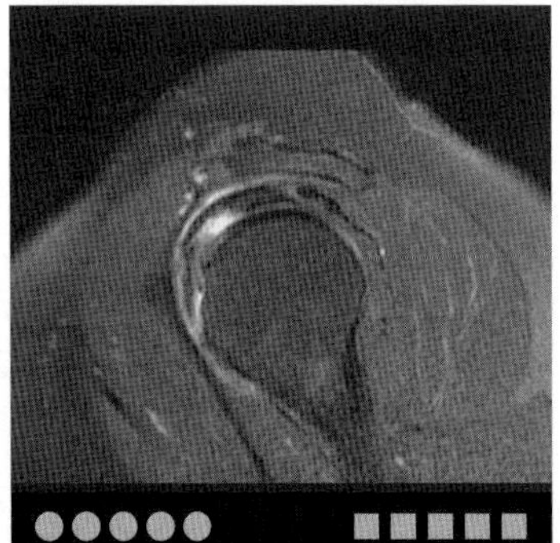

D. Partial-thickness tear of supraspinatus: Sagittal proton density SPIR image shows an intrasubstance bright signal in the anterior aspect of supraspinatus tendon. This intrasubstance tear extends to articular surface but not bursal surface.

DIFFERENTIAL DIAGNOSES IMAGES

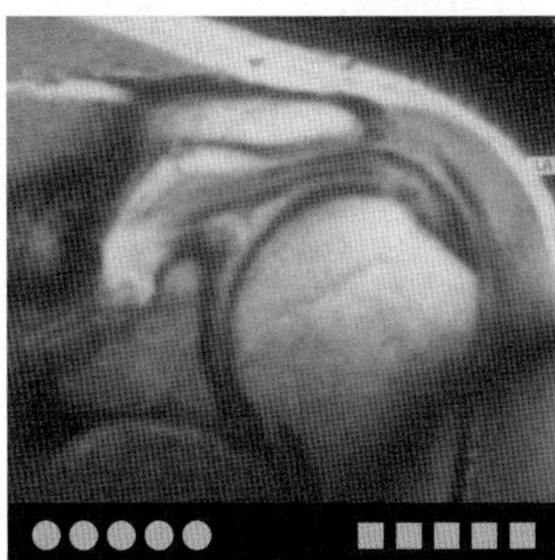

E. Tendinosis of supraspinatus tendon: Coronal oblique Proton density image shows intermediate to increased signal in the supraspinatus tendon.

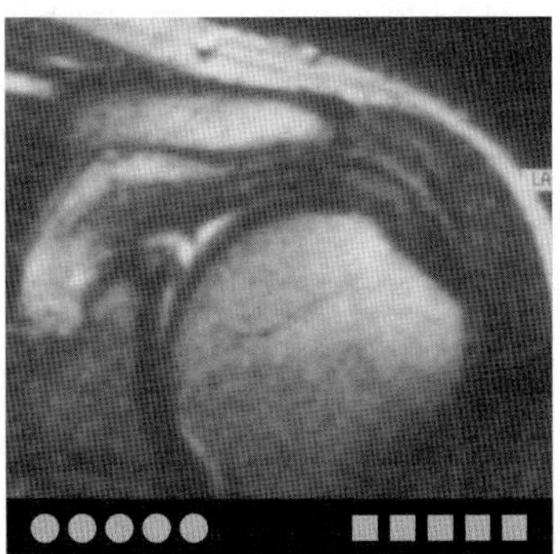

F. Tendinosis of supraspinatus tendon: Coronal oblique T2-weighted image shows intermediate signal in the supraspinatus tendon.

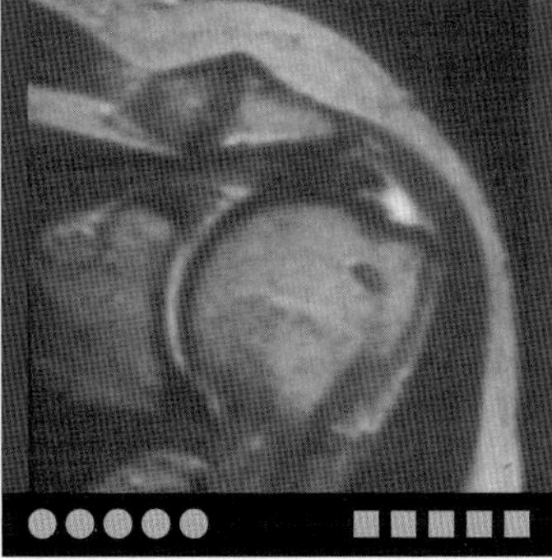

G. Full-thickness tear of supraspinatus: Coronal oblique T2-weighted image shows focal bright (fluid) signal in the supraspinatus tendon because of full thickness supraspinatus tear at the insertion site.

IMAGE KEY

Common ●●●●● ●●●● ●●● ●● ● Rare

Typical ■■■■■ ■■■■ ■■■ ■■ ■ Unusual

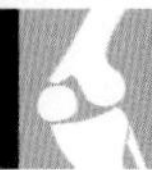

1–8 Sonographic Appearance of Tear of the Subscapularis and Supraspinatus Tendons

Mélanie Morel, Nathalie Boutry, and Anne Cotten

PRESENTATION

Pain and weakness with shoulder use

FINDINGS

Sonography exhibits anterior full-thickness rupture of the supraspinatus tendon, associated with complete detachment of the upper margin of the subscapularis tendon.

DIFFERENTIAL DIAGNOSES

- *Rotator cuff tendinosis (tendon degeneration):* The tendon shows ill-defined diffuse heterogeneous hypoechogenicity without any anechoic focal area representative of a tear.
- *Calcific tendonitis:* This is caused by the deposition of calcium apatite crystals in the rotator cuff tendons. It may become symptomatic when the calcium undergoes resorption. In ultrasonography (US), calcium deposits may appear as well-circumscribed calcifications with posterior shadowing or may have a fluffy appearance, with echogenic foci without posterior shadowing.
- *Subacromial subdeltoid bursitis:* US exhibits a hypoechoic collection located superficially to the supraspinatus tendon. Hyperemia of the walls of the inflamed bursa may be demonstrated on Doppler study.

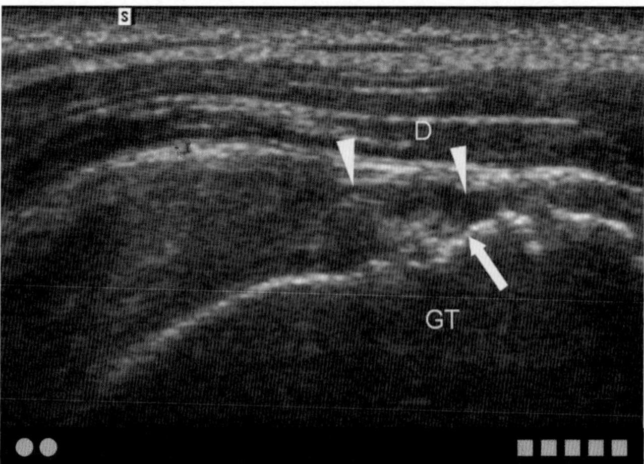

A. Supraspinatus tendon full-thickness tear: Longitudinal US image of the supraspinatus tendon shows hypoechoic area (between arrowheads) instead of the distal fibers of the supraspinatus tendon. Note dipping of the deltoid muscle (D) into the tendon gap, loss of the outward convexity of the tendon, and cortical irregularity of the greater tuberosity (GT) (arrow).

COMMENTS

This is the case of a 56-year-old woman complaining of chronic pain in the shoulder and weakness at abduction and internal rotation, diagnosed as full-thickness rupture of the subscapularis and supraspinatus tendons. Most rotator cuff tears occur at the site of insertion of the supraspinatus tendon on the greater tuberosity. Supraspinatus tear may extend anteriorly to the anterosuperior subscapularis tendon, which is far more frequent than the isolated subscapularis tear (mainly encountered in shoulder dislocation). US criteria for full-thickness supraspinatus tear are the following: Nonvisualization of the tendon or focal tendon defect filled with fluid and debris, with loss of the normal outward convexity of the tendon and dipping of the deltoid muscle into the tendon gap. The uncovered cartilage sign or naked cartilage sign is the hyperechoic interface between the joint fluid and the cartilage covering the humeral head. Other US signs are bone irregularity of the greater tuberosity, joint effusion, and fluid in the subdeltoid bursa. Articular-side partial-thickness tear is manifested as a hypoechoic or a mixed hyper/hypoechoic defect of the articular side of the tendon. Bursal-side partial-thickness tear interrupts the superficial aspect of the supraspinatus tendon, with flattening of this bursal surface. Lesions of the subscapularis tendon may be limited to the upper margin (grade 1), involve more than one-quarter of the craniocaudal diameter (grade 2), or be a complete detachment of the tendon from the lesser tuberosity (grade 3). Rotator interval injury (lesions of the coracohumeral ligament, superior glenohumeral ligament, and adjacent borders of the supraspinatus and subscapularis tendons) may be diagnosed on MR-arthrogram.

PEARLS

- **Prevalence of rotator cuff partial- and full-thickness tears increases with age, particularly after 50 years.**
- **Supraspinatus tendon is most often affected. Its tear may extend posteriorly to the infraspinatus tendon, and anteriorly to the subscapularis tendon.**
- **Full-thickness tear of the supraspinatus tendon is defined by anechoic disruption of the tendon. Hyperintense defect in the tendon is found on T2-weighted fat-saturated images.**
- **Partial-thickness tear may be located on the articular or on the bursal side of the tendon.**

ADDITIONAL IMAGES

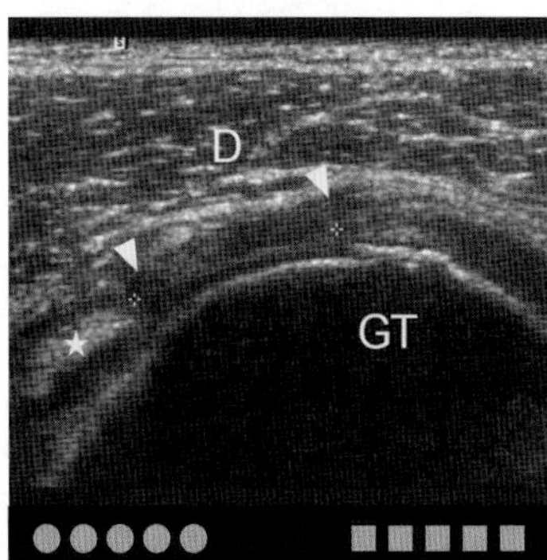

B. Supraspinatus tendon full-thickness tear: Transverse sonogram of the supraspinatus tendon demonstrates the absence of visualization of the distal supraspinatus tendon (between arrowheads) (star: long head of biceps tendon; D: deltoid muscle; GT: greater tuberosity).

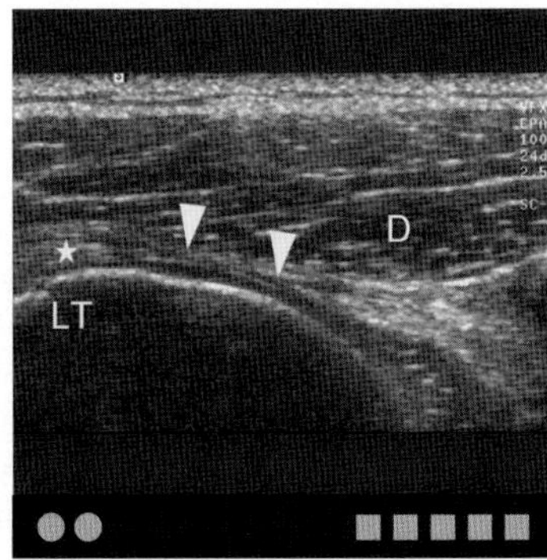

C. Subscapularis tendon detachment: Transverse US image of the subscapularis tendon shows that a large part of the subscapularis tendon fibers is missing (arrowheads). Some fibers (star) remain attached to the lesser tuberosity (LT). Note dipping of the deltoid muscle into the tendon gap (D).

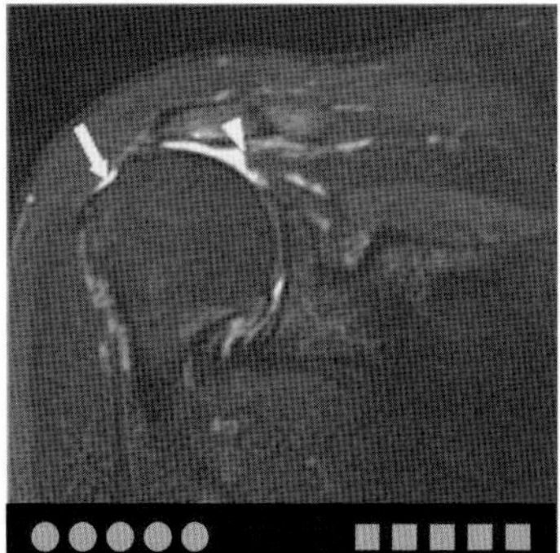

D. Supraspinatus tendon full-thickness tear: T2-weighted fat-saturated coronal oblique image exhibits high-signal fluid in the defect of the supraspinatus tendon (arrow). Note also retraction of the supraspinatus tendon (arrowhead).

E. Supraspinatus tendon full-thickness tear: T2-weighted fat-saturated sagittal oblique view confirms the nonvisualization of the supraspinatus tendon (arrow).

IMAGE KEY

Common

Rare

Typical

Unusual

DIFFERENTIAL DIAGNOSES IMAGES

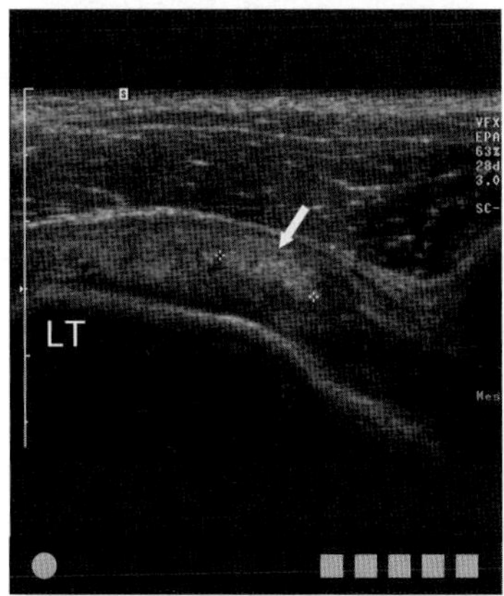

F.Calcific tendonitis of the subscapularis tendon: A dense calcification (arrow) is seen within the subscapularis tendon on this axial view (LT: lesser tuberosity).

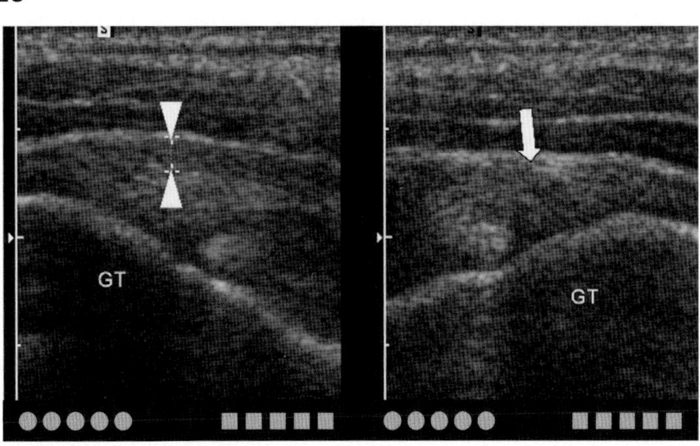

G. Subacromial subdeltoid bursitis: Bilateral longitudinal sonogram of the supraspinatus tendon exhibits hypoechoic thickening of the subacromial bursa (arrowheads) comparatively to the other side (arrow) (GT: greater tuberosity).

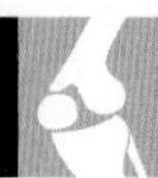

1–9 Isolated Full-Thickness Infraspinatus Tear

Peyman Borghei and Jamshid Tehranzadeh

PRESENTATION

Shoulder pain

FINDINGS

MRI shows fluid signal at the insertion site of the infraspinatus tendon on T2-weighted image. Small fluid is also noted in subacromial-subdeltoid bursa.

DIFFERENTIAL DIAGNOSES

- *Infraspinatus tendinosis:* On MRI the signal intensity of a normal rotator cuff tendon is low and homogeneous in all sequences. In tendinosis an intermediate to slightly increased signal intensity within the tendon is observed on T1-weighted and proton density images.
- *Supraspinatus tendinosis:* An intermediate to slightly increased signal intensity within the supraspinatus tendon is observed on T1-weighted and proton density images.
- *Supraspinatus tear:* An intratendinious tear depicts a region of intermediate signal intensity paralleling the long axis of the tendon in both T1-weighted and proton density weighted images, which increases to fluid signal intensity on T2-weighted image.
- *Teres minor tear:* An intratendinious tear depicts a region of intermediate signal intensity paralleling the long axis of the tendon in both T1-weighted and proton density weighted images, which increases to fluid signal intensity on T2-weighted image.

COMMENTS

The patient is a 61-year-old female with history of right shoulder pain diagnosed with isolated infraspinatus tear. The rotator cuff is made up of tendons from four muscles: the supraspinatus, infraspinatus, teres minor, and subscapularis. The tendon fibers of the supraspinatus, infraspinatus, and teres minor blend over their lateral 1.5 cm before they insert on the greater tuberosity, with the bulk of the latter two inserting along the posterior aspect of the greater tuberosity. The infraspinatus and teres minor muscles assist in external rotation of the shoulder and also provide an inferior pull upon the humeral head, assisting in its centering during overhead activity. The role of the MRI is to detect the presence of a rotator cuff pathology including tendonitis, partial versus full thickness and complete tear. The most common appearance of a full-thickness tear is high fluid signal on a T2-weighted image extending from the articular surface of the cuff to the subacromial/subdeltoid bursa. In chronic cuff tears where the shoulder joint has little or no effusion, the humeral head may be high riding such that little high signal is seen at the tear site. Acute tears can have hemorrhage at the tear site that can mimic some intact fibers. It is important to distinguish the smoothly curving, low-signal surfaces of the cuff from the disorganized low signal of fibrin and other blood products. Partial tears often appear on T1-weighted image as intermediate signal, isointense to muscle, which is bright on T2-weighted image; however, it does not fully extend from articular surface to subacromial subdeltoid bursa.

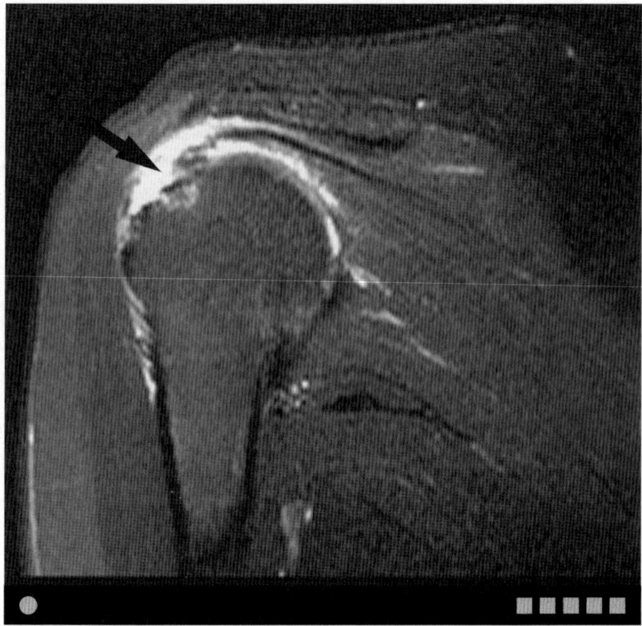

A. Isolated full-thickness infraspinatus tear: Posterior slice of coronal oblique T2 SPIR image shows fluid is replacing the distal tendon of infraspinatus tendon at the insertion site (arrow).

PEARLS

- **Infraspinatus muscle assists in external rotation and inferior pulling of the humeral head.**
- **Full thickness tear appears as a high fluid signal focus, which extends from the articular surface to the subacromial/subdeltoid bursa.**
- **Partial tears often appear on T1-weighted image as intermediate signal, isointense to muscle, which is bright on T2-weighted image; however, it does not fully extend from articular surface to subacromial subdeltoid bursa.**

ADDITIONAL IMAGES

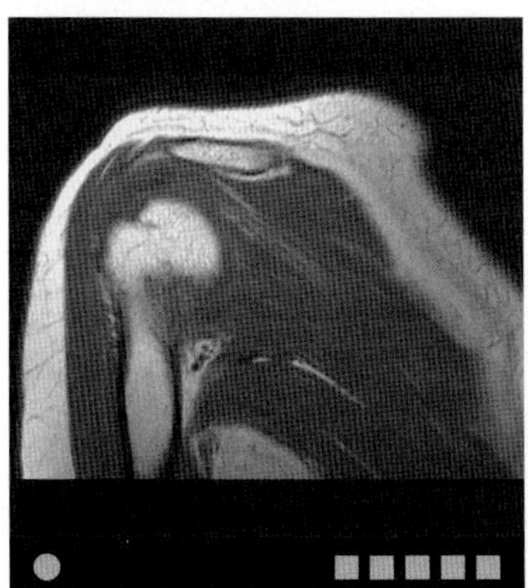

B. Isolated full-thickness infraspinatus tear: Posterior slice of coronal oblique T1-weighted image shows intermediate signal in the infraspinatus tendon.

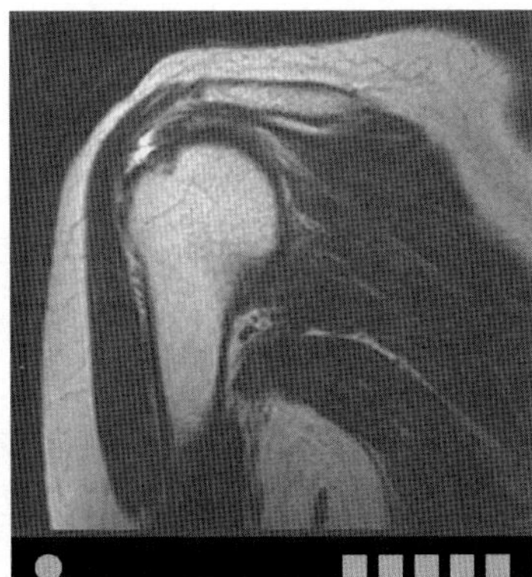

C. Isolated full-thickness infraspinatus tear: Posterior slice of coronal T2 image shows fluid is replacing the distal tendon on infraspinatus tendon at the insertion site.

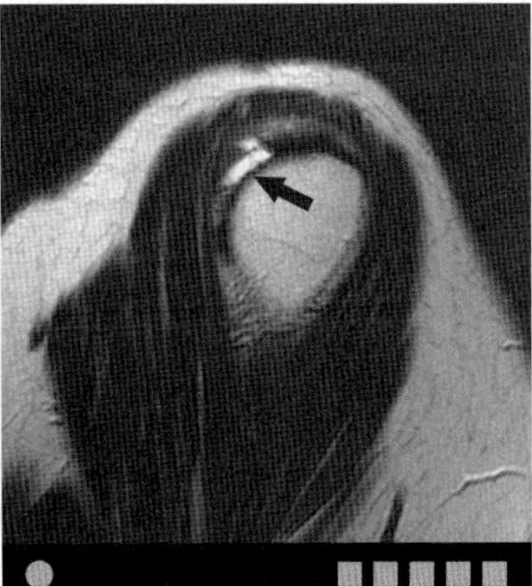

D. Isolated full-thickness infraspinatus tear: Sagittal T2-weighted image shows fluid signal replacing infraspinatus tendon representing full-thickness tear (arrow).

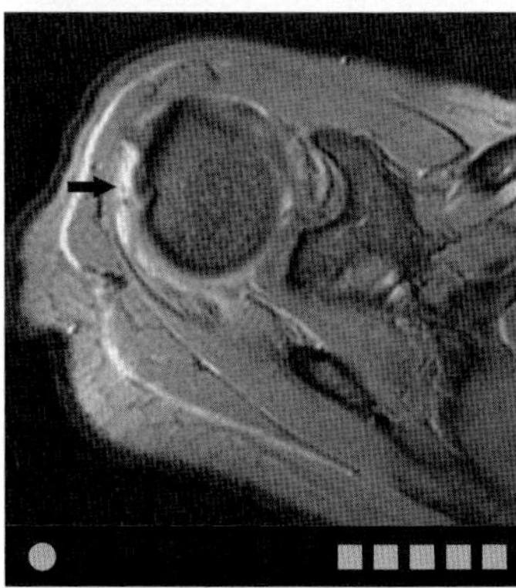

E. Isolated full-thickness infraspinatus tear: Axial T2-weighted image shows fluid is replacing the infraspinatus tendon at the site of insertion representing full-thickness tear (arrow).

IMAGE KEY

Common

Rare

Typical

Unusual

DIFFERENTIAL DIAGNOSES IMAGES

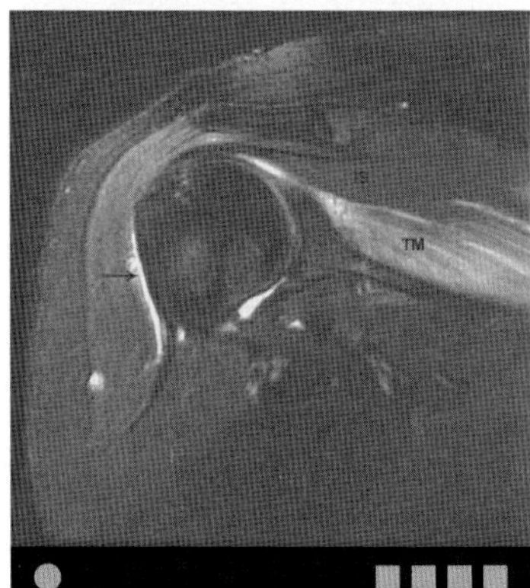

F. Teres minor tear: Coronal oblique fat-saturated T2-weighted image shows acute edematous change of the teres minor muscle (TM) throughout. The overlying infraspinatus muscle and tendon are intact. Abnormal subdeltoid fluid is again noted (arrow).

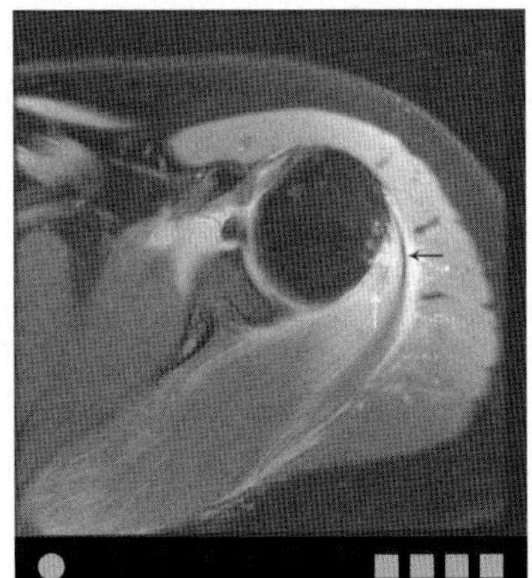

G. Teres minor tear: Axial fat-saturated proton density image demonstrates tear of the teres minor tendon (white arrow). Overlying infraspinatus tendon is intact (black arrow). Anterior labral tear is incidentally noted.

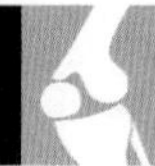

1-10 Rotator Interval Injury

Scott Kingston

PRESENTATION

Anterior shoulder pain and limited external rotation

FINDINGS

MRI shows irregular soft tissue surrounding the long head of the biceps tendon.

DIFFERENTIAL DIAGNOSES

- *Rotator cuff tear:* Tears of the anterior supraspinatus or superior subscapularis tendons without extension to the rotator interval.
- *Calcific bursitis/Tendinosis:* Calcium hydroxyapatite deposition in the surrounding soft tissues associated with inflammation, edema, and pain.
- *Hidden lesion:* Tendinosis and partial tears of the distal subscapularis tendon with medial subluxation of the long head of the biceps tendon.
- *Adhesive capsulitis:* Frozen shoulder syndrome often following trauma with fibrosis and contracture of the axillary pouch of the inferior glenohumeral ligament leading to restricted motion.

COMMENTS

The patient is an athlete with anterior shoulder pain and limited external rotation following trauma. The rotator interval (RI) is defined as the space between the anterior supraspinatus and superior subscapularis tendons from the intra-articular biceps tendon origin off the supraglenoid tubercle laterally to the bicipital groove. Injuries may occur within the RI range from rotator cuff tears of the anterior fibers of the supraspinatus and superior fibers of the subscapularis tendons to injuries of the anterior capsule and supporting ligaments. Anterior capsular tears of the RI may result in extravasation of intra-articularly injected contrast into the overlying subdeltoid bursa in the presence of a normal rotator cuff. Supporting structures such as the coracohumeral and superior glenohumeral ligament (CHL/SGL) complex help contribute to posterior/inferior shoulder stability and also help form a sling providing stability for the biceps tendon within the bicipital groove. Tears of the CHL/SGL complex in conjunction with injuries to the distal deep subscapularis tendon may result in medial subluxation of the biceps tendon. Subcoracoid impingement from an elongated coracoid process may be recognized by hyperintense subcortical cysts of the lesser tuberosity and

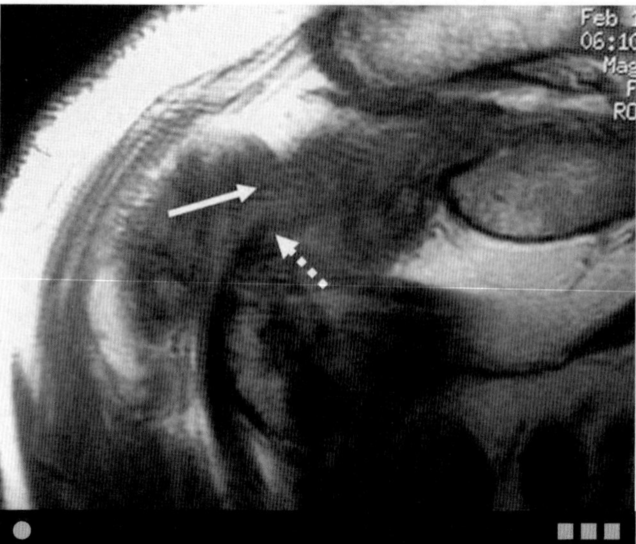

A. Rotator interval injury with fibrosis: Coronal T1-weighted image shows isointense soft tissue (solid arrow) from adhesions surrounding the long head of the biceps tendon (dashed arrow) within the RI.

may also contribute to chronic tendinosis of the subscapularis tendon with medial subluxation of the biceps tendon as well. Posttraumatic synovitis and tears to the RI soft tissues may lead to irregular granulation tissue with fibrosis appearing as intermediate to hyperintense signal tissue on proton density or T2-weighted image. Because of the fibrosis and contracture of the anterior capsular soft tissues, patients may have limited external rotation from adhesive capsulitis and symptoms related to the involved biceps tendon.

PEARLS

- **MR arthrography will help delineate the RI soft tissues including the capsule, CHL/SGL complex, and long head of the biceps tendon.**
- **Tears of the RI may result in extravasation of intra-articularly injected contrast in the presence of an intact rotator cuff.**
- **Biceps tendon subluxations may occur with tears of the deep subscapularis tendon with injury to the supporting sling from the CHL/SGL complex.**
- **Irregular soft tissue within the RI may be caused by synovitis and fibrosis leading to contractures and adhesive capsulitis with limited external rotation.**
- **Subcoracoid impingement may be recognized by lesser tuberosity subcortical cysts and tendinosis of the underlying subscapularis tendon.**

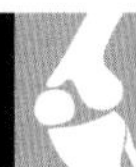

ADDITIONAL IMAGES

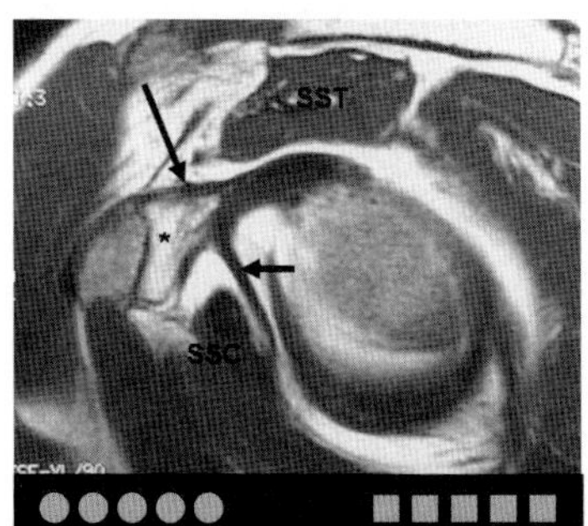

B. Normal rotator interval: Sagittal T1 arthrogram image of normal RI shows supraspinatus (SST), subscapularis (SSC), middle glenohumeral ligament (short arrow), coracohumeral ligament (long arrow), and normal subcoracoid fat (star).

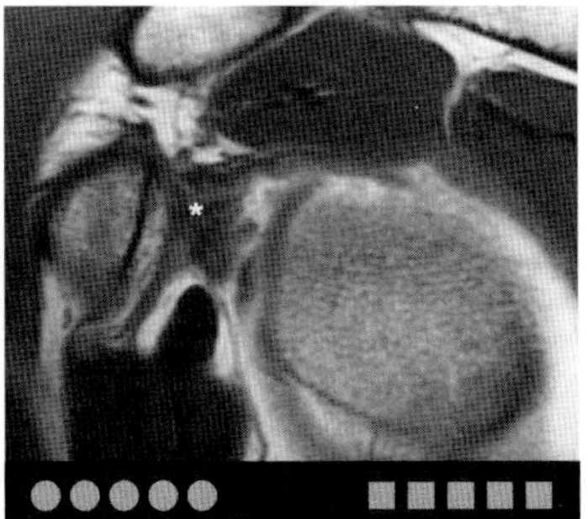

C. Rotator interval injury with fibrosis: Sagittal T1 MR arthrogram image demonstrates irregular scar tissue (star) from adhesions obliterating the normal subcoracoid fat within the rotator interval.

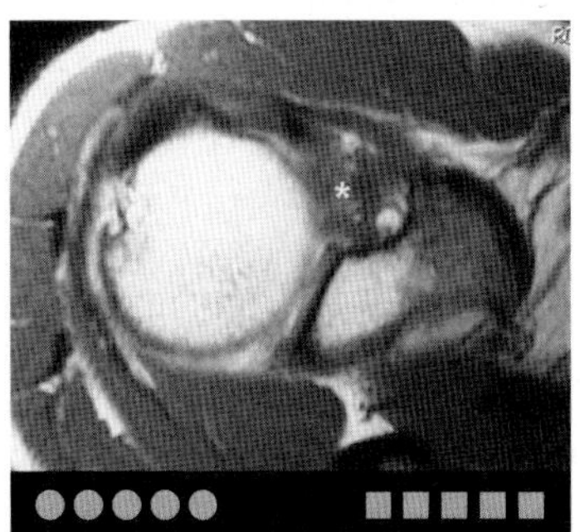

D. Rotator interval injury with fibrosis: Axial T1 MR arthrogram image showing irregular synovial adhesions (star) within the RI.

IMAGE KEY

Common
●●●●●
●●●●
●●●
●●
●
Rare

Typical
■■■■■
■■■■
■■■
■■
■
Unusual

DIFFERENTIAL DIAGNOSES IMAGES

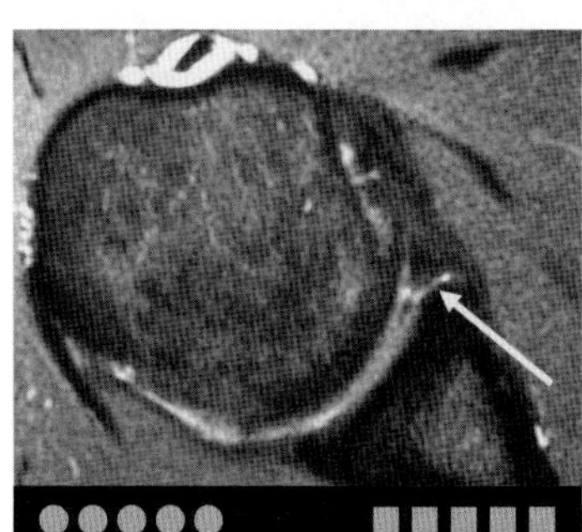

E. Labral tear: Axial proton density MR image shows a tear (arrow) at the base of the high anterior labrum.

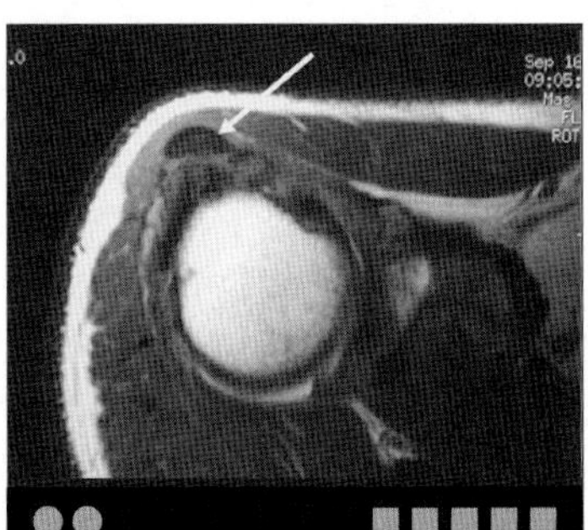

F. Calcific bursitis: Axial T1-weighted image demonstrates signal void from calcium hydroxyapatite deposition (arrow) because of calcific bursitis within the anterior subdeltoid bursa.

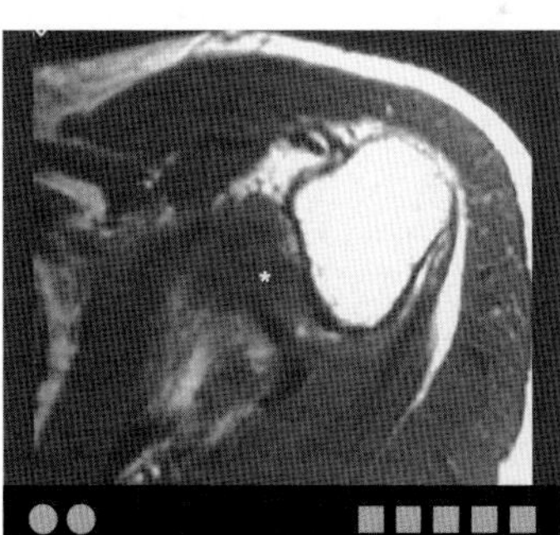

G. Adhesive capsulitis: Axial T1-weighted image demonstrates irregular soft tissue (star) from adhesive capsulitis at the inferior glenohumeral ligament level obliterating the axillary pouch.

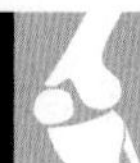

1–11 Teres Minor Muscle Tear

Eli J. Bendavid

PRESENTATION

Pain, status post twisting

FINDINGS

MRI demonstrates teres minor muscle edema, with nonvisualization of the tendinous insertion. Associated calcified body and anterior labral tear are also noted.

DIFFERENTIAL DIAGNOSES

- *Acute calcific tendinitis:* Manifests as calcified bodies along the course of the tendon. Associated musculotendinous edema is frequently present. Tendinous insertion, however, is intact.
- *Denervation atrophy:* Diffuse musculotendinous edema typically precedes size diminution and fatty replacement of the muscle. Tendinous insertion, again, is intact.
- *Infraspinatus tendon tear:* Isolated type is uncommon. Usually associated with supraspinatus tear.
- *Parsonage–Turner syndrome:* This is an acute brachial neuritis.

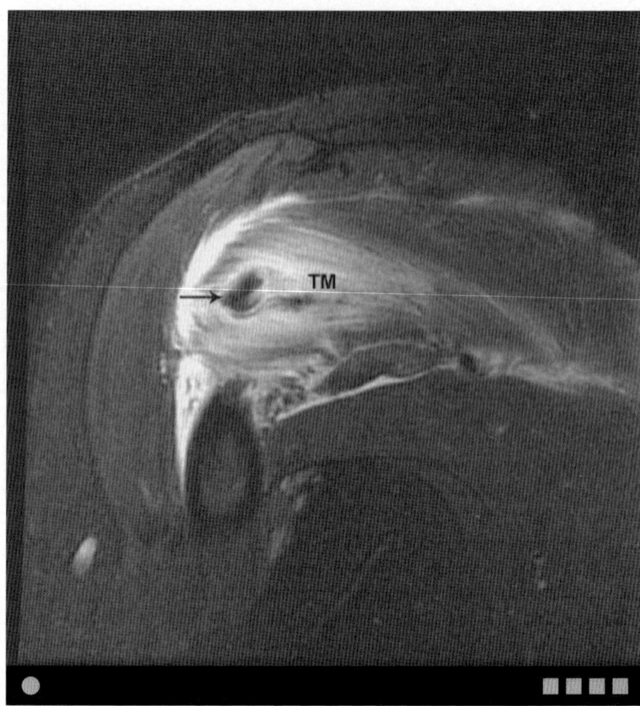

A. Teres minor tear: Coronal oblique fat-saturated T2 image shows disruption of the teres minor tendon (TM) at the humeral insertion site. A small calcified body within the tendon is partially visualized (arrow).

COMMENTS

The patient is a 65-year-old female with a history of acute left shoulder pain. Loss of normal low-signal intensity along the course of the teres minor tendinous insertion is noted, which is compatible with a rotator cuff tear. Anatomically, the rotator cuff includes musculature of the supraspinatus, infraspinatus, teres minor, and subscapularis. Both the supraspinatus and infraspinatus tendons extend to the superior facet of the greater tuberosity of the humerus. In contrast, the teres minor inserts to the inferior facet of the greater tuberosity. The subscapularis tendon extends anteriorly to the lesser tuberosity. Pain, weakness, and limited range of motion are the most common presentations associated with rotator cuff tears. Underlying tendinous calcification represents calcific tendonitis and is indicative of chronic underlying repetitive stress or degenerative trauma to the tendon, which often precedes a tear. Initially, edematous change of the tendon results in thickening and increased T2 or STIR signal intensity, which over time may progress to fibrosis. Finally, tendinous degeneration results in partial- or full-thickness tears. A full-thickness tear oftentimes results in musculotendinous retraction, which may demonstrate muscle belly edema acutely. Over time, atrophy of the associated muscle belly may result in the diminution of size and fatty replacement. Associated fluid within the subacromial/subdeltoid bursa is also a common finding of rotator cuff tears. Rotator cuff tears (versus tendinopathy) are more common with advancing age.

PEARLS

- **Rotator cuff muscles consist of the supraspinatus, infraspinatus, teres minor, and subscapularis.**
- **Disruption of the tendinous insertion, either partial- or full-thickness, is indicative of tear.**
- **Tears are often preceded by tendinous edema/inflammation.**
- **Tears may be associated with underlying calcific tendonitis.**
- **Massive full-thickness tears frequently demonstrate retraction of the musculotendinous junction, with muscle belly edema (acute) or atrophy (chronic).**

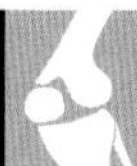

ADDITIONAL IMAGES

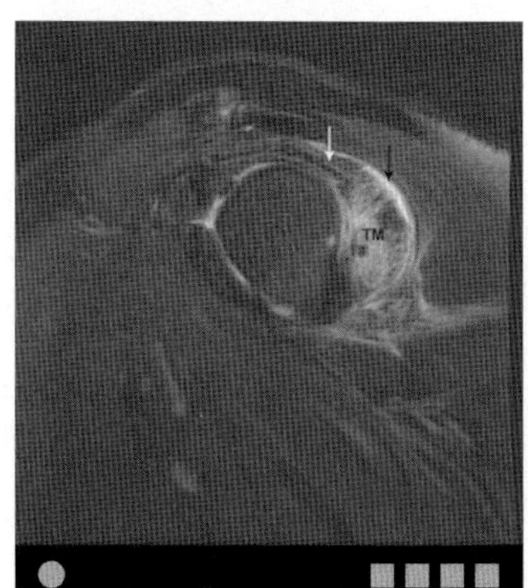

B. Teres minor tear: Sagittal oblique fat-saturated T2 image re-demonstrates the tear (TM), with associated fluid within the subdeltoid bursa (black arrow). The adjacent infraspinatus tendon is intact (white arrow).

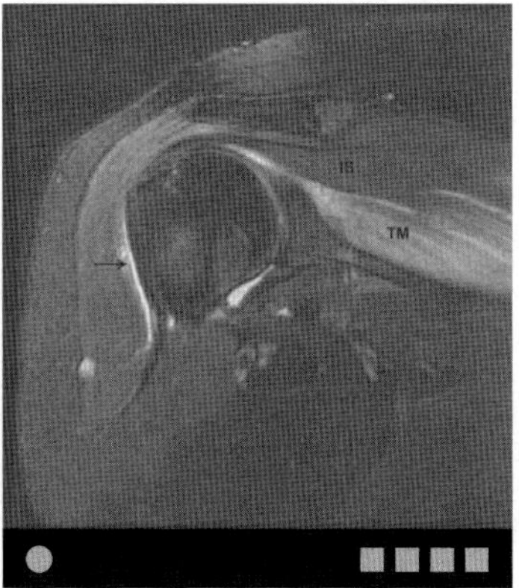

C. Teres minor tear: Coronal oblique fat-saturated T2 image shows acute edematous change of the teres minor muscle (TM) throughout. The overlying infraspinatus muscle and tendon (IS) are intact. Abnormal subdeltoid fluid is again noted (arrow).

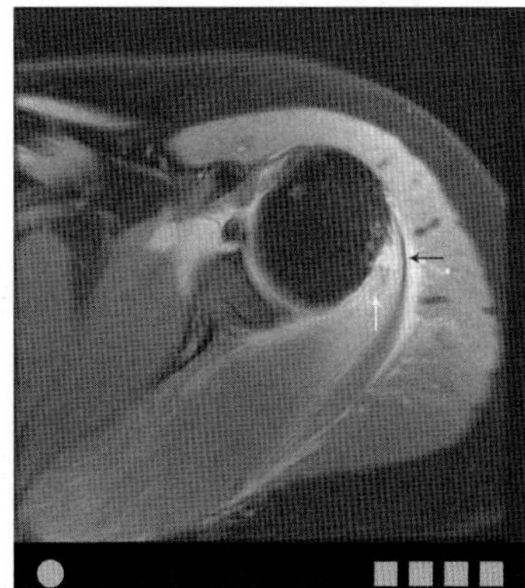

D. Teres minor tear: Axial fat-saturated proton density image demonstrates tear of the teres minor tendon (white arrow). Overlying infraspinatus tendon is intact (black arrow). Anterior labral tear is incidentally noted.

DIFFERENTIAL DIAGNOSES IMAGES

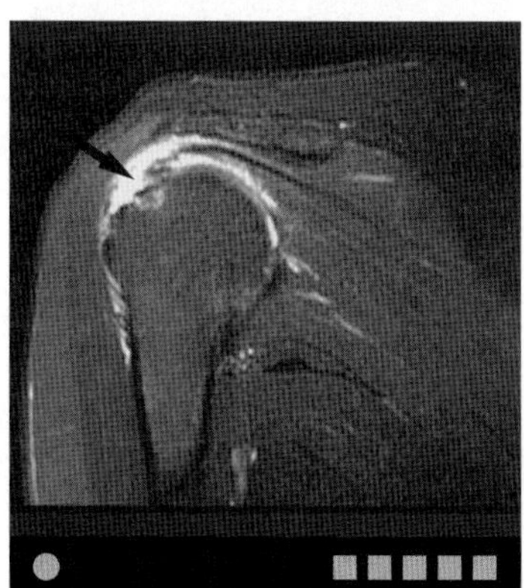

E. Isolated full-thickness infraspinatus tear: Posterior slice of coronal oblique T2 SPIR image shows fluid is replacing the distal tendon of infraspinatus tendon at the insertion site (arrow).

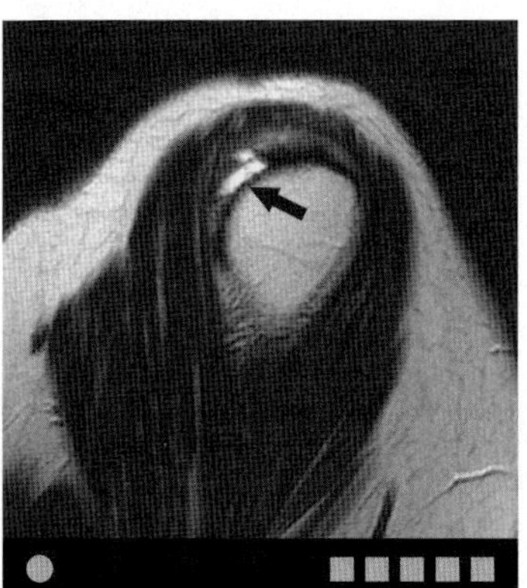

F. Isolated full-thickness infraspinatus tear: Sagittal T2-weighted image shows fluid signal replacing infraspinatus tendon representing full-thickness tear (arrow).

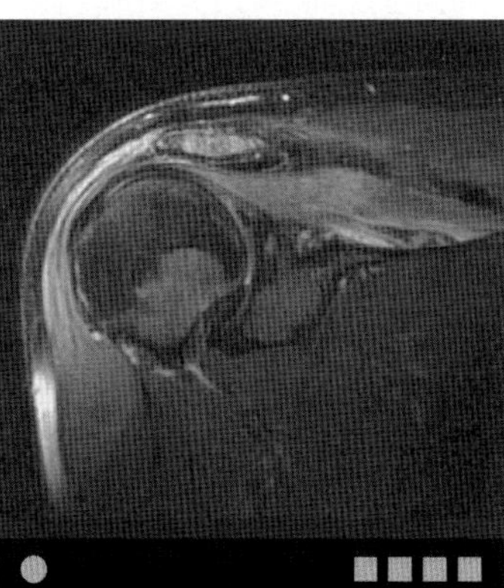

G. Parsonage-turner syndrome: Coronal fat-suppressed T2-weighted fast spin echo image shows intramuscular edema in the supraspinatus and deltoid muscles.

IMAGE KEY

Common

Rare

Typical

Unusual

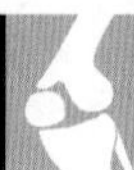

1–12 Subscapularis Tendon Tear with Biceps Dislocation

Lynne Steinbach and Jeffrey N. Masi

PRESENTATION

Impaired abduction, anterior dislocation

FINDINGS

Disruption of subscapularis tendon continuity, dislocated biceps tendon.

DIFFERENTIAL DIAGNOSES

- *GLOM sign:* Retracted labral Bankart lesion has appearance of biceps tendon in rotator interval.
- *Torn biceps tendon:* Empty biceps groove unrelated to dislocation; no tendon seen in area of tear on axial images.
- *Gas bubble:* Arthrogram gas that rises to nondependent location of the shoulder joint.

COMMENTS

Fibers from the subscapularis tendon course over the bicipal groove, and in conjunction with the superior glenohumeral and coracohumeral ligaments, offer structural support for the biceps tendon. Therefore, in roughly half of subscapularis tendon tears (partial and full thickness), there is also an associated dislocation of the biceps tendon. These tears often occur secondary to shoulder dislocation (usually anterior, especially in older patients), subcoracoid impingement, or from trauma and are more likely in patients older than 40 years. They may be restricted to the tendon alone or expand into the subscapularis muscle. Clinically, patients often experience difficulty or pain with internal rotation. Diagnosis is best made using MRI, visualizing the course of the tendon on axial images. Sagittal and coronal images are also helpful. As in other tendon injuries, the tendon may be avulsed, retracted, or in the case of partial tear, thinned or interrupted by fluid signal intensity. Narrowing of the space between the coracoid process and humerus (subcoracoid impingement) can produce subscapularis tendon tears. Avulsion fractures and lesser tuberosity cysts may be present. There is also an increased incidence of rotator interval and supraspinatus tears in shoulders with subscapularis tendon tears. Subcoracoid bursitis may cause anterior pain, mimicking subscapularis tendon pathology.

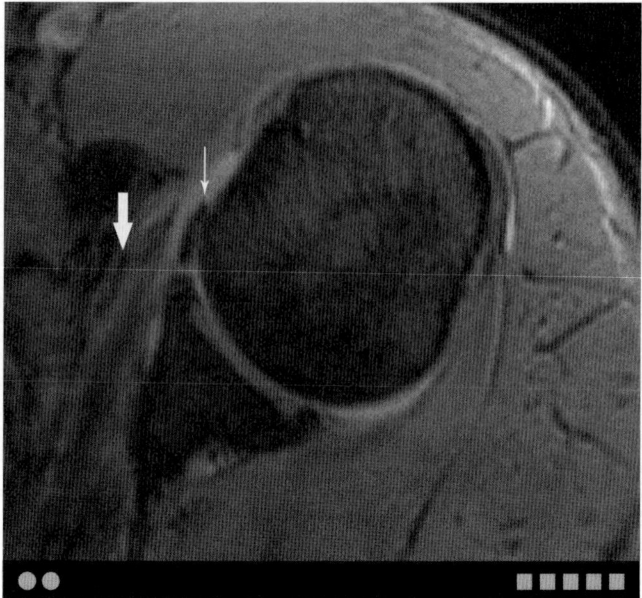

A. Tear of subscapularis tendon with biceps tendon dislocation: There is a full-thickness tear with medial retraction of the subscapularis tendon (large arrow) on this axial gradient echo MR image. The biceps is dislocated in front of the glenohumeral joint (small arrow).

PEARLS

- **Check the biceps tendon in the presence of a subscapularis tendon tear.**
- **The biceps tendon can sublux or dislocate into a partial tear of the subscapularis tendon.**
- **The biceps tendon can sublux anterior to the subscapularis tendon even if the tendon is not torn.**
- **Most subscapularis tendon tears are in the superior portion of the tendon.**
- **Use a fluid-sensitive sequence in the axial and sagittal plane to detect these tears.**

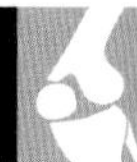

ADDITIONAL IMAGE

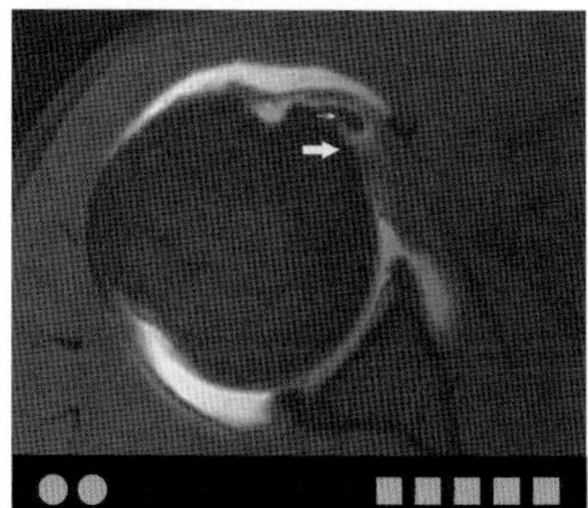

B. Partial tear of subscapularis tendon with biceps tendon dislocation: The biceps tendon (small arrow) is dislocated into a partial tear of the subscapularis tendon (large arrow) on this fat-suppressed axial T1-weighted MR arthrogram image.

DIFFERENTIAL DIAGNOSES IMAGES

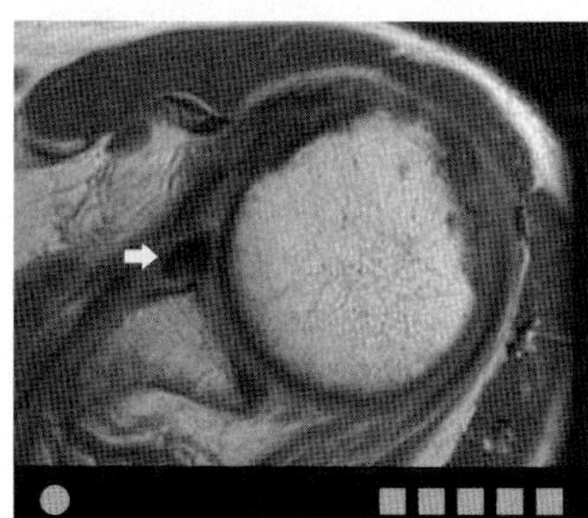

C. Glenoid labrum ovoid mass (GLOM) sign: This represents a superiorly retracted anterior labrum from a Bankart lesion that simulates a dislocated biceps medial to the coracoid (arrow) on this axial T1-weighted MR image.

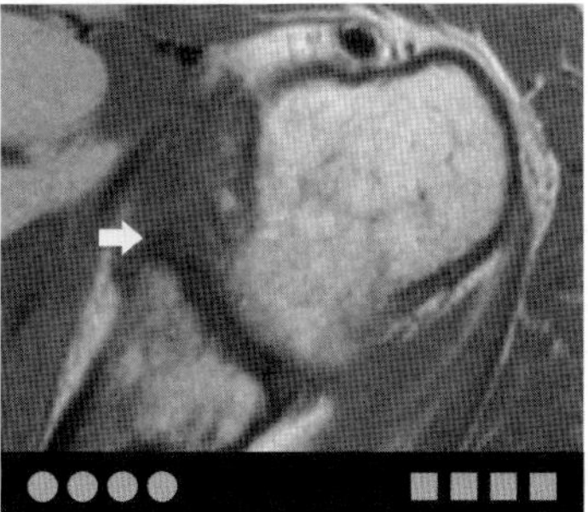

D. Bankart lesion: Axial T1-weighted MR image of the Bankart lesion (arrow) in the patient shown in image C.

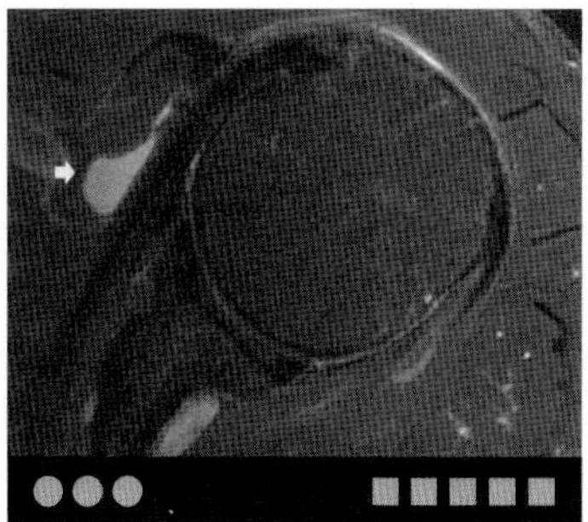

E. Subcoracoid bursa: This bursa lies anterior to the subscapularis tendon (arrow) on an axial fat-suppressed T2-weighted MR image. The pain from this bursa can mimic a subscapularis tendon problem.

IMAGE KEY

Common

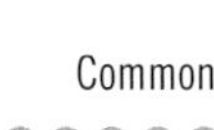

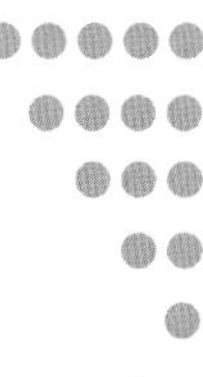

Rare

Typical

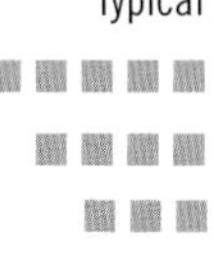

Unusual

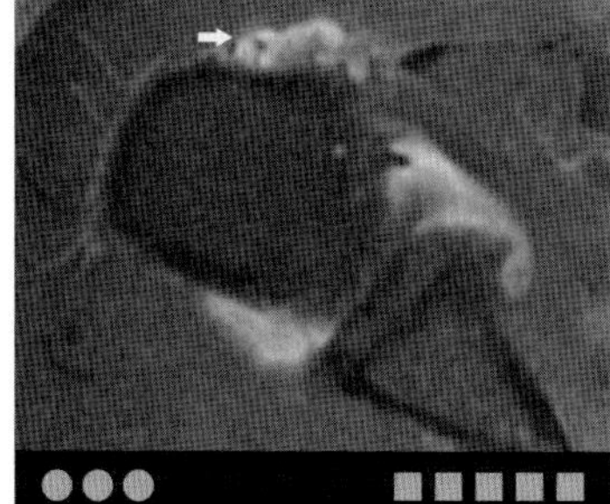

F. Biceps tendon tear: No biceps is seen in the intertubercular groove (arrow) on this axial fat-suppressed T2-weighted MR image. Unlike the first case, this resulted from a biceps tendon tear, not subluxation.

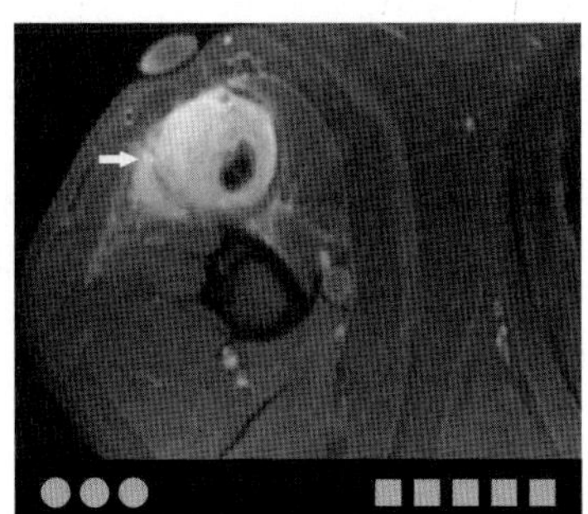

G. Biceps tendon tear: Same patient as in image 6. The fat-suppressed axial T2-weighted image distal to the glenohumeral joint shows the retracted biceps tendon.

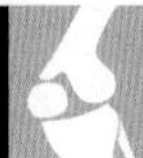

1–13 Hidden Lesion

Scott Kingston

PRESENTATION

Impingement symptoms and anterior shoulder pain

FINDINGS

MR image demonstrating thickening and hyperintensity of distal subscapularis tendon.

DIFFERENTIAL DIAGNOSES

- *Subcoracoid impingement:* Narrowing of the subcoracoid space, resulting in impaction on the lesser tuberosity with subcortical cysts.
- *Rotator cuff tear:* Partial or complete anterior tear of the supraspinatus or superior tear of the subscapularis tendons demonstrating focal high signal fluid intensity.
- *SLAP tear:* Superior labral tear with or without involvement of biceps labral anchor. Presents with anterior shoulder pain with biceps symptoms if biceps tendon is torn or degenerated.
- *Calcific bursitis/Tendinosis*: Presents with anterior shoulder pain with focal signal void from calcium hydroxyapatite deposition with surrounding edema of bursa or involved tendon.

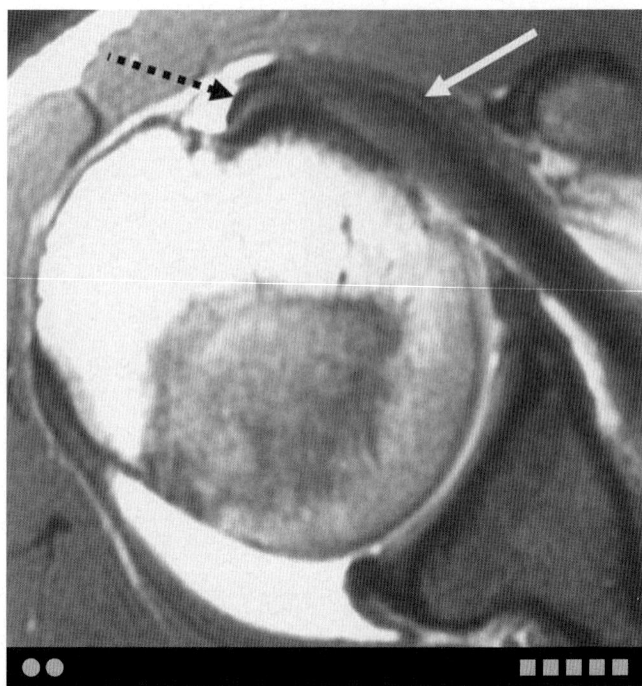

A. Hidden lesion: Axial MR arthrogram image of the shoulder demonstrates thickening of distal subscapularis tendon (solid white arrow) with mild medial location of biceps tendon (dashed black arrow) within upper groove.

COMMENTS

This patient presented with impingement symptoms with anterior shoulder pain on flexion and supination of forearm. Hidden lesions occur in the lateral aspect of the rotator interval and are difficult for the arthroscopist to visualize, and thus the term "hidden." Pathology ranges from partial tears to chronic degeneration/tendinosis of the distal upper subscapularis tendon at its attachment to the lesser tuberosity with or without accompanying injury to the adjacent superior glenohumeral (SGL) and coracohumeral ligaments (CHL). These ligaments form a sling around the long head of the biceps tendon, thus providing biceps stability within the upper bicipital groove. Injury to the subscapularis tendon may result in soft tissue thickening with intermediate signal intensity on T1-weighted images and hyperintensity on T2-weighted images. Tears of the distal subscapularis are usually partial, and if there is injury to the supporting SGL/CHL complex, then the biceps tendon may demonstrate hypermobility within the upper bicipital groove with subsequent medial subluxation into the torn fibers of the subscapularis tendon. If the medial fibers of the deep subscapularis tendon are still intact with an intact or lax SGL/CHL complex, the biceps may simply sublux in an extra-articular location. With complete rupture of the subscapularis tendon and SGL/CHL complex, the biceps may dislocate completely into the glenohumeral joint. The biceps tendon may also demonstrate tendinosis and appear thickened and isointense on T1-weighted images from subcoracoid impingement in conjunction with subcortical cystic changes of the lesser tuberosity.

PEARLS

- **Best depicted on axial MR images.**
- **Thickened distal subscapularis tendon demonstrates isointense signal to muscle on T1-weighted image and hyperintense signal on T2-weighted image. May have accompanying partial longitudinal tears.**
- **Long head of biceps tendon may appear flattened with medial subluxation from upper bicipital groove into partial tears of subscapularis tendon.**
- **Normal long head of biceps tendon appears medial in location above upper bicipital groove and superior aspect of subscapularis tendon.**

ADDITIONAL IMAGES

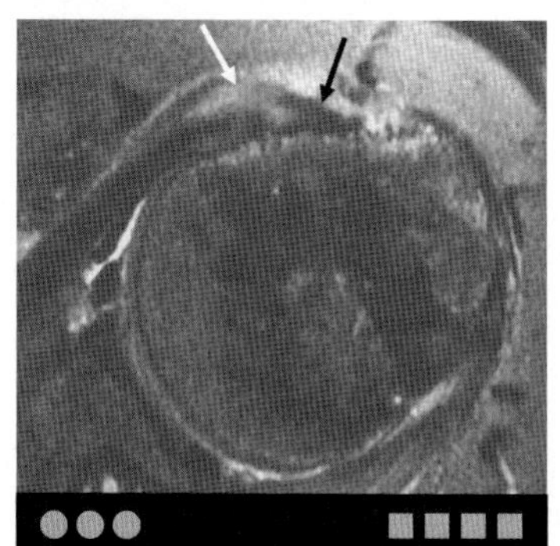

B. Hidden lesion: Axial fat-saturated contrast-enhanced PD image shows hyperintense partial superficial subscapularis tendon tear (white arrow) with mild medial subluxation of biceps tendon (black arrow).

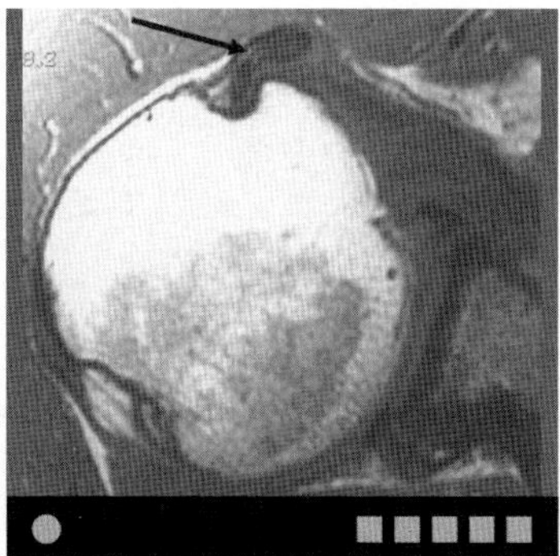

C. Hidden lesion: Axial T1-weighted image shows tendinosis of distal subscapularis tendon with degenerating biceps tendon (arrow) subluxing medially in an extracapsular fashion from the bicipital groove.

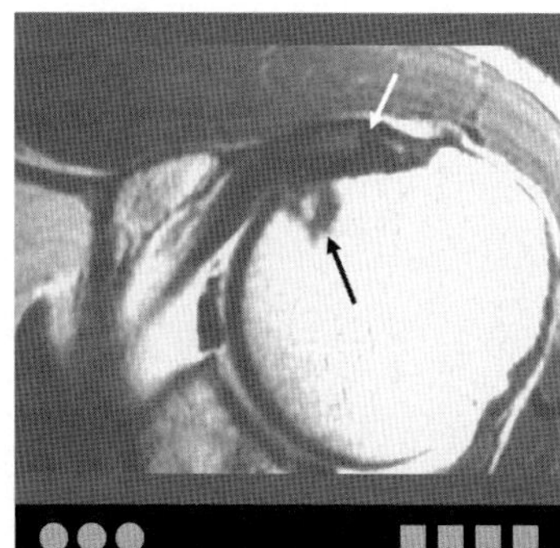

D. Hidden lesion: Axial T1-weighted image demonstrates medially subluxing biceps tendon (white arrow) into partial subscapularis tendon tear. Note lesser tuberosity subcortical cyst (black arrow) from subcoracoid impingement.

IMAGE KEY

DIFFERENTIAL DIAGNOSES IMAGES

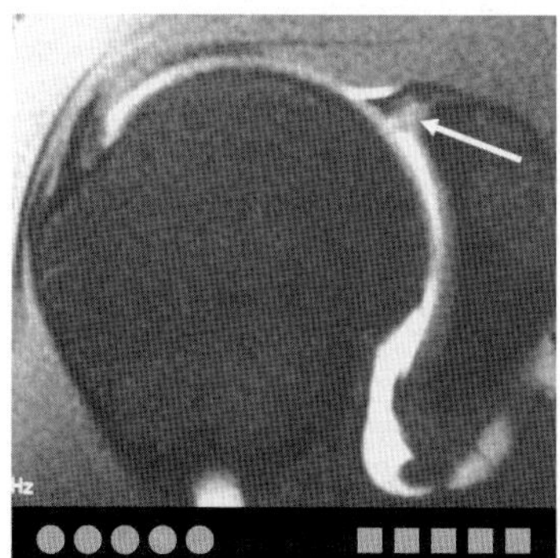

E. SLAP lesion: Coronal T1-weighted image with intra-articular gadolinium demonstrates a SLAP lesion (arrow) with contrast undermining the base of the superior labrum.

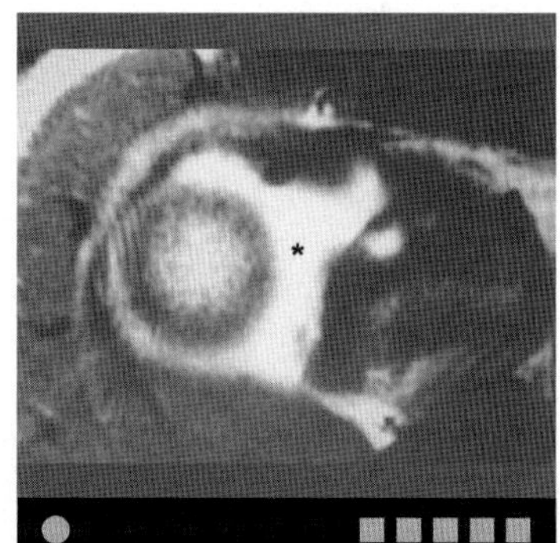

F. Biceps tendon rupture: Axial T1-weighted image with intra-articular gadolinium shows absence (star) of the intra-articular portion of the long head of biceps tendon secondary to tendon rupture from supraglenoid tubercle.

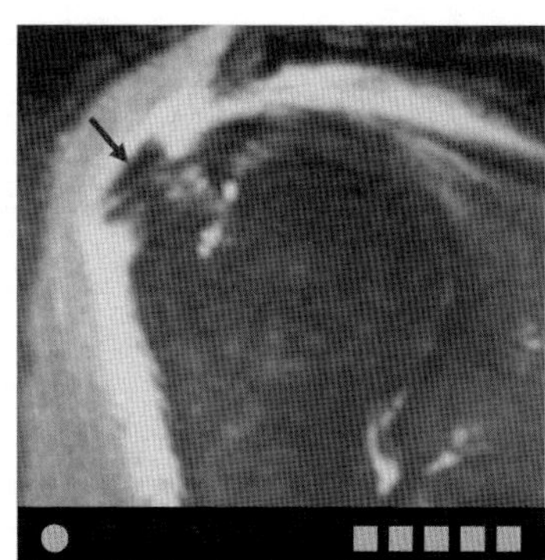

G. Calcific bursitis: Coronal STIR image shows signal void (arrow) secondary to calcium hydroxyapatite deposition within the subdeltoid bursa with surrounding edema.

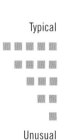

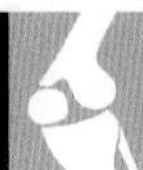

1–14 Quadrilateral Space Syndrome

Ashkan Afshin and Jamshid Tehranzadeh

PRESENTATION

Shoulder pain and numbness

FINDINGS

The MR findings in T1-weighted and T2-weighted images in triplane show fatty infiltration of teres minor muscle.

DIFFERENTIAL DIAGNOSES

- *Parsonage-turner syndrome:* A rare condition characterized by inflammation of the lower motor neurons of the brachial plexus innervating the muscles of the chest, shoulders, and arms.
- *Labral cyst:* Ganglion cysts of the shoulder that may cause suprascapular entrapment neuropathy resulting in shoulder pain and infraspinatus muscle weakness.

COMMENTS

The quadrilateral space syndrome is musculotendinous formation bounded by the teres minor muscle (superiorly), the teres major muscle (inferiorly), the Humerus (laterally), and the long head of triceps (medially). This space contains the axillary nerve and the posterior humeral circumflex artery (PHCA). Quadrilateral space syndrome is an infrequent condition that results from compression of the axillary nerve and posterior humeral circumflex artery (PHCA) in quadrilateral space. Presence of a fibrous band within the space is one of the most common causes of this disorder. Symptoms result from compression of the axillary nerve, not from PHCA occlusion. Patients with quadrilateral space syndrome complain of shoulder pain aggravated by abduction, extension, and external rotation. They also experience paresthesia radiating down the arm and forearm in a nondermatomal distribution and tenderness on palpation of the quadrilateral space. The diagnosis is clinical and is documented by subclavian arteriography or angio-MR imaging. A positive arteriogram reveals occlusion of the posterior humeral circumflex artery with the arm in abduction and external rotation. Isolated atrophy of the teres minor muscle, which is innervated by the axillary nerve, in MR images is suggestive of quadrilateral space syndrome. Treatment is usually conservative and operative management is considered for selected patients.

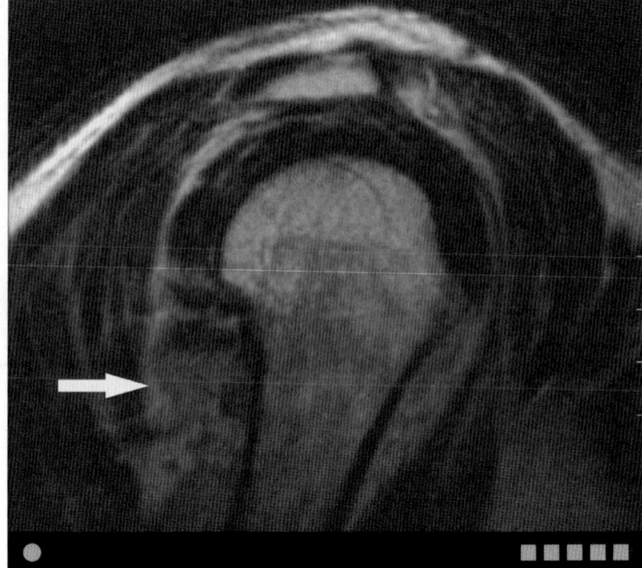

A. Quadrilateral space syndrome: Sagittal T2-weighted image shows fatty atrophy of the most of teres minor muscle. Note the increased signal of this muscle compared to other muscles (arrow).

PEARLS

- **Compression of the axillary nerve**
- **Shoulder pain with abduction, extension, and external rotation**
- **Paresthesia in a nondermatomal distribution and point tenderness**
- **Selective atrophy of the teres minor muscle**
- **Clinical diagnosis and confirmation with MR angiogram**
- **Posterior humeral circumflex artery occlusion in arteriogram**

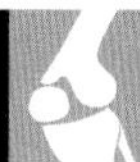

ADDITIONAL IMAGES

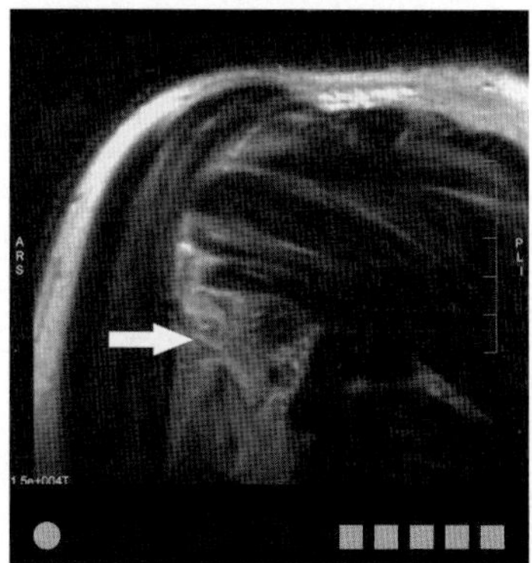

B. Quadrilateral space syndrome: Coronal T2-weighted image shows fatty atrophy of teres minor muscle (arrow).

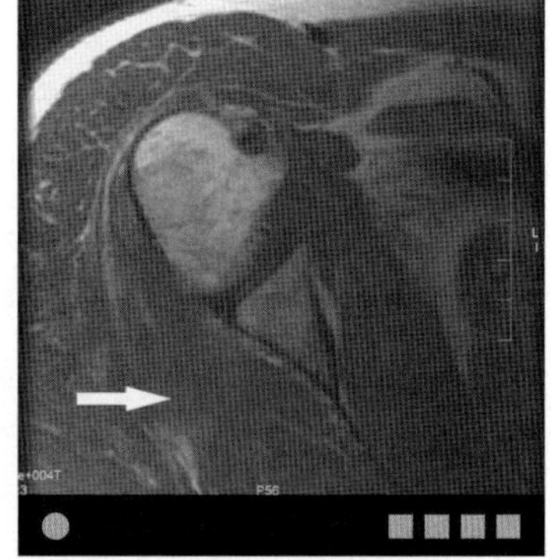

C. Quadrilateral space syndrome: Axial T1-weighted image shows intermediate instead of dark signal in teres minor muscle (arrow).

DIFFERENTIAL DIAGNOSES IMAGES

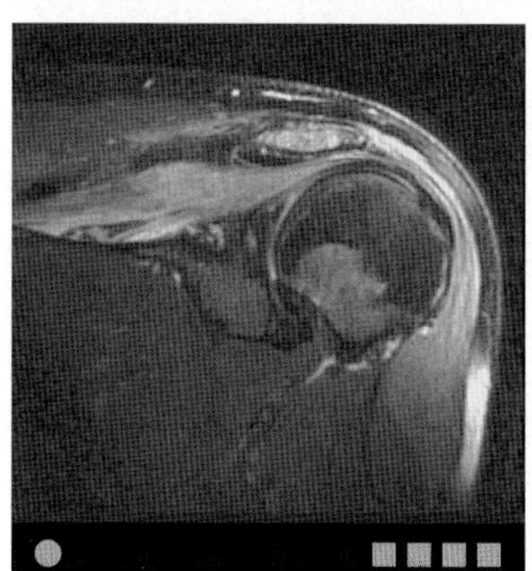

D. Parsonage–Turner syndrome: Coronal fat-suppressed T2-weighted fast spin echo image shows intramuscular edema in the supraspinatus and deltoid muscles.

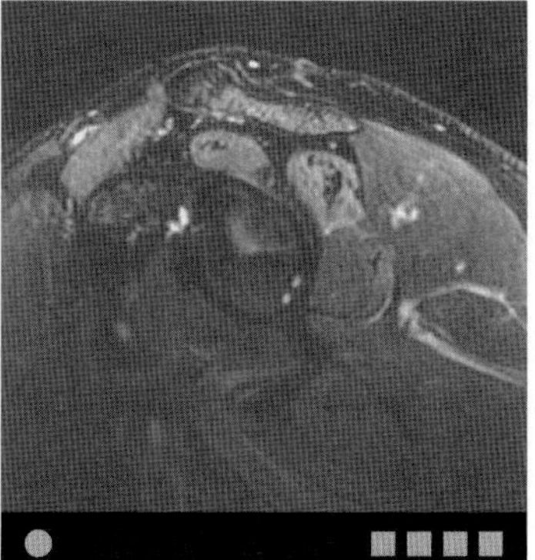

E. Parsonage–Turner syndrome: Sagittal fat-suppressed T2-weighted fast spin echo image shows intramuscular edema in the supraspinatus and infraspinatus musculature.

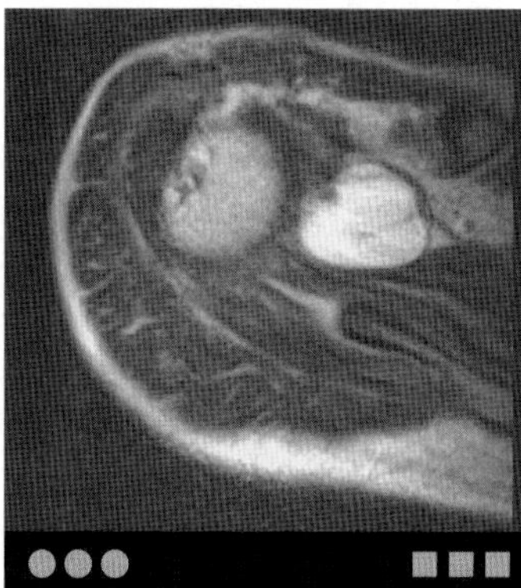

F. Labral cyst: Axial T2-weighted image demonstrates high signal intensity mass in the suprascapular notch leading to atrophy of infra-spinatus muscle.

IMAGE KEY

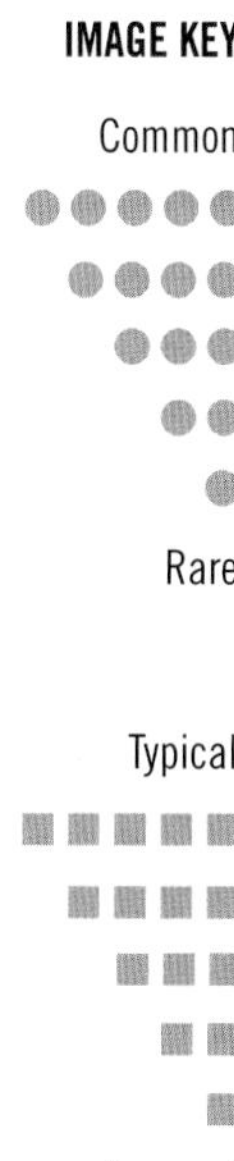

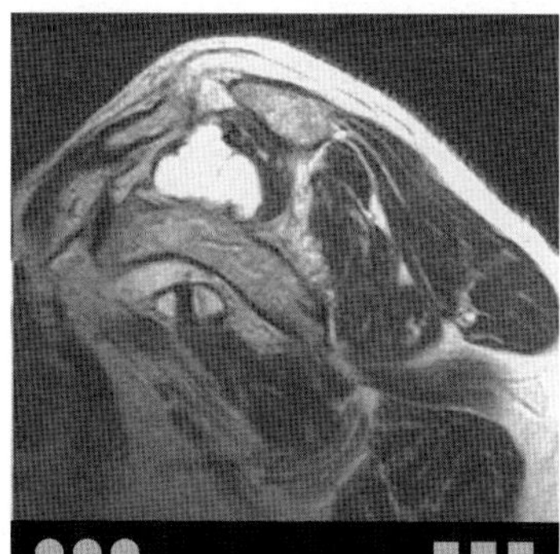

G. Labral cyst: Sagittal T2-weighted image shows high signal intensity mass in the suprascapular notch leading to atrophy of infraspinatus muscle.

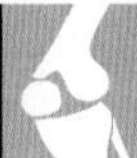

1–15 Posterior Shoulder Dislocation

Stephen E. Ling and William R. Reinus

PRESENTATION

Pain, swelling, limited range of motion

FINDINGS

Posteriorly displaced humeral head fixed in internal rotation.

DIFFERENTIAL DIAGNOSIS

- *Anterior shoulder dislocation:* Most common form of shoulder dislocation. This may result in Hill-Sachs and Bankart deformity. The humeral head is located anterior to the glenoid process on transscapular Y-view.

COMMENTS

Posterior glenohumeral dislocation is an uncommon type of shoulder dislocation, accounting for less than 5% of shoulder dislocation cases. There are three subtypes: subacromial (most common), subglenoid, and subspinous. Posterior dislocation is often seen in the clinical setting of seizure, electric shock, and electroconvulsive therapy, and it is not uncommonly bilateral. In addition, glenoid retroversion and deficiency of either the bony or fibrocartilagenous glenoid are predisposing risk factors. The injury mechanism involves sudden axial loading of the arm when in internal rotation and adduction. During the dislocation, an impaction injury occurs between the anteromedial humeral head and posterior glenoid rim, resulting in a humeral head compression fracture known as a Trough fracture or Reverse Hill-Sachs fracture (eventually noted in approximately 75% of cases) and possibly also a fracture of the posterior glenoid called a Reverse Bankart lesion, respectively. Despite the clinical findings, fewer than 50% of patients with posterior dislocation are correctly diagnosed at initial presentation. Radiographs show a shoulder fixed in internal rotation, as the humeral head is locked behind the posterior rim of the glenoid. There may also be loss of the normal "crescent sign," an ellipse-shaped radiodensity resulting from superimposition of the glenoid and humeral head in normal patients. Another sign of posterior dislocation that is best seen on radiographs is peaking of Maloney's arc, the line formed by the medial border of the humerus and the lateral border of the scapula.

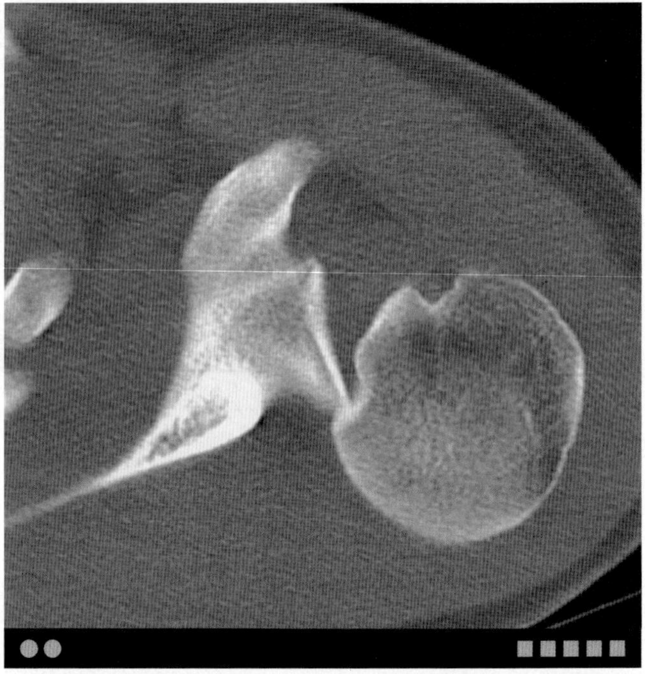

A. Posterior shoulder dislocation: Axial CT image of the shoulder shows the humeral head locked behind the posterior glenoid rim, and adjacent deformity of the anteromedial humeral head indicating a Reverse Hill-Sachs impaction fracture (Trough sign).

PEARLS

- **Check radiographs to be sure that the patient can move their shoulder into external rotation. Failing this, a posterior dislocation should be suspected.**
- **Evaluate the study for preservation/absence of the normal overlap of the glenoid and humeral head (i.e., the "crescent sign").**
- **The "trough sign" indicating impaction compression fracture of the anteromedial humeral head is highly suspicious for posterior dislocation.**
- **In a patient with severe pain, a CT facilitates diagnosis.**

ADDITIONAL IMAGES

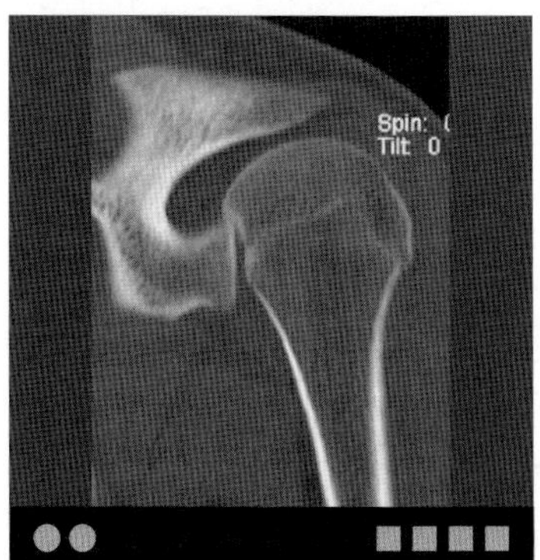

B. Posterior shoulder dislocation: Coronal CT image shows a Reverse Hill-Sachs compression fracture of the anteromedial humeral head caused by the nearby posterior rim of the glenoid.

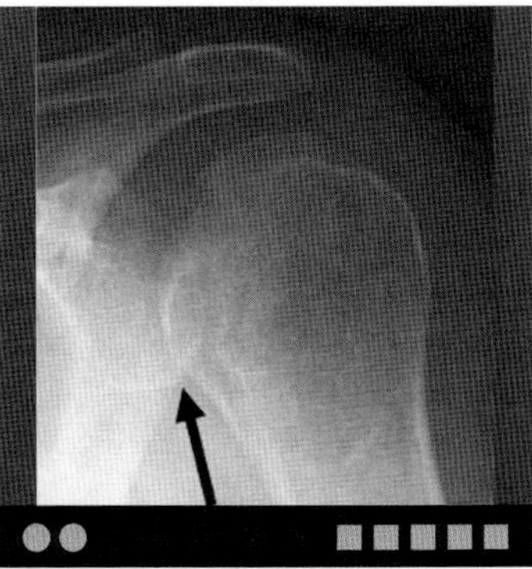

C. Posterior shoulder dislocation: AP radiograph in a different patient shows the shoulder fixed in internal rotation with a Reverse Hill-Sachs lesion of the humeral head. Note the peaking of Maloney's arc (arrow).

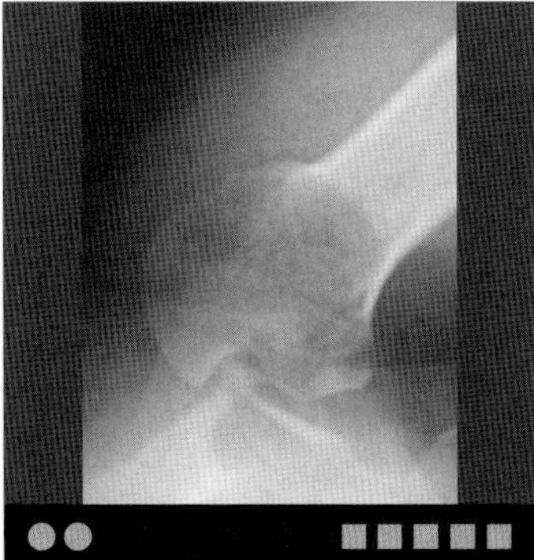

D. Posterior shoulder dislocation: Axillary radiograph shows posterior dislocation of the humeral head and Reverse Hill-Sachs fracture that locks the humeral head behind the glenoid.

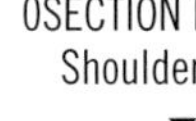

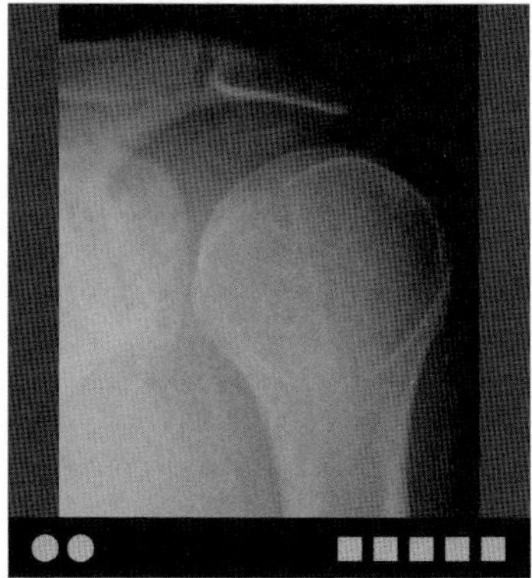

E. Posterior shoulder dislocation: AP radiograph in another patient shows loss of the normal "crescent sign," an ellipse-shaped radiodensity resulting from superimposition of the posterior glenoid and the humeral head. Note the fixation of the shoulder in internal rotation.

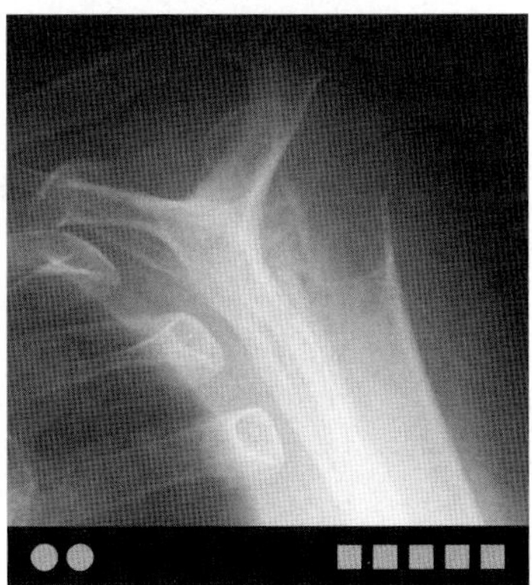

F. Posterior shoulder dislocation: Transscapular-Y view of the shoulder shows the humeral head located posterior to the glenoid fossa and under the spine of the scapula.

IMAGE KEY

Common

Rare

Typical

Unusual

DIFFERENTIAL DIAGNOSES IMAGES

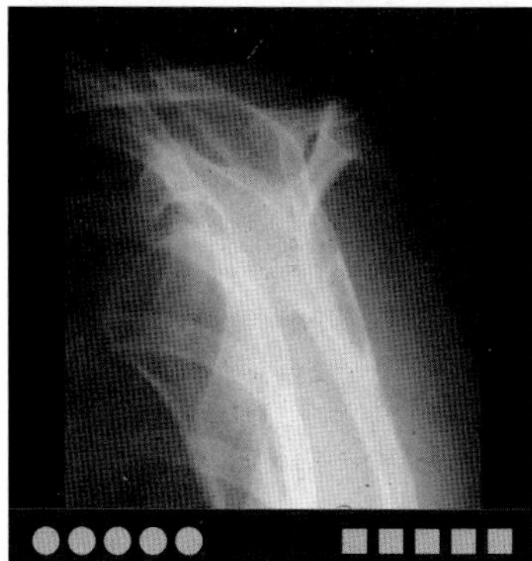

G. Anterior shoulder dislocation: Transscapular-Y view shows the humeral head is anterior to the glenoid fossa and under the coracoid process.

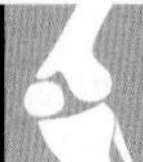

1–16 Buford Complex

Raymond Kuo and Rajeev K. Varma

PRESENTATION

Asymptomatic

FINDINGS

MR imaging is characterized by an absent anterosuperior labrum and thickened, cord-like middle glenohumeral ligament that originates at the superior labrum.

DIFFERENTIAL DIAGNOSES

- *SLAP tear:* Involvement of the biceps tendon insertion on the superior glenoid. May extend below 2- to 3-o'clock position. Secondary changes of inflammation with possible cartilage defects.
- *Bankart-type labral detachment:* May extend below the 2- to 3-o'clock position. Secondary changes of inflammation with possible cartilage defects.
- *Sublabral foramen:* Defect follows contour of bony cortex; no thickened middle glenohumeral ligament.

COMMENTS

This anatomic variant was found in several studies to be present in 1.5% to 6.1% of shoulders. The area of absent labral tissue extends from the 1-o'clock to 3-o'clock position (right shoulder). The cord-like middle glenohumeral ligament is of the same thickness or greater than the biceps tendon. Mistaking the middle glenohumeral ligament as a torn, detached labrum may lead to erroneous diagnosis of a SLAP lesion. If the Buford complex is mistakenly reattached to the neck of the glenoid, severe painful restriction of rotation and elevation occurs.

In a Buford complex, the labral tissue of the remaining three glenoid quadrants should be normal. A tear involving the biceps insertion site is inconsistent with the Buford complex and represents a SLAP lesion. In most cases, a SLAP tear will also show inflammatory changes around the biceps tendon origin. The underlying articular cartilage and its transition to the labrum should be examined for trauma or reparative tissue to help delineate pathology. A related anatomic variant, the sublabral foramen, is more common and has been reported in 12% to 40% of shoulders. Congenital labral detachment of varying sizes is observed in the anterosuperior quadrant. Again, this finding is not pathologic and should not be surgically repaired. A general rule is that the labral findings in both the Buford complex and sublabral foramen should not extend inferior to the 2- to 3-o'clock position.

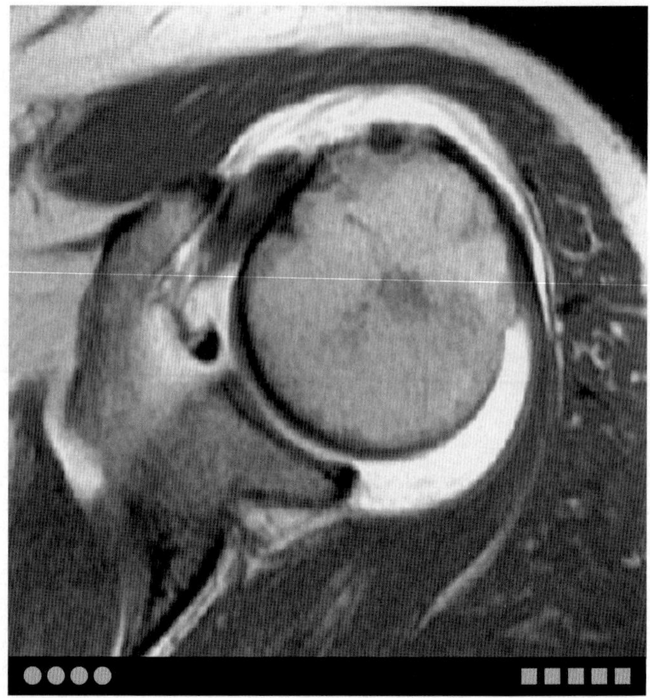

A. Buford complex: Axial T1-weighted image of MR arthrogram shows a cord-like middle glenohumeral ligament (MGHL) and no visible anterior labrum. Note that in this image the MGHL can be confused with a detached labrum.

PEARLS

- **Secondary signs of inflammation at the biceps tendon origin, reparative tissue, or cartilage lesions should be absent**
- **Cord-like middle glenohumeral ligament**
- **Labral defect should not extend inferior to the 2- to 3-o'clock position**

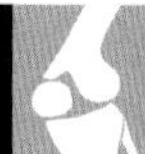

ADDITIONAL IMAGES

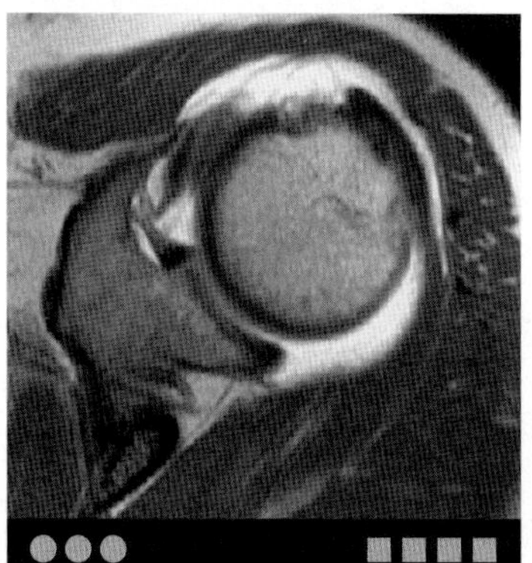

B. Buford complex: Axial T1-weighted image just superior to image A, showing the thickened glenohumeral ligament.

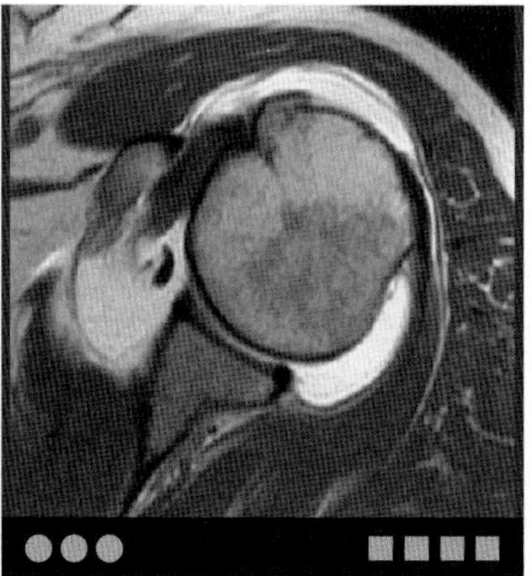

C. Buford complex: One slice inferior to image A demonstrating reappearance of the anterior labrum and the distinctly separate MGHL.

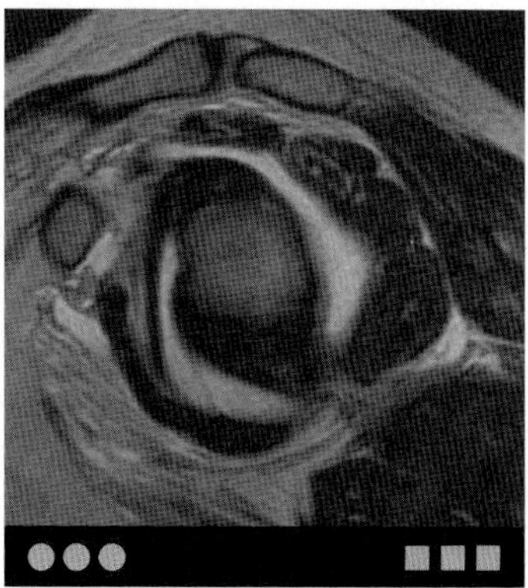

D. Buford complex: Sagittal T2-weighted image (anterior on left) showing a thickened MGHL and absence of the anterosuperior labrum.

DIFFERENTIAL DIAGNOSES IMAGES

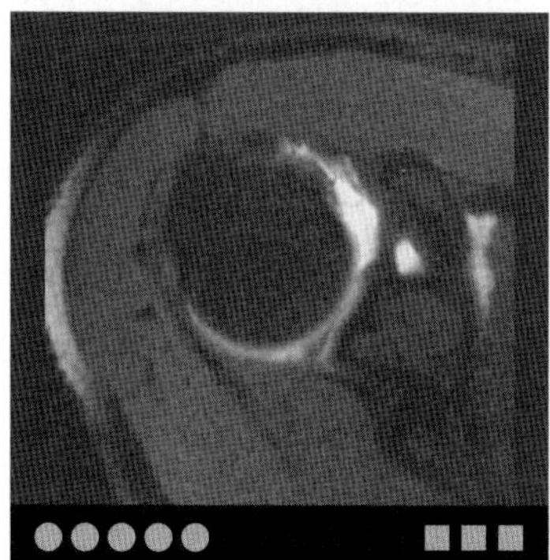

E. Superior labral tear: Axial T2-weighted image of MR arthrogram demonstrating a truncated antero-superior labrum representing a tear.

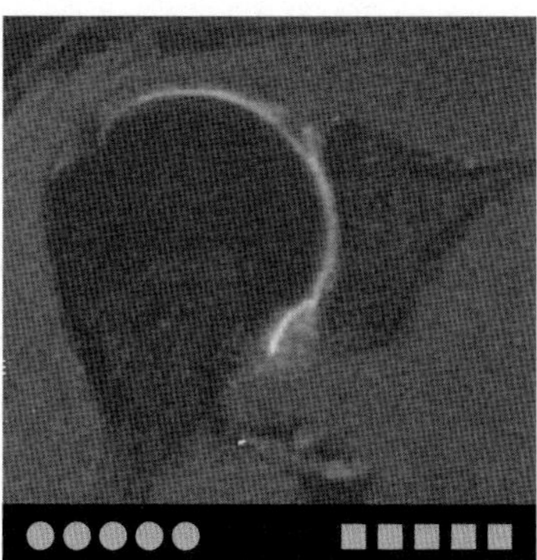

F. Superior labral tear: Coronal T2 image shows abnormal linear signal through the superior labrum from a SLAP tear.

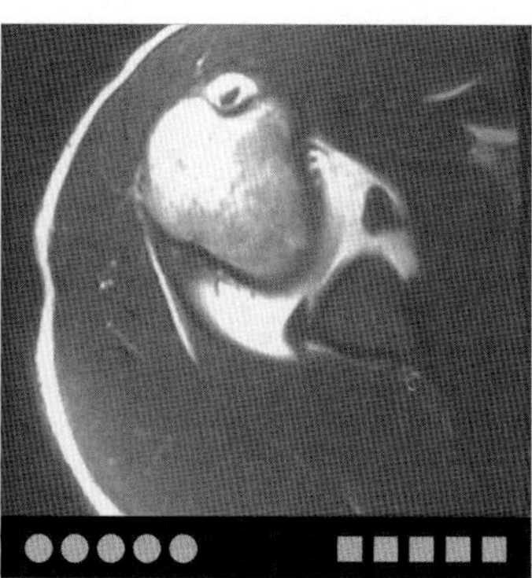

G. Anteroinferior labral tear: Axial T1-weighted MR arthrogram image shows anteroinferior labral tear and separation (Bankart deformity).

IMAGE KEY

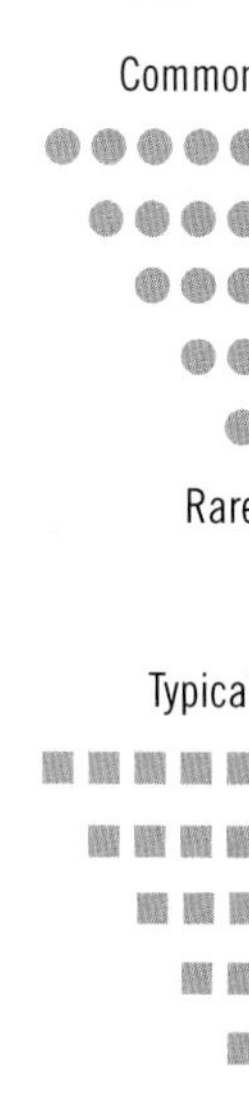

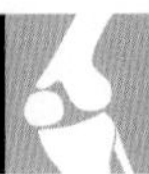

1–17 Osteocartilaginous Bankart Lesion and Hill-Sachs Deformity

Hamidreza R. Torshizy and Jamshid Tehranzadeh

PRESENTATION

Shoulder pain, tenderness, and instability

FINDINGS

MR images demonstrate a compression fracture of the posterolateral humeral head, corresponding to a Hill-Sachs deformity associated with avulsion fracture of the osteocartilaginous labrum from the glenoid bone with a lifted and torn scapular periosteum.

DIFFERENTIAL DIAGNOSES

- *Anterior labroligamentous periosteal sleeve avulsion (ALPSA) lesion:* ALPSA lesion is a variant of a classic Bankart lesion in which there is an avulsion of the anteroinferior labrum from the glenoid and an intact periosteum that is detached from the scapula anteriorly. The labral–ligamentous complex is usually displaced anteroinferiorly.
- *Perthes lesion:* An incompletely avulsed and minimally displaced anteroinferior labrum with a medially stripped but intact periosteum.

COMMENTS

The patient is a 19-year-old male with shoulder pain, tenderness, and instability. Hill-Sachs deformity is a compression fracture of the posterolateral humeral head, which occurs upon impaction against the anterior rim of the glenoid bone, occurring most commonly in patients younger than 30 years of age with a history of traumatic anterior dislocation of the glenohumeral joint. Hill-Sachs deformities are a clue to previous anterior glenohumeral dislocation. In about 75% of patients, Hill-Sachs deformities are associated with Bankart lesions. Bankart lesions can be cartilaginous or osseous in nature. A cartilaginous or classic Bankart lesion refers to an anteroinferior avulsion of the labrum from the glenoid bone with a lifted and torn scapular periosteum. Bankart lesions are found in the 3- to 6-o'clock position. At this position on axial T1 sequences, the avulsed labrum appears as if floating in the anterior joint space. This is because of the extravasation of contrast between glenoid and labrum with separation of the periosteum. The free labroligamentous tissue is attached to the anterior band of the inferior glenohumeral complex and to the disrupted scapular periosteum. An osseous or bony Bankart lesion refers to a fracture of the osseous anteroinferior glenoid rim in conjunction with the cartilaginous findings characteristic of a classic Bankart lesion. Of note, both the free labroligamentous complex, as well as the osseous segment of the glenoid, may migrate outside the 3- to 6-o'clock position, complicating diagnosis. MR arthrography imaging in the abduction and external rotation (ABER) view has been shown to enhance detection of Bankart lesions.

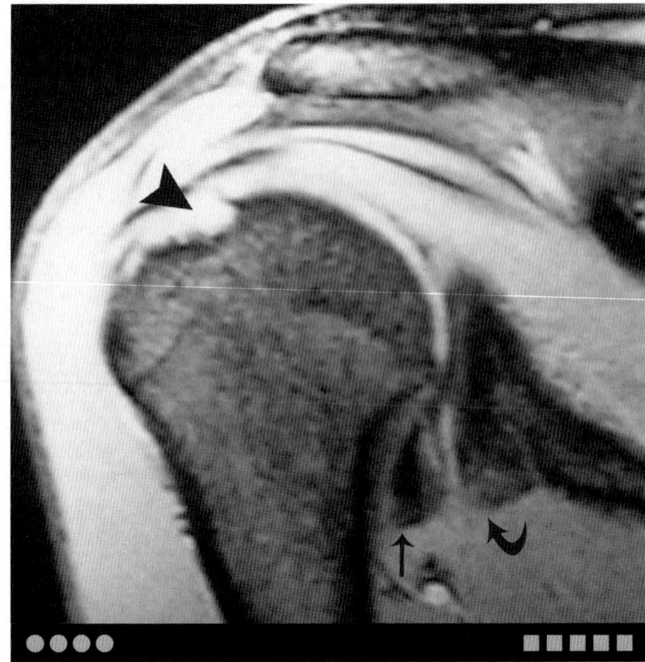

A. Osteocartilaginous Bankart lesion: Coronal T2-weighted MR arthrogram image demonstrating a compression fracture of the posterolateral humeral head (arrowhead), so-called Hill-Sachs deformity. An avulsion of the anteroinferior labrum with bony detachment (arrow) from the glenoid fossa (curved arrow), and accompanying discontinuity of the scapular periosteum is also noted.

PEARLS

- **Hill-Sachs deformity and Bankart lesions are manifestations of anterior glenohumeral joint instability.**
- **Hill-Sachs lesion is a compression fracture of the posterolateral humeral head.**
- **In 75% of times, it is associated with a cartilaginous or osseous Bankart lesion.**
- **A classic or cartilaginous Bankart lesion refers to anteroinferior avulsion of the labrum from the glenoid fossa with a lifted and torn scapular periosteum at 3- to 6-o'clock position.**
- **An osseous or bony Bankart lesion refers to an accompanying fracture of the osseous anteroinferior glenoid rim.**
- **Often, MR arthrography and ABER technique is necessary to differentiate Bankart lesions from its other variants.**

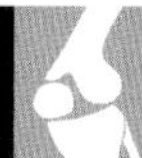

ADDITIONAL IMAGE

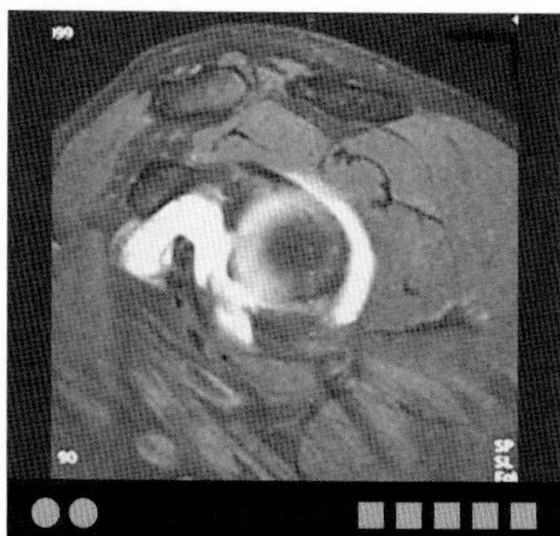

B. Osteocartilaginous Bankart lesion: Sagittal T1-weigthed MR arthrogram image demonstrating avulsion of the anteroinferior labrum from the glenoid bone, with interposed contrast extravasation.

DIFFERENTIAL DIAGNOSES IMAGES

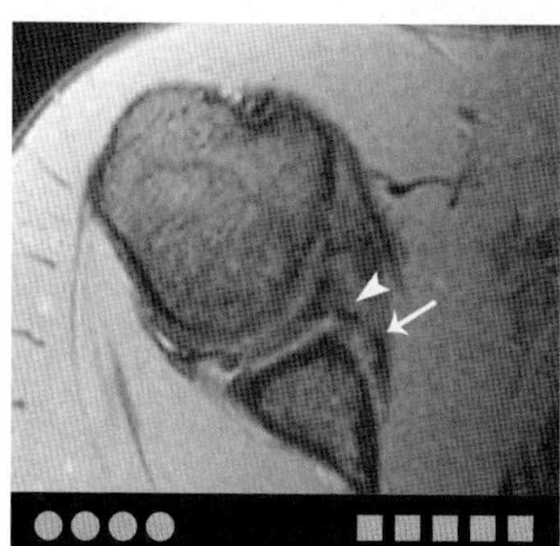

C. Cartilaginous Bankart lesion: Axial T2-weighted image demonstrating avulsion of the anteroinferior labrum (white arrowhead), with accompanying discontinuity of the scapular periosteum (white arrow) also noted.

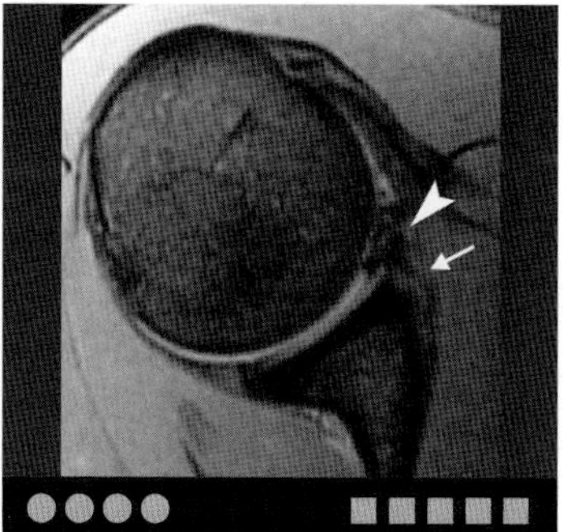

D. Cartilaginous Bankart lesion: Axial T2-weighted image demonstrating avulsion of the anteroinferior labrum (white arrowhead), with accompanying discontinuity of the scapular periosteum (white arrow) also noted.

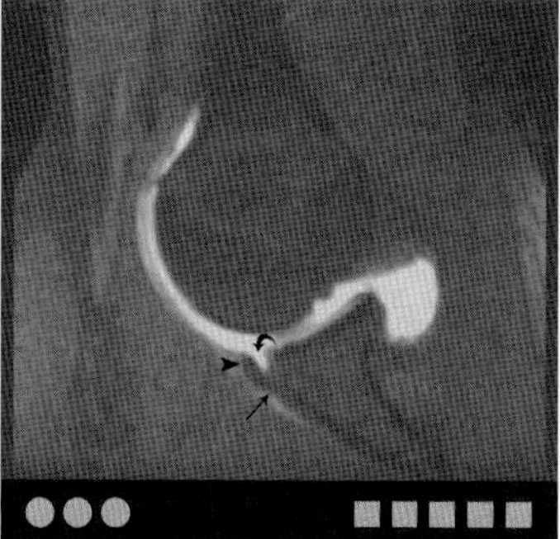

E. ALPSA lesion: ABER view including coronal fat-saturated T1-weighted post-MR arthrogram image demonstrating avulsion and lifting of the anteroinferior labrum (arrowhead) from the glenoid fossa and intervening extravasation of contrast (curved arrow). Note an intact scapular periosteum (arrow).

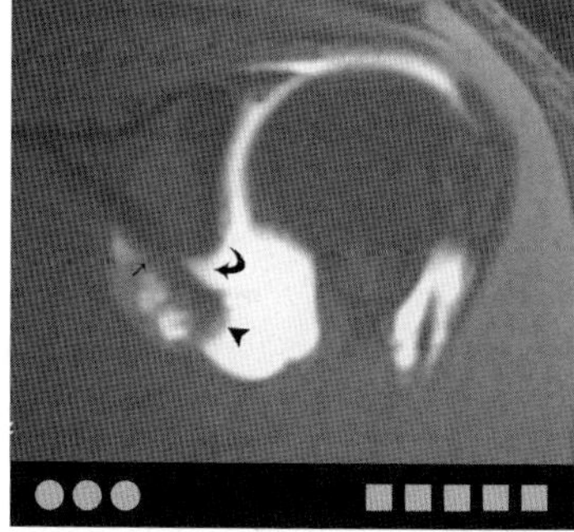

F. ALPSA lesion: Coronal T1-weighted fat-saturated post-MR arthrogram image demonstrating avulsion of the anteroinferior labrum (arrowhead) from the glenoid fossa and intervening extravasation of contrast (curved arrow). Note an intact scapular periosteum (arrow).

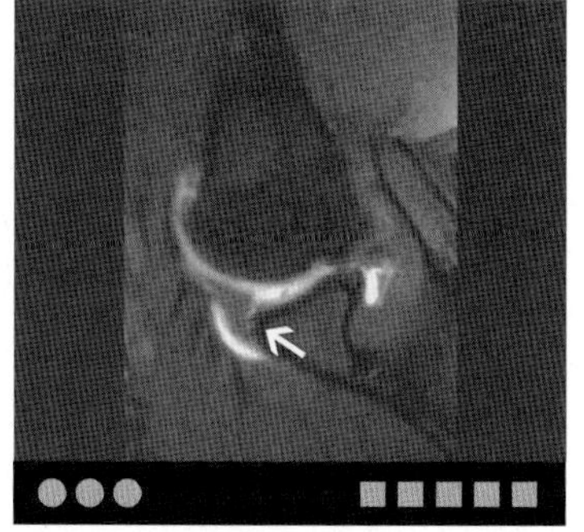

G. Perthes lesion: ABER view T1-weighted fat-saturated post-MR arthrogram image demonstrating a partially avulsed scapular periosteum with an anteroinferior labrum that is attached but not displaced. Note arrow is pointing to the site of the avulsion (arrow).

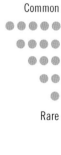

IMAGE KEY

Common

Rare

Typical

Unusual

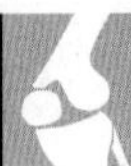

1–18 Glenoid Labral Articular Disruption (GLAD) Lesion

Hamidreza R. Torshizy and Jamshid Tehranzadeh

PRESENTATION

Shoulder pain and tenderness

FINDINGS

MR images demonstrate an anteroinferior labral tear associated with a defect in the glenoid hyaline articular cartilage.

DIFFERENTIAL DIAGNOSES

- *Delaminating glenoid articular cartilage lesion:* Surface defect in the integrity of the glenoid articular cartilage with peeling.
- *Bankart lesion:* Avulsion of the labroligamentous complex from the anteroinferior glenoid, with lifting and disruption of the scapular periosteum.
- *Anterior labroligamentous periosteal sleeve avulsion (ALPSA) lesion:* Avulsion of anteroinferior labrum from the glenoid, with an accompanying periosteum that is intact, but detached and lifted from the scapula anteriorly.

COMMENTS

The glenoid labral articular disruption (GLAD) lesion is an anteroinferior labral lesion associated with a defect in the glenoid hyaline articular cartilage. Torn labrum remains attached to the anterior scapular periosteum. GLAD lesions are most commonly the result of forced abduction injury to the shoulder from an abducted and external rotated position. Patients usually report anterior shoulder pain. However, no signs of anterior glenohumeral joint instability are present on physical examination. Differentiating GLAD lesions from delaminating cartilage lesions as well as the different variants of anteroinferior labral pathology (i.e., Bankart lesion, ALPSA lesion, and Perthes lesion) can be challenging and difficult. An advanced understanding of the inherent complex and intricate anatomy of the anteroinferior labrum is required to differentiate normal anatomical variations from pathological induced changes. Abduction and external rotation (ABER) positioning of the arm may be required to properly visualize the labral component. In addition, MR arthrography can help depict the extent of the cartilage damage. Articular cartilage defects can best be appreciated on fat-suppressed T2-weighted fast spin-echo sequences or fat-suppressed sequences post arthrography. Arthroscopic debridement of the labral tear, with subsequent glenoid articular chondroplasty or abrasion arthroplasty, has been shown to relieve symptoms.

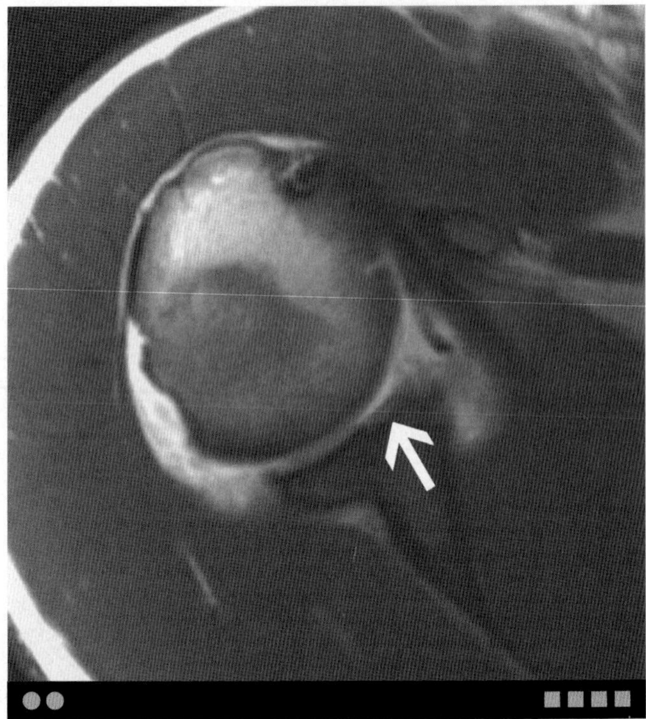

A. GLAD lesion: Axial T1-weighted post-MR arthrography image showing a tear of the articular cartilage and anteroinferior labrum (arrow). (From Torshizy H. *Appl Radiol.* Nov 2006 (suppl):14-21.)

PEARLS

- **GLAD lesion is an anteroinferior labral tear associated with a defect in the articular cartilage. Torn labrum remains attached to the anterior scapular periosteum.**
- **ABER position may be required to visualize the labral component, whereas articular cartilage defects are best seen on fat-suppressed T2-weighted fast spin-echo sequences or fat-suppressed arthrography.**

ADDITIONAL IMAGE

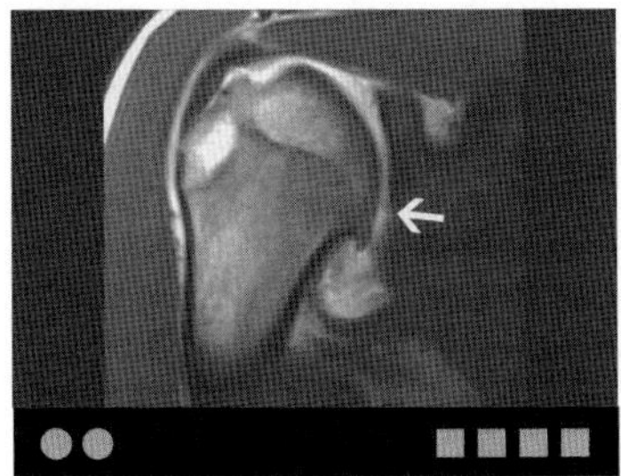

B. GLAD lesion: Coronal T1-weighted post-MR arthrography image showing a tear of the articular cartilage and anteroinferior labrum (arrow). Also note the presence of the Hill-Sachs deformity of humeral head. (From Torshizy H. *Appl Radiol.* Nov 2006 (suppl):14–21.)

DIFFERENTIAL DIAGNOSES IMAGES

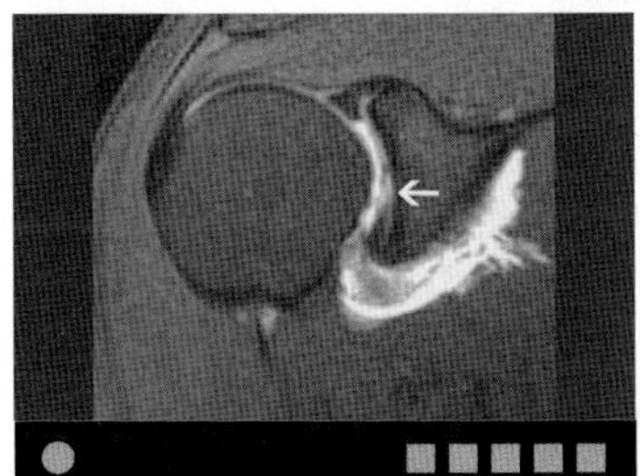

C. Delaminating glenoid cartilage lesion: Coronal oblique T2 fat-saturated post-MR arthrography image demonstrating a defect in the glenoid cartilage with fluid tracking under the articular cartilage, creating a delaminating phenomenon (arrow). (From Torshizy H. *Appl Radiol.* Nov 2006 (suppl):14–21.)

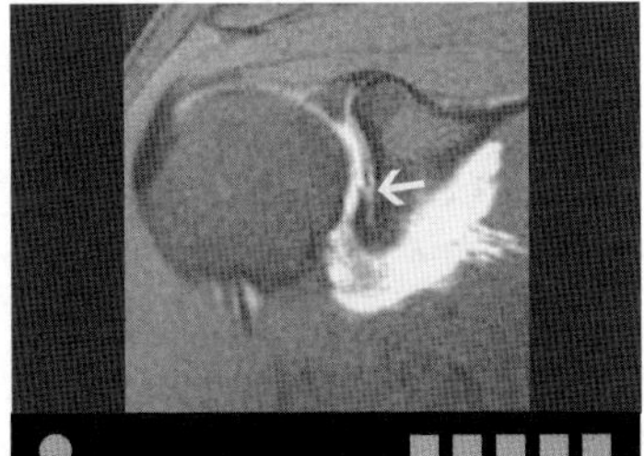

D. Delaminating glenoid cartilage lesion: Coronal oblique fat-saturated T1-weighted post-MR arthrography image demonstrating a defect in the glenoid cartilage with fluid tracking under the articular cartilage, creating a delaminating phenomenon (arrow). (From Torshizy H. *Appl Radiol.* Nov 2006 (suppl):14–21.)

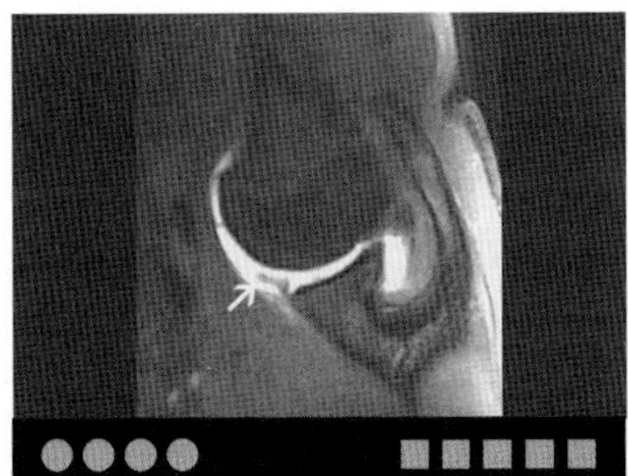

E. Bankart lesion: Fat-saturated T1-weighted post-MR arthrography image in the ABER view demonstrating a lifted and torn scapular periosteum (arrow). (From Torshizy H. *Appl Radiol.* Nov 2006 (suppl):14–21.)

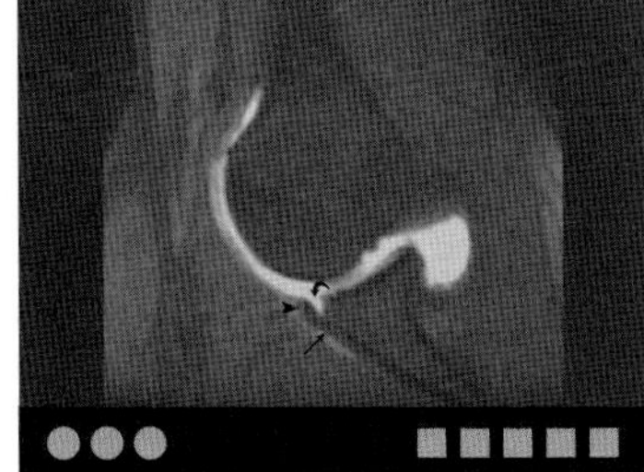

F. ALPSA lesion: Fat saturated T1-weighted post-MR arthrogram image in the ABER view demonstrating avulsion of the anteroinferior labrum (arrowhead) from the glenoid fossa, as evidenced by extravasation of contrast in between the labrum and glenoid fossa (curved arrow). Avulsion of the scapular periosteum is also noted (arrow). (From Torshizy H. *Appl Radiol.* Nov 2006 (suppl):14–21.)

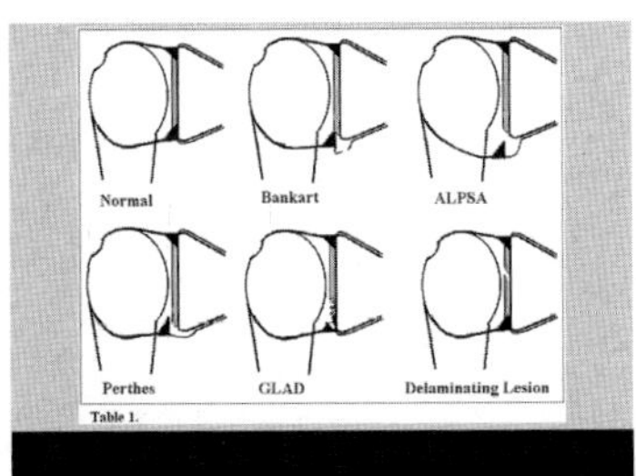

G. Diagram illustrating glenoid cartilage lesions. ALPSA, anterior labral periosteal sleeve avulsion; GLAD, glenoid labral articular disruption; Delaminating lesion,delamination of glenoid hyaline articular cartilage. (From Torshizy H. *Appl Radiol.* Nov 2006 (suppl):14–21.)

IMAGE KEY

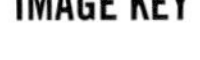

Common

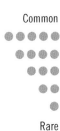

Rare

Typical

Unusual

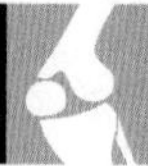

1–19 Perthes Lesion

Hamidreza R. Torshizy and Jamshid Tehranzadeh

PRESENTATION

Shoulder pain, tenderness, and instability

FINDINGS

MR images demonstrate an incompletely avulsed anteroinferior labrum from the glenoid and a medially stripped but intact scapular periosteum.

DIFFERENTIAL DIAGNOSES

- *Bankart lesion:* Avulsion of the labroligamentous complex from the anteroinferior glenoid, with lifting and disruption of the scapular periosteum.
- *Anterior labroligamentous periosteal sleeve avulsion (ALPSA) lesion:* Avulsion of anteroinferior labrum from the glenoid, with an accompanying periosteum which is intact, but detached and lifted from the scapula anteriorly.
- *Chronic ALPSA:* Similar to an acute ALPSA, with additional formation of scar tissue in the region of the labroligamentous complex.

COMMENTS

The image is of a 43-year-old patient with shoulder pain, tenderness, and instability. Patient demonstrates a Perthes lesion. A Perthes lesion is a variant of a classic Bankart lesion. It is characterized by an incompletely avulsed anteroinferior labrum with a medially stripped but intact periosteum. Given the inherent intricate and complex anatomy of the glenohumeral joint, differentiating among the different types of Bankart lesions can be challenging and difficult, as differences among variants (i.e., classic Bankart lesion, Perthes lesion, ALPSA lesion) are subtle. A Perthes lesion can be differentiated from the classic Bankart lesion by evaluating the anteroinferior labrum and the scapular periosteum. In the classic Bankart lesion, there is avulsion of the anteroinferior labrum from the underlying glenoid fossa, with displacement and disruption of the scapular periosteum. Perthes lesion is similar to an ALPSA lesion where in both there is avulsion of the anteroinferior labrum from the underlying glenoid fossa with an intact scapular periosteum. However, the amount of displacement of periosteal labral avulsed is less pronounced in Perthes lesion. MR arthrography and magnetic resonance imaging with the arm in the abduction and external rotation (ABER) position increase sensitivity in the detection of Perthes lesions. MR arthrography distends the joint and affords enhanced contrast outlining of intraarticular structures and accentuation of abnormalities. ABER positioning tauts the anterior inferior glenohumeral ligament at its insertion on the labrum.

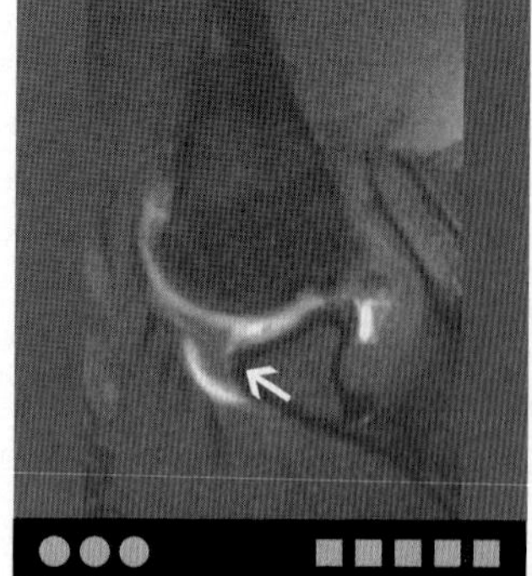

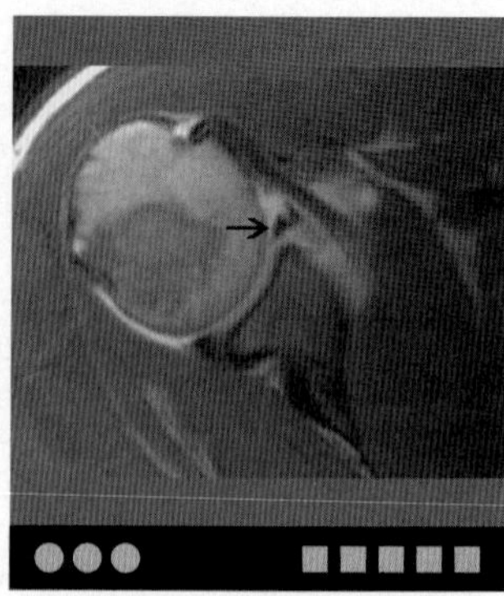

A. Perthes lesion: ABER view of T1-weighted fat-saturated post-MR arthrogram image demonstrating a partially avulsed scapular periosteum with an anteroinferior labrum that is attached but not displaced. Note arrow is pointing to the site of the avulsion (arrow). (From Torshizy H. *Appl Radiol.* Nov 2006 (suppl):14–21.)
B. Perthes lesion: Axial T1-weighted image from the same shoulder arthrogram shows an avulsed but nondisplaced anteroinferior labrum (arrow). (From Torshizy H. *Appl Radiol.* (suppl), Nov 2006:14–21.)

PEARLS

- **Perthes lesion is a variant of a classic Bankart lesion in which there is incomplete avulsion of the anteroinferior labrum from the glenoid and a medially stripped but intact periosteum.**
- **The labral periosteal avulsion is less pronounced in Perthes lesion as compared to ALPSA lesion.**
- **MR arthrography and ABER positioning allow enhanced detection and differentiation of Perthes lesions from other variants.**

DIFFERENTIAL DIAGNOSES IMAGES

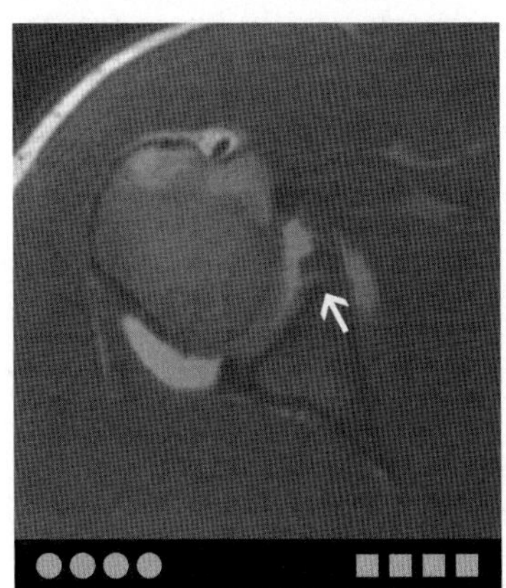

C. Bankart lesion: Fat-saturated axial T1-weighted post-MR arthrogram image depicting an anteroinferior labral tear (arrow). (From Torshizy H. *Appl Radiol.* Nov 2006 (suppl):14–21.)

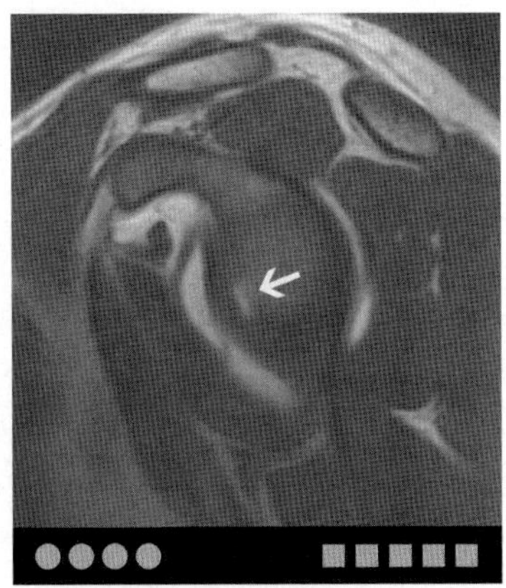

D. Bankart lesion: Sagittal T1-weighted post-MR arthrogram image depicting an anteroinferior labral tear (arrow). (From Torshizy H. *Appl Radiol.* Nov 2006 (suppl):14–21.)

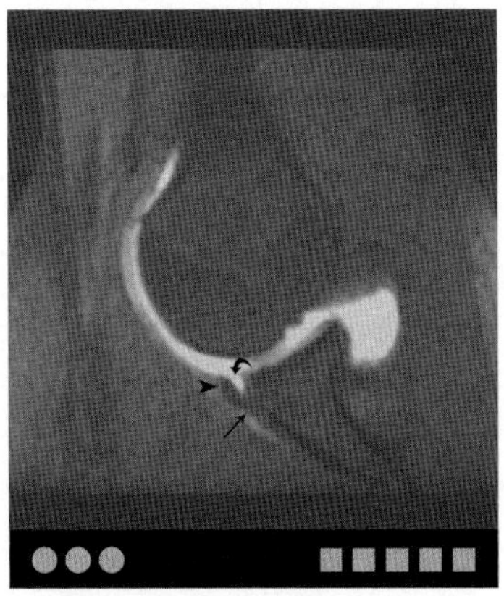

E. ALPSA lesion: Fat-saturated T1-weighted post-MR arthrogram image in the abduction and external rotation (ABER) view demonstrating avulsion of the anteroinferior labrum (arrowhead) from the glenoid fossa, as evidenced by extravasation of contrast in between the labrum and glenoid fossa (curved arrow). Avulsion of the scapular periosteum is also noted (arrow).

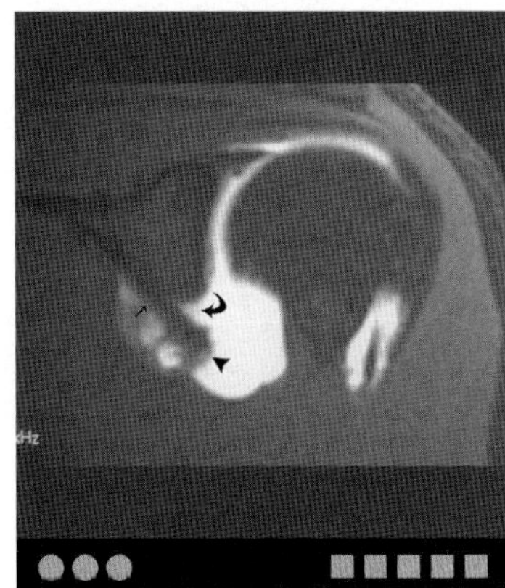

F. ALPSA lesion: Coronal T1-weighted fat-saturated post-MR arthrogram image demonstrating avulsion of the anteroinferior labrum (arrowhead) from the glenoid fossa with intervening extravasation of contrast (curved arrow). Note an intact scapular periosteum (arrow).

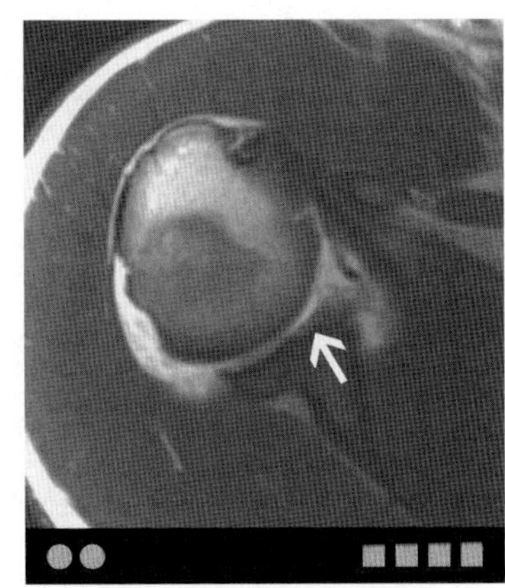

G. GLAD lesion: Axial T1-weighted post-MR arthrography image showing a tear of the articular cartilage and anteroinferior labrum (arrow). (From Torshizy H. *Appl Radiol.* Nov 2006 (suppl):14–21.)

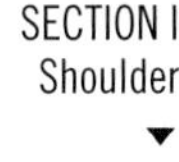

IMAGE KEY

Common

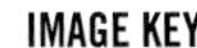

Rare

Typical

Unusual

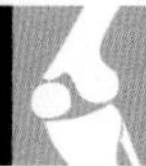

1–20 Anterior Labral Periosteal Sleeve Avulsion (ALPSA)

Hamidreza R. Torshizy and Jamshid Tehranzadeh

PRESENTATION

Shoulder pain, tenderness, and instability

FINDINGS

MR images demonstrate avulsion of anteroinferior labrum from the glenoid, with an accompanying periosteum that is intact, but detached and lifted from the scapula anteriorly.

DIFFERENTIAL DIAGNOSES

- *Bankart lesion:* Avulsion of the labroligamentous complex from the anteroinferior glenoid, with lifting and disruption of the scapular periosteum.
- *Perthes lesion:* An incompletely avulsed and minimally displaced anteroinferior labrum with a medially stripped but intact periosteum.
- *Chronic ALPSA:* Similar to an acute ALPSA, with additional formation of scar tissue in the region of the labroligamentous complex.

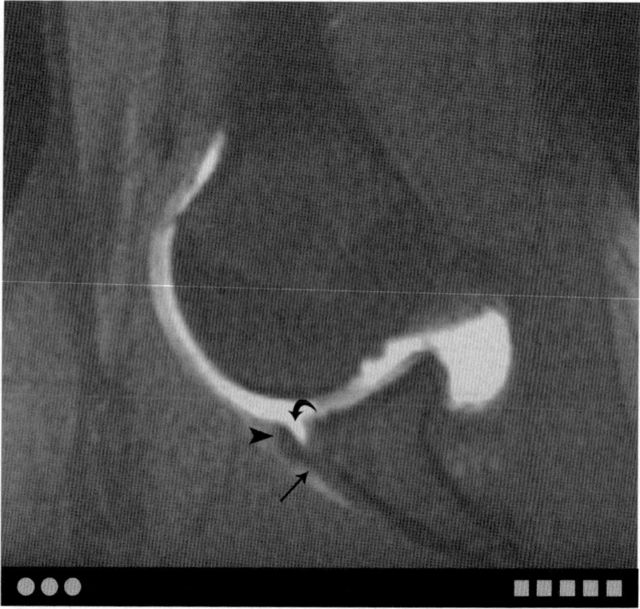

A. ALPSA lesion: ABER view including coronal fat-saturated T1-weighted post-MR arthrogram image demonstrating avulsion and lifting of the anteroinferior labrum (arrowhead) from the glenoid fossa and intervening extravasation of contrast (curved arrow). Note an intact scapular periosteum (arrow).

COMMENTS

This image is of a 28-year-old patient with shoulder pain, tenderness, and instability. Anterior labral periosteal sleeve avulsion (ALPSA) lesion is a variation of the classic Bankart lesion that is associated with recurrent unidirectional anterior instability and subsequent dislocation of the glenohumeral joint because of an incompetent anterior inferior glenohumeral ligament. This lesion is most common in patients younger than 30 years of age with a history of traumatic anterior dislocation of the glenohumeral joint. It is characterized by an anteroinferior labrum, which is avulsed from the glenoid margin, with an accompanying scapular periosteum that is intact and continuous, but detached and lifted from the scapula anteriorly. The entire labroligamentous complex is usually displaced anteroinferiorly. ALPSA lesions can be differentiated from Bankart lesions in that the anterior scapular periosteum remains intact in ALPSA lesions, whereas it is discontinuous or disrupted in Bankart lesions. ALPSA lesions also differ from Perthes lesions in that the labrum is displaced from the glenoid margin (usually in an inferomedial fashion) with the ALPSA lesions, whereas the labrum remains relatively nondisplaced in a Perthes lesion. MR imaging is preferred, given its superior soft tissue contrast and multi-planar capabilities. MR arthrography best allows identification and differentiation of ALPSA lesions from other variants. In addition, abduction and external rotation (ABER) positioning of the upper extremity further enhances detection and differentiation of lesions.

PEARLS

- **ALPSA lesion is a variant of a classic Bankart lesion in which there is avulsion of the anteroinferior labrum from the glenoid and an intact periosteum that is detached from the scapula anteriorly. The labral–ligamentous complex is usually displaced anteroinferiorly.**
- **It is associated with recurrent anterior dislocation and instability of the glenohumeral joint because of an incompetent anterior inferior glenohumeral ligament.**
- **MR arthrography and ABER positioning allow enhanced detection and differentiation of ALPSA lesions from Bankart and Perthes lesions.**

ADDITIONAL IMAGES

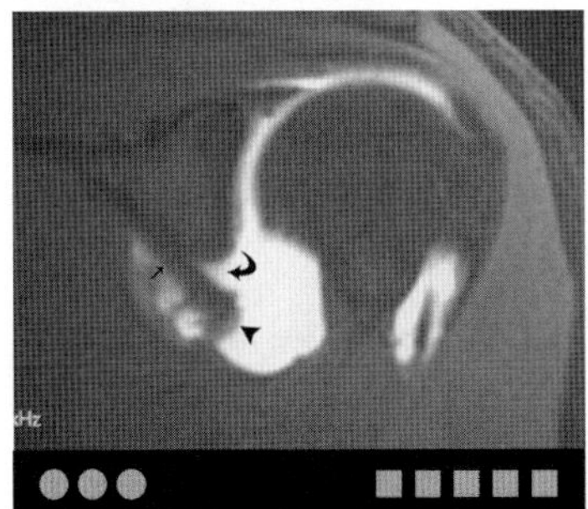

B. ALPSA lesion: Coronal T1-weighted fat-saturated post-MR arthrogram image demonstrating avulsion of the anteroinferior labrum (arrowhead) from the glenoid fossa and intervening extravasation of contrast (curved arrow). Note an intact scapular periosteum (arrow).

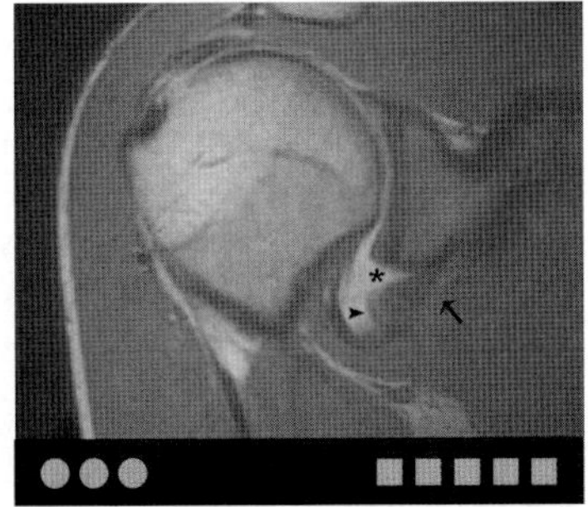

C. ALPSA lesion: Coronal T1-weighted image post-MR arthrogram in another patient demonstrating avulsion of the anteroinferior labrum (arrowhead) from the glenoid fossa and intervening extravasation of contrast (*). Note an intact scapular periosteum (arrow).

DIFFERENTIAL DIAGNOSES IMAGES

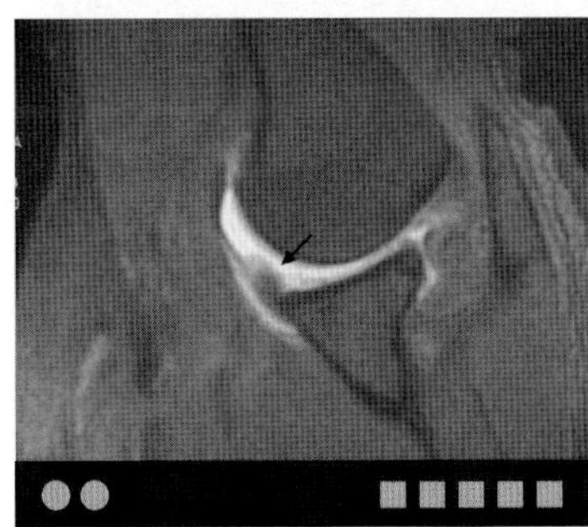

D. Chronic ALPSA lesion: ABER view T1-weighted fat-saturated image post-MR arthrogram demonstrating healing and fibrosis in the region of the anteroinferior labrum (arrow).

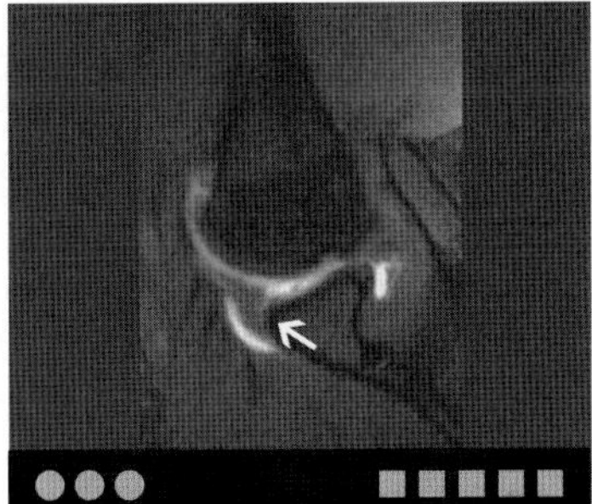

E. Perthes lesion: ABER view T1-weighted fat-saturated post-MR arthrogram image demonstrating a partially avulsed scapular periosteum with an anteroinferior labrum that is attached but not displaced. Note arrow is pointing to the site of the avulsion (arrow).

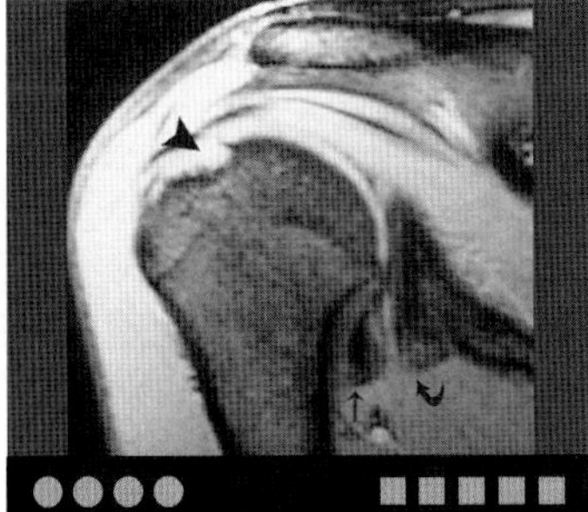

F. Bony Bankart lesion: Coronal T2-weighted image demonstrating a compression fracture of the posterolateral humeral head (arrowhead), so-called Hill-Sachs deformity. An avulsion of the anteroinferior labrum with bony detachment (arrow) from the glenoid fossa (curved arrow), and accompanying discontinuity of the scapular periosteum is also noted.

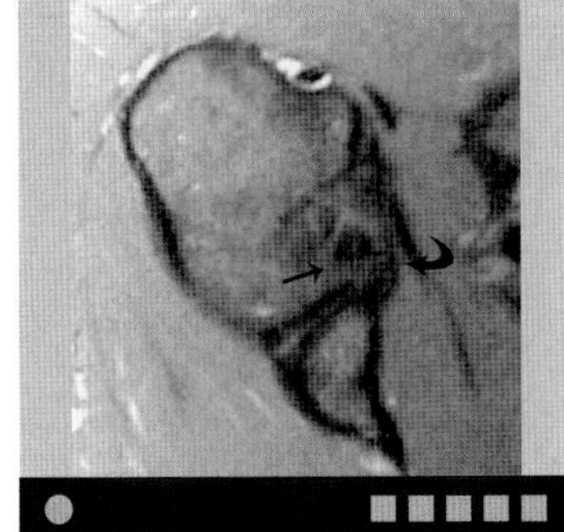

G. BHAGL lesion: Axial FSE T2-weighted image demonstrating an osseous fragment separating from the proximal humerus corresponding to a humeral avulsion fracture (arrow), with accompanying disruption of the anterior band of the inferior glenohumeral ligament (curved arrow).

IMAGE KEY

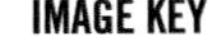

Common

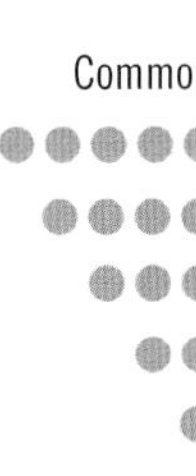

Rare

Typical

Unusual

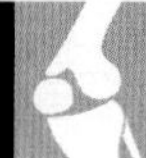

1–21 Bennett Lesion of the Shoulder

James Coumas

PRESENTATION

Pain in the posterior shoulder

FINDINGS

CT and MR imaging show a crescent-shaped calcification localized to the extra-articular posterior glenoid.

DIFFERENTIAL DIAGNOSES

- *Posterior labral tear:* May present as posterior shoulder discomfort but remains an intra-articular injury easily diagnosed by CT arthrogram or MR imaging.
- *Posterior glenoid fracture/degenerative disease:* Typically associated with a posterior dislocation or instability with or without reverse Hill-Sachs lesion or reverse Bankart lesion. This abnormality can be differentiated from a Bennett lesion because the posterior bony fragment represents a fracture of the posterior glenoid in contrast to mineralization posterior to an intact glenoid.
- *Posterior loose body:* Mimics injury to the posterior capsule and synovium as well as a posterior labral injury.

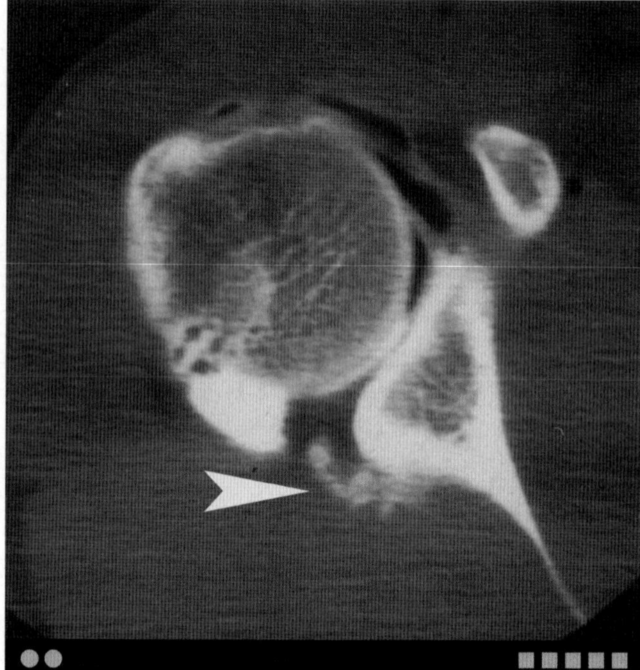

A. Bennett lesion: Axial CT arthrogram section shows extra-articular soft tissue mineralization posterior to the bony glenoid (arrowhead). No associated labral tear is noted.

COMMENTS

A 23-year-old baseball pitcher presented with progressive posterior shoulder pain exacerbated by pitching. The Bennett lesion is a posterior extracapsular injury associated with throwing and seen principally in baseball players. The most commonly cited etiology is repetitive microtrauma. This injury is thought to result from recurrent traction of the posterior capsule of the shoulder at or adjacent to the attachment of the posterior band of the inferior glenohumeral ligament to the posterior bony glenoid. The traction force is caused by the rapid deceleration of the arm after ball release in the throwing athlete. The etiology, treatment, and outcome of this injury remain controversial. Some believe the pathognomonic posterior soft tissue mineralization is an adaptive response to competitive pitching rather than a true injury. Curiously a prevalence of 12% was noted in a single small study of asymptomatic professional pitchers. There is a high association of posterior labral tears and partial thickness undersurface rotator cuff tears noted in symptomatic pitchers with a Bennett lesion. Conservative therapy appears to be more common for the isolated Bennett lesion but associated intra-articular injuries are treated by arthroscopy. CT imaging is especially helpful for the diagnosis and assessment of the pathognomonic posterior mineralization. The mineralization appears dense, solid, and bridged to the adjacent glenoid in the chronic (asymptomatic) lesion. Intra-articular contrast is necessarily for assessment of associated injuries. MR imaging is helpful in the assessment of marrow edema and hemorrhagic/inflammatory soft tissue changes seen in the acute and subacute (symptomatic) Bennett lesion.

PEARLS

- **Inflammatory changes of the bony glenoid or adjacent soft tissues may help in establishing symptomatic from asymptomatic Bennett lesion.**
- **Benign asymptomatic Bennett lesion will show a solid bridged mineralized process firmly attached to the bony glenoid.**
- **Intra-articulate injuries are commonly associated with a Bennett lesion and careful scrutiny of posterior glenoid labrum and rotator cuff is necessary.**

ADDITIONAL IMAGES

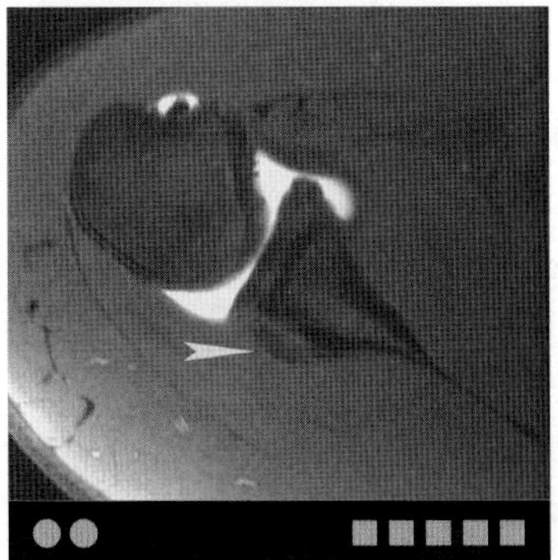

B. Bennett lesion: Axial T2-weighted MR image of Bennett lesion (arrowhead) without associated labral tear.

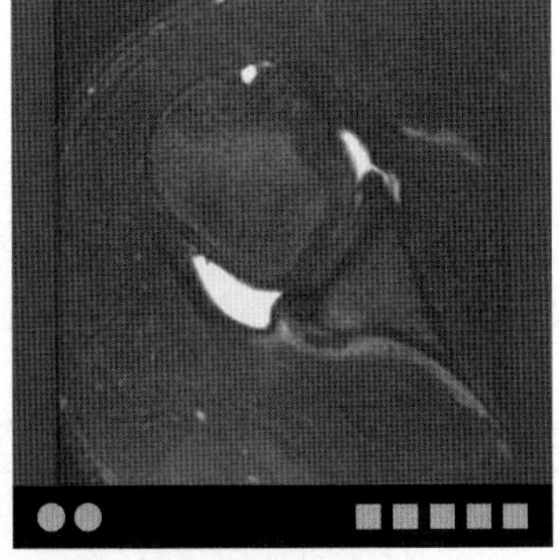

C. Bennett lesion: Axial T2-weighted MR image of symptomatic lesion with marrow edema in bony glenoid and extra-articular soft tissue edema.

DIFFERENTIAL DIAGNOSES IMAGES

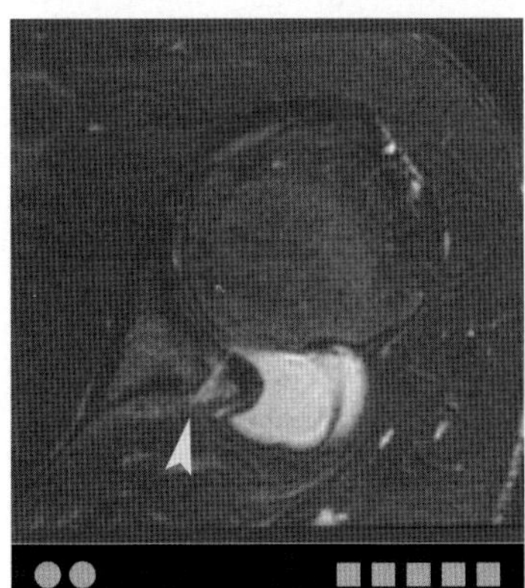

D. Fracture of posterior glenoid: Axial MR image shows a fracture of the posterior glenoid and labrum (arrowhead).

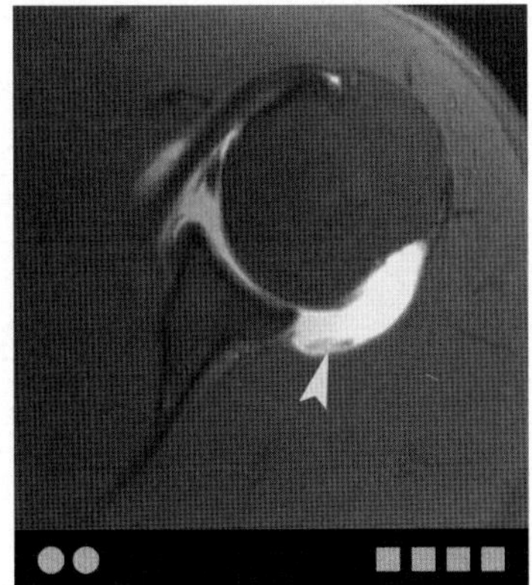

E. Loose body: Axial MR image T2-weighted shows intra-articular loose body (arrowhead) in the posterior capsular recess from a previous anterior repair.

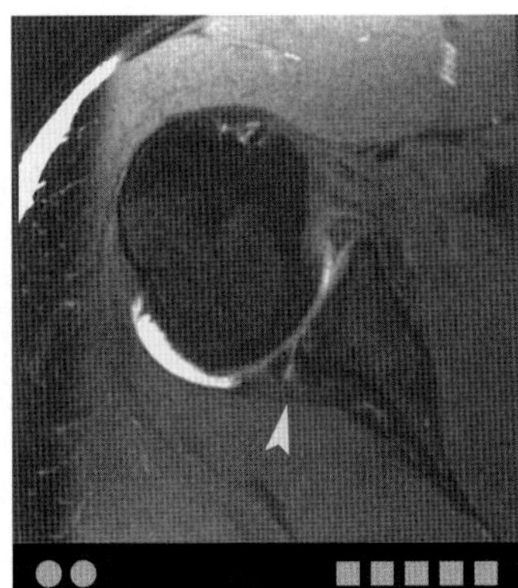

F. Posterior labral tear with associated Bennett lesion: MR image axial T2-weighted image. Mature Bennett lesion (arrowhead) with symptomatic labral tear and secondary degenerative change to articular glenoid.

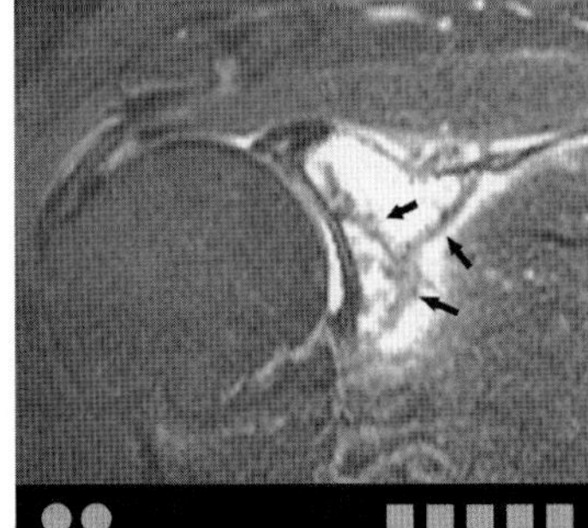

G. Insufficiency fracture of glenoid process: Coronal T2 SPIR image shows bone marrow edema of the glenoid with increased signal intensity. Note multiple insufficiency fracture lines with low signal intensities (arrows).

IMAGE KEY

Common

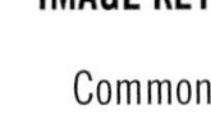

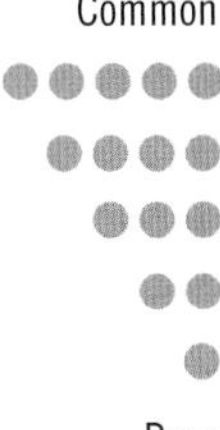

Rare

Typical

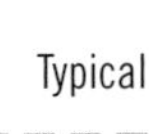

Unusual

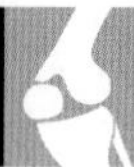

1–22 Glenohumeral Internal Rotational Deficit (GIRD Lesion)

Arash Tehranzadeh

PRESENTATION

Shoulder pain aggravated by throwing

FINDINGS

MR images show thickening of the posteroinferior glenohumeral ligament, posterosuperior subluxation of the humeral head, SLAP tear of the superior labrum, and articular-sided partial tear of the infraspinatus.

DIFFERENTIAL DIAGNOSES

- *Bennett lesion:* The Bennett lesion is a posterior extracapsular injury associated with throwing and also seen principally in baseball players. The mineralization appears dense, solid, and bridged to the adjacent glenoid in the chronic (asymptomatic) lesion. This lesion appears as calcified mineralization of the posterior joint capsule as a chronic consequence of an extra-articular posterior capsular avulsive injury. The mechanism is from traction of the posterior band of the inferior glenohumeral during decelerating phase of pitching. This lesion is also associated with posterior rotator cuff undersurface abnormalities and labral tears.
- *Posterior glenoid fracture/degenerative disease:* Typically associated with a posterior dislocation or instability with or without reverse Hill-Sachs lesion or reverse Bankart lesion. This abnormality can be differentiated from a Bennett lesion because the posterior bony fragment represents a fracture of the posterior glenoid in contrast to mineralization posterior to an intact glenoid.

COMMENTS

The patient is a 22-year-old professional baseball player with shoulder pain especially when throwing. The clinical entity of glenohumeral internal rotational deficit has been applied particularly to throwing athletes, who experience pain and instability attributed to posterior impingement. Symptoms of posterior impingement and instability are experienced by athletes during the "early cocking" phase of the throwing cycle specifically when the shoulder is in 90 degree abduction and greater than 90-degree external rotation (ABER position). Consequently, chronic thickening of the posterior band of the inferior glenohumeral ligament develops and sets forth a cascade of events. As a consequence of a thickened posterior joint capsule, the humeral head is subluxed posterosuperiorly resulting in a wider rotational arc of the greater tuberosity during the throwing cycle. The widened arc of the greater tuberosity causes impingement of the articular surface of the rotator cuff between the greater tuberosity and the posterosuperior portion of the glenoid labrum. Coexistent increased rotational torque of the biceps tendon and anchor may result in SLAP tears. Associated subchondral cyst formation in the superolateral humeral head may develop. MR imaging demonstrates thickened posterior capsule by a dark and thickened band of the IGHL near its glenoid attachment. Near the associated region of subchondral cyst formation in the humeral head, articular sided tears of the supraspinatus and infraspinatus may be appreciated. Tears or fraying of the posterosuperior labrum may be appreciated as a continuum of a SLAP tear. In the appropriate clinical setting, the constellation of these MR findings may be consistent with the clinical entity of GIRD.

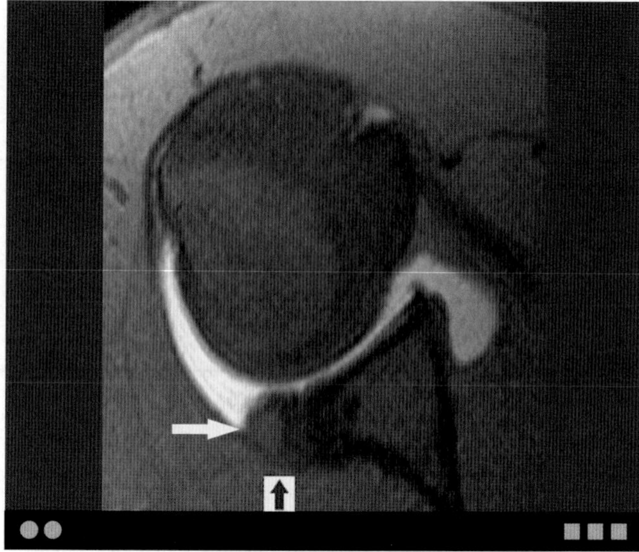

A. GIRD: Axial T1 spin-echo fat saturation MR arthrographic image demonstrates a thickened posterior capsule at the posterior capsular labral junction (arrow). The humeral head is shifted to a new equilibrium in this patient and is manifested by posterior subluxation of the humeral head with respect to the glenoid. (From Tehranzadeh A. *Clin Imaging*. 2007;31(5):343–348.)

PEARLS

- **Thickening of the posterior band of the inferior glenohumeral ligament**
- **Posterosuperior or SLAP tears of the labrum**
- **Articular-sided tear of the supraspinatus or infraspinatus**
- **Associated subchondral cysts in the superolateral aspect of the humeral head**

ADDITIONAL IMAGES

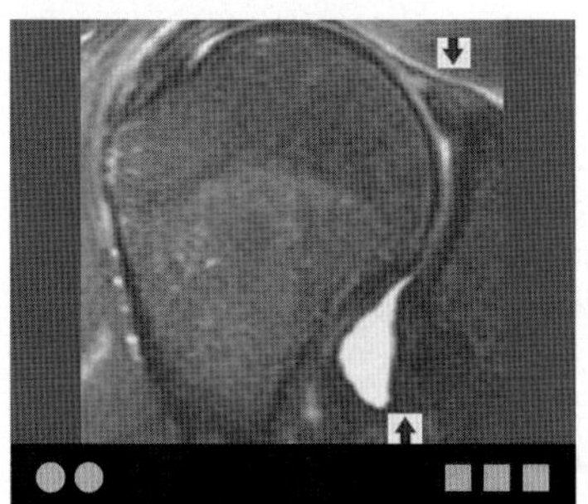

B. GIRD: Coronal oblique T2 turbo spin-echo fat saturation MR arthrographic coronal oblique image of the same patient shows thickening of the axillary pouch (bottom arrow) and a frayed appearance of the posterosuperior labrum (top arrow).

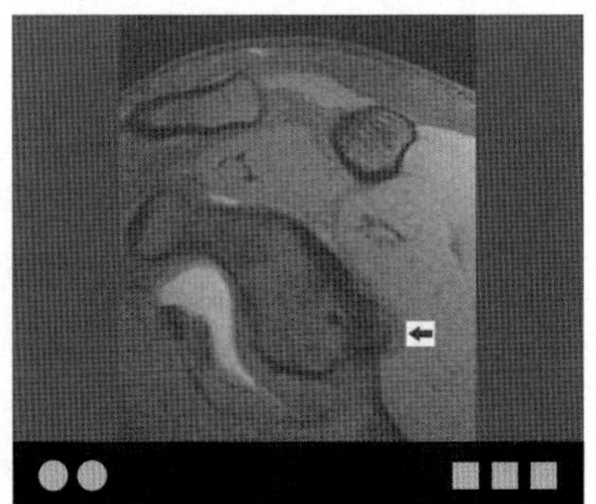

C. GIRD: Sagittal oblique T1 spin-echo MR arthrographic image with fat saturation shows a thickened posterior capsule (arrow).

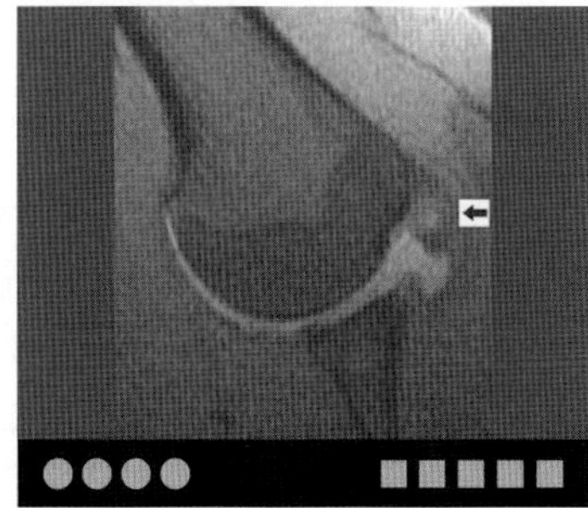

D. GIRD: ABER T1 spin-echo fat saturation MR arthrographic image demonstrates an arthroscopically proven undersurface partial tear of the infraspinatus tendon (arrow).

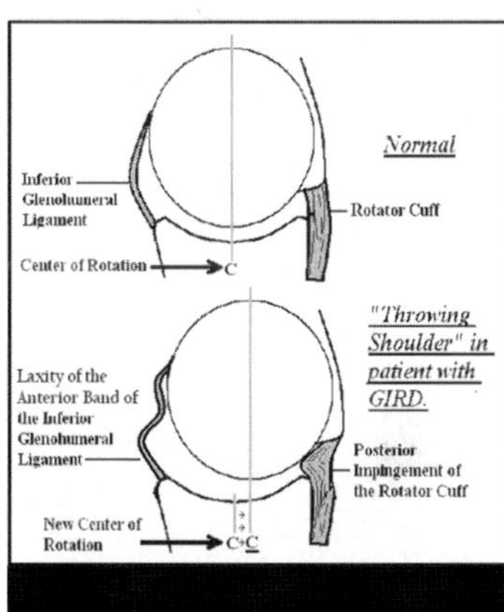

E. GIRD: ABER view shows posterior superior subluxation with migration of center of rotation (C), internal impingement of the rotator cuff, and laxity of the anterior band of the IGHL.

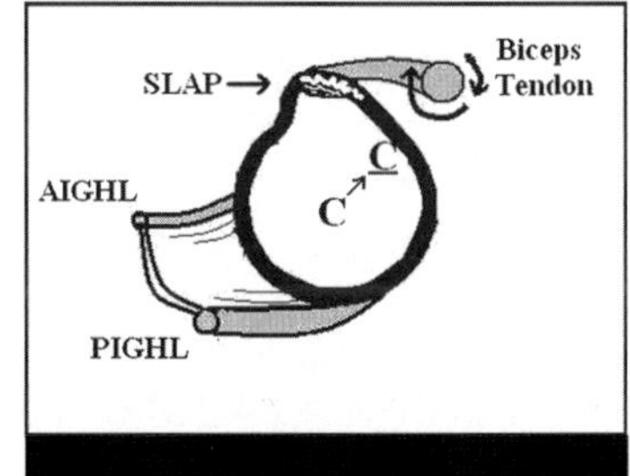

F. GIRD: Schematic of GIRD in this sagittal-oblique view of the glenoid fossa that shows a thickened posteroinferior glenohumeral ligament (PIGHL), posterosuperior migration of the center of humeral head rotation (C), and rotational torque on the proximal biceps tendon and anchor leading to a SLAP tear.

IMAGE KEY

Common

Rare

Typical

Unusual

DIFFERENTIAL DIAGNOSES IMAGES

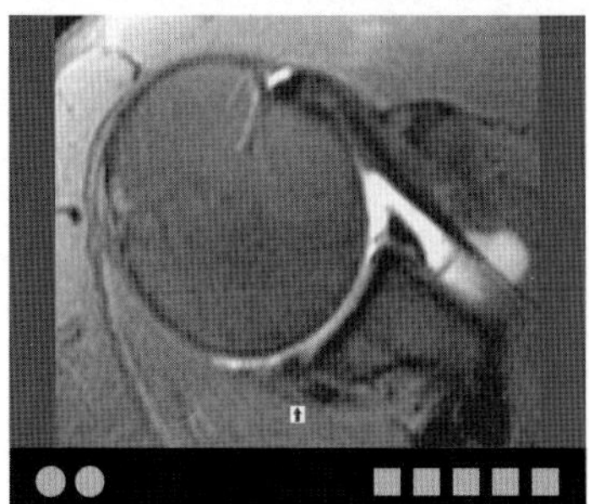

G. Bennett lesion: Axial T1 fat-suppressed MR arthrographic image. Dark signal at the posterior joint capsule confluence with the glenoid corresponds to the calcium deposits at posterior labral capsule.

Images A-F from Tehranzadeh A. *Clin Imaging*. 2007;31(5):343–348.

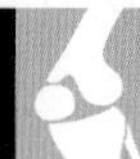

1–23 Slap Tear, Type II

Scott Kingston

PRESENTATION

Sudden anterior shoulder pain

FINDINGS

MR image shows linear contrast collection undermining the base of the superior labrum.

DIFFERENTIAL DIAGNOSES

- *Rotator cuff tear:* Tendinosis or partial articular sided tears are usually within the anterior supraspinatus.
- *Sublabral recess:* Normal sublabral sulcus is not associated with abnormal detachment of the superior labrum from underlying glenoid.
- *Biceps labral complex variation:* Contrast is outlining the base of the superior labrum and forming a normal large sublabral sulcus resulting in a meniscoid superior labrum.
- *Sublabral foramen:* Normal anatomical variation presenting in the anterosuperior quadrant where the labrum is not firmly attached to the underlying bony glenoid.

COMMENTS

The image is of a baseball player, who fell on an outstretched arm. SLAP lesions refer to tears of the superior labrum from anterior to posterior. Although they may acutely occur from falling on an outstretched arm, they often result from the repetitive motion of overhand throwers in baseball and other sports secondary to the chronic traction on the biceps labral complex. Originally classified into four different subtypes ranging from mild degeneration and undersurface fraying (type I), detachment of the superior labrum from the underlying glenoid (type II), bucket handle variety (type III), to superior labral detachment with extension into the biceps anchor or tendon with or without tendon rupture (type IV); other varieties exist depending if there is further propagation of the tear into the anterior or posterior labra, glenohumeral ligaments, or circumferential labral extension. The classic type II SLAP lesion may have associated partial undersurface tears of the rotator cuff as in the SLAC subtype (superior labrum/anterior cuff) or posterior peel back lesion with posterior tears of the superior labrum associated with chronic internal posterior superior impingement and undersurface partial tears of the posterior supraspinatus or anterior infraspinatus tendons. Occasionally, posterior superior paralabral cysts develop as a result of labral tear. With MR arthrography of the shoulder, high signal tears from the base of the superior labrum are best depicted in the coronal plane. One should be cautious not to confuse certain anatomical variations such as a prominent sublabral sulcus, meniscoid labrum, and sublabral hole or foramen with SLAP tears.

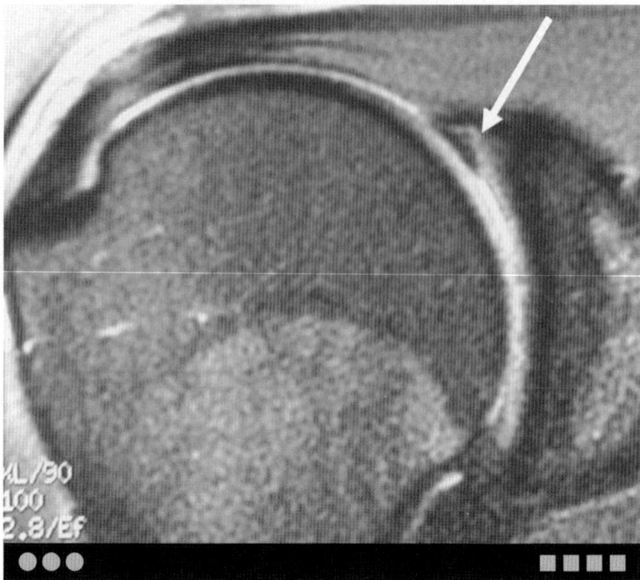

A. SLAP tear, type II: Coronal PD with fat saturation MR arthrogram image shows contrast intravasating into superior labrum away from the glenoid toward the labral tip.

PEARLS

- **SLAP, type II tears are often seen in overhand throwing sports from either acute trauma or from chronic traction forces on the biceps labral complex.**
- **Linear high signal on coronal T2-weighted image or MR arthrogram images should extend up into the superior labrum away from the underlying bony glenoid.**
- **Posterosuperior paralabral cysts are usually associated with SLAP, type II tears. If large enough, compressive neuropathy of the suprascapular nerve may occur.**
- **Sublabral foramina or holes occur in the high anterosuperior quadrant and do not extend posterior to the biceps labral anchor nor below the equator.**
- **SLAP, type II tears may be associated with partial undersurface rotator cuff tears (SLAC and posterior peel back varieties).**

ADDITIONAL IMAGES

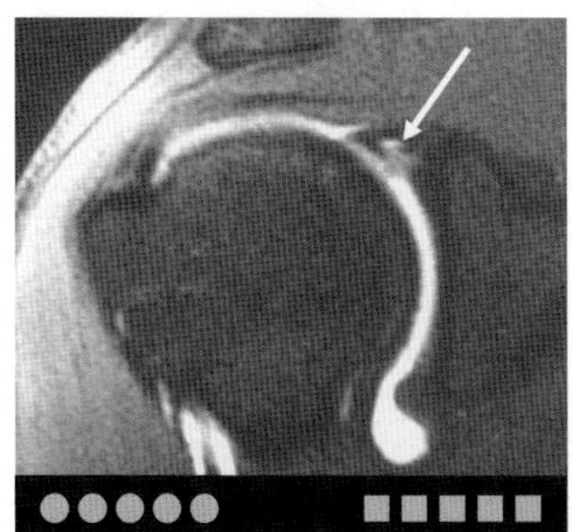

B. SLAP tear, type II: Coronal T1-weighted image with fat saturation MR arthrogram demonstrates better delineation of the irregular superior labral tear (arrow) from the normal hypointense labrum.

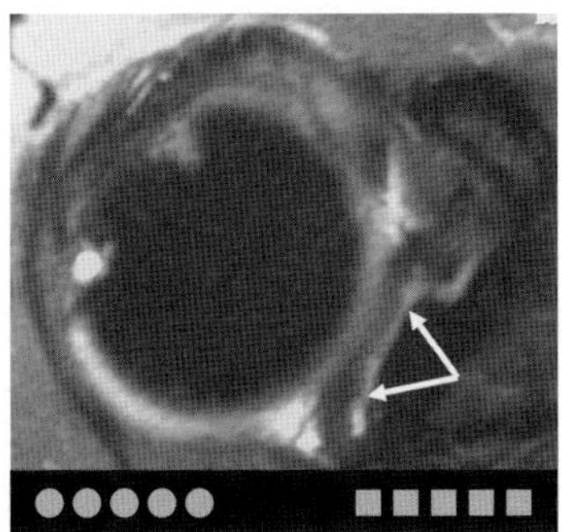

C. SLAP tear, type II: Axial T1-weighted image with fat saturation MR arthrogram shows the anterior to posterior extent (arrows) of the SLAP tear.

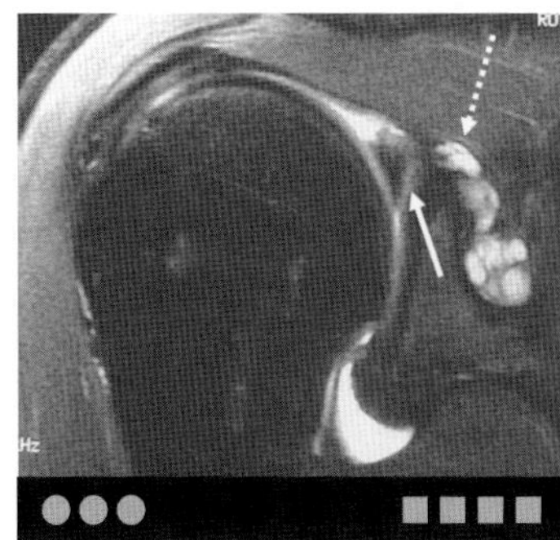

D. SLAP tear, type II: Coronal fat-saturated PD MR arthrogram image shows multiple small posterosuperior paralabral cysts (dashed arrow) associated with a SLAP, type II tear (solid arrow).

DIFFERENTIAL DIAGNOSES IMAGES

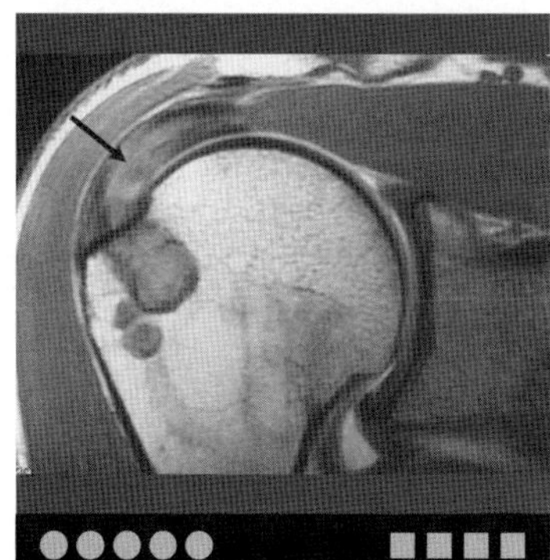

E. Tendinosis: Coronal T1-weighted MR arthrogram image shows a normal superior labrum but a thickened and hyperintense supraspinatus tendon consistent with tendinosis. Note the large subcortical cysts at the greater tuberosity base.

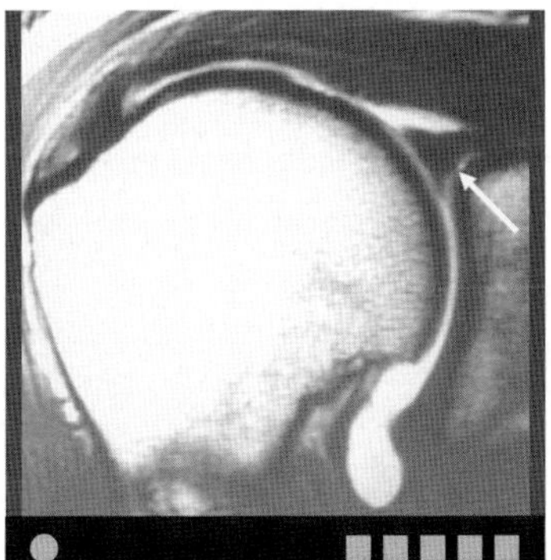

F. Meniscoid labrum: Coronal T1-weighted MR arthrogram image shows a normal meniscoid superior labrum with a thin curvilinear contrast collection (arrow) undermining the superior labral base while curving over the glenoid.

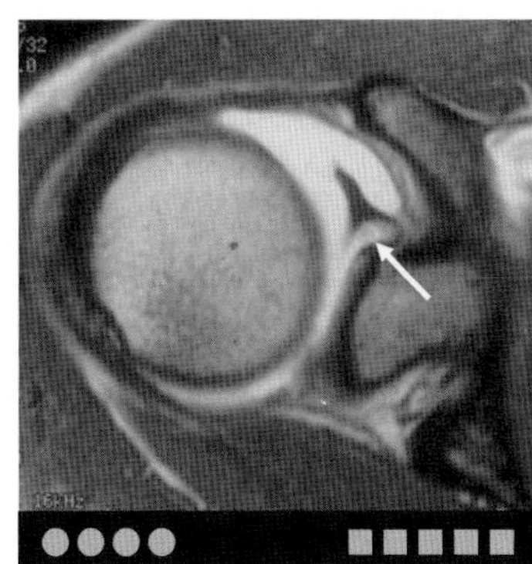

G. Sublabral foramen: Axial T1-weighted MR arthrogram image of a normal sublabral foramen (arrow) or hole in the anterosuperior quadrant. Note its smooth margins and location at the coracoid process level.

IMAGE KEY

Common

Rare

Typical

Unusual

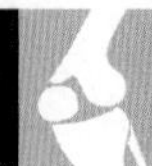

1–24 Perilabral Ganglion Cyst

Gideon Strich

PRESENTATION

Shoulder pain and weakness

FINDINGS

MRI shows a well-defined cyst in the suprascapular notch with edema of the infraspinatus muscle.

DIFFERENTIAL DIAGNOSES

- *Mass:* Other masses that may occur in this area are cysts of other etiologies and solid masses arising from the muscles, scapula, or connective tissue.
- *Rotator cuff tear:* Tears of the rotator cuff often involve the infraspinatus as well as the supraspinatus. The clinical presentation of pain and weakness may be indistinguishable.

COMMENTS

The image is of a middle-aged male with progressive shoulder pain and weakness. Perilabral ganglion cysts around the shoulder are often associated with tears of the glenoid labrum. The etiology is thought to be similar to the development of meniscal cysts around the knee, specifically a ball valve mechanism by which fluid escapes from the joint through a tear in the labrum and is trapped in the cyst, which then slowly enlarges. The cysts may cause entrapment neuropathies of the suprascapular nerve branches supplying the supraspinatus muscle if they arise in the supraspinatus fossa and similarly may impinge upon the branch of the nerve supplying the infraspinatus muscle if they occur in the spinoglenoid fossa. Rarely, entrapment neuropathies of the axillary nerve may occur as a result of cysts or masses occurring in the quadrilateral space, the denervated muscle may demonstrate edema or late fatty atrophy. Communication with the joint and the tear in the labrum may be demonstrated by MR arthrography following intra-articular injection of gadolinium; however, the communication with the cyst may not always be demonstrated. Treatment usually involves resection of the ganglion with repair of the adjacent labrum. Imaging-guided aspiration of the cyst has been reported, although the cyst may recur if the labrum is not repaired. The presence of a perilabral cyst is most often an incidental finding when performing routine MRI of the shoulder for diagnosis.

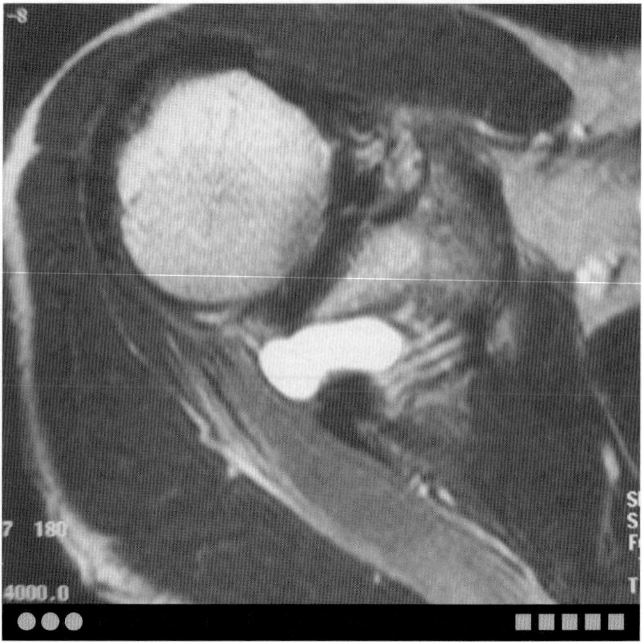

A. Perilabral cyst: Axial T2-weighted image shows a well-defined ganglion cyst in the suprascapular notch adjacent to branches of the suprascapular artery and nerve. There is edema of the infraspinatus muscle.

PEARLS

- **Perilabral ganglion cysts most commonly result from tears of the adjacent glenoid labrum. The tears may be demonstrated by MR arthrography although communication with a cyst is not always seen.**
- **Entrapment neuropathies and subsequent muscle edema and atrophy may affect the supraspinatus, infraspinatus, or teres minor muscles depending upon the location of the cyst relative to the anatomy of the underlying suprascapular nerve.**
- **Clinical symptoms may be indistinguishable from findings associated with rotator cuff pathology or unsuspected bone pathology or soft tissue tumors.**

ADDITIONAL IMAGES

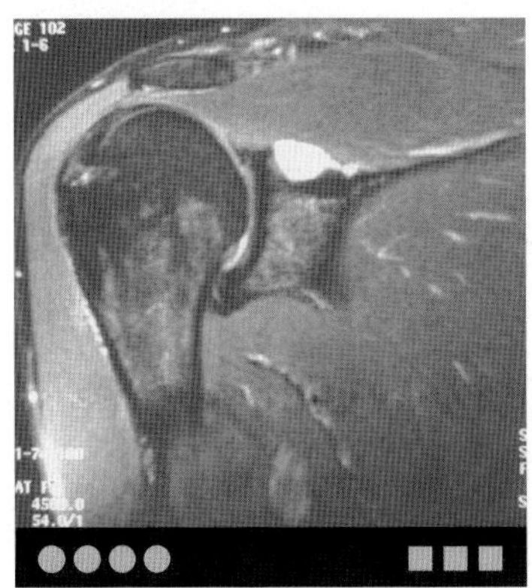

B. Perilabral cyst: Coronal proton density image with fat saturation shows the perilabral cyst in the suprascapular notch with an intact supraspinatus tendon. The labral tear is not seen.

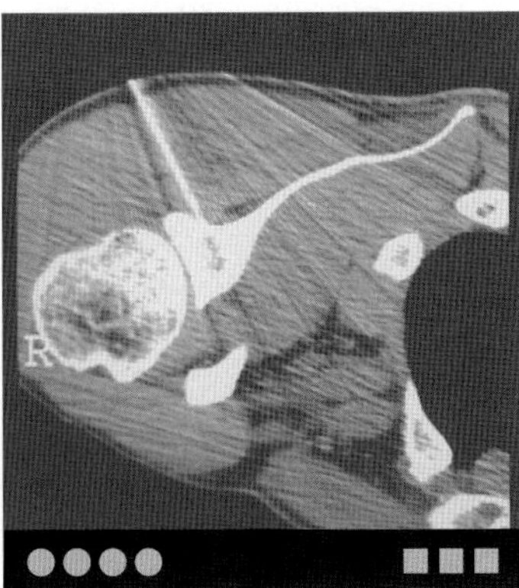

C. Perilabral cyst: Axial CT obtained during image-guided aspiration of the cyst.

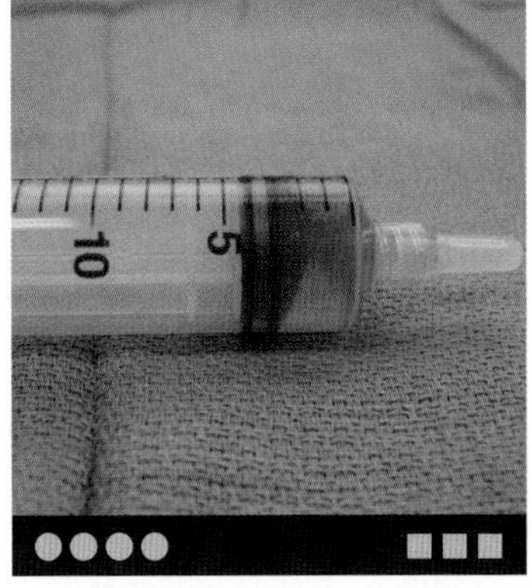

D. Perilabral cyst: Thick synovial fluid removed during the cyst aspiration.

DIFFERENTIAL DIAGNOSES IMAGES

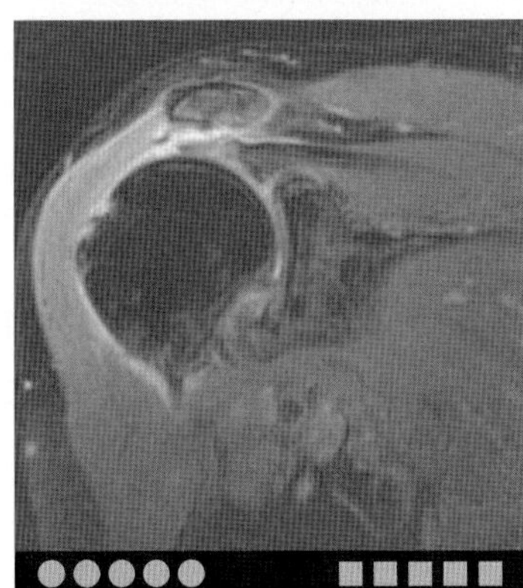

E. Rotator cuff tear: Coronal proton density image with fat saturation shows typical full thickness tear of the supraspinatus tendon with retraction.

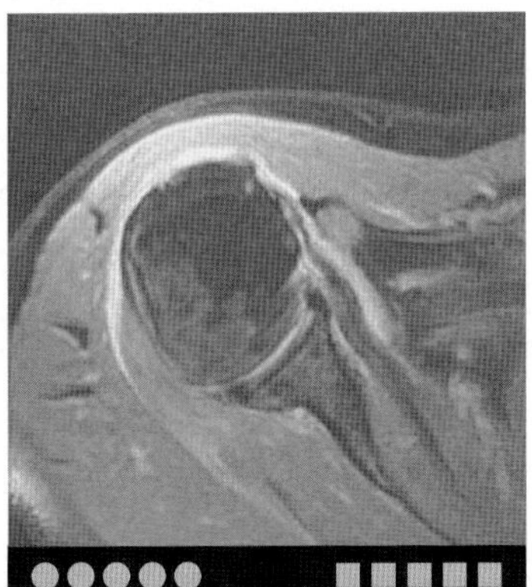

F. Rotator cuff tear: Axial proton density image with fat saturation in the same patient shows involvement of both the infraspinatus and subscapularis muscles with edema.

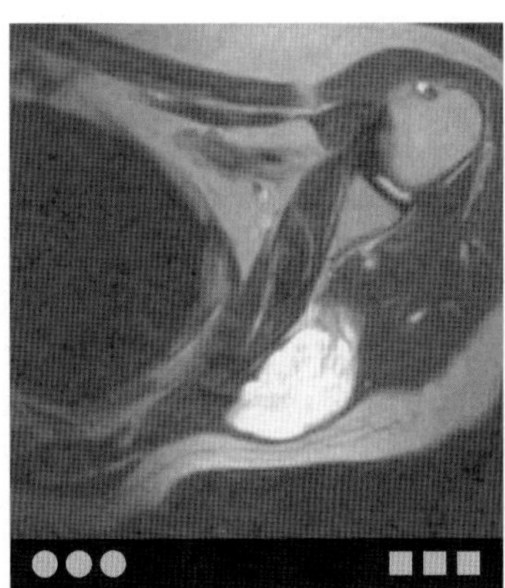

G. Malignant fibrous histiocytoma (MFH): Axial T2-weighted image shows a small soft tissue tumor in the infraspinatus muscle mimicking symptoms of pain and weakness.

IMAGE KEY

Common

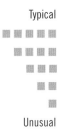

Rare

Typical

Unusual

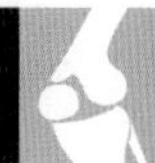

1–25 Suprascapular Nerve Entrapment Syndrome from Ganglion Cyst

Sulabha Masih

PRESENTATION

Chronic shoulder pain

FINDINGS

MR images show large ganglion cyst in the suprascapular notch.

DIFFERENTIAL DIAGNOSES

- *Atypical synovial cyst:* It shows as fluid filled cavity with extension to the joint.
- *Varices in suprascapular or spinoglenoid notch:* Presents as tubular high signal structure on T2-weighted images.
- *Tumor in suprascapular or spinoglenoid notch:* Shows variable appearance on MR. It may show contrast enhancement.
- *Chronic rotator cuff tear:* May cause supraspinatus, infraspinatus muscle atrophy.

COMMENTS

The image is of a 45-year-old man with chronic shoulder pain. Suprascapular nerve arises from upper trunk of the brachial Plexus, runs through the posterior triangle of neck, under the trapezius, and then courses in the anteroposterior direction to the suprascapular notch. It provides sensory innervation to glenohumeral and acromioclavicular joints. As it traverses through the suprascapular notch, it provides motor innervation to supraspinatus and infraspinatus muscles. Then it runs inferiorly to the spinoglenoid notch, supplying motor innervation only to infraspinatus muscle. Suprascapular ligament crosses over the upper margin of suprascapular notch. Entrapment of suprascapular nerve between the ligament and the tight bony notch can cause compression and dennervation of supraspinatus and/or the infraspinatus muscles, depending on the exact location. The most common etiology causing suprascapular nerve impingement is ganglion cyst. Other causes include enlarged veins, tumors, and fracture in the scapula in suprascapular and/or spinoglenoid notches. Usually, this entity is associated with superior labral tear. Cyst in the suprascapular notch compresses the nerve proximally and causes denervation of both suprascapular and infrascapular muscles. Cysts located inferiorly in the spinoglenoid notch compress the nerve distal to the branch innervating the supraspinatus, and selectively cause denervation of only infraspinatus muscle. Chronic muscle compression causes atrophy. MRI shows round or oval septated mass with low signal on T1-weighted and high signal intensity on T2-weighted images. Mass remains in the low signal intensity, with a thin line of peripheral enhancement on T1-weighted, after gadolinium injection. Muscle atrophy has high signal intensity on T1-weighted images.

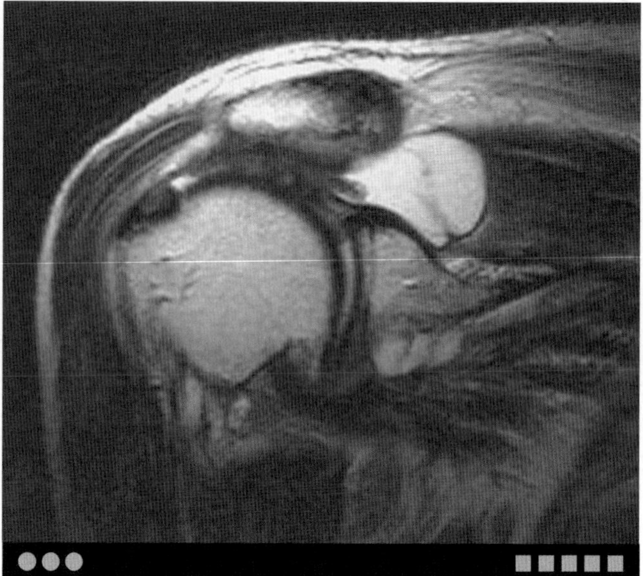

A. Ganglion cyst: Coronal T2-weighted image shows high signal intensity mass in the suprascapular notch.

PEARLS

- **Ganglion cyst in the suprascapular notch, compresses the nerve proximally and causes denervation of both suprascapular and infrascapular muscles.**
- **Cyst located inferiorly in the spinoglenoid notch compresses the nerve distal to the branch innervating the supraspinatus, and selectively causes denervation of only infraspinatus muscle.**
- **MRI shows mass with low signal intensity on T1-weighted and high signal intensity on T2-weighted images.**
- **After gadolinium injection, cyst presents as a low signal with a thin peripheral enhancement on T1-weighted image. Muscle atrophy will be high signal intensity on T1-weighted images.**

ADDITIONAL IMAGES

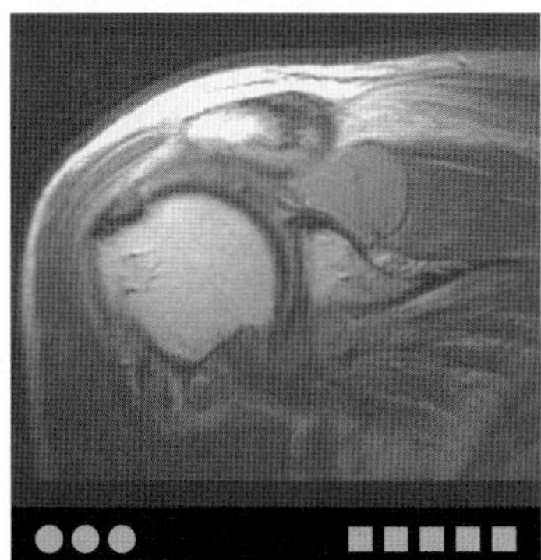

B. Ganglion cyst: Coronal PD-weighted image demonstrates low intermediate signal intensity mass in the suprascapular notch.

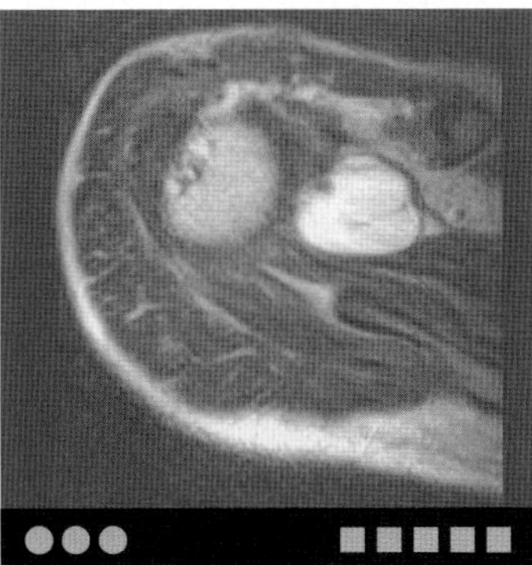

C. Ganglion cyst: Axial T2-weighted image demonstrates high signal intensity mass in the suprascapular notch.

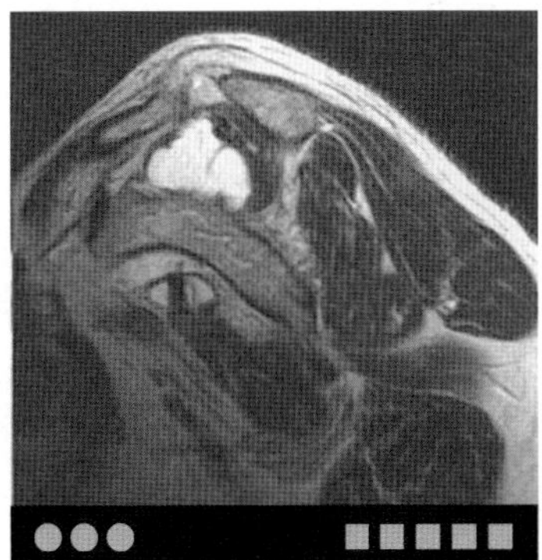

D. Ganglion cyst: Sagittal T2-weighted image shows high signal intensity mass in the suprascapular notch.

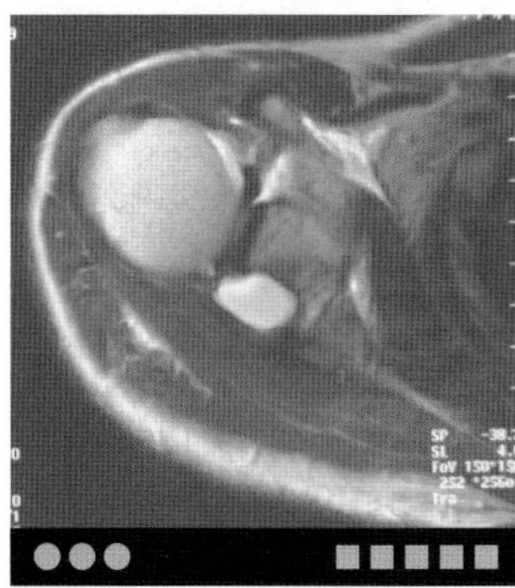

E. Ganglion cyst: Axial T2-weighted image shows cyst in the spinoglenoid notch.

IMAGE KEY

Common

●●●●●
●●●●
●●●
●●
●

Rare

Typical

■■■■■
■■■■
■■■
■■
■

Unusual

DIFFERENTIAL DIAGNOSES IMAGES

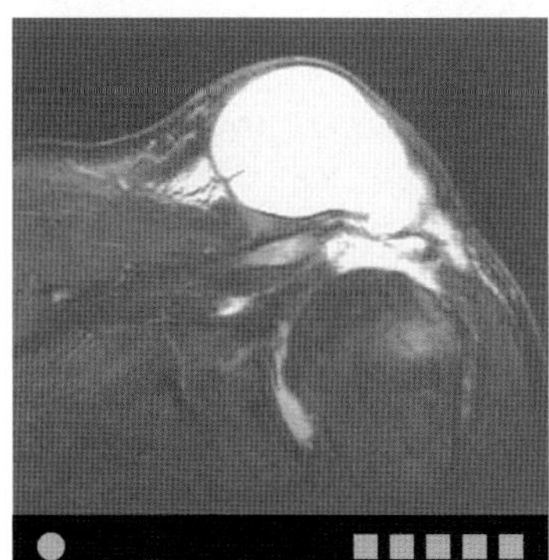

F. Synovial cyst: Coronal T2-weighted image shows high signal intensity fluid-filled cavity superior to the AC joint, with extension to the shoulder joint (Geyser phenomenon associated with rotator cuff tear).

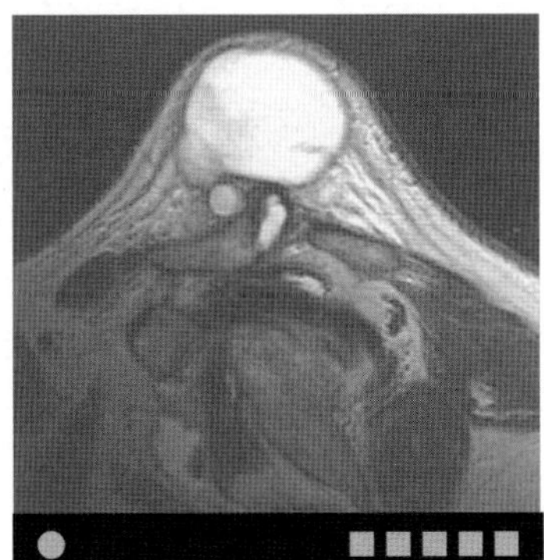

G. Synovial cyst: Sagittal T2-weighted image shows synovial cyst extending from the acromioclavicular joint.

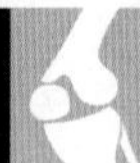

1–26 Humeral Avulsion of Anteroinferior Glenohumeral Ligament (HAGL)

John C. Hunter

PRESENTATION

Instability following two anterior shoulder dislocations

FINDINGS

Arthrogram performed prior to MR showed irregularity of the normally smooth axillary recess. The MR arthrogram showed HAGL lesion—humeral avulsion of the inferior glenohumeral ligament (IGL).

DIFFERENTIAL DIAGNOSES

- *ALPSA lesion (anterior labral periosteal sleeve avulsion)*: This avulsion at the anteroinferior glenoid is associated with remarkable displacement of labral cartilage. Although the periosteum is avulsed and the labrum is displaced, the periosteum is not torn.
- *Perthes lesion:* This avulsion at the anteroinferior glenoid is associated with minimal or mild displacement of labral cartilage. Although the periosteum is avulsed and the labrum is displaced, the periosteum is not torn.
- *Bankart lesion:* Anteroinferior labral tear is associated with tear or disruption of periosteal sleeve.
- *GLAD (glenoid labral articular defect):* This labral tear is associated with a defect in hyaline articular cartilage of the glenoid.
- *Hammock tear:* The IGL with the joint capsule at the axillary recess forms a hammock. Hammock tear leads to extravasation of fluid or contrast agent at axillary pouch.

COMMENTS

This image is of a 33-year-old male with shoulder instability following two anterior shoulder dislocations. The HAGL deformity (humeral avulsion of the glenohumeral ligament) results from anterior shoulder dislocation. The anterior band of IGL is disrupted at its humeral insertion. If an osseous fragment is avulsed, a bony HAGL (BHAGL) lesion would result. At arthrography and MR arthrography, the normally smooth axillary pouch is irregular with variable contrast extravasation inferiorly. There are various lesions associated with anterior dislocation and anterior shoulder instability. Resnick divides these lesions into three categories depending on the site of disruption. Humeral-sided lesions include the HAGL and BHAGL and account for 15% to 20% of such injuries. Bankart variants such as GLAD, ALPSA, Perthes, etc., account for up to 75% of injuries to the IGL. However, pure capsular failure can be seen in up to 20% of cases. These findings at arthrography and MR are pathognomonic of the HAGL lesion. The differential diagnosis involves mainly the various causes of anterior shoulder instability. The basic pathology is failure of the IGL. The challenge at MR arthrography is to identify the site of this failure. While the HAGL lesion represents failure at the humeral attachment, the Bankart and its variants represent failure at the glenoid attachment of the ligament. Pure capsular injury is less common.

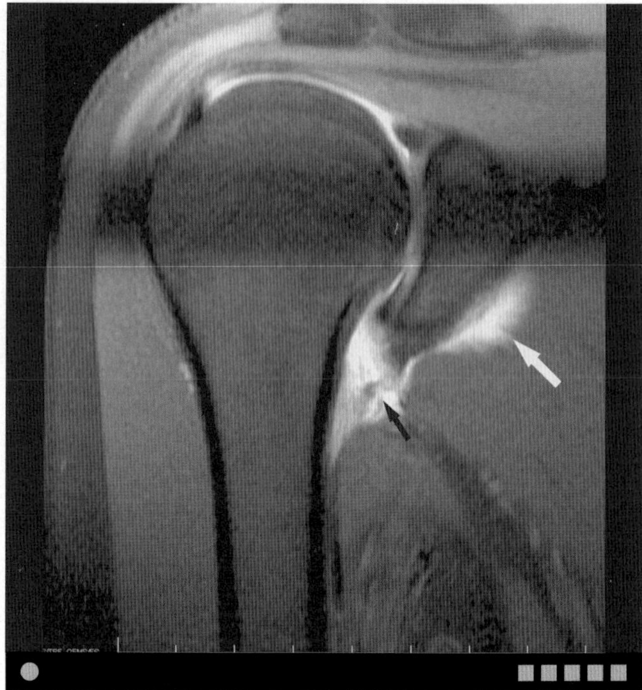

A. HAGL: Oblique coronal T1-weighted image with fat saturation following arthrogram shows extravasation of contrast outside the axillary pouch (white arrow) and tear of the IGL (black arrow).

PEARLS

- **Without arthrography to distend the joint, there is rarely enough fluid in a shoulder joint to evaluate labral and capsular structures. The exception is a recent dislocation where hemarthrosis may provide adequate distension.**
- **The axillary recess should be smooth in contour. Careful evaluation of conventional radiograph for a small piece of bone adjacent to the proximal humerus (BHAGL) is important to detect this rare variant.**
- **While most are familiar with other residuals of anterior dislocation such as the Hill-Sachs deformity and Bankart variants, evaluation of the humeral attachment of the IGL is important in evaluating shoulder instability.**

ADDITIONAL IMAGES

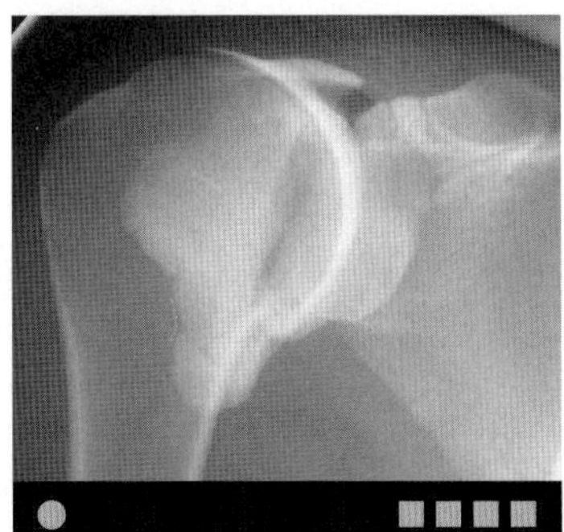

B. HAGL: Conventional arthrogram shows an outpouching inferiorly from the axillary pouch as the only abnormality.

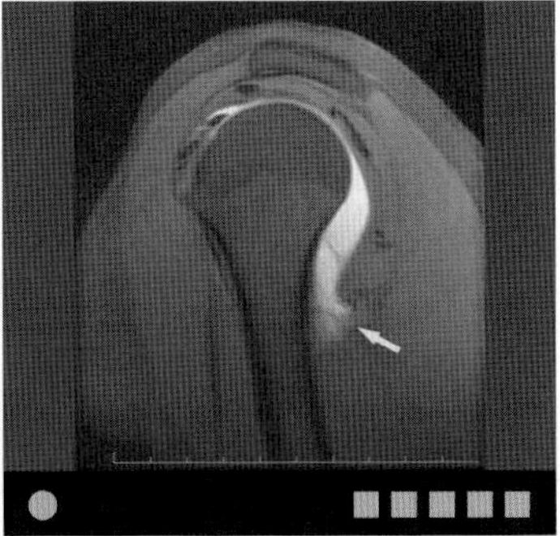

C. HAGL: Sagittal T1-weighted image with fat saturation shows extravasation of injected contrast through tear in the IGL (arrow).

DIFFERENTIAL DIAGNOSES IMAGES

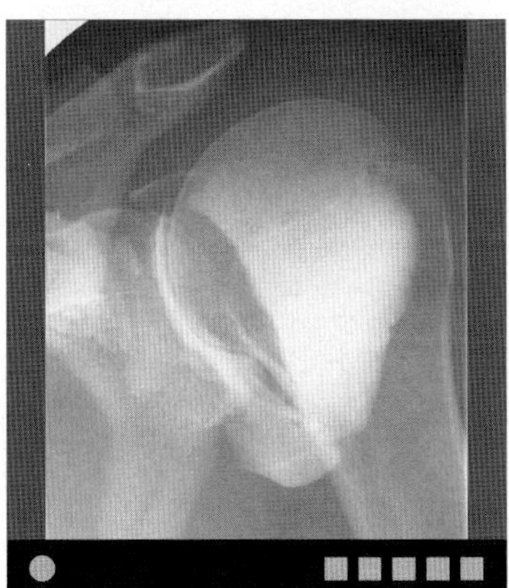

D. Hammock tear: This image is of a 29-year-male who was injured in a parasailing crash. The spot film during arthrography shows irregularity of the axillary recess.

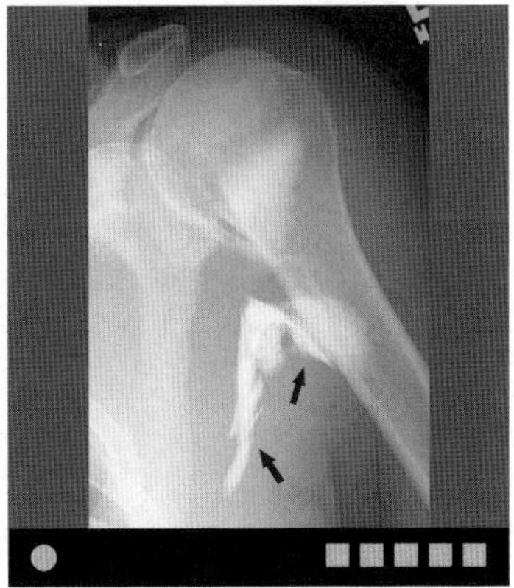

E. Hammock Tear: Overhead radiograph obtained approximately 5 minutes later (same patient shown in image D) shows inferior extravasation of contrast agent (arrows).

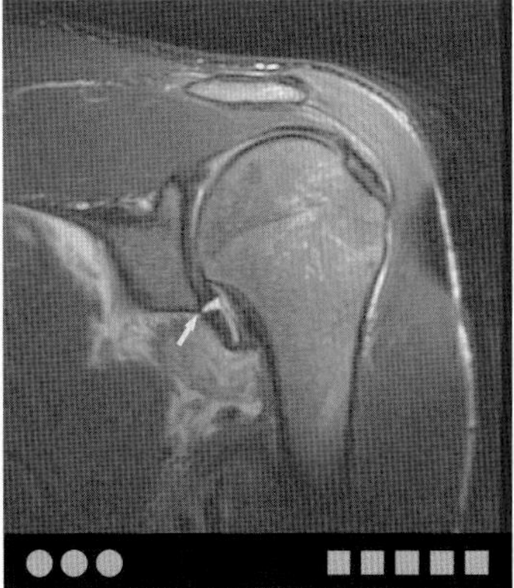

F. Perthes Lesion: A coronal T2-weighted image with fat saturation shows detachment of the labrum (arrow). This image is of a 19-year-male collegiate basketball player with anterior dislocation in a game. This study was performed within 24 hours without arthrography utilizing the hemarthrosis that usually accompanies this injury.

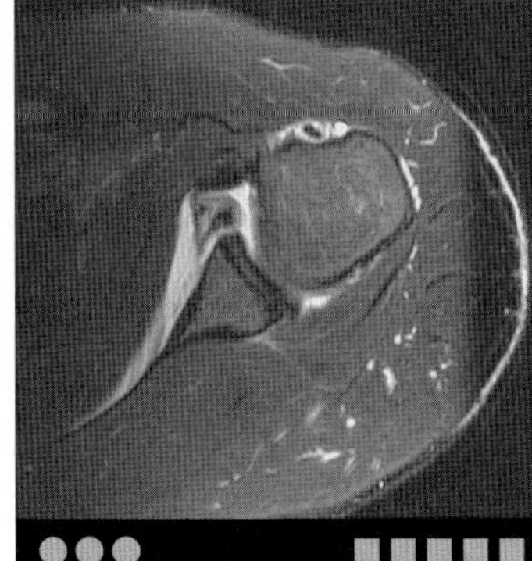

G. Perthes Lesion: An axial T2-weighted image with fat saturation (same patient shown in image F) shows avulsion tear of labrum and mild displacement with an intact periosteal attachment to the glenoid neck compatible with a Perthes lesion.

IMAGE KEY

Common

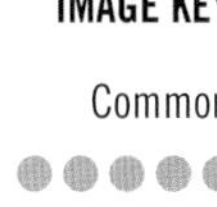

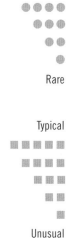

Rare

Typical

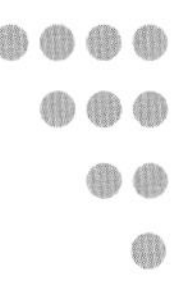

Unusual

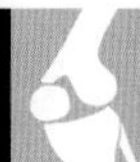

1–27 Bony Humeral Avulsion of the Anterior Glenohumeral Ligament (BHAGL)

Hamidreza R. Torshizy and Jamshid Tehranzadeh

PRESENTATION

Pain and tenderness upon abduction and lateral rotation

FINDINGS

MR imaging findings include bony humeral avulsion of the humerus by anterior band of the inferior glenohumeral ligament. Often a tear of the subscapularis tendon is also present.

DIFFERENTIAL DIAGNOSES

- *Humeral avulsion of the glenohumeral ligament (HAGL):* This lesion is similar to BHAGL except that there is no fracture of humerus. In this lesion the anteroinferior glenohumeral ligament is avulsed without bony avulsion.
- *Isolated avulsion of subscapularis tendon from lesser tuberosity of humerus*: In this condition the anteroinferior glenohumeral ligament may or may not be involved.

COMMENTS

This image is of a 34-year-old male with shoulder pain, tenderness, and instability. The pain and tenderness was localized to the anterior portion of the shoulder, mostly upon abduction and lateral rotation. Decreased external rotation, general laxity of the joint, and crepitus were also noted. The inferior glenohumeral ligament labral complex is the main anterior stabilizer of the shoulder upon abduction and prevents anterior dislocation during external rotation. The anterior glenohumeral ligament comprises of the three bands, including superior, middle, and inferior ligaments. These are part of the anterior joint capsule of the shoulder. A BHAGL lesion is consistent with HAGL, accompanied by a humeral avulsion fracture. In addition, a tear of the subscapularis tendon can also be present. Normally, the axillary pouch of the joint capsule assumes the shape of a hammock. However, with tear of the anteroinferior glenohumeral ligament, the axillary pouch of the joint capsule assumes a "J" shape. Patients, typically adult males, present with a history of anterior shoulder instability following a traumatic dislocation or prior episode of anterior dislocation that has been reduced. These lesions are often overlooked upon arthroscopy, and thus radiological evaluation becomes invaluable.

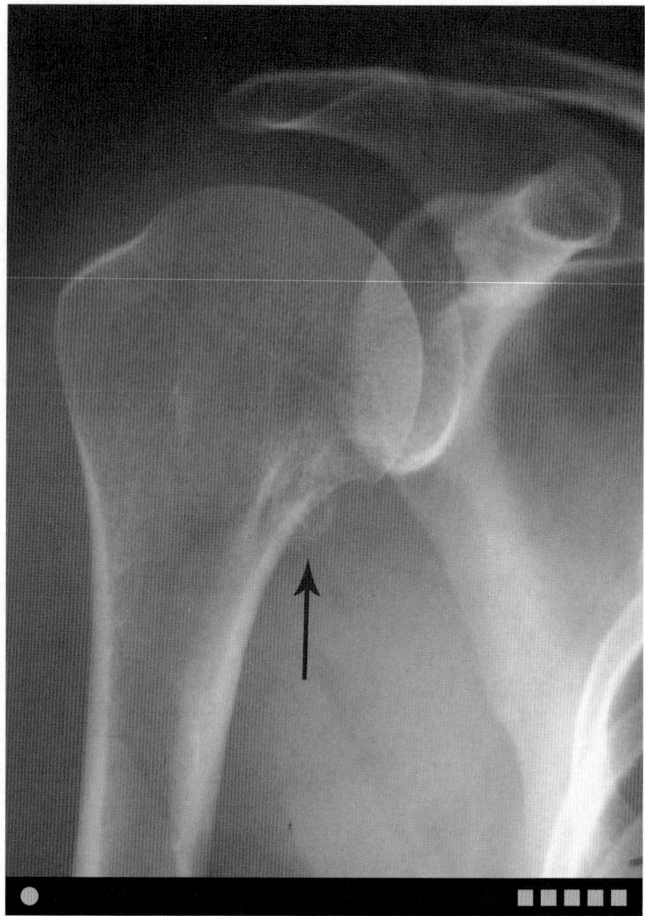

A. BHAGL: AP radiograph demonstrating an osseous avulsion of the humeral neck (arrow).

PEARLS

- **MR findings of a BHAGL lesion include HAGL and a humeral avulsion fracture.**
- **Disruption of the subscapularis tendon is often noted.**
- **Although a limited differential exists, differentiation from a HAGL lesion is important.**

ADDITIONAL IMAGES

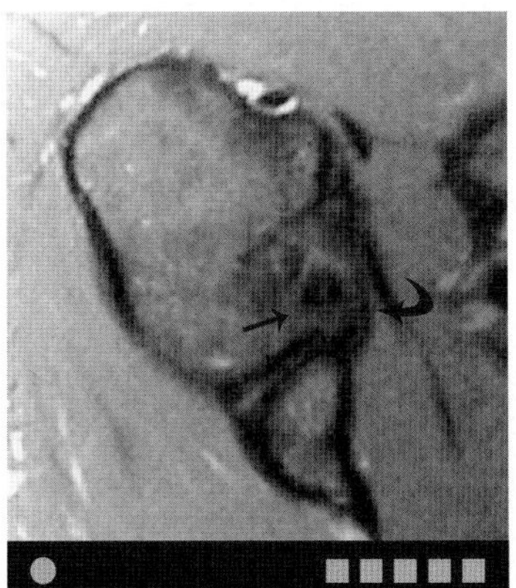

B. BHAGL lesion: Axial FSE T2-weighted image demonstrating an osseous fragment separating from the proximal humerus corresponding to a humeral avulsion fracture (arrow), with accompanying disruption of the anterior band of the inferior glenohumeral ligament (curved arrow).

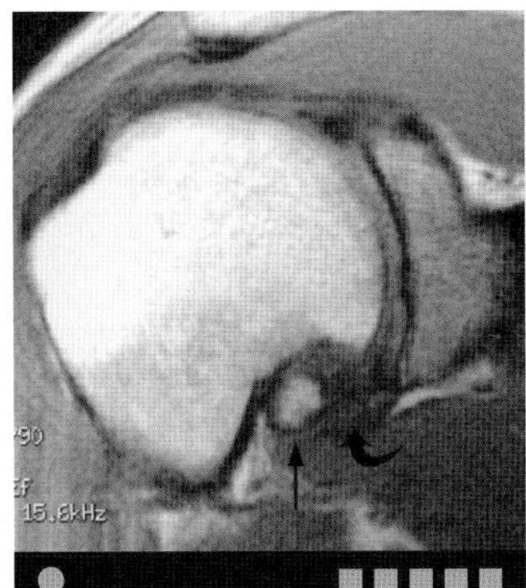

C. BHAGL lesion: Coronal FSE T1-weighted image demonstrating an osseous fragment corresponding to a humeral avulsion fracture (arrow), with accompanying disruption of the anterior band of the inferior glenohumeral ligament (curved arrow).

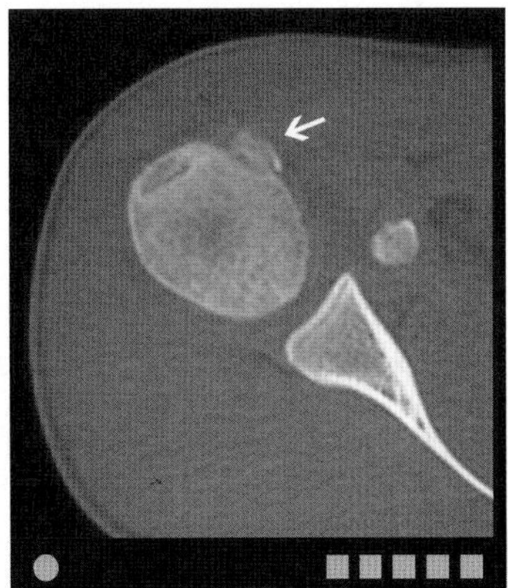

D. BHAGL lesion with subscapularis tendon avulsion: Axial CT of another patient with avulsion fracture of insertion site of the subscapularis tendon (arrow).

DIFFERENTIAL DIAGNOSES IMAGES

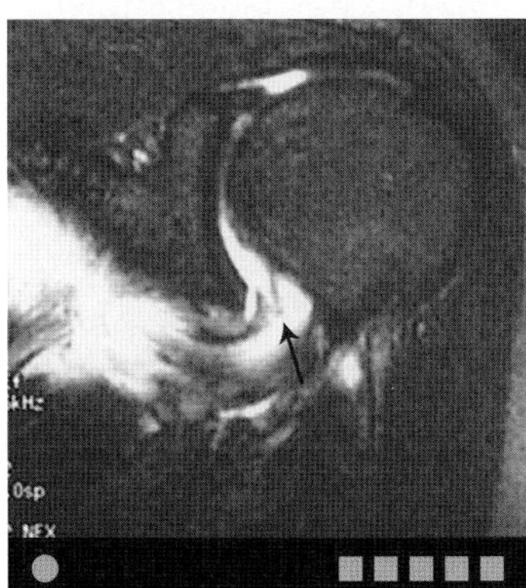

E. HAGL lesion: Coronal fat-saturated T2-weighted image of shoulder MR arthrogram shows tear of the anteroinferior glenohumeral ligament and partial tear of subscapularis tendon.

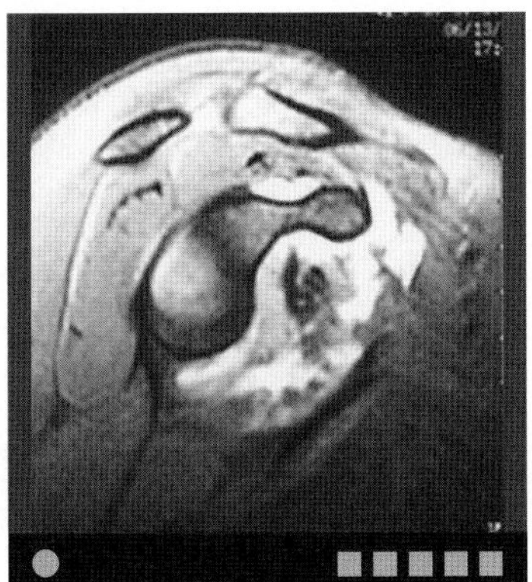

F. HAGL lesion: Sagittal fat-saturated T1-weighted shoulder MR arthrogram image shows tear of the of all anterior glenohumeral ligaments.

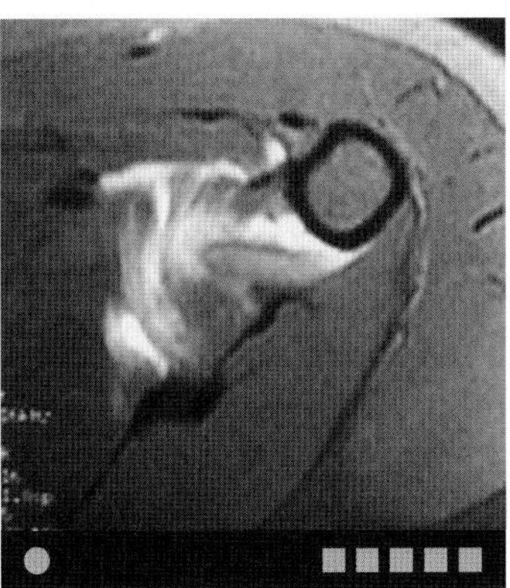

G. HAGL lesion: Axial fat-saturated T1-weighted shoulder MR arthrogram image shows tear of anteroinferior glenohumeral ligament at the region of the hammock.

IMAGE KEY

Common

Rare

Typical

Unusual

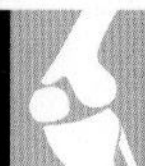

1–28 Insufficiency Fracture of Glenoid

Melitus Maryam Golshan and Jamshid Tehranzadeh

PRESENTATION

Shoulder pain

FINDINGS

MR imaging shows bone marrow edema and fracture lines in glenoid process.

DIFFERENTIAL DIAGNOSES

- *Osteomyelitis*: Shows low signal intensity marrow changes on T1-weighted and high signal intensity on T2-weighted images and marked postcontract enhancement. There is no fracture line in isolated infections.
- *Avascular necrosis*: Shows characteristic double line sign and marrow edema.
- *Post-traumatic fracture*: Patient has history of trauma and usually has joint effusion, extensive bone marrow, and soft tissue edema.

COMMENTS

This image is of a postmenopausal female with history of 1-month shoulder pain and limitation of motion. Insufficiency-type stress fractures occur in structurally weakened bone that cannot withstand the stresses of normal activity. The predisposing condition for an insufficiency fracture is usually osteoporosis; other metabolic diseases, long-term exposure to corticosteroids, and bone atrophy after irradiation may also be contributing factors. It is more common in postmenopausal females. The extent of marrow signal abnormalities exceeded the size of corresponding radiographic findings of fracture in most cases. The insufficiency fractures typically appear as hypointense lines or fissures in both the T1-weighted and T2-weighted sequences. Besides the hypo intense fissures, there are areas of hyperintensity on T2-weighted images adjacent to these hypointense fissures in some cases and absent in others. These represent active and chronic phases of the disease, respectively. In chronic insufficiency fractures, the hypointense lines may result from persisting sclerosis at the fracture site. STIR images shows superior contrast between normal and abnormal marrow. Intramedullary lines of hypointensity extending to the inner cortical margin were identified within the hyperintense marrow abnormality on STIR images. MRI with T1-weighted spin echo image and STIR sequence demonstrates prominent signal abnormalities at fracture sites including those in which radiographic signs are subtle.

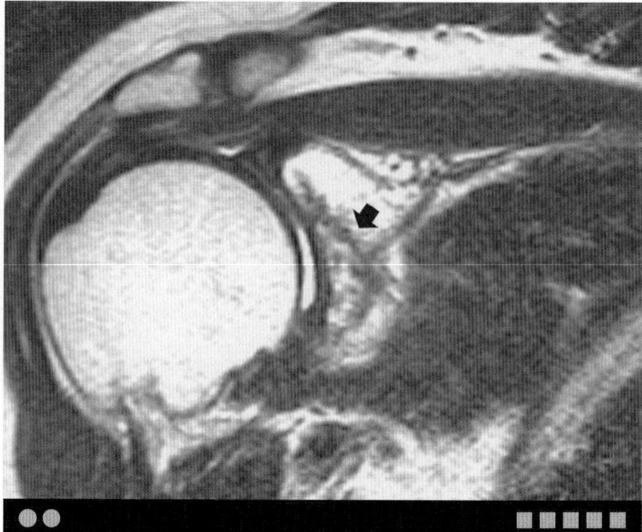

A. Insufficiency fracture of glenoid process: Coronal oblique proton density image shows a low signal intensity dark line crossing the glenoid process representing fracture line (arrow).

PEARLS

- **Insufficiency-type stress fractures occur in structurally weakened bone that cannot withstand the stresses of normal activity.**
- **The insufficiency fractures typically appeared as hypointense lines or fissures in both the T1-weighted and T2-weighted sequences.**
- **In acute insufficiency fracture MRI shows high signal intensity in marrow adjacent to fracture line on T2-weighted image and STIR. In chronic phase due to sclerosis of fracture line, MRI shows persistent low signal intensity line on T1 and T2 and absent of marrow changes.**

ADDITIONAL IMAGES

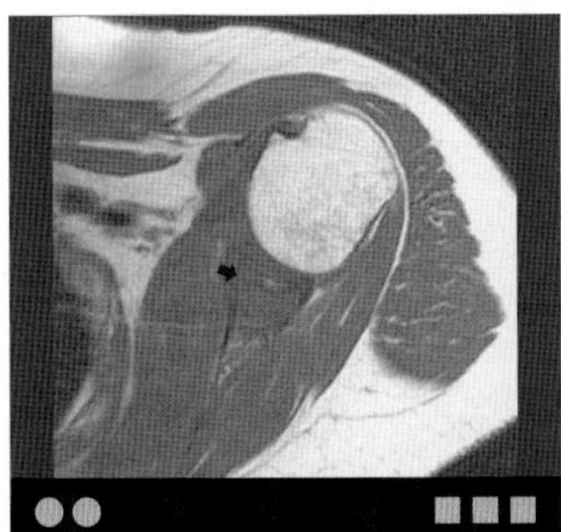

B. Insufficiency fracture of glenoid process: Axial T1-weighted image shows low signal intensity of the bone marrow indicating marrow edema of the glenoid process. In addition, a very dark line represents fracture line.

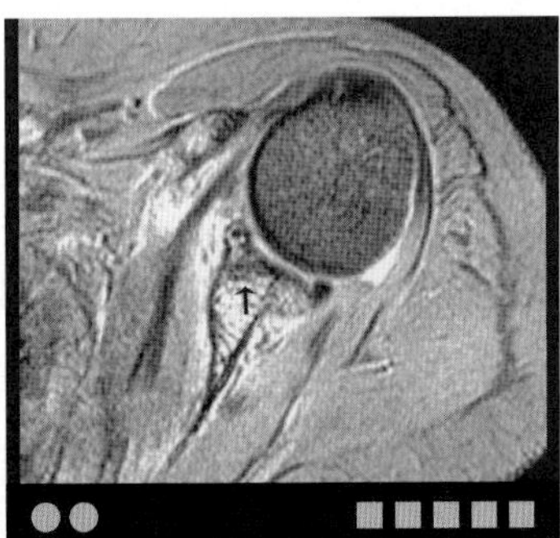

C. Insufficiency fracture of glenoid process: Axial T2-weighted image shows bone marrow edema of the glenoid process. Note oblique dark line indicating glenoid process insufficiency fracture (arrow).

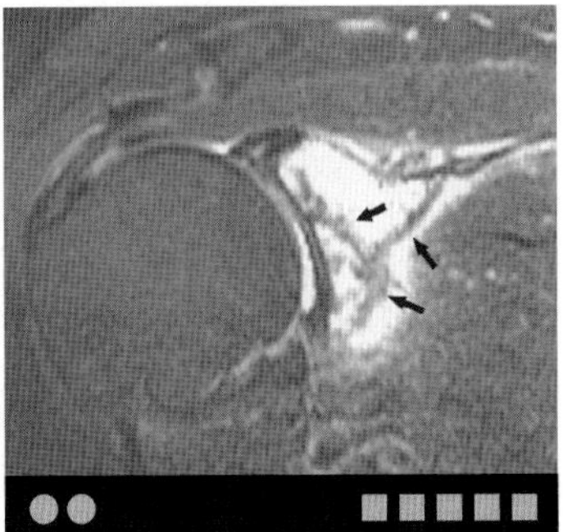

D. Insufficiency fracture of glenoid process: Coronal T2 SPIR image shows bone marrow edema of the glenoid with increased signal intensity. Note multiple insufficiency fracture lines with low signal intensities (arrows).

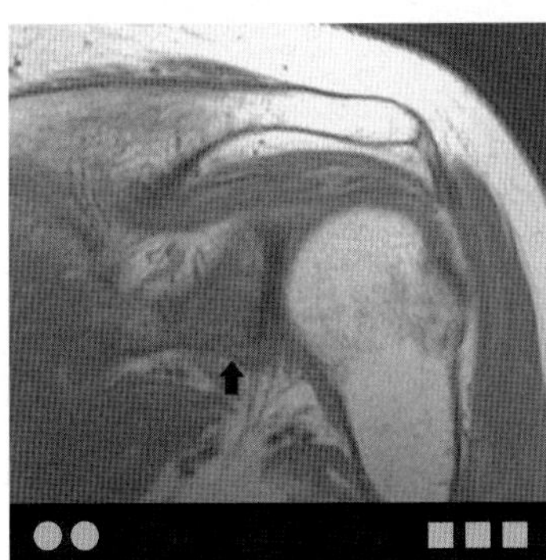

E. Insufficiency fracture of glenoid process: Coronal obliqueT1-weighted image shows low signal intensity of the glenoid process because of marrow edema. A darker line representing fracture in the lower corner of the glenoid process is seen.

DIFFERENTIAL DIAGNOSES IMAGES

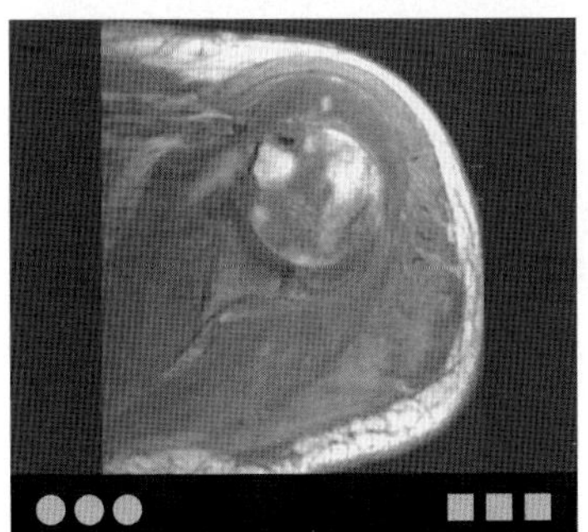

F. Septic arthritis and osteomyelitis: Axial T1 FSE image shows significant increase signal in glenoid and humeral head representing marrow edema. Joint effusion and low signal fluid collection in anterior arm are noted.

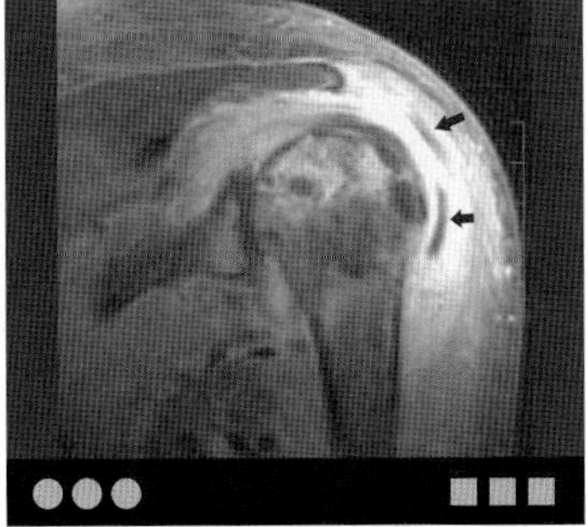

G. Septic arthritis and osteomyelitis: Coronal oblique fat saturated post-contrast T1-weighted image shows extensive marrow enhancement in glenoid and humeral head representing marrow edema. Note areas of low signal intensity in humeral head corresponding to necrotic tissue. There are fluid collections with wall enhancement in subcutaneous region representing abscesses (arrows).

IMAGE KEY

Common

Rare

Typical

Unusual

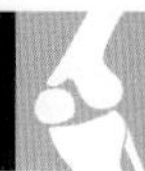

1–29 Intramuscular Rotator Cuff Cyst

Marcia F. Blacksin

PRESENTATION

Shoulder pain

FINDINGS

MRI shows longitudinal cyst in infraspinatus muscle ending as a partial, interstitial rotator cuff tear.

DIFFERENTIAL DIAGNOSIS

- *Paralabral cyst*: This is a cystic appearing mass found adjacent to the glenoid labrum, which may arise from extrusion of joint fluid through a labral tear, into the soft tissue.

COMMENTS

Identification of an intramuscular cyst should prompt a search for a rotator cuff tear. It is thought that the defect in the rotator cuff may allow joint fluid to dissect along tendon fibers and form this cyst. These cysts are associated with both full- and partial-thickness tears. Approximately 50% of the tears are partial, and they are found in three of the rotator cuff tendons, excluding the teres minor. The most frequently affected tendons are the supra- and infraspinatus tendons. Paralabral cysts can be round shaped, oval, or multiloculated. The site of origination may be from the anterior, posterior, or superior labrum. Sometimes the cyst is large enough to extend into the spinoglenoid or suprascapular notches. Cysts in the spinoglenoid notch can compress the distal suprascapular nerve, with resultant denervation of the infraspinatus muscle. When located in the suprascapular notch, these cysts can compress the proximal aspect of the suprascapular nerve and cause pain and denervation of both the supra- and infraspinatus muscles. Discovery of such cysts should lead to a search for labral tears as well as search for muscle abnormalities. Labral tears are seen with 100% of these types of cysts. Muscle edema or fatty atrophy can be seen and these findings are associated with the early and late manifestations of denervation, respectively.

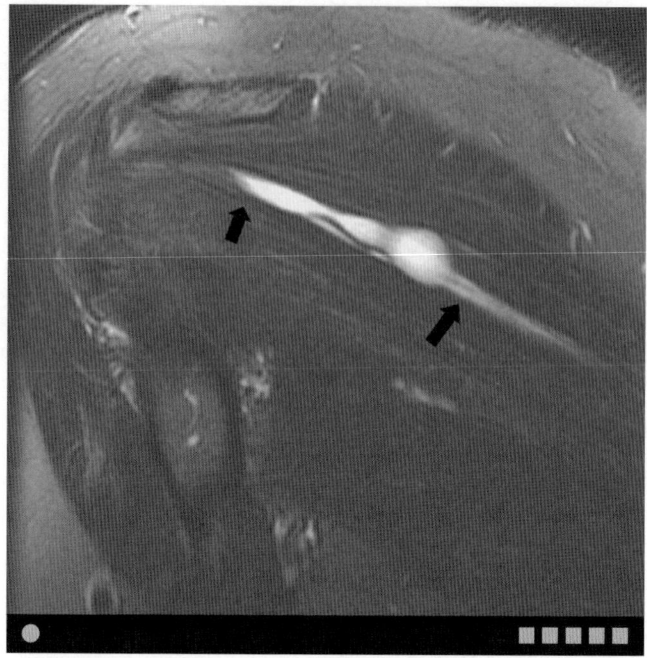

A. Intramuscular rotator cuff cyst: Coronal oblique fat-saturated T2-weighted MR images showing longitudinal cyst in infraspinatus muscle (arrows).

PEARLS

- **Intramuscular rotator cuff cysts are associated with both full and partial rotator cuff tears.**
- **Rotator cuff cysts are associated most frequently with tears in the supraspinatus and infraspinatus tendons.**
- **Paralabral cysts can cause compression neuropathy of the suprascapular nerve.**
- **Paralabral cysts are always associated with labral tears.**

ADDITIONAL IMAGES

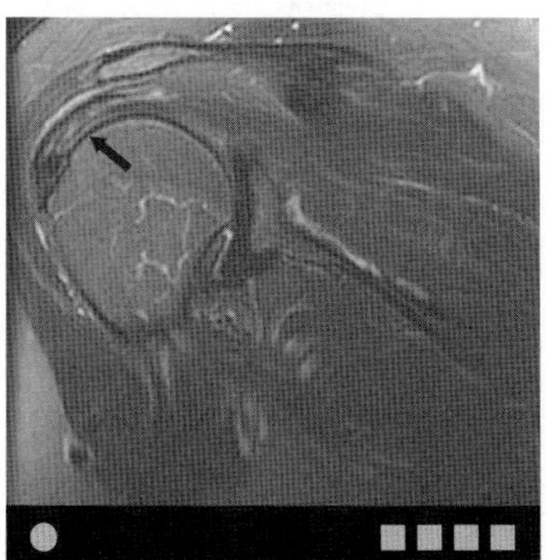

B. Intramuscular rotator cuff cyst: Coronal oblique fat-saturated T2-weighted MR image shows end of cyst as it elongates into the partial infraspinatus tendon tear (arrow).

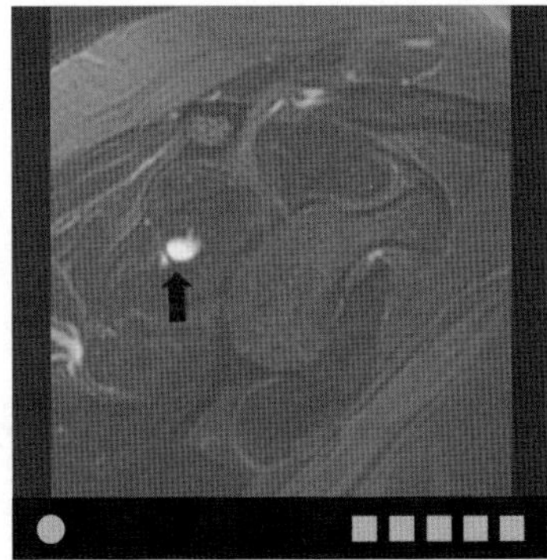

C. Intramuscular rotator cuff cyst: Sagittal oblique fat-saturated T2-weighted MR image shows cyst in infraspinatus muscle (arrow).

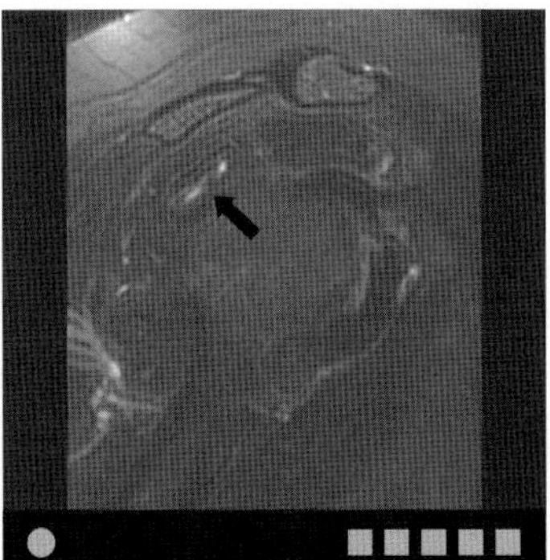

D. Intramuscular rotator cuff cyst: Sagittal oblique fat-saturated T2-weighted MR image shows elongation of cyst (arrow) as it approaches musculo-tendinous junction.

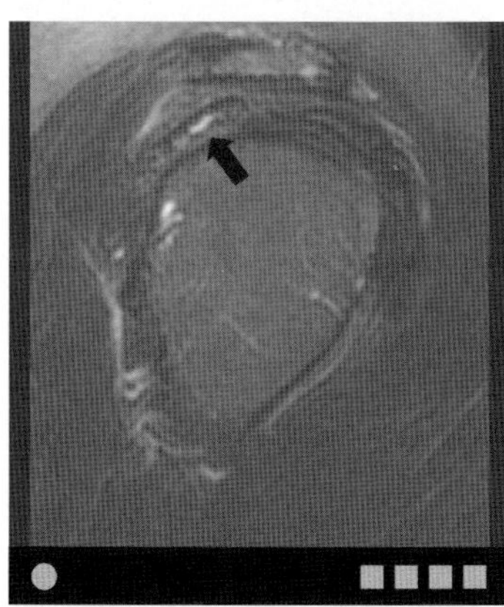

E. Intramuscular rotator cuff cyst: Sagittal oblique fat-saturated T2-weighted MR image shows termination of cyst as partial infraspinatus tendon tear (arrow).

DIFFERENTIAL DIAGNOSES IMAGES

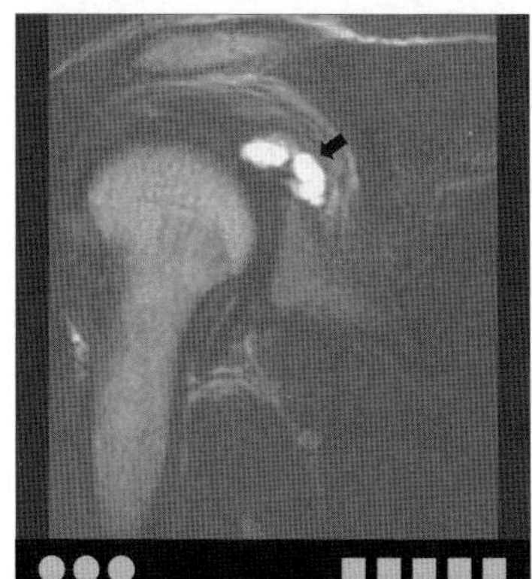

F. Paralabral cyst: Coronal oblique fat-saturated T2-weighted image shows multiloculated paralabral cyst adjacent to posterior glenoid rim (arrow).

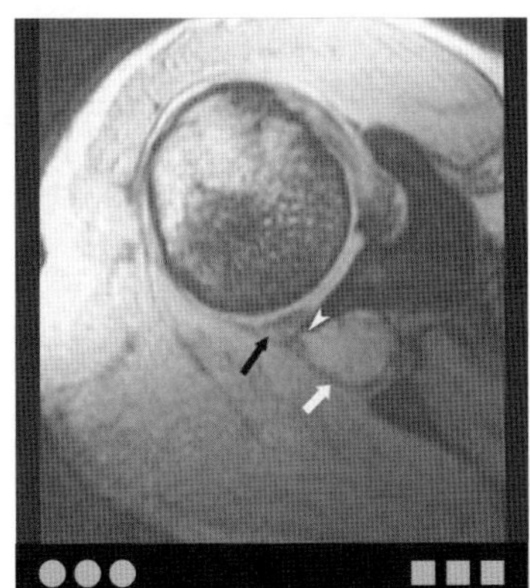

G. Paralabral cyst: Axial T2-weighted gradient echo image shows neck of cyst (arrowhead) leading to high signal area in posterior labrum (black arrow) consistent with a tear. Note paralabral cyst (white arrow).

IMAGE KEY

Common

●●●●●
●●●●
●●●
●●
●

Rare

Typical

■■■■■
■■■■
■■■
■■
■

Unusual

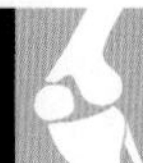

1–30 Adhesive Capsulitis

John C. Hunter

PRESENTATION

Progressive pain and gradual loss of range of motion

FINDINGS

The arthrogram showed a joint capacity of 6cc with loss of normal axillary and subscapularis recesses.

DIFFERENTIAL DIAGNOSIS

- *Scar tissue at rotator cuff interval:* This is the space between the supraspinatus and subscapularis muscle. Scar tissue formation in this space may create another focus in the shoulder joint for adhesive capsulitis.

COMMENTS

This image is of a 42-year-old female presenting with 6-month history of progressive pain and gradual loss of range of motion. Adhesive capsulitis or frozen shoulder is an inflammatory process leading to progressive scarring of the capsule, pain, and loss of range of motion. Although there may be no definite preceding incident, trauma, immobilization, hemiplegia, diabetes, and cervical disc disease have been implicated. The limited range of motion is nonspecific and can be seen with calcific tendonitis or rotator cuff tear and/or tendinopathy. Arthrography confirms diagnosis and can be combined with injection of steroids or anesthetics with joint distension for treatment. Normal joint volume is 10 to 12cc. Characteristic findings at arthrography include a joint capacity of less than 7cc, nonfilling of normal recesses (axillary and subscapular is recesses), irregularity of the normally smooth capsular surfaces, and visualization of lymphatics. Conventional MR is limited, but separation of the axillary portion of the capsule from the medial humeral cortex by more than 4 mm has been described in adhesive capsulitis with a sensitivity of 70% and a specificity of 95%. Enhancement of the pericapsular soft tissues following intravenous gadolinium administration has been reported as a sign of adhesive capsulitis. A study by Manton et al. (2001) found no additional information from MR or MR arthrography and that the conventional arthrogram was the gold standard for diagnosis. The findings of decreased joint capacity and loss of normal recesses is pathognomonic for adhesive capsulitis. Arthrography is the gold standard for diagnosis.

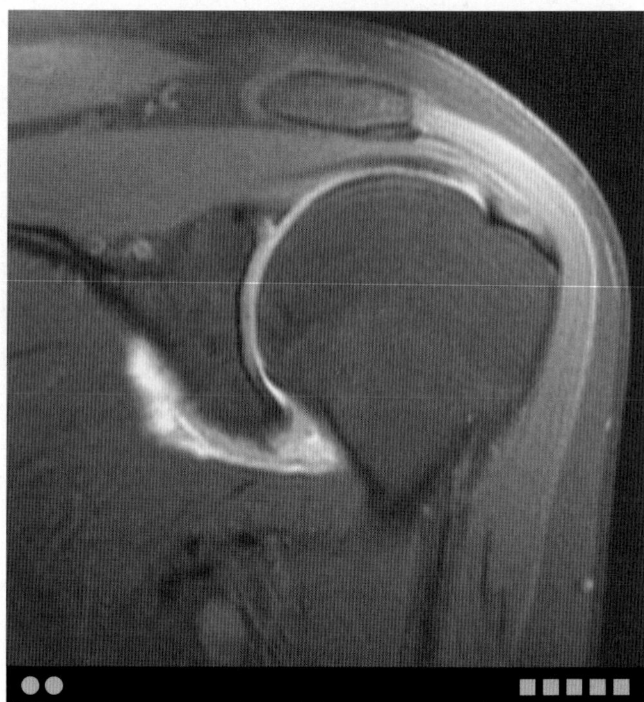

A. Adhesive capsulitis: Coronal oblique T1-weighted image with fat saturation shows loss of normal axillary and subscapularis recesses. Similar findings are seen with the conventional arthrogram (next image). The supraspinatus tendon is intact.

PEARLS

- **Arthrography is the gold standard for diagnosis, with loss of key recesses and a joint capacity of less than 7cc noted.**
- **Careful arthroscopic monitoring during the injection is important. Extravasation of contrast may occur at injection site, down biceps tendon sheath, or through capsular rents giving misleading joint volumes.**
- **Another advantage of arthrography is having joint access to inject steroids for treatment or local anesthetics to assess pain response and evaluate the true degree of loss of motion without the pain factor.**
- **Despite studies proposing the value of conventional MR, MR arthrography, and IV contrast enhanced MR, the results have been inconsistent.**

ADDITIONAL IMAGES

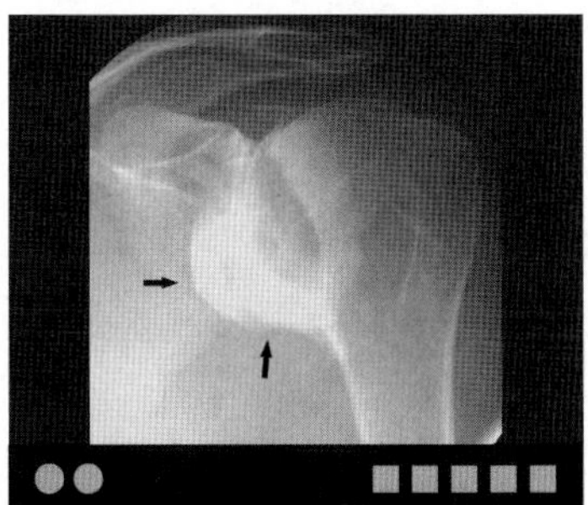

B. Adhesive capsulitis: Conventional arthrogram shows loss of normal axillary and subscapularis recesses (arrows). Joint capacity was only 6 mL.

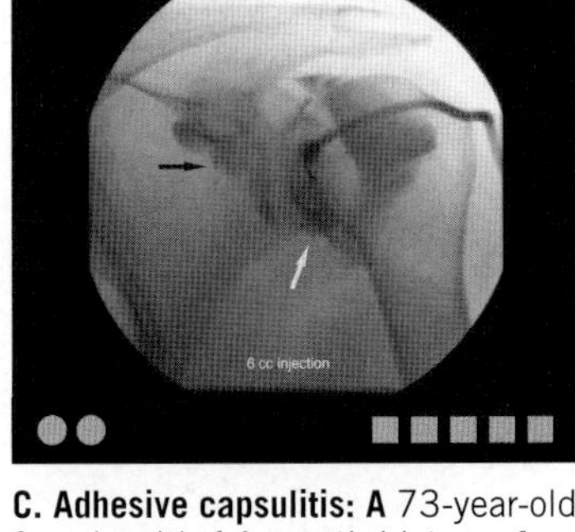

C. Adhesive capsulitis: A 73-year-old female with 14-month history of pain and decreased motion. Arthrogram showed 7-cc volume with loss of axillary recess (white arrow) and irregularity of the subscapularis bursa (black arrow).

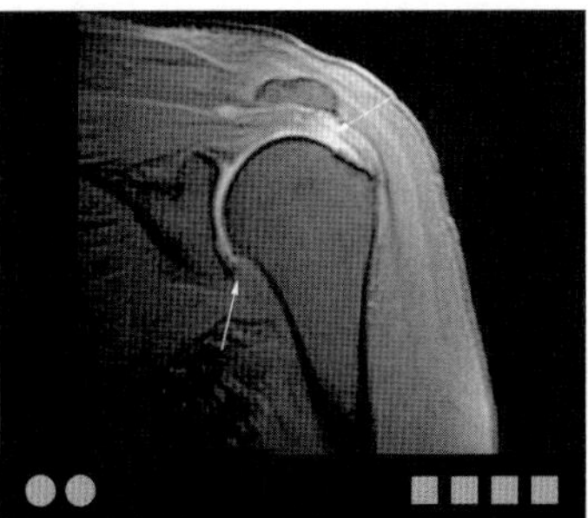

D. Adhesive capsulitis: T1-weighted fat-saturated coronal oblique image (same patient as in image C) shows loss of axillary recess and high-grade partial thickness tear of the supraspinatus tendon (arrow).

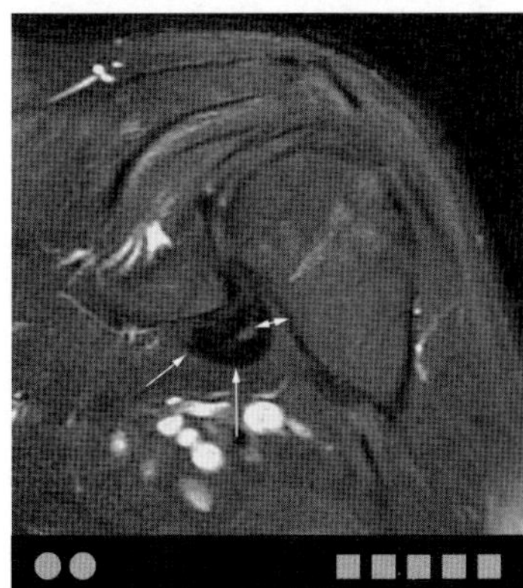

E. Adhesive capsulitis: A 62-year-old male with 8-month history of pain and loss of motion with clinical diagnosis of adhesive capsulitis. Coronal oblique T2-weighted image with fat saturation shows marked thickening of the IGL (arrow) and a distance between the fluid in the axillary recess and the medial humeral cortex to exceed 4 mm (double arrows).

DIFFERENTIAL DIAGNOSES IMAGES

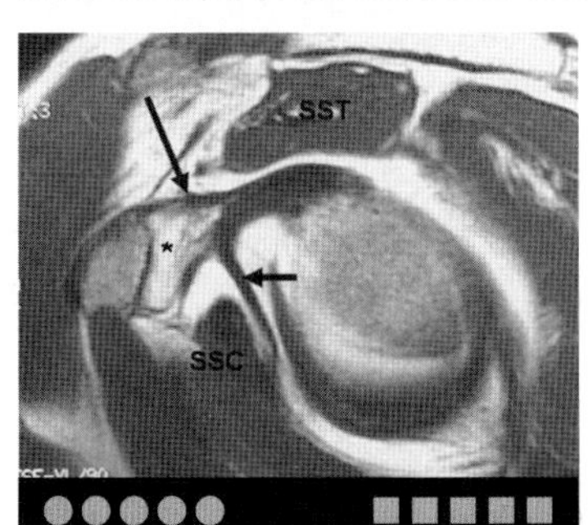

F. Normal rotator cuff interval: Sagittal T1-weighted image following arthrogram shows normal rotator cuff interval. Note coracohumeral ligament (long arrow), middle glenohumeral ligament (short arrow), supraspinatus (SST), and subscapularis muscles (SSC).

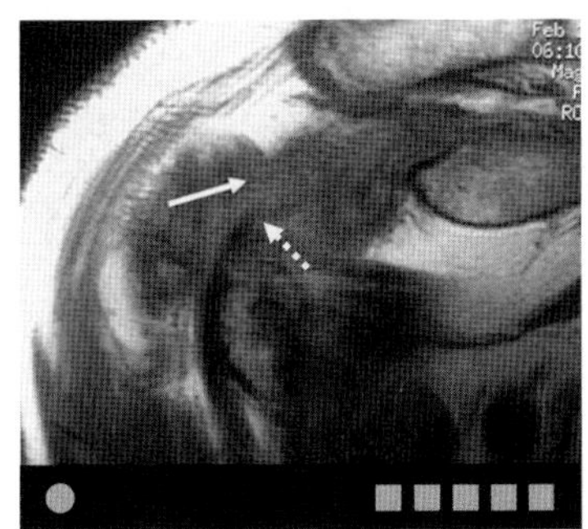

G. Scar tissue in rotator cuff interval: Coronal oblique T1-weighted image following arthrogram shows scar tissues at the rotator cuff interval (arrow) and near biceps tendon (interrupted arrow).

IMAGE KEY

Common

Rare

Typical

Unusual

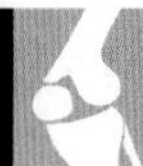

1–31 Proximal Rupture of the Biceps Tendon

Ibrahim F. Abdelwahab and Stefano Bianchi

PRESENTATION

Pain with tenderness over the bicipital groove

FINDINGS

MRI demonstrated empty bicipital groove in all three planes.

DIFFERENTIAL DIAGNOSES

- *Greater tuberosity bone trabecular fracture*: Visualized fracture fragment, hypointense fracture line on T1-weighted image, and hyperintense edema on T2-weighted image.
- *Biceps tenodesis*: Absent biceps in the rotator interval, micrometalic artifact, and surgical history.
- *Subscapularis rupture*: Secondary to anterior or posterior dislocation, edema of the lesser tuberosity, Bankart, reversed Bankart, Hill Sachs, or reversed Hill Sachs.

COMMENTS

This image is of a 45-year-old man with dull anterior shoulder pain felt especially during lifting, pushing, or pulling without preceding history of acute traction to his shoulder. On physical examination, he had severe tenderness over the bicipital groove. The etiology of the tear of the tendon of the long head of the biceps is chronic overuse and microtrauma. It usually accompanies impingement (rotator cuff tear). Other associated abnormalities are subacromial, subcoracoid impingement, lesser tuberosity degenerative changes and subarticular cysts, biceps tenosynovitis, and hooked acromion. The most common location of the tear is the rotator interval adjacent to the biceps anchor. The size of the gap varies from millimeter range to several centimeters. The muscle belly may retract inferiorly leading to "Popeye sign," which is less obvious than in distal tendon tear because of the anchor of the short head tendon preventing retraction. MRI findings reveal hypointense filling gap in the tendon on T1-weighted image, which intensifies on T2-weighted image. Reactive fluid of the subacromial and subcoracoid bursa may also occur. It is important to check the empty bicipital groove in all three planes. An empty groove may either result from a torn or a dislocated tendon. One must also identify whether the tear is intra- or extra-articular and to check both the proximal and distal stumps for fraying, thickening, and signal intensification to identify the etiology. MRI is the best modality to evaluate this lesion and the suggested protocol is fat-saturated fast spin echo proton density and T2-weighted images in the axial and coronal planes. When diagnosis is not certain images obtained in a caudal location to show the retracted muscle which would confirm a tendon tear.

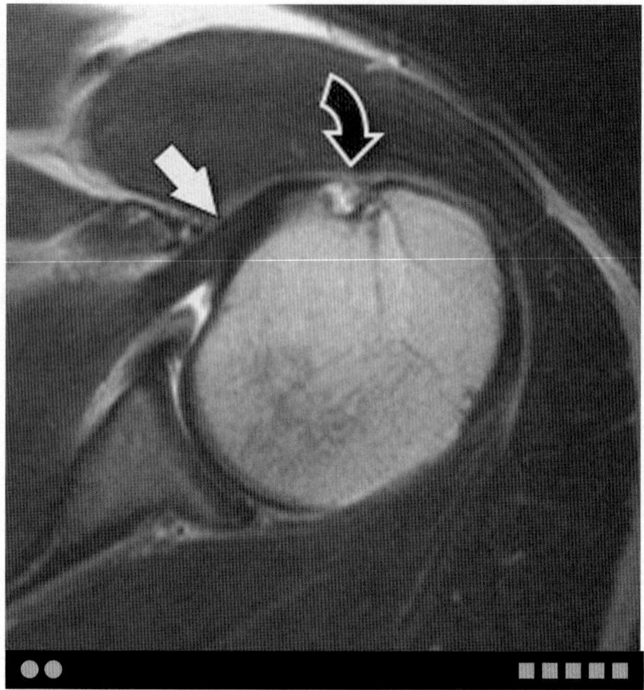

A. Proximal biceps tendon tear: Axial FS PD FSE at the level of the proximal part of the bicipital groove reveals an empty bicipital groove with fluid hyperintense signal (curved black arrow). The subscapularis tendon is intact (arrow).

PEARLS

- **To check the empty bicipital groove in all three planes. An empty groove may either result from a torn or a dislocated tendon.**
- **To identify whether the tear is intra- or extra-articular and to check both the proximal and distal stumps for fraying, thickening, and signal intensification to identify the etiology.**
- **Best imaging tool is MRI and the suggested protocol is FS PD FSE/FS/T2-WI FSE in the axial and coronal planes. When diagnosis is not certain images obtained in a caudal location to show the retracted muscle which would confirm a tendon tear.**

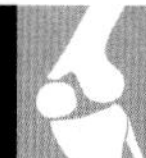

ADDITIONAL IMAGES

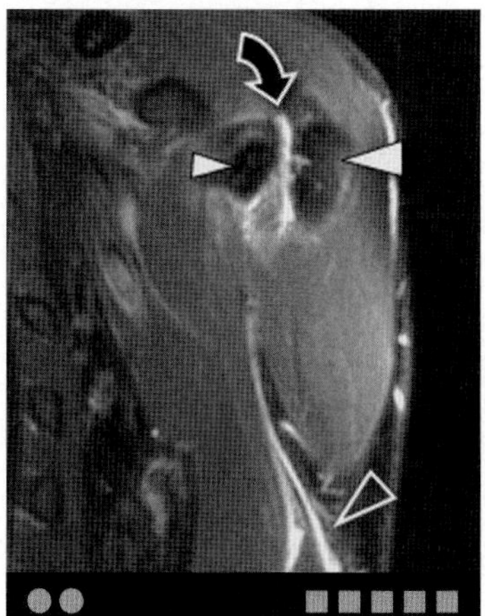

B: Proximal bicipital tendon tear: Coronal FS PD FSE showing the empty groove replaced by fluid hyperintense signal (curved black arrow). The groove is demonstrated between the lesser and greater tuberosities (arrow heads). Note caudal hyperintense fluid signal (void arrowhead).

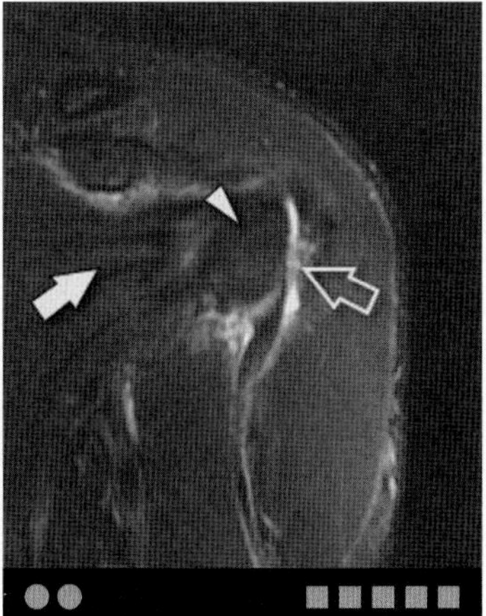

C. Proximal bicipital tendon tear: Coronal FS T2WI FSE again showing the empty groove replaced by fluid hyperintense signal lateral to the lesser tuberosity (arrow head). The fluid signal is filling almost the whole groove (open arrow). The subscapularis muscle is normal (arrow).

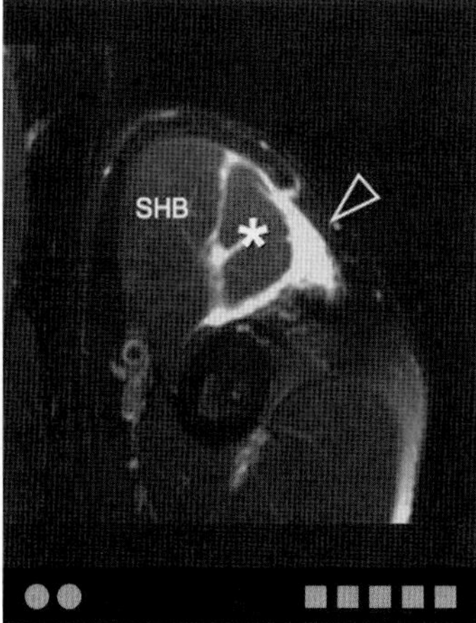

D. Proximal bicipital tendon tear: Axial FS T2WI FSE showing the long head of biceps muscle belly (asterisk) distal to the tear with fluid intensified signal (hemorrhage) adjacent to the lateral aspect of the muscle (open arrow head). The short head belly (SHB) is normal.

IMAGE KEY

Common

Rare

Typical

Unusual

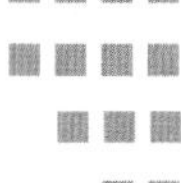

DIFFERENTIAL DIAGNOSES IMAGES

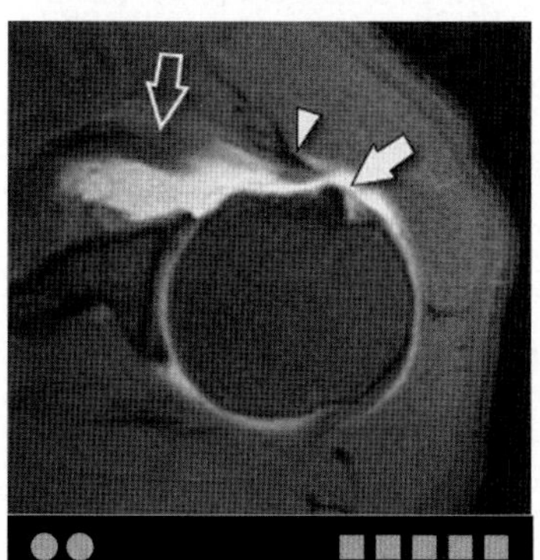

E. Acute tear of the subscapularis tendon: Axial T1-weighted MRI arthrogram showing a complete tear of the suscapularis tendon (void arrow), appearing retracted medially at the level of the glenohumeral joint. The tendon of the short head of the biceps (arrowhead) is normal. Note the normal tendon of the long head of the biceps (arrow) located inside the biceps groove. This is consistent with a continuous coracohumeral ligament.

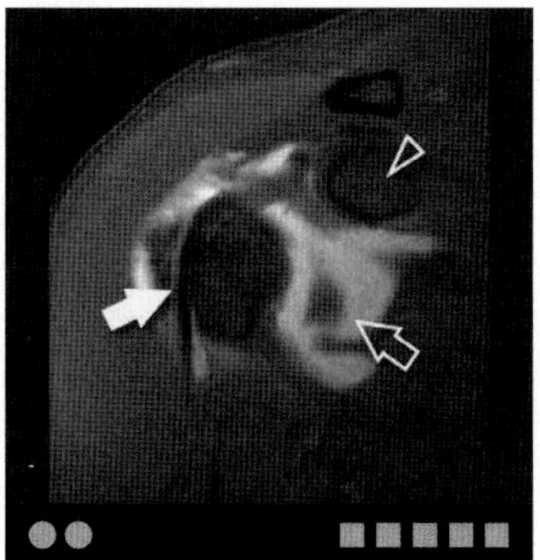

F. Acute tear of the subscapularis tendon: Coronal T1-weighted MRI arthrogram confirming complete tear of the suscapularis tendon (void arrow). The normal tendon of the long head of the biceps (arrow) is seen within the biceps sulcus. Arrowhead = coracoid process.

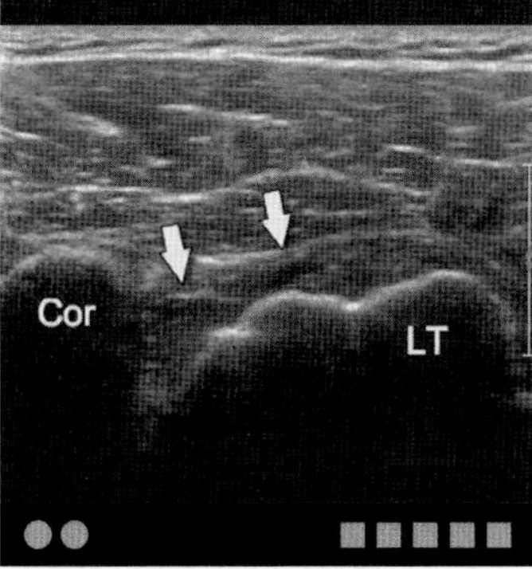

G. Acute tear of the subscapularis tendon: Axial sonogram obtained over the anterior aspect of the glenohumeral joint shows the tear of the subscapularis tendons (arrows). Cor, coracoid process; LT, lesser tuberosity.

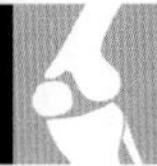

1–32 Distal Clavicular Osteolysis

Kambiz Motamedi

PRESENTATION

Shoulder pain

FINDINGS

CT shows loss of distal clavicular cortex at the acromioclavicular joint.

DIFFERENTIAL DIAGNOSES

- Distal clavicular resorption due to rheumatoid arthritis (RA) or hyperparathyroidism: The resorption is usually more aggressive. There is bone loss in addition to just cortical thinning or loss. The classical radiographic appearance in hyperparathyroidism and rheumatoid arthritis has been described as pencil tip shaped.
- Weight Lifters' clavicle: Chronic stress at distal clavicle results in bone resorption. Unlike RA or hyperparathyroidism; these patients lack osteoporosis.
- Acromioclavicular osteoarthritis: It usually affects the distal clavicle and the proximal acromion on both sides of the joint. Yet it may be more prominent on one side. MRI readily displays a combination of findings such as edema, subchondral cyst formation, synovial hypertrophy or joint effusion.
- Acromioclavicular septic arthritis: MRI reveals large joint effusion with edema of both distal clavicle and proximal acromion. There may be diffuse edema of the adjacent soft tissues as well.
- Prior clavicular resection: The MRI demonstrates artifact from suture material. Within the first few months following the Mumford procedure (distal clavicular resection) there may be bone marrow edema, which gradually disappears. There may be additional callus formation.

COMMENTS

This image is of a 27-year-old male who complains of a 3-week history of shoulder pain. He is an avid weightlifter. The pain, with an insidious onset, localizes to the acromioclavicular joint. Osteolysis of the distal clavicle is a pathologic process involving resorption of the subchondral bone of the distal clavicle. This entity is usually posttraumatic or caused by the repetitive microtrauma of weight lifting. Pain localized to the acromioclavicular joint and imaging showing pathology in the distal clavicle is diagnostic. The isolated edema of the distal clavicle is thought to be secondary to microfractures of the trabeculae due to increased stress. Thus the edema is usually patchy and ill-defined. This causes mild to moderate high signal on fluid sensitive sequences, while there may be no abnormal signal on T1-weighted (T1W) images. Alternatively one may see patchy areas of marrow replacement on T1W images. There may or may not be a tiny acromioclavicular joint effusion. Lack of synovial hypertrophy or other findings associated with osteoarthritis is paramount. On CT the loss of distal cortical definition along with adjacent osteopenia is a common finding. The radiographs may be normal in the initial stage. Bone scintigraphy is a very sensitive diagnostic mean to evaluate early stages.

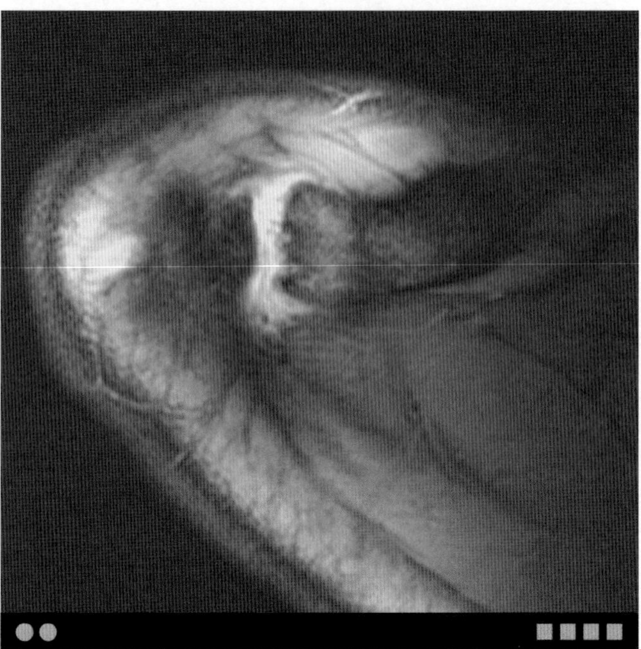

A. Distal clavicular osteolysis: Axial gradient echo image shows edema of the distal clavicle with cortical irregularity.

PEARLS

- **Affects only the clavicle side of the acromioclavicular articulation.**
- **Patchy ill-defined edema on T1W, and loss of distal cortex on CT imaging.**
- **Caveat of field inhomogeneity. The acromioclavicular joint may often be affected by field inhomogeneity because of the inherent peripheral location of the shoulder joint in the gantry. This artifact is usually bandlike and affects more than just the distal clavicle.**

ADDITIONAL IMAGES

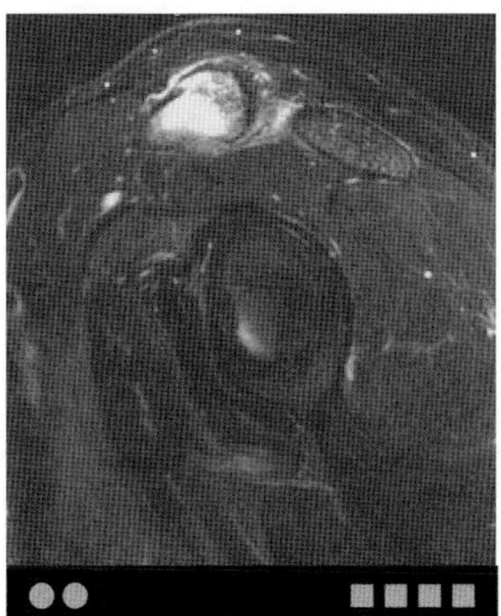

B. Distal clavicular osteolysis: Sagittal fat-saturated T2W FSE image demonstrates the marrow edema of the distal clavicle. Note the normal appearance of the acromion.

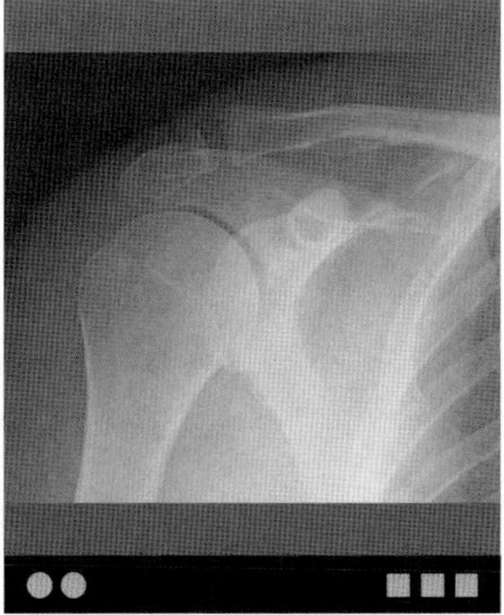

C. Distal clavicular osteolysis: The AP radiograph shows distal clavicular osteopenia and irregular cortex of the distal clavicle with a normal acromion.

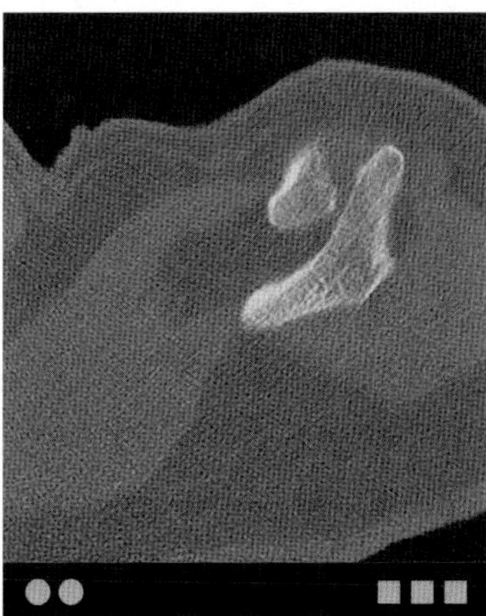

D. Distal clavicular osteolysis: The axial CT in another patient shows a similar finding with irregular cortex of the distal clavicle and a normal acromion.

DIFFERENTIAL DIAGNOSES IMAGES

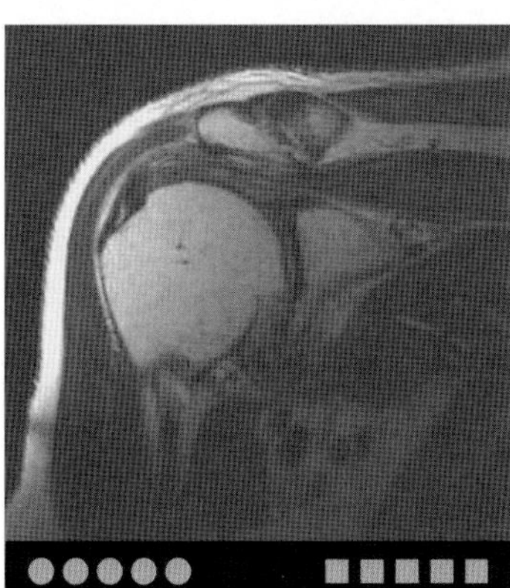

E. Acromioclavicular osteoarthritis: Coronal oblique PD image reveals the degenerative changes of the acromioclavicular joint affecting both distal clavicle and proximal acromion.

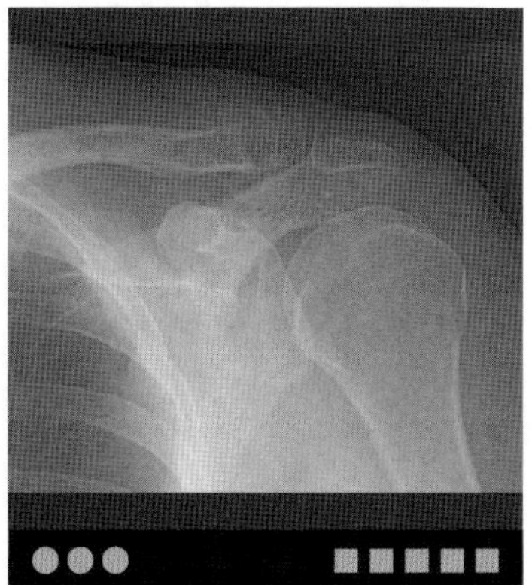

F. Distal clavicle fracture: AP radiograph demonstrates a healing fracture of the distal clavicle with callus formation.

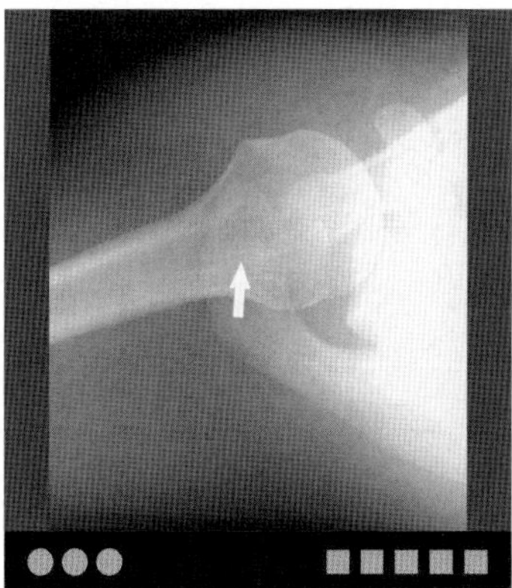

G. Os acromiale: Axially radiograph reveals an os acromiale (arrow).

IMAGE KEY

Common

Rare

Typical

Unusual

Chapter 2

Congenital, Systemic and Metabolic Diseases

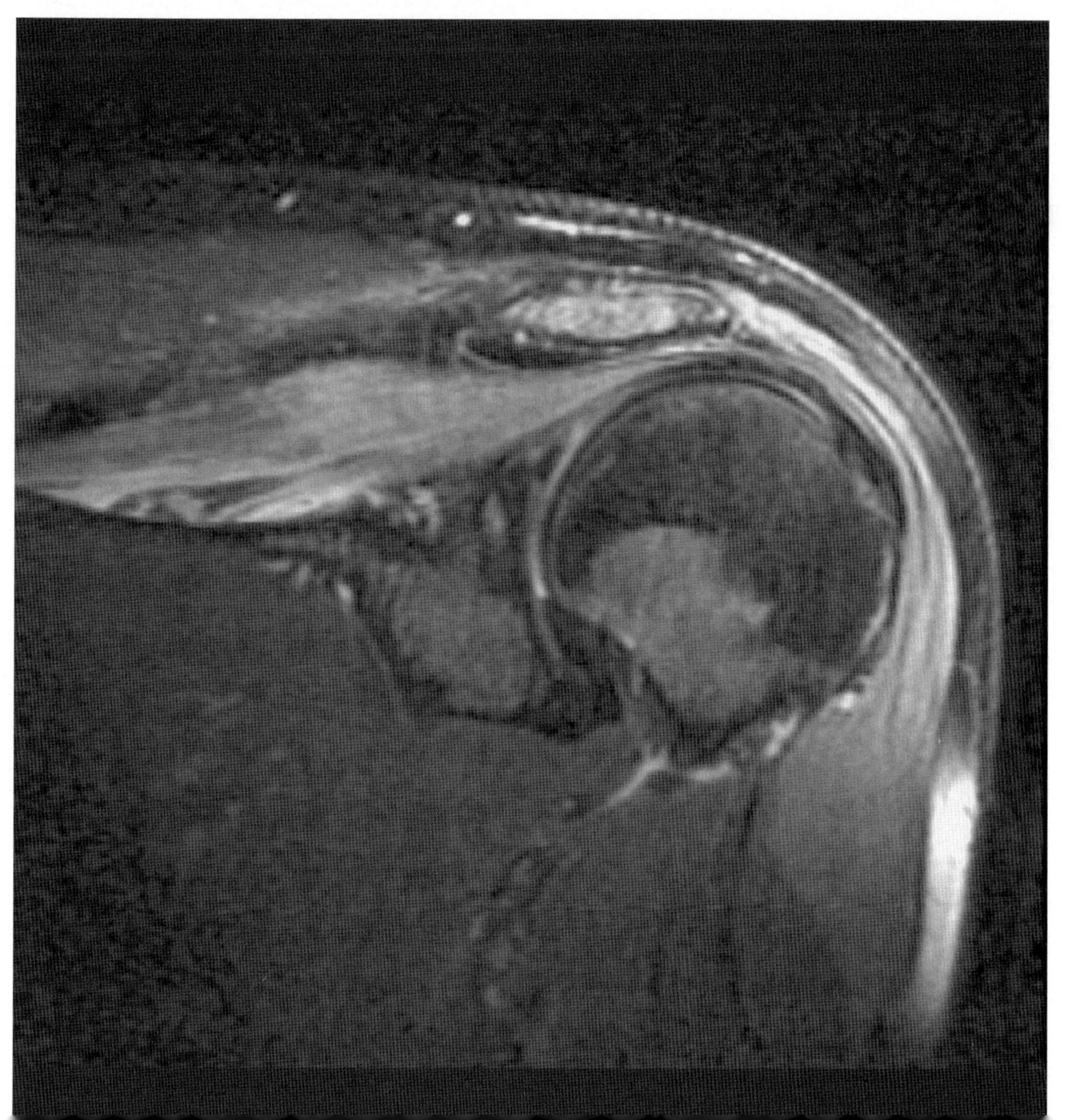

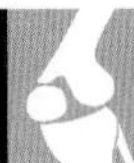

2–1 Parsonage-Turner Syndrome

Arash Tehranzadeh

PRESENTATION

Acute onset of shoulder pain

FINDINGS

MR images show edema in the supraspinatus, infraspinatus, and deltoid muscles.

DIFFERENTIAL DIAGNOSES

- *Rotator cuff tendinosis:* May be attributed to overuse or caused by deposit of hydroxyapatite and shows intermediate intensity signal on proton density image, which may remain the same or decrease in intensity with T2-weighted image.
- *Complete rotator cuff tear:* Symptoms may mimic those of Parsonage-Turner syndrome in the setting of acute onset of pain with a tear. The tendon is ruptured and retracted and fluid replaces the ruptured tendon site.
- *Adhesive capsulitis:* Clinically it may mimic Parsonage-Turner syndrome; however, MR imaging shows synovial inflammation. The joint capacity is markedly decreased and scar and adhesions fills the joint space.
- *Suprascapular nerve entrapment:* Paralabral cyst or ganglion cyst secondary to adjacent labral tear compress the suprascapular nerve leading to infraspinatus muscle atrophy.
- *Calcific tendinosis or bursitis:* Low-signal hydroxyapatite crystal deposits are found in the tendon or the bursa thus causing pain and edema.

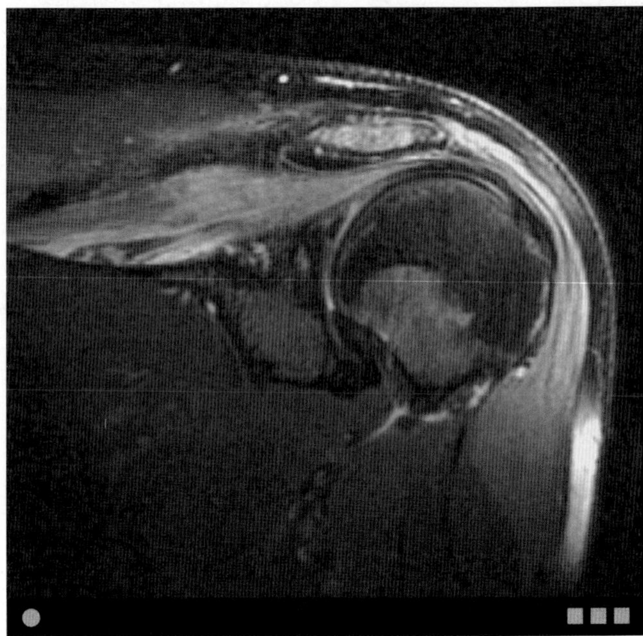

A. Parsonage-Turner syndrome: Coronal fat-suppressed T2-weighted fast spin echo image shows intramuscular edema in the supraspinatus and deltoid muscles.

COMMENTS

This is an image of a 43-year-old woman who presented with an acute onset of left shoulder pain. Parsonage-Turner syndrome is an acute brachial neuritis. Its cause is not known however; speculative associations have been made about its onset subsequent to viral illness and immunization. Trauma is not typically an inciting event. Although affected patients are typically male, the age range of patients involved is wide. The distribution of nerve involvement has included the suprascapular, axillary, long thoracic, and phrenic nerves. Bilateral and multinerve involvement is also a possibility. Affected patients often present with an acute onset of pain in the shoulder girdle, followed by weakness. The illness is self-limited and gradual recovery of muscle strength occurs in 2 to 3 months. This syndrome can be a diagnostic challenge and may be confused with rotator cuff pathology, adhesive capsulitis, cervical radiculopathy, peripheral nerve compression, spinal cord tumors, amyotrophic lateral sclerosis, and acute poliomyelitis. MR imaging features of Parsonage-Turner typically demonstrate intramuscular edema manifested by increased signal on T2 weighted and inversion recovery sequences. The muscles presenting with edema typically correlate with the pattern of denervation on EMG studies. Hence, MR imaging plays an important role as it demonstrates the pattern of edema and excludes other shoulder disorders such as impingement syndrome, rotator cuff tears, and ganglions, which may compress the suprascapular nerve.

PEARLS

- **Self-limited condition that presents with an acute onset of pain followed by weakness.**
- **The pattern of edema on MR T2-weighted images is manifested as high signal in the involved musculature, for example, in the suprascapular, and axillary nerve distributions.**
- **Presence of muscular edema in the absence of rotator cuff pathology or impingement, adhesive capsulitis, or ganglion formation.**

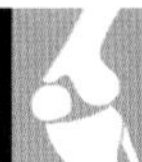

ADDITIONAL IMAGES

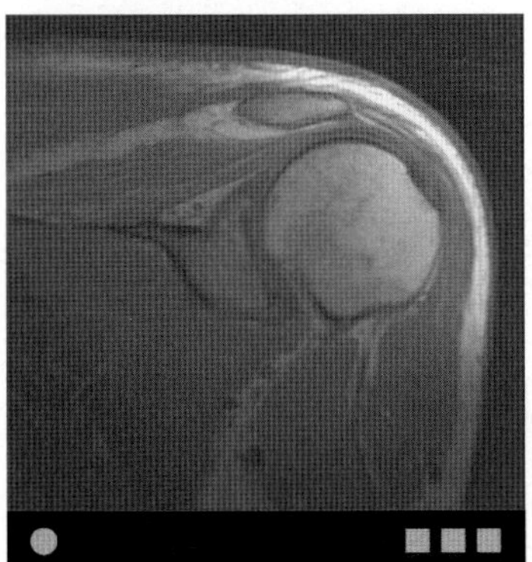

B. Parsonage-Turner syndrome: Coronal T1-weighted image shows no evidence of significant rotator cuff tear or evidence of impingement.

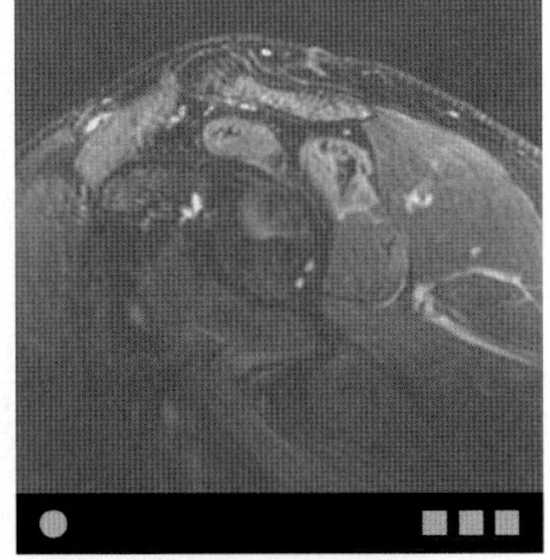

C. Parsonage-Turner syndrome: Sagittal fat-suppressed T2-weighted fast spin echo image shows intramuscular edema in the supraspinatus and infraspinatus musculature.

DIFFERENTIAL DIAGNOSES IMAGES

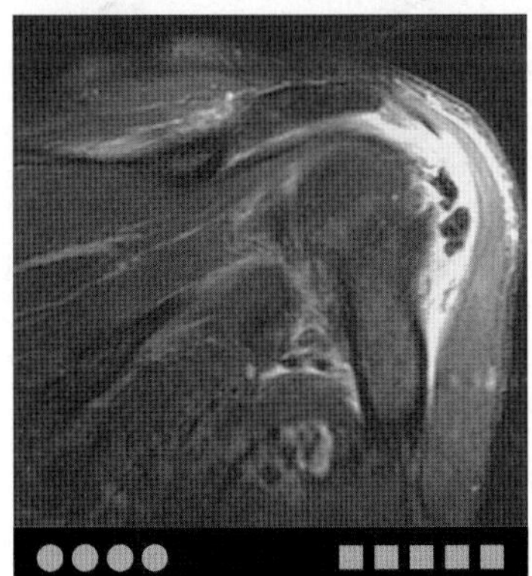

D. Hydroxyapatite deposition: Coronal fat-suppressed T2-weighted fast spin echo image demonstrates multiple dark foci of hydroxyapatite deposition in the supraspinatus tendon with tendinosis and bursal surface fraying.

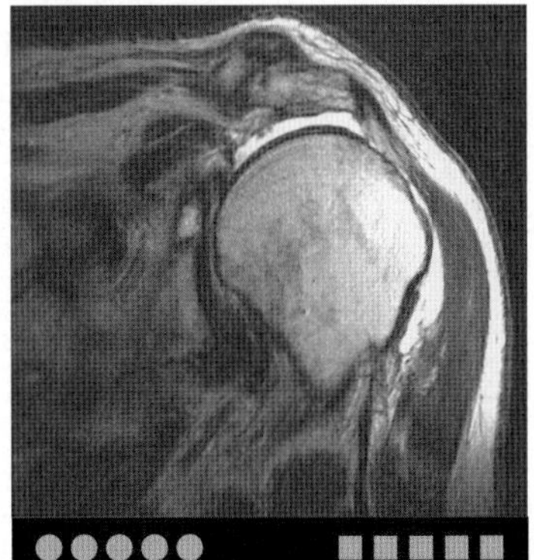

E. Complete rotator cuff tear: Coronal T2-weighted image shows a complete tear of the supraspinatus with retraction. Note fluid-filled decreased acromion-humeral space.

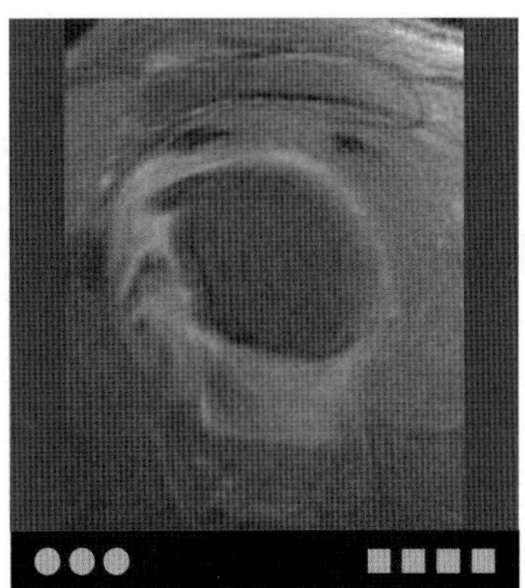

F. Adhesive capsulitis: Sagittal fat-suppressed T1-weighted image status post-IV contrast demonstrates synovial enhancement consistent with adhesive capsulitis.

IMAGE KEY

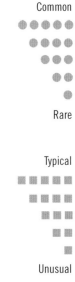

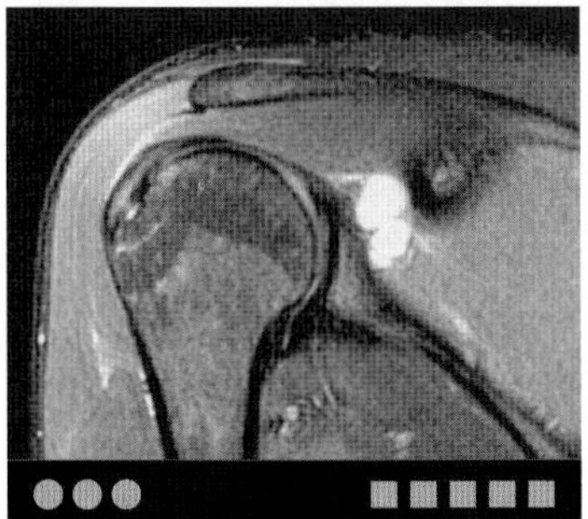

G. Suprascapular nerve entrapment: Coronal T2-weighted image with fat suppression demonstrates a ganglion cyst in the suprascapular notch.

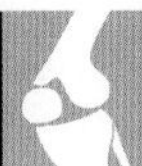

2–2 Avascular Necrosis of Shoulder Due To Sickle Cell Disease

Peyman Borghei and Melitus Maryam Golshan

PRESENTATION

Shoulder pain

FINDINGS

MRI shows serpentine regions of high signal intensity surrounded by low signal intensity, consistent with bone infarct.

DIFFERENTIAL DIAGNOSES

- *Osteomyelitis:* Imaging differentiation of osteomyelitis from infarction is not reliable; indeed, osteomyelitis may not be suspected until the signs and symptoms of a typical painful crisis have failed to resolve after 1 to 2 weeks of standard therapy.
- Enchondroma or low-grade chondrosarcoma often presents with punctuate calcifications.
- Nonossifying fibroma shows osteolytic lesion with single marginal sclerotic cortex.
- *Other causes of avascular necrosis (AVN):* Past history and laboratory evaluation can help to reach the definite diagnosis. Also the lesions seen in sickle cell disease (SCD) may be larger than those with other etiologies.

COMMENTS

This is an image of a 28-year-old man who presented with history of SCD with AVN of both shoulders. AVN represents a compromised circulation of blood to an area of bone. Risk factors include use of oral corticosteroid, alcohol abuse, systemic lupus erythematosus, SCD, Gaucher disease, trauma, cancer, dysbaric conditions (Caisson disease), and some idiopathic cases. SCD is the most common cause of AVN worldwide. Increased blood viscosity secondary to the sludging of the sickled red blood cells is the leading cause for ischemia and infarction in SCD. The most common skeletal sites involved are the head of femur and humerus. Symptomatic patients complain of painful, limited motion of the affected joint, occasionally with pain at rest. Findings from radiography can identify only the later stages of the disease, which show increased density of the epiphysis, subchondral lucent areas consistent with fracture (crescent sign), and flattening/collapse of the articular surfaces. MR imaging is the most sensitive diagnostic method that can be used in early stages. AVN shows a classic "double-line sign" representing a high-signal-intensity line within two parallel rims of decreased signal intensity on a T2-weighted MR image.

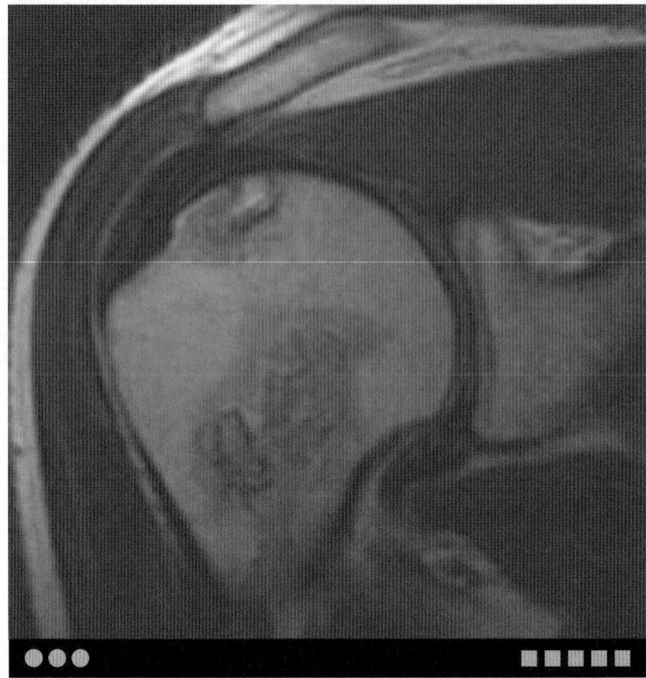

A. AVN: Coronal T2-weighted image shows focal double line sign at subchondral bone of humeral head. A second focus of infarct is noted in humeral metaphysis.

PEARLS

- **SCD is the most common cause of AVN worldwide, while in the United States, alcohol abuse is the leading cause.**
- **In every patient with SCD, development of an acute pain should always be suspected for an ischemia and/or infection.**
- **Radiograph is normal on early stages of AVN and shows sclerosis (snow cap) appearance on second stage.**
- **MRI is the most sensitive modality for the diagnosis of AVN, and classic feature is "double-line sign" on T2-weighted image.**

ADDITIONAL IMAGES

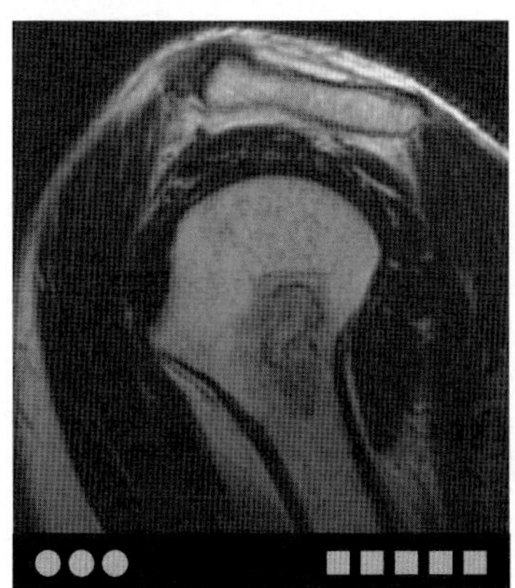

B. AVN: Sagittal T1-weighted image shows nonhomogenous low signal intensity of the metaphysis of right humerus.

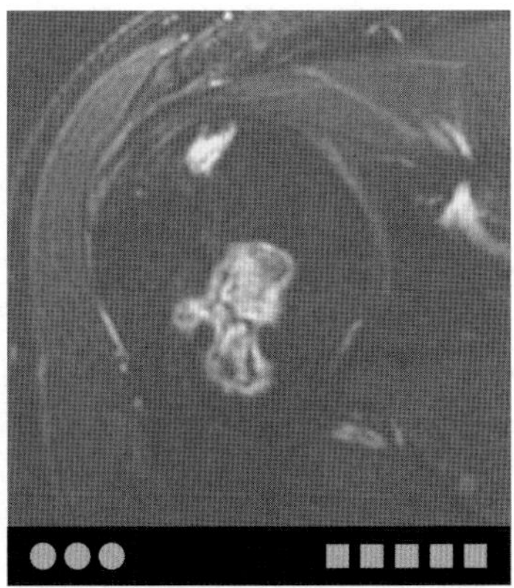

C. AVN: Coronal T2-weighted fat-saturated image shows high-signal-intensity lesions with focal foci of low signal intensity inside, consistent with bone infarct.

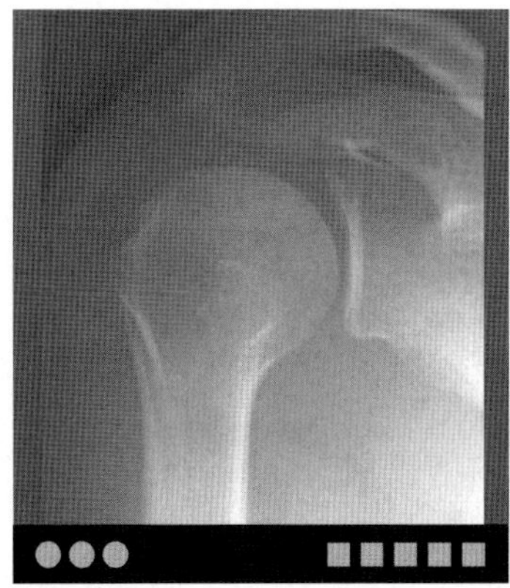

D. AVN: Right shoulder radiograph is normal.

DIFFERENTIAL DIAGNOSES IMAGES

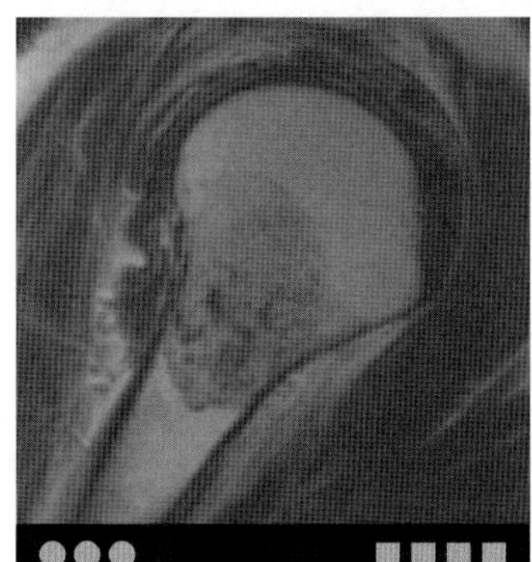

E. Low-grade chondrosarcoma: Sagittal T2-weighted image shows low-grade chondrosarcoma of left shoulder with low signal foci of punctuate calcification.

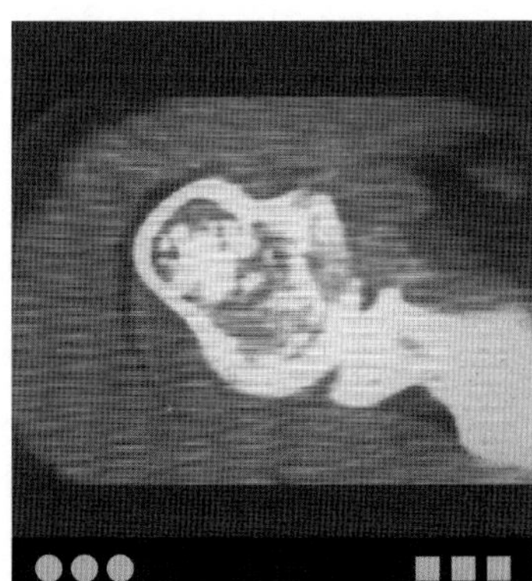

F. Enchondroma: Axial CT scan of the humerus shows chondral calcification in the proximal metaphysis of the humerus.

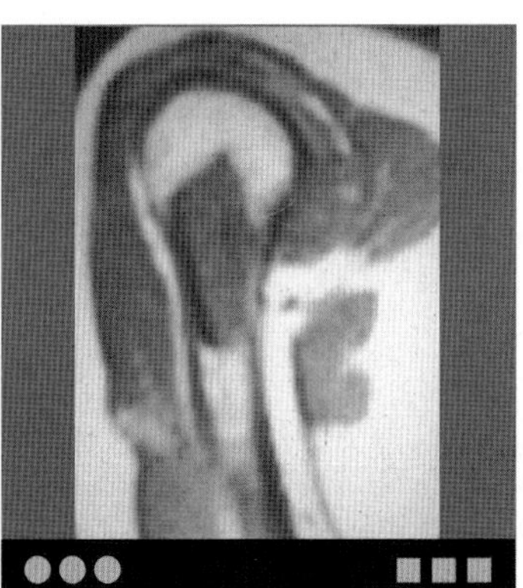

G. Enchondroma: Coronal T1-weighted image showing an area of low signal intensity in the proximal humerus with central calcification.

IMAGE KEY

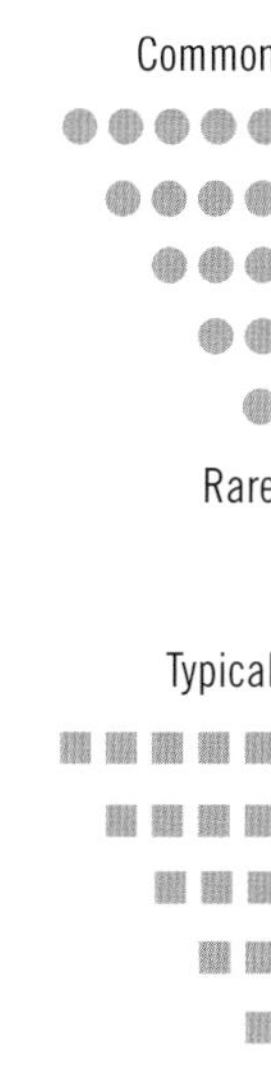

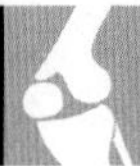

2–3 Osteopoikilosis

Mélanie Morel, Nathalie Boutry, and Anne Cotten

PRESENTATION

Mild shoulder pain

FINDINGS

Shoulder radiograph reveals multiple well-defined sclerotic lesions. Other similar radiodense foci are found in periarticular regions.

DIFFERENTIAL DIAGNOSES

- *Enostosis (bone island):* This isolated ovoid osteosclerotic focus has well-defined, spiculated margins. Its long axis is oriented parallel to the major bony trabeculae.
- *Osteoblastic metastases:* Osteosclerotic foci are less dense, ill-defined, and circular or ovoid. No symmetric distribution is seen. Bone scan reveals an abnormal uptake.
- *Osteoma:* This benign tumor made of compacted cortical bone arises from periosteum at the surface of the bone. Its homogeneous radiodensity is distinctive.
- *Tuberous sclerosis:* Skeletal manifestations of this phakomatosis include oval sclerotic foci involving the spine, pelvis, and ribs. Bone scan shows an increased uptake. Growth disturbance and pseudo-cystlike lesions of the phalanges and metacarpal bones are also found.
- *Osteopathia striata:* It is a rare sclerosing dysplasia of bilateral distribution. Regular, linear, and vertical oriented bands of increased radiodensity extend from the metaphases into the diaphysis.

COMMENTS

This is an image of a 32-year-old man who complained of intermittent pain in his right shoulder. Shoulder radiograph followed by skeletal survey leads to the diagnosis of osteopoikilosis. Osteopoikilosis is a benign sclerosing bone dysplasia, transmitted as an autosomal dominant fashion. It may be associated with dermatofibrosis lenticularis disseminate (Buschke-Ollendorff syndrome), organ abnormalities (coarctation of the aorta, double urether), endocrine dysfunction, spinal stenosis, and multiple disc protrusions of the spine. Patients are typically asymptomatic, although 15% to 20% may have mild articular pain and joint effusion. It is most often an incidental radiographic finding. Each lesion, similar to an enostosis, consists of compacted trabeculae of mature lamellar bone. Numerous circular or ovoid osteosclerotic foci measuring between 2 and 10 mm are found in the metaphyses and epiphyses of long bones, carpus, tarsus, pelvis, and scapulae. Involvement of small tubular bones of hands and feet has also been reported. The distribution is typically symmetric and periarticular. These lesions cannot be found before the age of three. Bone scintigraphy typically does not reveal any uptake. Laboratory studies are normal. The resulting combination of osteopoikilosis, melorheostosis, and osteopathia striata is called "mixed sclerosing bone dystrophy." Melorheostosis is sclerosing dysplasia with peripheral cortical hyperostosis resembling "flowing candle wax" and is found on the surface of long bones. Its distribution is typically hemimelic.

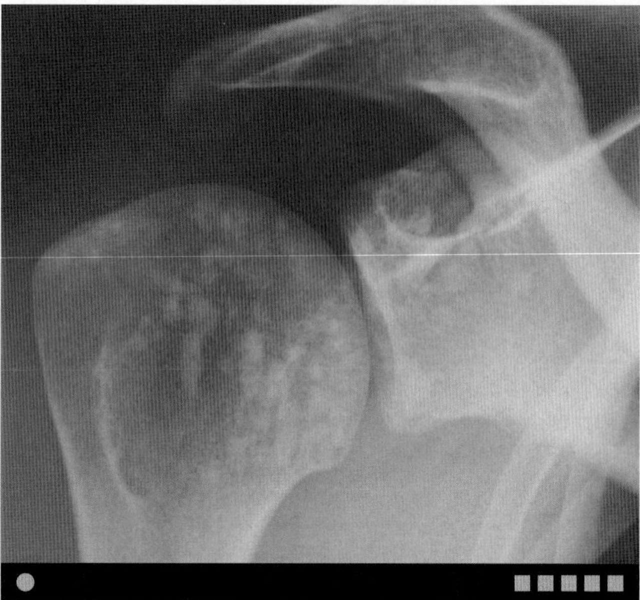

A. Osteopoikilosis: AP radiograph of the shoulder reveals multiple ovoid and round sclerotic lesions in the humeral head and the glenoid of the scapula.

PEARLS

- **Osteopoikilosis is a rare benign sclerosing dysplasia.**
- **It is genetically transmitted, but is often an incidental radiographic finding.**
- **Almost 15% to 20% of the patients have mild articular pain and joint effusion.**
- **It can be associated with other abnormalities.**
- **Multiple small round or ovoid radiodense foci are located symmetrically in periarticular osseous regions.**
- **Bone scintigraphy and laboratory studies are usually normal.**

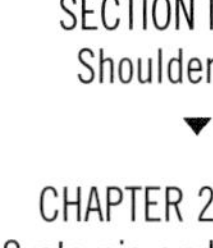

ADDITIONAL IMAGES

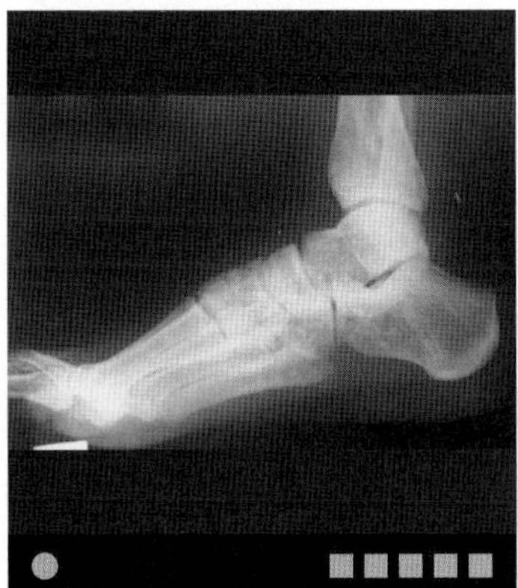

B. Osteopoikilosis: Lateral view of the foot shows several discrete radiodense foci in the tibial metaphysis, tarsal, and metatarsal bones.

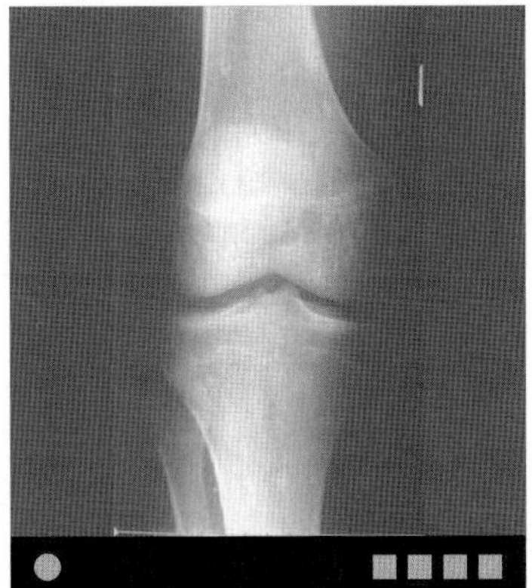

C. Osteopoikilosis: AP radiograph of the knee also exhibits multiple ovoid or circular sclerotic periarticular foci.

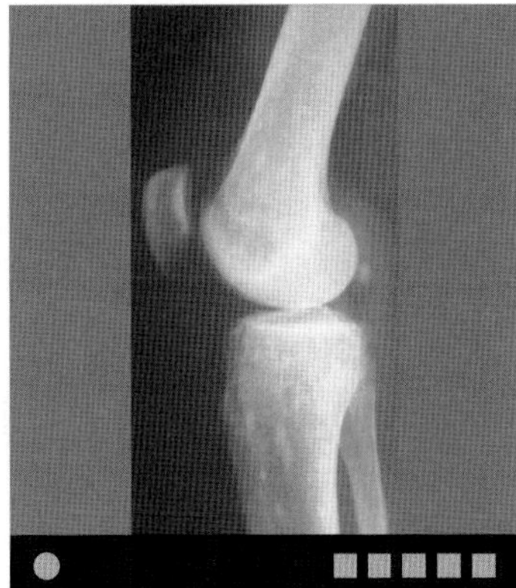

D. Osteopoikilosis: Lateral radiograph of the knee shows the epiphysometaphyseal distribution of the lesions in the distal femur and proximal tibia.

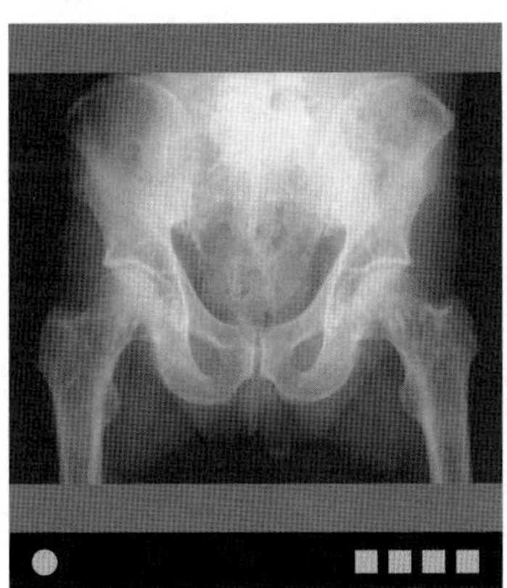

E. Osteopoikilosis: AP view of the pelvis reveals multiple symmetric radiodense lesions in the proximal femurs and pelvis.

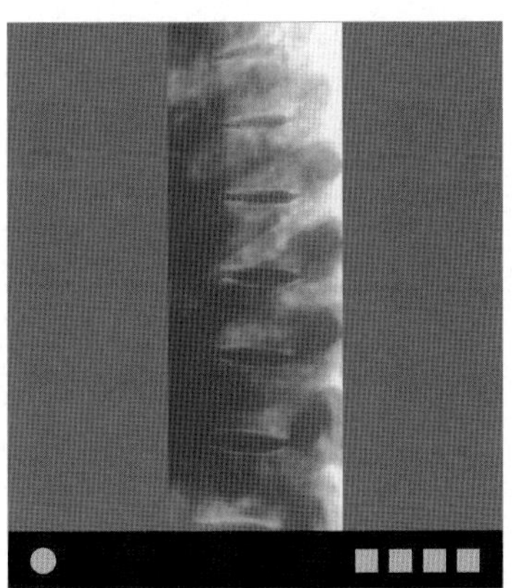

F. Osteopoikilosis: Small sclerotic lesions in vertebrae bodies can also be found on this thoracic spine radiograph.

DIFFERENTIAL DIAGNOSES IMAGES

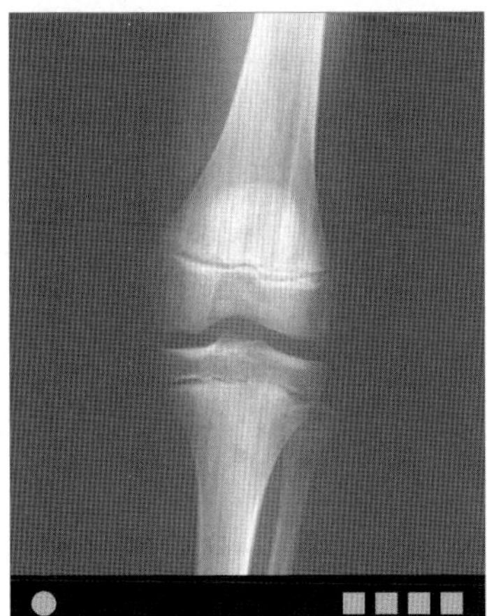

G. Osteopathia striata: AP radiograph of the knee exhibits linear bands of increased radiodensity in the distal femur and proximal tibia.

IMAGE KEY

Common

Rare

Typical

Unusual

Chapter 3

Arthritis, Connective Tissue and Crystal Deposition Disorders

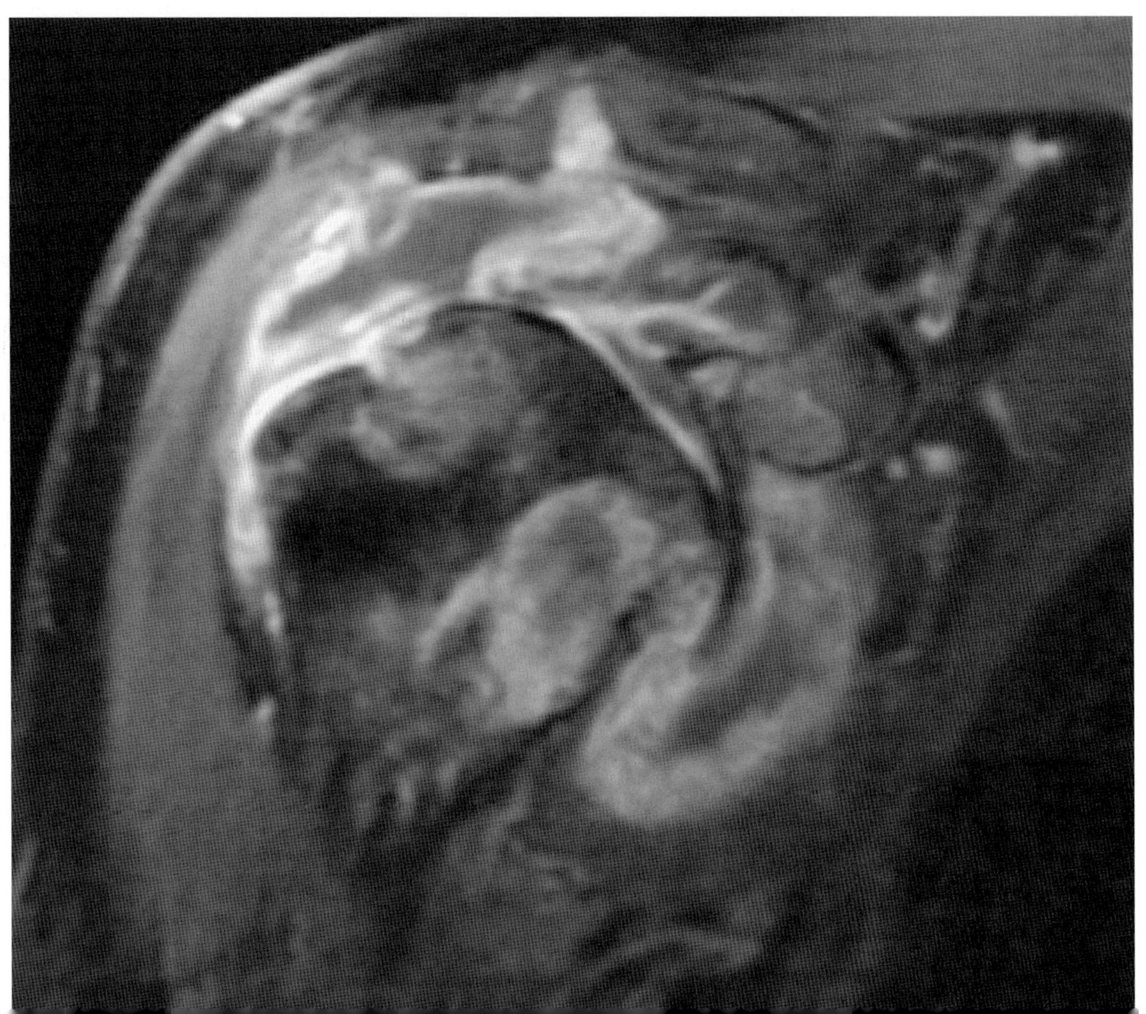

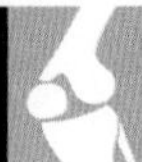

3–1 Rheumatoid Arthritis of the Shoulder

Edward Mossop and Jamshid Tehranzadeh

PRESENTATION

Worsening shoulder pain and reduced range of motion

FINDINGS

MRI shows joint narrowing erosions and synovial proliferation of the glenohumeral joint. Note joint effusion, muscle atrophy, and full-thickness tear of the supraspinatus and subscapularis tendons.

DIFFERENTIAL DIAGNOSES

- *Septic arthritis and osteomyelitis: Staphylococcus aureus* is the leading cause. The course of the disease is much more acute and rapidly progressive.
- *Psoriatic arthritis:* Erosions are more central in the joint and can be associated with enthesopathy and new bone formation. Patients often have the cutaneous or nail changes of psoriasis.
- *Reactive arthritis:* It occurs more commonly in young men with urethritis and uveitis and is associated with enthesopathy and erosions that have indistinct margins and are surrounded by periosteal new bone formation.
- Other inflammatory arthritides may simulate rheumatoid arthritis (RA) changes.

COMMENTS

This is an image of a 63-year-old female patient who presented with recent worsening of proven (RA). RA is a chronic systemic inflammatory disease of undetermined etiology involving primarily the synovial membranes and secondarily articular structures of multiple joints. The disease is often progressive and results in pain, stiffness, and swelling of joints. Prevalence is approximately 1% in the United States and affects women (between the ages of 25 to 50 years) three times more than men. The chronic inflammation leads to vascular proliferation of synovium into folds known as "pannus." This invades the joint causing destruction of cartilage and bone. Multiple joints are affected and 40 to 50% of patients have shoulder involvement. MRI shows hypertrophied synovium as a soft tissue mass adjacent to the joint. This is seen as low signal on T1-weighted images, which enhances after contrast, and mixed signal on T2-weighted images. Small fibrinated areas of pannus known as rice bodies may be visualized. Marginal erosions of the bone and cartilage appear as areas of low signal on T1-weighted images and as regions of heterogeneous signal on T2-weighted images. Cystic bone erosions are viewed as low signal on T1-weigted images and high signal on T2-weighted images and may enhance after contrast. Rotator cuff rupture is seen in approximately 20%. Other findings include effusions and loss of joint space.

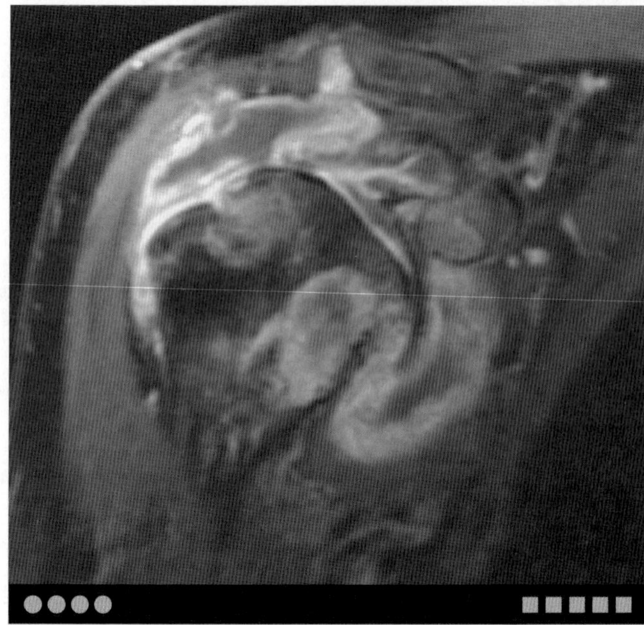

A. RA: Coronal T1 fat-saturated postcontrast image shows supraspinatus tear and low signal fluid in the glenohumeral and acromioclavicular joints and subdeltoid subacromial bursae. Note large erosive changes of the shoulder and synovial enhancement by contrast.

PEARLS

- **RA is a chronic systemic inflammatory disease of undetermined etiology involving primarily the synovial membranes and secondarily articular structures of multiple joints.**
- **Prevalence is approximately 1% in the United States and affects women three times more than men.**
- **MRI shows proliferation of inflamed synovium as low signal on T1-weighted images, which enhances after contrast, and mixed signal on T2-weighted images.**
- **Marginal erosions of the bone and cartilage appear as areas of low signal on T1-weighted images, which enhance with contrast, and as regions of highsignal on T2-weighted images.**
- **Other changes include cystlike changes, joint effusions, and rotator cuff atrophy and tears.**

ADDITIONAL IMAGES

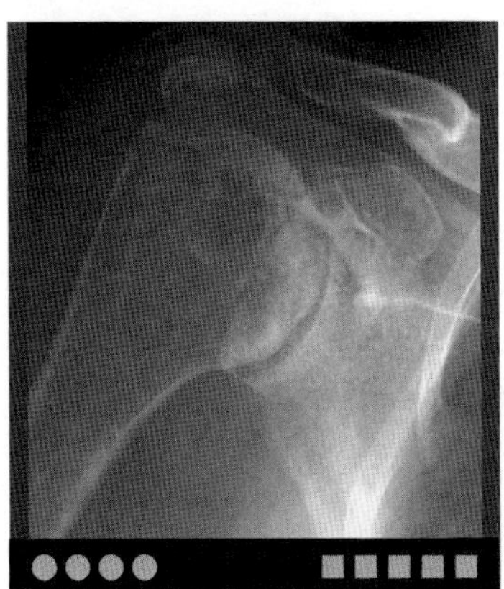

B. RA: AP radiograph of the shoulder shows severe joint narrowing with large erosion of the humeral head and small erosion of the subchondral glenoid.

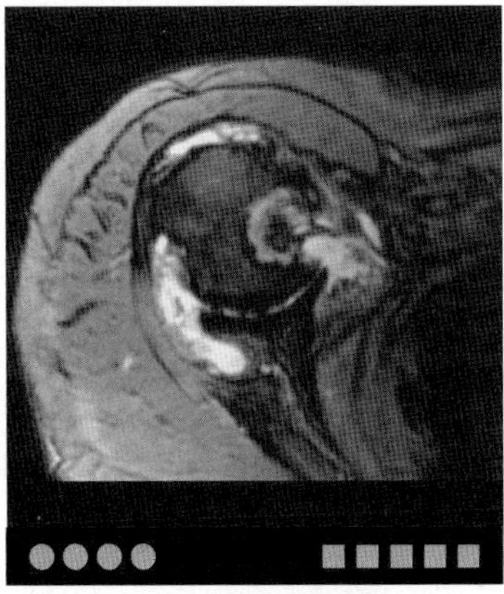

C. RA: Axial T2 fat-saturated image shows rotator cuff tear and joint fluid with large erosive changes.

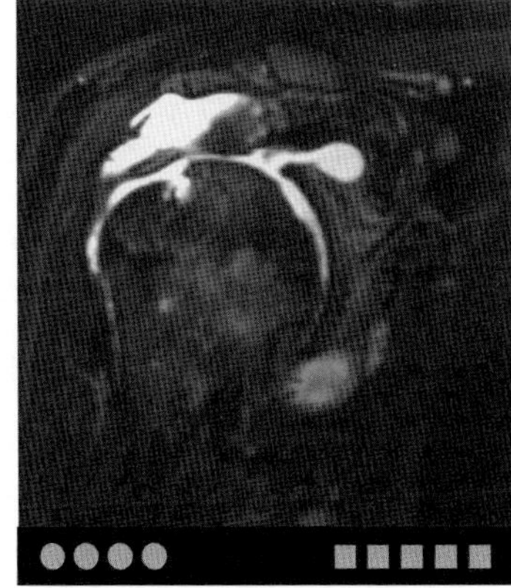

D. RA: Coronal T2 fat-saturated image shows rotator cuff tear and joint fluid with large erosive changes.

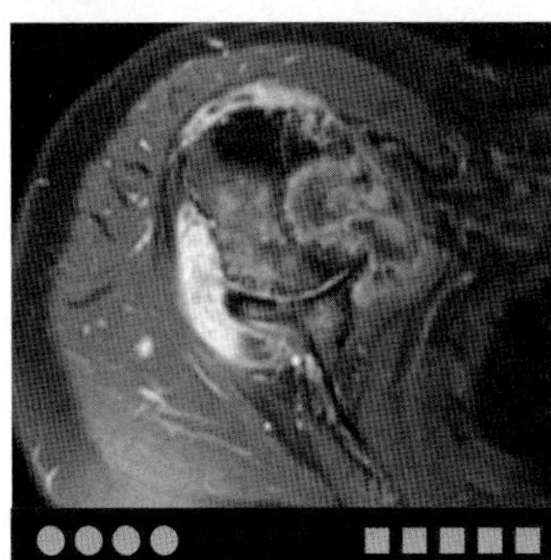

E. RA: Axial T1 fat-saturated postcontrast image shows RA with joint fluid and a large erosion of the humeral head. Note fluid in the subdeltoid bursa and rice bodies inside the joint.

IMAGE KEY

Common

Rare

Typical

Unusual

DIFFERENTIAL DIAGNOSES IMAGES

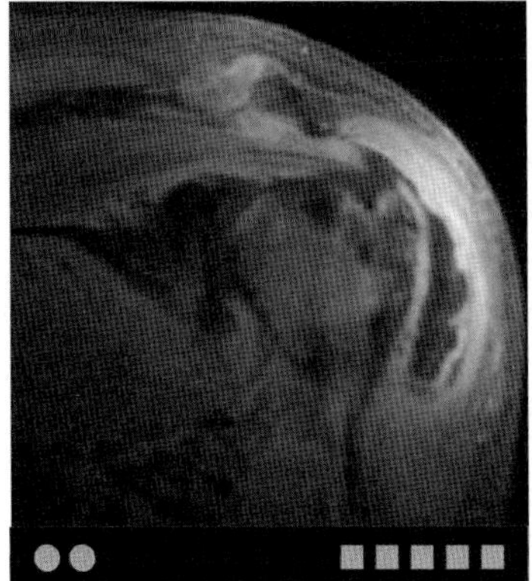

F. Septic Arthritis: Coronal T1 fat-saturated postcontrast image shows fluid within subacromial, subdeltoid bursa with marginal synovial enhancement consistent with septic arthritis and osteomyelitis.

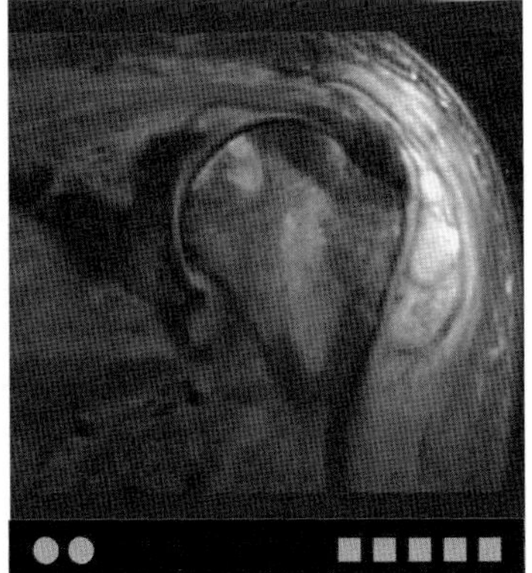

G. Septic Arthritis: Coronal T2 fat-saturated image shows septic arthritis and osteomyelitis with fluid within the subdeltoid bursa, inhomogeneous marrow signal, and erosions of the humeral head.

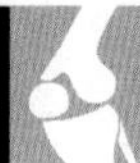

3–2 Neuropathic Osteoarthropathy with Syringomyelia

James Coumas

PRESENTATION

Painless, slow-growing chest wall mass

FINDINGS

Radiograph shows resorption of the humeral head, pseudosurgical amputation of proximal humeral shaft, erosions of the glenoid with intra-articular debris, and capsular mineralization.

DIFFERENTIAL DIAGNOSES

- *Diabetic osteoarthropathy:* Today's leading cause of neuropathic osteoarthropathy is a sequela to long-term diabetes mellitus and shows a strong predilection for the lower extremities. Isolated upper extremity involvement would be unusual.
- *Tabes dorsalis:* This disease has a male predominance with 20% of cases involving the axial skeleton. Radiographic findings include sclerosis, fragmentation, and fracture involving a joint, which make it difficult to differentiate from other causes of neuropathic osteoarthropathy.
- *Osteonecrosis:* This includes sclerosis of bone and subchondral collapse of the articular surface. However, extensive bony resorption and glenoid involvement would be difficult to explain.
- *Pott's disease:* Extensive humeral bony resorption, absence of discrete erosions at the articulation, or bony involvement of the spine would be atypical.

COMMENTS

This is an image of a 59-year-old female who presents with an enlarging anterior and lateral chest wall mass. Although controversial, three types of syringomyelia are described. Two of the three types are associated with a syrinx of the central canal of the spinal cord. The syrinx formed is in communication with the central canal and contains CSF-like fluid. The etiology of these two subtypes is based upon abnormalities of the CSF circulation. The term syringohydromyelia is commonly used to describe these two types. The third type does not arise from the central canal of the cord, but is localized to the spinal cord parenchyma. It is not lined by ependymal cells as in the prior two subtypes. The etiology is controversial but attributed to trauma, infection, or infarct. Approximately 20% to 25% of patients with syringomyelia develop neuropathic osteoarthropathy typically in the later stages of the disease. The upper extremity is involved in 75% to 80% of cases. Neuropathic osteoarthropathy is associated with diabetes, tabes dorsalis, and syringomyelia in 90% of cases. Clinical presentation includes painless swelling or pseudomass secondary to progressive joint effusion. Spontaneous dislocation is not an uncommon initial presentation. Radiographic hallmarks include sclerosis, fragmentation, and debris about an articulation. Isolated upper extremity involvement with a knifelike demarcation of bony resorption (pseudosurgical amputation) should suggest the diagnosis.

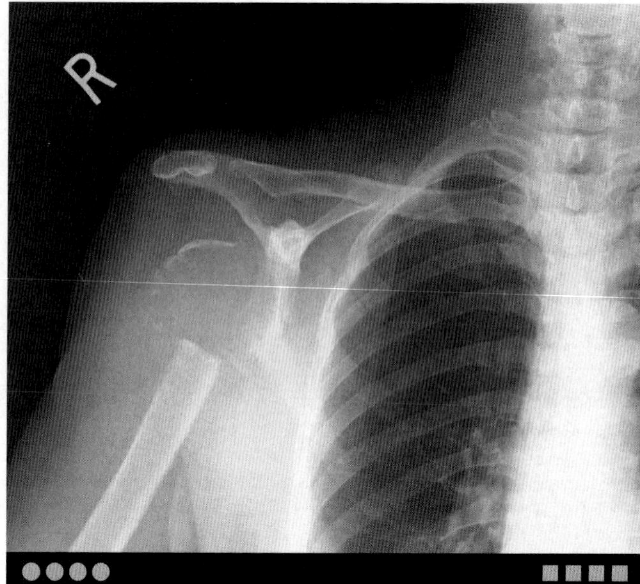

A. Neuropathic osteoarthropathy: AP radiograph of shoulder shows a sharp knifelike resorption (pseudosurgical amputation) of proximal humerus.

PEARLS

- **Radiographic hallmarks include sclerosis, fragmentation, and debris about an articulation. Isolated upper extremity involvement with a knifelike demarcation of bony resorption (pseudosurgical amputation) should suggest the diagnosis.**
- **MR or CT assessment of the cervical and thoracic spine is recommended.**
- **Contrast is necessary to exclude an underlying spinal cord neoplasm.**

ADDITIONAL IMAGES

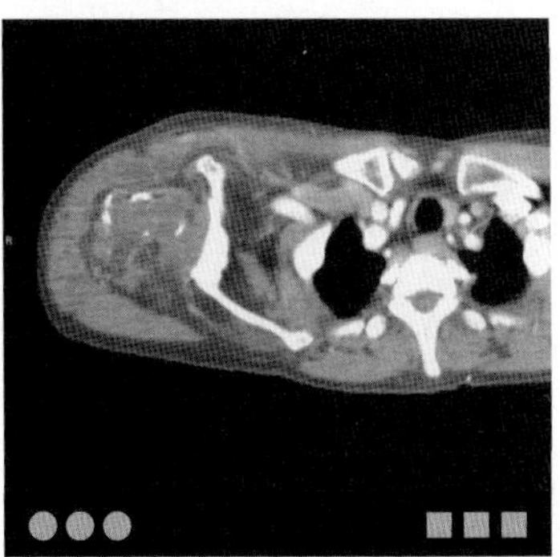

B. Neuropathic osteoarthropathy: Axial CT scan shows an absent humeral head and broad-based erosion of the glenoid.

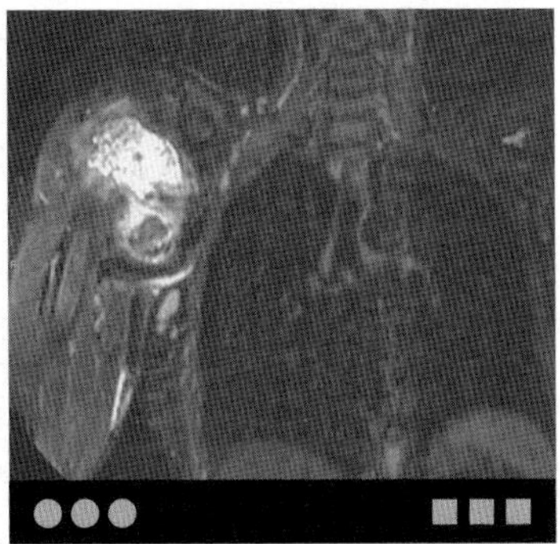

C. Neuropathic osteoarthropathy: Coronal T2-weighted image shows a large joint effusion with debris.

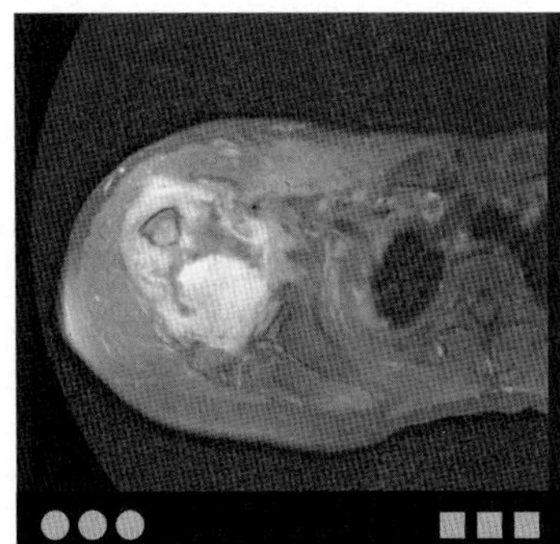

D. Neuropathic osteoarthropathy: Axial T2-weighted MR image with fat saturation shows a large joint effusion and sharp demarcation at the proximal humeral resorption site. Note enlarged, asymmetric right chest wall.

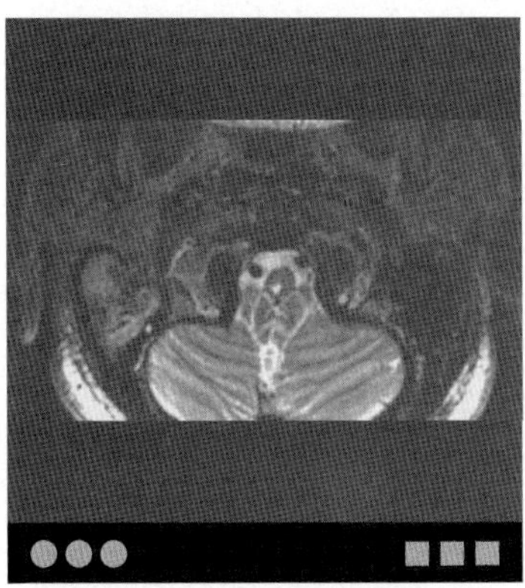

E. Neuropathic osteoarthropathy associated with syringomyelia: Axial T2-weighted image shows a parenchymal lesion in the upper cervical spinal cord. This is the same patient as in image A.

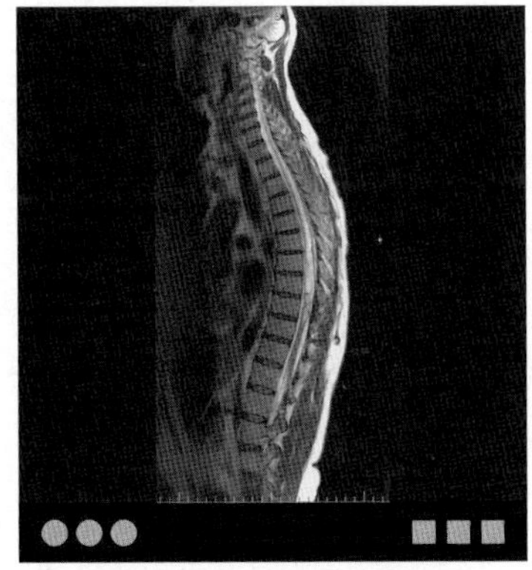

F. Neuropathic arthropathy associated with Syringomyelia: Sagittal T2-weighted image shows associated syrinx in the lower thoracic spine. This is the same patient as in image A.

DIFFERENTIAL DIAGNOSES IMAGES

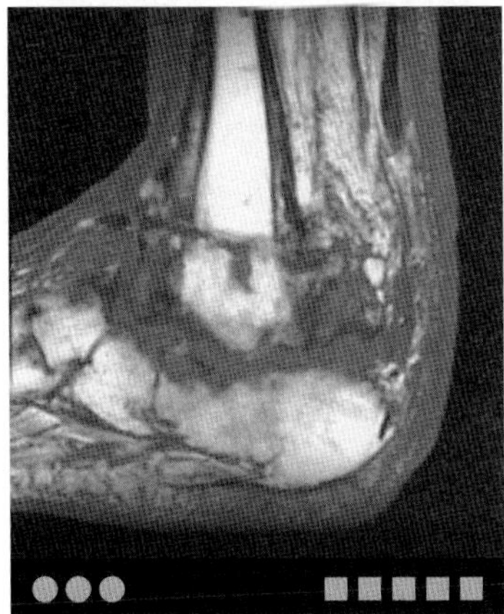

G. Diabetic neuropathic osteoarthropathy: Sagittal T1-weighted image shows destruction and fragmentation of the ankle joint.

IMAGE KEY

Common

Rare

Typical

Unusual

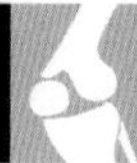

3–3 Granuloma in Calcium Pyrophosphate Dihydrate Deposition Disease

Oganes Ashikyan and Jamshid Tehranzadeh

PRESENTATION

Shoulder pain for 2 years

FINDINGS

Lytic lesion with sclerotic rim and cortical destruction is seen in the proximal humerus. The lesion is heterogeneous, but predominantly hyperintense on T2-weighted images and hypointense on T1-weighted images. Cartilage calcification, severe joint narrowing, and degenerative changes are noted.

DIFFERENTIAL DIAGNOSES

- *Rheumatoid geode:* This lesion can be differentiated from granuloma associated with CPPD crystal deposition disease by other related findings in rheumatoid arthritis, such as characteristic erosions, synovial proliferation, and lack of osteophytes.
- *Intraosseous tophi of gouty arthritis:* Gouty arthritis is associated with marginal erosion with overhanging edges.
- *Giant cell tumor:* These lytic tumors present most commonly at 20 to 40 years of age and often demonstrate lack of sclerotic rim. Most are seen in subarticular locations.
- *Metastatic disease:* Prostate metastases usually present as multiple osteoblastic lesions. Screening the skeleton with bone scan is helpful.

COMMENTS

This is an image of a 77-year-old male who presented with a 2-year history of pain in the right shoulder. Patient also had a history of prostate cancer. Subchondral cysts at this age can present in a variety of diseases, such as osteoarthritis, rheumatoid arthritis, osteonecrosis, and calcium pyrophosphate dihydrate (CPPD) crystal deposition disease. Pathologists may use a variety of terms describing these lesions, which include granulomas, geodes, cysts, and pseudocysts. While the exact etiology of the formation of such cysts is still under debate, some of the proposed theories include pressure-induced intrusion of the synovial fluid, bone necrosis from mechanical stress, or a combination of both. CPPD crystal deposition disease is a general term used to describe the presence of CPPD crystals in the joint or in the surrounding structures. This is a predominant finding in pseudogout, hyperparathyroidism, and hemochromatosis. Articular and periarticular calcifications are commonly found in CPPD crystal deposition disease; however, in some cases the crystals may be microscopic and not detectable by imaging modalities. Arthropathy is usually encountered in weight-bearing joints. However, wrist, elbow, and glenohumeral joints may also be involved. In a setting of CPPD crystal deposition disease, the subchondral cysts usually demonstrate lesion of giant size. Intraosseous lesions in pseudogout may rarely occur similar to intraosseous tophi in the cases of gouty arthritis. The margins may be sclerotic and indistinct. These features distinguish CPPD crystal deposition disease associated cysts from giant cell tumors, where margins are usually not sclerotic.

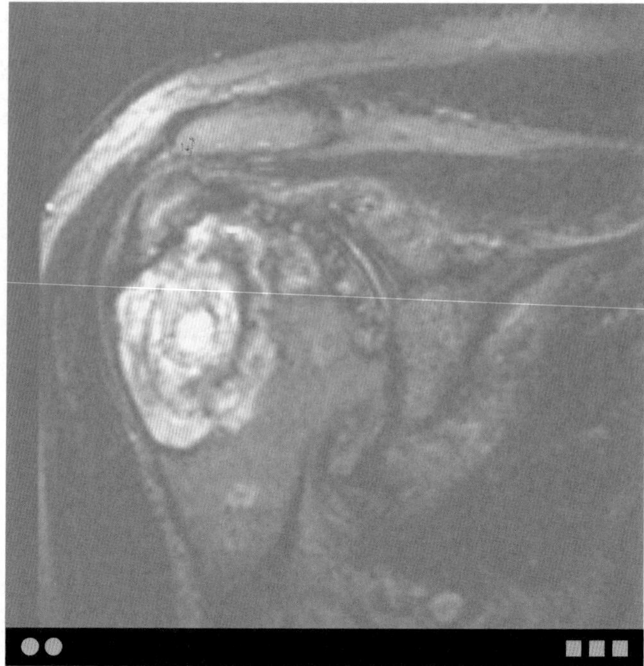

A. Humerus granuloma in a patient with calcium pyrophosphate deposition disease: Coronal T2-weighted image presents with fat saturation demonstrating heterogeneous lesion in the proximal humerus. Note that there is no soft-tissue involvement.

PEARLS

- **Although chondrocalcinosis is seen in many conditions, it is most commonly caused by CPPD crystal deposition disease.**
- **CPPD is a predominant finding in pseudogout, hyperparathyroidism, and hemochromatosis.**
- **Cysts associated with CPPD crystal deposition disease usually have indistinct, sclerotic margins.**
- **CPPD crystals may not be detected on any imaging modalities in cases of microscopic deposition.**

ADDITIONAL IMAGES

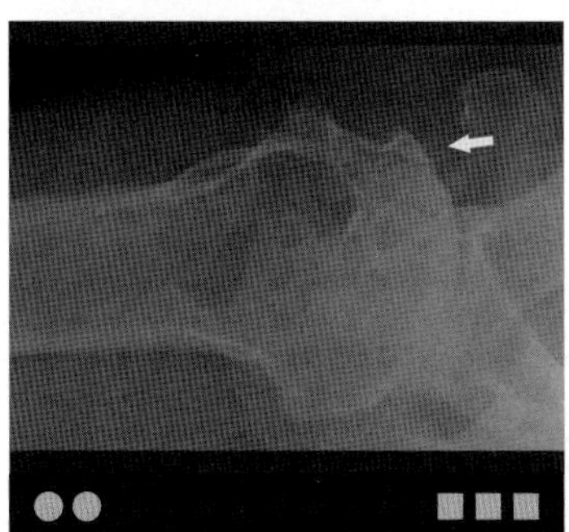

B. Humerus granuloma in patient with calcium pyrophosphate deposition disease: Axillary view of the right shoulder demonstrates nonexpansile, predominantly lytic lesion in the proximal humerus with narrow zone of transition. Note the presence of chondrocalcinosis.

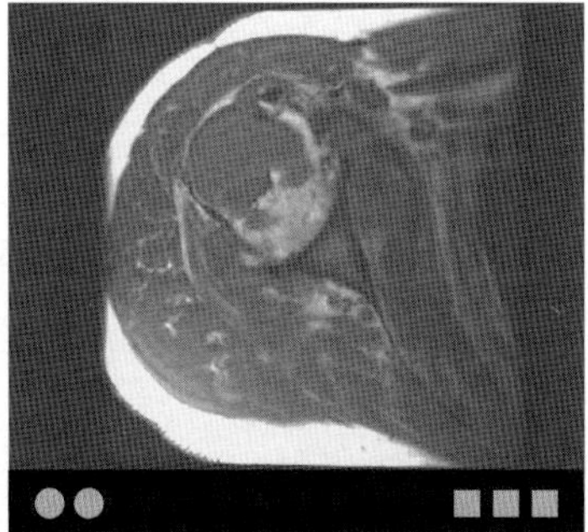

C. Humerus granuloma in patient with calcium pyrophosphate deposition disease: Axial T1-weighted image demonstrates low signal intensity of the lesion in the proximal humerus. Note the significantly more hypointense rim around the lesion corresponding to the calcifications.

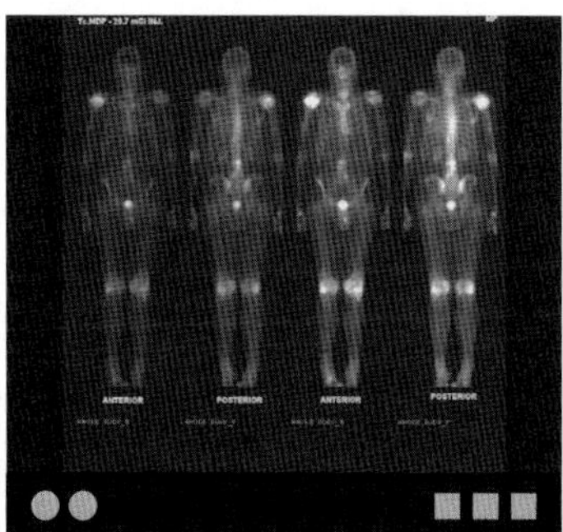

D. Humerus granuloma in patient with calcium pyrophosphate deposition disease: Whole body bone scan obtained after injection of Tc99m-MDP demonstrates nonspecific increased uptake in the lesion of the right proximal humerus. Increased uptake in both knees and lumbar spine is related to degenerative changes.

E. Humerus granuloma in patient with calcium pyrophosphate deposition disease: Axial CT image of the proximal right humerus demonstrates mixed lytic and sclerotic lesion in the anterolateral aspect of the humeral neck. Note the cortical disruption and microfractures. Note the presence of chondrocalcinosis.

DIFFERENTIAL DIAGNOSES IMAGES

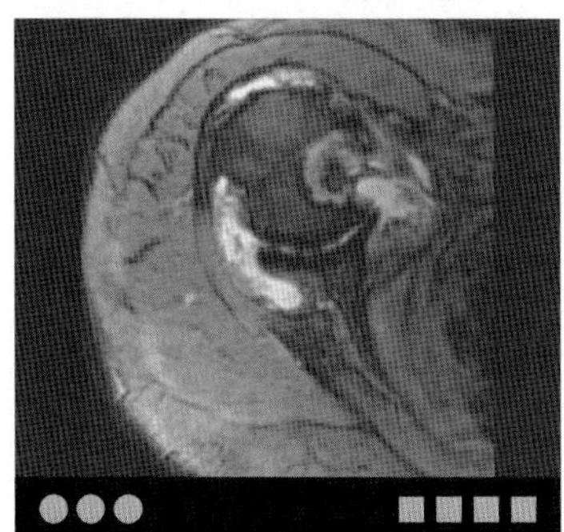

F. Erosion in the humeral head in a patient with rheumatoid arthritis: Axial T2-weighted image with fat saturation demonstrates large erosion in the humeral head.

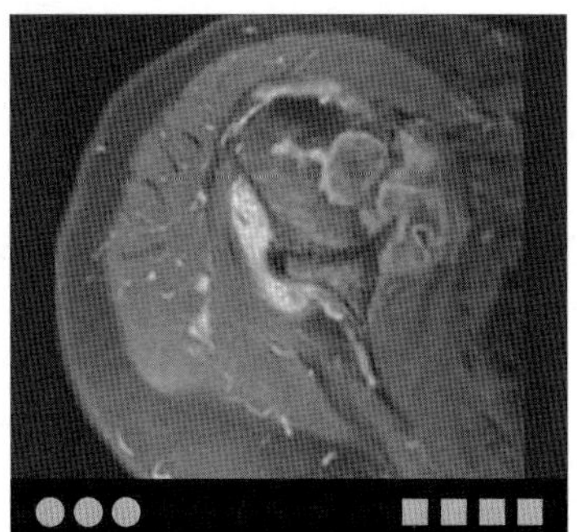

G. Erosion in the humeral head in a patient with rheumatoid arthritis: Axial T1-weighted image obtained after gadolinium contrast administration demonstrates large enhancing erosion in the humeral head. Enhancing synovium of the glenohumeral joint can also be seen.

IMAGE KEY

Common

Rare

Typical

Unusual

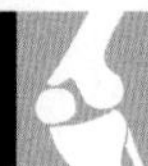

3–4 Polymyositis

Gideon Strich

PRESENTATION

Upper arm and thigh pain

FINDINGS

MRI shows diffuse edema of the proximal muscles of the arm and thigh progressing to fatty atrophy.

DIFFERENTIAL DIAGNOSES

- *Dermatomyositis:* MRI findings are similar to polymyositis with additional clinical findings of dermatologic features, particularly a rash on the face and torso. "Sheetlike" calcifications may occur late along the planes of the intermuscular fascia.
- *Connective tissue disease:* Polymyositis and subcutaneous calcifications may be seen in various connective tissue diseases including systemic lupus erythematosus, Sjogren syndrome, and mixed collagen vascular disease. Joint erosions and subluxations are more common in these entities.
- *Denervation atrophy:* Although early edema may occur, fatty atrophy predominates and is in the distribution of the affected nerve.
- *Muscle strain:* Findings are localized to specific muscles involved in exertional activity, typically hamstrings, biceps brachii, and gastrocnemius muscles. Muscle edema and fascial fluid collections predominate although hemorrhage may be present.

COMMENTS

This is an image of a middle-age female who presented with an onset of diffuse muscle soreness in the proximal muscles of the thigh and subsequently the upper arm. She had no dermatologic manifestations. Polymyositis and dermatomyositis are part of the spectrum of idiopathic inflammatory myopathies, which are characterized by inflammation of striated muscle, particularly the proximal muscles of the upper arm and thigh. Clinically, polymyositis is characterized by pain, muscle fatigue or weakness, and late muscle atrophy. In addition, dermatomyositis includes dermal manifestations, particularly on the face, chest, and extensor surfaces of the arm. There is an association with other autoimmune connective tissue diseases, including scleroderma, as well as an increased incidence of coexistent malignancies. Other organs may be involved including the heart, lungs, and gastrointestinal tract. Typical findings on imaging include early edema involving the proximal muscle groups of the thigh and upper arm with late fatty atrophy that may be difficult to distinguish from denervation atrophy. Imaging findings of edema are usually more localized and may show abscesses, abnormal fluid collection, and bone marrow edema. Rarely soft tissue gas is seen. In addition to imaging and laboratory findings of increased serum creatinine kinase, diagnosis may ultimately be made by biopsy which also helps differentiate polymyositis from other rare forms of myositis including inclusion body myositis, eosinophilic myositis, and myositis related to AIDS or drug toxicity. MRI may be helpful in guiding location for biopsy.

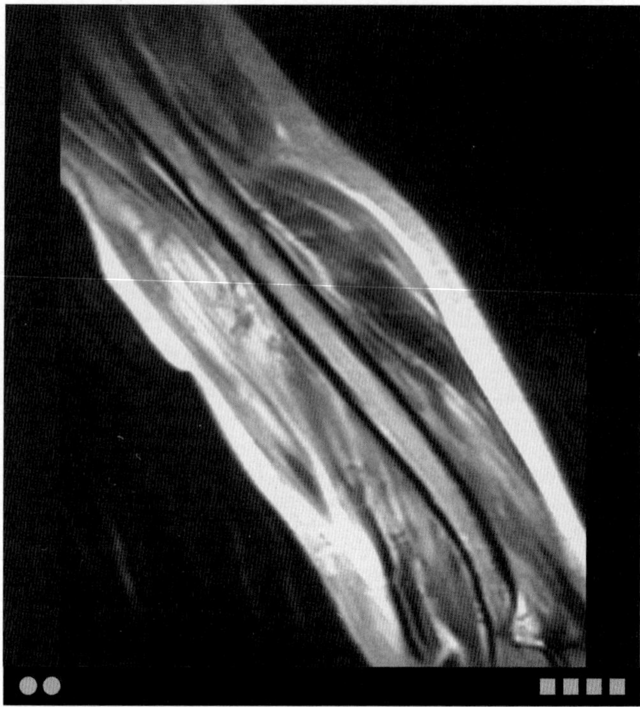

A. Polymyositis: Sagittal T2-weighted FSE image of the upper arm demonstrates abnormal signal intensity in the muscles of the proximal arm caused by edema.

PEARLS

- **Polymyositis most commonly affects the proximal muscles of the leg and arm and is most common in middle-age women.**
- **MRI demonstrates muscle edema and later atrophy.**
- **In association with dermatomyositis, radiograph may demonstrate late sheetlike soft tissue calcification in the planes of the muscles or fascia. Bony erosion or subluxation is rare.**
- **Radiographs may show avascular necrosis as a late complication of steroid treatment for polymyositis.**

ADDITIONAL IMAGES

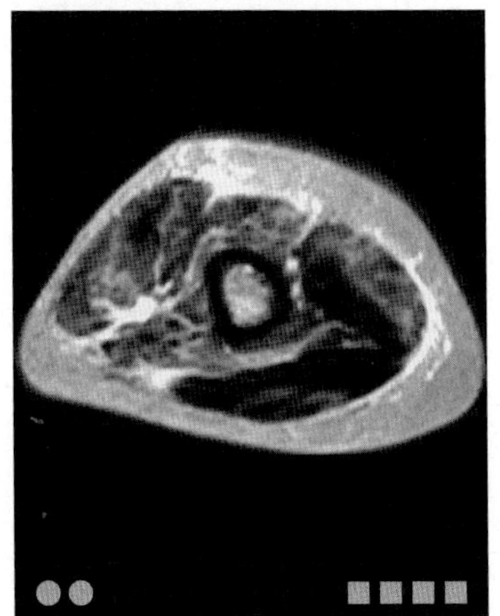

B. Polymyositis: Axial T2-weighted images demonstrates edema of the muscles of the upper arm with extensive fluid within the fascial planes.

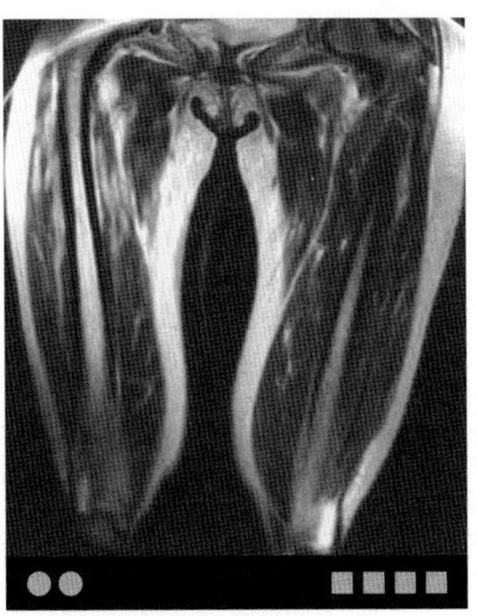

C. Polymyositis: Coronal T1-weighted image of the lower extremities demonstrates late muscle atrophy in the muscles of the right thigh.

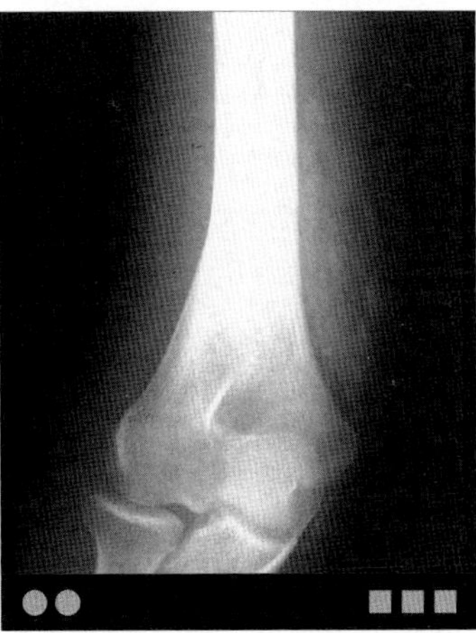

D. Polymyositis: Radiograph shows calcification in the fascial planes.

IMAGE KEY

Common

Rare

Typical

Unusual

DIFFERENTIAL DIAGNOSES IMAGES

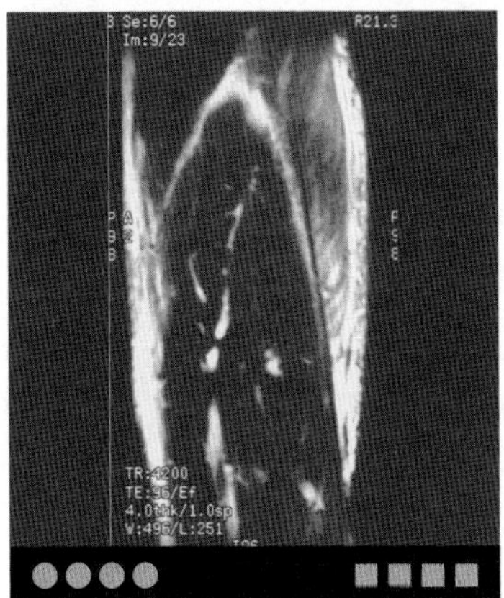

E. Muscle strain: Coronal T2-weighted image shows edema of gastrocnemius muscle.

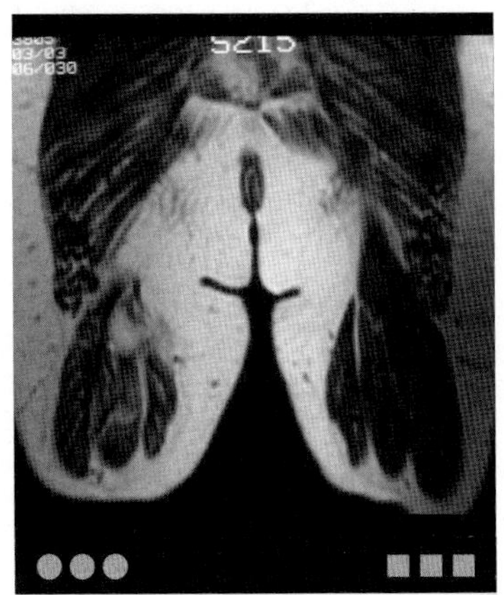

F. Denervation atrophy: Coronal T1-weighted image shows posttraumatic atrophy of the hamstrings and gluteal muscle on the right side.

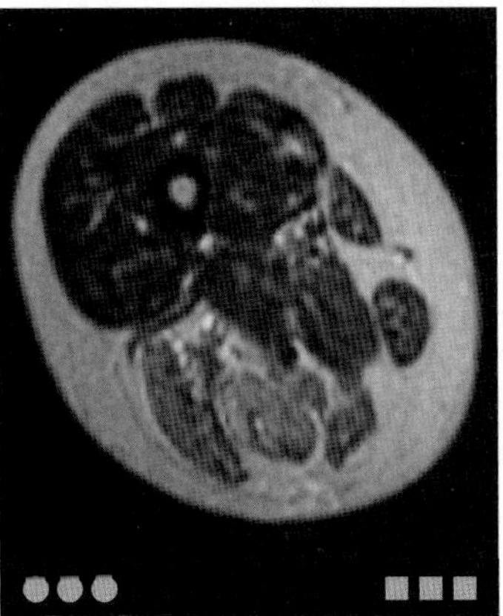

G. Denervation atrophy: Axial T1-weighted image shows fatty atrophy of hamstring muscles caused by previous injury.

Chapter 4

Infections

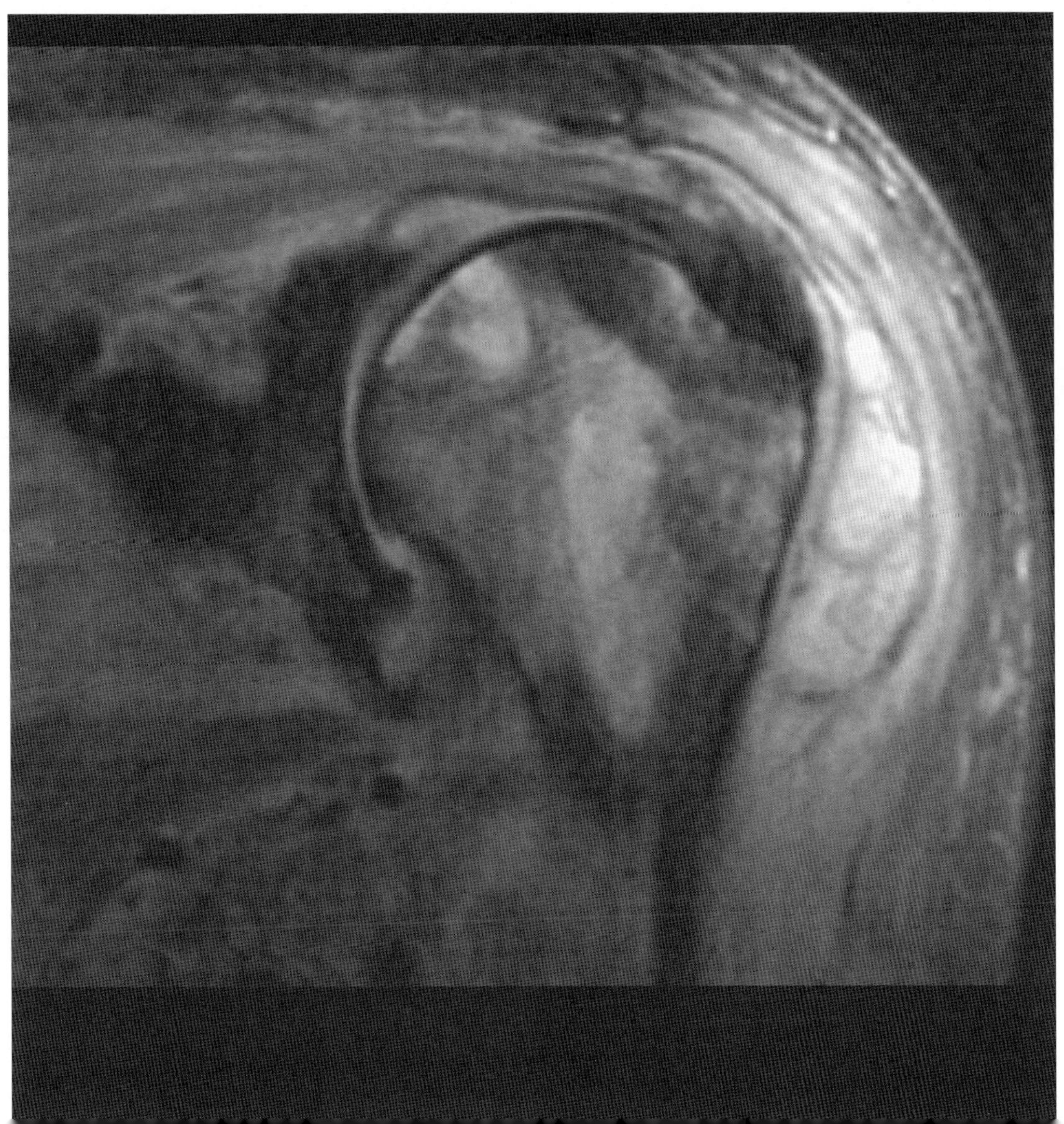

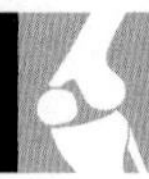

4–1 Septic Arthritis and Osteomyelitis of the Shoulder

Edward Mossop and Jamshid Tehranzadeh

PRESENTATION

Shoulder pain, reduced range of movement, fever, and malaise

FINDINGS

T2-weighted MRI shows large erosion, joint fluid, osteomyelitis, soft tissue edema, and rotator cuff tear.

DIFFERENTIAL DIAGNOSES

- *Rheumatoid arthritis:* Inflammation and proliferation of synovial tissue causes joint effusions, loss of cartilage, and subchondral erosions. Acute inflamed pannus is hypointense on T1-weighted images and enhances with contrast.
- *Reactive arthritis:* It occurs more commonly in young men with urethritis and uveitis and is associated with enthesopathy and erosions that have indistinct margins and are surrounded by periosteal new bone.
- *Psoriatic arthritis:* Erosions are more central in the joint and can be associated with enthesopathy and new bone formation. Patients often have the cutaneous or nail changes of psoriasis.
- *Crystal deposition disease:* Calcium pyrophosphate deposition diseases such as pseudogout, hyperparathyroidism, and hemochromatosis are associated with chondrocalcinosis and premature degenerative changes in joints.

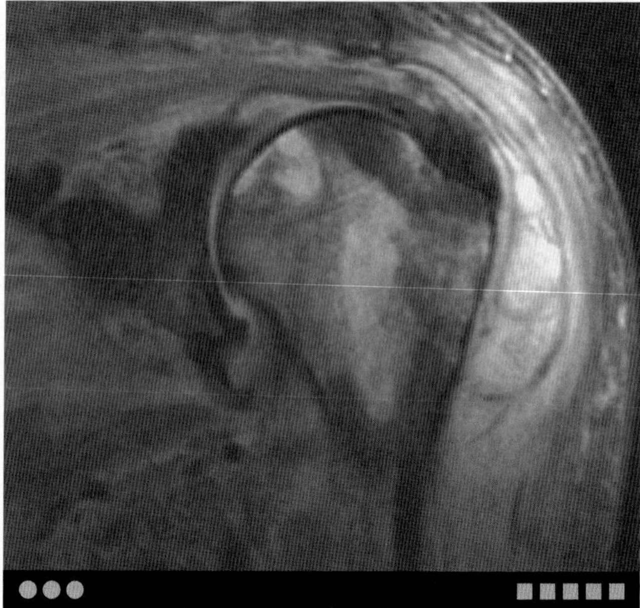

A. Septic Arthritis: Coronal T2 fat-saturated image shows septic arthritis and osteomyelitis with fluid within the subdeltoid bursa, inhomogeneous marrow signal, and erosions of the humeral head. Note rotator cuff tear.

COMMENTS

This is an image of a 57-year-old man with proven septic arthritis. Septic arthritis is an inflammation of the joint space, synovium, and articular cartilage caused by microorganisms. *Neisseria gonorrhoeae* remains the most frequent pathogen among younger, sexually active individuals; however, *Staphylococcus aureus* is the commonest overall cause. Joints become infected by direct injury or by blood-borne infection from a local or distant source. Bacterial invasion damages the joint cartilage secondary to the release of proteolytic enzymes. This process may extend into the underlying bone, leading to osteochondral erosions and osteomyelitis. Risk factors for septic arthritis include rheumatoid arthritis, steroids, joint prosthesis, and immunosuppression. MRI shows joint fluid as low signal on T1-weighted images and high signal on fat-suppressed T2-weighted images. Thickened synovium is seen on T1-weighted images and an enhancing rim of synovial membrane may be seen on contrast-enhanced images. Soft tissue inflammation appears as poorly defined areas of high signal on T2-weighted images and enhanced areas after contrast administration. Bone marrow appears as diffused poorly defined areas of low signal on T1-weighted images, which enhance after contrast administration and high signal on T2-weighted and STIR images. This represents marrow edema, exudates, and ischemia from osteomyelitis. Infected bone is frequently surrounded by a well-defined low signal periosteum on all sequences which forms the involucrum.

PEARLS

- **Septic arthritis is an inflammation of the joint space, synovial fluid, synovium, and articular cartilage caused by microorganisms.**
- ***S. aureus* is the most common cause of septic arthritis.**
- **MRI shows a combination of joint effusions, soft tissue changes, and bone marrow changes representing associated osteomyelitis.**
- **Thickened synovium is seen on T1-weighted images and an enhancing rim of synovial membrane may be seen on contrast-enhanced images.**
- **Bone marrow appears as diffused poorly defined areas of low signal on T1-weighted images, which enhance after contrast administration and high signal on T2-weighted and STIR images.**

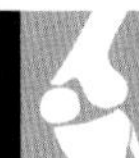

ADDITIONAL IMAGES

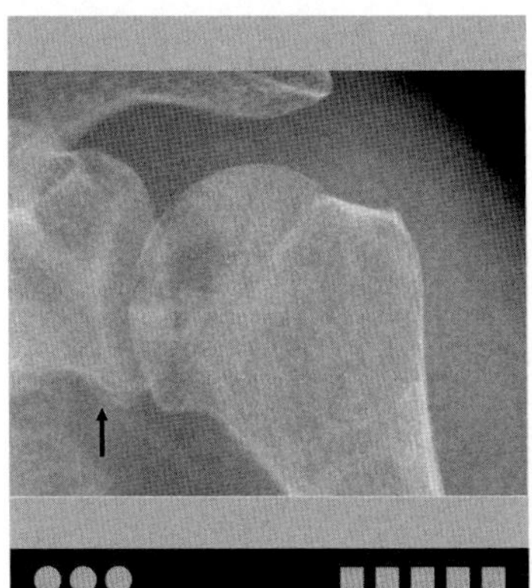

B. Septic Arthritis: AP radiograph of the shoulder shows osteoporosis and osteolytic lesion of subchondral bone. Note periosteal reaction (arrow).

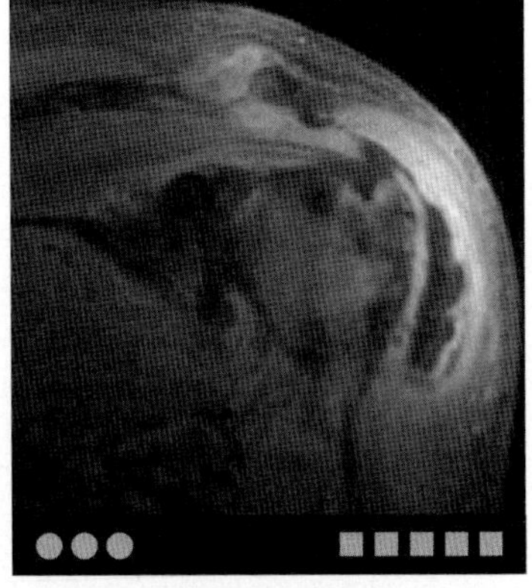

C. Septic Arthritis: Coronal T1 fat-saturated postcontrast image shows fluid within subacromial, subdeltoid bursa with marginal synovial enhancement consistent with septic arthritis and osteomyelitis.

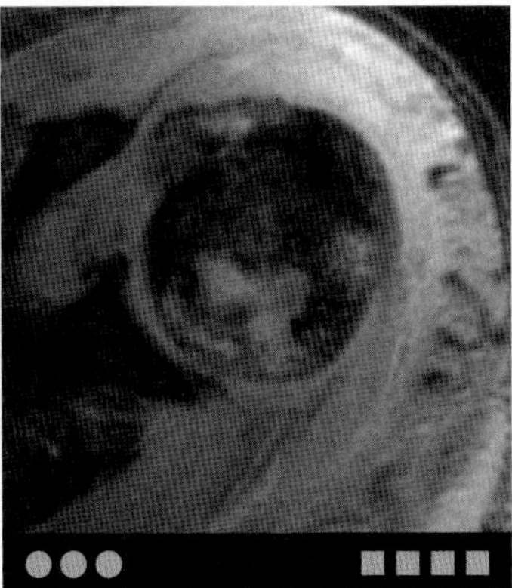

D. Septic Arthritis: Axial gradient echo image shows multiple erosions in the humeral head representing osteomyelitis.

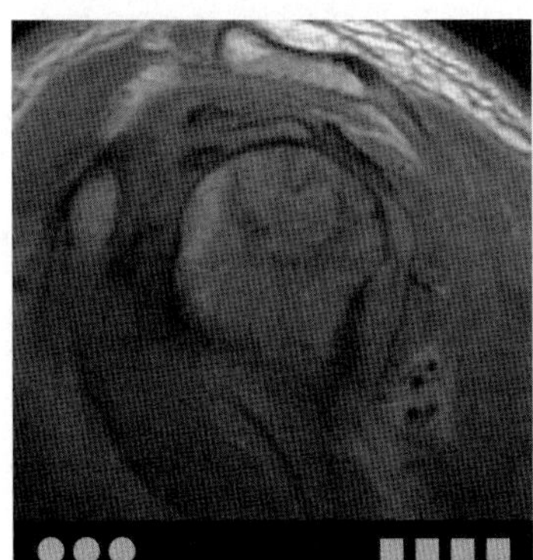

E. Septic Arthritis: Sagittal proton density image shows erosions of the humeral head caused by septic arthritis and osteomyelitis.

IMAGE KEY

Common

Rare

Typical

Unusual

DIFFERENTIAL DIAGNOSES IMAGES

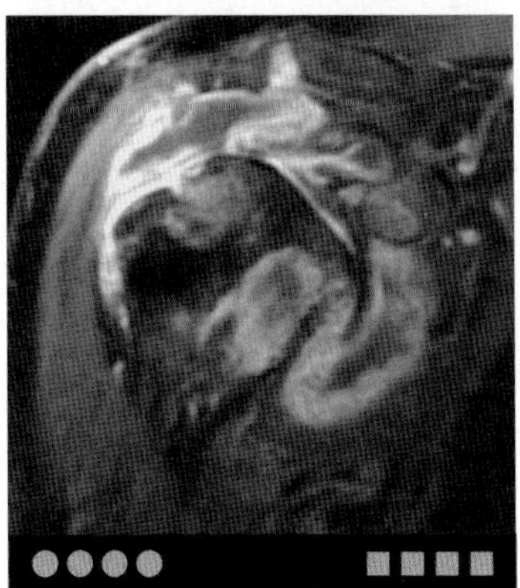

F. Rheumatoid Arthritis: Coronal T1 fat-saturated postcontrast image shows rheumatoid arthritis with massive inflammation and erosions of the glenohumeral joint. Note rotator cuff tear and fluid in the subacromial, subdeltoid bursa with marginal synovial enhancement.

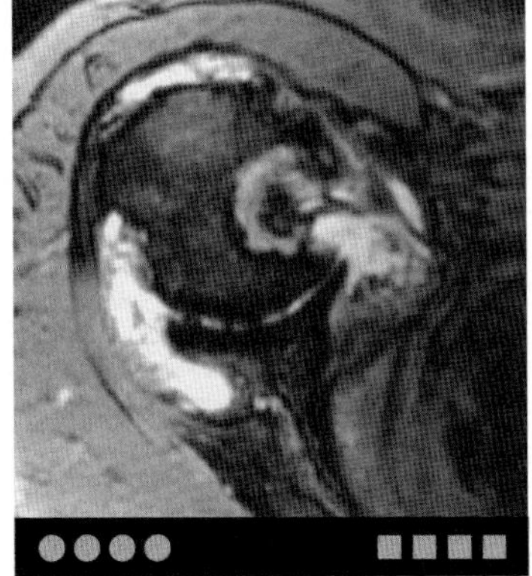

G. Rheumatoid Arthritis: Axial T2-weighted gradient echo image shows rheumatoid arthritis with massive inflammation and erosions of the glenohumeral joint. Note rotator cuff tear and fluid in the subacromial, subdeltoid bursa with marginal synovial enhancement.

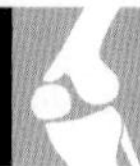

4–2 Osteomyelitis with Subperiosteal Abscess

Sailaja Yadavalli

PRESENTATION

Acute onset of severe arm pain, swelling, and fever

FINDINGS

MRI shows heterogeneous marrow signal with periosteal elevation extending from the proximal metaphysis to diaphysis. The epiphysis is not involved.

DIFFERENTIAL DIAGNOSES

- *Subperiosteal hemorrhage:* It may be seen with metaphyseal fractures and in conditions such as scurvy.
- *Tumors:* Periostitis maybe seen with malignant tumors, such as Ewing sarcoma and osteosarcoma.
- *Lymphoma:* Serpiginous areas of osteonecrosis may be seen with bone marrow changes and possible associated soft tissue mass.

COMMENTS

This is an image of a 6-year-old girl who presented with an acute onset of severe arm pain, swelling, and fever.

Hematogenous osteomyelitis is most common in the metaphyseal region in children between the ages of 3 and 15 years. In infants, some of the blood vessels in the metaphysis penetrate the growth plate and anastamose with the vessels in the epiphysis. Therefore, osteomyelitis in an infant may involve the epiphysis and the joint. After appoximately 1 year, the capillaries in the metaphysis are the terminal vessels and form loops that join the sinusoidal veins. Blood flow through these is sluggish. The epiphysis now has a separate blood supply. There is also a relative paucity of phagocytosis in the metaphysis of a child. These conditions result in the metaphysis being the most common site of infection in a child between the ages of 3 and 15 years. As the infectious process progresses in the bone, it penetrates the cortex and lifts the periosteum, which has a relatively loose attachment to the underlying bone in the immature skeleton. The infected fluid then collects under the periosteum forming a subperiosteal abscess. Changes of acute osteomyelitis and subperiosteal abscess become easily apparent on contrast enhanced MRI, whereas the radiographic findings lag the onset of infection by 1 to 2 weeks. On T1-weighted, fluid sensitive, and postcontrast images, nonenhancing subperiosteal fluid is seen. Decompression of the subperiosteal abscess to a soft tissue abscess may be seen. Later radiographs may show periostitis. Subsequently cortical necrosis can occur with formation of sequestrum.

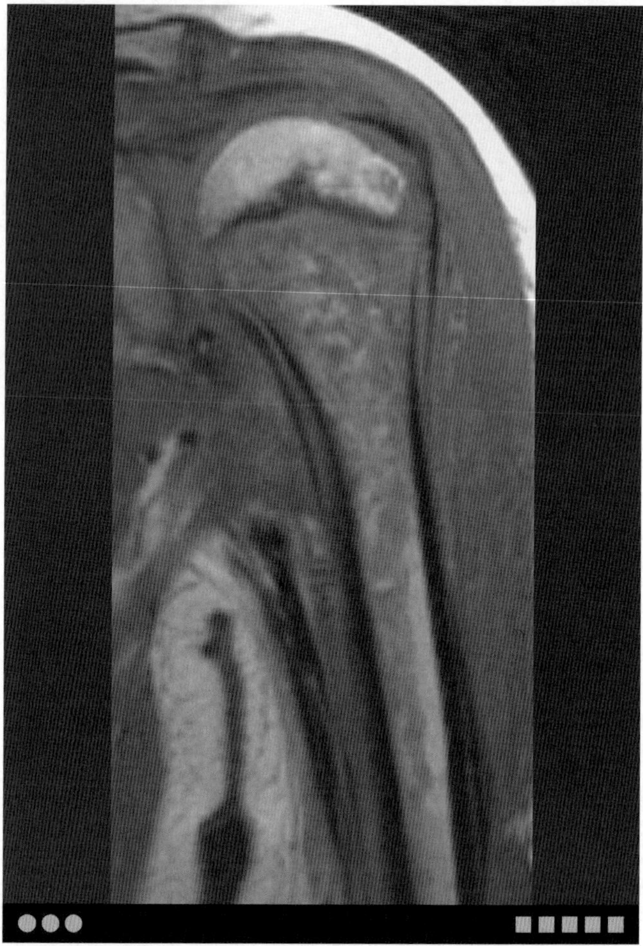

A. Osteomyelitis and subperiosteal abscess: Coronal T1-weighted image shows heterogeneous bone marrow signal with raised periosteum and subperiosteal abscess. Abnormal bone marrow signal does not cross the growth plate.

PEARLS

- **Hematogenous spread of infection is most commonly seen in children.**
- **Osteomyelitis of the metaphysis with subperiosteal abscess is seen in children older than 12 months.**
- **Both the epiphysis and metaphysis are involved with osteomyelitis in infants. This increases the risk of joint infection.**
- **Areas of osteonecrosis and periostitis are not unique to osteomyelitis with subperiosteal abscess.**
- **Radiographs do not exhibit the changes of subperiosteal abscess for a week or two after the onset of infection. MRI will show early changes.**

ADDITIONAL IMAGES

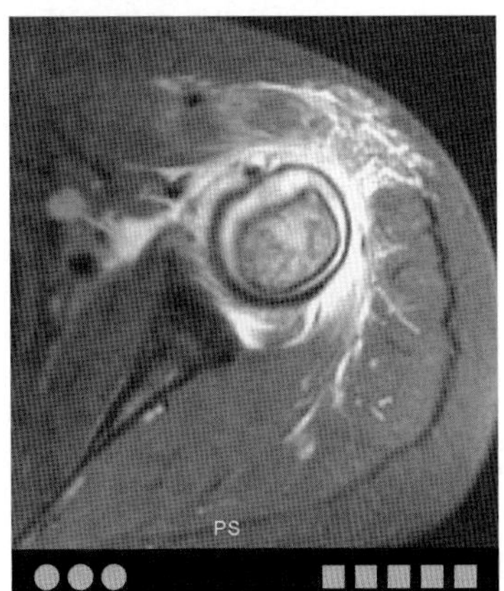

B. Osteomyelitis and subperiosteal abscess: Axial STIR image shows high signal in the bone marrow and in the subperiosteal region. Extensive soft tissue edema is also seen.

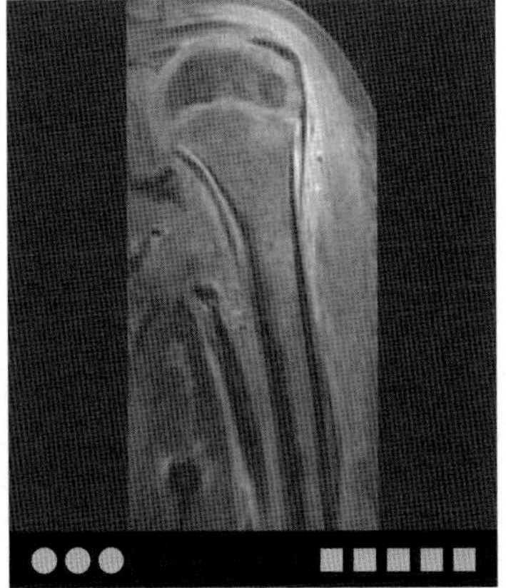

C. Osteomyelitis and subperiosteal abscess: Coronal T1-weighted fat-saturated postcontrast image shows enhancement of the bone marrow and nonenhancing subperiosteal abscess extending from the proximal metaphysis to the diaphysis.

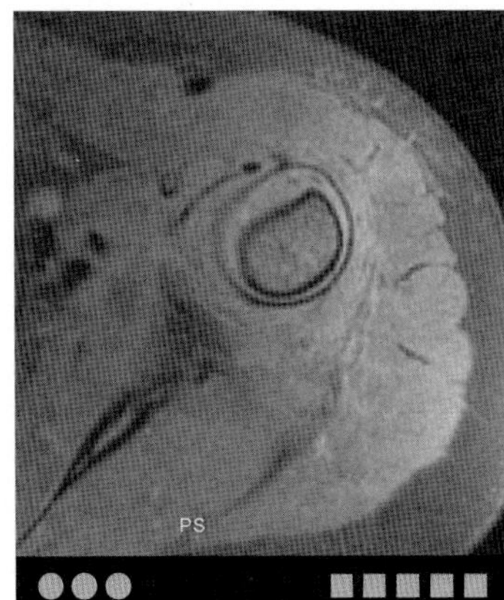

D. Osteomyelitis and subperiosteal abscess: Axial T1-weighted fat-saturated postcontrast image shows the periosteal elevation with underlying nonenhancing fluid collection.

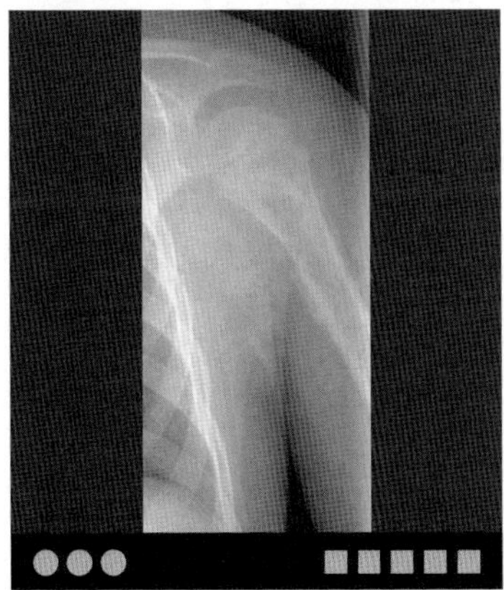

E. Osteomyelitis and subperiosteal abscess: Radiograph 20 days after presentation and drainage of the abscess shows periostitis, which was not seen on radiographs obtained at presentation.

DIFFERENTIAL DIAGNOSES IMAGES

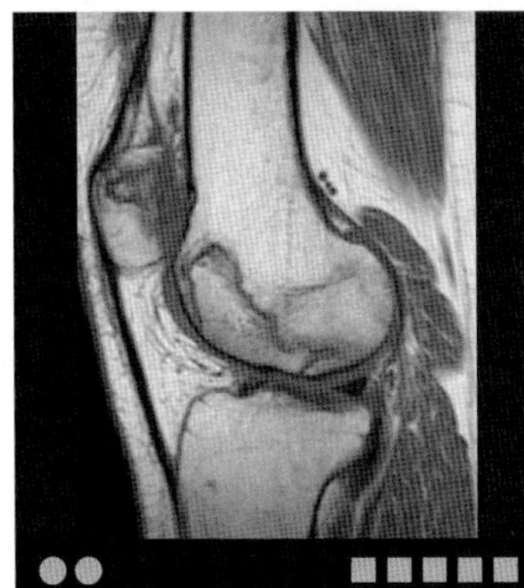

F. Osteonecrosis in lymphoma: Sagittal T1-weighted image shows bone infarcts with serpiginous low signal in the distal femur and patella with the typical bone-in-bone appearance.

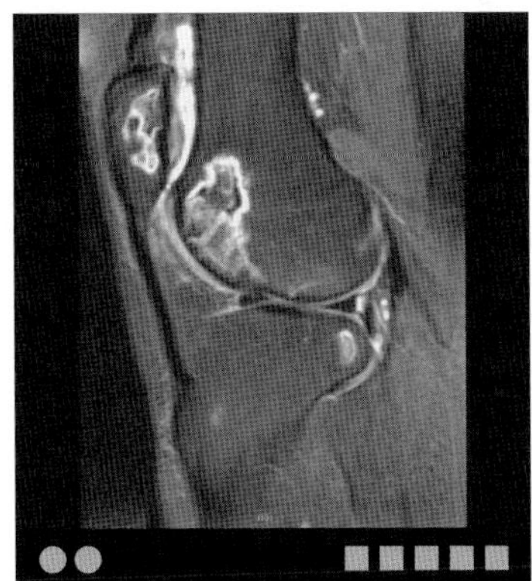

G. Osteonecrosis in lymphoma: Sagittal fat-saturated fluid sensitive image shows typical curvilinear abnormal signal compatible with osteonecrosis. Posterior tibia is also involved.

IMAGE KEY

Common

Rare

Typical

Unusual

Chapter 5

Tumors and Tumor Like Lesions

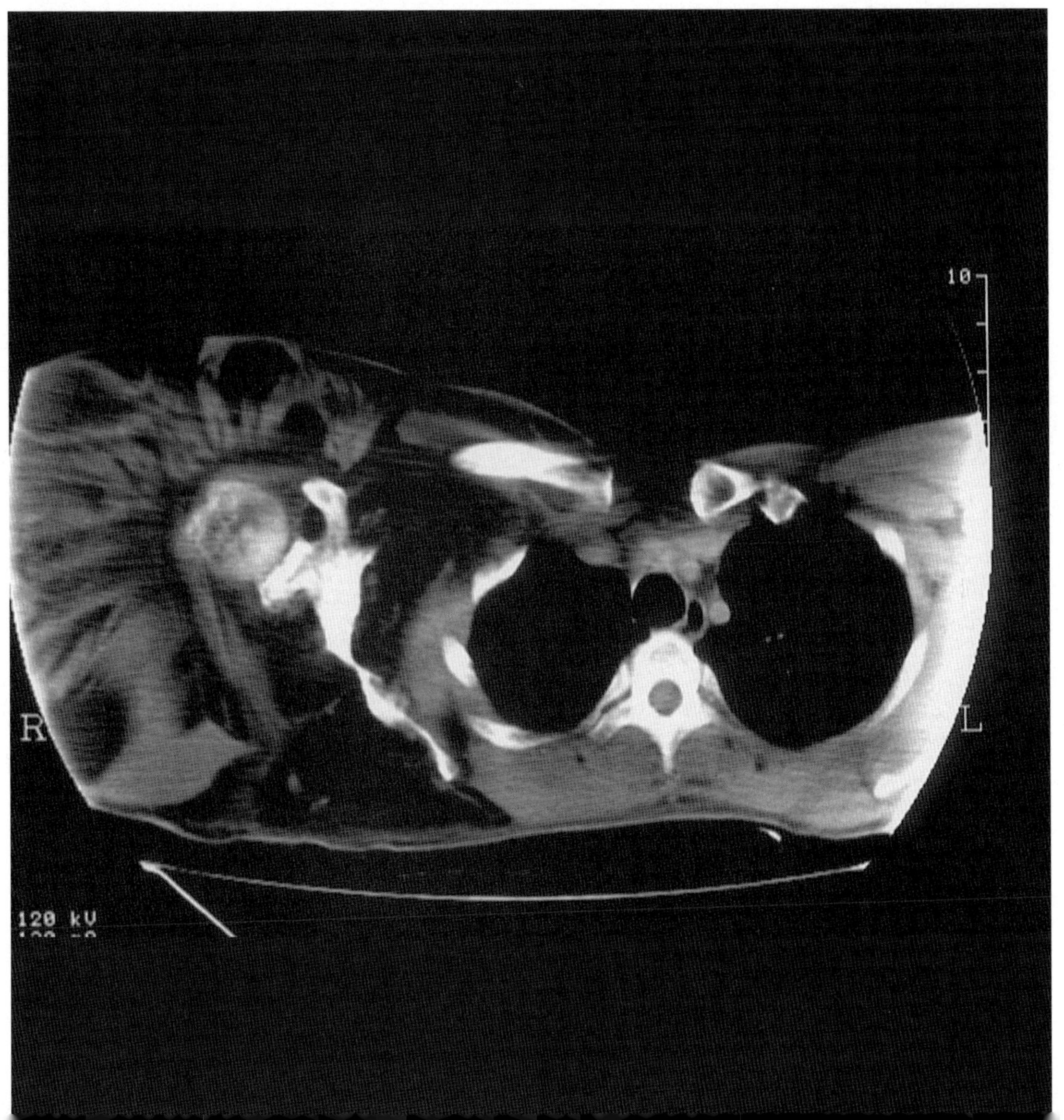

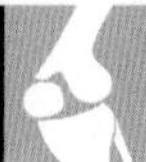

5–1 Soft Tissue Lipomatosis of Shoulder

Kambiz Motamedi

PRESNTATION

Longstanding hypertrophy of the upper extremity

FINDINGS

A CT scan of the humerus demonstrates a diffused and infiltrative fatty mass of the arm.

DIFFERENTIAL DIAGNOSES

- *Focal gigantism/macrodactyly/macrodystrophia lipomatosa:* Cross-sectional imaging reveals three-dimensional enlargement of fibro-fatty tissue of toes or fingers.
- *Lymphedema of the upper extremity:* Cross-sectional imaging shows edema of the upper extremity most prominent in the subcutaneous compartment
- *Neurofibromatosis:* Lobular or sheathlike soft tissue masses (neurofibromas) mostly along the major nerves, but also anywhere in the soft tissues.

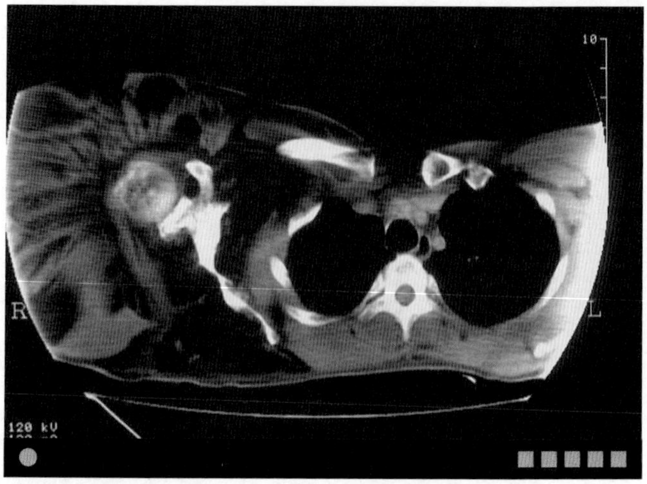

A. Lipomatosis: Nonenhanced CT section of upper thorax and right upper extremity at the level of the shoulder joint demonstrates the diffused fatty hypertrophy of the upper arm affecting the subcutaneous and the muscle compartments. The underlying bony structures are normal at this level. Note the diffuse involvement of the shoulder girdle with fatty hypertrophy affecting the deep tissues anterior to scapula.

COMMENTS

This is an image of a 57-year-old man with longstanding history of upper extremity enlargement. Congenital infiltrating lipomatosis is a rare clinical entity characterized by infiltrating lipomatous tumors. These tumors tend to reoccur, despite their benign histology. The patients have no other associated congenital anomalies. There is no familial predisposition, and there is a usual lack of neurofibromatosis stigmata. There is a predilection for the extremities and the trunk with few reported cases in the neck and face. There is common overgrowth of the bones along with the fatty tissue. The treatment is surgical excision. The common involvement of nerves with hypertrophy (digital nerves) or fibro-fatty proliferation (median nerve) seen in the cases of isolated finger macrodactyly may not be present in cases of lipomatosis. A variant of this clinical presentation may be the familial multiple lipomatosis. This clinical entity is characterized by several, small, well-demarcated, encapsulated lipomas that commonly involve the extremities. They typically appear during or soon after adolescence. The neck and shoulders are usually spared, and there is usually a family history of multiple lipomas. An autosomal dominant mode inheritance has been suggested for this entity. The congenital infiltrating lipomatosis is to be differentiated from multiple angiolipomas. The angiolipomas are usually tender, soft, and subcutaneous nodules that are frequently multilobulated. They are usually firmer than the ordinary lipomas and may be associated with vague pain.

PEARLS

- **Characteristic involvement of bones with periosteal thickening and enlargement.**
- **Lipomatosis affects upper extremity and trunk.**
- **Radiographs suggest the presence of fatty tissue by prominent radiolucency of the hypertrophied soft tissues. Advanced imaging with MRI or CT scan confirms the findings.**

ADDITIONAL IMAGES

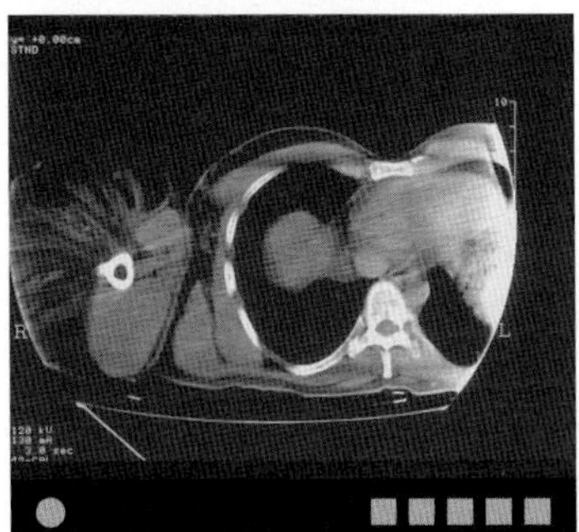

B. Lipomatosis: Nonenhanced CT section at the level of humeral mid shaft reveals the involvement of the subcutaneous tissue and the flexor muscles. The chest wall appears normal.

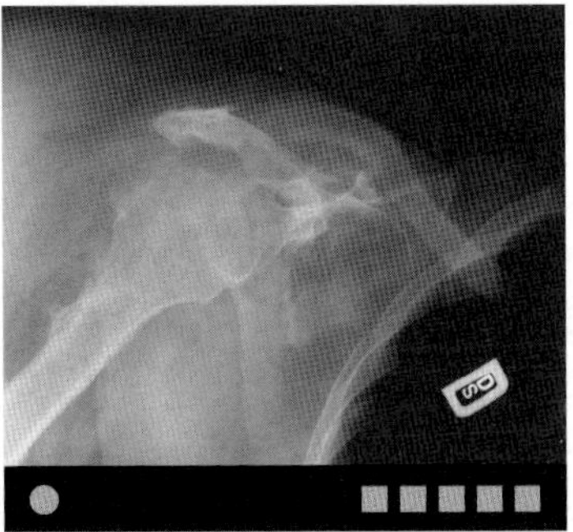

C. Lipomatosis: AP radiograph of shoulder shows the generalized soft tissue hypertrophy with interspersed lucent strands. There is irregular and bizarre periosteal thickening on the involved bony structures.

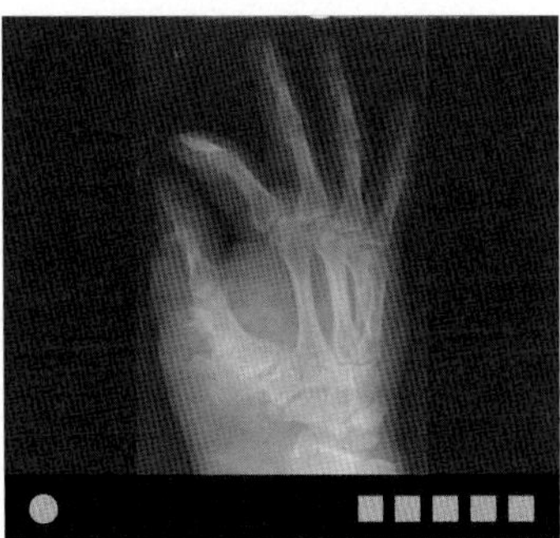

D. Lipomatosis: Oblique radiograph the hand demonstrates soft tissue hypertrophy along the radial aspect of the hand with bizarre hypertrophic changes of the underlying bony structures. Note the absence of second and third- digit involvement.

DIFFERENTIAL DIAGNOSES IMAGES

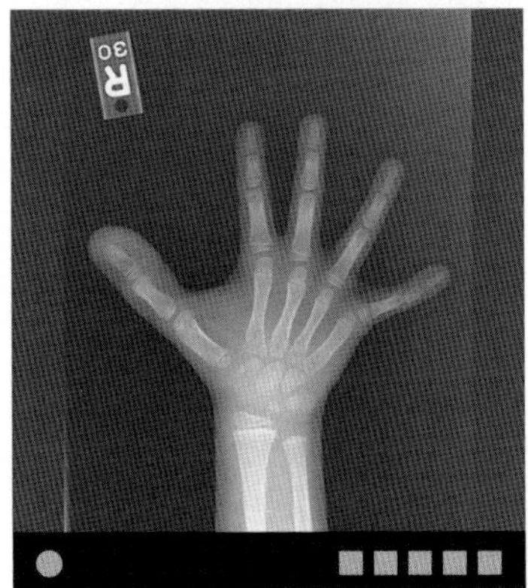

E. Macrodactyly: AP radiograph of the hand shows isolated soft tissue hypertrophy of the thumb.

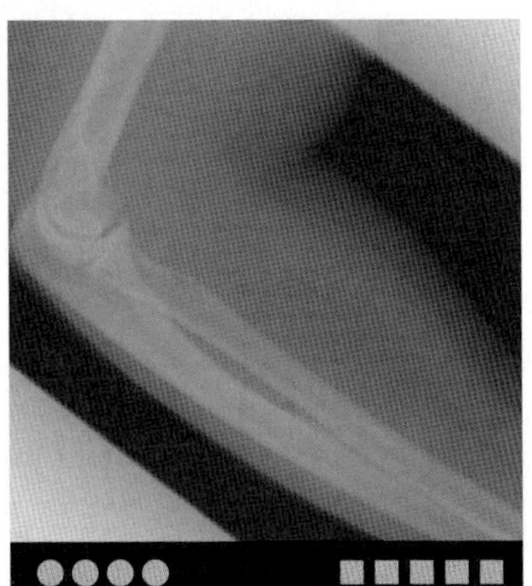

F. Lipoma: Lateral radiograph of the forearm shows a lucent, spindle-shaped soft tissue mass.

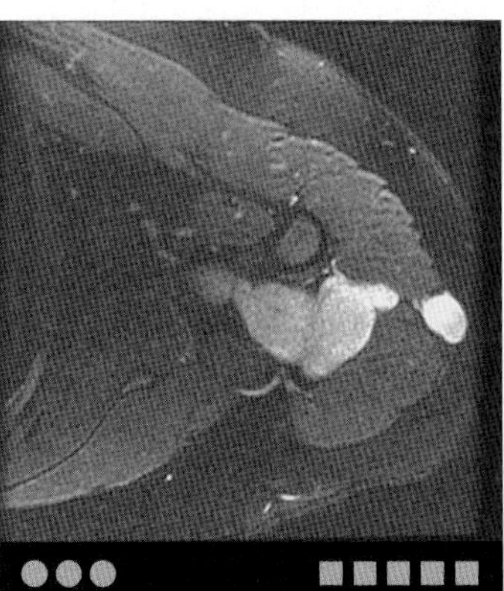

G. Neurofibromatosis: Axial fat-saturated T2-weighted FSE image shows a hyperintense mass of the axilla extending to the deltoid muscle and superficial subcutaneous compartment.

IMAGE KEY

Common

Rare

Typical

Unusual

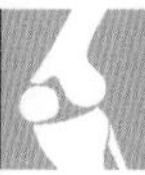

5–2 Subdeltoid Lipoma of the Shoulder

Wilfred CG Peh

PRESENTATION

Painless, slowly growing mass

FINDINGS

MR images show large fusiform soft tissue lipoma with bright signal on T1-weighted image and dark signal on fat-saturated T2-weighted image.

DIFFERENTIAL DIAGNOSES

- *Subcutaneous lipoma:* This is the most common type of lipoma and may blend with subcutaneous fat and therefore may be difficult to see if there is no surface marker placed.
- *Intramuscular deltoid lipoma:* Also known as infiltrating lipoma, this lipoma is located within a large muscle and may produce a striated appearance on MR imaging.
- *Liposarcoma:* Usually affects elderly patients. Well-differentiated liposarcoma is seen as a predominantly fatty mass with irregularly thickened or nodular septa on MR imaging. Other types of liposarcoma generally do not contain large amounts of fat.

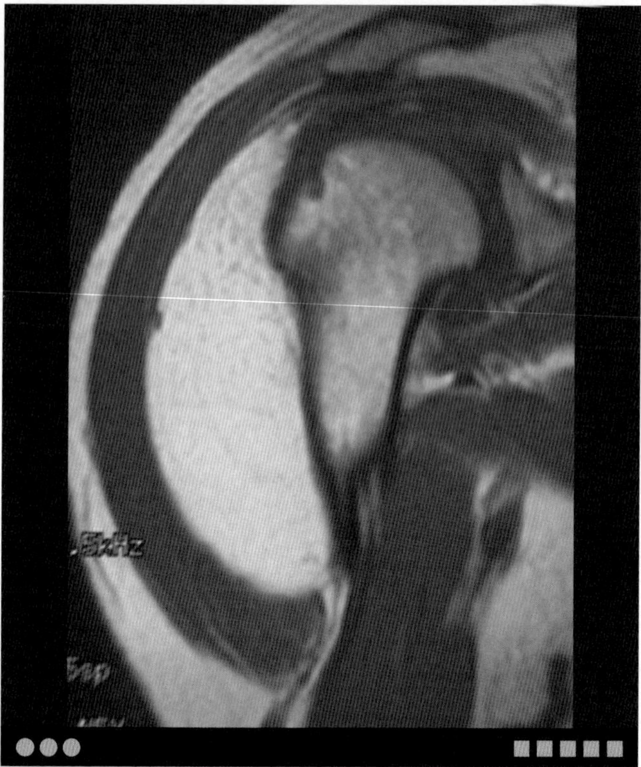

A. Subdeltoid lipoma: Coronal SE T1-weighted MR image of the right shoulder shows a well-defined lobulated mass located deep to the deltoid muscle. The mass is homogeneously hyperintense and is identical in signal characteristics to adjacent normal subcutaneous fat. The overlying deltoid muscle and underlying humerus are uninvolved.

COMMENTS

This is an image of a 40-year-old woman who noticed a painless mass over her right shoulder. The mass was slowly growing and was associated with occasional local pain and tenderness. Lipoma is the most common soft tissue tumor in the musculoskeletal system. It is a benign lesion that is composed of mature adipose tissue. They are usually divided into superficial and deep lipomas, with superficial lipomas being much more common. Lipomas are usually encapsulated and have a distinct lobular pattern. Radiographs are usually nondiagnostic, although occasionally a mass of fatty density may be seen. Lipomas are best characterized on CT scan and MR imaging. On CT scan the lesion is well-defined and homogeneous, with a low attenuation coefficient of approximately minus 100 HU. On MR imaging, the signal intensity of a lipoma is identical to that of normal subcutaneous fat on all sequences, being T1-hyperintense and T2-hypointense. Placement of a surface marker is useful as a lipoma situated in the subcutaneous fat layer may be difficult to identify as a distinct mass on MR images. MR imaging with inherently superior anatomic capability is able to precisely show the precise lesion extent. Intra- and intermuscular lipomas are members of a subgroup called heterotopic lipomas that arise in intimate association with nonadipose tissue. Intermuscular lipomas are less common than intramuscular lipomas. Brown fat is another form of adipose tissue with different cellular pattern than white fat. Hibernoma is a rare type of benign neoplasm in human beings consisting of brown fat, which resembles fat in certain hibernating animals.

PEARLS

- **MR imaging is the modality of choice for detection and diagnosis of lipomas.**
- **MR imaging is able to show the exact location of the lipoma, e.g. intermuscular lipoma.**
- **Placement of a surface marker aids in identification of superficial lipomas.**

ADDITIONAL IMAGES

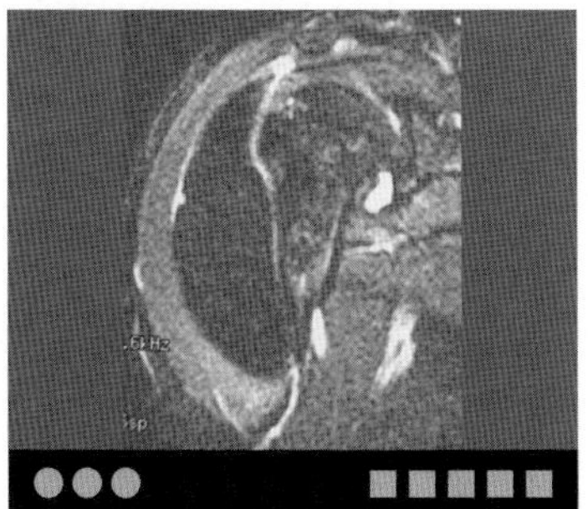

B. Subdeltoid lipoma: Coronal fat-suppressed FSE T2-weighted MR image of the right shoulder shows that the mass is homogeneously hypointense. Its signal intensity remains identical to that of normal fat.

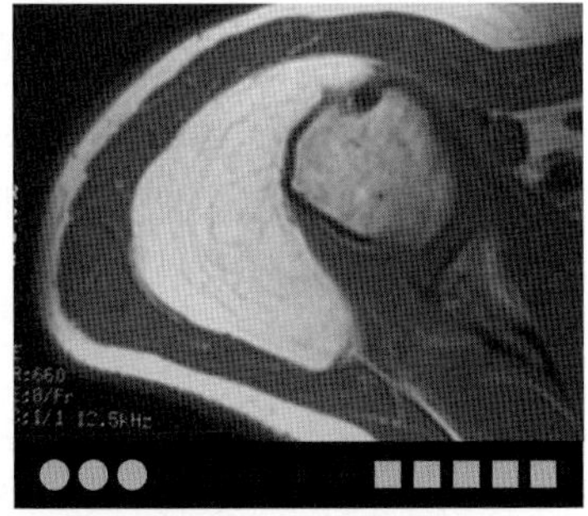

C. Subdeltoid lipoma: Axial SE T1-weighted MR image of the right shoulder shows a well-defined fatty mass located in the plane deep to the deltoid muscle. It contains fine internal septations.

DIFFERENTIAL DIAGNOSES IMAGES

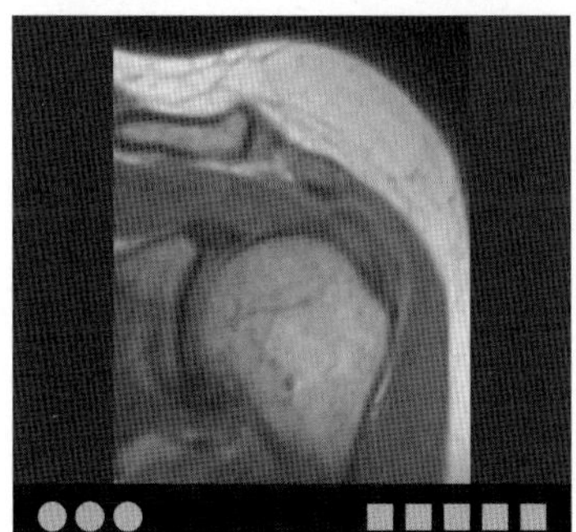

D. Subcutaneous lipoma: This is an image of a 46-year-old woman. Coronal SE T1-weighted MR image of the left shoulder shows the lipoma as an area of subcutaneous thickening overlying the acromioclavicular joint and lateral deltoid muscle. It has numerous fine septations.

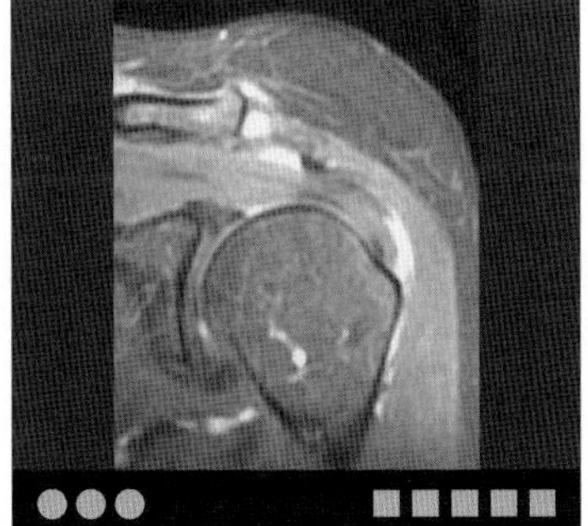

E. Subcutaneous lipoma: This is the same image of a 46-year-old woman as image D. Contrast-enhanced coronal fat-suppressed SE T1-weighted MR image shows near-uniform hypointense signal within the subcutaneous lipoma, similar to that of adjacent normal subcutaneous fat. Note mild enhancement of the septal strands.

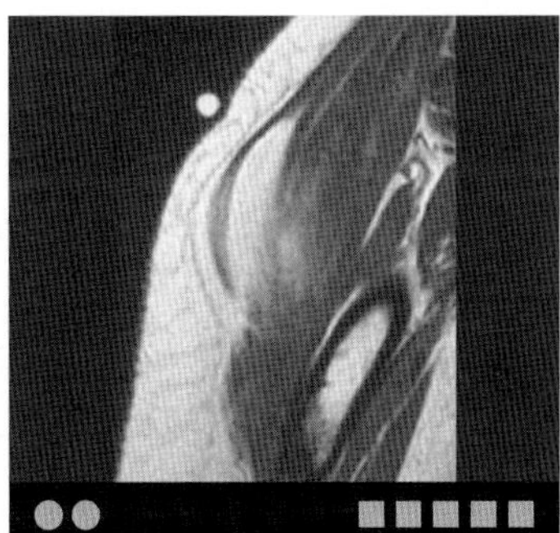

F. Intramuscular lipoma: This is an image of a 69-year-old man. Coronal SE T1-weighted MR image shows a well-defined lens-shaped mass within the anterior deltoid muscle. The mass is homogeneously hyperintense, with signal characteristics identical to those of normal fat. There is some infiltration between muscle fibers giving rise to a striated appearance.

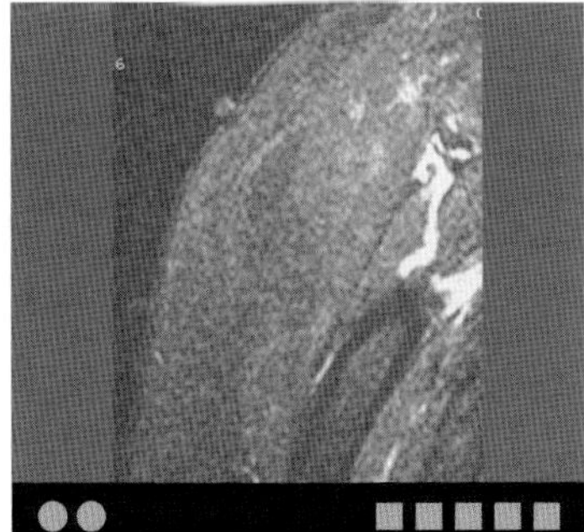

G. Intramuscular lipoma: This is the same image of a 69-year-old man as shown in image F. Contrast-enhanced coronal fat-suppressed SE T1-weighted MR image shows that the lesion is completely hypointense, indicating it is composed of mature fat in deltoid muscle.

IMAGE KEY

Common

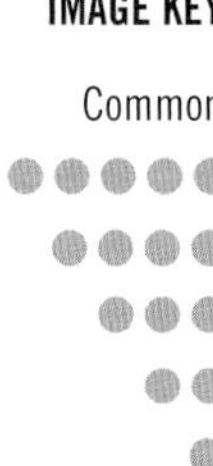

Rare

Typical

Unusual

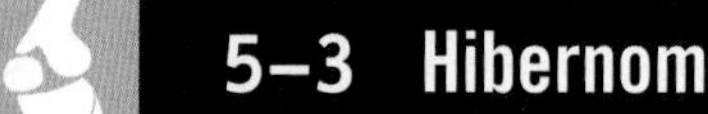

5–3 Hibernoma

Sulabha Masih

PRESENTATION

Right shoulder pain

FINDINGS

MRI shows heterogeneous signal intensity mass, with increased fat signal, similar to liposarcoma, but it is distinguished by demonstrating branching, serpentine low signal vascular structures.

DIFFERENTIAL DIAGNOSES

- *Atypical lipoma:* It presents as homogeneous, fatty radiolucent mass on radiographs. MR imaging shows homogenous fatty increase signal on T1-weighted image.
- *Liposarcoma:* Most common soft tissue malignancy, with poorly defined mass. It does not represent branching vascular pattern on MRI.
- *Angiolipoma:* Radiogrphs and CT scanning demonstrate inhomogeneous fat and water density, with phleboliths and infiltration into adjacent tissue.
- *Hemangioma:* Vascular lesion with fat, which is associated with overlying skin abnormalities.

COMMENTS

This is a case of 60-year-old female who presented with right shoulder pain for 4 months. Hibernoma is extremely rare, benign soft tissue tumor of brown fat and presents as a slow growing, vascular movable mass. Hibernoma is more frequently seen in 30- to 50-year-old adults. Common anatomic locations include thigh, shoulder, back, neck, and arm. Frequently hibernoma may not be diagnosed clinically. Imaging and core needle biopsy make the final diagnosis. The tumor contains brown fat, which histologically resembles immature white adipose tissue. Most tumors are composed of coarsely multivacuolated fat cells with small central nuclei and no atypia. Four morphological variants of hibernoma are identified: typical, myxoid, spindle cell, and lipomalike. Typical hibernoma contains eosinophilic cell, pale cell, and mixed cell type. Myxoid variant demonstrates loose basophilic matrix. Spindle cell variant contains features of spindle cell lipoma and hibernoma. Lipoma variant contains only scattered hibernoma cells. Immunohistologically majority are positive for S-100. On physical exam, the mass may feel warm because of hypervascularity. Patient exhibits no symptoms. Tumor size ranges from 1 to 24 cm. On radiograph and CT scan, Hibernoma resembles atypical lipoma or liposarcoma. This tumor usually appears as a well-circumscribed mass, without osseous involvement. On MR, the lesion is heterogeneous with increase signal similar to fat and branching with serpentine vasculature, which shows low signal intensity. Doppler sonography and angiography will demonstrate hypervascularity.

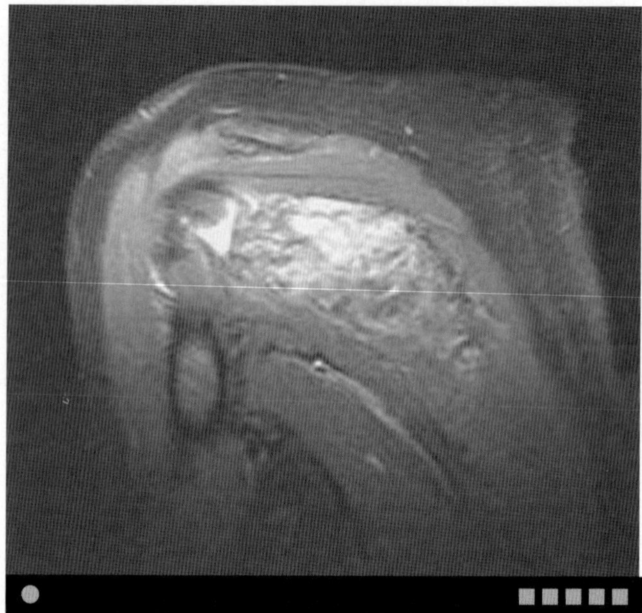

A. Hibernoma: Coronal STIR-weighted image exhibits fat suppression and branching vascular pattern.

PEARLS

- **Hibernomas are benign; slow growing, vascular, fatty tumor resembling atypical lipoma vs. liposarcoma.**
- **Important distinguishing features of this tumor from liposarcoma are branching and serpentine vascular structures, which are low signal intensity on all sequences.**
- **Core needle biopsy makes the final diagnosis. Histologically, brown fat resembles immature white adipose tissues.**

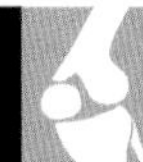

ADDITIONAL IMAGES

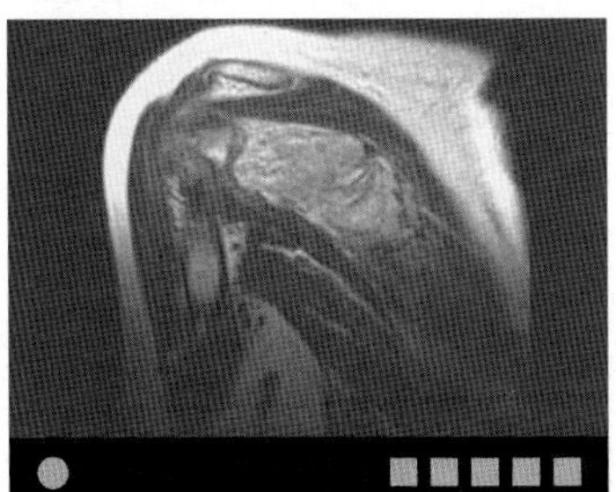

B. Hibernoma: Coronal T2-weighted image shows 6.6 × 3.4 × 2.8 cm mass deep to the subscapularis muscle and anterior to the glenoid.

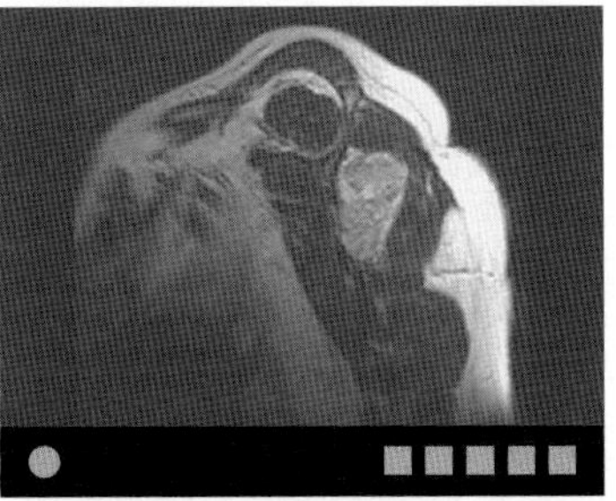

C. Hibernoma: Sagittal T2-weighted image demonstrates heterogeneous mass with fat and branching low signal vascular structures. Note few areas of low signal intensity which are calcified phleboliths.

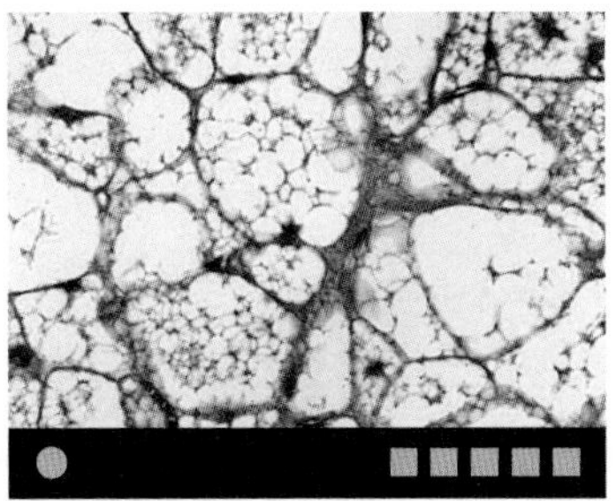

D. Hibernoma: Histologically, brown fat resembles immature white adipose tissues.

DIFFERENTIAL DIAGNOSES IMAGES

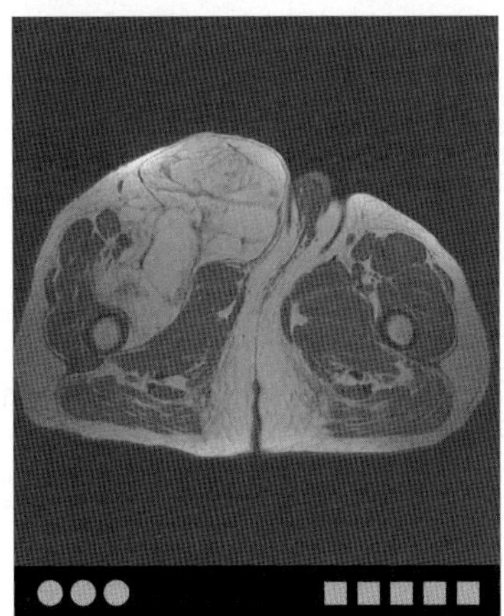

E. Liposarcoma: Axial T1-weighted image shows inhomogeneous fatty high signal intensity mass of upper thigh.

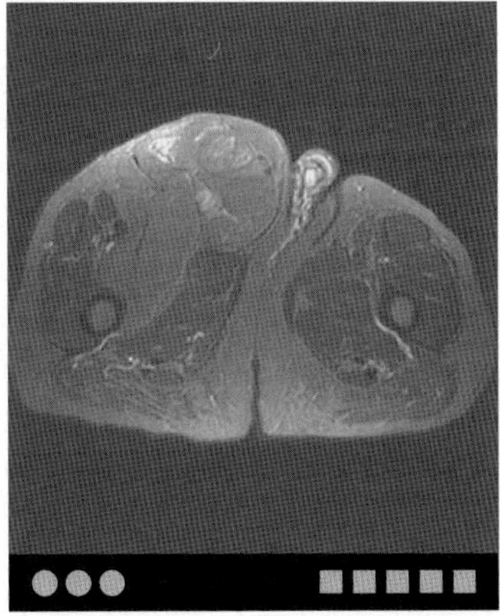

F. Liposarcoma: Axial fat sat proton density image shows inhomogeneous fat suppression and patchy high signal necrosis.

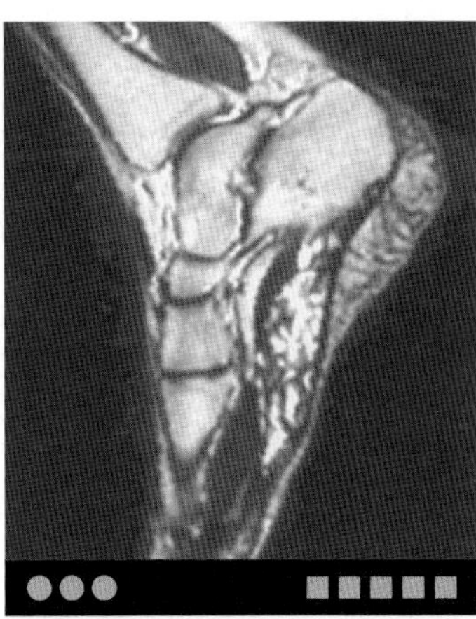

G. Hemangioma: Axial T2-weighted image shows serpigenous high signal intensity, with foci of decreased signal intensity caused by calcified phleboliths.

IMAGE KEY

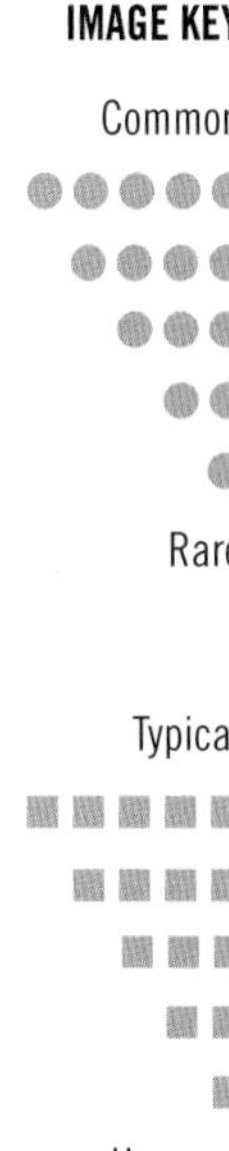

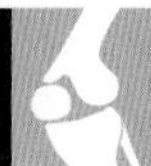

5–4 Malignant Fibrous Histiocytoma of Deltoid Muscle

Shahla Modarresi and Daria Motamedi

PRESENTATION

Mass of the shoulder

FINDINGS

MR imaging shows heterogeneous, subcutaneous mass with areas of low and high signal on T1-weighted image.

DIFFERENTIAL DIAGNOSES

- *Liposarcoma:* It may have differentiated fat with MR showing high signal in T1-weighted image. Otherwise, the lesion shows low signal on T1-weighted image and high signal on T2-weighted images.
- *Other soft tissue sarcoma:* MR is nonspecific with usually low T1 and high T2 signal. Tumor may contain fat or become necrotic and bleed showing high signal on T1-weighted image.
- *Metastatic melanoma:* MR may show increased signal intensity on T1-weighted image and some decreased signal on T2-weighted image because of paramagnetic compounds within the lesion. It demonstrates intense contrast enhancement.
- *Hemangioma:* MR imaging shows variable amount of increased signal intensity in T1-weighted image from fat content and very high T2 signal from stagnant blood.

COMMENTS

This is an image of a 60-year-old male who presented with enlarging mass in the right shoulder. Malignant fibrous histiocytoma (MFH) accounts for 20% to 24% of soft tissue sarcomas, making it the most common soft tissue sarcoma occurring in late adult life. MFH occurs more commonly in Caucasians and men. The tumor peak incidence is in the fifth and sixth decades. MFH occurs most commonly in the extremities (70%–75%), followed by the retro peritoneum. Tumors are typically large arising in deep fascia or skeletal muscle but can occur anywhere. MFH usually present as enlarging, painless soft tissue mass that often cause pathologic fracture because of adjacent bony destruction. Prognosis is poor. MFH has been associated with hematopoietic diseases such as lymphoma, multiple myeloma, and malignant histiocytosis. MRI is the imaging method of choice and typically reveals an intramuscular mass with low T1-weighted, low to intermediate T2 signal from fibrous component, and intense contrast enhancement. Tumor margins appear relatively well defined on MR. A low signal intensity margin may be observed as pseudocapsule.

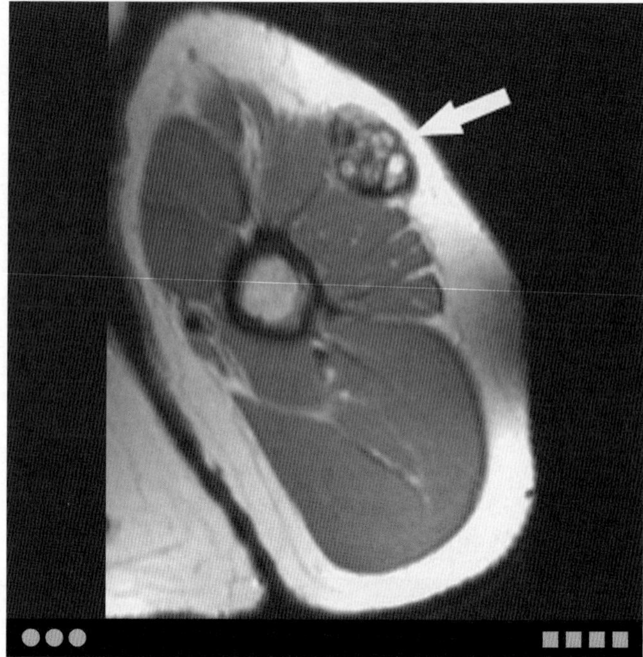

A. MFH: Axial T1-weighted image showing heterogeneous, subcutaneous mass (arrow) with high signal intensity on T1-weighted image in a case of MFH.

CT scan can provide adequate information regarding the location, calcification, and gross extent of the mass, although with less tissue contrast than MR. No single imaging technique can provide a specific diagnosis of MFH and biopsy is usually necessary. After biopsy of a potentially malignant soft tissue mass, the biopsy tract must be removed with the mass and orthopedic consultation for presurgical image-guided biopsy is recommended.

PEARLS

- **Enlarging soft tissue mass in an extremity of an otherwise healthy older patient is statistically likely to represent MFH.**
- **MR and CT scan findings are nonspecific. MR typically reveals an intramuscular mass with low T1 and low to intermediate T2-weighted signal.**
- **Many malignant and several benign soft tissue tumors may have imaging appearances identical to MFH.**
- **After biopsy of a potentially malignant soft tissue mass, the biopsy tract must be removed with the mass. Orthopedic consultation for presurgical image-guided biopsy is recommended to avoid more extensive surgery.**

ADDITIONAL IMAGE

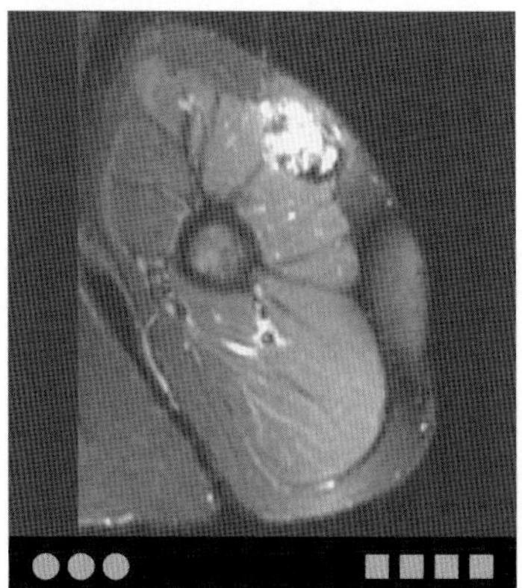

B. MFH: Axial postcontrast fat-saturated T1-weighted image shows intense, nonspecific enhancement of the mass.

DIFFERENTIAL DIAGNOSES IMAGES

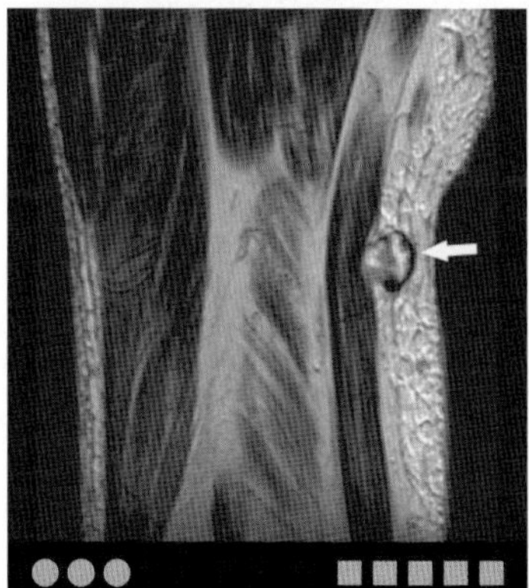

C. Metastatic melanoma: Sagittal T1-weighted image shows a small superficial mass (arrow) with areas of increased signal intensity because of paramagnetic compounds within this lesion consistent with metastatic melanoma.

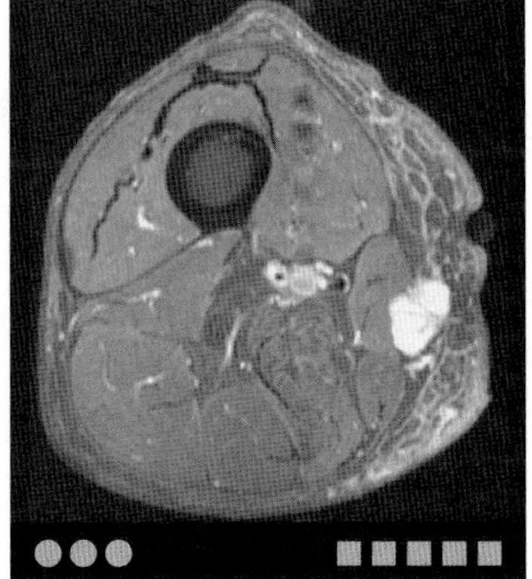

D. Metastatic melanoma: Axial fat-saturated postcontrast T1-weighted image showing intense contrast enhancement of this malignant metastatic melanoma lesion.

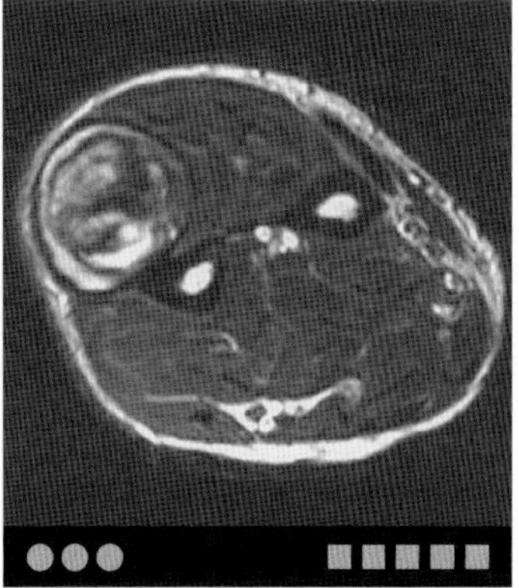

E. Liposarcoma: Axial T1-weighted image shows heterogeneous fat content soft tissue mass with scattered areas of nonfatty components demonstrating mixed increase and decrease signal in T1-weighted image consistent with liposarcoma.

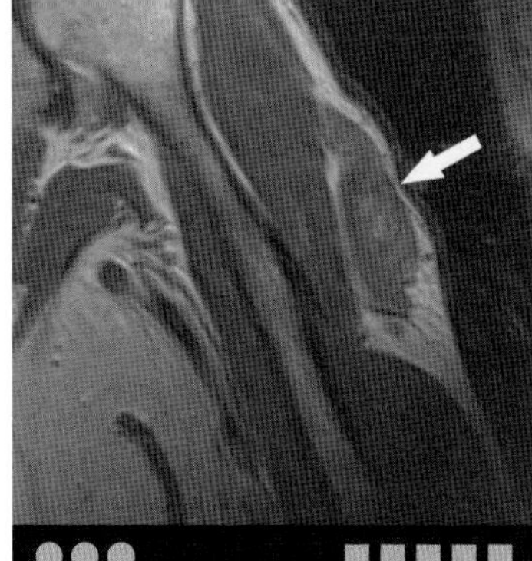

F. Soft tissue sarcoma: Coronal T1-weighted image shows soft tissue mass (arrow) slightly higher signal than muscle because of fat or blood without surrounding edema consistent with soft tissue sarcoma.

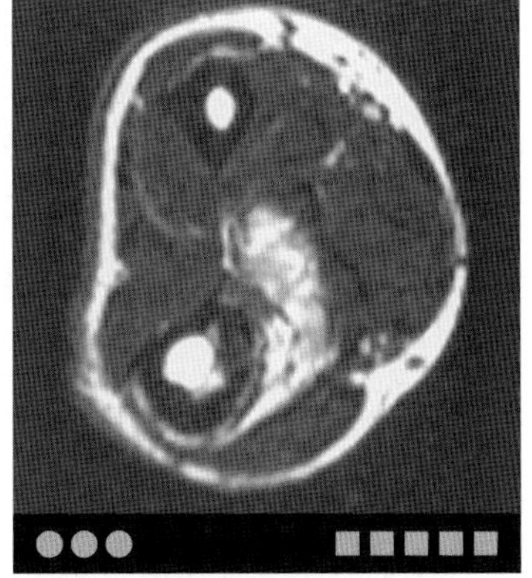

G. Hemangioma: Axial T2-weighted image shows intramuscular hemangioma with very high T2 signal from stagnant blood within the lesion. The lesion can have lobular margin with high T1 signal from fat content resembling our case

IMAGE KEY

Common

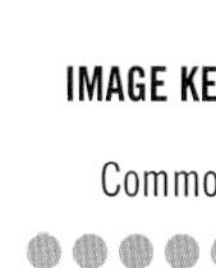

Rare

Typical

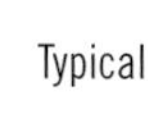

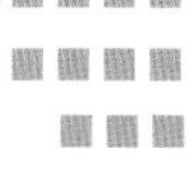

Unusual

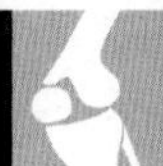

5–5 Rhabdomyosarcoma of the Bicep Muscle

Roy C. Kwak and Rajeev K. Varma

PRESENTATION

Enlarging upper arm mass

FINDINGS

MRI shows an enhancing soft tissue mass arising from the biceps muscle with areas of necrosis.

DIFFERENTIAL DIAGNOSES

- *Malignant fibrous histiocytoma:* This spindle cell neoplasm is the most common soft tissue sarcoma of late adult life. It can occur in any organ, but is most often found in the extremities.
- *Other pleomorphic sarcomas:* Dedifferentiated sarcomas have very similar imaging and histological characteristics. Immunohistochemical stains for desmin and myoglobin can help to differentiate the rhabdomyosarcoma.
- *Osseous or chondroid tumors:* These tumors are suggested by areas of calcification, which will show up on MR as signal voids on all pulse sequences.
- *Lymphoma:* A true primary lymphoma of the soft tissues is rare. Lymphoma is usually suggested by adjacent lymph node involvement or involvement of bony structures. Imaging characteristics is similar to other soft tissue tumors.

COMMENTS

This is an image of a 31-year-old female who presented with alveolar rhabdomyosarcoma arising from the right bicep. Rhabdomyosarcoma is the most common soft tissue malignancy of childhood and is classified into three types: embryonal, alveolar, and pleomorphic. The different subtypes can arise in any age and in any location, except the bone. The embryonal type is the most common, compromising 55% to 70% of cases. It usually arises in children during the first decade of life and is most commonly located in the head and neck region, especially the orbit. The botryoid subtype of embryonal rhabdomyosarcoma manifests as grapelike growths that arise from mucosal surfaces, often in the GU system. The alveolar type is common in adolescents and young adults. It often arises from skeletal muscle in the extremities. The pleomorphic type is uncommon and is seen in older adults. It may be difficult to differentiate from other sarcomatous tumors histologically and is often found in the large muscles of the extremities. Rhabdomyosarcoma metastasizes hematogenously usually to the lungs and

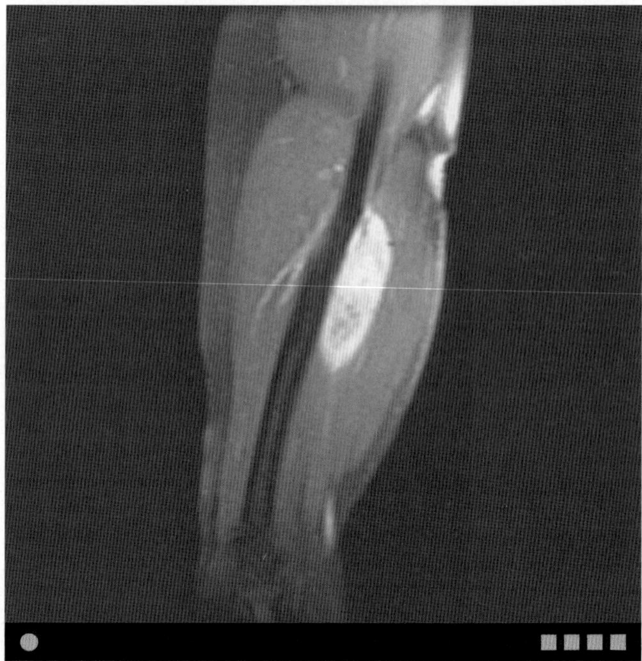

A. Rhabdomyosarcoma: Sagittal T1-weighted postcontrast image with fat saturation shows diffused enhancement.

pleura but also to the bone, bone marrow, liver, and lymph nodes. There is an increased incidence of rhabdomyosarcoma in patients with neurofibromatosis. The imaging features are not specific. As with other small round blue cell tumors, conventional radiograph may demonstrate soft tissue density with permeative bone destruction and expansile remodeling. MR usually shows a mass that is isointense to muscle on T1-weighted image and predominantly high signal on T2-weighted images.

PEARLS

- **It is the most common malignant soft tissue tumor in children.**
- **The embryonal type is the most common and is usually located in the head, neck, or genitourinary regions.**
- **The alveolar and pleomorphic types often arise in skeletal muscle.**
- **MR typically shows mass that is isointense to muscle on T1-weighted imaging and hyperintense on T2-weighted imaging; however, the imaging findings are not specific.**

ADDITIONAL IMAGES

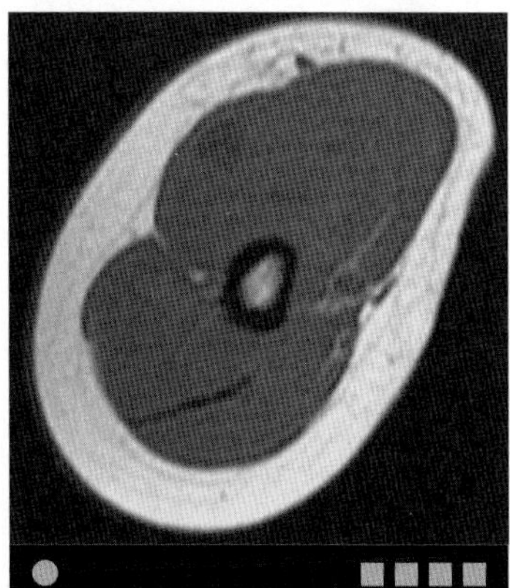

B. Rhabdomyosarcoma: Axial T1-wighted image shows a subtle, faintly heterogeneous, intramuscular mass with signal isointense to the muscle.

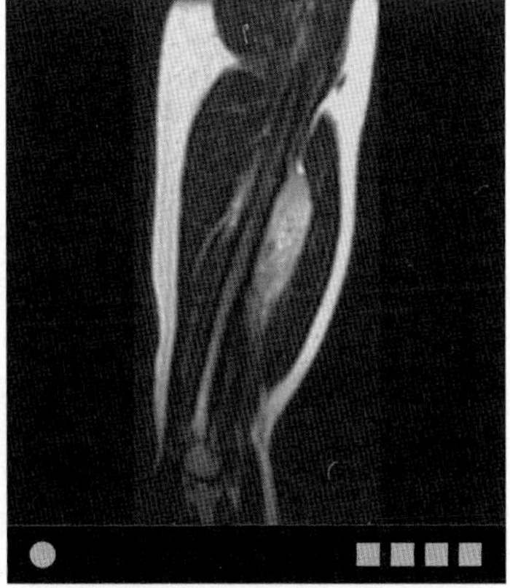

C. Rhabdomyosarcoma: Sagittal T2-weighted image shows an oval heterogeneous mass arising from the biceps muscle. It is adjacent to the humerus, but the cortex is intact.

DIFFERENTIAL DIAGNOSES IMAGES

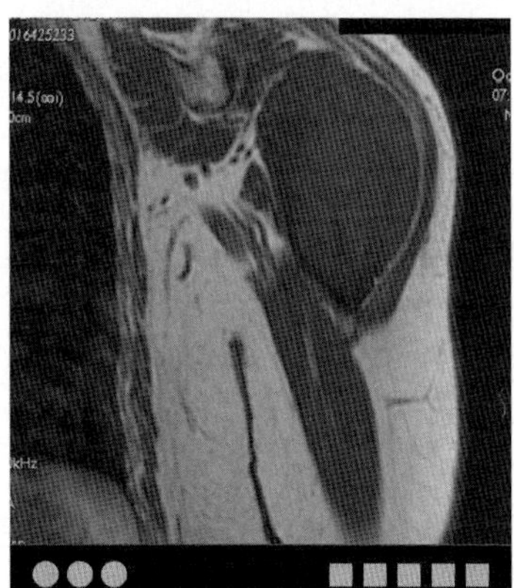

D. Osteosarcoma of humerus: Coronal T1-weighted image shows a mass isointense to muscle arising from left deltoid region.

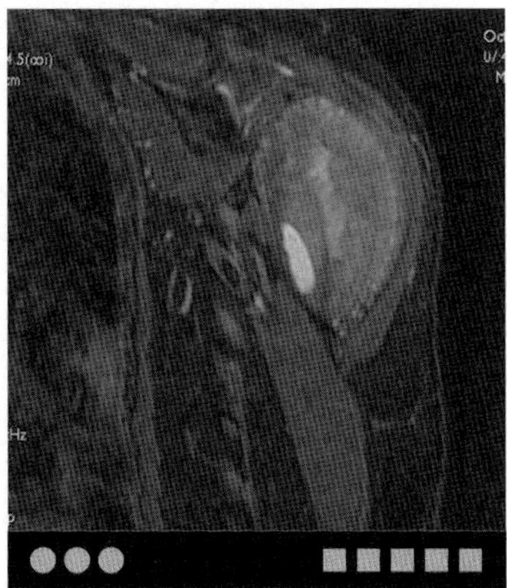

E. Osteosarcoma of humerus: A STIR image shows the mass more clearly as heterogeneously high signal with areas of necrosis.

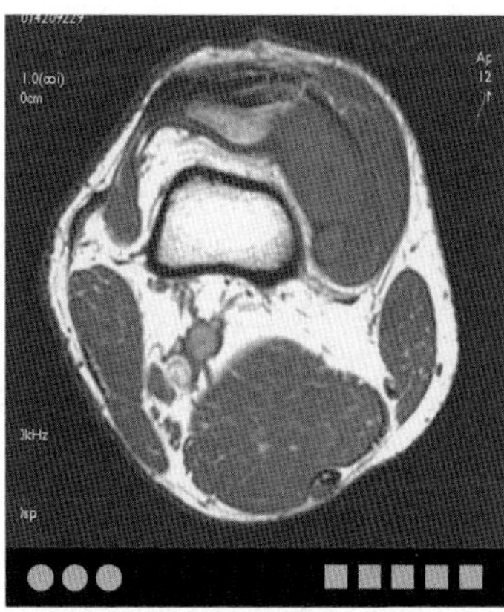

F. Malignant fibrous histiocytoma: Axial T1-weighted image shows a soft tissue mass isointense to muscle arising around the knee.

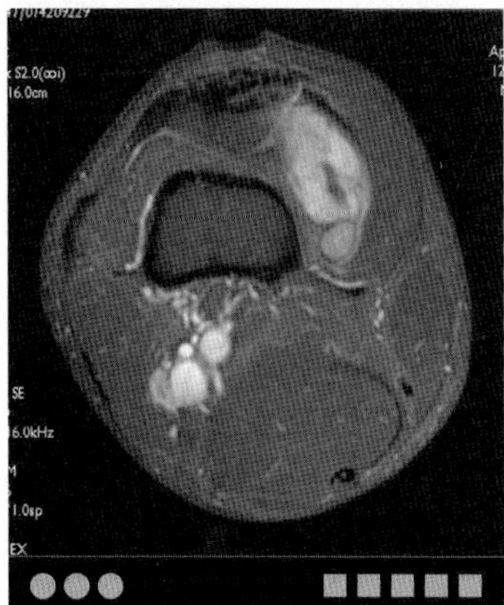

G. Malignant fibrous histiocytoma: Axial T1-weighted postcontrast image with fat saturation shows the enhancing mass more clearly.

IMAGE KEY

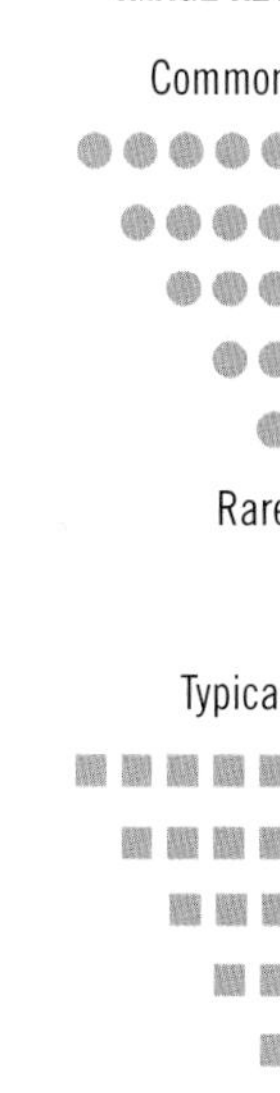

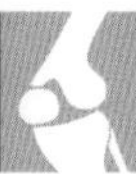

5–6 Malignant Peripheral Nerve Sheath Tumor of Shoulder

Janis Owen

PRESENTATION

Pain at rest, weakness, and a mass

FINDINGS

There is a heterogeneous septated mass in the region of the left brachial plexus that is low/intermediate signal on T1-weightedand high onT2-weighted sequences. There in enhancement of the lesion with gadolinium and an area of central necrosis.

DIFFERENTIAL DIAGNOSES

- *Benign peripheral nerve sheath tumor:* There is a low signal central area on T2-weighted sequences (target sign).
- *Pleomorphic sarcoma:* This may occasionally appear cystic on MRI. Generally, it is not associated with a large nerve.
- *Differentiated soft tissue sarcoma:* These are usually not associated with a large nerve.

COMMENTS

This is an image of a 88-year-old female who presented with a painful left supraclavicular mass. Malignant peripheral nerve sheath tumors involve major nerves in the body, particularly, the brachial plexus, sacral plexus, or sciatic nerve. They account for 10% of soft tissue neoplasms. The lesions may be sporadic; however, 50% are associated with neurofibromatosis-I (Von Recklinghausen's disease). Neurofibromatosis-1, also known as peripheral neurofibromatosis is characterized by café-au-lait spots, neurofibromas, and iris nodules (Lisch nodules). The neurofibromas in neurofibromatosis will undergo malignant degeneration on an average of 5%, with a range of 2% to 29%. The lesions associated with neurofibromatosis in 2% to 13% of patients may be multiple. Malignant peripheral nerve sheath tumors are usually diagnosed in the fourth decade, but occur in the third decade with neurofibromatosis. Malignant peripheral nerve sheath tumors are isointense to muscle on T1-weighted sequences, high on T2-weighted sequences, and enhance following gadolinium administration. Malignant peripheral nerve sheath tumors may be differentiated from its benign counterpart by the lack of a central low signal area on T2-weighted sequences (target sign). The tumor's association with major nerves may aid in differentiation from other soft tissue neoplasm. CT scan findings are not as specific; however, low attenuation areas, either central or peripheral, in a higher attenuation mass associated with a major nerve is suggestive of malignant degeneration.

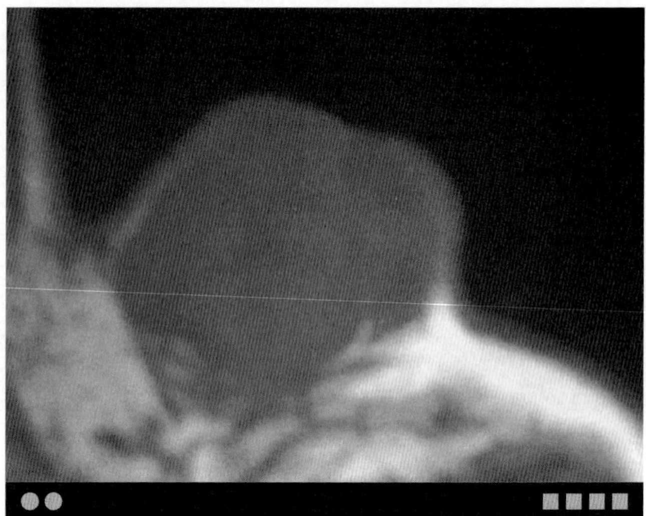

A. Malignant peripheral nerve sheath tumor: Coronal T1-weighted image shows a heterogeneous intermediate signal mass attached to the brachial plexus in the left supraclavicular region.

PEARLS

- **Associated with large nerves.**
- **No central low signal area (target sign) on MRI.**
- **Sporadic or associated with Neurofibromatosis-I (Von Recklinghausen's disease).**

ADDITIONAL IMAGES

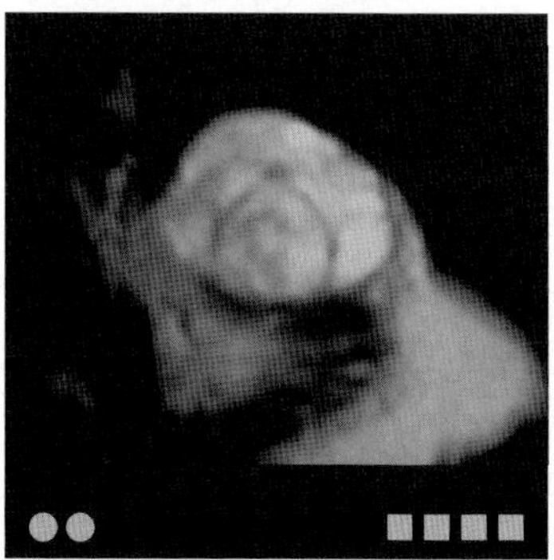

B. Malignant peripheral nerve sheath tumor: Coronal T2-weighted sequence shows the high signal mass with internal septations.

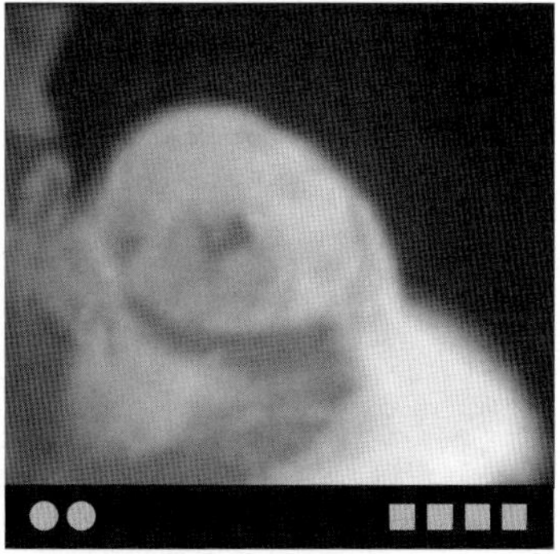

C. Malignant peripheral nerve sheath tumor: Coronal T1-weighted sequence postgadolinium shows enhancement of the lesion with an area of central necrosis.

DIFFERENTIAL DIAGNOSES IMAGES

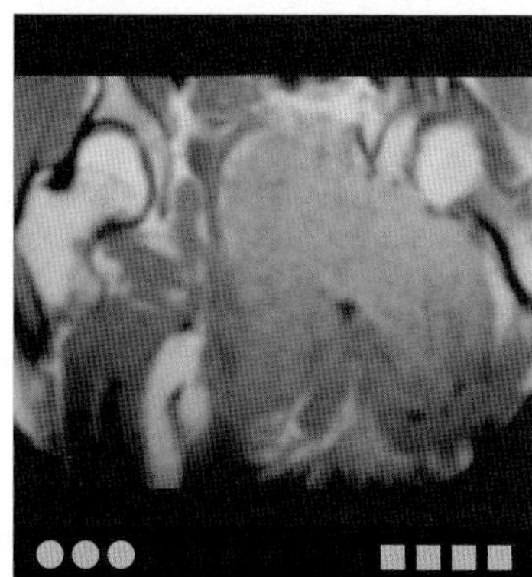

D. Benign peripheral nerve sheath tumor: Coronal T1-weighted sequence of pelvis shows a large intermediate signal mass within the left hemipelvis.

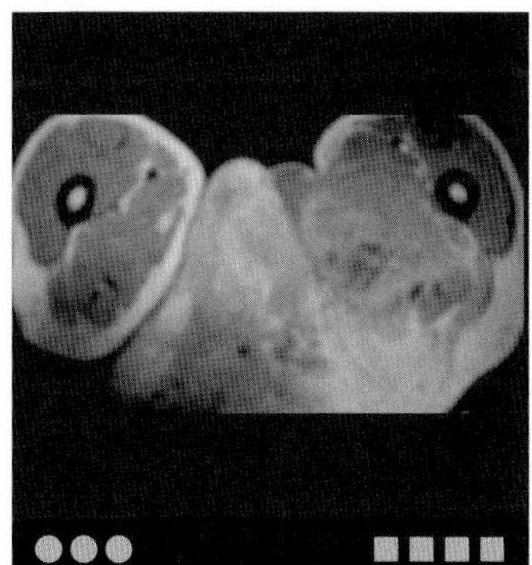

E. Benign peripheral nerve sheath tumor: Axial proton density sequence shows the intermediate/ high signal mass with central low signal areas (target sign).

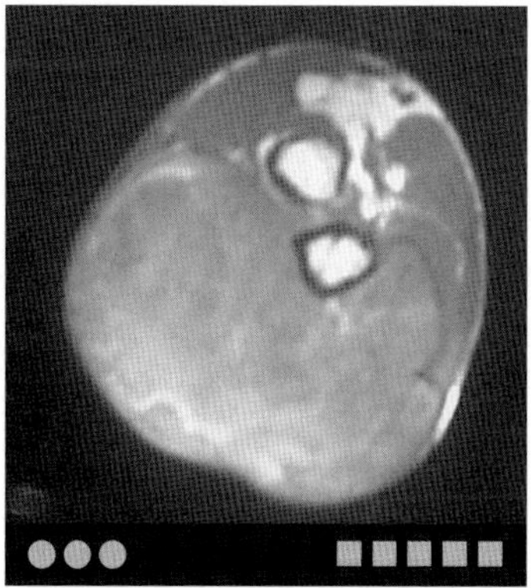

F. Malignant fibrous histiocytoma: Axial T1-weighted sequence of fore arm shows a heterogenous intermediate signal mass along the dorsal proximal forearm.

IMAGE KEY

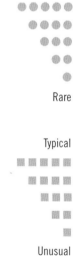

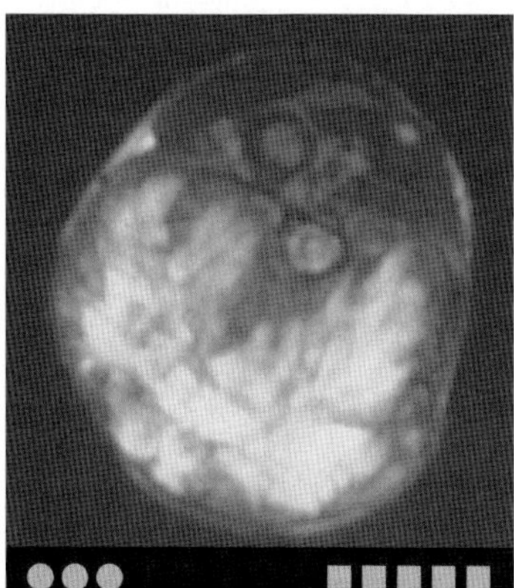

G. Malignant fibrous histiocytoma: Axial T2-weighted sequence of forearm shows the heterogenous high signal mass with central necrosis.

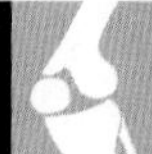

5–7 Elastofibroma Dorsi

Stefano Bianchi and Ibrahim F. Abdelwahab

PRESENTATION

Slightly tender soft tissue mass

FINDINGS

CT scan shows a well-circumscribed, crescentlike mass located between the serratus anterior muscle and the chest wall. The mass presents an internal striated appearance made by alternating hypodense and hyperdense stripes.

DIFFERENTIAL DIAGNOSES

- *Lipoma:* It presents in CT scan as a uniform hypodense mass with well-defined borders. No striated appearance is usually seen.
- *Rib tumors:* These are usually associated with local pain. CT scan would easily demonstrate local bone destruction.
- *Malignant fibrous histiocytoma:* CT scan exhibits a hypodense mass without any layered appearance. The attenuation is higher than fat.

COMMENTS

This is an image of a 68-year-old female who presented with a slightly tender, well-localized, slowly growing mass located adjacent to the inferior angle of the right scapula. Elastofibroma dorsi (ED) is a slowly growing tumorlike condition localized at the posterolateral aspect of the thoracic wall. It most frequently affects the elderly patients, with prevalence for females. It is usually bilateral and is commonly associated with hard manual work. Repeated mechanical friction between the tip of the scapula and the chest wall has been implicated in its pathogenesis. Some pathologic data suggest that it may result from fibroblasts with deranged elastogenesis. Pathology shows a peculiar appearance made by alternating stripes of fat and fibrous tissue. Most patients are asymptomatic and seek medical attention because of a mass. Sometimes, a slight local pain is present. At physical examination, a firm mass adherent to the chest wall is found and may suggest a tumor infiltrating the deep planes. Since ED does not contain internal calcifications, standard radiographs are normal or can rarely show an ill-defined soft tissue mass on tangential views. Ultrasound (US), CT scan, and MR can appreciate a lenticular mass adherent to the outer chest wall. All these modalities appreciate the peculiar multilayered internal structure of ED. CT scan and MRI allow a more panoramic evaluation compared with US and can simultaneously discover the presence of a contralateral lesion.

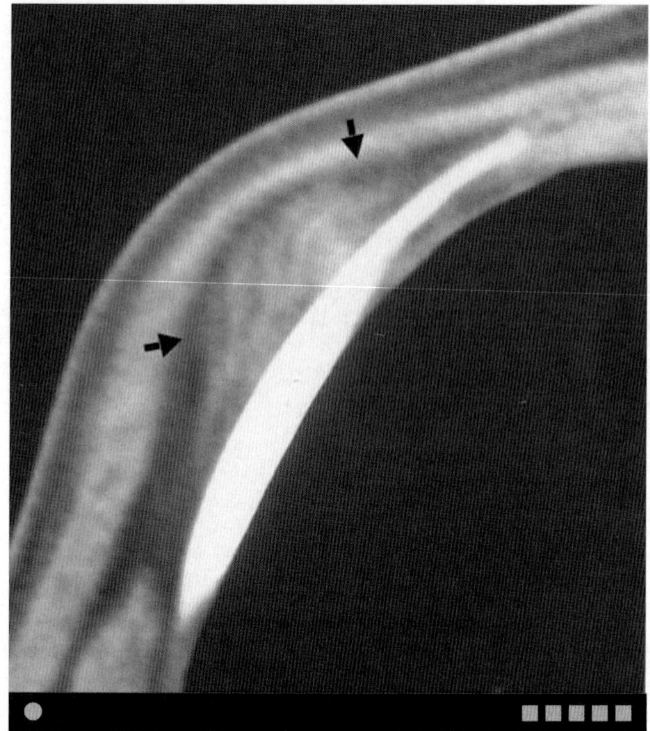

A. Elastofibroma dorsi: Axial CT scan image is obtained in the prone position. Image shows ED as a well-circumscribed, crescent lesion (arrows) located between a rib and the inferior aspect of the serratus anterior muscle. Note the typical internal striated appearance made by alternating hypo- and hyperdense stripes.

PEARLS

- **ED is a frequently bilateral benign condition affecting the posterolateral aspect of the chest wall. It presents a typical striated appearance made by alternating fat and fibrous tissue.**
- **Clinical appearance can suggest an aggressive condition.**
- **US, CT, and MRI can accurately detect ED and assess its peculiar internal multilayered texture.**
- **Imaging findings, particularly when the mass is bilateral, strongly suggest the diagnosis and can obviate the need for biopsy**

ADDITIONAL IMAGES

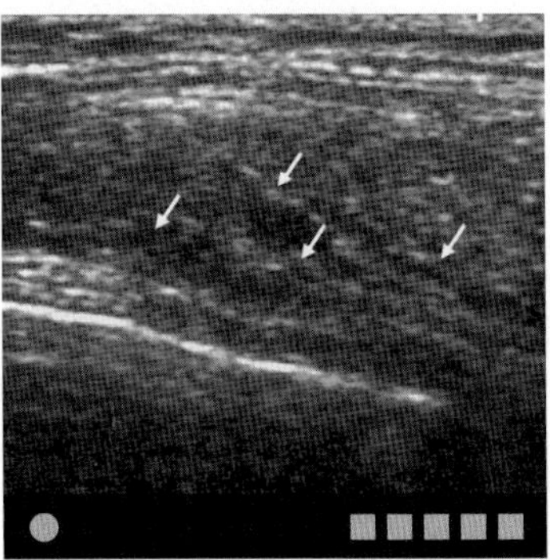

B. Elastofibroma dorsi: US axial image obtained in a patient with ED shows a mass containing internal striations (arrows) made by alternating hypo- and hyperechoic stripes.

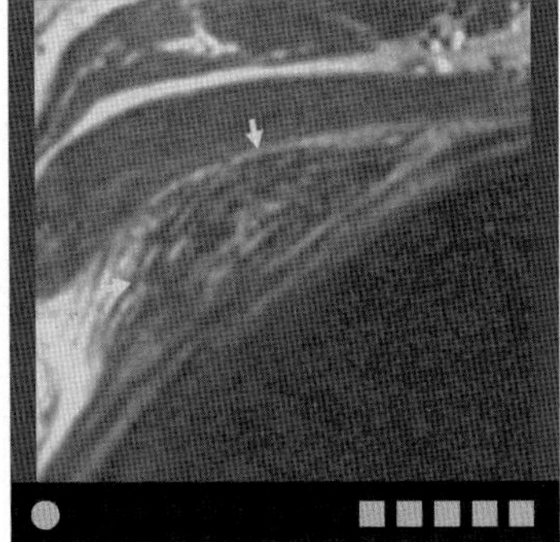

C. Elastofibroma dorsi: Axial T1-weighted MRI image obtained in a patient with ED shows a lenticular mass made by a bulk of hypointense fibrous tissue containing hyperintense fat stripes. Note the deep location of ED.

DIFFERENTIAL DIAGNOSES IMAGES

IMAGE KEY

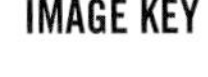

Common

Rare

Typical

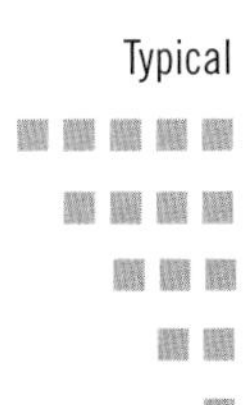

Unusual

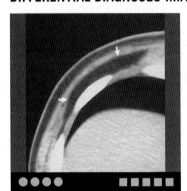

D. Chest wall lipoma: Axial CT scan image obtained at approximately the same level as image A shows a homogeneous, hypodense crescent lesion (arrows) located between the serratus anterior and the rib plane. The CT scan findings are typical of a lipoma.

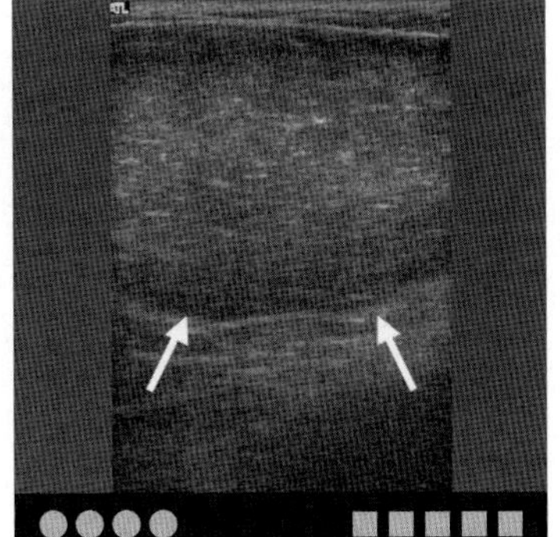

E. Subcutaneous lipoma: Axial US image demonstrates a homogeneous, hypoechoic, well-delineated mass (arrows) located inside the subcutis.

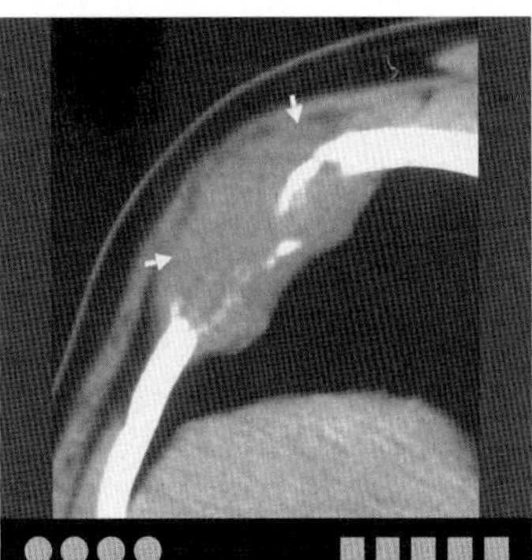

F. Chest wall metastasis: Axial CT image obtained at approximately the same level, then image A shows a hypodense mass (arrows) originating from the osteolytic lesion of a rib. The CT scan findings are typical of an osteolytic metastasis extending to the adja cent soft tissue.

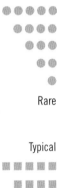

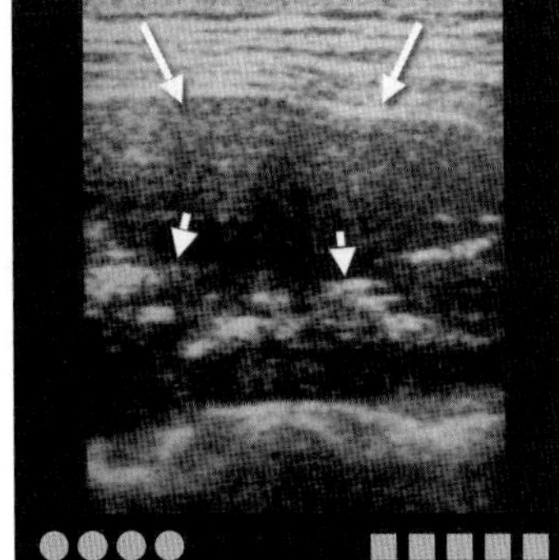

G. Chest wall metastasis: Axial US image obtained in the same patient of image F shows a hypoechoic mass (large arrows) originating from the osteolytic lesion of a rib (small arrows).

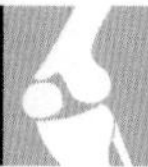

5–8 Chondroblastoma of the Humeral Head

Neerjana Doda and Wilfred CG Peh

PRESENTATION

Pain, tenderness, and limited joint movement

FINDINGS

Frontal radiograph shows a well-defined osteolytic lesion located in the epiphysis of the humeral head. CT scan confirms the epiphyseal location of this expanded lesion and further shows small punctate calcifications.

DIFFERENTIAL DIAGNOSES

- *Simple bone cyst:* Patients younger than 30 years. The lesion is usually metaphyseal in location and asymptomatic unless fractured. "Fallen Fragment sign" may be present and is diagnostic. Commonest sites are the proximal humerus and proximal femur.
- *Giant cell tumor:* Mature patients aged 20 to 40 years. At presentation, the lesion is expansile and larger in size. Typically subarticular in position and extends to the metaphysis with no matrix calcification.
- *Enchondroma*: This is an osteolytic often metaphyseal or metadiaphyseal in location with cartilaginous calcification.
- *Osteomyelitis:* Clinical features of infection are present and the lesion appears osteolytic with less well-defined and variable margins. In the case of brodie's abscess fuzzy, sclerotic margin fades to the normal bone.

COMMENTS

This is an image of a 16-year-old girl who complained of pain and limited range of movement in the right shoulder joint. Chondroblastoma, also known as Codman tumor is an uncommon, benign, cartilaginous tumor. It typically occurs in epiphyses or apophysis of a long bone and may straddle the growth plate. Approximately 90% affect patients aged between 5 to 25 years. The male to female ratio is 2:1. It is most commonly seen in epiphyses of long bones, especially the femur, humerus, and tibia (80%). Histologically, the presence of "chicken wire" appearance in the matrix of this lesion is diagnostic. Bones in the lower extremity are more commonly affected than those in the upper extremity. Affected patients present with pain, tenderness, and limited joint movement. Radiographs show a well-defined, ovoid or spherical, osteolytic lesion that is centrally or eccentrically located in an epiphysis or apophysis.

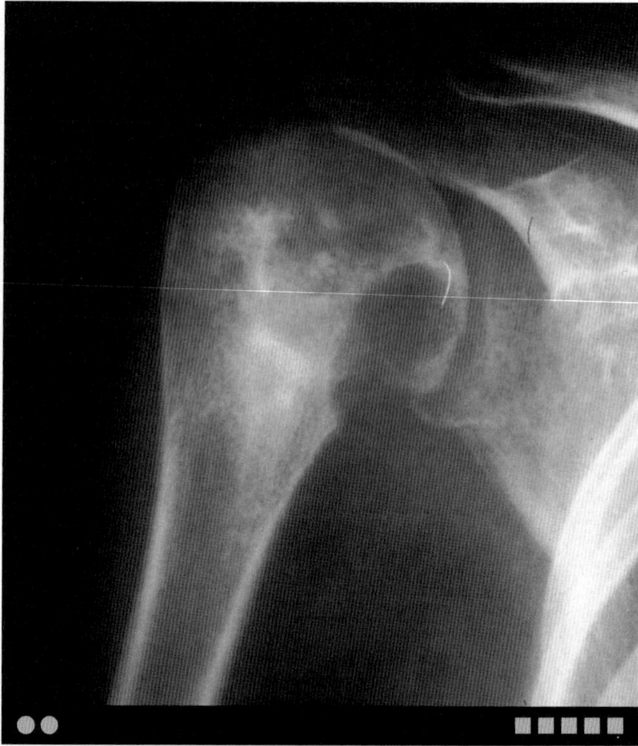

A. Chondroblastoma of the humeral head: Frontal radiograph shows an osteolytic lesion with well-defined borders. It is located in the humeral head epiphysis.

The lesion is usually bordered by the thin sclerotic rim. Lesion extension to subarticular bone and metaphyseal involvement are well-recognized. Thirty to fifty percent show central punctate or irregular calcification. Linear periosteal reaction in the adjacent metaphysis or diaphysis may also occur. CT scan is useful in assessing the extent, mineralization, and cortical integrity of the lesion. Soft tissue masses and pathologic fractures are rare. They may rarely become locally aggressive and may metastasize.

PEARLS

- **Site is characteristic—almost always occur in epiphyses or apophyses of a long bone.**
- **Age group is typical, affecting children and adolescents, mostly in the second decade of life.**
- **Well-defined osteolytic lesion, with thin sclerotic rim, which has matrix calcifications and often an intact cortical border.**

ADDITIONAL IMAGES

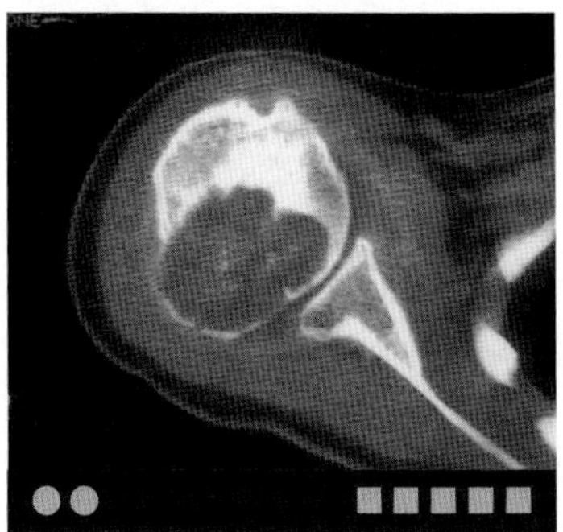

B. Chondroblastoma of the humeral head: Axial CT scan image shows an expanded osteolytic lesion in the posteromedial humeral head. It contains small punctate calcifications and has a thin, well-defined sclerotic rim. A small joint effusion is noted.

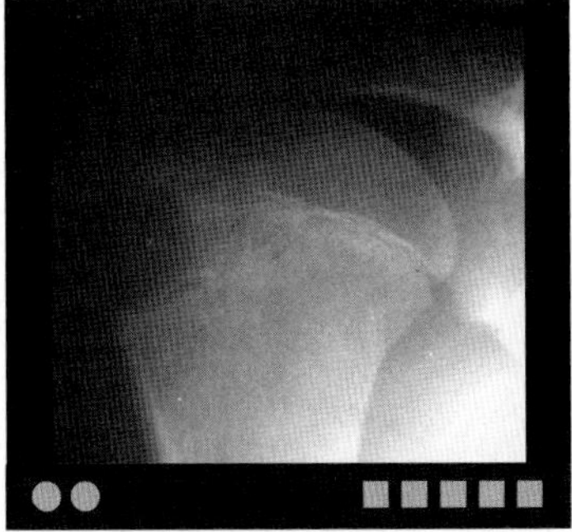

C. Chondroblastoma of the greater tuberosity: This is another image of a patient who is a 15-year-old boy. Frontal radiograph shows a rounded osteolytic lesion in the greater tuberosity apophysis.

DIFFERENTIAL DIAGNOSES IMAGES

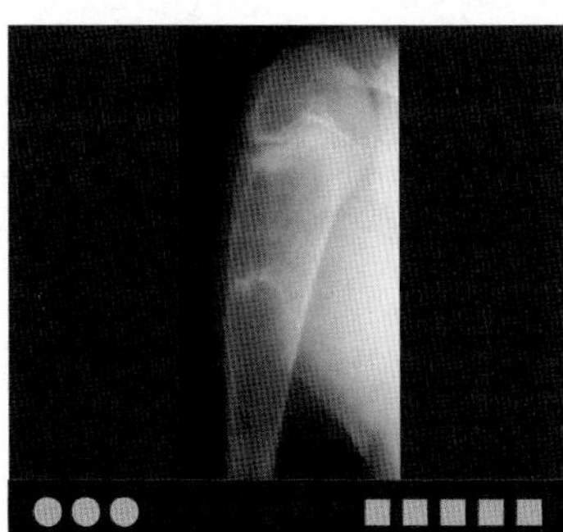

D. Simple bone cyst of the humerus: This is an image of a 14-year-old boy. Frontal radiograph shows a well-defined, slightly expanded, osteolytic lesion that is centrally located in the upper shaft of the humerus. Its upper border abuts the physeal plate.

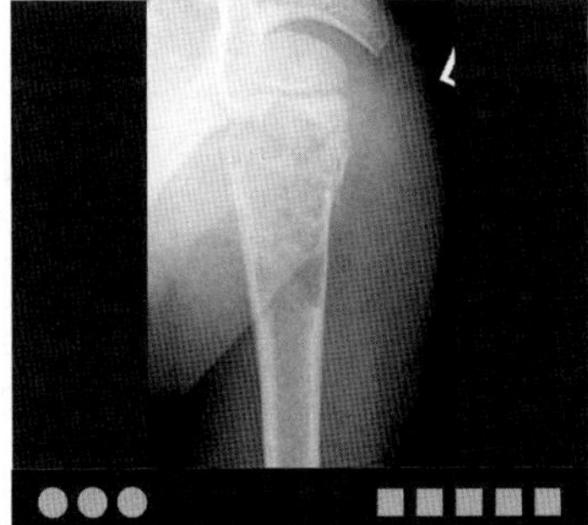

E. Simple bone cyst with fracture: Frontal radiograph of another patient's humerus shows a simple bone cyst complicated by a pathologic fracture in this 5-year-old boy.

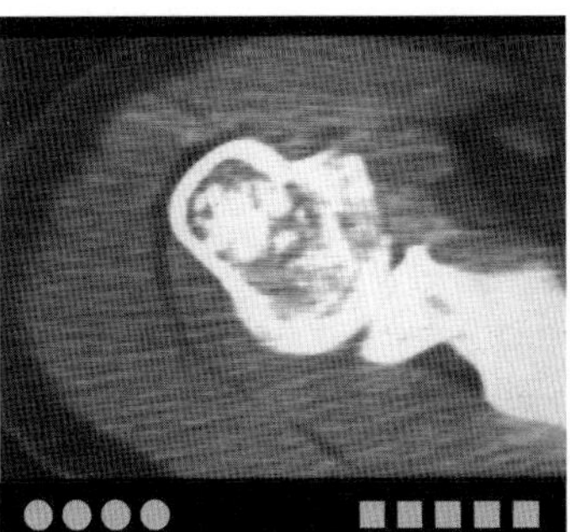

F. Enchondroma of proximal humerus: Axial CT scan of the humerus shows an osteolytic lesion of humeral metaphysis with central calcification and cortical erosion.

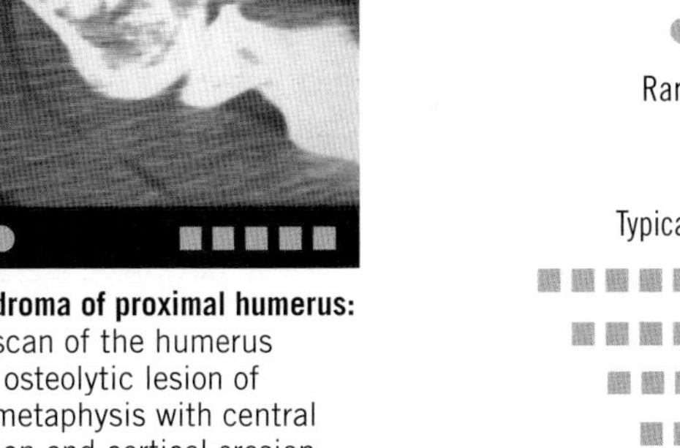

IMAGE KEY

Common

Rare

Typical

Unusual

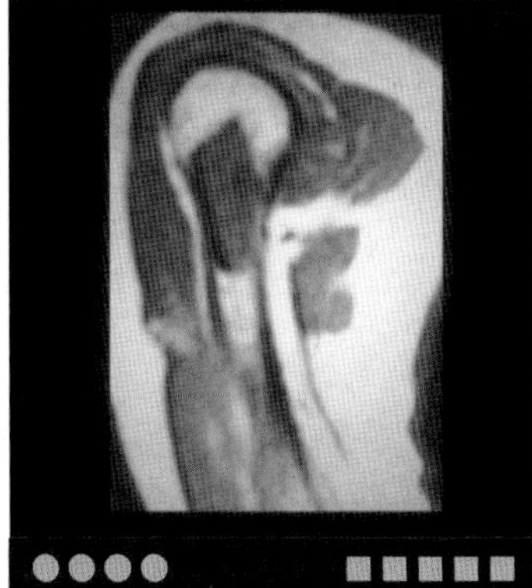

G. Enchondroma of proximal humerus: Sagittal T1-weighted MR image (same patient as in image F) shows a low signal intensity lesion of the proximal humerus.

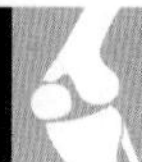

5–9 Enchondroma of the Humerus

Janis Owen

PRESENTATION

Asymptomatic, painless swelling, or pain

FINDINGS

There is a lobular intramedullary, lobular metaphyseal mass with endosteal scalloping. The mass is low/intermediate signal on T1-weighted sequences, high signal on the T2-weighted sequences with amorphus low signal mineralization. A satellite lesion is seen in the greater tuberosity of the humerus.

DIFFERENTIAL DIAGNOSES

- *Bone infract:* The mineralization occurs on the periphery of the lesion instead of occuring internally.
- *Fibrous dysplasia:* Ground-glass mineralization or thick sclerotic rim (rind sign) is seen.
- *Chondrosarcoma:* "Hot" lesion on bone scan is noted.

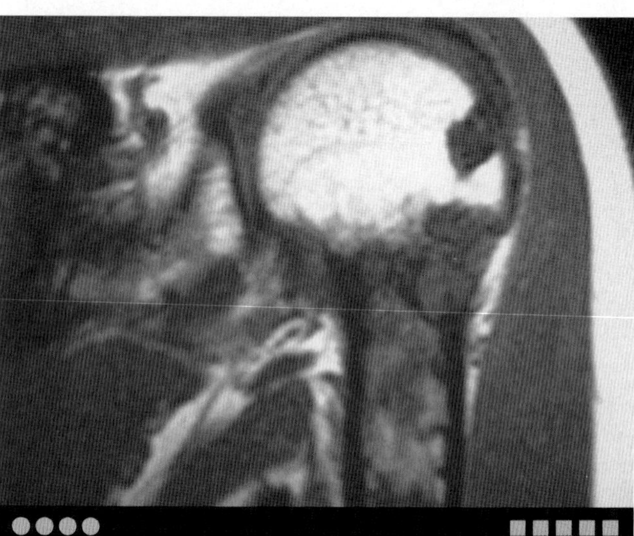

A. Enchondroma: Coronal T1-weighted sequence shows a low signal peripheral rim around an intermediate signal mass with internal low signal calcifications in the left proximal humerus. There is a satellite lesion seen in the greater tuberosity.

COMMENTS

This is an image of a 45-year-old female who presented with left shoulder pain. Enchondroma is a benign neoplasm of bone composed of lobules of hyaline cartilage. Enchondromas are usually asymptomatic or present as a painless swelling. It is a lytic intramedullary lesion with endosteal scalloping usually diagnosed in the third of fourth decade. Enchondromas are generally solitary (40%–60%) and occur in the hand, but may be multiple in syndromes such as Ollier's disease or Maffucci's syndrome. Twenty five percent of the lesions occur in long tubular bones. When they occur in small tubular bones, they are diaphyseal lesions. Those that occur in long bones are metaphyseal lesions. The lesions close to the axial skeleton (pelvis, hips, and shoulders) have a 2% to 3% risk of conversion to chondrosarcoma. The development of pain may be a sign of malignant transformation. Other signs of malignant transformation are change in size, development of a soft tissue mass, or change in the appearance of preexisting calcifications. On MRI, the lesions are lobular and frequently have satellite lesions. Enchondromas are low(intermediate signal on T1-weighted sequences and high signal on the T2-weighted or STIR sequences. The mineralized areas are low signal on all sequences. It may be difficult to differentiate enchondroma from low-grade chondrosarcoma on MRI. Enchondromas tend to be "warm" lesions on bone scintigraphy, whereas chondrosarcomas tend to be "hot" lesions. CT scan is beneficial for the assessment of the mineralized areas.

PEARLS

- **Geographic lobular mass with or without chondroid type mineralization and endosteal scalloping.**
- **Most common neoplasm of the hand.**
- **Diaphyseal in small tubular bones and metaphyseal in long tubular bones.**

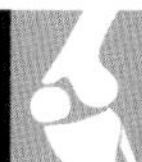

ADDITIONAL IMAGES

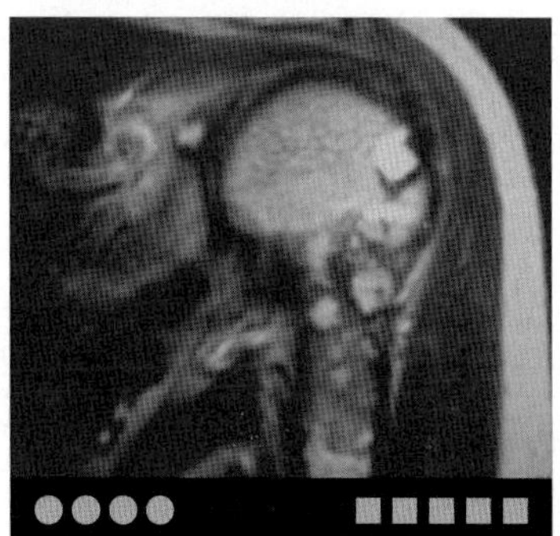

B. Enchondroma: Coronal T2-weighted sequence shows the high signal mass and the internal low signal calcifications.

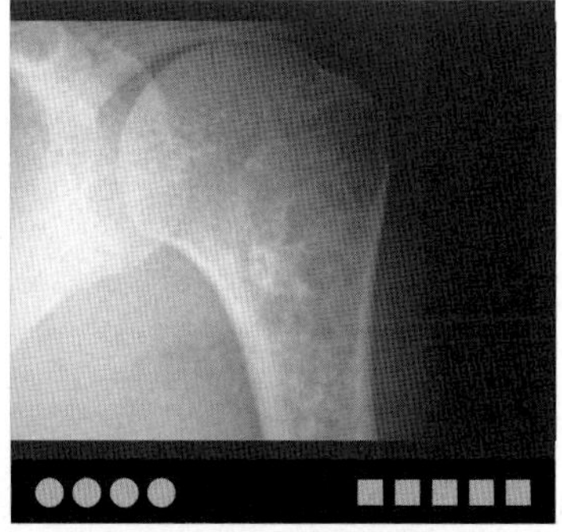

C. Enchondroma: AP radiograph of shoulder shows a geographic lytic lesion with internal chondroid calcifications.

DIFFERENTIAL DIAGNOSES IMAGES

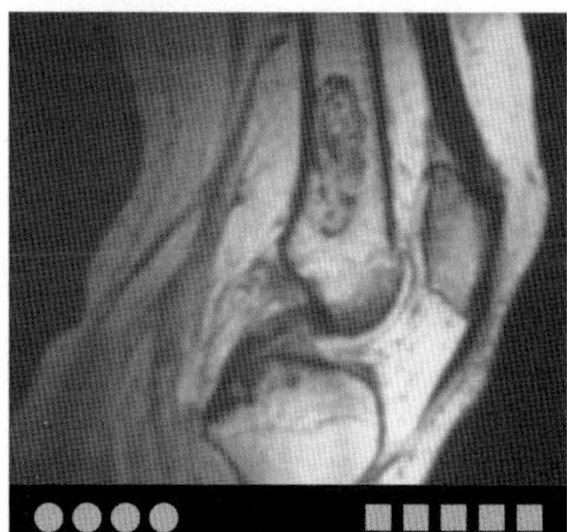

D. Bone infarct: Sagittal T2-weighted sequence shows a low signal peripheral rim around the intermediate signal bone marrow with internal low signal calcifications.

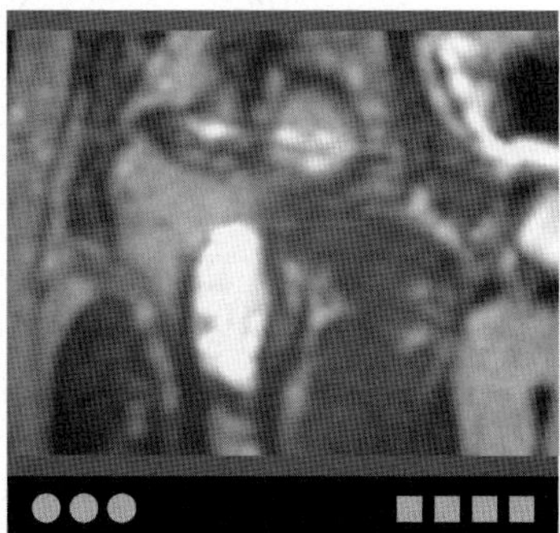

E. Fibrous dysplasia: Coronal T2-weighted sequence shows the high signal mass with internal low signal areas and the peripheral low signal rim.

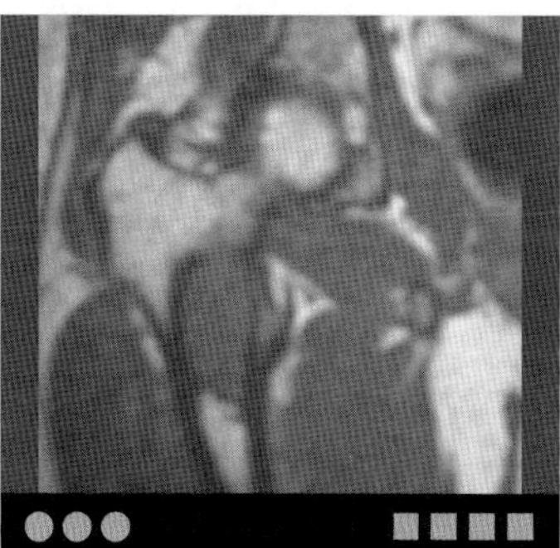

F. Fibrous dysplasia: Coronal T1-weighted sequence shows an intermediate signal mass and the peripheral low signal rim.

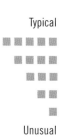

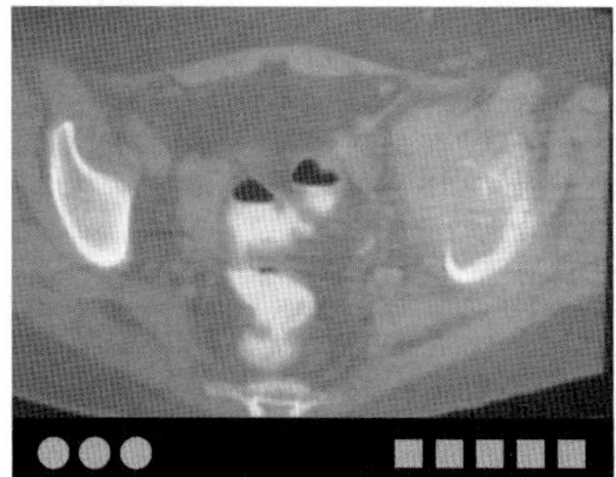

G. Chondrosarcoma: CT scan shows the isointense to muscle mass arising from the distal ilium with internal chondroid calcifications.

IMAGE KEY

Common

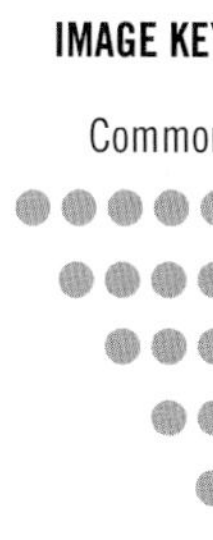

Rare

Typical

Unusual

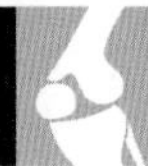

5–10 Chondrosarcoma of Proximal Humerus Arising in an Enchondroma

John C. Hunter

PRESENTATION

Shoulder pain

FINDINGS

An expansile lesion of the proximal humerus was noted with high intensity on T2-weighted images, low intensity on T1-weighted image with inhomogeneous enhancement on fat-saturated T1-weighted images postcontrast images. Cortical breakthrough was also noted.

DIFFERENTIAL DIAGNOSES

- *Benign enchondroma:* One would expect the benign version of this lesion to be well-defined with sharp margins and no cortical or soft tissue invasion. However, it is difficult on imaging criteria alone to exclude a low-grade chondrosarcoma in these lesions.
- *Metastatic lesion:* In this age group, metastatic tumor and myeloma must be considered. Typical "mini-brain" enhancement pattern, lobulated margins, and presence of typical calcification on radiograph makes these diagnoses unlikely.
- *Simple bone cyst/aneurysmal bone cyst:* While location is good for simple bone cyst, both the age and solid pattern of contrast enhancement would make poor choices.
- *Bone infarct:* Typical "serpigenous" margins, diaphyseal location, and history help to differentiate.
- *Chondroblastoma:* A lesion of an epiphysis or epiphyseal equivalent typically seen in the first two decades of life.

COMMENTS

This is an image of a 53-year-old female with shoulder pain who represented a degeneration of a benign enchondroma into a chondrosarcoma. Enchondromas are benign lesions composed of lobules of hyaline cartilage. They are metaphyseal lesions, centrally located, and frequently seen in the long bones. The small bones of the hands and feet account for more than 50% of lesions. Male and female incidence are equal, and patients are typically in the third or fourth decade. Radiographs show a lytic, at times expansile lesion with frequent cartilaginous calcification consisting of rings and arcs. Mild endosteal scalloping is often noted and characteristic. The lesions in the hands and feet frequently lack calcification. Enhancing pattern of the rings and arcs on MRI, no doubt accounts for the designation by Health and Environment Library Modules as the mini brain pattern with enhanced images resembling the gyri and sulci seen on fluid sensitive images of the cerebral cortex. When presents, the cartilaginous matrix is characteristic for a cartilage lesion. However, the common problem is to distinguish enchondroma from low-grade chondrosarcoma. This can be difficult on imaging and on histologic examination. Central lesions are more likely to undergo malignant transformation, while the lesions of the hands and feet rarely do so. Features suggesting malignancy on imaging include cortical breakthrough, soft tissue mass, soft tissue hyperintensity or enhancement, and the "two-thirds" rule (scalloping of greater than two-third of the cortical thickness, scalloping spanning greater than two-third of the length of the lesion, and matrix calcification in less than two-third of the lesion).

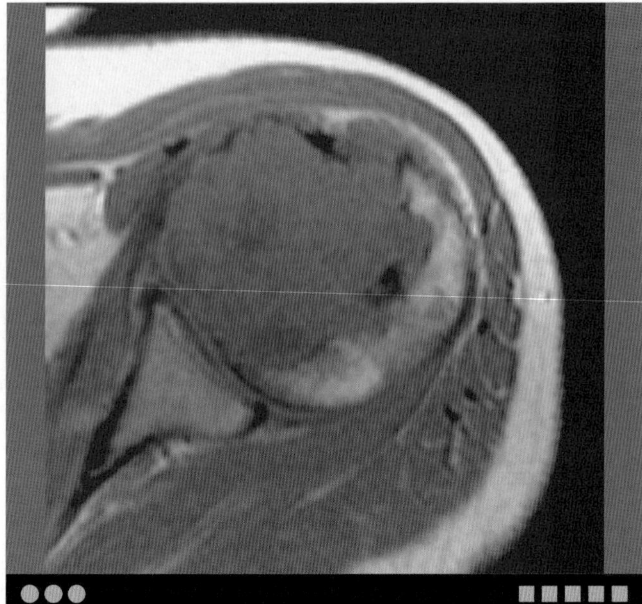

A. Chondrosarcoma arising in an enchondroma: Axial T1-weighted image shows low signal intensity mass of proximal humeral head.

PEARLS

- **Enchondromas and low-grade chondrosarcomas may be difficult to differentiate.**
- **More aggressive lesions tend to be seen in long bones; in the axial skeleton, such lesions may show cortical breakthrough and soft tissue masses.**
- **Pain is a worrisome symptom when following an apparent benign enchondroma and should prompt a work-up to rule out malignant transformation.**
- **Many painful joints with incidental enchondromas nearby turn out to be secondary to the usual internal derangements rather than malignant transformation.**

ADDITIONAL IMAGES

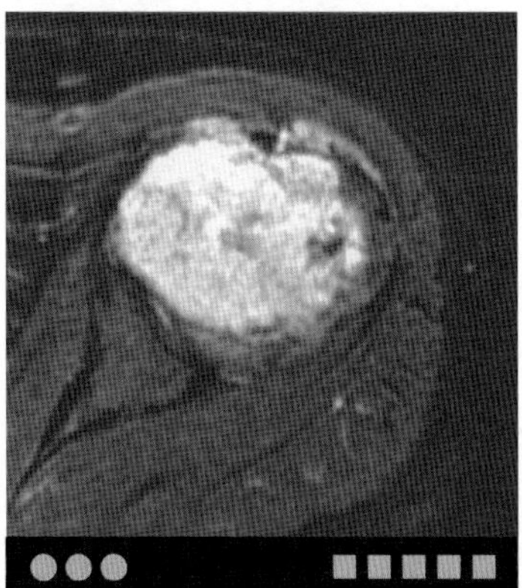

B. Chondrosarcoma arising in an enchondroma: Axial STIR image shows the boarders are scalloped with zones of low intensity representing calcium.

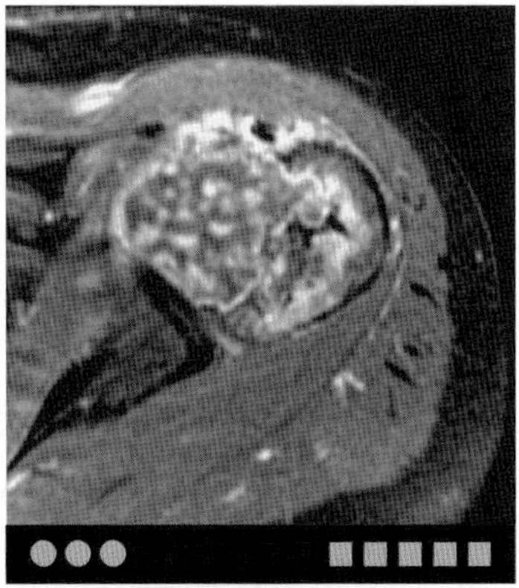

C. Chondrosarcoma arising in an enchondroma: Axial FS T1-weighted postcontrast image demonstrates the mini-brain enhancement pattern. Cortic breakthrough is noted on all images (arrows).

DIFFERENTIAL DIAGNOSES IMAGES

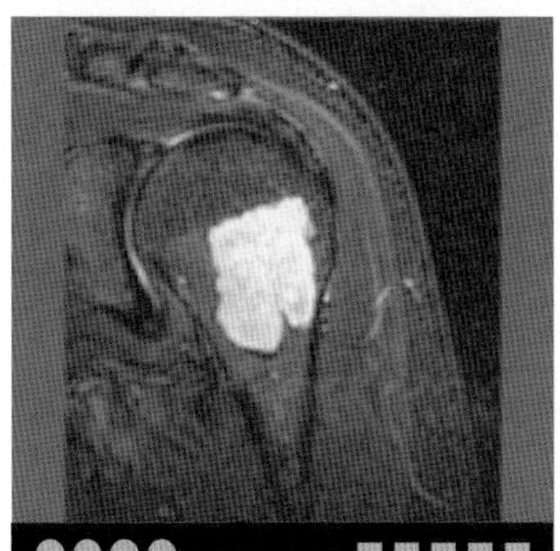

D. Benign enchondroma: Coronal STIR image in this 43-year-old man shows a high signal, well-defined lobulated lesion in the proximal humerus.

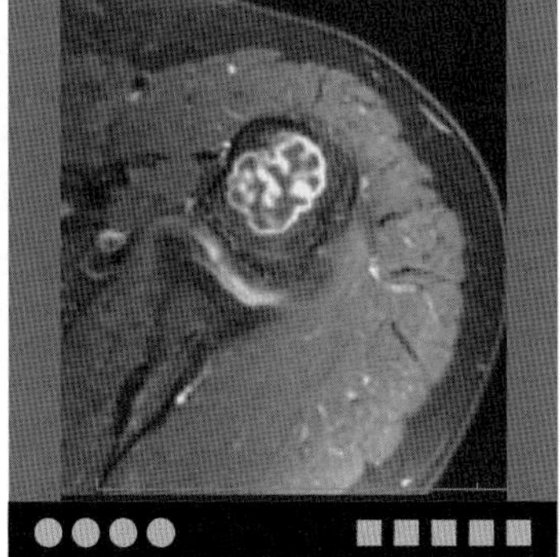

E. Benign enchondroma: Axial fat-saturated T1-weighted images postcontrast (same patient as in image D) showing mini-brain pattern of enhancement.

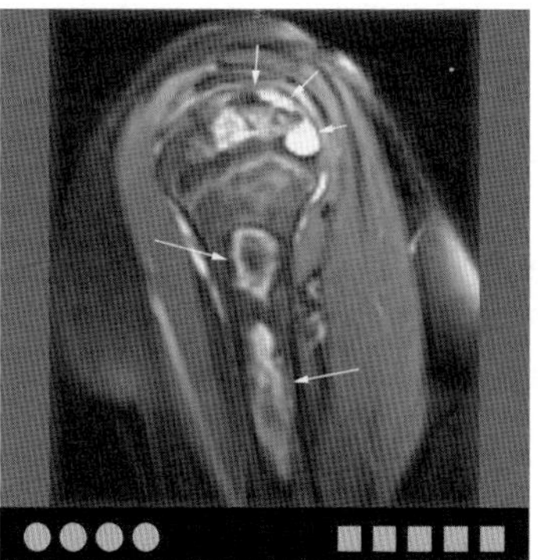

F. Bone infarct: This image shows a 13-year-old boy with acute lymphocytic leukemia. T2-weighted sagittal image with fat saturation demonstrates avascular necrosis of the humeral head and bone infarcts of the proximal humeral diaphysis (arrows).

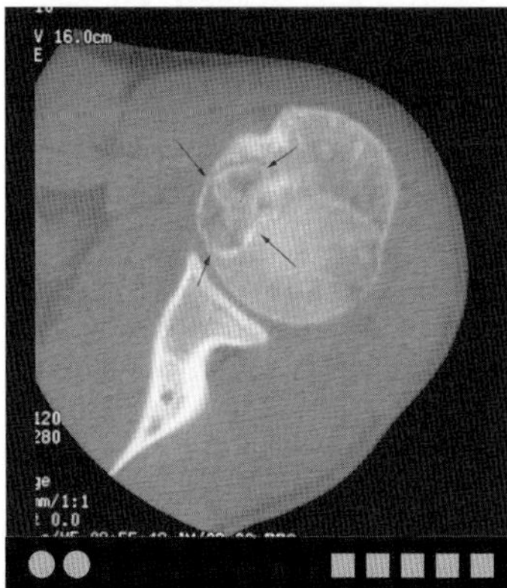

G. Chondroblastoma: This is an image of a 18-year-old male with incidentally noted lesion. Axial CT scan demonstrates a well-defined lytic lesion with central calcification in an epiphyseal equivalent of the lesser tuberosity of the humerus (arrows).

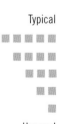

IMAGE KEY

Common

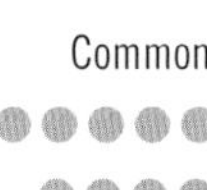

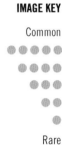

Rare

Typical

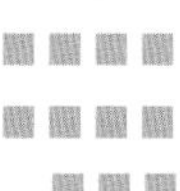

Unusual

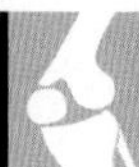

5–11 Lymphoma of Shoulder

Peyman Borghei and Jamshid Tehranzadeh

PRESENTATION

Shoulder pain

FINDINGS

MRI shows large lesions of the humeral head because of marrow infiltration with joint fluid and soft tissue mass.

DIFFERENTIAL DIAGNOSES

- *Metastatic disease:* It is very hard to distinguish from lymphoma, although it tends to be more destructive with less soft tissue mass.
- *Giant cell tumor:* This lesion often starts in epiphysis or subchondral area of long bones in adults and extends to metaphysis and is mostly solitary.
- *Other round cell tumors such as plasma cell cytoma or myeloma:* These are expansile osteolytic lesions with cortical destruction.
- *Osteomyelitis:* Presents with soft tissue inflammation and edema with clinical setting of fever, redness, high erythrocyte sedimentation rate, and leukocytosis.

COMMENTS

This is an image of a 19-year-old female diagnosed with non-Hodgkin B-cell lymphoma of left humeral head. Bone marrow involvement in lymphoma is microscopically identical to its nodal counterpart, but presents as bone mass. Histologically, most of these lesions represent non-Hodgkin lymphoma (NHL). The majority of primary bone lymphomas fall into the category of diffuse large B-cell type with mixed small and large cells, while follicular lymphomas are very unusual. In the literature there are several reports presenting trauma-related bone lymphomas, possibly because of an inflammatory response eventually leading to local carcinogenesis. Primary lymphoma of bone most often involves the diametaphysis of major long bones and has an aggressive pattern of osteolytic destruction with soft tissue mass. CT scan and MR imaging can suggest the diagnosis, particularly when a large soft tissue mass and abnormal marrow attenuation or signal intensity is seen without extensive cortical destruction. Common appearances are osteolytic (70%) or mixed density (28%) with most cases showing a permeative or moth-eaten pattern (74%), which is the hallmark of the round cell tumors. Periosteal reaction is also reported in half of the involved bones. The lesion usually manifests hypointense on T1-weighted and hyperintense on T2-weighted images, while inhomogeneity of the lesion is noted on all sequences. STIR sequence is more sensitive than T2-weighted images in discriminating the lesion from red marrow.

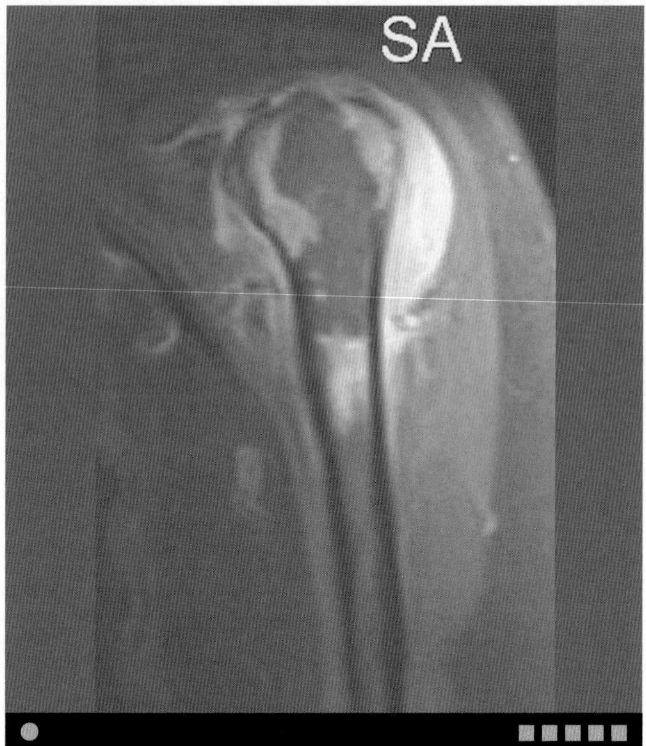

A. Lymphoma: Coronal fat-saturated T1-weighted image postcontrast shows focal areas of bright marrow enhancement in proximal humerus. Note homogeneous circumferential enhancing soft tissue mass.

PEARLS

- **Bone marrow lymphoma mostly involves the diaphysis and metaphysis of a major long bone.**
- **It usually has a permeative, moth-eaten pattern presenting with osteolytic destruction.**
- **Presence of soft tissue mass with abnormal marrow signal, without major cortical destruction favors the diagnosis**
- **MRI of osseous lymphoma presents low signal intensity on T1-weighted and usually high signal intensity on T2-weighted images.**

ADDITIONAL IMAGES

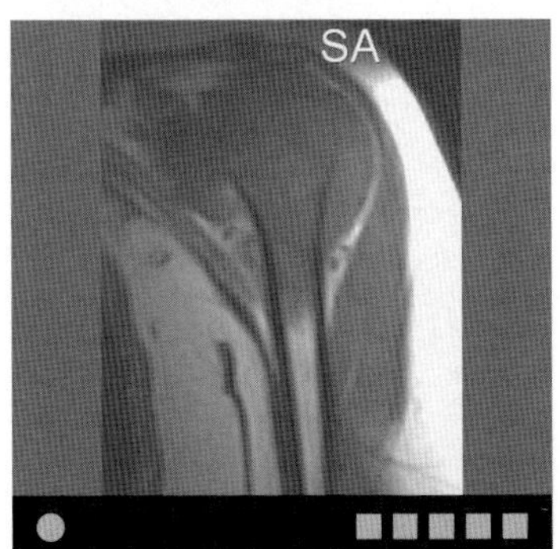

B. Lymphoma: Coronal T1-weighted image of the left shoulder shows low signal intensity lesion of proximal humerus with soft tissue mass, with possible involvement of glenoid process.

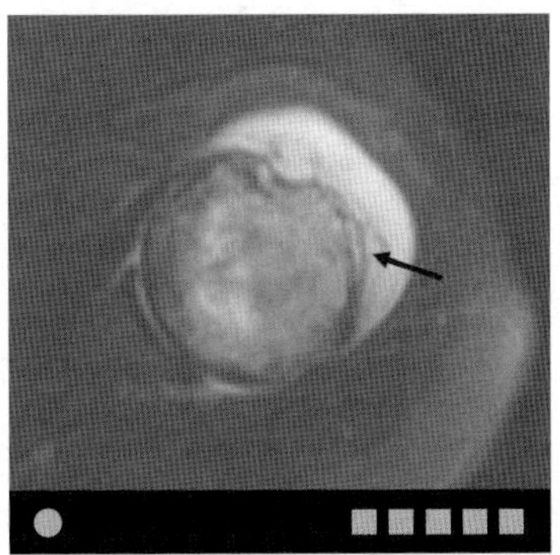

C. Lymphoma: Axial fat-saturated T2-weighted image shows intermediate to high signal intensity lesion in bone marrow and high signal intensity soft tissue mass. Note periosteal elevation at humeral head (arrow).

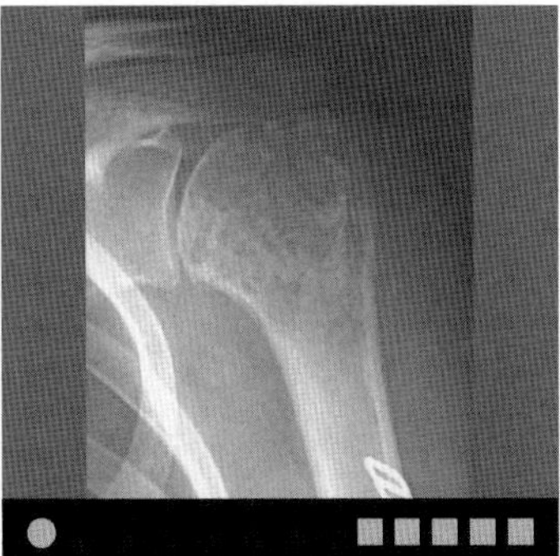

D. Lymphoma: Frontal view of the left shoulder shows permeative moth-eaten osteolytic lesion. Note wide zone of transition of the lesion in the humeral head with nondisplaced greater tuberosity fracture.

E. Lymphoma: Bone scintigraphy shows multiple areas of increased uptake of radiotracer in the left side of the skull, left proximal humerus, right hip including acetabulum and femur, distal half of the left femur, and left side of S1 vertebrae.

DIFFERENTIAL DIAGNOSES IMAGES

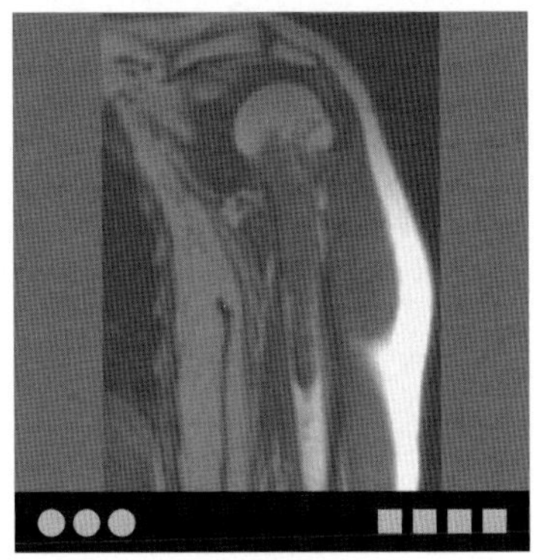

F. Metastatic melanoma: Coronal T1-weighted image shows low signal intensity intramedullary lesion consistent with metastasis.

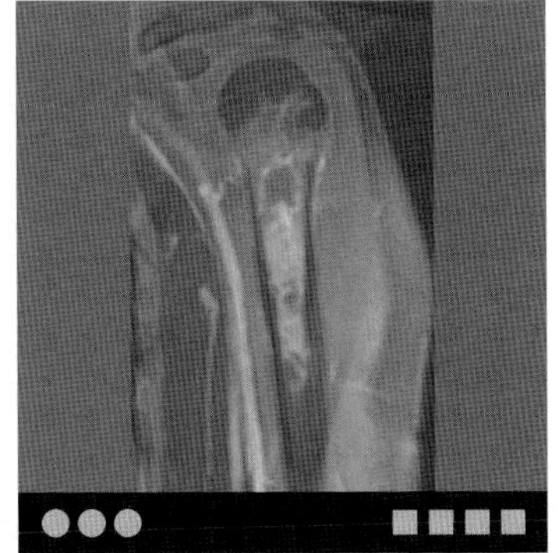

G. Metastatic melanoma: Coronal postcontrast fat-saturated T1-weighted image shows heterogeneous contrast enhancement of the metastatic lesion.

IMAGE KEY

Common

Rare

Typical

Unusual

Chapter 6

Miscellaneous

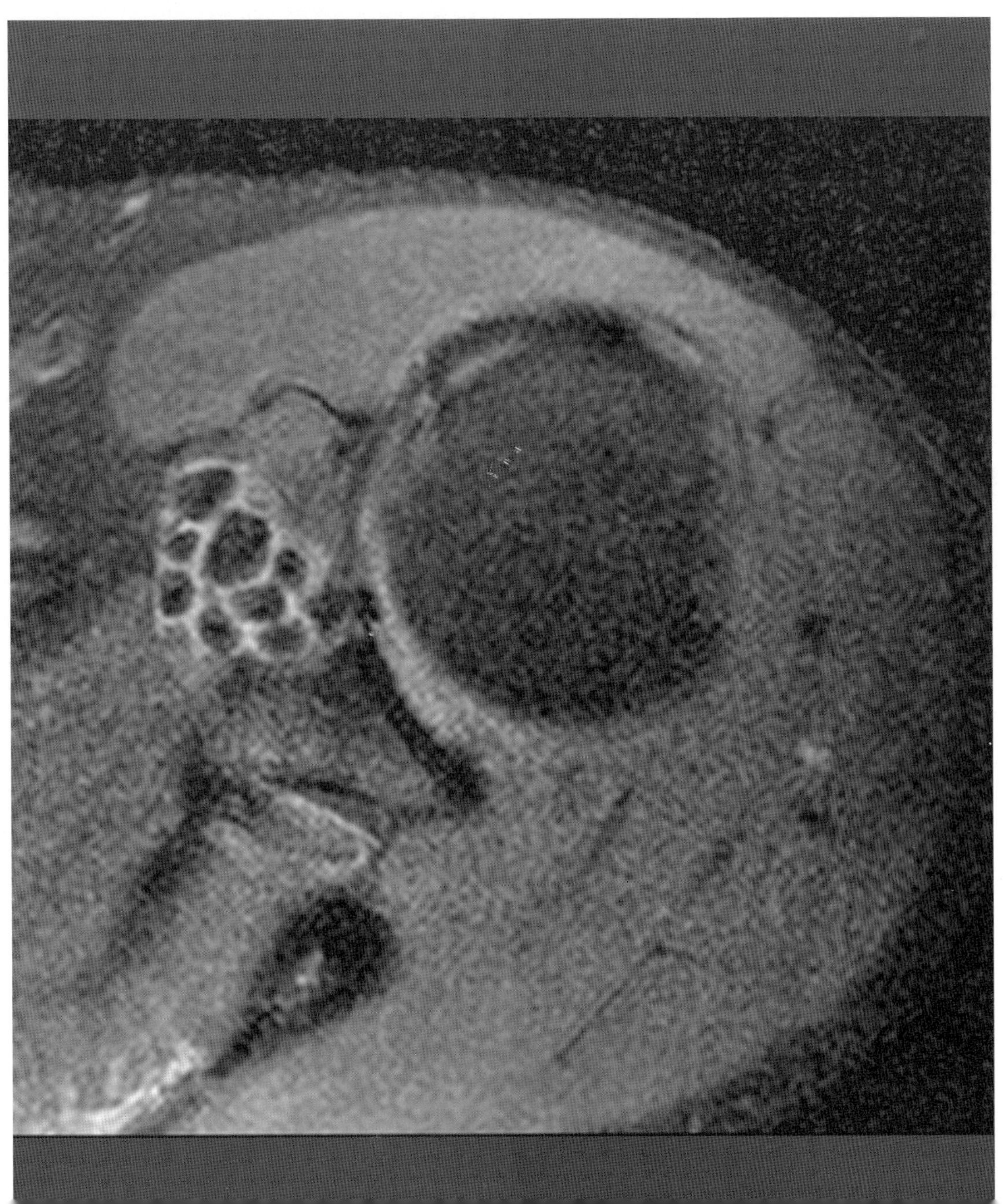

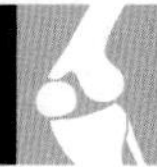

6–1 Synovial Osteochondromatosis of the Shoulder

Michael A. Bruno

PRESENTATION

Longstanding pain and limited range of motion

FINDINGS

MRI shows the characteristic appearance of synovial osteochondromatosis in the subscapularis bursa.

DIFFERENTIAL DIAGNOSES

- *Rheumatoid arthritis:* Synovial proliferation and expansion with the presence of rice bodies may mimic this condition.
- *Pigmented villonodular synovitis (PVNS):* This condition is associated with synovial villi with hemosiderin deposits and has low signal in all MR sequences.
- *Chondrosarcoma:* This condition whether arising from bone or joint has more aggressive features.
- *Osteopoikilosis:* This is associated with multiple bone islands around the joint. No bone island in joint or soft tissues is noted.

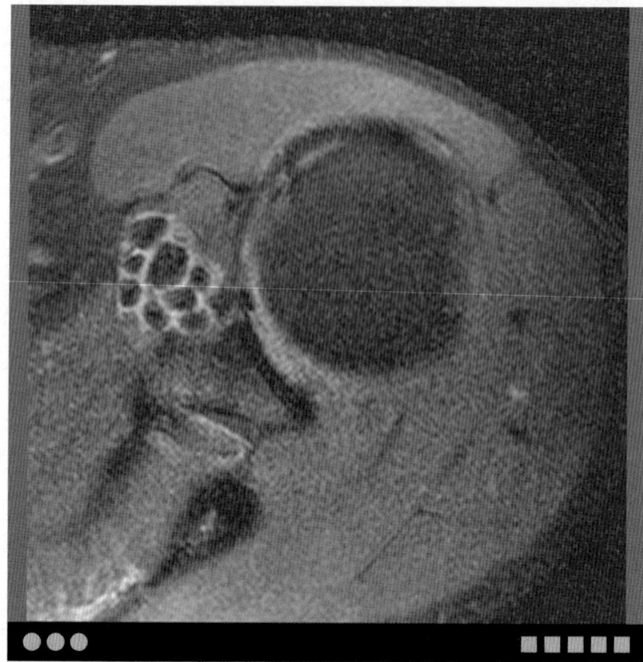

A. Synovial osteochondromatosis: Axial T2-weighted MRI image shows characteristic appearance of the lesion. Note dark signal (caused by calcification) of the loose bodies, their characteristic shape, and their apparent immersion in bright signal joint fluid within the subscapularis bursa.

COMMENTS

This patient presented with the classic appearance of synovial osteochondromatosis in the subscapularis bursa, as shown on MRI. There was no antecedent imaging. Synovial osteochondromatosis may appear in two forms: The primary form having characteristic appearance, with longstanding calcified osteochondral loose bodies with a faceted or squared-off appearance within the bursa or joint capsule, and the secondary form, which is seen as the result of osteoarthrosis. The primary type is a benign condition felt to occur as a result of benign synovial metaplasia. The degree of calcification is variable, the size of the loose bodies may be variable, and the number of these loose bodies are often numerous. These loose bodies themselves are essentially free within the joint or bursal cavity, where they tend to grind against one another and produce the characteristic appearance. This condition is easily differentiated from PVNS by its appearance and signal characteristics on MRI. The appearance is pathognomonic. The presence of pressure erosion is quite common in this benign condition and should not create any warning for malignancy. Malignant degeneration to chondrosarcoma is extremely unusual. Early osteoarthritis may be associated in joint hosting synovial osteochondromatosis. Longstanding loose bodies in the joint result in synovial expansion of the joint capsule leading to dissection of the joint into the adjacent soft tissues.

PEARLS

- **Male-to-female ratio is 4:1.**
- **Often this is associated with several years' history of joint pain, presenting with locking/clicking and intermittent swelling as well as limited range of motion.**
- **It can occur in any joint or bursa; the subscapularis location, as in this case, it is fairly common.**
- **It can usually be diagnosed on conventional radiographs.**

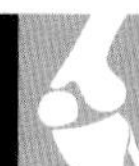

ADDITIONAL IMAGES

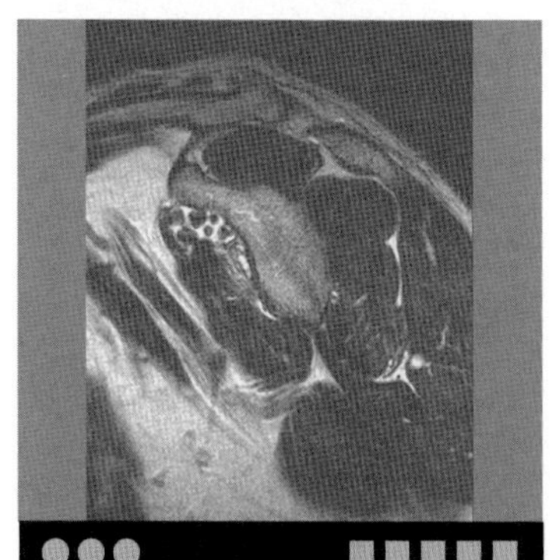

B. Synovial osteochondromatosis: Sagittal STIR sequence; this image plane better delineates the location of the loose bodies within the subscapularis bursa, anterior to the glenoid fossa.

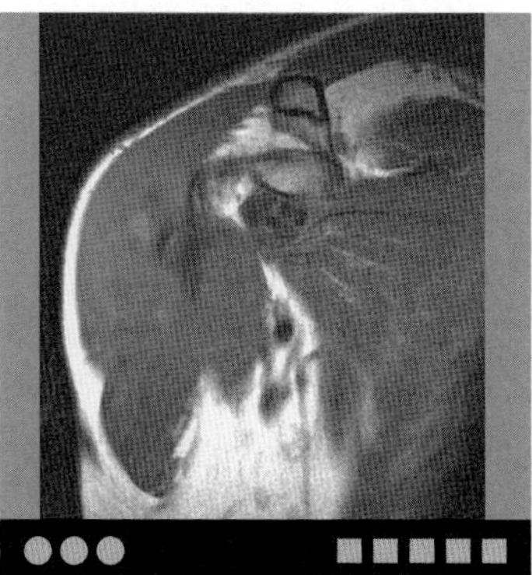

C. Synovial osteochondromatosis: Coronal T1-weighted image in the same patient.

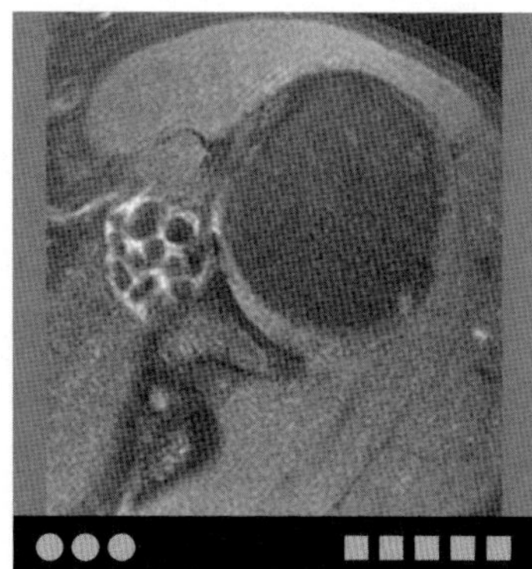

D. Synovial osteochondromatosis: Another axial T2-weighted image in the same patient, caudad to image A.

DIFFERENTIAL DIAGNOSES IMAGES

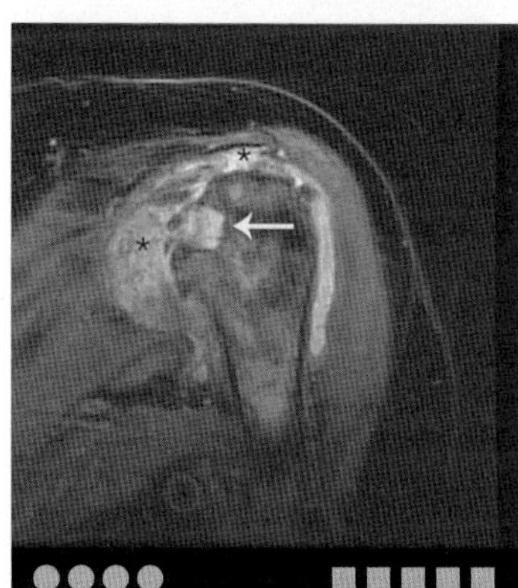

E. Rheumatoid arthritis: Coronal oblique T2-weighted FS image shows erosion (arrow) and synovial proliferation (*).

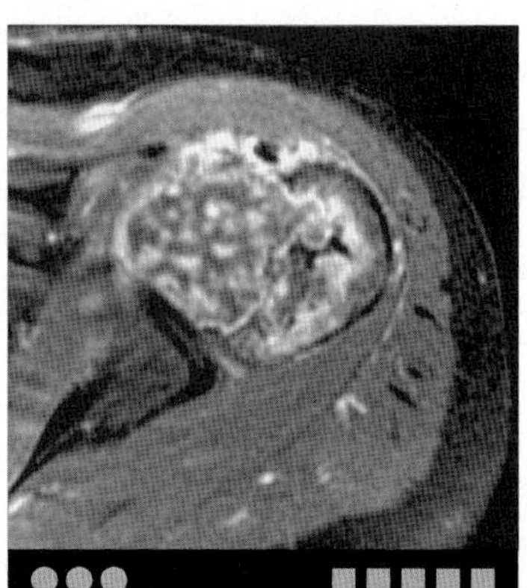

F. Chondrosarcoma of the humeral head: Axial T2-weighted FS image shows large expansile lesion with cortical destruction and soft tissue extension in the humeral head.

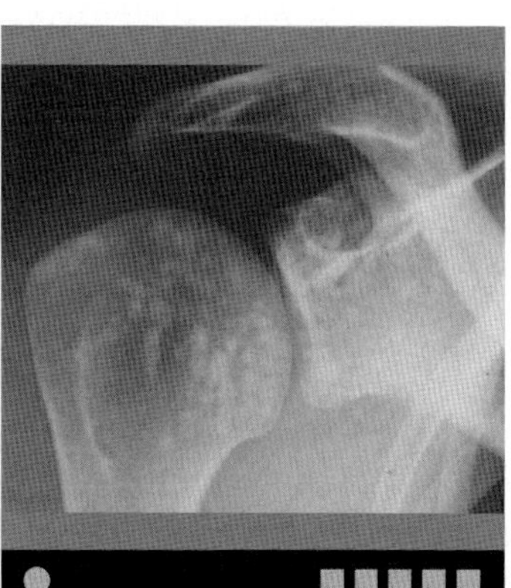

G. Osteopoikilosis: External oblique radiograph of the shoulder shows multiple bone islands of humeral head and glenoid.

IMAGE KEY

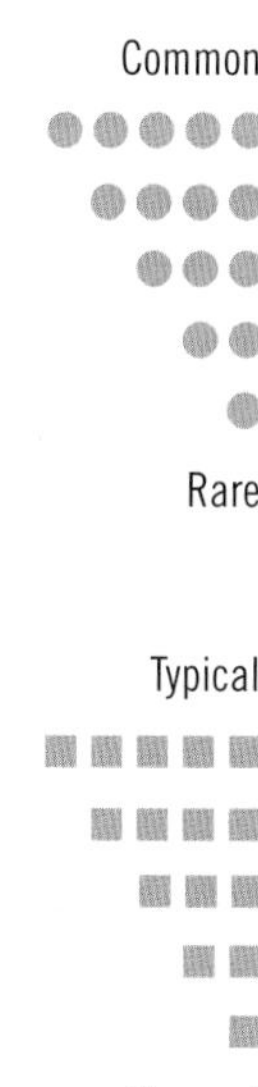

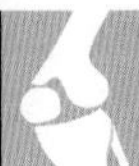

6–2 Synovial Osteochondromatosis of Biceps Tendon Sheath

Peyman Borghei and Jamshid Tehranzadeh

PRESENTATION

Left shoulder pain

FINDINGS

Radiograph of left shoulder shows a string of calcific densities on the medial side of humeral neck. MRI shows synovial osteochondromatosis of the left biceps tendon sheath.

DIFFERENTIAL DIAGNOSES

- *Synovial osteochondroma of shoulder:* On MRI, the effusion conforming to a distended joint capsule and multiple round bodies are seen, which follow the signal of the bone or cartilage.
- *Calcific tendinitis:* MRI shows a focus of low signal intensity in the tendon on all sequences.
- *Soft tissue hemangiomas with phleboliths:* A congregation of phleboliths may be seen, which is characteristic on radiograph. On CT scan and MRI, a characteristic "can of worms" could be identified.
- *Heterotopic ossification:* It follows a soft tissue injury, a new bone formation in the lesion merges to the adjacent bone.

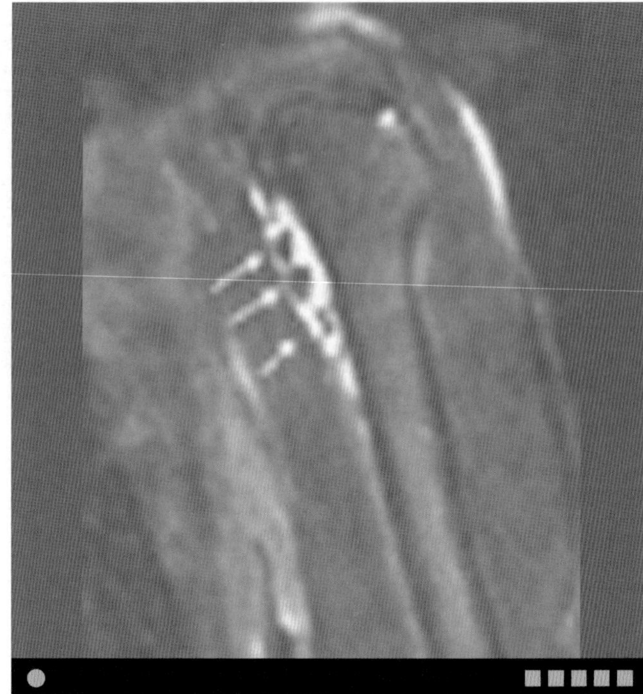

A. Coronal T2-weighted image shows low signal intensity bodies within the biceps tendon sheath surrounded by fluid (arrow) representing synovial osteochondromas of the biceps tendon sheath.

COMMENTS

This is an image of a 92-year-old male who presented with a long history of left shoulder pain diagnosed with synovial osteochondromatosis of left biceps tendon sheath. Synovial osteochondromatosis is a benign, rare disorder of synovial joints, which can also be seen in the tendon sheaths and bursae. Histologically, synovial cells undergo metaplasia to chondrocytes, which produce multiple nodules of cartilage, with the chondroid matrix frequently undergoing calcification and ossification. The process is most frequently seen radiographically as multiple round bodies of similar size and variable in mineralization. The individual body size may range from 1 mm to 2 cm, but generally is uniform. Although there is usually not an associated arthritis, mechanical or pressure erosion can eventually be formed by the bodies and secondary osteoarthritis may occur. It is seen more frequently in males than females and generally in the third through fifth decades. Symptoms include pain, limited motion, intermittent locking, and crepitation. Radiography may reveal soft tissue prominence, specks of calcification, peripherally dense lesion, or mature central ossified trabeculation. In the 15% that do not ossify, MR imaging is diagnostic, which shows multiple round bodies in the tendon sheath.

PEARLS

- **Synovial osteochondromatosis can rarely develop in the tendon sheaths.**
- **The patient usually complains of pain and limited range of motion.**
- **Most of the cases can be diagnosed on radiography; otherwise, MR imaging can detect rounded and sharp loose bodies in the tendon sheath often surrounded by fluid.**

ADDITIONAL IMAGES

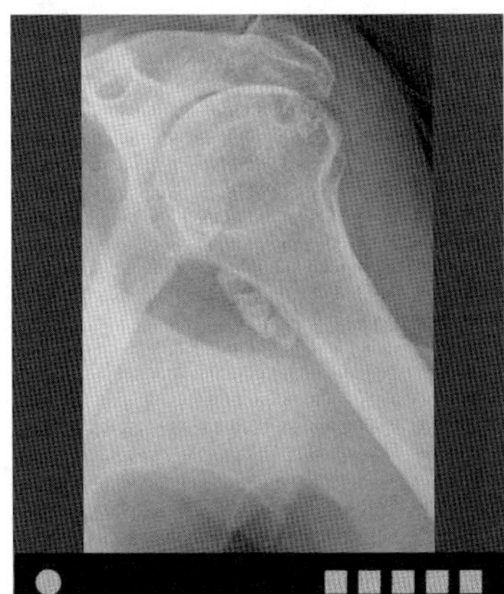

B. AP radiograph of left shoulder shows a string of osseous bodies along the medial side of humeral neck.

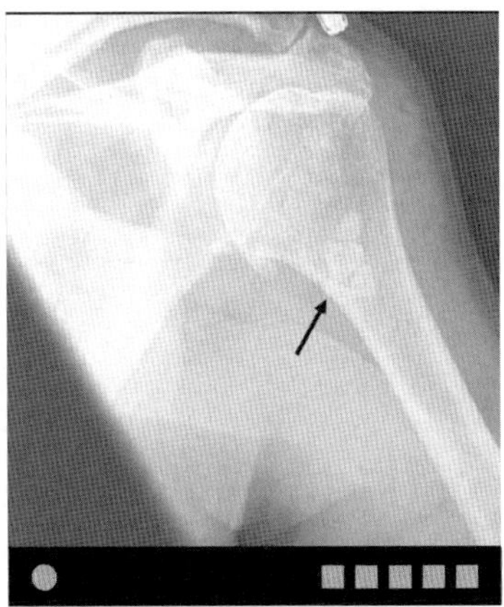

C. External rotation radiograph of the shoulder shows osteoarthritis of the glenohumeral joint. Four osseous bodies are projected on the proximal humerus (arrow).

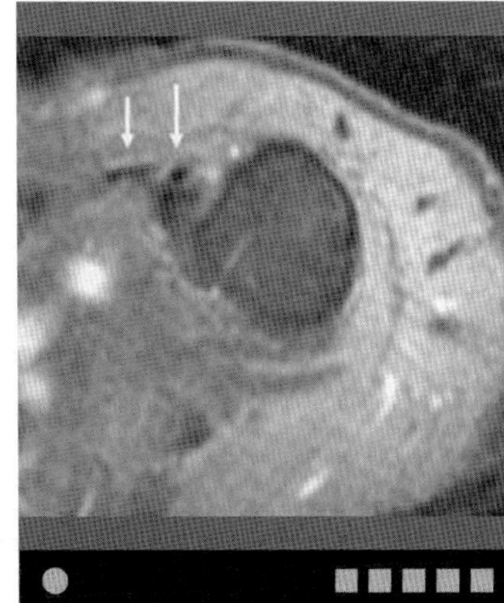

D. Axial T1-weighted fat-saturated MR image shows multiple uniform low signal foci within the biceps tendon sheath (arrows).

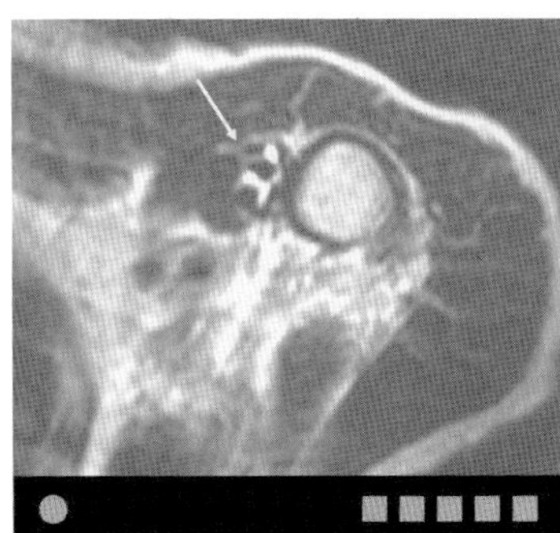

E. Axial T2-weighted SE image shows osteochondral bodies in the synovial sheath of the biceps tendon surrounded by small fluid.

DIFFERENTIAL DIAGNOSES IMAGES

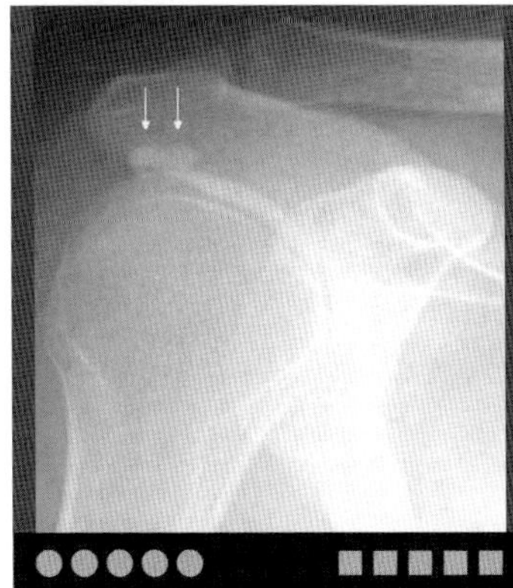

F. Calcific tendonitis: Radiograph of the shoulder shows a focus of calcific density (arrows) in the supraspinatus tendon caused by calcific tendonitis.

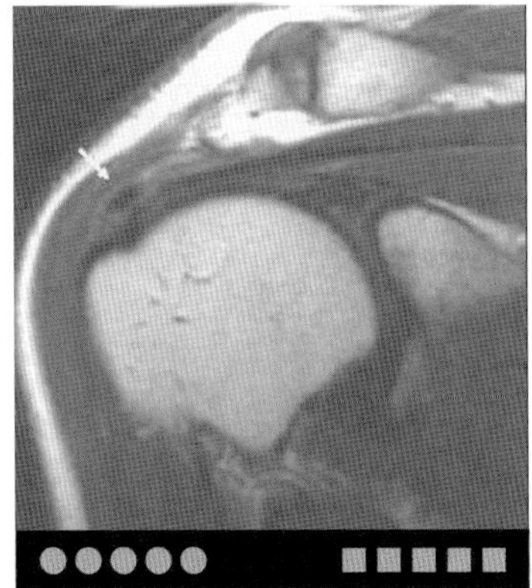

G. Calcific tendonitis: Coronal oblique T2-weighted proton density MR image of the shoulder shows a focus of calcific density (arrow) in the supraspinatus tendon caused by calcific tendonitis.

IMAGE KEY

Common

Rare

Typical

Unusual

SECTION II

ELBOW

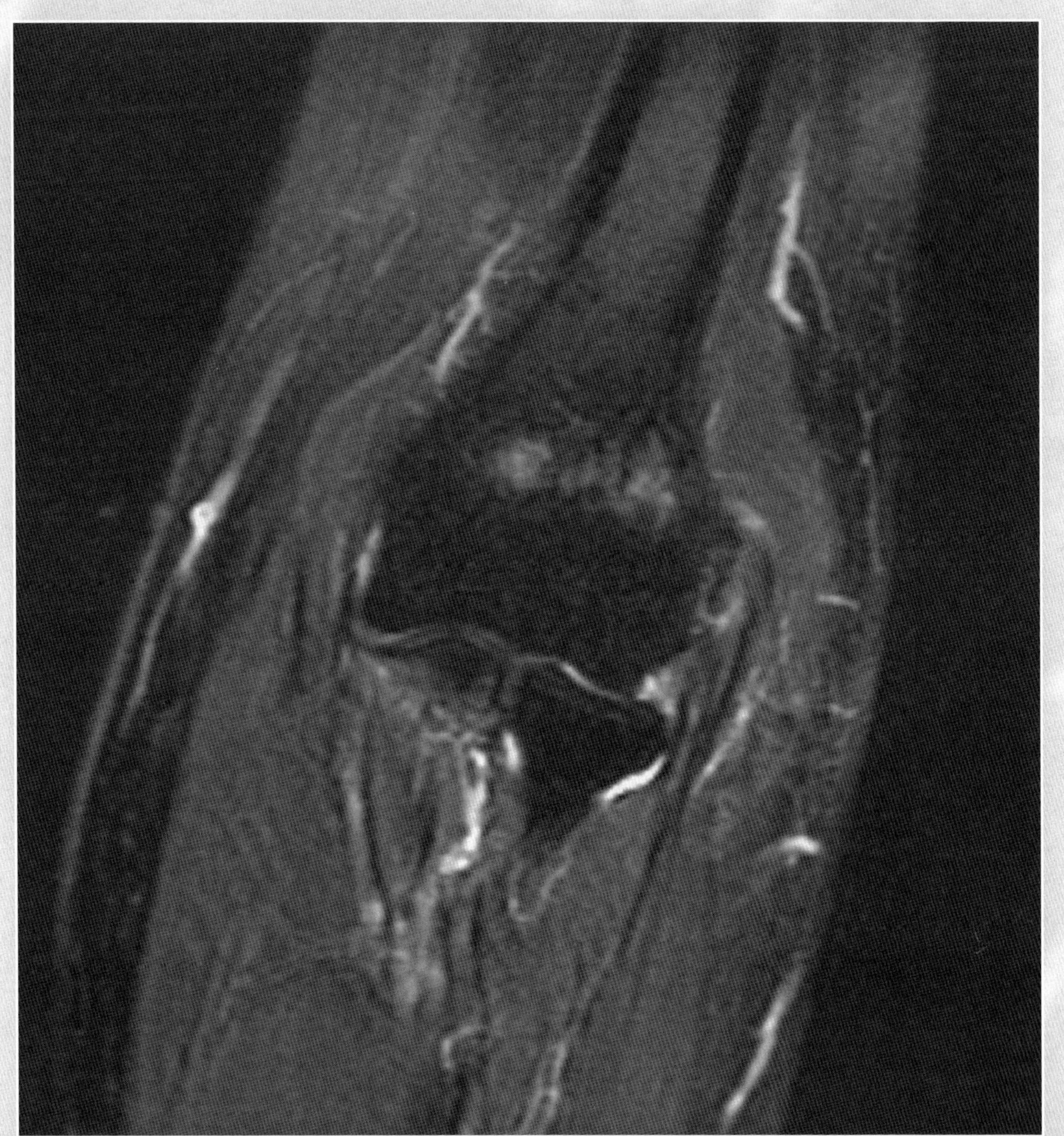

Chapter 7

Sport Medicine and Trauma

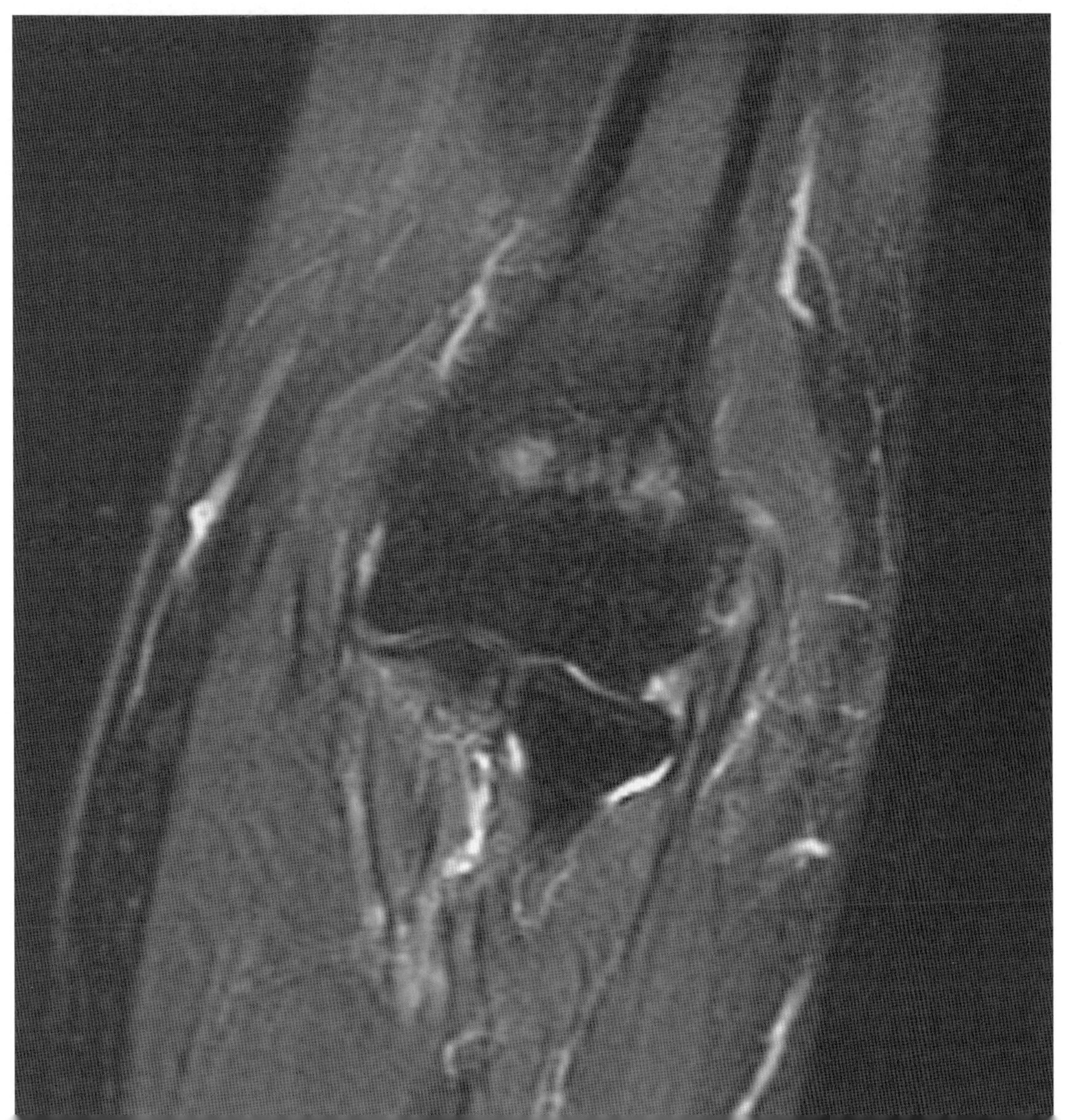

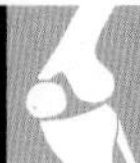

7–1 Advanced Lateral Epicondylitis with Common Extensor Tear of the Elbow

Gregory T. Lee and Rajeev K. Varma

PRESENTATION

Lateral elbow pain

FINDINGS

MR images show thickening and increased T1 and T2W signal intensity of the common extensor tendon and soft tissue edema around the common extensor tendon.

DIFFERENTIAL DIAGNOSES

- *Synovitis of the radio-humeral joint:* Synovial inflammation and joint fluid are noted. A common cause is rheumatoid arthritis.
- *Radial tunnel syndrome:* Pain in the radial side of elbow should be evaluated by MRI.
- *Posterior interosseous nerve palsy:* The nerve compression may be caused by masses such as bursa or hemangioma and diagnosis can be made by ultrasound, nerve conduction study, or MRI.
- *Neuralgic amyotrophy:* This condition is regarded as being associated with viral conditions or immunization, though commonly no antecedent event is identified.

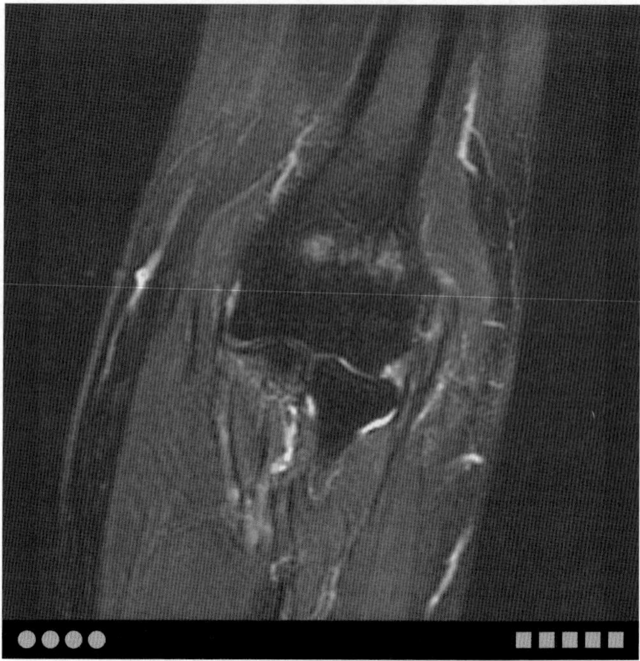

A. Lateral Epicondylitis with tear of common extensor tendon: Coronal T2WI shows increased signal in the area of the common extensor tendons origin.

COMMENTS

This case is a 66- year-old woman with 1- year history of lateral elbow pain. Lateral epicondylitis is the most common cause of elbow pain and is commonly known as tennis elbow. It is an overuse injury affecting anyone who regularly participates in rigorous activities involving wrist extension and/or supination. Men or women are affected and generally are between 35 to 55 years of age. Patients complain of lateral elbow pain and tenderness at the origin of the wrist extensor tendon complex from the lateral epicondyle. Although the term epicondylitis suggests an inflammatory process, histologic samples reveal angiofibroblastic hyperplasia tendinosis and fibrillary degeneration of collagen rather than an inflammatory reaction. This represents a healing response to chronic microtraumatic and possibly macrotraumatic injury. The extensor carpi radialis brevis (ECRB) tendon is almost always involved with involvement of the extensor digitorum communis about a third of the time. MR shows increased intra-tendon signal intensity on T1WI and T2WI as well as increased signal on fat-saturated FSE and fast STIR images. Tendon thickening is also a common finding on MRI. Intense T2 signal in the tendon can represent a full-thickness tear of the common extensor tendon as in the patient in this case. Anconeus edema and periostitis has been documented to occur in lateral epicondylitis, though likely infrequently. Most patients respond to conservative therapy. Patients who are refractory to 6 months to a year of conservative therapy including corticosteroid injections are candidates for surgery.

PEARLS

- **Lateral epicondylitis or tennis elbow is the most common cause of elbow pain.**
- **The most common MR finding is increased signal in the extensor carpi radialis brevis tendon on both T1WI and T2WI.**
- **Intense T2 signal in the tendon can represent frank tear of the tendon.**
- **Anconeus edema and periostitis have been documented to occur.**

ADDITIONAL IMAGES

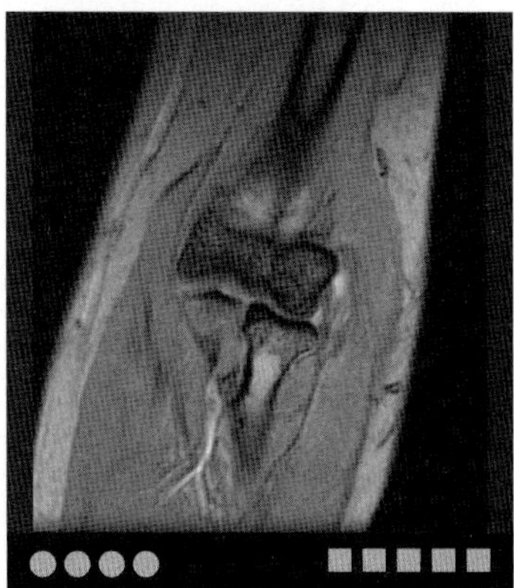

B. Lateral Epicondylitis with tear of common extensor tendon: Coronal T2* GE image shows intense signal in the region of the lateral epicondyle.

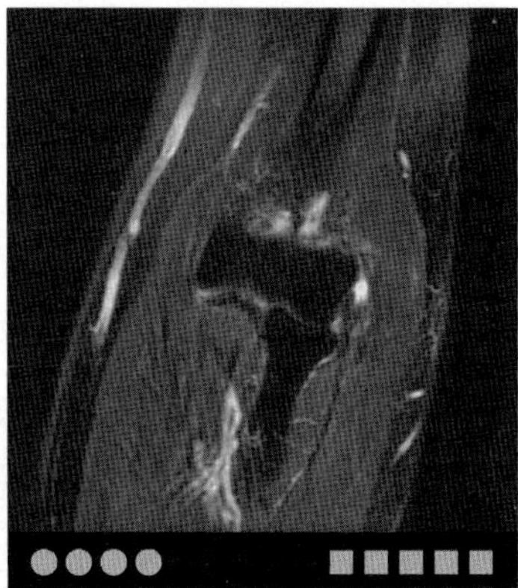

C. Lateral Epicondylitis with tear of common extensor tendon: Coronal T2WI with fat saturation shows a gap with increased signal in the common extensor tendons origin consistent with a full thickness tear.

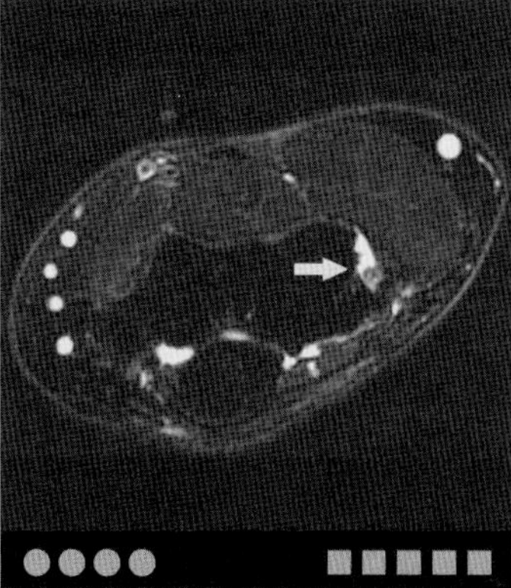

D. Lateral Epicondylitis with tear of common extensor tendon: Axial STIR image shows high intensity fluid signal at lateral epicondyle (arrow).

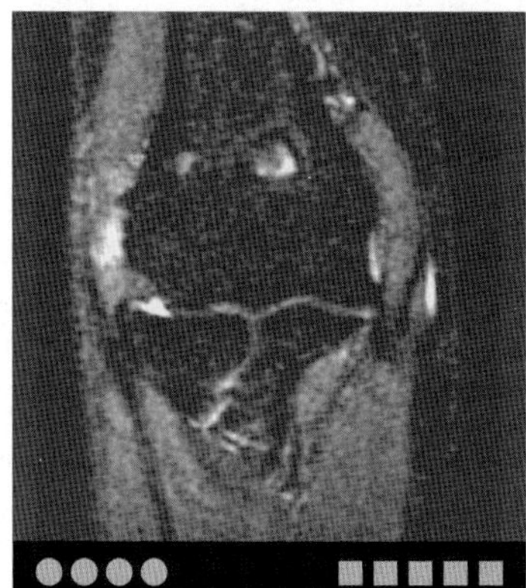

E. Tear at origin of common extensor tendon: Coronal STIR image in a different patient shows tear at the origin of common extensor tendons.

IMAGE KEY

Common

Rare

Typical

Unusual

DIFFERENTIAL DIAGNOSES IMAGES

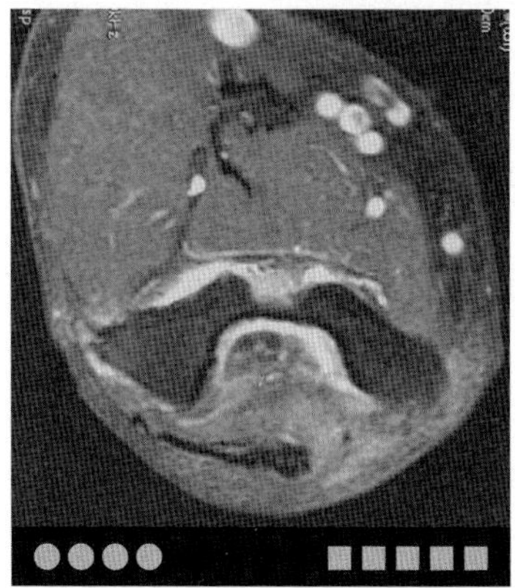

F. Synovitis: Contrast enhanced T1W image with fat saturation in a different patient shows increased enhancement in and partly around the joint indicating inflammation.

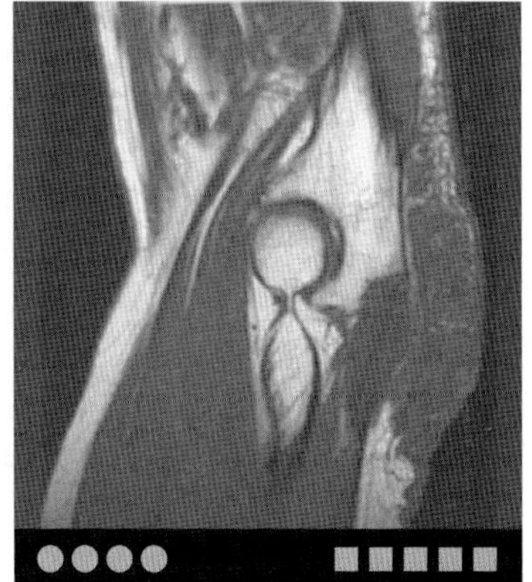

G. Rheumatoid arthritis: Sagittal T1W image shows low signal synovial proliferation at olecranon bursa.

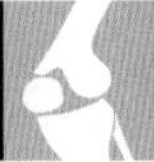

7–2 Occult Radial Head Fracture

Kambiz Motamedi

PRESENTATION

Pain following rollerblading accident with fall

FINDINGS

MRI shows edema of the radial head.

DIFFERENTIAL DIAGNOSES

- *Lymphoma:* MRI of lymphoma in early stage may just show marrow replacement, an edema of the bone without a soft tissue mass. Later there may be decreasing edema and increased sclerosis.
- *Multiple myeloma:* The initial lytic lesion without bone extension and soft tissue mass may present on MRI as high signal lesion on fluid-sensitive sequences commonly accompanied by homogenous marrow replacement of T1W images.
- *Metastatic disease:* An array of primary neoplasms may metastasize to bone. The primary cancers include lung, breast, and prostate. The MRI appearance is nonspecific and includes high-signal on fluid-sensitive sequences and marrow replacement on T1WI often with a soft tissue component.

COMMENTS

The patient is a 24-year-old male who suffered a recent fall while rollerblading. The MRI showed a stress fracture of the radial head. Radial head fractures and dislocations are traumatic injuries. They may be isolated just to the radial head and the lateral elbow, or they may be part of a combined complex fracture injury pattern involving the other structures. Radial head fractures and dislocations are the result of trauma, usually from a fall on the outstretched arm with the force of impact transmitted up the hand through the wrist and forearm to the radial head, which is forced into the capitellum. A variant may be radial head stress reaction. Stress fractures result from repetitive loads on normal bone. Stress fractures are particularly common among athletes, military recruits, healthy people who have recently started new or intensive physical activity and elderly patients. Stress fractures and stress injuries are most common in the lower extremities, but have been reported in nearly every bone in the body. Stress fractures are frequently occult on early radiographs. Radiographic findings associated with stress fractures include ill definition of the affected cortex, periosteal reaction, trabecular sclerosis, and cortical break. The utility of MRI in diagnosis of stress fractures has long been known, and has since become a reliable technique for diagnosing stress fractures not visible by radiography or CT.

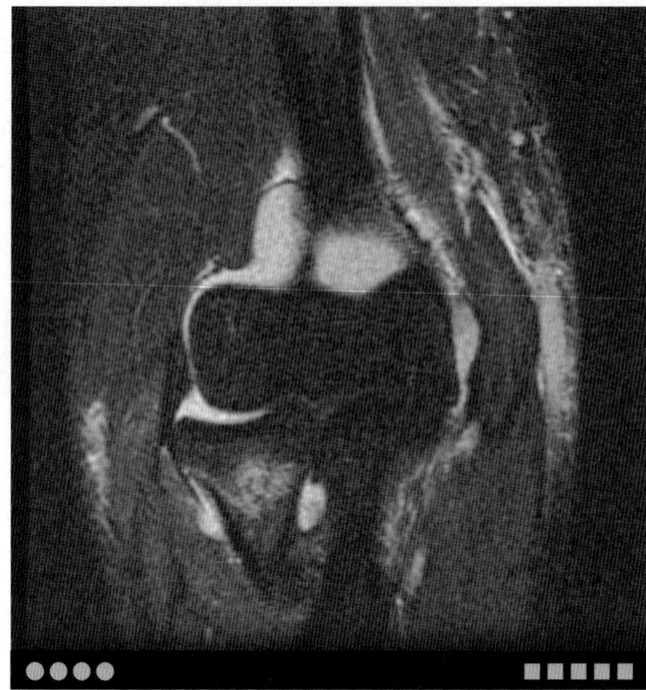

A. Occult radial head contusion: Coronal inversion recovery MRI image shows edema of the radial head.

PEARLS

- **Radial head fractures are common in adults with elbow injury. They may be occult on radiographs.**
- **MRI readily shows the edema on fluid-sensitive sequences. The T1WI may show patchy ill-defined marrow replacement.**
- **Look for the linear fracture line on MRI specifically on T1WI.**
- **Lack of a soft tissue component suggests absence of a neoplastic process.**

ADDITIONAL IMAGES

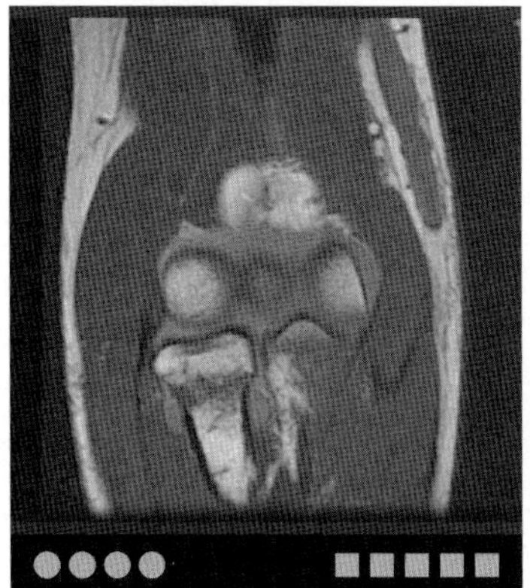

B. Occult radial head contusion: Coronal T1WI show the low signal linear fracture line across the radial neck.

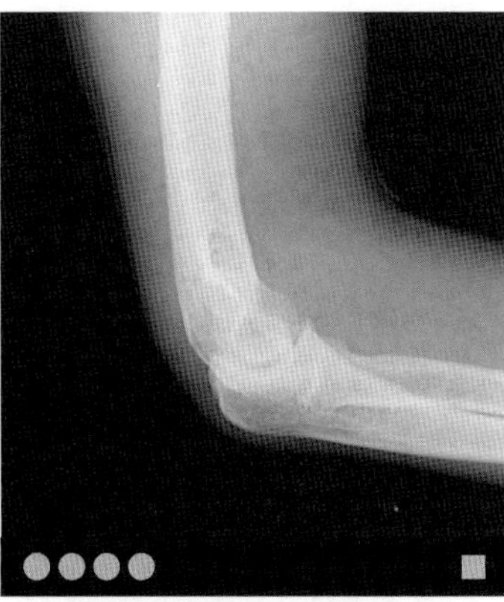

C. Occult radial head contusion: Lateral elbow radiographs reveal fat pad elevation because of joint effusion.

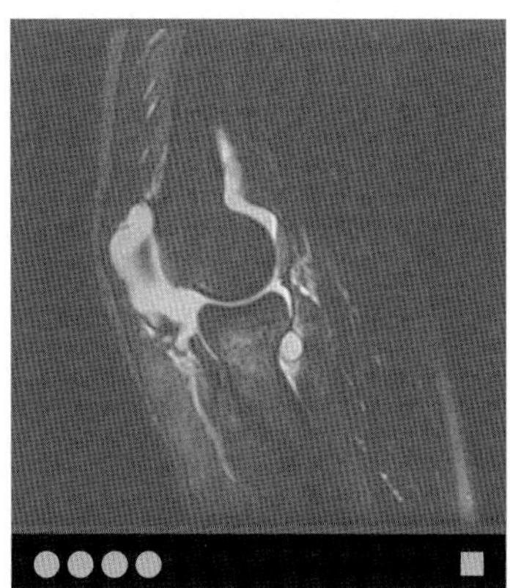

D. Occult radial head fracture: Sagittal inversion recovery image demonstrate a small joint effusion as well.

DIFFERENTIAL DIAGNOSES IMAGES

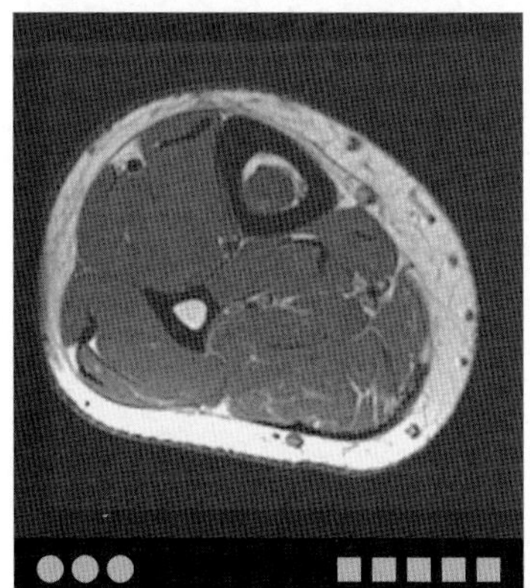

E. Enchondroma: Axial T1WI through mid tibia shows a well delineated concentrated lesion distinct from the patchy edema of a stress fracture.

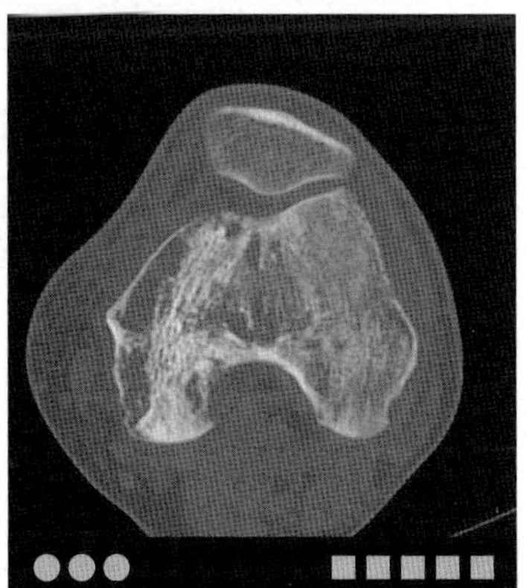

F. Treated Lymphoma: Axial CT scan through the condylar region of the femur demonstrates the increased marrow sclerosis in a case of treated lymphoma.

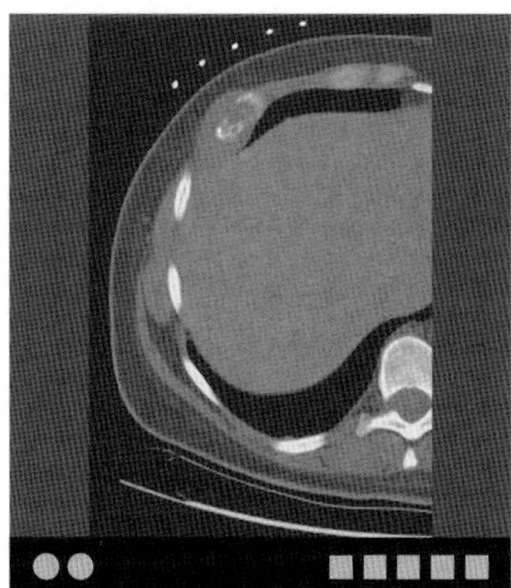

G. Lymphoma: Axial CT scan through a lymphoma lesion of the rib readily reveals an associated soft tissue mantel.

IMAGE KEY

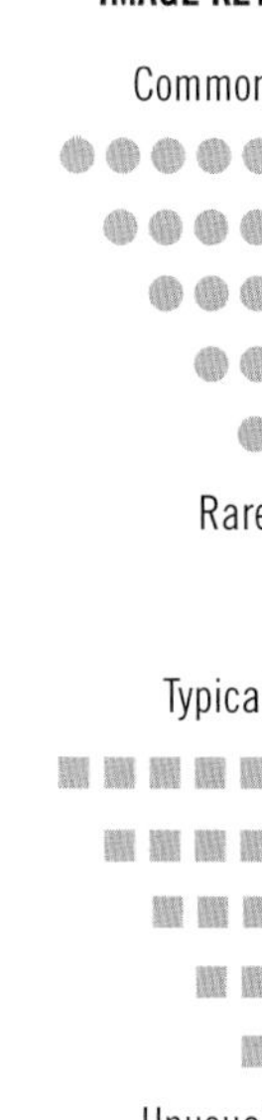

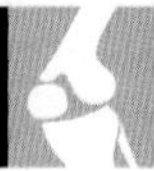

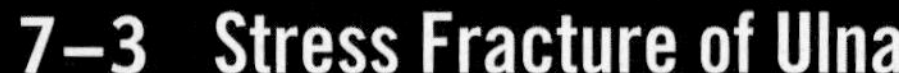

7–3 Stress Fracture of Ulna

Hakan Ilaslan

PRESENTATION

Gradually worsening forearm pain, no history of trauma

FINDINGS

MR images show abnormal bone marrow signal in a long segment of ulnar diaphysis with a focal area of cortical thickening and irregularity.

DIFFERENTIAL DIAGNOSES

- *Osteoid osteoma:* Usually a nidus is visible. Presence of fracture line excludes this diagnosis.
- *Osteomyelitis:* Osteomyelitis usually demonstrates marked reactive edema like signal in the adjacent soft tissues along with marrow changes. Clinical history might be helpful. Similar to osteoid osteoma, presence of fracture line excludes this differential as well.
- *Lymphoma:* Marrow signal abnormality on MRI may simulate an infiltrating process such as lymphoma. Radiographs usually help in demonstrating the fracture line and solid periosteal reaction.

COMMENTS

This is a 27-year-old healthy male with gradually increasing pain in the forearm. He has no history of trauma, but he plays volleyball a few times every week. Osseous structures undergo constant remodeling in response to applied stresses. Cortical or trabecular micro injuries occur as a result of physical activities, and normally osteoclastic resorption of the injured bone is followed by osteoblastic bone production, resulting in equilibrium. However, with new or sudden increase in physical activity, the degree of remodeling increases and bone resorption outpaces bone. During this "period of vulnerability," the imbalance between resorption and new bone formation results in a localized weakening of the bone, and if the offending activity is not stopped, the microdamage will begin to increase. At this stage in the stress reaction, periosteal and endosteal new bone is produced in an attempt to strengthen the temporarily weakened cortex. If MRI is performed during this period, bone marrow edema can be seen without fracture line. Ultimately, if the activity is continued, further weakening of the bone will lead to mechanical failure and the development of a full-blown stress fracture. Numerous athletic activities have been associated with these injuries, the two most common are gymnastics and throwing sports, such as baseball and softball. In some cases fracture line may not be evident initially on MRI, in which case, a short-term follow-up with radiograph might help to show fracture line and differentiate this entity from osteoid osteoma or osteomyelitis.

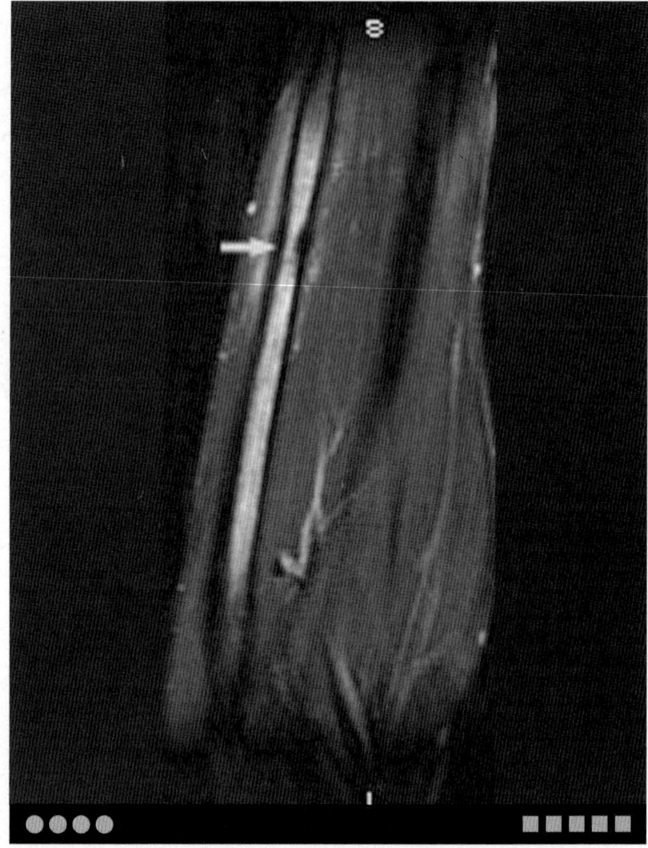

A. Stress fracture of ulna: Coronal STIR of right forearm demonstrate abnormal bright bone marrow signal in a long segment of ulnar diaphysis with a subtle focal area of cortical thickening and irregularity in the mid diaphysis (arrow)

PEARLS

- **Marked bone marrow edema on MRI, which can obscure the fracture line.**
- **Periosteal reaction is frequently present.**
- **If fracture line is not seen initially on MRI, a follow-up radiograph in 2 weeks might help to establish the diagnosis.**

ADDITIONAL IMAGES

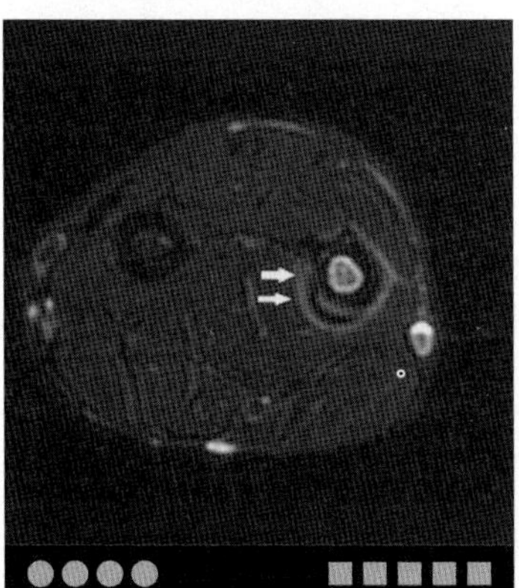

B. Stress fracture of ulna: Axial STIR image of the right forearm shows thickened cortex and abnormal marrow signal. Note the active periostitis (arrows).

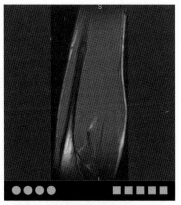

C. Stress fracture of ulna: Sagittal T1WI of the right forearm demonstrate abnormal bone marrow signal in a long segment of ulnar diaphysis with a focal area of cortical thickening and irregularity.

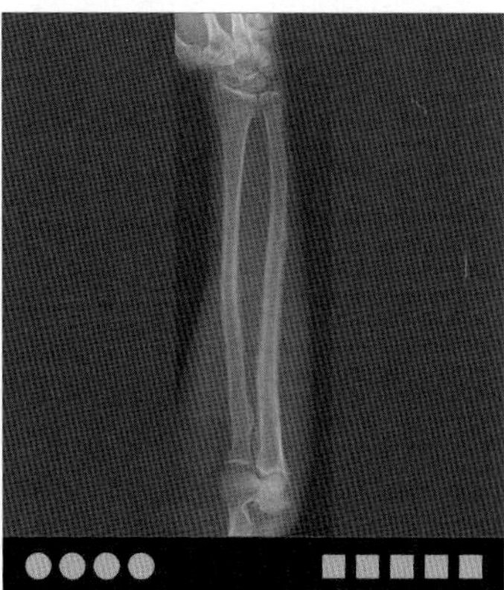

D. Stress fracture of ulna: AP radiograph shows mature periosteal thickening along the mid ulnar diaphysis.

IMAGE KEY

Common

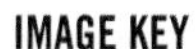

Rare

Typical

Unusual

DIFFERENTIAL DIAGNOSES IMAGES

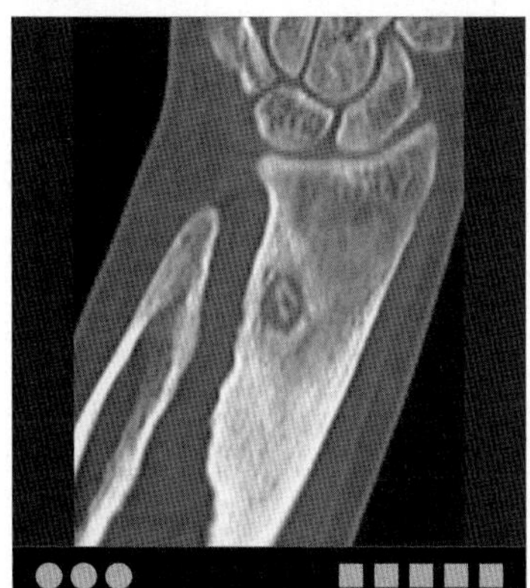

E. Distal radial osteoid osteoma: Coronal CT reconstruction demonstrates cortical thickening and typical nidus.

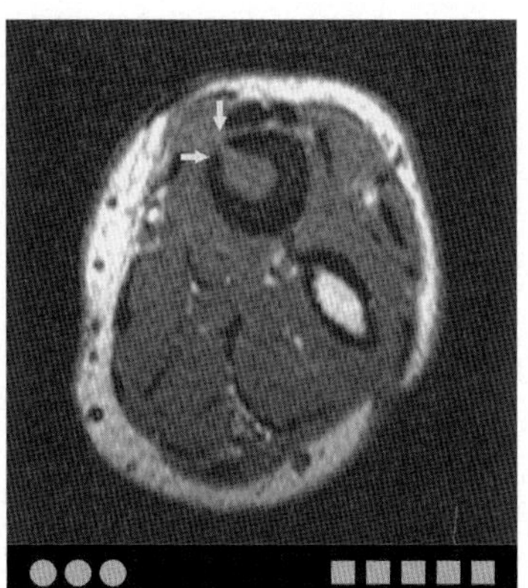

F. Radial diaphysis Brodie's abscess: Axial T1WI shows a focal area of cortical destruction (arrows) and thickening of adjacent cortices. Enhancing phlegmon extends from the marrow cavity into adjacent subcutaneous tissues.

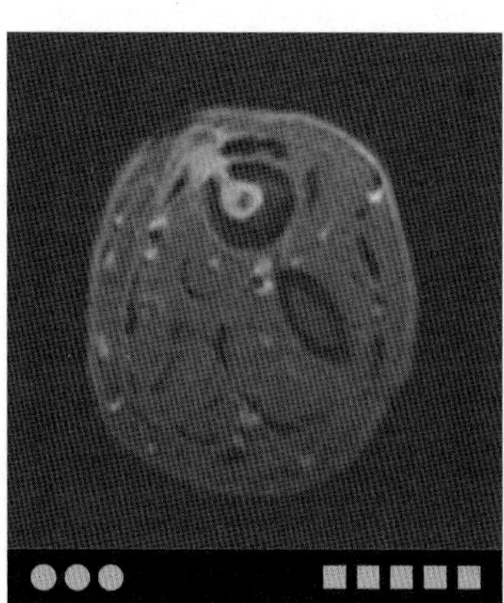

G. Radial diaphysis Brodie's abscess: Axial T1WI after the administration of intravenous gadolinium shows a focal area of cortical destruction and thickening of adjacent cortices. Enhancing phlegmon extends from the marrow cavity into adjacent subcutaneous tissues.

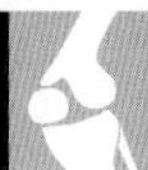

7–4 Avulsion of Distal Biceps Tendon from Radial Tuberosity

Arash Tehranzadeh

PRESENTATION

Pain and tumefaction in the forearm

FINDINGS

There is osseous proliferation and marrow edema of the radial tuberosity because of subacute avulsion. MRI shows a tear of the distal biceps brachii tendon at its distal attachment.

DIFFERENTIAL DIAGNOSES

- *Complete biceps tendon tear:* The distal biceps tendon injury may vary in range from tendinosis to a complete tear.
- *Common flexor tendinosis:* In the posttraumatic setting, differential considerations should include other causes of elbow pain. Although the common flexor tendon attaches to the medial humeral condyle, this is a cause of medial joint line pain.
- *Medial epicondylitis:* Also known as Little Leaguer's elbow, this is another cause of medial joint line tenderness and is manifested by marrow edema in the medial epicondyle and associated common flexor tendinosis may also be seen.

COMMENTS

An injury to the biceps brachii tendon most commonly occurs in the proximal aspect of the long head of the biceps, occurring in 96% of cases. The least common site of tendon injury is the short head of the biceps, occurring in 1% of cases. Injury of the distal biceps brachii tendon occurs in 3% of cases. A distal tendon injury is classically described as a consequence of a single traumatic event. The mechanism of injury involves contraction of the biceps brachii muscle in an attempt to resist forcible extension. When the biceps muscle contracts while it is lengthening; the biceps tendon may rupture from the bone at its attachment to the radial tuberosity. At the time of injury, this often elicits an audible popping sound subsequently followed by antecubital ecchymosis and weakness on supination and elbow flexion. Radiographs are typically normal. However, a small bone fragment may avulse from the radial tuberosity. MRI evaluation demonstrates bone marrow edema, and in some cases, avulsion of the radial tuberosity. Tendinosis manifested by increased intrasubstance T2W signal intensity is commonly seen in the distal biceps tendon. In more severe cases, partial and complete rupture may be observed by discontinuity of the distal tendon with surrounding edema. Management options may include conservative care or surgical re-attachment.

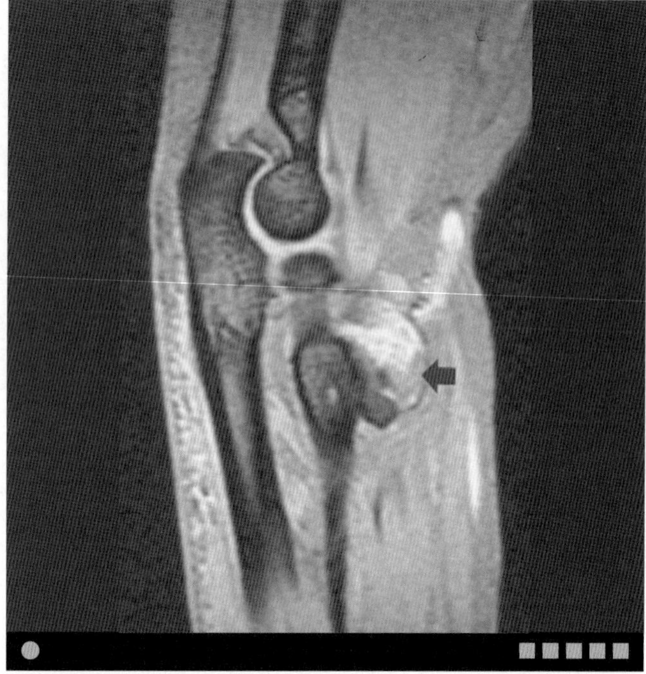

A. Avulsion of distal biceps tendon: Sagittal T2 shows radial tuberosity proliferative changes and marrow edema due to avulsion and distal biceps tendon tear (arrow).

PEARLS

- **Avulsion of distal biceps brachii tendon is rare, occurring in approximately 3% of cases.**
- **The injury may present as either tendinosis or partial versus complete tear.**
- **The radial tuberosity may be avulsed.**

ADDITIONAL IMAGES

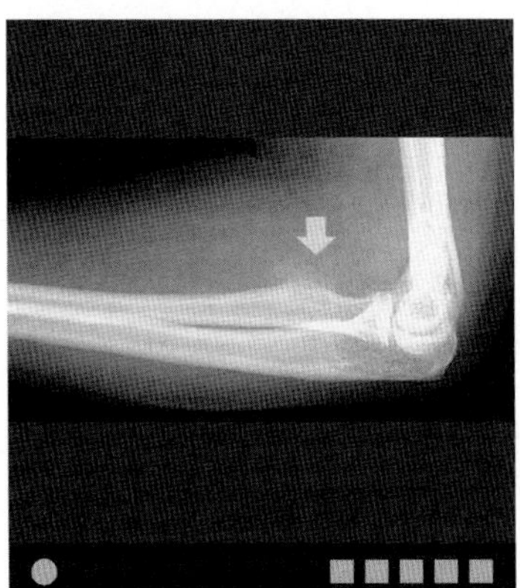

B. Avulsion of distal biceps tendon: Lateral plain film radiograph of the elbow demonstrates proliferation of the radial tuberosity (arrow) as a consequence of avulsion from a distal biceps tendon.

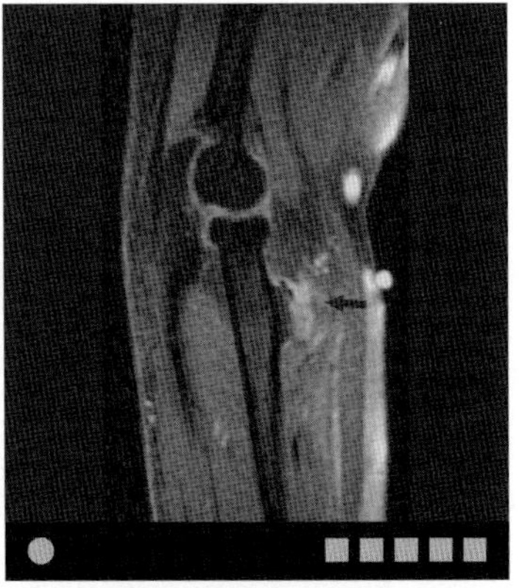

C. Avulsion of distal biceps tendon: Sagittal T1 fat saturation with intravenous gadolinium shows tendinosis, tear, and enhancement of the distal biceps tendon (arrow).

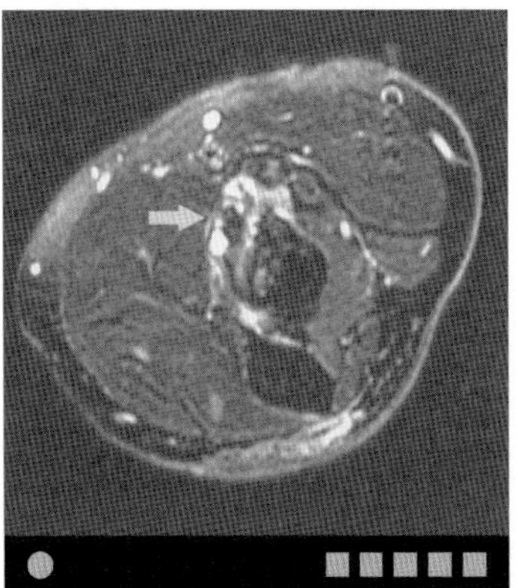

D. Avulsion of distal biceps tendon: Axial T2 fat saturation shows distal biceps brachii tendinosis, tear, surrounding edema, and radial tuberosity proliferation from chronic avulsion (arrow).

IMAGE KEY

Common

Rare

Typical

Unusual

DIFFERENTIAL DIAGNOSES IMAGES

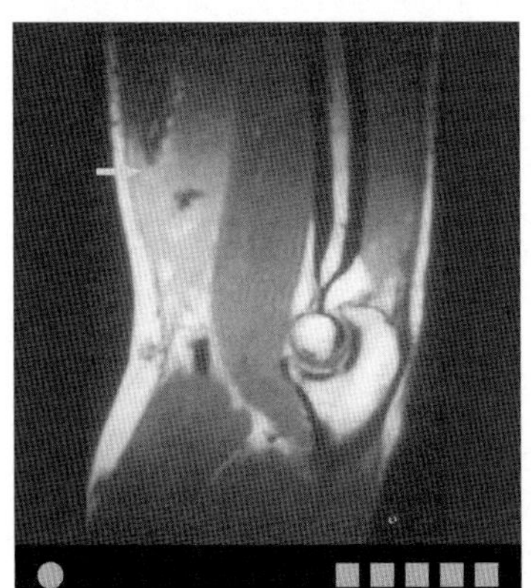

E. Complete biceps tendon tear: Sagittal spin echo T2WI shows a complete tear of biceps tendon. Note retracted biceps tendon (arrow).

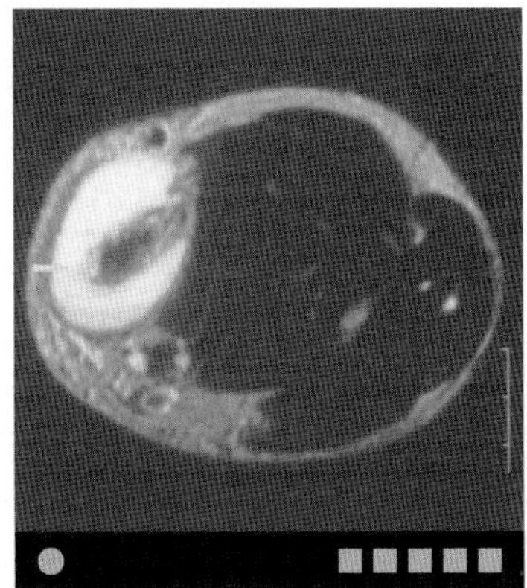

F. Complete biceps tendon tear: Axial T2W spin echo image shows a complete distal tear of the biceps tendon (arrow) surrounded by fluid.

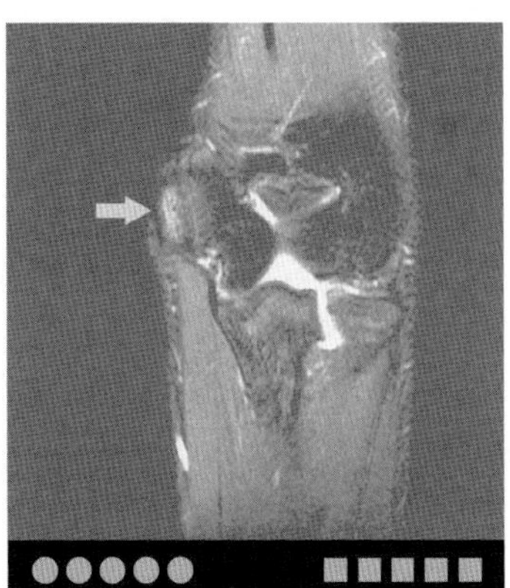

G. Medial epicondylitis: Coronal T2 fat saturation. Medial epicondylitis (arrow) manifested by increased edema in the medial epicondyle and tendinosis in the common flexor tendon.

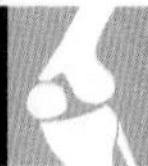

7–5 Rupture of the Distal Biceps Tendon

Atul Agarwal and Thomas Learch

PRESENTATION

A palpable mass in the anterior arm with limitation of elbow flexion

FINDINGS

MRI shows torn and retracted biceps tendon and surrounding high-signal-intensity edema and hemorrhage.

DIFFERENTIAL DIAGNOSES

- *Tenosynovitis:* This condition is associated with tendinopathy and presence of fluid in tendon sheath.
- *Bicipitoradial bursitis:* Accumulation of fluid in this bursa appears as an antecubital mass.
- *Biceps tendon tear:* Hemorrhage following biceps tendon tear may create a mass at antecubital area.
- *Soft tissue tumors:* Present as a mass in this region.
- *Cat scratch disease:* Presents with an inflammatory mass.

COMMENTS

This is a 27-year-old football player who was on anabolic steroids and reported recent elbow injury. On examination he had a palpable mass in the anterior aspect of the arm with decreased ability to flex forearm. Ruptures of the distal tendon are rare and account for only 3% of all biceps tendon ruptures. Most biceps tendon tears occur proximally near the shoulder joint. A history of tendinitis, overuse, or anabolic steroid abuse predisposes tendons to rupture typically at the tendon insertion onto the radial tuberosity. The mechanism of injury is usually forced extension against a flexed elbow. It is usually easily diagnosed on physical examination, presenting as a palpable defect in the antecubital fossa, a palpable mass in the anterior aspect of the arm corresponding to the retracted muscle and tendon, and a weakness of flexion and supination. Failure of active supination while the biceps muscle is squeezed is a simple physical finding to aid in diagnosing distal biceps tendon ruptures. Sonographic and MR features of complete rupture are absence of tendon in the expected location, fluid collection in a typical tendon gap, and a retracted, edematous muscle in the anterior arm. Sagittal scanning is better for showing tendon discontinuity and estimation of the amount of tendon retraction because both the torn retracted tendon edge and the radial tuberosity can be depicted on a single image. The MR technologist should be advised to extend the scan to include the radial tuberosity to evaluate the entire extent of the tendon.

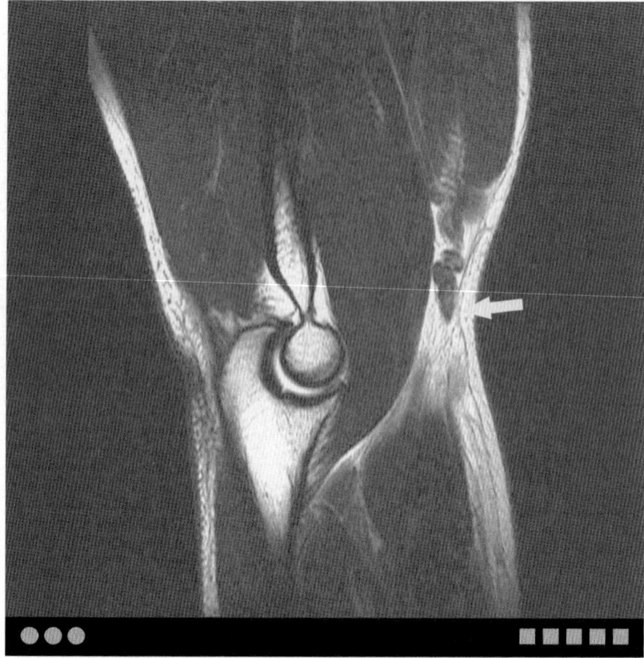

A. Rupture of distal biceps tendon: Sagittal T2W MR image of affected left elbow shows torn and retracted tendon (arrow) and biceps muscle.

PEARLS

- **Presents with history of forced extension against a flexed elbow.**
- **A history of tendinitis, overuse, or anabolic steroid abuse predisposes tendons to rupture at the insertion onto the radial tuberosity.**
- **Sonographic and MR features are absence of tendon in the expected location, fluid collection in a typical tendon gap, and retracted, edematous muscle in the anterior arm.**
- **Ruptures of the distal biceps tendon are rare, accounting for only 3% of all biceps tendon ruptures.**
- **The technologist should include the radial tuberosity to evaluate the integrity of the entire bicipital tendon.**

ADDITIONAL IMAGES

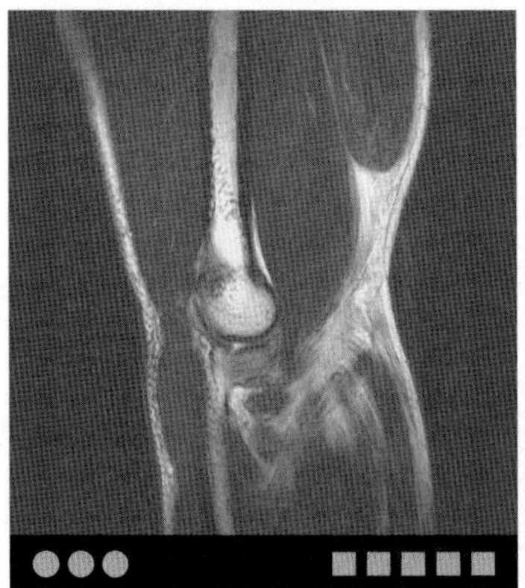

B. Rupture of distal biceps tendon: Sagittal T2W MR image of affected left elbow shows torn and retracted biceps muscle with a rounded border instead of a pointed taper.

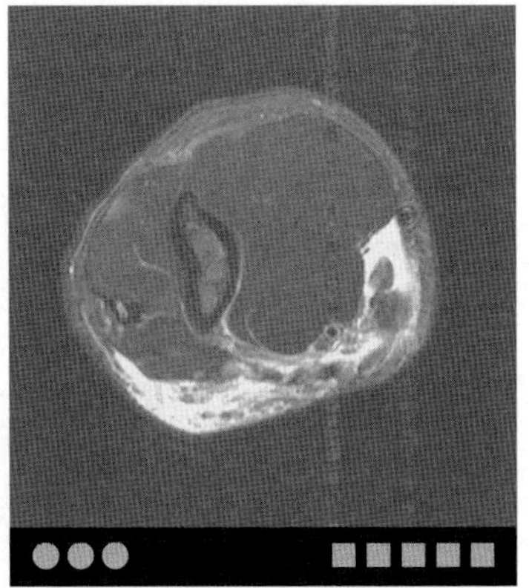

C. Rupture of distal biceps tendon: Axial T2-weighted STIR MR shows torn and retracted tendon and biceps muscle.

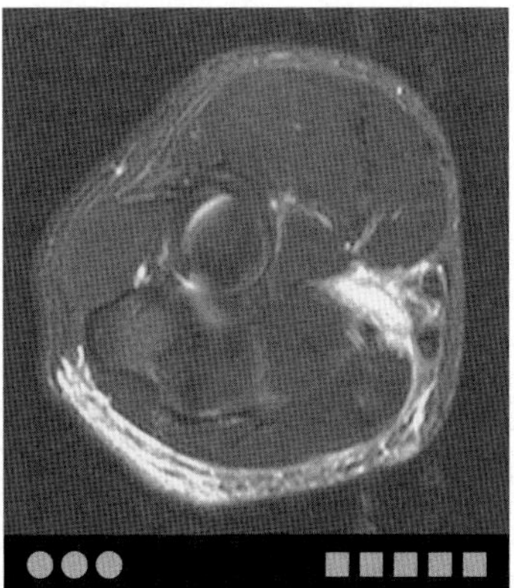

D. Rupture of distal biceps tendon: Axial T2-weighted STIR MR obtained more distal shows high-signal-intensity edema and hemorrhage in the expected area of the distal biceps tendon.

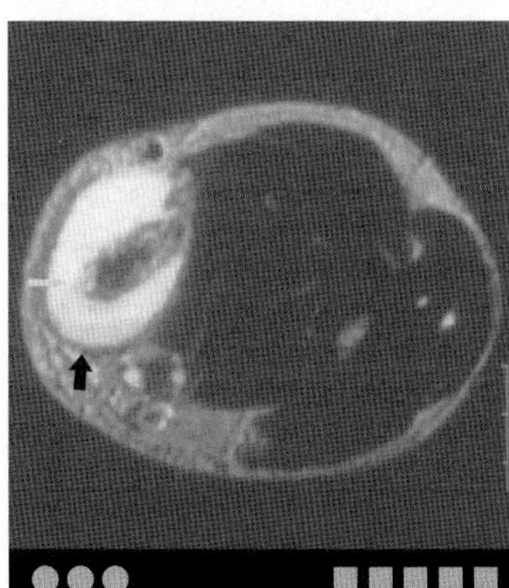

E. Rupture of distal biceps tendon: Axial T2W image in another patient shows hemorrhage (black arrow) around torn biceps tendon (white arrow).

DIFFERENTIAL DIAGNOSES IMAGES

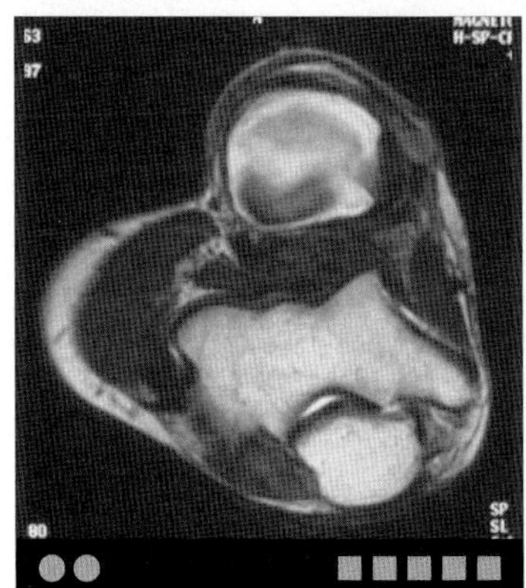

F. Pseudoaneurysm of brachial artery: Axial T2 MRI shows a large high signal cystic pseudoaneurysm with central low signal pertaining to flow void from fast moving blood. A second smaller pseudoaneurysm with low signal is noted adjacent.

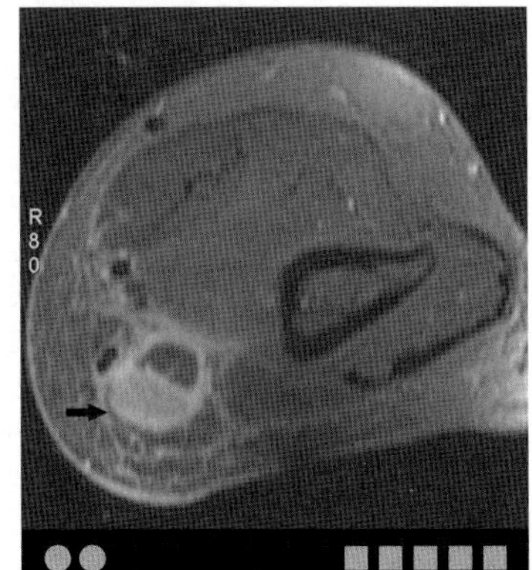

G. Cat scratch disease: Axial fat saturated T1W image shows enhancement of inflammatory mass (arrow) in elbow.

IMAGE KEY

Common

Rare

Typical

Unusual

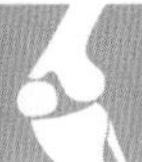

7–6 Bicipitoradial Bursitis

Brian Yue and Rajeev K. Varma

PRESENTATION

Painful mass in the antecubital fossa

FINDINGS

MRI of the right elbow demonstrates fluid surrounding the distal biceps tendon sheath with enhancement.

DIFFERENTIAL DIAGNOSES

- *Rupture of the distal biceps tendon:* Distal biceps tendon appears wavy due to retraction and depicts an irregular contour with thickening. High T2 signal intensity within the torn tendon and adjacent soft tissues and bone is usually present because of peritendinous hemorrhage, posttraumatic edema, and hemorrhage.
- *Chronic biceps tendinosis:* Intermediate signal intensity within the tendon on all pulse sequences, which may be associated with osseous proliferation at the radial tuberosity in addition to inflammation of the bicipitoradial bursa.
- *Interosseous bursitis:* Located medial to the bicipitoradial bursa adjacent to the median nerve. Does not abut the biceps tendon, but sometimes the two bursae may communicate.
- *Synovial cyst:* Communicates with the synovial joint.

COMMENTS

This is a 72-year-old female with a 2-month history of right arm pain and swelling in the antecubital fossa diagnosed with bicipitoradial bursitis. The bicipitoradial bursa is a subtendinous bursa that surrounds and sometimes ensheaths the distal biceps tendon, which inserts onto the posterior portion of the radial tuberosity. Its role is to reduce friction between the tendon and the radius over a limited range of pronation and supination of the forearm. Bicipitoradial bursitis is uncommon and most frequently results from repetitive mechanical trauma, but can also be caused by infection, inflammatory arthropathy, chemical synovitis, bone proliferation, or synovial chondromatosis. Symptoms include pain, mass, and limited range of motion. Pain may increase on pronation because of stretching and compression of the bicipital bursa upon posterior rotation of the radius. The presence of sensory and motor symptoms resulting from compression of the radial or median nerves may confound the diagnosis and increase suspicion for a tumor, but the MRI appearance is definitive. Fluid signal with enhancement surrounding an intact distal biceps tendon is diagnostic. Chronic inflammation may cause thickening of the wall of the bursa and surrounding soft tissues. An inflamed subtendinous bursa can be differentiated from an elbow joint effusion by the absence of fluid in the anterior elbow compartment.

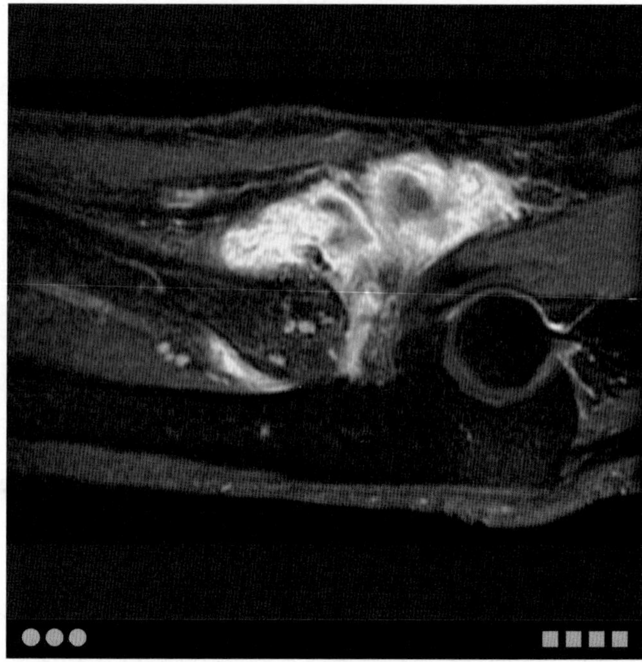

A. Bicipitoradial bursitis: Sagittal T1W fat-saturated post-contrast image shows enhancement of the soft tissues around the radial head.

PEARLS

- **The patient usually complains of pain, antecubital mass, and limited range of motion.**
- **An intact distal biceps tendon differentiates tendon rupture from bicipitoradial bursitis.**
- **Chronic biceps tendinosis is associated with bicipitoradial bursitis and may be a precursor.**

ADDITIONAL IMAGES

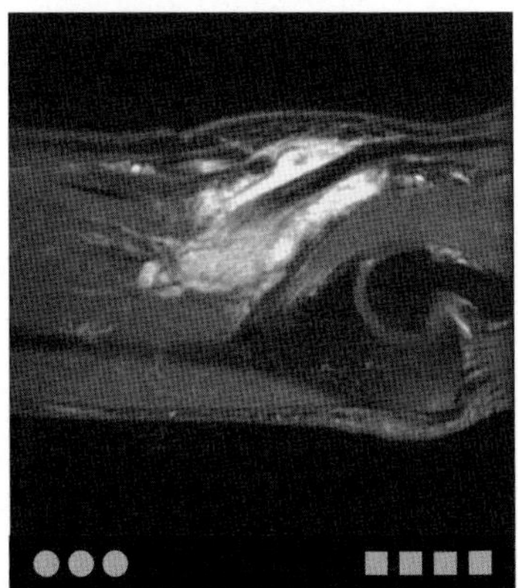

B. Bicipitoradial bursitis: Sagittal T1W fat-saturated post-contrast image shows a large region of enhancement surrounding the distal biceps tendon insertion in the area of the bicipitoradial bursa.

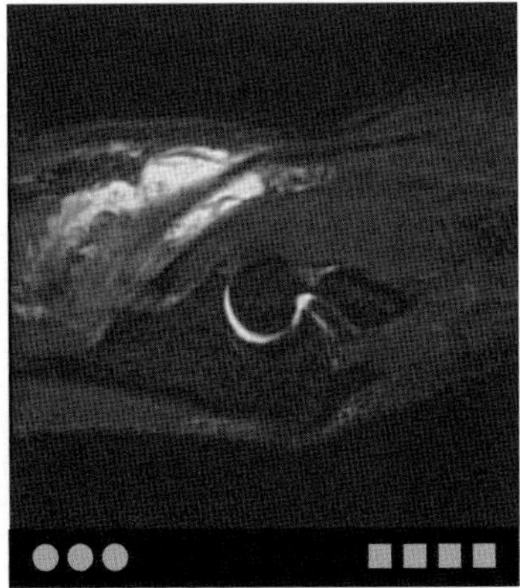

C. Bicipitoradial bursitis: Sagittal STIR image at the level of the biceps tendon insertion shows bright fluid signal around an intact tendon.

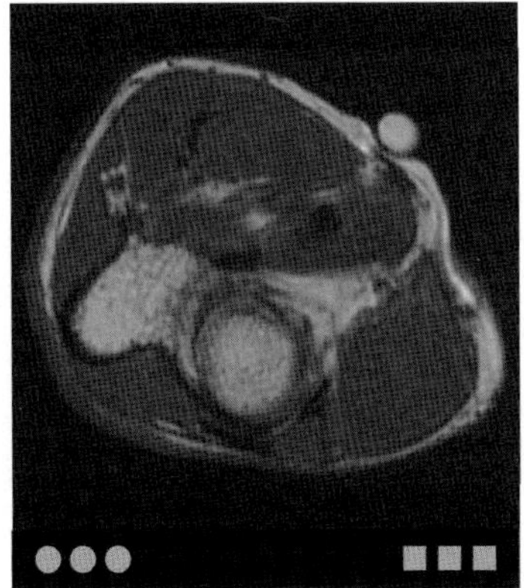

D. Bicipitoradial bursitis: Axial T1WI through the biceps tendon and olecranon shows intermediate signal around the tendon insertion.

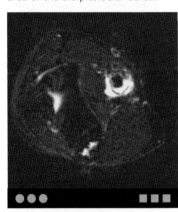

E. Bicipitoradial bursitis: Axial FSE T2WI through the capitellum shows bright fluid signal in an enlarged bursa posterior and surrounding the biceps tendon.

IMAGE KEY

Common

Rare

Typical

Unusual

DIFFERENTIAL DIAGNOSES IMAGES

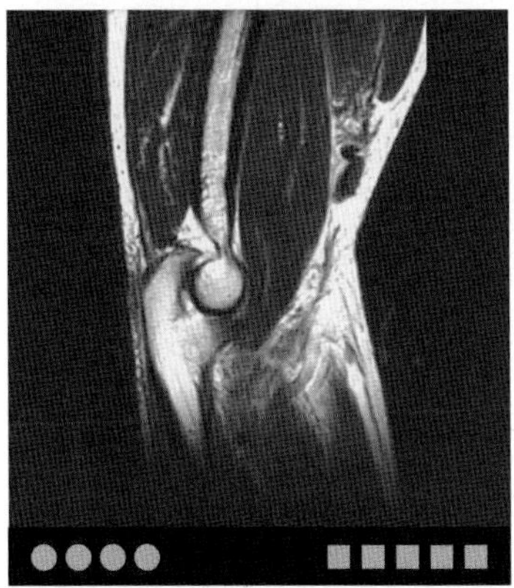

F. Distal biceps tendon rupture: Sagittal FSE T2WI similarly demonstrates a ruptured biceps tendon with peritendinous hemorrhage and edema.

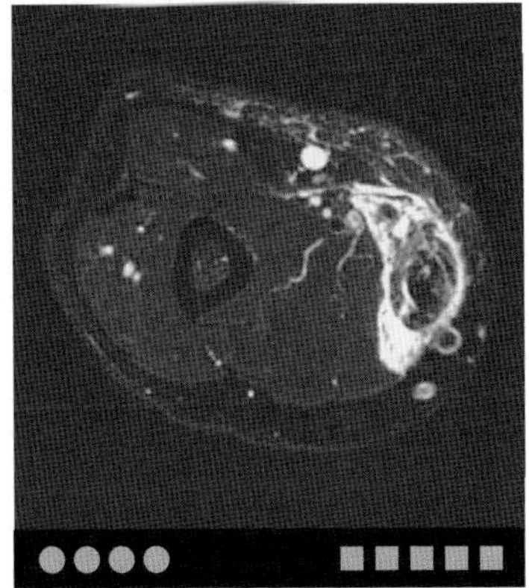

G. Distal biceps tendon rupture: Axial FSE T2W fat saturated image through the distal biceps demonstrates fluid signal surrounding the distal biceps with a wavy, retracted ruptured biceps tendon.

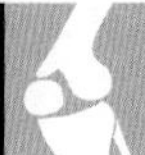

7–7 Medial Collateral Avulsion at Sublime Tubercle

Arash Tehranzadeh

PRESENTATION

Acute onset of elbow pain

FINDINGS

MR images show marrow edema in the sublime tubercle avulsion that is attached to the injured ulnar collateral ligament.

DIFFERENTIAL DIAGNOSES

- *Medial Epicondylitis:* Also known as Little Leaguer's elbow, this is another cause of medial joint line tenderness and is manifested by marrow edema in the medial epicondyle and may be associated with common flexor tendinosis.
- *Tendinosis of the common flexor tendon:* In the post-traumatic setting, differential considerations should include other causes of elbow pain. Although the common flexor tendon attaches to the medial humeral condyle, this is a cause of medial joint line pain.
- *Ulnar stress fracture:* Stress fractures of the olecranon may occur as a consequence of repetitive abutment of the olecranon into the olecranon fossa or traction of the triceps tendon, which may be seen in baseball players, gymnasts, or javelin throwers. These may occur in conjunction with medial collateral ligament injuries.

COMMENTS

The patient is a 16-year-old baseball player with right elbow overuse by pitching and throwing. The ulnar collateral ligament is composed of three parts, which include the anterior and posterior bundles and the transverse band. The anterior bundle arises from the anterior—inferior surface of the medial epicondyle of the humerus and inserts onto sublime tubercle of the ulna. Injuries to the ulnar collateral ligament most commonly present as a mid substance tear. Less common presentations include avulsion of the epicondylar attachment and avulsion of the ulnar attachment at the sublime tubercle. Avulsion of the sublime tubercle is common in throwing athletes or those involved in sports requiring overhead arm positions as sequelae of either acute traumatic or repeated valgus stress to the elbow. Such sports may include baseball and tennis. The anterior bundle is the primary stabilizing structure when the elbow is exposed to valgus stress. The repeated valgus stress can cause attenuation or rupture of the ulnar collateral ligament and result in functional medial elbow pain and instability. On MRI, the ulnar collateral ligament will appear attenuated and will demonstrate increased intrasubstance signal isointense to fluid. Discontinuity of the band of the ulnar collateral ligament may be seen. With avulsion of the sublime tubercle, the avulsed fragment may be separate or attached to the ulnar collateral ligament. Increased signal intensity consistent with marrow edema is seen in the avulsed sublime tubercle fragment and in the corresponding ulna.

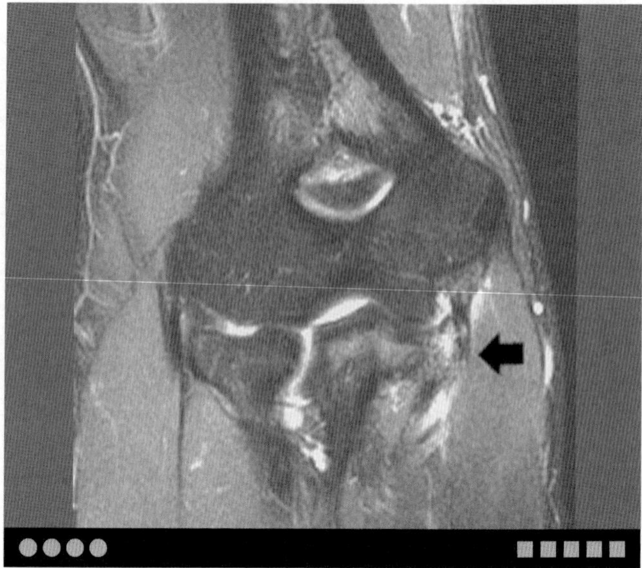

A. MCL avulsion at sublime tubercle (this image shows edema in the avulsed sublime tubercle and ulna): Coronal T2W fat-saturated image shows marrow edema in the ulna and in the avulsed sublime tubercle (arrow) which is attached to an attenuated anterior band of the ulnar collateral ligament.

PEARLS

- **The course of the anterior band of the ulnar collateral ligament is from the anterior—inferior surface of the medial epicondyle of the humerus to the sublime tubercle of the ulna.**
- **Avulsion of the sublime tubercle related to ulnar collateral ligament injury occurs as a consequence of either acute or chronic repetitive valgus stress in throwing athletes.**
- **The ulnar collateral ligament will appear attenuated and may show increased intrasubstance signal isointense to fluid.**
- **Marrow edema is visualized in the avulsed fragment and in the corresponding ulna.**

ADDITIONAL IMAGES

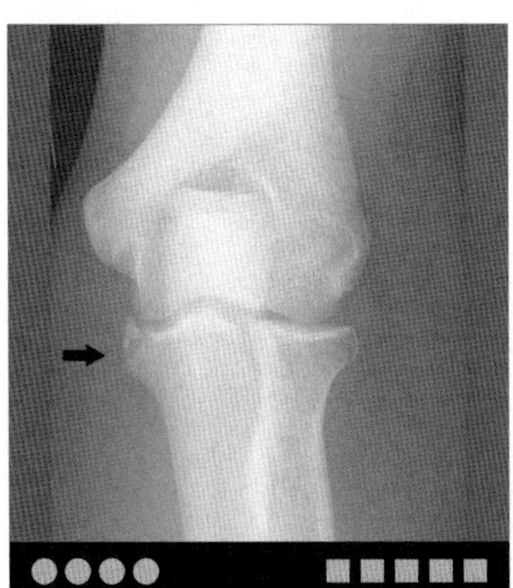

B. MCL avulsion at sublime tubercle: AP radiograph demonstrates an avulsion of the sublime tubercle of the ulna (arrow).

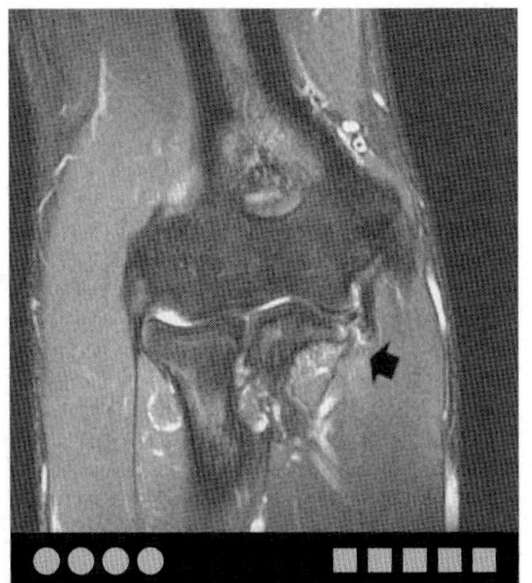

C. MCL avulsion at sublime tubercle: (this image depicts the anterior band of ulnar collateral ligament): Coronal T2W fat-saturated sequence demonstrates an attenuated anterior band of the ulnar collateral ligament with intrasubstance signal at its distal attachment to the avulsed sublime tubercle of the ulna (arrow).

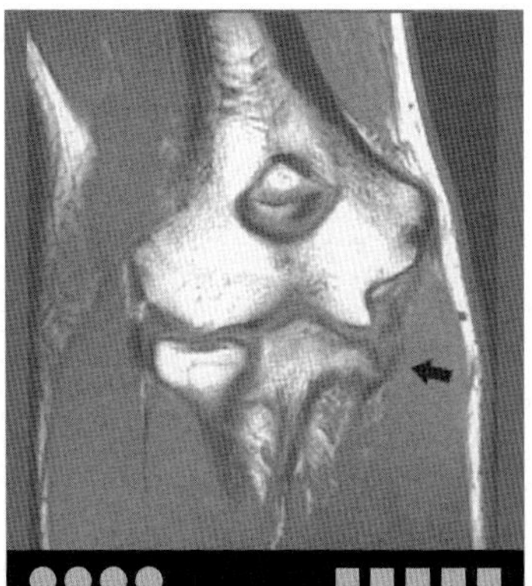

D. MCL avulsion at sublime tubercle: (this image depicts attenuated anterior band of the ulnar collateral ligament): Coronal T1W fast spin echo show the anterior band of the ulnar collateral ligament is attenuated with an avulsion at its ulnar attachment (arrow).

IMAGE KEY

Common

Rare

Typical

Unusual

DIFFERENTIAL DIAGNOSES IMAGES

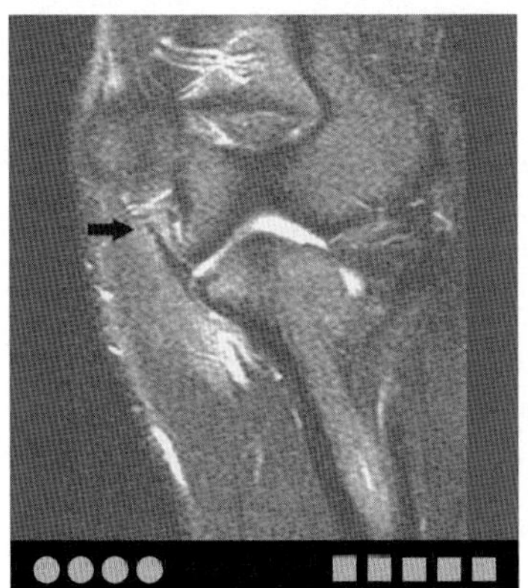

E. Medial collateral ligament midsubstance tear: Coronal fat-saturated T2W sequence. A more common presentation of an ulnar collateral ligament tear involves a midsubstance tear manifested by an attenuated ligament with intrasubstance signal isointense to fluid (arrow).

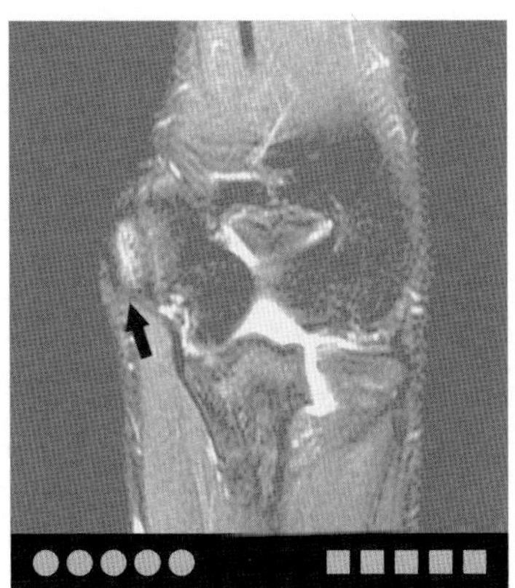

F. Medial epicondylitis: Coronal fat-saturated T2WI shows medial epicondylitis as increased edema in the medial epicondyle (arrow) and there is tendinosis in the common flexor tendon.

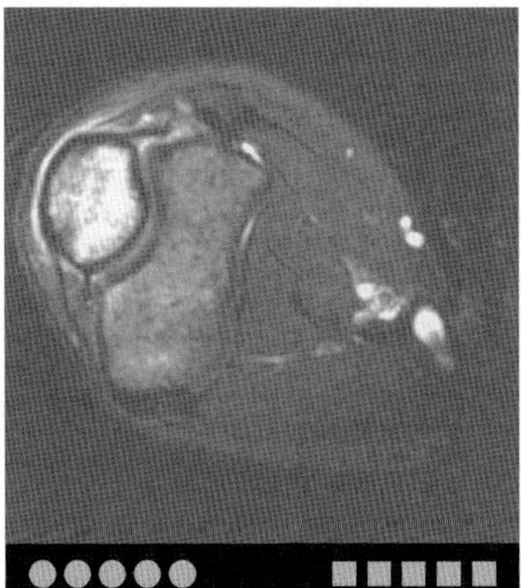

G. Ulnar stress fracture: Axial fat-saturated T2WI in a gymnast shows a chronic stress fracture manifested by marrow edema. There is also a disruption of the posterior band of the ulnar collateral ligament.

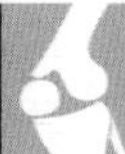

7–8 Olecranon Bursitis

Shahla Modarresi and Daria Motamedi

PRESENTATION

Pain and swelling at the posterior aspect of the elbow

FINDINGS

MR image shows intermediate PD signal mass in the olecranon bursa.

DIFFERENTIAL DIAGNOSES

- *Rheumatoid arthritis (RA):* Patients with RA show synovial proliferation and pannus formation in and about the joints. MR shows soft tissue mass isointense with muscle and fluid in the joint.
- *Crystal induced arthropathy (e.g., gout, pseudogout):* Gouty tophi when present show low signal in both T1W and T2W MR images. Soft tissue calcification and well-defined erosions with overhanging edge are typical radiographic findings of gout.
- *Trauma, Hematoma:* History of trauma with or without olecranon fracture. MR imaging shows mass of varying signal in the olecranon fossa depending on the duration of hematoma.
- *Synovial abscess:* MR imaging shows low signal intensity on T1W and high signal on T2W images. Postcontrast image shows rim enhancement, with the center of the mass that contains the pus remaining low signal.

COMMENTS

Olecranon bursitis is an inflammation of the bursa overlying the olecranon process at the proximal aspect of the ulna. The bursa is located between the ulna and the skin at the posterior tip of the elbow. Bursal inflammation may be caused by a variety of mechanisms. This bursa, because of its superficial location, is susceptible to inflammation from either acute or repetitive (cumulative) trauma. Less commonly, the inflammation may be caused by infection (septic bursitis). This condition is relatively common with focal swelling and at times pain at the posterior elbow noticed by the patient which may cause morbidity, limiting some functional activities such as writing. Complications after aspiration or injection include recurrence, infection, and persistent drainage. Chronic recurrent swelling is usually not tender. Onset may be sudden if the condition is secondary to infection or acute trauma. Onset is gradual when the bursitis is secondary to chronic irritation. Single joint involvement always suggests infection, crystal-induced arthritis, trauma, or rarely tumor. With septic bursitis, redness, heat over the bursa, and a purulent tap are noted. MR imaging shows a low signal mass on T1WI and intermediate to high signal mass on T2WI posterior to olecranon process. Septic olecranon bursitis can be excluded in the absence of bursal and soft tissue enhancement on contrast-enhanced MR imaging.

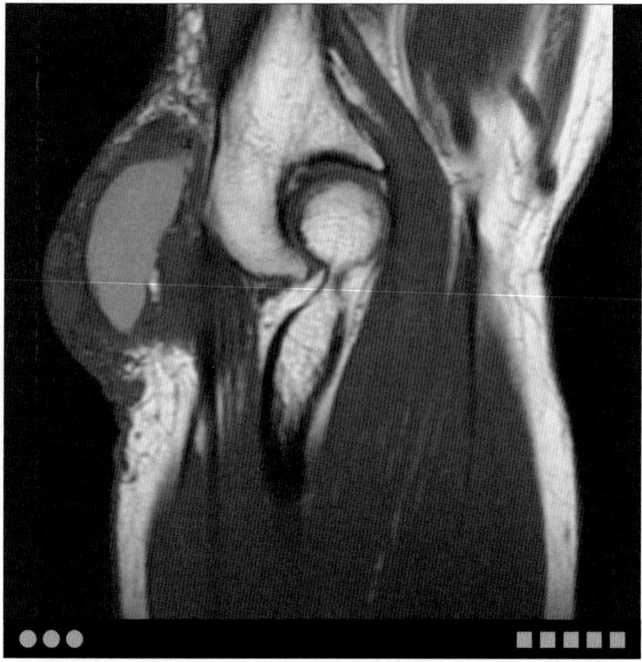

A. Olecranon bursitis: Sagittal PD image shows intermediate signal mass in the olecranon bursa.

PEARLS

- **Olecranon bursitis is inflammation of the bursa overlying the olecranon process at the proximal aspect of the ulna.**
- **Most common cause is chronic repeated microtrauma and prior infection.**
- **MR imaging shows a low signal mass on T1WI and intermediate to high signal mass on T2WI posterior to olecranon process.**
- **Septic olecranon bursitis can be excluded in the absence of bursal and soft tissue enhancement on contrast-enhanced MRI.**

ADDITIONAL IMAGE

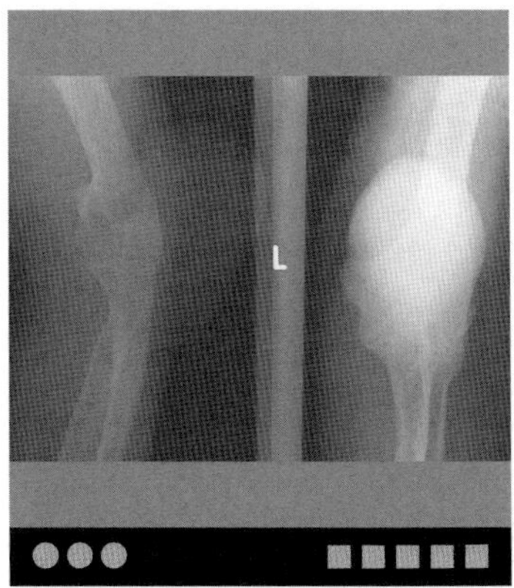

B. Olecranon bursitis: AP and lateral radiographs show olecranon bursitis with large soft tissue mass posterior to olecranon process.

DIFFERENTIAL DIAGNOSES IMAGES

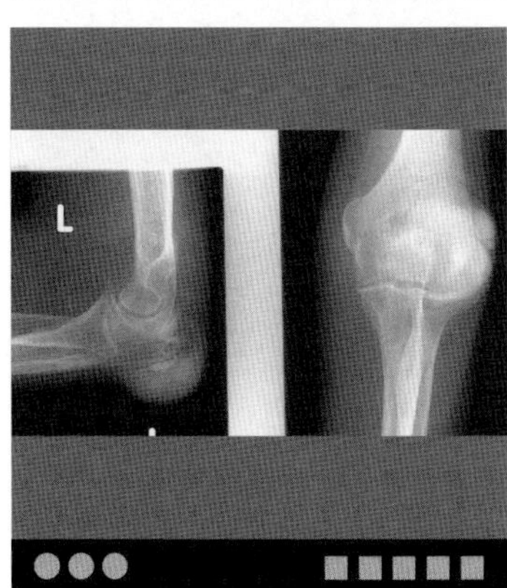

C. Gout with bursitis: Plane film shows soft tissue mass posterior to olecranon process with synovial calcification and olecranon erosion consistent with history of gouty arthritis and olecranon bursitis.

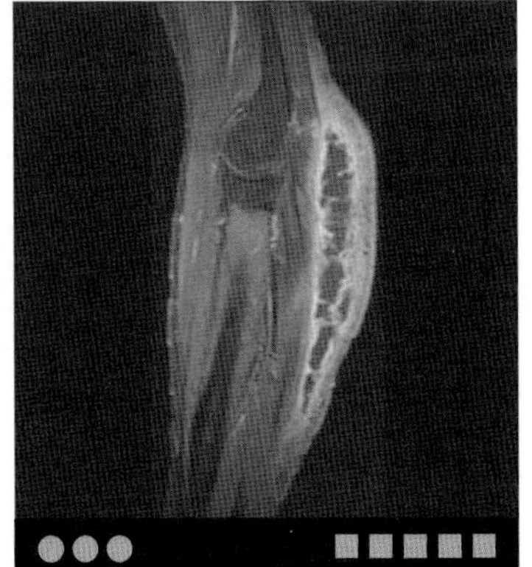

D. Abscess: Sagittal fat-saturated postcontrast T1W MR image shows multiloculated low signal fluid collection in the olecranon fossa with rim enhancement consistent with clinical evidence of abscess.

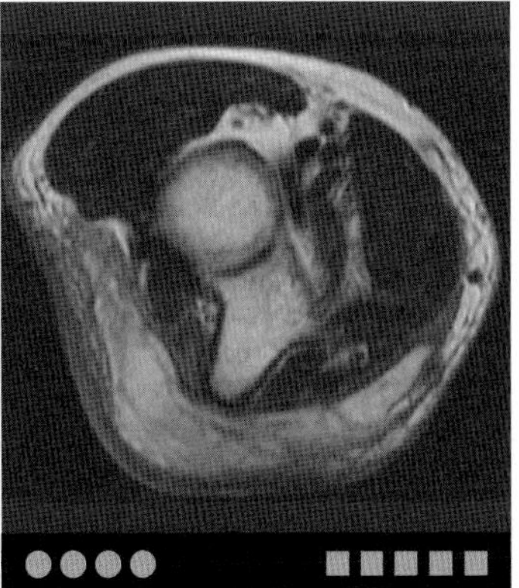

E. Subacute hematoma: Axial T2WI shows high signal fluid in the olecranon fossa with history of recent fall consistent with subacute hematoma.

IMAGE KEY

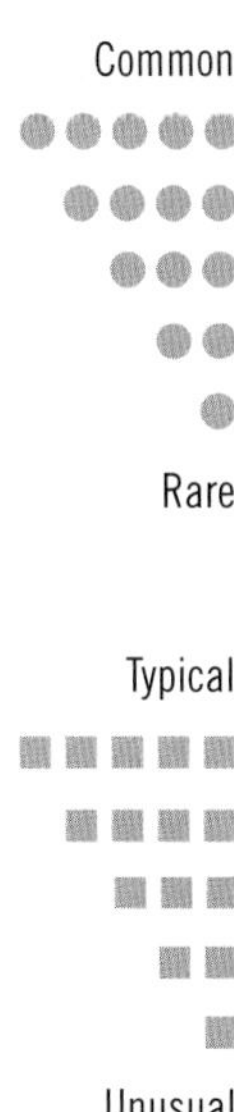

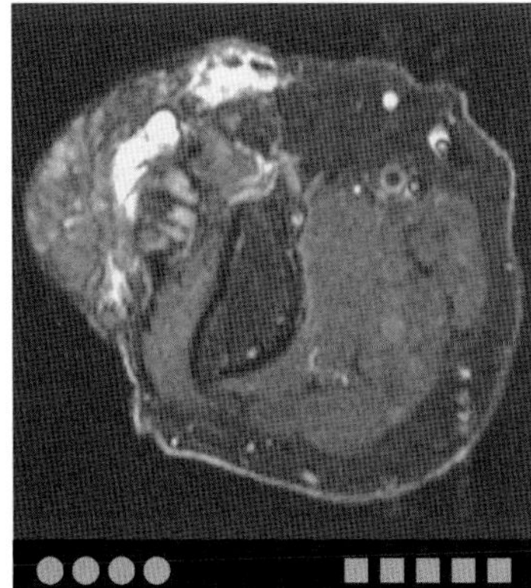

F. RA: Axial STIR image shows intermediate signal intensity pannus and high signal fluid in the olecranon fossa in patient with Rheumatoid arthritis.

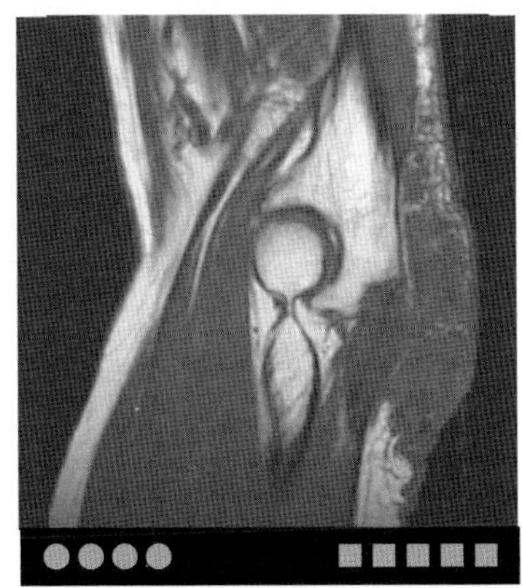

G. RA: Sagittal T1WI shows low signal mass in the olecranon fossa consistent with pannus in patient with rheumatoid arthritis.

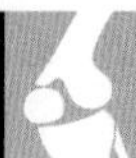

7–9 Common Extensor Tendonitis of Elbow

Kambiz Motamedi

PRESENTATION

Lateral elbow pain.

FINDINGS

MRI shows edema surrounding the insertion site of the common extensor tendons to the lateral humeral epicondyle.

DIFFERENTIAL DIAGNOSES

- *Strain of the common extensor tendon:* The MRI will show more extensive edema of the tendon and the musculotendinous junction. The edema typically tracks along the muscle fibers. In case of a tug lesion there may be a bony fragment as well.
- *Partial or complete tear of the lateral collateral ligament:* An MR arthrogram would show leak of contrast through the lateral aspect of the joint space with a complete tear. A partial tear would reveal contrast undercutting the radial (distal) attachment site of the ligament.
- *Cellulitis:* The MRI shows the edema to be limited to the subcutaneous compartment.

COMMENTS

This is a 50-year-old female patient with several month history of lateral elbow pain. The MRI shows mild edema of the common wrist extensor insertion site to the lateral humeral epicondyle. This is readily visualized on fluid-sensitive sequences, and may appear normal on T1WI. The sensitive planes to evaluate this entity are coronal and axial. There may be a subtle patchy marrow replacement of lateral humeral epicondyle marrow as well because of reactive edema. Radiographs are commonly normal, although are useful to exclude other pathologies, such as calcific tendinitis. Ultrasound may be useful to show the edematous tendon and possible adjacent hyperemia. Lateral epicondylitis is an overuse injury involving the extensor/supinator muscles that originate on the lateral epicondylar region of the distal humerus. Lateral epicondylitis has been demonstrated to occur in up to 50% of tennis players. However, this condition is not limited to tennis players and has been reported to be the result of overuse from many activities. Any activity involving wrist extension and/or supination can be associated with overuse of the muscles originating at the lateral epicondyle. The cause is attributed to microscopic tearing with formation of reparative tissue (i.e., angiofibroblastic hyperplasia) in the origin of the extensor carpi radialis brevis (ECRB) muscle. This microtearing and repair response can lead to macroscopic tearing and structural failure of the origin of the ECRB muscle.

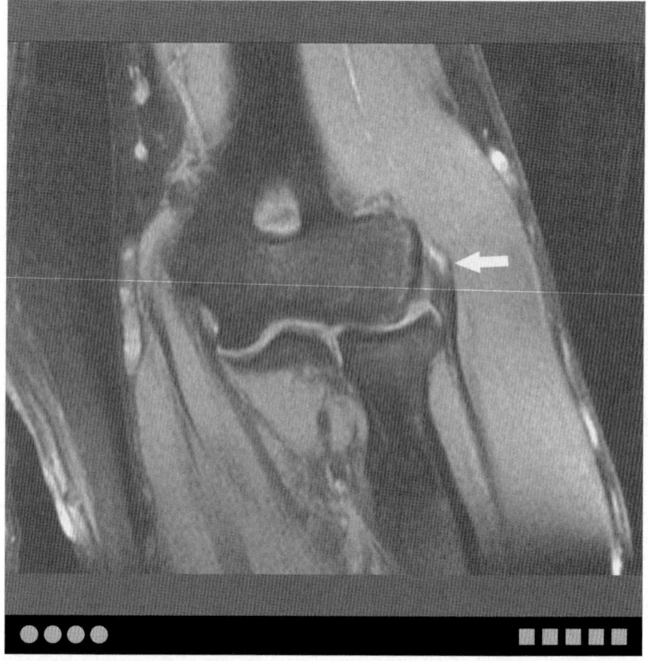

A. CET. Coronal PD MR image shows thickening of the common extensor tendon and intermediate signal at the attachment site (arrow).

PEARLS

- **MRI shows the edema concentrated around the insertion site of the tendon to the lateral humeral epicondyle.**
- **Positioning of the elbow in the middle of the gantry (outstretched) and use of appropriate coil are paramount to avoid common field inhomogeneity, when using fat saturation. Inversion recovery pulse sequence may be used as an alternative.**
- **Edema extending to the musculotendinous junction and spreading along the muscle fibers are more likely to result from strain.**

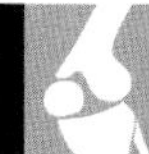

ADDITIONAL IMAGES

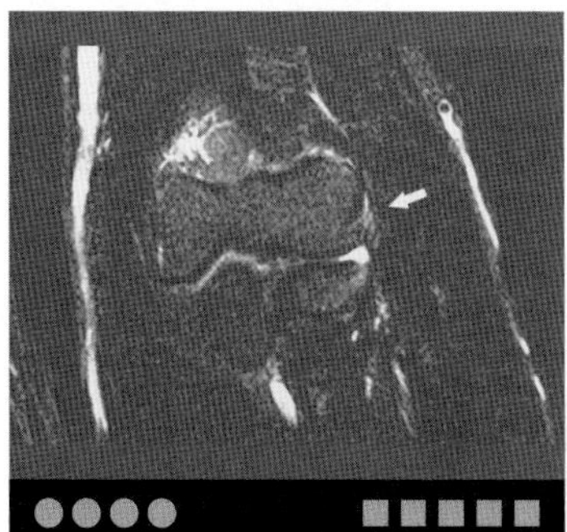

B. Common extensor tendonitis: Coronal inversion recovery MR image shows fluid signal at the attachment site of common extensor tendon the lateral epicondyle (arrow). There is no bone edema.

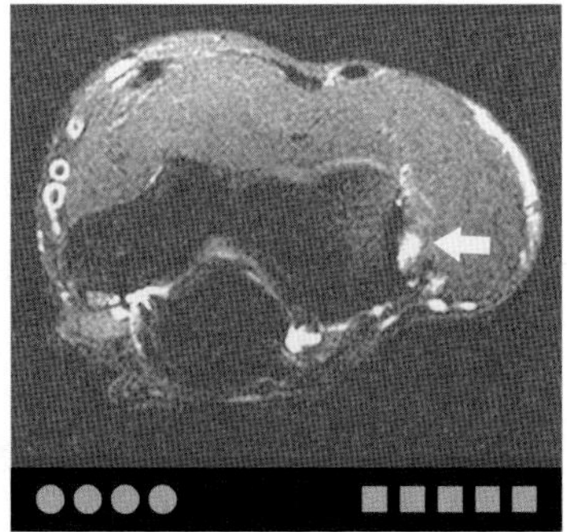

C. Common extensor tendonitis: Axial fat-saturated T2WI confirms the edema of the tendon at the attachment site (arrow). There is no joint effusion.

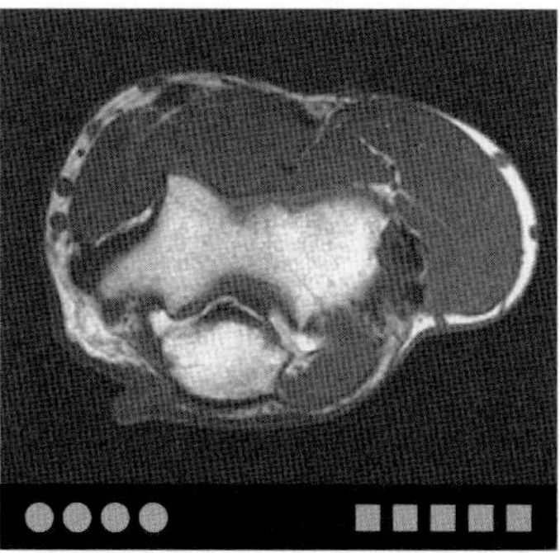

D. Common extensor tendonitis: Axial T1WI shows minimal thickening of the tendon with intermediate signal consistent with tendinosis.

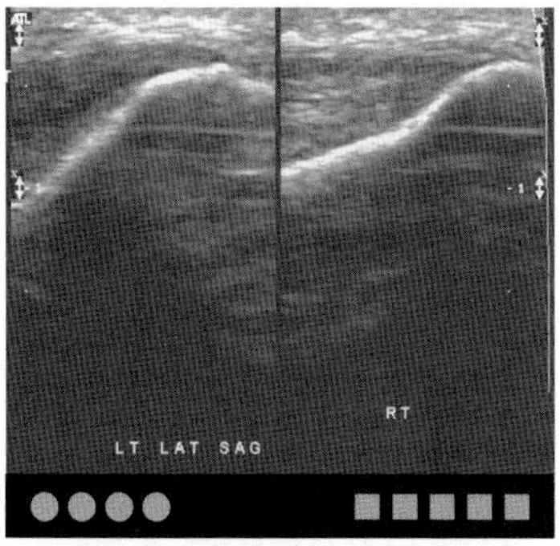

E. Common extensor tendonitis: A longitudinal ultrasound in a different patient with common extensor symptoms shows thickening of the left tendon fibers at the attachment site to the lateral humeral epicondyle. This becomes more apparent when directly compared to the contralateral side.

IMAGE KEY

Common

Rare

Typical

Unusual

DIFFERENTIAL DIAGNOSES IMAGES

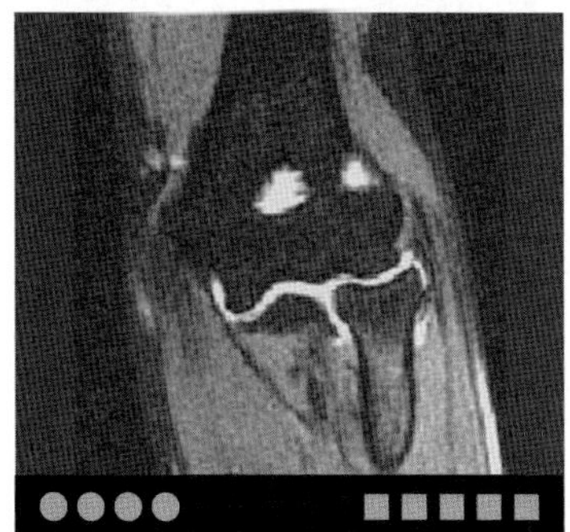

F. Partial radial collateral ligament tear: Coronal fat-saturated T1WI of the elbow following intra-articular injection of diluted gadolinium shows the contrast undercutting the radial attachment of the lateral collateral ligament, consistent with a tear.

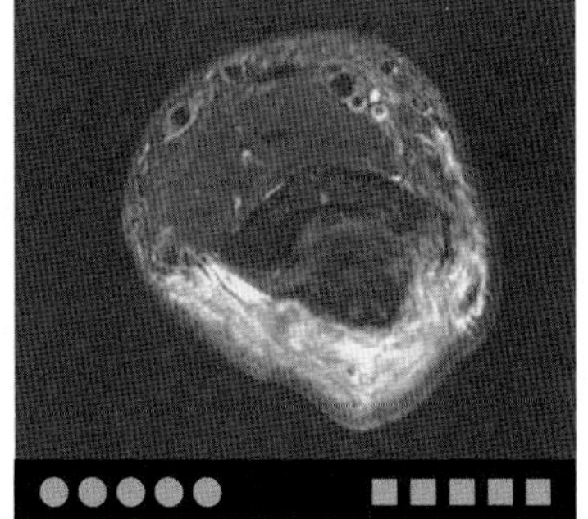

G. Cellulitis: Axial fat-saturated T2W FSE image demonstrates diffuse edema of the posterior, medial, and lateral predominantly subcutaneous compartment consistent with cellulitis.

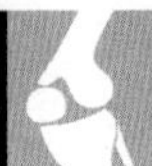

7–10 Tendinosis of Common Flexors of Elbow

Mohammad Reza Hayeri and Robert J. Ward

PRESENTATION

Medial elbow pain

FINDINGS

MRI shows low to intermediate signal change in common flexor tendon of the elbow.

DIFFERENTIAL DIAGNOSES

- *Ulnar neuritis:* This is the compression of the ulnar nerve at the level of the elbow and presents with tingling and numbness in ring and little fingers.
- *Medial collateral ligament elbow injury:* It is an injury to medial collateral ligament of elbow because of valgus stress and injury to the elbow.
- *Medial epicondylar avulsion:* Also know as Little Leaguer's elbow, this is traction apophysitis of medial epicondyle because of valgus overload or overstress injury that occurs as a result of repetitive throwing motions.
- *Avulsion of UCL graft:* Continued overuse or bad mechanics may lead to degeneration and retear of the UCL graft and may be recognized on MRI by edema, high signal fluid within the graft substance or focal discontinuity of the graft.
- *MCL avulsion at sublime Tubercle:* It is a less common presentation of MCL tear. Avulsion of the sublime tubercle is common in throwing athletes as sequelae of either acute traumatic or repeated valgus stress to the elbow.

COMMENTS

Tendinosis of the common flexor tendons also known as medial epicondylitis or "golfer's elbow" is an overuse injury of flexor/pronator muscles, especially with valgus stress at the medial epicondyle of the humerus. Tendinosis is defined as tendon degeneration without clinical or histological signs of an inflammatory response and as most patients lack these findings, it is more accurate to address these tendinopathies as "tendinosis" rather than "tendinitis" or "epicondylitis." The tendinosis that occurs is primarily the result of failure of the damaged tendon to heal. The medial condyle of the humerus gives origin to pronator teres, the flexor carpi radialis, the humeral head of flexor ulnaris, the Palmaris longus, ulnar head of the flexor digitorum superficialis. The pronator teres and the flexor carpi radialis share a conjoined tendon that is regarded as the primary site of origin of this condition. With repetitive stress loading of this conjoined tendon and the subsequent degenerative changes, medial elbow pain occurs. Decreased grip strength may also be noted. In one third of patient the disease develops subsequent to an injury. A male-to-female ratio of 2:1 is reported and patients usually present in the third through fifth decades. Ulnar neuropathy is an associated complain in over one half of the cases. On MRI, tendons demonstrate poorly defined low to intermediate signal change on T1WI, with a relative increase in signal on T2WI. Cystic changes with focal areas of high signal seen within the tendon on T2 are findings in later stages.

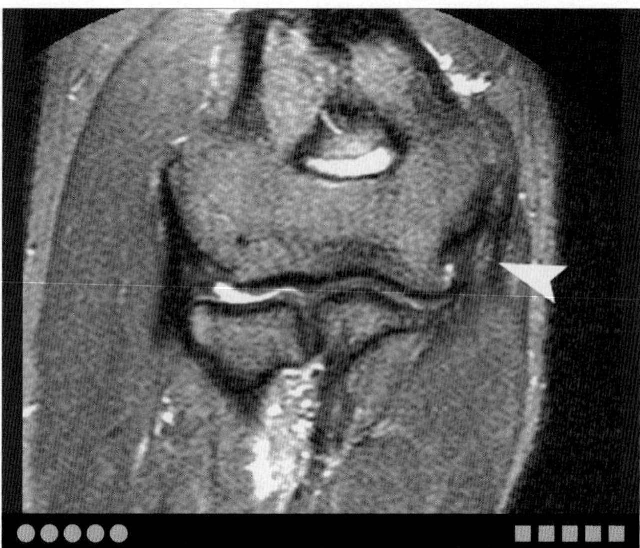

A. Tendinosis of common flexor tendon of elbow: Coronal T2W fat-saturated image shows intermediate signal in common flexor tendon (arrowhead). (Courtesy of Thomas L Huang.)

PEARLS

- **Tendinosis of the common flexor tendons is an overuse injury of flexor/pronator muscles, especially with valgus stress at the medial epicondyle of the humerus.**
- **The medial condyle of the humerus gives origin to pronator teres, the flexor carpi radialis, the humeral head of flexor ulnaris, the Palmaris longus, and ulnar head of the flexor digitorum superficialis.**
- **Patients may present with pain, decreased grip strength, and ulnar neuropathy.**
- **On MRI tendons demonstrate poorly defined low to intermediate signal change on T1WI, with a relative increase in signal on T2WI**

ADDITIONAL IMAGES

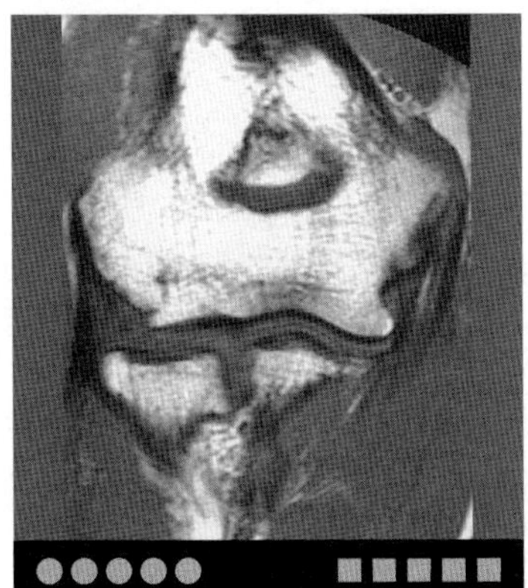

B. Tendinosis of common flexor tendon of elbow: Coronal T1WI shows intermediate signal in common flexor tendon. (Courtesy of Thomas L Huang.)

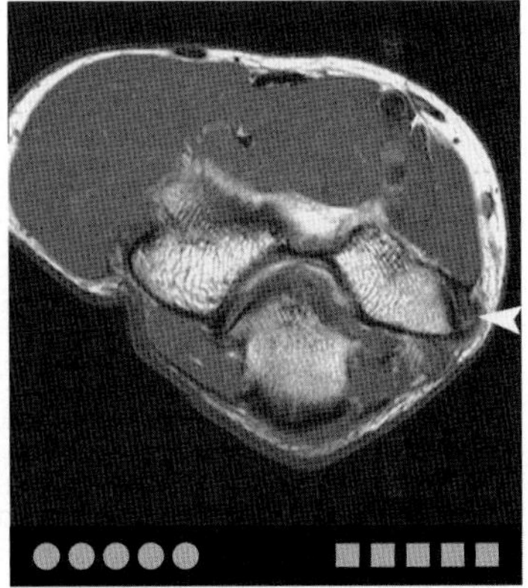

C. Tendinosis of common flexor tendon of elbow: Axial T1WI shows intermediate signal in common flexor tendon (arrowhead). (Courtesy of Thomas L Huang.)

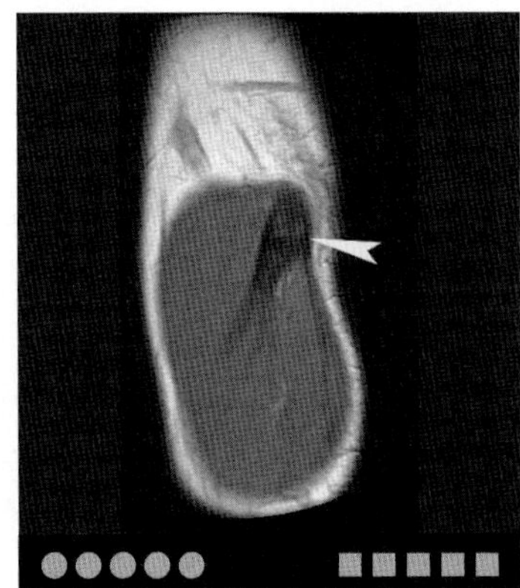

D. Tendinosis of common flexor tendon of elbow: Sagittal T1WI shows intermediate signal in common flexor tendon (arrowhead). (Courtesy of Thomas L Huang.)

IMAGE KEY

Common

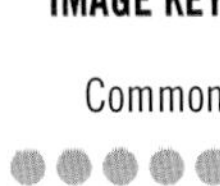

Rare

Typical

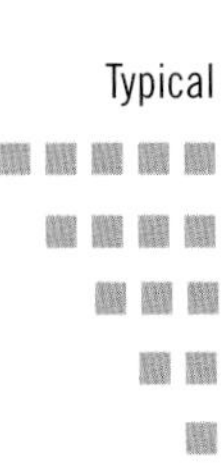

Unusual

DIFFERENTIAL DIAGNOSES IMAGES

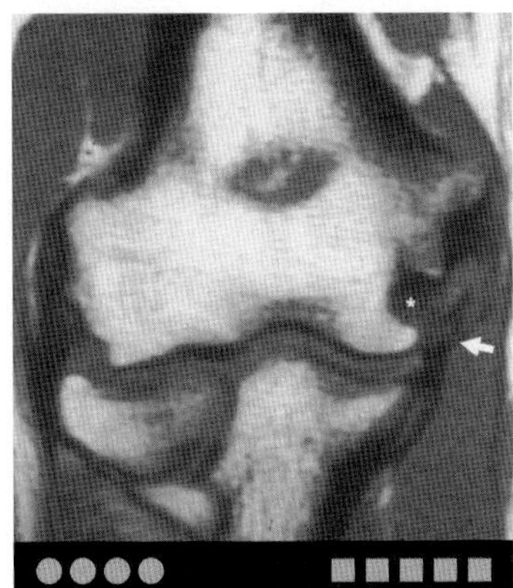

E. Ulnar collateral ligament injury: Coronal T1WI showing a torn and frayed proximal UCL (arrow). Note isolntense edema (star) obliterating the normal fat pad between the ligament and trochlea.

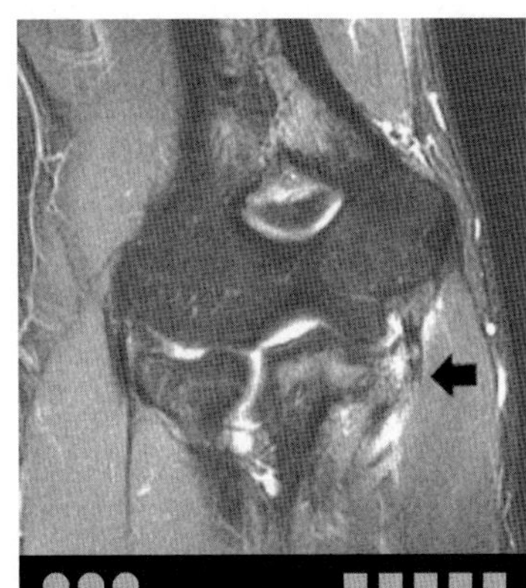

F. MCL avulsion at sublime Tubercle (this image shows edema in the avulsed sublime tubercle and ulna): Coronal T2W fat-saturated image shows marrow edema in the ulna and in the avulsed sublime tubercle (arrow) which is attached to an attenuated anterior band of the ulnar collateral ligament.

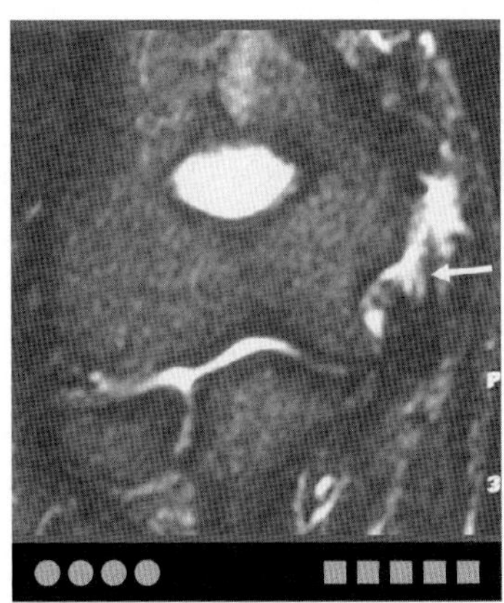

G. Avulsion of UCL graft: Coronal STIR image demonstrates acute avulsion of the proximal UCL graft with high signal fluid at the tear site.

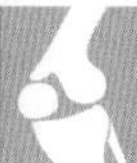

7–11 Tear of Common Flexor Tendon of Elbow

Mohammad Reza Hayeri and Robert J. Ward

PRESENTATION

Medial elbow pain

FINDINGS

MRI shows high signal intensity on T2W or fluid-sensitive sequences within the substance of a tendon. In complete tears, a focal area of discontinuity and retraction may be observed.

DIFFERENTIAL DIAGNOSES

- *Tendinosis of common flexor tendon:* Tendinosis of the common flexor tendons is an overuse injury of flexor/pronator muscles, especially with valgus stress at the medial epicondyle of the humerus. Tendinosis has intermediate signal on T2WI.
- *Medial collateral ligament elbow injury:* It is injury to medial collateral ligament of elbow resulting from valgus stress and injury to the elbow. Fluid signal in ulnar collateral ligament is seen on T2WI.
- *Medial epicondylar avulsion:* Also known as Little Leaguer's elbow is traction apophysitis of medial epicondyle resulting from valgus overload or overstress injury that occurs as a result of repetitive throwing motions. There is bony avulsion of medial distal humeral epicondyle.

COMMENTS

The medial condyle of the humerus gives origin to pronator teres, the flexor carpi radialis, the humeral attachment of flexor ulnaris, the Palmaris longus, and ulnar head of the flexor digitorum superficialis. The pronator teres and the flexor carpi radialis share a conjoined tendon that is regarded as the primary site of origin of this condition. Common flexor tendon (CFT) provides a dynamic support to valgus stress in throwing elbow. CFT injuries occur in 1% to 3% of adults who are 35 to 55 years old. Common flexor tendon tear is more common in golfers, high-performance throwers, swimmers, racquetball squash players, and bowlers. Common flexor tear can be one of the findings at MRI in medial epicondylitis, an overuse tendinopathy of flexor pronator group. Patient usually presents with pain in the medial aspect of the elbow. The diagnosis of partial tears is critical to throwing athletes, because these patients will likely undergo surgery. On MR sagittal images, common flexor tendon is seen on the most medial images as a hypointense band of signal parallel to the lung axis of ulna coursing to insert on the medial epicondyle. Abnormal morphology (attenuation or thickening) can be seen in tendinosis or tear. Partial tears are depicted by thinning or partial disruption of the tendon, and increased T2W signal within and adjacent to the tendon origin. Complete rupture of the tendons will lead to a tendinous gap containing fluid signal, and distal retraction of the involved muscle(s).

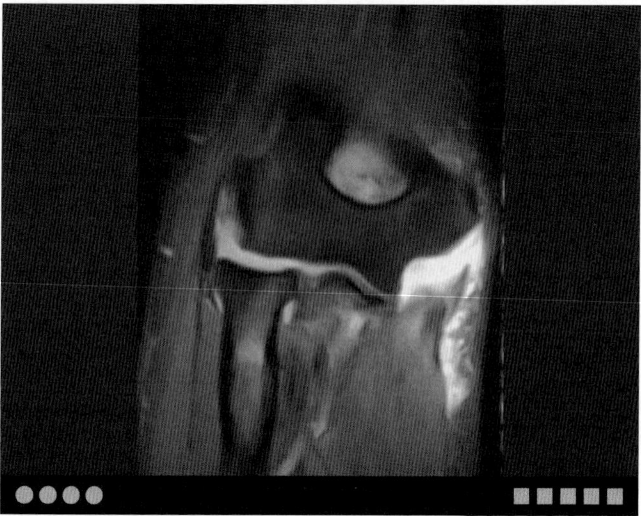

A. Tear of common flexor tendon of elbow: Coronal fat-saturated T2WI shows tear of common flexor tendon. The fluid extends in the medial subcutaneous tissue. Medial collateral ligament tear is also noted. (Courtesy of Adam Zoga.)

PEARLS

- **The medial condyle of the humerus gives origin to pronator teres, the flexor carpi radialis, the humeral head of flexor ulnaris, the Palmaris longus, and ulnar head of the flexor digitorum superficialis.**
- **Common flexor tendon tear is more common in golfers, high-performance throwers, swimmers, racquetball squash players, and bowlers.**
- **Partial tears are depicted by thinning or partial disruption of the tendon, and increased T2W signal within and adjacent to the tendon origin.**
- **Complete rupture of the tendons will lead to a tendinous gap containing fluid signal and distal retraction of the involved muscle(s).**

ADDITIONAL IMAGES

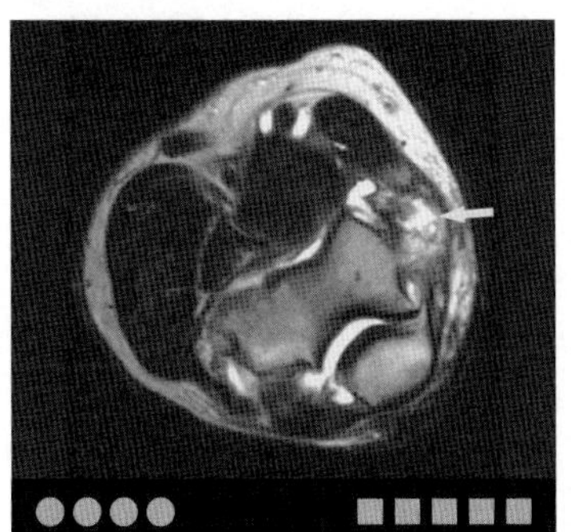

B. Tear of common flexor tendon of elbow: Axial T2WI of the same patient as image A shows tear of common flexor tendon. Fluid collection is seen in common flexor tendon (arrow). (Courtesy of Adam Zoga.)

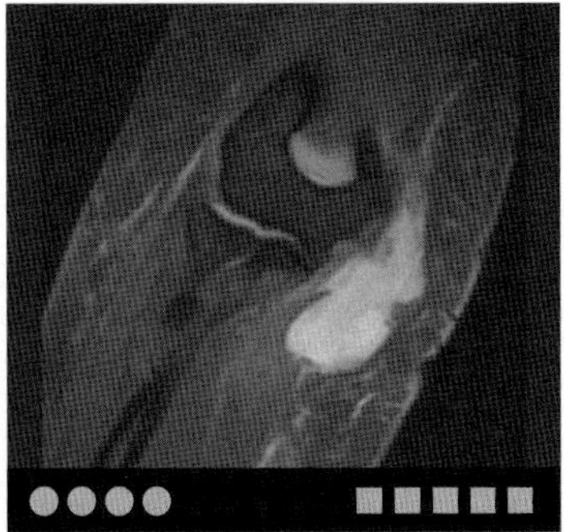

C. Tear of common flexor tendon of elbow: Coronal T2 fat-saturated image of another patient shows large fluid collection in the medial side of elbow joint as a result of complete tear and retraction of common flexor tendon. (Courtesy of Adam Zoga.)

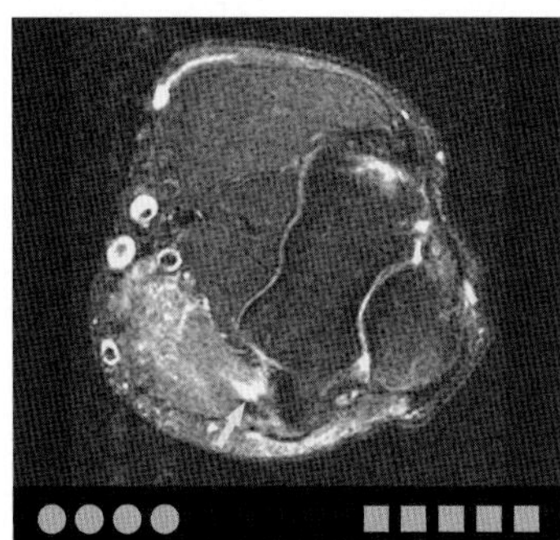

D. Tear of common flexor tendon of elbow: Axial T2 fat-saturated image of the same patient (as in image C) shows tear of the common flexor tendon (arrow) with muscle edema. (Courtesy of Adam Zoga.)

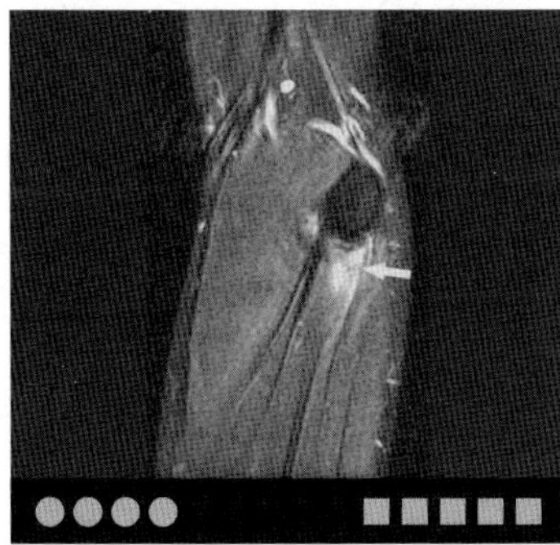

E. Tear of common flexor tendon of elbow: Sagittal T2 fat-saturated image of another patient shows tear of the common flexor tendon (arrow). (Courtesy of Adam Zoga.)

IMAGE KEY

Common

●●●●●
●●●●
●●●
●●
●

Rare

Typical

■■■■■
■■■■
■■■
■■
■

Unusual

DIFFERENTIAL DIAGNOSES IMAGES

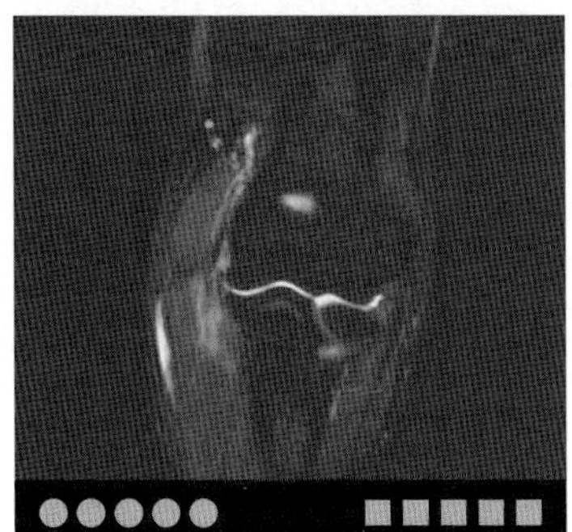

F. Tendinosis of common flexor tendon of elbow: Coronal T2 weighted fat saturated image shows intermediate to bright signal in the medial aspect of elbow because of tendinosis of common flexor tendon. (Courtesy of Adam Zoga.)

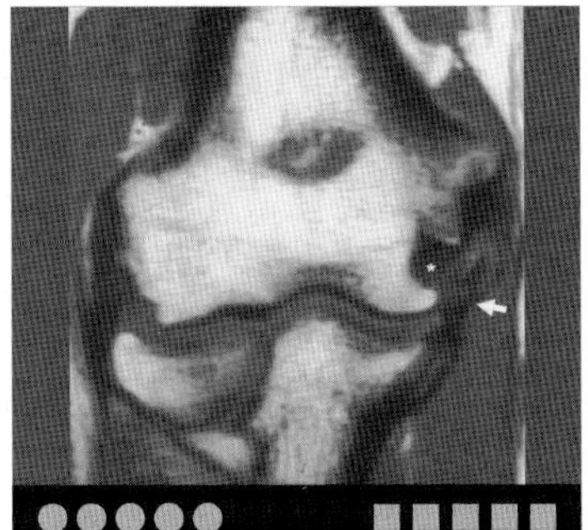

G. Ulnar collateral ligament injury (UCL): Coronal T1WI showing a torn and frayed proximal UCL (arrow). Note isointense edema (star) obliterating the normal fat pad between the ligament and trochlea.

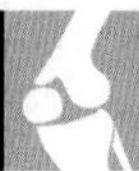

7–12 Lateral Ulnar Collateral Ligament Tear

Ashkan Afshin and Jamshid Tehranzadeh

PRESENTATION

Elbow pain

FINDINGS

MR findings show disruption of the ligamentous fibers with fluid signal intensity.

DIFFERENTIAL DIAGNOSES

- *Tear of the radial collateral ligament:* MR images demonstrate disruption of the fibers of radial collateral ligament. Fluid signal intensity replaces this ligament in fluid-sensitive images.
- *Common extensor tendon tear:* MR images show disruption of the common extensor tendons with the gap and area of increased signal in the origin of the tendon.

COMMENTS

Lateral ligament complex consists of radial collateral ligament (RCL), lateral ulnar collateral ligament (LUCL), the accessory lateral collateral ligament, and the annular ligament. The LUCL originates from the lateral epicondyle of the humerus and extends through a diagonal course along the posterior aspect of the radius to inserts to the tubercle of the supinator crest of the ulna. Visualization of LUCL is often difficult and it may be possible in only 50% of the cases in routine MRI studies. LUCL provides the primary ligamentous constraint to varus stress in the elbow. Excessive posterolateral rotatory force can result in rupture of the lateral ulnar collateral ligament. Fall on outstretched hand is a common mechanism of LUCL injury. Disruption of LUCL leads to posterolateral rotatory instability (PLRI) of the elbow. The instability manifests in a spectrum of severity from mild subluxation to recurrent dislocation. Patients with mild forms complain of intermittent symptoms such as pain, clicking, or catching on the lateral side of the elbow associated with supination of the forearm. Some patients may experience even more sever symptoms including locking, sensations of elbow instability or recurrent dislocation of the elbow. MR imaging provides the best diagnostic tool for LUCL injuries. MR findings show disruption of the ligamentous fibers with fluid signal intensity. Disruption usually occurs at the radial side under the surface of lateral epicondyle beneath the radial neck.

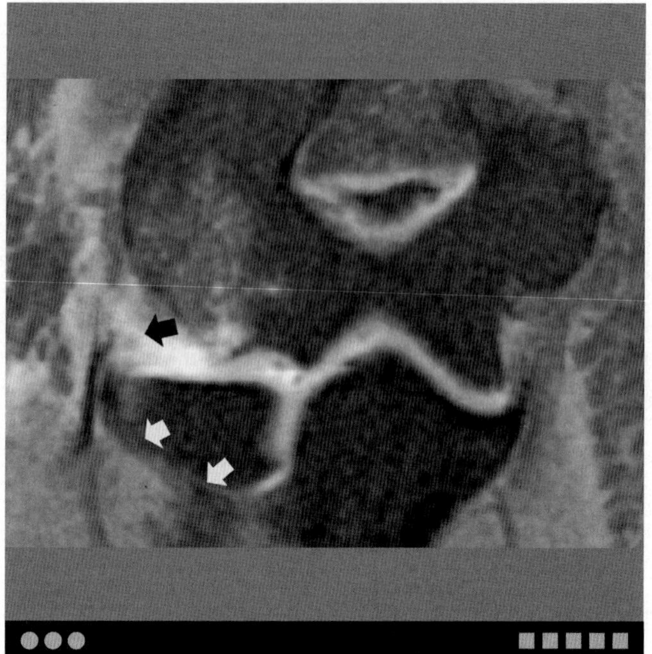

A. Complete tear of the lateral ulnar collateral ligament: Coronal T2W fat-saturated image shows complete tear of the LUCL (black arrow).The oblique course of this ligament which attaches to the lateral side of ulna is shown by white arrows. Note the bone contusion of the capitellum. (Courtesy of Mark Schweitzer.)

PEARLS

- **LUCL originates from the lateral epicondyle of the humerus and inserts to the tubercle of the supinator crest of the ulna.**
- **Fall on outstretched hand is a common mechanism of injury.**
- **Its tear may result in posterolateral rotatory instability.**
- **Disruption of the ligamentous fibers with fluid signal intensity are shown on MR images.**

ADDITIONAL IMAGE

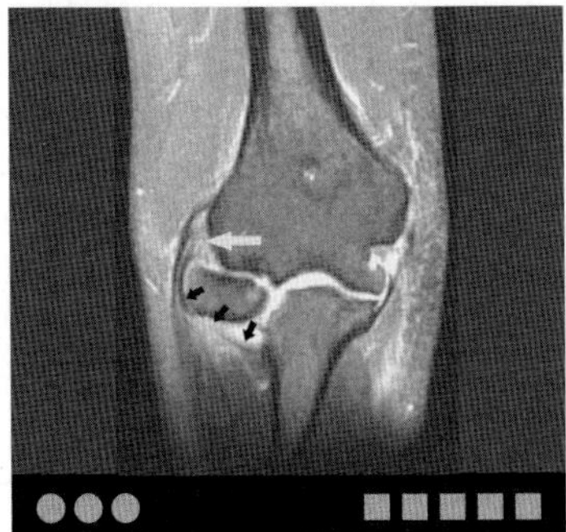

B. Partial tear of the lateral ulnar collateral ligament: Coronal T2W fat-saturated image in another patient shows partial tear of the LUCL (large white arrow). The black arrows show the oblique course of this ligament, which inserts to lateral aspect of the ulna. There is a small bone contusion and flattening of the medial aspect of radial head. There is also tearing of medial collateral ligament. (Courtesy of Mark Schweitzer.)

IMAGE KEY

Common

●●●●●
●●●●
●●●
●●
●

Rare

Typical

■■■■■
■■■■
■■■
■■
■

Unusual

DIFFERENTIAL DIAGNOSES IMAGES

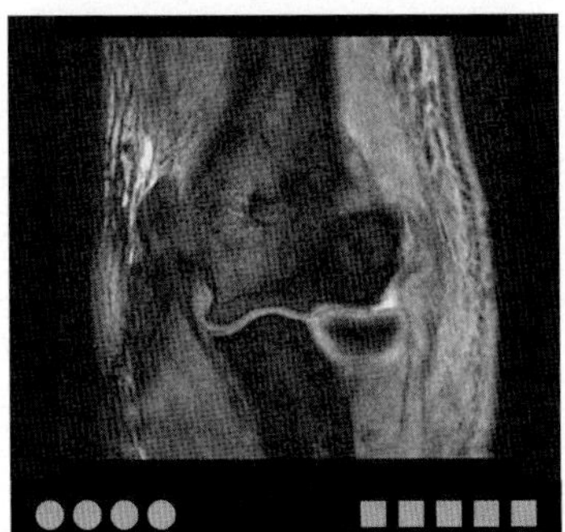

C. Tear of the radial collateral ligament: Coronal T2W fat-saturated image shows complete tear and absence of the radial collateral ligament.

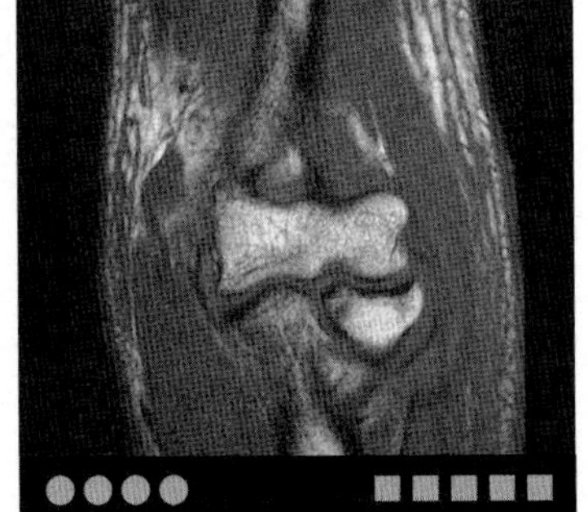

D. Tear of the radial collateral ligament: Coronal T1WI in the same patient (as in image C) shows complete tear of the radial collateral ligament.

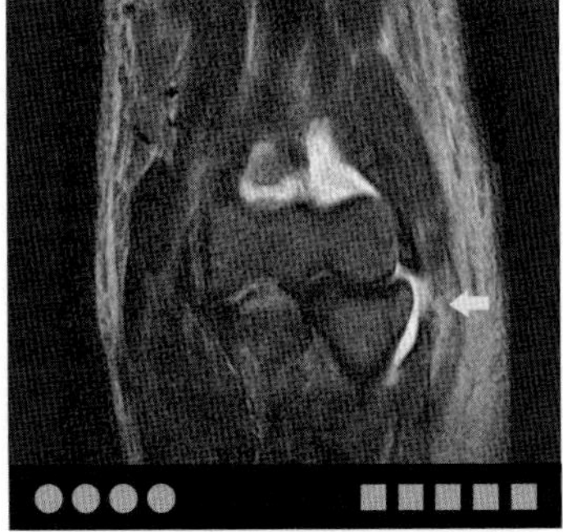

E. Common extensor tendon tear: Coronal T2WI shows tear of the common extensor tendon (arrow).

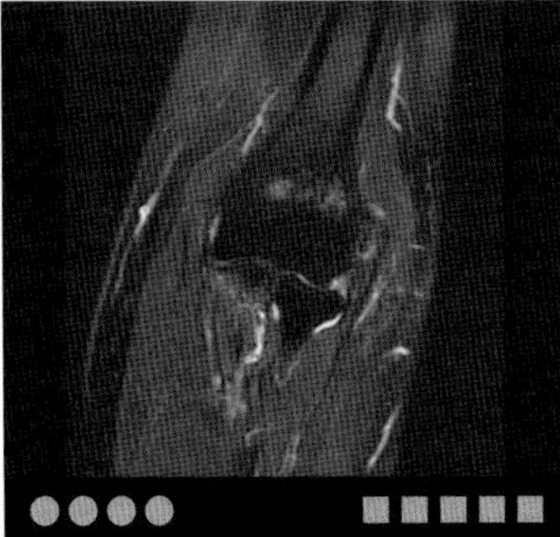

F. Lateral epicondylitis with tear of common extensor tendon: Coronal T2WI shows increased signal in the area of the common extensor tendons origin.

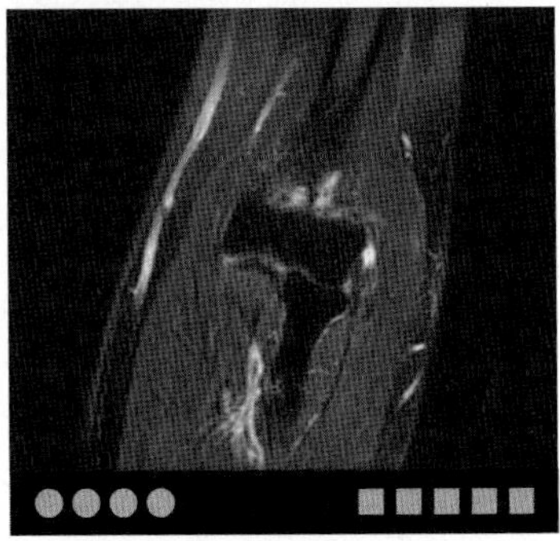

G. Lateral epicondylitis with tear of common extensor tendon: Coronal T2WI with fat saturation shows a gap with fluid increased signal in the common extensor tendons origin consistent with a full thickness tear.

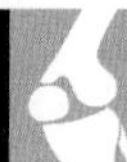

7–13 Posterolateral Instability of the Elbow

Ashkan Afshin and Robert J. Ward

PRESENTATION

Elbow pain

FINDINGS

MR images show tear of the lateral collateral, lateral ulnar collateral, and medial collateral ligaments. Posterior disruption of the joint capsule is also observed.

DIFFERENTIAL DIAGNOSES

- *Avulsion fracture of triceps tendon:* The lateral radiograph of the elbow may show the presence of flecks of avulsed osseous fragment from the olecranon process ("flake sign"). MR images show separation of the triceps tendon from olecranon process and fluid signal is observed between the distal end of the tendon and olecranon.
- *Tear of the radial collateral ligament:* MR images show disruption of the fibers of the radial collateral ligament. Fluid signal intensity replaces the ligament in fluid sensitive images.
- *Lateral epicondylitis:* MR images demonstrate increased signal in lateral collateral ligament on T1WI and intermediate signal on T2WI.

COMMENTS

Posterolateral instability is the most frequent form of elbow instability. It results from disruption of the lateral collateral and annular ligaments. Lateral ulnar collateral tear in association with rupture of the medial collateral ligament may also be observed. However, when the annular ligament is intact, either the radial collateral ligament or the lateral ulnar collateral ligament can be transected without inducing posterolateral instability of the elbow. This condition can be associated with conditions like elbow dislocation, radial head excision, and coronoid fracture. Posterolateral instability manifests in a spectrum of severity from mild subluxation to recurrent dislocation. Patients with mild forms complain of intermittent symptoms such as pain, clicking, or catching on the lateral side of the elbow associated with supination of the forearm. Some patients may experience even more sever symptoms including locking, sensations of elbow instability, or recurrent dislocation of the elbow. These symptoms are particularly marked in near-extension with the forearm supinated. An extension deficit is seen in one third of the patients. The most sensitive physical examination is the lateral pivot-shift test. The lateral pivot-shift is enhanced if the lateral collateral ligament is transected, or if all the collateral ligaments are cut. MR imaging is an effective tool in the preoperative, noninvasive diagnosis of posterolateral instability.

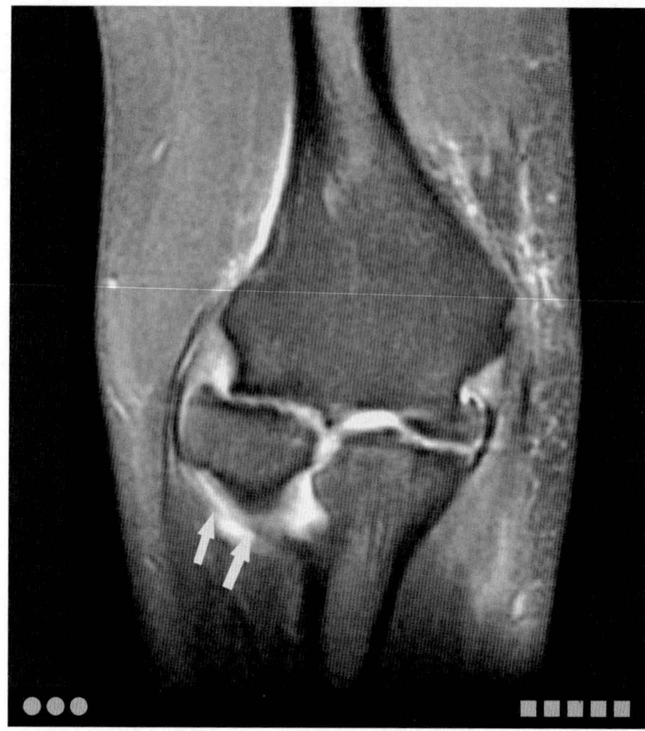

A. Posterolateral instability of the elbow: Sagittal T2WI demonstates posterior subluxation of radius relative to the capitellum indicative of lateral ulnar collateral ligament tearing. Obvious trauma is present as evidenced by increased interstitial muscle signal as well as the obvious effusion. (Courtesy of Adam Zoga.)

PEARLS

- **It results from disruption of the lateral collateral and annular ligaments.**
- **Lateral ulnar collateral tear in association with rupture of the medial collateral ligament may be observed.**
- **It can be can be associated with conditions like elbow dislocation, radial head excision, and coronoid fracture.**
- **It manifests in a spectrum of severity from mild subluxation to recurrent dislocation.**
- **Patients have pain and report a sensation of snapping or catching.**
- **The most sensitive physical examination is the lateral pivot-shift test.**

ADDITIONAL IMAGES

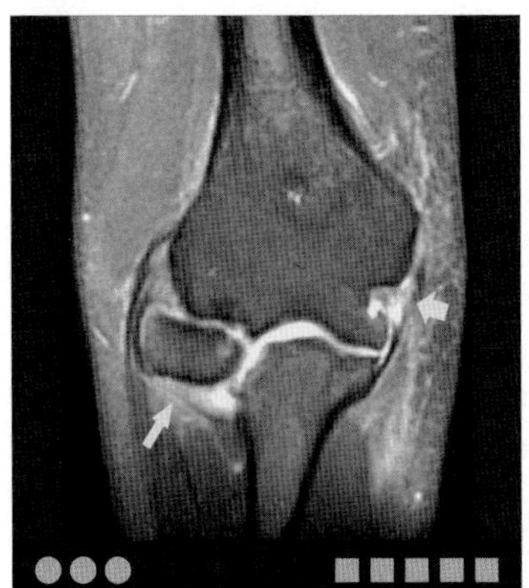

B. Posterolateral instability of elbow: Coronal fat-saturated T2WI shows tear of the lateral ulnar collateral ligament (long arrow) and medical collateral ligament (short fat arrow). Osteochondral injury of the capitellum and radial head resulting in narrowing of the capitellum-radial head joint is noted. (Courtesy of Adam Zoga.)

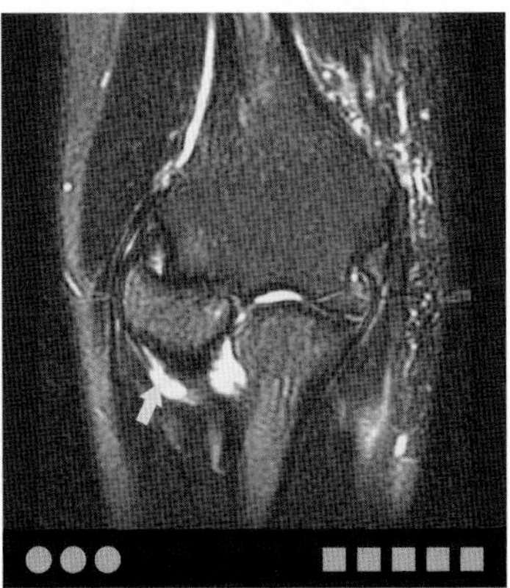

C. Posterolateral instability of elbow: Coronal fat-saturated T2WI shows tear of the lateral ulnar collateral ligament (arrow) and medical collateral ligament. Osteochondral injury of the capitellum and radial head resulting in narrowing of the capitellum-radial head joint is noted. (Courtesy of Adam Zoga.)

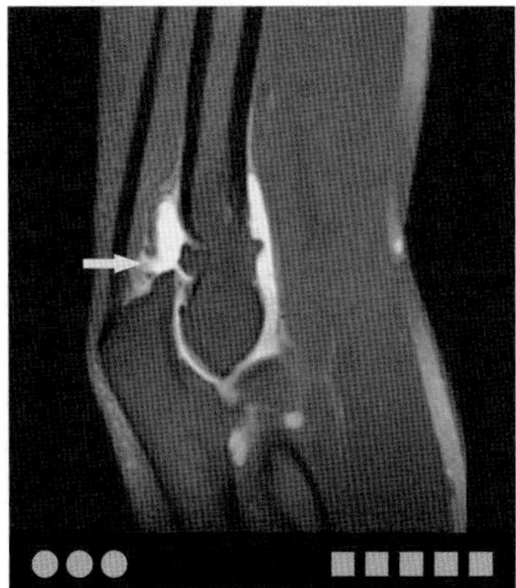

D. Posterolateral instability of elbow: Sagittal fat-saturated T2WI in the same patient (as in images A to C) shows posterior disruption of the joint capsule (arrow). (Courtesy of Adam Zoga.)

IMAGE KEY

Common

●●●●●
●●●●
●●●
●●
●

Rare

Typical

■■■■■
■■■■
■■■
■■
■

Unusual

DIFFERENTIAL DIAGNOSES IMAGES

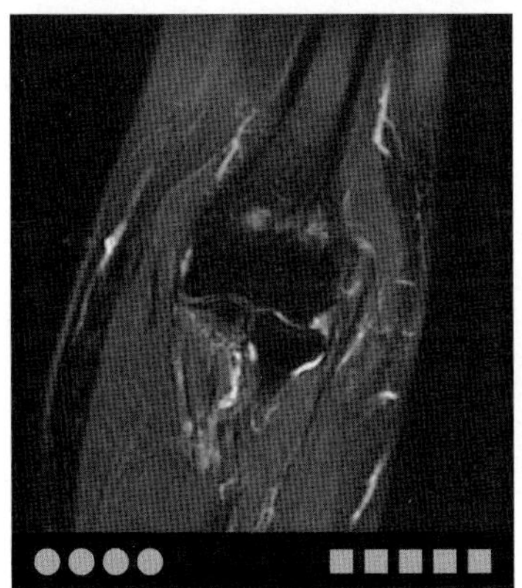

E. Lateral epicondylitis with tear of common extensor tendon: Coronal T2WI shows increased signal in the area of the common extensor tendons origin.

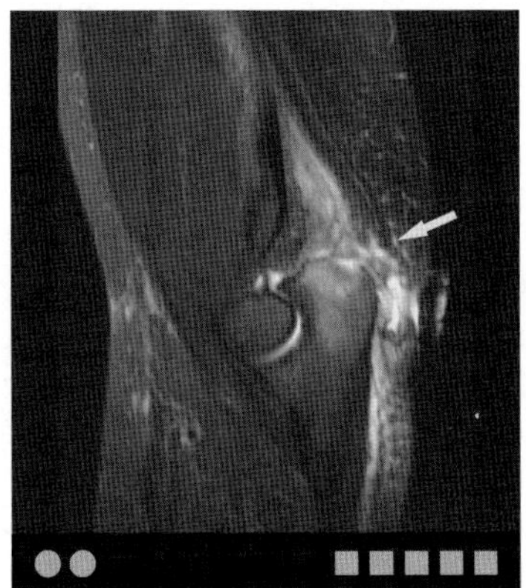

F. Avulsion fracture of triceps tendon: Sagittal T2W fat-saturated image shows avulsion of the triceps tendon from olecranon process. Note fluid is intervening between the distal end of the tendon (arrow) and olecranon. There is bone and soft tissue edema at the avulsion fracture site of the olecranon with a notch at the tip of olecranon process created as a result of fracture. The patient has the infection of the bone and soft tissue.

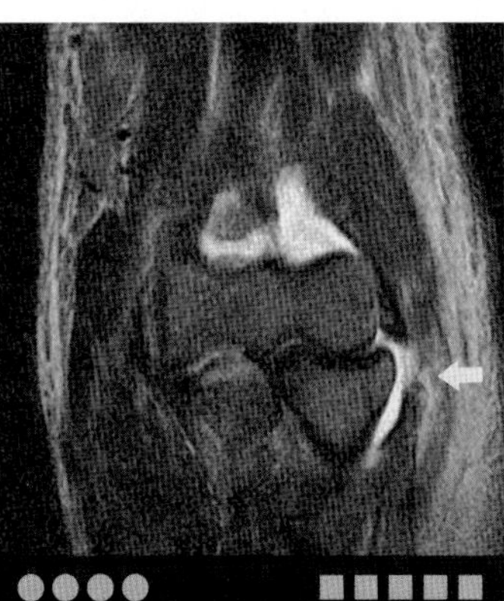

G. Tear of the radial collateral ligament and common extensor tendon: Coronal T2WI shows tear of radial collateral ligament and common extensor tendon (arrow).

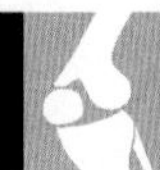

7–14 Radial Collateral Ligament Tear

Ashkan Afshin and Jamshid Tehranzadeh

PRESENTATION

Elbow pain

FINDINGS

MR images demonstrate disruption of the fibers of radial collateral ligament and common extensor tendon. This patient also has tear of lateral ulnar collateral ligament. Fluid signal intensity replaces these ligaments and tendon in fluid sensitive images.

DIFFERENTIAL DIAGNOSES

- *Tear of the lateral ulnar collateral ligament:* MR findings show disruption of the fibers of lateral ulnar collateral ligament with fluid signal intensity.
- *Common extensor tendon tear:* MR images show disruption of the common extensor tendons with the gap and area of increased signal in the origin of the tendon.
- *Lateral epicondylitis:* Increased signal in radial collateral ligament on T1W with intermediate signal in T2W images.

COMMENTS

Lateral ligament complex consists of radial collateral ligament (RCL), Lateral Ulnar Collateral ligament (LUCL), the accessory lateral collateral ligament, and the annular ligament. The radial collateral ligament is a thick and roughly triangular band of fibrous tissue which originates from the lateral epicondyle of the humerus and extends along the posterior aspect of the radius to inserts to annular ligament along with the fibers of capsule. RCL reinforces the lateral side of the elbow articular capsule. Rupture of the radial collateral ligament is relatively uncommon and may be associated with conditions such as lateral epicondylitis, common extensor tendon tear or lateral ulnar collateral ligament tear. Acute varus injury and subluxation/dislocation are common mechanisms of injury. Radial collateral injury is less common that medial collateral injury. Disruption of RCL may lead to posterolateral rotatory instability (PLRI) of the elbow. However, it seems that when the annular ligament is intact, either the radial collateral ligament or the lateral ulnar collateral ligament can be transected without inducing posterolateral rotatory instability of the elbow. Patients usually complain of pain on the lateral side of the elbow associated with supination of the forearm. On physical examination patient are often guarding which makes the diagnosis difficult. The have a positive pivot shift test.

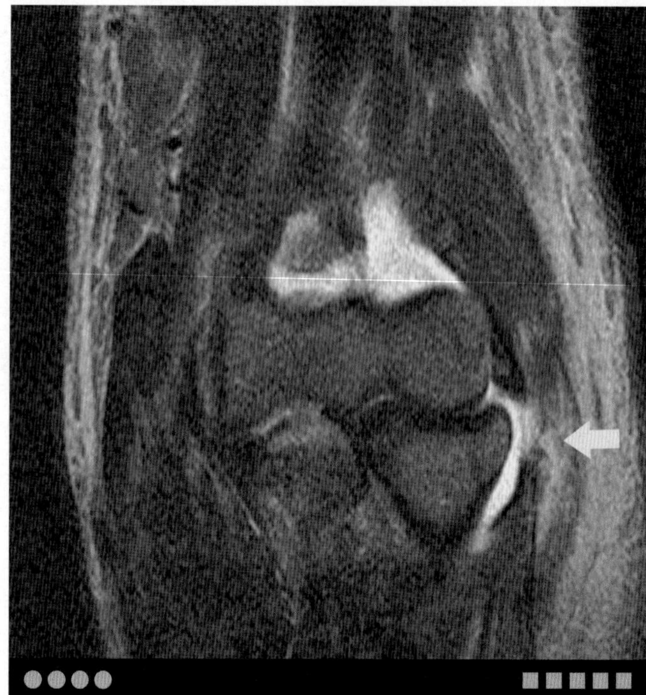

A. Tear of the radial collateral ligament and common extensor tendon: Coronal T2WI shows tear of radial collateral ligament and common extensor tendon (arrow).

MR imaging provides the best diagnostic tool for RCL injuries. MR findings show disruption of the ligament with fluid signal intensity on fluid sensitive sequences.

PEARLS

- **RCL originates from the lateral epicondyle of the humerus and inserts to annular ligament along with the fibers of capsule**
- **Acute varus injury and subluxation/dislocation are common mechanisms of injury**
- **RCL tear may be associated with lateral epicondylitis, common extensor tendon tear or lateral ulnar collateral tear**
- **RCL rupture may result in posterolateral rotatory instability.**
- **Pain on the lateral side of the elbow associated with supination of the forearm, guarding and positive pivot shift test are common clinical findings.**
- **Disruption of the Ligament with fluid signal intensity is shown on fluid sensitive sequences.**

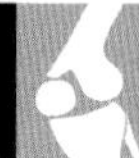

ADDITIONAL IMAGES

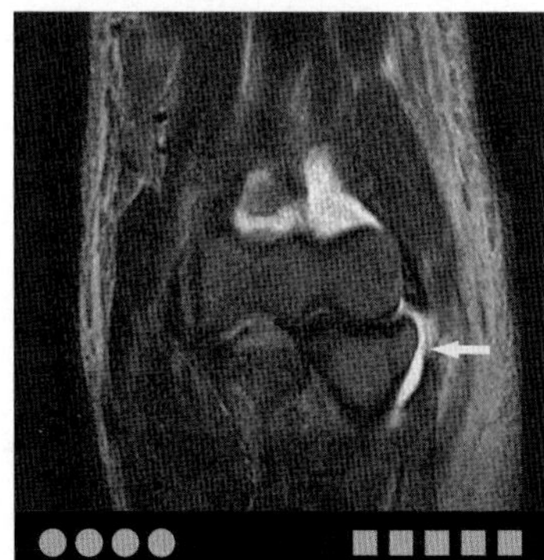

B. Tear of the radial collateral ligament and common extensor tendon: Coronal STIR image shows tear of radial collateral ligament (arrow) and common extensor tendon.

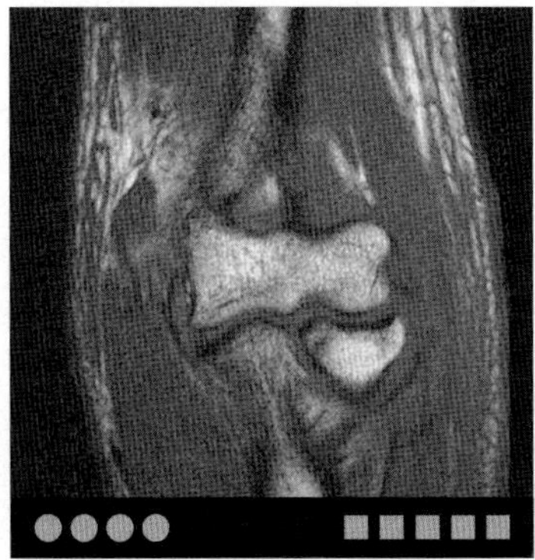

C. Tear of the radial collateral ligament and common extensor tendon: Coronal T1WI shows tear of the radial collateral ligament and common extensor tendon.

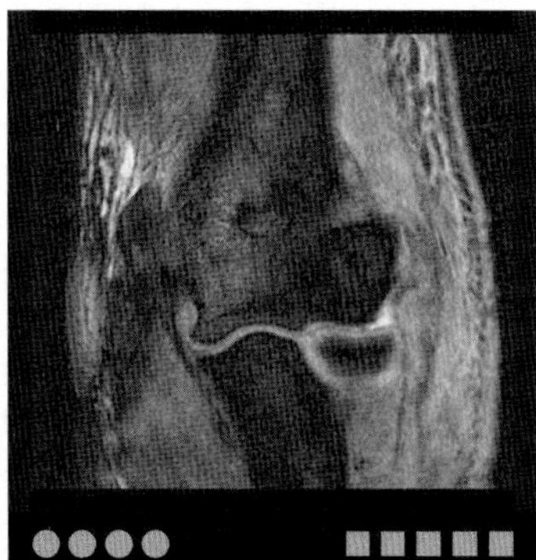

D. Tear of the radial collateral ligament and common extensor tendon: Coronal T2W fat-saturated image shows complete tear of the radial collateral ligament and common extensor tendon.

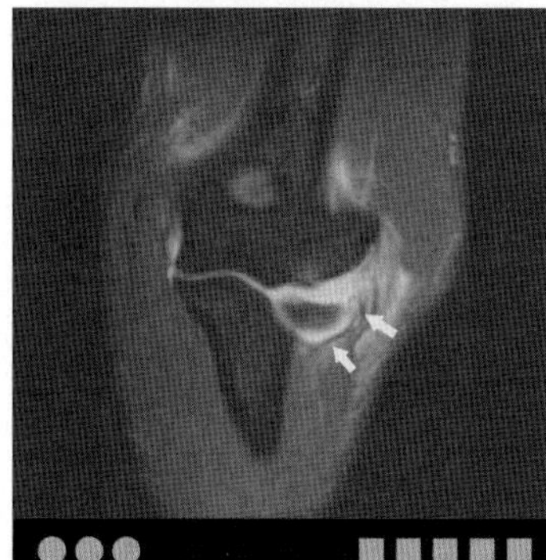

E. Tear of the radial collateral ligament and lateral ulnar collateral ligament: Coronal T2W fat-saturated image shows tear of the lateral ulnar collateral ligament (arrows) associated with radial collateral ligament tear.

DIFFERENTIAL DIAGNOSES IMAGES

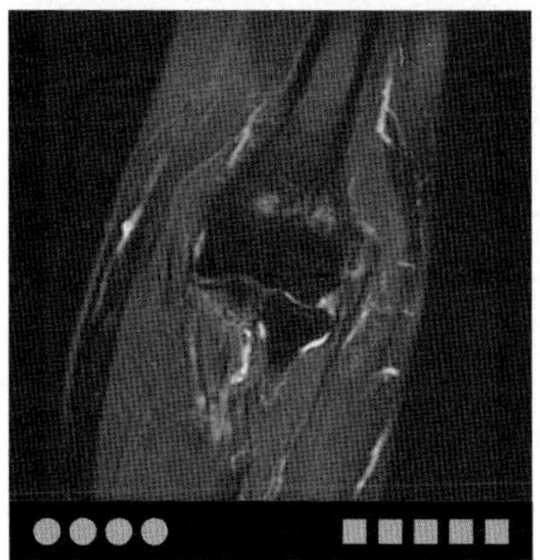

F. Lateral epicondylitis with tear of common extensor tendon: Coronal T2WI shows increased signal in the area of the common extensor tendons origin.

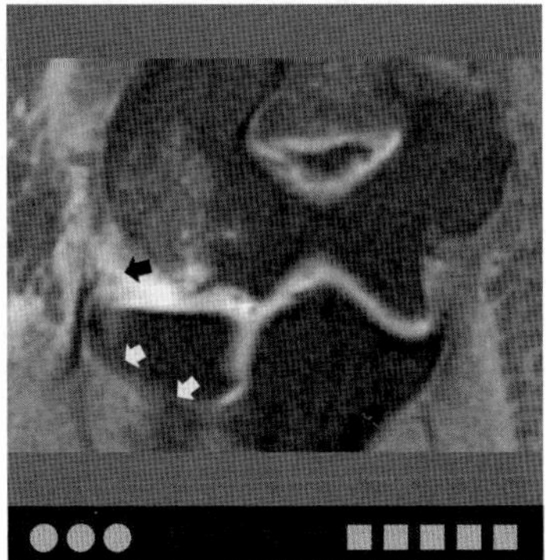

G. Complete tear of the lateral ulnar collateral ligament: Coronal T2W fat-saturated image shows complete tear of the LUCL (black arrow). The oblique course of this ligament which attaches to the lateral side of ulna is shown by white arrows. Note the bone contusion of the capitellum. (Courtesy of Mark Schweitzer.)

IMAGE KEY

Common

Rare

Typical

Unusual

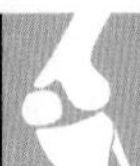

7–15 Tendinosis of the Triceps Tendon with Avulsion Fracture of

Ashkan Afshin and Adam Zoga

PRESENTATION

Elbow pain

FINDINGS

Intermediate to increased signal of triceps tendon in T1 and proton density weighted images, which slightly decrease in intensity in T2WI. A bony chip is noted posterior to elbow.

DIFFERENTIAL DIAGNOSES

- *Partial tear of triceps tendon:* MR images show intermediate signal intensity inside the triceps tendon on T1 or proton density weighted images. Bright fluid signal is also observed in the triceps tendon in fluid sensitive images.
- *Complete tear of triceps tendon:* The tendon is disrupted and fluid signal replaces the torn segment. The tendon is retracted proximally.
- *Avulsion fracture of triceps tendon:* MR examination shows avulsion fracture of triceps tendon with separation of the tendon from the insertion site and with a piece of bone fragment detached from olecranon process.

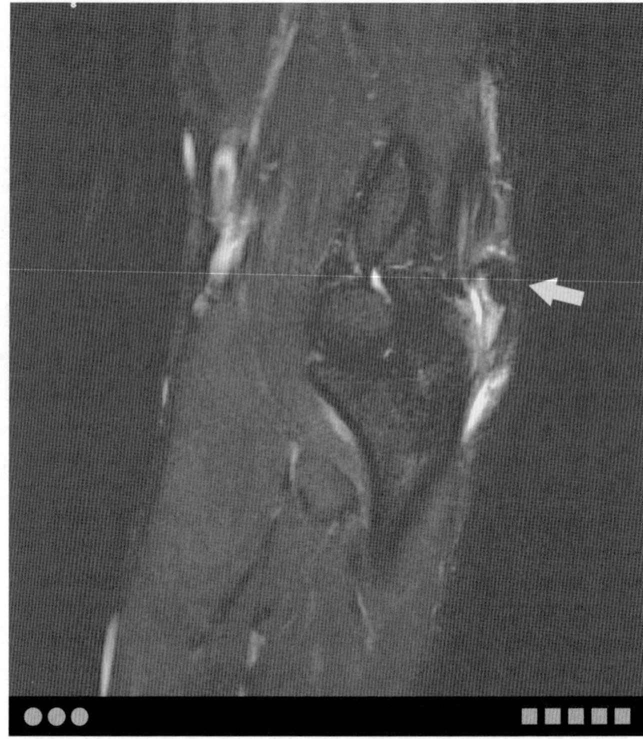

A. Tendinosis of the triceps tendon with avulsion fracture of olecranon process: Sagittal fat-saturated T2W image shows intermediate signal in the triceps tendon. There is an avulsion fracture of the olecranon process (arrow) with the edema at the fracture site.

COMMENTS

Tendinosis of the triceps tendon sometimes is referred to as posterior tennis elbow or boxer's elbow. This uncommon injury is an overuse syndrome, which is caused by repetitive elbow extension against resistance and has been associated with overuse related to occupational and sporting activities, posterior impingement, and intra-articular osteocartilaginous bodies. Rapid extension of the elbow such as during throwing, punching, and serving motions are implicated in the pathology, as is weightlifting. Patients with triceps tendinosis often present with pain over the triceps tendon. Physical examination of the patients reveals point tenderness just superior to the attachment on the olecranon process, which is provoked with extension performed under resistance. Resisted elbow extension with the elbow in flexion and forearm fully supinated is a key test to the clinical diagnosis of tendinosis of the triceps tendon. Conventional radiographs are usually normal in these patients. However, in the presence of the osteoarthritis, the radiographs may show calcifications within the tendon, traction spurs, and hypertrophy of the ulna or loose bodies. MRI is valuable for diagnosis of this injury. MR images show intermediate to increased signal of triceps tendon in T1 and proton density weighted images, which slightly decrease in intensity in T2WI.

PEARLS

- **It is also referred to as posterior tennis elbow or boxer's elbow and is an uncommon injury.**
- **It is associated with overuse related to occupational and sporting activities, posterior impingement, and intra-articular osteocartilaginous bodies.**
- **Pain over the triceps tendon is a common symptom.**
- **Resisted elbow extension is the key to the clinical diagnosis.**
- **Conventional radiographs are usually normal.**
- **MR images show intermediate to increased signal of triceps tendon in T1 and proton density weighted images, which slightly decrease in intensity in T2WI.**

ADDITIONAL IMAGES

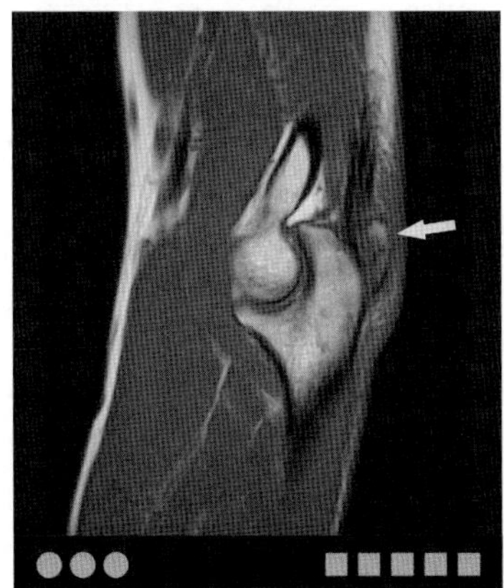

B. Tendinosis of the triceps tendon with avulsion fracture of olecranon process: Sagittal T1WI shows avulsion fracture of the olecranon process (arrow). Intermediate signal of the triceps tendon at the insertion site representing tendinosis is noted.

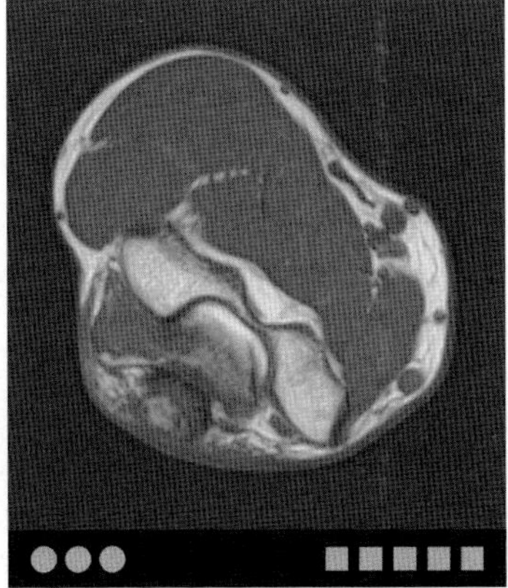

C. Tendinosis of the triceps tendon with avulsion fracture of olecranon process: Axial T1WI shows avulsion fracture of the olecranon process. Intermediate signal of the triceps tendon at the insertion site representing tendinosis is noted.

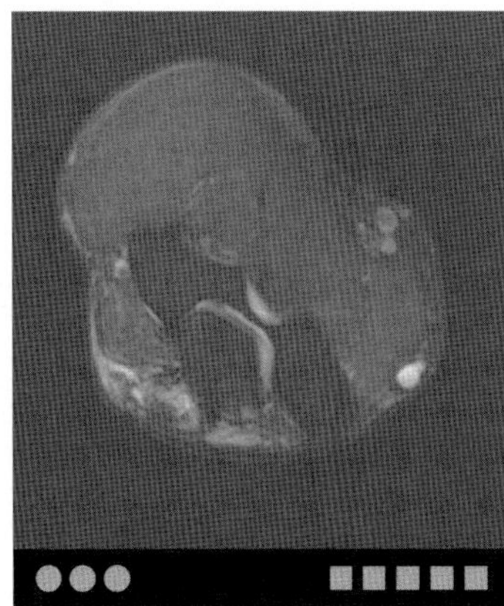

D. Tendinosis of the triceps tendon with avulsion fracture of olecranon process: Axial fat-saturated T2WI shows a bony fragment at the posterior olecranon representing avulsion fracture of the olecranon process.

IMAGE KEY

Common

Rare

Typical

Unusual

DIFFERENTIAL DIAGNOSES IMAGES

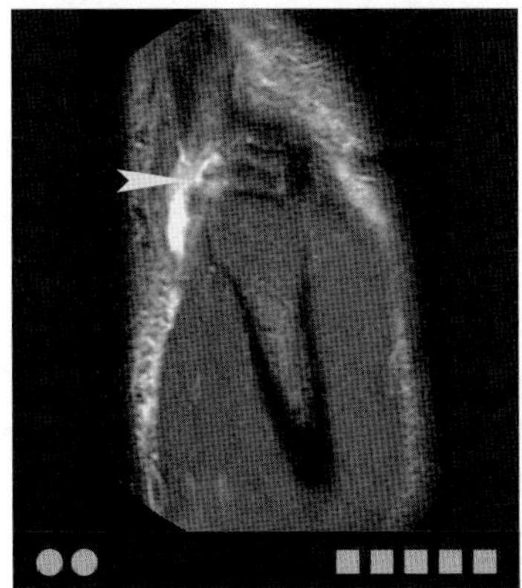

E. Partial tear of triceps tendon: Coronal proton density fat-saturated image shows bright fluid signal in the triceps tendon (arrowhead), proximal to the insertion site to olecranon process. (Courtesy of Thomas L. Huang.)

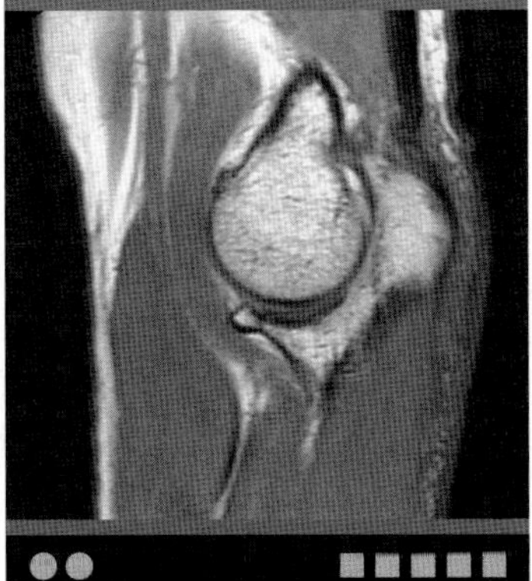

F. Partial tear of triceps tendon: Sagittal T1WI shows intermediate signal intensity inside the triceps tendon, just proximal to the insertion site to olecranon process. (Courtesy of Thomas L. Huang.)

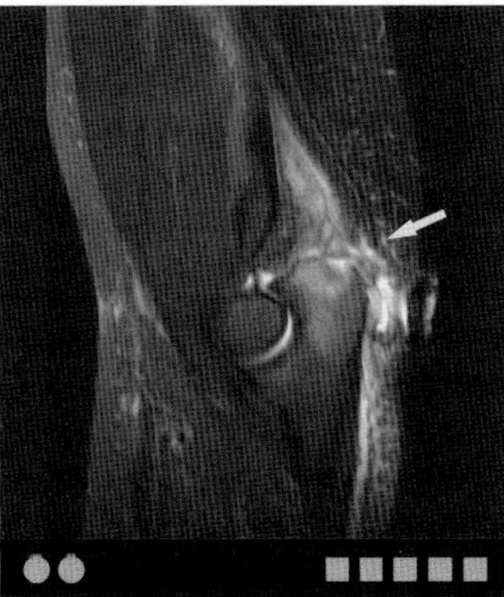

G. Avulsion fracture of triceps tendon: Sagittal T2W fat-saturated image shows avulsion of the triceps tendon from olecranon process. Note fluid is intervening between the distal end of the tendon (arrow) and olecranon. There is bone and soft tissue edema at the avulsion fracture site of the olecranon with a notch at the tip of olecranon process created as a result of fracture. The patient has the infection of the bone and soft tissue.

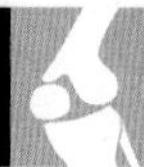

7–16 Partial Tear of Triceps Tendon

Ashkan Afshin and Thomas L. Huang

PRESENTATION

Posterior elbow pain

FINDINGS

MR images show intermediate signal on T1WI and partial bright fluid signal in T2WI in the triceps tendon, proximal to the insertion site to olecranon process with no retraction of tendon.

DIFFERENTIAL DIAGNOSES

- *Complete tear of triceps tendon:* This is associated with tendon retraction proximally.
- *Avulsion fracture of triceps tendon:* This is a rare condition that manifests as detachment of triceps tendon and may be associated with detachment of a piece of bone from its insertion site at superior–posterior surface of the olecranon process of the ulna. Lateral radiograph shows presence of the flecks of avulsed osseous material. Small fluid filled gap which separates the distal triceps tendon from the olecranon are observed on MR images
- *Tendinosis of triceps tendon:* This condition results in intermediate signal on T1WI and T2WI. There is absence of fluid signal in the tendon.

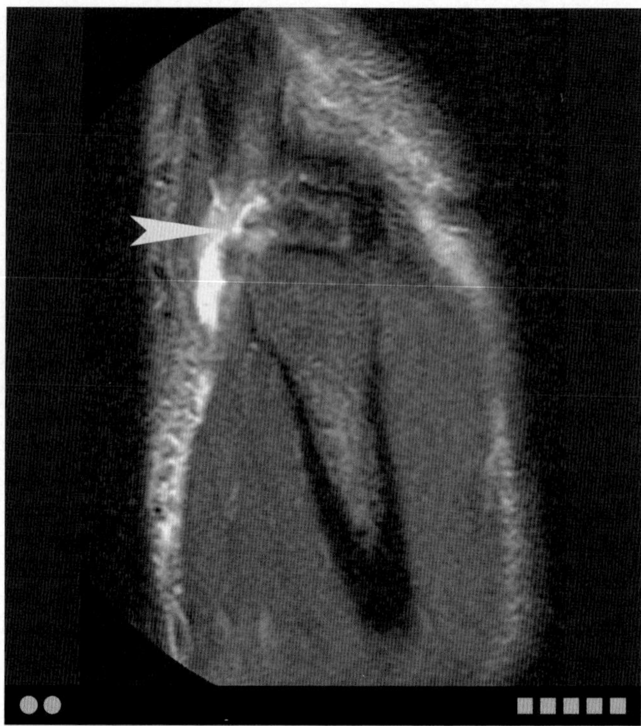

A. Partial tear of triceps tendon: Coronal proton density fat-saturated image shows bright fluid signal in the triceps tendon (arrowhead), proximal to the insertion site to olecranon process.

COMMENTS

Distal triceps begins in the middle of the muscle and form the tendon that insert to superior–posterior surface of the olecranon process of the ulna. Rupture of the distal triceps tendon is an uncommon injury that can be complete or partial. Partial tear is less common and usually occurs in the central third of the tendon, adjacent to the olecranon. Renal failure, steroid use, and olecranon bursitis are predisposing factors for rupture of the triceps tendon. However, the majority of injuries occur in healthy tissue after a fall onto an outstretched hand or after a direct blow to the arm. In patient with the history of falling on the outstretched hand, triceps tendon rupture may be associated with radial head fracture. Patients with rupture of triceps tendon usually complain of pain and swelling at the posterior elbow, at the level of olecranon insertion of the triceps, which limit the physical examination. Partial tear of the triceps is more difficult to be diagnosed clinically. MR imaging is useful for diagnosis of triceps tendon tear and differentiation between complete tears that require surgery and partial tears that may heal well with protection and rehabilitation. MR images show partially discontinuous tendon with presence of partial bright fluid signal in the triceps tendon without proximal retraction.

PEARLS

- **It is a rare injury and usually occurs in the central third of the tendon.**
- **Renal failure, steroid use, and olecranon bursitis are the predisposing factors.**
- **Fall onto an outstretched hand and direct blow to the arm are common mechanisms of injury.**
- **Pain and swelling at the posterior elbow are common symptoms.**
- **It may be associated with radial head fracture.**
- **MR images show partially discontinuous tendon with presence of partial bright fluid signal in the triceps tendon without proximal retraction.**

ADDITIONAL IMAGES

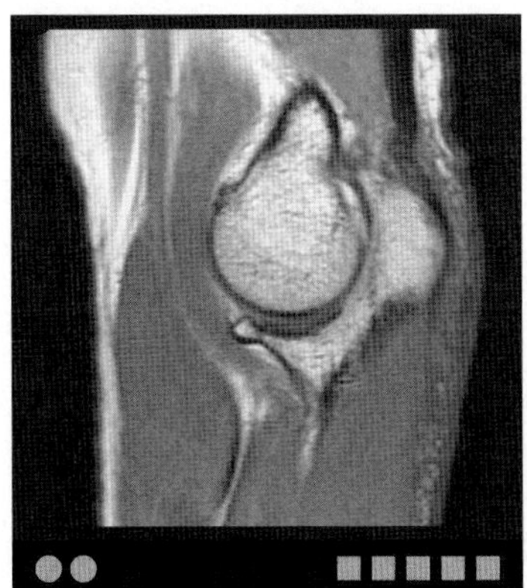

B. Partial tear of triceps tendon: Sagittal T1WI shows intermediate signal intensity inside the triceps tendon, just proximal to the insertion site to olecranon process.

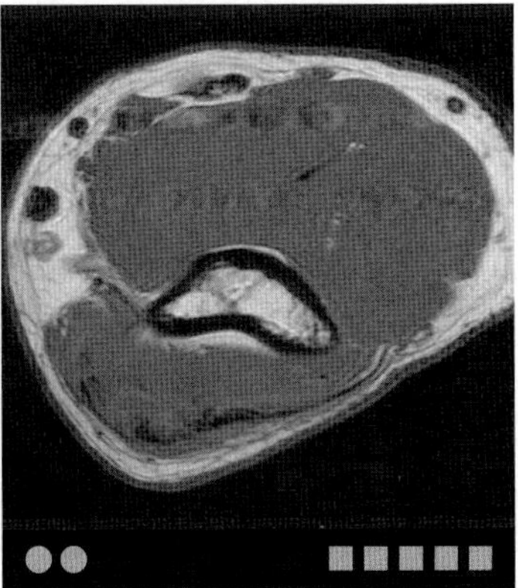

C. Partial tear of triceps tendon: Axial T1WI shows intermediate signal intensity inside the triceps tendon, just proximal to the insertion site to olecranon process.

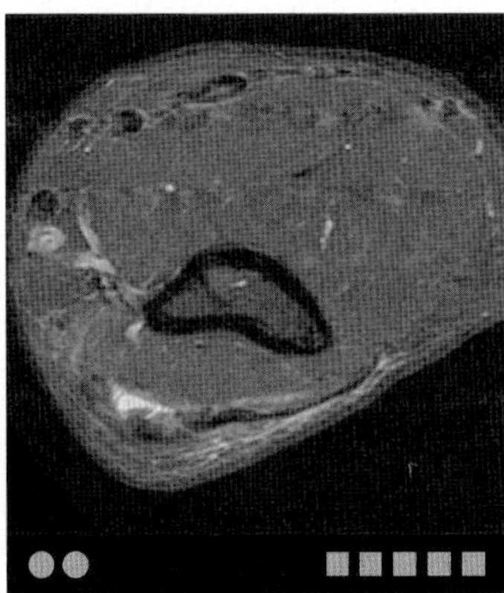

D. Partial tear of triceps tendon: Axial T2 fat-saturated image shows fluid bright signal in the substance of triceps tendon.

IMAGE KEY

Common

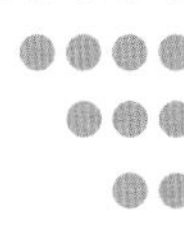

Rare

Typical

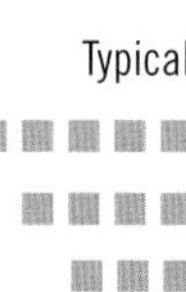

Unusual

DIFFERENTIAL DIAGNOSES IMAGES

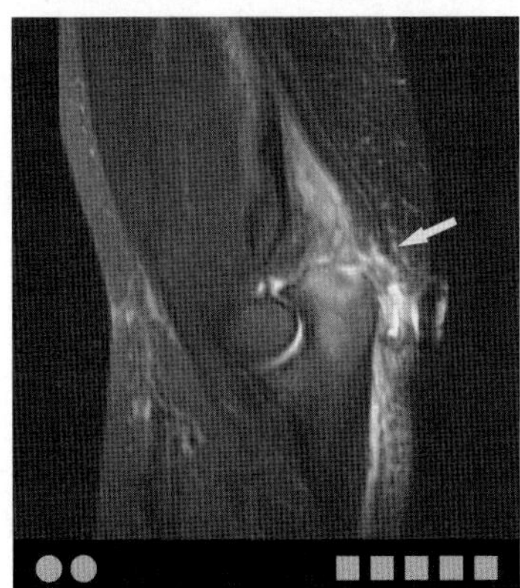

E. Avulsion fracture of triceps tendon: Sagittal T2W fat-saturated image shows avulsion of the triceps tendon from olecranon process. Note fluid is intervening between the distal end of the tendon (arrow) and olecranon. There is bone and soft tissue edema at the avulsion fracture site of the olecranon with a notch at the tip of olecranon process created as a result of fracture. The patient has the infection of the bone and soft tissue.

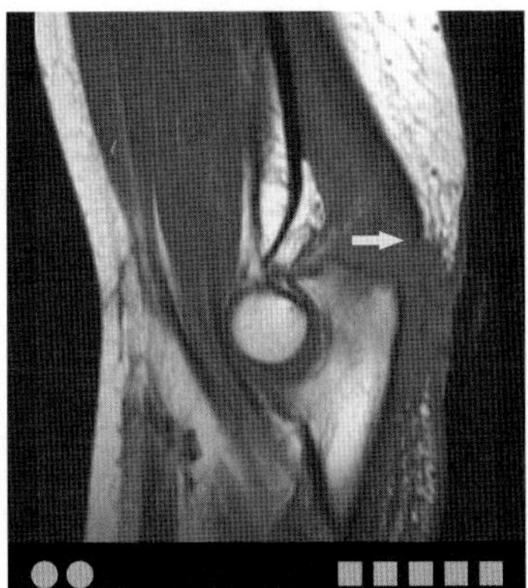

F. Avulsion fracture of triceps tendon: Sagittal T1WI shows a wide gap between the avulsed and detached distal triceps tendon (arrow) and the edematous bone of olecranon.

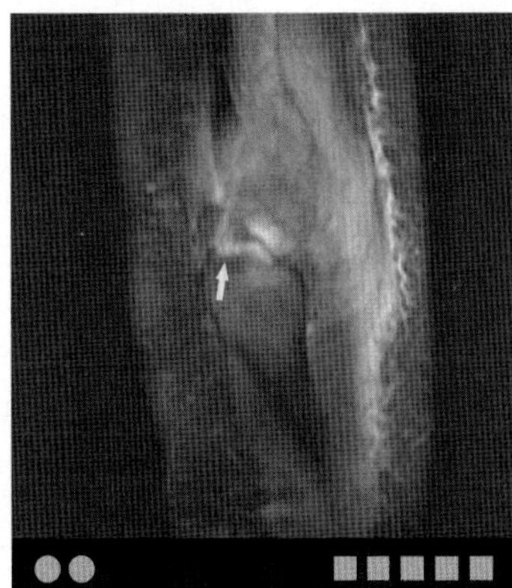

G. Avulsion fracture of triceps tendon: Posterior section of a coronal T2W fat saturated image at the olecranon process level shows fluid intervening between olecranon process and the triceps tendon. The arrow is pointing to the defect created by avulsion fracture of the tip of olecranon process.

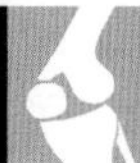

7–17 Avulsion Tear of Triceps Tendon

Ashkan Afshin and Jamshid Tehranzadeh

PRESENTATION

Pain of the elbow

FINDINGS

MR examination shows avulsion fracture of triceps tendon with separation of the tendon from the insertion site and with a piece of bone fragment detached from olecranon process

DIFFERENTIAL DIAGNOSES

- *Gout:* Radiograph of the joint in early stages of gout shows soft tissue swelling. The initial bony changes appear as punch-out lesions with overhanging edges in intermediate phase of gout. In the late phase of the disease, radiographs may show intraosseous tophi and joint narrowing.
- *Rheumatoid Nodule:* It results from granulomatous reaction in patients with RA. Rheumatoid nodule is usually found on extensor surfaced of the body and on MR images manifest as low signal intensity mass in soft tissue.
- *Tendinosis of the triceps tendon:* Increased signal of triceps tendon in T1 and proton density weighted images, which slightly decrease in intensity in T2WI.

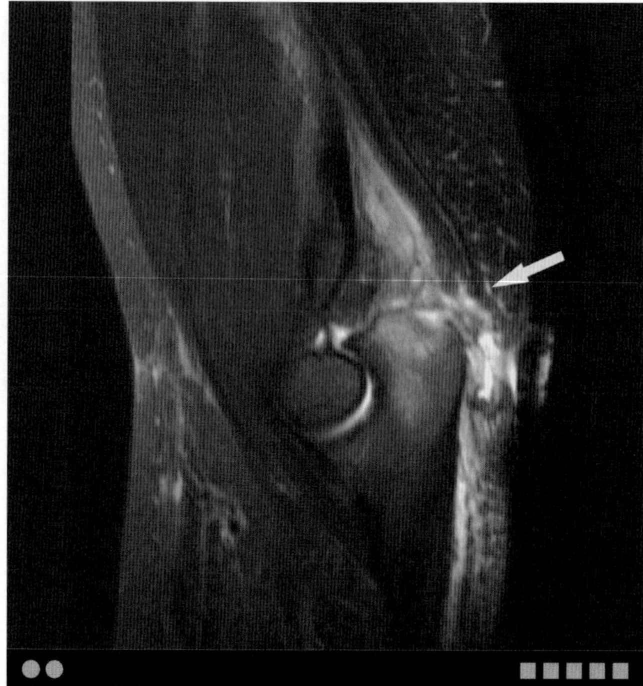

A. Avulsion fracture of triceps tendon: Sagittal T2W fat-saturated image shows avulsion of the triceps tendon from olecranon process. Note fluid is intervening between the distal end of the tendon (arrow) and olecranon. There is bone and soft tissue edema at the avulsion fracture site of the olecranon with a notch at the tip of olecranon process created as a result of fracture. The patient has the infection of the bone and soft tissue.

COMMENTS

This is a 19-year-old female who had an ulcer with purulent discharge on her left elbow. She developed the osteomyelitis of the olecranon and avulsion fracture of the triceps tendon. Avulsion of the triceps tendon is a rare condition that usually manifests as detachment of tendon and may be associated with detachment of a piece of bone from its insertion site at the superior–posterior surface of the olecranon process of the ulna. This condition usually results from falling on the outstretched elbow, with sudden contraction of the triceps muscle. Anabolic steroid abuse (e.g., in athletes), local steroid injections (e.g., in olecranon bursitis) and hyperparathyroidism may increase the risk of the tear. Avulsion tear of triceps can also be associated with the fracture of the radial head. Patients with this lesion usually complain of pain in the elbow region. Physical examination of the patients reveals swelling and a palpable depression just proximal to the olecranon and functional impairment of the muscle in the form of inability to extend the elbow against gravity. Lateral radiograph may show the presence of flecks of avulsed osseous material lying posterior to the distal end of the Humerus ("flake sign"), which is almost pathognomonic of this lesion. The diagnosis can be suggested by the physical findings and radiographs. MR images show small fluid-filled gap, which separate the distal triceps tendon from the olecranon and can be useful in confirming the diagnosis.

PEARLS

- **Caused by falling on the outstretched elbow.**
- **Can be associated with the fracture of the radial head.**
- **Pain, swelling, and a palpable depression proximal to the olecranon and inability to extend the elbow against gravity are common clinical findings.**
- **Presence of the flecks of avulsed osseous material on lateral radiograph ("flake sign").**
- **Small fluid-filled gap, which separate the distal triceps tendon from the olecranon on MR images.**

ADDITIONAL IMAGES

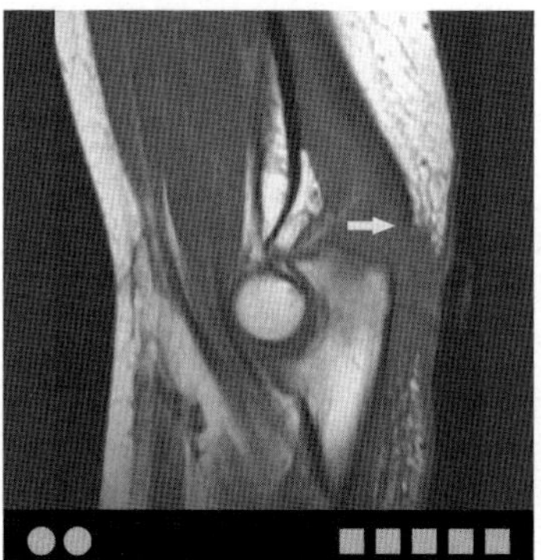

B. Avulsion fracture of triceps tendon: Sagittal T1WI shows a wide gap between the avulsed and detached distal triceps tendon (arrow) and the edematous bone of olecranon.

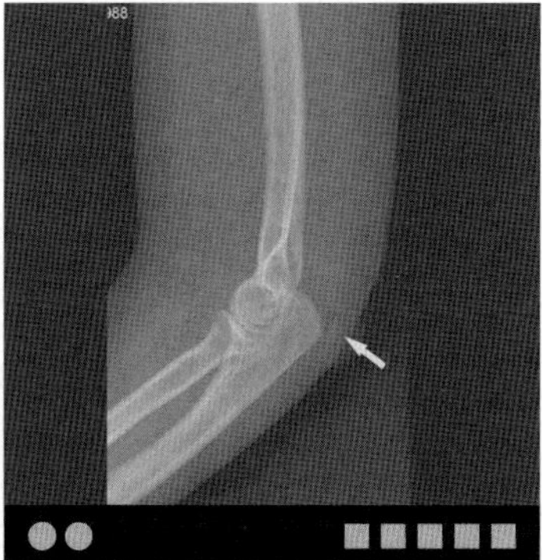

C. Avulsion fracture of triceps tendon: Lateral radiograph of the elbow shows detached bone fragment (arrow) with soft tissue swelling adjacent to olecranon process.

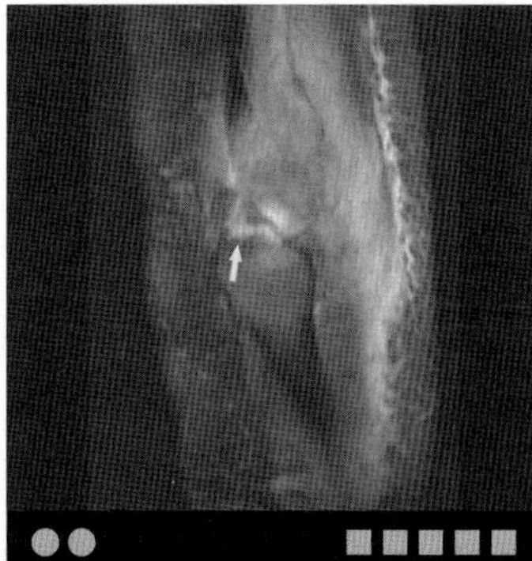

D. Avulsion fracture of triceps tendon: Posterior section of a coronal T2W fat-saturated image at the olecranon process level shows fluid intervening between olecranon process and the triceps tendon. The arrow is pointing to the defect created by avulsion fracture of the tip of olecranon process.

E. Avulsion fracture of triceps tendon: Axial T2W fat-saturated image shows edema and fluid at the site of the avulsed triceps tendon, olecranon process, and the adjacent soft tissue.

IMAGE KEY

Common

Rare

Typical

Unusual

DIFFERENTIAL DIAGNOSES IMAGES

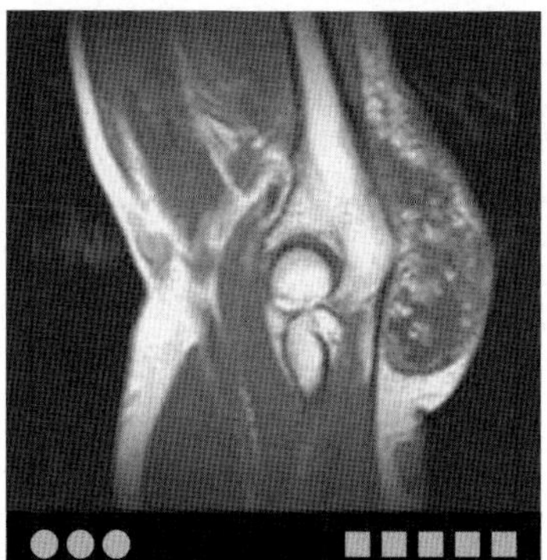

F. Gout of olecranon bursa: Sagittal T1WI shows a large heterogeneous, but predominantly low signal, lobulated structure in the region of the olecranon bursa with adjacent lower signal pertaining to tophaceous material and bursal effusion.

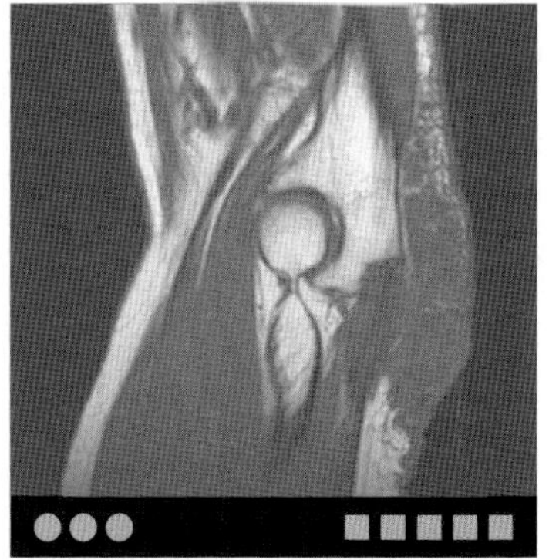

G. Rheumatoid nodule: Sagittal T1WI shows low signal intensity mass in olecranon soft tissue representing rheumatoid nodule.

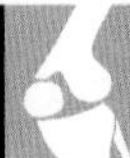

7–18 Radial Tunnel Syndrome

Mohammad Reza Hayeri and Thomas L. Huang

PRESENTATION

Lateral elbow pain

FINDINGS

MRI shows lipoma anterior to the proximal radius in supinator muscle with entrapment of posterior interosseous nerve.

DIFFERENTIAL DIAGNOSES

- *Posterior interosseous nerve syndrome:* This is differentiated from the radial tunnel syndrome (RTS) by the presence of motor abnormalities (complete loss of function to partial weakness).
- *Ganglion cyst:* It can be a cause of RTS at the proximal radioulnar joint.
- *Lateral antebrachial neuritis:* This is impingement of the lateral antebrachial cutaneous nerve from the lateral edge of the biceps, just above the elbow.
- *Hemangioma:* Intramuscular hemangiomas can cause pain and swelling although most of them are asymptomatic.
- *Bicipitoradial bursitis:* The bicipitoradial bursa is a thin and delicate structure lined by a synovial membrane and is located between the radial insertion of the biceps tendon and the cortex of the radial tuberosity.

COMMENTS

RTS also known as radial pronator syndrome is a pain syndrome arising from compression of posterior interosseous nerve (PIN) in proximal forearm. The radial tunnel originates near the level of the radiocapitellar joint where the nerve lies against the joint capsule. The tunnel's medial border is the brachialis muscle proximally and the biceps tendon distally. The roof and lateral border of the tunnel comprises of the extensor carpi radialis longus and the extensor carpi radialis brevis. The tunnel continues to the distal border of the supinator. The compression occurs in the proximal forearm where the radial nerve splits into the PIN (main trunk) and the sensory branch of the radial nerve (minor trunk). Compression can occur either before or after this split. There are five sites of potential compression of the PIN: Proximal origin of the extensor carpi radialis brevis (ECRB) or fibrous bands within the ECRB, radiocapitellar capsule, "leash of Henry" (radial recurrent vessels), distal boarder of the supinator muscle, and "arcade of Froshe" (proximal border of the supinator muscle). Of these, the arcade of Froshe is the most frequent site for RTS. Pain over the lateral forearm with repetitive elbow extension is the major presentation of RTS. RTS is frequently misdiagnosed as lateral epicondylitis because of the similarity of pain distribution and mechanism. MRI may show atrophy, edema, and fatty infiltration of the musculature innervated by PIN, particularly supinator muscle. MRI can also detect other causes of entrapment such as tumors, ganglia, radiocapitellar synovitis, bicipital bursitis, fractures, and dislocation of the radial head.

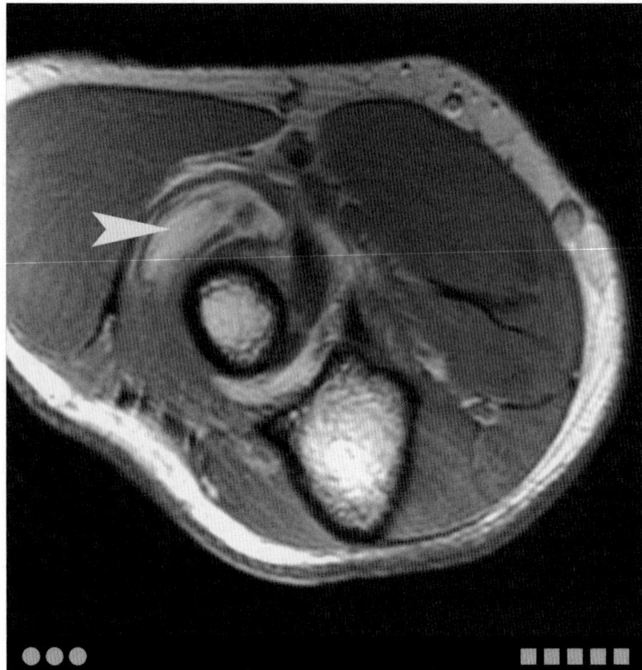

A. Radial tunnel syndrome: Axial proton density image shows lipoma anterior to the proximal radius in supinator muscle (arrowhead).

PEARLS

- **RTS also known as radial pronator syndrome is a pain syndrome arising from compression of posterior interosseous nerve (PIN) in proximal forearm.**
- **Arcade of Froshe (proximal border of the supinator muscle) is the most frequent site of compression in RTS.**
- **RTS is frequently misdiagnosed as lateral epicondylitis because of the similarity of pain distribution and mechanism.**
- **MRI may show atrophy, edema, and fatty infiltration of the musculature innervated by PIN, particularly supinator muscle.**

ADDITIONAL IMAGES

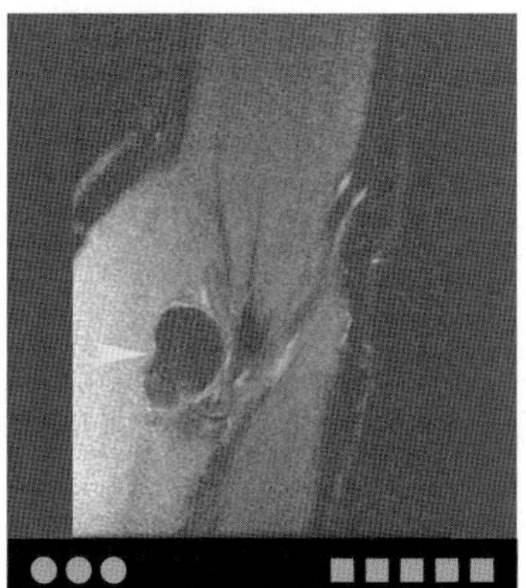

B. Radial tunnel syndrome: Coronal proton density fat saturated image of the same patient as image A shows low signal mass in supinator muscle representing lipoma (arrowhead).

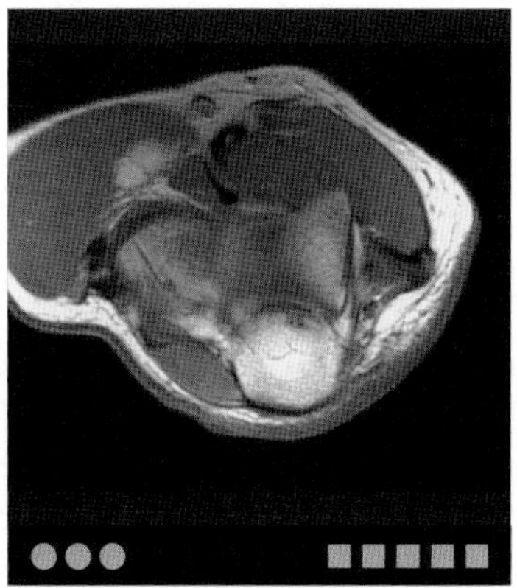

C. Radial tunnel syndrome: Axial proton density image (same patient as in images A and B) shows bright to intermediate signal in the supinator muscle representing lipoma.

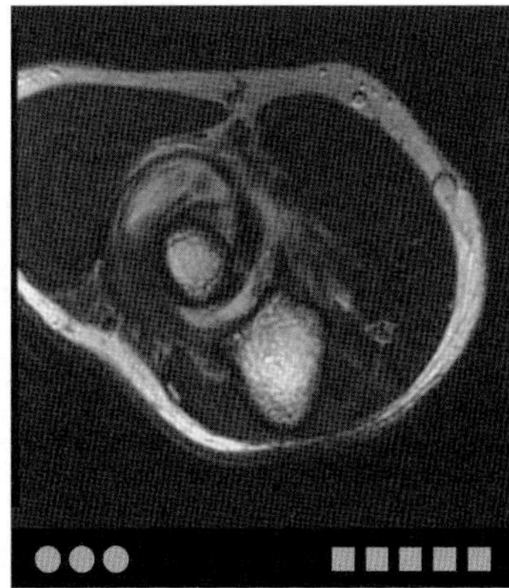

D. Radial tunnel syndrome: Axial T2WI shows this lipoma (same patient as in images A, B, and C) with intermediate signal in the supinator muscle.

IMAGE KEY

Common

Rare

Typical

Unusual

DIFFERENTIAL DIAGNOSES IMAGES

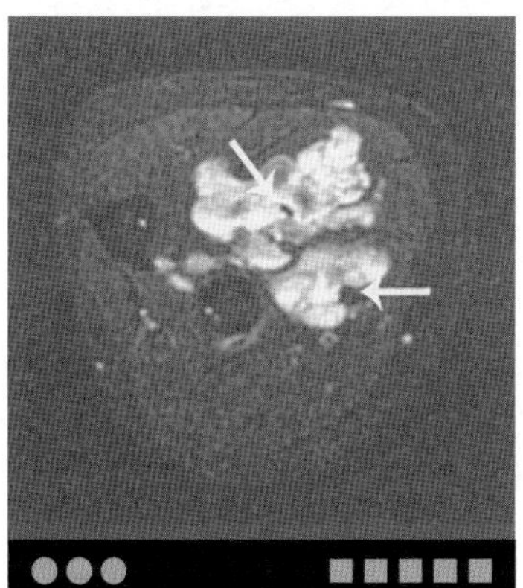

E. Hemangioma: Axial STIR image demonstrates a hyperintense lobulated septated mass with several hypointense foci (arrow).

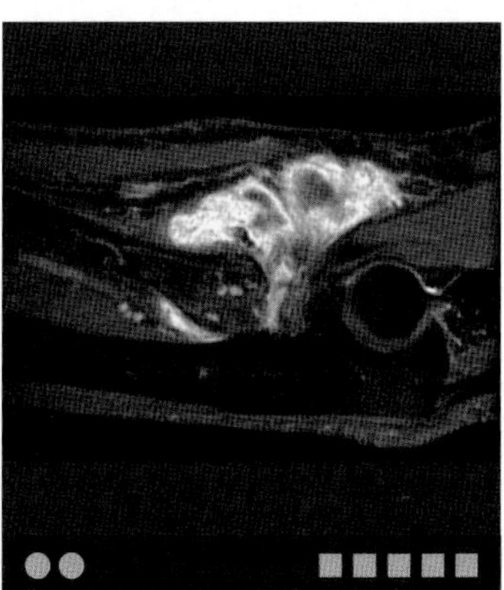

F. Bicipitoradial bursitis: Sagittal T1W fat-saturated postcontrast image shows enhancement of the soft tissues around the radial head.

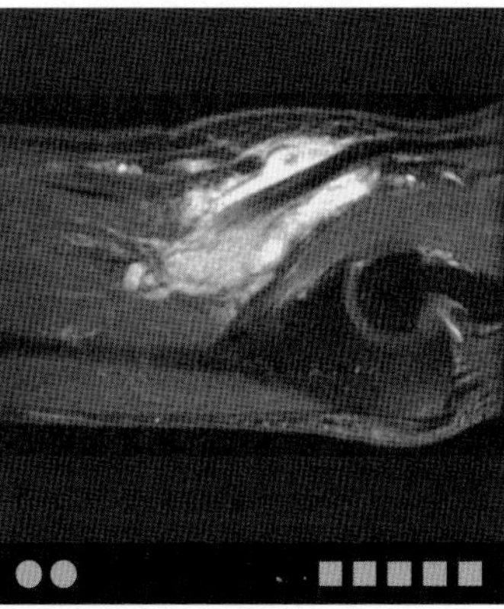

G. Bicipitoradial bursitis: Sagittal T1W fat-saturated postcontrast image shows a large region of enhancement surrounding the distal biceps tendon insertion in the area of the bicipitoradial bursa.

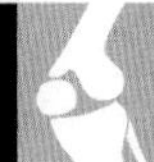

7–19 Cubital Tunnel Syndrome

Mohammad Reza Hayeri and Jamshid Tehranzadeh

PRESENTATION

Tingling and numbness in ring and little fingers

FINDINGS

MRI shows enlargement of the ulnar nerve with intermediate signal on T1WI and high signal on T2WI at the region of cubital tunnel indicating cubital tunnel syndrome.

DIFFERENTIAL DIAGNOSES

- *Olecranon bursitis:* Olecranon bursitis is the inflammation of the bursa overlying the olecranon process at the proximal aspect of the ulna.
- *Stress fracture:* Stress fractures result from repetitive subthreshold loading on the bones that overtime exceeds the bone's intrinsic ability to repair itself.
- *Medial epicondylitis:* Also known as golfer's elbow is the most common cause of medial elbow pain and is an overuse injury of the medial epicondyle of the humerus, where flexor-pronator muscle originate.
- *Ulnar nerve transposition:* Ulnar nerve transposition is removing the ulnar nerve from posterior elbow to a new place in front of the elbow to take the pressure off the nerve. The transposition could be subcutaneous, submuscular, or intramuscular.

COMMENTS

Ulnar nerve compression is encountered as the second most common compression neuropathy in the arm. Arcade of Struther, medial intermuscular septum, cubital tunnel, arcade of the flexor carpi ulnaris, and the flexor–pronator aponeurosis are the principal locations where ulnar nerve may be trapped around the elbow; of these cubital tunnel is by far the most common. The ulnar tunnel is a fibro-osseous canal containing the ulnar nerve whose roof is formed by a fascial band called the cubital tunnel retinaculum, which extends from the tip of the olecranon to the medial epicondyle. Most of the time the cause of ulnar neuropathy at the elbow is uncertain but may be caused by constricting fascial bands, subluxation of the ulnar nerve over the medial epicondyle, bony spurs, tumor, ganglia, cubitus valgus, or direct compression activities. The cubital tunnel syndrome occurs most commonly between 30 and 60 years and is exceptionally uncommon in children under 15 years. Concomitant disorders like thoracic outlet syndrome in up to 1/3 of patients and carpal tunnel syndrome in up to 40% of patients may exist. Patients often experience tingling and numbness along little and ring finger usually accompanied by weakness of grip. Compression of the nerve for a long time may lead to irreversible muscle wasting. T1WI show diffuse swelling with intermediate signal and enlargement of the ulnar nerve. T2W or STIR images show hyperintense signal within the ulnar nerve best demonstrated on axial plane. Associated mass lesion in the cubital tunnel may be present.

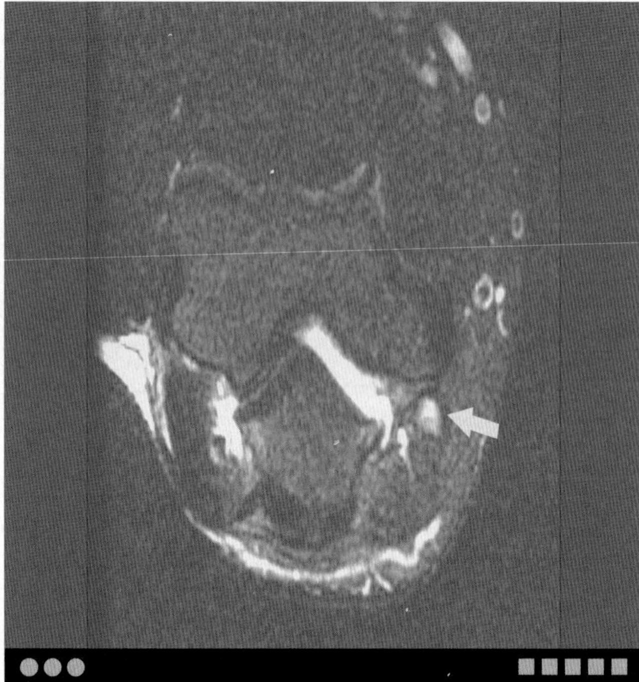

A. Cubital tunnel syndrome: Axial T2 fat-saturated image shows enlargement of the ulnar nerve (arrow) with bright signal indicating cubital tunnel syndrome. (Courtesy of Mark Schweitzer.)

PEARLS

- **Cubital tunnel syndrome is the second most common compression neuropathy in the arm.**
- **Ulnar neuropathy at the elbow is uncertain but may be caused by constricting fascial bands, subluxation of the ulnar nerve over the medial epicondyle, bony spurs, tumor, ganglia, cubitus valgus, or direct compression activities.**
- **Patients often experience tingling and numbness along little and ring finger usually accompanied by weakness of grip.**
- **On MRI ulnar nerve entrapment is shown by increased signal intensity and swollen bright nerve in the tunnel.**

ADDITIONAL IMAGES

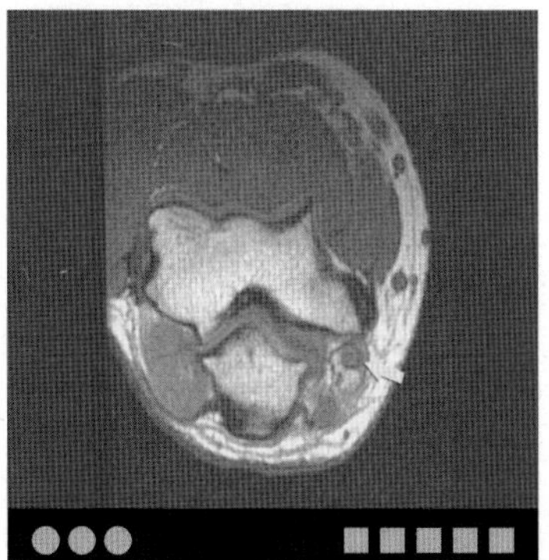

B. Cubital tunnel syndrome: Axial spin echo T1WI shows enlarged ulnar nerve (arrow) with intermediate signal indicating cubital tunnel syndrome. (Courtesy of Mark Schweitzer.)

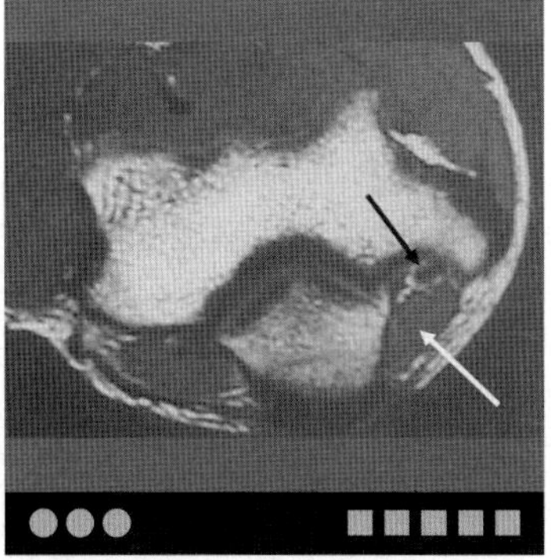

C. Cubital tunnel syndrome due to accessory muscle: Axial T1WI demonstrates ulnar nerve (black arrow) in cubital tunnel with an accessory muscle (white arrow, anconeus epitrochlearis) resulting in compressive ulnar neuropathy.

DIFFERENTIAL DIAGNOSES IMAGES

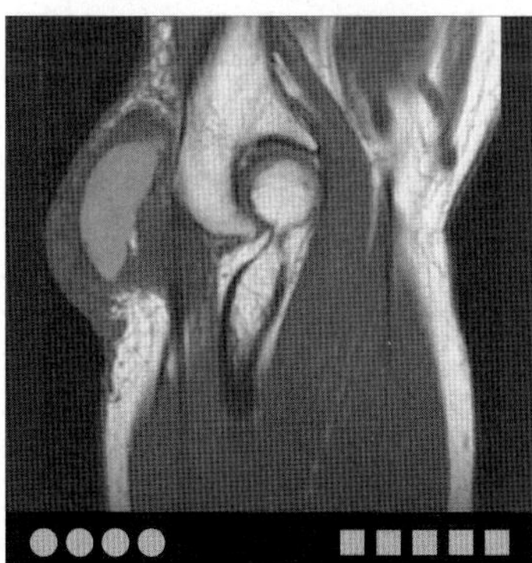

D. Olecranon bursitis: Sagittal PD image shows intermediate signal mass in the olecranon bursa.

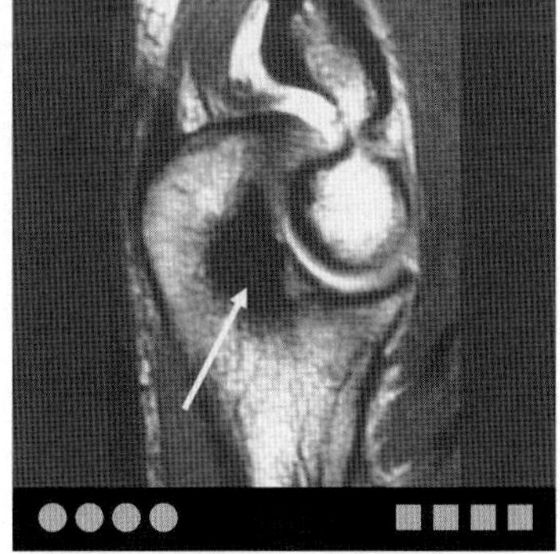

E. Stress fracture: Sagittal T1WI shows marked signal void area (arrow) secondary to reactive bony sclerosis from a healing olecranon stress fracture. Note the fracture line is not visible because of the sclerosis.

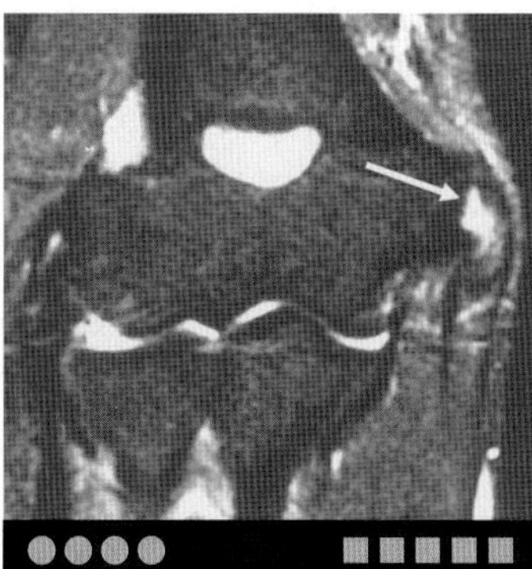

F. Medial epicondylitis: Coronal STIR image demonstrates hyperintense signal from fluid within the base of the common flexor tendon (arrow) secondary to medial epicondylitis.

IMAGE KEY

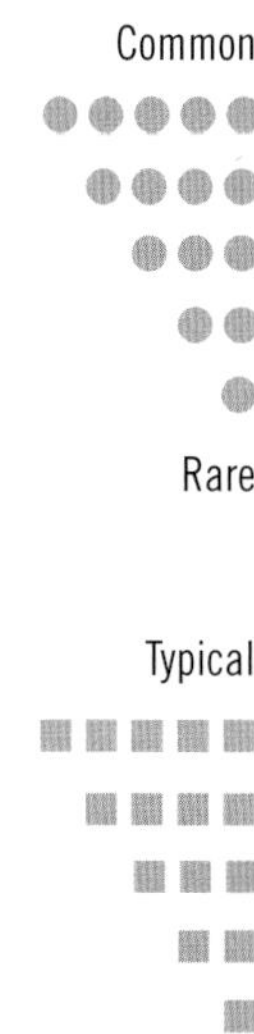

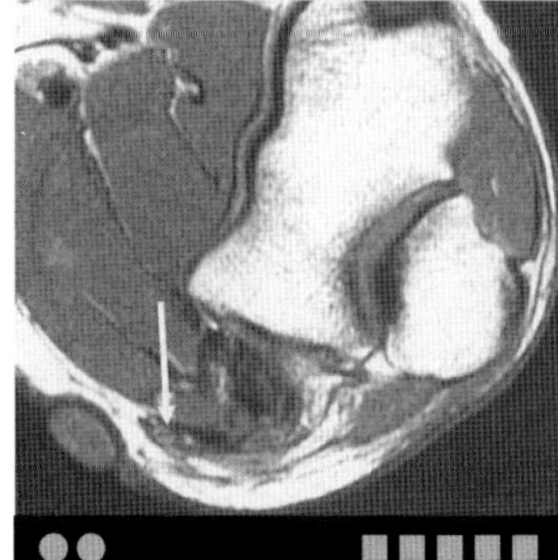

G. Ulnar nerve transposition: Axial T1WI shows an anteriorly relocated ulnar nerve (white arrow) with adjacent scar tissue in a patient with medial elbow pain.

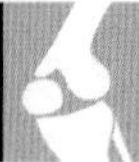

7-20 Anterior Interosseous Nerve Syndrome

Mohammad Reza Hayeri and Zehava Sadka Rosenberg

PRESENTATION

70-year-old male with dull pain in the forearm

FINDINGS

On T2 MRI increased signal intensity is seen in the flexor digitorum profundus, flexor pollicis longus, and pronator quadratus muscles while on T1W images fatty changes corresponding to muscle atrophy are noted.

DIFFERENTIAL DIAGNOSES

- *Lipoma:* Lipoma can be a cause of anterior interosseous nerve compression with associated signs and symptoms.
- *Hemangioma:* Hemangioma may present as a mass in forearm with characteristic vascular pattern.
- *Intersection syndrome:* It is the tenosynovitis of the second extensor compartment of distal forearm.
- *Fibrolipomatous hamartoma of the median nerve:* It is a benign rare tumor that in more than 80% arise exclusively in the median nerve.

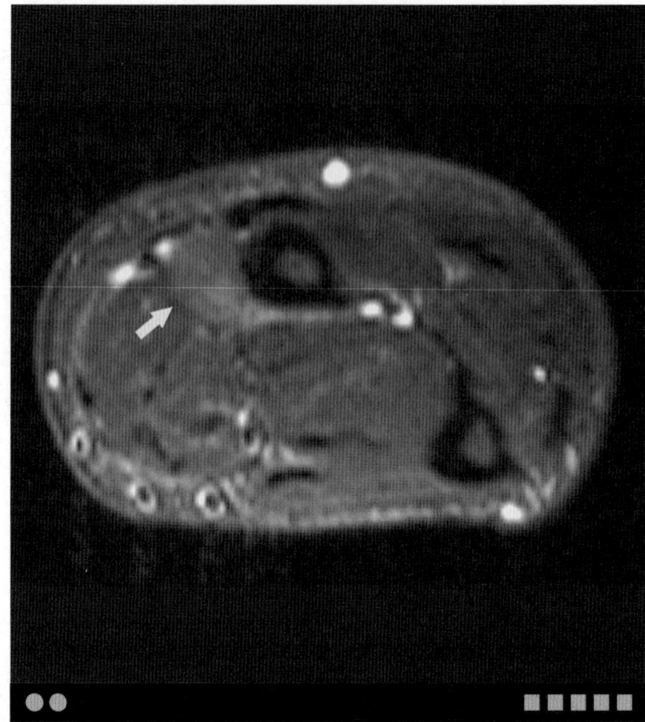

A. Anterior interosseous nerve syndrome: Axial T2 fat-saturated image shows increased signal intensity in the flexor pollicis longus (arrow).

COMMENTS

Anterior interosseous nerve syndrome (also called Kiloh-Nevin syndrome) is caused by entrapment or compression of the anterior interosseous nerve (AIN) in the proximal part of the forearm. AIN is a branch of the median nerve arising from approximately 6 cm below the elbow. It is principally a motor nerve. It passes between two heads of the pronator teres, descends vertically in front of interosseous membrane between flexor digitorum profundus (FDP) and flexor pollicis longus (FPL), supplies these 2 muscles, and finally terminates in pronator quadratus near wrist joint. Patients with AIN syndrome experience a dull pain in the volar aspect of the forearm, combined with an acute onset of muscle weakness. The muscle weakness affects the thumb, the index finger, and occasionally the middle finger. Patients with AIN syndrome have a decreased pinch grip and are not able to form an "O" with the thumb and index finger. Direct trauma and external compression are the main cause of AIN syndrome. External compression can be caused by various anomalies, including a tendinous origin of the deep head of the pronator teres muscle, a soft-tissue mass such as lipoma or ganglion, an accessory muscle including accessory head of FPL (Gantzer's muscle), a fibrous band originating from the superficial flexor, or a vascular abnormality. T2-weighted fat-suppressed or STIR images depict denervation related increased signal intensity in the FDP, FPL, and pronator quadratus muscles. T1-weighted MR images may show fatty atrophy in the above mentioned muscles.

PEARLS

- **AIN syndrome is caused by entrapment or compression of the AIN in the proximal part of the forearm.**
- **AIN is a motor nerve that supplies flexor pollicis longus, pronator quadratus and lateral half of flexor digitorum profundus.**
- **Patients with AIN syndrome are not able to form an "O" with the thumb and index finger.**
- **T1 weighted images may show fatty atrophy in FPL, FDP and pronator quadratus while T2 weighted images show high signal intensity in the mentioned muscles.**

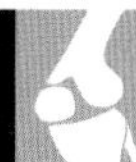

ADDITIONAL IMAGE

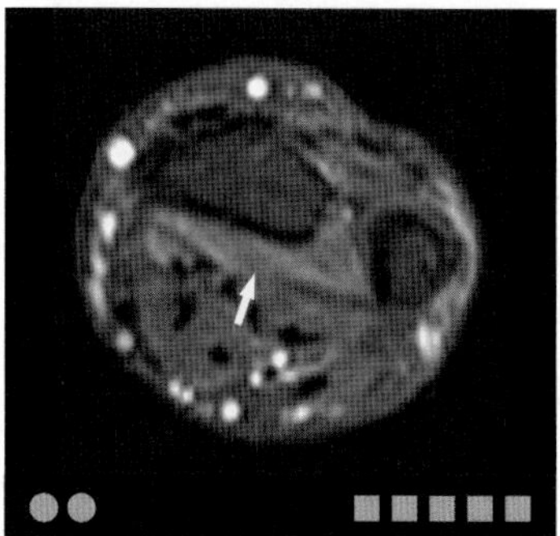

B. Anterior interosseous nerve syndrome: Axial T2W fat-saturated image in the distal forearm in the same patient shows intermediate signal in the pronator quadratus muscle (arrow).

DIFFERENTIAL DIAGNOSES IMAGES

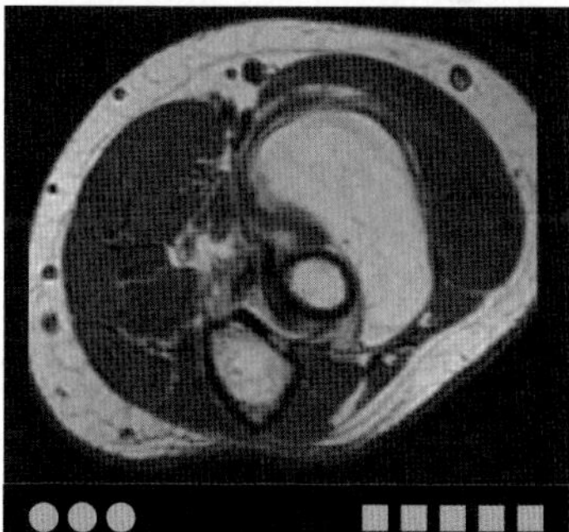

C. Lipoma: Axial T1WI shows a lipoma compressing the AIN.

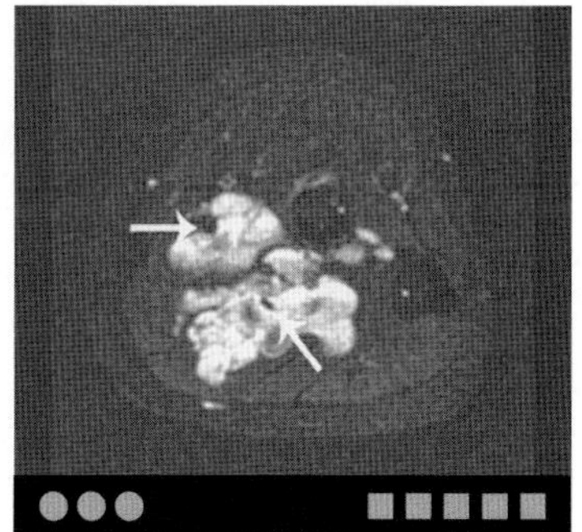

D. Hemangioma: Axial STIR image demonstrates a hyperintense lobulated septated mass with several hypointense foci (arrow).

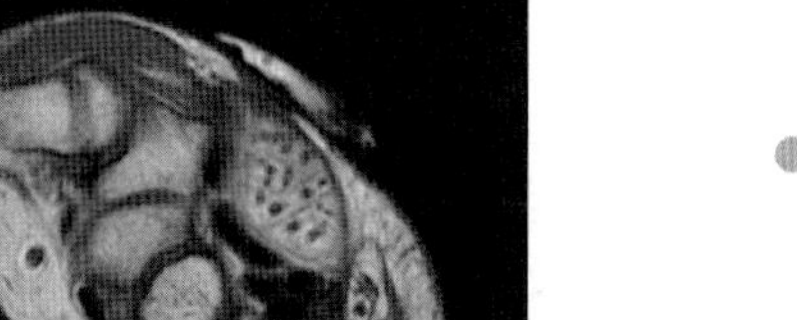

E. Fibrolipomatous hamartoma of the median nerve: Axial T1WI demonstrates a fatty mass infiltrating median nerve, separating out the low signal nerve fascicles.

IMAGE KEY

Common

Rare

Typical

Unusual

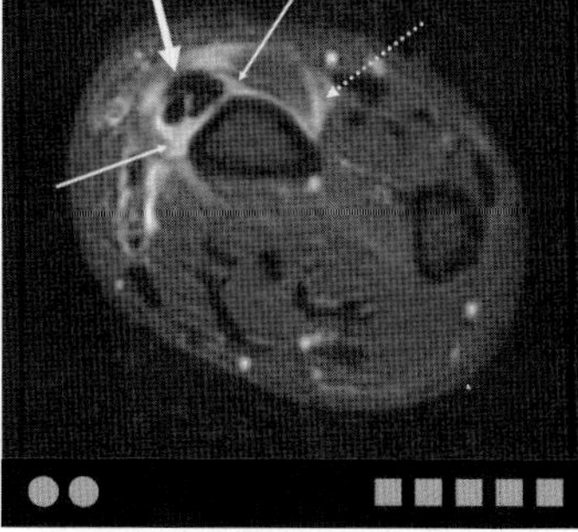

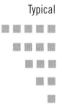

F. Intersection syndrome: Axial T2-weighted image with fat saturation (T2WFS) shows fluid distention of the extensor carpi radialis longus and extensor carpi radialis brevis tendon sheaths of the second compartment (thin arrows) and abductor pollicis longus and extensor pollicis brevis tendon sheaths of the first compartment (thick arrow) at the crossover point of the two compartments. There is also fluid around the first compartment musculature (dotted arrow).

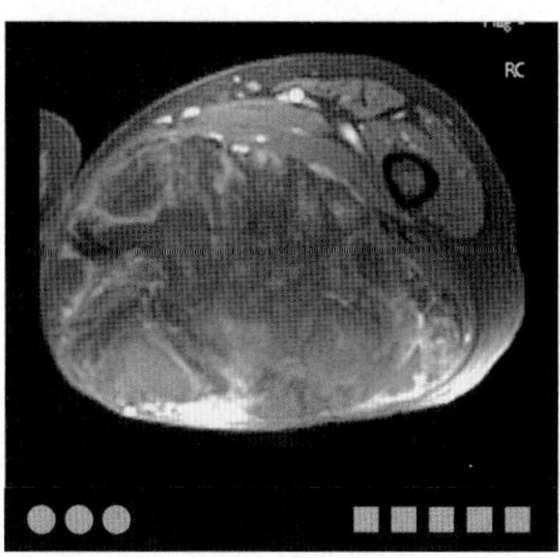

G. Liposarcoma: Axial T1WI with fat suppression after IV contrast injection demonstrates a mass with septal enhancement favoring malignant transformation.

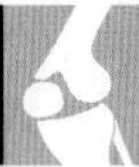

7–21 Ulnar Collateral Ligament Injury

Scott Kingston

PRESENTATION

Acute medial elbow pain and valgus instability

FINDINGS

MR image demonstrates focal disruption with avulsion of the proximal ulnar collateral ligament (UCL).

DIFFERENTIAL DIAGNOSES

- *Medial epicondylitis:* Chronic overuse of the flexor pronator tendon mass from repeated valgus stress resulting in tendinosis. Sometimes referred to as golfer's or pitcher's elbow.
- *Ulnar neuritis:* Ulnar neuropathy due to impingement from osseous spurs, synovial processes, compression from accessory muscle (anconeus epitrochlearis), or other cubital tunnel masses.
- *Little Leaguer's elbow:* Acute or chronic valgus stress elbow injury resulting in edema, avulsion, or stress fracture of the medial epicondyle. Seen in young adolescents involved with throwing sports.

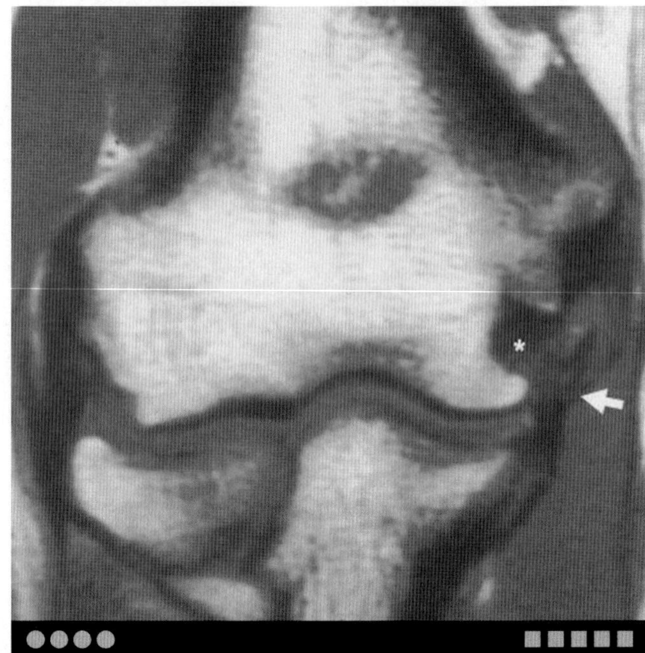

A. Ulnar collateral ligament injury: Coronal T1WI showing a torn and frayed proximal UCL (arrow). Note isointense edema (star) obliterating the normal fat pad between the ligament and trochlea.

COMMENTS

This baseball pitcher is presenting with acute medial elbow pain and valgus instability with applied stress. The UCL is the main soft tissue restraint to valgus stress of the elbow. Repetitive throwing motion in the athlete causes undue stress on the ligament during the late cocking and acceleration phases resulting in an overuse syndrome leading to degeneration of the ligament, microtears, and subsequent complete ligament failure. Minor sprains appear as an intact ligament with adjacent soft tissue edema with partial and complete tears demonstrating discontinuity of the ligament's fibers. High signal from fluid on T2WI is seen at the site of the tear, most commonly occurring in its midportion, followed by its distal attachment onto the sublime tubercle of the ulnar coronoid process. The UCL is composed of an anterior bundle, being the strongest of its three components and most responsible for elbow joint stability. This originates from the anterior undersurface of the medial humeral epicondyle and courses obliquely to its insertion onto the coronoid process. The other less important components of the ligament are the posterior bundle and transverse ligament. Coronal T1WI and T2WI are most useful in observing the normal ligament that often fans out from its proximal humeral origin to its thin linear hypointense insertion onto the sublime tubercle. Chronic tears of the UCL may appear as a diffusely thickened and poorly defined but continuous ligament without hyperintensity on T2WI. If there is doubt about the ligament's integrity, MR arthrography is helpful.

PEARLS

- **Anterior bundle component of the UCL is the major stabilizing restraint of the elbow from valgus forces and is often injured in throwing sports.**
- **UCL sprains will demonstrate an intact ligament with adjacent edema with tears portraying discontinuity of its fibers or avulsion from its origin or insertion.**
- **Chronic UCL tears may appear as a continuous but diffusely thickened and poorly defined ligament.**
- **Normal fat pad between the proximal UCL and underlying trochlea demonstrates high signal intensity on T1WI in the presence of a normal UCL.**
- **Partial tears of the UCL may demonstrate a "T" sign when fluid outlines the corner of the sublime tubercle without frank extravasation.**

ADDITIONAL IMAGES

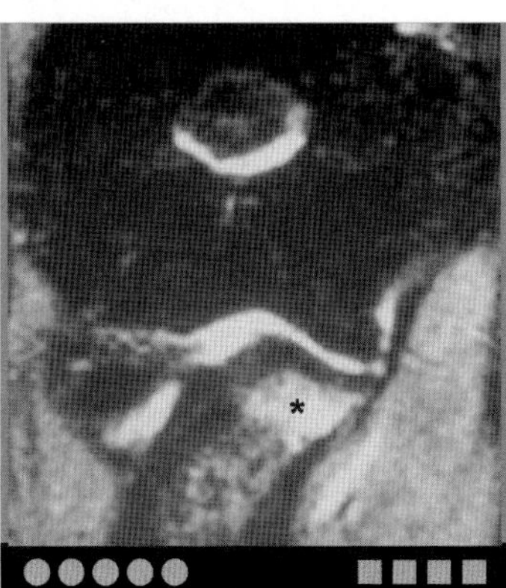

B. Ulnar collateral ligament injury: Coronal STIR image demonstrates reactive bone marrow edema (star) in the coronoid process due to chronic tensile stress from valgus forces of the elbow.

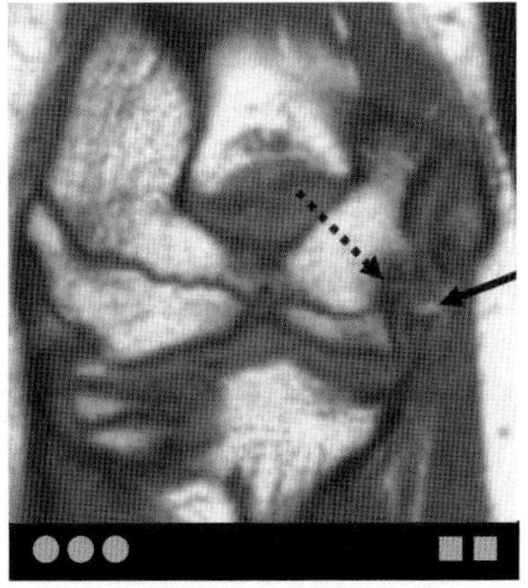

C. Ulnar collateral ligament injury: Coronal T1WI shows torn proximal UCL with small bony avulsion (solid black arrow) and edema (dashed arrow) obliterating normal fat pad deep to the ligament.

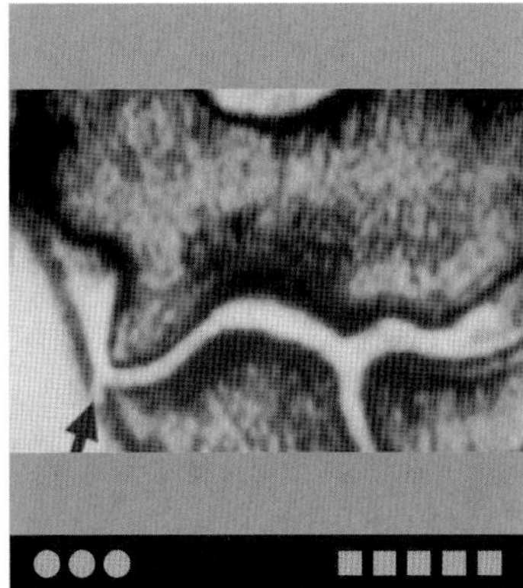

D. Ulnar collateral ligament injury: Coronal contrast assisted gradient MR arthrogram image shows small partial distal tear at sublime tubercle insertion ("T" sign).

DIFFERENTIAL DIAGNOSES IMAGES

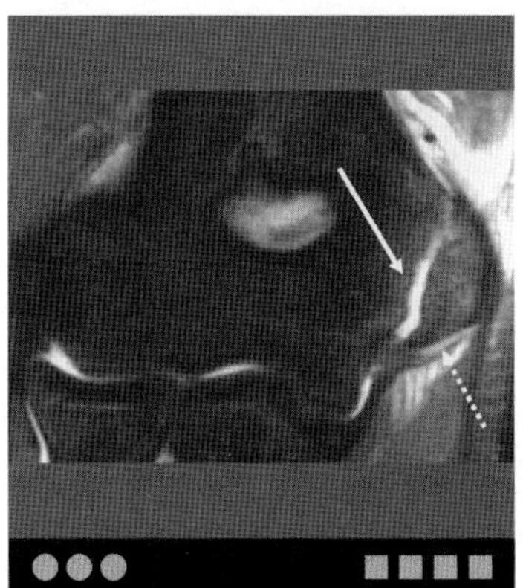

E. Little Leaguer's elbow: Coronal STIR image shows avulsion of the medial epicondyle with fluid in widened apophyseal growth plate (solid arrow). Note stripping of the proximal UCL (dashed arrow) from the epicondyle.

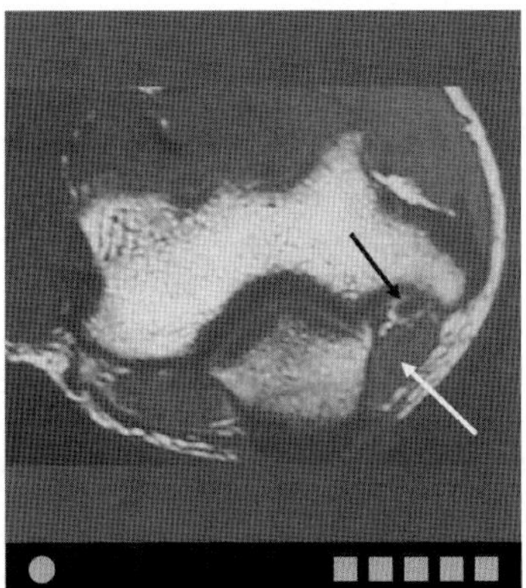

F. Accessory muscle: Axial T1WI demonstrates ulnar nerve (black arrow) in cubital tunnel with an accessory muscle (white arrow, anconeus epitrochlearis) resulting in compressive ulnar neuropathy.

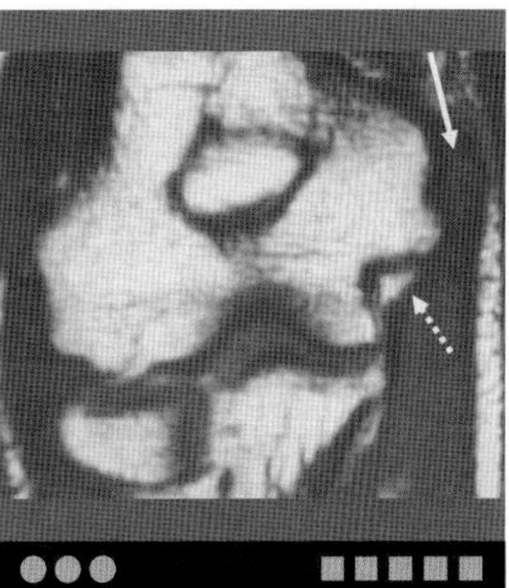

G. Medial epicondylitis: Coronal T1WI demonstrates thickening and hyperintensity of common flexor tendon (solid arrow) secondary to medial epicondylitis in the presence of a normal UCL (dashed arrow). Note normal underlying fat pad.

IMAGE KEY

Common ●●●●● ●●●● ●●● ●● ● Rare

Typical ■■■■■ ■■■■ ■■■ ■■ ■ Unusual

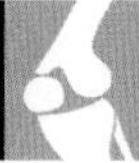

7–22 Ulnar Collateral Ligament Reconstruction Injury

Scott Kingston

PRESENTATION

Baseball pitcher felt a pop and elbow pain

FINDINGS

MR image demonstrates high signal fluid from an acute retear of his ulnar collateral ligament (UCL) graft.

DIFFERENTIAL DIAGNOSES

- *UCL graft sprain:* Soft tissue edema adjacent to an intact UCL graft. High signal bone marrow edema may be observed from chronic tensile forces on the coronoid process.
- *Medial epicondylitis:* Tendinosis or partial to complete tears of the common flexor tendon from chronic valgus forces demonstrating high signal intensity on T2WI.
- *Stress fracture:* Chronic overuse syndrome resulting in occult bony stress fractures with mixed areas of signal void from sclerosis and hyperintensity from marrow edema.
- *Ulnar neuropathy:* Impingement on the ulnar nerve from bone spurs or other cubital tunnel masses may result in an enlarged and hyperintense nerve with medial elbow pain.

COMMENTS

This is a baseball pitcher with past ulnar collateral ligament (UCL) reconstruction (Tommy John reconstruction) who felt a pop and elbow pain. In certain professional athletes, repetitive overhand throwing produces a chronic valgus strain on the UCL of the elbow and may exceed the normal strength of the ligament resulting in a torn anterior bundle leading to medial elbow pain, instability, and a reduction in throwing performance. Such career-ending injuries are now surgically corrected after the first surgical procedure was performed on a professional baseball pitcher, Tommy John, in 1974 by Dr. Frank Jobe. Reconstruction of the torn UCL is often accomplished by harvesting a tendon from either the forearm (palmaris longus), hamstrings (semitendinosus), or calf (plantaris) and weaving the tendon-graft in a figure-eight fashion through bone tunnels drilled in the medial epicondyle of the distal humerus and coronoid process of the ulna. The new interwoven graft consists of several strands of tendon and appears thicker on MRI. After a long rehabilitation program, the player may begin throwing at 6 to 7 months and pitching by 1 year and may achieve the same or better level of throwing or pitching with an overall success rate approaching 90% to 95%. Continued overuse or bad mechanics may still lead to degeneration and retear of the UCL graft and may be recognized on MRI by edema, high signal fluid within the graft substance or focal discontinuity of the graft. MR arthrography with coronal fat saturated T1W images while observing for partial or complete tears is often recommended.

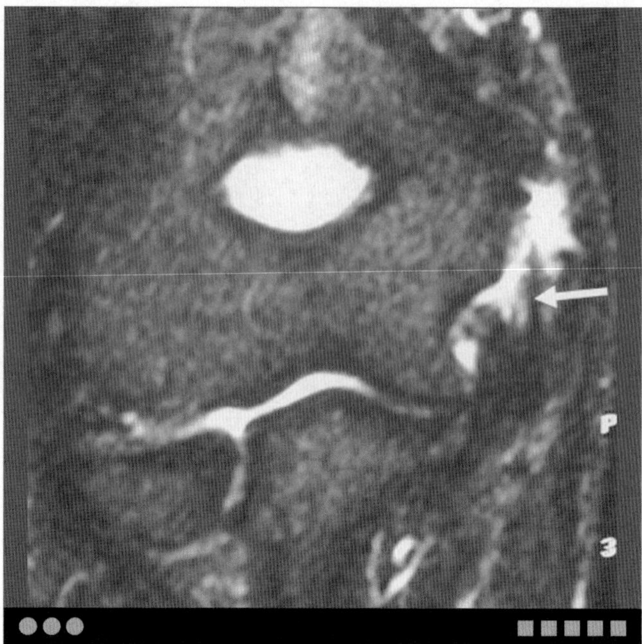

A. Avulsion of UCL Graft: Coronal STIR image demonstrates acute avulsion of the proximal UCL graft with high signal fluid at the tear site.

PEARLS

- **Normal Tommy John UCL graft reconstructions appear thickened and hypointense on all imaging sequences.**
- **Normal postsurgical magnetic susceptibility artifacts occurring near the intact graft and bone tunnels should not be mistaken for focal tears or edema.**
- **Sprains and retears are recognized by high signal intensity on T2-weighted fat-saturated proton density or STIR images and disruptions in the graft.**
- **Intra-articular injection of contrast with coronal fat saturated T1WI is quite helpful in looking for partial ("T" sign) or complete tears.**
- **Earlier surgical procedures with anterior transposition of the ulnar nerve have been replaced with newer techniques no longer requiring nerve relocation.**

ADDITIONAL IMAGES

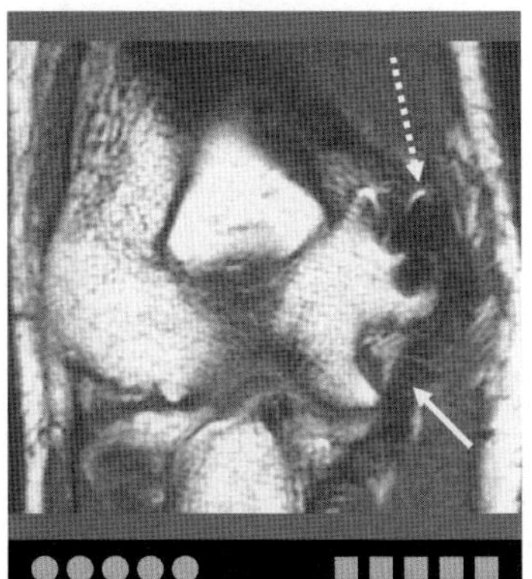

B. Thickened normal UCL graft: Coronal T1WI shows a hypointense and thickened normal UCL graft (arrow). Note magnetic susceptibility artifacts (dashed arrow) from surgical bone tunnels in the medial epicondyle.

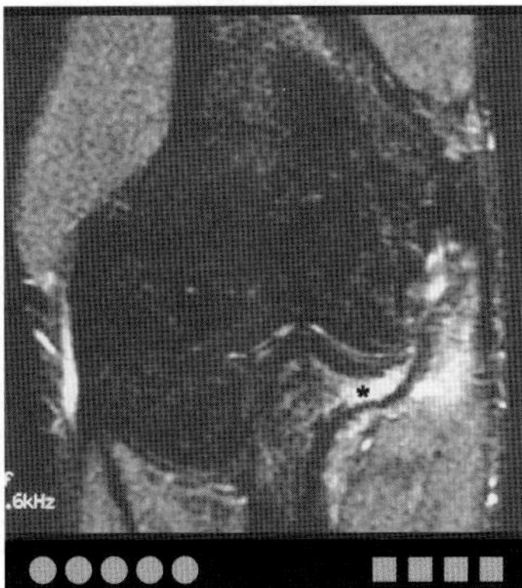

C. Bone marrow edema: Coronal STIR image shows reactive bone marrow edema (star) within the coronoid process and soft tissue edema adjacent to the acutely sprained UCL graft.

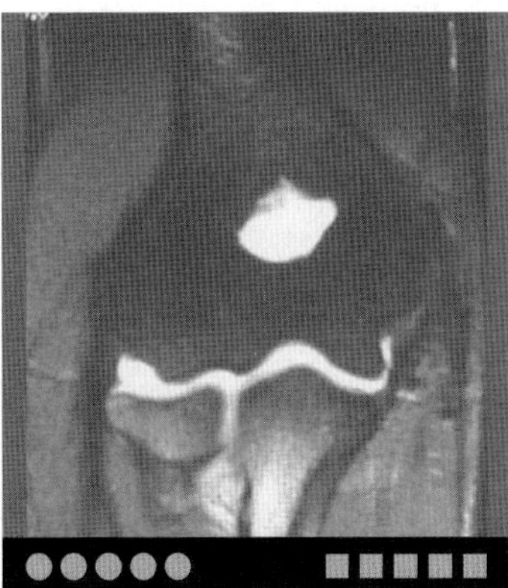

D. Normal ulnar collateral ligament: Coronal fat saturated T1W MR arthrogram image demonstrates the normal articular side of an intact UCL graft, excluding any recurrent tear.

SECTION II
Elbow

CHAPTER 7
Sport Medicine and Trauma

CASE
Ulnar Collateral Ligament Reconstruction Injury

IMAGE KEY

Common

Rare

Typical

Unusual

DIFFERENTIAL DIAGNOSES IMAGES

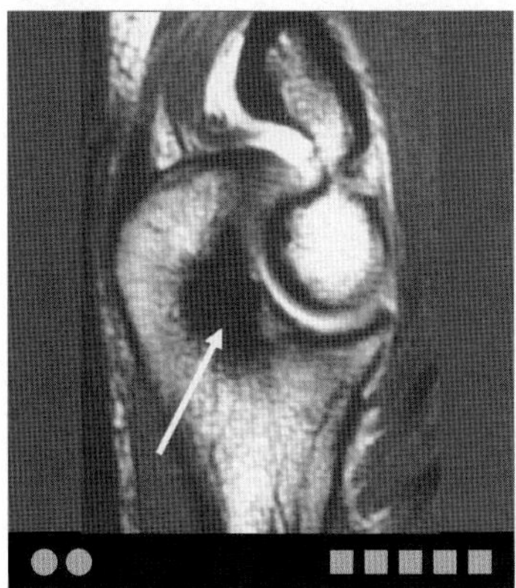

E. Stress fracture: Sagittal T1WI shows marked signal void area (arrow) secondary to reactive bony sclerosis from a healing olecranon stress fracture. Note the fracture line is not visible due to the sclerosis.

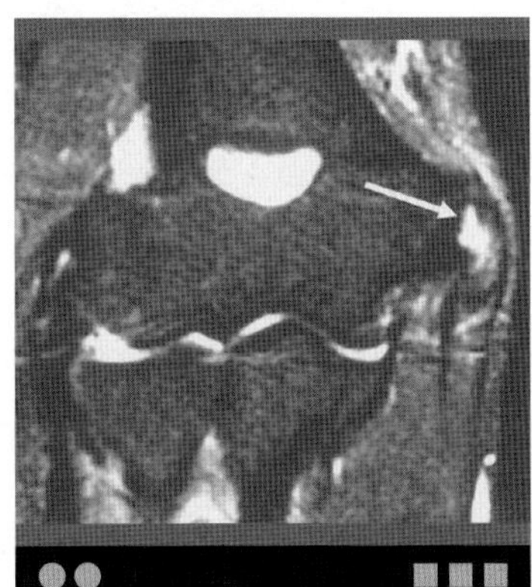

F. Medial epicondylitis: Coronal STIR image demonstrates hyperintense signal from fluid within the base of the common flexor tendon secondary to medial epicondylitis/partial tear.

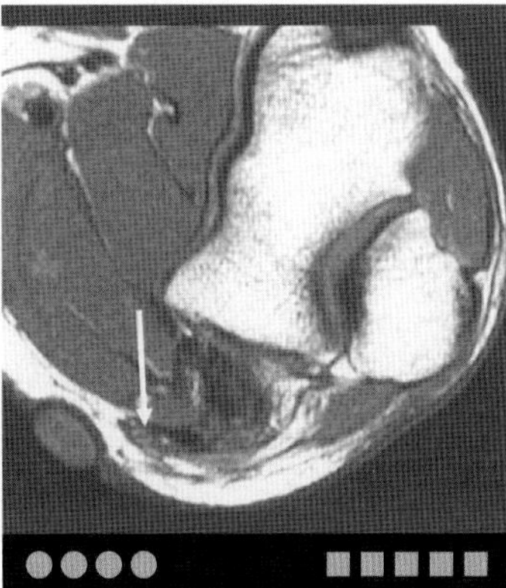

G. Ulnar nerve transposition: Axial T1WI shows an anteriorly relocated ulnar nerve (white arrow) with adjacent scar tissue in a patient with medial elbow pain.

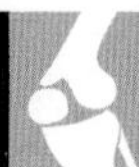

7–23 Large Pseudoaneurysm of Brachial Artery

Atul Agarwal and Thomas Learch

PRESENTATION

Growing, pulsatile mass in the antecubital fossa

FINDINGS

MRI shows a large high signal cystic pseudoaneurysm with central low signal pertaining to flow void from fast moving blood. A second smaller pseudoaneurysm with low signal is noted adjacent.

DIFFERENTIAL DIAGNOSES

- *Ganglion cyst:* These are cystic swellings that are closely connected to joint or tendon sheaths and contain mucinous material.
- *Biceps tendon tear:* Hemorrhage following biceps tendon tear may create a mass at antecubital area.
- *Soft tissue tumors:* Presents as a mass in this region including benign or malignant neoplasms.
- *Cat scratch disease:* Presents with an inflammatory mass.

COMMENTS

This is a 24-year-old female who was an intravenous drug abuser and developed this pseudoaneurysm as a sequela of chronic attempts at vascular access. A pseudoaneurysm is defined as an aneurysmatic sac surrounded by fibrous tissue instead of other vascular layers. Blunt or penetrating trauma and vascular access attempts are the most common etiologic factors. Penetrating trauma (gunshot and stab wounds) accounts for 70% to 90% of vascular injuries, whereas, iatrogenic trauma related to endovascular procedures accounts for less than 10% of all cases. Hemodialysis patients carry a high risk of pseudoaneurysm because of inadvertent puncture of the brachial artery during venous cannulation for hemodialysis. Regarding blunt trauma, the axilla, medial/anterior upper arm, and antecubital fossa are particularly considered high-risk areas because of the superficial location of the axillary and brachial arteries in these regions. Angiography remains the gold standard for evaluation of vascular injuries in trauma patients presenting with "hard signs" such as, bruit and thrills, active or pulsatile hemorrhage, pulsatile or expanding hematoma, signs of limb ischemia, and diminished or absent pulses. It aids in determining the precise location of injury, especially when surgical access is difficult or when atherosclerosis limits the pulse exam. Duplex ultrasonography plays a role in the evaluation of patients presenting with "soft signs" of injury such as, neurological deficit caused by primary adjacent nerve injury, stable, nonpulsatile or small hematoma, and history of hypotension or shock. Helical CT and MR are also highly sensitive methods of diagnosing arterial injuries.

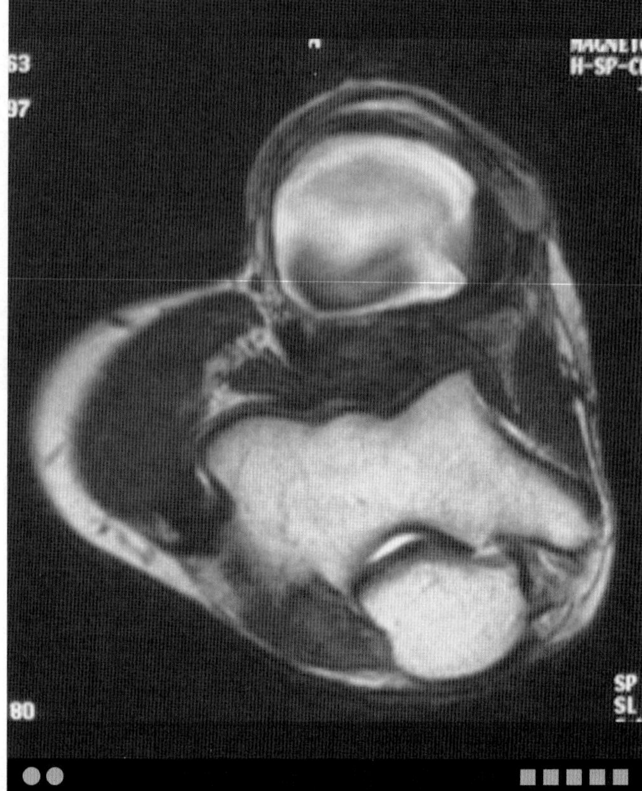

A. Pseudoaneurysm of brachial artery: Axial T2 MRI shows a large high signal cystic pseudoaneurysm with central low signal pertaining to flow void from fast moving blood. A second smaller pseudoaneurysm with low signal is noted adjacent.

PEARLS

- **A pseudoaneurysm is defined as an aneurysmatic sac surrounded by fibrous tissue.**
- **Blunt or penetrating trauma and vascular access attempts are the most common etiologic factors.**
- **Angiography demonstrates a saccular structure arising from an artery with brisk and dense opacification upon contrast administration.**
- **Ultrasonography demonstrates a typical "yin yang" color Doppler signal.**

ADDITIONAL IMAGES

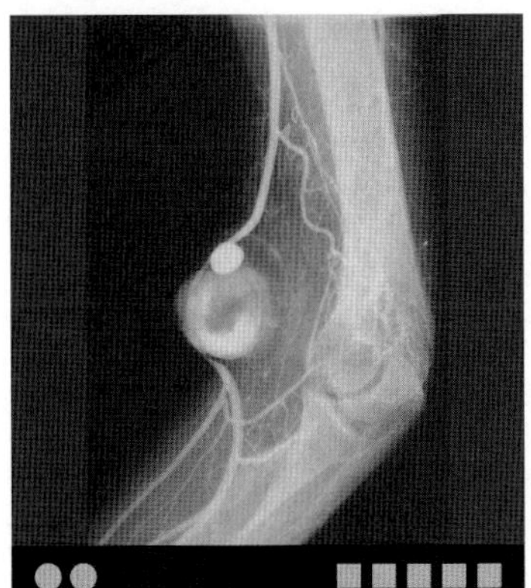

B. Pseudoaneurysm of brachial artery: Angiography of the lateral elbow demonstrates these two pseudoaneurysms in the antecubital fossa with dense contrast opacification within them.

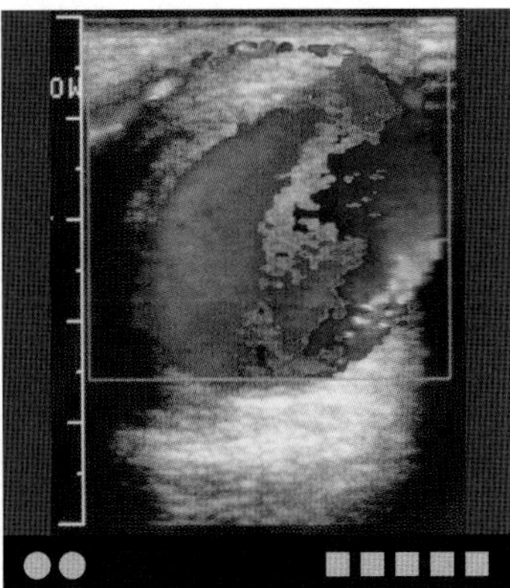

C. Pseudoaneurysm of brachial artery: Color Doppler sonographic image of the larger pseudoaneurysm shows a "yin yang" appearance due to rapid blood flow changing directions.

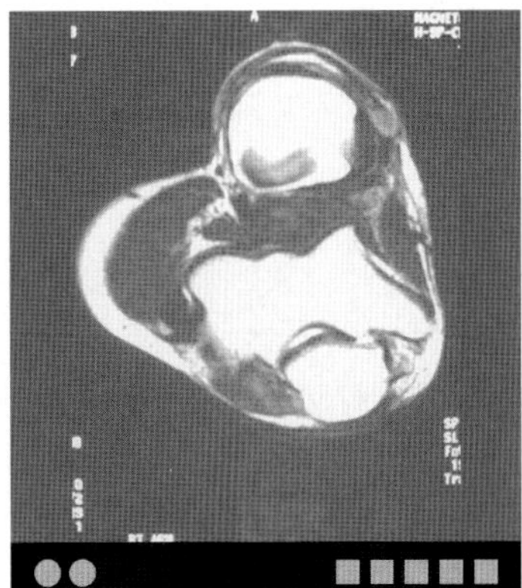

D. Pseudoaneurysm of brachial artery: This axial T2 MRI with wider window width also shows reverberation artifact, in an anterior to posterior direction, from the rapid blood flow in the pseudoaneurysms.

IMAGE KEY

Common

Rare

Typical

Unusual

DIFFERENTIAL DIAGNOSES IMAGES

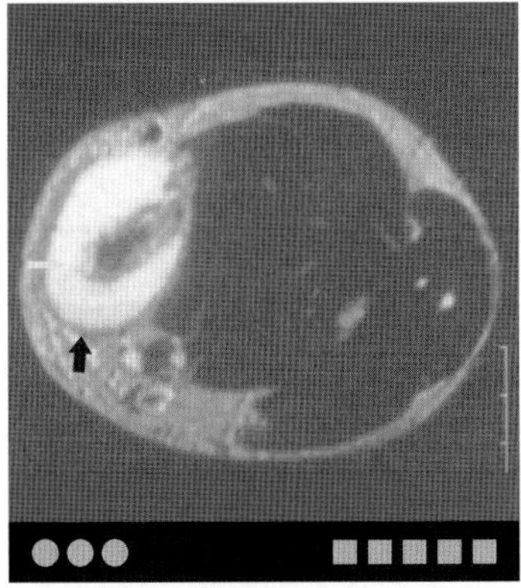

E. Tear of biceps tendon: Axial T2WI shows hemorrhage (black arrow) around torn biceps tendon (white arrow).

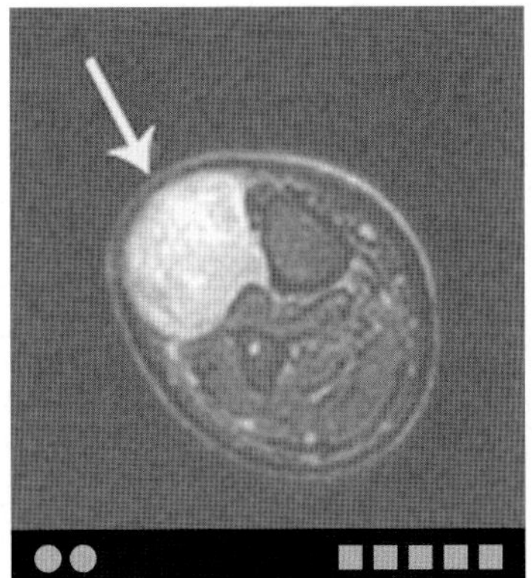

F. Leiomyosarcoma: Axial fat saturated post contrast T1WI shows enhancement of this soft tissue sarcoma (arrow).

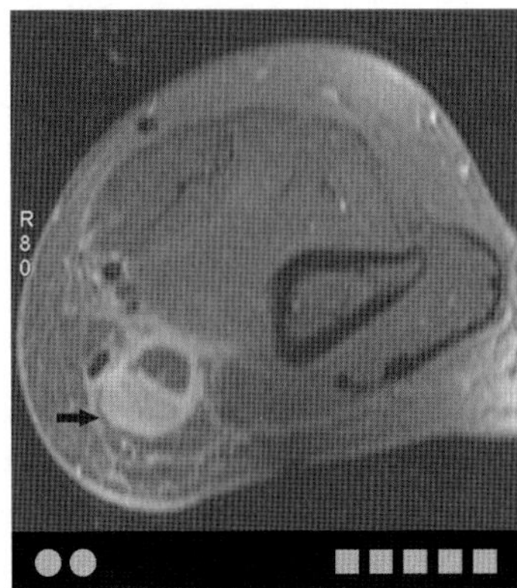

G. Cat scratch disease: Axial fat saturated T1WI shows enhancement of inflammatory mass (arrow) in elbow.

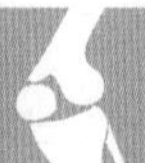

7-24 Osteochondritis Dissecans of Elbow (OCD)

Mohammad Reza Hayeri and Jamshid Tehranzadeh

PRESENTATION

Pain, tenderness, and swelling over the lateral aspect of elbow

FINDINGS

MRI shows high signal changes at the subchondral bone with osteochondral defect of capitellum on fluid sensitive sequences. The osteochondral fragment is seen as a loose body in the joint.

DIFFERENTIAL

- *Panner's disease:* Osteochondrosis of capitulum because of interference in blood supply to growing epiphysis of distal humerus, which results in resorption and eventual repair and replacement of the ossification center.
- *Multiple epiphyseal dysplasias:* It is a common form of osteochondrodysplasia inherited as an autosomal dominant trait and characterized by disturbance in enchondral ossification of multiple epiphyses and physes.
- *Normal posterior capitellum irregularity:* There is a normal posterior capitellum osteochondral irregularity that may mimic osteochondral injury. This finding is considered normal variant.

COMMENT

Humeral capitellum osteochondritis dissecans (OCD) occurs after the capitellum has ossified and is the result of compressive valgus forces to the subchondral bone like in pitchers, which leads to adaptive changes in subchondral blood supply of the humeral capitellum. The initial appearance is consistent with avascular necrosis, which leads to loss of support for adjacent cartilaginous structures. The natural history of some OCD lesion is the separation of these structures from the capitellum leading to the development of a free osteochondral fragment of articular cartilage on the underlying bone at the superficial surface of the diarthrodial joint (stage IV). OCD is rare in individuals younger than 10 years or older than 50 years and is primarily observed in children aged 10 to 15 years. OCD is an uncommon cause of elbow pain. The main findings are pain, tenderness, and swelling over the lateral aspect of elbow with intermittent limitations with range of motion that are worse with activity. Joint effusion, crepitus with motion, muscle atrophy, and catching and locking of the elbow are late findings. In AP radiograph with elbow at 45 degrees flexion sclerotic rim of subchondral bone adjacent to the articular surface, irregular ossification, and/or a bony defect adjacent to the articular surface are seen. Lateral radiographs may show flattening of the capitellum. Early detection, size, and extent of the lesion can be done with MRI; T1WI shows a focus of low-signal change at the surface of the capitellum; on T2W and STIR images focus of bright signal with osteochondral irregularity of subchondral bone are noted.

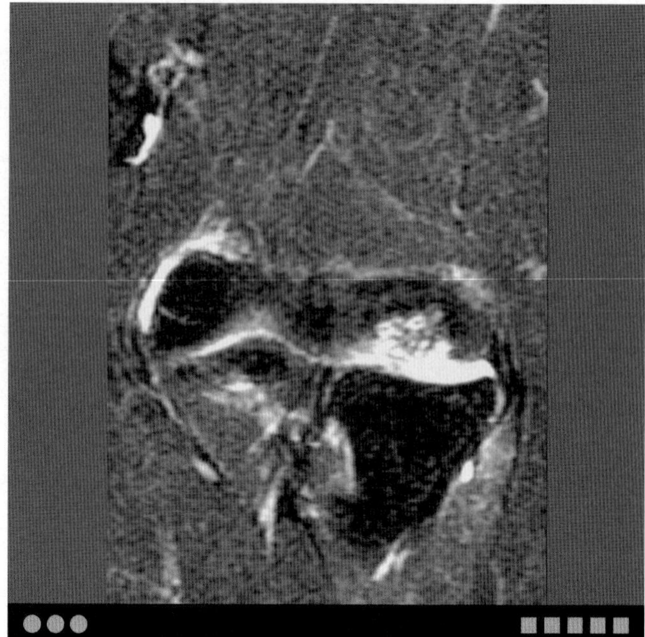

A. Osteochondritis dissecans of capitellum: Coronal fat-saturated T2WI shows high signal in the subchondral bone of capitellum with osteochondral irregularity. (Courtesy of Mark Schweitzer.)

PEARLS

- **The early findings of OCD are pain, tenderness, and swelling over the lateral aspect of the elbow.**
- **Lateral radiographs may show flattening of the capitellum.**
- **In later stages of OCD (stage IV), compressive valgus forces cause articular cartilage and associated bone becomes partially or totally detached and form joint loose bodies.**
- **T1WI shows low-signal changes at the surface of the capitellum on T2W and STIR images focus of bright signal with osteochondral irregularity of subchondral bone is noted. Free osteochondral fragment may be seen.**

ADDITIONAL IMAGES

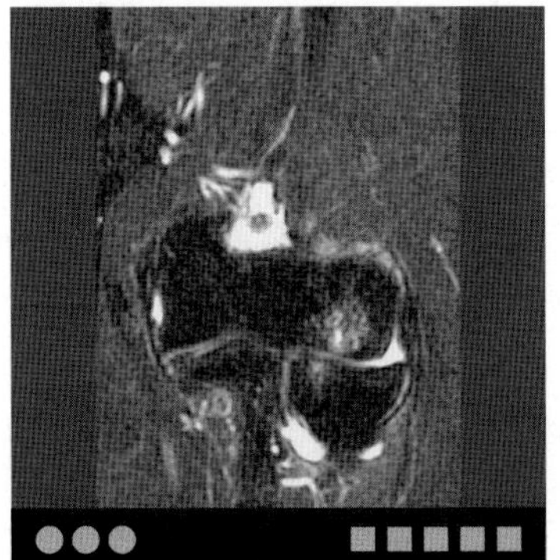

B. Osteochondritis dissecans of capitellum: Coronal fat-saturated T2WI of the same patient shows kissing marrow edema and contusion of capitellum and radial head. (Courtesy of Mark Schweitzer.)

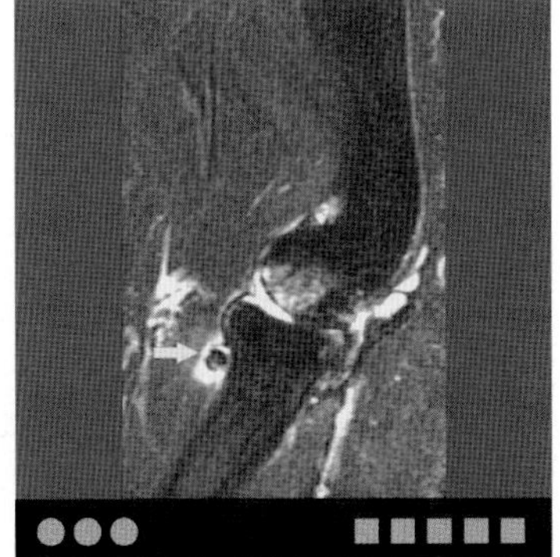

C. Osteochondritis dissecans of capitellum: Sagittal fat-saturated T2WI shows marrow edema of the capitellum and loose bony fragment separated from capitellum, which is seen in the anterior joint space next to radial head (arrow). (Courtesy of Mark Schweitzer.)

DIFFERENTIAL DIAGNOSES IMAGES

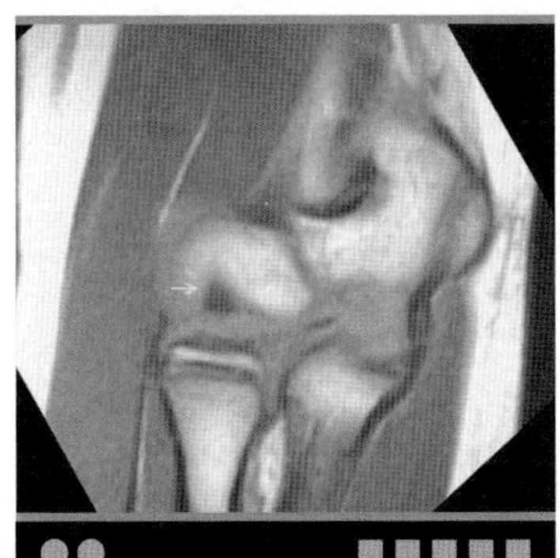

D. Panner's disease: Coronal T1WI shows a focal area of low signal in the capitellum (arrow). (Courtesy of Mark Schweitzer.)

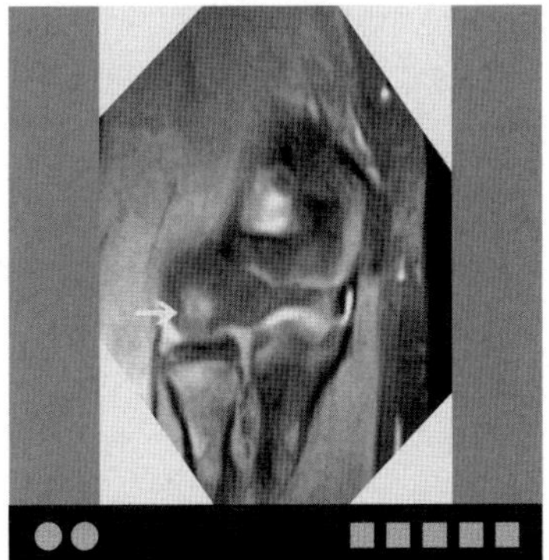

E. Panner's disease: Coronal T2WI shows a focal area of high signal in the capitellum (arrow). (Courtesy of Mark Schweitzer.)

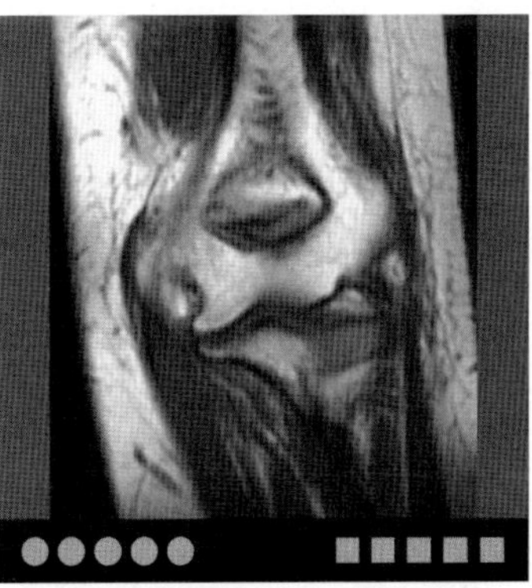

F. Normal capitellum irregularity: Coronal T1WI shows normal irregularity of the posterior capitellum (normal variant).

IMAGE KEY

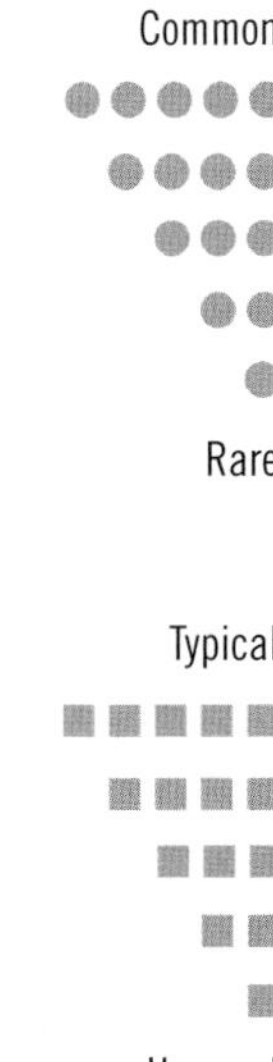

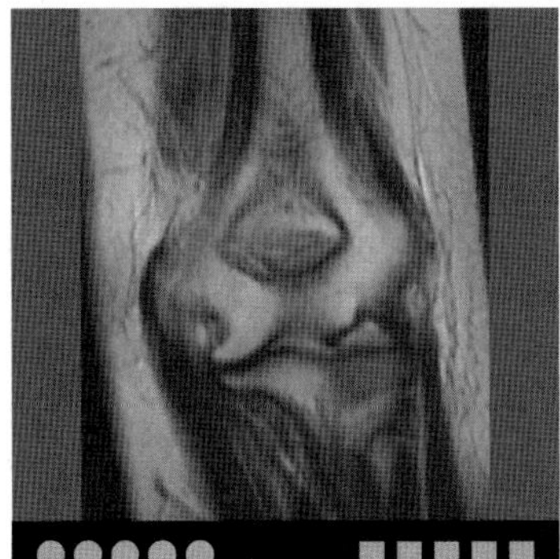

G. Normal capitellum irregularity: Coronal T2WI shows normal irregularity of the posterior capitellum (normal variant).

Chapter 8

Congenital, Systemic and Metabolic Diseases

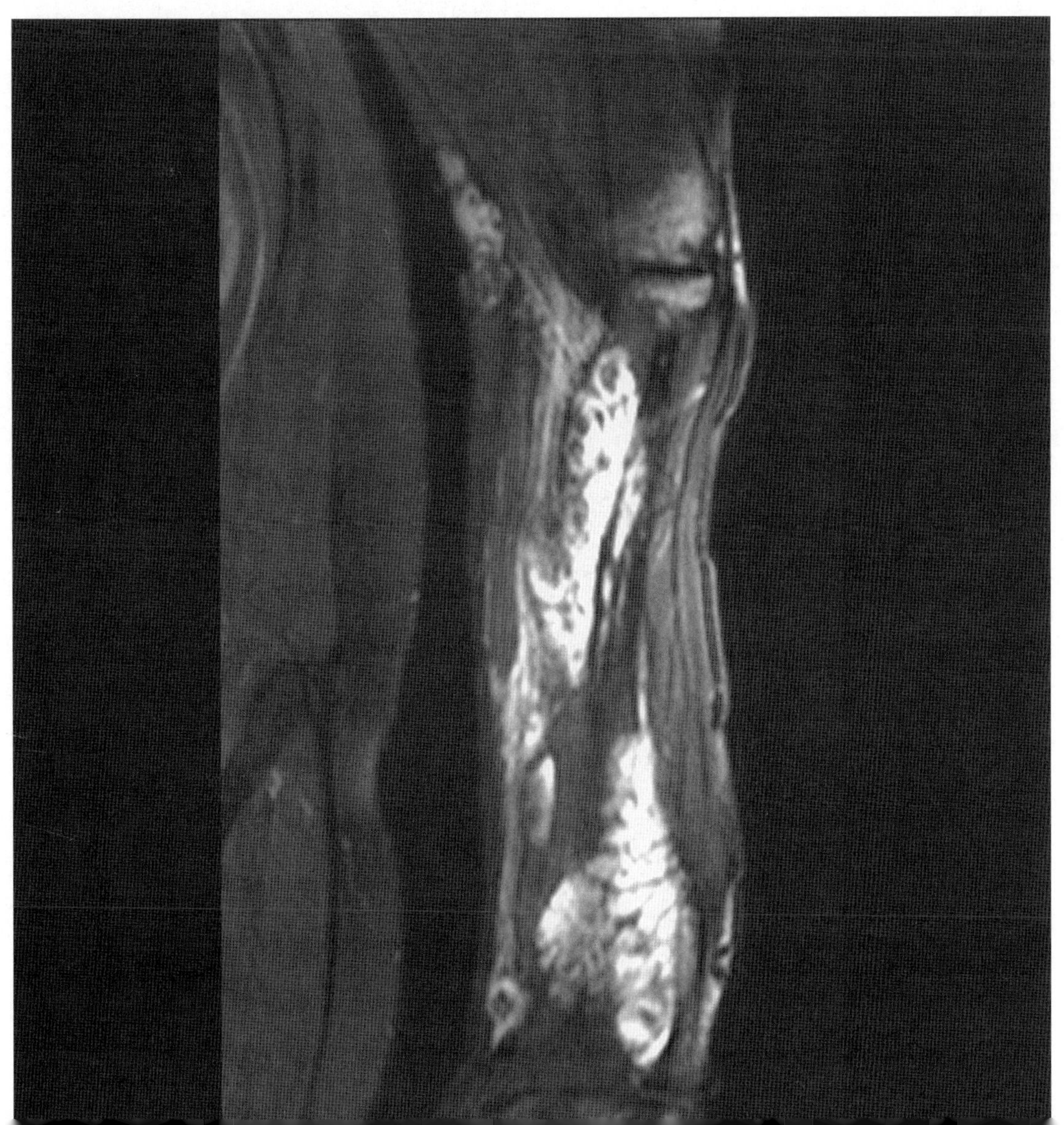

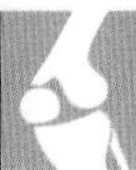

8–1 Arteriovenous Malformation of the Forearm

Oganes Ashikyan and Jamshid Tehranzadeh

PRESENTATION

Arm numbness

FINDINGS

Poorly defined mass, which has low to intermediate signal intensity on T1-weighted images and high signal intensity on T2-weighted and contrast-enhanced images. Signal voids are present in vessels with high flow velocities.

DIFFERENTIAL DIAGNOSES

- *Capillary, cavernous, or venous hemangioma:* These entities will present similar to arteriovenous malformation. Histologic diagnosis is necessary to make the distinction.
- *Lymphangioma:* High fat content of this lesion results in increased signal intensity on T-weighted and nonfat-saturated T-weighted sequences.
- *Resolving hematoma or infectious abscess:* Flow voids would be absent in these lesions. Clinical context can be useful in differentiating these entities from arteriovenous malformation involving soft tissues.
- *Angiosarcoma:* This predominantly involves long bones. Large portion of the bone is usually involved with adjacent areas of reactive sclerosis.

COMMENTS

The patient is a 27-year-old male who presented with arm numbness. Vascular malformations arise from abnormal embryological development of vascular tissues. Persistence of venous capillary beds results in abnormal communications between arterial and venous beds, which are characteristic of arteriovenous malformations. Arteriovenous malformations have been categorized as a subtype of hemangioma with capillary, cavernous, and venous hemangiomas, constituting remaining varieties. However, other authors consider arteriovenous malformation to be a separate lesion, which is not a part of hemangioma continuum. A mixture of lesions can be present. Hereditary hemorrhagic telangiectasia also known as Osler-Weber-Rendu syndrome is characterized by presence of multiorgan arteriovenous malformations. Association of extensive hemangiomas with thrombocytopenia is termed Kasabach-Merrit syndrome. Arteriovenous malformations can present as incidental findings or as a catastrophic event such as cerebral hemorrhage. Arteriovenous malformations are demonstrated as ill-defined masses of low to intermediate signal intensity on T-weighted images. Areas of high signal intensity maybe present, which correspond to fatty components of the mass. Important aspect of decision making related to therapeutic approach is flow velocity within the lesion. Slow-flowing serpentine channels demonstrate high signal intensity on T2-weighted images. Areas with high flow rates demonstrate flow voids on T2-weighted images.

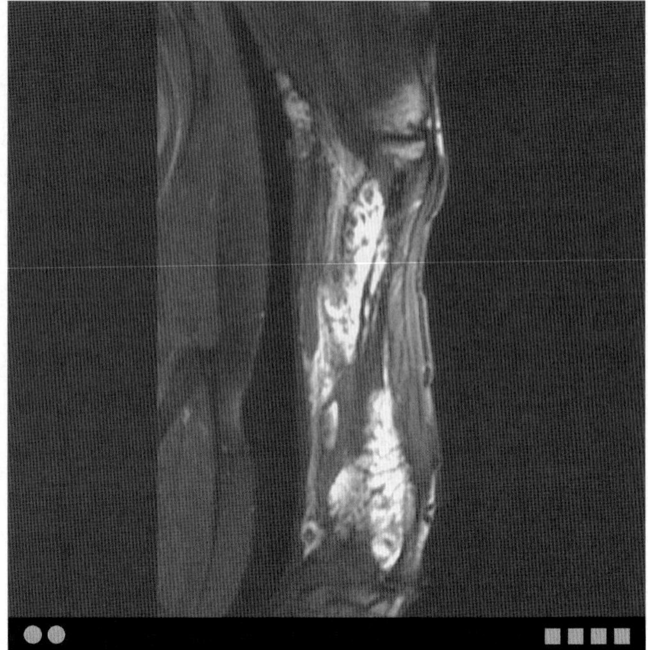

A. Arteriovenous malformation of the forearm: Coronal spin echo T2-weighted image with fat saturation demonstrates high signal intensity mass with serpentine channels, which extensively involves soft tissues of left forearm.

PEARLS

- **Arteriovenous malformation is a congenital malformation.**
- **T-weighted images demonstrate ill-defined low to intermediate signal intensity mass.**
- **T2-weighted images demonstrate high signal intensity mass with serpentine channels.**
- **Channels that have high flow rates demonstrate flow void on all sequences.**

ADDITIONAL IMAGES

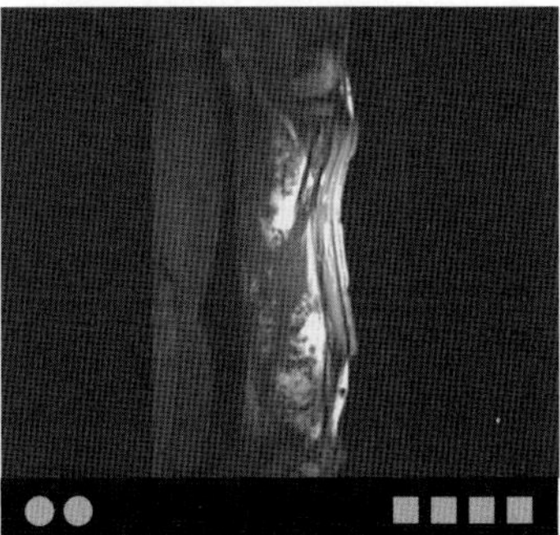

B. Arteriovenous malformation of the forearm: Coronal T1-weighted image obtained after gadolinium contrast administration demonstrates high signal intensity mass with serpentine channels, which extensively involves soft tissues of left arm.

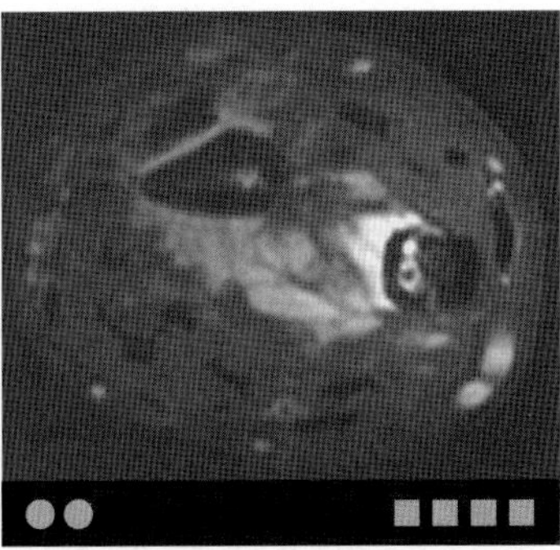

C. Arteriovenous malformation of the forearm: Axial T1-weighted image obtained after gadolinium contrast administration also demonstrates high signal intensity mass. Also note vascular channels with flow voids, which correspond to areas with high flow velocities.

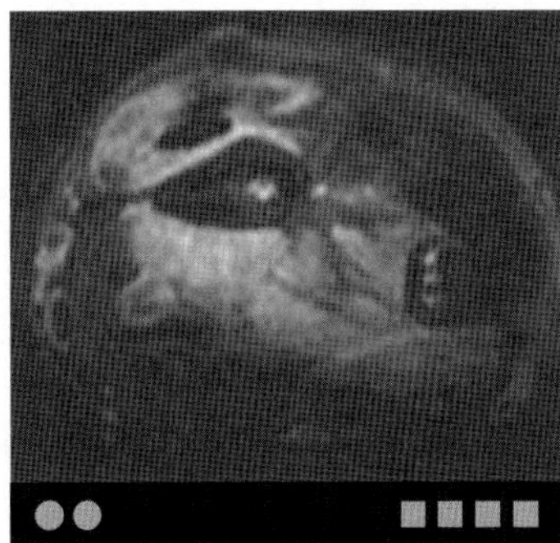

D. Arteriovenous malformation of the forearm: Axial spin echo T2-weighted image with fat saturation also demonstrates high signal intensity mass.

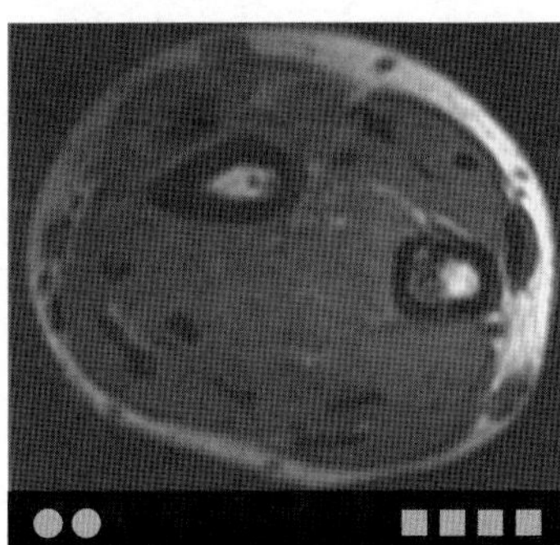

E. Arteriovenous malformation of the forearm: Axial spin echo T1-weighted image shows only a subtle area of abnormal signal intensity in the region of the arteriovenous malformation.

DIFFERENTIAL DIAGNOSES IMAGES

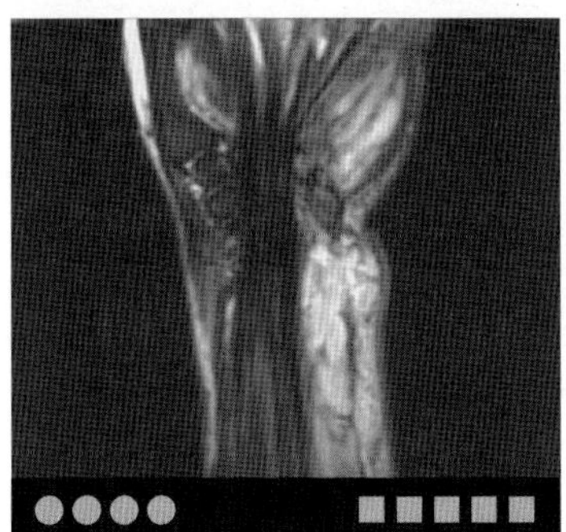

F. Large abscess in the soft tissues of the wrist: Coronal T2-weighted image with fat saturation demonstrates a large abscess in the lateral soft tissues of the wrist. Note lack of flow voids in the abscess.

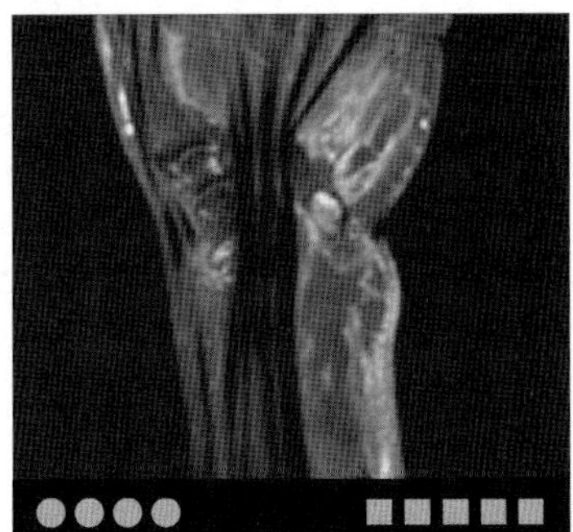

G. Large abscess in the soft tissues of the wrist: Coronal T1-weighted image with fat saturation obtained after gadolinium contrast administration demonstrates a large abscess in the lateral soft tissues of the wrist with peripheral enhancement. Note lack of flow voids in the abscess.

IMAGE KEY

Common

Rare

Typical

Unusual

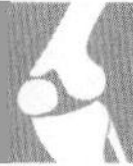

8–2 Anconeus Epitrochlearis

Rajeev K. Varma

PRESENTATION

Weakness in the ulnar nerve distribution

FINDINGS

MR images show high signal around the ulnar nerve on T2-weighted images and evidence of an anomalous muscle on all sequences.

DIFFERENTIAL DIAGNOSES

- *Malignancy:* Soft tissue masses may compress ulnar nerve.
- *Compression by enthesophyte:* Enthesopathy may be responsible for compression.
- *Pigmented villonodular synovitis:* This infiltrating mass has characteristic low signal on MR sequences and results in cystic bone erosion.
- *Ulnar neuritis:* MRI would be helpful to exclude mechanical compression causes. Neuritis shows contrast enhancement and bright signal of nerve on T2-weighted images.

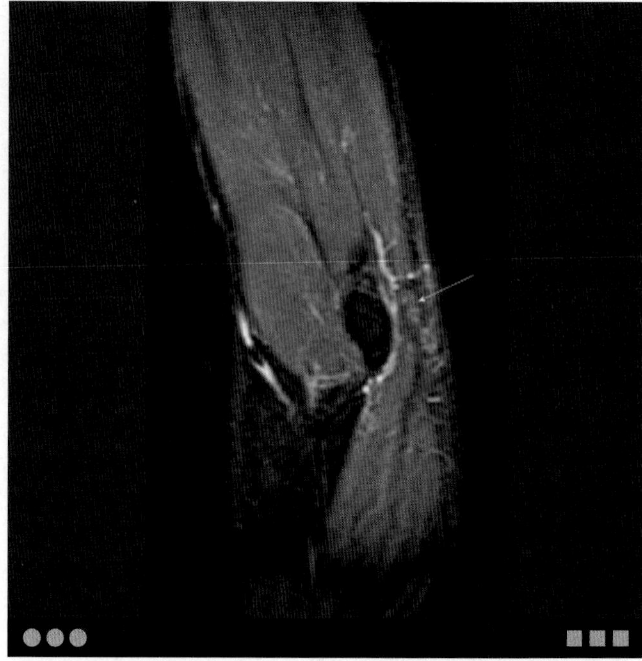

A. Anconeus epitrochlearis: T1-weighted oblique coronal image of the posterior elbow shows the ulnar nerve and another structure (small arrow), isointense to surrounding muscle, in the expected position of an *anconeus epitrochlearis.* The adjacent high signal structure is the ulnar nerve.

COMMENTS

This is the case of a 49-year-old male with weakness in the left ulnar nerve distribution (C8, T1). Clinical diagnosis of left ulnar nerve entrapment was made, and the patient was sent for confirmatory imaging. The ulnar nerve passes through the cubital tunnel of the elbow, through a groove in the posterior surface of the medial humeral epicondyle, and then deep to the heads of the flexor carpi ulnaris muscle. The cubital tunnel retinaculum covers the medial epicondyle and olecranon and creates the tunnel. The cubital tunnel is second only to the carpal tunnel as the most frequent site of nerve compression in the upper extremity. Nerve compression at this site can be due to several causes, as listed above, but rarely the anconeus epitrochlearis muscle replaces the cubital tunnel retinaculum, causing compression within the tunnel. The ulnar nerve normally shows high signal on T1 imaging. The nerve will often appear enlarged and with abnormally elevated T2-weighted signal in abnormal states. Other masses, benign or malignant, such as soft tissue tumor, enthesopathy, and neuritis in the cubital tunnel may simulate signs and symptoms created by anconeus epitrochlearis.

PEARLS

- **The ulnar nerve is easily identified as a bright oval structure on T1-weighted images.**
- **Enlargement and abnormally elevated T2 signal of the ulnar nerve within the region of the cubital tunnel may be caused by several processes.**
- **The anconeus epitrochlearis is an anomalous muscle that replaces the carpal tunnel retinaculum and may cause compression.**

ADDITIONAL IMAGES

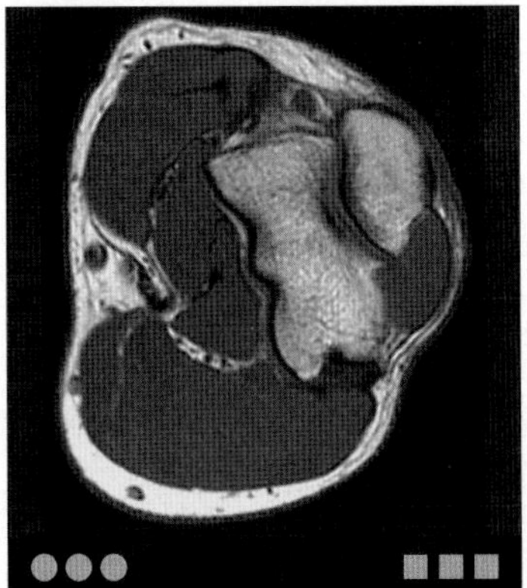

B. Anconeus epitrochlearis: Axial T1 image of the elbow shows the ulnar nerve and its position within the cubital tunnel at this level.

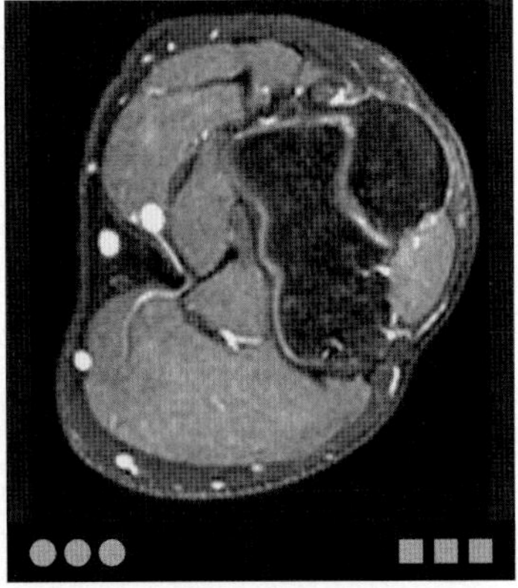

C. Anconeus epitrochlearis: Axial T1 image of the elbow with fat suppression and gadolinium contrast enhancement shows evidence of enhancement of the ulnar nerve sheath.

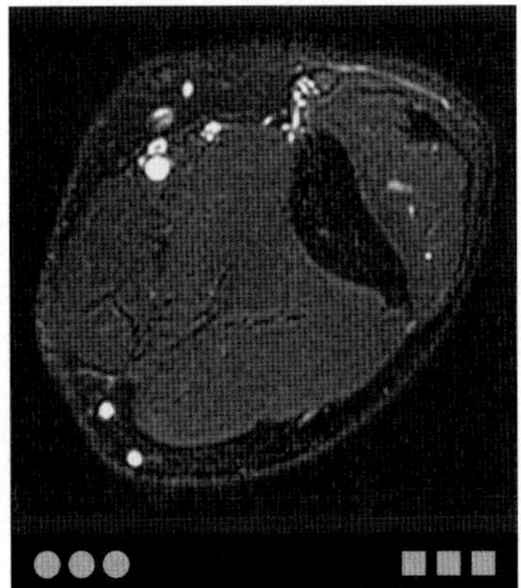

D. Anconeus epitrochlearis: Axial T2-weighted image of the elbow shows abnormally elevated signal within and around the ulnar nerve.

DIFFERENTIAL DIAGNOSES IMAGES

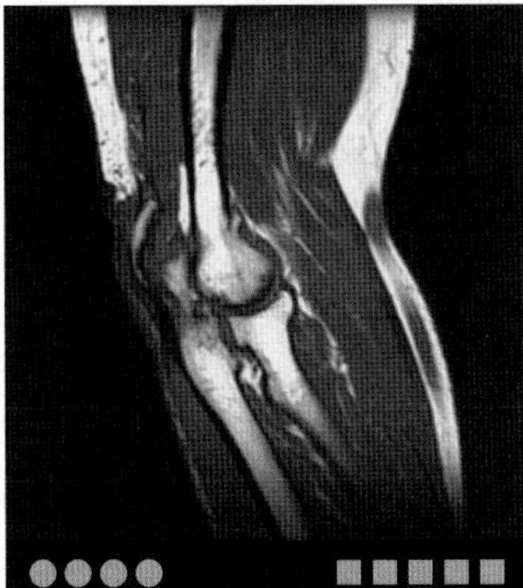

E. Enthesophyte: Sagittal oblique T1-weighted image through the elbow shows the dark cortical signal surrounding bright marrow signal of an enthesophyte projecting off the proximal ulna, another common cause of nerve compression.

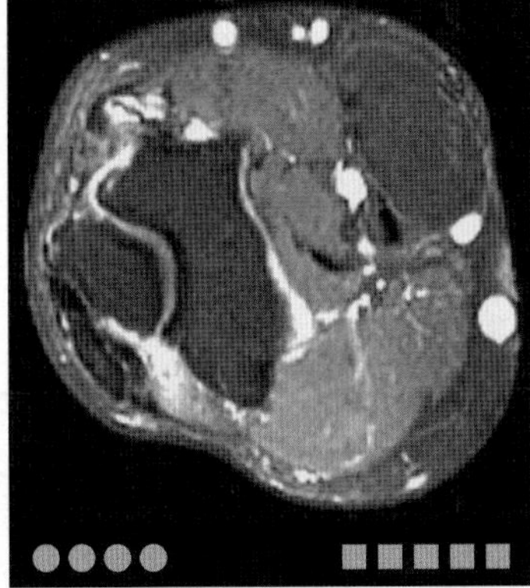

F. Enthesophyte: Axial T1 image through the elbow again shows the large enthesophyte off the proximal ulna.

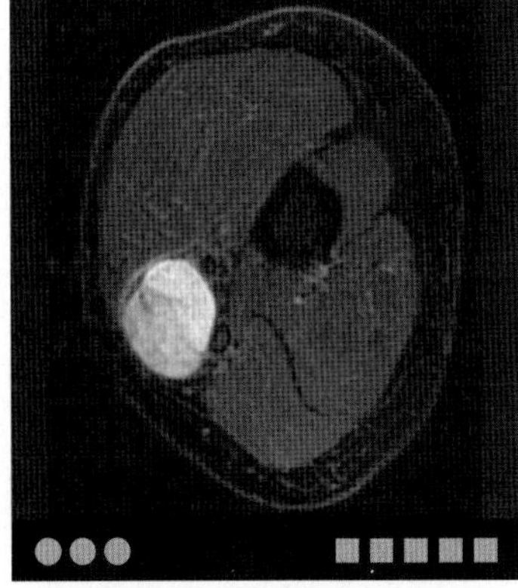

G. Neoplasm: Axial STIR images through the distal humerus show a very high signal, slightly heterogeneous mass along the expected course of the ulnar nerve, likely a schwannoma or neurofibroma.

IMAGE KEY

Common

Rare

Typical

Unusual

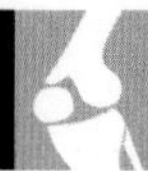

8–3 Reversed Palmaris Longus Muscle

Stefano Bianchi and Ibrahim F. Abdelwahab

PRESENTATION

Localized swelling of anterior aspect of the distal forearm

FINDINGS

Ultrasound (US) demonstrated a solid hypoechoic mass located under the superficial fascia.

DIFFERENTIAL DIAGNOSES

- *Volar wrist ganglion:* It presents as a nonechogenic mass, sometimes with lobulated margin. Usually lies in a deeper position
- *Lipoma of the flexor tendon sheath:* This appears as an echogenic mass located close to the tendon. Lipoma follows tendon movements during flexion extension of the fingers
- *Flexor tendon tenosynovitis:* It presents as an echogenic or mixed-echogenic area surrounding the tendons.

COMMENTS

This 14-year-old girl consulted because of a painless lump of the anterior aspect of the left wrist. Physical examination showed normal skin overlying an ill-defined fusiform mass. The mass was not attached to the skin. Variations of the palmaris muscle belly can be found as a symptomatic or asymptomatic anatomic variation. Normally the muscle belly is located proximally at the level of the proximal third of the forearm and continues with a very thin tendon that inserts in the proximal edge of the transverse carpal ligament. The palmaris tendon is located in the subcutaneous tissues just anterior to the median nerve and flexor digitorum tendons. Occasionally, the muscle is aberrant and found located in a central or distal position. When located distally, the muscle continues with a proximal long tendon, giving the appearance of a "reversed" palmaris muscle. In these patients, the anomalous muscle can have a mass effect on the median nerve and flexor tendons lying immediately deep to it. US and MRI can easily show the superficially located anomalous muscle in both the axial and sagittal plane. Because of its superficial location, US is superior to MRI in the evaluation of the size and shape of the adjacent median nerve. Both techniques allow accurate evaluation of the synovial fluid inside the flexor tendon sheath. Standard radiographs and CT appear useless in this field.

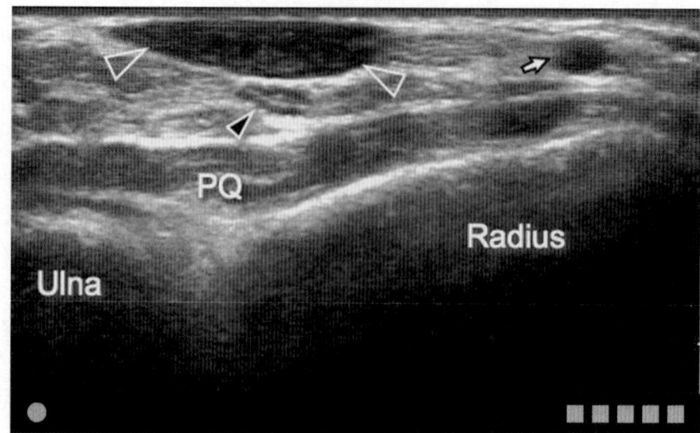

A. Reversed palmaris longus muscle: Axial US image, over the anterior aspect of the wrist, shows a hypoechoic oval mass (ope arrowheads) located under the superficial fascia. The mass presents well-marginated border and a quite homogeneous internal structure. The median nerve (black arrowhead) lies between the mass and the pronator quadratus muscle (PQ). Arrow = radial artery.

PEARLS

- **The reversed palmaris longus muscle lies in the distal third of the forearm between the superficial fascia and the median nerve.**
- **This accessory muscle can be asymptomatic or cause compression on the median nerve.**
- **US is accurate in its detection and characterization. It allows a differential diagnosis with lipomas and ganglia as well as tenosynovitis of the flexor tendons or other masses. MRI must be obtained in the rare cases, in which differentiation from a tumor is not evident by US.**

ADDITIONAL IMAGES

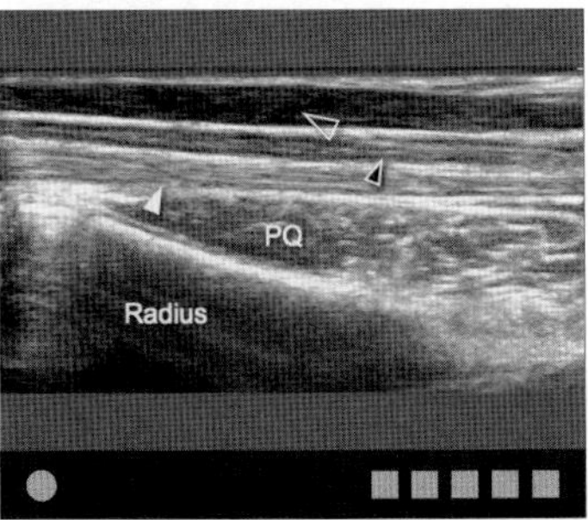

B. Reversed palmaris longus muscle: Sagittal US image over the anterior aspect of the distal forearm. Image confirms the diagnosis of reversed palmaris longus muscle (ope arrowhead). The internal fascicular structure of the median nerve (black arrowhead), made by hypoechoic nerve fascicles, is readily evident. Note the flexor tendons (white arrowhead) running in a deeper location.

IMAGE KEY

Common

Rare

Typical

Unusual

DIFFERENTIAL DIAGNOSES IMAGES

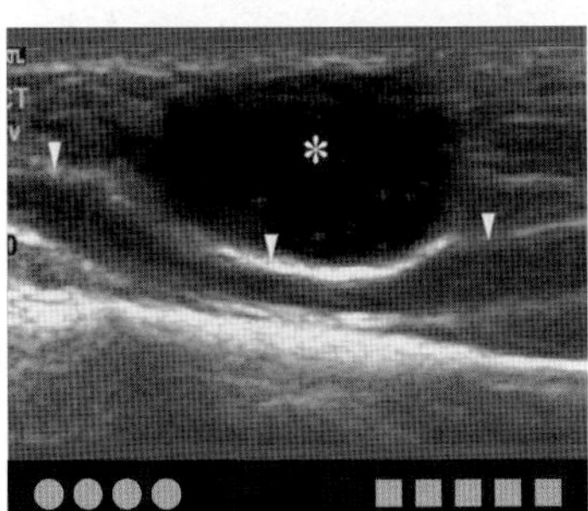

C. Palmar wrist ganglion: Sagittal US image, obtained over the volar aspect of the wrist, shows a mass (asterisk) with well-marginated border. The internal structure is anechoic, corresponding to fluid. Some small internal septa appear as hyperechoic spots. The mass is located in the subcutaneous tissues between the skin and the radial artery (arrowheads).

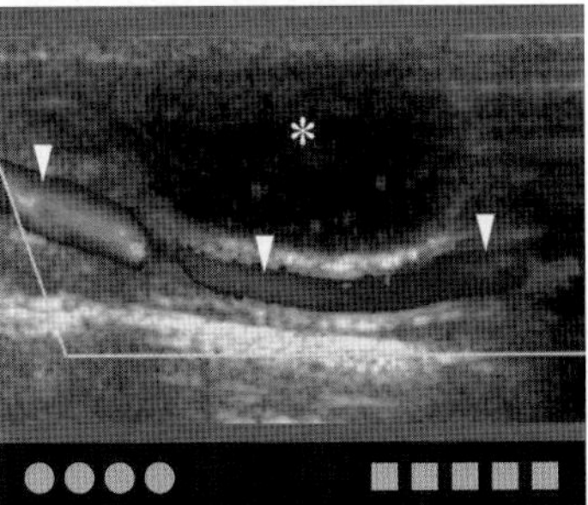

D. Palmar wrist ganglion: Sagittal color Doppler image corresponding to image C. Image shows absence of flow signals inside the cystic mass (asterisk). Note normal flow signals inside the radial artery (arrowheads) that appears inferiorly dislocated by the ganglion.

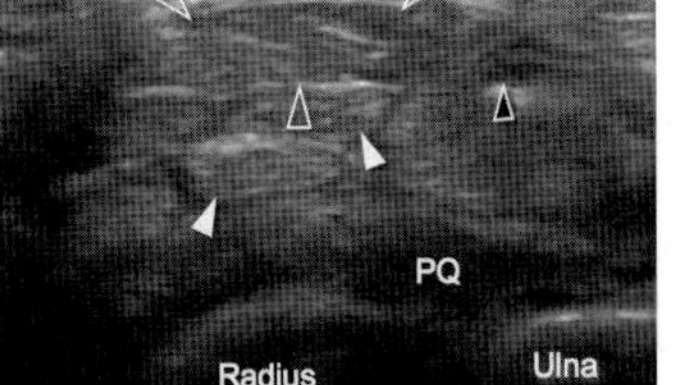

E. Lipoma of the flexor tendons sheath: Axial US image, over the anterior aspect of the wrist, shows an echogenic oval mass (open arrowheads) located under the superficial fascia. The mass presents an ill-defined border and a heterogeneous internal structure. The median nerve (black arrowhead) lies medial to the mass. The flexor tendons (white arrowhead) and the PQ are normal.

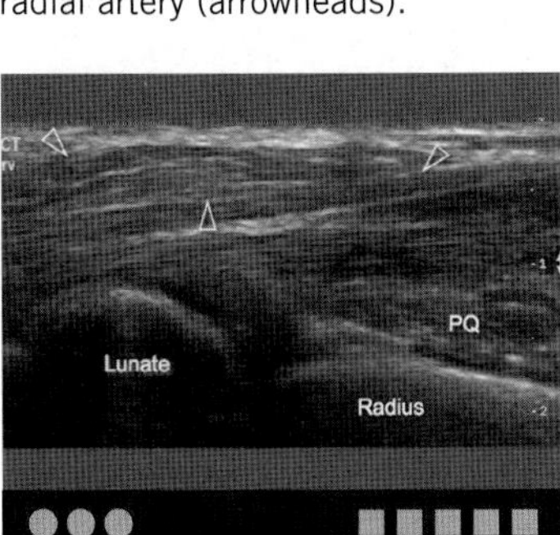

F. Lipoma of the flexor tendons sheath: Sagittal US image over the anterior aspect of the wrist obtained with the fingers extended. The lipoma (arrowheads) lies at the level of the radiolunate joint.

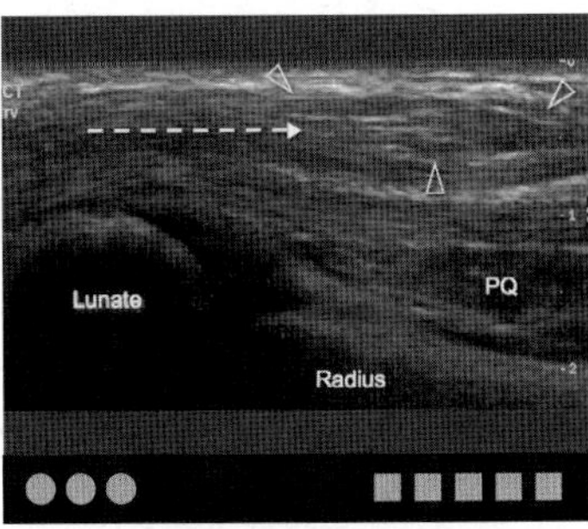

G. Lipoma of the flexor tendons sheath: Sagittal US image over the anterior aspect of the wrist obtained with the fingers flexed. Note cranial displacement (arrow) of the lipoma (arrowheads).

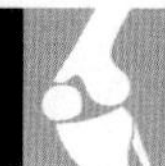

8–4 Panner Disease

Sailaja Yadavalli

PRESENTATION

Persistent elbow pain

FINDINGS

MRI of the elbow shows abnormal morphology of the capitulum and associated bone marrow edema in a skeletally immature patient.

DIFFERENTIAL DIAGNOSES

- *Osteochondritis dissecans:* Similar in appearance to Panner disease but seen in adolescents between 12 and 16 years of age and is associated with intra-articular bodies.
- *Pseudodefect of the capitulum:* Irregularity along the posterior aspect of the capitulum mimics a defect mainly in the coronal plane on MRI. No bone marrow edema is seen.
- *Septic arthritis:* Erosions, bone marrow, and soft tissue edema with joint fluid suggests an infectious or inflammatory process.

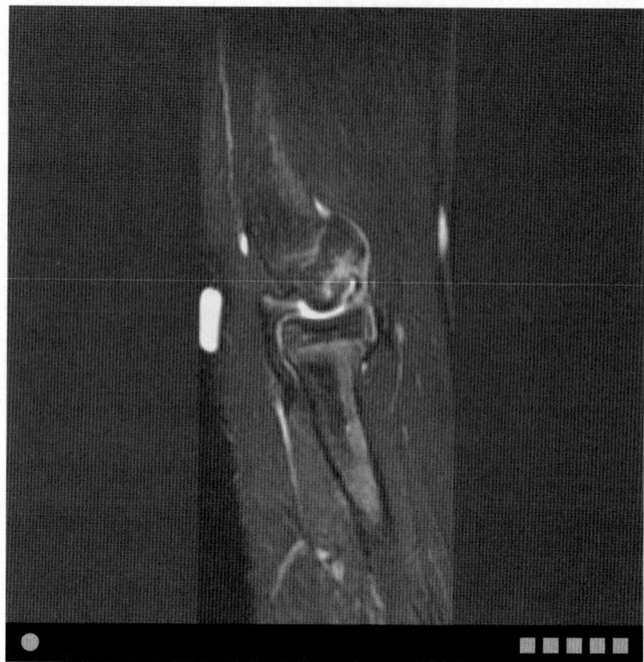

A. Panner disease: Sagittal T2-weighted fat-saturated image shows irregularity and edema in the mid to anterior aspect of the capitulum.

COMMENTS

Panner disease is osteochondrosis of the capitulum of the humerus and is seen in patients between the ages of 5 and 10 years. This is not associated with long-term deformity or intra-articular bodies. Patients present with mild pain and slightly decreased extension. It is often related to trauma in baseball pitchers and gymnasts and is rarely bilateral. Radiographs show fragmentation and increased density of capitulum especially when compared to the contralateral side. MRI findings include abnormal contour of the capitulum, low signal on T1-weighted images, and high signal on fluid sensitive sequences. Follow-up studies show resolution of these changes with no residual deformity. Panner's disease can be differentiated from osteochondritis dissecans mainly by the age of the patient. Osteochondritis dissecans is seen in adolescents and young adults with ossified capitulum. Affected patients are again involved in throwing activities or gymnastics. Radiographs show flattening, sclerosis, and cystic changes of the capitulum along the anterior aspect. Fragmentation may lead to intra-articular bodies. Unstable lesions may need surgical treatment. MR arthrography can be useful to assessthe stability of the lesion. Air-contrast CT arthrogram or MR arthrogram may aid in the detection of intra-articular bodies. These conditions should be distinguished from the pseudodefect of the capitulum seen on the posterior slices on coronal MR images with no associated bone marrow edema.

PEARLS

- **Panner disease occurs between ages 5 and 10 years.**
- **Osteochondritis dissecans is seen between ages 12 and 16 years.**
- **Both are typically seen in baseball pitchers and gymnasts.**
- **Panner disease resolves, whereas osteochondritis dissecans is associated with fragmentation and intra-articular bodies.**
- **Pseudodefect of the capitulum is a normal irregularity seen along the posterior aspect on coronal MR images.**

ADDITIONAL IMAGES

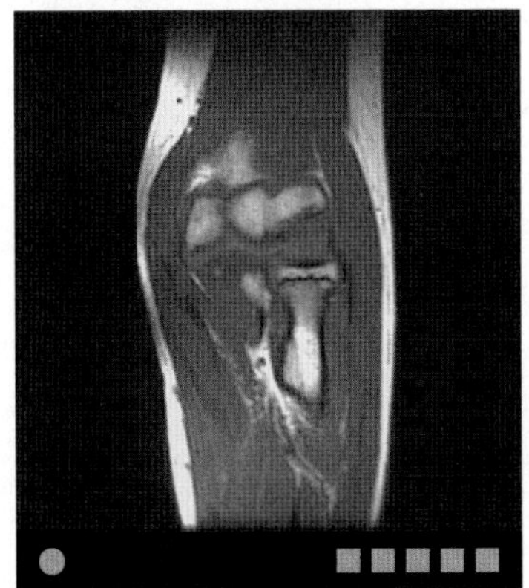

B. Panner disease: Coronal T1-weighted image shows irregularity and abnormal signal in the capitulum.

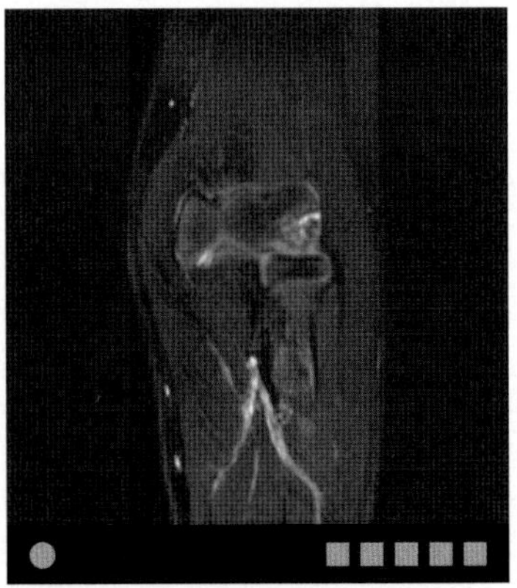

C. Panner disease: Coronal T2-weighted fat-saturated image shows bone marrow edema in the capitulum.

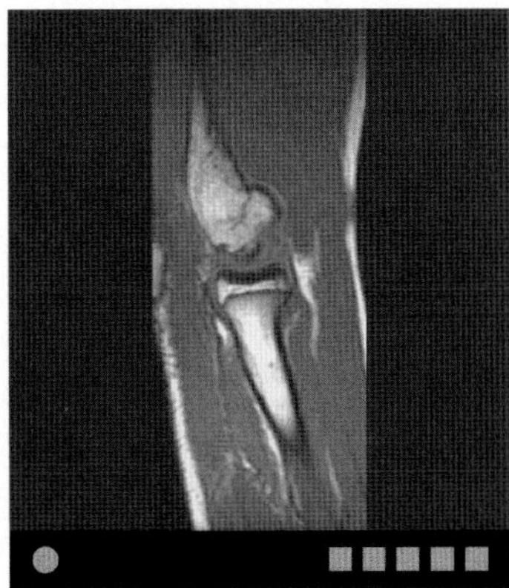

D. Panner disease: Sagittal T1-weighted image shows abnormal signal in the mid to anterior aspect of the capitulum.

DIFFERENTIAL DIAGNOSES IMAGES

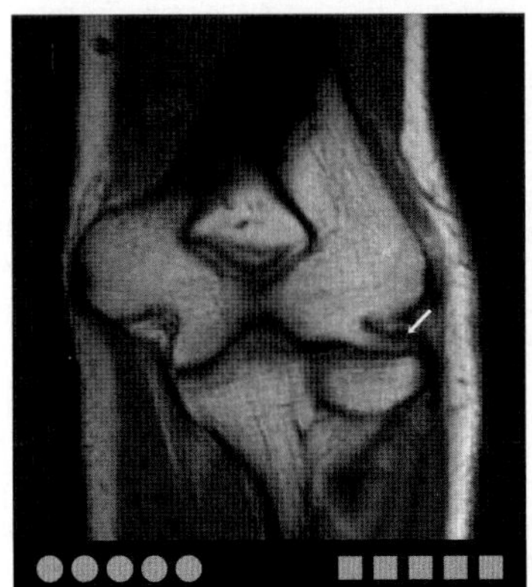

E. Pseudodefect of the capitulum: Coronal T1-weighted image shows irregularity (arrow) of the posterior aspect of the capitulum which is a normal finding.

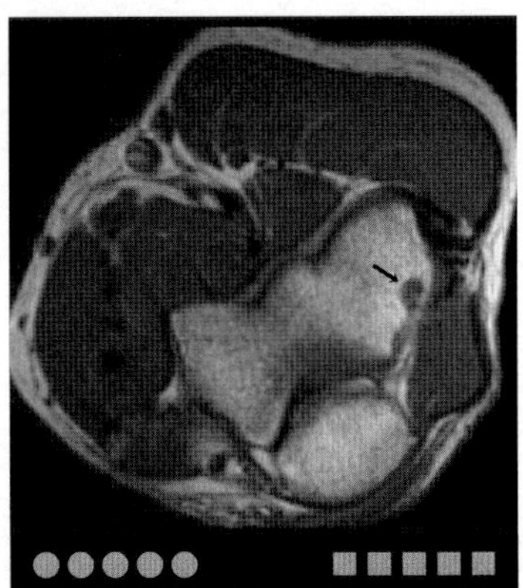

F. Pseudodefect of the capitulum: Axial T1-weighted image shows irregularity (arrow) of the contour of the capitulum along the posterior margin; a normal finding.

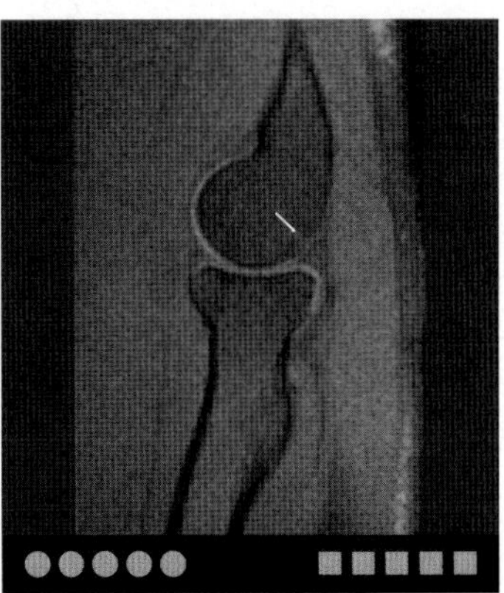

G. Pseudodefect of the capitulum: Sagittal fluid sensitive image shows the normal margin (arrow) of posterior aspect of capitulum and no bone marrow edema.

IMAGE KEY

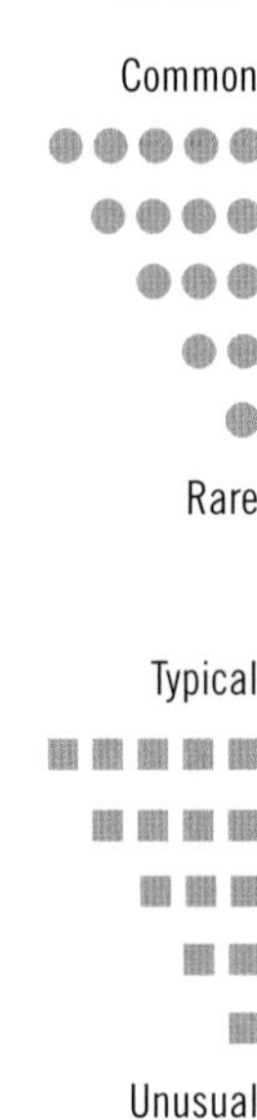

Chapter 9

Arthritis, Connective Tissue and Crystal Deposition Disorders

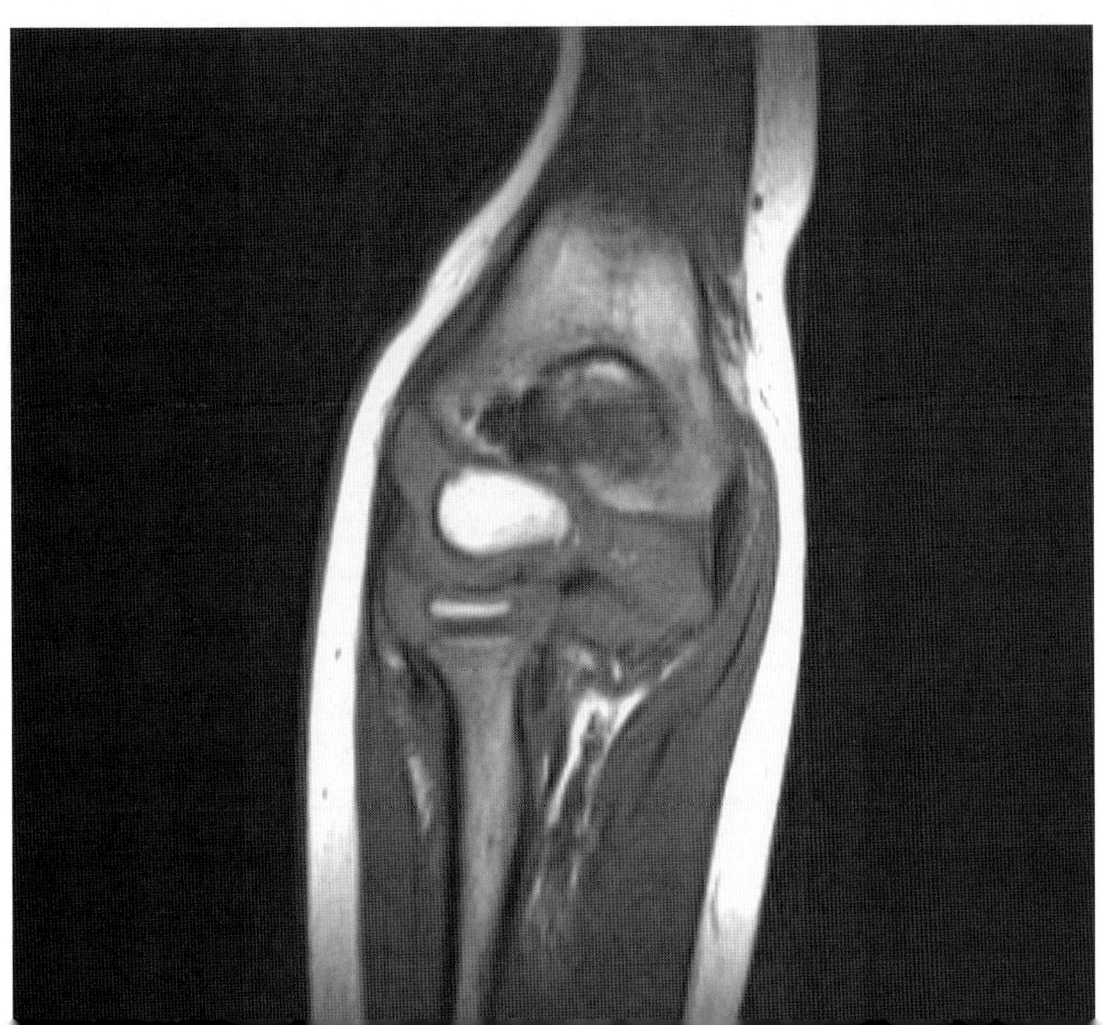

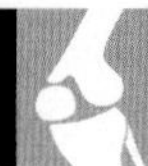

9–1 Hemophilic Arthropathy

Oganes Ashikyan and Jamshid Tehranzadeh

PRESENTATION

Pain, swelling, erythema, and color

FINDINGS

Heterogeneous dark material (hemosiderin) is seen in the elbow joint that has low signal intensity on T1-weighted and T2-weighted images consistent with hemorrhagic byproducts. Osseous erosions are also present.

DIFFERENTIAL DIAGNOSES

- *Hemarthrosis caused by trauma:* This diagnosis should be evident from patient's history and concomitant osseous findings.
- *Pigmented villonodular synovitis:* This presents as monoarticular process with cystic changes on both sides of the joint and intra-articular synovial villi, which demonstrates low signal intensity on all MR sequences.
- *Joint infection:* The joint fluid would demonstrate high signal intensity on T2-weighted images. Concomitant findings related to osteomyelitis such as bone edema, soft tissue swelling, and periosteal reaction are usually present.
- *Juvenile rheumatoid arthritis:* It shows synovial proliferation, joint effusion, erosions, and bone marrow edema.

COMMENTS

The patient is a 5-year-old boy with hemophilia A, who presented with elbow swelling. Acute hemophilic joint hemorrhage originates from subsynovial venous plexus and results in pain, edema, erythema, and heat in the joint. If untreated or frequently recurrent, chronic hemophilic hemorrhage into the joint space leads to destruction of cartilage and formation of osseous cysts and erosions. The osseous erosions are likely related to increased intra-articular and intramedullary pressure. Enlargement of olecranon fossa in the elbow and widening of intercondylar notch in the knee will occur. Destruction of cartilage and formation of osseous cysts and erosions result from inflammatory response, which has been created secondary to recurrent or untreated hemophilic hemorrhage. Epiphyseal hypertrophy and osteoporosis may also be seen and are thought to be related to hyperemia. Radiography may underestimate the degree of joint and osseous involvement. MRI is the most sensitive modality that can be used for the follow up of the disease. MRI is especially useful when serial examinations can be performed. The presence of hemosiderin in the joint space results in low signal intensity of the joint fluid on T1-weighted and T2-weighted images. Osseous erosions can also be easily seen on MR images.

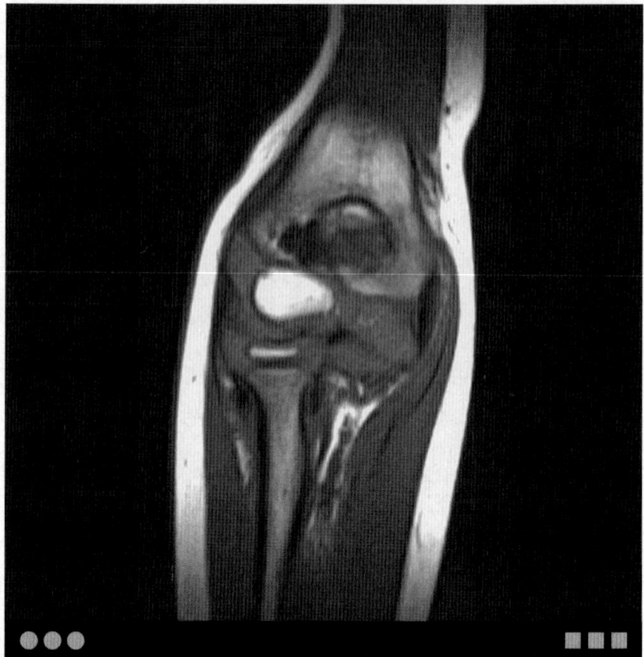

A. Hemophilic arthropathy: Coronal T1-weighted image shows heterogeneous joint fluid that has low signal intensity on T1-weighted images.

PEARLS

- **Repeated hemorrhage into the joint space leads to hemophilic arthropathy.**
- **Presence of hemosiderin in the joint space results in low signal intensity deposits in the joint.**
- **Destruction of cartilage and formation of osseous cysts and erosions result from inflammatory response, which has been created secondary to recurrent or untreated hemophilic hemorrhage.**
- **Enlargement of olecranon fossa in the elbow and widening of intercondylar notch in the knee can occur.**

ADDITIONAL IMAGES

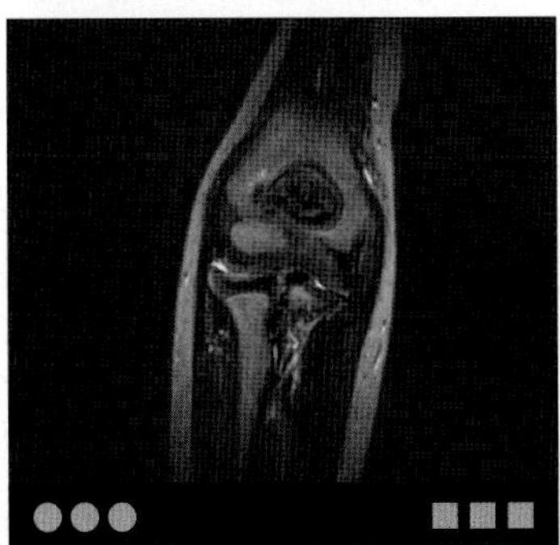

B. Hemophilic arthropathy: Coronal T2-weighted image also shows heterogeneous joint fluid that has predominantly low signal intensity on T2-weighted images.

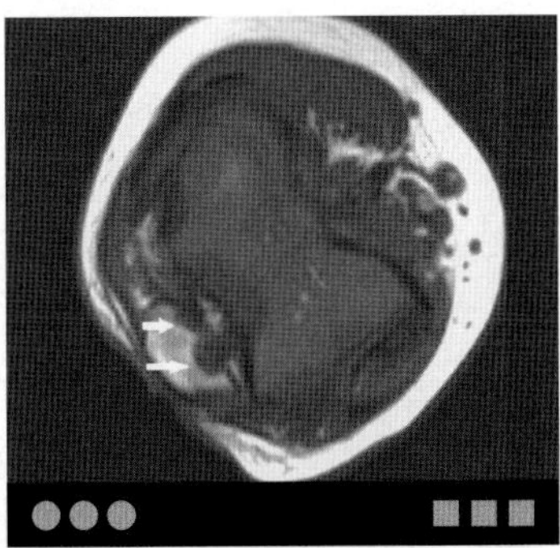

C. Olecranon erosions in hemophilic arthropathy: Axial T1-weighted image demonstrates osseous erosions in the olecranon process (arrows) of the ulna, in addition to the heterogeneous joint effusion.

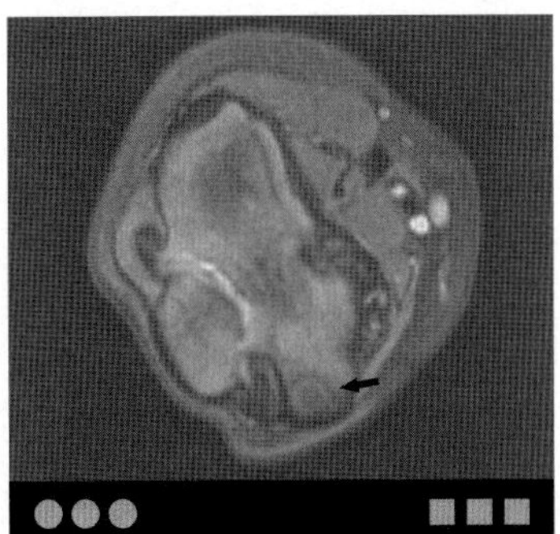

D. Humerus erosion in hemophilic arthropathy: Axial proton density image demonstrates osseous erosion (arrow) in the medial humeral epicondyle.

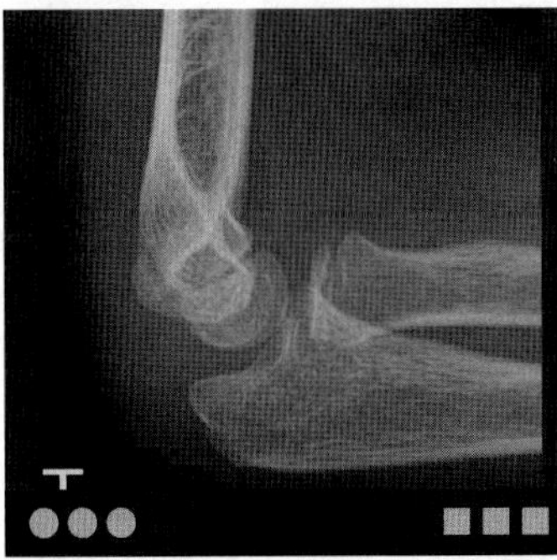

E. Hemophilic arthropathy: Lateral radiograph of the elbow obtained 5 months after the MRI study shows posterior fat pad, which is indicative of effusion in the joint. Frontal and oblique views (not shown) were unremarkable.

DIFFERENTIAL DIAGNOSES IMAGES

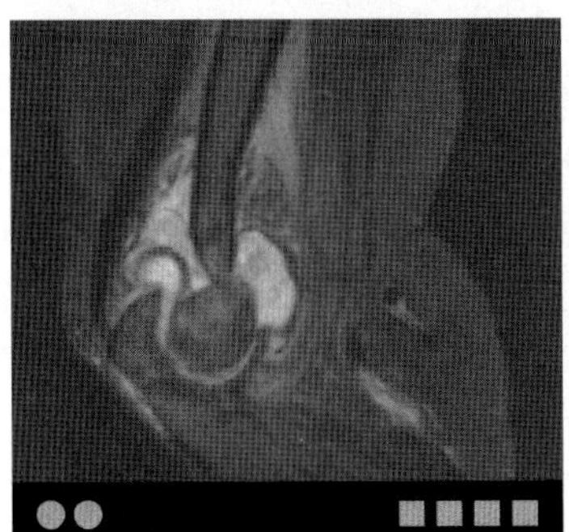

F. Acute septic arthritis of the elbow: Sagittal fat-saturated T2-weighted image of the elbow demonstrates hyperintense elbow joint effusion in a patient with septic arthritis.

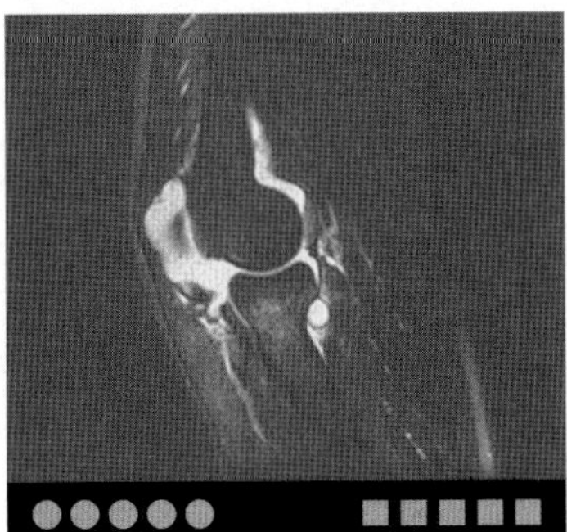

G. Elbow joint effusion related to radial head fracture: Sagittal T2-weighted image of the elbow demonstrates bone marrow edema, which is adjacent to the radial head fracture. The joint effusion is hyperintense.

IMAGE KEY

Common

●●●●●
●●●●
●●●
●●
●

Rare

Typical

■■■■■
■■■■
■■■
■■
■

Unusual

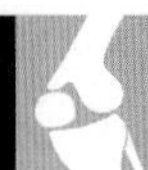

9–2 Gout of Olecranon Bursa

Atul Agarwal and Thomas Learch

PRESENTATION

Posterior elbow swelling

FINDINGS

MRI shows a large heterogeneous, lobulated structure in the region of the olecranon bursa areas of predominantly low signal.

DIFFERENTIAL DIAGNOSES

- *Fracture of the olecranon process with local hematoma:* History of trauma is present.
- *Pannus secondary to rheumatoid arthritis:* It is the so-called rheumatoid nodule. Patient has history of rheumatoid arthritis.
- *Calcium pyrophosphate dehydrate disease:* This condition is associated with chondrocalcinosis
- *Xanthofibromas:* This is associated with family history of hypercholesterolemia.
- *Olecranon bursitis:* There is fluid consistency present with olecranon mass.

COMMENTS

The patient is a 52-year-old male with a long history of gout. He presented with progressive swelling and inflammation of the posterior elbow. Olecranon bursitis is inflammation of the bursa overlying the olecranon process at the proximal aspect of the ulna. Pain often is exacerbated by pressure, such as when the patient leans on the elbow or the elbow rubs against the table. Tophaceous deposits may be palpable in the free wall of bursae. Physical findings can be similar to infectious bursitis and aspiration is required for diagnosis, which is made by finding monosodium urate (MSU) crystals in bursal aspirate detected by polarizing microscopy. Conventional radiography may be used to evaluate gout; however, findings generally do not appear until after at least 1 year of uncontrolled disease. The presence of erosions with overhanging edges helps confirm the diagnosis. On T1-weighted images, the signal intensity of tophaceous lesions is similar to that of muscles. T2-weighted SE images demonstrate extremely variable signals, ranging from homogeneous high signal intensity to near-homogeneous low signal intensity, because of the differences in calcium concentration within a tophus. Vascularized granulation tissue surrounding the tophus center enhance after intravenous application of contrast agents. The inflamed tophus is associated with local edema, causing high signal intensity on T2-weighted images. MRI is superior to plain radiography for early detection of intraosseous tophi. Involvement of anatomical structures such as ligaments and tendons can additionally be evaluated.

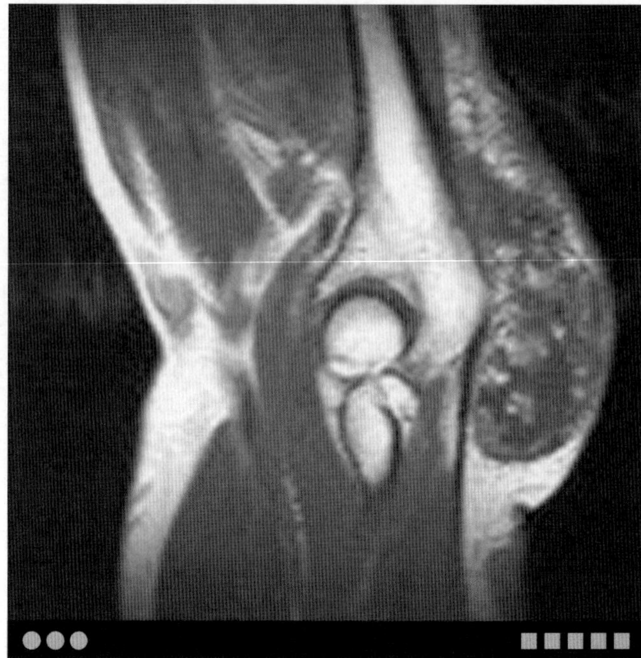

A. Gout of olecranon bursa: Sagittal T1 MRI shows a large heterogeneous, but predominantly low signal, lobulated structure in the region of the olecranon bursa with adjacent lower signal pertaining to bursal effusion.

PEARLS

- **Tophaceous deposits tend to be palpable in the free wall of bursae.**
- **Physical findings can be similar to infectious bursitis and aspiration is required for diagnosis.**
- **Tophaceous deposits present as masses with low to intermediate signal intensity on both T1- and T2-weighted images, but may display high signal intensity in the presence of associated inflammation.**
- **Conventional radiography may help in later stages of the disease, but is generally negative earlier in the course.**

ADDITIONAL IMAGES

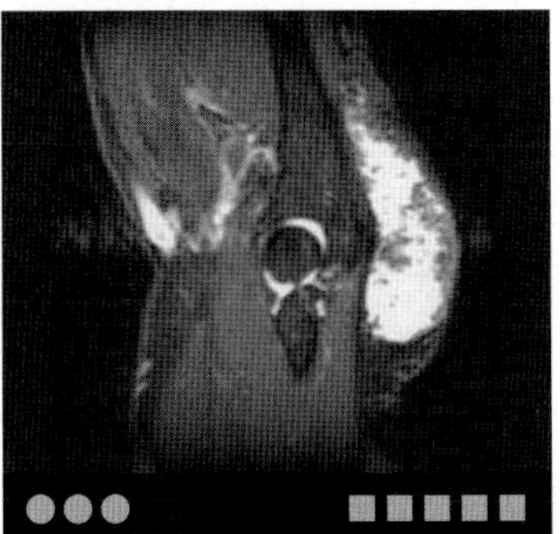

B. Gout of olecranon bursa: Sagittal T2 fat-suppressed MRI shows an intermediate to low signal lesion in the olecranon bursa with high signal corresponding to bursal effusion.

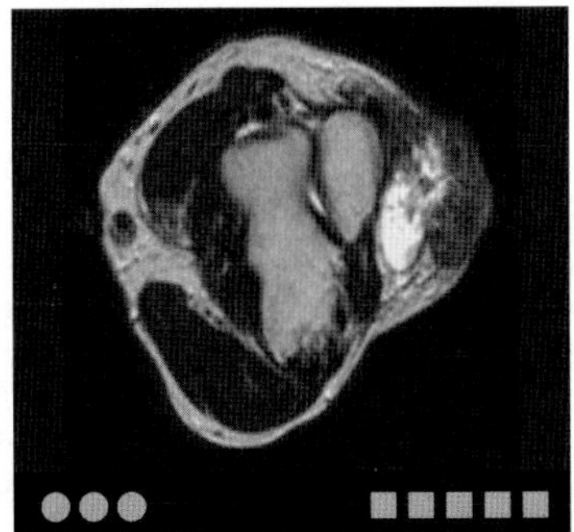

C. Gout of olecranon bursa: Axial T2 MRI demonstrates low to intermediate signal in the region of the olecranon bursa with surrounding high signal because of inflammation.

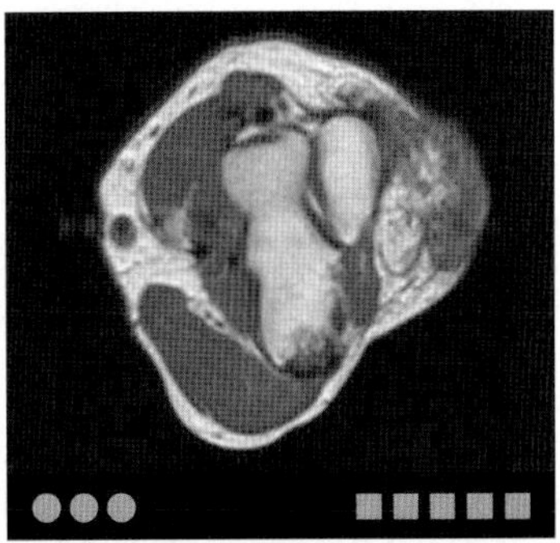

D. Gout of olecranon bursa: Axial proton density MRI shows intermediate signal in the region of the olecranon bursa with surrounding higher signal because of inflammation.

E. Gout of olecranon bursa: Lateral radiograph of the elbow demonstrates soft tissue swelling over the olecranon process with punctate calcifications in the tophaceous deposit. The joint space is not narrowed. Erosion with overhanging edge is present in the olecranon (arrow).

IMAGE KEY

Common

Rare

Typical

Unusual

DIFFERENTIAL DIAGNOSES IMAGES

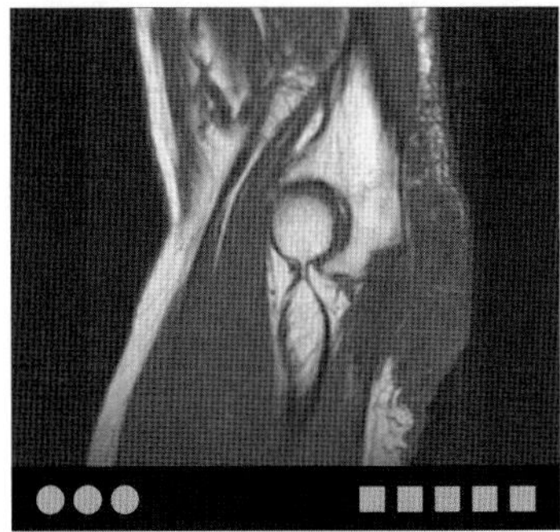

F. Rheumatoid nodule: Sagittal T1-weighted image shows low signal intensity mass in olecranon soft tissue representing rheumatoid nodule.

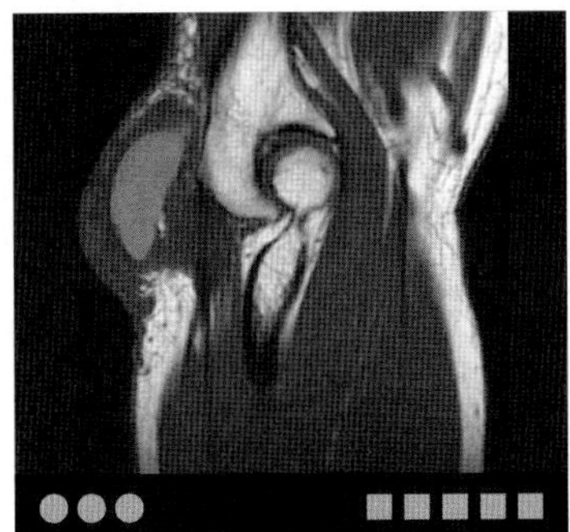

G. Olecranon bursitis: Sagittal T1-weighted image shows a fluid-filled bursa having low signal because of olecranon bursitis.

Chapter 10

Infections

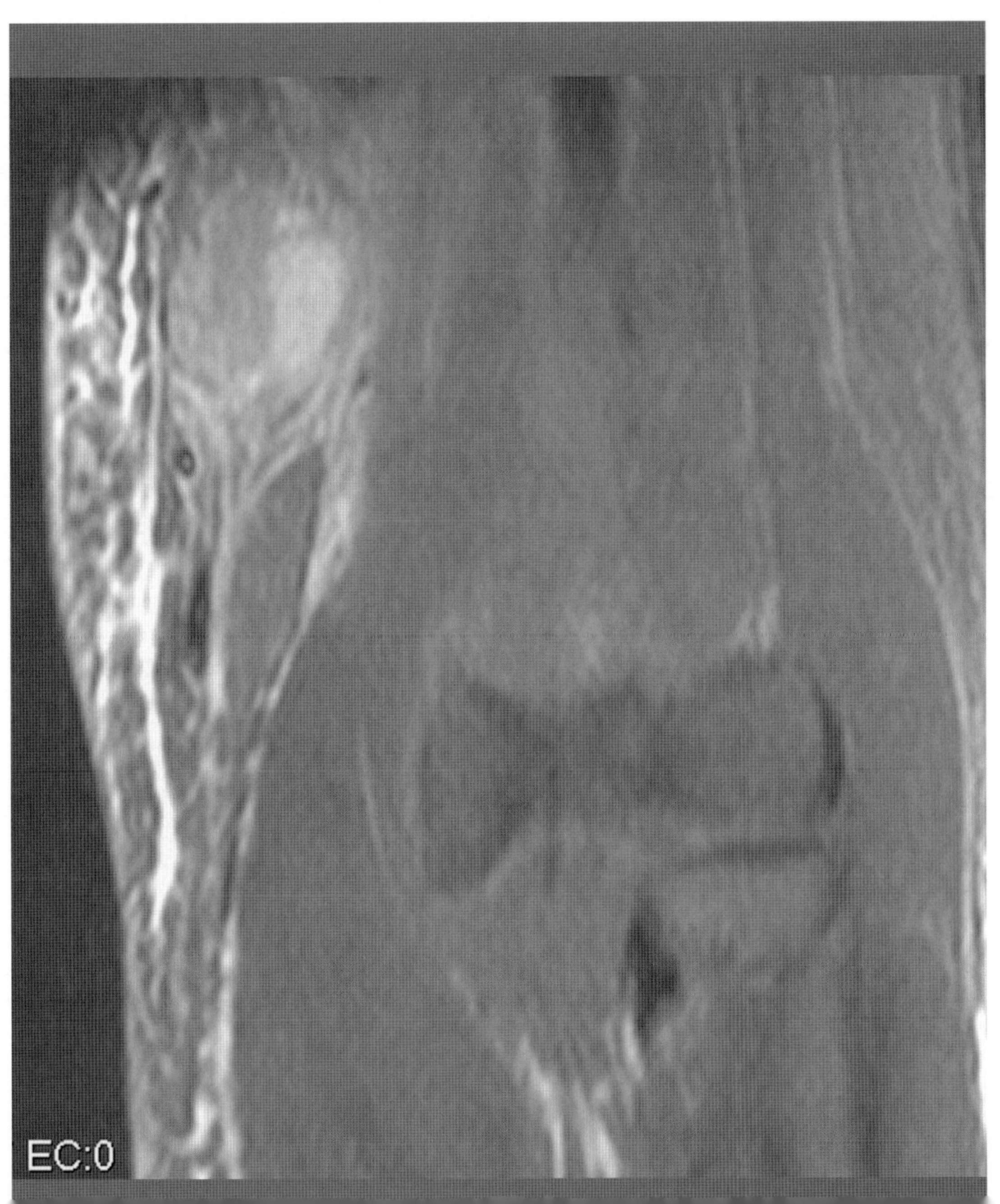

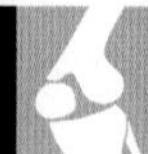

10–1 Cat Scratch Disease

Ingrid B. Kjellin

PRESENTATION

Tender mass in the medial aspect of the elbow

FINDINGS

MRI of the elbow shows a rounded mass with mild surrounding soft tissue edema.

DIFFERENTIAL DIAGNOSES

- *Rheumatoid nodules:* These are present in about 25% of patients with rheumatoid arthritis, typically those with positive rheumatoid factor. The nodules are usually seen between the skin and a bony prominence, such as the olecranon and the proximal portion of the ulna.
- *Septic arthritis:* Typically presents with localized pain, tenderness, redness, heat, and soft tissue swelling. Involvement of the elbow can occur with or without preexisting articular abnormality. In the setting of rheumatoid arthritis, it may be difficult to differentiate the changes related to the purulent infection from those of chronic synovitis.
- *Tendon tear or avulsion about the elbow:* It may present like a lump as the tendon retracts. Avulsion of the common flexor-pronator tendon group ("little league elbow") is seen in children, while biceps and triceps tendon ruptures are seen after the age of 40.
- *Supracondylar process:* It is a bony outgrowth at the anterior medial aspect of the distal humerus in about 3% of the general population. It may be clinically significant as it may fracture or cause median nerve compression.

COMMENT

This is an image of a 54-year-old man who presented with a recent exposure to cats. Cat scratch disease usually presents as a chronic regional lymphadenopathy in the upper extremity, with or without fever. It is caused by *Bartonella henselae*, which is a gram-negative bacillus. Most patients are young and have a history of exposure to cats. In some patients there is a transient rash, consisting of papules or pustules. Within a few weeks after the exposure, regional lymphadenopathy develops. The diagnosis can be established by enzyme immunoassay serology or polymerase chain reaction of lymph node aspirates. The disease is usually self-limited, but may become disseminated in immunocompromised patients and cause bacillary angiomatosis, abscesses, osteomyelitis, and encephalitis. Imaging studies should be considered when the diagnosis is in question. Radiographs and ultrasound may show soft tissue edema and one or more focal soft tissue masses, ranging in size from 1 cm to 5 cm, in the epitrochlear region. On MR imaging, the mass is intermediate in signal on T1-weighted images and hyperintense on T2-weighted images with irregular margins. Regions of necrosis within the mass, presenting as low echogenicity on ultrasound or absence of enhancement on gadolinium-enhanced MR images, are often encountered. Bone involvement in cat scratch disease is rarely seen.

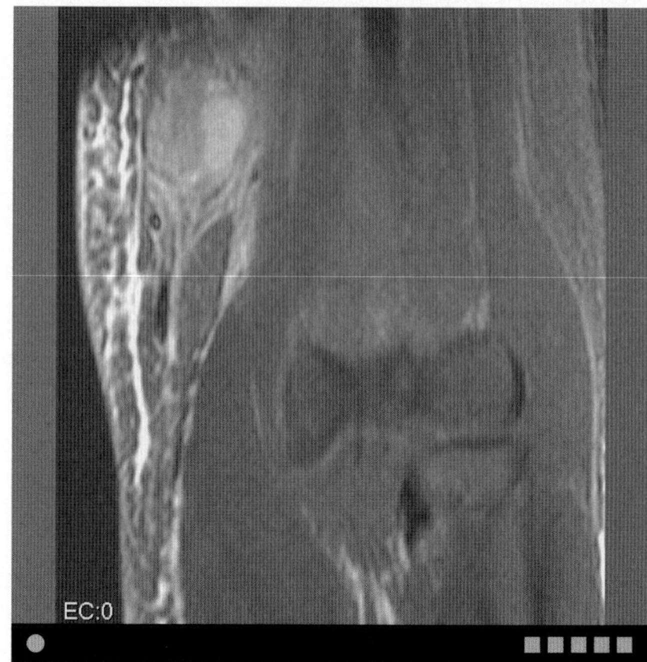

A. Cat scratch disease. Coronal STIR image shows a round, mildly heterogeneous mass in the medial aspect of the elbow, with adjacent subcutaneous edema.

PEARLS

- **Cat scratch disease commonly presents with epitrochlear and axillary lymphadenopathy.**
- **The etiologic agent is *Bartonella henselae*.**
- **MR imaging of the elbow typically depicts an epitrochlear mass, which is surrounded by subcutaneous edema.**
- **Necrosis within lymph nodes can be present and is best imaged with ultrasound or gadolinium-enhanced MRI.**

ADDITIONAL IMAGES

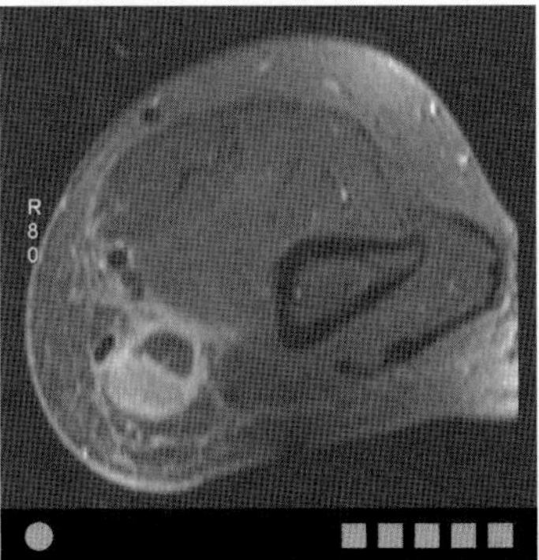

B. Cat scratch disease. Axial T1-weighted fat-saturated postcontrast image shows enhancement of a portion of the mass and the adjacent fascia and subcutaneous fat. The nonenhancing portion of the mass represents necrosis.

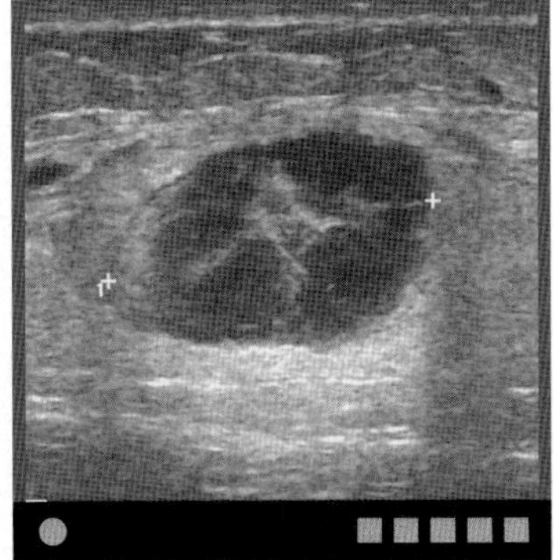

C. Cat scratch disease. A transverse ultrasound image of the medial aspect of the elbow shows a round, well-defined heterogeneous mass located along a vein.

DIFFERENTIAL DIAGNOSES IMAGES

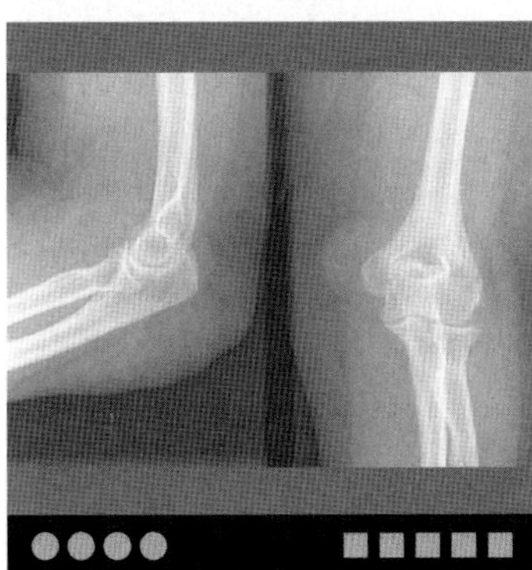

D. Rheumatoid nodules: Radiographs of the elbow show rounded soft tissue masses in the medial and posterior aspects of the elbow. Mild radiocapitellar arthritis is present in this patient with chronic rheumatoid arthritis.

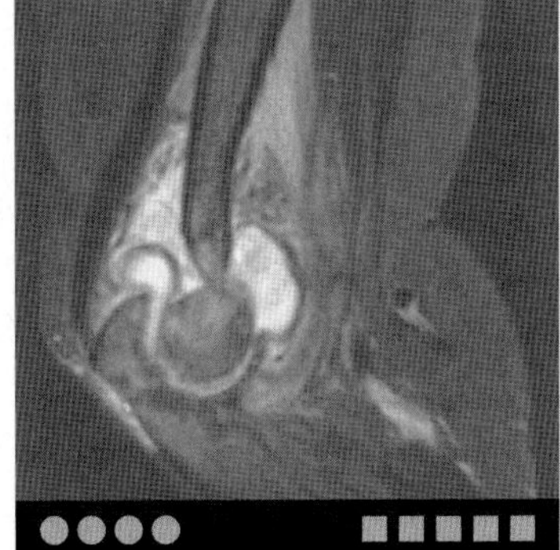

E. Septic arthritis: A T2-weighted sagittal image of the elbow shows extensive synovial thickening and a large effusion.

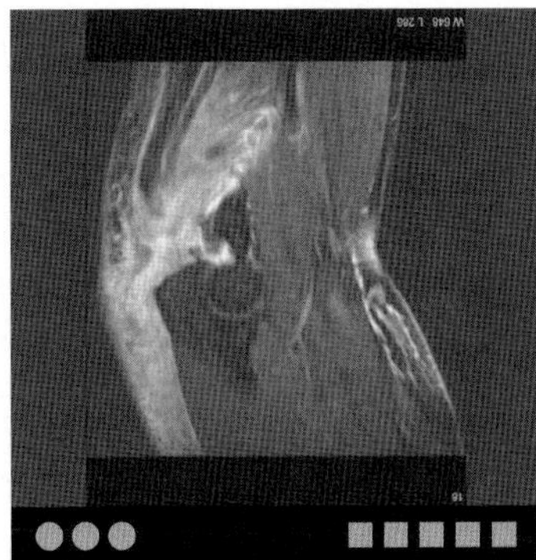

F. Tendon tear: A sagittal gradient echo image of the elbow shows a tear of the triceps tendon with 2cm to 3 cm tendon retraction in a weight lifter. There is extensive contusion and edema in the surrounding soft tissues.

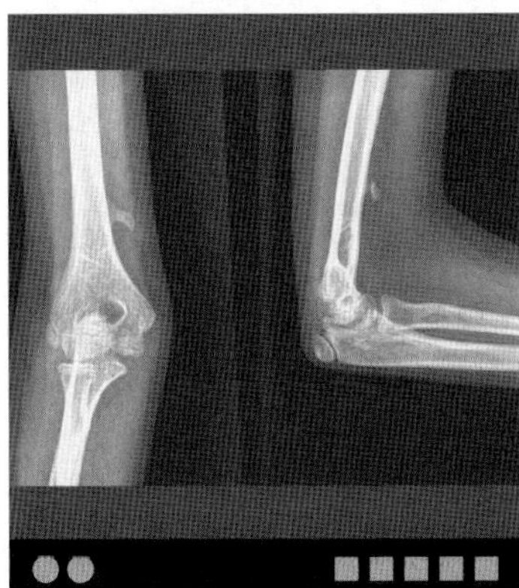

G. Supracondylar process: A lateral radiograph of the elbow shows a small exostosis along the anterior medial aspect of the distal humerus. A lucency through its base represents a fracture.

IMAGE KEY

Common

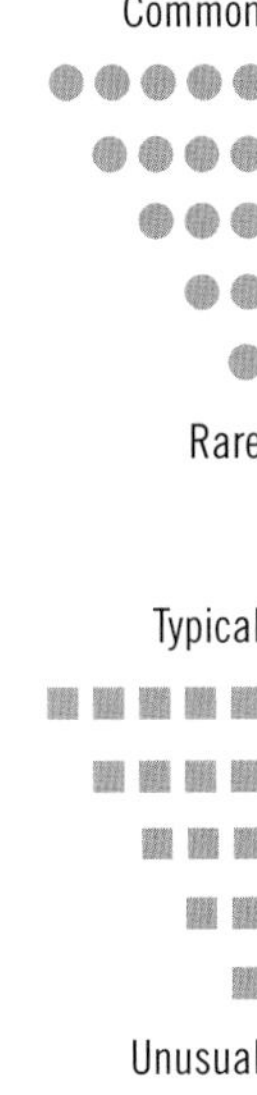

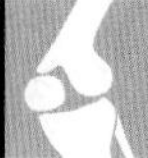

10–2 Tuberculous Arthritis

Oganes Ashikyan and Jamshid Tehranzadeh

PRESENTATION

Long-term pain and edema

FINDINGS

MRI shows osseous erosions and joint effusion.

DIFFERENTIAL DIAGNOSES

- *Septic arthritis:* This includes blastomycosis and other fungal and bacterial arthritis. Differentiation based on imaging alone is very difficult. If clinical picture is equivocal, aspiration or biopsy is required for definitive diagnosis.
- *Inflammatory arthritis:* Pattern of joint involvement and patient's clinical history are usually helpful in making the differentiation between infectious and other inflammatory arthritides.
- *Post-traumatic and hemophilic joint effusion:* Clinical history and other concomitant osseous findings will be helpful for establishing correct diagnosis.

COMMENTS

This is an image of a 63-year-old male who presented with tuberculous arthritis of the elbow. Osteoarticular tuberculosis is less common than pulmonary form; however, it is still frequently encountered in developing countries. More than 50% of the osteoarticular tuberculosis is extraspinal. Tuberculosis (TB) can involve intra-articular and extra-articular osseous structures, synovium, or soft tissues. Multiple osteolytic lesions in spine may mimic multiple myeloma and metastases. Involvement of joints and osseous structures is most often secondary to primary disease in the lungs; however, the primary focus may not be evident in some patients with osteoarticular tuberculosis. Extra-articular lesions may remain silent for long periods of time, until a complication occurs. Soft tissue or articular involvement usually leads to clinically detectable signs and symptoms, which may present as long-term complaints. The joint involvement may result from hematogenous spread via synovial membrane. The infection initially involves the bone near the synovial membrane attachment and later spreads into the joint. Direct spread into the joint from adjacent osseous lesions can also occur. In children, the destruction of bone is rapid and extensive, while in older patients there is only minimal bone destruction. Osseous erosions present as low signal intensity lesions on T1-weighted images and high signal intensity lesions on T2-weighted images. Areas of caseating necrosis have intermediate signal intensity on T2-weighted images.

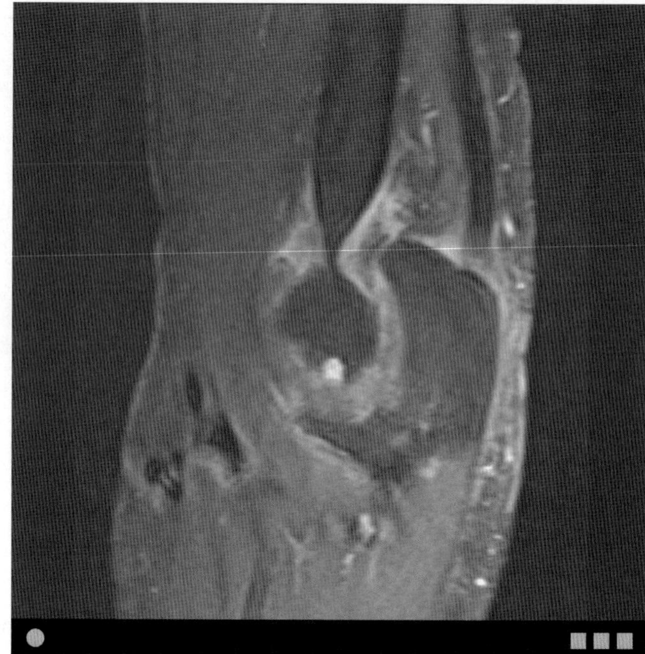

A. Tuberculous arthritis: Sagittal T1-weighted image with fat saturation obtained after gadolinium contrast administration demonstrates low signal joint effusion and small enhancing erosion in the trochlea.

PEARLS

- **Osteoarticular tuberculosis should be included in the differential diagnosis of osteomyelitis and arthritis.**
- **The symptoms, such as pain and swelling, may be a chronic phenomenon in TB and are associated with osteoporosis.**
- **Osseous erosions with areas of caseating necrosis may present as lesions with intermediate signal intensity on T2-weighted images.**

ADDITIONAL IMAGES

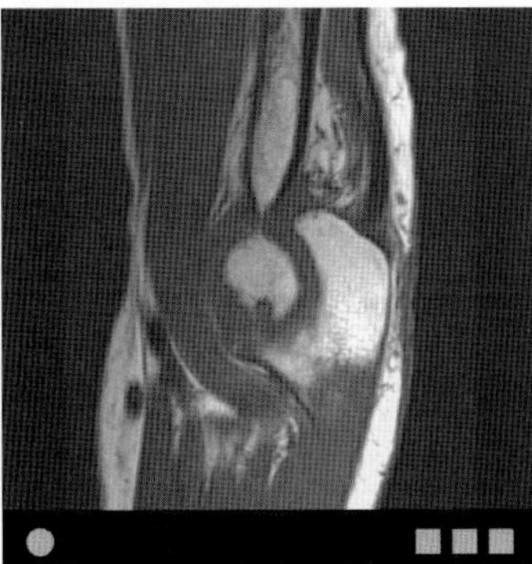

B. Tuberculous arthritis: Sagittal T1-weighted image also demonstrates erosion in the trochlea, which has low signal intensity on this sequence.

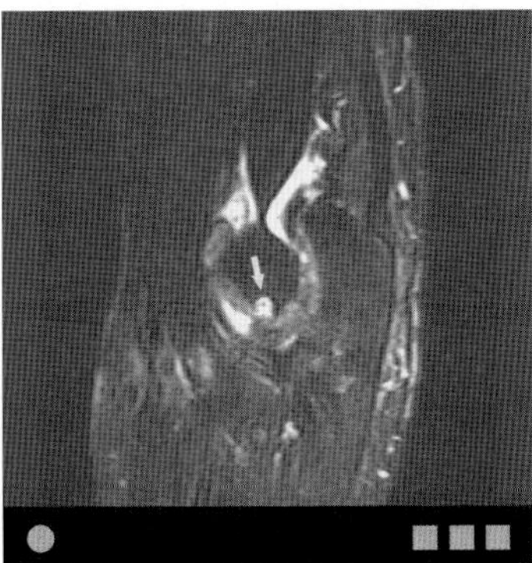

C. Tuberculous arthritis: Sagittal T2-weighted image also demonstrates bright signal joint fluid and erosion in the trochlea, which has high signal intensity reflecting granulomatous erosion (arrow).

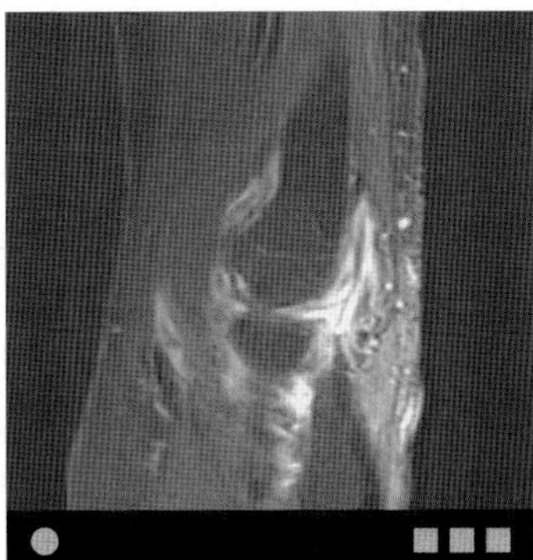

D. Tuberculous arthritis: Sagittal T1-weighted image obtained after gadolinium contrast administration demonstrated enhancing left elbow synovium with low signal joint effusion.

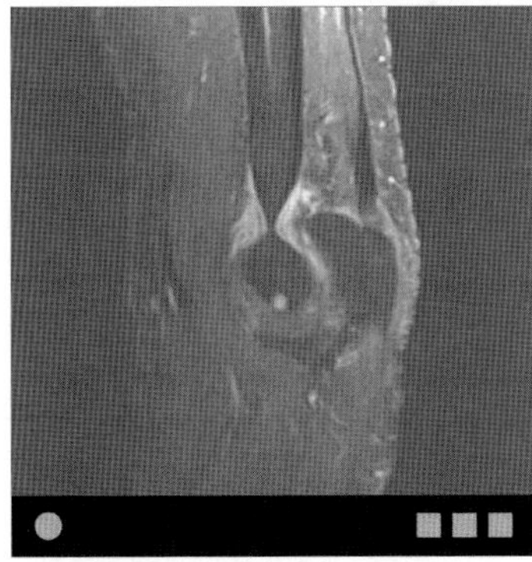

E. Tuberculous arthritis: Sagittal T1-weighted image with fat saturation and contrast enhancement obtained at 3 months follow-up demonstrates persistent erosion in the trochlea.

DIFFERENTIAL DIAGNOSES IMAGES

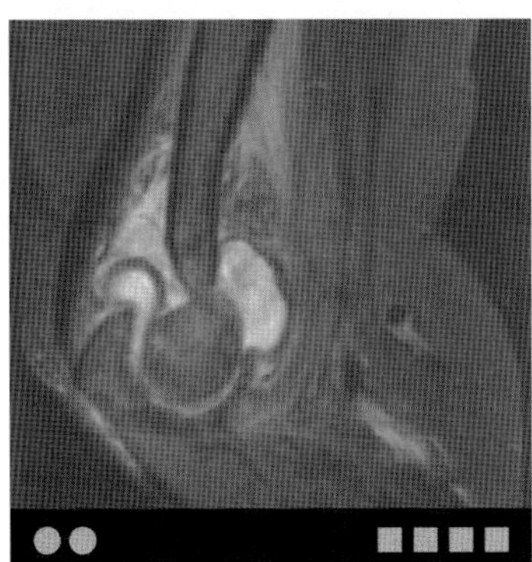

F. Acute septic arthritis of the elbow: Sagittal fat-saturated T2-weighted image of the elbow demonstrates hyperintense elbow joint effusion in a patient with septic arthritis.

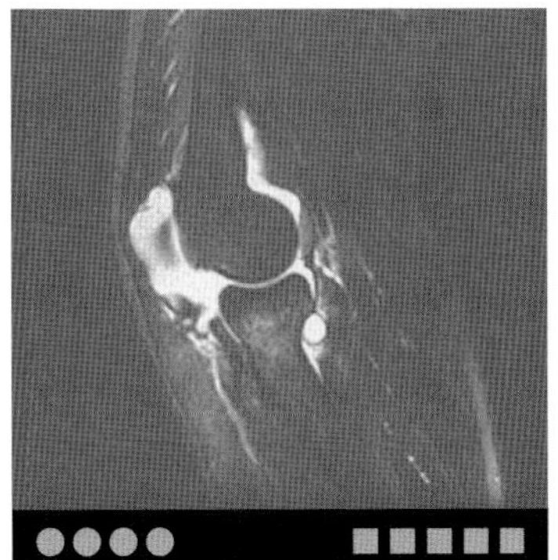

G. Elbow joint effusion related to radial head fracture: Sagittal T2-weighted image of the elbow demonstrates bone marrow edema, which is adjacent to the radial head fracture. The joint effusion is hyperintense.

IMAGE KEY

Common

Rare

Typical

Unusual

Chapter 11

Tumors and Tumor Like Lesions

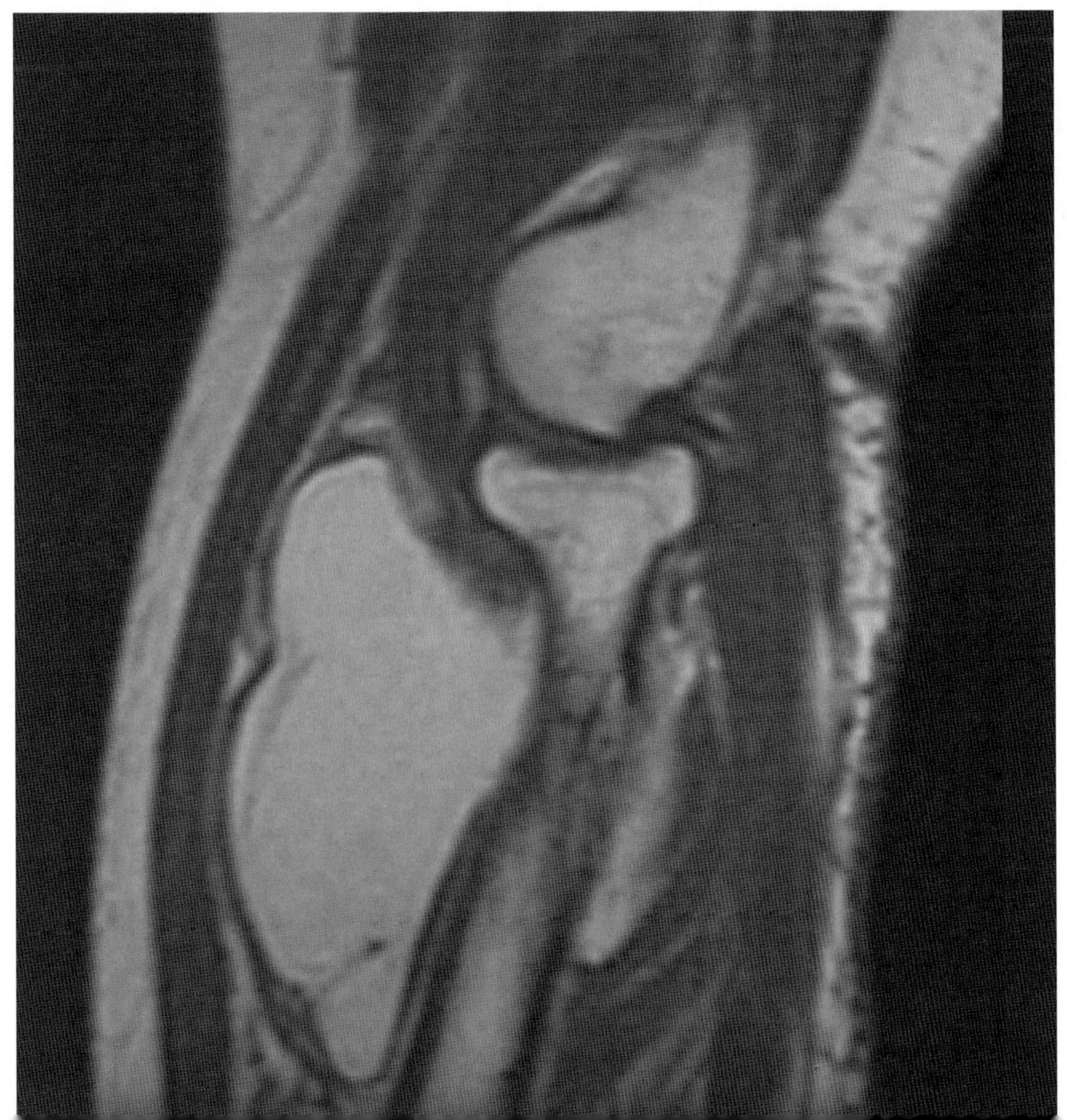

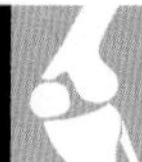

11–1 Lipoma of Elbow

Binh-To Tran and Rajeev K. Varma

PRESENTATION

Elbow mass and forearm paresthesias

FINDINGS

A well-defined 7 cm × 4 cm cystlike structure with hyperintense signal on T1-weighted image, with septa is seen anterior to the radius. No extension is demonstrated into the surrounding soft tissue, tendon, nerves, or bone.

DIFFERENTIAL DIAGNOSES

- *Lipomatosis:* Affects mainly toddlers and are rare in adulthood. Lipomatosis represent extensive overgrowth of adipose tissue into the surrounding subcutaneous tissue and muscle. Neuropathies associated with these lesions affect more than 50% of cases.
- *Liposarcoma:* Second most common soft tissue sarcoma in adults. It has similar age distribution as lipomas and is rare in children.
- *Lipoblastoma or lipoblastomatosis:* Occurs in infancy and early childhood. They are tumors of embryonal white fat containing varying amounts of adipose and myxoid stroma. It has a lobular imaging appearance with internal septations.
- *Angiolipoma:* Occurs predominantly in male patient aged between 10 -and 30 years. Lesions are painful to palpation, typically superficial in location, and always encapsulated with evidence of internal vascularization.

COMMENTS

This is an image of a 55-year-old woman who presented with a mass in her elbow and paresthesias in the forearm. Lipomas are benign tumors of mature adipose cells. Lipomas develop in adulthood and are most noticeable among middle-aged adults. They represent almost 50% of all soft tissue tumors and have characteristic imaging findings. Lesions are similar or identical to subcutaneous fat, they are encapsulated, and homogeneous in appearance. They commonly affect the upper back, neck, proximal extremities, and abdomen. Lipomas are rare on the face and scalp, and uncommon on the hands and feet. Lesions can be superficial or deep, and it is uncommon to exceed 10 cm in size. Hounsfield unit measurement is between −65 and −120. Lipomas are isointense to subcutaneous fat in all MR pulse sequences. Only the fibrous capsule may enhance with contrast on CT scan or MR imaging. Few thin septa are characteristic; however, soft tissue lipomas may

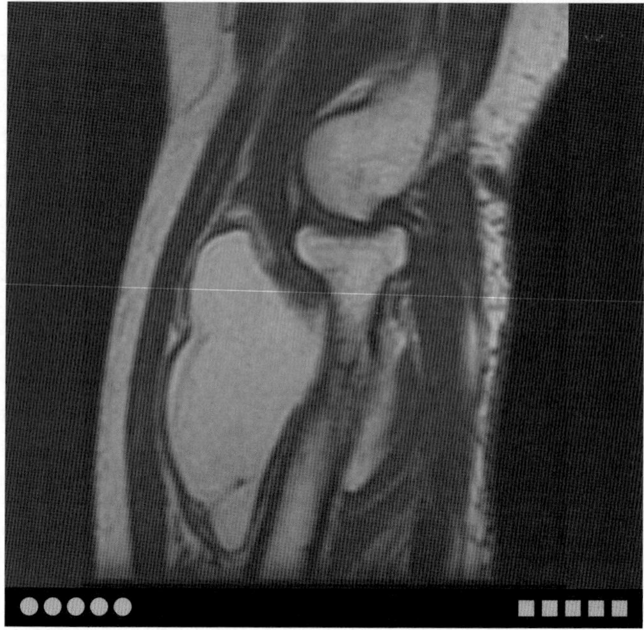

A. Lipoma: Sagittal T1-weighted image shows a hyperintense lesion in antecubital fossa.

have thick septa with regions of nonadipose tissue. Intramuscular lipomas may demonstrate a striated appearance secondary to interdigitations with skeletal muscle. This feature distinguishes it from liposarcoma. Their transformation to liposarcoma is very rare. Liposarcoma contains both soft tissue and adipose component. They frequently arise from deep stroma rather than subcutaneous fat. The more differentiated the tumor becomes, the more it is similar to fat on MR and CT scan imaging. These tumors are hyperintense on T2-weighted images and demonstrate faint or no enhancement after contrast administration.

PEARLS

- **Lipomas are easily palpable as mobile, soft, and spongy masses that may grow slowly without producing symptomatology.**
- **Lipomas can vary in size with weight gain but not with weight loss.**
- **Solitary lipomas are seen predominately in women. Multiple lipomas occur more frequently in men.**
- **Subcutaneous lipomas may not demonstrate a capsule on CT scan or MR imaging.**
- **Deep lipomas are commonly intramuscular, especially when found in the extremities or the retroperitoneum.**

ADDITIONAL IMAGES

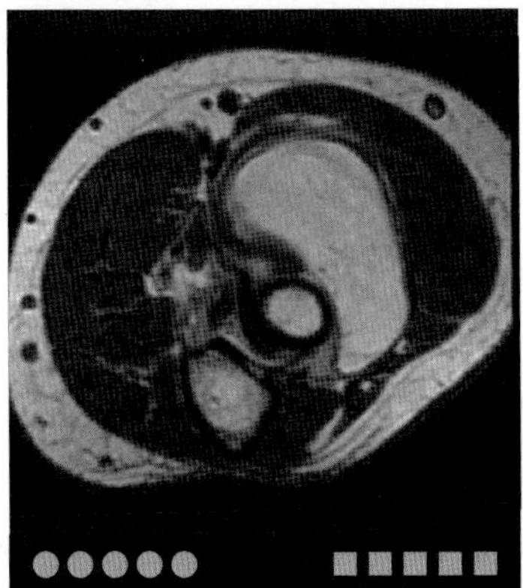

B. Lipoma: Axial T1-weighted image of the same lesion likely compressing the anterior interosseous nerve.

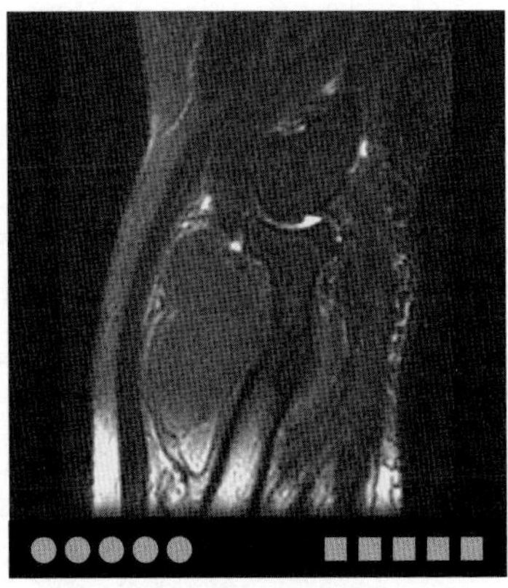

C. Lipoma: Sagittal T2-weighted image with fat suppression shows hypointensity in the mass confirming it is a lipoma.

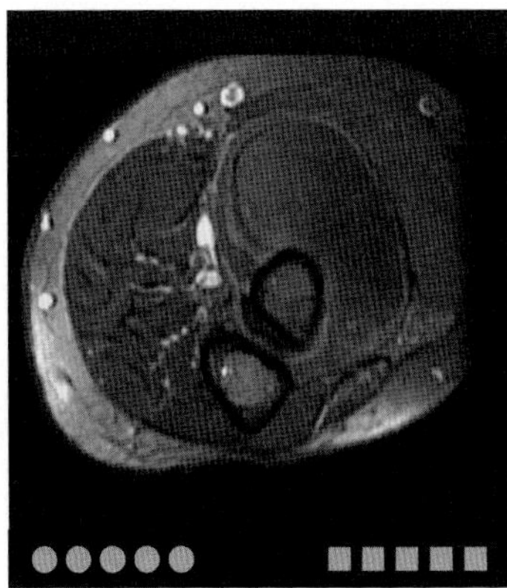

D. Lipoma: Sagittal T1-weighted image after IV contrast shows no significant contrast uptake.

DIFFERENTIAL DIAGNOSES IMAGES

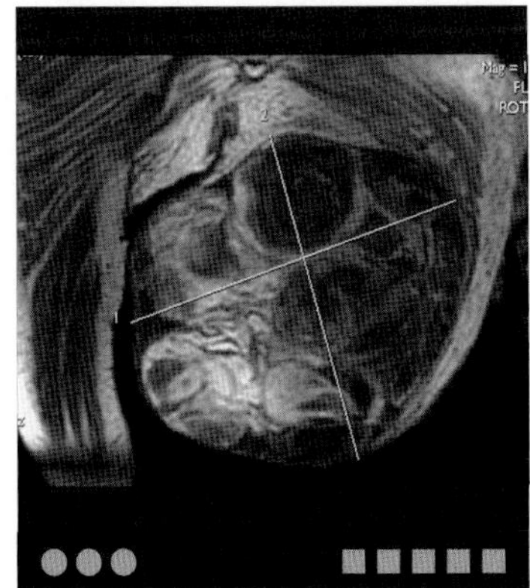

E. Liposarcoma: Coronal T1-weighted image shows a lesion with mixed signal in thigh. The hyperintense areas denote it is primarily a lipoma type lesion, but hypointense foci indicate necrotic or fluid density zones in the lesion.

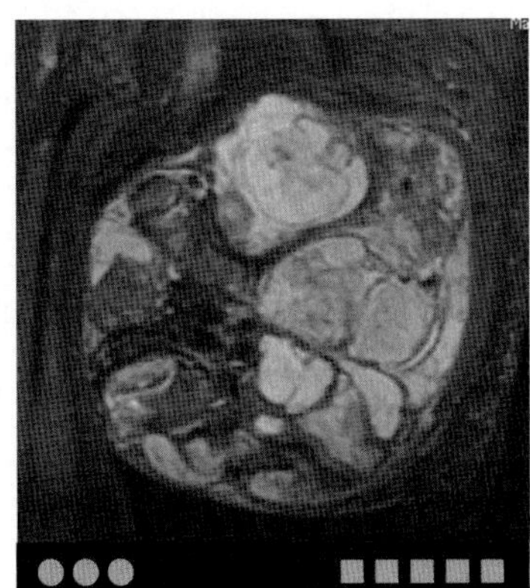

F. Liposarcoma: Coronal STIR image with inhomogeneous fat suppression makes this lesion's transformation into liposarcoma more suspicious.

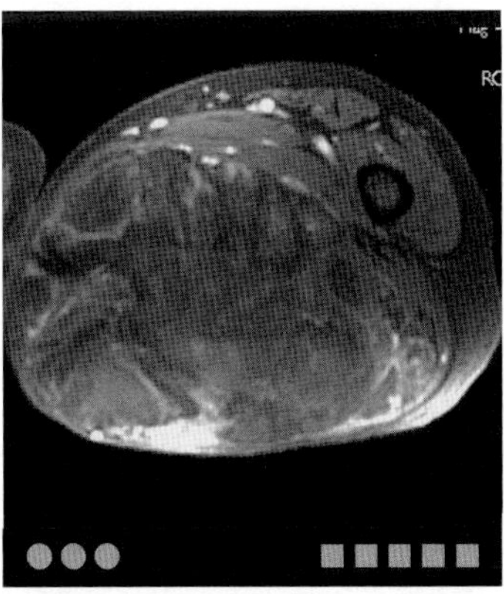

G. Liposarcoma: Axial T1-weighted image with fat suppression after IV contrast injection demonstrates enhancement in the septa favoring malignant transformation (compare with image D).

IMAGE KEY

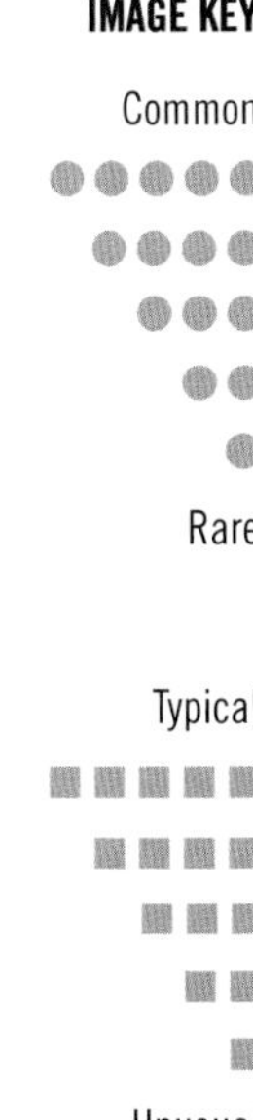

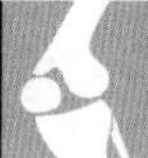

11–2 Hemangioma of Forearm

Ayodale S. Odulate and Piran Aliabadi

PRESENTATION

Chronic intermittent pain and a palpable mass

FINDINGS

Vascular tumor of the proximal forearm with multiple venous channels and calcifications.

DIFFERENTIAL DIAGNOSES

- *Sarcoma:* Heterogeneously enhancing T2 hyperintense mass without defined vascular structures.
- *Intramuscular lipoma:* Well-defined hyperintense T1-weighted mass.
- *Hematoma:* Calcifications around the peripheral margin of a hematoma.
- *Cysticercosis:* Multiple oval (cigar-shaped) calcifications within skeletal muscle.

COMMENTS

This is an image of a 35-year-old man who presented with chronic right forearm pain. Soft tissue hemangiomas are benign tumors composed of vessels. Five subtypes of vascular lesions exist and include capillary, cavernous, arteriovenous, venous, and mixed type histology. Cavernous hemangiomas tend to be larger compared to the capillary type and are often intramuscular. Treatment is limited to symptomatic patients and involves surgical resection for patients with tumors that do not involute or grow. Calcifications can be seen as a result of the slow flow of blood in the tumors. Venous hemangiomas have thicker walled vessels containing smooth muscle cells. Radiograph of cavernous hemangiomas can appear normal if no calcifications are present, which are more common with this subtype of hemangiomas. The tumor may appear as an otherwise undefined soft tissue mass. CT scan examinations may reveal phleboliths that are not seen on radiographs and enhance avidly. Technetium-99 delayed, tagged red blood cell study will demonstrate blood pooling in the mass. MR imaging is the modality of choice and demonstrates nonspecific, heterogeneous, and isointense signal to muscle on T1-weighted images and hyperintensity on T2-weighted images. Often these benign tumors are lobulated, septated, and have punctate foci of hypointensity. Following administration of gadolinium, significant enhancement is seen. Angiography of hemangiomas is usually limited to embolization or sclerotherapy of arteriovenous hemangiomas prior to surgical excision. Needle biopsies are often read as a false negative with blood products and vessels histologically. The imaging characteristics are often pathognomic such that biopsies can be avoided.

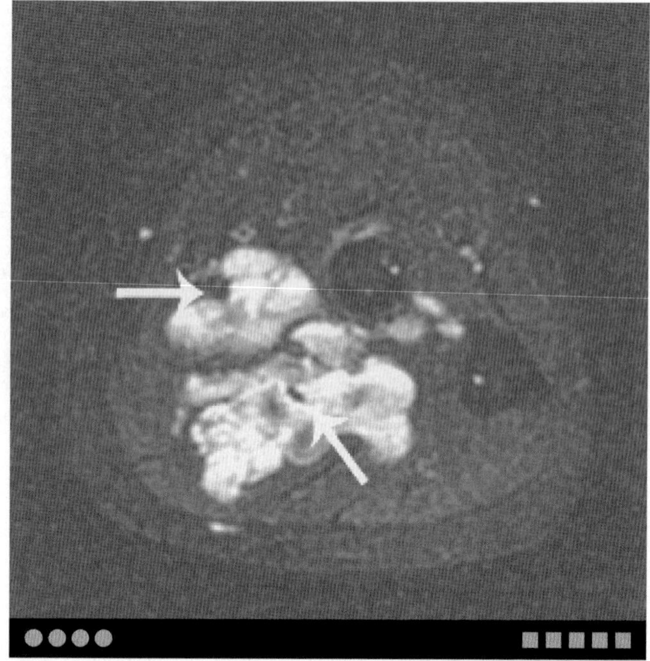

A. Hemangioma: Axial STIR image demonstrates a hyperintense lobulated septated mass with several hypointense foci (arrow).

PEARLS

- **Calcifications are associated with slow flow vascular lesions.**
- **Multiple signal voids on MRI and interspersed fat within a mass suggest a vascular lesion.**

ADDITIONAL IMAGES

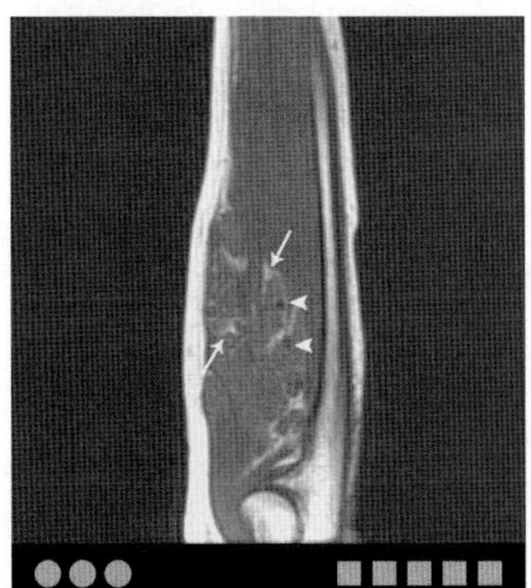

B. Hemangioma: Sagittal T1-weighted image demonstrates an isointense mass to muscle with interspersed hyperintensity representing fat (arrow). Calcifications (arrowheads) are seen within the mass.

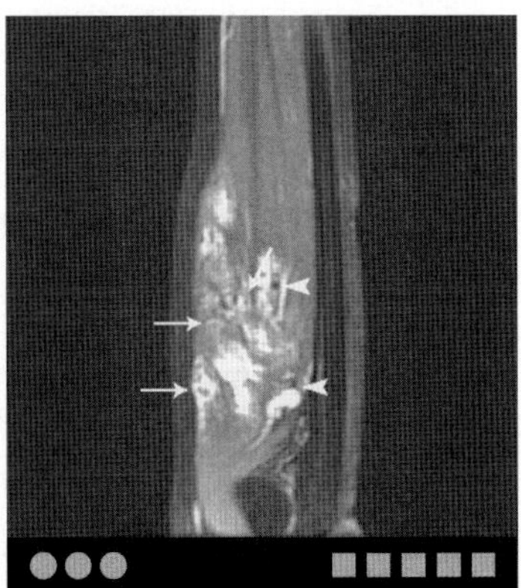

C. Hemangioma: Sagittal fat-saturated T2-weighted image shows tubular structures (arrows) within the heterogeneous, hyperintense mass. Circular regions of hypointensity (arrowheads) represent phleboliths.

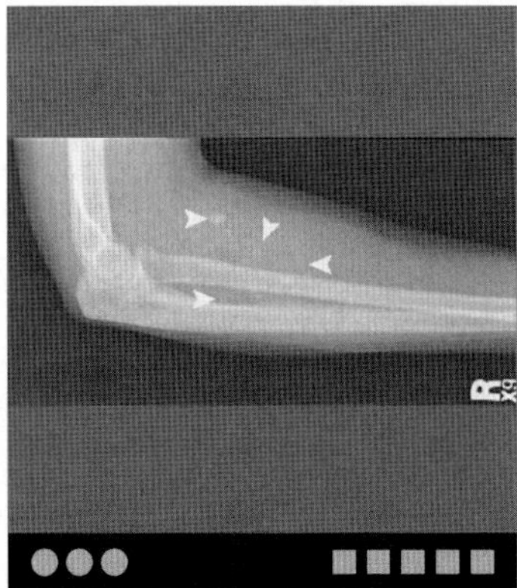

D. Hemangioma: Lateral radiograph shows multiple clustered smooth calcifications (arrowheads), a suggestion of a soft tissue mass in the proximal forearm. No bony involvement is seen.

DIFFERENTIAL DIAGNOSES IMAGES

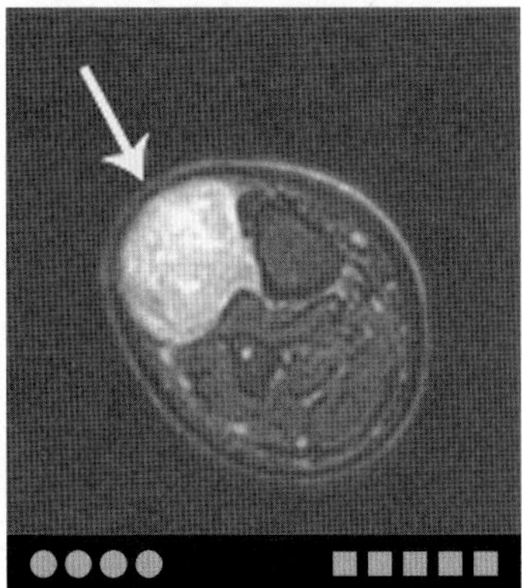

E. Soft tissue sarcoma: Axial fat-saturated T2-weighted image shows a hyperintense mass (arrow) relative to muscle. The mass abuts the lateral tibia without cortical involvement.

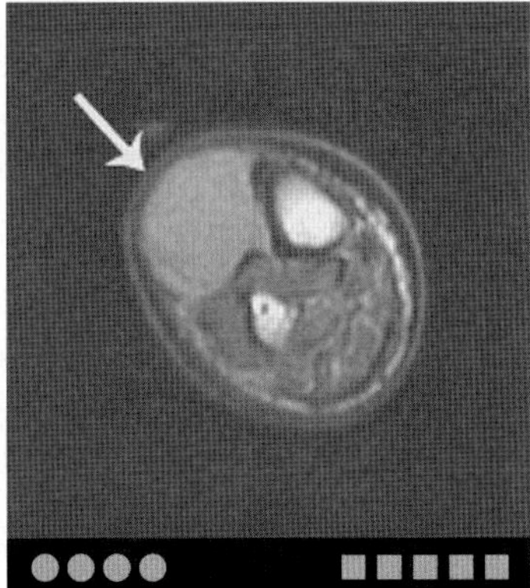

F. Soft tissue sarcoma: Axial proton density image demonstrates a mass (arrow) that is hyperintense compared to muscle in this patient with histology proven leiomyosarcoma.

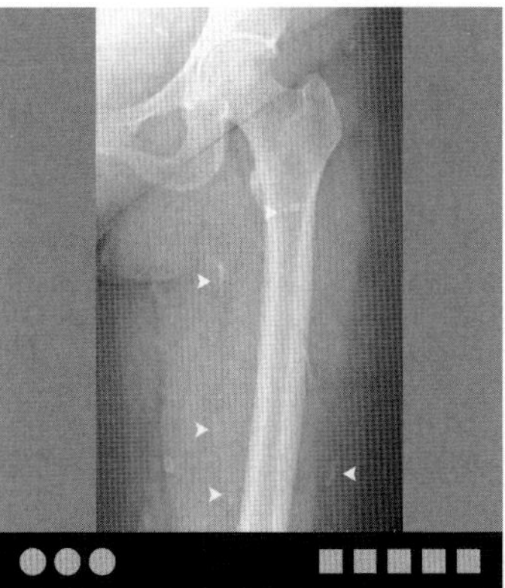

G. Cysticercosis: Frontal view of the hip shows multiple scattered oval calcifications (arrowheads) that lie along the orientation of muscle fibers in the thigh.

IMAGE KEY

Common

●●●●●
●●●●
●●●
●●
●

Rare

Typical

■■■■■
■■■■
■■■
■■
■

Unusual

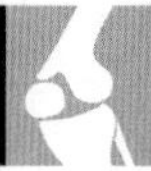

11–3 Osteochondroma of the Radius

Oganes Ashikyan and Jamshid Tehranzadeh

PRESENTATION

Painless swelling

FINDINGS

MRI shows exophytic distal radius lesion with cartilaginous cap and adjacent pressure erosion in the distal ulna. The cortex of the lesion is continuous with adjacent normal bone cortex.

DIFFERENTIAL DIAGNOSES

- *Soft tissue tumors:* Tumors such as lipoma or lipohemangioma of soft tissue may mimic these lesions. Hemangiomas are associated with phleboliths.
- *Juxtacortical chondroma:* Commonly located near metaphysis, but with no stalk or peduncle connecting this lesion to the adjacent bone. Location and appearance of this lesion is similar to periosteal osteosarcoma.
- *Parosteal osteosarcoma:* This lesion is usually seen around the knee, but may occasionally be seen at the proximal humerus. There is a stalk connecting this to the bone with absence of cleavage plane.
- *Diaphyseal aclasis (hereditary multiple exostoses):* Hereditary condition that is characterized by multiple exostosis (osteochondromas) involving long bones. This condition has up to 10% chance of malignant degeneration.

COMMENTS

Osteochondroma (osteocartilagenous exostosis) is the most common benign skeletal neoplasm. Osteochondromas occur only in the bones that undergo enchondral ossification (developed from cartilage). The etiology of the osteochondroma formation is thought to be related to trauma of the perichondrium with resultant herniation of a portion of the epiphyseal growth plate. Osteochondromas may have sessile or stalklike (pedunculated) appearance. The structure of the lesion consists of bone marrow core covered by cortex, periosteum, and cartilaginous cap. The bone marrow of the tumor is continuous with the marrow of the adjacent bone. The appearance of the marrow of the lesion and the marrow of the adjacent bone is identical. The cartilaginous portion of the tumor functions as a growth plate, which undergoes enchondral ossification to produce exostosis. The tumors usually become inactive after closure of the epiphyseal plates. Solitary osteochondroma has less than 1% chance of malignant degeneration. Growth activity in the adult life should raise the suspicion for malignant degeneration. The patient may present with pain if adjacent structures are compressed. However, the remnants of the benign cartilaginous cap can show renewed benign growth activity years after epiphyseal plate closure. Bursitis may develop adjacent to exostosis because of pressure effect. Radiographs are usually sufficient for diagnoses of osteochondroma. MRI can be helpful in demonstrating continuity between marrow and osseous components of the lesion with the adjacent normal bone. MRI can also help in evaluating the thickness of the cartilaginous cap.

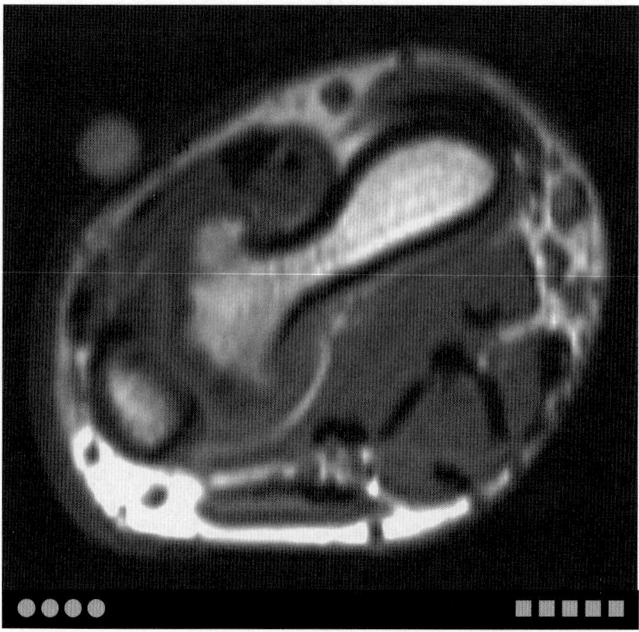

A. Osteochondroma of the distal radius: Axial T1-weighted image demonstrates pedunculated lesion of the distal radius. The cortex of the lesion is continuous with the cortex of adjacent bone. Cartilaginous cap can be seen at the most medial aspect of the lesion.

PEARLS

- **Osteochondroma is the most common benign osseous tumor.**
- **The diagnosis of osteochondroma can be established by demonstrating continuity of the cortex of the lesion with cortex of adjacent bone.**
- **Growth of the tumor during adult life maybe related to the reactivation of the growth of the cartilaginous cap remnants; however, malignant degeneration should be the working diagnosis until proven otherwise.**
- **Benign osteochondroma should have a cartilaginous cap, which measures less than one centimeter thick.**

ADDITIONAL IMAGES

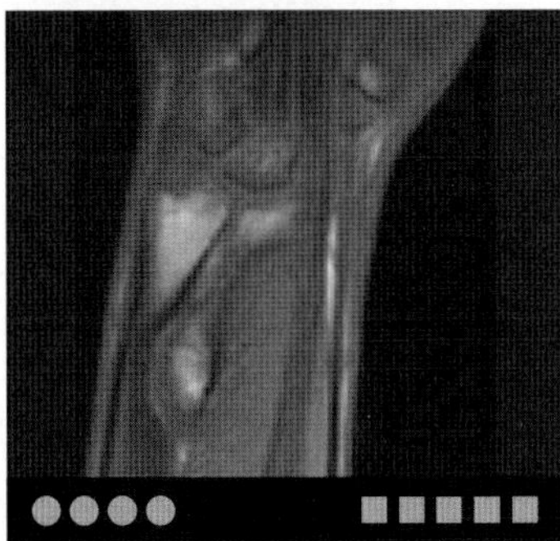

B. Osteochondroma of the distal radius: Coronal T1-weighted image of the distal radius and ulna demonstrates cartilaginous cap at the leading edge of the lesion. Note that the axis of the lesion is oriented away from the nearest (wrist) joint.

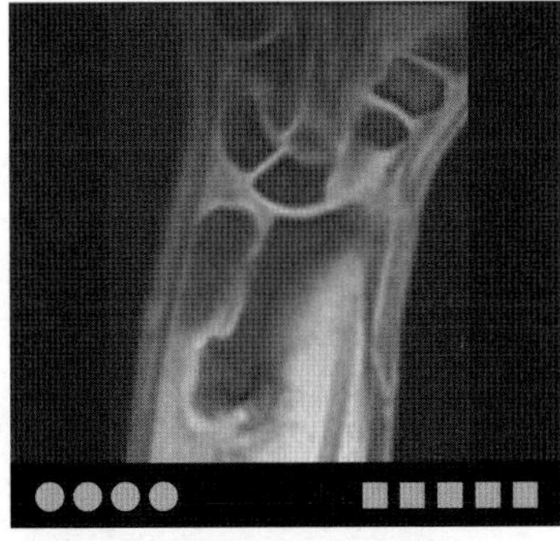

C. Osteochondroma of the distal radius: Coronal T1-weighted image with fat saturation demonstrates that the signal characteristics of the lesion are identical to the signal characteristics of the adjacent bone.

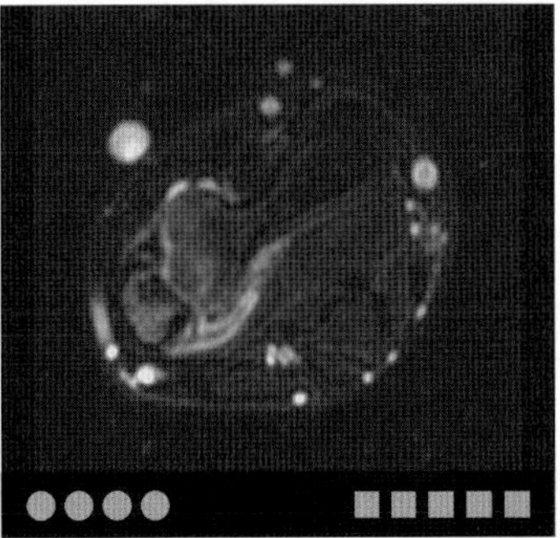

D. Osteochondroma of the distal radius: Axial T2-weighted image with fat saturation demonstrates bright cartilage cap surrounding the osteochondroma.

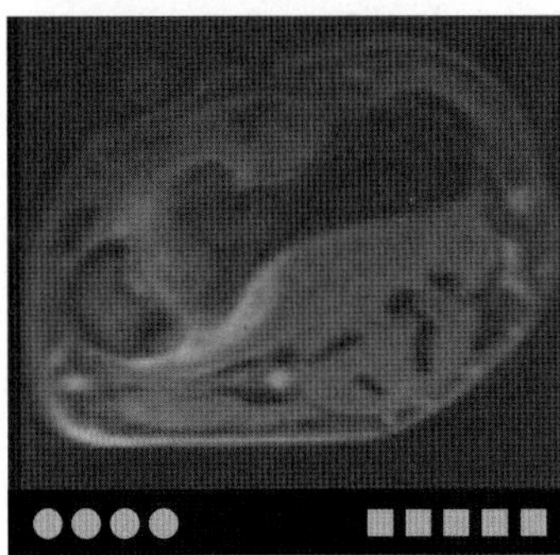

E. Osteochondroma of the distal radius: Axial 3D VIBE (volumetric interpolated breath-hold examination) image obtained after contrast administration demonstrates mild enhancement of the surrounding cartilaginous cap. Enhancing erosion, which resulted from mass effect by the lesion, can be seen in the distal ulna.

IMAGE KEY

Common

Rare

Typical

Unusual

DIFFERENTIAL DIAGNOSES IMAGES

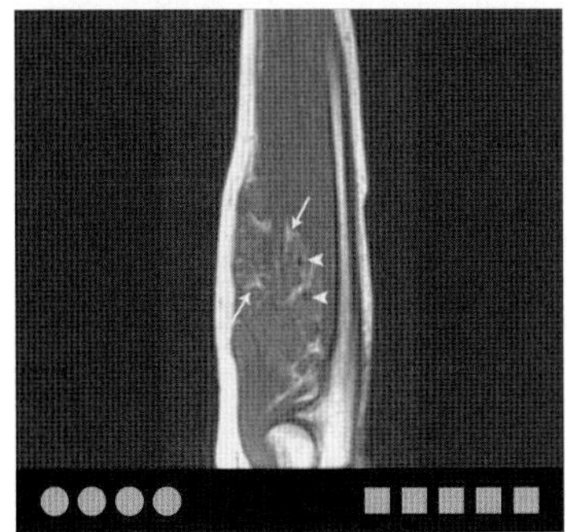

F. Hemangioma of forearm: Sagittal T1-weighted image shows increased vascularity (arrows) in soft tissues associated with the phleboliths seen as dark signal dots (arrowheads).

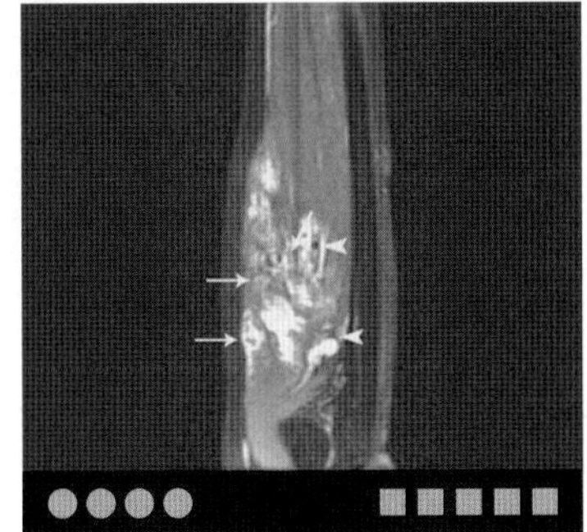

G. Hemangioma of forearm: Sagittal T2-weighted image with fat saturation shows increased vascularity (arrows) in soft tissues associated with the phleboliths seen as dark signal dots (arrowheads).

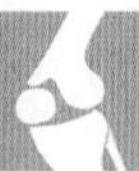

11–4 Aneurysmal Bone Cyst of Humerus

Kambiz Motamedi

PRESENTATION

Elbow pain

FINDINGS

MRI shows a cystic mass of the distal humerus.

DIFFERENTIAL DIAGNOSES

- *Chondroblastoma:* MRI shows a lobular mass of the epiphysis with high signal on fluid sensitive sequences because of cartilage contents. There is usually surrounding edema.
- *Telangiectatic osteosarcoma:* MRI shows a cystic expansile mass with fluid-fluid levels.
- *Metastatic renal cell carcinoma:* MRI reveals an expansile cystic lesion of the bone.

COMMENTS

This is an image of a 16-year-old female patient who presented with a cystic lesion of the distal humerus displaying fluid-fluid levels on MRI, and biopsy revealed an aneurysmal bone cyst (ABC). ABC is an expansile cystic lesion that most often affects children and adolescents during their second decade of life. The ABC may occur in any bone in the body. In a published review of 897 cases of ABC, 9.1% were located in the humerus. Although benign, the ABC can be locally aggressive and cause extensive weakening of the bony structure and impinge on surrounding tissues. The true etiology and pathophysiology remain a mystery. The mainstay of treatment has been intralesional curettage; however, recurrence is not uncommon. As defined by the World Health Organization, the ABC is a benign tumor-like lesion. It is described as "an expanding osteolytic lesion consisting of blood-filled spaces of variable size separated by connective tissue septa containing trabeculae or osteoid tissue and osteoclast giant cells." Although benign, the ABC can be a rapidly growing and destructive bone lesion. The expansile nature of the lesions can cause pain, swelling, deformity, disruption of growth plates, neurologic symptoms, and pathologic fracture. ABC is one of the few bony lesions where CT scan and MRI may actually further aid in diagnosis as the fluid levels within the cystic lesion become apparent. Up to 40% of ABC lesions are secondary. The common primary accompanying lesions are giant cell tumors, fibrous dysplasia, chondroblastoma, osteoblastoma, and osteosarcoma.

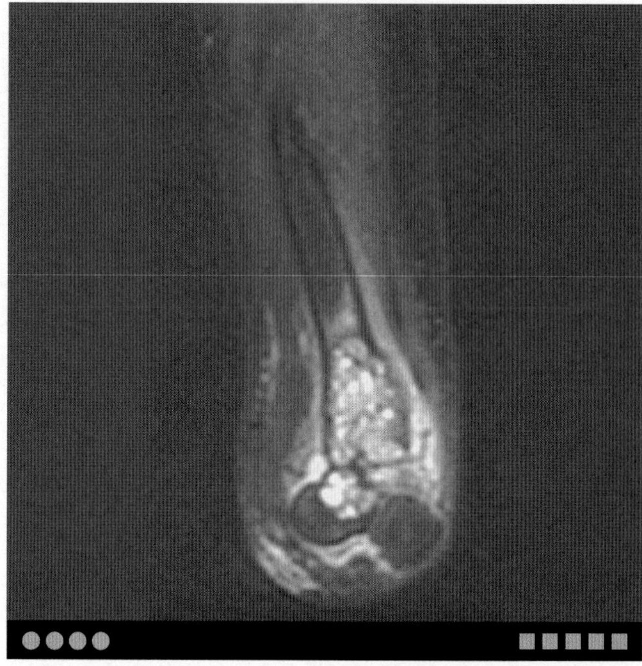

A. ABC: Sagittal inversion recovery image shows a cystic lesion of the lateral, humeral epicondyle.

PEARLS

- **ABC accounts for 5% of primary bone tumors with most common locations in the lower extremities, pelvis, and spine.**
- **MRI and CT scan readily show fluid levels within the cystic lesions and may show a focus of soft tissue mass, likely the primary lesion.**
- **ABC may also arise in an area of prior trauma.**

ADDITIONAL IMAGES

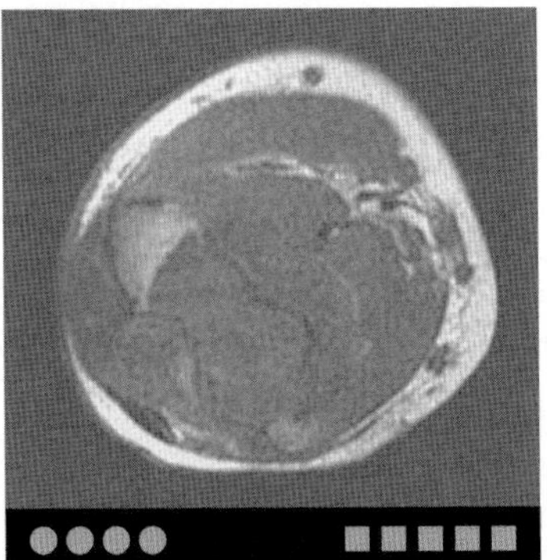

B. ABC: Axial T1-weighted image shows the extent of the lesion. The cysts are rather small and fluid levels are not readily visible.

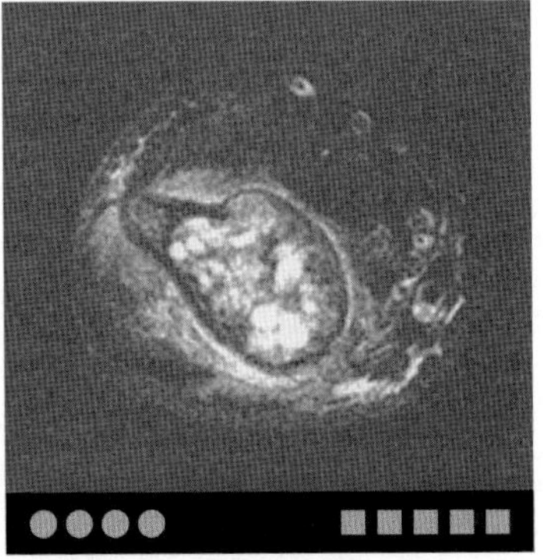

C. ABC: Axial fat-saturated T2-weighted image demonstrates the small cysts with fluid levels. The surrounding edema is caused by a pathologic fracture.

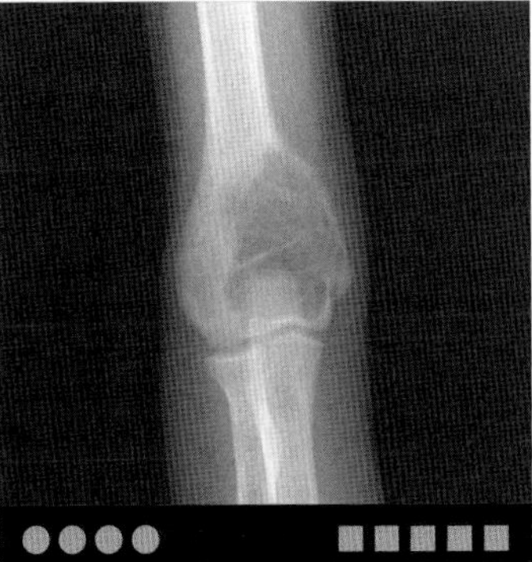

D. ABC: AP radiograph of the elbow shows the lytic expansile lesion of the medial humeral epicondyle. Note the pathologic fracture of the superior aspect of the lesion.

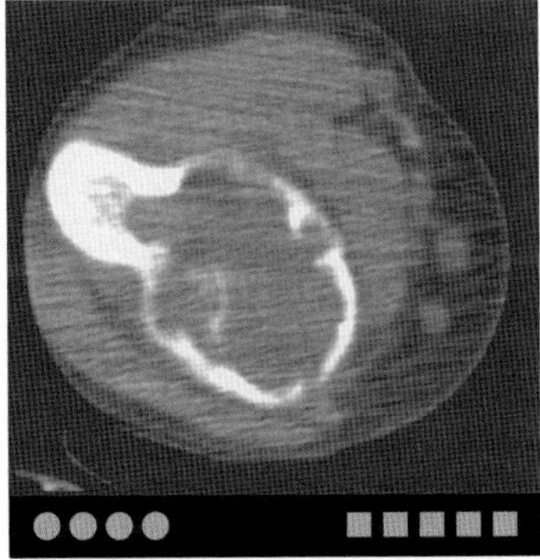

E. ABC: Axial CT (bone window) shows the expansile lytic lesion of the medial humeral condyle. There is no matrix mineralization. There are bony fragments related to the pathologic fracture.

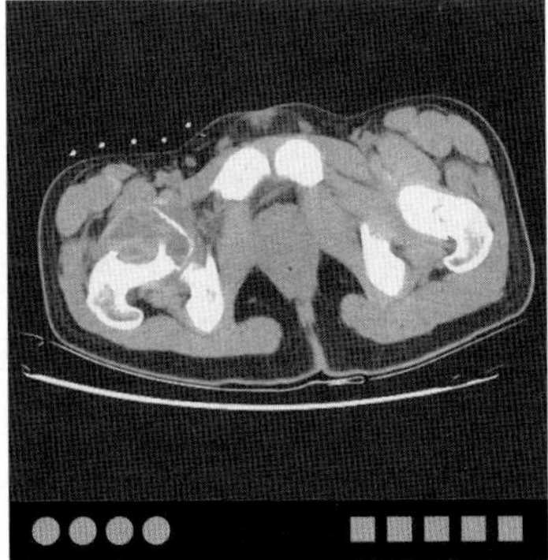

F. ABC: Axial CT (bone window) of proximal femur in another patient shows an expansile lesion of the femoral neck with fluid levels and no matrix mineralization.

DIFFERENTIAL DIAGNOSES IMAGES

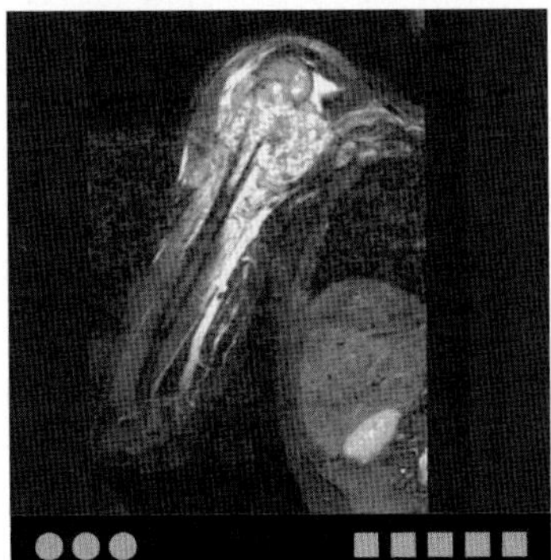

G. Telangiectatic osteosarcoma: The sagittal inversion recovery image of the humerus shows a large destructive expansile mass with a large soft tissue mass and several fluid-filled cysts.

IMAGE KEY

Common

Rare

Typical

Unusual

SECTION III

HAND AND WRIST

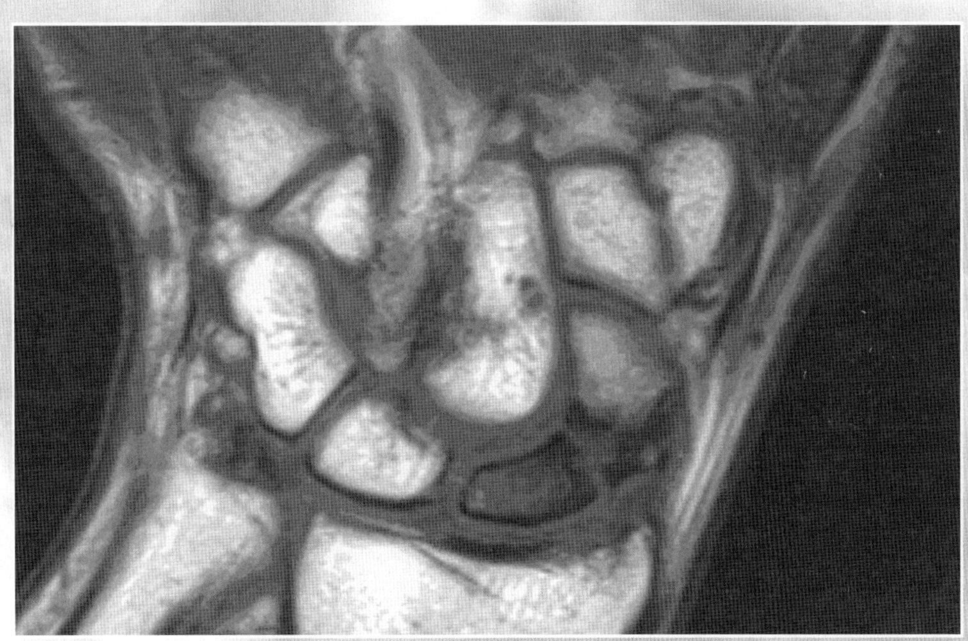

Chapter 12

Sport Medicine and Trauma

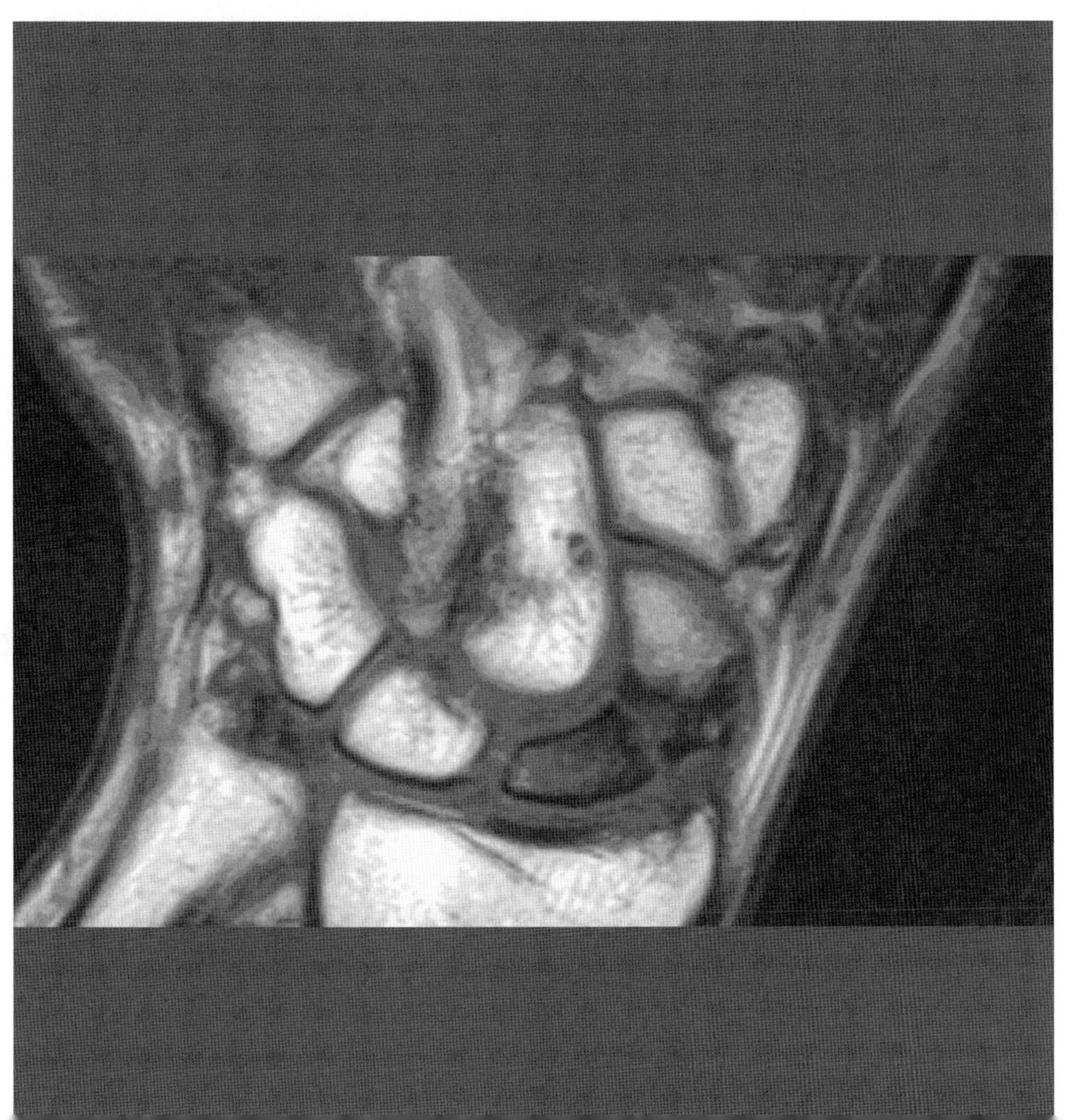

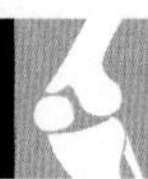

12–1 Scaphoid Fracture with Avascular Necrosis

Edward Mossop and Jamshid Tehranzadeh

PRESENTATION

Left wrist pain

FINDINGS

MRI shows fracture of the carpal scaphoid with avascular necrosis seen on T1WI as low signal intensity in proximal fragment.

DIFFERENTIAL DIAGNOSES

- *Arthritis with sclerosis:* Severe osteoarthritis may cause diffuse sclerosis.
- *Idiopathic avascular necrosis (AVN) of the scaphoid:* Preiser's disease, also known as osteochondrosis of the scaphoid, is not associated with fracture.
- *Scaphoid fracture with nonunion:* This is associated with sclerosis at the cortical margin at the fracture site.
- *Osteomyelitis:* Healing phase of osteomyelitis may cause diffuse sclerosis.
- Normal for comparison.

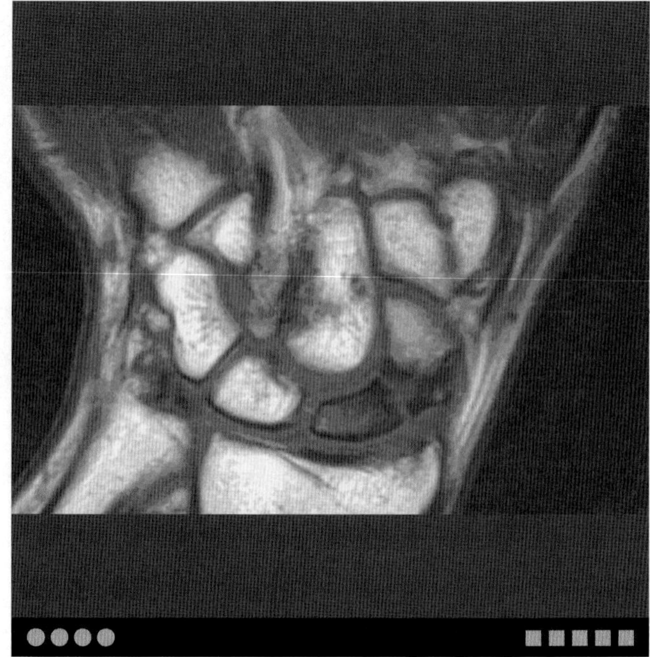

A. Scaphoid fracture with AVN: Coronal T1WI shows scaphoid fracture with low signal at the proximal fracture fragment.

COMMENTS

The scaphoid is the most frequently fractured carpal bone, accounting for 71% of all carpal bone fractures, and 5% of all wrist injuries. Fall on an outstretched hand when the wrist is laterally deviated is the most common cause. Patients present with dull deep pain in the radial side of the wrist. A scaphoid fracture may disrupt the dorsal branches of the radial artery, which feed the proximal fragment by retrograde flow. This accounts for up to 80% of the entire blood supply and as much as 100% of the supply to the proximal segment. Five percent of scaphoid fractures result in nonunion, and many patients develop osteoarthritis and AVN. Initial radiographs do not always detect scaphoid fractures. The pattern on MRI is a linear focus of decreased signal intensity on T1WI. Increased signal intensity in a distribution similar to that of the T1W is seen with T2W. The fracture line may be more difficult to see on T2WI. Short-tau inversion recovery or fat-suppressed T2WI are very sensitive to edema. For AVN radiographic findings include cystic and sclerotic changes in the scaphoid. The MRI shows dark signal on T1WI and increased signal on T2WI within the proximal pole of the scaphoid fragment. IV Gadolinium contrast has been used to evaluate healing versus nonunion and/or AVN.

PEARLS

- **Scaphoid fractures are the most common carpal bone fractures.**
- **The scaphoid fracture may be complicated by AVN and/or nonunion.**
- **The proximal segment of the scaphoid is dependent on endosteal retrograde blood flow from a recurrent branch of the radial artery.**
- **AVN of the scaphoid is characterized by a low signal area on T1WI and a high-signal area on T2WI.**

ADDITIONAL IMAGES

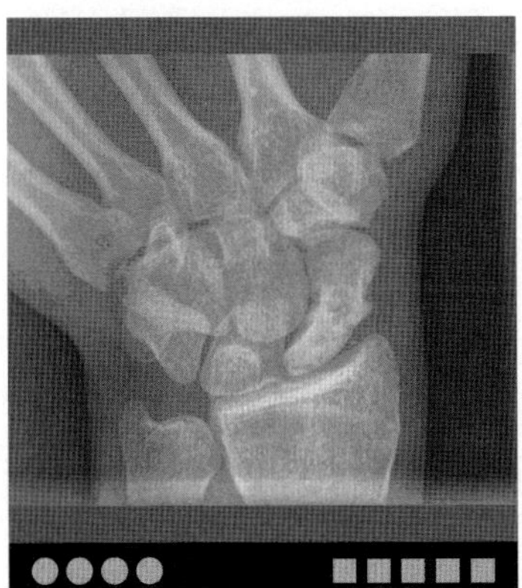

B. Scaphoid fracture with AVN: AP radiograph of the wrist shows scaphoid fracture and sclerosis of proximal fragment with small cystic change at the fracture site.

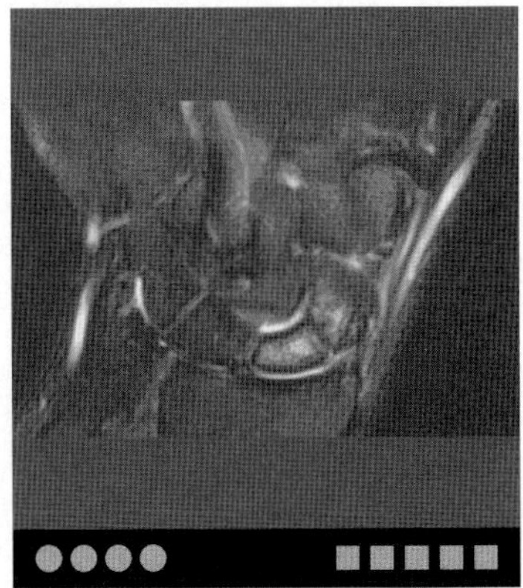

C. Scaphoid fracture with AVN: Coronal fat-saturated T2WI shows bright signal representing marrow edema within the proximal and distal fragments.

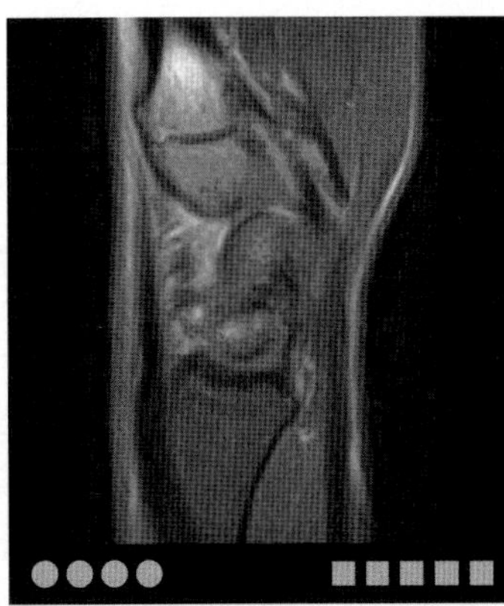

D. Scaphoid fracture with AVN: Sagittal fat-saturated T2WI shows bright signal representing marrow edema within the proximal and distal fragments.

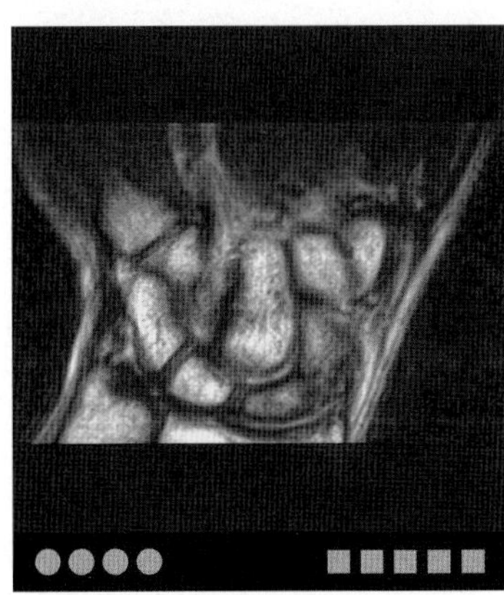

E. Scaphoid fracture with AVN: Coronal T2WI shows mixed signal on fracture fragments.

DIFFERENTIAL DIAGNOSIS IMAGES

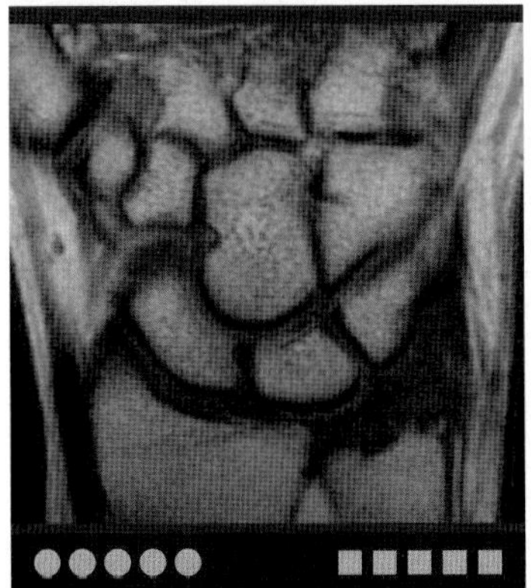

F. Normal Scaphoid: Coronal T2WI of normal scaphoid.

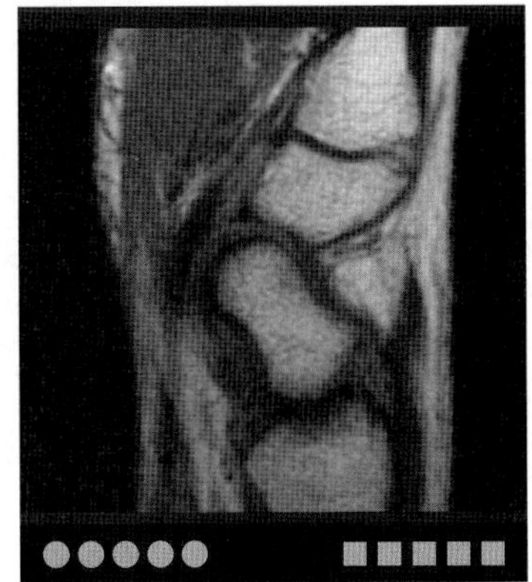

G. Normal Scaphoid: Sagittal T2WI of normal scaphoid.

IMAGE KEY

Common

Rare

Typical

Unusual

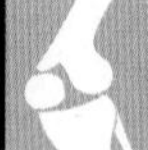

12–2 Kienbock's Disease

Shahla Modarresi and Daria Motamedi

PRESENTATION

Wrist pain, swelling, and decreased motion

FINDINGS

MRI shows diffuse decreased signal intensity of the lunate bone in coronal T1WI.

DIFFERENTIAL DIAGNOSES

- *Fracture:* MRI shows low T1 and high T2 marrow signal intensity. Fracture lines, soft tissue edema, and joint effusion may exist.
- *Infection:* MRI shows marrow edema with low signal on T1W, high signal on T2W, and bright signal on STIR image, soft tissues edema, and joint effusion. Other bones may be involved.
- *Intraosseous ganglion cyst:* Shows intraosseous lesion of lunate, which is low signal on T1W and high signal on T2WI consistent with cyst.
- *Arthritis:* MRI shows erosive changes in the lunate and other carpal bones, showing patchy or well-defined low T1W and high T2W signal intensity lesions, which enhance with contrast.

COMMENTS

Kienbock's disease is an avascular necrosis (AVN) of the lunate bone also called lunatomalacia occurring most often in adults between 15 and 40 years and males more than females. The patient presents with pain, swelling, and tenderness of lunate bone. The disease is usually unilateral, likely caused by repeated microfractures disrupting the blood supply to the lunate. Patients with negative ulnar variance, sickle cell anemia, diabetes, and type II or IV hyperlipidemia are at increased risk. The radiograph may initially be normal or show negative ulnar variance. Gradually sclerosis of the lunate develops with progressive loss of height and eventual fragmentation and collapse of the lunate. This can lead to carpal instability, degenerative joint disease, and cyst formation within lunate and ultimately osteoarthrosis of the entire wrist joint. Two different radiographic staging classification for the Kienbock's disease exists, which is based on the shape and density of the lunate: (1) Modified Stahl's classification. (2) Lichtman's radiographic classification. Early diagnosis and treatment of Kienbock's disease are important to decrease the compressive force on the lunate and increase revascularization before collapse can occur. MR imaging shows low signal of the lunate on T1W and increased or decreased signal on T2WI depending on the stage of the disease. Contour deformity, cyst formation and loss of height of the lunate may also be noted. Treatment is primarily for symptomatic relief with better results if picked up early.

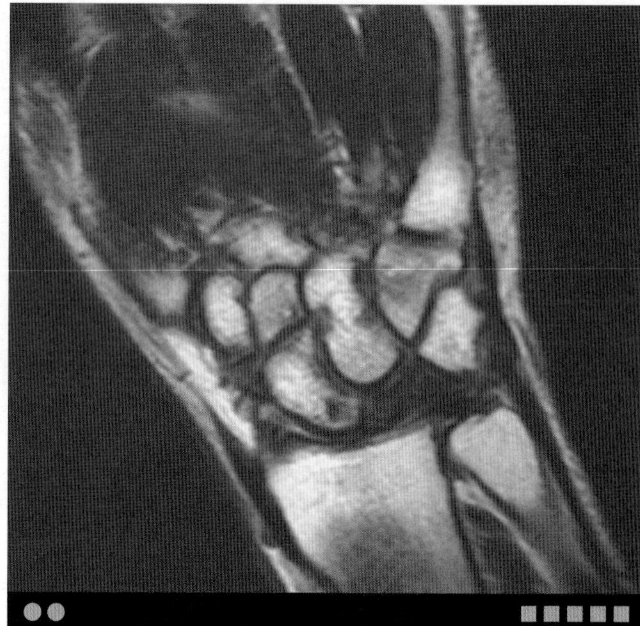

A. Kienbock's disease: Coronal T1WI of the wrist shows AVN of the lunate with diffuse decreased signal intensity.

PEARLS

- **Kienbock's disease is an avascular necrosis of the lunate, likely caused by repeated microfractures disrupting the blood supply to the lunate bone.**
- **Patients with negative ulnar variance, sickle cell anemia, diabetes, and type II or IV hyperlipidemia are at increased risk.**
- **Radiograph may show sclerosis of the lunate, progressive loss of height, and eventual fragmentation and collapse leading to carpal instability and osteoarthrosis.**
- **MRI shows low T1W and increased or decreased T2W signal depending on the stage of the disease.**

ADDITIONAL IMAGES

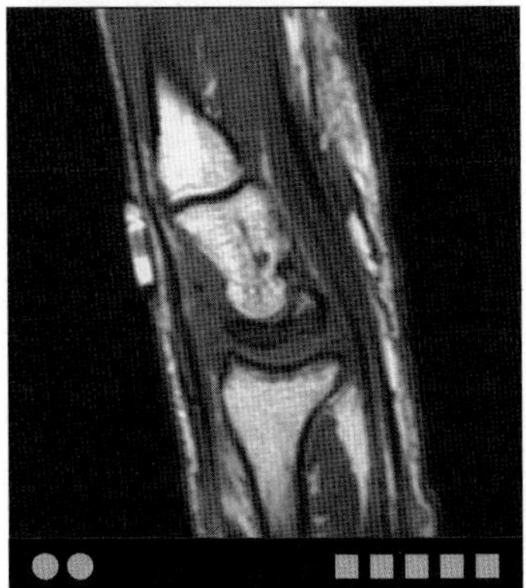

B. Kienbock's disease: Sagittal T2WI of the wrist shows AVN of the lunate with diffuse decreased signal intensity.

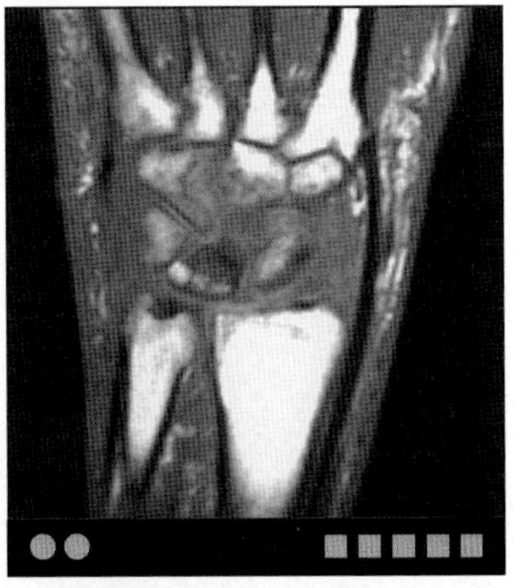

C. Kienbock's disease: Coronal T1WI shows AVN of lunate with heterogeneous signal intensity from focal marrow sparing.

DIFFERENTIAL DIAGNOSIS IMAGES

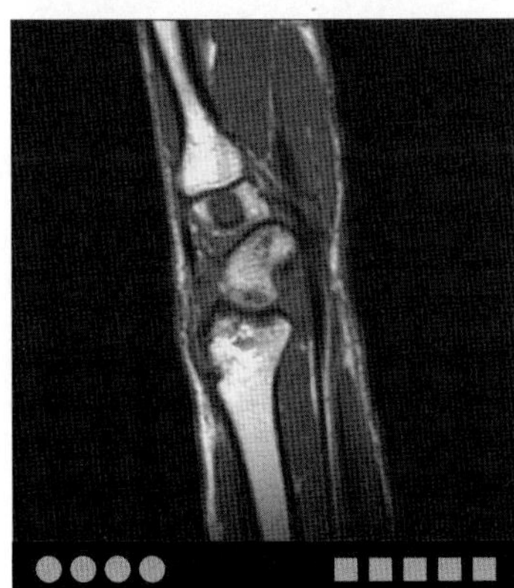

D. Ganglion cyst: Sagittal T1WI shows small rounded low T1W signal lesion of trapezium consistent with ganglion cyst.

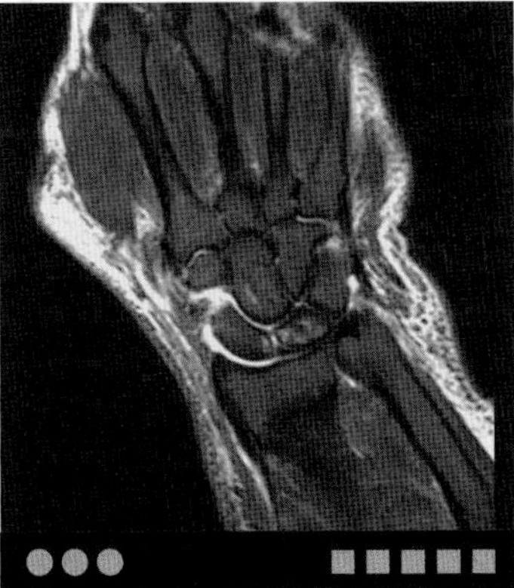

E. Osteomyelitis: Coronal STIR image shows fluid in the joint from septic arthritis and marrow edema of lunate consistent with osteomyelitis.

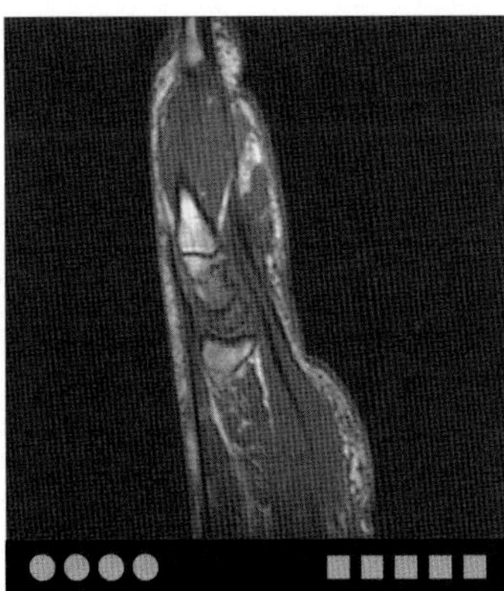

F. Bone contusion: Sagittal PD image shows low signal of lunate and proximal capitate with fracture line consistent with bone bruise and history of trauma.

IMAGE KEY

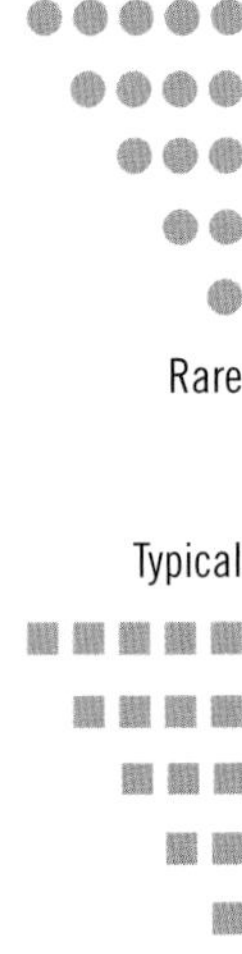

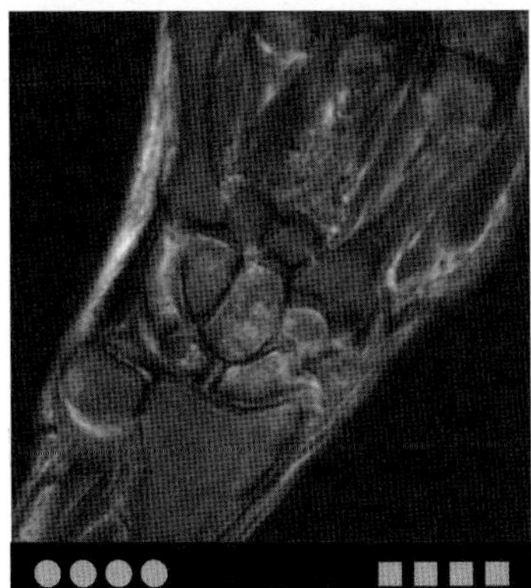

G. Gout: Coronal STIR image shows high signal erosion and edema of the carpal bones in this patient with history of gouty arthritis.

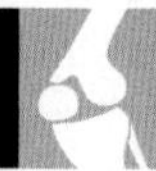

12–3 Scaphoid Nonunion Advanced Collapse (SNAC)

Stephen E. Ling and William W. Reinus

PRESENTATION

Pain, swelling, carpal instability

FINDINGS

The images show widening of the scapholunate articulation with proximal migration of the capitate and radioscaphoid osteoarthritis.

DIFFERENTIAL DIAGNOSIS

- *Kienbock disease:* Avascular necrosis of the lunate is associated with loss of marrow signal on MR sequences, which finally leads to lunate collapse.

COMMENTS

Tear of the scapholunate ligament can be caused by trauma, calcium pyrophosphate deposition disease (CPPD), and inflammatory arthropathies such as rheumatoid arthritis. Once torn, the dissociation of the scaphoid and lunate (SLD) allows palmar flexion by the scaphoid with concomitant posterior displacement of the proximal pole. The resulting gap between the two bones in the coronal plane/projection was originally termed the "Terry Thomas" sign after the famous British comedic actor. Management of scapholunate ligament tears is somewhat controversial, and ligamentous repair/reconstruction, surgical pinning, dorsal capsulodesis, and triscaphe (STT) and scaphocapitate arthrodesis have all been advocated. If left untreated or not adequately addressed, scapholunate dissociation (SLD) may lead to dorsal intercalated segmental instability (DISI). This entity manifests itself by dorsal tilt of the lunate with respect to the distal radial articular surface and dorsal displacement of the capitate in relation to the lunate. Both the scapholunate and lunocapitate angles are increased. Furthermore, loss of congruence between the scaphoid and lunate with resulting DISI predisposes the patient to develop scapholunate advanced collapse (SLAC). In this disorder, the capitate migrates proximally resulting in secondary osteoarthritis of the radioscaphoid and lunocapitate joints. Classically, the radiolunate joint space is preserved. Surgical treatment for SLAC can be either motion preserving (i.e., four-corner fusion, proximal row carpectomy) or nonmotion preserving (i.e., total wrist arthrodesis). Scaphoid nonunion advanced collapse (SNAC) is a variant of SLAC characterized by scaphoid fracture nonunion instead of scapholunate tear. Here too proximal migration of the capitate leads to radioscaphoid and lunocapitate osteoarthritis, and DISI.

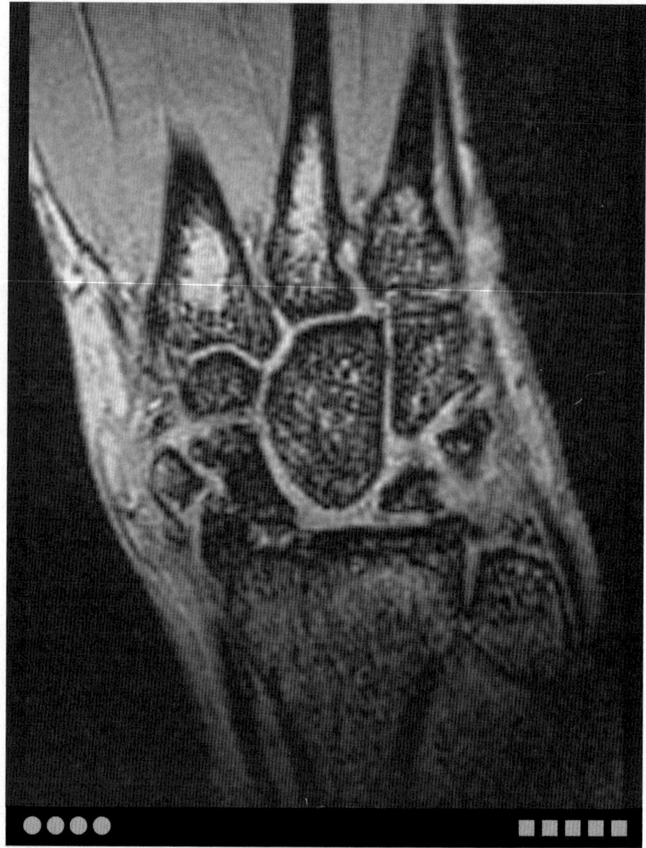

A. Scaphoid nonunion advanced collapse: Coronal gradient recalled acquisition (GRE) image shows marked widening of the scapholunate joint space with extensive proximal migration of the capitate. Note the diffuse hypointense marrow signal in the proximal portion of the scaphoid. Note also the characteristic radiocarpal osteoarthritis and elongation of the radial styloid as well as the small ossicle lateral to the distal scaphoid.

PEARLS

- **The "Terry Thomas" sign has been updated as the "David Letterman" sign and "Madonna" sign.**
- **The earliest finding in the radioscaphoid osteoarthritis occurring with SLAC and SNAC is elongation and pointing of the radial styloid.**
- **Radioscaphoid and lunocapitate osteoarthritis is the most common pattern of arthritis in the wrist.**
- **In addition to ligamentous tear, scaphoid fracture may function as the equivalent of a tear and lead to SLD.**

ADDITIONAL IMAGES

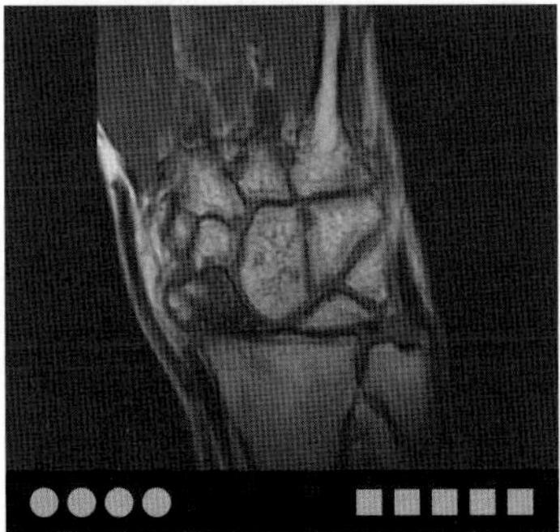

B. Scaphoid nonunion advanced collapse: Coronal T1WI at the same level as image A again shows severe widening of the scapholunate articulation as well as marked proximal capitate migration. Note the diffuse marrow hypointensity in the proximal scaphoid consistent with osteonecrosis.

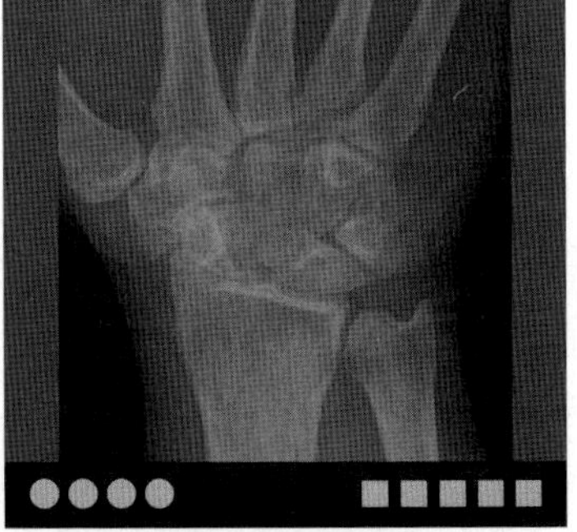

C. Scaphoid nonunion advanced collapse: PA radiograph of the wrist in the same patient as in images A and B shows the fracture this is the cause of the osteonecrosis shown above, in this patient with severe SLAC with evidence of secondary osteoarthritis and fragmentation of the distal scaphoid.

DIFFERENTIAL DIAGNOSIS IMAGES

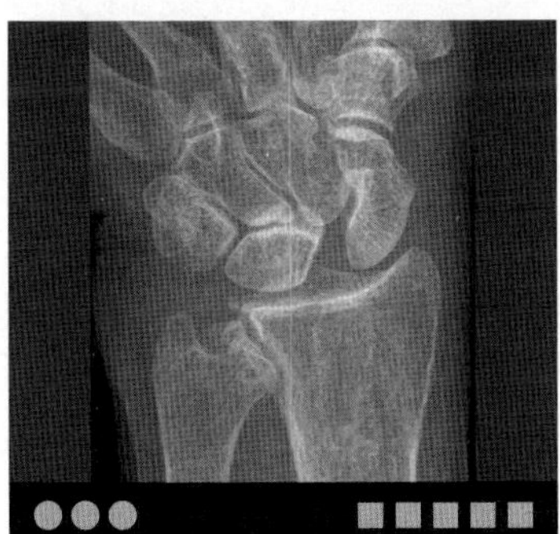

D. Early scaphoid-lunate advanced collapse: PA radiograph of the wrist in another patient shows SLD as manifested by widening of the scapholunate joint space, in this patient with early SLAC. Note that there thus far has been only been mild migration of the capitate proximally and radiocarpal osteoarthritis has yet to develop.

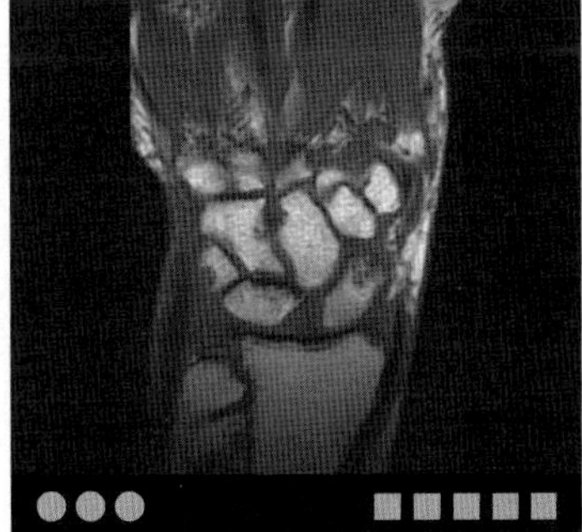

E. Early scaphoid-lunate advanced collapse: Coronal T1WI in the same patient as in image D also shows scapholunate joint widening with limited accompanying proximal migration of the capitate.

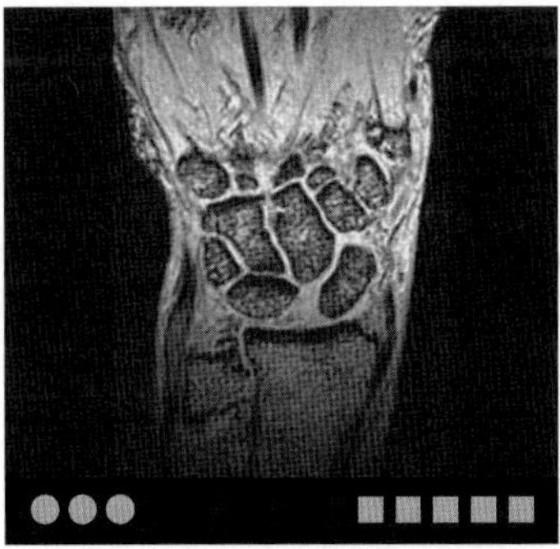

F. Early scaphoid-lunate advanced collapse: Coronal fat saturation GRE image at the same level as in image E shows the same findings.

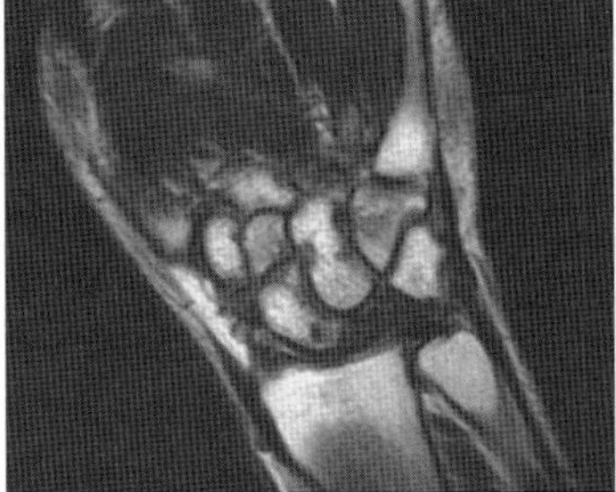

G. Kienbock disease: Coronal SE T2W MR image shows total loss of signal within the lunate bone due to avascular necrosis or Kienbock's disease.

IMAGE KEY

Common

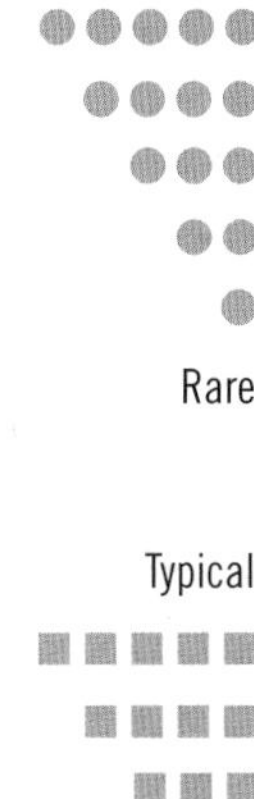

Rare

Typical

Unusual

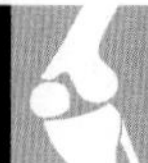

12–4 Multidetector Computed Tomography Evaluation of Scaphoid Fracture

Joshua Farber

PRESENTATION

Wrist pain after a fall

FINDINGS

Initial coronal and sagittal reformatted images (MPRs) of the left wrist from a MDCT demonstrate the patient to be status postcasting for a fracture through the waist of the scaphoid. Notice the step-off on the sagittal images. Coronal and sagittal images taken 3 months after Herbert screw placement demonstrate osseous bridging across the fracture line and reduction of the step-off.

DIFFERENTIAL DIAGNOSES

- *Fractural nonunion:* Nonunion of a fracture, involving the scaphoid or any bone, results in persistent visualization of the fracture line. With time, the nonhealed bone develops cortication on both sides of the fracture. Ultimately, nonunion is a clinical diagnosis that is confirmed by radiological evaluation.
- *Osteonecrosis of the scaphoid:* Osteonecrosis of the scaphoid can occur after fracture if the blood supply to the proximal pole is disrupted and remains so. Osteonecrosis of the scaphoid causes the proximal pole to become sclerotic, and it may eventually collapse.

COMMENTS

This 16-year-old male suffered a left scaphoid fracture after falling. Because the blood supply to the proximal pole of the scaphoid travels from a distal portion of the bone, osteonecrosis of the proximal pole is a frequent occurrence from waist (50%) and proximal pole (80%) fractures. To prevent scaphoid osteonecrosis, anatomic opposition of the fracture after reduction is essential. In this case the initial MDCT showed a step-off with poor opposition. The Herbert screw placement corrected the alignment and opposition and allowed for good osseous bridging. MRI is more sensitive than MDCT for the evaluation of osteonecrosis, especially if gadolinium is administered. The presence of the Herbert screw, however, would make MR scanning difficult at this point. The MDCT technique for scanning the scaphoid, with or without the presence of a Herbert screw *in situ*, uses the highest spatial resolution parameters possible. In this case axial 0.6-mm slices were obtained at 0.2-mm intervals. The pitch was less then 1 and the mAs was 200. The patient was scanned with his wrist over his head. The combination of extremely thin slices with at least 50% overlap creates an essentially isotropic data set, which in turn allows coronal and sagittal MPRs to be produced that are indistinguishable from direct acquisition images. The appropriate pitch and mAs prevent significant metallic artifact. Note also that this technique allows scanning through casting material. Similar MDCT technique can be used for scanning other small osseous structures as well, even if small fixation devices or casting material is present.

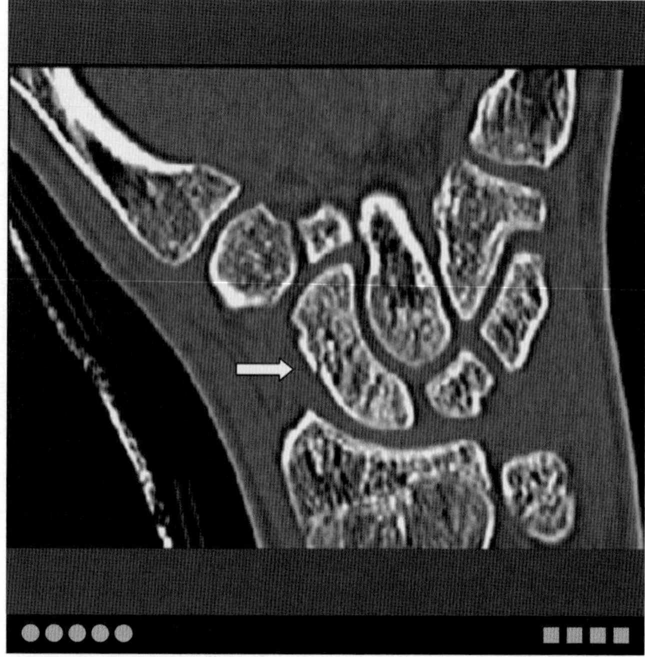

A. Scaphoid Fracture after Casting: Coronal MPR image from a MDCT of the left wrist demonstrates a fracture through the waist of the scaphoid (arrow). Thin axial slices with appropriate overlap produce robust MPRs.

PEARLS

- **Scaphoid fractures through the waist and body of the scaphoid frequently lead to osteonecrosis of the proximal pole.**
- **Anatomic alignment and good fracture opposition reduce the incidence of scaphoid osteonecrosis.**
- **MDCT allows accurate assessment of fracture alignment and healing, even when metallic fixation screws are present.**
- **Thin slices with at least 50% overlap create essentially isotropic data set that produces robust MPRs.**

ADDITIONAL IMAGES

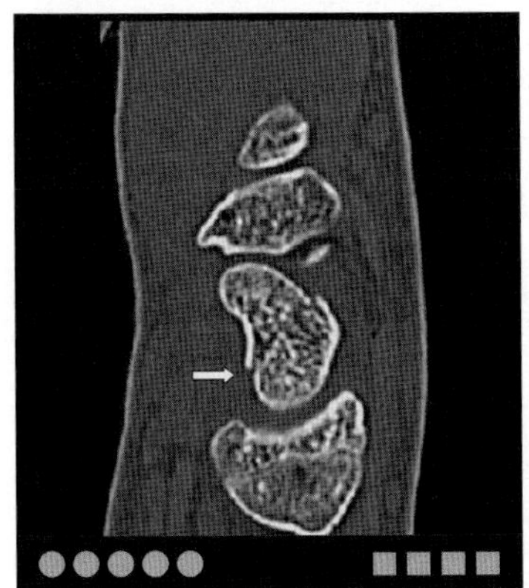

B. Scaphoid fracture after casting: Sagittal MPR image from a MDCT of the left wrist demonstrates a fracture through the waist of the scaphoid (arrow). With appropriate mAs the scan is acquired easily through cast material.

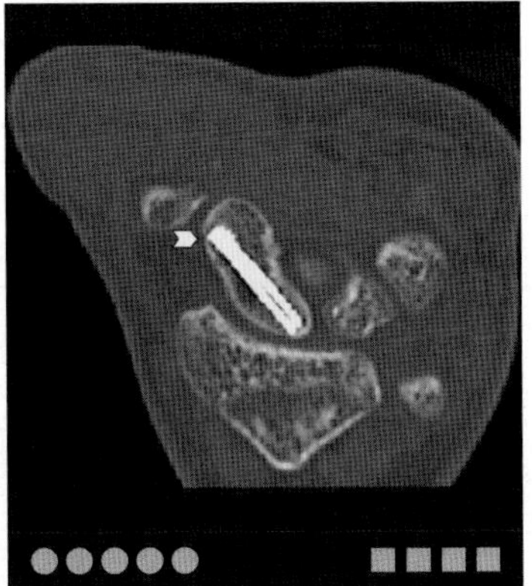

C. Healed scaphoid fracture after Herbert screw placement: Coronal MPR image from a MDCT of the left wrist demonstrates a Herbert screw *in situ* (arrow head). Significant metallic artifact is absent with appropriate scanning technique.

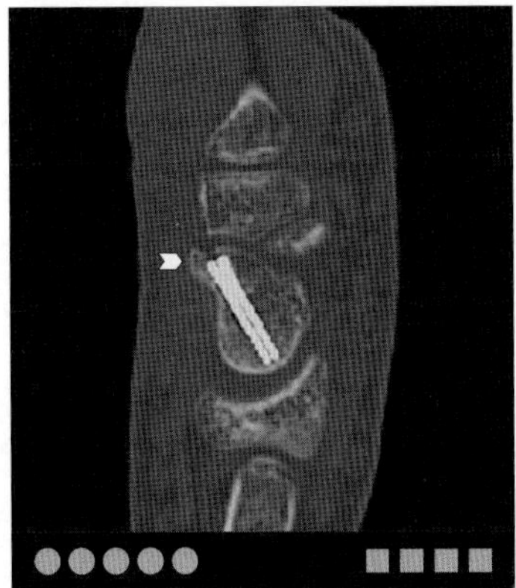

D. Healed scaphoid fracture after Herbert screw placement: Sagittal MPR image from a MDCT of the left wrist demonstrates osseous bridging across the fracture and anatomic alignment with Herbert screw *in situ* (arrow head). Note the lack of sclerosis in the proximal pole.

IMAGE KEY

Common

Rare

Typical

Unusual

DIFFERENTIAL DIAGNOSES IMAGES

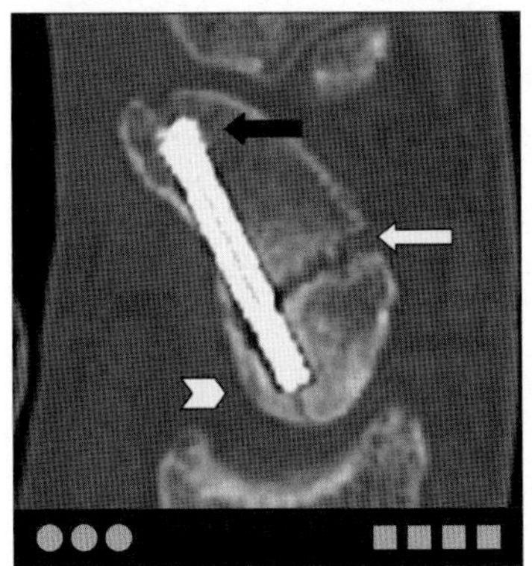

E. Scaphoid Nonunion and ischemic change after Herbert screw placement: Sagittal MPR image from a MDCT of the right wrist demonstrates a Herbert screw in situ (black arrow). The screw was placed six months prior to this scan for a scaphoid fracture. Note that the fracture is still visible (white arrow) and that the fracture lines are corticated. These are radiological signs of nonunion. Note also that the proximal pole is sclerotic (white arrow head). This sclerosis indicates osteonecrosis.

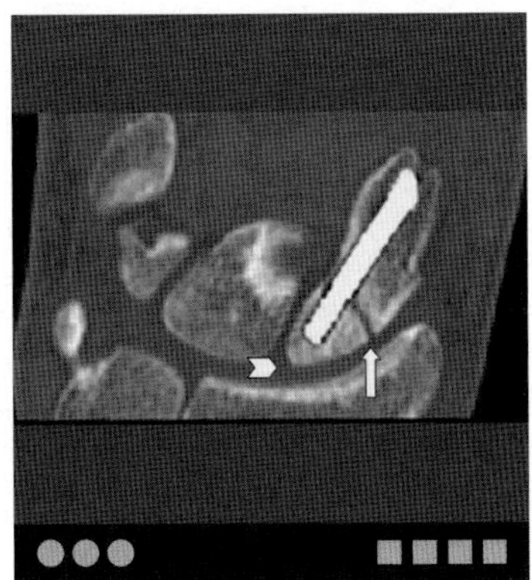

F. Scaphoid nonunion and ischemic change after Herbert screw placement: Coronal MPR image from a MDCT of the right wrist demonstrates cortication about the fracture site (arrow), which indicates nonunion. Note the sclerosis of the proximal pole (arrow head), which is a sign of ischemic changes.

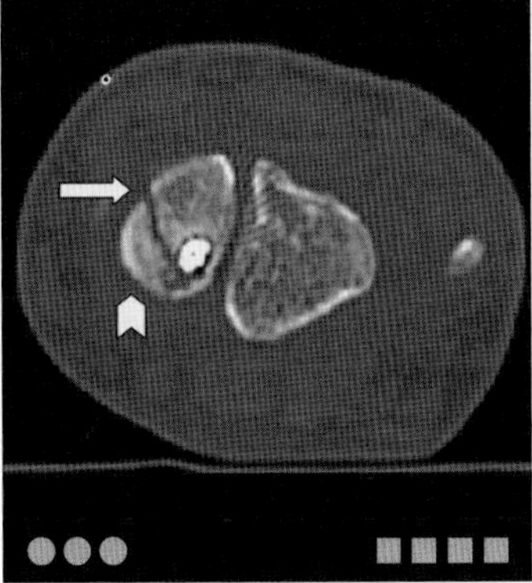

G. Scaphoid nonunion and ischemic change after Herbert screw placement: Axial source image from a MDCT of the right wrist demonstrates a persistent fracture line with cortication (arrow) despite Herbert screw placement. Note the increase in bone density (sclerosis) between the proximal pole of the scaphoid (white arrow head) and the adjacent lunate. The findings indicate nonunion and ischemic changes.

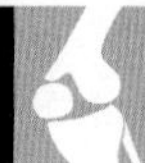

12–5 Hook of Hamate Fracture

Neerjana Doda and Wilfred CG Peh

PRESENTATION

Dorsal wrist pain

FINDINGS

Frontal radiograph does not show any fracture. Axial CT shows a nondisplaced transverse fracture across the base of the hook of hamate.

DIFFERENTIAL DIAGNOSES

- *Scaphoid fractures:* Most common carpal bone fracture. These are classified according to location. Delayed union or nonunion is most frequent in fracture of the proximal pole.
- *Intraarticular fractures:* Isolated fractures of other carpal bones are much less frequent. These may be difficult to detect on radiographs alone and may require special projections or preferably, CT with multiplanar reconstruction.
- *Avascular necrosis:* In the carpal bones, avascular necrosis is most frequently documented in the proximal pole of the scaphoid. This well-known complication develops following a fracture, with a frequency of 10% to 15%. Other carpal bones that may undergo avascular necrosis are the capitate (proximal pole) and the lunate (Kienbock's disease).

COMMENTS

This is a 28-year-old man who fell onto his wrist and complained of persistent pain dorsal wrist pain, diminished grip strength, and ulnar nerve paraesthesia. The hook of the hamate is situated slightly distal and radial to the pisiform. It forms the lateral border of Guyon's canal, which transmits the ulnar nerve and artery to the hand. Fractures of hook are the most common type of hamate fracture, and represent 2% to 4% of carpal fractures. These usually result from fall on the dorsiflexed wrist or from direct impact, e.g., in athletes such as golfers, tennis players, and batters. Clinically, in affected individuals, pain and tenderness occur on the ulnar side of palm. These symptoms may be aggravated by grasp, and result in ulnar nerve weakness and mild carpal tunnel syndrome. Complications of hamate hook fractures include nonunion, ulnar or median nerve injury, and tendon rupture. Avascular changes may follow if this fracture is not treated and immobilized on time. On the frontal radiograph, three radiographic signs have been described: "absence" of the hook of hamate, "sclerosis" of the hook, and lack of cortical density of the hamulus. Presence of these signs may help increase the index of suspicion for a fractured hook of hamate. The carpal tunnel view and special oblique radiograph taken with the wrist supinated are other recommended additional views. Axial 2-mm fine-cuts CT with sagittal and coronal reconstructions have a diagnostic accuracy of 97%, and are the imaging procedure of choice.

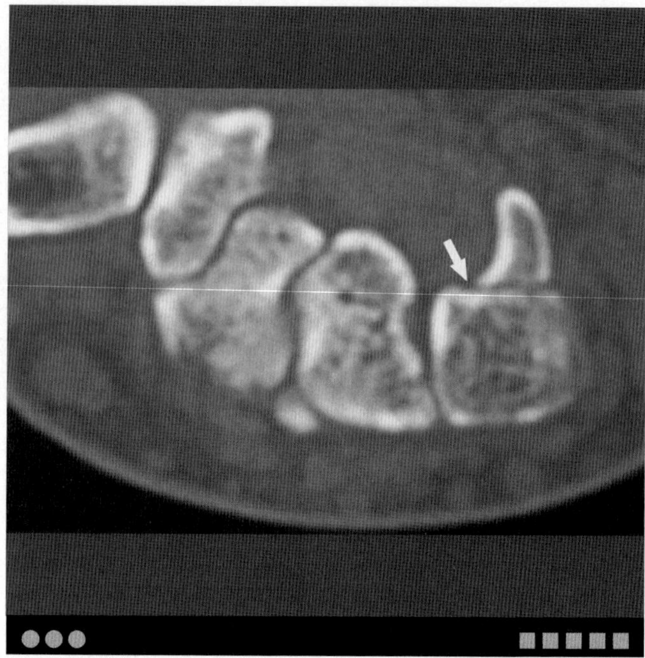

A. Hook of hamate fracture: Hook of hamate fracture. Axial CT image shows a nondisplaced transverse fracture through the base of the hamate (arrow).

PEARLS

- **Usually sports related, particularly in golfers, tennis players, and batters.**
- **Present with dorsal and ulnar wrist pain, diminished grip strength, ulnar nerve paraesthesia.**
- **The diagnosis is often difficult on PA radiographs.**
- **Axial CT, with option of sagittal and coronal reconstruction capability, is the imaging modality of choice.**

ADDITIONAL IMAGE

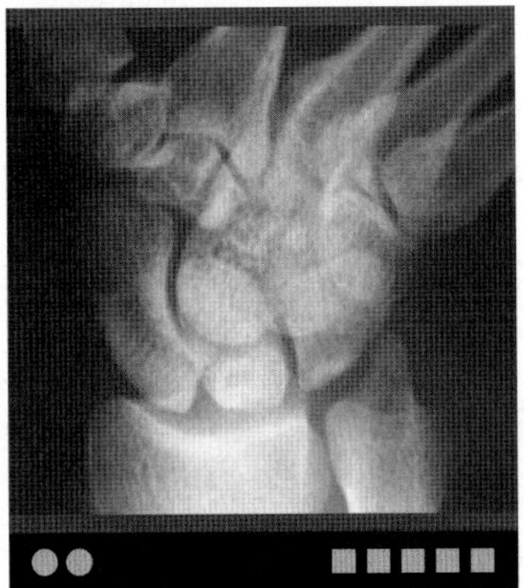

B. Hook of hamate fracture: Frontal radiograph fails to show any carpal bone fracture.

DIFFERENTIAL DIAGNOSES IMAGES

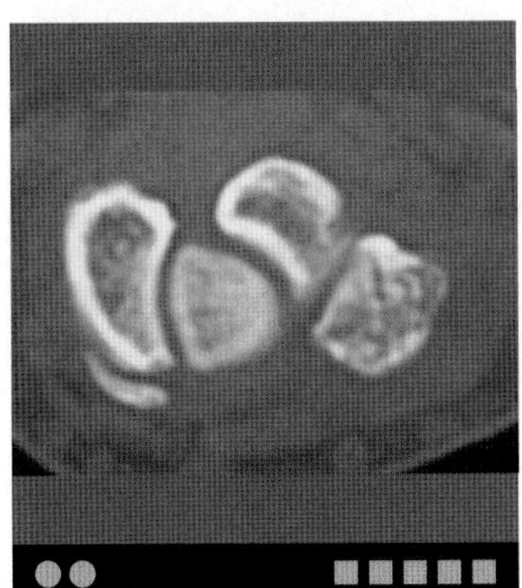

C. Isolated dorsal fracture of the scaphoid: This is a 56-year-old woman. Axial CT image shows a curvilinear bony fragment located dorsal to the scaphoid.

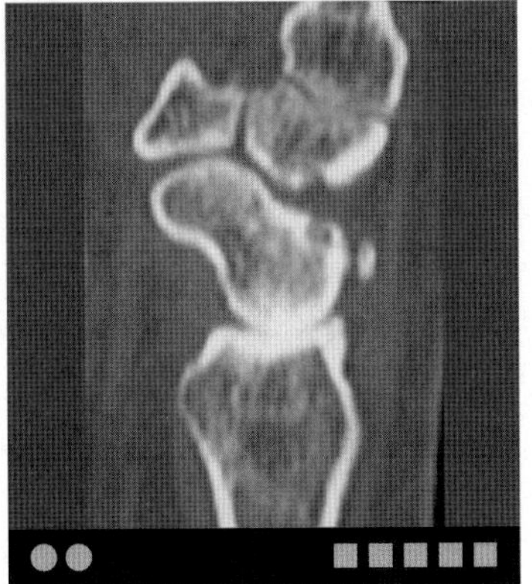

D. Isolated dorsal fracture of the scaphoid: This is a 56-year-old woman. Reconstructed sagittal CT image shows a curvilinear bony fragment located dorsal to the scaphoid.

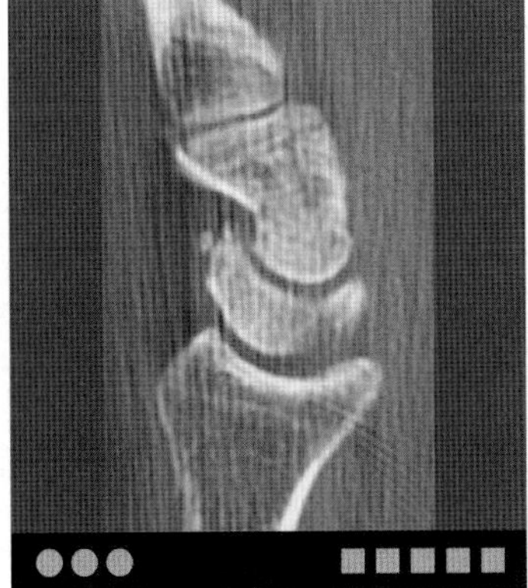

E. Lunate and triquetral fractures: This is a 57-year-old man. Reconstructed sagittal CT image shows a small fracture fragment at the dorsal aspect of the lunate.

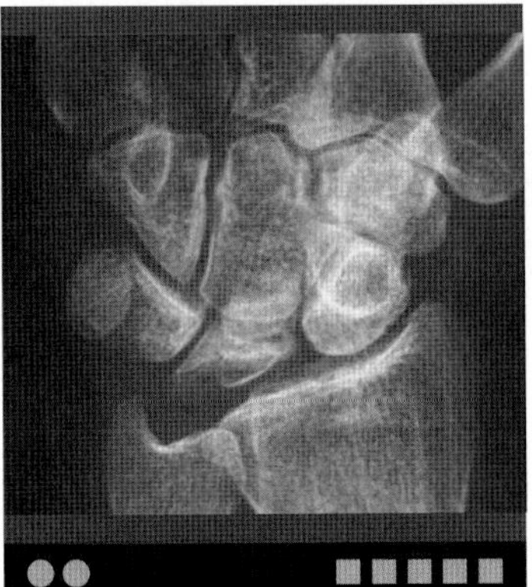

F. Kienbock's disease of the lunate: This is a 23-year-old man. Frontal radiograph shows an irregular sclerotic lunate.

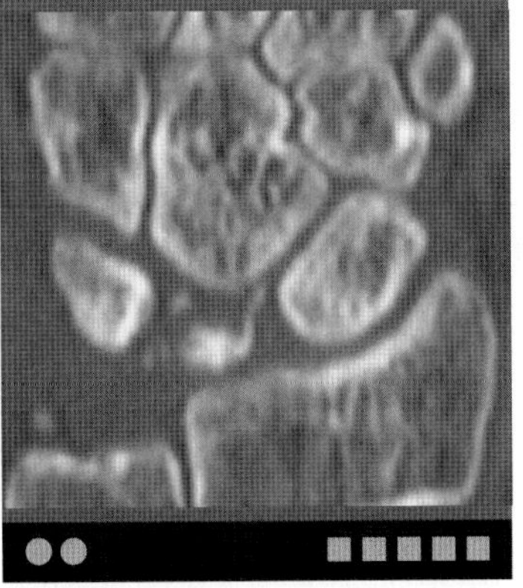

G. Kienbock's disease of the lunate: This is a 23-year-old man. Reconstructed coronal CT image better shows the extent of the sclerotic, collapsed and fragmented lunate.

IMAGE KEY

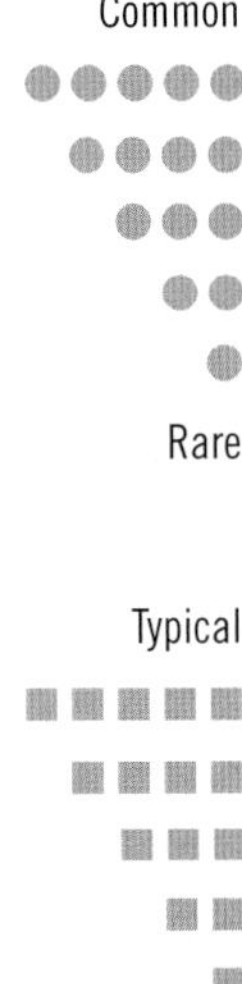

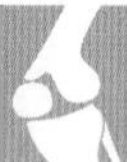

12–6 Hamate Fracture

Amita Sapra and Thomas Learch

PRESENTATION

Ulnar volar wrist pain

FINDINGS

Low signal intensity curvilinear line on T1WI and T2WI with bone edema and adjacent inflammatory change on STIR images.

DIFFERENTIAL DIAGNOSES

- *Bone contusion:* Carpal bone contusion on the ulnar side of the wrist may cause similar pain.
- *Tear of Triangular fibrocartilage:* Creates pain in the ulnar side of the wrist.
- *Kienbock's disease:* Shows low signal on T1WI and may be associated with compression.

COMMENTS

This is a 22-year-old football player who fell with his hand in dorsiflexion. He presented with point tenderness over the medial volar aspect of the distal wrist, with increased pain elicited with palmar flexion or gripping. This is one of the two common mechanisms for a hamate fracture, the other resulting from direct trauma usually secondary to athletic activity using dorsiflexion of the wrist such as baseball, golf, or tennis. Clinically, the patient may describe an immediate pain over the hypothenar eminence. Hamate fractures account for only 2% to 4% of all wrist bone fractures. Fractures of the hamate bone may occur anywhere within this bone although greatest clinical concern is reserved for the hook of hamate fractures as these injuries have high associations with tendon injuries, avascular necrosis, and nonunion. Anatomically, the ulnar artery runs just under the hook of the hamate and evaluation should be performed for possible associated vascular injury. This is a very difficult diagnosis to make clinically as it is rare and radiographs are frequently normal, even with carpal tunnel views.MRI has the capacity to identify the most subtle of fracture lines. T1WI and T2WI show a dark fracture line. At times, a fracture line may not be appreciated even on MRI. STIR or T2 fat suppressed images are ideal for demonstrating focal bone edema within the hamate. Soft tissue edema and high signal intensity fluid may be present in the joint spaces indicating an ongoing inflammatory process.

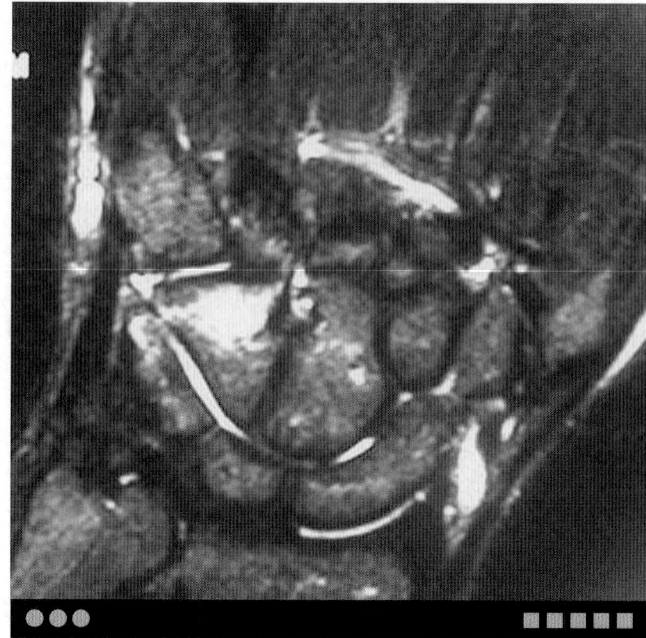

A. Hamate fracture: The coronal STIR image shows marked bone edema and surrounding soft tissue edema.

PEARLS

- **The mechanism of injury is very specific, repetitive athletic activity or fall with a dorsiflexed wrist.**
- **Hook of hamate fractures have a higher incidence of AVN, tendon injury, and nonunion.**
- **T2W, STIR, or fat-suppressed images are ideal for detection of focal bone edema and inflammatory fluid.**

ADDITIONAL IMAGES

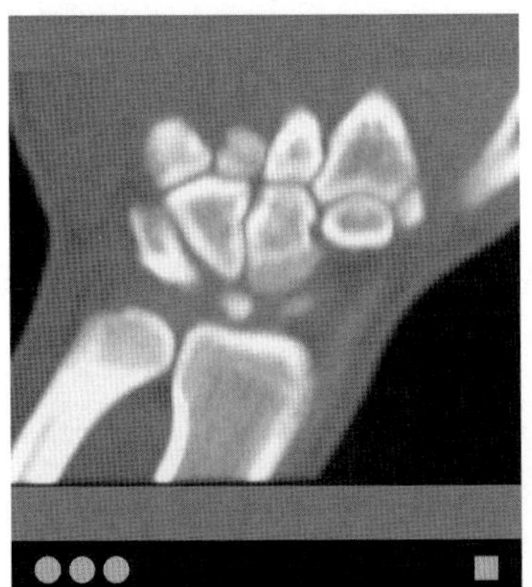

B. Hamate fracture: Coronal CT image is unremarkable.

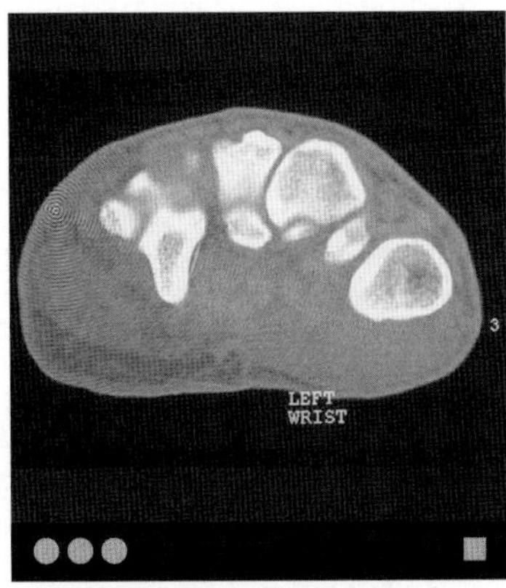

C. Hamate fracture: Axial CT shows no fracture line through the hook of the hamate.

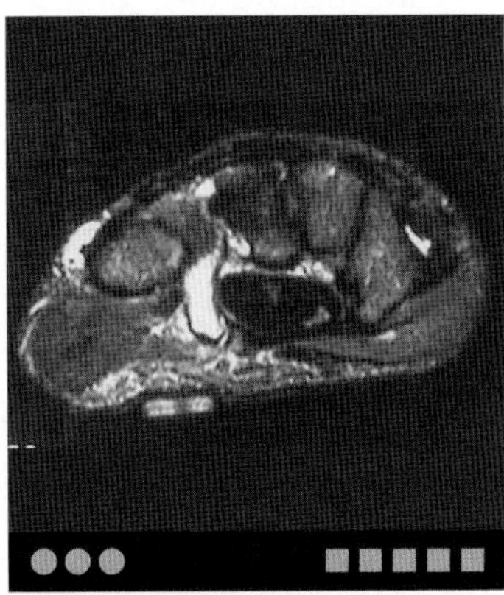

D. Hamate fracture: Axial STIR demonstrates marked bone marrow edema in the hook of the hamate with surrounding soft tissue edema.

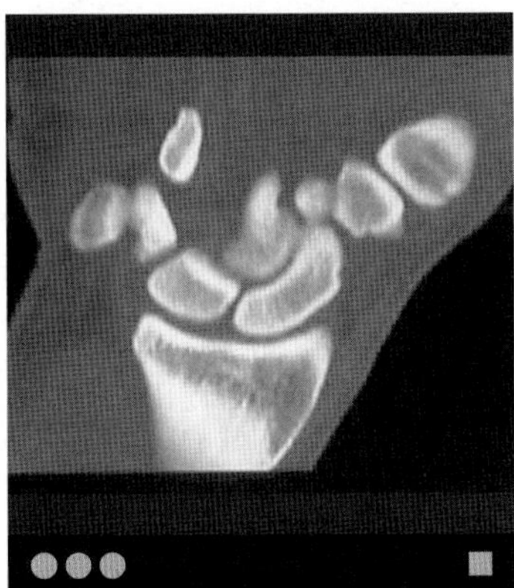

E. Hamate fracture: Coronal CT appears normal.

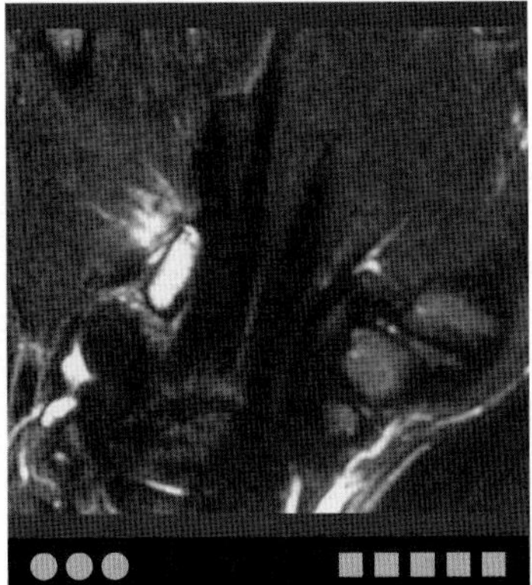

F. Hamate fracture: Coronal STIR image more palmer slice demonstrates bone edema and adjacent inflammatory fluid.

IMAGE KEY

Common

Rare

Typical

Unusual

DIFFERENTIAL DIAGNOSIS IMAGE

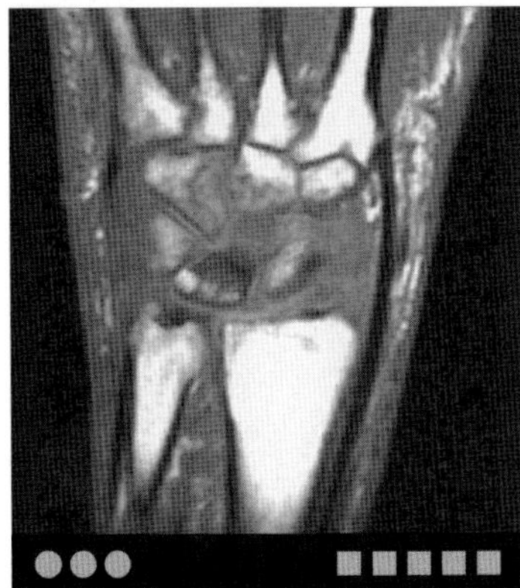

G. Kienbock's disease: Coronal T1WI shows low signal in lunate indicating avascular necrosis.

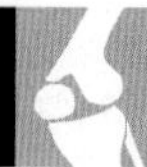

12–7 Scapholunate Ligament Dissociation with DISI

Ashkan Afshin and Shahla Modarresi

PRESENTATION

Wrist pain

FINDINGS

Coronal and sagittal MR images show a wide gap between scaphoid and lunate with intervening fluid signal between scaphoid and lunate indicating tear of scapholunate ligament and rotation of the lunate with the concave surface facing dorsally suggesting dorsal intercalated segmental instability (DISI).

DIFFERENTIAL DIAGNOSES

- *Lunotriquetral ligament tear:* Contrast or fluid in the radiocarpal joint will enter the common carpal joint through the tear of lunotriquetral ligament.
- *TFCC tears:* Arthrogram shows contrast injected in the radiocarpal joint to leak into distal radioulnar recess.
- *Distal radioulnar joint (DRUJ) injury:* Injuries to distal radioulnar ligament with subluxation are best detected by CT or MRI.
- *Ulnar impaction:* This may lead to TFCC tear or osteochondrosis of lunate. Positive ulnar variance and ulnar impaction can be associated with LTL tear and can be seen on radiograph.
- *Scapholunate advanced collapse (SLAC):* A pattern of severe osteoarthritis and malalignment that results from radial-sided wrist pathologies such as scapholunate dissociation with rotatory subluxation of the scaphoid. Other etiologies include inflammatory arthritis such as idiopathic calcium pyrophosphate dihydrate (CPPD) crystal deposition disease.

COMMENTS

The scapholunate ligament connects the proximal pole of scaphoid to lunate and stabilizes the palmar rotation force of the scaphoid against the dorsal rotation force of the lunate allowing relative motion between the two bones. This ligament is composed of three main ligamentous structures: volar, membranous, and dorsal (strongest). The scapholunate ligament tear is the most significant and most common type of ligament injury of wrist. Repetitive wrist rotations in sports such as tennis and baseball and fall on the outstretched hand with the wrist in extension are common mechanisms of this injury. Scapholunate ligament disruption (scapholunate dissociation) can be partial or complete.

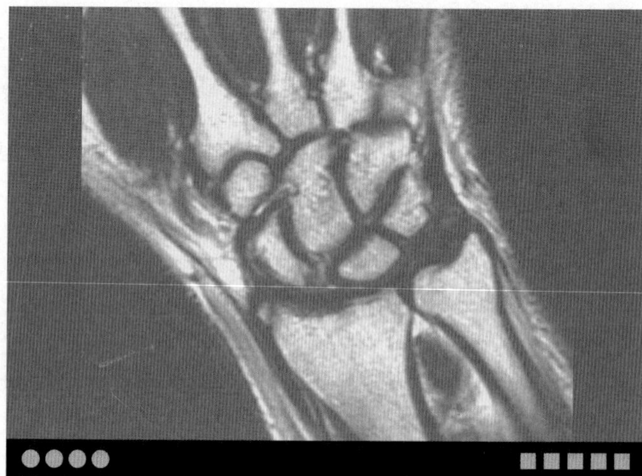

A. Scapholunate ligament dissociation: Coronal proton density image shows fluid signal in the wide gap between scaphoid and lunate.

Complete tear of the scapholunate ligament results in palmar flexion of the scaphoid and dorsiflexion of the lunate. This condition is called scapholunate ligament tear with DISI; the diagnosis of which is normally done on lateral radiograph, when lunate concave surface is facing dorsally. In contrast in volar intercalated segmental instability (VISI) the lunate concave surface is facing anteriorly. Pain and localized tenderness over the anatomical snuffbox are common clinical findings in the patient with scapholunate ligament tear. These patients may also have audible click when rotating the wrist. The association of the ligament tear and distal radial fracture is relatively common. On lateral radiograph of patient with DISI deformity, the scapholunate angle is greater than 70 degree. Radiograph and MRI findings in complete tear of the scapholunate ligament show increased scapholunate gap (Terry Thomas sign), and dorsal tilting of the lunate.

PEARLS

- **The most common type of ligament injury of wrist.**
- **Complete tear results in DISI, which is normally diagnosed on lateral radiograph.**
- **Pain and localized tenderness.**
- **Associated with distal radial fracture.**
- **Scapholunate angle is greater than 70 degrees.**
- **Dissociation between scaphoid and lunate and dorsal tilting of the lunate on MRI.**

ADDITIONAL IMAGES

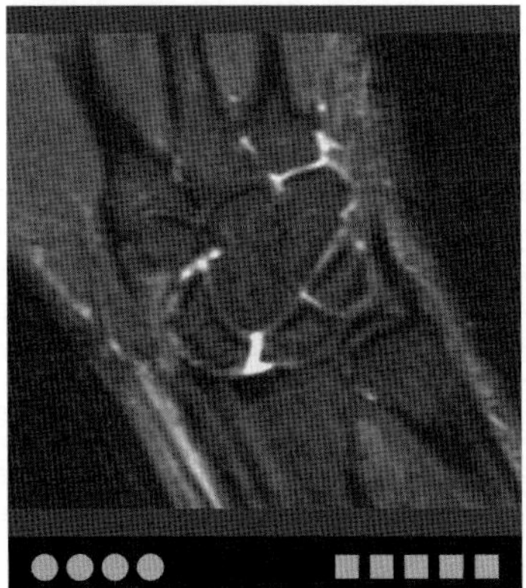

B. Scapholunate ligament dissociation: Coronal fat-saturated T2WI shows fluid signal between scaphoid and lunate.

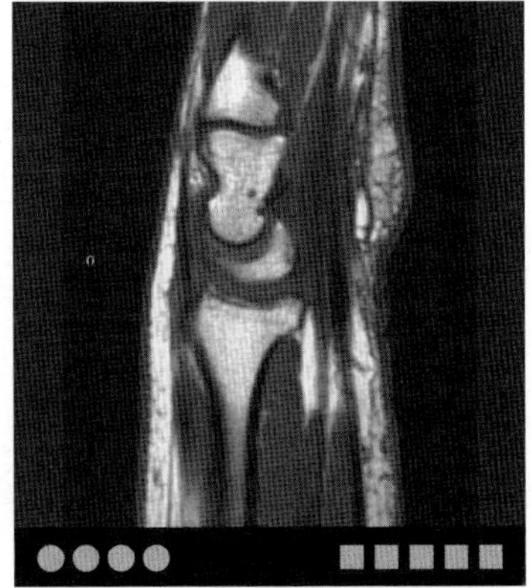

C. Scapholunate ligament dissociation: Sagittal proton density image shows rotation of the lunate with the concave surface facing dorsally suggesting dorsal intercalated segment instability.

DIFFERENTIAL DIAGNOSES IMAGES

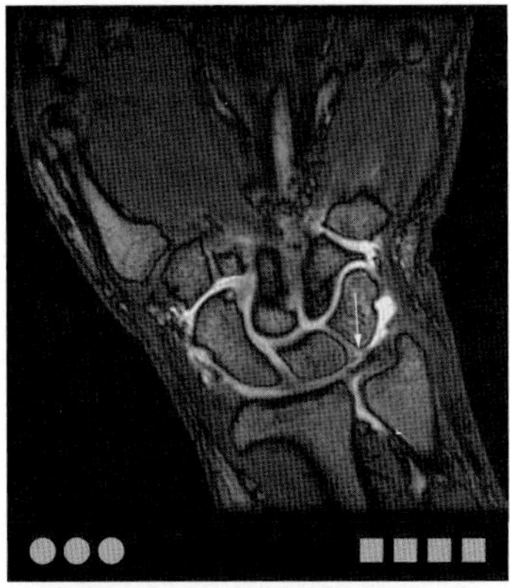

D. Lunotriquetral ligament tear: Coronal 3D gradient echo images at 2-mm intervals show the tear of the lunotriquetral ligament (arrow). The TFCC was intact (arrow).

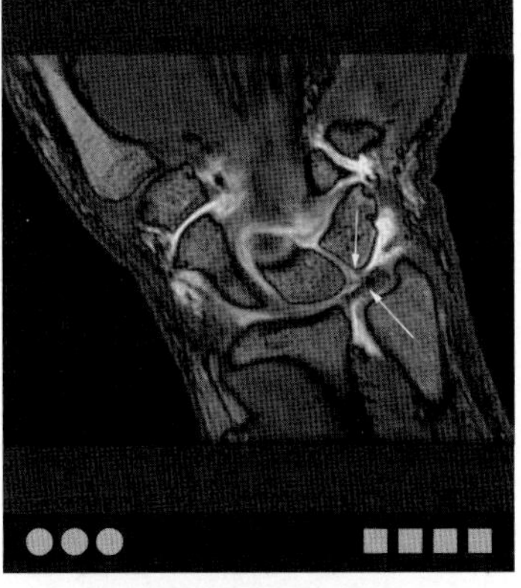

E. Lunotriquetral ligament tear: Coronal 3D gradient echo images at 2-mm intervals show the tear of the lunotriquetral ligament (arrow). The TFCC was intact (arrow).

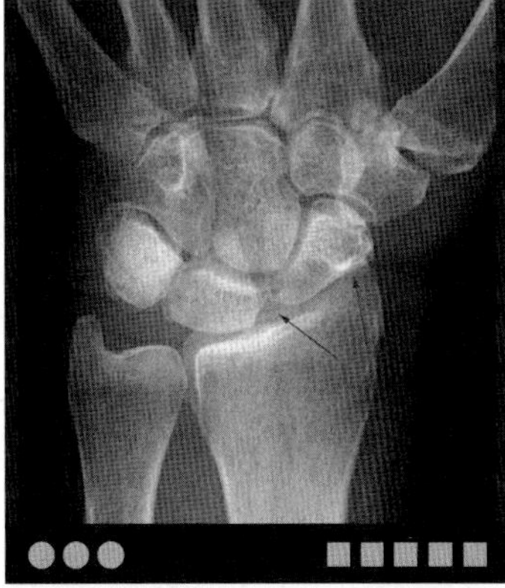

F. Scapholunate advanced collapse (SLAC): A 48-year-old male with remote history of wrist trauma. AP radiograph of the wrist shows typical scapholunate advanced collapse (SLAC) because of chronic SLL tear. Arthritic changes at the radioscaphoid articulation and widening of the scapho-lunate ligament are typical of SLAC (arrows).

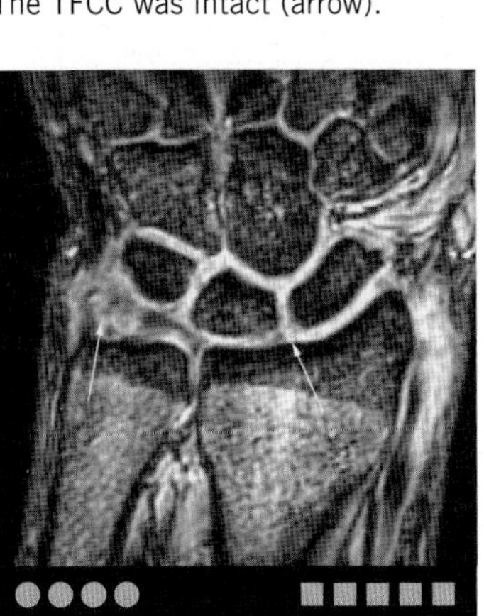

G. Scapholunate advanced collapse (SLAC): Coronal 3D gradient echo image (same patient as in image D) shows tear of the SLL and ulnar attachment of the TFCC (arrows).

IMAGE KEY

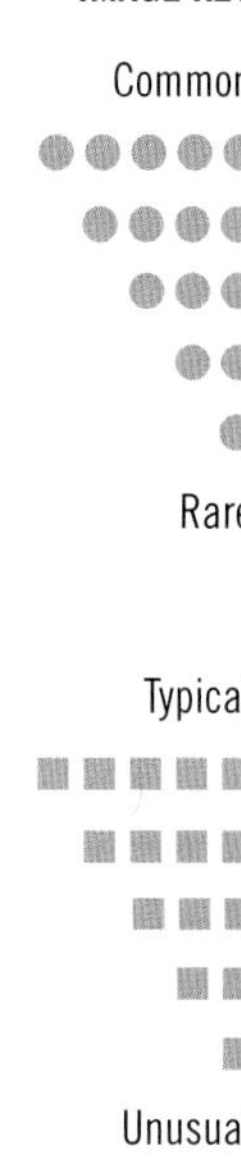

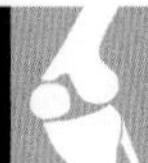

12–8 Lunotriquetral Ligament Tear

John C. Hunter

PRESENTATION

Ulnar-sided wrist pain

FINDINGS

Middle carpal row arthrogram shows extravasation of contrast into the radiocarpal joint via the lunotriquetral space. MR confirms lunotriquetral (LT) ligament tear and sparing of the triangular fibrocartilage (TFCC).

DIFFERENTIAL DIAGNOSES

- *TFCC tears:* Arthrogram shows contrast injected in the radiocarpal joint to leak into distal radioulnar recess.
- *Distal radioulnar joint (DRUJ) injury:* Injuries to distal radioulnar ligament with subluxation are best detected by CT or MRI.
- *Ulnar impaction:* This may lead to TFCC tear or osteochondrosis of lunate. Positive ulnar variance and ulnar impaction can be associated with LTL tear and can be seen on plain films.
- *Extensor carpi ulnaris (ECU) ligament partial tear(subluxation*: This is best detected by MRI.

COMMENTS

This is a 66-year-old male with ulnar-sided wrist pain and no history of antecedent trauma. The lunotriquetral ligament (LTL) is one of the intrinsic ligaments of the wrist. Along with the scapholunate ligament (SLL) and extrinsic ligaments, they insure a smooth, coordinated motion typical of the human wrist joint. This ligament is smaller than the SLL and inserts either on the bone or articular cartilage at the proximal margins of the lunate and triquetrum. The LTL tear is usually secondary to trauma, most often an acute injury although chronic repeated stress may lead to disruption as well. Degenerative processes associated with positive ulnar variance and ulnar impaction syndrome can lead to LTL tear. Small perforations need to be distinguished from clinically significant tears. This distinction can be difficult on imaging alone and require expert clinical correlation. Some have advocated bilateral imaging with MR or conventional arthrography to detect perforation in the opposite, asymptomatic wrist. Unlike the SLL, which can usually be successfully imaged with conventional arthrography, the smaller LTL requires MR arthrography for reliable assessment. While SLL injury may be associated with rotary subluxation of the scaphoid and a dorsal intercalated segmental instability (DISI) deformity, the LTL injury may be associated with a volar intercalated segmental instability (VISI) deformity. Imaging abnormalities of the LTL are generally seen on arthrography and MR with intra-articular contrast. Lateral conventional radiograph may demonstrate VISI deformity. Arthrography may reveal extravasation of injected contrast through the LT space. MRI may reveal disruption of the ligament.

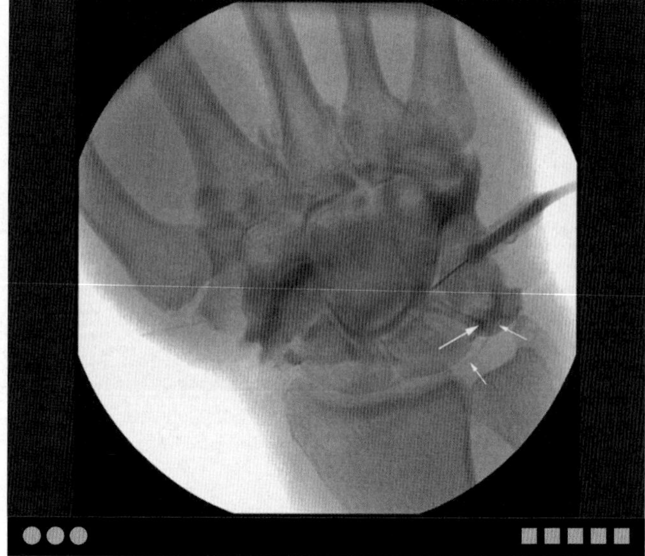

A. Lunotriquetral ligament tear: Middle carpal arthrogram shows extravasation of contrast along the LT space and into the radiocarpal joint.

PEARLS

- **Arthrography is the gold standard for evaluation of the intrinsic ligaments, LTL and SLL.**
- **Contrast injected in the middle carpal row does not normally flow into the radiocarpal space. Contrast injected into the radiocarpal or DRUJ spaces should not extravasate into other spaces.**
- **Ulnar-sided wrist pain has a variety of causes. The combination of arthrography and MR can distinguish tears of the LTL and TFCC. Occult osseous injury and tendon pathology in the ulnar side of the joint can be detected with MR.**
- **Careful attention to the DRUJ is essential in this evaluation: Tears of the TFCC, intrinsic ligaments of this joint and the ECU can be difficult to distinguish clinically.**

ADDITIONAL IMAGES

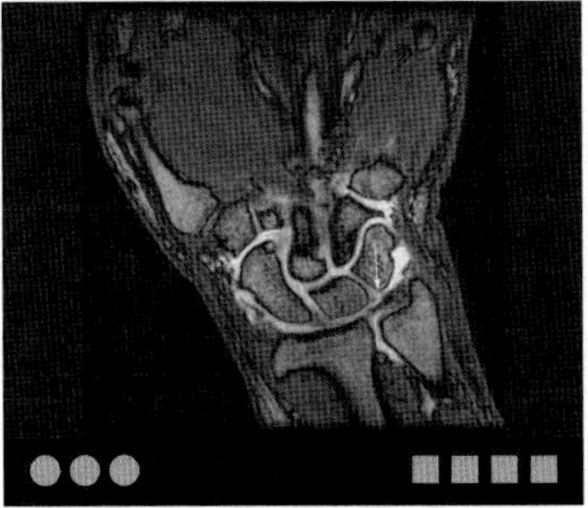

B. Lunotriquetral ligament tear: Coronal 3D gradient echo images at 2-mm intervals show the tear of the LTL (arrow). The TFCC was intact (arrow).

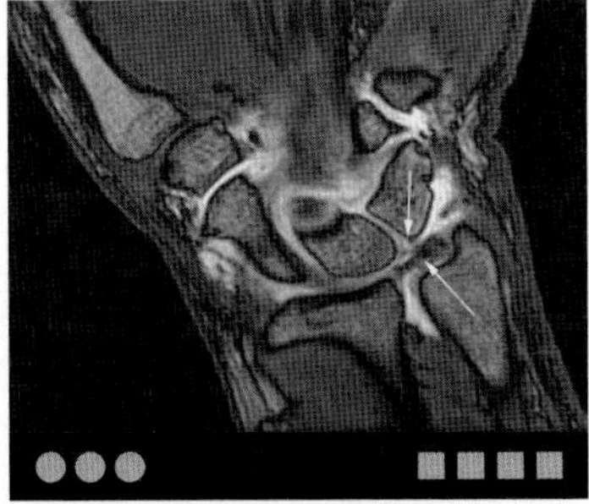

C. Lunotriquetral ligament tear: Coronal 3D gradient echo images at 2-mm intervals show the tear of the LTL (arrow). The TFCC was intact (arrow).

DIFFERENTIAL DIAGNOSES IMAGES

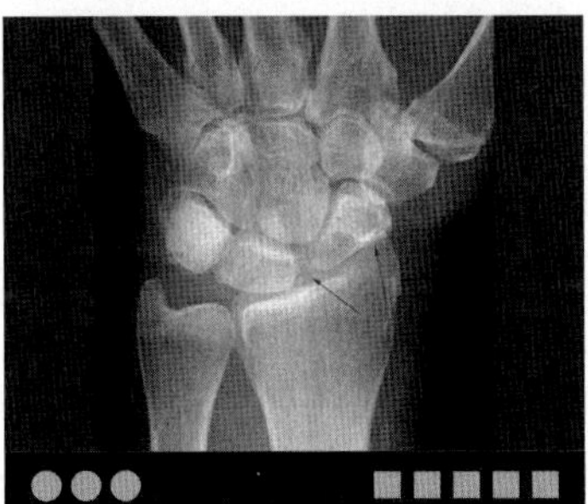

D. Scapholunate advanced collapse: A 48-year-old male with remote history of wrist trauma. AP radiograph of the wrist shows typical scapholunate advanced collapse (SLAC) because of chronic SLL tear. Arthritic changes at the radioscaphoid articulation and widening of the scapho-lunate interval are typical of SLAC (arrows).

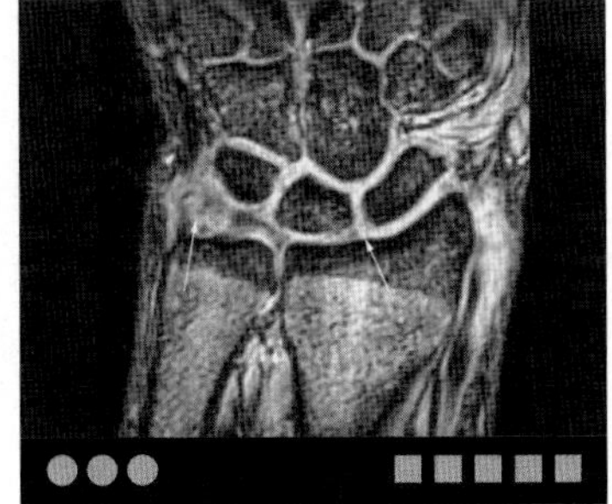

E. Scapholunate advanced collapse: Coronal 3D gradient echo image (same patient as in image D) shows tear of the SLL and ulnar attachment of the TFCC (arrows).

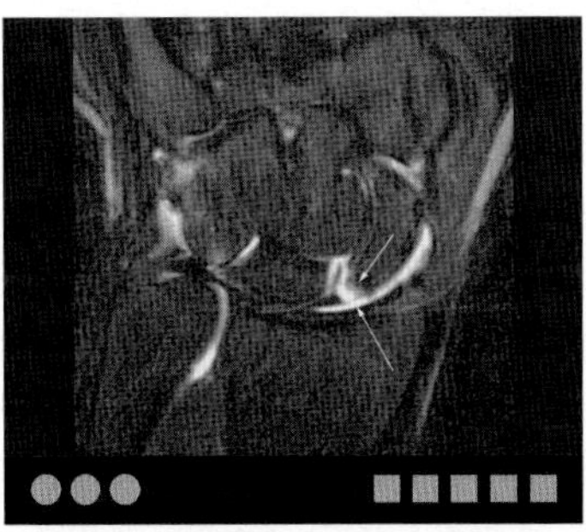

F. Tear of the scapholunate ligament: This is a 30-year-old female with wrist pain following trauma 6 months prior. T2WI with fat saturation shows a tear of the SLL (arrow).

IMAGE KEY

Common

Rare

Typical

Unusual

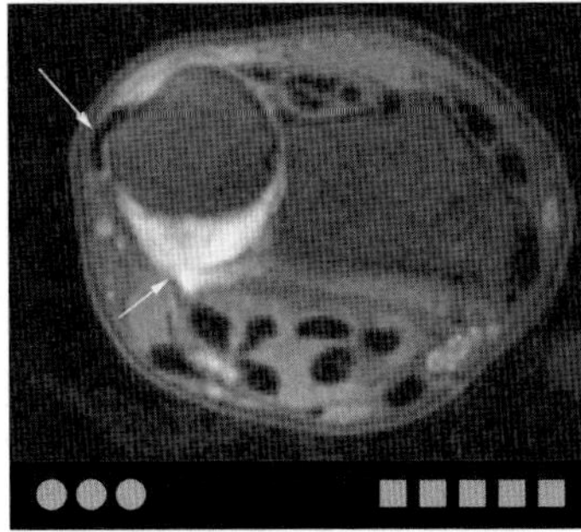

G. Tear of volar radioulnar ligament: This is a 38-year-old male with ulnar-sided pain and "snapping" following injury to wrist. Axial T1WI with fat saturation shows dorsal subluxation of the ulna because of tear of the volar radioulnar ligament (arrows) as well as subluxation of the ECU ligament out of its groove in the dorsum of the ulna (arrow).

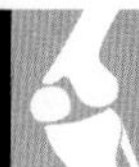

12–9 Triangular Fibrocartilage Complex (TFCC) Tear

Edward Mossop and Jamshid Tehranzadeh

PRESENTATION

Persistent pain in the wrist following trauma

FINDINGS

The defect in TFCC is manifested by contrast fluid crossing over from radiocarpal joint into the distal radioulnar recess.

DIFFERENTIAL DIAGNOSES

- *Ulnar impaction syndrome:* Ulnar impaction can progress from TFCC wear to frank tears, triquetral chondromalacia, and lunotriquetral instability. Radiographs show an ulnar positive variant and, often, cysts in the triquetrum and medial one half of the proximal lunate. MRI reveals signal change and edema in the ulnar head, triquetrum, and lunate.
- *Scapholunate advanced collapse (SLAC):* This refers to a specific pattern of osteoarthritis and subluxation, which results from untreated chronic scapholunate (SL) dissociation or from chronic scaphoid nonunion. MRI shows widening of the SL articulation and may show associated fluid or osteonecrosis.
- Distal radial ulnar joint (DRUJ) arthritis can be associated with TFCC tear. Plain radiographs may reveal osteophytes, joint space narrowing, deformity, or subchondral cysts. When radiographic findings are negative, a CT scan of the DRUJ may reveal degenerative changes of the ulnar head.

COMMENTS

This is a 26-year-old female with persistent left wrist pain. The TFCC is composed of the articular disc (triangular fibrocartilage), meniscus homologue (ulnocarpal), ulnocarpal ligament, dorsal and volar radioulnar ligament, and extensor carpi ulnaris sheath. The function of the TFCC is to provide an articular sling for the lunate and triquetrum as the cartilage rotates over the head of the ulna. The mechanism of injury to the TFCC is generally compression between the lunate and the ulna. Traumatic injury can occur with acute rotational force or from an axial compression(distraction force to the ulnar carpus. Degenerative lesions may develop a repetitive loading of the TFCC secondary to forearm rotation. The most common site of tears in the TFCC is parallel to the sigmoid notch of the radius; second most common, central perforation of the triangular fibrocartilage (TFC) disk proper; third, parallel to the dorsal capsular attachment; and the fourth, parallel to the volar capsular attachment. Only the peripheral 15% to 20% TFCC has a blood supply therefore tears can be repaired. In contrast, tears in the central avascular area must be debrided, as they have no potential for healing. MR arthrography is a valuable tool in the evaluation of tears of the TFCC. Discontinuity of the TFCC and leakage of contrast material into the distal radioulnar joint indicates TFCC perforation. However, clinical correlation is essential in the diagnosis. On fat-saturated T1WI this appears as bright signal fluid crossing the TFCC and extending into the distal radioulnar recess.

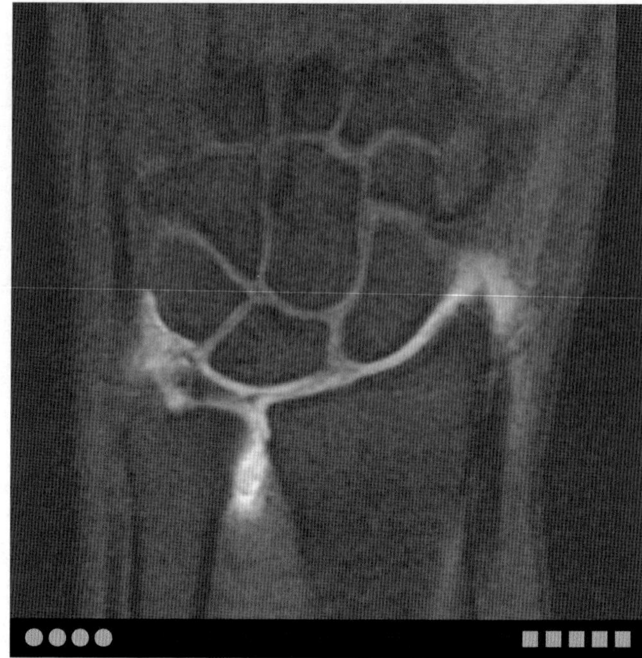

A. TFCC tear: Coronal T1 fat-saturated postcontrast arthrogram shows bright signal contrast fluid extending from the radiocarpal joint into the distal radioulnar recess indicating perforation of the TFCC.

PEARLS

- **The function of the TFCC is to provide an articular sling for the lunate and triquetrum as the cartilage rotates over the head of the ulna.**
- **The most common site of tears in the TFCC is parallel to the sigmoid notch of the radius.**
- **Only the peripheral 15% to 20% TFCC has a blood supply therefore tears can be repaired.**
- **Discontinuity of the TFCC and leakage of contrast material into the distal radioulnar joint indicates TFCC tear or perforation.**

ADDITIONAL IMAGES

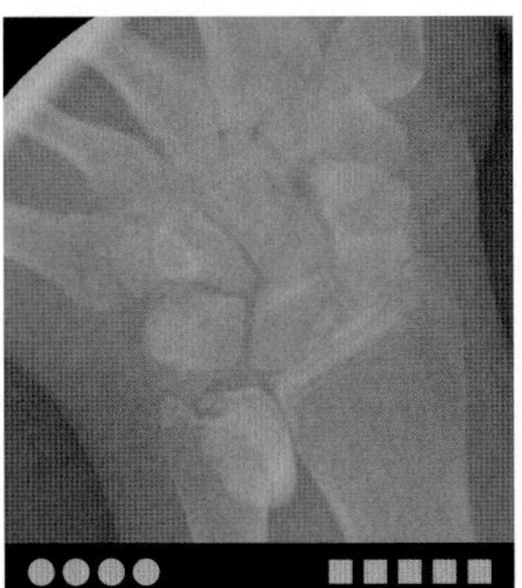

B. TFCC tear: AP radiograph following arthrogram of the radiocarpal joint shows filling of the distal radioulnar recess indicating tear of the TFCC.

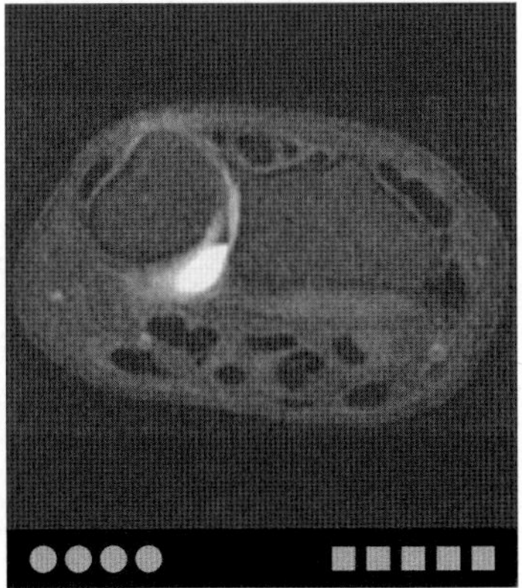

C. TFCC tear: Axial T1 postcontrast image at the level of the distal radioulnar recess shows presence of bright contrast fluid in the distal radioulnar recess.

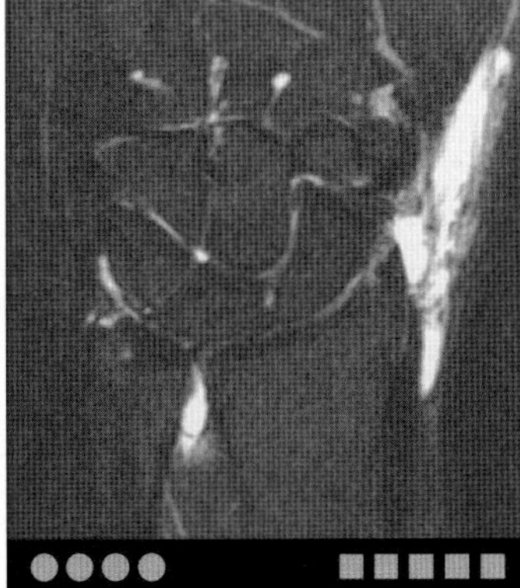

D. TFCC tear: Coronal T2 fat-saturated image shows presence of fluid in the radiocarpal joint and distal radioulnar recess indicating tear of TFCC.

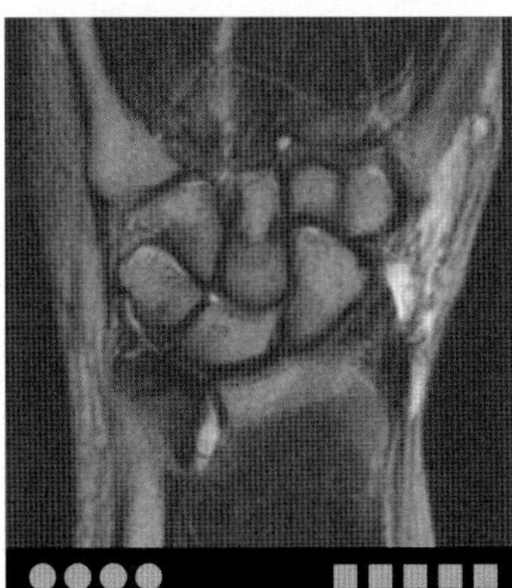

E. TFCC tear: Coronal T2WI shows presence of fluid in the radiocarpal joint and distal radioulnar recess indicating tear of TFCC.

IMAGE KEY

Common

Rare

Typical

Unusual

DIFFERENTIAL DIAGNOSES IMAGES

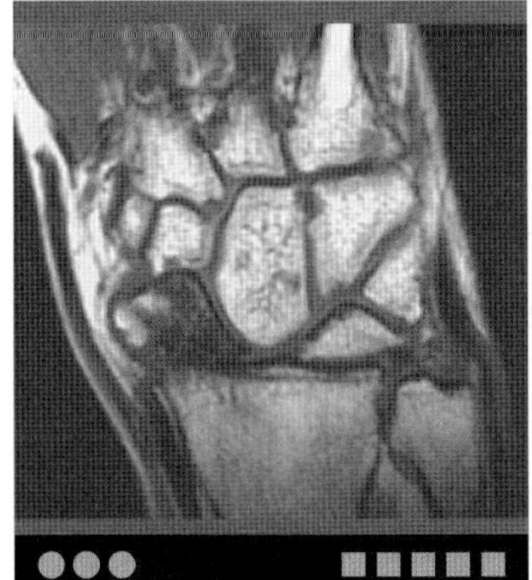

F. SLAC wrist: Coronal T1WI shows severe widening of the scapholunate articulation as well as marked proximal capitate migration. Note the diffuse marrow hypointensity in the proximal scaphoid consistent with osteonecrosis.

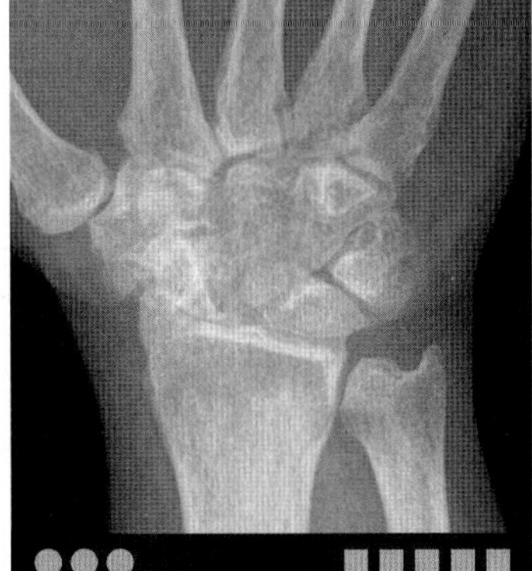

G. SLAC wrist: PA radiograph of the wrist in the same patient as image F shows the fracture is the cause of the osteonecrosis shown above. There is evidence of secondary osteoarthritis and fragmentation of the distal scaphoid.

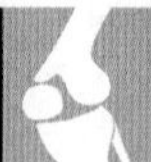

12–10 Ulnar Impaction Syndrome

Amilcare Gentili

PRESENTATION

Wrist pain

FINDINGS

MR images show erosion ulnar plus, tear of the triangular fibrocartilage, and bone marrow changes in the triquetrum and lunate.

DIFFERENTIAL DIAGNOSES

- *Kienböck disease:* Bone marrow changes in the lunate are more extensive and usually involve also the radial side of the lunate.
- *Ulnar styloid impaction:* The lunate is spared, proximal pole of the triquetral bone and the ulnar styloid process are involved.
- *Intraosseous ganglia:* Limited to the lunate or triquetrum, often with well defined border on radiographs.

COMMENTS

This is a 60-year-old man with malunion of distal radius fracture with ulnar impaction syndrome after fracture of the distal radius, resulting in radial shortening. Ulnar impaction syndrome, also known as ulnar abutment or ulnar-carpal loading, is a degenerative condition characterized by chronic ulnar wrist pain caused by impaction of the distal ulna against the proximal lunate and triquetrum. The pain is exacerbated by activity and relieved by rest. Ulnar impaction is often associated with positive ulnar variance, but rarely can be seen with normal and even negative ulnar variance. Common predisposing factors include congenital positive ulnar variance, malunion of the distal radius, premature physeal closure of the distal radius, and previous radial head resection. MR imaging demonstrates cartilage abnormalities in the ulnar head lunate and triquetrum. Bone marrow changes are often present in the ulnar side of the lunate less frequently in the radial side of the triquetrum and distal ulna. These bone marrow changes range from bone hyperemia, characterized by low signal intensity on T1-weighted images and high signal intensity on T2WI, to bone sclerosis manifested by low signal intensity on both T1WI and T2WI, to subchondral cyst formation. MR imaging is also useful in demonstrating tears of the triangular fibrocartilage and lunotriquetral ligament. Ulnar impaction syndrome is treated by means of mechanical decompression of the distal radioulnar articulation by either an ulnar-shortening osteotomy or resection of portion of the radial head. After treatment bone marrow changes may revert to normal.

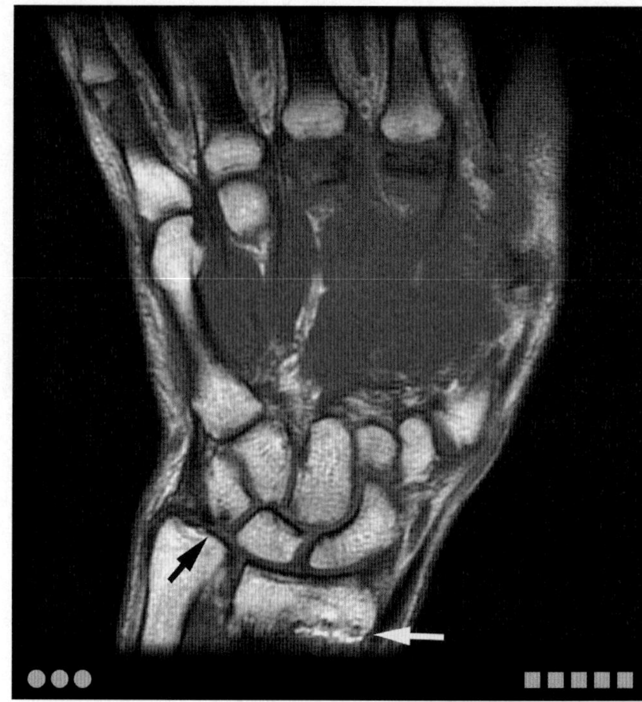

A. Ulnar impaction syndrome: Coronal T1W MR image shows positive ulnar variance, tear of the triangular fibrocartilage (black arrow), and bone marrow changes in the triquetrum. Note fracture of the distal radius (white arrow).

PEARLS

- **Usually is associated with positive ulnar variance.**
- **The ulnar side of the lunate is most commonly involved.**

ADDITIONAL IMAGES

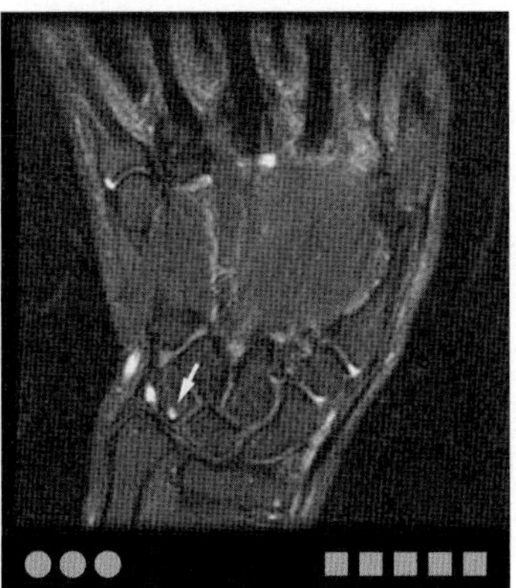

B. Ulnar impaction syndrome: Coronal T2 fat-saturated MR image shows positive ulnar variance, bone marrow changes in the triquetrum (white arrow).

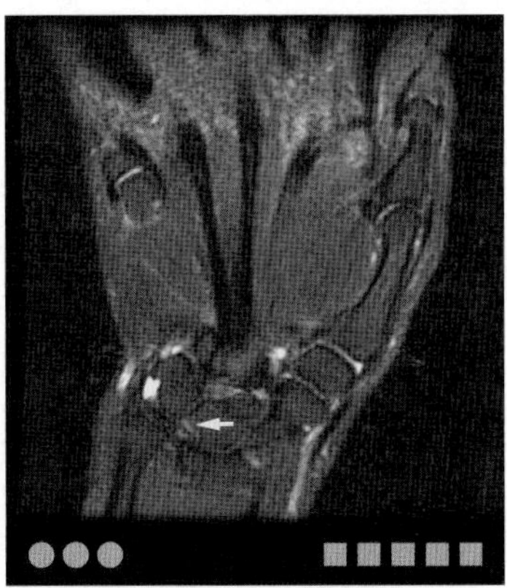

C. Ulnar impaction syndrome: Coronal T2 fat-saturated MR image shows positive ulnar variance, bone marrow changes in the ulnar side of the lunate (white arrow).

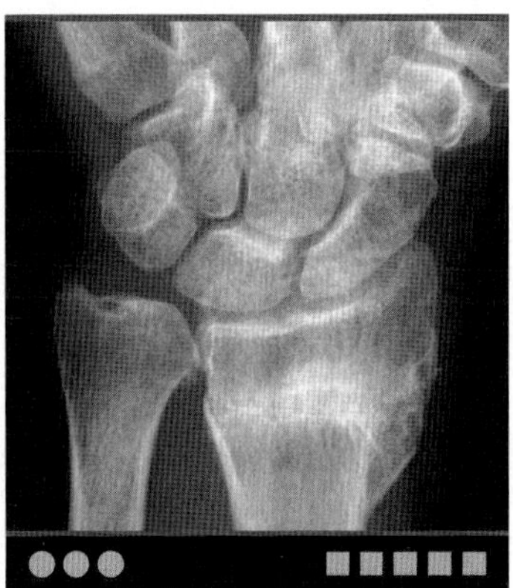

D. Ulnar impaction syndrome: Radiograph of the wrist shows an old fracture of the radius and small subchondral cyst in the triquetrum and lunate.

DIFFERENTIAL DIAGNOSES IMAGES

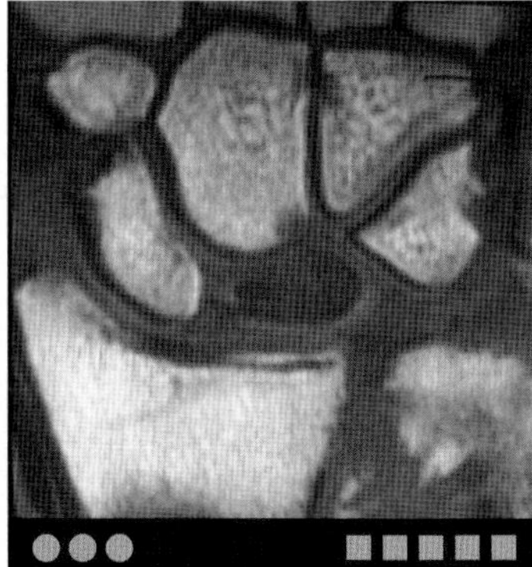

E. Kienböck disease: Coronal T1W MR image shows low signal intensity in the entire lunate.

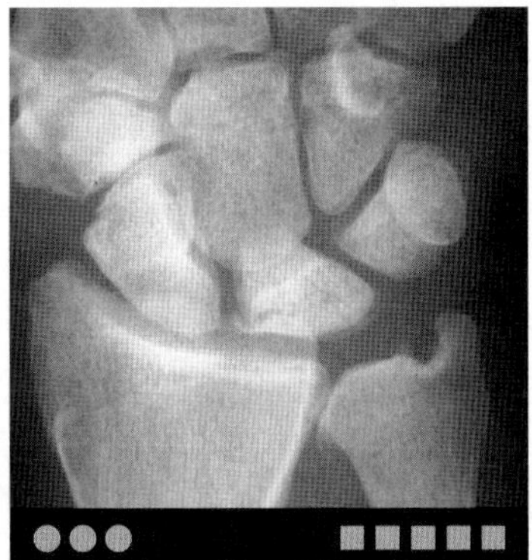

F. Kienböck disease: Radiograph of the wrist shows a dense lunate with collapse.

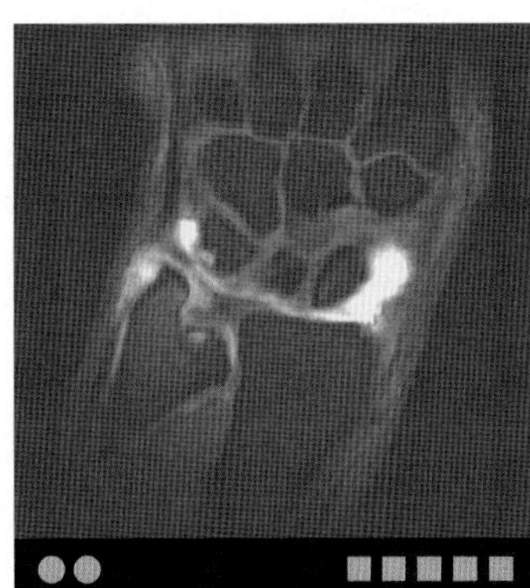

G. Ulnar styloid impaction: Coronal T2 fat saturated MR image shows ulnar minus, an enlarged ulnar styloid, and bone marrow changes in the triquetrum.

IMAGE KEY

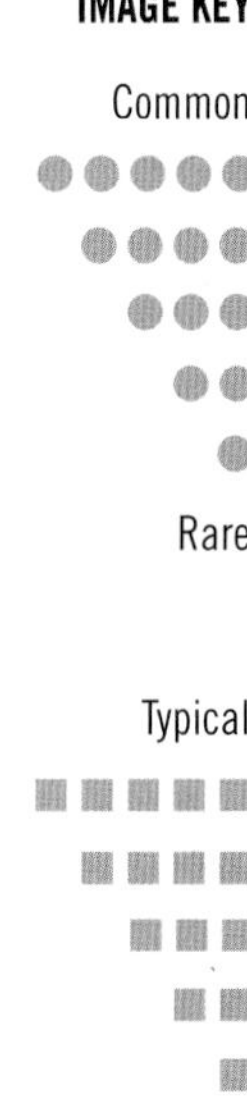

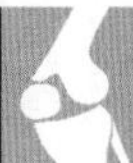

12–11 Ganglion Cyst with Compression of Ulnar Artery

Joseph C. Giaconi and Thomas Learch

PRESENTATION

Wrist pain

FINDINGS

MRI shows large, fluid filled mass in the wrist with medial deviation of ulnar artery.

DIFFERENTIAL DIAGNOSES

- *Giant cell tumor of tendon sheath:* Differs from ganglion cyst in that giant cell tumors are solid. Giant cell tumors are low signal on T2W sequences.
- *Palmar fibromatosis:* Solid mass in palmar soft tissues with low signal on T2W sequences.

COMMENTS

This is a 35-year-old man who complained of wrist pain. MR angiogram was performed initially because of pulsatile wrist mass on physical examination. MRA demonstrates intact arteries of the hand and wrist, with medial deviation of the ulnar artery due to extrinsic mass effect. There was no tumor blush. A ganglion cyst is a mucin filled cyst occurring adjacent to a joint capsule or tendon sheath and is the most common soft tissue mass of the hand. The most common sites of occurrence are on the dorsum of the wrist (60%–70%) over the scapholunate ligament, the volar wrist (20%), the flexor tendon sheath of the fingers (10%), or at the fingertip just below the cuticle where they are known as "mucous cysts." Ganglion cysts are more common in women and 70% are found in people 20 to 40 years old. The exact cause of ganglion cysts is unknown, but theories suggest they result from trauma or tissue irritation. These cysts consist of an outer fibrous coat comprised of collagen. The content of the cyst is a viscous mucin consisting of hyaluronic acid, albumin, globulin, and glucosamine. Ganglion cysts usually appear singly, but may be multifocal. MRI findings demonstrate a fluid-filled structure with smooth margins, which is low signal on T1 and high signal on T2 sequences. The walls of the cyst are thin and fibrous, which are low signal on both T1 and T2 sequences. There is no contrast enhancement, which is critical in differentiating it from other tumors.

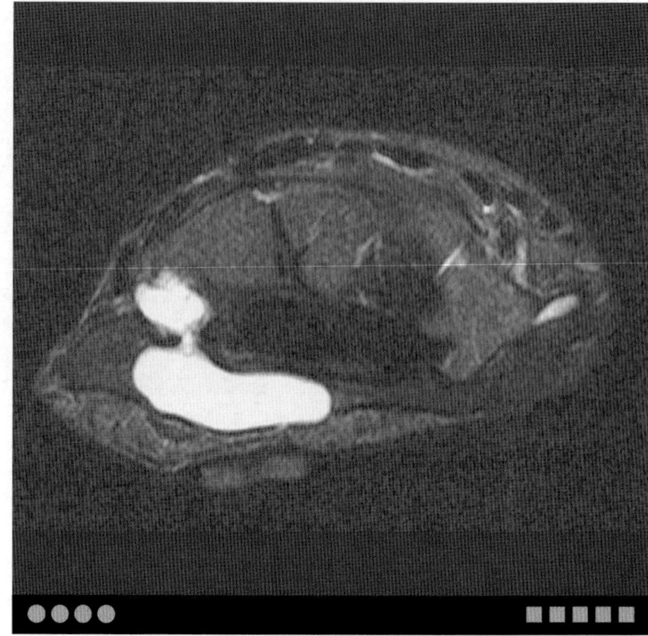

A. Ganglion cyst: Transverse STIR demonstrates large fluid-filled mass arising from pisiform- triquetral articulation, consistent with ganglion cyst.

PEARLS

- **Most common soft tissue mass in wrist.**
- **On physical exam, may feel very hard and firm because of high pressure inside the cyst.**
- **MRI findings are pathognomonic: well-marginated mass next to a joint or tendon sheath which follows fluid signal.**
- **Treatment consists of immobilization, aspiration, or surgical excision.**

ADDITIONAL IMAGES

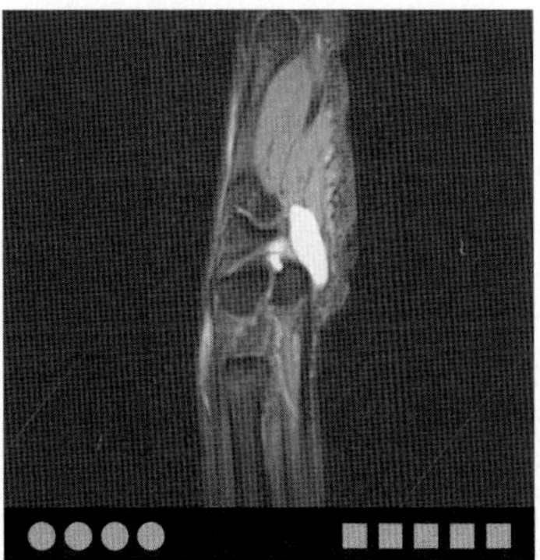

B. Ganglion cyst: Sagittal gradient echo again demonstrates the ganglion cyst as a fluid filled mass, which is high signal.

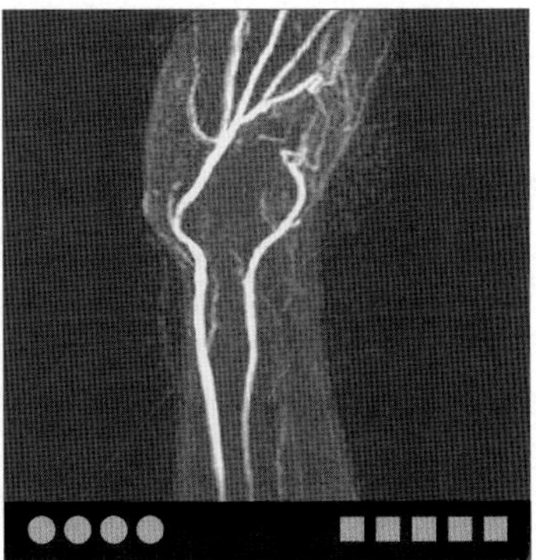

C. Ganglion cyst: Coronal MRA of wrist. MR angiogram was initially ordered in this patient because of pulsatile wrist mass. MRA demonstrates displacement and deviation of ulnar artery from mass, with no tumor blush, consistent with ganglion cyst.

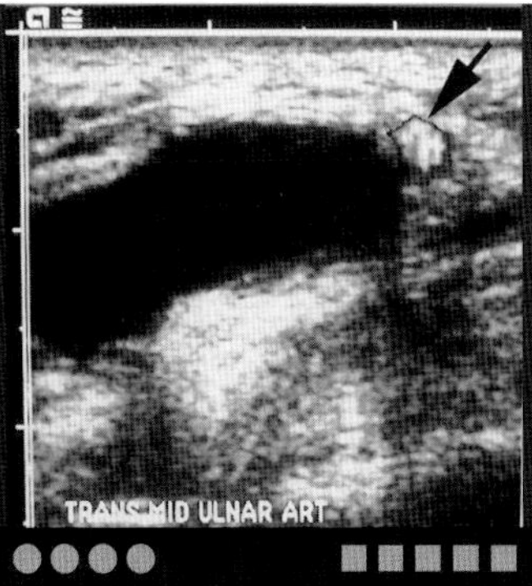

D. Ganglion cyst: Transverse Doppler ultrasound of ganglion cyst. Note posterior acoustic enhancement. The ulnar artery (arrow) is displaced medially by the cyst.

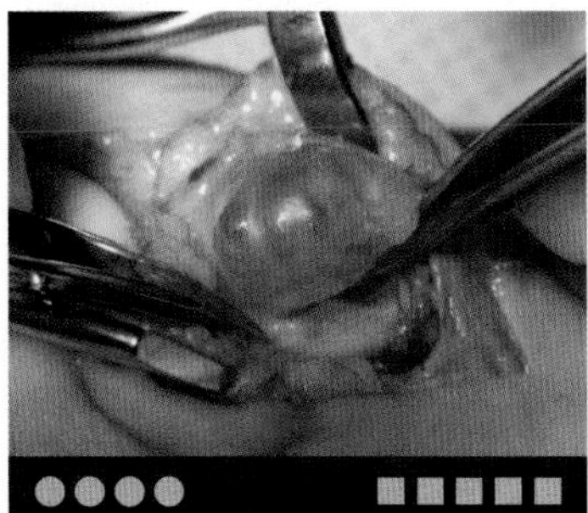

E. Ganglion cyst: Operative photograph during removal of ganglion cyst.

DIFFERENTIAL DIAGNOSES IMAGES

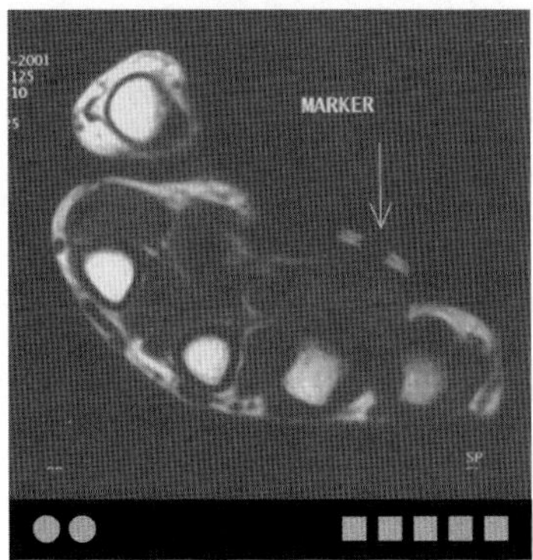

F. Palmar fibromatosis: Transverse T1WI of hand demonstrates mass in subcutaneous tissues with low signal on T1 sequence, consistent with palmar fibromatosis.

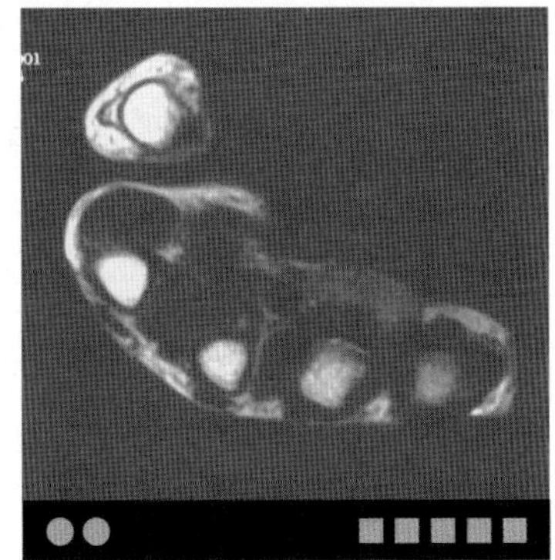

G. Palmar fibromatosis: Transverse T2WI of the hand demonstrates mass in subcutaneous tissues with low signal on both T1 (image F) and T2 sequences, consistent with palmar fibromatosis.

IMAGE KEY

Common

Rare

Typical

Unusual

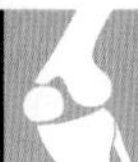

12–12 De Quervain Tenosynovitis

Peyman Borghei and Jamshid Tehranzadeh

PRESENTATION

Wrist pain

FINDINGS

MRI shows thickening of abductor pollicis longus (APL) and extensor pollicis brevis (EPB) tendons and enhancement of tendon sheath on postcontrast fat-saturated T1WI.

DIFFERENTIAL DIAGNOSES

- *Schwannoma:* Manifests as a well-defined lesion with oval- or spindle-shaped appearance. MRI shows low-to-intermediate signal on T1WI and high signal on T2WI.
- *Ganglion cyst:* Is a soft tissue mass usually attached to tendon sheath or bone surface and may be associated with periosteal new bone formation.
- *Giant cell tumor of tendon sheath:* MRI shows lobulated lesion with decreased signal intensity on both T1WI and T2WI.
- *Pseudoaneurysm:* Fusiform or saccular mass often complicated with hemorrhage and thrombosis. Thrombosis manifests as dark lesions on both T1WI and T2WI.

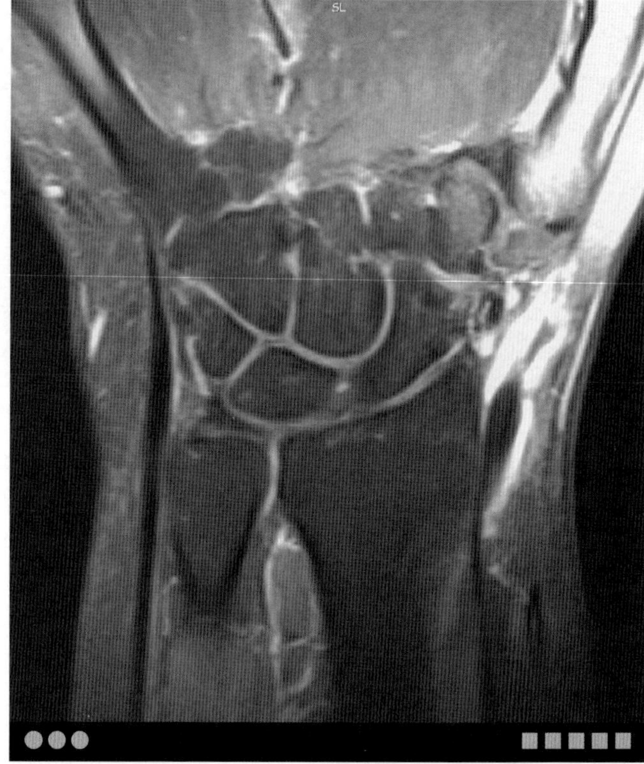

A. De Quervain tenosynovitis: Coronal T1W fat-saturated postcontrast image shows enhancement of synovial sheath of EPB and APL tendons.

COMMENTS

This is a 36-year-old female with the complaint of wrist pain diagnosed with De Quervain tenosynovitis. De Quervain tenosynovitis is usually seen in the women between the ages of 35 and 50 years because of repetitive movements of the hands such as grasping and pinching. It involves the tendons of APL and EPB while on their pathway passing side to side through the first dorsal compartment tunnel or extensor retinaculum. The walls of the tendon sheath becomes inflamed which causes the patient's symptoms which is gradual onset of pain over the radial styloid. The pain might radiate to the thumb or to the forearm. Physical examination may reveal tenderness and thickness of the mentioned tendons. The thickness of the tendon might limit the motion of the hand at the wrist level sometimes associated with "stop and go" sensation or a squeaking sound while moving the thumb. Frankelstein test (bending of the wrist toward the little finger while the patient makes a fist with the fingers over the thumb) usually provokes pain and is diagnostic. MRI shows thickening of APL and EPB tendons and enhancement of tendon sheath on post-contrast fat-saturated T1WI. Fluid signal would be detected in tendon sheath on T2WI. MRI also demonstrates the extent of the lesion and rules out other anatomic lesion.

PEARLS

- **De Quervain tenosynovitis usually occurs in 35- to 50-year-old women who have repetitive motion of the hand.**
- **It involves the APL and EPB tendons at the level of first dorsal compartment tunnel.**
- **MRI shows thickening of APL and EPB tendons and enhancement of tendon sheath on postcontrast fat-saturated T1WI. Fluid signal would be detected in tendon sheath on T2WI.**

ADDITIONAL IMAGES

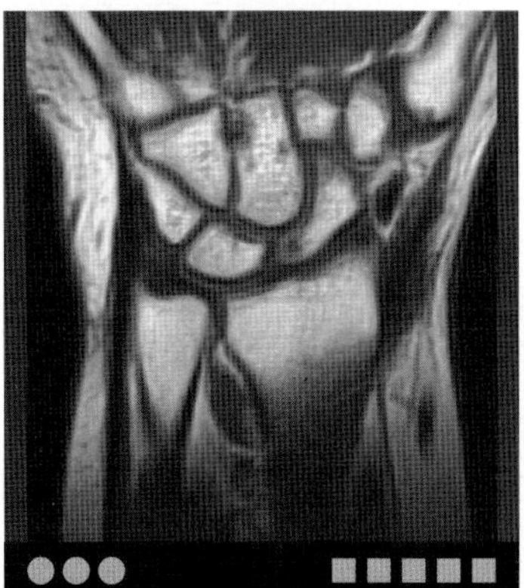

B. De Quervain tenosynovitis: Coronal T1WI shows decreased signal intensity around the tendons of EPB and APL indicating thickening of the tendon sheath right over the radial styloid process.

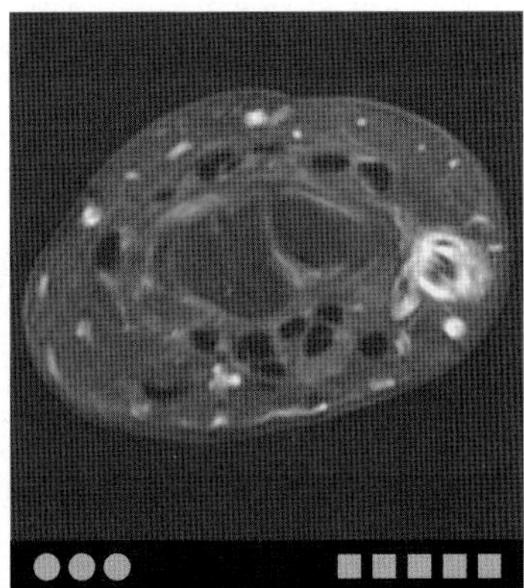

C. De Quervain tenosynovitis: Axial T1W fat-saturated postcontrast image shows enhancement of synovial sheath of EPB and APL tendons in the first dorsal extensor compartment.

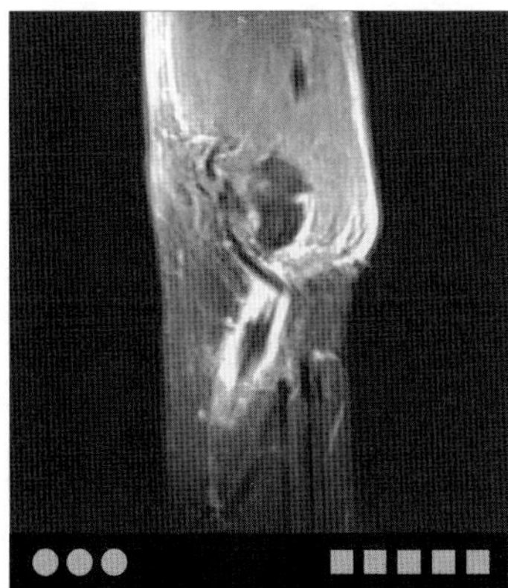

D. De Quervain tenosynovitis: Sagittal T1W fat-saturated postcontrast image shows thickening of the tendon and tendon sheath of EPB and APL with surrounding soft tissue inflammation.

DIFFERENTIAL DIAGNOSES IMAGES

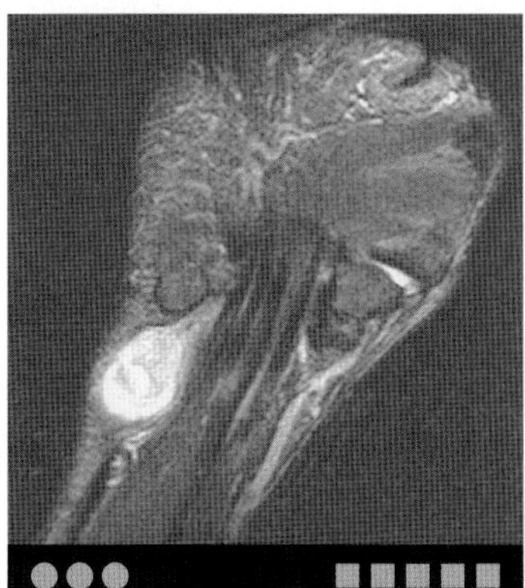

E. Schwannoma: Coronal STIR images demonstrates high signal intensity mass with central low signal intensity with positive "String" sign and " Target" sign.

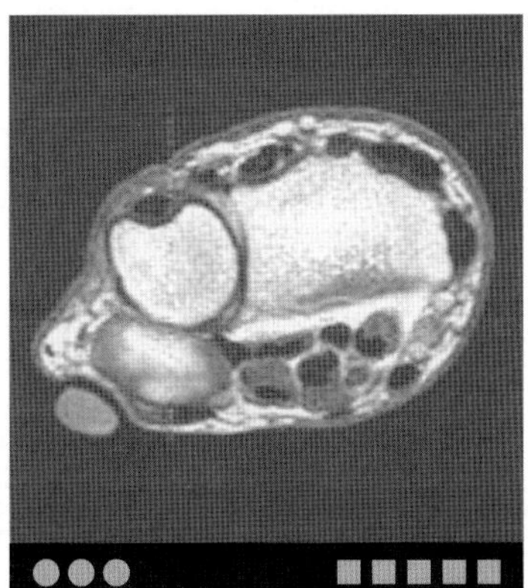

F. Schwannoma: Axial T1WI shows inhomogeneous fatty signal mass.

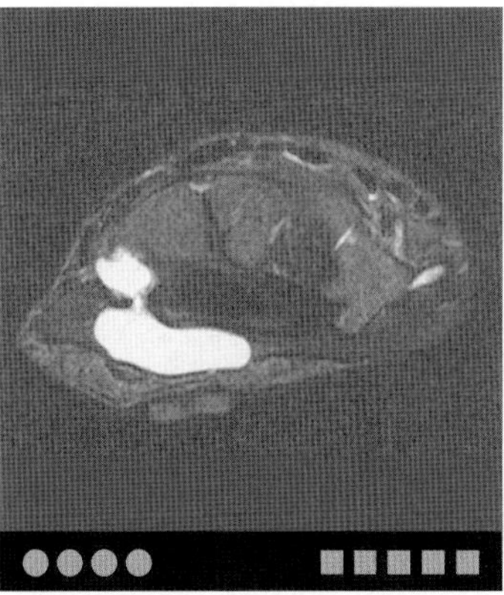

G. Ganglion cyst: Transverse STIR demonstrates large fluid-filled mass arising from pisiform-triquetral articulation, consistent with ganglion cyst.

IMAGE KEY

Common

Rare

Typical

Unusual

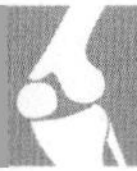

12–13 Flexor Digitorum Profundus Avulsion

Eli J. Bendavid

PRESENTATION

Limited ring finger motion

FINDINGS

MRI demonstrates absence of tendinous low signal intensity along the volar aspect of the distal ring finger.

DIFFERENTIAL DIAGNOSES

- *Flexor digitorum superficialis tear:* Tendinous disruption is noted along the volar aspect of the proximal interphalangeal joint. Tendon along the distal interphalangeal joint is intact.
- *Flexor tenosynovitis:* Abnormal fluid signal intensity surrounds the intact flexor tendon. There is enhancement of tendon sheath.

COMMENTS

This is a 68-year-old male with a history of limited ring finger range of motion. Loss of normal (low T1 and low T2/IR) tendinous signal intensity is noted along the volar aspect of the distal interphalangeal (DIP) joint. Finding represents avulsion at the insertion of the flexor digitorum profundus (FDP) tendon. In this case, a normal insertion of the flexor digitorum superficialis (FDS) is identified at the level of the proximal interphalangeal (PIP) joint. Most commonly, FDP tendon tears occur from sudden traumatic hyperextension at the DIP joint, during active contraction of the FDP. Less commonly, the tendon tear may result from chronic degenerative change, as seen with friction of the tendon against bony osteophytes. On physical examination, patient is unable to flex at the DIP joint, while the PIP joint is held in fixed position. The ring finger is most commonly involved with flexor tendon ruptures. Furthermore, the FDP is more susceptible to rupture than the FDS. The avulsed FDP may retract to the palm (type I), retract to the PIP joint (type II), or is associated with an avulsed segment of the distal phalangeal base (type III). Surgical repair, aimed at reattaching the retracted tendon, is most successful when retraction is only to the PIP joint and repair is performed within 14 days of the tear.

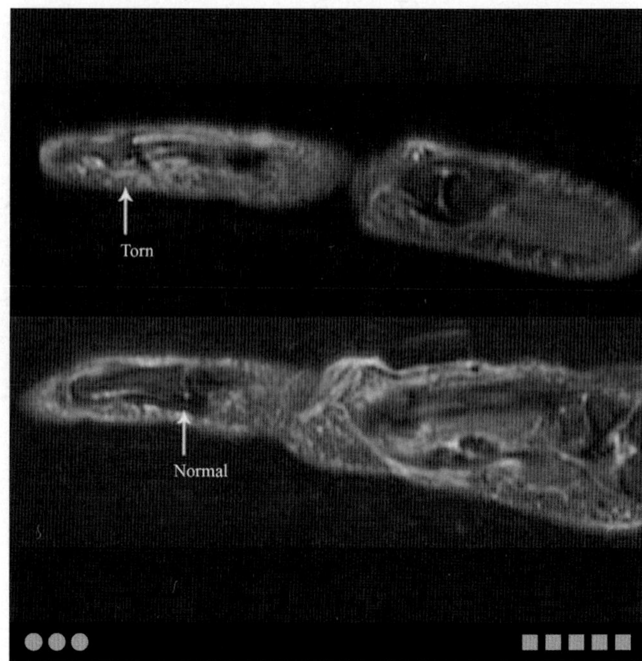

A. FDP avulsion (top): Sagittal inversion recovery image of the ring finger at the DIP joint shows absence of FDP tendon in the region of the edematous volar soft tissues (arrow). Marrow edema of the distal aspect middle phalanx is noted, compatible with avulsion of the associated vinculum breve. **Bottom (normal):** In contrast, sagittal inversion recovery image of the middle finger at the DIP joint demonstrates normal insertion of the FDP tendon to the base of the distal phalanx (arrow).

PEARLS

- **Disruption of tendon signal along volar aspect of DIP joint.**
- **Loss of DIP joint flexion, when PIP held fixed.**
- **Ring most common finger for flexor tendon tears.**
- **FDP more commonly torn than the FDS.**
- **Sagittal imaging plane is most sensitive for diagnosis.**

ADDITIONAL IMAGES

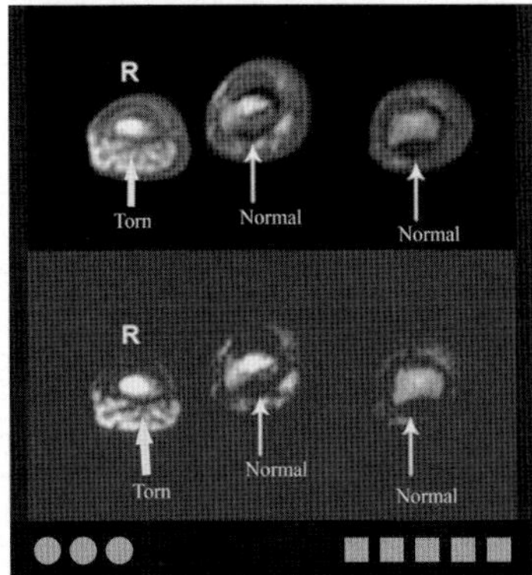

B. FDP avulsion: Axial T1 image (top) and axial fat-saturated T2 image(bottom) at the level of the DIP joint demonstrate absence of normal low signal intensity along the expected course of the ring finger (R) FDP tendon (thick arrows). The corresponding middle and index finger FDP tendons are intact (thin arrows).

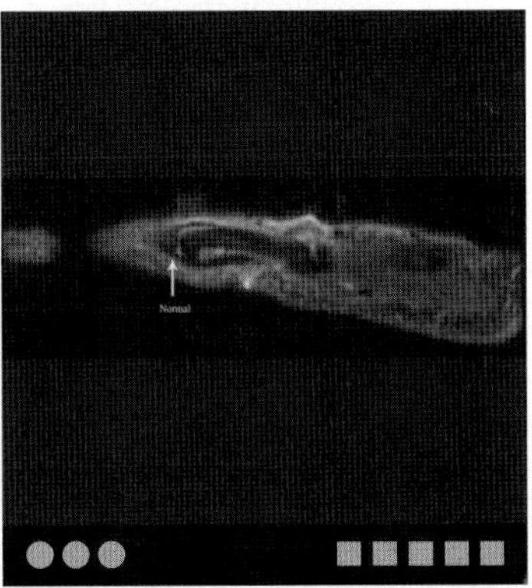

C. Normal flexor tendon (comparison): Sagittal inversion recovery image of the ring finger at the PIP joint demonstrates a normal insertion of the FDS tendon to the base of the middle phalanx (arrow).

DIFFERENTIAL DIAGNOSES IMAGES

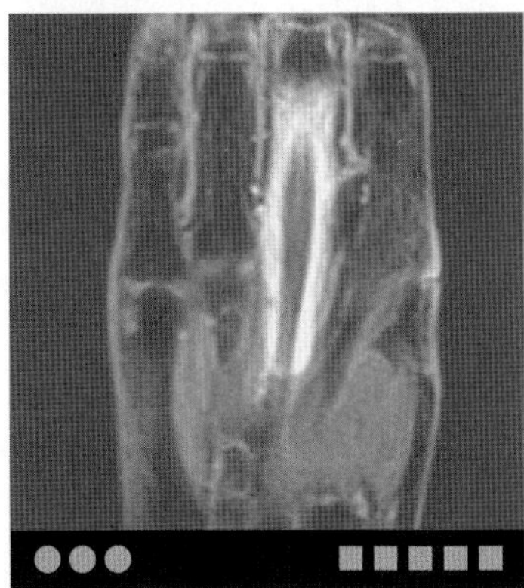

D. Flexor tenosynovitis: Sagittal T1W postcontrast image shows marked enhancement of flexor tendon sheath of the third finger.

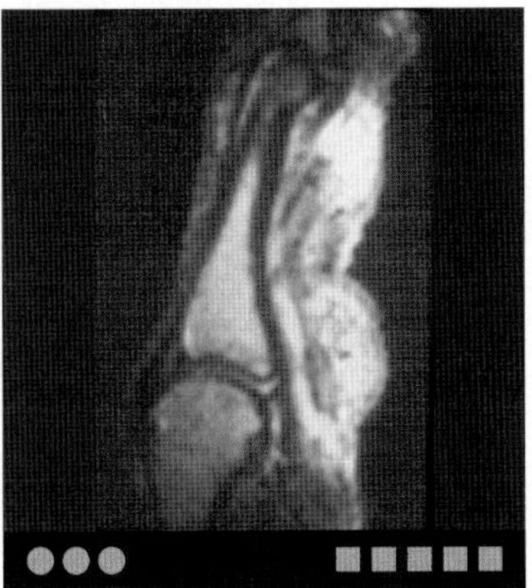

E. Flexor hallucis superficialis tear: Sagittal T2WI in another patient with recurrent tear of flexor tendon. Note absence of normal flexor tendon. Fluid and scar tissue has replaced the flexor tendon.

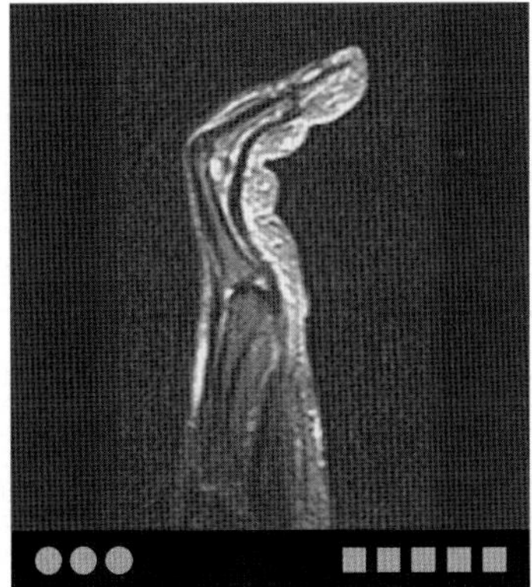

F. Pulley injury: Sagittal STIR image of the ring finger in another patient shows the bowstring appearance characterized by increased AP distance between the proximal phalanx and flexor tendon because of A2 pulley injury.

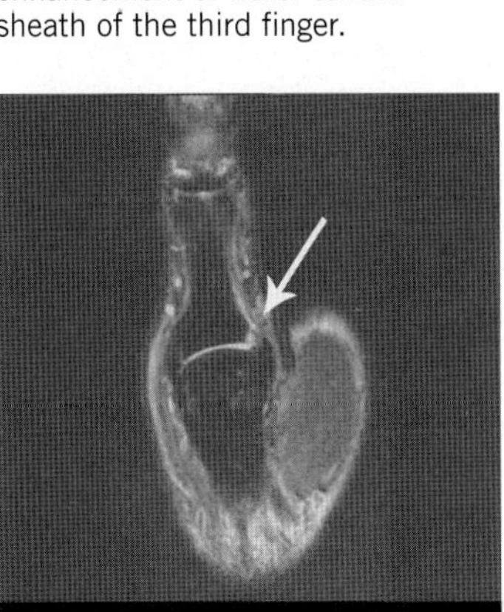

G. Gamekeeper thumb: Sagittal fat-saturated T2WI demonstrates a complete rupture of the ulnar collateral ligament (arrow).

IMAGE KEY

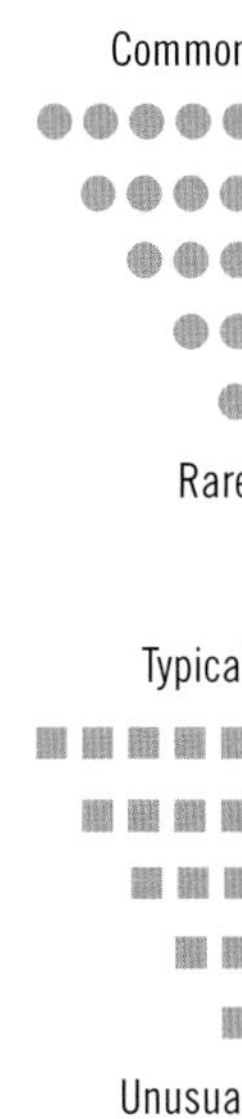

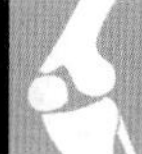

12–14 Gamekeeper Thumb

Piran Aliabadi

PRESENTATION

Weakened grip after skiing accident

FINDINGS

Tear of the ulnar collateral ligament of the thumb.

DIFFERENTIAL DIAGNOSES

- *Gamekeeper fracture:* Avulsion fracture of the ulnar aspect of the proximal phalanx.
- *Stener lesion:* Interposition of the adductor aponeurosis and ulnar collateral ligament.

COMMENTS

This is a 45-year-old male with acute thumb pain after planting a ski pole during a fall. The common cause of this injury is a fall onto an outstretched hand causing valgus force with the thumb abducted. Historically, this injury occurred with game handlers. Today, this injury is often associated with athletic activities such as skiing. An associated bony injury called gamekeeper's fracture involves an avulsion fracture of the ulnar aspect of the base of the proximal phalanx. A Stener lesion may be an associated finding because of the interposition of the adductor aponeurosis and ulnar collateral ligament. A Stener lesion requires surgical correction. The ulnar collateral ligament originates from the metacarpal head and travels obliquely to insert on the lateral tubercle of the proximal phalanx. MR imaging can demonstrate a gradation of injuries to the ulnar collateral ligament in the region of the metacarpal-phalangeal joint, which results in instability of the joint. Edema within the ulnar collateral ligament is seen on fluid sensitive sequences and represents a partial tear. Partial tears are treated conservatively. Increased signal intensity, discontinuity, and recoil of the ulnar collateral ligament are seen with ligament disruption. Surgical correction is necessary with complete disruption. Conventional radiographs taken in stress or pinch maneuver may demonstrate instability of the ligament with subluxation. Cortical bone may be seen with fractures and an intact ligament. These types of injuries inevitably lead to arthritis of the metacarpal-phalangeal joint.

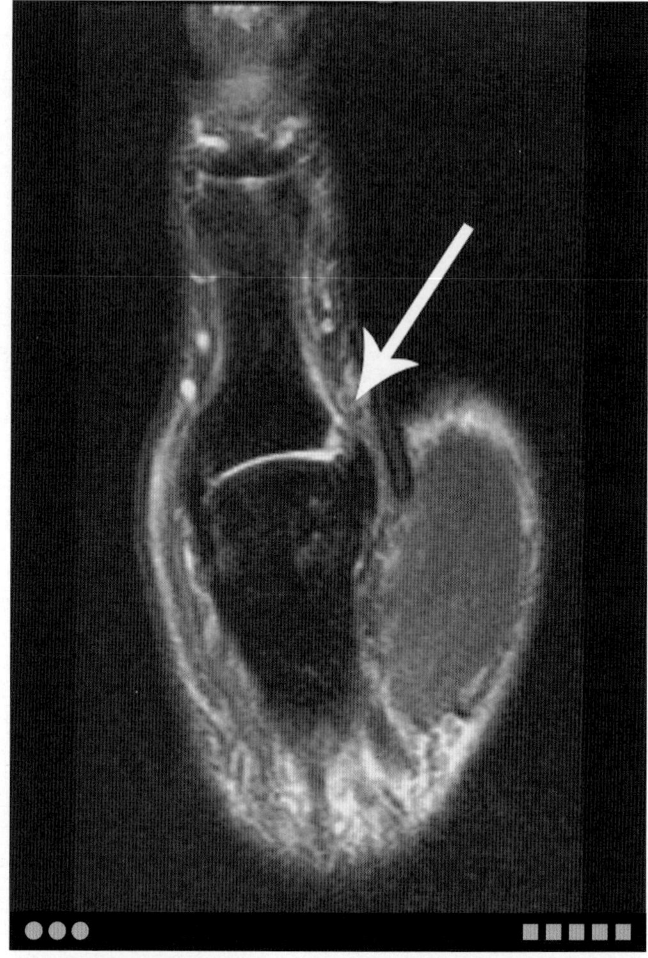

A. Gamekeeper thumb: Sagittal fat-saturated T2WI demonstrates a complete rupture of the ulnar collateral ligament (arrow).

PEARLS

- **Common injury of the thumb in skiers.**
- **Conventional radiographs demonstrate subluxation in stressed or pinch maneuvers.**
- **Stener lesion is a complication of the ulna collateral ligament tear with interposition of the adductor aponeurosis and ulnar collateral ligament. Surgical reduction is indicated.**

ADDITIONAL IMAGE

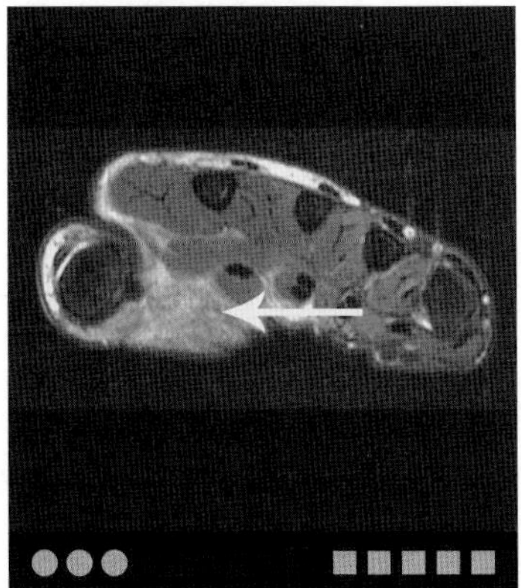

B. Gamekeeper thumb: Axial, fat-saturated T2WI shows edema in the thenar eminence (arrow).

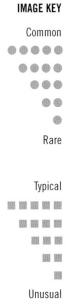

DIFFERENTIAL DIAGNOSES IMAGES

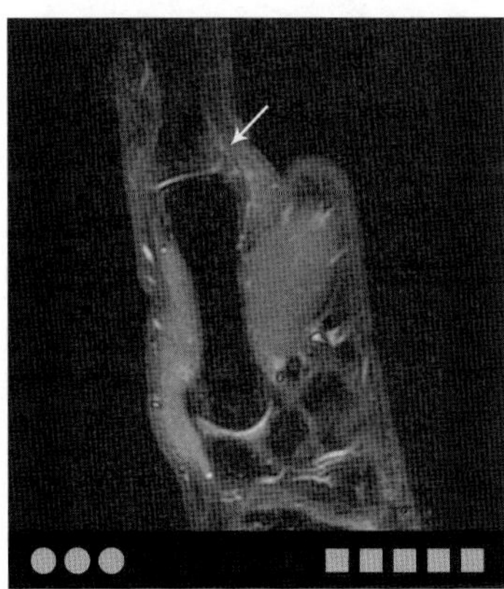

C. Gamekeeper fracture: Sagittal STIR image demonstrates an avulsion fracture of the base of the proximal phalanx (arrow) with disruption of the ulnar collateral ligament.

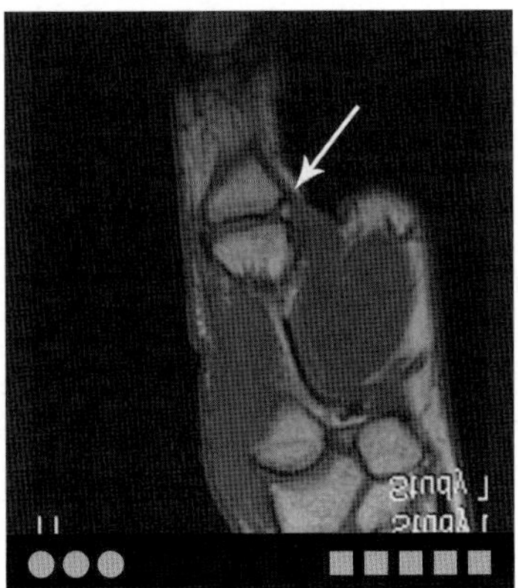

D. Gamekeeper fracture: Sagittal T1WI shows a linear hypointense signal of the base of the proximal phalanx representing the avulsion fracture (arrow).

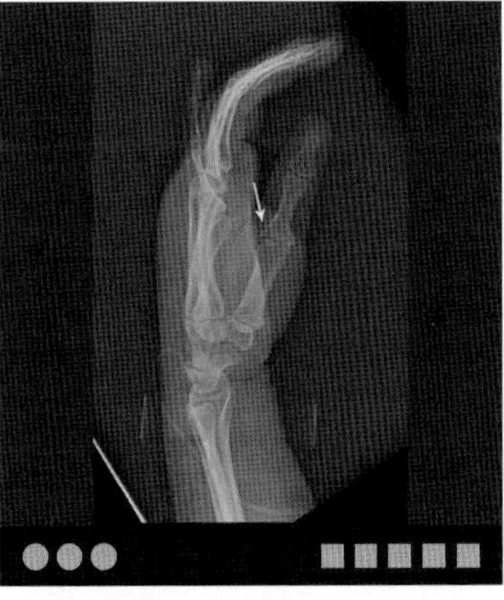

E. Gamekeeper fracture: Radiograph from the same patient demonstrates the gamekeeper fracture (arrow).

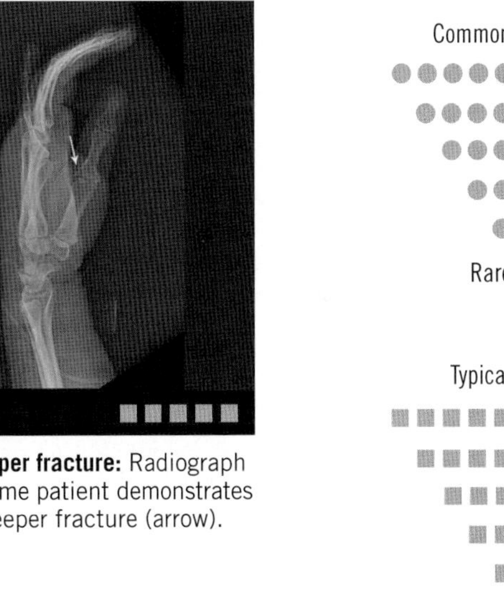

IMAGE KEY

Common

Rare

Typical

Unusual

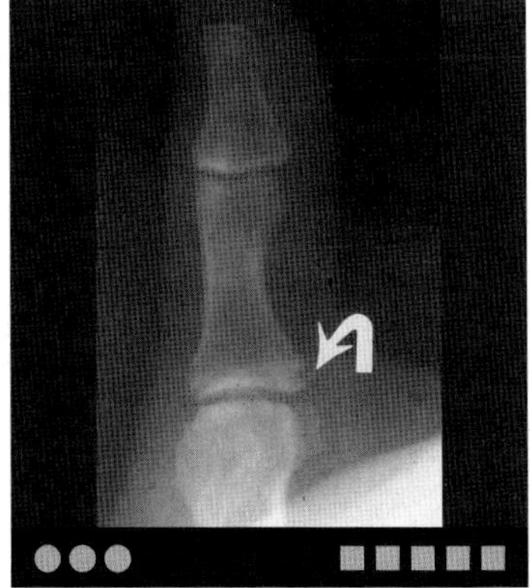

F. Gamekeeper fracture: Radiograph from another patient demonstrates the gamekeeper fracture (arrow).

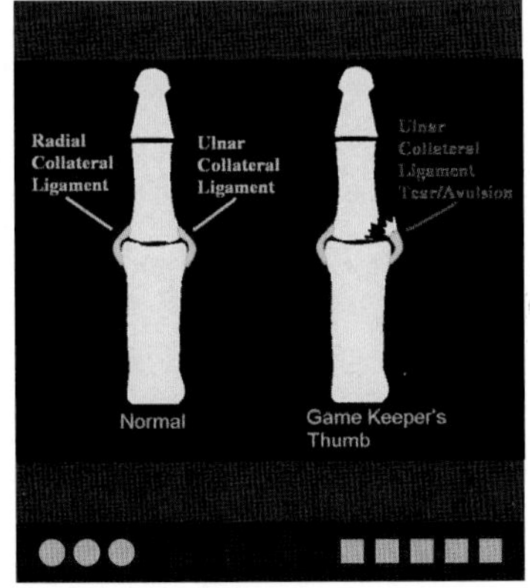

G. Gamekeeper fracture: Diagram of normal thumb compared with gamekeeper fracture. (Courtesy of Arash Tehranzadeh from Los Angeles.)

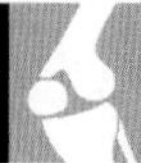

12–15 Pulley Injury

Piran Aliabadi

FINDINGS

Acute ring finger pain

DIFFERENTIAL DIAGNOSES

- *Pulley strain:* Edema within intact tendon sheaths.
- *Rheumatoid trigger finger:* Inflammation causing nodular thickening of the tendon sheath.
- *Trigger/locked finger:* Audible clicking with flexion of the finger. Often a nodule is palpable on the volar aspect of the finger.

COMMENTS

This is a 28-year-old male rock climber with an episode of acute pain and difficulty flexing the ring finger. Injuries to the pulley system are often seen in rock climbers or associated with activities that require significant weight loading on the fingers. The flexor tendon system is a complex arrangement of annular tendon sheath thickenings that allow the tendons to glide around anchor points otherwise known as cruciate ligaments. The most common injury is to the A2 pulley followed by combined A2 and A3 injuries. The A2 pulley measures approximately 20 mm in length along the volar aspect of the proximal phalanx and does not cross the joint. It is the most important pulley in terms of functional loss when injured. Diagnosis of annular pulley ruptures can be made by physical examination showing bowstringing of the flexor tendon in restrained active flexion. MR, CT, and ultrasound imaging is helpful in grading injuries of the pulley system with four defined grades. Grade I injuries are sprains. Grade II injuries describe partial rupture of A2 or A3 pulley or complete rupture of the A4 pulley. Grade III injuries describe complete rupture of A2 or A3 with a protracted recovery period. Grade IV injuries represent complex injuries involving multiple pulleys, ligament, and lumbricalis muscle injuries requiring surgical repair. Disruption of the tendon sheath can be appreciated on axial images by discontinuity of the sheath. Sagittal images will show increased distance between the volar plate and tendon.

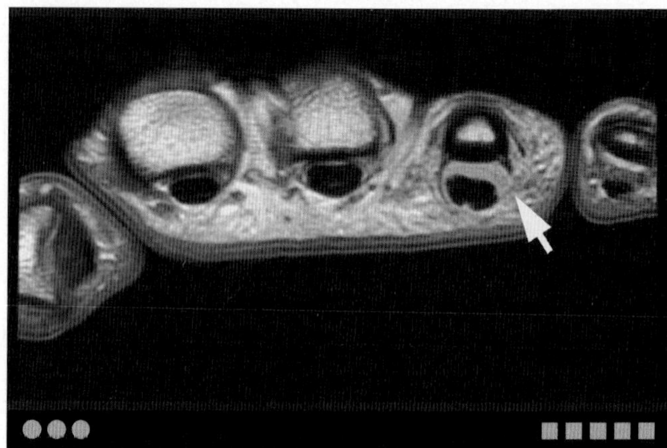

A. Pulley injury: Axial PD image shows disruption of the ulnar aspect of the tendon sheath (A2 pulley Injury) (arrow).

PEARLS

- **Common injury to the fingers of rock climbers. Presents as bowing of the flexor tendon in restrained flexion.**
- **A2 pulley is the most commonly injured with significant loss of function.**

ADDITIONAL IMAGE

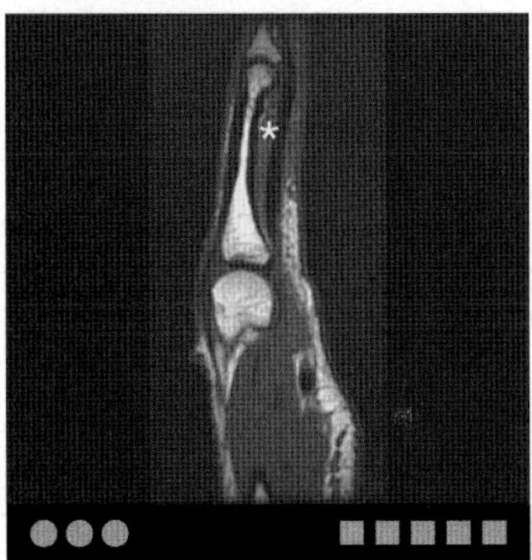

B. Pulley injury: Sagittal PD image of the ring finger shows the bowstring appearance characterized by increased AP distance (asterisk) between the proximal phalanx and flexor tendon because of A2 pulley injury.

DIFFERENTIAL DIAGNOSES IMAGES

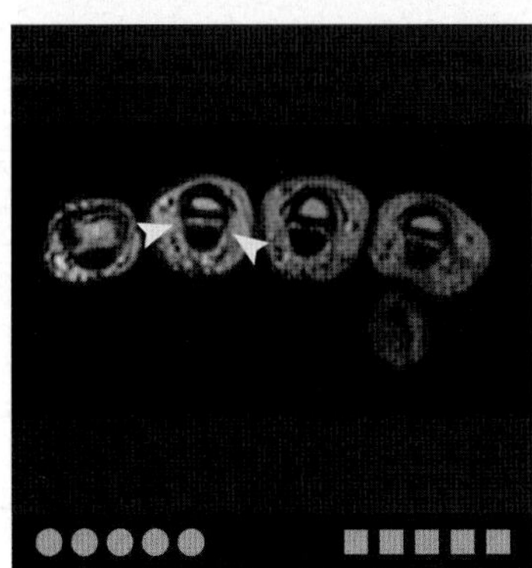

C. Normal A2 pulley: For comparison, a normal A2 pulley is shown in this axial T1WI. The A2 tendon sheath (arrowheads) completely surrounding the flexor tendon.

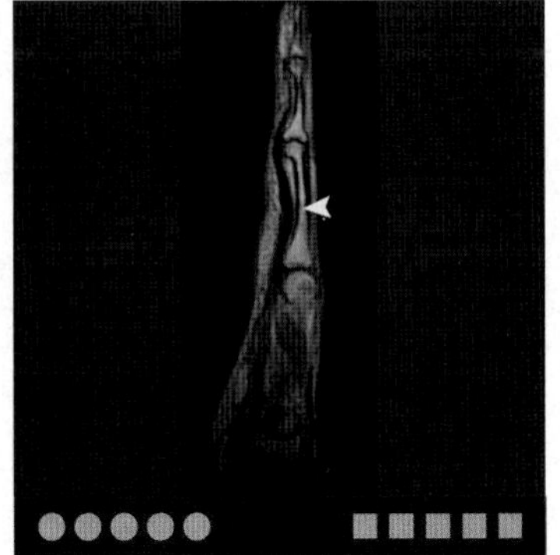

D. Normal A2 pulley: Sagittal T1WI, note the close approximation of the flexor tendon to the volar aspect of the proximal phalanx (arrowhead).

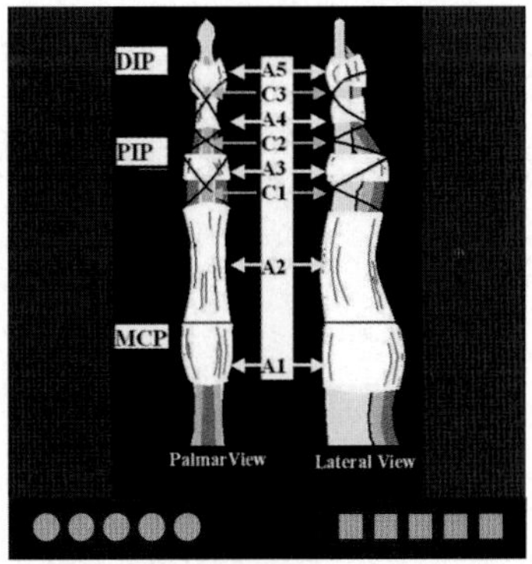
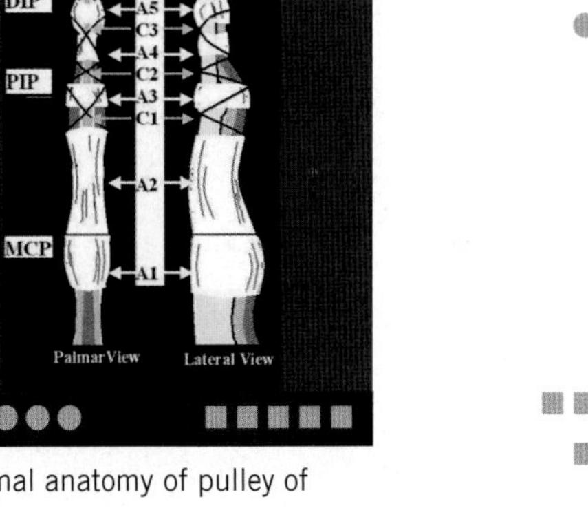

E. Normal anatomy of pulley of finger.

IMAGE KEY

Common

Rare

Typical

Unusual

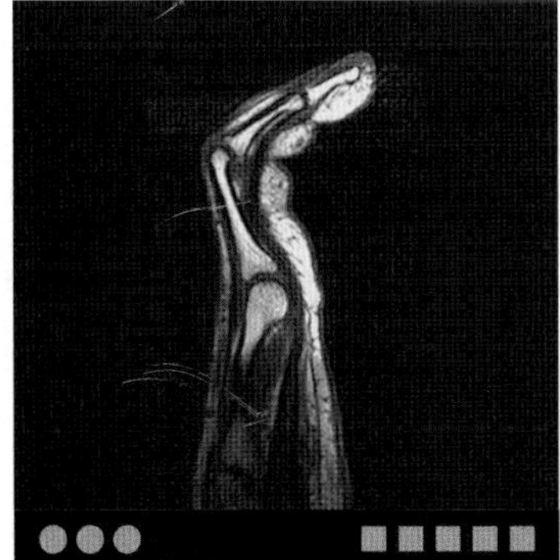

F. Pulley injury: Sagittal T1 image of the ring finger in another patient shows the bowstring appearance characterized by increased AP distance between the proximal phalanx and flexor tendon because of A2 pulley injury.

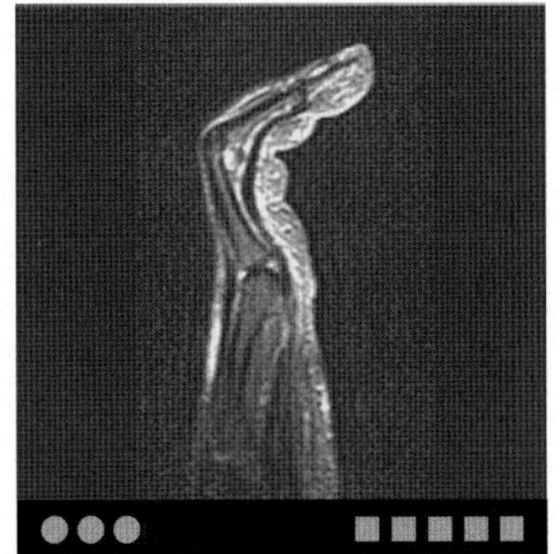

G. Pulley injury: Sagittal STIR image of the ring finger (in the same patient as in image F) shows the bowstring appearance characterized by increased AP distance between the proximal phalanx and flexor tendon because of A2 pulley injury.

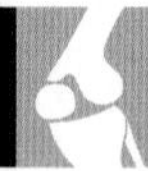

12–16 Intersection Syndrome

Stephen E. Ling and William R. Reinus

PRESENTATION

Pain, swelling, crepitus in the dorsal radial forearm

FINDINGS

Second extensor compartment tenosynovitis and/or peritendinitis.

DIFFERENTIAL DIAGNOSES

- *De Quervain's tenosynovitis:* Pain at wrist radial styloid region instead of distal forearm, first extensor compartment tendons always affected. Inflammation includes tendons of the extensor pollicis brevis and the abductor pollicis longus.
- *Decussation (distal intersection) syndrome:* Cross over of second compartment and extensor pollicis longus (third compartment) occurs more distally at the level of Lister's tubercle of the radius.
- *Extensor pollicis longus tendinosis/tenosynovitis:* This includes tenosynovitis of the extensor pollicis longus.
- *First carpal–metacarpal osteoarthritis:* Trapezium first metacarpal joint is the target joint of osteoarthritis.

COMMENTS

Intersection syndrome is a relatively uncommon tenosynovitis affecting the dorsal radial-sided tendons of the distal forearm. It is most often seen in patients involved in sports-related activities, such as rowing, canoeing, racket sports, horseback riding, hockey, skiing, and weightlifting. The syndrome has been referred to by numerous other terms, including peritendinitis crepitans, abductor pollicis longus bursitis, crossover syndrome/tendinitis, oarsman's wrist, squeaker's wrist, and bugaboo forearm. The first extensor compartment of the distal forearm and wrist contains two tendons: the abductor pollicis longus (APL) and the extensor pollicis brevis (EPB). The second extensor compartment contains extensor carpi radialis longus (ECRL) and the extensor carpi radialis brevis (ECRB). As the muscles of these two compartments travel down the forearm, the APL and the EPB are medial to the ECRL and the ECRB until 4 to 5 cm proximal to Lister's tubercle at the proximal margin of the extensor retinaculum. Here, the EPB and APL cross over (intersect) the ECRB and the ECRL as the former move laterally toward the first compartment. Two main hypotheses have been described. One is chronic trauma through a friction mechanism involving repetitive wrist extension and radial deviation leading to peritendinitis and scarring in the tendon sheaths of the ECRB and the ECRL. The second mechanism is stenosis of the tendon sheaths and tendon entrapment. MR is the imaging modality of choice and shows abnormalities of the second compartment at the crossover point in the dorsoradial distal forearm and often extend proximally 3 to 4 cm. At times, there may be concomitant first compartment muscle pathology.

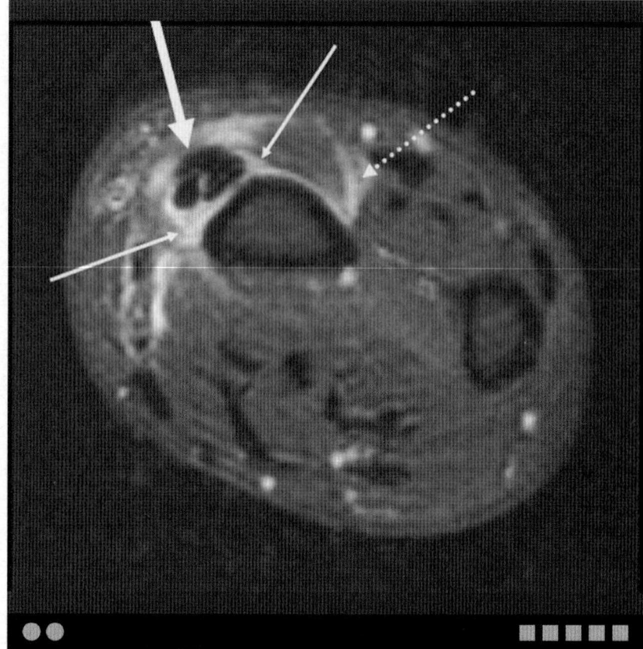

A. Intersection syndrome: Axial T2WFS shows fluid distention of the extensor carpi radialis longus and extensor carpi radialis brevis tendon sheaths of the second compartment (thin arrows) and abductor pollicis longus and extensor pollicis brevis tendon sheaths of the first compartment (thick arrow) at the crossover point of the two compartments. There is also fluid around the first compartment musculature (dotted arrow).

PEARLS

- **Peritendinous edema and/or enhancement are sufficient to make the MR diagnosis of intersection syndrome, with tendon sheath fluid distention not required.**
- **Decussation (distal intersection) syndrome is a similar, less well-known overuse disorder involving the second compartment (extensor carpi radialis longus (ECRL) and brevis (ECRB)) and third compartment (extensor pollicis longus).**
- **Clinical and imaging findings in intersection syndrome are more proximal as well as medial and dorsal to those seen in De Quervain's tenosynovitis.**

ADDITIONAL IMAGES

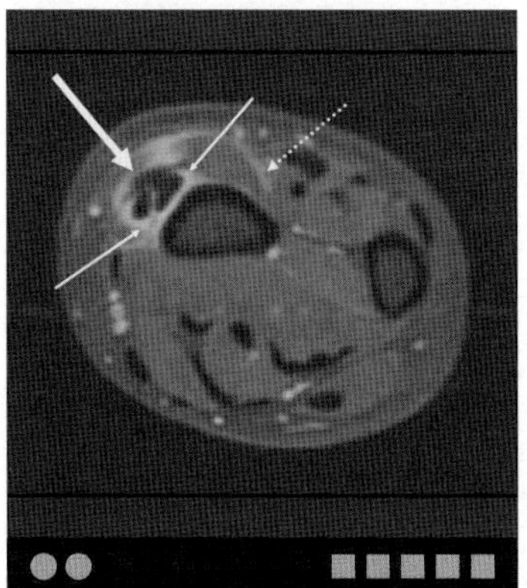

B. Intersection syndrome: Axial T1WFS with contrast at the same level as image A shows peritendinous enhancement involving the tendons of the second compartment (thin arrows) and first compartment (thick arrow) at their crossover point. There is also enhancement around the first compartment musculature (dotted arrow).

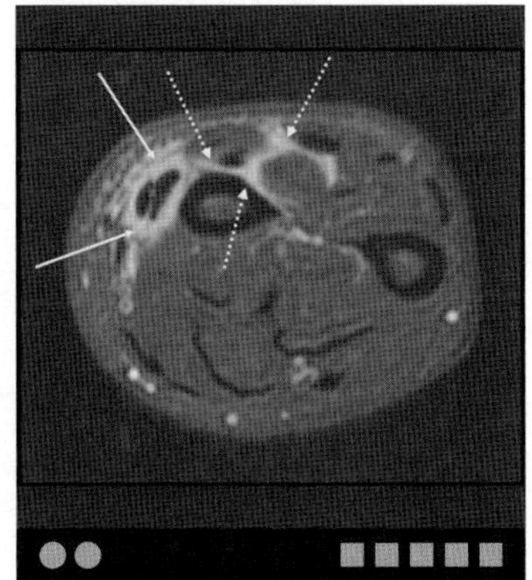

C. Intersection syndrome: Axial T2WFS at a level proximal to images A and B shows additional fluid distention of the second compartment tendon sheaths (solid arrows). Additional fluid is also seen around the first compartment musculature myotendinous junction (dotted arrows).

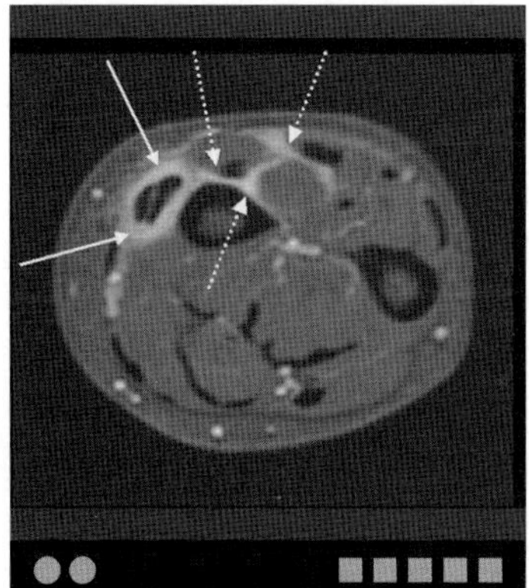

D. Intersection syndrome: Axial T1WFS with contrast at a level proximal to images A and B and at the same level as image C shows additional peritendinous enhancement involving the second compartment tendons (solid arrows). Additional enhancement is also seen around the first compartment musculature myotendinous junction (dotted arrows).

IMAGE KEY

DIFFERENTIAL DIAGNOSES IMAGES

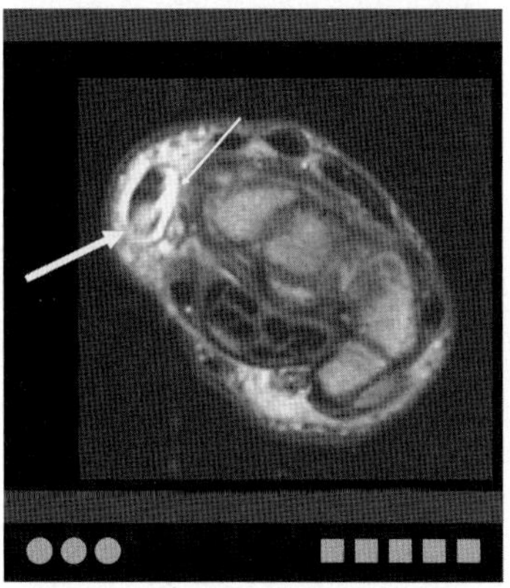

E. De Quervain's tenosynovitis: Axial T2WFS in another patient shows conspicuous fluid distention of the abductor pollicis longus (APL) and extensor pollicis brevis (EPB) tendon sheaths of the first compartment (thin arrow), as well as intrasubstance mild T2 hyperintensity of the APL tendon (thick arrow), at the level of the radial styloid.

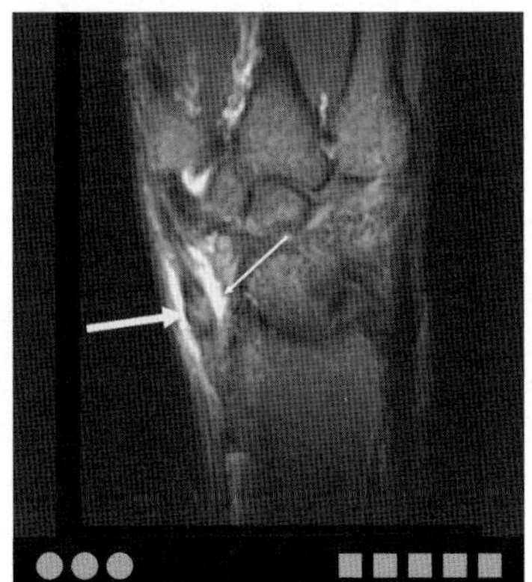

F. De Quervain's tenosynovitis: Coronal T2WFS (in the same patient as in image E) again shows tendon sheath fluid distention (thin arrow) and APL tendon mild T2 hyperintensity (thick arrow) of the first compartment.

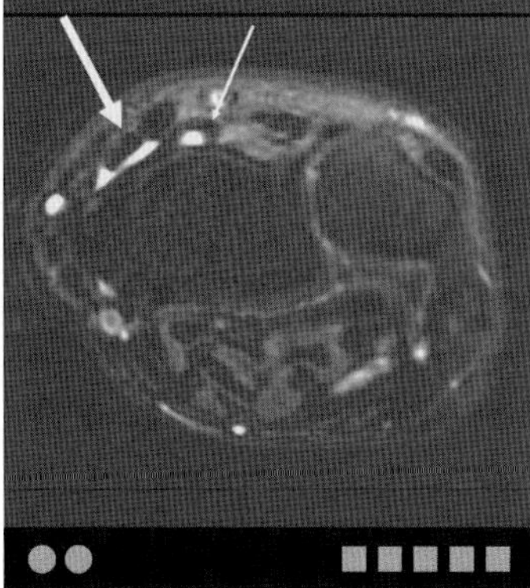

G. Decussation syndrome: Axial T2WFS in a third patient at about the level of Lister's tubercle shows mild fluid distention of the tendon sheaths of the second compartment (thick arrow) and of the extensor pollicis longus tendon (third compartment) (thin arrow).

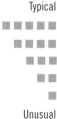

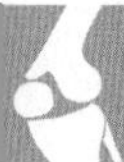

12–17 Lunate Dislocation

Ashkan Afshin and Jamshid Tehranzadeh

PRESENTATION

Wrist pain following injury

FINDINGS

Radiographic images reveal "pie-shaped" lunate on AP view and volar dislocation of lunate in relation to radius and other carpal bone on the lateral view.

DIFFERENTIAL DIAGNOSES

- *Perilunate dislocation:* Radiographic findings show normal alignment of the lunate with distal radius while other carpal bones are posteriorly dislocated.
- *Transscaphoid perilunate dislocation:* Perilunate dislocation may be associated with carpal bone fracture often scaphoid.
- *Hook of hamate fracture:* Hook of hamate is obscured on AP radiograph of the wrist and the fracture is best detected on CT study.
- *Kienbock disease:* Ischemic changes of lunate are best diagnosed on MR study. This may be associated with injury or conditions such as positive and negative variances of distal ulna.

COMMENTS

Anterior lunate dislocation is the most frequent type of carpal dislocation. This condition usually results from falling on outstretched hand and other conditions that cause acute dorsiflexion and ulnar deviation of the wrist. Anterior dislocation of the lunate should be differentiated from perilunate dislocation in which the lunate remains normally in the lunate fossa of the radius and the entire carpus except lunate dislocate. Patient with lunate dislocation usually complain of the wrist pain. On physical examination, they have diffuse pain on palpitation, which makes it difficult to differentiate the diagnosis from other causes of the wrist pain. Anterior dislocation of the lunate may cause compression of the median nerve, which, if not treated by emergency reducing, may lead to permanent palsy. Radiographs of the wrist, both anteroposterior and lateral, are of diagnosis value. Lateral radiograph of a normal wrist shows distal radius to be aligned with lunate, capitate and third metacarpal. In lunate dislocation lateral radiograph demonstrates volar displacement of the lunate, which results in a break in the longitudinal alignment of third metacarpal, the capitate over the distal surface of the radius at the site of lunate. Anteroposterior radiograph demonstrates the disruption of the arc II, which is described by concave surface of the scaphoid, the lunate, and the triquetrum. Furthermore, normal rectangular profile of lunate on AP images changes to triangular shape "pie shape" after dislocation because of its tilt. While lunate dislocation is isolated event; perilunate dislocation is often associated with a fracture of carpal bone often scaphoid.

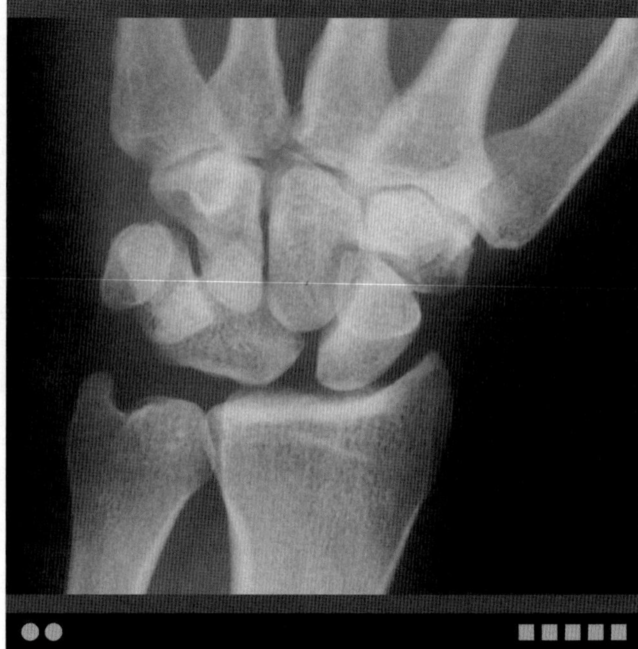

A. Lunate dislocation: AP radiograph of the wrist shows triangular or "pie shape" lunate suggesting lunate dislocation.

PEARLS

- **Most frequent type of carpal dislocation.**
- **Falling on outstretched hand is the most common mechanism of injury.**
- **Wrist pain is the most common symptom.**
- **Median nerve compression is the complication, which needs emergency intervention.**
- **Volar displacement of the lunate on lateral radiograph.**
- **Triangular or "pie shape" appearance of the lunate on AP radiograph of the wrist and disruption of the arc II on anteroposterior radiograph.**

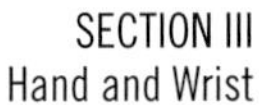

ADDITIONAL IMAGE

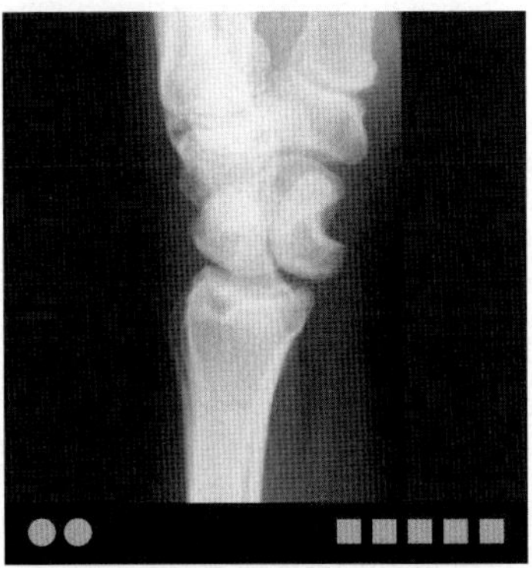

B. Lunate dislocation: Lateral radiograph of the wrist shows lunate is not aligned with the radius and capitate and is located volar to the other carpal bones.

DIFFERENTIAL DIAGNOSES IMAGES

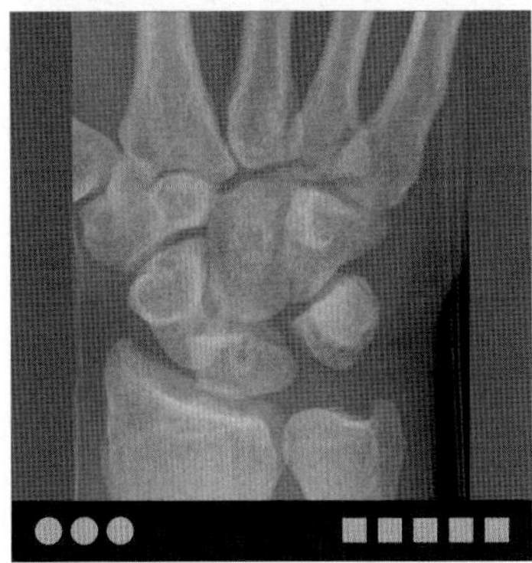

C. Perilunate dislocation: AP radiograph of the wrist shows abnormal overlapping of the lunate and scaphoid bones.

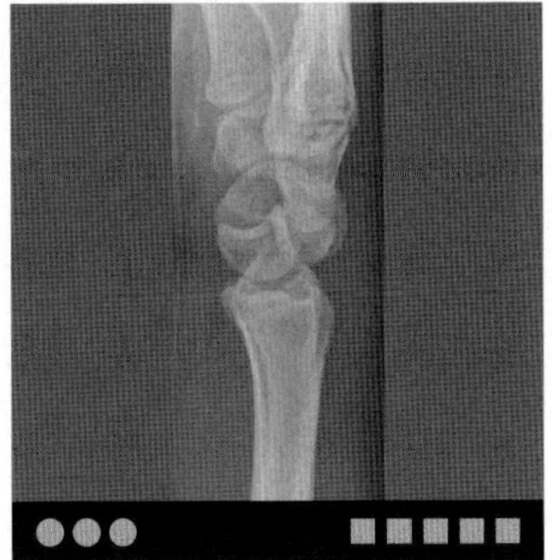

D. Perilunate dislocation: Lateral radiograph of the wrist shows lunate is aligned with the distal radius; however, capitate and other carpal bones are posteriorly dislocated, so called Perilunate dislocation.

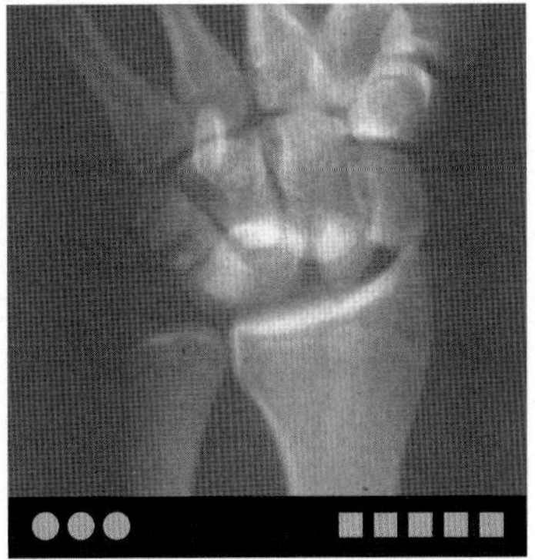

E. Transscaphoid perilunate dislocation: AP radiograph shows fracture of the scaphoid waist and abnormal overlapping of the lunate on other carpal bones with a gap between the lunate and scaphoid. Lateral view (not shown) revealed lunate in good alignment with radius but other carpal bones were posteriorly dislocated.

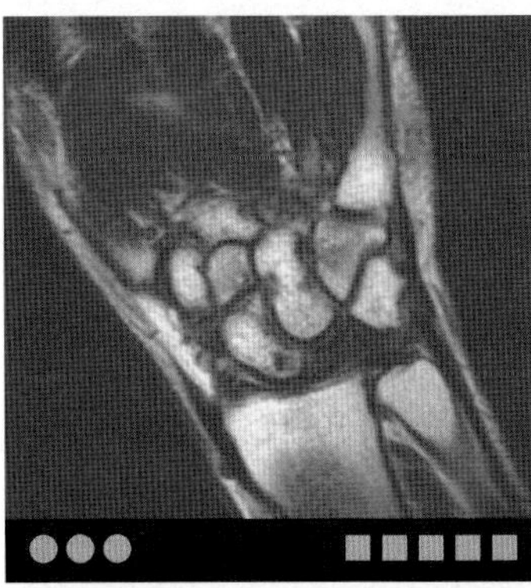

F. Kienbock's disease: Coronal T1WI of the wrist shows avascular necrosis of the lunate with diffuse decreased signal intensity.

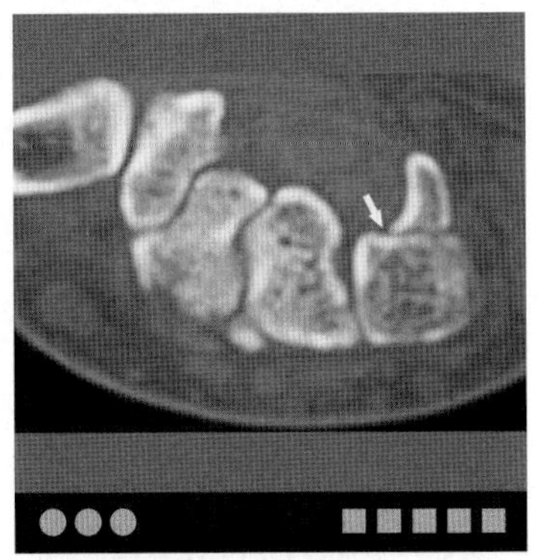

G. Hook of hamate fracture: Hook of hamate fracture. Axial CT image shows a nondisplaced transverse fracture through the base of the hamate (arrow).

IMAGE KEY

Common

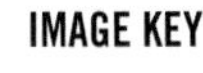

Rare

Typical

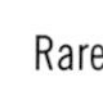

Unusual

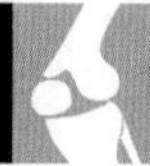

12–18 Carpometacarpal Fracture Dislocation

Ashkan Afshin and Jamshid Tehranzadeh

PRESENTATION

Wrist pain

FINDINGS

Conventional radiographs demonstrate incongruity of metacarpophalangeal joint associated with fracture of hamate and base of fifth metacarpal. There is overriding of fractured carpometacarpal bones.

DIFFERENTIAL DIAGNOSES

- *Gamekeeper thumb:* This condition results from rupture of the ulnar collateral ligament. MR images show discontinuity of the ulnar collateral ligament attachment to proximal phalanx of the thumb.
- *Hamate fracture:* Fluid-sensitive MR image shows marrow edema, which may be associated with hypointense fracture line in the body of the hamate.
- *Hook of hamate fracture:* Hook of hamate is obscured on conventional PA radiograph. CT image shows lucent fracture line in the hook of hamate with or without displacement. Loss of the normal osseous concavity of the hook may also be observed.

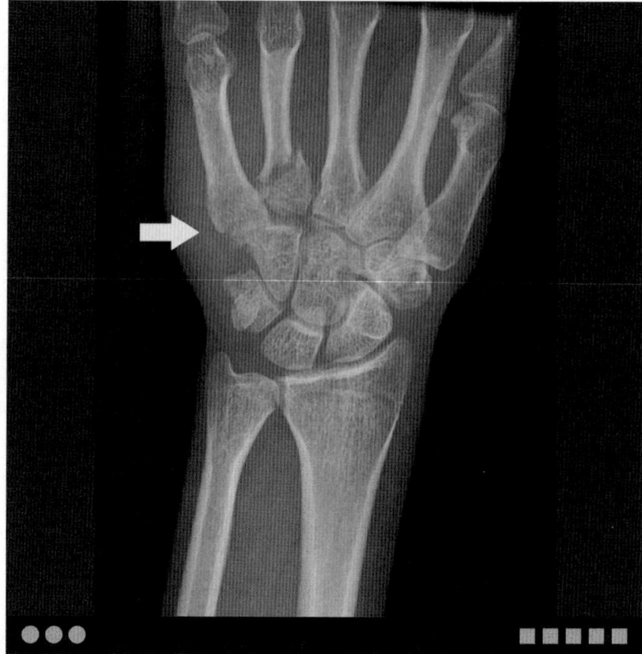

A. Carpometacarpal fracture dislocation: PA radiograph of the left wrist shows fracture dislocation of the fifth metacarpal. The base of the fifth metacarpal is fractured, dislocated, and overlapping the hamate bone (arrow). There is also fracture of the hamate and proximal shaft of the fourth metacarpal. Note the congruity of the carpometacarpal joint is disrupted on medial side.

COMMENTS

Carpometacarpal fracture dislocation is a relatively rare injury caused by the force acting along the longitudinal axis of the metacarpal. The impact of a clenched hand on an immobile object is a common mechanism of the injury. The dislocation can be volar or dorsal. Patients are usually presented with the wrist pain following an accident. Physical examination of the patients reveals swelling, tenderness, and crepitation over the affected joints. Deep motor branch of the ulnar nerve is located volar to the fifth carpometacarpal joint and may be compressed on volar dislocation of the fifth metacarpal. Diagnosis requires a high index of suspicion, careful examination, and appropriate radiography. Three radiographic views including PA, lateral, and oblique are usually required. Conventional radiograph reveals lack of congruity between carpal and metacarpal articulations. These joints, which are arranged in zigzag orientation, should always appear parallel (congruent) on PA radiograph. Overlap of the joint surfaces and loss of the normal carpometacarpal alignment are common radiographic findings in these patients. Roentgenograms may also exhibit fracture of the carpal or metacarpal bones. Fracture of the base of the metacarpals or of the hamate should increase the suspicion of carpometacarpal dislocation in the patients. CT images show the full extent of the injury and provide adequate insight in the relation of fractured and dislocated parts. CT images may demonstrate the facture of the carpal and metacarpal bones and malalignment of the Carpometacarpal joints.

PEARLS

- **Rare injury caused by a force acting along the longitudinal axis of the metacarpal.**
- **Swelling, tenderness, and crepitation over the affected joints are common clinical findings.**
- **Compression of the deep motor branch of the ulnar nerve may occur in volar dislocation of the fifth metacarpal.**
- **Loss of the parallel joint surface, overlap of the joint surfaces, loss of the normal carpometacarpal alignment, and fracture of the carpal or metacarpal bone may be seen on radiographs.**
- **CT images more clearly show the extent of injury.**

ADDITIONAL IMAGES

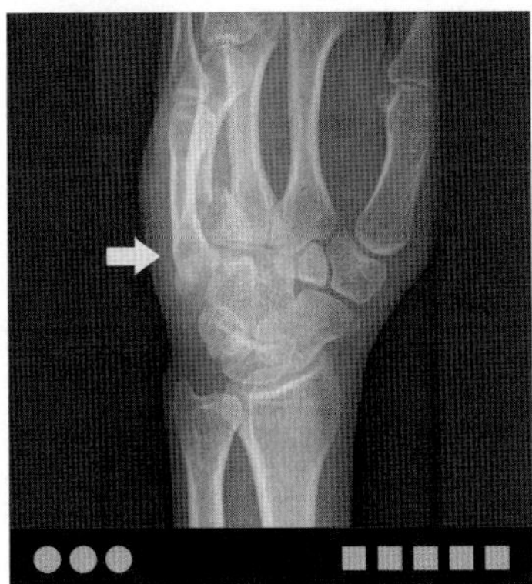

B. Carpometacarpal fracture dislocation: Oblique view of the left wrist shows fracture dislocation of the fifth metacarpal (arrow). Fracture of the hamate and proximal shaft of the fourth metacarpal is also seen.

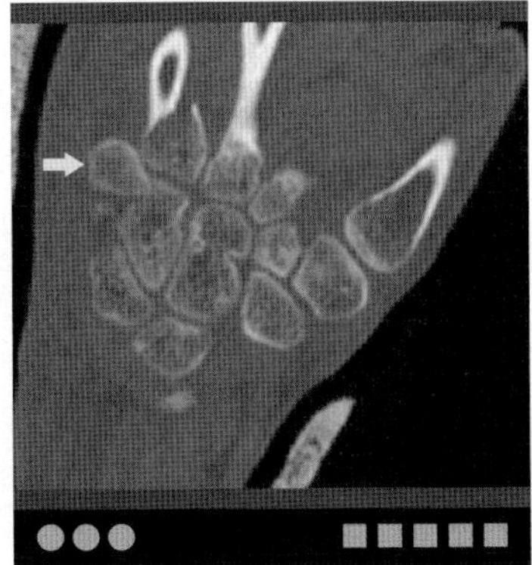

C. Carpometacarpal fracture dislocation: Coronal CT reformatting of the left wrist shows fracture of the base of the fifth metacarpal (arrow), which is overlapping the fractured hamate. There is also fracture of the proximal shaft of the fourth metacarpal.

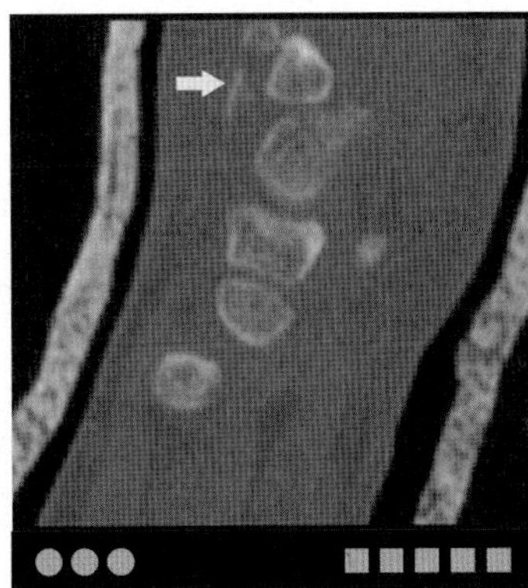

D. Carpometacarpal fracture dislocation: Sagittal CT reformatting of the left wrist through the plaster cast shows fractured and malaligned base of the fifth metacarpal (arrow). Note hamate is also fractured and it is not aligned with fifth metacarpal.

IMAGE KEY

Common

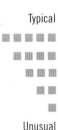

Rare

Typical

Unusual

DIFFERENTIAL DIAGNOSES IMAGES

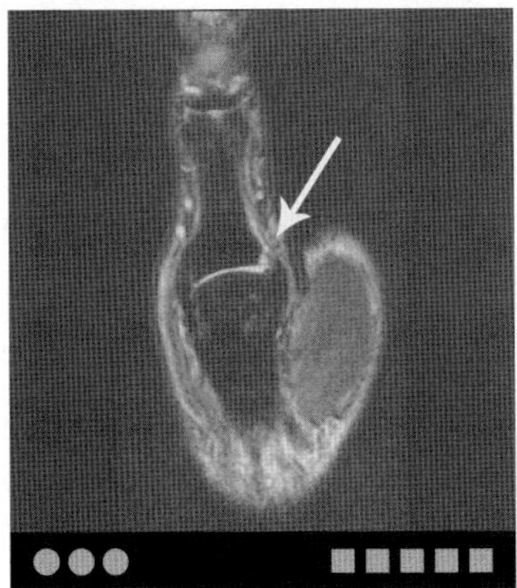

E. Gamekeeper thumb: Sagittal fat-saturated T2WI demonstrates a complete rupture of the ulnar collateral ligament (arrow).

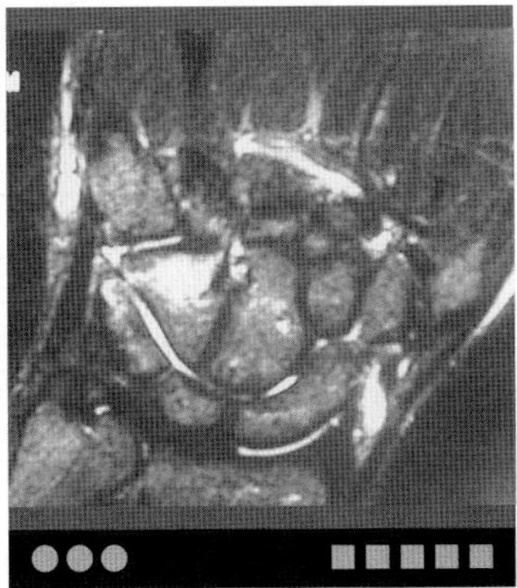

F. Hamate fracture: The coronal STIR image shows marked bone edema and surrounding soft tissue edema.

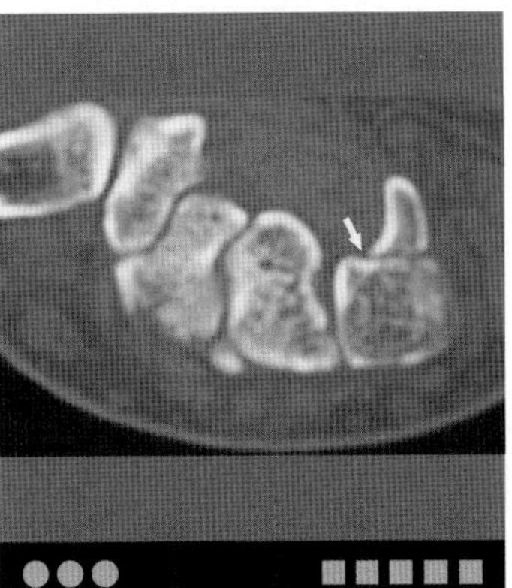

G. Hook of hamate fracture: Hook of hamate fracture. Axial CT image shows a nondisplaced transverse fracture through the base of the hamate (arrow).

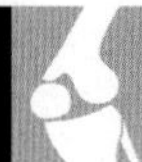

12–19 Distal Radioulnar Subluxation

Ashkan Afshin and Jamshid Tehranzadeh

PRESENTATION

Wrist pain

FINDINGS

Radiographs show widening of distal radioulnar joint and distal ulnar displacement. This case also shows comminuted intraarticular fracture of distal radius and ulnar styloid fracture.

DIFFERENTIAL DIAGNOSES

- *Ulnar impaction syndrome:* This condition results from increased pressure in the ulnocarpal joint. It usually occurs following distal radial fractures with radial shortening. Radiographs show a positive ulnar variance.
- *Triangular fibrocartilage complex (TFCC) tear:* MR or arthrogram images show extension of the fluid across the Triangular fibrocartilage complex into the distal radioulnar bursa.
- *SLAC wrist:* Scapholunate advanced collapse (SLAC) is a specific pattern of wrist malalignment that has been attributed to posttraumatic or spontaneous osteoarthritis of the wrist. Radiographs show nearly identical changes to those occurring in calcium pyrophosphate deposition disease (CPPD).

COMMENTS

This is a 38-year-old female with history of the fall and comminuted intraarticular fracture of distal radius with radioulnar subluxation. Radioulnar subluxation usually results from fractures of forearm bones specially fractures of the radius (Galeazzi's Fracture, Colles fracture, radial head fracture). However, it may occur as an isolated injury. This condition may also be seen in patients with inflammatory arthritis such as rheumatoid arthritis. Triangular fibrocartilage complex (TFCC) is almost always injured in radioulnar subluxation. Dislocation can be either dorsal or palmar. Dorsal subluxation is more frequent and occurs as a result of falling on pronated hand. Palmar subluxation caused by forced supination. Patients usually complain of wrist pain. Physical examination of the patients reveals limitation and pain in rotation. In dorsal dislocation, patients are unable to perform supination while pronation is blocked by palmar dislocation. Radiographic findings in these patients show widening of distal radioulnar joint on AP view. Fracture at base of ulnar styloid and significant shortening of the radius may also be observed. Subluxation and dislocation can accurately be diagnosed from a lateral radiograph of the wrist with the forearm in neutral rotation. Minimal supination or pronation of the forearm leads to inaccurate diagnosis. Lateral view must be taken with proper technique so that the radial styloid process overlies the proximal pole of the scaphoid, lunate, and triquetrum. When proper positioning is ensured, dorsal or palmar subluxation is noted by the relative position of the ulna above or below the radius. CT may be used for subtle cases and reveals radioulnar joint incongruity.

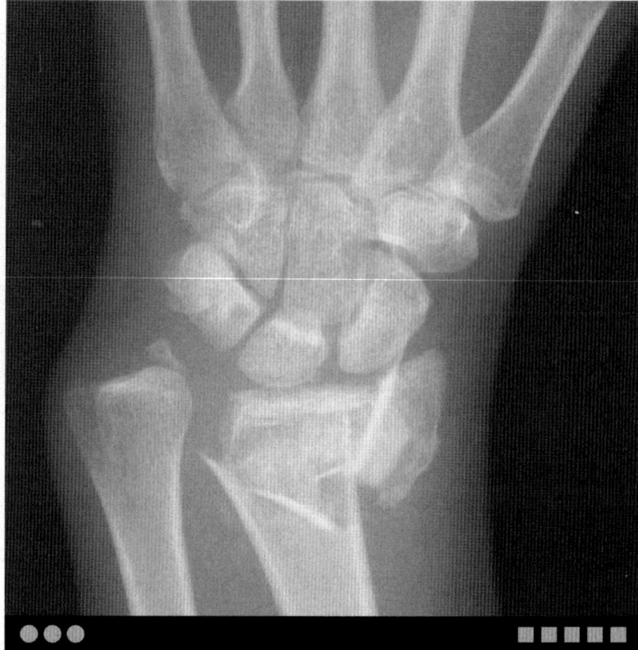

A. Distal radioulnar subluxation: PA radiograph of the wrist shows widening of the distal radioulnar joint. There are comminuted intra-articular impacted fracture of the distal radius and the ulnar styloid fracture. Positive ulnar variance as a result of impaction and foreshortening of the distal radius is noted.

PEARLS

- **Occurs as an isolated injury or is associated with forearm bone fractures.**
- **Dorsal dislocation is more frequent than palmar dislocation.**
- **Wrist pain and limited and painful wrist rotation are common clinical findings.**
- **Supination block is noted in dorsal dislocation and pronation block is seen in palmar dislocation.**
- **Widening of radioulnar joint is noted on AP view and displacement of the head of the ulna is seen on lateral view.**

ADDITIONAL IMAGES

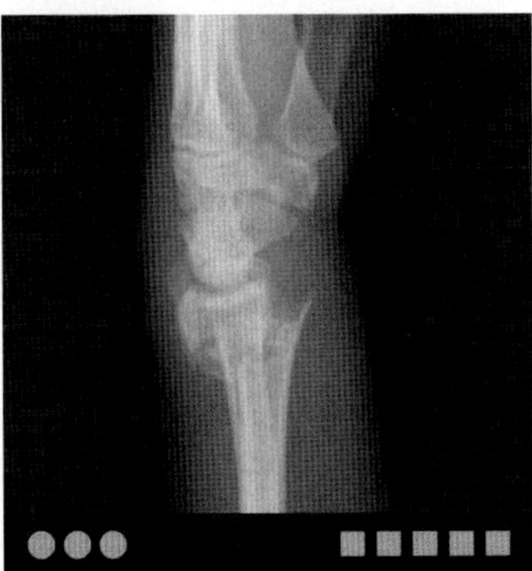

B. Distal radioulnar subluxation: Lateral radiograph of the wrist (same patient as in image A) shows distal radioulnar bones are not aligned and are not properly superimposed.

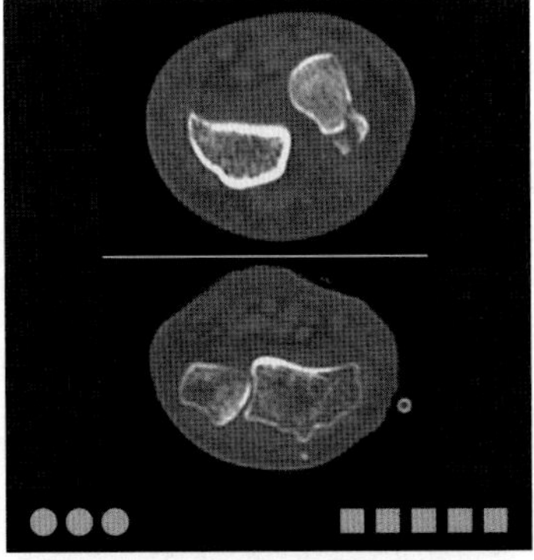

C. Distal radioulnar fracture dislocation: Top image shows CT of a wrist in a different patient with fracture of distal radius and dislocation of distal radioulnar joint. Bottom image shows CT of the other wrist of the same patient which is normal for comparison.

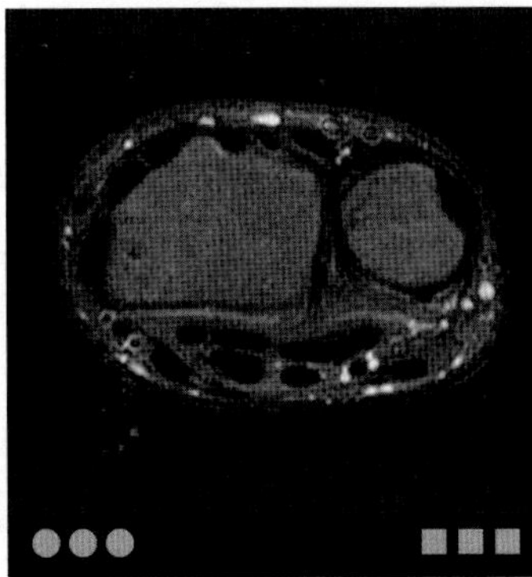

D. Distal radioulnar subluxation: Axial STIR imaging in another patient. MR in this 15-year-old boy with the distal radioulnar instability shows subtle dorsal subluxation of ulna due to chronic tear of the volar segment of distal radioulnar ligament.

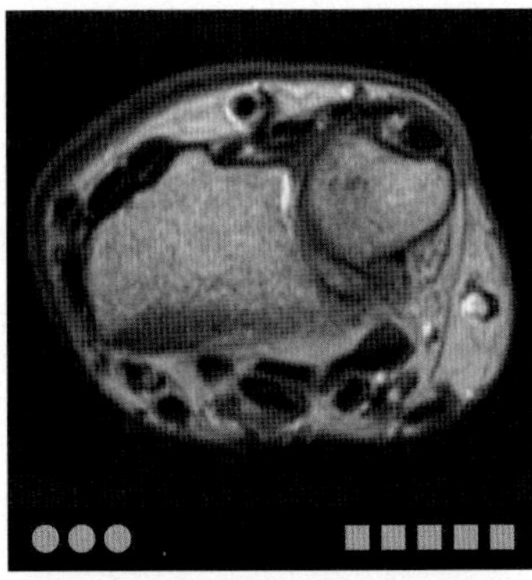

E. Distal radioulnar subluxation due to rheumatoid arthritis: Axial T2W image shows dorsal subluxation of distal ulna in relation to radius. Tenosynovitis of extensor carpi ulnaris and common extensors are also noted.

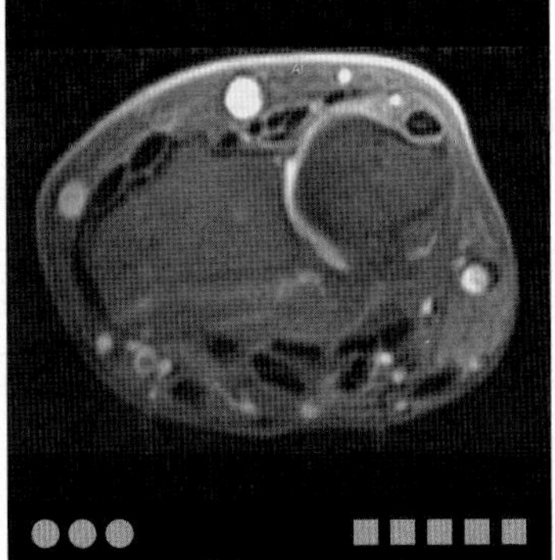

F. Distal radioulnar subluxation due to rheumatoid arthritis: Axial T1 fat-saturated postcontrast image (same patient as in image E) shows dorsal subluxation of distal ulna in relation to radius. Tenosynovitis of extensor carpi ulnaris and common extensors are also noted.

IMAGE KEY

Common

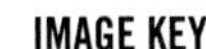

Rare

Typical

Unusual

DIFFERENTIAL DIAGNOSIS IMAGE

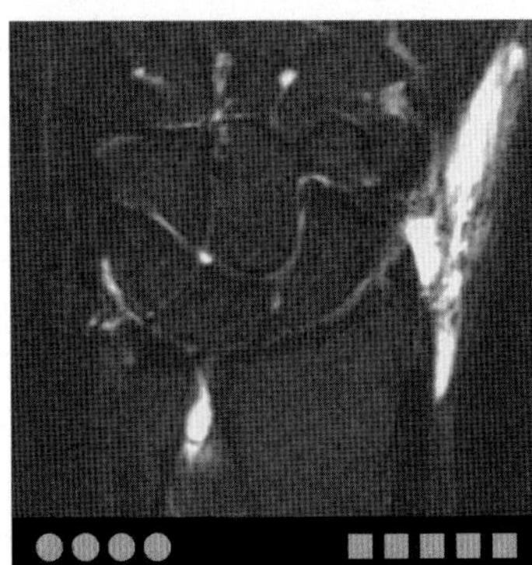

G. TFCC tear: Coronal T2 fat-saturated image shows presence of fluid in the radiocarpal joint and distal radioulnar recess indicating tear of TFCC.

Chapter 13

Congenital, Systemic and Metabolic Disorders

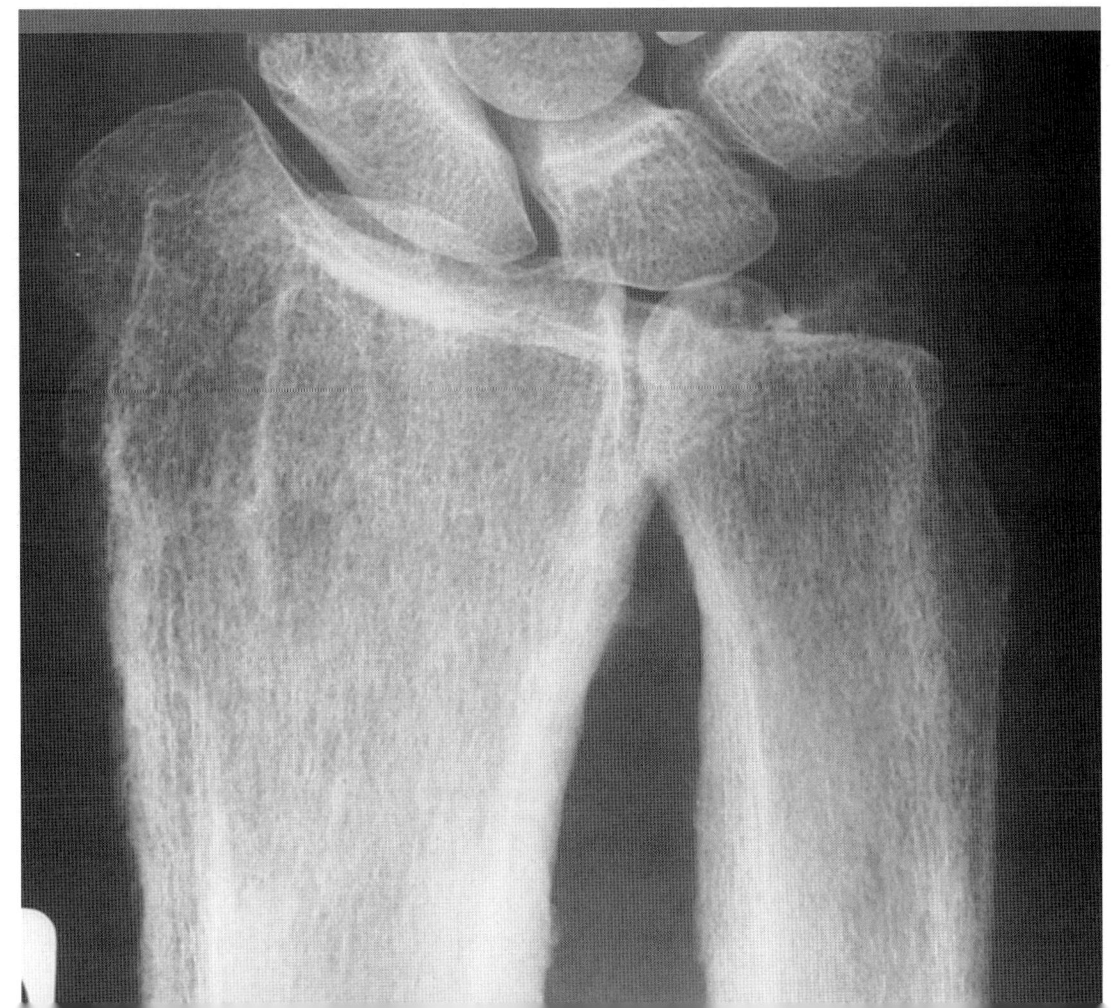

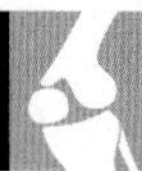

13–1 Pachydermoperiostosis

Mélanie Morel, Nathalie Boutry, and Anne Cotten

PRESENTATION

Progressive broadening of the wrists and hands with clubbing digits

FINDINGS

Radiographs of the extremities show thick, chronic, and irregular periostitis along the entire bone length.

DIFFERENTIAL DIAGNOSES

- *Secondary hypertrophic osteoarthropathy:* Most of them are linked with a pulmonary disease (epidermoid lung cancer, bronchiectasis) so called hypertrophic pulmonary osteoarthropathy (Pierre Marie syndrome).
- *Chronic venous insufficiency:* Thick, undulating periosteal reaction occurs along the shafts of tibia and fibula. Soft tissue calcifications and ossifications are also found.
- *Hypervitaminosis A:* It causes undulating diaphyseal periostitis of the tubular bones. Severe cases include premature fusion of the growth plates and cone-shaped epiphyses.
- *Thyroid acropachy:* Irregular speculated periosteal bone production is asymmetric and seen at the mid diaphyses of metacarpal, metatarsal bones, and phalanges (mainly on radial or tibial sides). Exophthalmia, soft tissue swelling, and pretibial myxedema are associated.
- *Osteomyelitis:* Acute osteomyelitis is accompanied by thin, linear periosteal bone constructions, whereas thick periosteal reaction and heterogeneous sclerosis mixed with osteolytic areas are encountered in the chronic phase.

COMMENTS

This is an image of a 40-year-old man presenting with clubbing deformity of the digits and thick facial skin. Pachydermoperiostitis represents the primary form of the hypertrophic osteoarthropathy (HOA). The secondary forms may be associated with multiple disorders, the most frequent one being lung cancer. HOA is a syndrome including clubbing of the digits, synovial effusion or painful joints, and periostitis. Periostitis is typically bilateral and symmetric and found mainly along the long bones of the upper and lower limbs. Periostitis located along the metaphysodiaphyses of long bones is painful. It is thin, linear with single or multilayer pattern. Bone scintigraphy demonstrates abnormal linear uptake along the outer side of the cortex. Active periostitis is clearly depicted on MRI images. Arthralgias are rather severe.

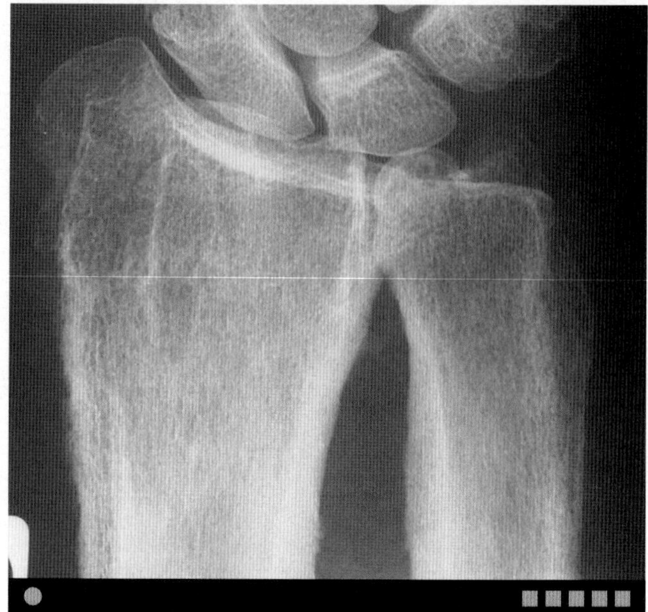

A. Pachydermoperiostosis: Prominent, irregular, and incorporated periostitis affects the entire length of the ulna and radius.

Pachydermoperiostosis is characterized by thickening of the skin, including massive cutaneous overgrowth of the scalp called cutis vertices gyrate. Primary HOA only accounts for 3% to 5% of all HOA. It is genetically transmitted and affects men more often. Periosteal proliferation is more prominent at the distal parts of the extremities. Radiographs reveal irregular, thick, and incorporated periosteal bone formation along the entire length of long bones (epiphysis, metaphysis, and diaphysis) of extremities, leading to widened bones. Such periostitis is not painful. Prominent osseous enthesophytes at the lower limbs are also commonly depicted. Digital clubbing is often prominent with bulbous hypertrophy of the soft tissues overlying the distal end of the digits,whereas bone production or acro-osteolysis may be found in association. Arthralgias are rarely encountered.

PEARLS

- **Pachydermoperiostosis is synonymous with primary HOA.**
- **It accounts for 3% to 5% of all HOA.**
- **Periosteal bone production is bilateral and mainly affects the entire length of long bones (epiphysis, metaphysis, and diaphysis) of extremities.**
- **Periostitis is thick and irregular.**
- **Osseous enthesophytes can be encountered.**

ADDITIONAL IMAGES

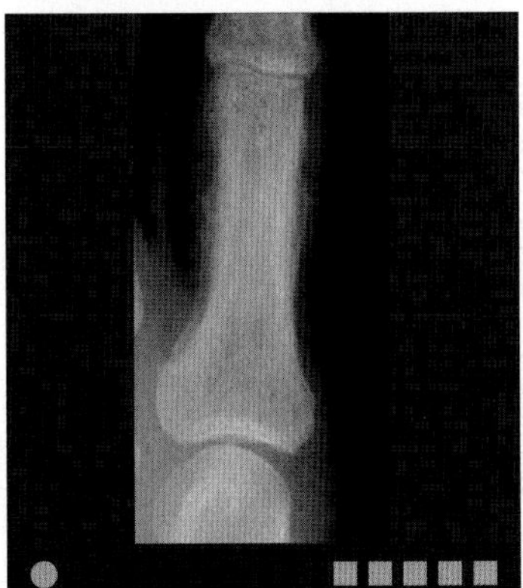

B. Pachydermoperiostosis: Thick, chronic, and irregular periostitis widens the metacarpal bone.

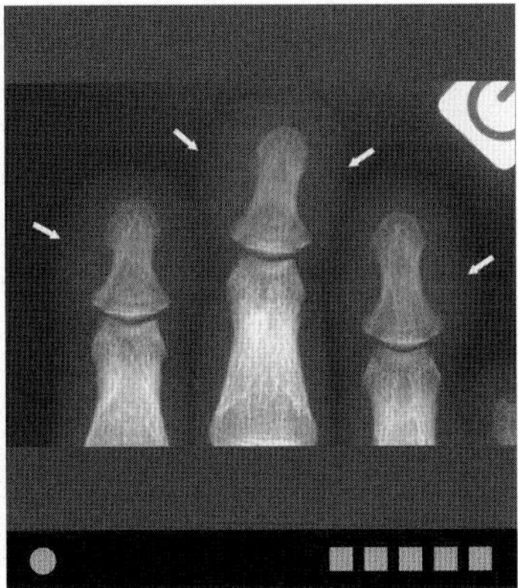

C. Pachydermoperiostosis: Bulbous hypertrophy of the soft tissue overlying the distal phalanges (arrows) leads to clinical clubbing digits.

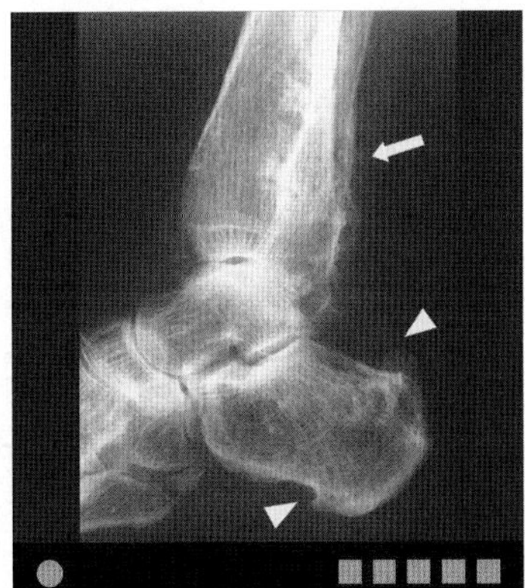

D. Pachydermoperiostosis: Prominent, calcaneal enthesophytes (arrowheads) are associated with thick, irregular periostitis along the posterior, tibial, and fibular entire length (arrow).

IMAGE KEY

Common

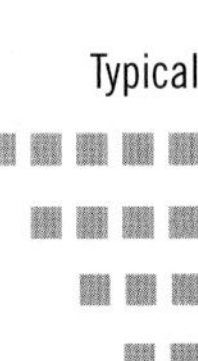

Rare

Typical

Unusual

DIFFERENTIAL DIAGNOSES IMAGES

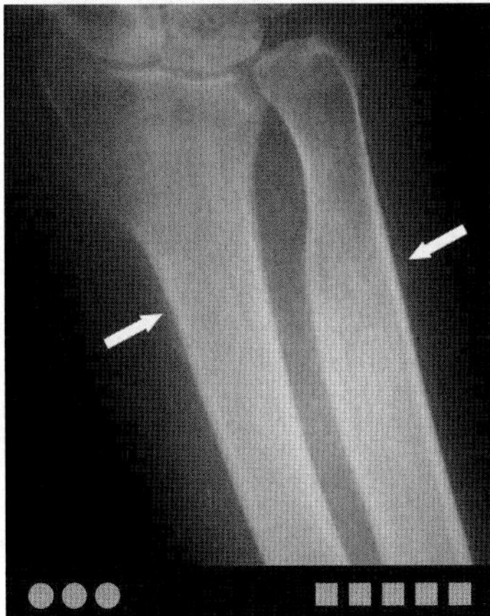

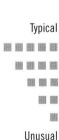

E. Secondary hypertrophic osteoarthropathy: Radiograph of the wrist exhibits thin, linear periostitis (arrows) along the metaphysodiaphyses of the radius and ulna.

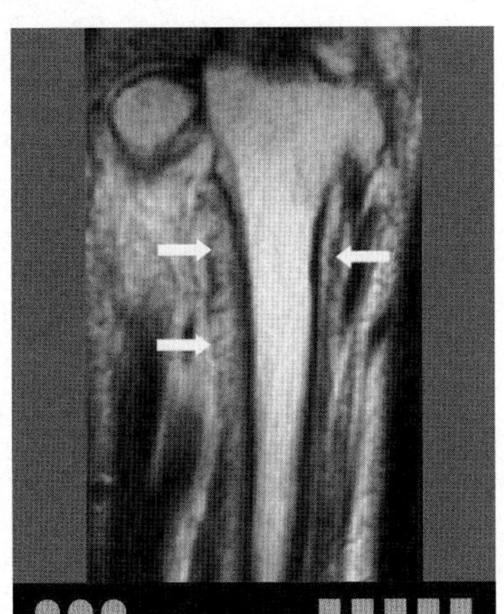

F. Secondary hypertrophic osteoarthropathy: Coronal T1-weighted postcontrast image shows enhancement of the bilateral, symmetric periostitis along the radial metaphysodiaphyses (arrows).

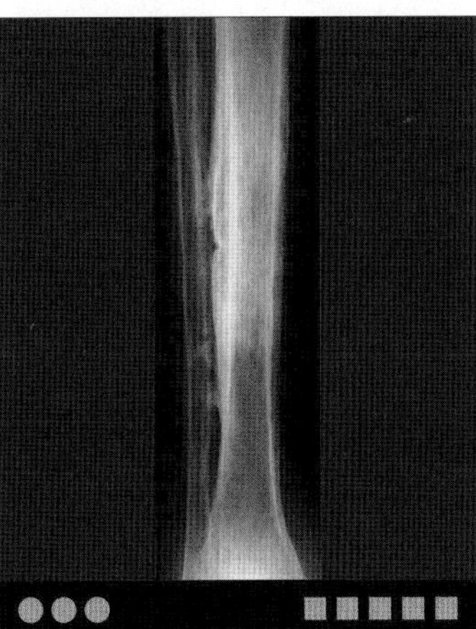

G. Chronic venous insufficiency: Radiograph exhibits a thick, undulating periosteal reaction along the shafts of the tibia and the fibula.

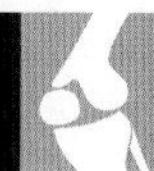

13–2 Arteriovenous Malformation of Digit

Peyman Borghei and Jamshid Tehranzadeh

PRESENTATION

Right fifth finger soft tissue mass

FINDINGS

MRI shows tangled, vascular structures with signal void in all sequences. Angiogram shows dilated vessels with the "bag of worms" appearance.

DIFFERENTIAL DIAGNOSES

- *Enchondroma:* The most common lesion of the digits, it usually appears as an osteolytic lesion with cartilaginous matrix calcification.
- *Glomus tumor:* It is seen in forth to fifth decades of life at the tips of the digits. It maybe associated with extrinsic bone erosion. MRI shows homogeneously hypo to isointense lesion on T1-weighted image.
- *Epidermal inclusion cyst:* Benign well-circumscribed cutaneous (subcutaneous) lesion, which is filled with keratin and/or cholesterol. This variation of content results in a variety of signal intensities on T1-weighted and T2-weighted images.
- *Capillary hemangioma:* A poorly marginated mass on both T1-weighted and T2-weighted image, which is isointense to muscle on T1-weighted and hyperintense on T2-weighted image. High signal intensity hemangioma on both T1-weighted and T2-weighted image indicates hemorrhage.

COMMENTS

This is an image of a 9-year-old patient who presented with a right fifth finger vascular mass diagnosed with arteriovenous malformation (AVM) of digit. AVMs are masses of abnormal blood vessels which consist of a blood vessel "nidus" (nest) through which arteries connect directly to veins, instead of connecting through the capillaries. Most of the cases are congenital; however, acquired AVM is also reported with a history of preceding trauma. The congenital forms are usually seen in the brain, spinal cord, and visceral organs and they grow with the child. However, the acquired forms are seen in areas susceptible to trauma, such as the extremities and especially in the fingers. They usually present with a small patch of AVM localized to the tip of one finger, and therefore are quite different from congenital AVM, which consists of a large pulsatile mass. Diagnosis can be made by the use of angiography, which provides the most accurate picture of the vessel structure. Of the noninvasive methods CT, MRI, and MRA are useful; however, the latter also provides information regarding pattern and velocity of blood flow through the vascular lesions. The role of MRI is to assess the extent of involvement of the vascular malformation with adjacent vital structures; MRA will determine if the lesion is a high-flow malformation. MRI shows soft tissue mass with marked edema in the surrounding tissue and flow void (imaging with GRASS gradient echo and long TR sequences).

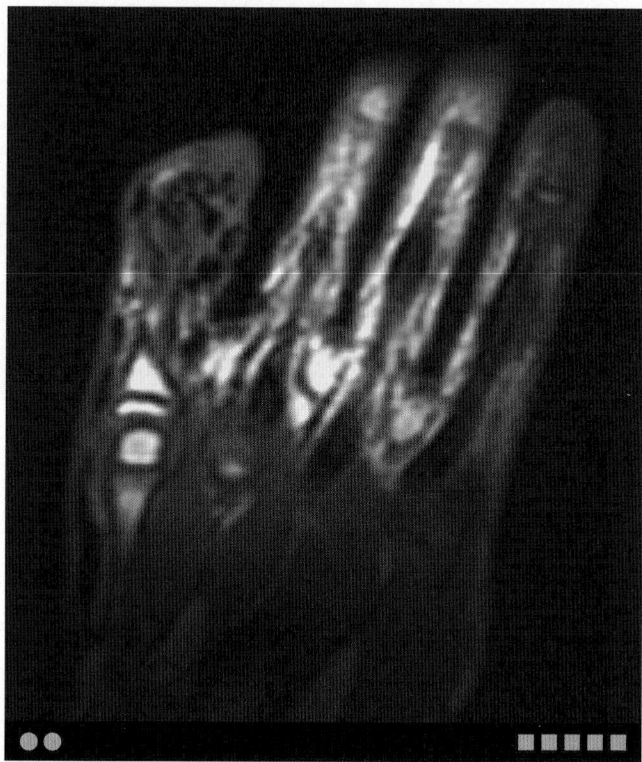

A. AVM: Coronal T1-weighted image shows serpiginous signal void, tubelike structure in the soft tissue of the fifth finger.

PEARLS

- **Acquired AVM is usually seen in digits and is preceded by a trauma.**
- **Angiography is the best invasive method for the diagnosis of AVM demonstrating the vascular structure.**
- **MRI is useful in determining the extent of the lesion; however, MRA shows the flow velocity.**
- **Characteristic MRI manifestation is flow void in all sequences.**

ADDITIONAL IMAGES

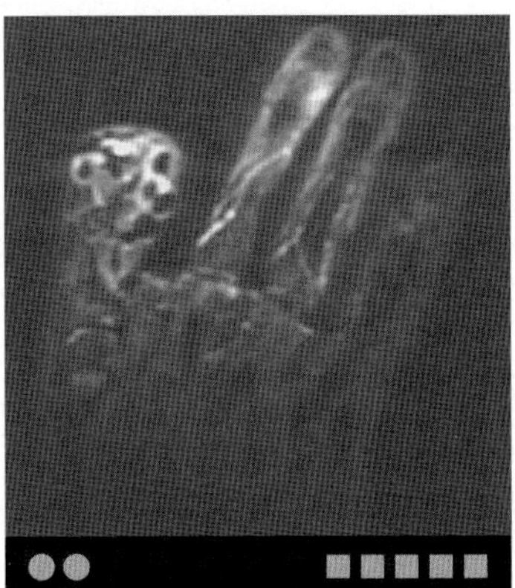

B. AVM: Coronal T2-weighted fat-saturated image shows focal round areas of signal void in the fifth finger surrounded by bright fluid signal.

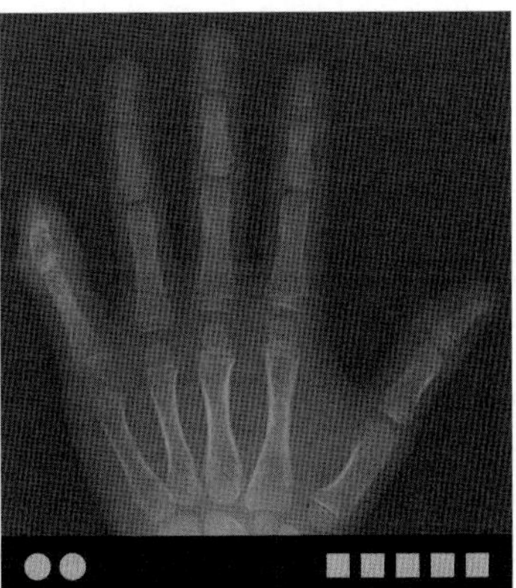

C. AVM: AP radiograph of the left hand shows soft tissue mass of the fifth finger with osteolytic changes in the middle and proximal phalanges.

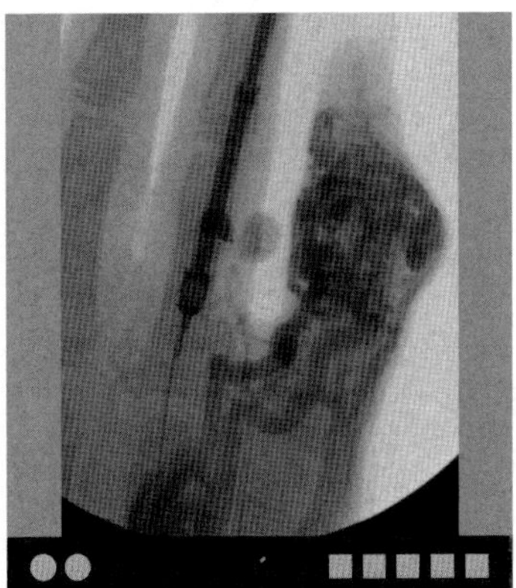

D. AVM: The angiogram of the digital artery shows bag of worms appearance with early venous drainage at the fifth finger.

DIFFERENTIAL DIAGNOSES IMAGES

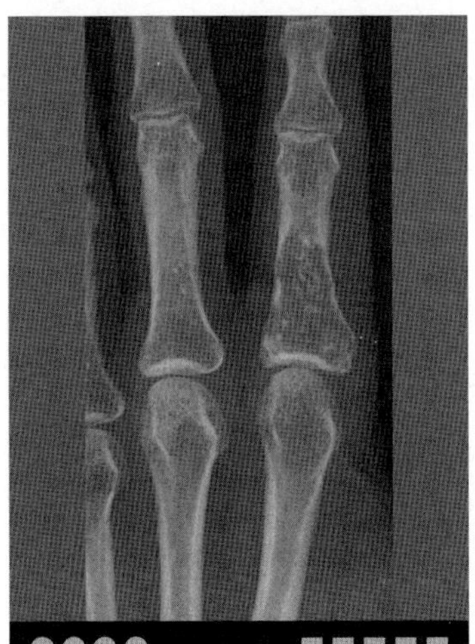

E. Enchondroma: AP radiograph of the index finger shows osteolytic lesion of the proximal phalanx of the middle finger with endocortical scalloping and punctuate microcalcification.

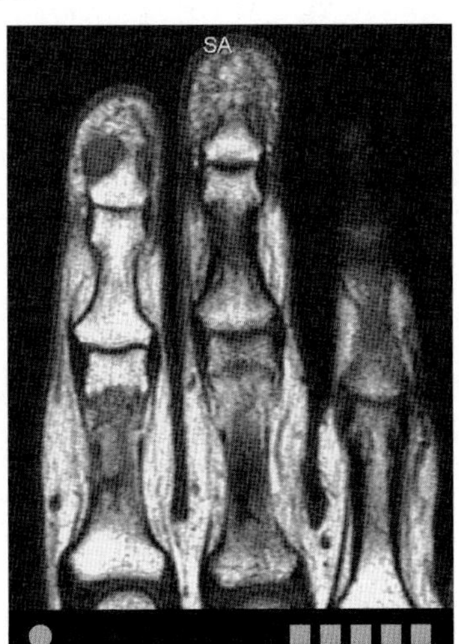

F. Glomus tumor: Coronal T1-weighted image shows oval, homogenous low signal intensity mass in the radial aspect of the distal phalanx of the third finger eroding into the bone.

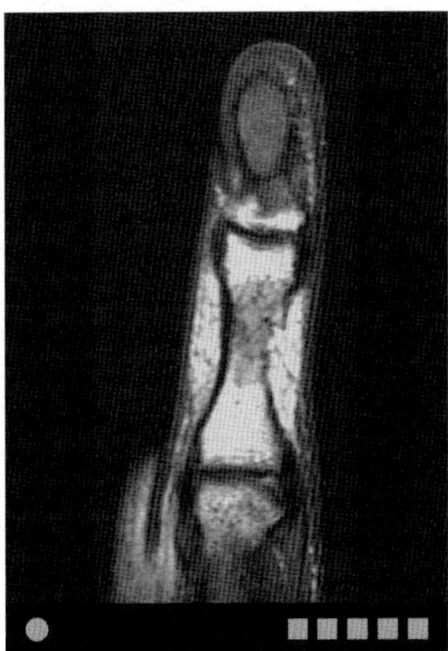

G. Epidermal inclusion cyst: Coronal T1-weighted image of the index finger showing expansile low signal oval-shaped lesion in the distal phalanx.

IMAGE KEY

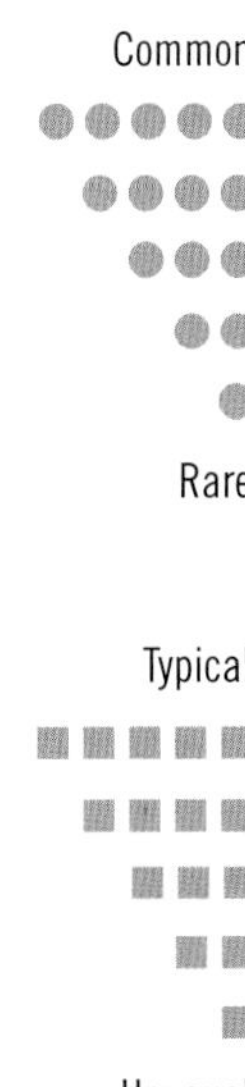

Chapter 14

Arthritis, Connective Tissue and Crystal Deposition Disorders

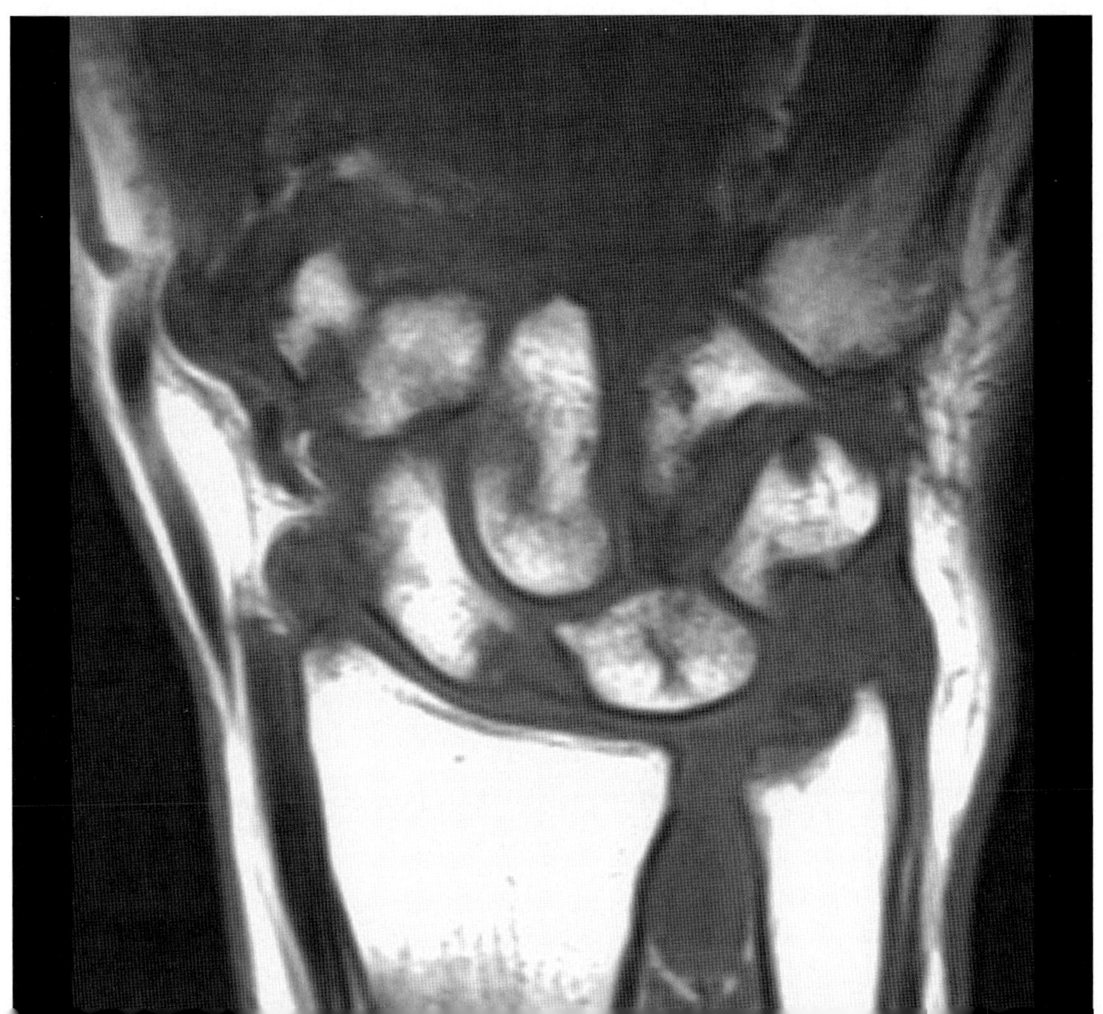

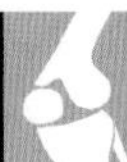

14–1 Rheumatoid Arthritis of the Hand and Wrist

Michael A. Bruno and Peyman Borghei

PRESENTATION

Progressive pain, swelling, and deformity

FINDINGS

Images show multimodality demonstration of the imaging manifestations of severe rheumatoid arthritis (RA). These include osteoporosis, synovitis, bone erosions, and subluxation deformities.

DIFFERENTIAL DIAGNOSES

- *Erosive inflammatory arthritides:* Psoriatic arthritis can mimic the clinical and imaging findings of rheumatoid disease. Unlike RA, which is often associated with osteoporosis, bone density is preserved in psoriatic arthritis.
- *Gouty arthritis:* This condition in the hands may be initially misdiagnosed as RA. Soft tissue masses around the joint and presence of erosions with overhanging edges are the hallmarks of gouty arthritis.

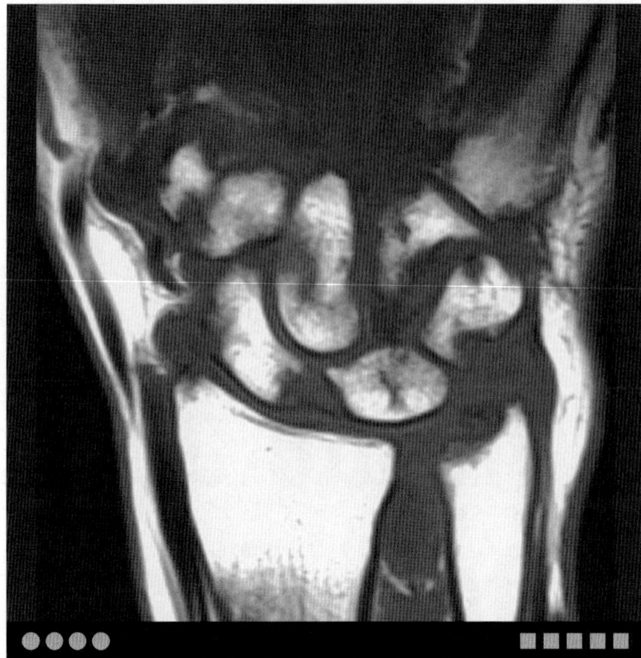

A. Rheumatoid arthritis: Coronal T1-weighted image shows erosive changes of all of the carpal bones and ulnar and radial styloid processes.

COMMENTS

This is a collection of images illustrating the typical findings of RA in the hands and wrists as seen on radiograph, MRI, and ultrasound (with Power Doppler). RA is actually a systemic disease that results in joint destruction, although there are also significant extra-articular manifestations of RA, most notably a characteristic pattern of interstitial lung disease. The overall adult prevalence of RA in the United States is estimated at ten million persons. Overall incidence is the same in all races, but there is an approximately 2–3:1 female-to-male ratio. Radiographically, osteopenia is the initial finding because of neovascularization and hyperemia/hyperplasia of the synovium. As the disease progresses, there is proliferation of a distinct and invasive inflammatory tissue known as pannus, which directly causes the erosion, joint destruction, and progressive deformity. This pannus can itself be distinctly imaged by MRI, and the hyperemia and neovascularity are easily identified (and can be quantified) on Power Doppler ultrasound. Erosive joint changes can be seen on radiograph, CT, MRI, or ultrasound, but are perhaps best seen and measured on MRI. Ultrasound is relatively limited in the detection of erosions because of limitations in probe placement; however, it can more reliably assess the degree of synovitis and hyperemia than can MRI.

PEARLS

- **Disease is characterized by a highly cellular inflammatory synovial tissue, the rheumatoid pannus, which causes progressive joint erosion, destruction, and deformity.**
- **A chronic, systemic, and life-threatening disease, with significant extra-articular manifestations and a high prevalence—more than 10 million affected persons in the United States alone.**
- **Radiographs are the historical standard for imaging, but MRI is highly sensitive to detect and characterize erosive changes.**
- **Ultrasound, especially supplemented by Power Doppler, is best suited to evaluate the inflammatory neovascularity and hyperemia.**

ADDITIONAL IMAGES

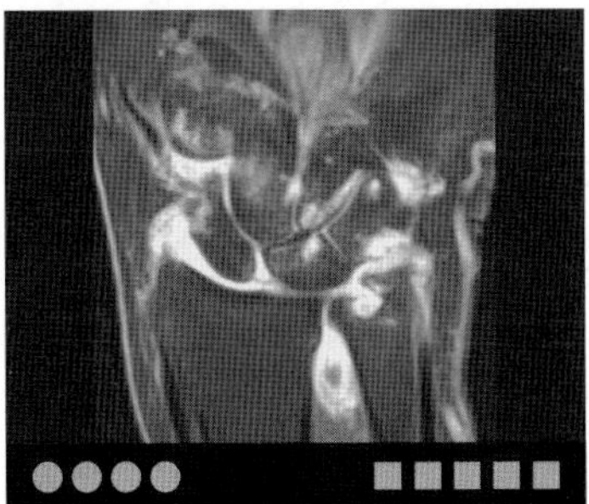

B. Rheumatoid arthritis: Postcontrast fat-saturated T1-weghted image shows enhancement of pannus surrounding the carpal bones and distal, radioulnar bursa. Also note enhanced foci of bony erosions in the carpal bones.

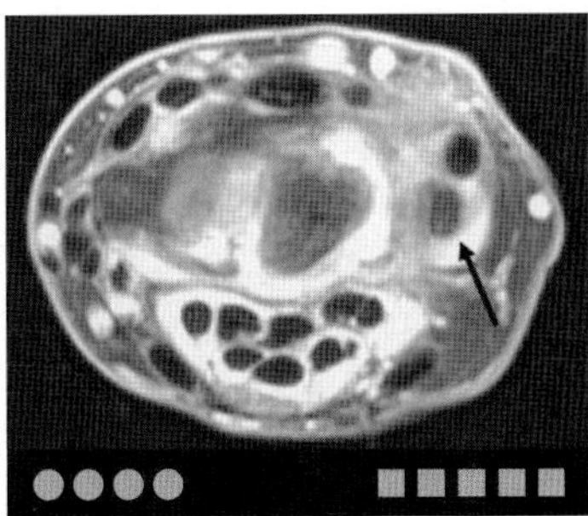

C. Rheumatoid arthritis: Axial T1 fat-saturated postcontrast MR image shows tenosynovitis of flexor and extensor tendons of the right wrist. Note synovial enhancement around the flexor tendons in the carpal tunnel area and tenosynovitis of extensor carpi ulnaris (black arrow).

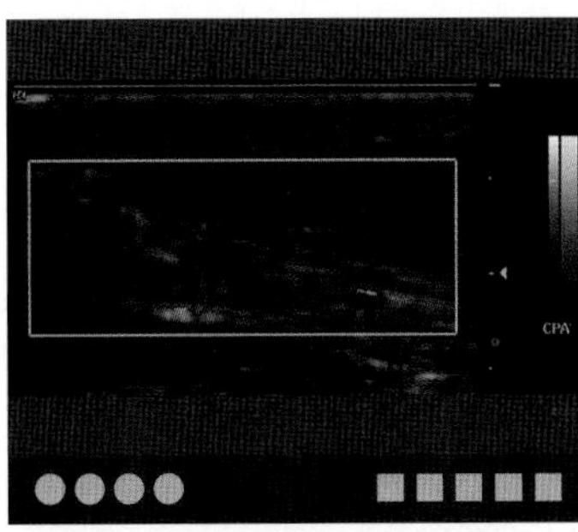

D. Rheumatoid synovitis, Power Doppler ultrasound: Image from another patient showing synovial hyperemia surrounding a hand tendon on this Power Doppler image.

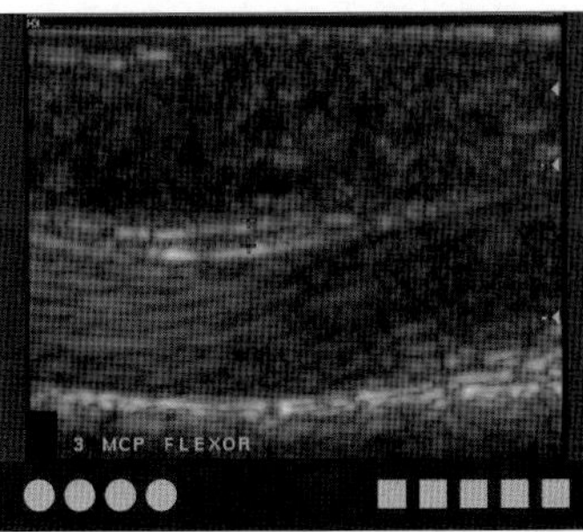

E. Rheumatoid synovitis, ultrasound: Another patient with RA of the hands showing a thin rim of fluid in the peritendinous sheath of the flexor tendon of the third digit near the MCP joint. Once thought to represent a pathognomonic feature of RA, such a small fluid collection, readily detectable on ultrasound (US), can be seen in any case of synovitis.

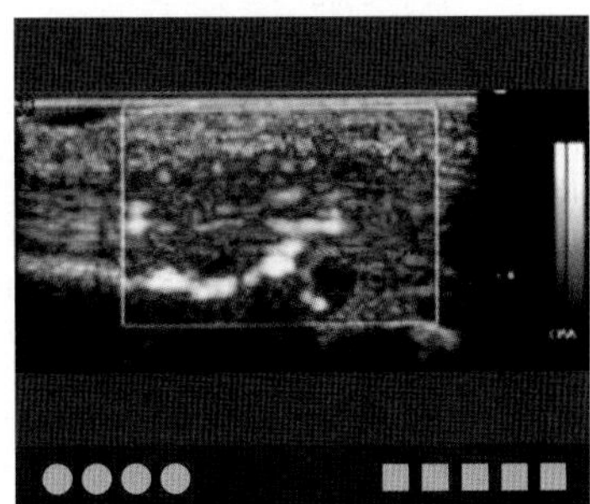

F. Rheumatoid arthritis, severe synovitis by Power Doppler ultrasound: Another patient with severe synovitis showing a very high degree of hyperemic signal in the synovial tissues of the flexor tendon on Power Doppler. The degree of signal on Power Doppler is quantifiably related to the severity of synovitis on clinical measures.

IMAGE KEY

Common

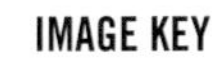

Rare

Typical

Unusual

DIFFERENTIAL DIAGNOSES IMAGE

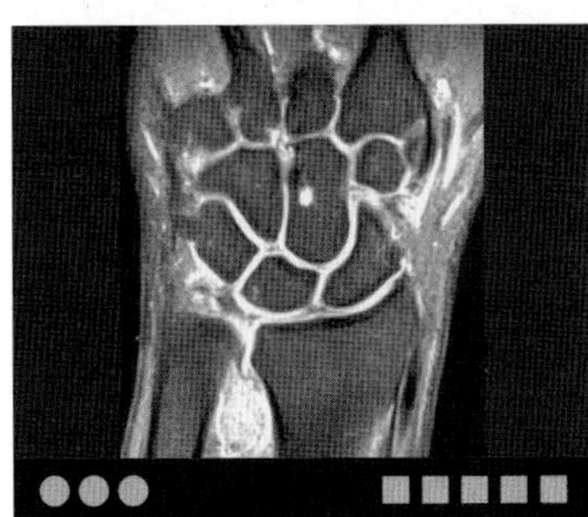

G. Gouty arthritis: Coronal T1-weighted fat-saturated postcontrast image shows erosion in the capitate and ulnar styloid, which enhances following contrast administration. Also note enhanced synovial proliferation at the distal, radioulnar joint and bursa.

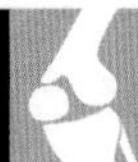

14–2 Juvenile Rheumatoid Arthritis of the Wrist

Edward Mossop and Jamshid Tehranzadeh

PRESENTATION

Worsening left wrist pain

FINDINGS

MRI shows multiple enhancing erosions with synovitis of the wrist and tear of the scapholunate ligament.

DIFFERENTIAL DIAGNOSES

- *Juvenile psoriatic arthritis:* An inflammatory arthritis occurring before the age of 16 with characteristic rash of psoriasis, nail pitting, dactylitis, and family history of psoriasis. Small joints of the hands are commonly involved.
- Septic arthritis is a purulent infection of joints usually caused by *Staphylococcus aureus*. The wrist is involved in 10% of cases. Patients are usually systemically unwell.
- *Reactive arthritis:* A transient, nonpurulent (reactive) arthritis appearing in the weeks following a digestive infection. Rarely this is polyarticular involving the wrist.
- *Systemic lupus erythematosus:* May cause less erosions and more deformity of the fingers.

COMMENTS

This is an image of a 19-year-old girl with proven juvenile rheumatoid arthritis (JRA). JRA represents a group of heterologous autoimmune diseases that have a common chronic inflammatory arthritis and a prevalence of approximately 1 in 1000 children. Chronic inflammation of synovium is characterized by B lymphocyte infiltration and expansion. The resulting thickened pannus causes joint destruction, pain, and loss of function. There are three main types of JRA; pauciarticular, polyartricular, and systemic. JRA commonly affects the knees, hands, and feet. Radiographic findings in the hands are often negative; however, these can include soft tissue swelling around the joints and periarticular demineralization. Joint space destruction and erosions ensue and eventually ankylosis of the carpal bones. MRI typically shows synovitis of the joints and tendon sheaths as low signal on T1-weighted images and mixed signal on T2-weighted images. Active synovium enhances after contrast helping to differentiate it from fluid. Marginal erosions of the bone and cartilage appear as areas of low signal on T1-weighted images and as regions of heterogeneous signal on T2-weighted images. Cystic bone erosions are viewed as low signal on T1-weighted images and high signal on T2-weighted images and often enhance after contrast. Other changes include subchondral sclerosis, damage to ligaments, and osteonecrosis. Measurement of synovial volumes with MRI can be used to monitor disease progression.

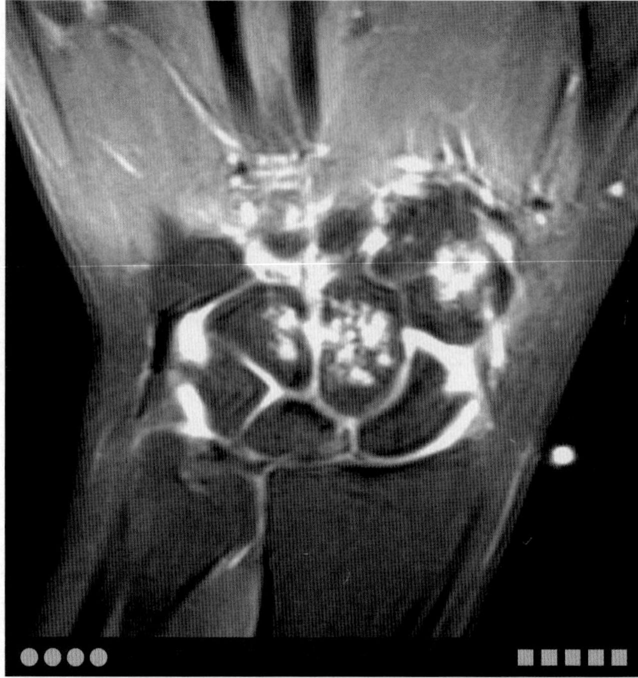

A. JRA: Coronal T1-weighted fat-saturated postcontrast image shows multiple bony erosions of the carpal bones. Note marked synovial enhancement.

PEARLS

- **JRA represents a group of heterologous autoimmune diseases that have a common chronic inflammatory arthritis.**
- **Prevalence is approximately 1 in 1000 children in the United States.**
- **Radiographic findings in the hands can include soft tissue swelling around the joints and periarticular demineralization.**
- **MRI typically shows synovitis of the joints and tendon sheaths as low signal on T1-weighted images and mixed signal on T2-weighted images.**
- **Erosion of joints will enhance with contrast and joint fusion may occur.**

ADDITIONAL IMAGES

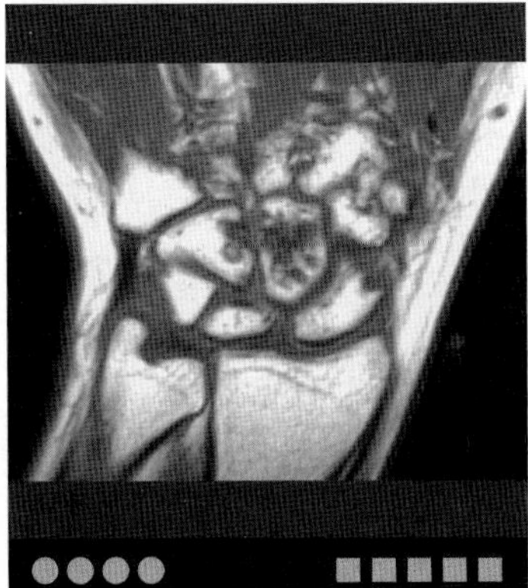

B. JRA: Coronal T1-weighted spin echo image shows multiple carpal bone erosions including capitate, hamate, trapezium, trapezoid, and scaphoid bones.

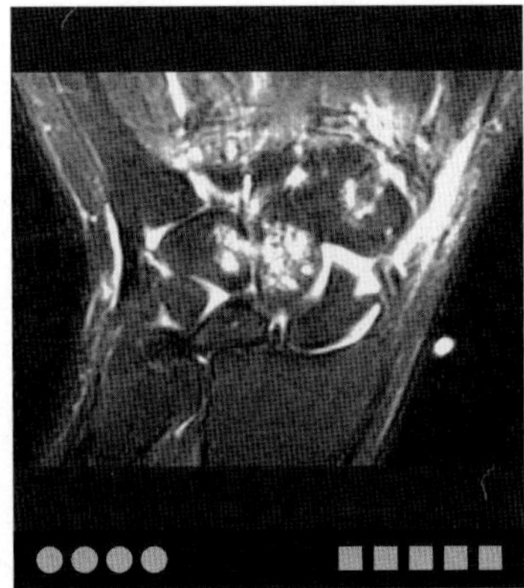

C. JRA: Coronal T2-weighted fat-saturated image shows multiple carpal bone erosions. Note fluid in the radio-carpal and common carpal joints.

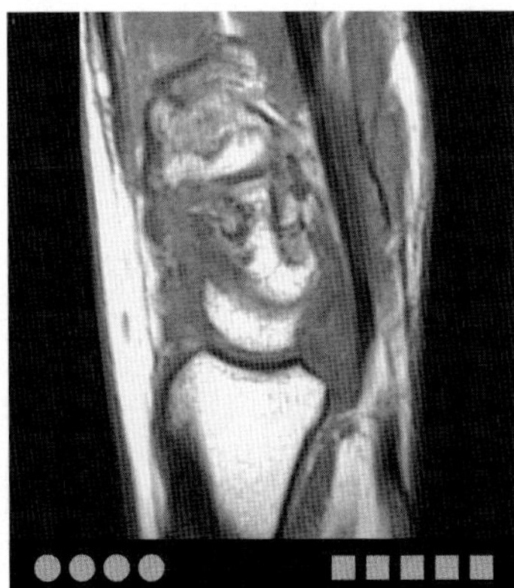

D. JRA: Sagittal T1-weighted spin echo image shows intermediate signal synovial proliferation surrounding the wrist joint with multiple capitate erosions.

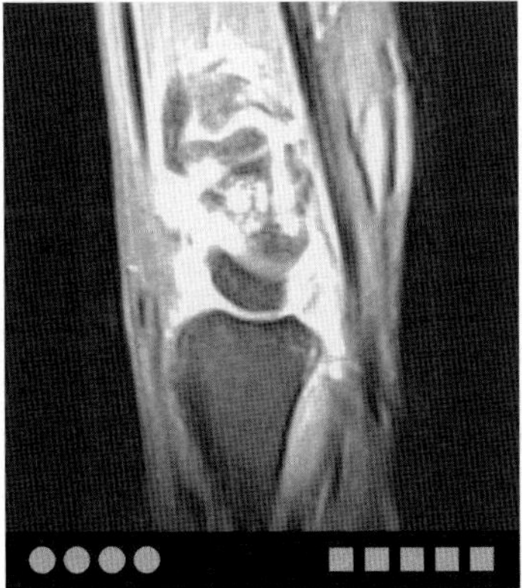

E. JRA: Sagittal T1-weighted fat-saturated postcontrast image shows multiple enhancing erosions of the capitate bone. Note diffuse synovial enhancement surrounding the wrist joint.

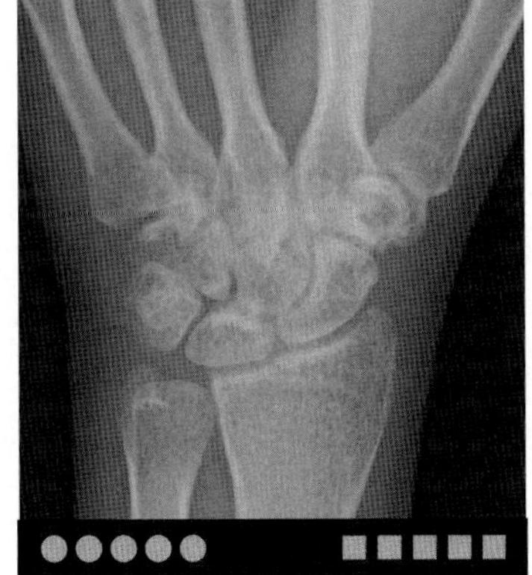

F. JRA: AP radiograph of the wrist may show questionable cystic changes in the capitate and hamate. However, it fails to show extensive erosions noted on MRI study.

DIFFERENTIAL DIAGNOSES IMAGE

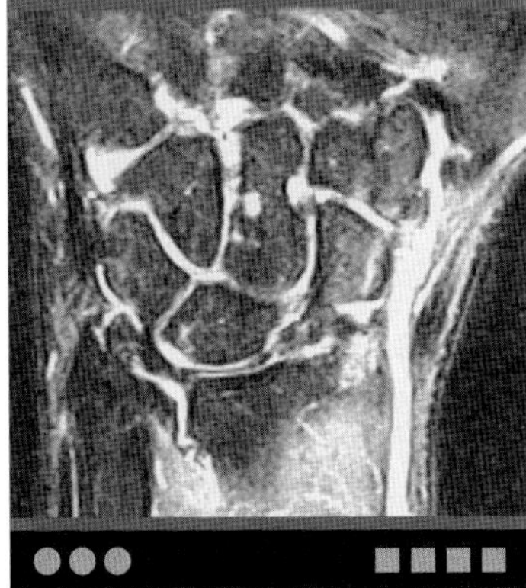

G. Psoriatic arthritis: Coronal T2-weighted fat-saturated image shows two small erosions in the capitate and a larger erosion in the radial styloid with joint fluid present.

IMAGE KEY

Common

Rare

Typical

Unusual

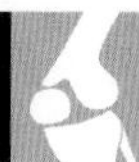

14–3 Carpal Tunnel Syndrome Caused By Rheumatoid Arthritis

Peyman Borghei and Jamshid Tehranzadeh

PRESENTATION

Hand paresthesia

FINDINGS

MR Image shows bulging of the flexor retinaculum and flattening of the median nerve consistent with carpal tunnel syndrome (CTS).

DIFFERENTIAL DIAGNOSES

- *Normal carpal tunnel:* Normally the flexor retinaculum is flat, and there is no abnormal signal around the flexor tendons and median nerve on T2-weighted image.
- CTS caused by other arthritidies such as psoriasis may be associated with cutaneous changes.
- CTS caused by infiltrating diseases and fibrosis such as gout and amyloidosis shows regions of low signal intensity within the carpal tunnel on T2-weighted image.
- CTS caused by edema related to trauma, pregnancy, or hypothyroidism manifests as high signal intensity foci on T2-weighted image.
- C6 radiculopathy caused by nerve root compression is associated with neck pain and decreased neck mobility. Sensory and motor deficits are usually of equivalent severity.

COMMENTS

This is an imag of a 77-year-old woman with long history of rheumatoid arthritis (RA) who presented with paresthesia of right hand diagnosed with CTS. CTS is median nerve dysfunction caused by increased pressure within the carpal tunnel. It usually affects women between ages 35 and 65, with a predilection for dominant hand and also individuals who have repetitive wrist motion, such as typists and cashiers. Other potential causes include RA and other arthritic and synovial diseases, trauma, hemorrhage, benign tumors (ganglion cyst, lipoma, haemangioma, and neuroma), amyloidosis, gout, diabetes, myxedema, acromegaly, and congenital anomalies such as carpal tunnel stenosis. The common MRI feature is the palmar bowing of the flexor retinaculum which extends from pisiform and hook of hamate medially to the scaphoid and hook of trapezium laterally, which is best seen on axial views. There is also flattening of median nerve. MRI might show increased signal intensity of the flexor tendon sheaths in RA because of edema and fluid accumulation (tenosynovitis) associated with carpal bone erosions. Gadolinium contrast may enhance the synovial or connective tissue around the flexor tendons. In acute cases, MRI shows enlarged median nerve with increased signal intensity on T2-weighted image because of edematous changes, while in chronic cases, median nerve may show decreased signal intensity because of ischemia and fibrosis.

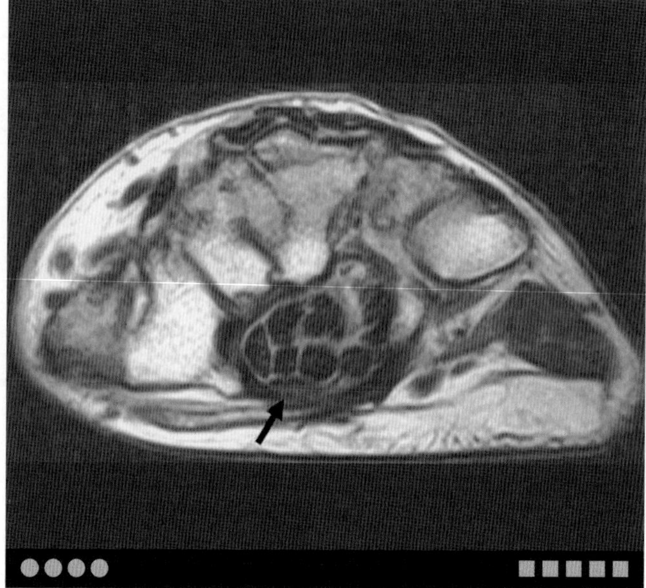

A. CTS in RA: Axial T2-weighted image shows low signal intensity foci in the median nerve caused by chronic pressure and ischemia (arrow). Note separation of flexor tendons caused by proliferation of connective tissue and synovium.

PEARLS

- **CTS is usually seen in women with a predilection for dominant hand.**
- **Risk factors include repetitive wrist motion and(or previous history of RA, infiltrative diseases, trauma, and other problems affecting carpal tunnel space.**
- **Axial MR image shows palmar bowing of flexor retinaculum with flattening of the median nerve.**
- **On MRI, median nerve may show high signal intensity because of neuritis and edema or low signal intensity caused by ischemia and fibrosis.**

ADDITIONAL IMAGES

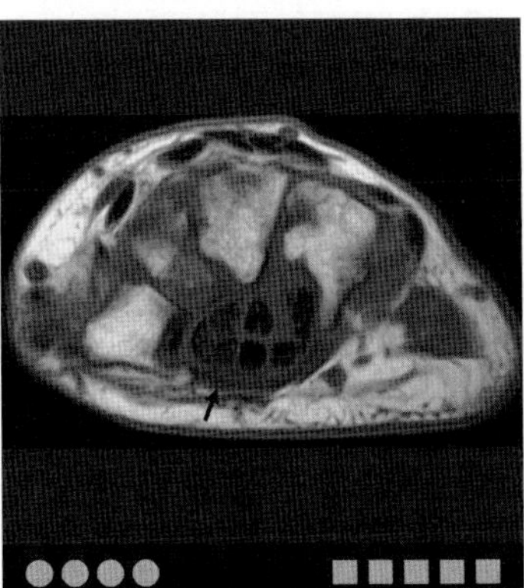

B. CTS in RA: Axial T1-weighted image at the level of hook of hamate and hook of trapezium shows bulging of the flexor retinaculum and also flattening of the median nerve (arrow).

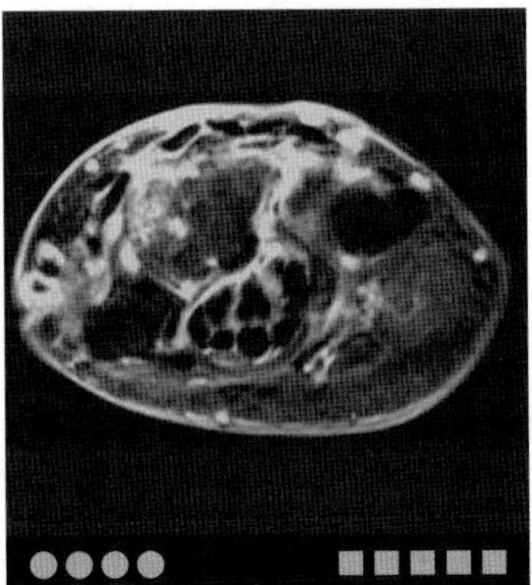

C. CTS in RA: Axial T1-weighted fat-saturated postcontrast image shows enhancement surrounding flexor tendons consistent with tenosynovitis at the level of carpal tunnel. Tenosynovitis of extensor tendons is also present.

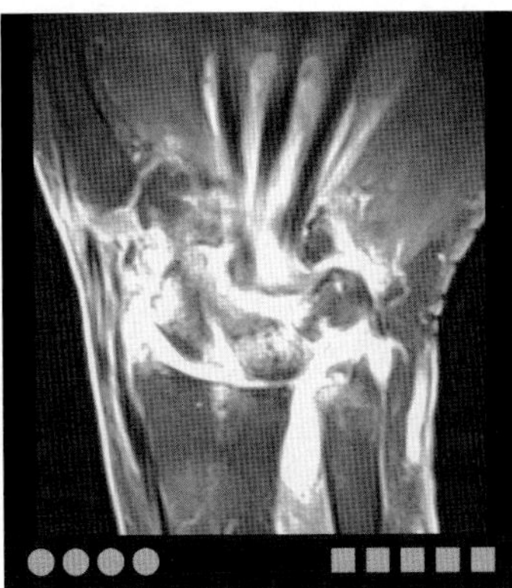

D. CTS in RA: Coronal T1-weighted fat-saturated postcontrast image shows enhancement surrounding flexor tendons. Note diffuse synovial enhancement and extensive bony erosions.

E. CTS in RA: Sagittal T1-weighted fat-saturated postcontrast image shows diffuse synovial enhancement around the wrist. Flexor and extensor tenosynovitis and bony erosions are noted.

DIFFERENTIAL DIAGNOSES IMAGES

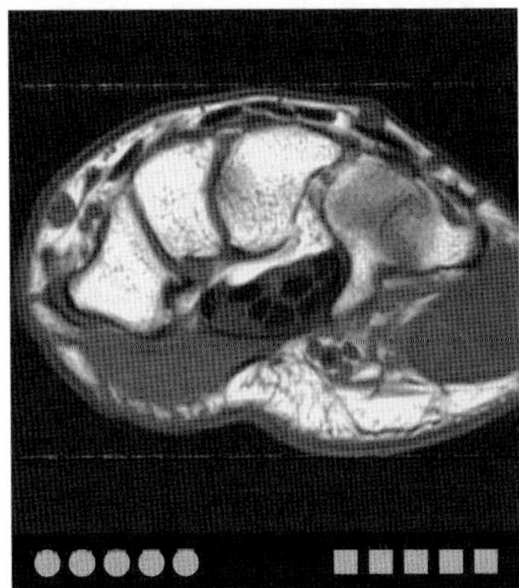

F. Normal carpal tunnel. Axial T1-weighted image shows flat flexor retinaculum and normal round or oval median nerve.

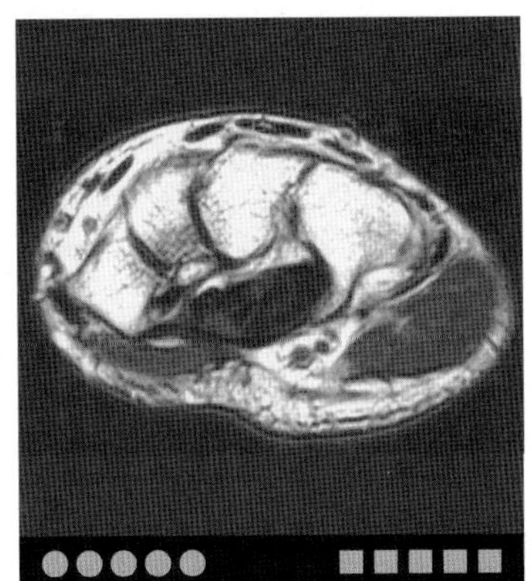

G. Normal carpal tunnel: Axial T2-weighted image shows flat flexor retinaculum and normal round or oval median nerve.

IMAGE KEY

Common

Rare

Typical

Unusual

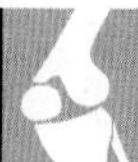

14–4 Psoriatic Arthritis

Joseph G. Giaconi and Thomas Learch

PRESENTATION

Swollen finger

FINDINGS

MRI shows distention of flexor synovial sheaths by fluid collection with limited joint involvement, with a bone edema at the enthesis.

DIFFERENTIAL DIAGNOSES

- *Flexor tendon sheath infection:* Fluid signal in flexor tendon sheath with clinical signs of infection. Clinical diagnosis made by exquisite pain upon passive extension of the involved finger. Incision and debridement will obtain definitive diagnosis based upon bacterial growth from surgical specimen.
- *Reiter's syndrome:* Dactylitis affects the toes more often than the fingers. This condition is similar to psoriatic arthritis in which there is enthesitis and periosteal reaction. Clinical triad of nongonococcal urethritis, conjunctivitis, and arthritis is diagnostic.
- *Tuberculous osteomyelitis:* The bones of the hands are usually affected more often than the feet, with the proximal phalanx of the index and middle fingers being the most common site. Radiographic features are of a cystic, expansile lesion with well-defined margins, with a large soft tissue mass, known as "spina ventosa." Affected individuals are usually less than 6 years.

COMMENTS

This is an image of a 35-year-old female who presented with a swollen finger, the "cocktail sausage digit," or dactylitis. Psoriatic dactylitis is a fusiform soft tissue swelling of a digit, which maybe acute or chronic. Dactylitis maybe the initial presentation of the disease, and it can be triggered by trauma. The digits of the feet are more often affected than of the hands, and it is usually asymmetric. Those digits which are affected are associated with a greater degree of radiological damage than those digits which are not affected by dactylitis. The imaging findings of psoriatic dactylitis are characteristic. Radiographs demonstrate fusiform soft tissue swelling. MRI demonstrates distention of the flexor synovial sheaths by fluid collection, which is manifested by high signal on STIR sequences. There is bone edema at the enthesis. Joint capsule distention is rare. There are five recognized patterns of psoriatic arthritis: oligoarticular (four or fewer joints affected), polyarticular, predominant distal interphalangeal (DIP) joint involvement, arthritis mutilans, and psoriatic spondylitis. The oligoarticular type accounts for more than 70% of cases. Radiographs in patients with psoriatic arthritis demonstrate erosive arthritis, with frequent DIP joint involvement, pencil-in-cup changes because of marked resorption of bone. Other findings include enthesitis with periosteal reaction, sacroiliitis, and spondylitis. Treatment with anti-TNF (Antitumor necrotizing factor) medication may halt radiological progression of disease. Injection of corticosteroid into the tenosynovial tendon sheath can produce some resolution of symptoms.

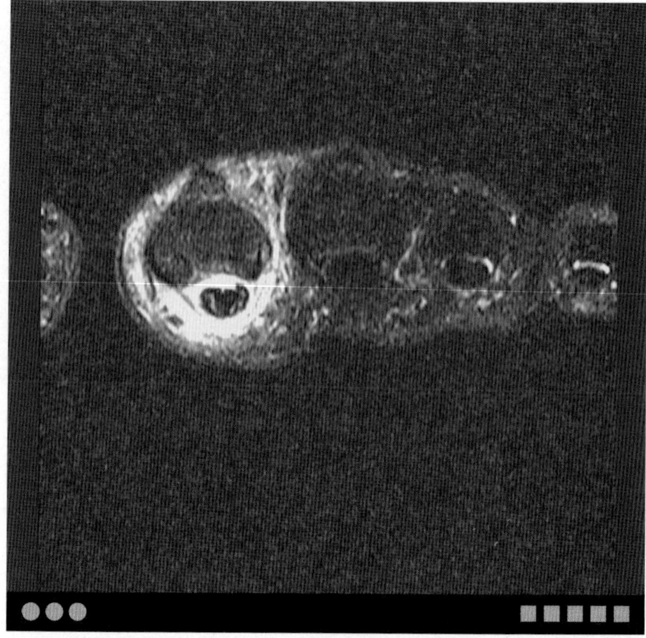

A. Psoriatic arthritis: Axial STIR sequence of hand demonstrates marked inflammation about the second digit.

PEARLS

- **Distention of flexor synovial sheaths by fluid collection with limited joint involvement appears as high signal on STIR sequences.**
- **Psoriatic dactylitis more often affects the toes than the fingers.**
- **Estimates of the frequency of arthritis in patients with psoriasis are in the range of 2% to 6%.**
- **Nail abnormalities are correlated most closely with articular disease.**

ADDITIONAL IMAGES

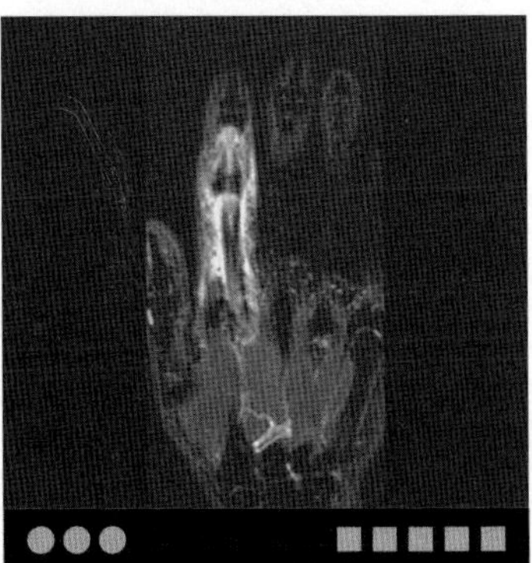

B. Psoriatic arthritis: Coronal STIR sequence of hand demonstrates marked inflammation about the second digit.

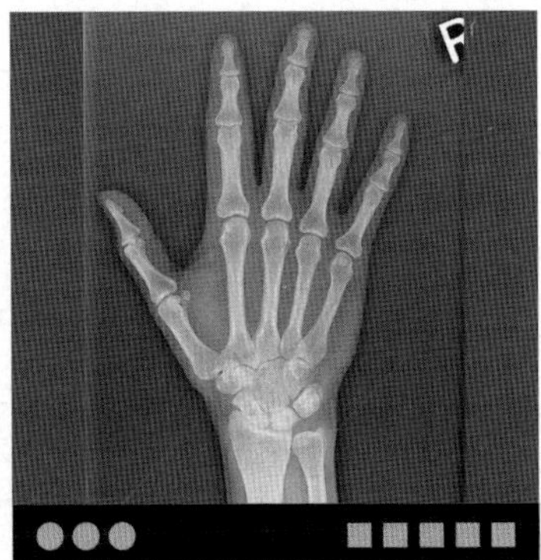

C. Psoriatic arthritis: Radiograph of hand demonstrates diffuse soft tissue swelling of second digit. Underlying bones and joints are normal.

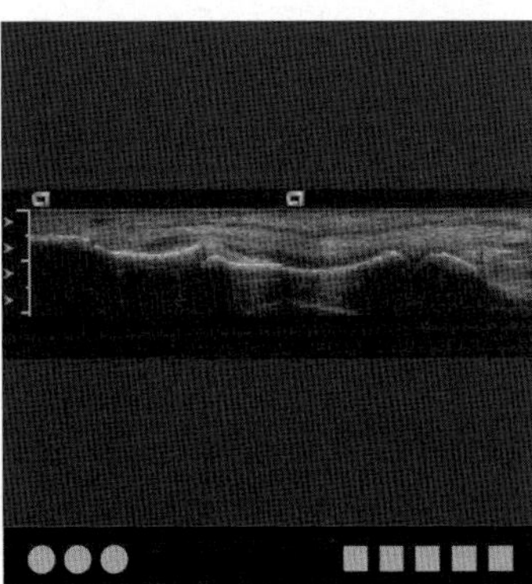

D. Psoriatic arthritis: Longitudinal ultrasound of second digit demonstrates extensive tenosynovitis of the flexor tendon.

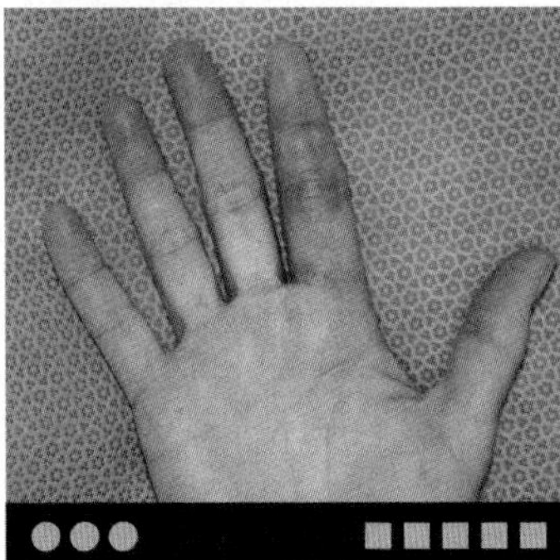

E. Psoriatic arthritis: Photograph of hand demonstrates diffuse swelling of entire second digit with erythema. Faint scar is visualized on third digit, where patient had prior incision and drainage with negative cultures for previous episode of swollen digit. Patient also reported similar episode involving a toe.

IMAGE KEY

Common

Rare

Typical

Unusual

DIFFERENTIAL DIAGNOSES IMAGES

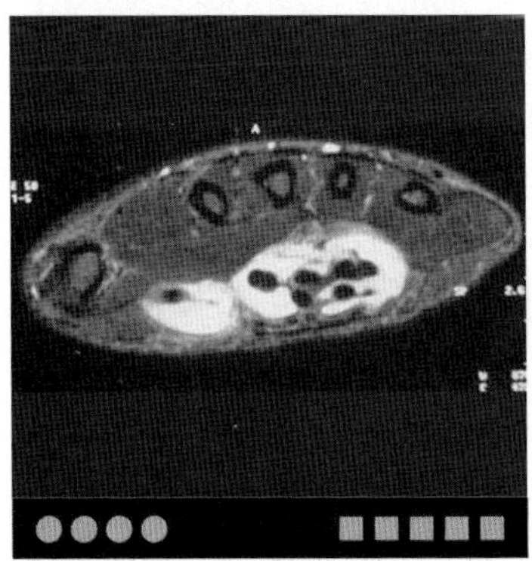

F. Flexor tendon sheath synovitis: Axial STIR image demonstrates high signal fluid in the flexor tendon sheaths. Culture was positive for *Mycobacterium marinum.*

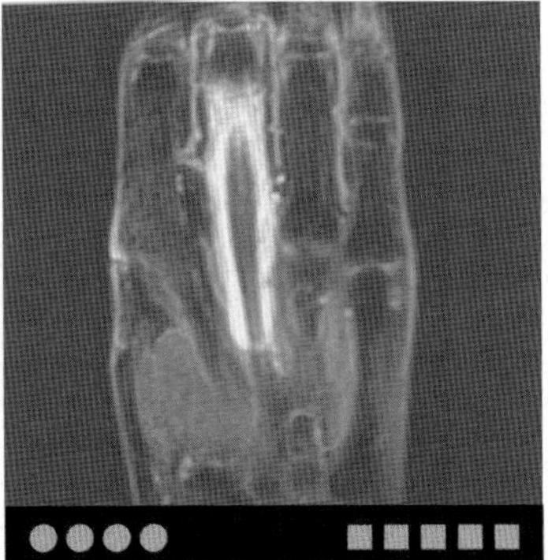

G. Tenosynovitis in inflammatory arthritis: Coronal fat-saturated T1-weighted postcontrast image in a 68-year-old female with systemic lupus erythematosus and enhanced synovial sheath of the flexor tendon of the third finger.

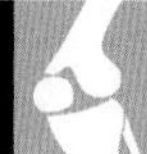

14–5 Pseudogout

Ashkan Afshin and Jamshid Tehranzadeh

PRESENTATION

Acute wrist pain

FINDINGS

Radiographic finding shows narrowing of the joint space and calcification in hyaline cartilages and triangular fibrocartilage of the wrist. Note significant joint narrowing at trapezium-scaphoid joint.

DIFFERENTIAL DIAGNOSES

- *Gout:* Radiograph of the joint in early stages of gout shows soft tissue swelling. The initial bony changes appear as punch-out lesions with overhanging edges in intermediate phase of gout. In the late phase of the disease, radiographs may show intraosseous tophi and joint narrowing.
- *Hyperparathyroidism:* Conventional radiographs show subperiosteal resorption of phalanges and digital tufts. Cystic lesions known as osteitis fibrosa cystica (brown tumor), chondrocalcinosis, and calcification of the soft tissues are other manifestations.
- *Hemochromatosis:* This condition results from iron deposition in multiple organs including liver, pancreas, heart, joints, and skin. Radiographic findings in patients with hemochromatosis may show osteoporosis, articular calcification, or structural joint damage (arthropathy) predominantly osteophytosis of metacarpophalangeal joints.

COMMENTS

Pseudogout results from deposition of the calcium pyrophosphate dihydrate (CPPD) in articular tissues. This condition may manifest as chondrocalcinosis, crystal-induced synovitis, and pyrophosphate arthropathy. It usually occurs in people over 60 years of age and affects female more than men. Articular deposition of CPPD crystals can have a variety of presentations, such as incidental radiographic finding, acute attack, and chronic arthritis. It most often involves the knee and the wrists but can occur at hips, shoulders, and other joints. Acute attack is characterized by sudden and severe pain, redness, warmth, and swelling (inflammation) in the joint, which can resemble a gout attack but dose not respond to usual treatment (colchicine) (hence the old term "pseudogout"). Chondrocalcinosis occurs from calcification of the hyaline cartilage or fibrocartilage. Chondrocalcinosis of the meniscus are common in old individuals and in association with several distinct metabolic disorders. It can be seen as linear densities in hyaline or fibrocartilage, which are parallel to and separate from subchondral bone. Evidence of the CPPD crystals often can be seen on conventional radiograph before symptoms are present. Although radiographic finding can be diagnostic, and the definitive clinical diagnosis requires identification of CPPD crystal from joint fluid. CPPD crystals are visualized under compensated polarized light microscopy.

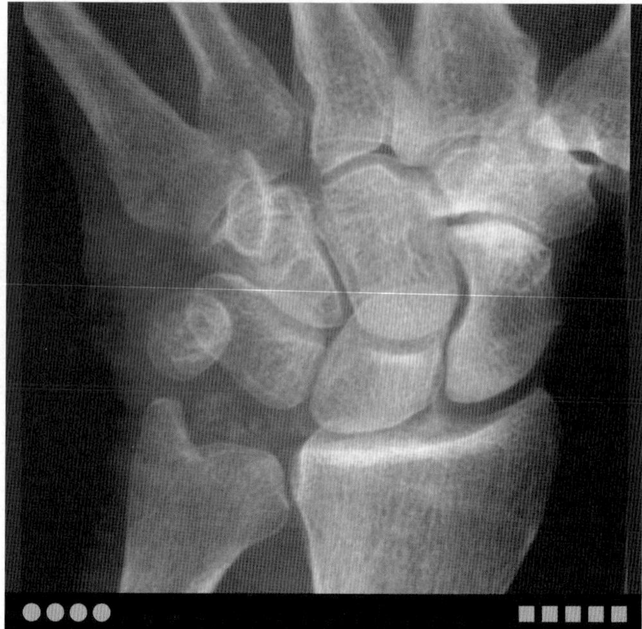

A. Pseudogout: PA radiograph of the wrist shows calcification of triangular fibrocartilage and articular cartilages consistent with pseudogout. Note significant joint narrowing at trapezium-scaphoid joint.

In the wrist joint, the target areas of significant joint narrowing includes trapezium-scaphoid and trapezium-first metacarpal joints. Characteristic remarkable femoropatellar joint narrowing is the hallmark of CPPD in the knee joint.

PEARLS

- **Deposition of the CPPD in articular tissue.**
- **Three main manifestations : chondrocalcinosis, crystal induced synovitis, and pyrophosphate arthropathy.**
- **Calcification of the hyaline cartilage or fibrocartilage results in chondrocalcinosis.**
- **Femoropatellar joint and trapezium-scaphoid, trapezium-first metacarpal joints and metacarpophalangeal joints are the target joints.**
- **Diagnosis requires identification of CPPD crystals from joint fluid**

ADDITIONAL IMAGES

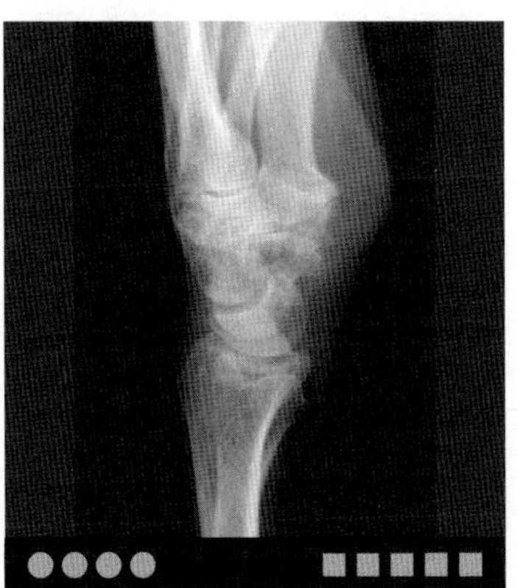

B. Pseudogout: Lateral radiograph of the wrist shows chondrocalcinosis of the wrist joint.

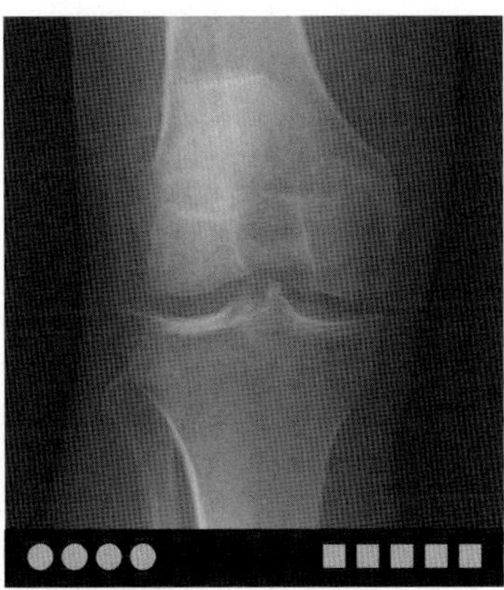

C. Pseudogout: AP radiograph of the knee shows chondrocalcinosis of the cartilages of the knee with secondary osteoarthrosis in another patient with pseudogout.

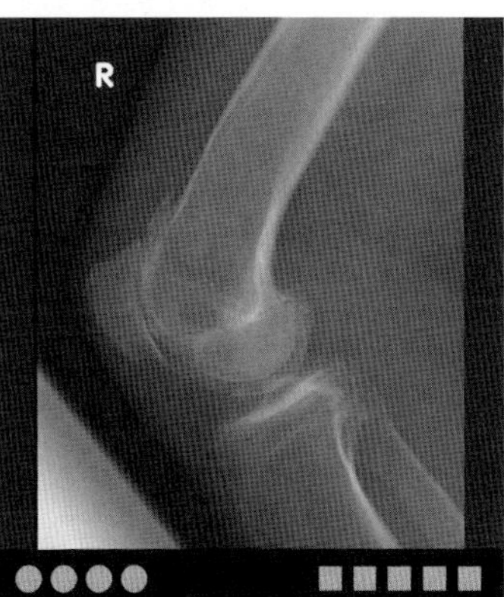

D. Pseudogout: Lateral radiograph of the knee of the same patient as in image C shows chondrocalcinosis with sever osteoarthrosis. Note marked narrowing of the femoropatellar joint, which is a target joint for pseudogout.

IMAGE KEY

Common

Rare

Typical

Unusual

DIFFERENTIAL DIAGNOSES IMAGES

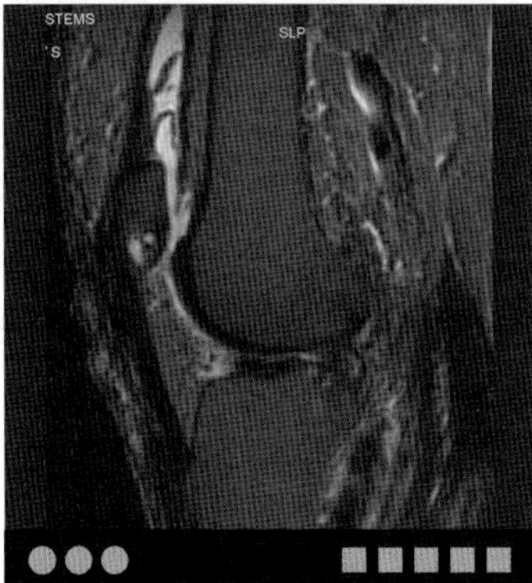

E. Gout: Sagittal fat-saturated T2-weighted image of the knee shows intraosseous erosions suggesting intraosseous tophi of the lower pole of patella. Joint effusion and thickening of suprapatellar plica is also noted.

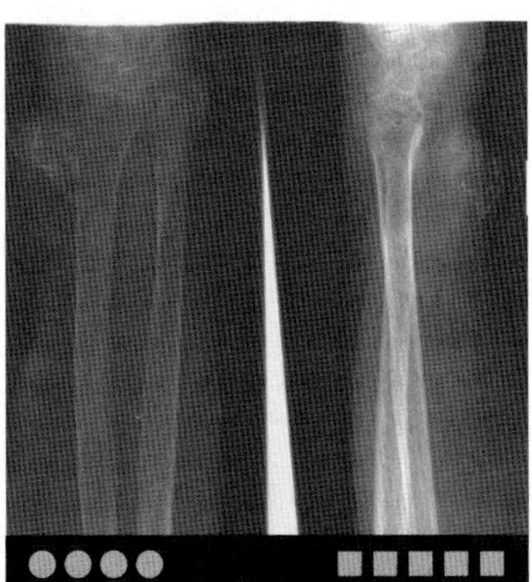

F. Hyperparathyroidism secondary to end-stage renal disease (ESRD) in a patient on dialysis: AP and lateral radiograph of the distal forearm shows chondrocalcinosis of the wrist as well as osteoporosis and vascular calcifications. Note typical ring calcification at the arteriovenous dialysis shunt level in the volar aspect of the wrist.

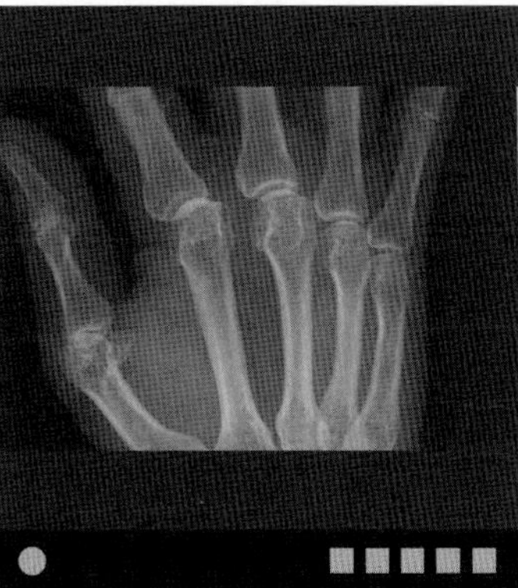

G. Hemochromatosis: Oblique radiograph of metacarpophalangeal joint in a patient with hemochromatosis shows osteoarthrosis and osteophyte formation of metacarpophalangeal joints in first, second, and third rays.

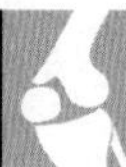

14–6 Hemochromatosis

Ashkan Afshin and Adam C. Zoga

PRESENTATION

Wrist Pain

FINDINGS

Radiographic imaging of both hands and wrists shows joint space narrowing, osteophytosis at the metacarpal heads, and osteoporosis. Chondrocalcinosis of the triangular fibrocartilage with periarticular calcifications can also be observed.

DIFFERENTIAL DIAGNOSES

- *Pseudogout:* This condition results from deposition of calcium pyrophosphate dihydrate (CPPD) crystals in the joints. Radiographic images show chondrocalcinosis, subchondral sclerosis, joint space narrowing, and subchondral cyst.
- *Rheumatoid arthritis:* This is a highly inflammatory polyarthritis often leading to joint destruction, deformity, and loss of function. Radiographs of the hands are often normal at presentation or may show swelling of soft tissue, loss of joint space, or periarticular osteoporosis. MRI can detect early erosion foci which are low signal on T1-weighted image, bright on T2-weighted image, and enhance with contrast.

COMMENTS

Hemochromatosis is an uncommon disorder which results from iron deposition in multiple organs including liver, pancreas, heart, joints, and skin. Primary hemochromatosis is an autosomal recessive disorder characterized by unrestricted absorption of the iron in the small intestine. Secondary hemochromatosis results from iron overload because of conditions such as transfusion or alcohol abuse. This disorder affects men 10 times more than women and is generally diagnosed between the fourth to seventh decades of life. Hemochromatosis has a wide range of clinical manifestations from completely asymptomatic, to cirrhosis, skin hyperpigmentation, bronze diabetes, degenerative joint disease, and restrictive cardiopathy. Laboratory findings in patients of hemochromatosis show increase in serum iron and decrease total iron-binding capacity. MR images of liver show abnormally decreased signal intensity, which indicates the iron accumulation in the liver. Biopsy of the liver or synovium confirms the diagnosis. Hemochromatosis may have four different types of bone and joint involvement, which can be classified as: osteoporosis, articular calcification, structural joint damage (arthropathy), and miscellaneous abnormality. Osteophytosis at the metacarpal heads is a characteristic finding in hemochromatosis. Osteoporosis secondary to hemochromatosis may involve axial bones resulting in deformities such as "fish vertebrate" or affect appendicular skeleton, with the diverse range of distribution. CPPD crystal deposition in patient with hemochromatosis is most frequently found in wrists, knees, and symphysis pubis. Involvement of symphysis pubis, prominent calcification of hyaline cartilage, and correlation between the severity of arthropathy and degree of chondrocalcinosis are characteristics of hemochromatosis, and may differentiate this condition from other causes of chondrocalcinosis such as pseudogout.

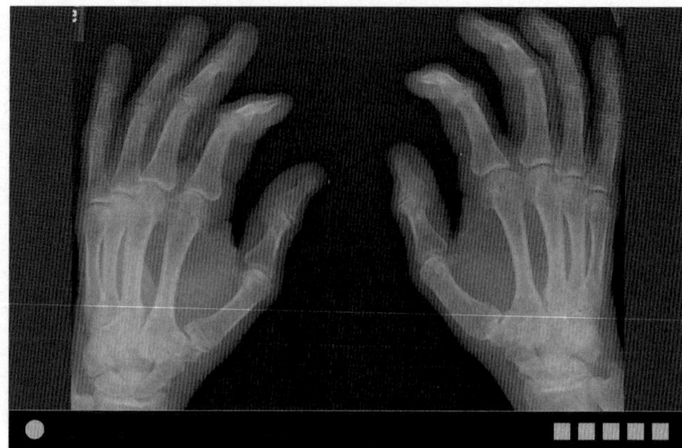

A. Hemochromatosis: Oblique radiograph of both hands shows chondrocalcinosis of the triangular fibrocartilage with periarticular calcifications. There are typical osteophytes noted at the metacarpal heads, best seen on the second and third metacarpals. Subchondral erosions on the second metacarpal heads are also noted.

PEARLS

- **Hemochromatosis is a rare condition resulting from iron deposition in multiple organs, which may be primary or secondary.**
- **Primary type is autosomal recessive and secondary type is caused by conditions such as transfusion or alcohol abuse.**
- **It has a wide range of clinical manifestations from no clinical symptom to cirrhosis, skin hyperpigmentation, bronze diabetes, degenerative joint disease, and restrictive cardiopathy.**
- **Liver MRI shows abnormally decreased signal intensity and biopsy of the liver or synovium confirms the diagnosis.**
- **Osteoporosis, articular calcification, structural joint damage (arthropathy), and miscellaneous abnormality are four different types of bone and joint involvement in hemochromatosis.**
- **Osteophytosis at the metacarpal heads is a characteristic finding.**

ADDITIONAL IMAGES

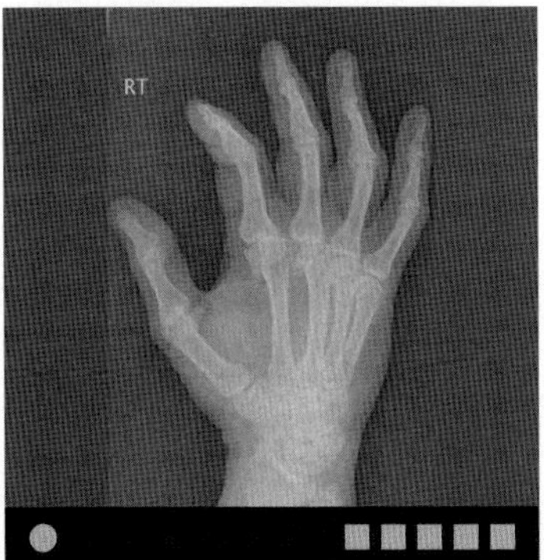

B. Hemochromatosis: Oblique radiograph of hand in another patient shows hypertrophic osteophytes in metacarpal heads with chondrocalcinosis (Courtesy of Adam Zoga).

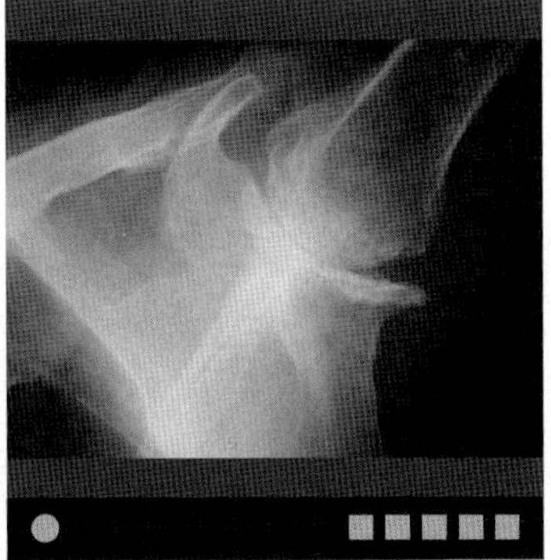

C. Hemochromatosis: Axillary radiograph of shoulder shows concentric joint narrowing with subchondral sclerosis and hypertrophic changes of glenohumeral joints (Courtesy of Adam Zoga).

DIFFERENTIAL DIAGNOSES IMAGES

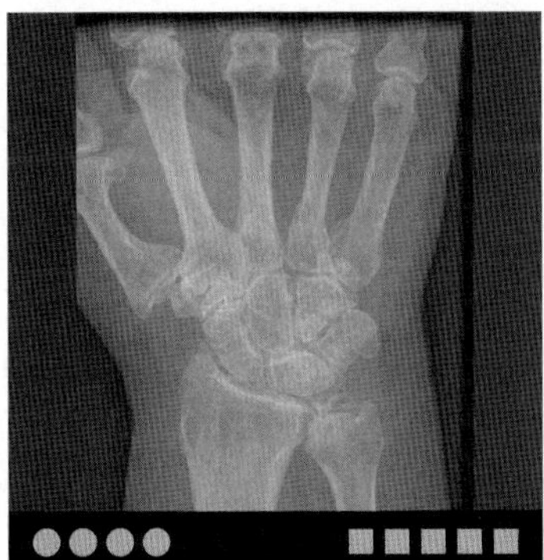

D. Pseudogout: AP radiograph of the wrist shows chondrocalcinosis with periarticular calcifications noted at the wrist joint and metacarpophalangeal joints.

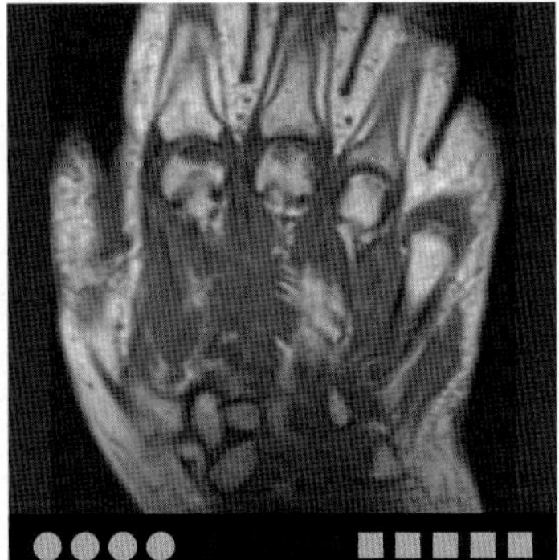

E. Pseudogout: Coronal T1-weighted image, in the same patient as in image C, shows synovial proliferation of the wrist and metacarpophalangeal joints. Note erosions at the metacarpal heads as foci of low signal intensity.

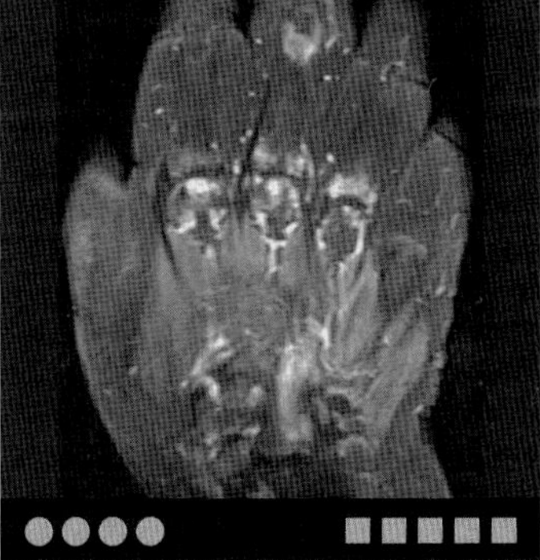

F. Pseudogout: Coronal T1 fat-saturated postcontrast image, in the same patient as in images D and E, shows synovial enhancement of the wrist joint as well as second, third, and forth metacarpal heads and proximal interphalangeal joints of the third finger. Note the erosion at the metacarpal head seen as fossae of low signal intensity.

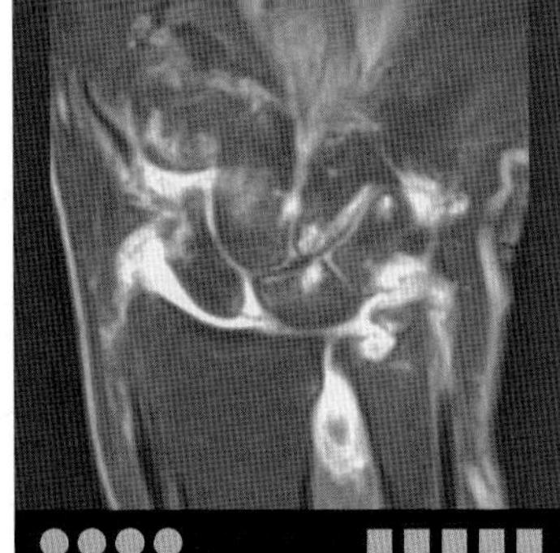

G: Rheumatoid arthritis: Coronal postcontrast fat-saturated T1-weighted image shows enhancement of pannus surrounding the carpal bones and distal radioulnar bursa. Also note enhanced foci of bony erosions in the carpal bones.

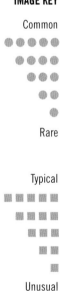

IMAGE KEY

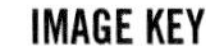

Chapter 15

Infections

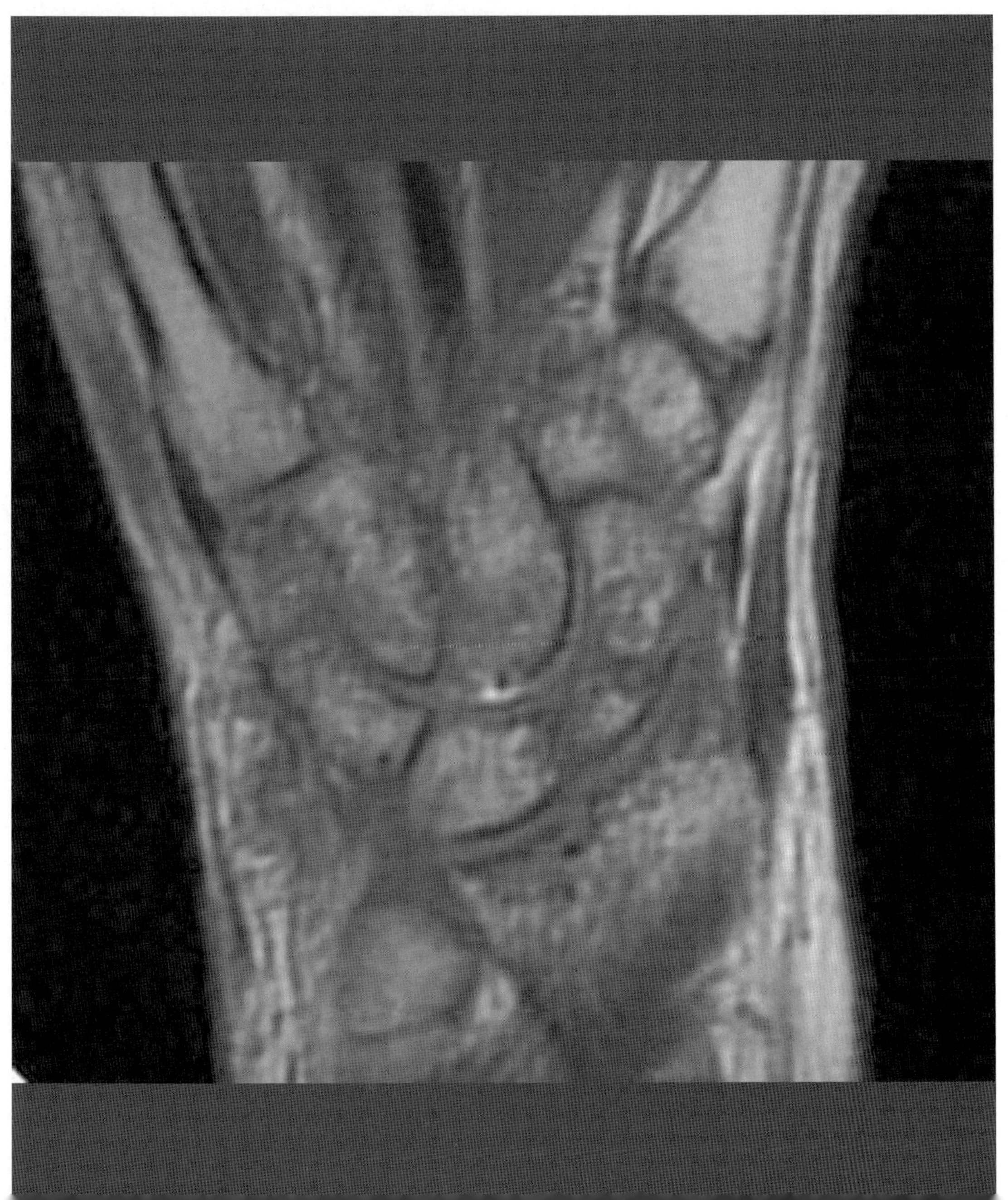

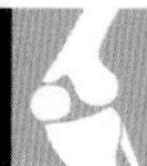

15–1 Septic Arthritis of the Wrist

Joseph C. Giaconi and Thomas Learch

PRESENTATION

Wrist pain

FINDINGS

MRI shows joint effusion, bone marrow edema, and periarticular bone erosions.

DIFFERENTIAL DIAGNOSES

- *Rheumatoid arthritis:* Characteristic symmetric joint involvement of wrist and metacarpophalangeal joints is the key to diagnosis and joint effusions and bone erosions may also be seen.
- *Juvenile rheumatoid arthritis:* It involves synovial proliferation associated with bony erosion, which may lead to joint fusion. Age is an important distinguishing factor.
- *Psoriatic arthritis:* Joint effusions and bone erosions are also seen in this disorder. However, fluid collection in the flexor tendon sheaths is characteristic.

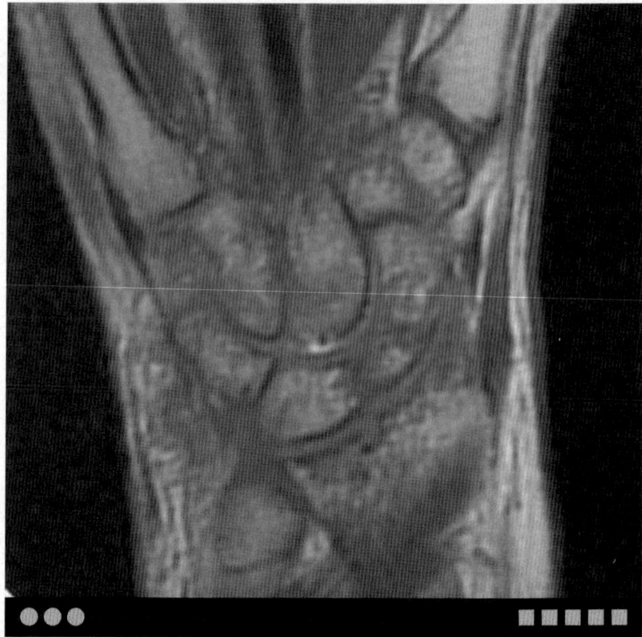

A. Septic arthritis of wrist: Coronal T1-weighted image demonstrates joint effusion and pancarpal and periarticular bone marrow edema, consistent with inflammatory arthritis.

COMMENTS

The patient is a 66-year-old female with wrist pain, initially thought to be due to fracture. Her wrist was immobilized with cast and radiographs were obtained, which were negative. MRI of the wrist was obtained after she did not improve postcasting. Septic arthritis is traditionally a clinical diagnosis based on an acute onset of monoarticular joint pain with erythema and warmth of the affected joint. Delays in diagnosis have been shown to be a major determinant in the final outcome. Therefore, prompt aspiration of the affected joint is essential. The most commonly affected joint is the knee, followed by the hip, ankle, and wrist. Most septic joints occur from hematogenous seeding of the highly vascular synovial membrane. Bacterial arthritis is the most common cause of joint infections. MRI is helpful in the diagnosis and evaluation of septic arthritis because of its sensitivity in detection of bone marrow abnormalities, soft tissue extent of disease, and the presence of fluid collections, which all appear as high signal on T2 or STIR sequences. Synovial inflammation and effusions are the earliest findings. Bone marrow signal abnormality occurs adjacent to the joint space, which, in the acute phase, usually represents reactive inflammation. The onset of osteomyelitis is difficult to determine prior to bone destruction. As the disease progresses, marginal and central erosions of articular areas develop into extensive destruction of large portions of articular surfaces, leading to diffuse joint space narrowing. Chronic septic arthritis will lead to osteomyelitis and a destroyed or ankylosed joint.

PEARLS

- **MRI findings of septic arthritis consist of joint effusion and bone marrow edema, which are high signal on T2 or STIR sequences, as well as periarticular erosions.**
- **MRI appearance of septic arthritis is nonspecific and is similar to other inflammatory arthritides. There are no pathognomonic MRI signs of joint infection.**
- **History, laboratory findings, and prompt joint aspiration are necessary for diagnosis.**
- **Radiography should be the initial imaging of septic arthritis.**

ADDITIONAL IMAGE

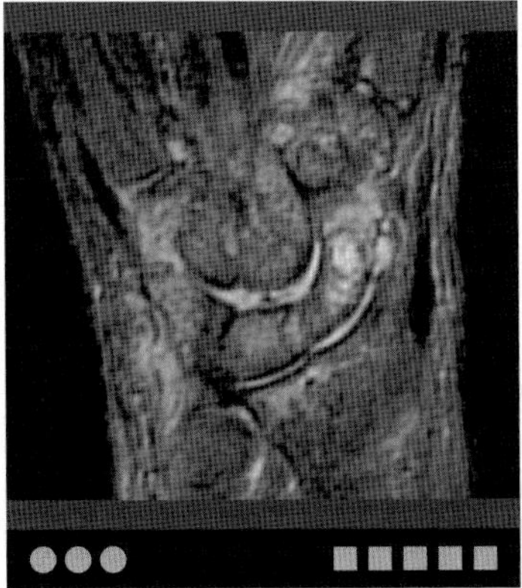

B. Septic arthritis of wrist: Coronal STIR image demonstrates joint effusion and pancarpal and periarticular bone marrow edema, consistent with inflammatory arthritis.

DIFFERENTIAL DIAGNOSES IMAGES

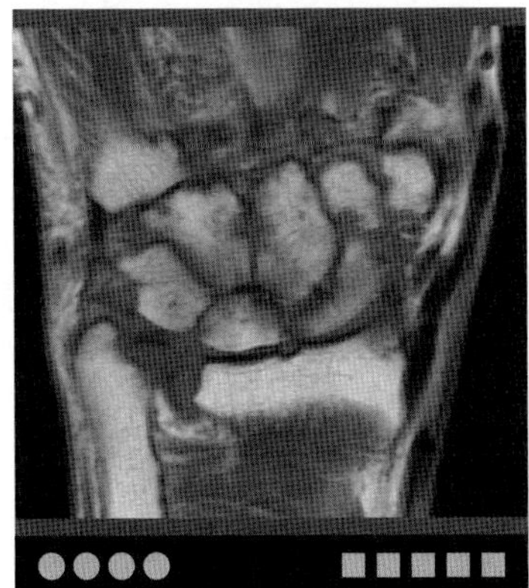

C. Rheumatoid arthritis of wrist: Coronal T1 demonstrates pancarpal synovitis and erosions in a patient with rheumatoid arthritis.

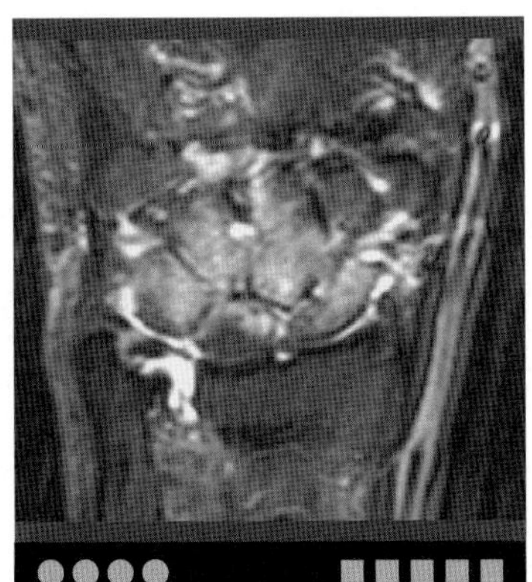

D. Rheumatoid arthritis of wrist: Coronal STIR demonstrates pancarpal synovitis and erosions in a patient with rheumatoid arthritis.

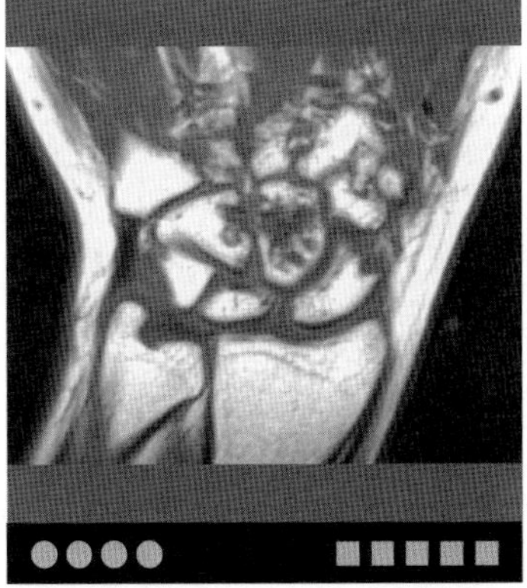

E. JRA: Coronal T1-weighted spin echo image shows multiple carpal bone erosions including capitate, hamate, trapezium, trapezoid, and scaphoid bones.

IMAGE KEY

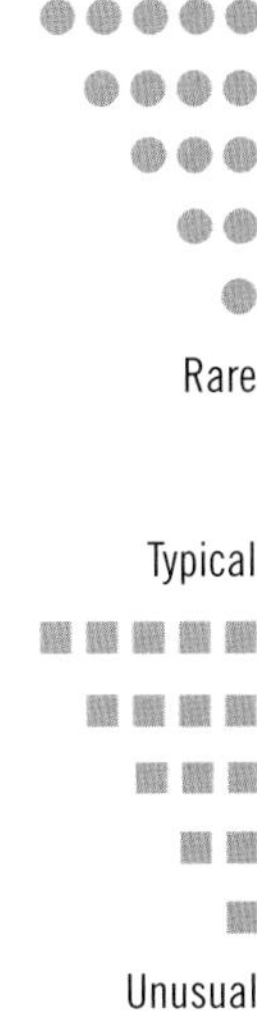

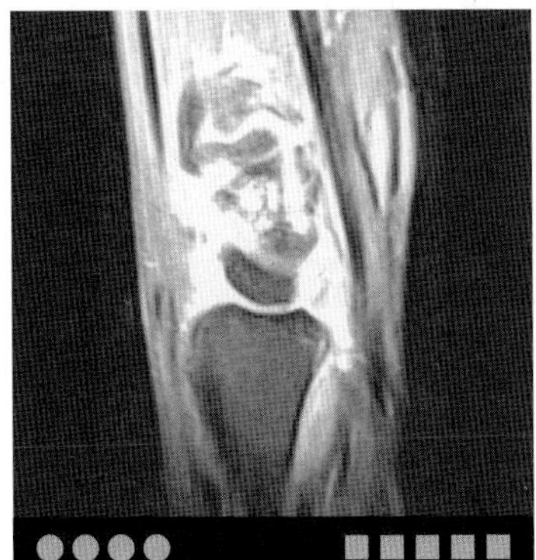

F. JRA: Sagittal T1-weighted fat-saturated postcontrast image shows multiple enhancing erosions of the capitate bone. Note diffuse synovial enhancement surrounding the wrist joint.

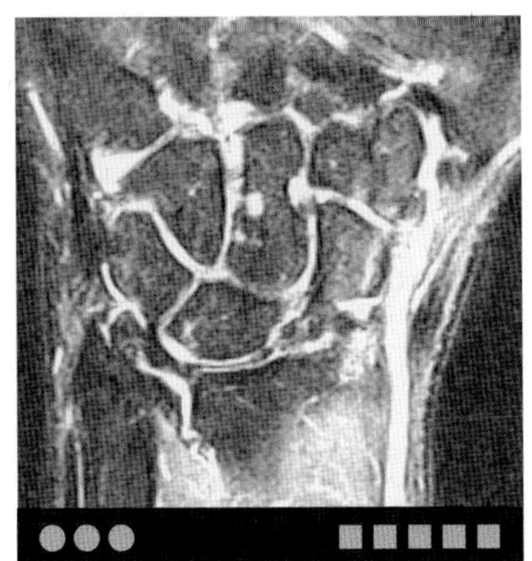

G. Psoriatic arthritis: Coronal T2-weighted fat-saturated image shows two small erosions in the capitate and larger erosion in the radial styloid with joint fluid present.

Chapter 16

Tumors and Tumor Like Lesions

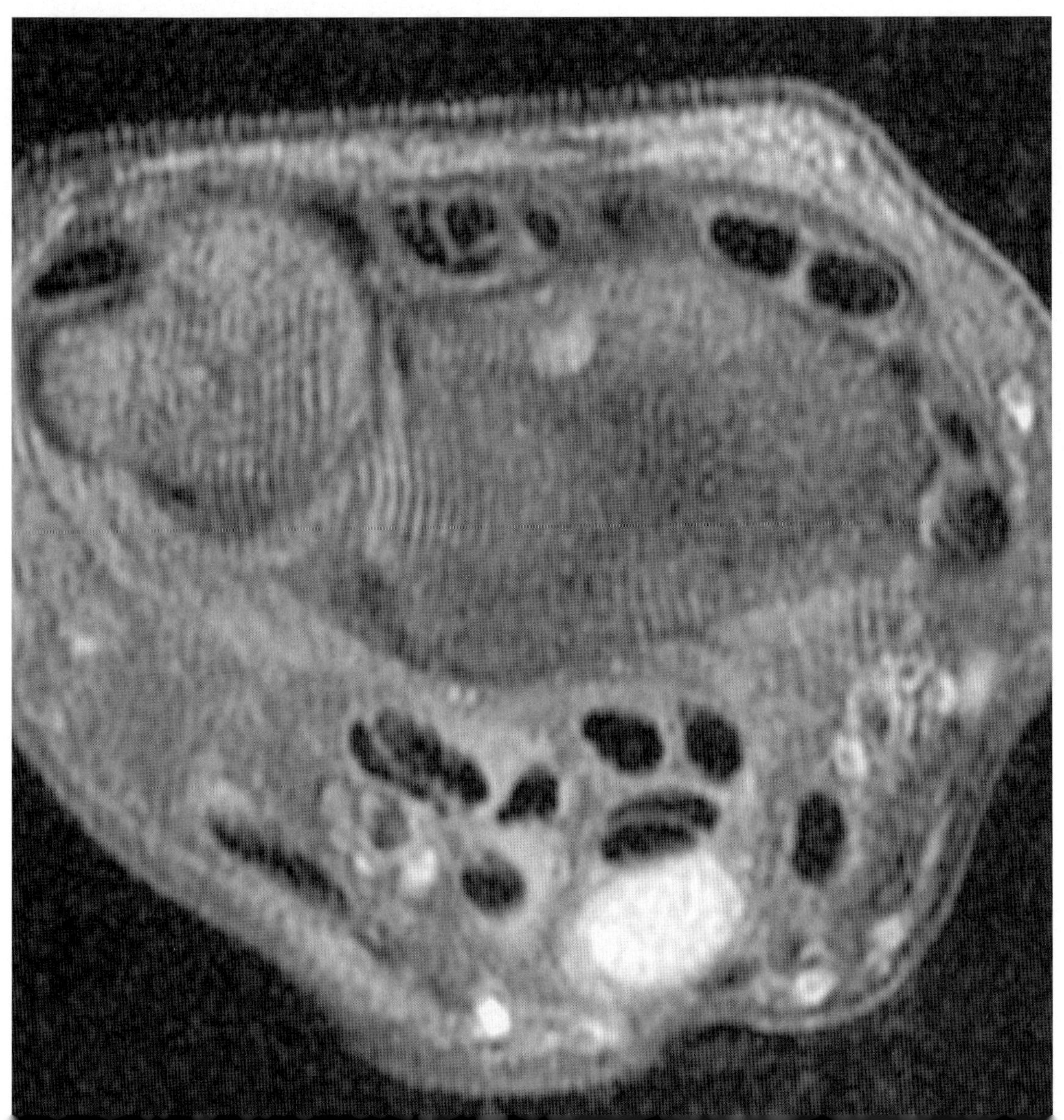

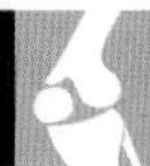

16-1 Median Nerve Schwannoma

Amilcare Gentili

PRESENTATION

Wrist mass for 10 years

FINDINGS

MR images show a mass in the carpal tunnel in the expected location of the median nerve.

DIFFERENTIAL DIAGNOSES

- *Ganglion cyst:* Usually extends to the joint capsule.
- *Giant cell tumor tendon sheet:* Often contains areas of intermediate or low signal intensity on fluid sensitive sequences because of hemosiderin deposits.
- *Fibrolipomatous hamartoma:* The nerve is enlarged and contains fatty tissue; often it is associated with macrodactyly.
- *Carpal tunnel syndrome:* The median nerve is often flattened.

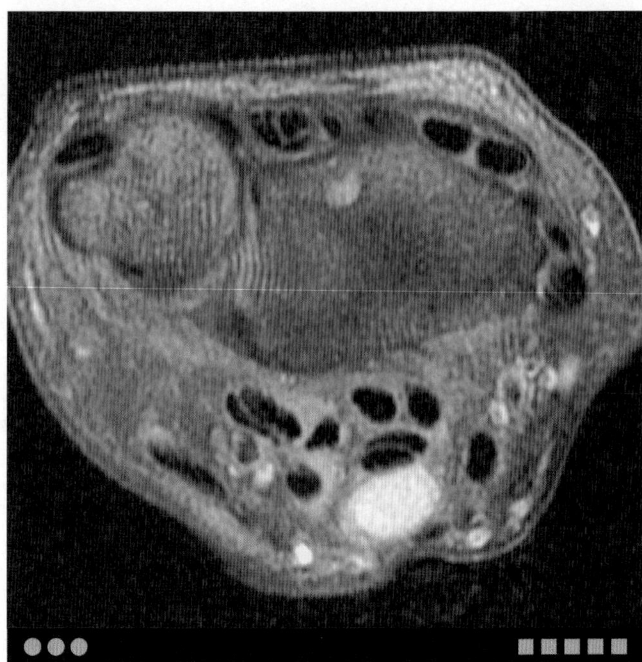

A. Median nerve schwannoma: Axial T2 fat-saturated MR image shows an elliptical high signal intensity lesion in the volar aspect of the wrist, superficial to the flexor tendons.

COMMENTS

This is an image of a 41-year-old male who presented with a wrist mass tender to palpation. Surgical resection confirmed the diagnosis of a schwannoma. Schwannoma, also called neurilemmoma, is a benign tumor developing in the sheath that surrounds the nerves. It is most common in patients between 20– and 30 years of age and represents approximately 5% of benign soft tissue tumors. It affects man and women equally. Schwannomas are often solitary and not associated with neurofibromatosis, but multiple schwannomas may be present in patients with neurofibromatosis type 1. Schwannoma develops as a fusiform mass localized eccentrically to the nerve and is often encapsulated. This capsule allows complete surgical removal of the tumor without injuring the underlying nerve. Schwannomas are composed of a richly cellular zone called Antoni type A, which is made up of compact spindle cells, and of a loose myxoid area zone, called Antoni type B. The MR appearance of schwannoma is often highly suggestive of a nerve sheet tumor, although the distinction between schwannoma and neurofibroma is often impossible. The most important imaging feature of neurogenic neoplasm is the appearance of a fusiform mass, with an entering and exiting tubular structure (a nerve) in a typical location of a nerve. The target sign, a center of low intermediate signal, surrounded by high signal intensity on T2-weighted images, has been described as typical for neurofibroma, but it is also often seen with schwannoma. The split fat sign, a rim of fat surrounding the lesion, is also commonly seen in both schwannoma and neurofibromas.

PEARLS

- **Schwannoma are usually fusiform with tapered ends continuing into the parent nerve.**
- **If a needle biopsy is attempted, it can be very painful.**

ADDITIONAL IMAGES

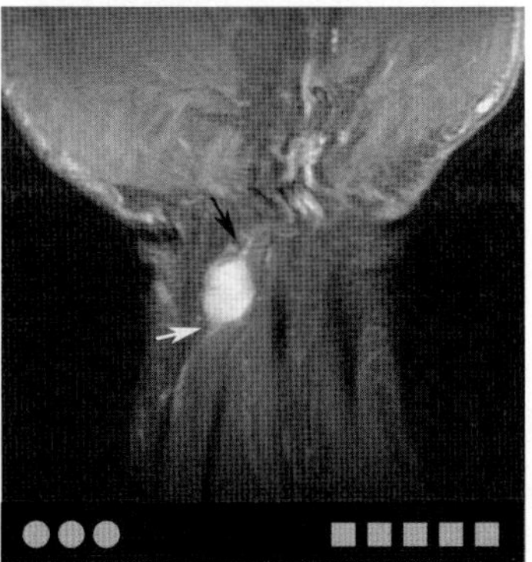

B. Median nerve schwannoma: Coronal T2 fat-saturated MR image shows an elliptical high signal intensity lesion in the volar aspect of the wrist. Note entering (white arrow) and exiting (black arrow) median nerve fibers.

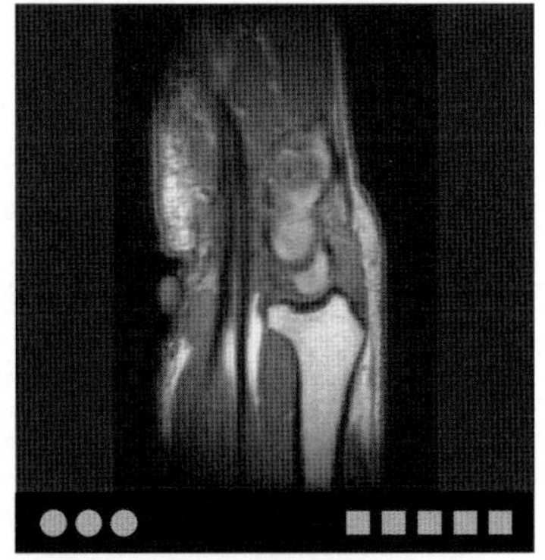

C. Median nerve schwannoma: Sagittal T1-weighted MR image shows a low intensity lesion in the volar aspect of the wrist, superficial to the flexor tendons.

DIFFERENTIAL DIAGNOSES IMAGES

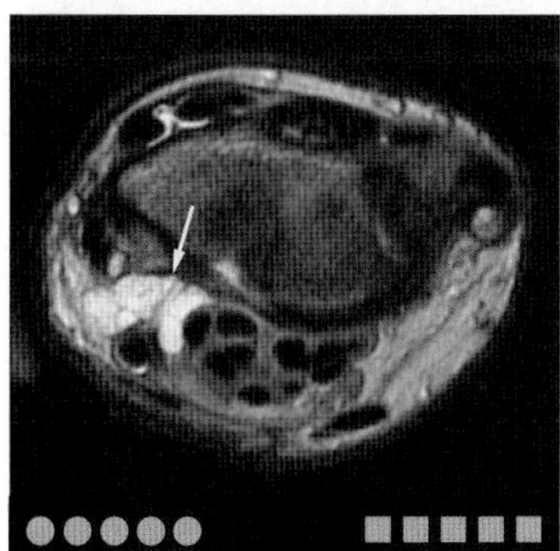

D. Ganglion cyst: Axial T2 fat-saturated MR image shows a multiloculated high signal intensity lesion (arrow) in the volar aspect of the wrist, deep to the flexor carpi radialis, and radial to the flexor tendons of the digits.

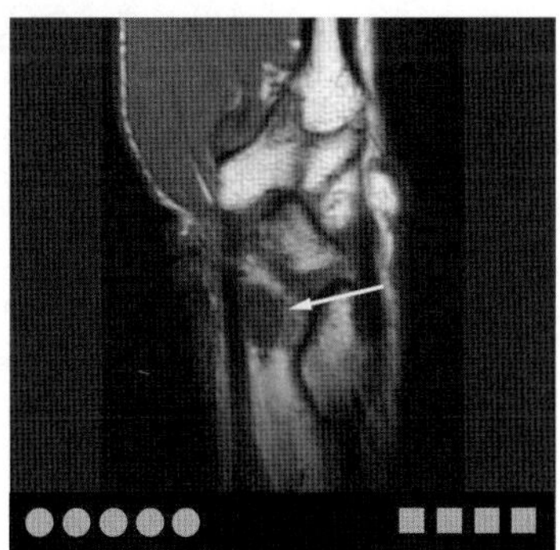

E. Ganglion cyst: Sagittal T1-weighted MR image shows a low intensity lesion (arrow) in the volar aspect of the wrist, deep to the flexor carpi radialis.

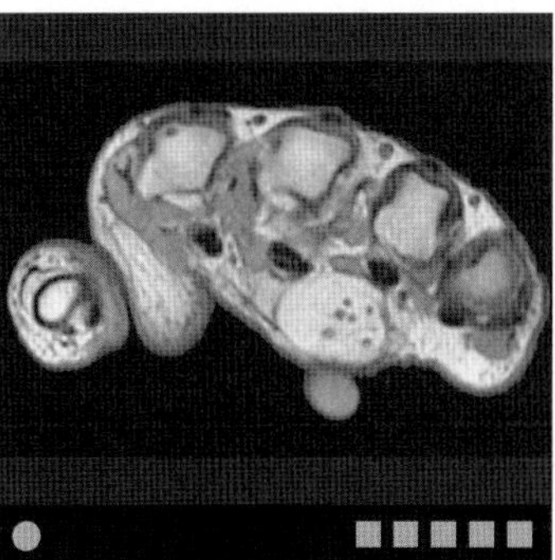

F. Fibrolipomatous hamartoma: Axial T1-weighted MR image shows fat tissue causing expansion of the median nerve. Note the nerve bundles within the adipose tissue.

IMAGE KEY

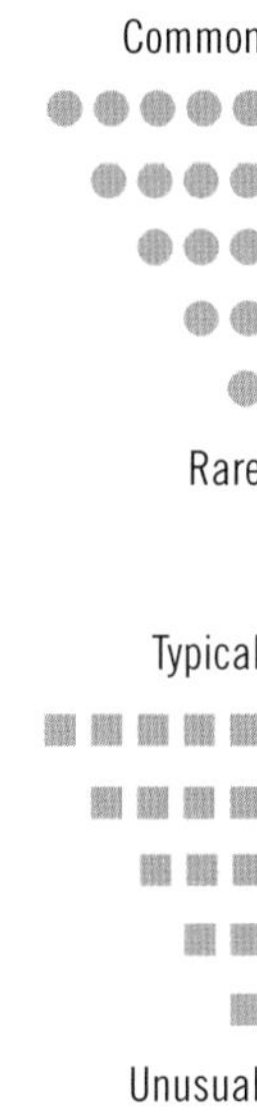

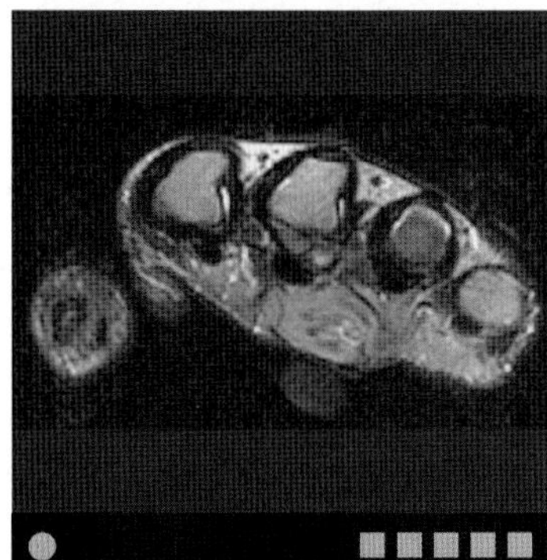

G. Fibrolipomatous hamartoma: Axial T2-weighted MR image shows fat tissue causing expansion of the median nerve.

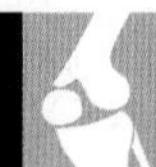

16–2 Lipoma of the Hand

Alipasha Adrangui and Jamshid Tehranzadeh

PRESENTATION

A palmar lump in the hand

FINDINGS

There is an oval shape lipoma with bright signal with a thin fibrous capsule anterior to flexor tendons of the fourth finger just under the subcutaneous tissue.

DIFFERENTIAL DIAGNOSES

- *Liposarcoma:* Well-differentiated liposarcoma or atypical lipoma resembles lipoma on both CT and MR imaging. These tumors are low-grade lesions containing a large amount of fat, usually more than 75% of their volume, and thorough pathologic examination of the tumor may be required to establish the diagnosis.
- *Hibernoma:* Is an uncommon tumor that arises from brown fat. This is also a benign but with a slightly greater tendency to bleed during excision and to recur if intralesional excision is performed.
- *Fibrolipoma of median nerve:* Fibrolipomatous hamartoma of nerve is a rare, benign, fibro fatty malformation of peripheral nerves.

COMMENTS

This image is of a 31-year-old man with a lump in the right hand and discomfort for several months. Palmar soft tissue lipomas are rare. Many lipomas contain fat visible on CT and MR imaging. On CT, areas of low attenuation have been accepted as evidence of fat within tissues. T1-weighted MR image shows bright signal for fatty tissue, which would be mildly suppressed on T2-weighted and finally totally saturated with STIR or fat-suppressed images. The use of contrast agents can be helpful in improving the delineation of tumors as well as revealing areas of viable vascularized tumors. MRI can also help surgical planning. A variety of different types of lipomas exist. Classic lipomas have CT and MR imaging signal characteristics similar to subcutaneous fat. The deep lesions tend to be variable in shape most likely because they tend to mold themselves around the surrounding tissues. The growth of lipomas in the hand may cause neurologic changes in the peripheral nerves of the hand. Compression of the median nerve causes a syndrome similar to carpal tunnel syndrome.

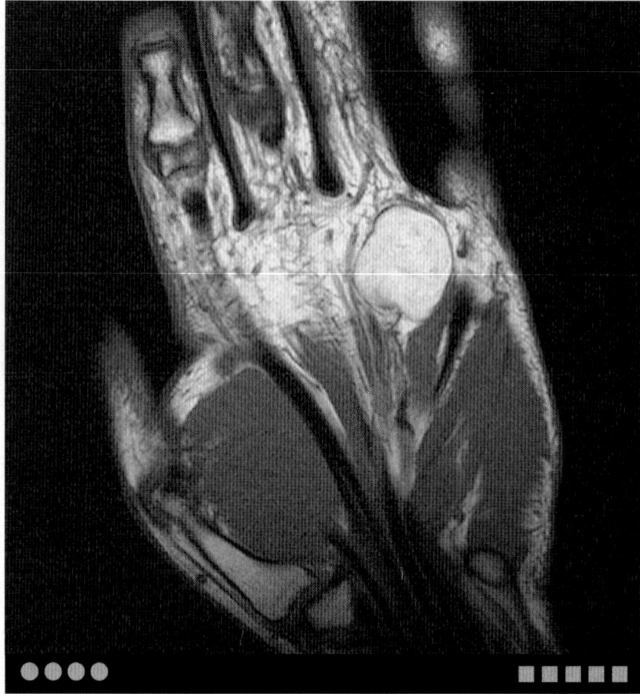

A. Lipoma of the hand: Coronal T1-weighted image shows an oval shape lipoma with bright signal with a thin fibrous capsule anterior to flexor tendon of the fourth finger just under the subcutaneous tissue.

Heterotopic lipomas are associated with nonadipose elements. The most common heterotopic lipoma is intramuscular lipoma. Another type of lipoma is infiltrating or lipomatosis, which is characterized by diffuse infiltrating adipose tissue and can be associated with neural symptoms. The other groups of lipomas are lipoma variants include angiolipoma, lipoblastoma, spindle cell lipoma and chondroid lipoma.

PEARLS

- **T1-weighted MR image shows bright signal for fatty tissue, which would be mildly suppressed on T2-weighted and finally totally saturated with STIR or fat suppressed images.**
- **The growth of lipomas in the hand may cause neurologic changes in the peripheral nerves of the hand. Compression of the median nerve causes a syndrome similar to carpal tunnel syndrome.**

ADDITIONAL IMAGES

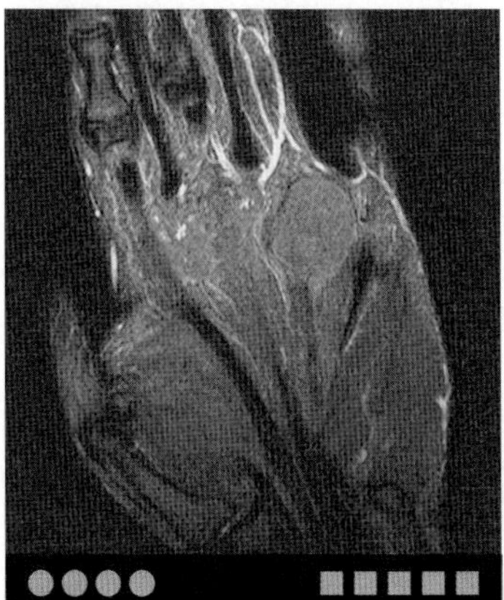

B. Lipoma of the hand: Coronal STIR imaging shows fat saturation of this lipoma.

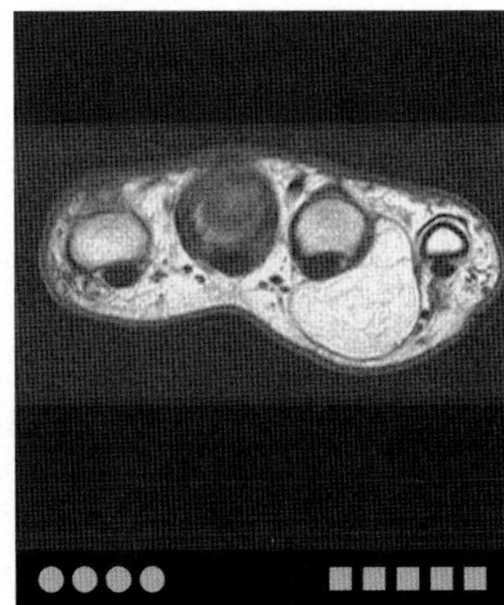

C. Lipoma of the hand: Axial T1-weighted image shows extension of the lipoma between the web of the fourth and fifth distal metacarpals.

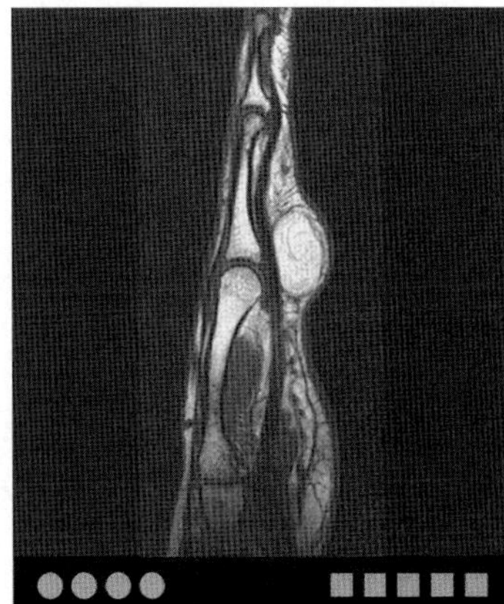

D. Lipoma of the hand: Sagittal T1 SE image shows the lipoma anterior to the flexor tendon of the fourth ray at the metacarpophalangeal region.

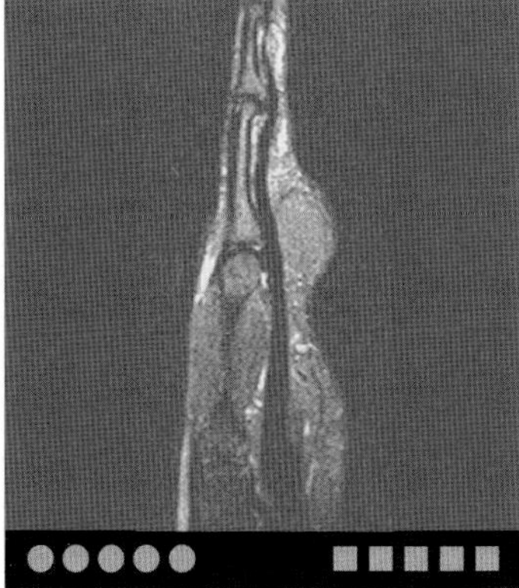

E. Lipoma of the hand: Sagittal STIR image shows fat saturation of this lipoma.

DIFFERENTIAL DIAGNOSES IMAGES

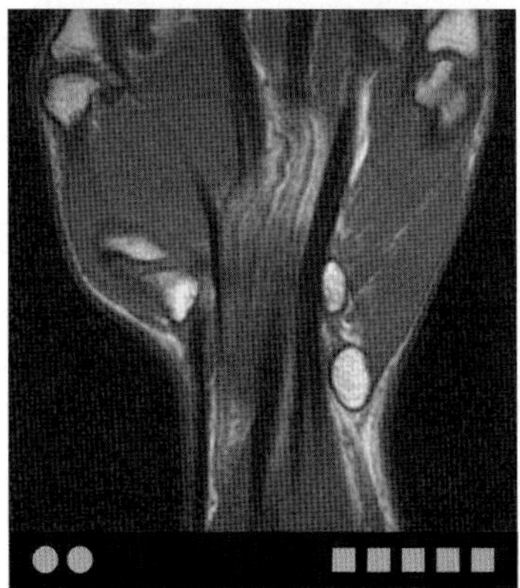

F. Fibrolipomatous hamartoma of the median nerve: Coronal T1-weighted SE image shows fibrofatty fibers of the mixed bright signal in between bundles of the median nerve at the carpal tunnel region.

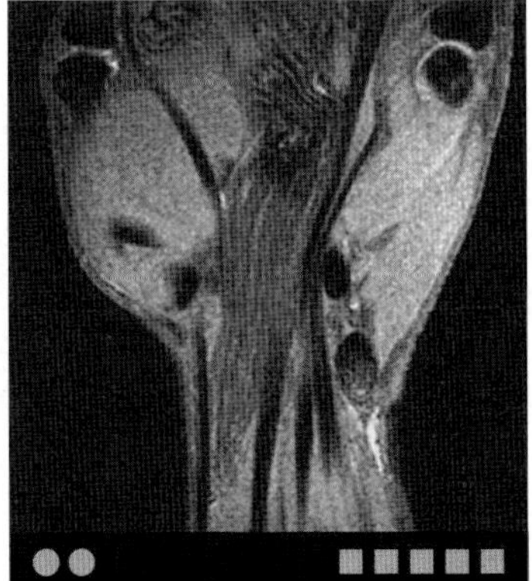

G. Fibrolipomatous hamartoma of the median nerve: Coronal STIR imaging of the palmar aspect of the wrist shows dark fibers of fibrolipoma between bundles of the median nerve at the carpal tunnel region.

IMAGE KEY

Common

●●●●●

●●●●

●●●

●●

●

Rare

Typical

■■■■■

■■■■

■■■

■■

■

Unusual

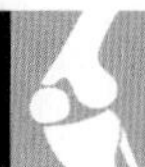

16–3 Vascular Leiomyoma

Kambiz Motamedi

PRESENTATION

Painless forearm mass

FINDINGS

Radiographs showed a calcified mass. MRI demonstrates a mass of the forearm flexor compartment with intermediate T1-weighted and high T2-weighted signal. There are several low-signal foci on all pulse sequences corresponding to the calcifications.

DIFFERENTIAL DIAGNOSES

- *Heterotopic ossification (HO):* MRI of HO shows characteristic findings depending on the stage of maturation. A CT scan would show the characteristic peripheral maturation and zone of calcification.
- *Metastatic calcification:* The diffuse or masslike calcium deposit in the soft tissues in the chronic renal failure appears masslike on cross-sectional imaging.
- *Synovial sarcoma:* The MRI may be very similar. But the clarifications, if present are pleomorphic, smaller in size, and better seen with radiography or CT scan.
- *Pseudoaneurysm:* The MRI may display the flow artifact from the arterial inflow. The appearance may be similar. The location would be similar as well as they arise from radial or ulnar arteries (prior arterial puncture).

COMMENTS

The patient is an image of a 72-year-old Asian male who presented with a large painless mass of the flexor aspect of the forearm. The mass was fixed and indurated. A biopsy was nondiagnostic, and excision of the tumor was performed. This tumor involved the ulnar artery and vein and compressed the ulnar nerve. The vascular leiomyoma or angiomyomas are usually solitary lesions, probably arising from the vascular wall. They are usually located in the subcutaneous compartment of the extremities. The lesion is usually small with two third of the cases found in adults in the fourth to sixth decades of life. Angiomyomas are more common in women than in men, with a ratio of 2:1. About 50% of angiomyomas are symptomatic. They may be initiated with changes in temperature or pressure, pregnancy, or menses. On physical examination, these lesions are usually firm and fixed. There is usually no pain or neuralgic deficit distally. Their location is commonly close to the neurovascular bundle. The imaging features are ruled by the presence of a soft tissue mass with varying amount of course calcifications. The calcifications are usually more apparent on radiography and CT scan. The MRI commonly shows the calcifications as foci of low signal. The close proximity to the neurovascular bundle of the extremity should point to the correct diagnosis.

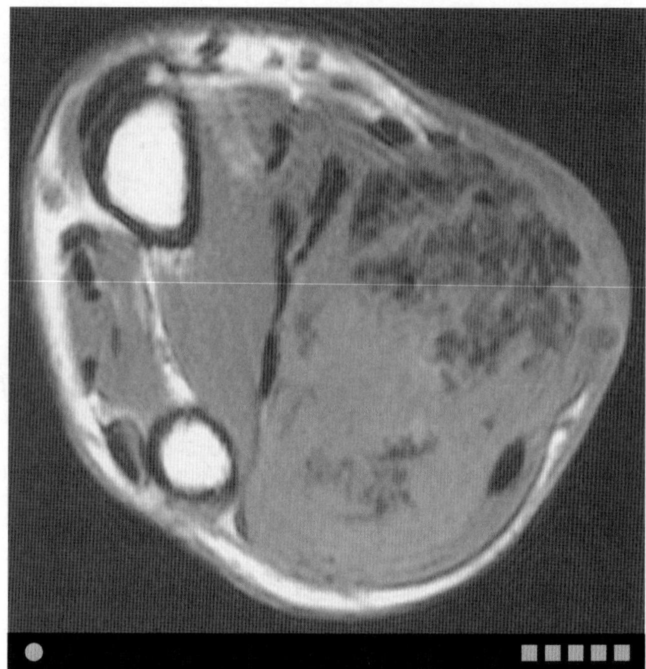

A. Vascular leiomyoma. Axial T1-weighted image shows a homogeneous mass of the flexor aspect with several low-signal foci.

PEARLS

- **Rare tumor along the major vascular pathways.**
- **It resembles a "misplaced" uterine leiomyoma.**
- **Calcifications are a hallmark.**

ADDITIONAL IMAGES

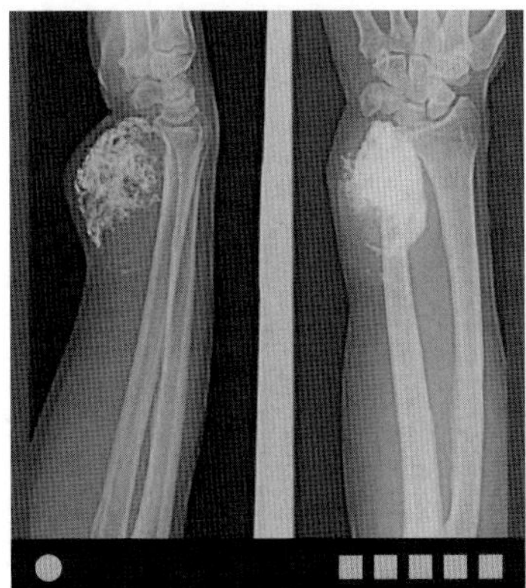

B. Vascular leiomyoma. AP and lateral radiographs show a partially calcified mass of the volar aspect of the distal forearm.

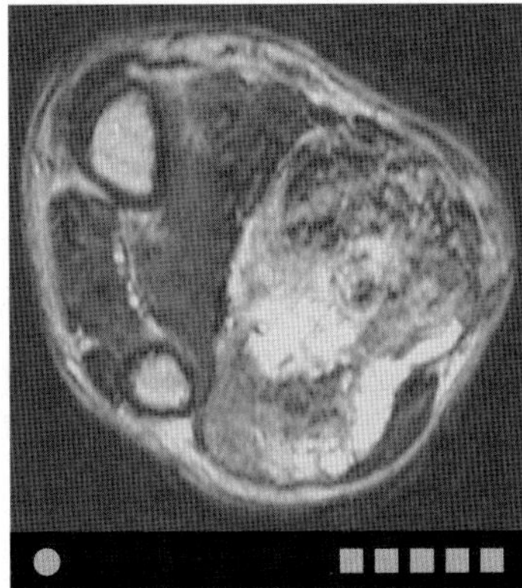

C. Vascular leiomyoma. Axial fat-saturated T2-weighted demonstrates predominant high signal with scattered low-signal foci.

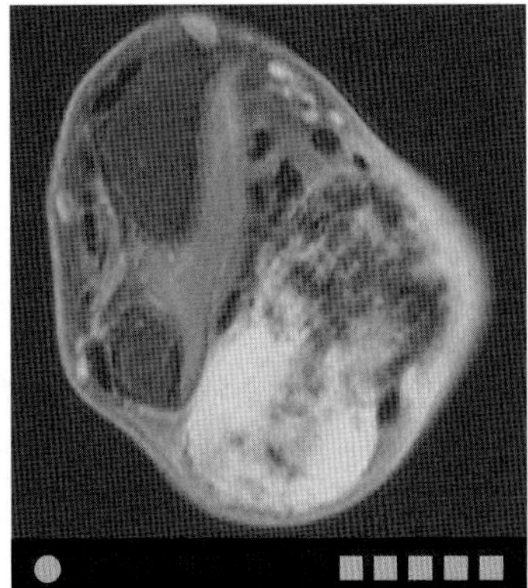

D. Vascular leiomyoma: Contrast-enhanced axial fat-saturated T1-weighted image shows intense enhancement of the solid portion of this mass. The calcific foci remain low signal.

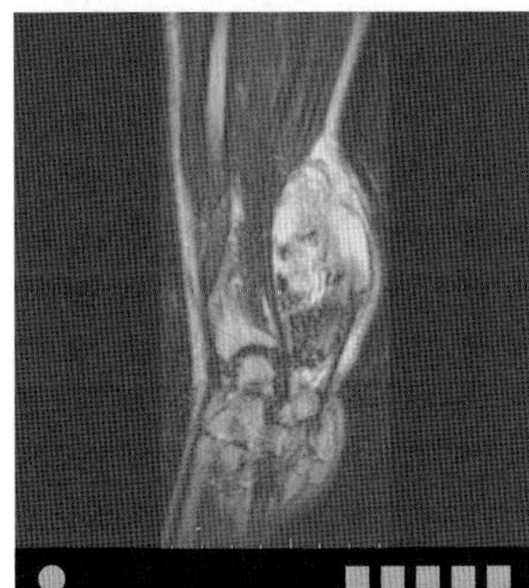

E. Vascular leiomyoma: Sagittal T2-weighted image demonstrates the bulging nature of the mass in the volar aspect of the forearm with low-signal calcific foci.

DIFFERENTIAL DIAGNOSES IMAGES

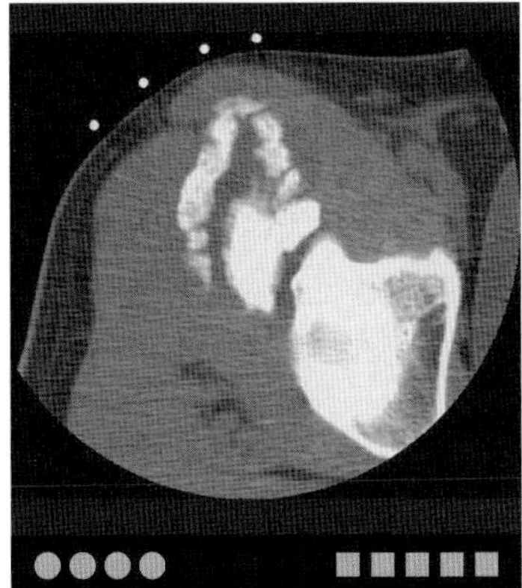

F. Heterotopic ossification: Axial nonenhanced CT scan section through the hip at the level of the inferior and anterior iliac spine reveals a partially ossified soft tissue mass consistent, with a large focus of heterotopic ossification from prior rectus femoris avulsion tear.

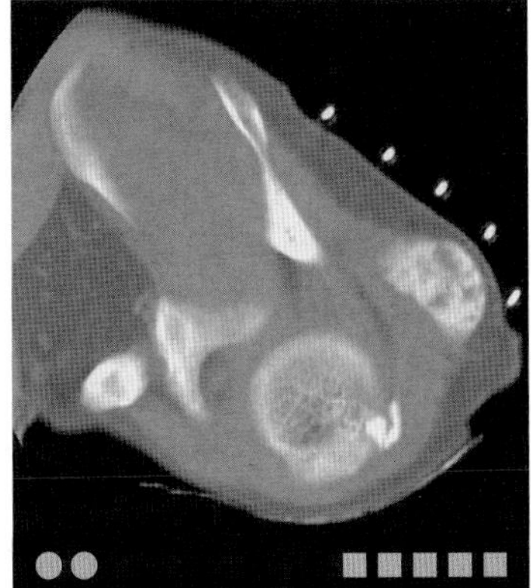

G. Metastatic calcification: Axial nonenhanced CT scan section obtained for biopsy guidance reveals a nonspecific, well-circumscribed mass in the deltoid muscle compartment.

IMAGE KEY

Common

Rare

Typical

Unusual

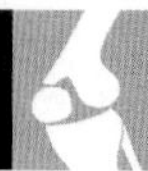

16–4 Fibrolipomatous Hamartoma of Median Nerve

Thomas Learch

PRESENTATION

Wrist mass with numbness and tingling in the first three digits

FINDINGS

MRI shows fusiform enlargement of the median nerve. The nerve fascicles are separated by fibrous and fatty tissue within the expanded nerve sheath.

DIFFERENTIAL DIAGNOSES

- *Mycobacterium marinum synovitis of the flexor sheaths:* Synovial mass involving flexor tendon sheaths. Key to diagnosis is the clinical history of individuals with occupational or recreational exposure to freshwater or saltwater.
- *Lipoma within the nerve sheath:* Focal masses that follow fat signal, which dislocate and compress normal nerve bundles. There is no fibrous component.
- *Neurofibromatosis:* Neurofibromas have MRI signal characteristics of soft tissue rather than fat. The nerve is studded by small tumors in plexiform neurofibromatosis.

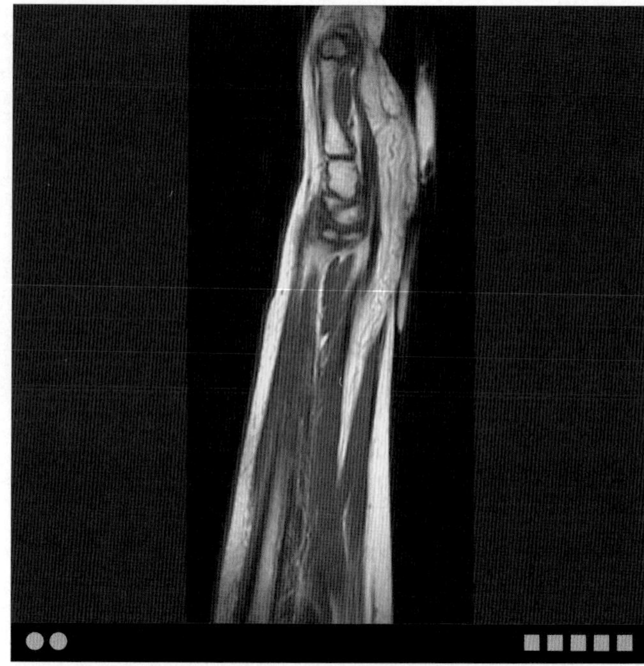

A. Fibrolipomatous hamartoma of the median nerve: Sagittal T1-weighted image demonstrates large, predominantly fatty mass in the forearm and carpal tunnel.

COMMENTS

This is an image of a 28-year-old female who presented wrist mass with numbness and tingling in the first three digits and was diagnosed with fibrolipomatous hamartoma of the median nerve. This lesion, thought to be congenital, usually presents in patients younger than 30 years as a volar wrist mass and carpal tunnel syndrome. The median nerve is affected in the majority of cases (~80%), but the radial, ulnar, peroneal, plantar, and cranial nerves have been reported as sites of occurrence. There is macrodactyly in approximately 50% of the cases because of bony overgrowth and progression of subcutaneous fat. Macrodactyly is associated with advanced degenerative joint disease in the affected digit. The MRI findings in fibrolipomatous hamartoma are pathognomomic. MRI shows fusiform enlargement of the median nerve. The nerve fascicles are separated by fibrous and fatty tissue within the expanded nerve sheath. There are serpentine form nerve fascicles surrounded and separated by fibrous and fatty tissue within an expanded nerve sheath. The nerve itself is hypointense on T1, indicating fibrous degeneration of the nerve. The fibrous components are hypointense, while the fatty components are hyperintense, on both T1- and T2-weighted sequences. Fibrolipomatous hamartoma is a benign tumor. Pathologic inspection reveals that the epineurium is expanded by fibrolipomatous tissue, and scattered nerve bundles are dissociated by perineurial and endoneurial fibrosis.

PEARLS

- **Fibrolipomatous hamartoma mostly affects the median nerve at the wrist.**
- **It is associated with macrodactyly and compressive neuropathy.**
- **MR imaging demonstrates both fibrous and fatty tissue with fusiform enlargement of the affected nerve, which has a serpentine-like appearance.**
- **It is a benign tumor.**

ADDITIONAL IMAGES

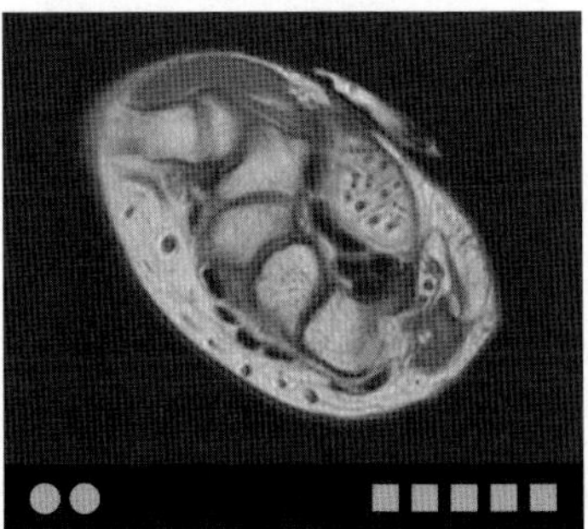

B. Fibrolipomatous hamartoma of the median nerve: Axial T1-weighted image demonstrates mass infiltrating median nerve, separating out nerve fascicles, which are low signal on T1.

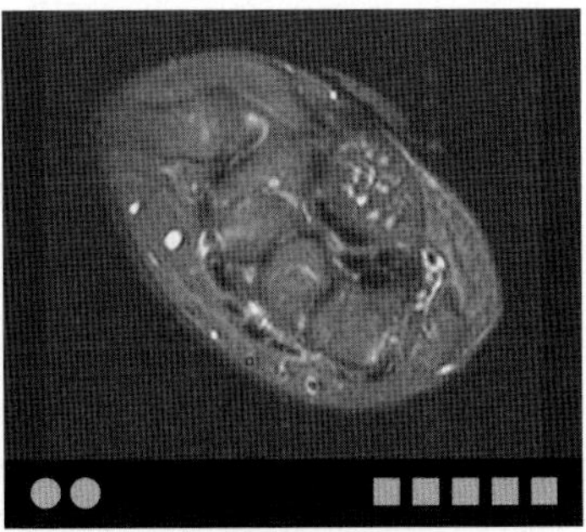

C. Fibrolipomatous hamartoma of the median nerve: Axial STIR demonstrates mass infiltrating median nerve. Nerve fascicles are high signal on STIR image.

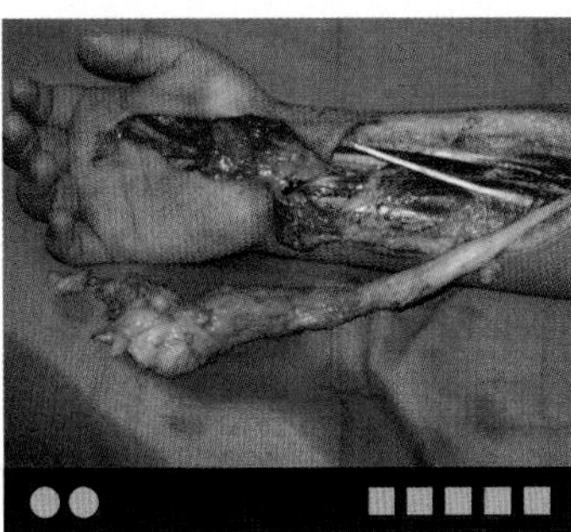

D. Fibrolipomatous hamartoma of the median nerve: Intraoperative imagedemonstrates resection of mass, which on gross inspection is fatty in appearance.

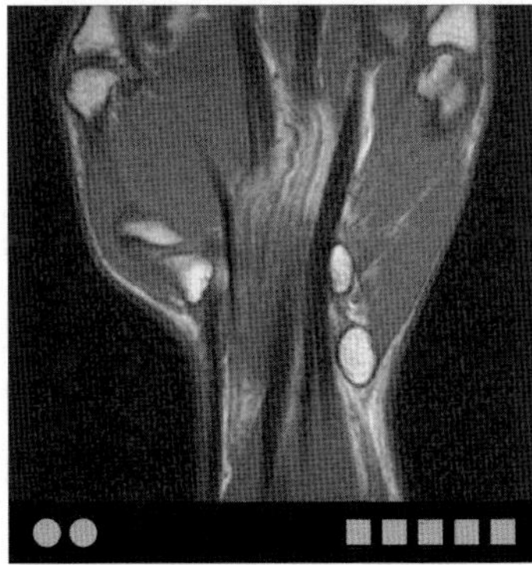

E. Fibrolipomatous hamartoma of the median nerve: Coronal T1-weighted image in a different patient shows strands of fibrolipoma of medial nerve.

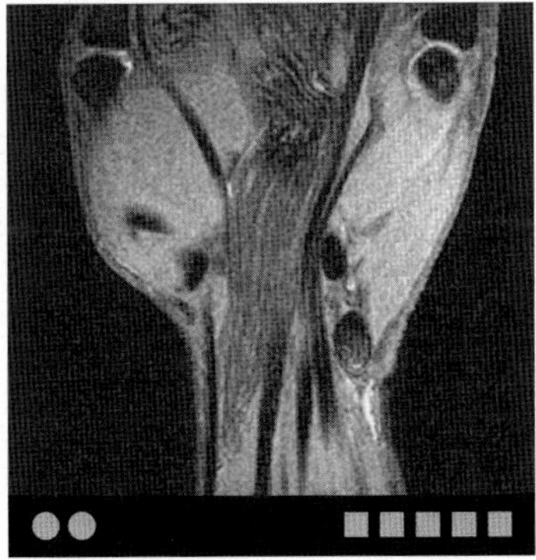

F. Fibrolipomatous hamartoma of the median nerve: Coronal STIR image, in the same patient as in image E, shows saturation of fatty tissue in this tumor.

DIFFERENTIAL DIAGNOSES IMAGES

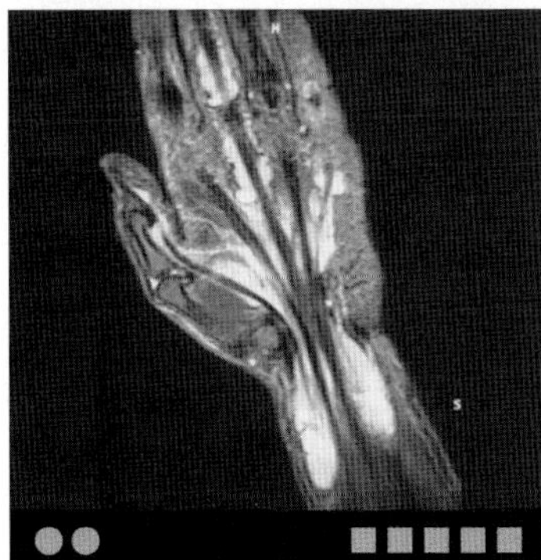

G. Mycobacterium marinum synovitis: Coronal STIR image of wrist and hand demonstrates extensive synovitis along flexor tendons in a patient who previously cut himself while cleaning his aquarium. Cultures were positive for *Mycobacterium marinum*.

IMAGE KEY

Common

Rare

Typical

Unusual

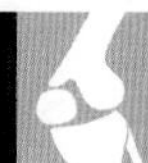

16–5 Glomus Tumor

Ingrid B. Kjellin

PRESENTATION

Pain, tenderness, and sensitivity to cold in the distal digit

FINDINGS

MRI shows a small, well-demarcated, and hyperintense tumor in the nail bed.

DIFFERENTIAL DIAGNOSES

- *Epidermal inclusion cyst:* This expansile osteolytic lesion is often in the volar aspect of the finger.
- *Enchondroma:* It may present with a pathologic fracture and calcified matrix.
- *Mucoid cyst:* This is sometimes seen in the digits in the region of a joint, which may or may not have arthritic changes.
- *Sarcoidosis:* The hand is the most common site of osseous involvement in sarcoidosis. The middle and distal phalanges are typically involved and may display a coarsened trabecular pattern and/or focal lytic (lacelike) lesions. Acro-osteolysis is also a reported finding.
- *Aneurysmal bone cyst:* This expansile osteolytic lesion often presents with fluid-fluid levels in CT scan and MRI.

COMMENTS

The glomus tumor is a benign tumor, which arises from the glomus body, also known as the neuromyoarterial glomus. It is an arteriovenous shunt composed of an afferent arteriole, an anastomotic vessel, a collecting vein, and a capsule portion. Glomus bodies are found in great numbers in the digital wall, where they help regulating blood flow in the skin. The glomus tumor is usually only a few millimeters in maximum dimension, and it is typically located in the extremities in the region of the fingertips or nail beds. Subungual lesions are much more common in females than males, and are seen between the ages of 20 and 40 years. In 10% of cases, there is more than one lesion. A pathologic variant is the very rare glomangiosarcoma. Pain, point tenderness, and cold sensitivity constitute the classic clinical triad of the glomus tumor, and are present in about one third of patients. The lesion is difficult to palpate, but may be seen as a small pink or blue nodule beneath the nail. A small focus of extrinsic erosion of bone can often be seen on radiographs. If there is a diagnostic dilemma, MRI or ultrasound may be helpful for further evaluation. On MRI, there is very high and homogeneous signal intensity exhibited on T2-weighted images within a rounded mass. On ultrasound, a well-defined hypoechoic mass with mildly increased through transmission may be identified.

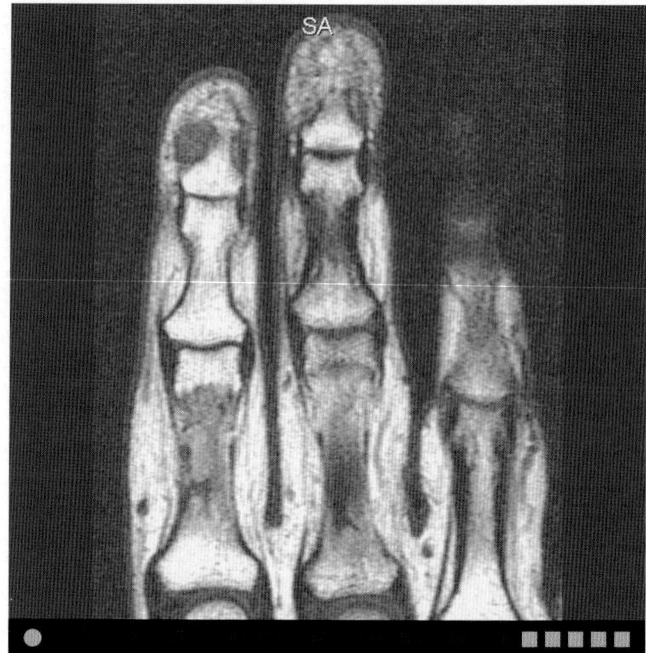

A. Glomus tumor: A coronal T1-weighted image of the hand shows a small, rounded isointense lesion in radial aspect of the distal phalanx of the index finger.

PEARLS

- **Glomus tumors may present with aching pain, point tenderness, and sensitivity to cold.**
- **It is usually located around the distal phalanx of the hand.**
- **Pressure erosions and sclerotic margins are sometimes seen on radiographs.**
- **MRI may be helpful for preoperative planning and in identification of tumor recurrence.**

ADDITIONAL IMAGE

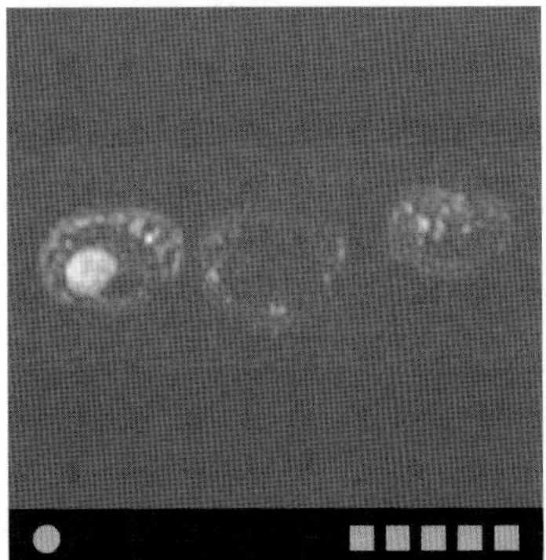

B. Glomus tumor: A T2-weighted axial image shows hyperintense signal of the lesion, which has eroded the bone.

DIFFERENTIAL DIAGNOSES IMAGES

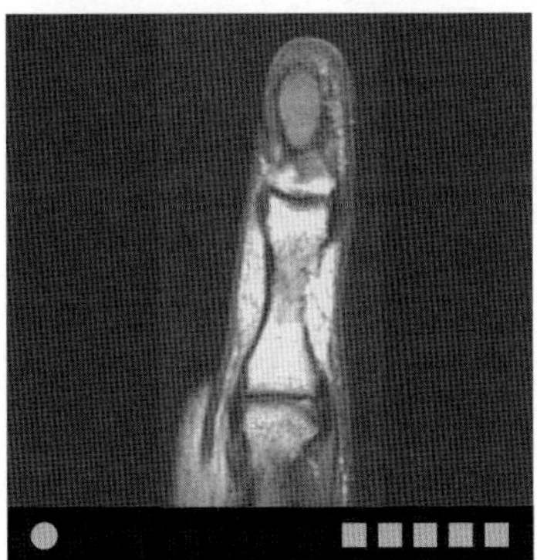

C. Epidermal inclusion cyst: A coronal T1-weighted image shows an oval, well defined lesion in the distal phalanx of the thumb.

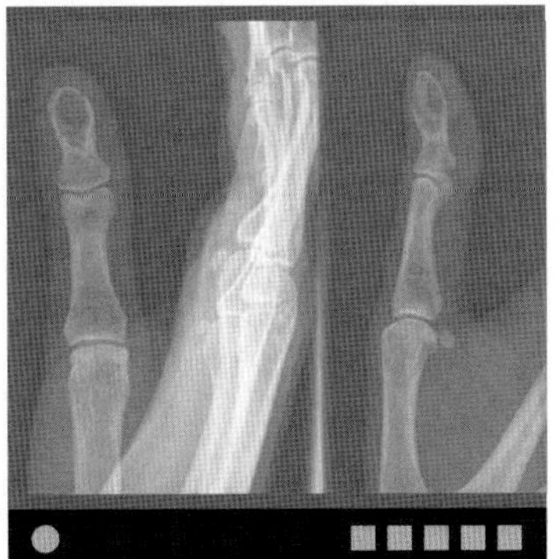

D. Epidermal inclusion cyst: Radiographs of the hand shows a lytic lesion with a nondisplaced cortical fracture.

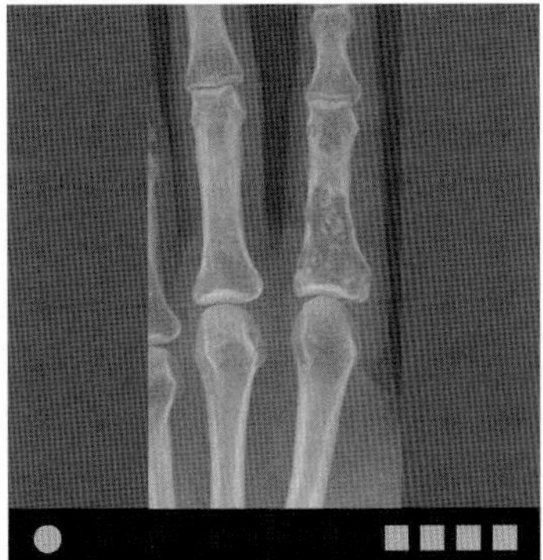

E. Enchondroma: A frontal radiograph of the hand shows a lytic, mildly expansile lesion in the proximal phalanx of the index finger with a nondisplaced acute cortical fracture. There is mildly calcified matrix within the lesion.

IMAGE KEY

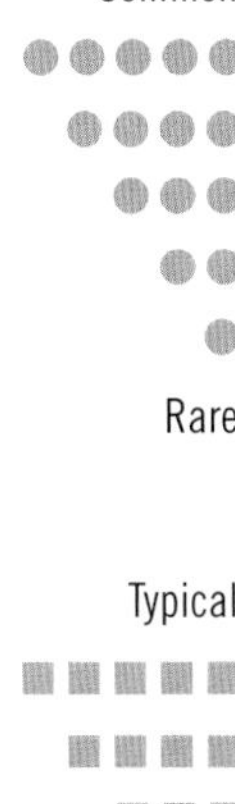

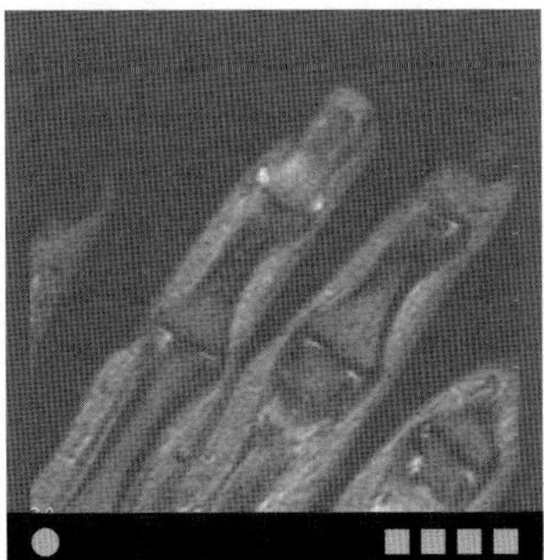

F. Mucoid cyst: A coronal STIR image of the hand shows mild subchondral edema in the distal interphalangeal joint of the fourth digit, consistent with arthritis. There is also a small, lobulated, and hyperintense lesion along the joint margin.

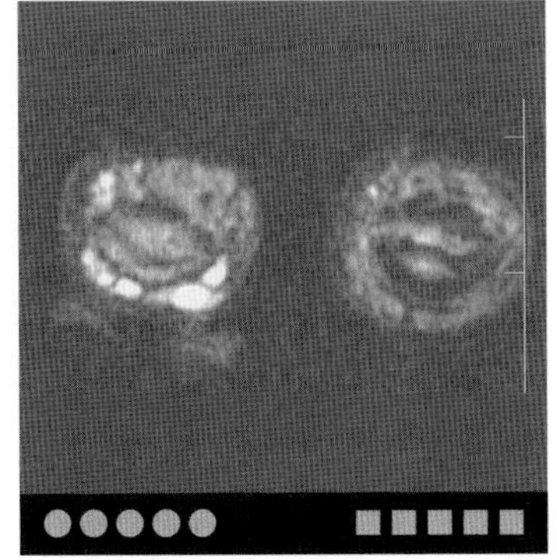

G. Mucoid cyst: A T2-weighted axial image shows the lesion extending along the dorsal margin of the distal interphalangeal joint.

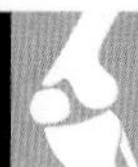

16–6 MRI Changes of Giant Cell Tumor of the Tendon Sheath

Marcia F. Blacksin

PRESENTATION

Mass palmar aspect of hand

FINDINGS

Soft tissue neoplasm is interdigitated between the flexor tendons. The mass has low signal intensity on T1-weighted and T2-weighted images.

DIFFERENTIAL DIAGNOSES

- *Fibromatosis*: Proliferation of benign fibrous tissue with deep and superficial locations in the extremities.
- *Soft tissue inflammatory masses*: From rheumatoid arthritis, gout, or amyloidosis. Rheumatoid nodules and gouty tophi can have high, low, or heterogeneous signal intensity on both T1- and T2-weighted sequences. Amyloid deposits may also have low signal on T2-weighted images secondary to histology of a fibrous nature.

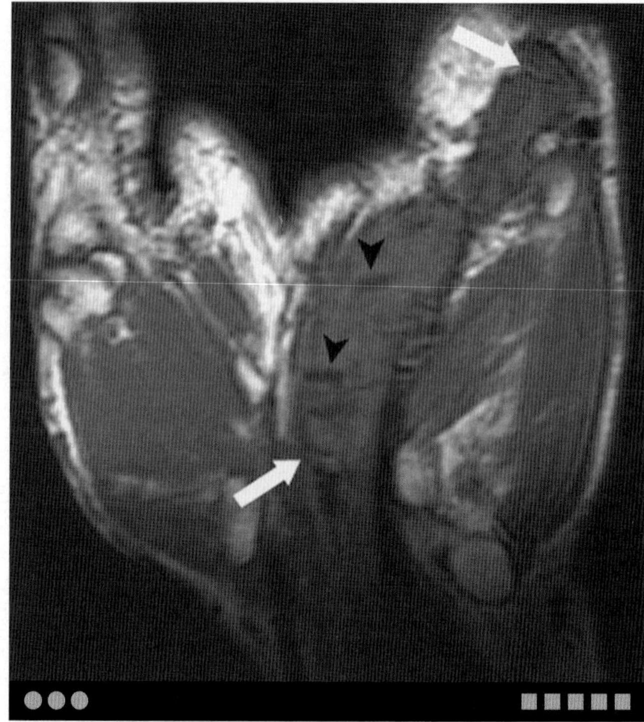

A. GCTTS: T1-weighted coronal image of hand with intermediate signal neoplasm (arrows) and low signal hemosiderin (arrowheads).

COMMENTS

Giant cell tumor of the tendon sheath (GCTTS) and Pigmented villonodular synovitis (PVNS) have similar histology. The presence of hemosiderin in these neoplasms will lower the signal intensity seen, particularly on T2-weighted images. The diffuse form of GCTTS develops predominately outside the joint, while the localized form is usually a polypoid mass in or adjacent to a joint. The localized form is easy to resect, with a low recurrence rate. The diffuse form has a recurrence rate between 40 percent and –50 percent. PVNS is purely intraarticular, and often requires total synovectomy. Fibromatosis is composed of fibrous tissue and collagen. These tumors have a variety of behaviors. The superficial forms are usually slow growing and the deeper forms may have more aggressive behavior. Signal intensity of these lesions is dependant on the degree of cellularity and the proportion of collagen in the tumor. The greater the degree of dense collagen and hypocellularity, the lower the signal intensity of the mass on T1- and T2-weighted images. The deep variety is often seen in young adults and is usually solitary. At initial presentation, tumor margins may be well-defined or infiltrative. Rheumatoid nodules and gouty tophi should be considered when multiple superficial nodular masses are seen in the hands and feet. Evaluation of radiographs can be key in making this diagnosis. Rheumatoid nodules are often seen at pressure points in the extremities. Amyloid deposition is usually seen in patients with chronic renal failure. Pressure erosions may be seen in the bones, and the most frequently affected site is the wrist.

PEARLS

- **Giant cell tumors of the tendon sheath and PVNS have similar histologies.**
- **Both lesions contain low signal intensity foci secondary to hemosiderin deposition.**
- **Fibromatosis may demonstrate low signal intensity because of hypocellularity and collagen matrix.**

ADDITIONAL IMAGES

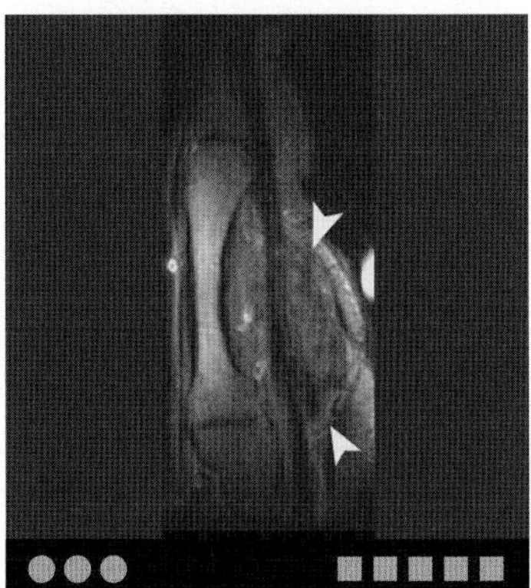

B. GCTTS: Sagittal T2-weighted image shows predominately low signal lesion (arrowheads) surrounding flexor tendon.

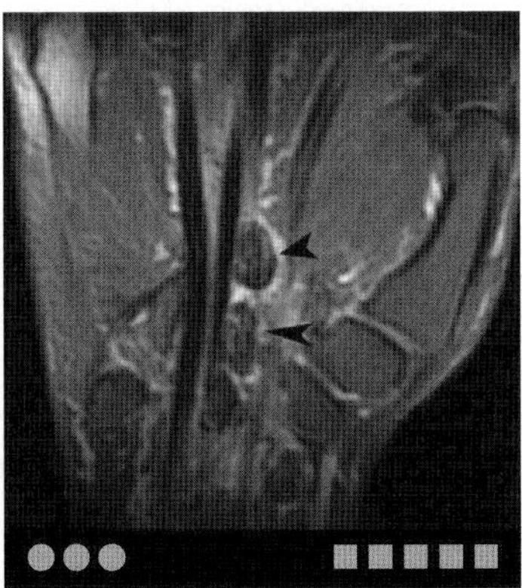

C. GCTTS: Coronal Fat Sat T1-weighted contrast-enhanced image after resection shows recurrence with low signal tumor nodules (arrowheads) adjacent to flexor tendons.

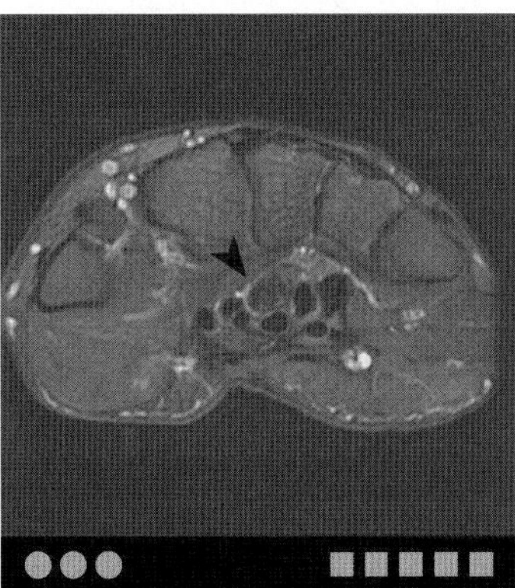

D. GCTTS: Axial Fat Sat T1-weighted contrast-enhanced image shows tumor nodule in carpal tunnel (arrowhead).

DIFFERENTIAL DIAGNOSES IMAGES

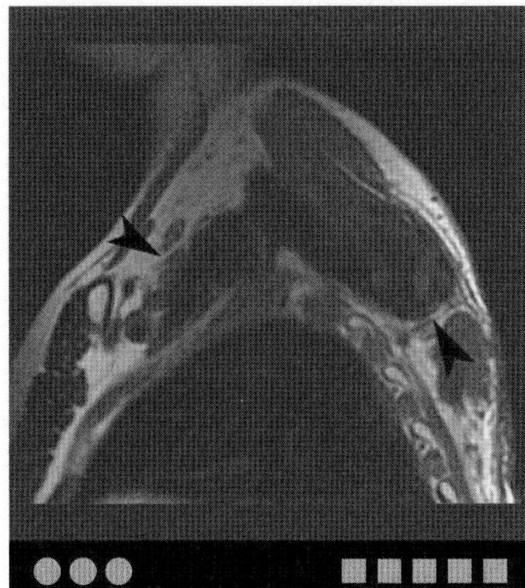

E. Fibromatosis: Sagittal T1-weighted image shows low signal deep fibromatosis crossing supraclavicular region (arrowheads).

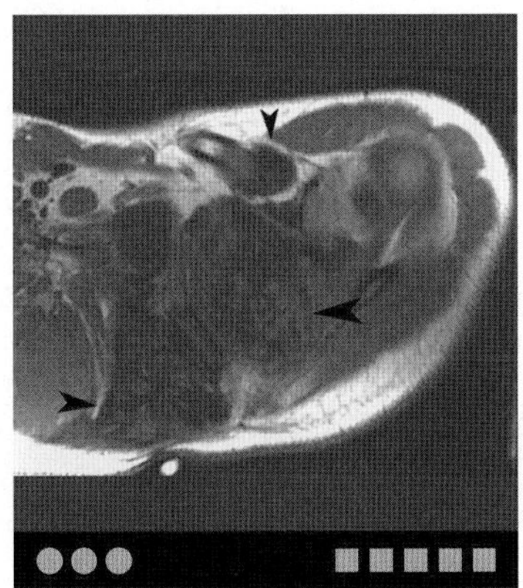

F. Fibromatosis: Axial T1-weighted image shows low signal neoplasm with infiltrating margins (arrowheads).

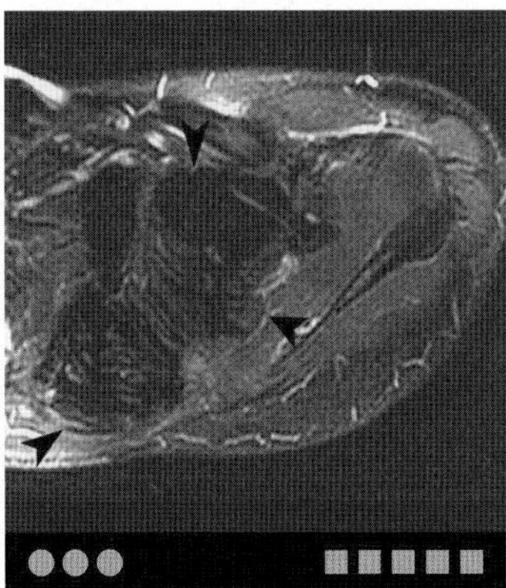

G. Fibromatosis: Axial T2-weighted image shows low signal intensity of neoplasm consistent with fibrous histology.

IMAGE KEY

Common

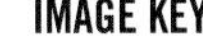

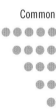

Rare

Typical

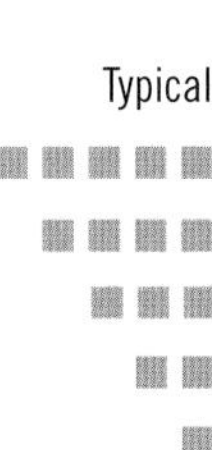

Unusual

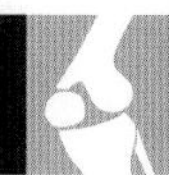

16–7 Sonographic Appearance of Giant Cell Tumor of the Tendon Sheath

Stefano Bianchi and Ibrahim F. Abdelwahab

PRESENTATION

Soft tissue tender mass

FINDINGS

Ultrasound (US) shows a well-circumscribed, slightly vascularized, and mass located palmar to the distal insertion of the flexor digitorum profundus tendon of the left little finger.

DIFFERENTIAL DIAGNOSES

- *Tendon ganglia:* US shows them as anechoic cystic lesions with posterior enhancement. Color Doppler does not display internal flow signals.
- *Glomus tumors:* Painful lesions. Pain is temperature dependent. Color Doppler shows internal hypervascularity.
- *Vascular lesions:* US exhibits posterior shadowing caused by internal blood and collapse under pressure of the transducer. Color Doppler shows low velocity internal flow signals.

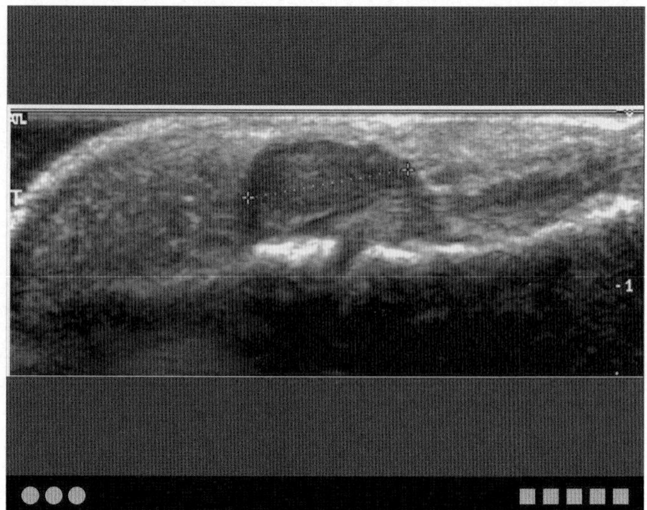

A. Giant cell tumor of the tendon sheath: Sagittal grey-scale US image obtained over the palmar aspect of the fifth digit shows GCTTS as a well-circumscribed hypoechoic nodule located adjacent to the distal insertion of the flexor digitorum profundus tendon.

COMMENTS

This 46-year-old male presented with a tender, well-localized, and slow growing mass located at the palmar aspect of the distal inter phalangeal (DIP) joint of the fifth finger. Pigmented villonodular synovitis (PVNS) is an uncommon benign proliferative disease of the synovium consisting of a fibrous stroma covered by hyperplastic lining cells, presence of histiocytes that contain fat or hemosiderin, and multinucleated giant cells. PVNS presents macroscopically as a diffuse or a nodular type. The diffuse type is characterized by hypertrophy of the joint or bursal synovium, large pressure erosions, and hemorragic effusion. The hips, knees, and ankles are mostly affected. The nodular type, also known as giant cell tumor of tendon sheath (GCTTS); it appears as a well-circumscribed synovial nodular mass, mainly found around tendons of the hand and foot. The condition is usually painless, but may recur following surgical excision. Standard radiographs can show an ill-defined increased density of peritendinous soft tissue. US can accurately evaluate the size of the nodule, its location, borders and relations with tendons and joints as well as the internal vascularity. A definite diagnosis can be only obtained by MRI that shows internal low signal in both T1- and T2-weighted sequences reflecting intralesional hemosiderin deposition.

PEARLS

- **Pigmented villonodular synovitis affects the synovium and can present as a diffuse or nodular form. The latter is also known as GCTTS and is more commonly found around hand and foot tendons.**
- **US can accurately detect GCTTS, assess its location, borders, internal vascularity, and relation with adjacent structures.**
- **The most accurate diagnostic imaging study is MRI that shows internal low signal in both T1- and T2-weighted sequences reflecting internal hemosiderin deposition.**

ADDITIONAL IMAGES

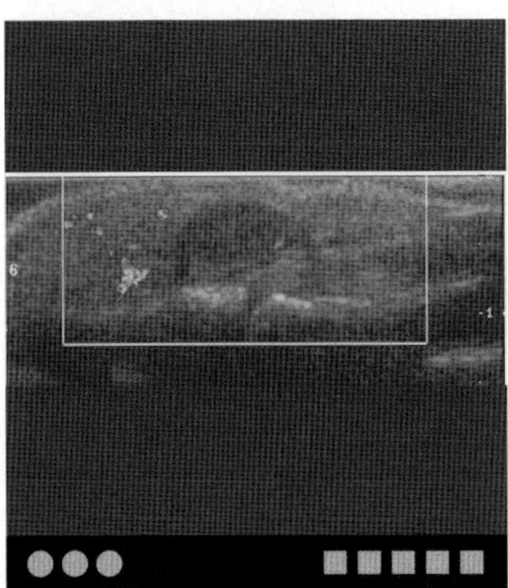

B. Giant cell tumor of the tendon sheath: Corresponding color Doppler US image demonstrates minimal, internal vascularization (cranial part).

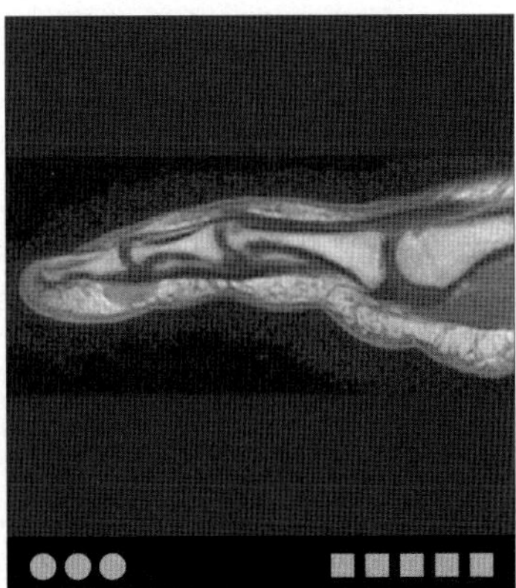

C. Giant cell tumor of the tendon sheath: Sagittal PD MRI image shows GCTTS as a isointense, well-delineated nodule.

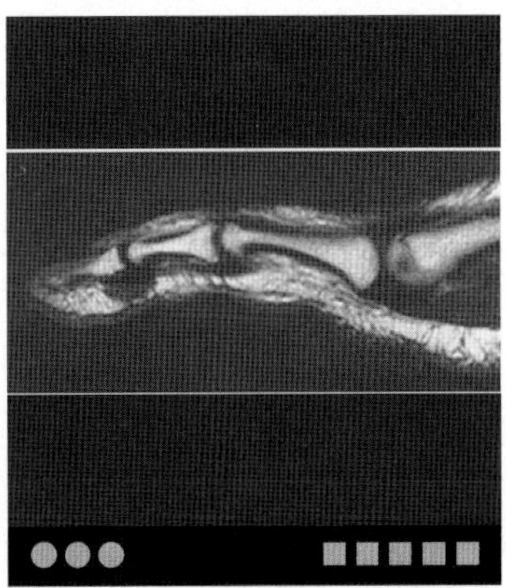

D. Giant cell tumor of the tendon sheath: Sagittal T2-weighted shows hypointense signal of the mass, typical of GCTTS.

IMAGE KEY

Common

Rare

Typical

Unusual

DIFFERENTIAL DIAGNOSES IMAGES

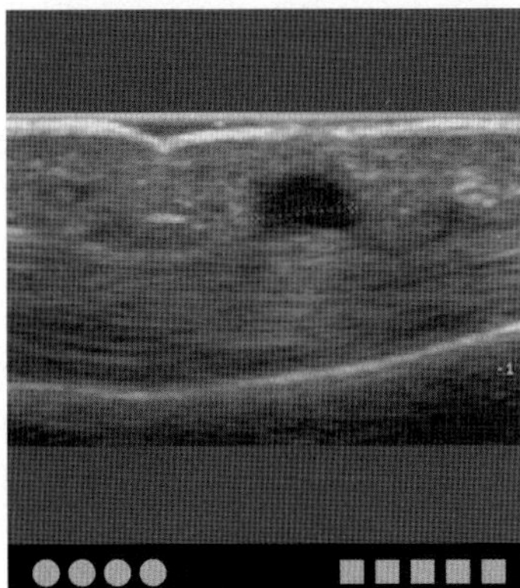

E. Ganglion: Sagittal US image shows an anechoic ganglion located palmar to the flexor tendons of a finger. Note presence of posterior enhancement.

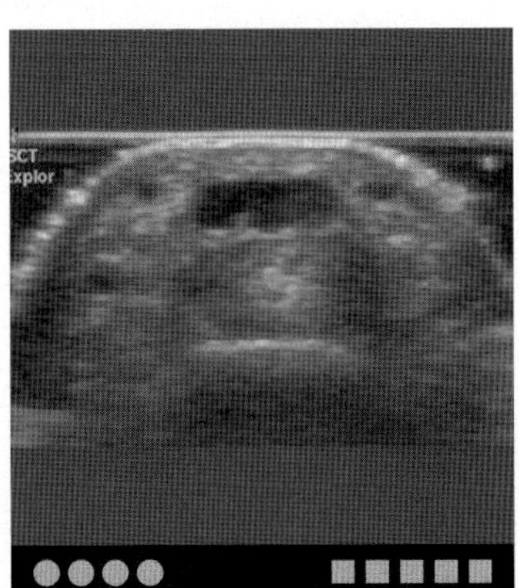

F. Ganglion: Transverse US image obtained during compression with the probe shows flattening of the fluid-filled ganglion.

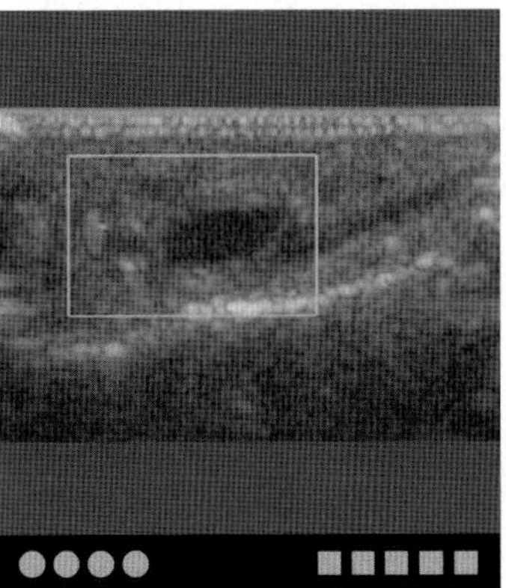

G. Ganglion: Sagittal color Doppler image, obtained in a different patient, demonstrates a ganglion located anterior to the insertion of the flexor digitorum profundus tendon. Note absence of internal flow signals.

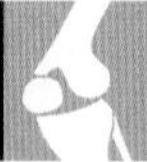

16–8 Giant Cell Tumor of a Metacarpal Bone

Ibrahim F. Abdelwahab and Stefano Bianchi

PRESENTATION

Painless swelling of dorsum of the hand

FINDINGS

Standard radiographs show an expansile lesion of the third metacarpal bone associated with cortical thinning.

DIFFERENTIAL DIAGNOSES

- *Aneurysmal bone cyst:* This is often in a younger age group.
- *Giant cell reparative granuloma (solid aneurysmal bone cyst):* This differentiation can be made on histology.
- *Chondromyxoid fibroma:* This lesion is also expansile, but often lobulated by internal septa.
- *Enchondroma:* This is the most common lesion of the short tubular bones of the hand and feet and may show internal calcification.

COMMENTS

This is an image of a 51-year-old man who presented with painless swelling of dorsum of the hand for 4 months. Giant cell tumor (GCT) of bone represents approximately 2% to 5% of primary bone tumors. GCT is most common in the third and fourth decade of life. Hand is involved in approximately 5% of cases. Hand involvement is seen usually in younger age group and tends to be multicentric (13%–18%) and often recurs (50%–70%). Pain and swelling are the most frequent presenting symptoms. Typical radiographic findings of GCT seen throughout the body are expansile, eccentric, and lytic lesion located in a subarticular position involving the epiphysis and metaphysis of long bone. GCT in hand tends to arise in central location with involvement of whole width of bone. Tc-99m bone scintigraphy shows intense uptake in the tumor. In approximately 50% of cases, uptake is primarily around periphery of tumor, with much less central activity representing a "doughnut" shape. Since multicentric involvement is more common in GCT of hand; bone scintigraphy is recommended in these patients. CT scan determines presence of cortical destruction, pathological fracture, periosteal reaction, and assessment of tumor mineralization. MRI shows low to intermediate T1-signal intensity and heterogeneous high signal intensity mass on T2-weighted image. GCT may show very low signal intensity on all pulse sequences in MRI, which is indicative of chronic hemosiderin deposition. The intramedullary extent of tumor is best appreciated on T1-weighted image. MRI is the best modality for follow-up given the high incidence of local recurrence rate in GCT of the hand.

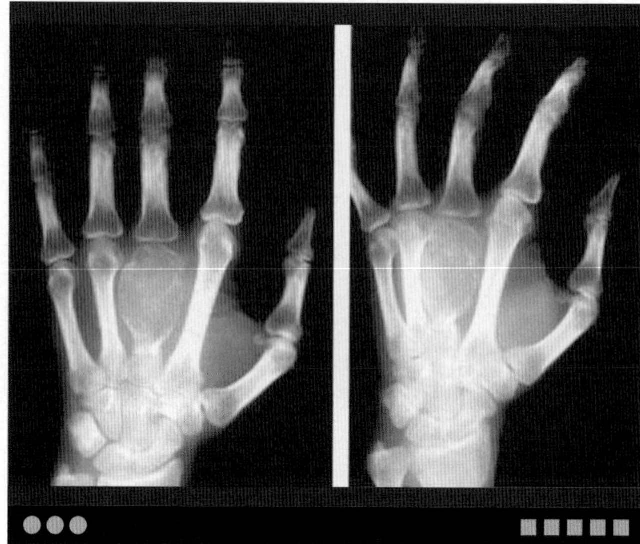

A. Giant cell tumor of a metacarpal bone: AP and oblique view of the left hand show an expansile lesion involving the distal two-thirds of the third metacarpal bone associated with cortical thinning.

PEARLS

- **The incidence of giant cell tumor in the hands is 2%–5%. It occurs in the metaepiphyseal region, and expansion of the involved bone is a prominent feature.**
- **There are two distinguishing features between giant cell tumor of the hands and feet and those arising elsewhere in the skeleton. One is the high rate of multicentric giant cell tumors (18%) when at least one giant cell tumor occurs in the hand. The other characteristic is that giant cell tumor of the hand and foot occurs 10 years younger than those with giant cell tumors in more common locations.**
- **Tc-99m bone scintigraphy shows intense uptake in GCT and in 50% of cases is doughnut shape. CT scan shows presence of cortical disruption, pathological fracture, periosteal reaction, and assessment of tumor mineralization.**
- **MRI shows low to intermediate T1-signal intensity and heterogeneous high signal intensity mass on T2-weighted image and is valuable in follow up of recurrence.**

ADDITIONAL IMAGES

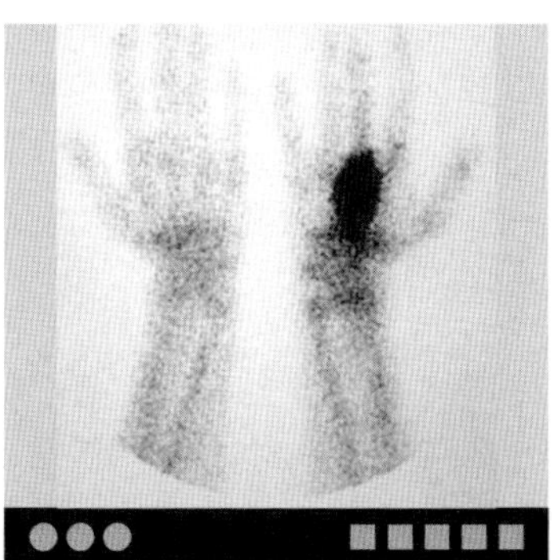

B. Giant cell tumor of a metacarpal bone: Bone scan shows marked local uptake of the radionuclide material.

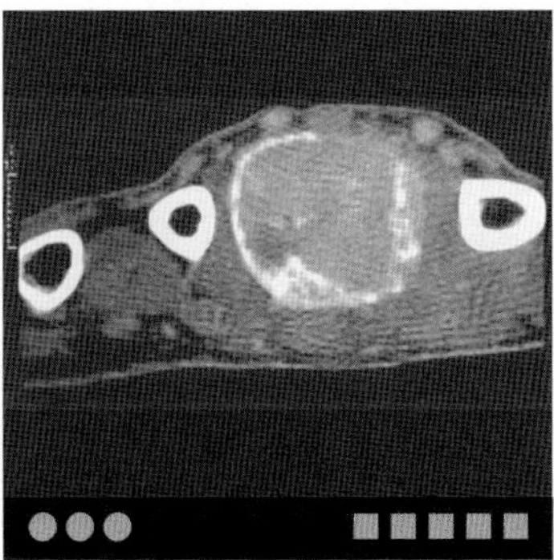

C. Giant cell tumor of a metacarpal bone: CT scan confirms massive expansion of the metacarpal bone, thinning and focal discontinuity of the cortex.

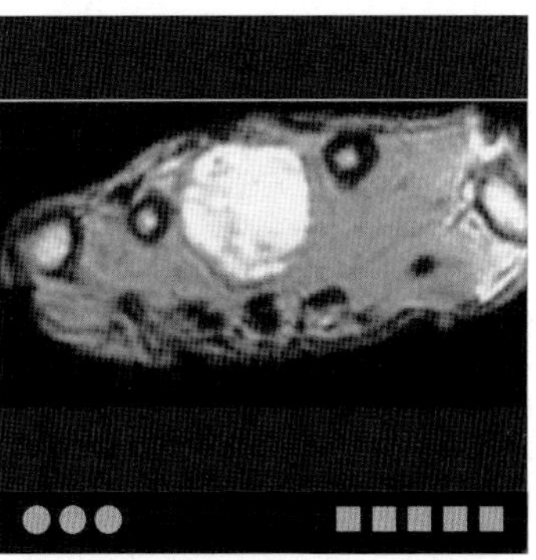

D. Giant cell tumor of a metacarpal bone: Axial T2-weighted MR image shows inhomogeneous hyperintensity signal of the mass.

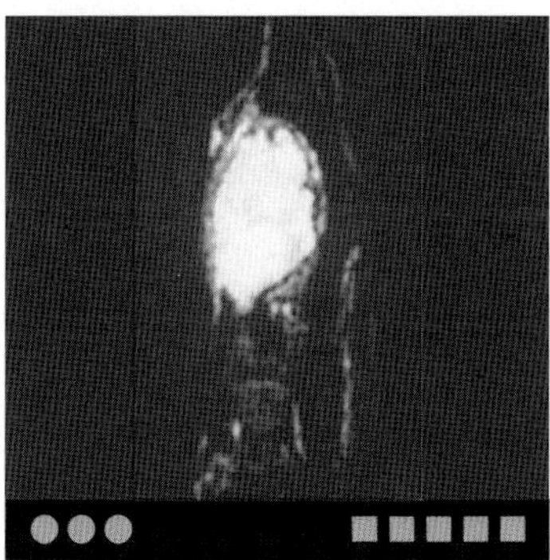

E. Giant cell tumor of a metacarpal bone: Sagittal STIR MR image shows the hyperintense tumor located in the distal two-thirds of the metacarpal bone.

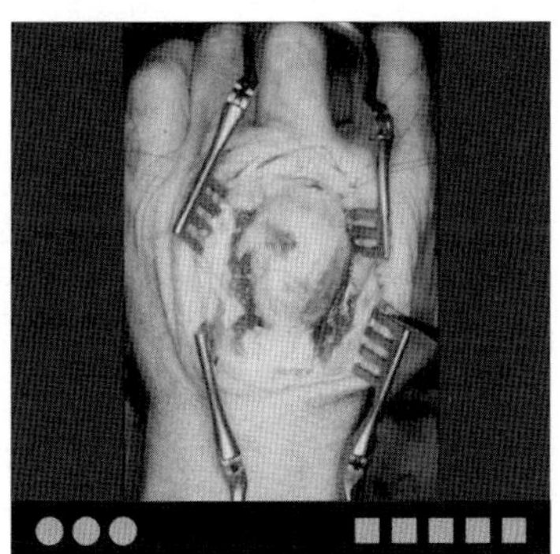

F. Giant cell tumor of a metacarpal bone: Operative image.

DIFFERENTIAL DIAGNOSES IMAGE

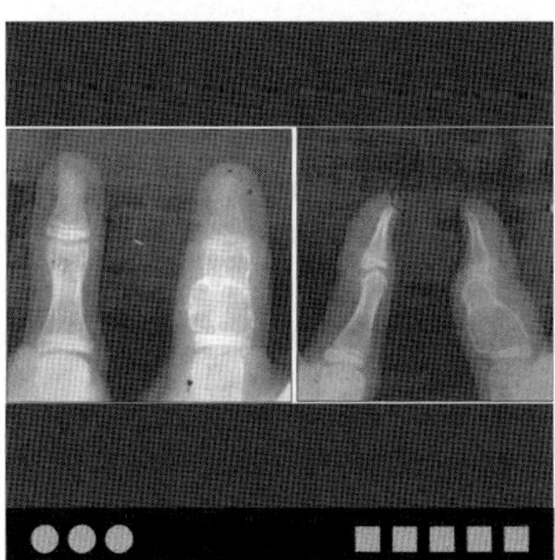

G. Giant cell reparative granuloma: AP and lateral view of the right and left thumb of a 14-year-old young female reveals a cystic expansion of the whole proximal phalanx of the left thumb. There is thinning of the cortex without interruption, permeation, or soft tissue extension. It mimics exactly giant cell tumor.

IMAGE KEY

Common

Rare

Typical

Unusual

SECTION IV

HIP AND PELVIS

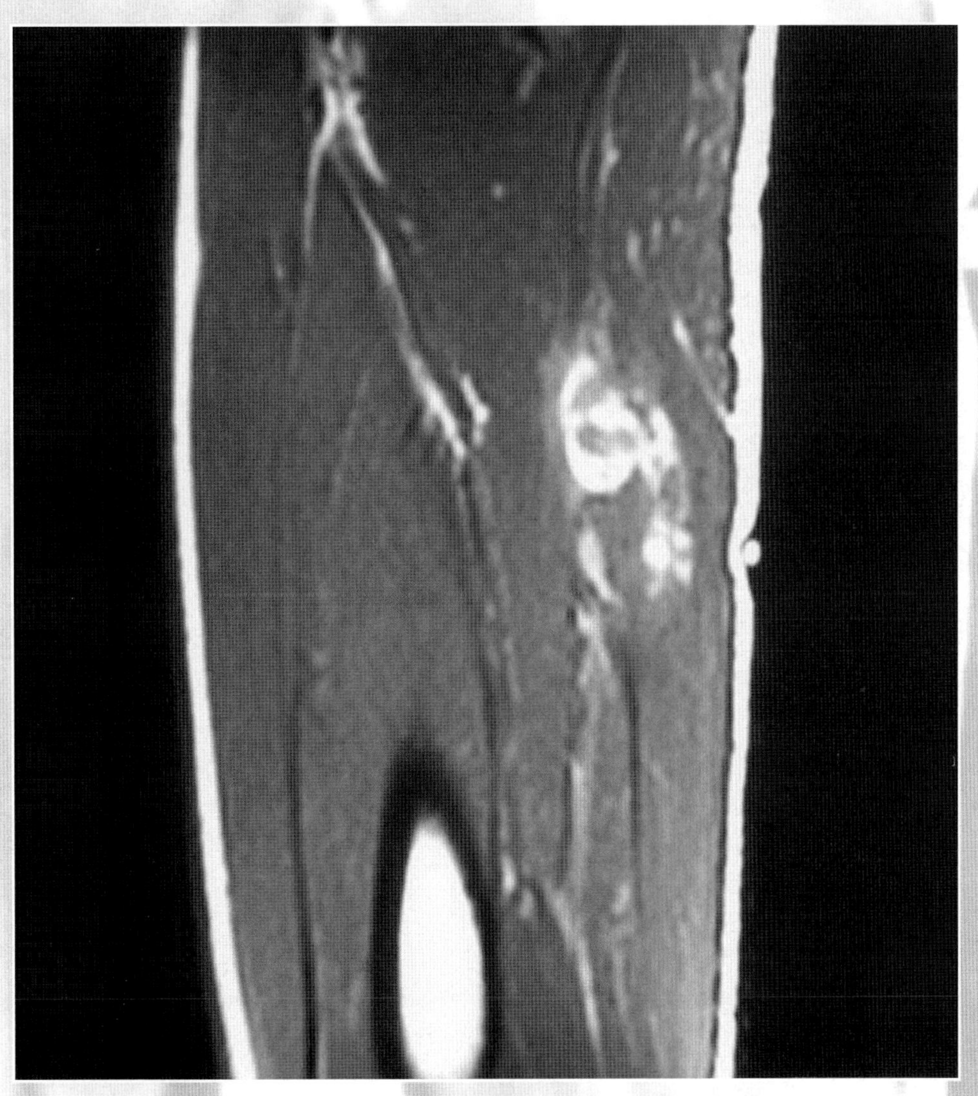

Chapter 17

Sport Medicine and Trauma

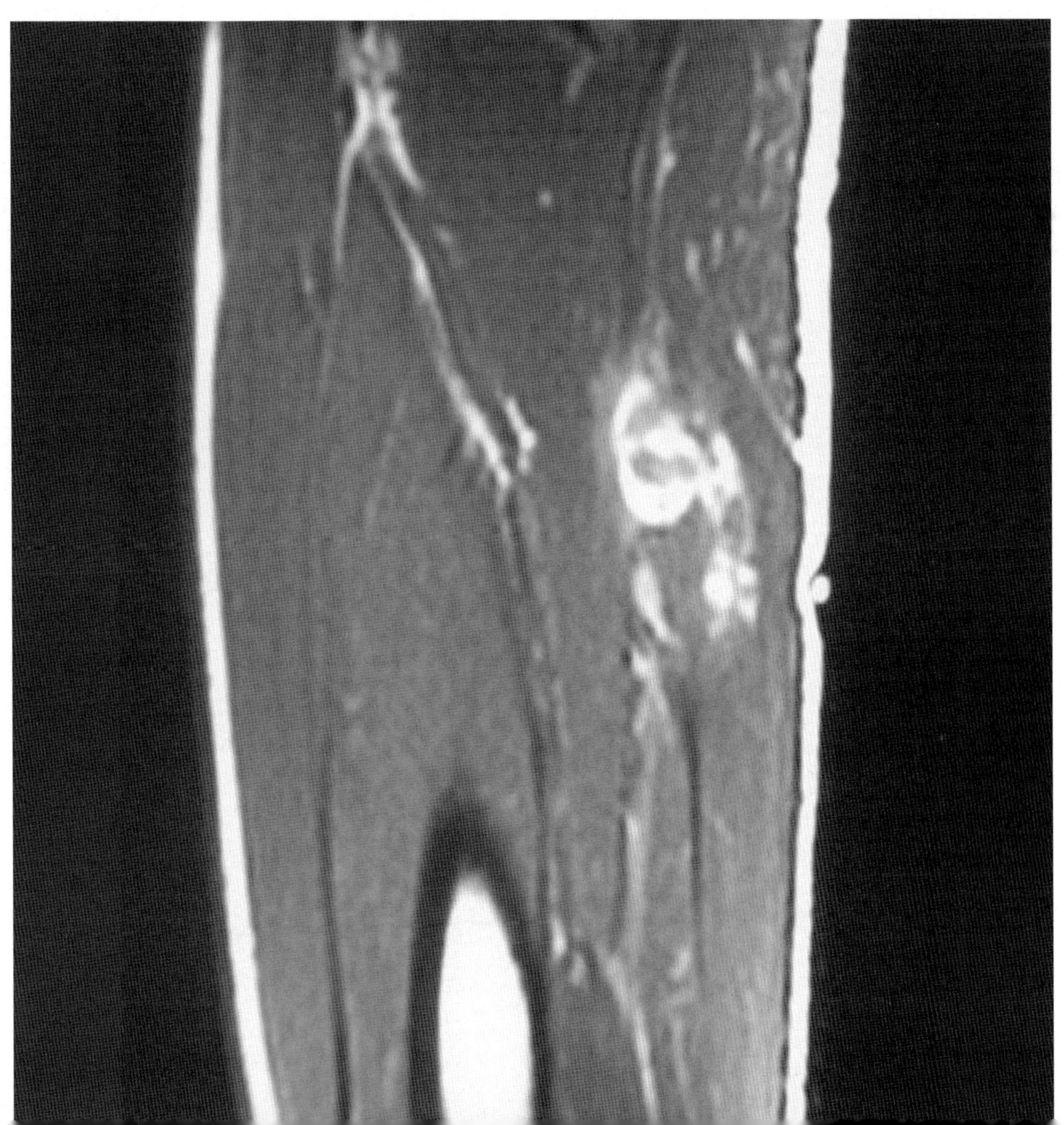

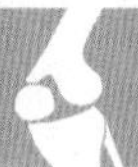

17–1 Subacute Intramuscular Hematoma of the Gluteus Maximus

Nuttya Pattamapasong and Wilfred CG Peh

PRESENTATION

Pain swelling and history of injury

FINDINGS

MR images show an irregular area within the distal gluteus maximus muscle that is hyperintense on both T1W and T2W MR images and show marked hypointensity and blooming on the GRE image.

DIFFERENTIAL DIAGNOSES

- *Pyomyositis:* Signs and symptoms of infection. On MR imaging, there are T2-hyperintense rim-enhancing pockets of abscesses within the diffusely edematous muscle.
- *Fat-containing tumor:* Bulky mass with a fat component in which signal intensity is similar to the subcutaneous fat in all pulse sequences. Use of fat suppression helps distinguish hematoma from other T1-hyperintense fat containing tumors such as lipoma well-differentiated liposarcoma or hemangioma.
- *Other intramuscular tumors:* Most soft tissue tumors are hypo- to isointense on T1W MR images, hyperintense on T2WI, and display moderate to marked enhancement.

COMMENTS

This is a 32-year-old man who sustained an injury to the right posterior thigh during a soccer game. Intramuscular hematomas usually result from injury or bleeding diatheses, but may sometimes occur spontaneously. The MR imaging appearances of intramuscular hematoma are variable, depending on the static field strength of the magnet, the timing of evaluation of the blood-containing tissue, and the relative degree of edema at the injury site. Several forms of blood product can alter signal intensity of MR images. If MR imaging is conducted within 48 hours of injury, interstitial hemorrhage and hematoma have signal intensity similar to muscle on T1WI and are hyperintense on T2WI. During the subacute stage (7 days to 1 month after injury), the hematoma has moderately decreased T1 and T2 relaxation times, producing a hyperintense signal on T1WI. The presence of oxyhemoglobin, deoxyhemoglobin, and red blood cells in tissues results in T1 shortening because of oxidative denaturation of hemoglobin and the production of methemoglobin. The increasing concentration of methemoglobin over 3 to 4 days produces progressive shortening of the T1 relaxation time. The intracellular deoxyhemoglobin and intracellular methemoglobin cause low signal intensity on T2-weighted images, while subsequent accumulation of extracellular methemoglobin results in hyperintense signal on T2-weighted images. In the last stage of evolution of hematoma, hemosiderin is formed, producing markedly low signal intensity on both T1WI and T2WI at the periphery of the hematoma. The rim of decreased signal intensity is better appreciated with time because of the of hemosiderin-laden macrophages.

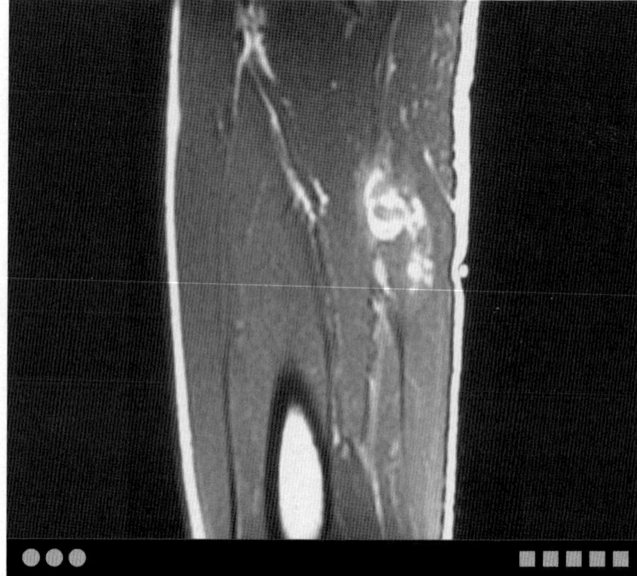

A. Subacute hematoma of the right gluteus maximus muscle: Sagittal SE T1W MR image shows a heterogeneous area of predominant hyperintense signal in the distal gluteus maximus muscle. The high signal intensity results from T1 shortening because of methemoglobin. Site of postinjury painful swelling is indicated by the surface marker.

PEARLS

- **Knowledge of a history of bleeding diathesis, injury, and anticoagulant therapy leads to diagnosis of intramuscular hematoma.**
- **The signal intensity of hematomas is variable, depending on the component of blood products.**
- **Presence of hyperintense signal on T1W MR images is a valuable clue to diagnosis but this finding is not present in all stages of hematoma.**
- **Use of fat suppression helps distinguish the T1 hyperintense signal found in hematoma from fat-containing masses.**
- **Use of gradient echo images produce a blooming effect because of the magnetic susceptibility properties of hemosiderin and help confirm the diagnosis of subacute and chronic hematomas.**

ADDITIONAL IMAGES

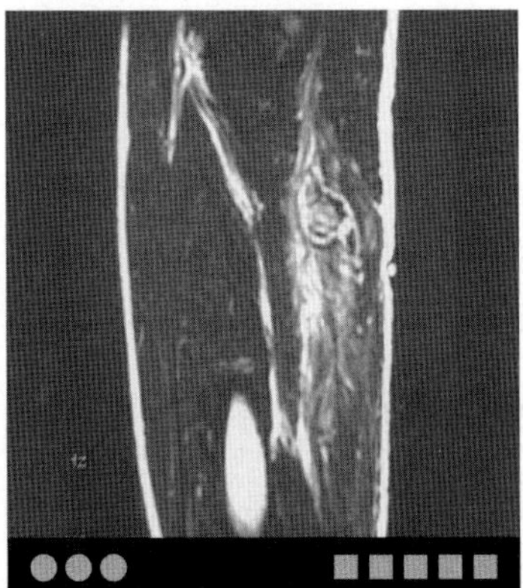

B. Subacute hematoma of the right gluteus maximus muscle: Sagittal FSE T2W MR image shows a heterogeneous area of hyperintense signal in the distal gluteus maximus muscle. Scattered areas of hypointense signal result from hemosiderin because of T2 shortening.

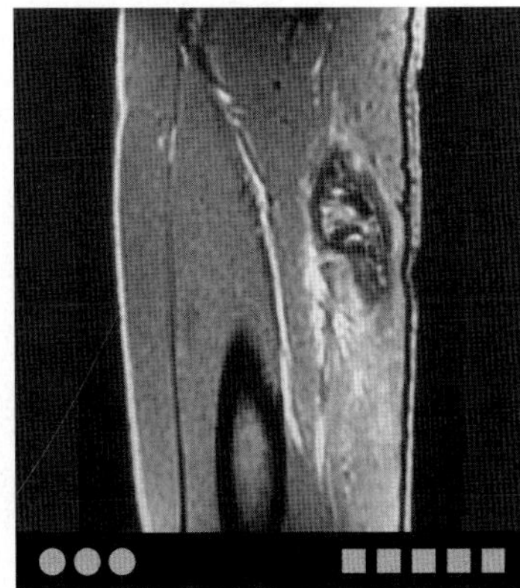

C. Subacute hematoma of the right gluteus maximus muscle: Sagittal GRE MR image shows further marked hypointensity and blooming, confirming the presence of hemosiderin.

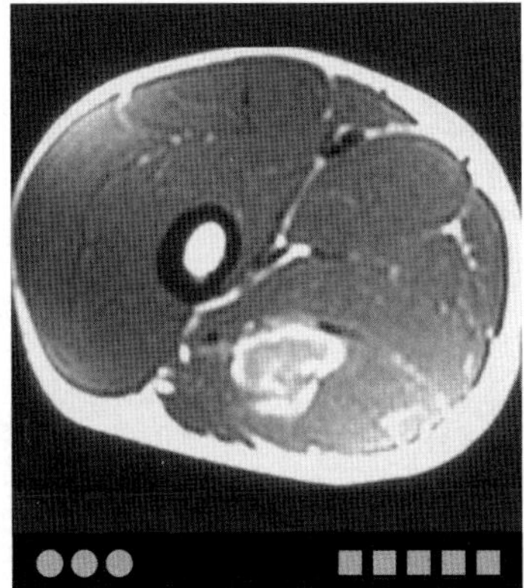

D. Subacute hematoma of the right gluteus maximus muscle: Axial SE T1W MR image shows a heterogeneous hematoma in the distal gluteus maximus muscle. The hyperintense area represents methemoglobin.

DIFFERENTIAL DIAGNOSES IMAGES

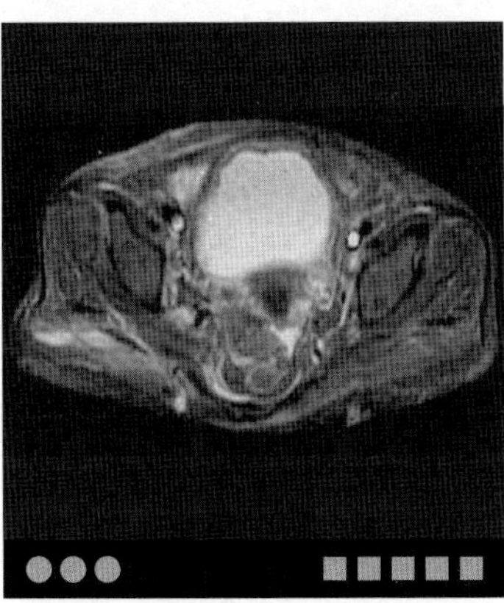

E. Pyomyositis of the right gluteus maximus muscle: Axial fat-suppressed FSE T2W MR image shows multiple pockets of increased signal intensity representing abscesses, with surrounding diffuse edema.

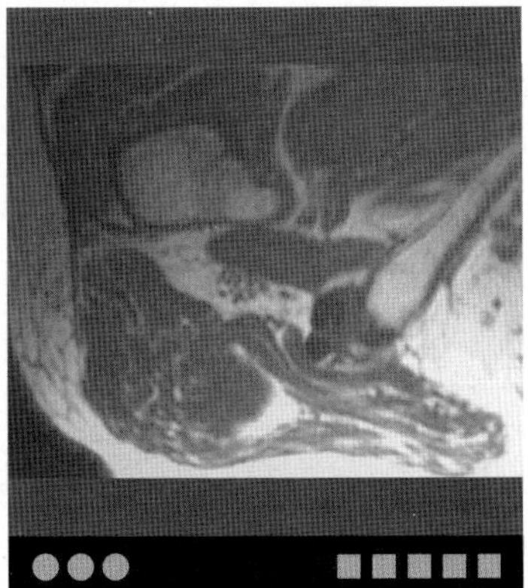

F. Neurofibroma of the right gluteus maximus muscle: Axial SE T1W MR image shows a rounded hypointense area in the gluteus maximus muscle.

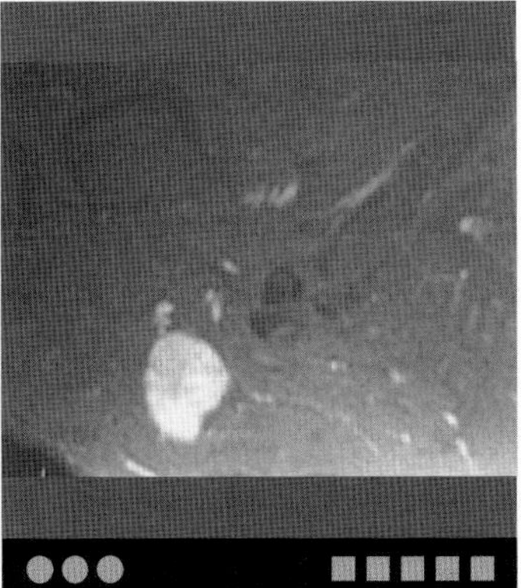

G. Neurofibroma of the right gluteus maximus muscle: Axial fat-suppressed FSE T2W MR image shows a hyperintense lesion.

IMAGE KEY

Common

Rare

Typical

Unusual

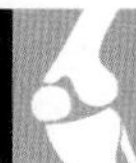

17–2 Obturator Externus Bursitis

Piran Aliabadi

PRESENTATION

Right hip pain

FINDINGS

Fluid-filled sac posteroinferior to the femoral head and anterior to the obturator externus muscle.

DIFFERENTIAL DIAGNOSES

- *Joint effusion:* Distended joint capsule with homogenous signal intensity on fluid sensitive sequence.
- *Iliopsoas bursitis:* Fluid-filled sac anterior to the femoral head. May communicate with the joint.
- *Synovitis:* May be septic or aseptic with thickened irregular margins.
- *Trochanteric bursitis:* Inflammation of the trochanter bursa, extra-articular.

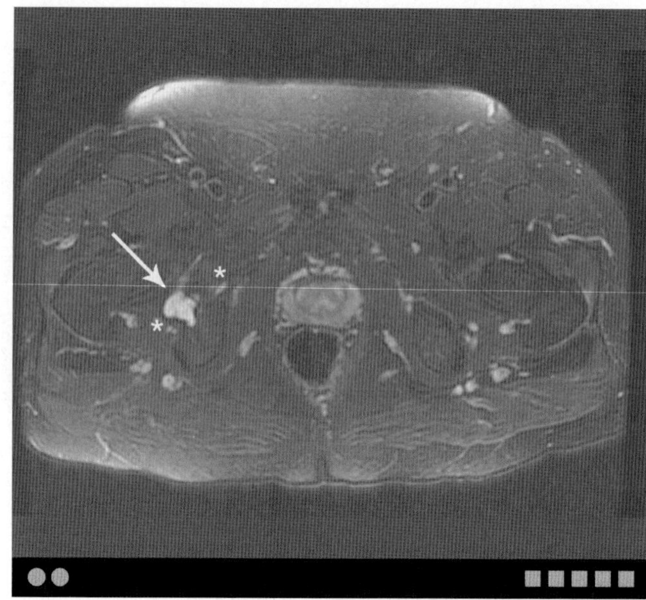

A. Obturator externus bursitis: Axial STIR image shows a homogenous fluid collection (arrow) posterior to the obturator externus muscle (asterisk).

COMMENTS

This is a 48-year-old woman with hip pain. The obturator externus bursa extends deep from the belly of the obturator externus and follows the tendon to its insertion onto the femur at the trochanteric fossa. It is hypothesized that constant friction between the obturator externus tendon and joint capsule can produce distension of the bursa along the tendon. The bursa then communicates with the joint capsule through weakening posteriorly along the ischiofemoral ligament portion of the joint capsule. This theory has been discussed in the more common iliopsoas bursa along the anteromedial portion of the joint capsule. The bursa itself can become inflamed as in a primary bursitis or become involved secondarily from an organic process in the hip joint. The bursa can be distinguished from the joint by its smooth sac and visualization of the joint capsule. However, when inflamed this margin may become irregular. The MR findings include a fluid-filled sac that follows fluid signal intensity on all sequences along the margin of the obturator externus muscle. Radiography will fail to show any abnormalities and ultrasonography will demonstrate a hypoechoic structure that communicates with the hip joint. A large joint effusion can be seen distending the joint. No medical treatment is indicated for this finding when it exists independently in an asymptomatic patient.

PEARLS

- **Obturator externus bursa is contiguous with the hip joint capsule but seen posterior to the joint.**
- **Can be an associated finding in patients with organic hip disease. May become secondarily inflamed.**

ADDITIONAL IMAGE

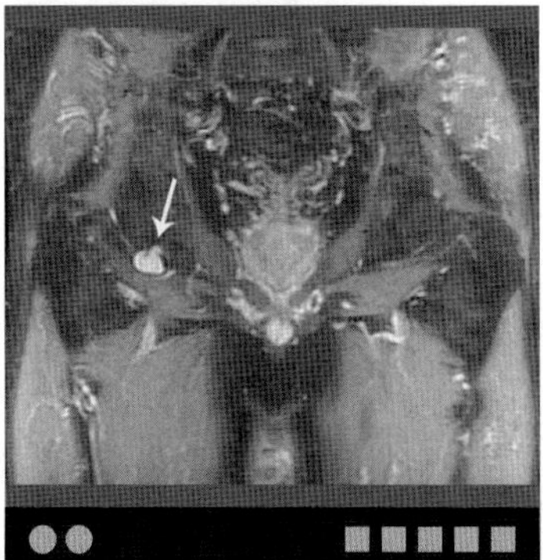

B. Obturator externus bursitis: Coronal fat-saturated T2WI demonstrates a discrete fluid-filled structure (arrow) superior to the obturator externus muscle. Note the walls are thin and smooth with homogeneous internal signal intensity.

DIFFERENTIAL DIAGNOSES IMAGES

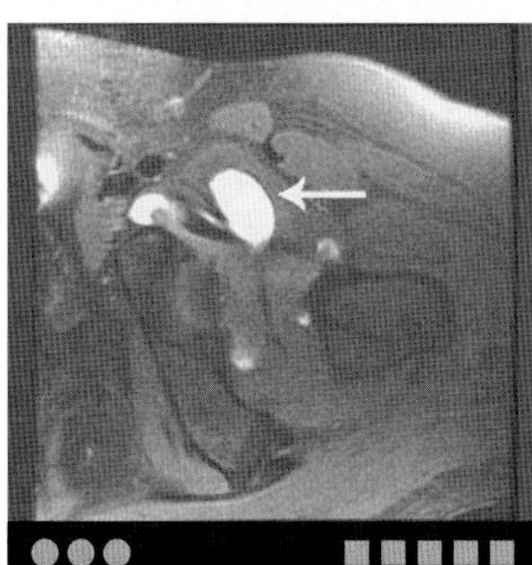

C. Iliopsoas bursitis: Axial fat-saturated T1WI demonstrates a smooth fluid-filled sac (arrow) following the iliopsoas tendon anterior to the femoral head.

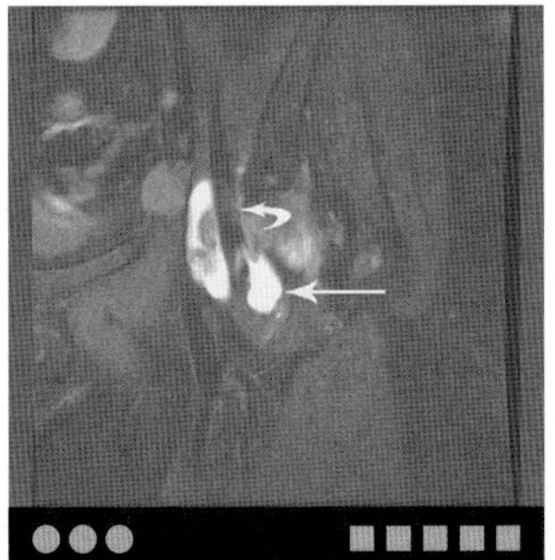

D. Iliopsoas bursitis: Coronal fat-saturated T1WI shows the iliopsoas tendon (curved arrow) bisecting the bursa (arrow).

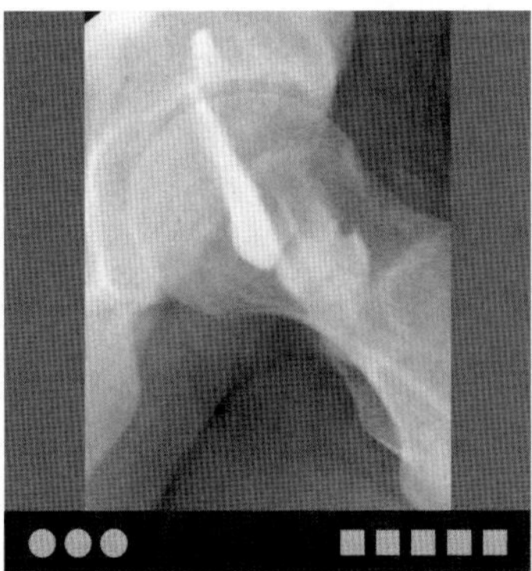

E. Iliopsoas bursitis: Iliopsoas bursogram shows contrast agent in the iliopsoas bursa.

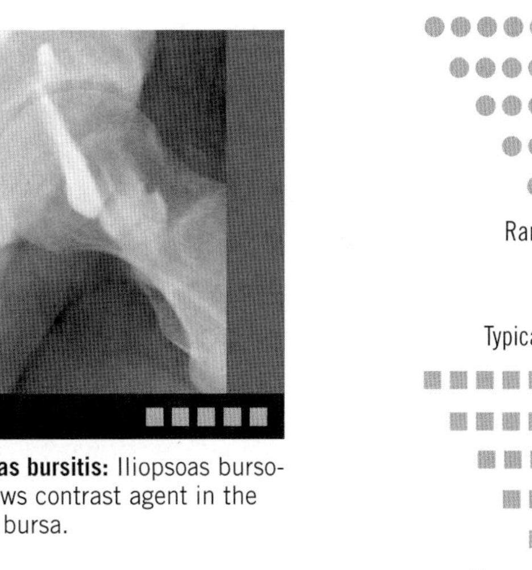

IMAGE KEY

Common

Rare

Typical

Unusual

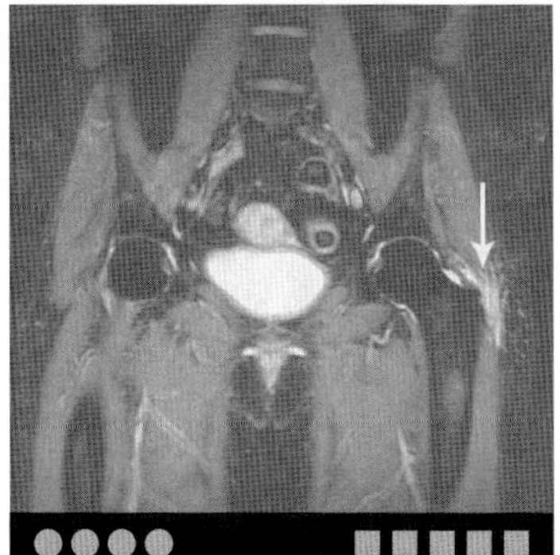

F. Greater trochanter bursitis: Coronal fat-saturated T2WI demonstrates fluid signal (arrow) within the greater trochanter bursa lateral to the greater trochanter.

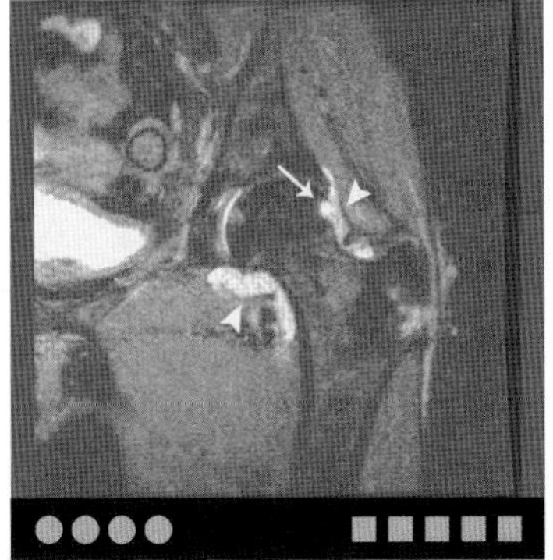

G. Rheumatoid arthritis: Coronal STIR image of the left hip shows a femoral head erosion (arrow) and cartilage loss. The signal intensity of the joint effusion is heterogeneous and represents thickened synovium (arrowheads).

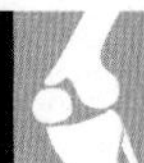

17–3 Iliopsoas Bursitis

Ibrahim F. Abdelwahab and Stefano Bianchi

PRESENTATION

Painful anterior groin mass

FINDINGS

MRI demonstrated an enlarged distended iliopsoas bursa in all planes.

DIFFERENTIAL DIAGNOSES

- *Paralabral cyst:* Associated with acetabular labral tear, it may project anteriorly.
- *Muscle strain:* Anterior abdominal muscle edema, for example, rectus abdominis, not associated with bursal fluid distension.
- *Malignancy:* Malignant fibrous histiocytoma, liposarcoma, synovial sarcoma, metastatic soft tissue mass.

COMMENTS

This is a 36-year-old woman who presented with progressive pain of the left groin for few months. MRI demonstrated an enlarged distended iliopsoas bursa in all planes. The pain precipitated with activity and then progressed to become constant and at rest. Physical examination revealed a tender anterior groin mass located in the femoral triangle. The pain was exacerbated by flexion, abduction, and external rotation. MR imaging of the iliopsoas tendon reveals hypointense to intermediate signal on T1WI. It demonstrates the lateral displacement of the iliopsoas tendon. The signal intensify on T2WI is usually homogeneous with sharp border. Axial MRI images show direct communication with hip with a tail-like extension medial to the iliopsoas tendon best seen on T2WI. Fat-saturated TIWI with contrast shows peripheral enhancement with no enhancement of the fluid unless the synovium is hypertrophied. Long axis of the bursa is oriented superior to inferior on coronal MR images. MR protocol suggested is fat-saturated proton density fast spin echo and fat-saturated T2W fast spin echo image in the coronal and axial planes. T1W postcontrast fat-saturated image is used if looking for synovial hypertrophy. US imaging is the most cost-effective test and reveals unechoic to hyperechoic fluid, well-circumscribed fluid collection, hyperechoic if hemorrhage is present. Treatment is usually conservative.

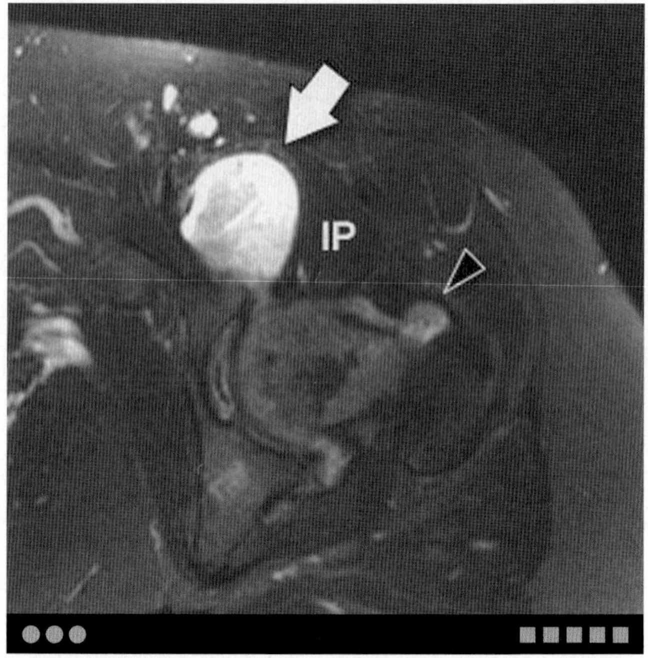

A. Iliopsoas bursitis: Axial fat-saturated T2W fast spin echo image showing a sharply defined hyperintense mass (arrow) medial to the iliopsoas muscle (IP) communicating with the hip joint. Note the joint effusion (arrow head).

PEARLS

- **Axial MRI images show direct communication with hip with a tail-like extension medial to the iliopsoas tendon best seen on T2WI.**
- **Long axis of the bursa is oriented superior to inferior on coronal MRI images.**
- **US imaging is the most cost-effective test.**
- **MR protocol suggested is fat-saturated proton density fast spin echo and fat saturated T2W fast spin echo images in the coronal and axial planes. T1W postcontrast fat-saturated image is used if looking for synovial hypertrophy.**

ADDITIONAL IMAGES

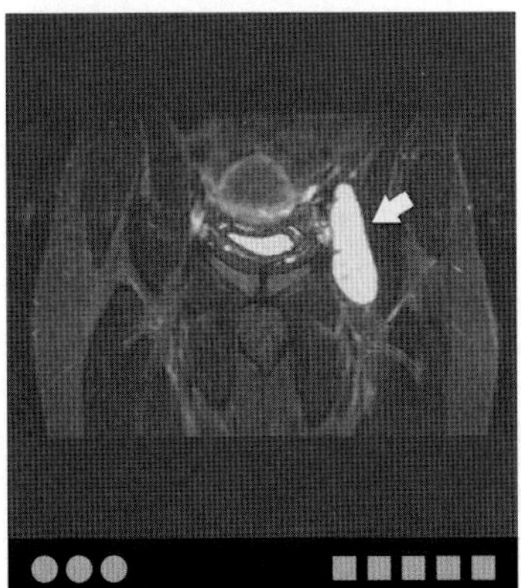

B. Iliopsoas bursitis: Coronal fat-saturated T2WI FSE demonstrating the long axis of the markedly distended bursa oriented superior to inferior (arrow).

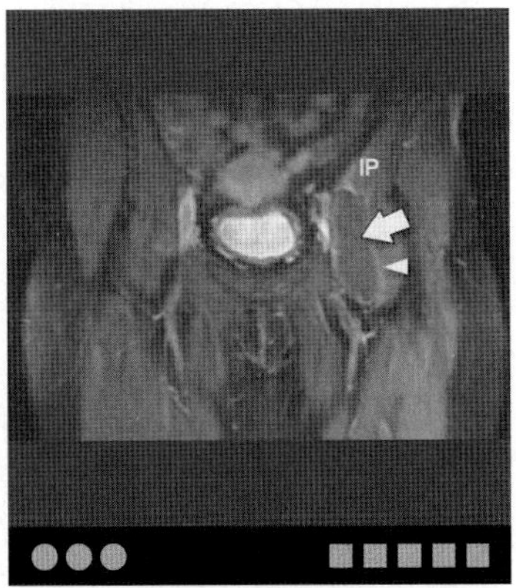

C. Iliopsoas bursitis: Coronal postcontrast fat-saturated T1WI reveals peripheral enhancement (arrow head) without enhancement of the mass lesion indicating its fluid consistency (arrow). Note that the bursa is medial to the iliopsoas (IP).

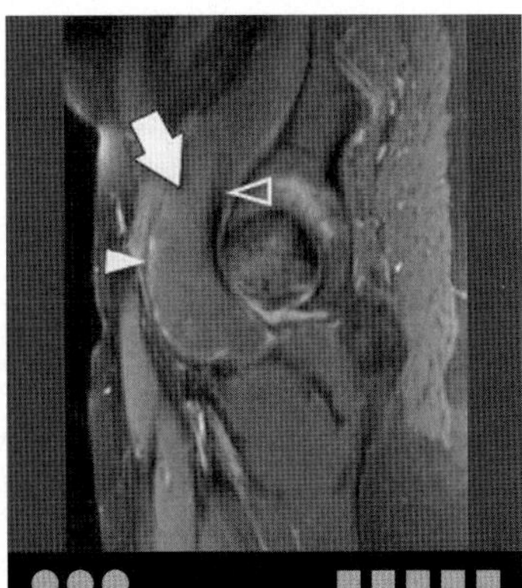

D. Iliopsoas bursitis: Sagittal fat-saturated postcontrast T1WI showing the distended bursa (arrow) with peripheral enhancement (white arrowhead). In this plane, the bursa has a C-shaped appearance with anterior convexity leaning on the rectus abdominis and posterior concavity anterior to the joint capsule and iliopsoas tendon (void arrowhead). The bursa is tapering inferiorly to accompany the iliopsoas tendon.

IMAGE KEY

Common

Rare

Typical

Unusual

DIFFERENTIAL DIAGNOSES IMAGES

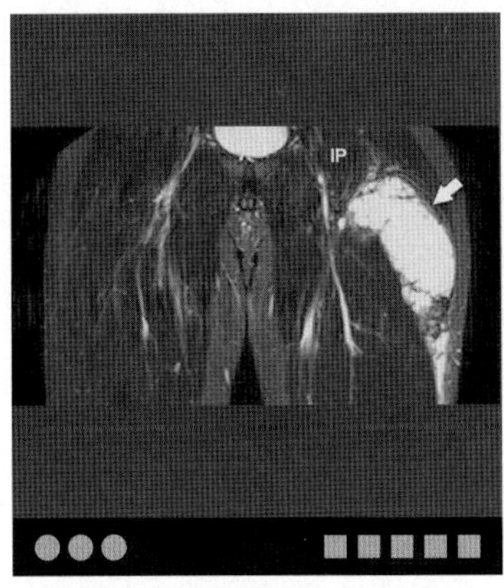

E. Tumor (malignant fibrous histiocytoma): Coronal STIR image demonstrating a hyperintense mass (arrow) located lateral to the iliopsoas muscle (IP).

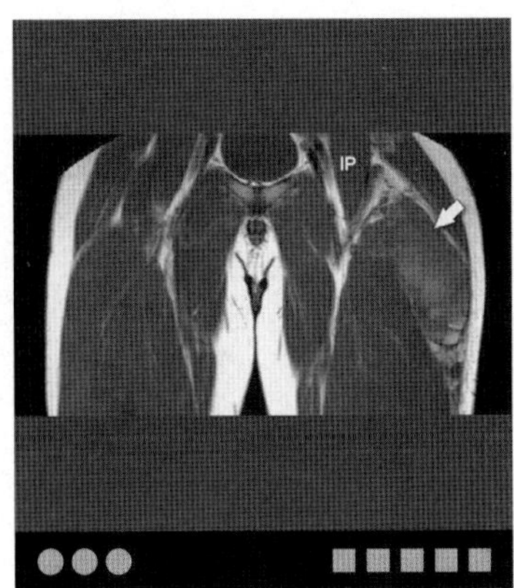

F. Tumor (malignant fibrous histiocytoma): Coronal T1 image reveals a hypointense mass containing some internal septa (arrow).

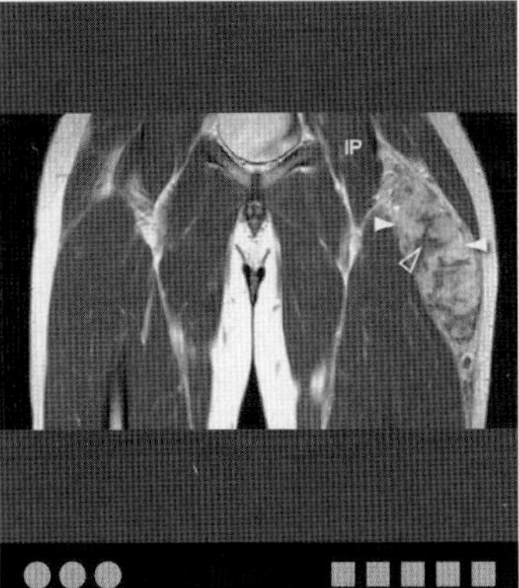

G. Tumor (malignant fibrous histiocytoma): Coronal fat-saturated T1WI postcontrast showing contrast enhancement of the mass (white arrowheads) and some internal necrotic area (void arrowhead).

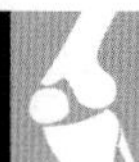

17–4 Calcific Tendinosis of the Gluteus Maximus Tendon

Tod G. Abrahams

PRESENTATION

Hip pain

FINDINGS

Lateral radiograph shows amorphous calcification in the posterior aspect of the femoral diaphysis (gluteal line).

DIFFERENTIAL DIAGNOSES

- *Adductors and hamstring avulsions:* The pain may simulate tendinosis.
- *Soft tissue tumor:* Masses may be confused with muscle strains.
- *Infection:* Myositis may mimic muscle strain.

COMMENT

This 50-year-old female presented with hip pain. Calcific tendinosis results from deposition of calcium hydroxyapatite crystals in periarticular muscular attachments. It is most common in the fourth to sixth decades. The clinical presentation is generally quite dramatic with acute onset of severe pain, decreased range of motion, and soft tissue swelling. There may be low-grade fever, mild leukocytosis, and acute-phase reactants. Involvement of unusual sites as in this case can create a diagnostic challenge to the clinician. The presentation of calcific tendinosis of the gluteus maximus tendon can be quite variable and includes acute hip pain, radicular symptoms, and more subacute to chronic hip or thigh discomfort. Key to the diagnosis is knowing the distal insertion, which is along the gluteal tubercle at the posterolateral aspect of the proximal femoral diaphysis within 6 cm of the lesser trochanter. Since this region projects over the femoral shaft on the AP view, areas of calcific tendinosis are seen best on lateral or "frog leg" lateral projections. The calcification is typically round and amorphous though it can be solid or stippled. Cortical erosion is common and periosteal reaction may be seen. The periosteal reaction is most commonly solid though can be lamellated. CT is the modality of choice and is helpful to better visualize and characterize these changes. MR imaging allows evaluation of marrow involvement, which is seen in about one third of cases. It also depicts the inflammation and edema in the adjacent soft tissues.

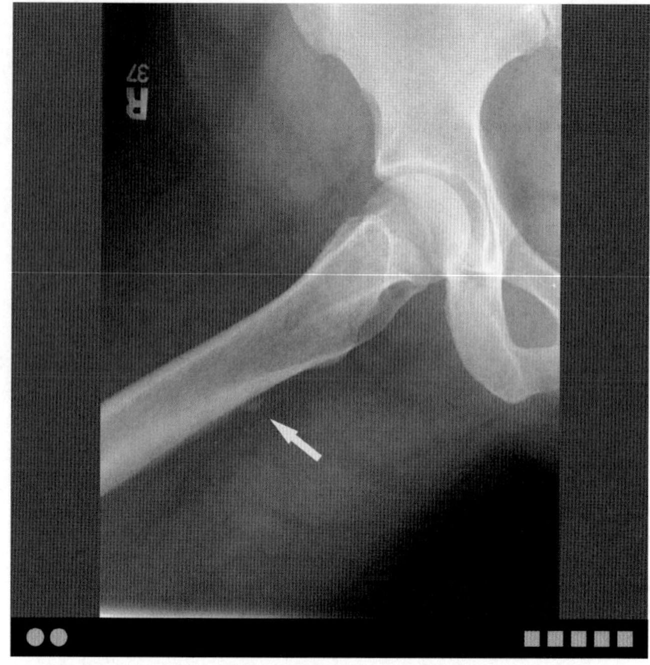

A. Calcific tendinosis of gluteus maximus tendon: Frog leg lateral view of the hip shows calcific deposit at the terminal insertion of the gluteus maximus tendon (arrow).

PEARLS

- **Calcific tendinosis in unusual sites presenting with soft tissue calcification, cortical erosion, periosteal reaction, and marrow changes can be misdiagnosed as neoplasm or infection clinically and radiographically.**
- **Calcific tendinosis of the gluteus maximus tendon requires recognition of the characteristic location of the deposit at the gluteal tubercle.**
- **Radiograph and CT are the cornerstones to the imaging diagnosis.**
- **MR imaging can be confusing and the radiologist must always correlate the MR findings with the radiograph or CT to prevent unnecessary biopsy.**

ADDITIONAL IMAGES

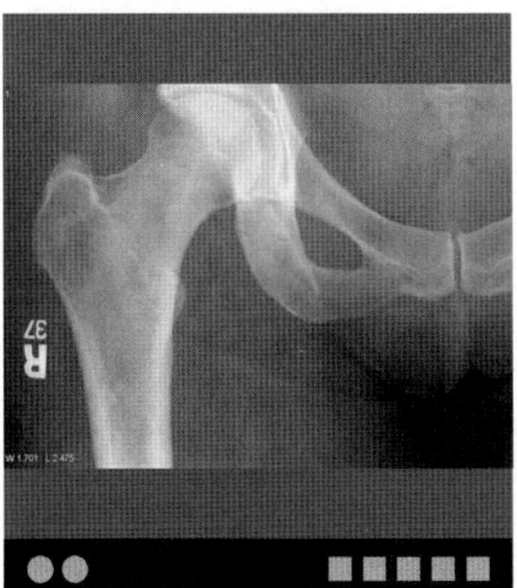

B. Calcific tendinosis of gluteus maximus tendon: The AP view shows subtle calcific density overlying the proximal femur.

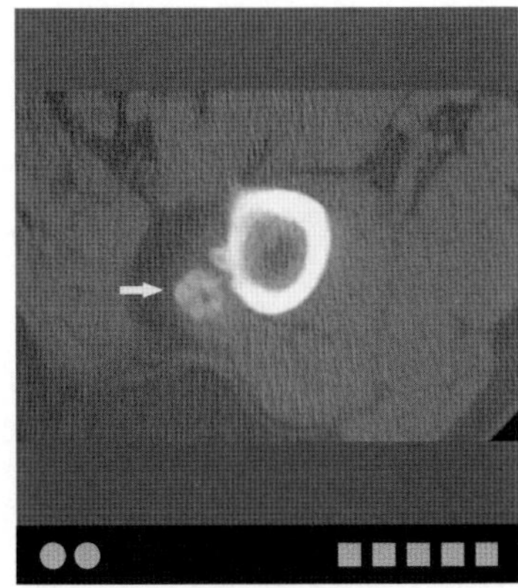

C. Calcific tendinosis of gluteus maximus tendon: Axial CT shows calcification at the gluteal tubercle, cortical erosion, and solid periosteal reaction.

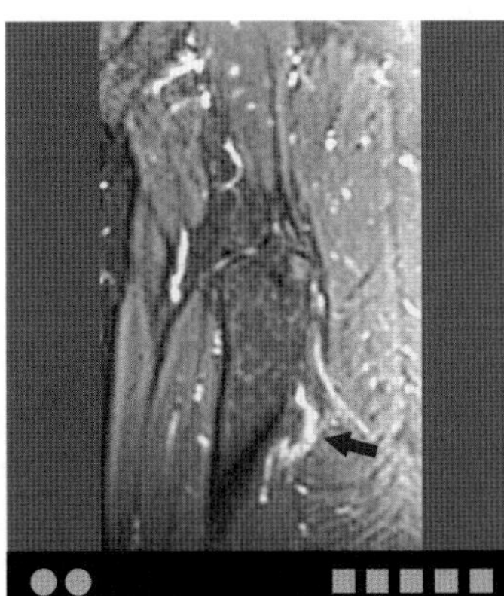

D. Calcific tendinosis of gluteus maximus tendon: Sagittal T2W fat-saturated MR image shows calcification at the distal termination of the tendon. Note presence of soft tissue edema (arrow).

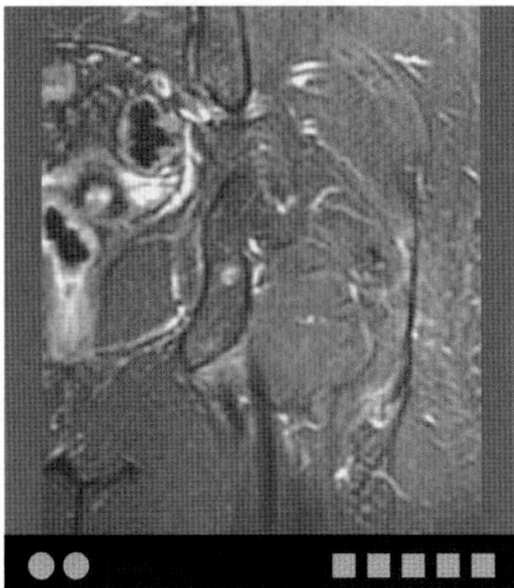

E. Calcific tendinosis of gluteus maximus tendon: Coronal T2W fat-saturated MR image shows calcification as decreased signal with mild surrounding edema.

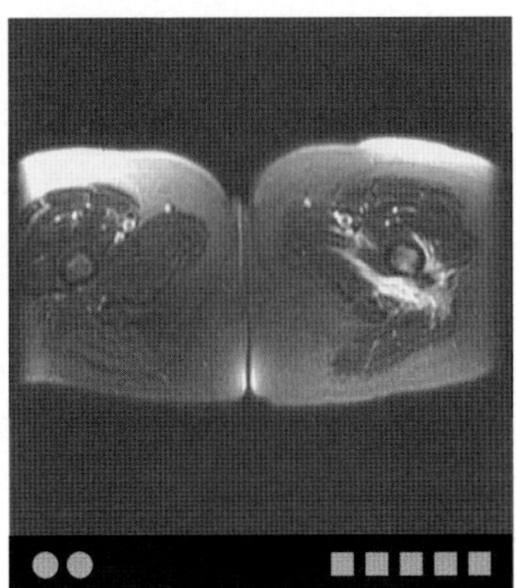

F. Calcific tendinosis of gluteus maximus tendon: Axial T2W fat-saturated MR image shows extensive edema that can be potentially confused with tumor or infection.

DIFFERENTIAL DIAGNOSIS IMAGE

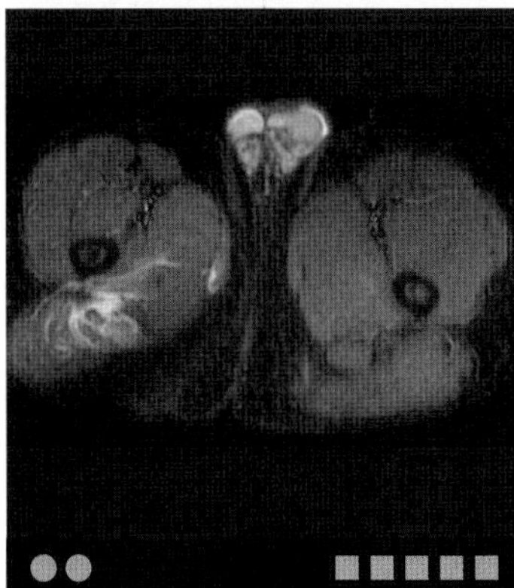

G. Hamstring avulsion: Axial STIR image shows edema at the site of hamstring avulsion.

IMAGE KEY

Common

Rare

Typical

Unusual

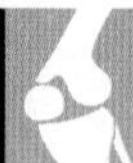

17–5 Occult Hip Fracture

Lynne Steinbach and Jeffrey N. Masi

PRESENTATION

Hip pain, weight-bearing difficulty

FINDINGS

Linear bands on T1W and T2W MR images at site of fracture is noted.

DIFFERENTIAL DIAGNOSES

- *Muscle injury:* High signal intensity in muscle on fluid sensitive sequence.
- *Insufficiency fracture:* Fracture in weakened bone in characteristic locations.
- *Bone contusion:* Bone marrow edema without fracture line; history of trauma.
- *Osteoarthritis:* Joint space narrowing, sclerosis, subchondral cysts, osteophytes.
- *AVN:* Abnormal signal femoral head, double line sign, predisposing factors (alcoholism, HIV, SS anemia).
- *Transient osteoporosis of the hip:* Diffuse edema pattern in femoral head/neck; no history of trauma.

COMMENTS

This is an elderly patient with hip pain and weight-bearing difficulty. On physical exam, occult hip fractures classically cause an abducted and externally rotated leg with leg-length discrepancy, localized hip pain, and reduced range of motion. Occult hip fractures may present with less specific symptoms, especially in patients who have underlying psychiatric disorders or dementia. Radiographs are a good first test although they are not always sufficient in detecting nondisplaced fractures. MR is the imaging procedure of choice. MRI can quickly detect the fracture along with bleeding and bone marrow edema as well as muscle injury that would be associated with occult, nondisplaced fractures of the proximal femur. Muscle injury may be present without fracture and mimic and occult fracture clinically. CT can miss occult fractures, unlike MRI, and is therefore not the best follow-up test to a negative radiograph for diagnosis. However, CT can help assess the orientation and extent of fractured bone segments in many cases when the fracture is not occult. Radionuclide scans are extremely sensitive, with the cost of turnaround times ranging from 24 to 48 hours in best-case scenarios and up to a week in patients older than 65 years.

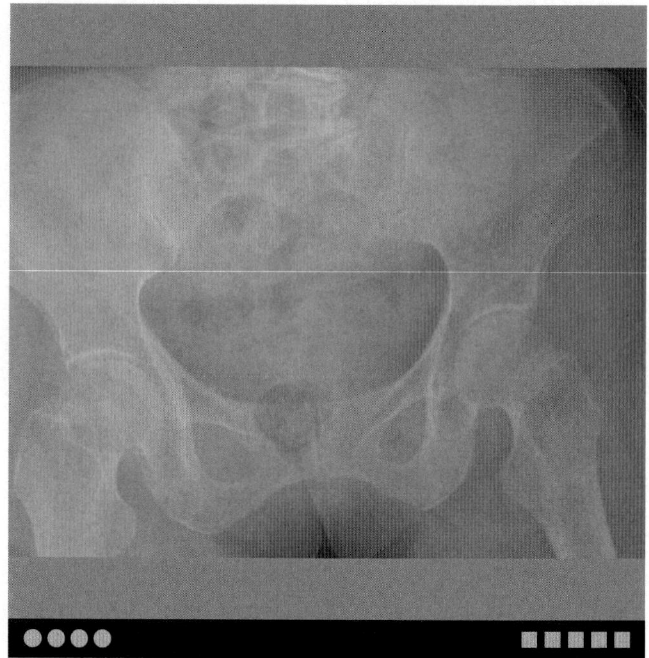

A. Occult hip fracture: AP radiograph of the pelvis in a patient who fell with left hip pain does not demonstrate a fracture. What test should be done next?

PEARLS

- **Multiple studies have shown expedited diagnosis of occult hip fractures with MR when compared to CT, with an ultimate outcome of quicker treatment and shorter hospital stays.**
- **CT may not demonstrate an occult fracture.**
- **Associated soft-tissue abnormalities may be seen in the majority of occult hip fractures on MR.**
- **It is important to use a fluid sensitive MR sequence to demonstrate muscle pathology in the presence or absence of a fracture as well as reactive changes around a fracture.**

ADDITIONAL IMAGE

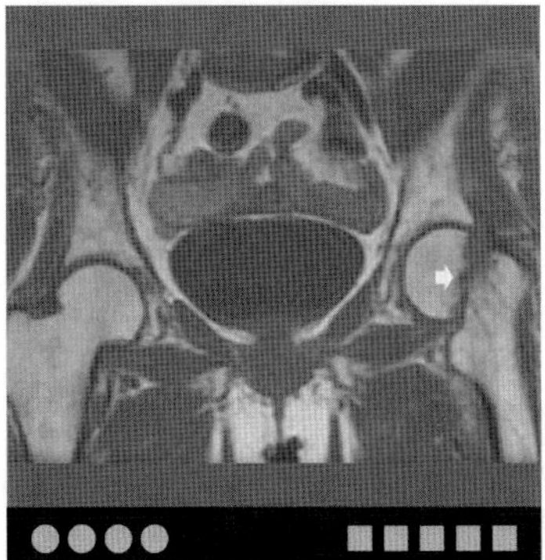

B. Occult hip fracture: Coronal T1W MR image of the left hip in the same patient (as in image A) obtained on the same day as the radiograph shows the high signal intensity fracture line in the subcapital region (arrow).

DIFFERENTIAL DIAGNOSES IMAGES

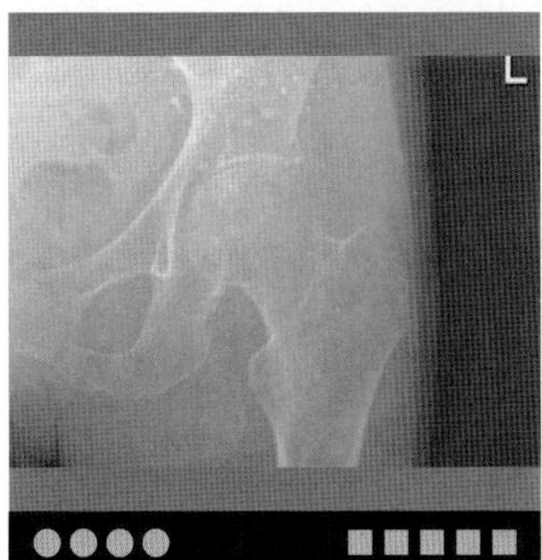

C. Incomplete fracture of the left greater trochanter: This woman fell and presented to the emergency room with left hip pain. AP pelvis radiograph does not demonstrate a fracture.

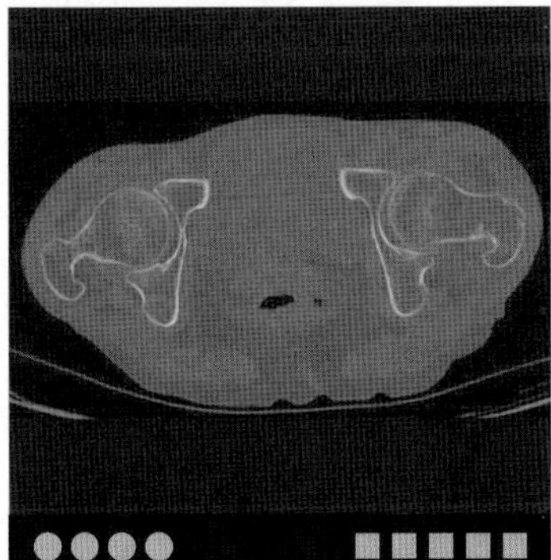

D. Incomplete fracture of the left greater trochanter: A CT was obtained on the same patient (as in image C). No fracture was identified.

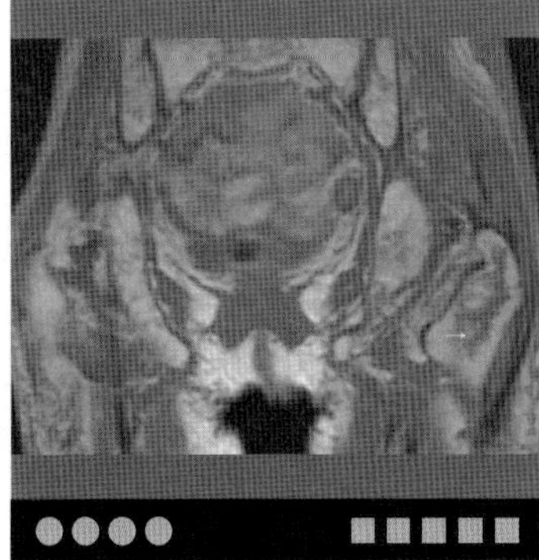

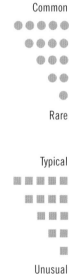

E. Incomplete fracture of the left greater trochanter: The following day, an MRI was performed on the patient depicted in images C and D. The MRI showed an incomplete fracture of the left greater trochanter (arrow).

IMAGE KEY

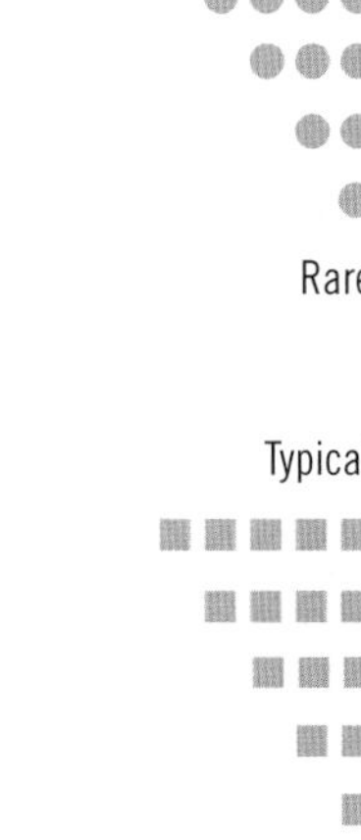

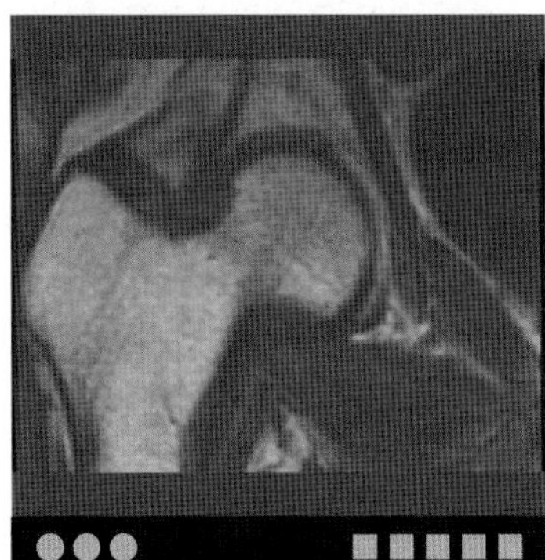

F. Adductor and obturator externus muscle strain: This woman fell the day before this MRI was obtained to exclude hip fracture. A T1W coronal MRI does not show a fracture.

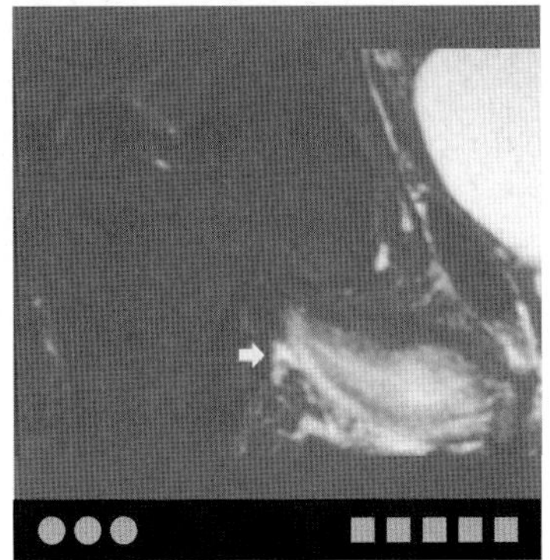

G. Adductor and obturator externus muscle strain: Coronal STIR image in the patient shown in image F. The muscle strain not seen on the T1W sequence is visible on this STIR image (arrow).

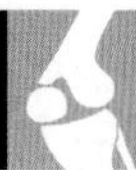

17–6 Fatigue Fracture of Femur

Peyman Borghei and Jamshid Tehranzadeh

PRESENTATION

Leg pain

FINDINGS

The radiograph of femur showed periosteal reaction of distal femoral shaft. MRI showed periosteal elevation, edema, and calcification with extensive marrow edema at fractured site.

DIFFERENTIAL DIAGNOSES

- *Osteosarcoma:* Presents with low signal intensity on T1W and mixed high signal intensity on T2WI with contrast enhancement. Aggressive periosteal reaction and soft tissue mass with calcification may be present.
- *Ewing sarcoma:* Presents with large soft tissue mass, osteolytic or mixed osteolytic, and osteoblastic lesions on radiograph with decreased signal intensity lesion on T1WI and increased signal intensity on T2WI.
- *Osteoid osteoma:* The lesion is less than 2 cm, surrounded by bone marrow and soft tissue edema and reactive sclerosis. The reactive sclerosis appears as low signal intensity on both T1 and T2WI.
- *Osteomyelitis:* Osteomyelitis demonstrates low signal intensity on T1W and high signal intensity on T2WI on bone marrow, which enhances with contrast. May be associated with cellulitis.

COMMENTS

This is 17-year-old female runner with a 5 to 6 months history of right leg pain. Stress related injuries to bone are common in athletes especially in women. These injuries comprise a wide spectrum ranging from bone edema to stress fracture. Stress fractures are divided into fatigue and insufficiency types. Fatigue fractures result from intense and repetitive activity without adequate period of rest in normal bone. The fatigue fractures usually demonstrate sports specificity, for example march fractures of metatarsal bones in soldier, coracoid process fracture in trap-shooters, and tibia fracture in ballet dancers. Although initial radiograph is normal, the earliest sign consists of a linear lucent fracture line which often remains occult and is not appreciable on radiograph. As healing occurs, a band of sclerosis perpendicular to the bone trabeculae, a periosteal reaction and callus will be formed in ten days to two weeks.

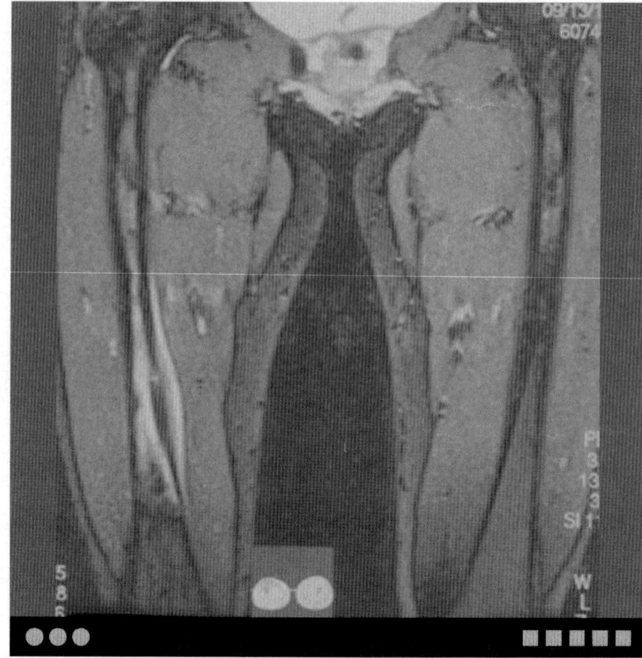

A. Fatigue fracture of femur: Coronal proton density fat saturated MR image shows marrow edema in middle to lower shaft of right femur with elevation of the periosteum by subperiosteal edema.

The MRI findings usually precede radiographic manifestations by several weeks, and are more specific than scintigraphy. The MRI changes of stress fracture includes a linear low signal focus surrounded by an area of intermediate signal intensity seen on T1W images and a low signal intensity line surrounded by a high signal intensity zone on T2W images. Marrow abnormalities are best evaluated with fat suppression techniques such as Short Tau Inversion Recovery (STIR) or Selective Partial Inversion Recovery (SPIR).

PEARLS

- **Fatigue fracture occurs when multiple and frequent stresses are placed over a normal bone.**
- **Follow up radiograph shows a sclerotic line and periosteal new bone formation at the site of injury.**
- **MRI findings precede changes on radiograph.**
- **MRI is highly sensitive for diagnosis as it shows low signal fracture line associated with surrounding bone marrow edema.**

ADDITIONAL IMAGES

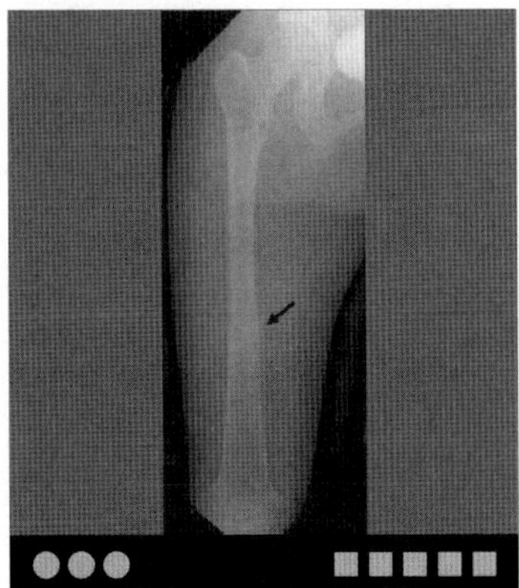

B. Fatigue fracture of femur: AP radiograph shows periosteal new bone in the mid to lower shaft of the right femur (arrow).

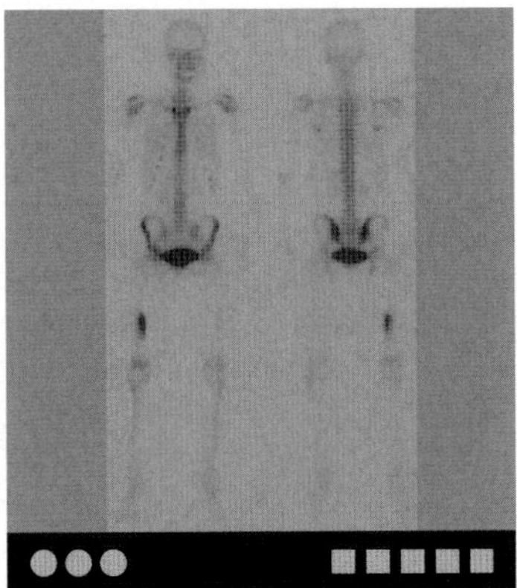

C. Fatigue fracture of femur: Anterior and posterior bone scan views show fusiform augmented uptake of radionuclide in the medial shaft of the right femur.

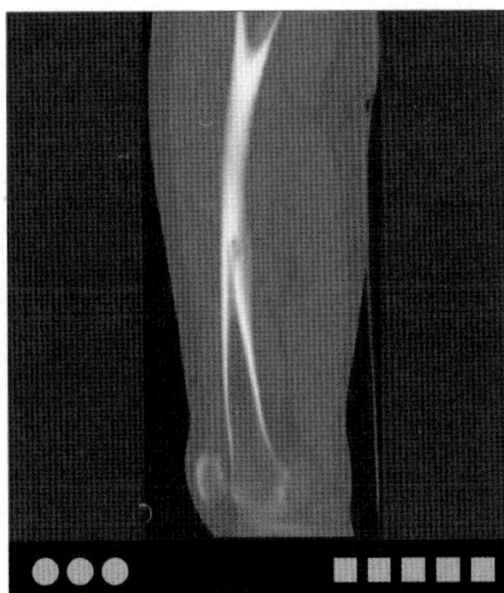

D. Fatigue fracture of femur: Sagittal bone CT scan shows a fracture line of the femoral shaft with laminated periosteal reaction and no soft tissue mass.

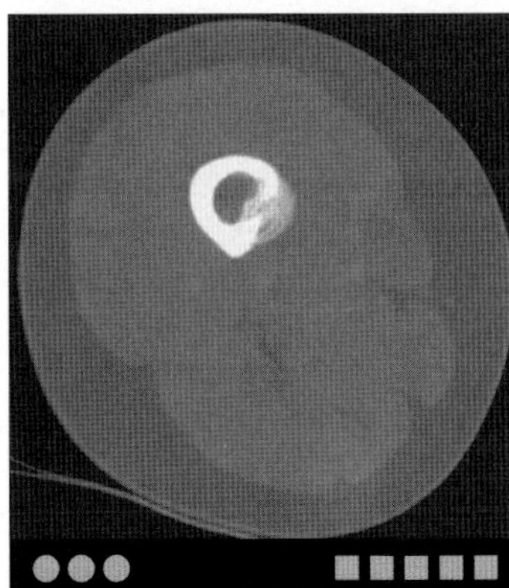

E. Fatigue fracture of femur: Axial bone CT scan shows a fracture line of the femoral shaft with laminated periosteal reaction and no soft tissue mass.

IMAGE KEY

Common

Rare

Typical

Unusual

DIFFERENTIAL DIAGNOSES IMAGES

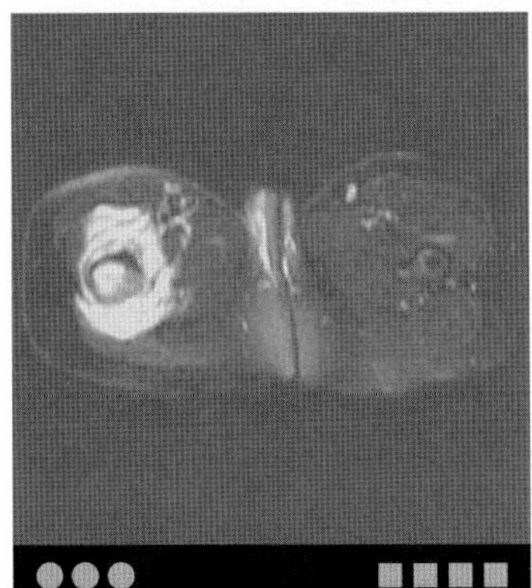

F. Osteosarcoma of femoral shaft: Axial fat saturated T2W image shows large soft tissue mass with periosteal reaction and inhomogeneity of femoral cortex and abnormal bright marrow signal.

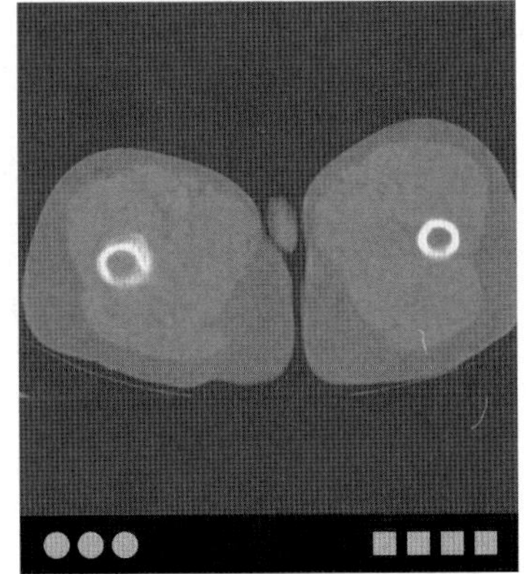

G. Osteosarcoma of femoral shaft: Axial CT-Scan shows inhomogeneous cortical density of the femoral shaft with periosteal new bone formation.

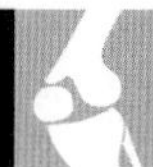

17–7 Slipped Capital Femoral Epiphysis (SCFE)

Michelle Chandler

PRESENTATION

Hip and knee pain and limp

FINDINGS

MR images show widening of the proximal femoral physis with associated marrow edema, malalignment, and smaller size of the femoral capital epiphysis.

DIFFERENTIAL DIAGNOSES

- *Avascular necrosis of the femoral head:* The alignment at the physis will be maintained and the predominance of signal abnormalities will be in the femoral head instead of the proximal femoral metaphysis. If advanced the femoral head may be flattened with associated degenerative changes of the hip.
- *Proximal focal femoral deficiency:* The proximal femur will be hypoplastic without associated signal abnormality in the marrow or widening of the physis.

COMMENTS

This is an 11-year-old boy with right hip pain. The slipped capital femoral epiphysis (SCFE) is actually a Salter I fracture of the proximal femur. This entity occurs most commonly in preteen and teen overweight males. The prominent, but weakened growth plate fails under changing mechanical stresses in the maturing hip. In younger patients it occurs in the setting of metabolic disorders. The patient presents with hip or knee pain or a limp. The symptoms may be acute or chronic. SCFE is more common on the left and is bilateral in a quarter of cases. Radiographs of both hips should be obtained. In subtle cases only widening of the growth plate is observed; in more severe cases the femoral capital epiphysis is displaced posteromedially, but not dislocated from the acetabulum. A line drawn along the lateral aspect of the femoral neck on an AP view of the pelvis should extend through a portion of the proximal femoral epiphysis or a "slip" should be suspected. Findings are often easier to detect on the frog leg view of the pelvis in which the femoral head is no longer centered on the femoral shaft or appears shorter on one side. This has been referred to as the "ice cream slipping off the cone." In cases of high risk or high suspicion if radiographs are normal MRI may be obtained. Marrow edema, metaphyseal widening, or slippage may be demonstrated. Treatment is surgical pinning and postoperative radiographs will show the femoral head unchanged in position.

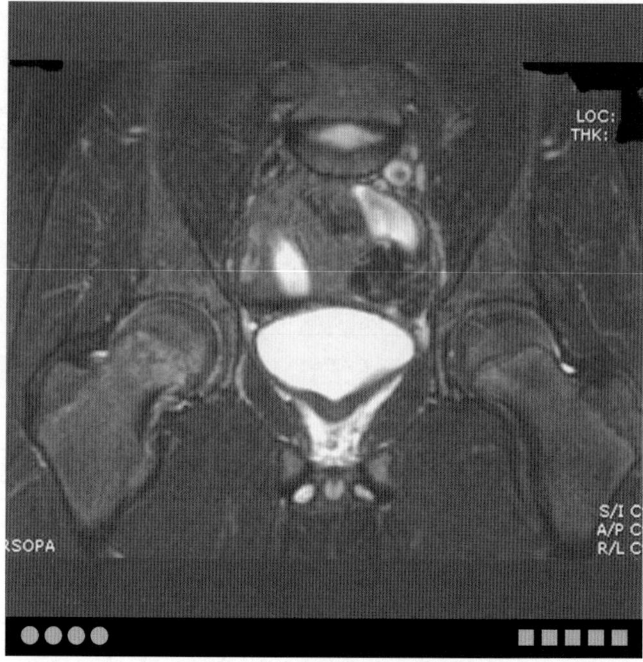

A. SCFE: Coronal T2 MR with fat saturation image shows metaphyseal edema of the right proximal femur with displacement or "slippage" of the right femoral capital epiphysis.

PEARLS

- **Both AP and frog leg views of the pelvis should be obtained to improve detection and to compare with the opposite hip. If clinical suspicion is high an MRI may be useful.**
- **Bilateral involvement is present in up to a quarter of the cases, either at initial presentation or following the first event.**
- **In classical patients presenting with knee pain the hip should also be imaged to seek out this diagnosis.**

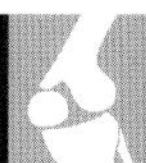

ADDITIONAL IMAGES

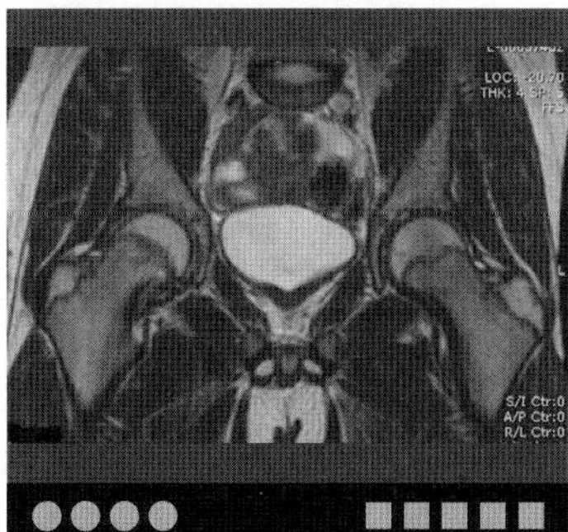

B. SCFE: Coronal T2 MR shows the widened right proximal femoral physis and the posterior and inferior slippage of the femoral capital epiphysis.

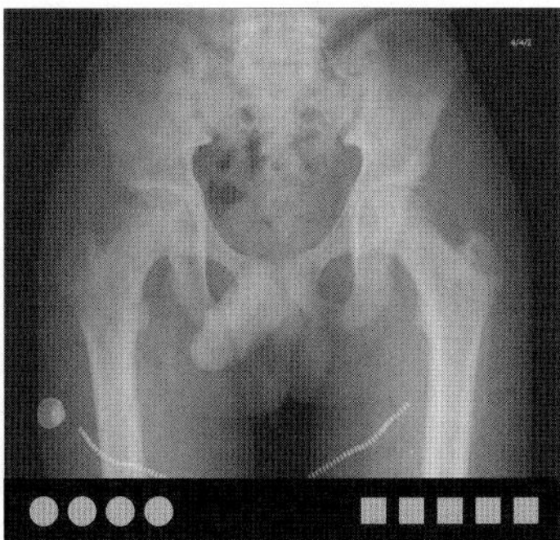

C. SCFE: AP radiograph of the pelvis in the same patient demonstrates subtle widening of the right proximal femoral physis and subtle displacement of the femoral capital epiphysis.

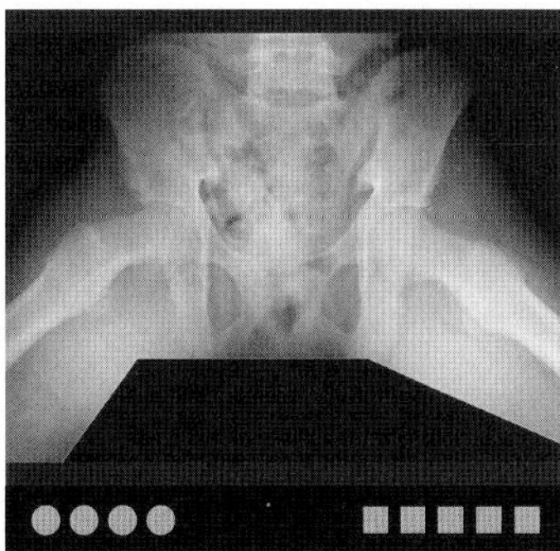

D. SCFE: Frogleg lateral radiograph of the pelvis shows the same "slippage" as the previous figure. This finding is much easier to detect in this view.

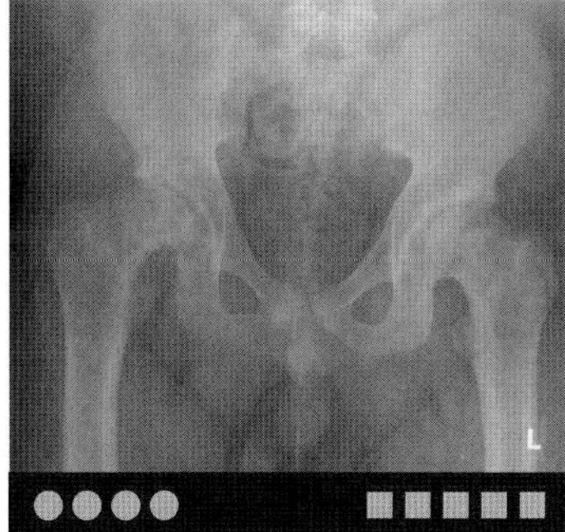

E. SCFE: An AP view of the pelvis in a different patient presenting with right hip pain acutely shows an acute right SCFE, but the patient also appears to have had a remote slippage on the left complicated by avascular necrosis, degenerative joint narrowing, and premature fusion of the physis.

DIFFERENTIAL DIAGNOSES IMAGES

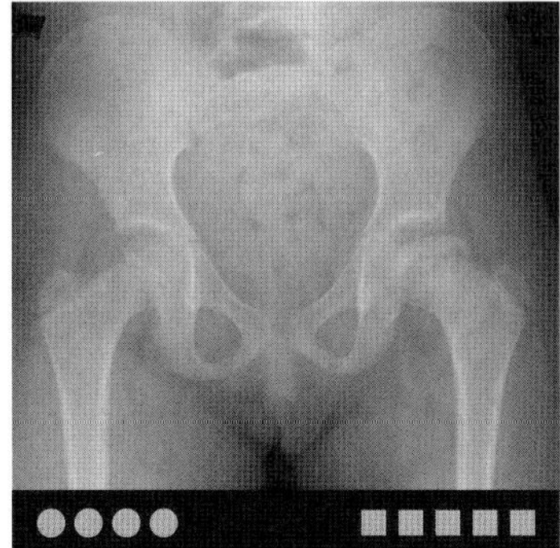

F. Avascular necrosis: An AP view of the pelvis shows flattening and heterogeneous mineralization of the left femoral capital epiphysis with maintenance of the position or relationship to the metaphysis compatible with advanced avascular necrosis.

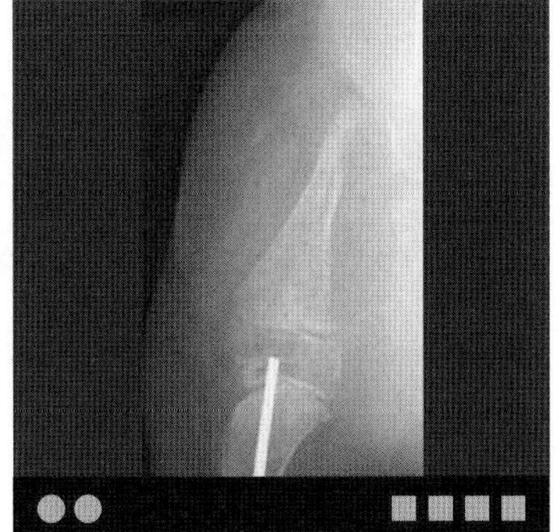

G. Proximal focal femoral deficiency: A frog leg view of the right hip shows a severe case of hypoplasia of the proximal right femur resulting in absence of the right femoral capital epiphysis, metaphysis, and proximal shaft.

IMAGE KEY

Common

Rare

Typical

Unusual

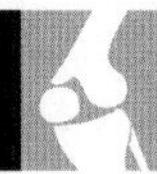

17–8 Insufficiency Fractures of the Pelvis

Gideon Strich

PRESENTATION

Back and pelvic pain

FINDINGS

MR imaging shows bilateral low signal sacral fracture lines and marrow edema.

DIFFERENTIAL DIAGNOSES

- *Neoplasms:* The pelvis is a common site for metastatic disease or less commonly primary tumor. MR signal characteristics of subtle tumor replacement may resemble edema of insufficiency fracture.
- *Sacroiliitis:* Edema of sacroiliitis may be unilateral or bilateral but more typically involves both sides of the joint rather than being confined to the sacrum.
- *Marrow transformation:* In patients with anemia, leukemia, lymphoma, and other myeloproliferative disease, bone marrow signal may be abnormal; however, the abnormality usually extends to involve the entire pelvis rather than being localized to the sacrum.
- *Paget's disease:* While early Paget's disease may have a lytic or osteoporotic phase, later stages shows characteristic cortical thickening and coarsened trabeculae. Paget's disease may also lead to insufficiency fractures as well.

COMMENTS

This is an elderly female with back, pelvic, and hip pain. The vast majority of insufficiency fractures occur in elderly patients as a result of osteoporosis and the most common fracture is the vertebral compression fracture. The most common extraspinal site is the pelvis followed by hip and occasionally other sites including the distal tibia. Fractures of the sacrum are often associated with coexisting insufficiency fractures of the ischium and pubis. The clinical presentation in these patients may be confusing and it may be difficult to differentiate a local source of pain, i.e., insufficiency fracture of the pelvis, from referred pain from osteoarthritis of the sacroiliac and hip joints or radicular pain due to disease of the lumbar spine. Findings on radiographs are subtle and may initially be missed. MR findings of decreased signal on T1WI and increased signal on T2WI may be nonspecific in the absence of a well-defined fracture line and may resemble those of tumor replacement. Typically however, extraosseous soft tissue mass or hemorrhage is not associated with sacral insufficiency fractures and may be a useful differentiating point. An H-shaped uptake pattern on bone scan ("Honda" sign) is typical and characteristic for sacral insufficiency fracture. The most specific modality is high resolution MDCT and oblique coronal reformatting in the plane of the sacrum may be helpful in diagnosis. DEXA scanning of the spine and hip is useful to confirm the presence of osteoporosis and monitor patients on drug therapy.

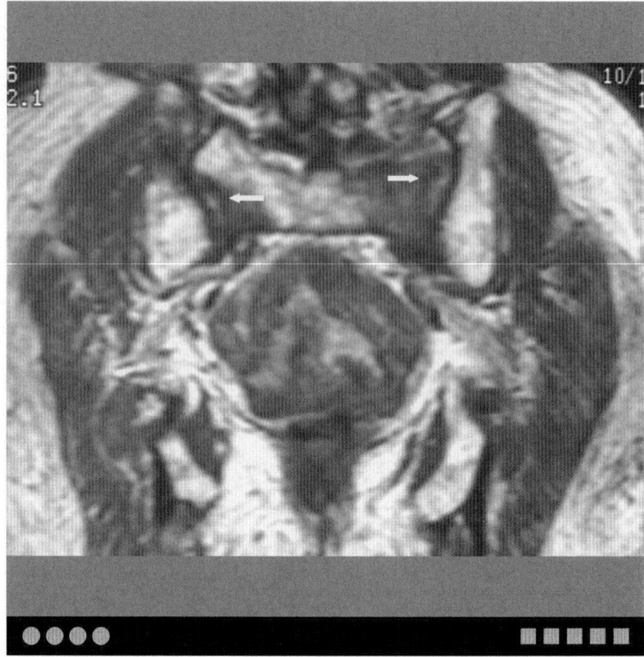

A. Insufficiency fracture: Coronal T1WI shows bilateral low signal intensity lines in the sacrum (arrows).

PEARLS

- **Insufficiency fractures of the pelvis most typically occur in elderly females with osteoporosis.**
- **Findings on radiograph are subtle and are often overlooked initially. MR imaging is more sensitive but may be nonspecific. CT and radionuclide bone scan may be more specific.**
- **The clinical presentation may be confusing, and coexisting degenerative joint disease of the sacroiliac joints and hips as well as degenerative disc disease of the lumbar spine may need to be evaluated clinically and with imaging.**
- **DEXA screening and preventative medical therapy may be helpful in reducing prevalence of insufficiency fractures.**

ADDITIONAL IMAGES

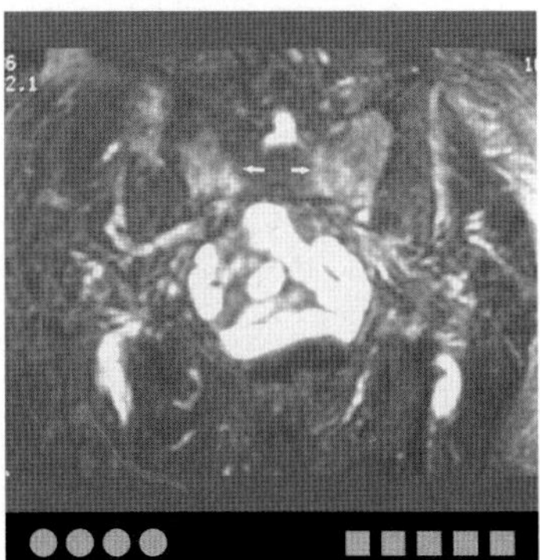

B. Insufficiency fracture: Coronal STIR image shows bilateral sacral edema with subtle nondisplaced fractures (arrows).

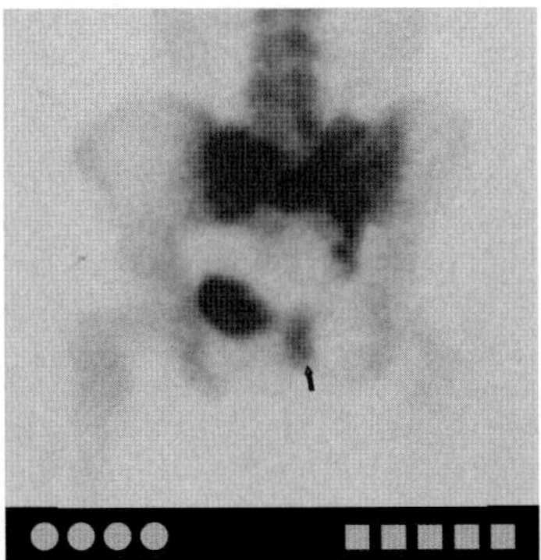

C. Insufficiency fracture: Bone scan (posterior view) shows H-shaped configuration of uptake in the sacrum, typical of insufficiency fracture, and uptake in the right pubic rami (arrow). The other hot area is the bladder.

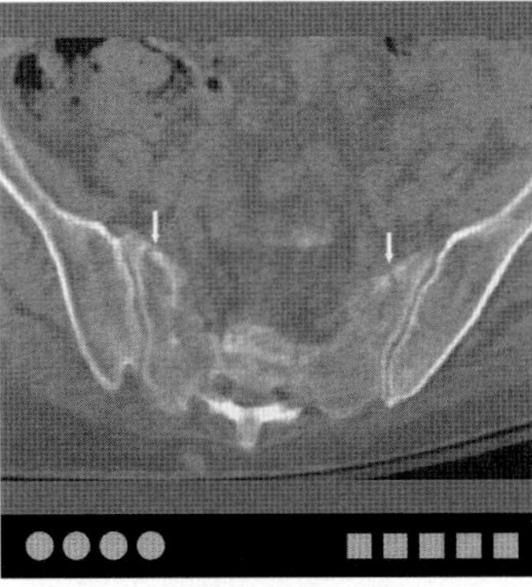

D. Insufficiency fracture: Axial CT scan shows subtle nondisplaced insufficiency fractures of the sacrum bilaterally (arrows).

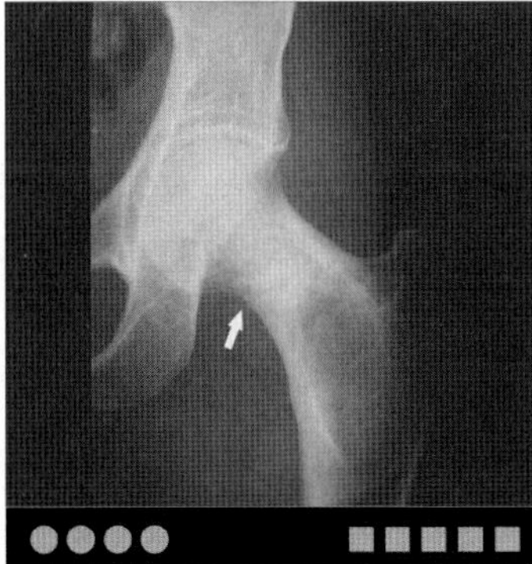

E. Insufficiency fracture: This is a different patient with AP radiograph showing another common location for insufficiency fracture (arrow) in the appendicular skeleton.

IMAGE KEY

Common

Rare

Typical

Unusual

DIFFERENTIAL DIAGNOSES IMAGES

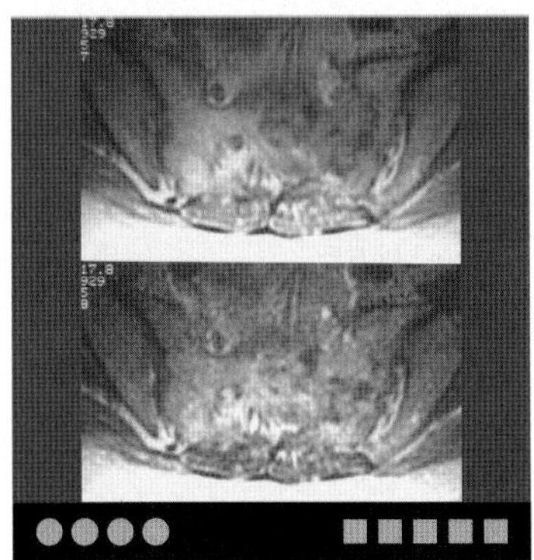

F. Metastatic disease: Axial proton density (top) and T2W (bottom) images shows subtle bone marrow signal abnormality in the sacrum with what appears to be a fracture line in this patient with metastatic breast carcinoma.

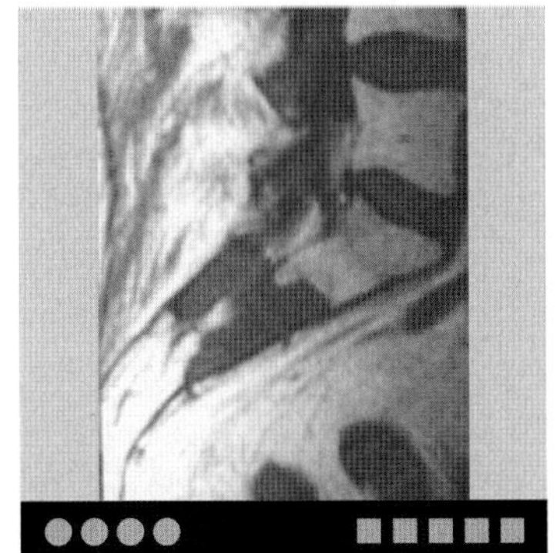

G. Metastatic disease: Sagittal T1WI in this breast cancer patient shows the mass in the sacrum to be focal and well defined, with some extraosseous extension consistent with tumor replacement.

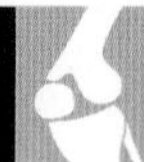

17–9 Pubic Stress Injury

Kira Chow

PRESENTATION

Groin pain

FINDINGS

Axial T2W fat-saturated MRI demonstrates edema about the symphysis pubis.

DIFFERENTIAL DIAGNOSES

- *Hyperparathyroidism:* Bone resorption with or without brown tumor.
- *Metastasis:* Bony metastasis may mimic these findings.
- *Insufficiency fracture:* Common in elderly post-menopausal women.

COMMENTS

Pelvic stress fractures account for 10% of all stress fractures. Women are at higher risk than men, and sports such as jumping and running place athletes at risk. These injuries have also been described in military recruits. Additionally, muscle fatigue, changes in foot gear and training, changes in intensity and/or duration of training, and nutritional or hormonal deficiencies resulting in decreased bone density may all play a role. As bone is subjected to high stress levels, osseous remodeling occurs. When osteoclastic activity outpaces osteoblastic new bone formation, the result is microfractures. These are usually radiographically occult, but are visualized on MRI as ill-defined T2 or inversion recovery hyperintensity without defined fracture line. If the stress is stopped, these abnormalities typically resolve in 6 to 12 weeks. With continued activity, however, stress injury can progress to stress fracture, in which the cortex is actually disrupted. The superior and inferior pubic rami, as well as the sacrum and proximal femur, are at high risk for stress fracture. Inferior pubic ramus fractures typically occur near the symphysis pubis and present as groin pain.

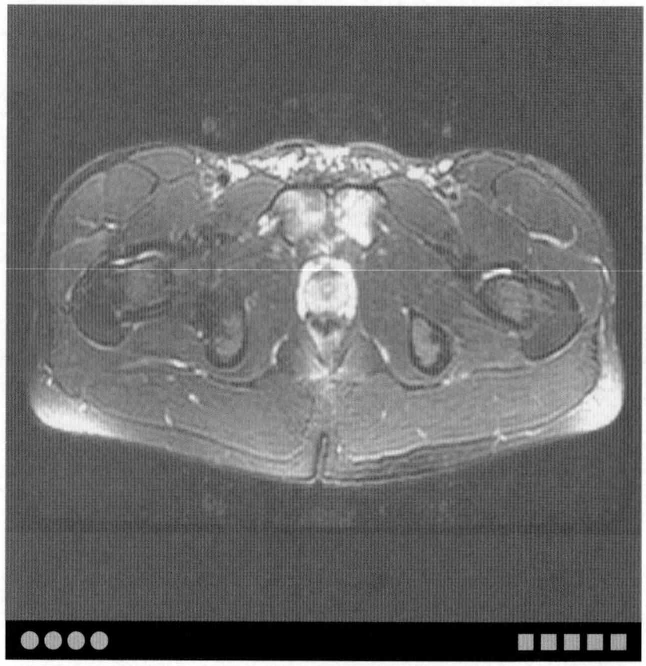

A. Stress injury: Axial T2W fat-saturated MRI demonstrates marrow edema in the medial pubic rami.

Radiographically, stress fractures may be subtle, with patchy sclerosis or periosteal reaction. On MRI, a stress fracture has a demonstrable T1 and T2 hypointense fracture line amidst marrow edema.

PEARLS

- **Stress fracture is differentiated from stress injury by visualization of a fracture line.**
- **The pubic rami are at high risk for stress injury and fractures in athletes and military recruits.**
- **Stress injury/fracture is usually radiographically subtle but can be seen on MRI as signal abnormality on fluid sensitive sequences.**

ADDITIONAL IMAGES

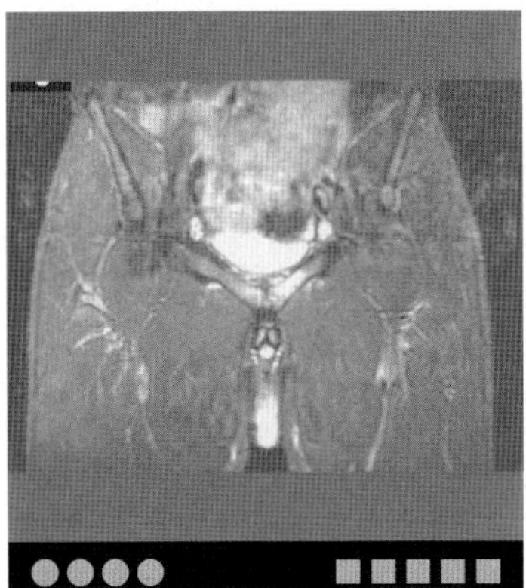

B. Stress injury: Coronal inversion recovery again demonstrates the abnormal signal in the medial pubic rami.

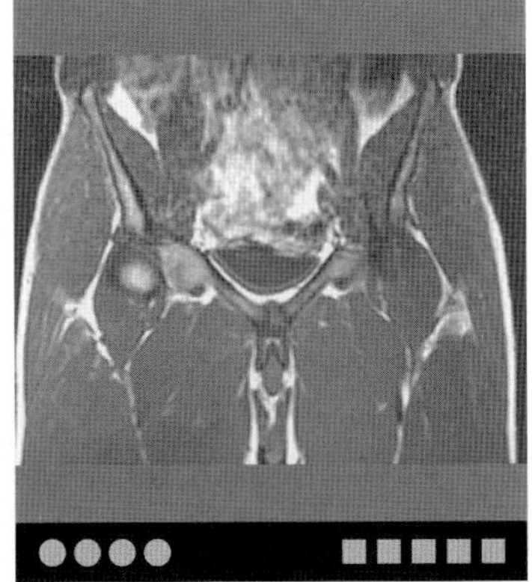

C. Stress injury: Coronal T1W MRI shows heterogeneous marrow signal in the medial pubic rami, compatible with edema.

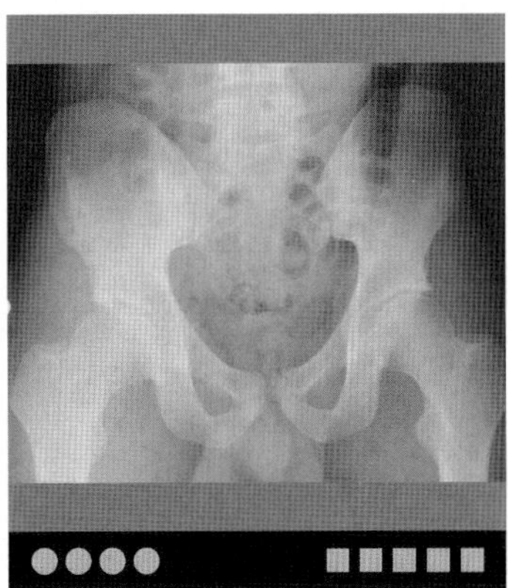

D. Stress injury: On this frontal radiograph of the pelvis, abnormality in the pubic bones cannot be appreciated with certainty.

DIFFERENTIAL DIAGNOSES IMAGES

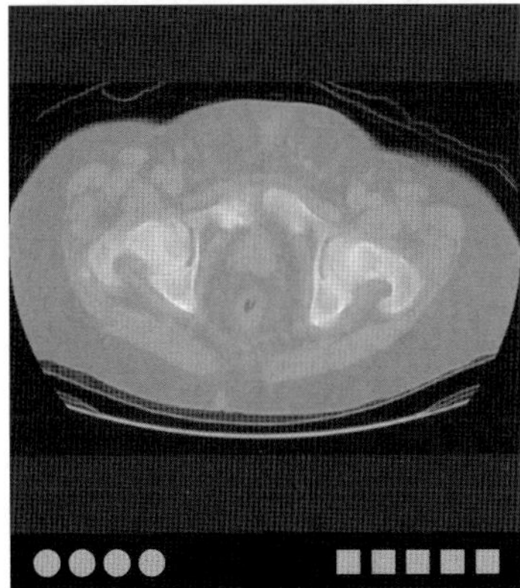

E. Hyperparathyroidism: Axial CT image demonstrates subchondral resorption commonly seen about the symphysis pubis in hyperparathyroidism.

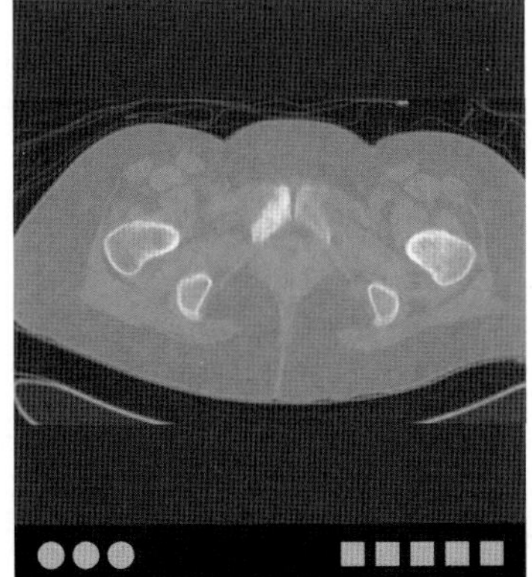

F. Metastatic adrenal carcinoma: Axial CT image shows sclerosis and destructive appearance along the medial right pubic bone.

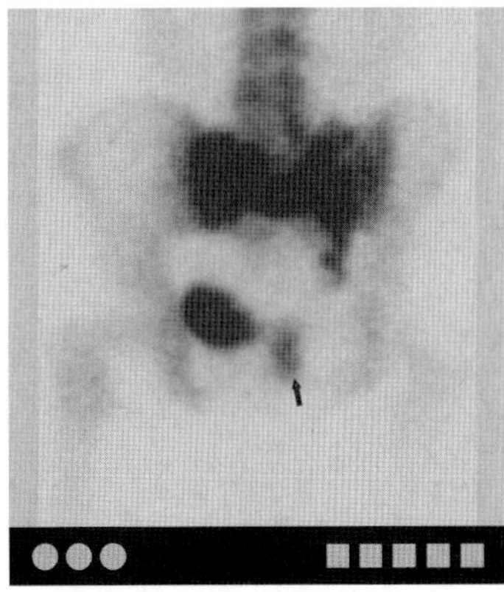

G. Insufficiency fractures: AP view of bone scan shows increased radionuclide uptake in left pubis (arrow) and sacrum due to insufficiency fractures.

IMAGE KEY

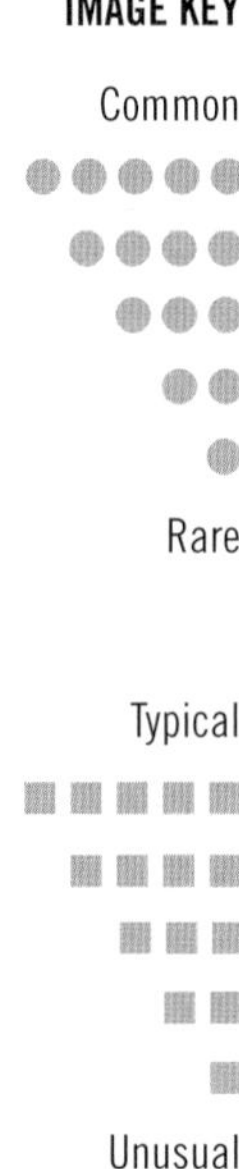

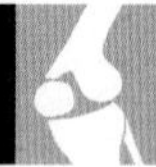

17–10 Hamstring Avulsion

Rosemary J. Klecker

PRESENTATION

Sudden pain in the posterior thigh

FINDINGS

MR image shows hemorrhage in the posterior compartment of the right thigh.

DIFFERENTIAL DIAGNOSES

- *Myositis:* The morphology of the muscle is preserved. The volume of the muscle may increase secondary to edema.
- *Intramuscular Hematoma:* Shows focal mass within the muscle.
- *Muscle contusion:* Demonstrates edema inside the muscle without tear.

COMMENTS

This is a 40-year-old man with sudden onset of pain in the posterior right thigh. The biceps femoris, semimembranosus and semitendinosus muscles make up the hamstring muscle complex (HMC). The biceps femoris and semitendinosus muscles share a conjoined insertion on the ischial tuberosity just inferomedial to the semimembranosus tendon insertion. Injuries of the HMC are more often seen after eccentric muscle contraction (contraction with passive stretching) than with concentric contraction. However, injury of the HMC has been associated with sudden flexion and a "push off" motion associated with athletic activities. Regardless of the mechanism, injury or tears typically occur in the region of the musculotendinous junction (MTJ) and may involve more than one muscle of the hamstring complex. Tendon avulsion with bone involvement necessitates prompt surgical repair and occurs more commonly at the ischial tuberosity than at the distal insertions. Injuries to the MTJ are seen on MR imaging as abnormal signal intensity in the muscle belly with a "featherlike" appearance because of edema and blood in the muscle. With high-grade partial or complete tears, blood and edema track along muscle bundles, distribution limited by the surrounding fascia (perimysium). Confinement of the hemorrhage by the fascia appears as a "rim" of blood and edema at the site of injury. The blood and edema will extravagate into the surrounding soft tissues when the fascia is disrupted. Some studies report that a large cross sectional area of involvement (>50%) is associated with a poorer prognosis and longer recovery time.

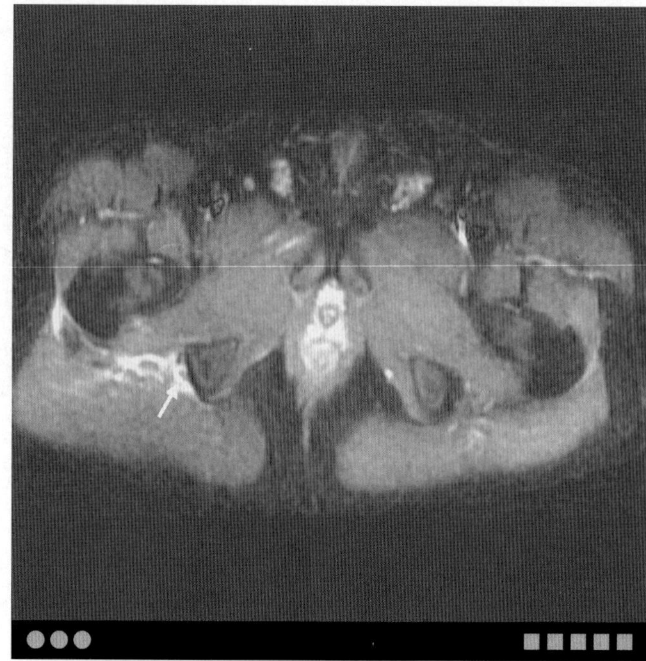

A. Hamstring muscle complex tear: Axial T2WI with fat saturation shows hemorrhage between the right ischial tuberosity and the semimembranosus and conjoined (biceps femoris and semitendinosus) tendons compatible with high-grade partial tear.

PEARLS

- **Hamstring muscular complex injuries are most often associated with eccentric contraction of the muscles.**
- **The biceps femoris is the most commonly injured hamstring muscle. The most common site of injury is at the proximal MTJ.**
- **Because each muscle is surrounded by a thick perimysium, injuries are commonly associated with a "rim" of blood and edema as fluid collects in a perifascial location.**
- **A large cross-sectional area of involvement (>50%) on MR imaging is associated with a longer period of convalescence.**

ADDITIONAL IMAGES

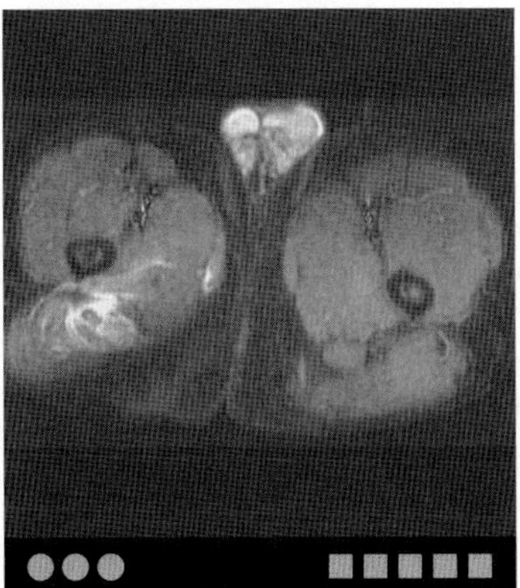

B. Hamstring muscle complex tear: Axial T2WI with fat saturation shows a rim of high signal intensity (representing perifascial fluid) around the biceps femoris, semimembranosus, and semitendinosus tendons in the posterior right thigh.

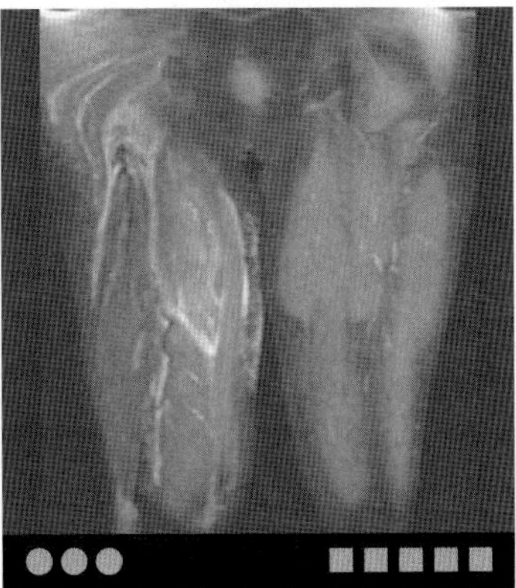

C. Hamstring muscle complex tear: Coronal STIR weighted image shows complete tear of the semitendinosus muscle and hemorrhage in the biceps femoris muscle.

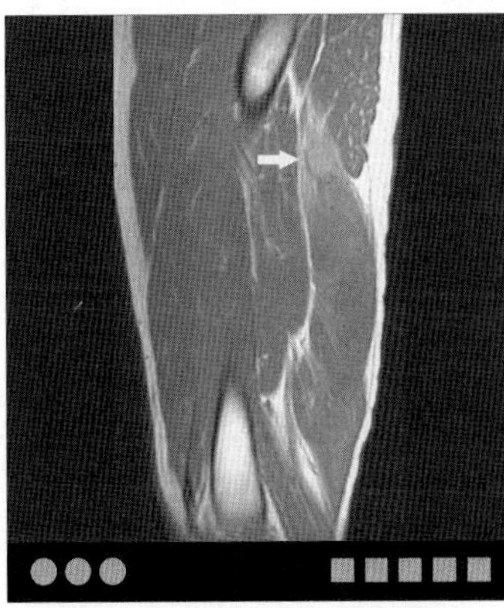

D. Hamstring muscle complex tear: Sagittal PD weighted image of hemorrhage at site of biceps femoris tendon tear (arrow).

IMAGE KEY

Common

Rare

Typical

Unusual

DIFFERENTIAL DIAGNOSES IMAGES

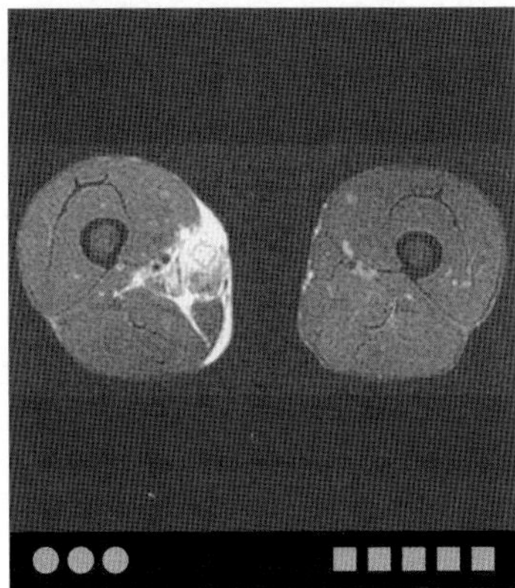

E. Myositis with abscess: Axial T2W fat saturation shows edema and fluid signal in the Gracilis muscle. Note that the muscle volume is preserved.

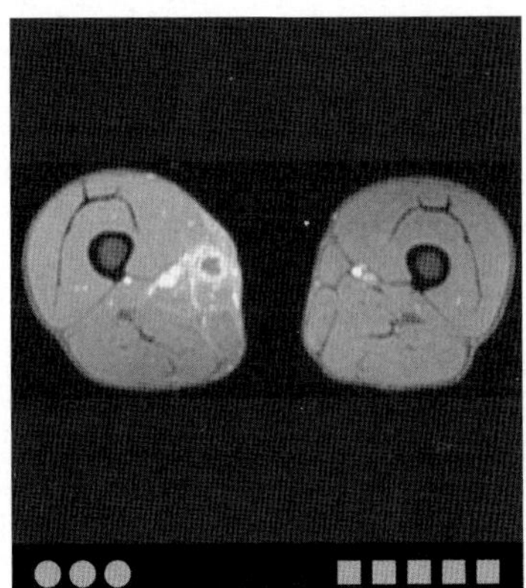

F. Myositis with abscess: Axial T1W fat saturation image with gadolinium shows enhancement of the Gracilis and Sartorius muscle fascia and rim enhancement of an intramuscular abscess in the Gracilis muscle.

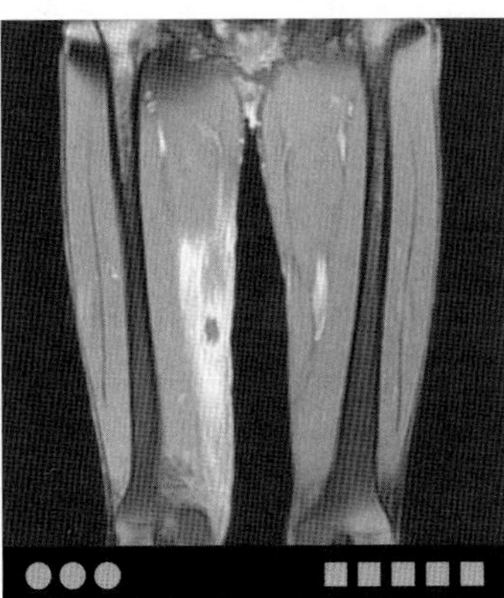

G. Myositis with abscess: Coronal T1W fat saturation with gadolinium contrast shows enhancement of the lateral muscles and an intramuscular abscess in the Gracilis muscle.

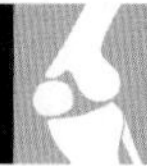

17–11 Hamstring Tendon Rupture

Kira Chow

PRESENTATION

Hip pain after fall.

FINDINGS

Axial T2W MRI demonstrates edema, without normal hamstring tendon attachment on the ischial tuberosity.

DIFFERENTIAL DIAGNOSES

- *Osteomyelitis of the ischial tuberosity:* Because of the common occurrence of decubitus ulcers overlying the ischial tuberosity, this region is frequently involved with cellulitis and/or osteomyelitis.
- *Ischial tuberosity bursal fluid:* This bursa is usually injured with fall on the buttocks.
- *Ischial tuberosity apophysitis:* The key to diagnosis of this entity is the lack of major trauma in the history. Radiographs demonstrate sclerosis and irregularity of the ischial tuberosity.
- *Gluteus maximus hemorrhage or hematoma:* High MRI signal hemorrhage following acute or subacute trauma more posterior to hamstring at gluteal muscle is noted.

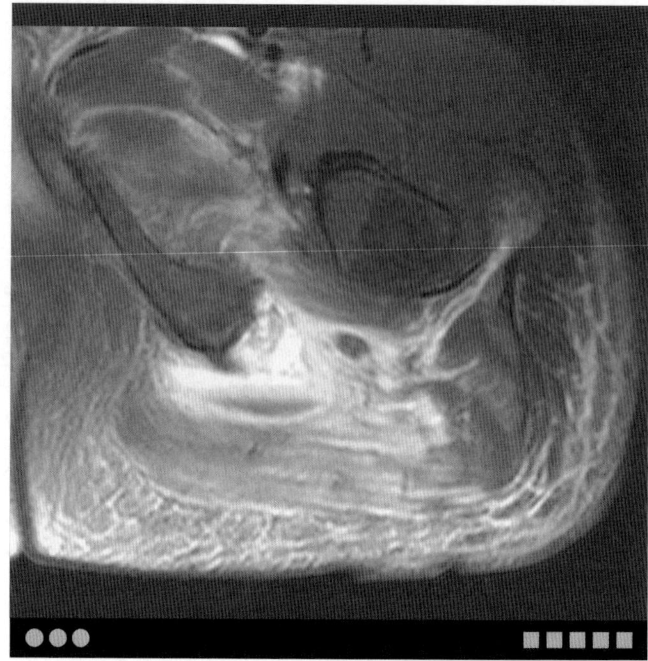

A. Hamstring tendon tear: Axial T2W fat-saturated image demonstrates extensive edema adjacent to the ischial tuberosity with T2 hypointense focus representing retracted torn end of the hamstrings tendon.

COMMENTS

The hamstring muscles consist of the semitendinosus, semimembranosus, and biceps femoris. All the hamstring muscles originate from the ischial tuberosity except the short head of the biceps, which comes off the linea aspera on the posterior cortex of the femur. On the axial view, the semimembranosus tendon is anterolateral while the conjoint tendon of the biceps femoris-semitendinosus is posteromedial. Hamstring injury can occur in three locations: tendon avulsion at the origin (as in this case), avulsion fracture of the ischial tuberosity, and musculotendinous junction injury or muscle strain within the muscle belly. Tendon avulsion typically involves both the semimembranosus and conjoint tendon of the biceps femoris-semitendinosus although sometimes only one tendon is torn. This injury is usually repaired acutely with suture anchor fixation of the torn tendons. Avulsion fracture occurs mostly in young age group before the physis is fused. Mechanism of injury in hamstring injuries is forceful muscle contraction or excessive passive lengthening with flexed hip and extended knee. Radiographically, a crescent-shaped piece of bone is noted adjacent to the ischial tuberosity. On MRI, there may be fluid or a hematoma at the tendinous attachment site with retraction or waviness of the torn tendons.

PEARLS

- **The hamstring muscles consist of the semitendinosus, semimembranosus, and biceps femoris.**
- **Hamstring injury can occur in three locations: tendon avulsion at the origin, avulsion fracture of the ischial tuberosity, musculotendinous junction injury, or muscle strain within the muscle belly.**
- **Avulsion fracture of ischial tuberosity occurs mostly in young age group before the physis is fused.**

ADDITIONAL IMAGES

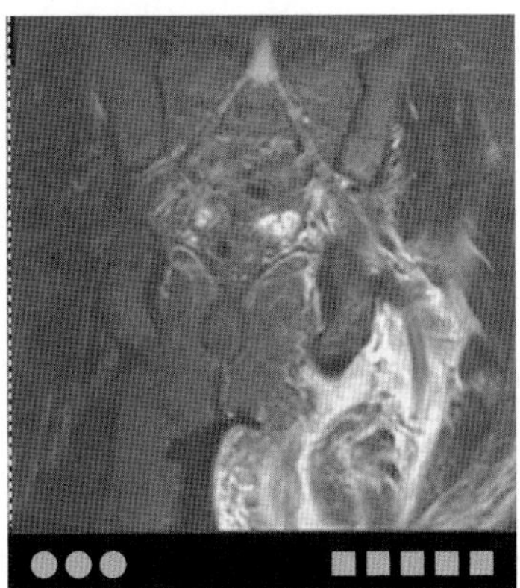

B. Hamstring tendon tear: Coronal inversion recovery sequence shows normal right hamstring tendon insertion and edema in the course of the left hamstring tendon insertion.

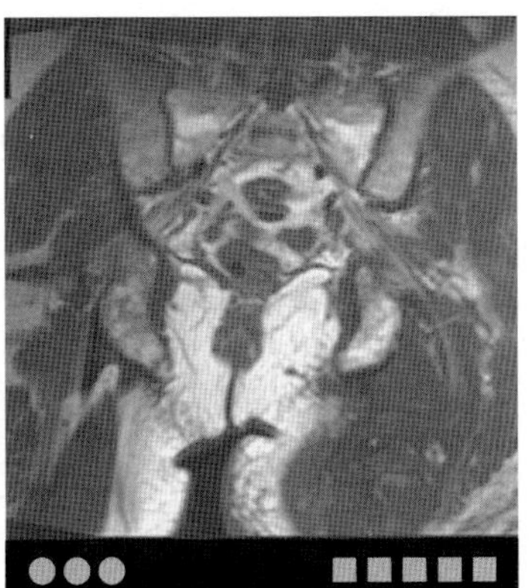

C. Hamstring tendon tear: Coronal T1W sequence better demonstrates the normal right hamstring tendon, T1 hypointense and outlined by adjacent fat, attaching to the ischial tuberosity.

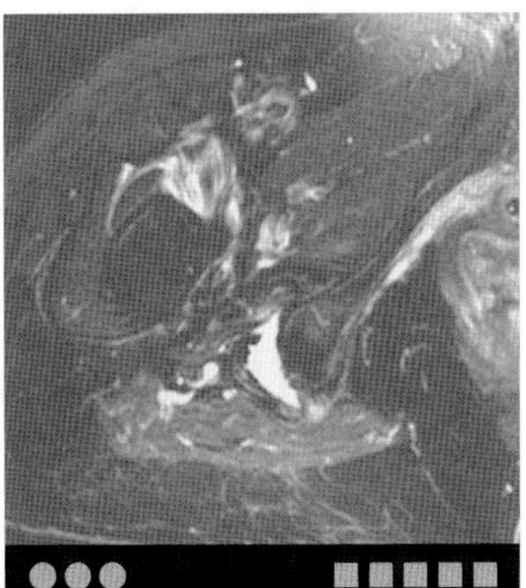

D. Hamstring tendon tear: Axial T2W fat-saturated MRI in another patient shows fluid replacing the normal origin of the hamstring muscles. The torn end of the semimembranosus tendon is seen with retraction.

DIFFERENTIAL DIAGNOSES IMAGES

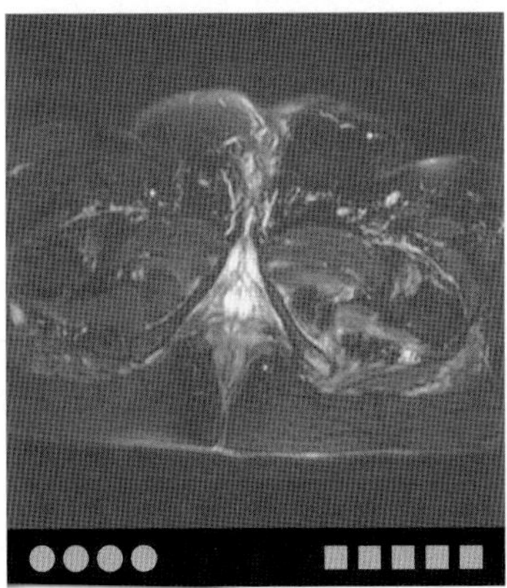

E. Osteomyelitis: Axial T2W MRI shows signal abnormality in the ischial tuberosity with abnormal soft tissue edema surrounding the hamstring tendon.

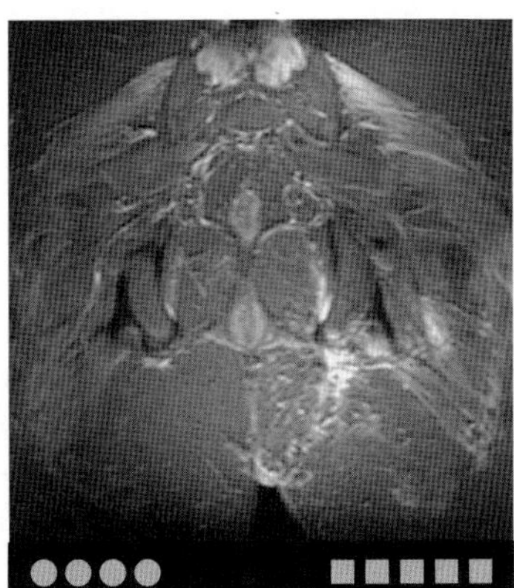

F. Osteomyelitis: Coronal STIR image (same patient as in image E) demonstrates the normal hamstring origins bilaterally on the ischial tuberosities. Signal abnormality on the left is adjacent to the hamstring origin and in the ischial tuberosity.

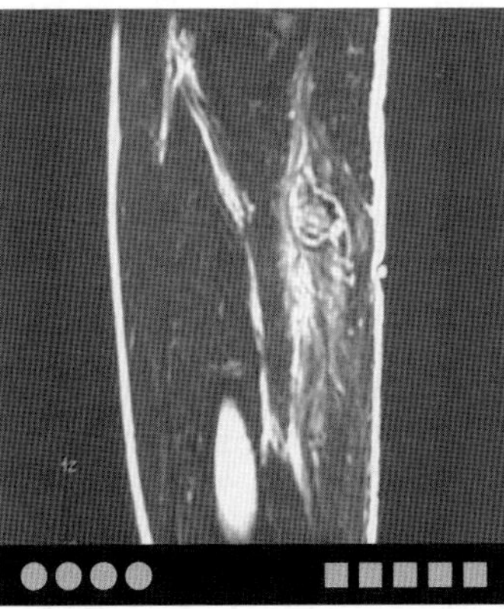

G. Subacute hemorrhage of gluteus maximus: Sagittal T2WI shows high signal hematoma in the gluteus maximus muscle. Low signal hemosiderin inside this hematoma is noted.

IMAGE KEY

Common

Rare

Typical

Unusual

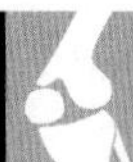

17–12 Femoroacetabular Impingement (FAI)

Stephen Thomas and Derek Armfield

PRESENTATION

Progressive hip pain

FINDINGS

Oblique axial T1W MR arthrogram image of the right hip showing loss of normal femoral head neck offset. Note anterosuperior intrasubstance labral tear.

DIFFERENTIAL DIAGNOSES

- *Type 2 FAI, pincer type:* This is associated with acetabular retroversion, which is not an abnormality of the femoral head and neck.
- *Hip Dysplasia:* FAI findings are subtle on radiographs unlike typical developmental dysplasia.
- *Osteoarthritis:* Cartilage damage in FAI usually occurs anteriorly and is not easily seen on radiographs.

COMMENTS

This is a 40-year-old active male with progressive hip pain. Femoroacetabular impingement (FAI) is a more recently recognized entity associated with hip pain, labral tears, and chondrosis. There are two basic types of impingement: Type 1 or cam impingement and type 2 or pincer impingement. Cam impingement occurs when the typical normal sphericity, or roundedness, of the femoral head is replaced with a bony bump or excrescence at the femoral head-neck junction. This bony bump can cause impingement of the labrum and cartilage with the acetabular rim particularly when the hip is flexed and internally rotated. The etiology of type 1 FAI is unclear: it could be related to a congenital anatomic defect, subclinical healed epiphyseal/SCFE, or bony reactive changes related to labral injury and biomechanical bony adaptation much like Fairbanks changes of the knee after meniscectomy. Radiographic findings require a keen eye to detect subtle abnormalities. FAI is associated with periacetabular ossicles and synovial herniation pits or impingement cysts. Oblique axial images parallel to the femoral neck on MR imaging best depict this abnormality. Type 2 FAI, pincer type, is associated with acetabular retroversion. Radiographically, pincer impingement is associated with a "cross-over" sign in which the anterior acetabular rim line crosses over the posterior acetabular rim line. Acetabular retroversion can also be evaluated with CT or MR when attention is directed to the superior aspect of the acetabulum.

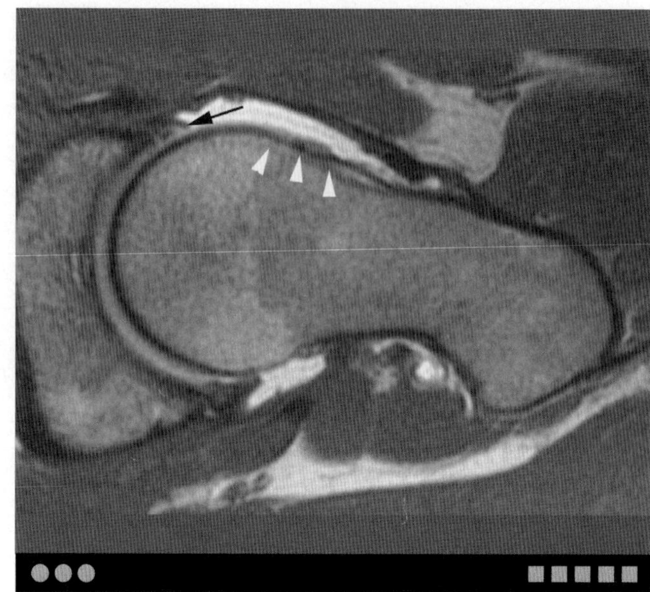

A. Femoroacetabular impingement, type 1 or cam type: Oblique axial T1W MR showing loss of normal head—neck offset (white arrowheads), which results in collision with the acetabular rim and labrum resulting in cartilage and labral damage (black arrow, labral tear).

PEARLS

- **FAI is recently recognized structural abnormality associated with labral tears and cartilage damage.**
- **Type 1 FAI (cam type) is associated impingements cysts and periacetabular ossicles.**
- **Oblique axial MR images show loss of femoral head–neck offset associated with type 1 FAI.**
- **Type 2 FAI (pincer type) is associated with acetabular retroversion.**

ADDITIONAL IMAGES

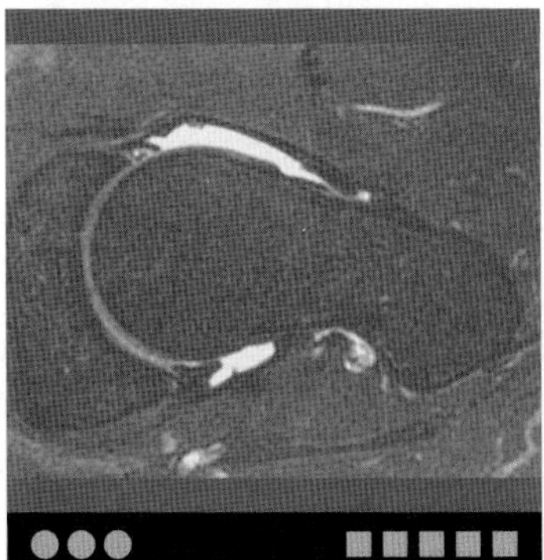

B. Femoroacetabular impingement, type 1 or cam type: Oblique axial T2W MR showing loss of normal head–neck offset, which results in collision with the acetabular rim and labrum resulting in cartilage and labral damage.

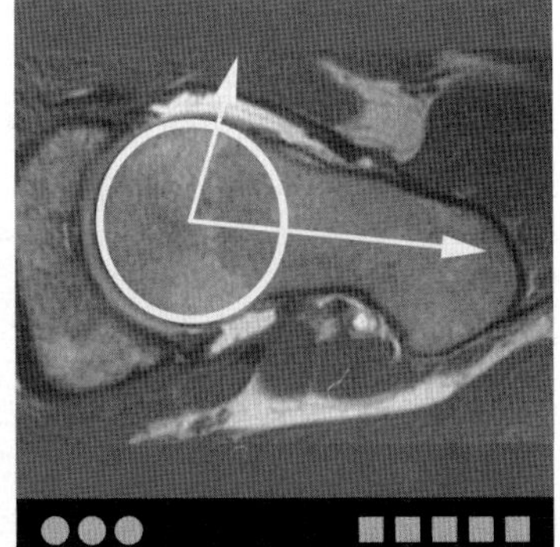

C. Femoroacetabular impingement, type 1 or cam type: Oblique axial T1WI shows method for quantifying degree of FAI using the alpha angle. A line parallel to the mid femoral neck is drawn along with a best-fit circle of the femoral head. An angle with a line parallel to the femoral neck is created by determining the point were the anterior femoral neck deviates from the best-fit circle. Values less than 50 to 55 are degrees considered abnormal.

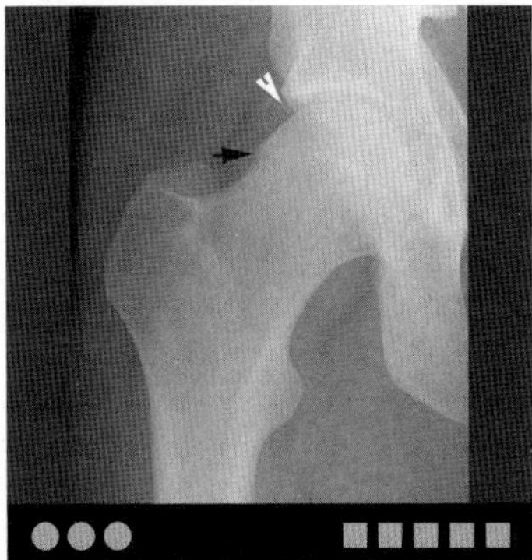

D. Femoroacetabular impingement, type 1 or cam type: AP radiograph shows subtle loss of femoral head sphericity (black arrow) and small periacetabular ossicle (white arrow) in this case of cam impingement.

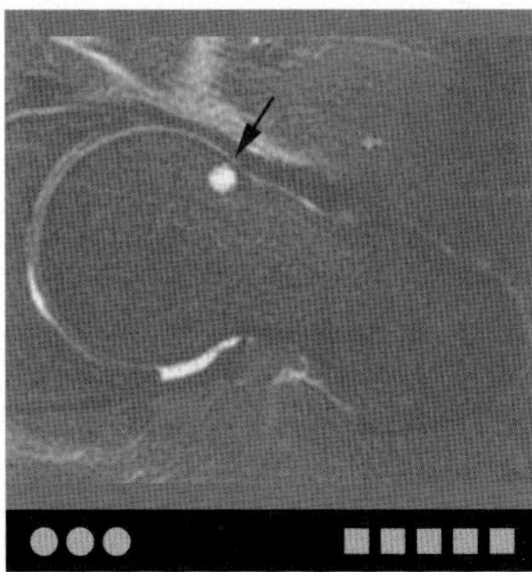

E. Femoroacetabular impingement, type 1 or cam type: Oblique axial T2 MRI shows loss of offset at femoral head—neck junction with focal T2 hyperintensity consistent with an impingement cyst (black arrow).

IMAGE KEY

Common

Rare

Typical

Unusual

DIFFERENTIAL DIAGNOSES IMAGES

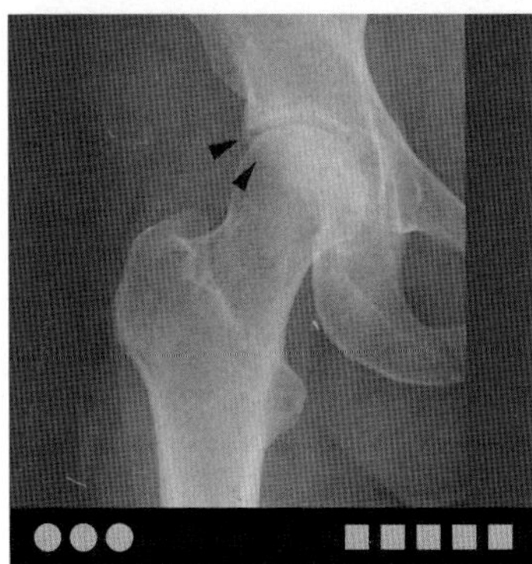

F. Femoroacetabular impingement, type 2 or pincer type: Type 2 FAI (pincer) with well-centered AP radiograph showing acetabular retroversion with "cross-over" sign (black arrows).

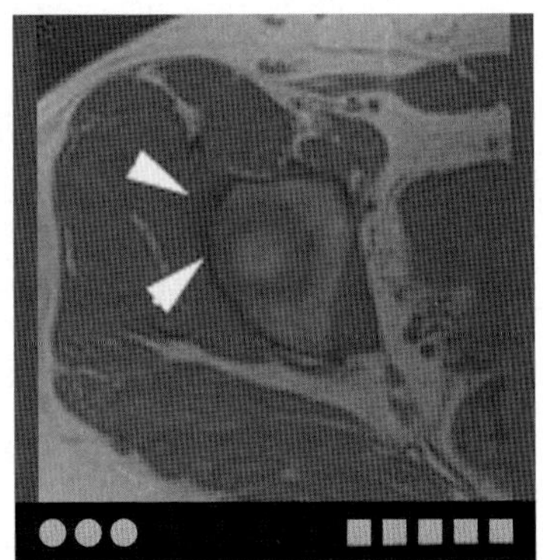

G. Femoroacetabular impingement, type 2 or pincer type: Axial T1WI image showing retroversion of anterior superior acetabular rim, which acts as source of impingement.

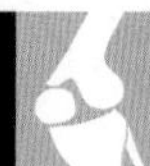

17–13 Anterior Labral Tear of Hip Joint

Mohammad Reza Hayeri and Jamshid Tehranzadeh

PRESENTATION

Hip pain often accompanied by clicking and giving way

FINDINGS

MR arthrogram shows contrast leaking into the labral tear. Tears may be associated with short, blunting, or irregular labral margins.

DIFFERENTIAL DIAGNOSES

- *Posterior labral tear:* Posterior labral tears are less common than anterior labral tears. In MR arthrogram tears are shown as contrast extension into the posterior labrum.
- *Acetabular para labral cyst:* Paralabral cyst arises adjacent to the acetabular labrum and frequently associates with labral tears. On MRI paralabral cyst shows low signal on T1W and high signal on T2W and rim enhancement after contrast administration.

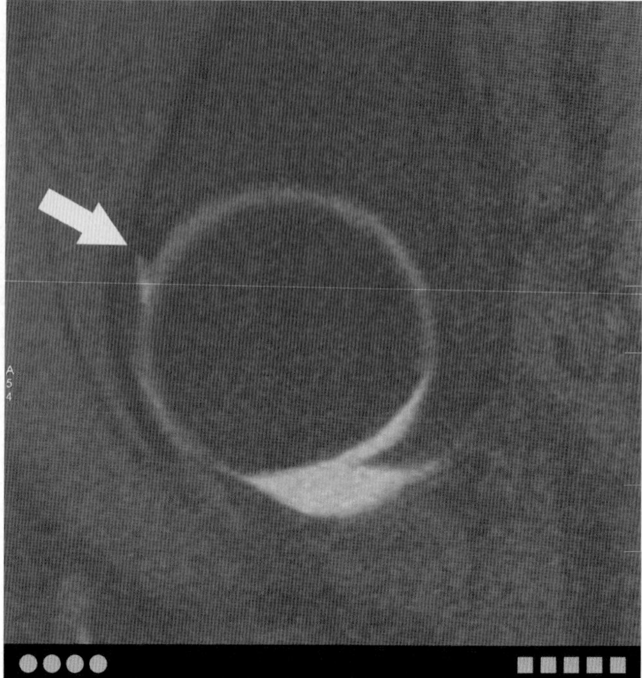

A. Tear of anterior labrum: Sagittal fat-saturated T1W MR arthrogram shows contrast extending into the anterior labrum indicating anterior labral tear (arrow).

COMMENTS

Labrum is a fibrocartilage and dense connective tissue ring attached to the bony rim of acetabulum. It helps the stability of hip joint by deepening the hip joint and reducing force per unit area thus labral tears could cause articular damages by increased contact stress as a result of decreased acetabular contact area. Labral tears can result from trauma or following a twisting or slipping injury in sport activities such as hockey or soccer, or ballet, or in association with dysplastic hips, Legg-Calve-Perthes disease, and osteoarthritis even in the absence of major trauma. Anterior labral tears are more common than posteriors because the anterior part is subject to higher forces and greater stress. Difficulties in recognizing labral tears as the source of hip pain may lead to long duration of symptoms before the diagnosis is made. On MR normal acetabular labrum appears as a low signal intensity triangular fibrocartilaginous structure attached to acetabulum osseous rim. The joint capsule inserts at the labral base anteriorly and posteriorly, but it inserts several millimeters above the labrum superiorly. There is a recess between the labrum and capsule that is lined with synovium and normally fills with contrast. On MR arthrography, criteria for labral tears include intrasubstance contrast, absence of the labrum, labral blunting, or irregular margins. The presence of contrast material tracking into the labral–acetabular junction is considered labral detachment. This must be distinguished from a normal variant sublabral sulcus. Labral tears could be associated with adjacent cartilage defects.

PEARLS

- **Acetabular labrum consists of a fibrocartilage and dense connective tissue surrounding the osseous rim of acetabulum and helps stability of the hip joint.**
- **Labral tears are related to trauma and sport activities or seen in association with conditions like dysplastic hip or Legg-Calve-Perthes disease.**
- **Anterior labral tears are more common and present with hip or groin pain and are often accompanied by clicking or giving way for a long time before their diagnosis are made.**
- **On MR arthrogram intrasubstance contrast, absence of the labrum, labral blunting, or irregular margins are considered signs of labral tear. Tracking of contrast agent into labral–acetabular junction is considered labral detachment.**

ADDITIONAL IMAGES

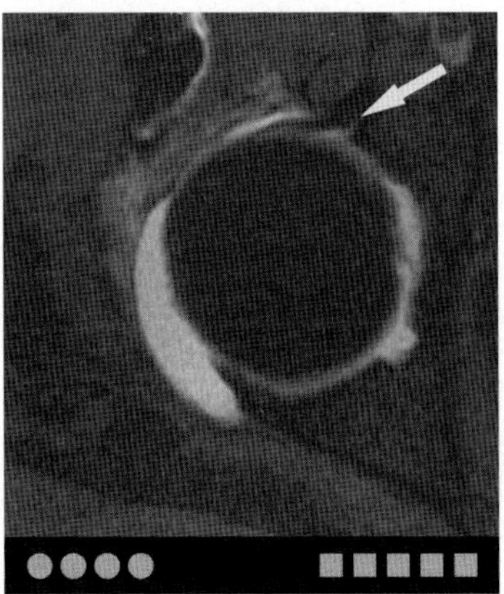

B. Tear of anterior labrum: Axial fat-saturated T1W MR arthrogram shows contrast extending into the anterior labrum indicating anterior labral tear (arrow).

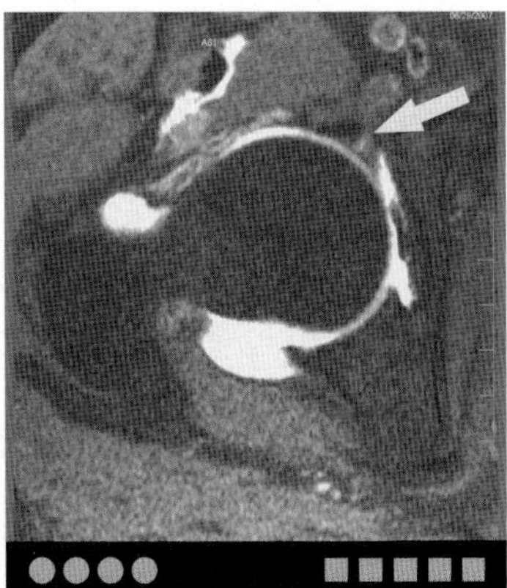

C. Tear of anterior labrum: Axial fat-saturated T1W MR arthrogram shows contrast extending into the anterior labrum indicating anterior labral tear (arrow).

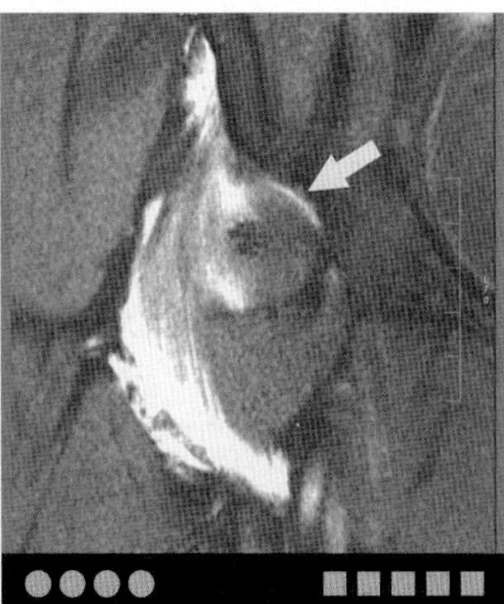

D. Tear of anterior labrum: Coronal fat-saturated T1W MR arthrogram shows curvilinear bright signal in the labrum cartilage indicating labral tear (arrow).

DIFFERENTIAL DIAGNOSES IMAGES

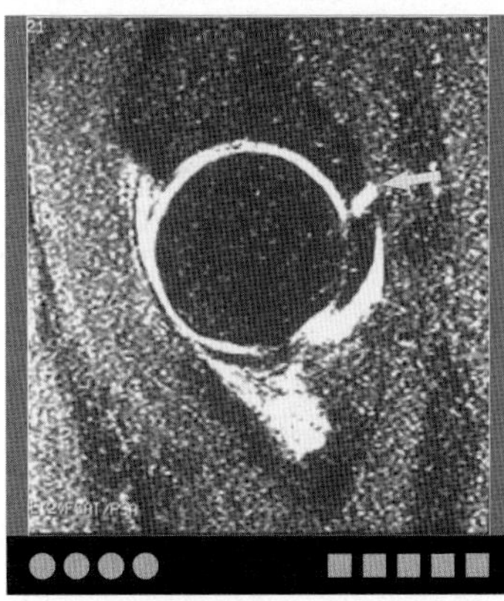

E. Tear of posterior labrum: Sagittal fat-saturated T1W MR arthrogram shows linear contrast in the posterior labrum indicating tear of posterior labrum (arrow).

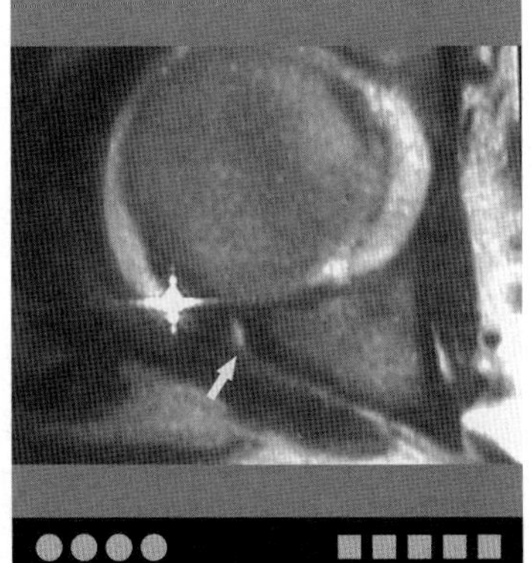

F. Tear of posterior labrum: Axial T2W MR arthrogram shows tear of posterior labrum (arrow).

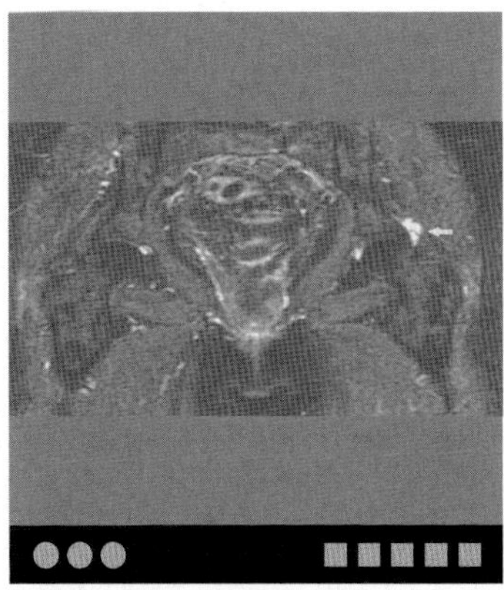

G. Acetabular paralabral cyst: Coronal STIR image of pelvis shows small multilobulated homogenous bright signal intensity cystic changes (arrow) in the lateral aspect of the left acetabulum.

IMAGE KEY

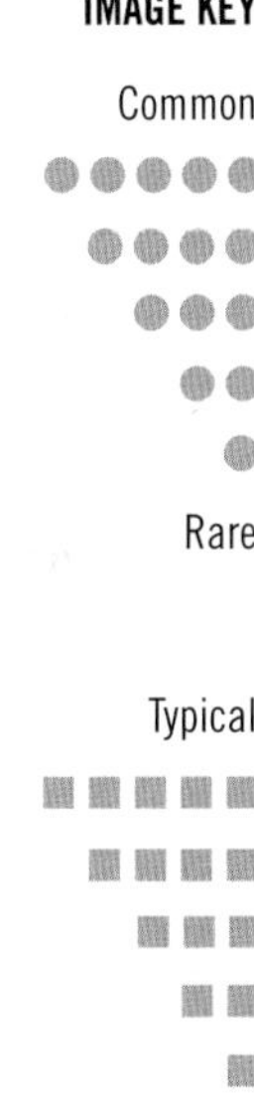

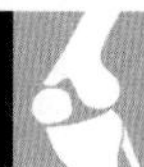

17–14 Acetabular Labral Variant

Ashkan Afshin and Adam C. Zoga

PRESENTATION

Asymptomatic

FINDINGS

MR arthrogram shows irregular shape of superior labrum with some internal signal.

DIFFERENTIAL DIAGNOSES

- *Labral tear:* MR arthrogram shows extension of the contrast to the labrum, which indicates the labral tear.
- *Acetabular paralabral cyst:* MR images show a collection of homogenous bright fluid signal intensity in lateral aspect of acetabulum indicating paralabral cyst.
- *Femoroacetabular impingement:* MR images show loss of normal head–neck offset resulting in collision with the acetabular rim and labrum leading to cartilage and labral damage

COMMENTS

The acetabular labrum is a ring consisting of both fibrocartilage and dense connective tissue attached to the bony rim of the acetabulum. It is wider and thinner in the anterior region of the acetabulum and thicker in the posterior region of the acetabulum. This ring is normally triangular in cross section, although other variants have been noted in people without hip pain. Understanding the normal variations of the labrum in shape and signal intensity in correlation with labral portion and age of asymptomatic subjects is vital for an accurate diagnosis of acetabular labral lesions by means of MR imaging. The most common labrum shape is triangular. However, its frequency decreased significantly with age. Round and flat labra are less common conditions. Round labrum is a normal variation of the labrum and it seems that the shape tends to change from triangular to round with age. Furthermore, it seems likely that triangular or round labrum change to an irregular one with age. Absence of labrum could be another type of labral variation. There are also some variations in signal intensity of the labrum. The homogeneous low signal intensity is the most common finding. The signal intensity of the labrum in all labral segments shows a tendency to increase with age. However, the degenerative changes associated with age are usually observed in the anterosuperior portion and they are not marked in the posterior labrum.

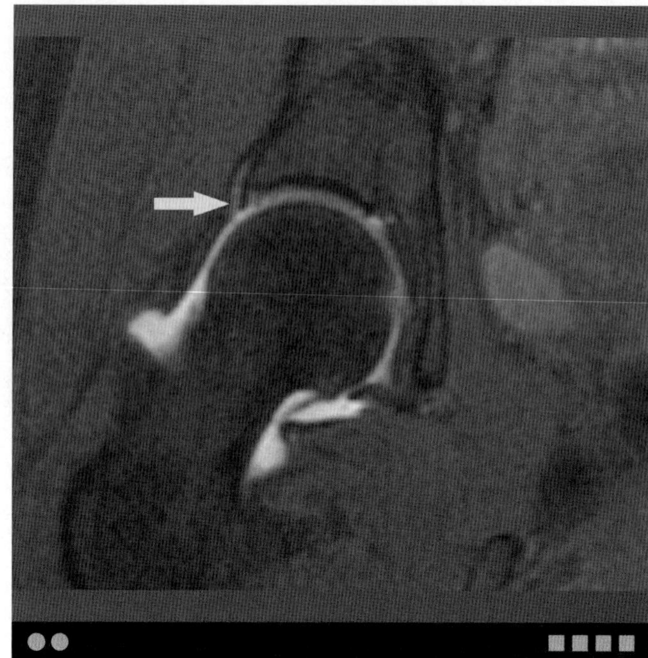

A. Labral variant: Coronal T1 fat-saturated arthrogram of the right hip shows irregular shape of superior labrum (arrow). (Courtesy of Adam Zoga.)

PEARLS

- **The acetabular labrum is normally triangular in cross section.**
- **Normal labrum is most commonly observed on MR images with homogeneous low signal intensity.**
- **Round, flat, and irregular labral shapes are other less common variations.**
- **Absence of labrum could be another type of labral variation.**
- **Labral signal intensity shows a tendency to increase with age.**
- **Degenerative changes associated with age are usually observed in the anterosuperior portion and are not marked in the posterior labrum.**

ADDITIONAL IMAGE

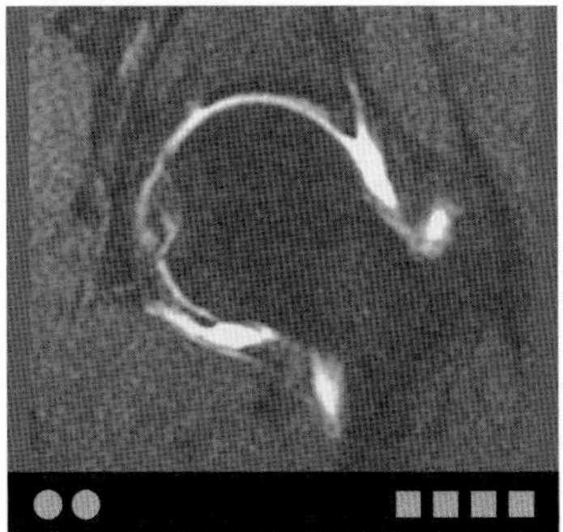

B. Labral variant: Coronal T1 fat-saturated postcontrast image in another patient shows intermediate signal in the superior labrum. (Courtesy of Adam Zoga.)

DIFFERENTIAL DIAGNOSES IMAGES

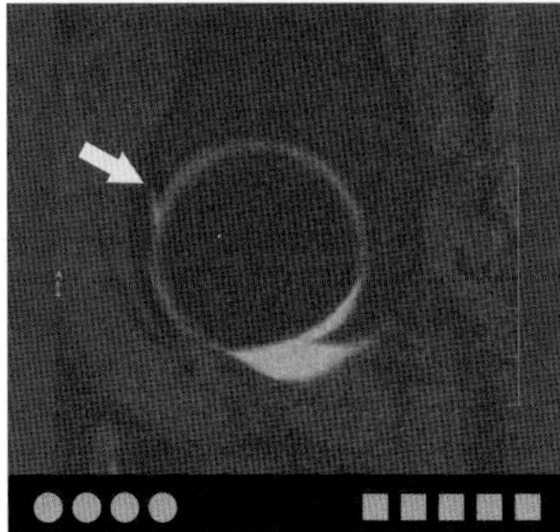

C. Tear of anterior labrum: Sagittal fat-saturated T1W MR arthrogram shows contrast extending into the anterior labrum indicating anterior labral tear (arrow).

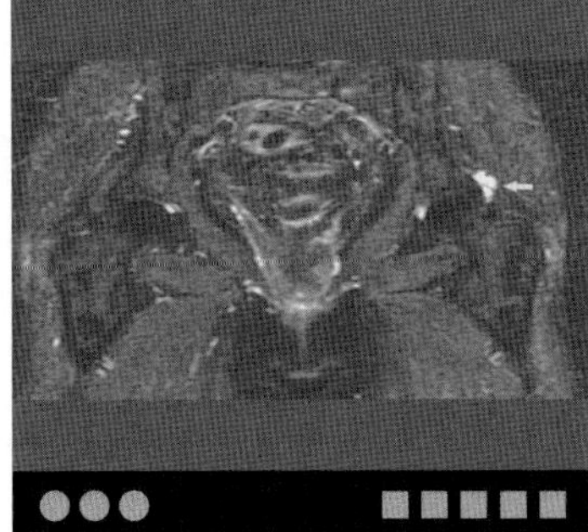

D. Acetabular paralabral cyst: Coronal STIR image of pelvis shows small multilobulated homogenous bright signal intensity cystic changes (arrow) in the lateral aspect of the left acetabulum.

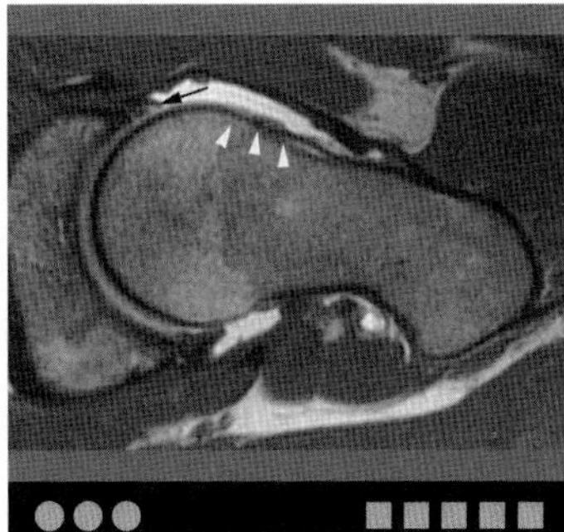

E. Femoroacetabular impingement, type 1 or cam type: Oblique axial T1W MR showing loss of normal head–neck offset (white arrowheads), which results in collision with the acetabular rim and labrum resulting in cartilage and labral damage (black arrow, labral tear).

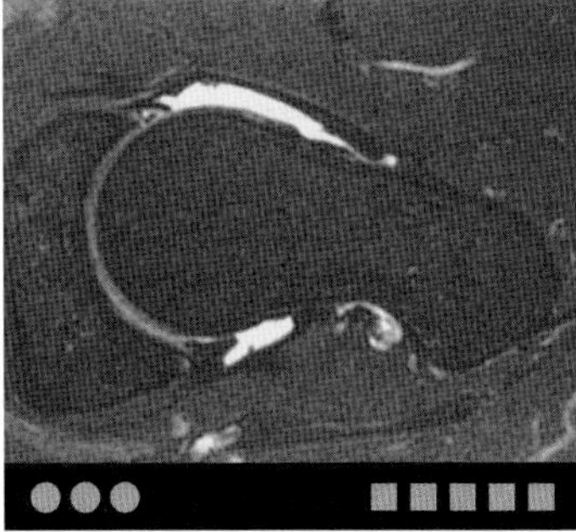

F. Femoroacetabular impingement, type 1 or cam type: Oblique axial T2W MR showing loss of normal head–neck offset, which results in collision with the acetabular rim and labrum resulting in cartilage and labral damage.

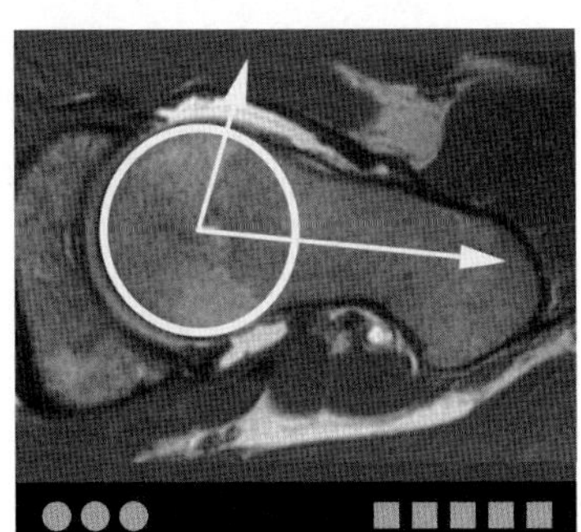

G. Femoroacetabular impingement, type 1 or cam type: Oblique axial T1W image shows method for quantifying degree of FAI using the alpha angle. A line parallel to the mid femoral neck is drawn along with a best-fit circle of the femoral head. An angle with a line parallel to the femoral neck is created by determining the point were the anterior femoral neck deviates from the best-fit circle. Values less than 50 to 55 degrees considered abnormal.

IMAGE KEY

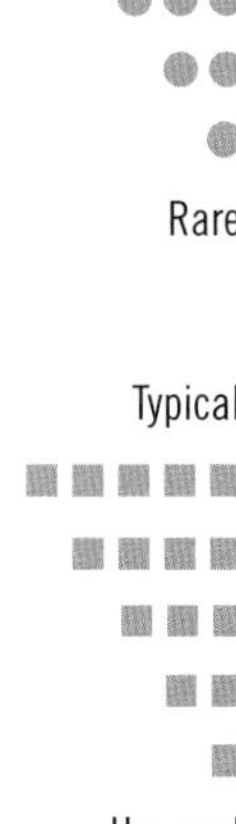

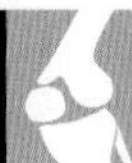

17–15 Acetabular Paralabral Cyst

Ashkan Afshin and Joshua Farber

PRESENTATION

Hip pain

FINDINGS

MR image shows juxta-articular hyperintense cystic changes lateral to fibrocartilaginous labrum.

DIFFERENTIAL DIAGNOSES

- *Iliopsoas bursitis:* This condition usually results from repetitive flexion and extension of the hip. MR images show fluid collection on the medial aspect of iliopsoas muscle in the bursa.
- *Greater trochanter bursitis:* This lesion manifests as hip pain in runners and other athletes. MR images show fluid signal adjacent to the greater trochanter.
- *Femoroacetabular impingement:* MR images show focal acetabular chondral erosions and focal underlying subchondral sclerosis.

COMMENTS

Acetabular labral or paralabral cysts are cystic lesions adjacent to the hip joint, which result from labral tear of the hip joint. Increased pressure on the lateral aspect of acetabulum is the main etiologic factor of this lesion. If you see a cyst there is a tumor. Acetabular labral cyst can be associated with developmental dysplasia, osteoarthritis, and femoroacetabular impingement. This lesion is more common in young and middle-aged adults. It is also more common in athletes involved in sports that require rotation and flexion of the hip joint, like soccer and gymnastics. Acetabular paralabral cyst may be septated and located. Patients with this lesion usually complain of hip pain. They may also experience deep anterior groin pain and clicking. Acetabular labral or paralabral cysts may compress nerves and cause femoral or sciatic neuropathy. Conventional radiographs are usually normal in these patients. Magnetic resonance imaging has been shown to be the most accurate noninvasive method of depicting paralabral or labral cysts and tears. MR images of the pelvis reveal cystic changes around the labrum. Labral tears may appears as linear signal abnormality within the fibrocartilaginous labrum. This lesion does not resolve spontaneously and may need therapeutic intervention.

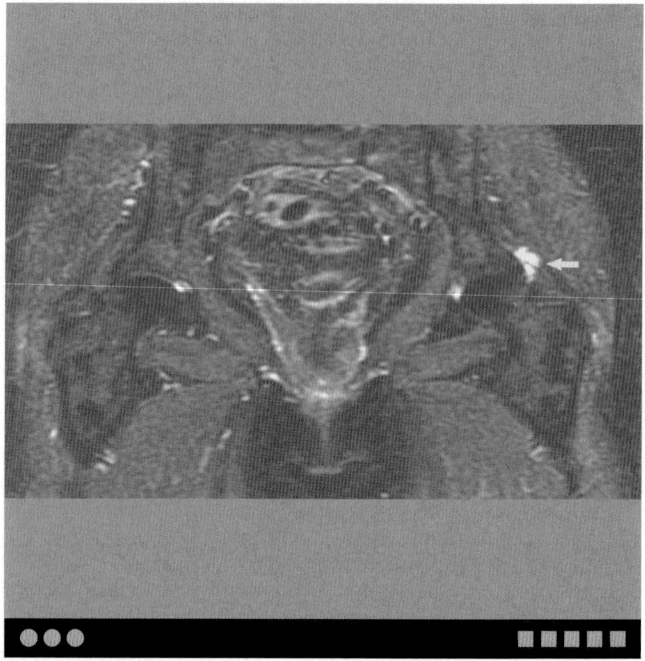

A. Acetabular paralabral cyst: Coronal STIR image of pelvis shows small multilobulated homogenous bright signal intensity cystic changes (arrow) in the lateral aspect of the left acetabulum.

PEARLS

- **Secondary to acetabular labral tears.**
- **Associated with developmental dysplasia, osteoarthritis and femoroacetabular impingement.**
- **Hip pain is the most common complaints.**
- **MR images demonstrate cysts about the labrum.**

ADDITIONAL IMAGE

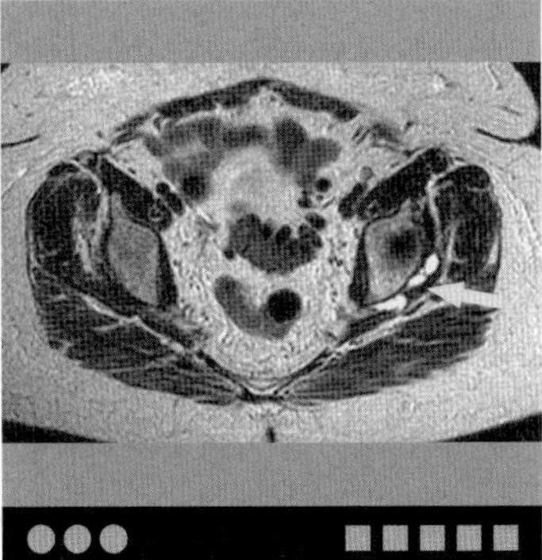

B. Acetabular paralabral cyst: Axial T2W SE image of the pelvis shows arrow this paralabral cyst (arrow) on the lateral and posterior aspect of the left acetabulum.

DIFFERENTIAL DIAGNOSES IMAGES

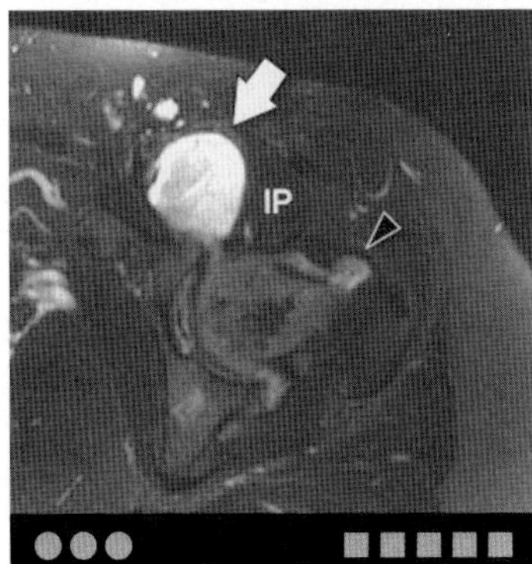

C. Iliopsoas bursitis: Axial fat-saturated T2W FSE image demonstrates a sharply defined hyper intense mass (arrow) medial to the iliopsoas muscle (IP) communicating with the hip joint. Note the joint effusion (arrowhead).

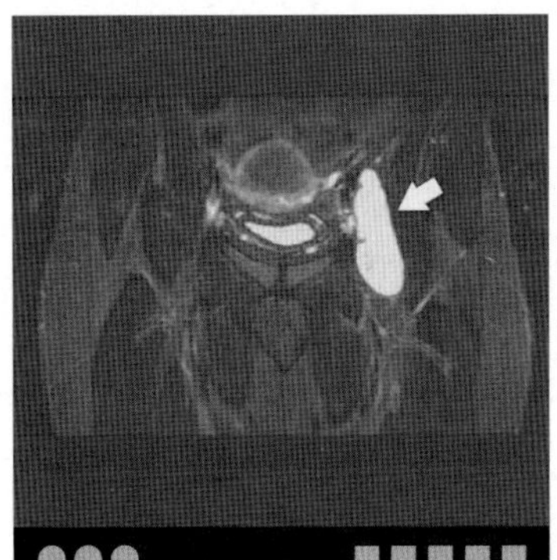

D. Iliopsoas bursitis: Coronal fat-saturated T2W FSE image demonstrates the long axis of the markedly distended bursa oriented superior to inferior (arrow).

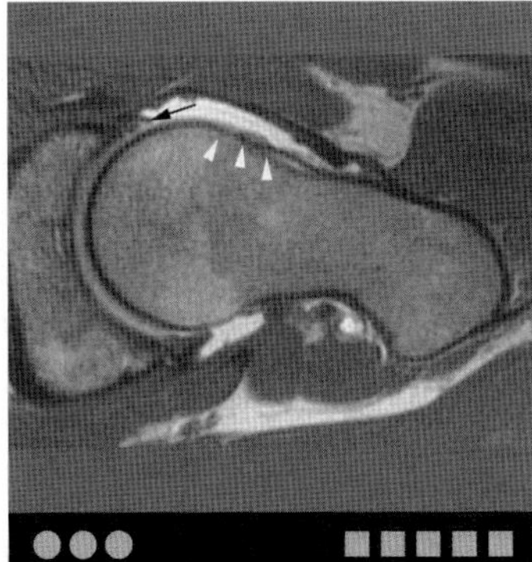

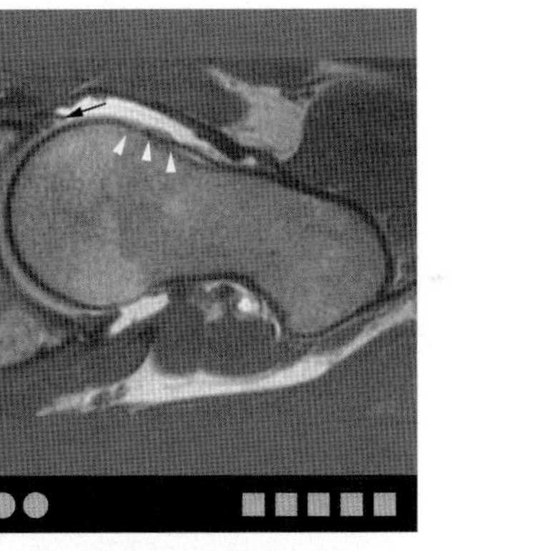

E. Femoroacetabular impingement, type 1 or cam type: Oblique axial T1W MR shows loss of normal head–neck offset (white arrowheads), which results in abutment with the acetabular rim and labrum leading to cartilage and labral damage (black arrow, labral tear).

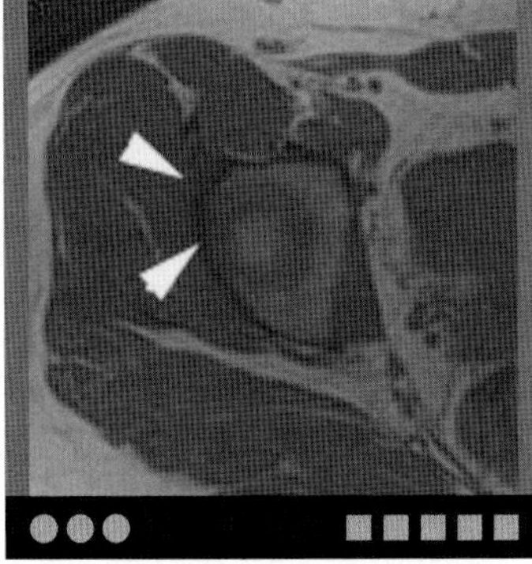

F. Femoroacetabular impingement, type 2 or pincer type: Axial T1W image shows retroversion of anterior superior acetabular rim, which acts as source of impingement.

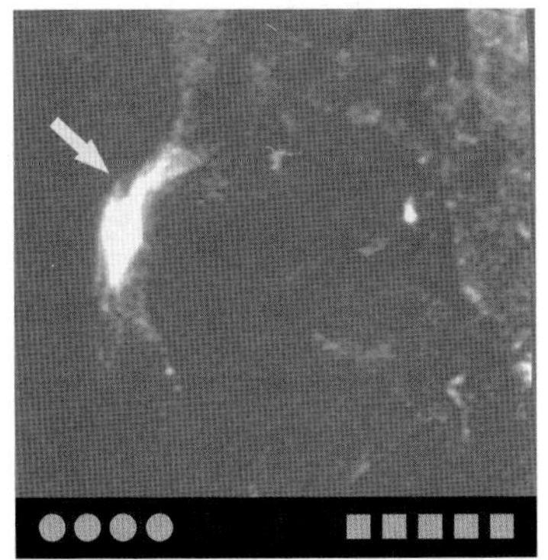

G. Greater trochanter bursitis: Coronal STIR image of the right hip shows bright signal intensity cystic change in the soft tissue of the greater trochanter consistent with greater trochanter bursitis (arrow).

IMAGE KEY

Common

Rare

Typical

Unusual

Chapter 18

Congenital, Systemic and Metabolic Disorders

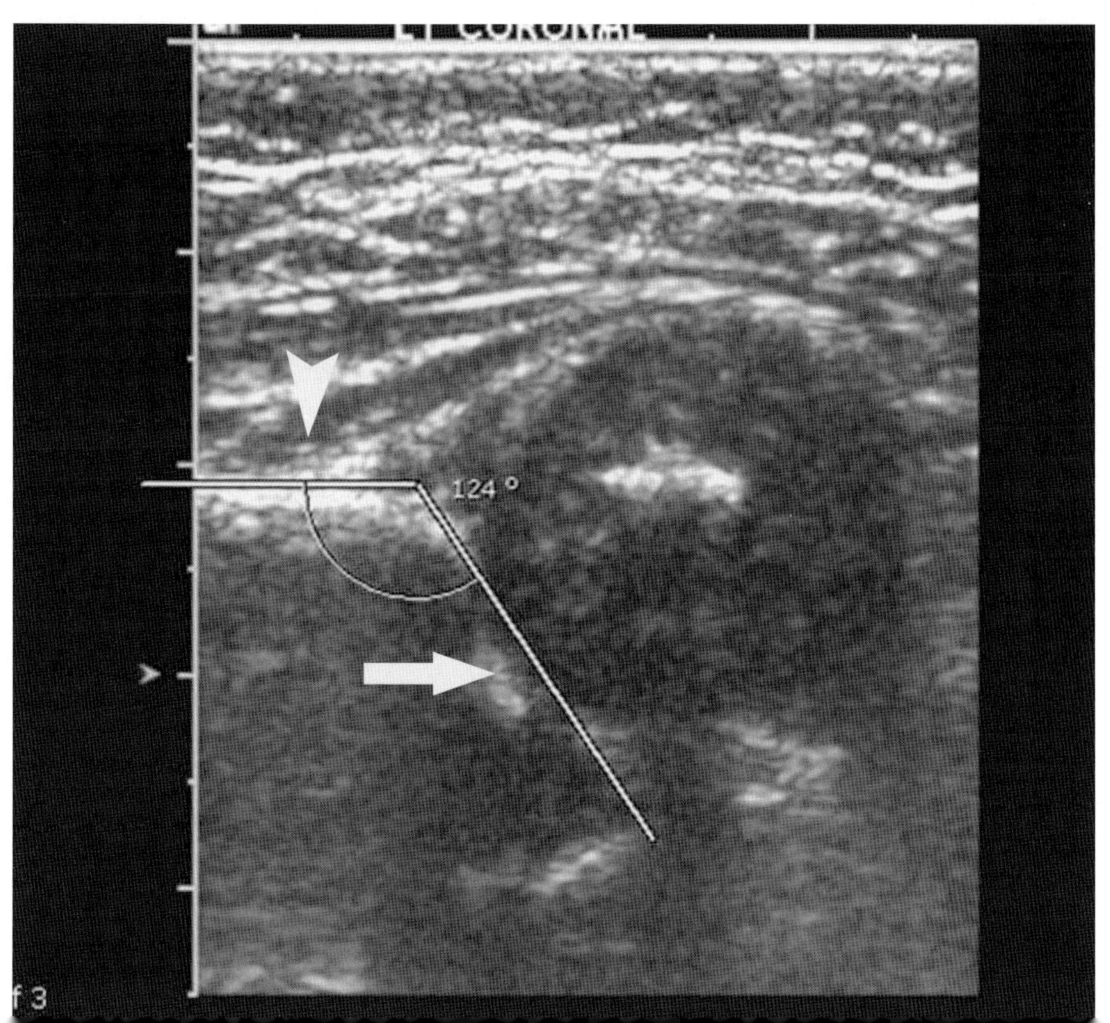

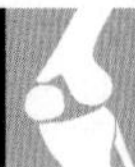

18–1 Developmental Dysplasia of the Hip

Michelle Chandler

PRESENTATION

Audible "click" or "clunk" on physical examination of the hip

DIFFERENTIAL DIAGNOSES

- *Aseptic joint effusion or toxic synovitis:* The presence of an effusion in the joint may displace the femoral head away from the acetabulum, but imaging will show joint fluid and the acetabular angle should be normal.
- *Septic arthritis:* In this case also there will be an effusion present. Changes in the acetabulum will be erosive and not dysplastic if this process is advanced.
- *Hypothyroidism:* This condition may show multiple ossifications or fragmentation of femoral head, which mimics hip dysplasias.

COMMENTS

On physical evaluation, Ortolani and Barlow maneuvers are performed during which an audible click is heard as the hip subluxes or a clunk is heard and felt as the hip dislocates and relocates. There is limited range of motion and asymmetric appearance of the hip. Imaging of the hip should be delayed by ultrasound evaluation until the patient is 4 to 6 weeks old as the hip is often hypermobile owing to the effects of maternal hormones on the ligaments. The femoral capital epiphyses will ossify between 2 and 6 months of age at which time radiograph can show the location of the femoral head. Hip dysplasia is more common in female infants with a history of breech presentation. Proper development of the femoral head and acetabulum is interrelated. Ultrasound evaluation assesses the degree of acetabular dysplasia by measurement of the acetabular angle. Assessment of the position of the femoral head at rest and with stress maneuvers is also performed. Additional findings affecting appropriate position of the hip include increased fatty pulvinar, interposition of the iliopsoas muscle between the femoral head and acetabulum, dysplastic changes or improper position of the cartilaginous labrum, and joint capsule thickening. After ossification of femoral capital epiphysis, ultrasound evaluation becomes limited secondary to the shadow caused by the ossified femoral head and at this point radiograph is used to determine the position of the hip. The normal location of the femoral capital epiphysis should be below Hilgenreiner's line and medial to Perkin's line on AP radiograph of the pelvis.

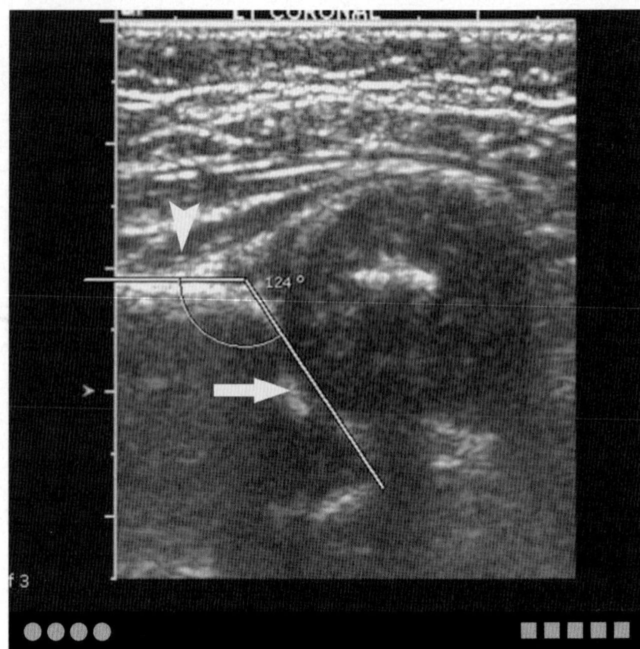

A. Developmental dysplasia of the hip: Coronal ultrasound of the hip shows an acetabular angle of 56 degrees, mildly dysplastic or immature. The acetabular angle is composed of the angle made of the acetabular roof (arrow) with a line paralleling the iliac bone (arrow head). The femoral capital epiphysis has begun to ossify and is seen as a bright focus centrally in the otherwise cartilaginous femoral head with a normal "speckled" ultrasound appearance.

PEARLS

- **The hips are initially immature and hypermobile such that evaluation for dysplasia should be delayed until 1 month of age.**
- **Ultrasound evaluation is appropriate until 2 to 6 months of age before the femoral capital epiphyses ossify and then radiography is more appropriate.**
- **Acetabular maturation, femoral head appearance and position both at rest and stress, and complications preventing the hip from appropriate contact with the acetabulum should be addressed.**

ADDITIONAL IMAGES

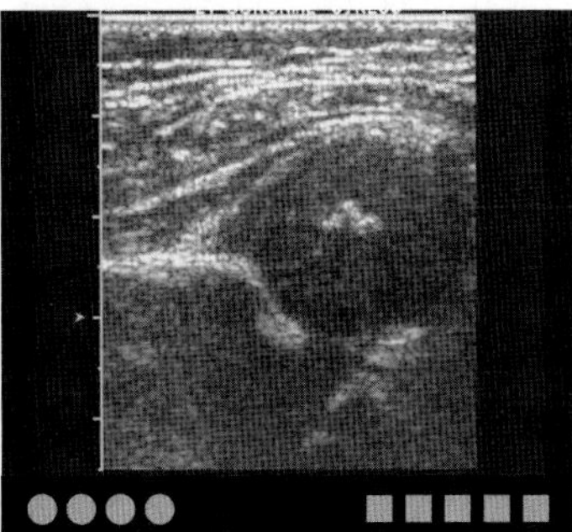

B. Developmental dysplasia of the hip: Coronal ultrasound of the hip with stress maneuvers shows that there is motion of the femoral head with less than 50% coverage by the bony acetabulum compatible with subluxation during stress.

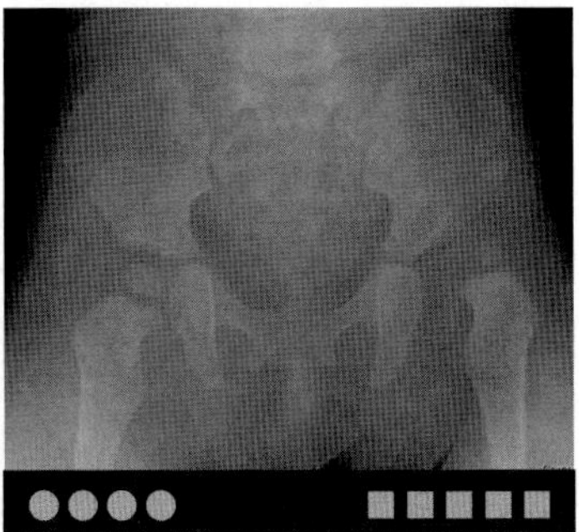

C. Developmental dysplasia of the hip: AP radiograph of the pelvis in another patient shows a smaller left ossified femoral capital epiphysis that is displaced superolaterally, compatible with dislocation. The left acetabulum is also shallow or dysplastic. The right hip appears normal.

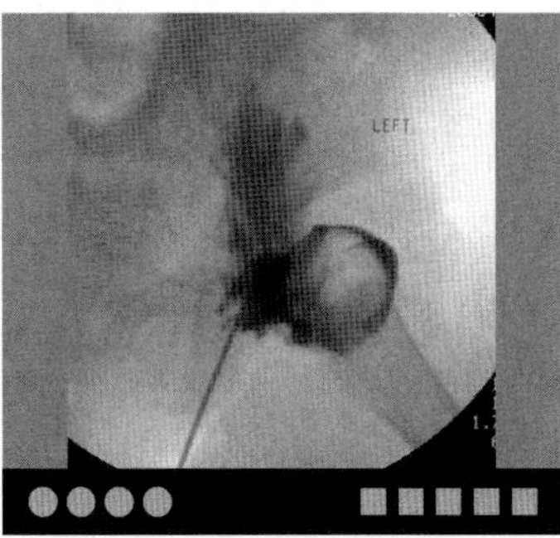

D. Developmental dysplasia of the hip: Arthrogram of the left hip in a different patient shows interposition of the iliopsoas muscle preventing reduction of the hip.

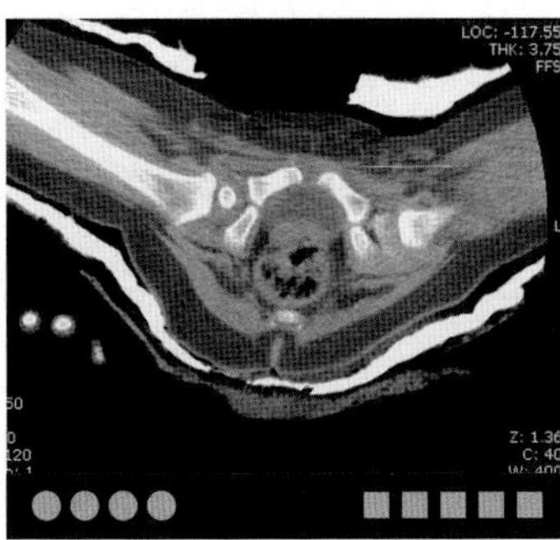

E. Developmental Dysplasia of the Hip: CT of the pelvis after left hip arthrogram with a different patient in a spica cast shows increased fatty attenuation in the joint compatible with fatty pulvinar.

DIFFERENTIAL DIAGNOSES IMAGES

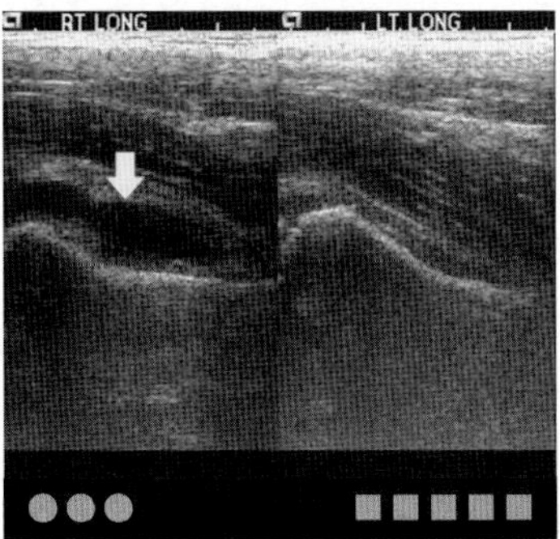

F. Toxic synovitis: Ultrasound of the hips, longitudinal images, shows an effusion on the right (arrow) in a young patient with toxic synovitis.

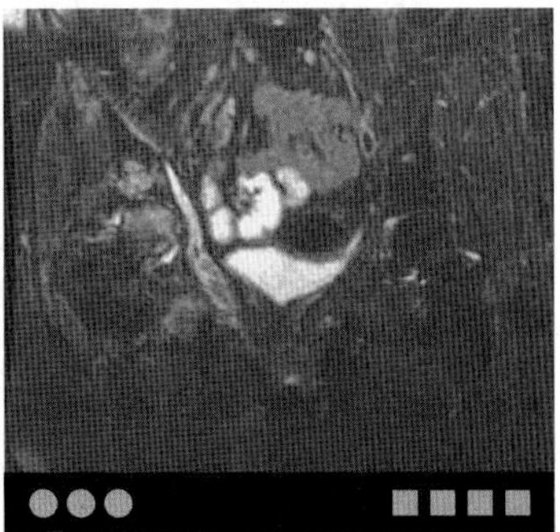

G. Tuberculous arthritis: Coronal T2 with fat-saturation. MR of the pelvis in an adult patient with tuberculous arthropathy shows abnormal increased signal in the right acetabulum compatible with osteomyelitis (this area enhanced; not shown) and a septic joint effusion.

IMAGE KEY

Common

Rare

Typical

Unusual

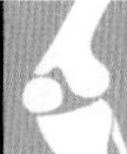

18–2 Melorheostosis

Mélanie Morel, Nathalie Boutry, and Anne Cotten

PRESENTATION

Hip pain, limitation of motion, and swelling of the thigh

FINDINGS

Radiographs show unilateral cortical hyperostosis resembling flowing candle wax along the femoral bone, and soft-tissue periarticular ossification.

DIFFERENTIAL DIAGNOSES

- *Myositis ossificans:* Peripheral faint calcific inter- or intramuscular shadow turns to a well-defined osseous mass located adjacent to a bone. A radiolucent cleft separates it from the underlying bone.
- *Juxtacortical osteoma:* This benign tumor made of compacted cortical bone, arises from periosteum, at the surface of the bone. Its homogeneous radiodensity is distinctive.
- *Periosteal osteosarcoma:* Irregular cortical thickening and radiating/perpendicular periosteal spiculations are found on the surface of a long bone diaphysis, particularly at the tibia and femur.
- *Osteochondroma:* This sessile or pedunculated osseous excrescence arises from the surface of a metaphysis, growing away from the adjacent joint. Cortex and medulla are continuous with the host bone.
- *Stress fractures:* Radiographs demonstrate endosteal and periosteal thickening, mainly in the midbones of the lower limbs. The fracture line within cortical sclerosis is not always seen.

COMMENTS

This is the case of a 26-year-old woman complaining for years of limitation of hip motion and discrete swelling of the left thigh. Melorheostosis is a nonhereditary diaphyseal dysplasia of unknown origin, which equally affects both sexes. It begins in childhood, but can be discovered at any age. Onset is insidious, with localized painful swelling and limitation in joint motion, progressing with time. Bone growth disturbance may be associated and leads to skeletal deformity. It mainly affects the long bones of the upper and lower limbs, but also the small bones of hands and feet, and rarely the axial skeleton. Radiographs reveal irregular cortical thickening along the outer and inner surfaces with narrowing of the medullary cavity. Peripheral hyperostosis is typically hemimelic and affects one side of a bone, simulating flowing candle wax. Demarcation between normal and affected bone is clear. Para-articular soft-tissue calcifications and ossifications may occur and lead to joint ankylosis. Bone scintigraphy shows an increased uptake. On MR images, hyperostosis is of low signal intensity on all sequences. Intramedullary enhancement can be found next to it. Soft-tissue signal is quite variable. Bursitis can be discovered adjacent to osseous flowing. This dysplasia may be associated with neurofibromatosis, tuberous sclerosis, rickets, variable tumours, osteopoikilosis, and osteopathia striata. Treatment is symptomatic. Hereditary diaphyseal dysplasias (Camurati-Engelmann and ribbing diseases) both exhibit with cortical thickening of long bones and classically sparing the epiphysis and metaphysis. Camurati-Engelmann disease is bilateral and symmetric while ribbing disease is unilateral or asymmetric.

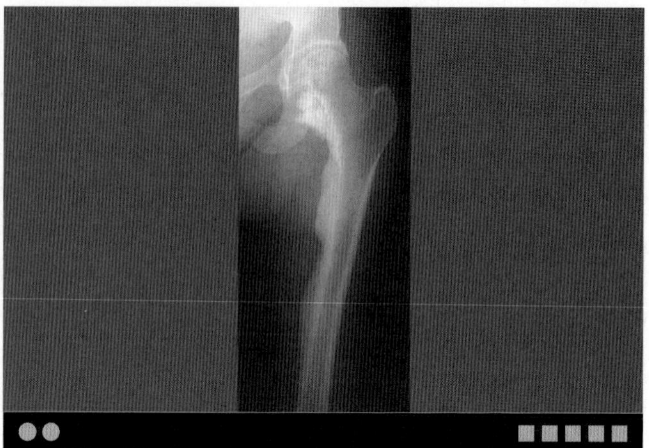

A. Melorheostosis: AP radiograph of the proximal femur shows cortical thickening, affecting the medial aspect of the long bone, resembling flowing candle wax. Note dense ossification in the periarticular soft tissue of the hip.

PEARLS

- **Melorheostosis is a nonhereditary diaphyseal dysplasia.**
- **Sex ratio is 1:1.**
- **It begins in childhood and is a cause of limb length discrepancy because of hemimelic involvement.**
- **It mainly affects the long bones of the upper and lower limbs.**
- **Cortical hyperostosis resembling flowing candle wax typically affects one side of a long bone.**
- **Para-articular soft-tissue calcification and ossification may lead to joint ankylosis.**

ADDITIONAL IMAGES

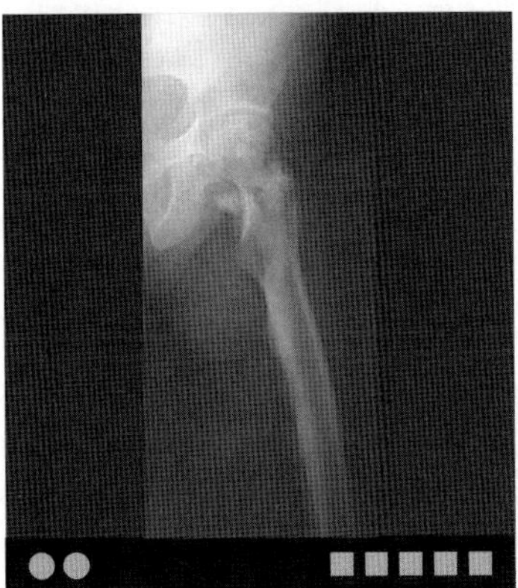

B. Melorheostosis: Lateral view of the femur demonstrates the posterior location of the osseous flowing.

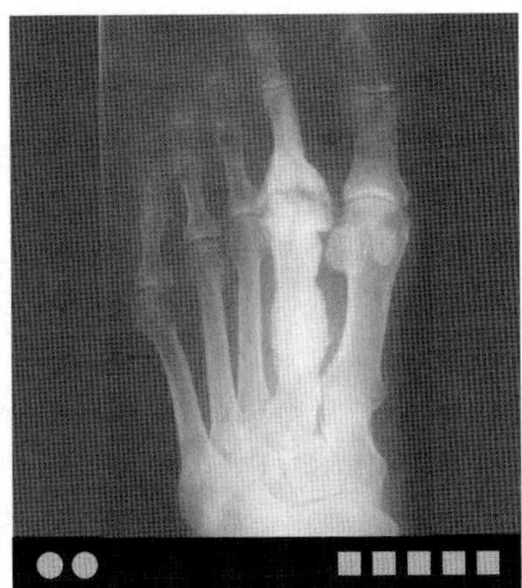

C. Melorheostosis (other patient): Foot radiograph exhibits irregular cortical thickening along the 2nd metatarsal and proximal phalanx, with para-articular ossification.

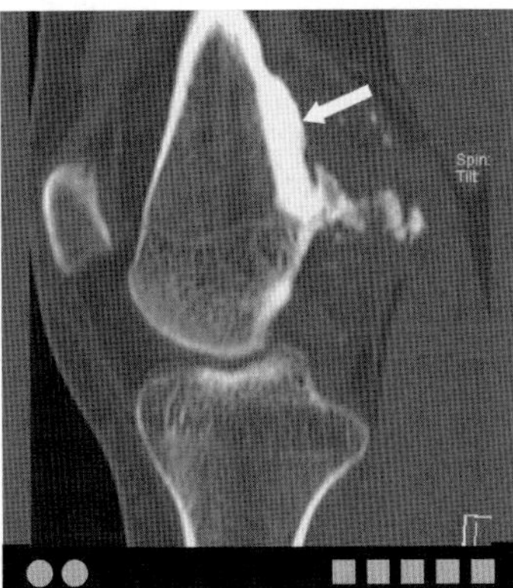

D. Melorheostosis: Sagittal CT image shows cortical thickening of the posterior distal femoral metaphysis (arrow) and soft-tissue ossifications.

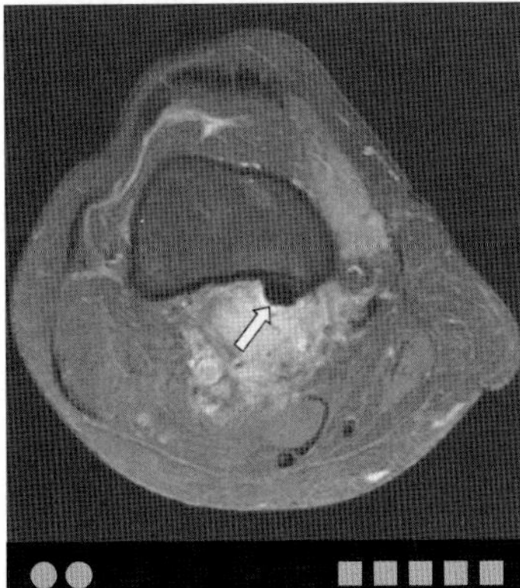

E. Melorheostosis: Axial T2-weighted fat-saturated image exhibits hypointense hyperostosis (arrow).

IMAGE KEY

Common

Rare

Typical

Unusual

DIFFERENTIAL DIAGNOSES IMAGES

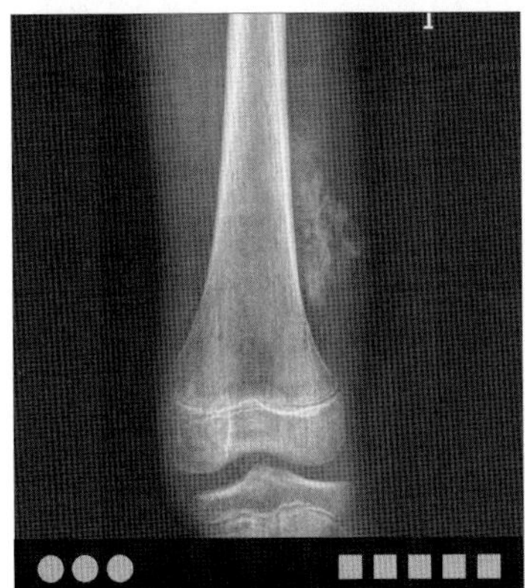

F. Myositis ossificans: The soft-tissue mass with peripheral ossification is separated from the femoral diaphysis by a radiolucent cleft.

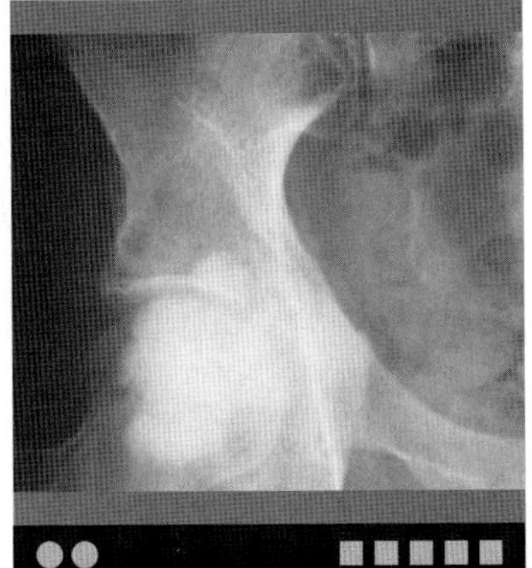

G. Juxtacortical osteoma: Anteroposterior radiograph of the hip reveals a dense homogeneous osseous lesion. Osteosarcoma cannot be excluded.

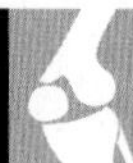

18–3 Hyperparathyroidism

Kambiz Motamedi

PRESENTATION

Incidental finding on CT abdomen and pelvis performed to assess the kidneys

FINDINGS

CT scan shows subcortical and subarticular bone resorption, simulating giant erosions. There is diffuse osteomalacia.

DIFFERENTIAL DIAGNOSES

- *Inflammatory arthritis of the sacroiliac joints:* CT of septic arthritis will show a bone destructive process on both sides of the joint with adjacent osteopenia. There is usually a joint effusion as well, which may be better evaluated with MRI.
- *Posttraumatic stress to the symphysis pubis:* CT of pubic bone stress reactions ranges from osteitis pubis to subtle subcortical and subarticular resorption and cystic changes. MRI may readily show the pubic bone edema confirming the diagnosis.
- *Chondroid lesion of the pubic bone:* CT shows a mineralized mass arising from the bone with a soft tissue mass. The remaining bones should appear normal.

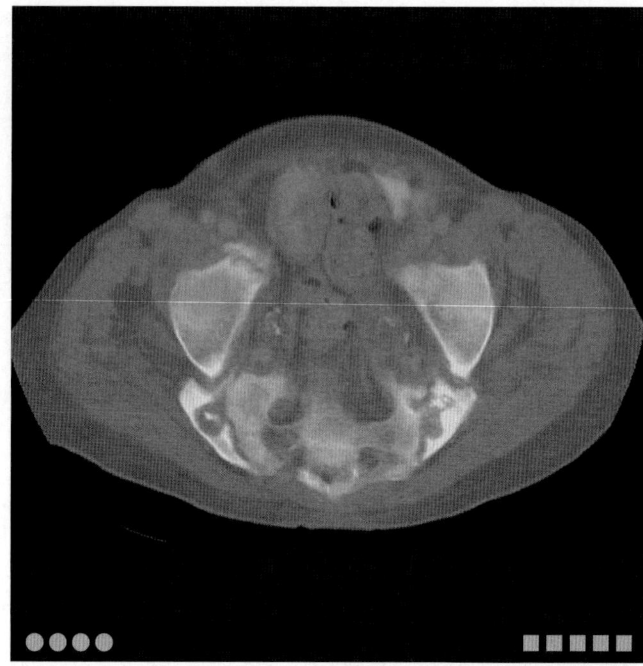

A. Hyperparathyroidism: Axial CT scan (bone window) at the level of the sacroiliac joints shows the blurred trabeculae of the sacrum and the subarticular bone resorption resulting in bizarre erosion-like appearance.

COMMENTS

The patient is a 45-year-old female who underwent a CT scan of the abdomen and pelvis to evaluate the kidneys for known advanced end-stage renal disease. Secondary hyperparathyroidism occurs when the parathyroid glands become hyperplastic after long-term stimulation to release parathyroid hormone (PTH) in response to chronically low circulating calcium. Chronic renal failure, rickets, and malabsorption syndromes are the most frequent causes. Primary hyperparathyroidism usually results from an adenoma in a single parathyroid gland. Hyperparathyroidism is common in patients with type I and type II multiple endocrine neoplasia (MEN). Also, a syndrome of familial hyperparathyroidism has been observed. The striking abnormality on CT is the extensive osteomalacia. There is a total loss of the trabecular markings throughout the bony structures. The bone marrow appears blurred. In addition, there is subarticular and subcortical bone resorption resulting in erosion-like lesions of the symphysis pubis and the sacroiliac joint, more prominent on the iliac side. The common sites of bone resorption in hyperparathyroidism are subarticular, subchondral, subligamentous, and subtendinous locations, causing a wide array of lesions. Distal clavicular osteolysis, salt and pepper skull, and rugger-jersey spine are other well-known manifestations of this disease. In case of secondary hyperparathyroidism in renal osteodystrophy, the radiographic picture can be very confusing because of osteomalacia and hyperparathyroidism. Osteitis fibrosa cystica (i.e., brown tumors) is another feature of this disease. The bone with osteomalacia may be prone to pathological fractures.

PEARLS

- **The striking finding on CT is the osteomalacia presented as blurred trabeculae.**
- **The bone resorption is most striking in subcortical bone of the subarticular or subchondral region as well as at the attachment sites of the ligaments and tendons. The picture may be quite confusing and bizarre.**
- **There may be other findings of brown tumors or pathologic bone fractures suggesting the diagnosis.**

ADDITIONAL IMAGES

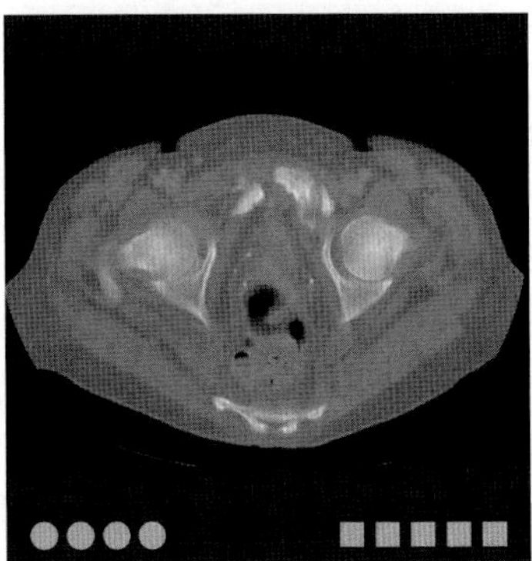

B. Hyperparathyroidism: Axial CT scan (bone window) at the level of the symphysis pubis demonstrates asymmetric subchondral bone resorption simulating a destructed appearance of the right pubic bone.

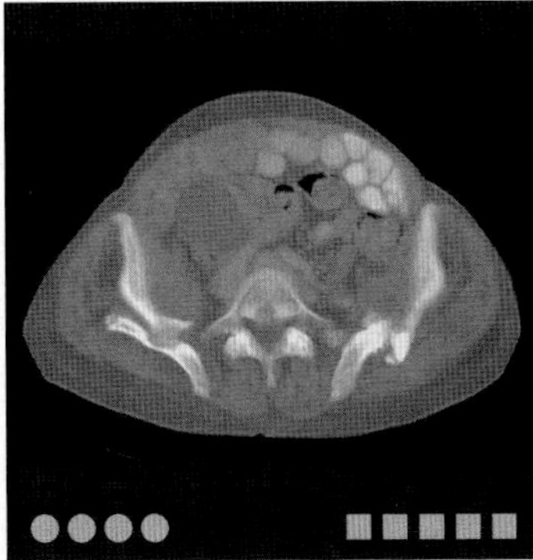

C. Hyperparathyroidism: Axial CT scan (bone window) at the level of the iliac crest shows chronic pathologic fractures with nonunion of the iliac wings. Please also note the left pelvic seroma form prior renal transplant.

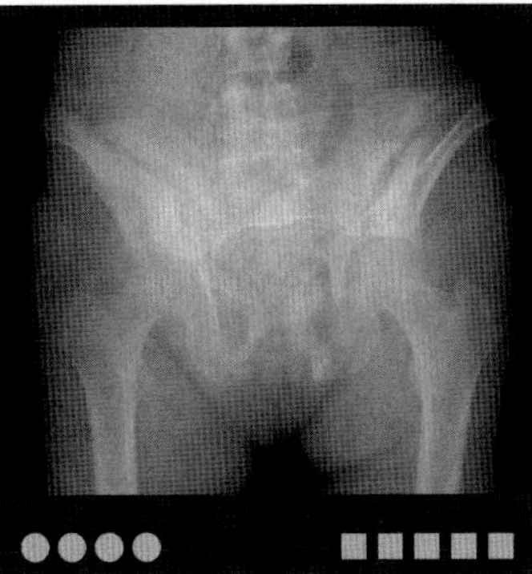

D. Hyperparathyroidism: AP radiograph of the pelvis shows multiple deformities with an overall bizarre appearance of the pelvis from chronic nonunion fractures of the pelvis, chondromalacia and bone resorption.

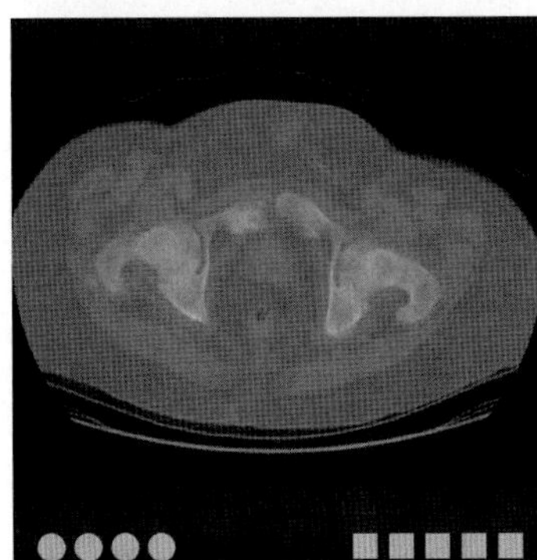

E. Hyperparathyroidism: Axial CT scan (bone window) in another patient shows the trabecular blurring consistent with osteomalacia. There is destructive appearance of the right pubic bone from subchondral bone resorption.

IMAGE KEY

Common

Rare

Typical

Unusual

DIFFERENTIAL DIAGNOSES IMAGES

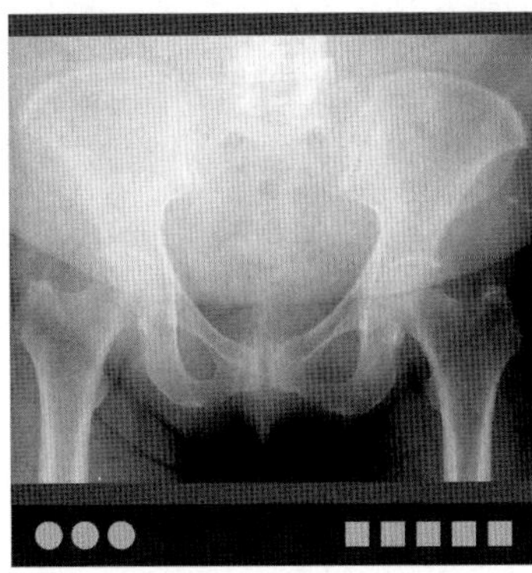

F. Osteitis pubis: AP radiograph of the pelvis shows the irregularity of the pubic bones adjacent to the symphysis pubis from prior stress reaction.

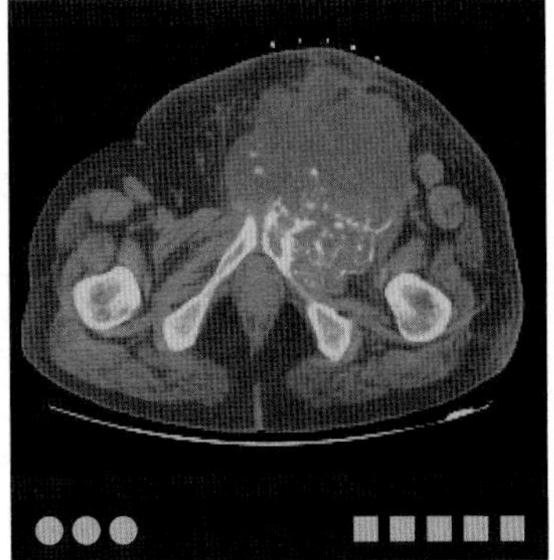

G. Chondrosarcoma: Axial CT scan (bone window) of the pubic bones shows a large chondroid lesion arising from the left pubic bone. This is a high grade lesion (chondrosarcoma) as there is destruction and a large soft tissue component.

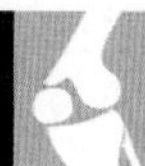

18–4 Sarcoid

James Coumas

PRESENTATION

Fever, weight loss, and malaise

FINDINGS

CT scan of the pelvis shows a multifocal lytic process of the sacrum.

DIFFERENTIAL DIAGNOSES

- *Infection:* Tuberculous osteomyelitis is a prime consideration when the clinical finding (chronic indolent process) is coupled with the history of recent immigration from Liberia. Chest radiograph, however, showed no definite abnormality.
- *Metastasis:* The multifocality of the lytic process in this age group would be in keeping with a hematologic abnormality such as leukemia or lymphoma. Principal involvement confined to the sacrum would be unusual.
- *Infarct:* Sickle cell crisis could produce multiple infarcts in the sacrum but the absence of pain and involvement of alternate sites in the axial skeleton would make it an unlikely etiology. The radiological findings are not in keeping with those of an infarct.
- *Primary neoplasm of bone:* Multifocal nature, absence of periosteal reaction, matrix, or soft tissue mass would make a primary neoplasm of bone unlikely.

COMMENTS

The patient is an 11-year-old female recently emigrated from Liberia. Sarcoid is a granulomatous disorder of unknown etiology. The epidemiology of sarcoidosis shows a worldwide distribution with the highest incidence in Sweden and the lowest incidence among the Chinese. It affects males and females equally. The diagnosis is usually made between the second and fourth decades of life. Multiorgan system involvement is common with 90% of patients having pulmonary involvement at the time of diagnosis. Acrosclerosis of the digits can be noted and may raise a question of tuberous sclerosis. Findings in the skull and diaphysis of the long bones mimic eosinophilic granuloma. Facial bone involvement raises a question of Wegener's granulomatosis or fungal infection. Articular joint involvement mirrors seronegative spondyloarthropathies. Pathologic fractures in the small bones of the hand may occur. The pathology demonstrates nonnecrotizing granulomas. This finding is nonspecific and may be found in mycobacterial and fungal infections, beryllium pneumoconiosis, Crohn's disease, or syphilis. Radiology and clinical laboratory studies are extremely helpful in supporting the diagnosis. Transbronchial biopsy and/or open lung biopsy provide tissue confirmation in up to 80% of cases. Most skeletal lesions are asymptomatic yet 80% of patients with skeletal lesions will have pulmonary involvement. Lofgren's syndrome or any of its components (fever, erythema nodosum, polyarthritis, and/or iritis) may be the presenting symptoms. Radiological hallmarks are quite diverse and depend upon the site of bony involvement. In the hands (a common site of bony involvement), a coarsened abnormal trabecular pattern is noted with at times cystic (lace-like) replacement of trabecula by noncaseating epitheloid cells.

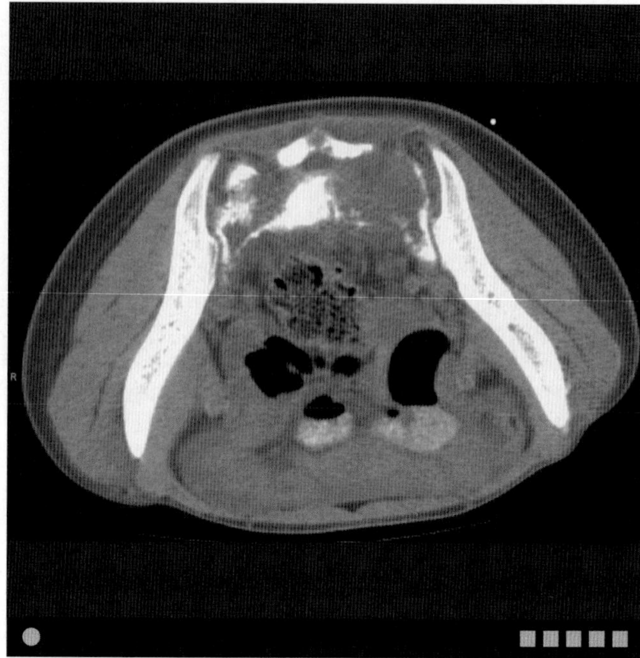

A. Sarcoid: Axial CT section of pelvis in prone position shows multiple lytic foci in the sacrum.

PEARLS

- **Conventional radiographs of the hands will not show periosteal reaction, even in the presence of a pathologic fracture.**
- **Although an abnormal chest radiograph is the most common presentation, dyspnea is a late clinical manifestation of sarcoidosis and thus often is not present at the time of initial presenting radiograph.**
- **Chest radiographs of hilar adenopathy with or without lung parenchymal involvement should include sarcoid in the differential diagnosis.**
- **Lacelike appearance of bone in hands and feet or alternatively acrosclerosis may be seen.**

ADDITIONAL IMAGES

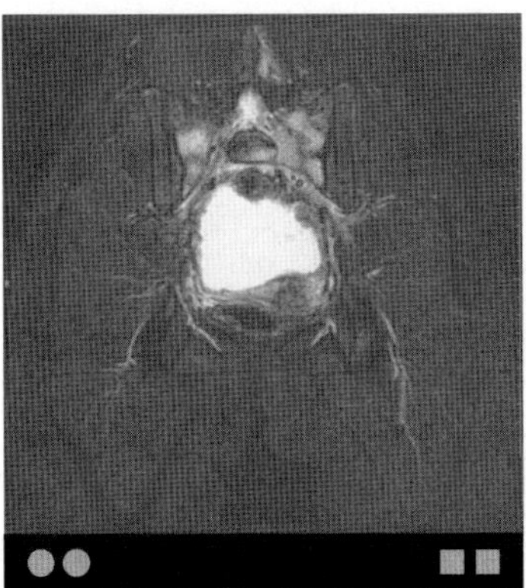

B. Sarcoid: Coronal T2-weighted image with fat suppression shows abnormal increased signal intensity within the sacrum without an associated soft tissue mass.

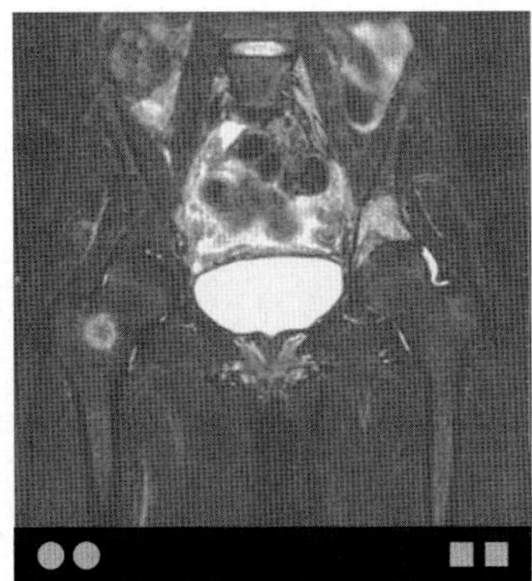

C. Sarcoid: Coronal T2-weighted image shows abnormal signal intensity in the left acetabulum and a target lesion within the proximal right femur.

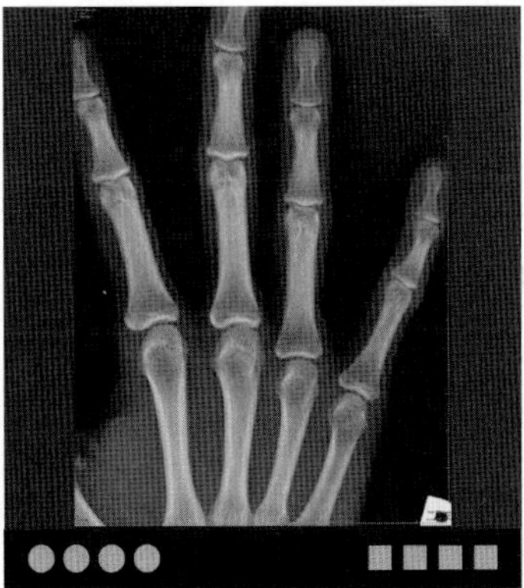

D. Sarcoid: Radiograph of the hand shows granulomatous replacement of normal bony trabecula in the heads of the 2nd through 5th proximal phalanges and 2nd through 4th intermediate phalanges.

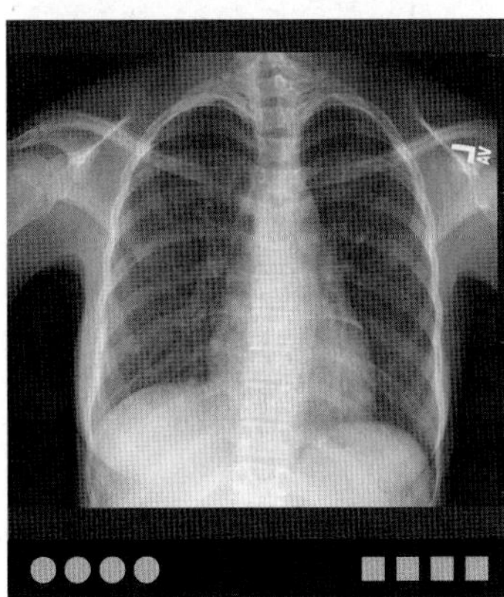

E. Sarcoid: Chest radiograph shows no focal infiltrate, effusion, or significant adenopathy.

IMAGE KEY

Common

Rare

Typical

Unusual

DIFFERENTIAL DIAGNOSES IMAGES

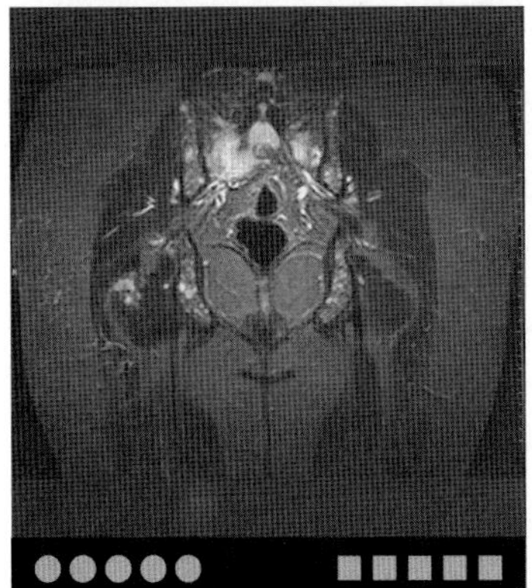

F. Metastatic multiple myeloma: Coronal T2-weighted image shows multiple foci of marrow replacement in the sacrum and in the iliac wings bilaterally.

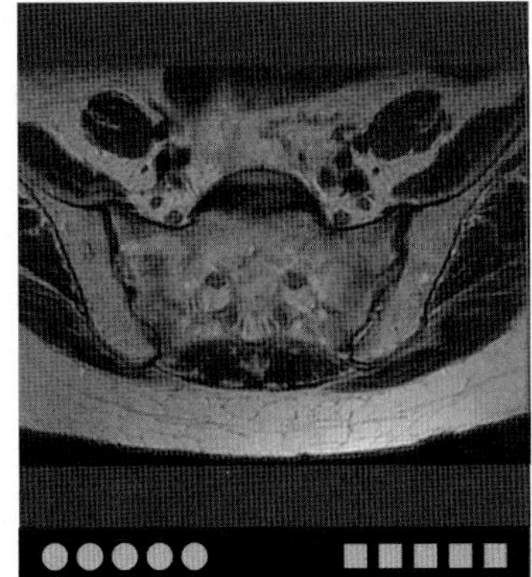

G. Stress fractures in the sacrum: Axial intermediate weighted image shows abnormal marrow signal confined to the sacrum.

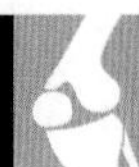

18–5 Rickets with Slipped Capital Femoral Epyphysis

Peyman Borghei and Jamshid Tehranzadeh

PRESENTATION

Generalized bone pain

FINDINGS

MR image shows widening and increased T2 signal of the physis of femoral head and neck junction bilaterally. Note the bilateral slippage of the capital femoral epiphysis.

DIFFERENTIAL DIAGNOSES

- *Slipped capital femoral epiphysis (SCFE) secondary to salter type I fracture:* Posttraumatic or poststress fracture of physis of the femoral head and neck junction.
- *Osteogenesis imperfecta:* Blue sclera, abnormal dentine and diffuse bony osteoporosis, deficient trabecular structure, cortical thinning, and multiple fractures are characteristic of this disease.
- *Scurvy:* Characteristic appearance is ground glass osteoporosis. Sclerotic ring around the epiphysis indicating severe osteoporosis of the epiphysis outlined by white cortical margin (Wimberger ring) and subperiosteal hematoma.
- *Hyperparathyroidism:* Subperiosteal, intracortical, and endocortical bone resorption is evident.

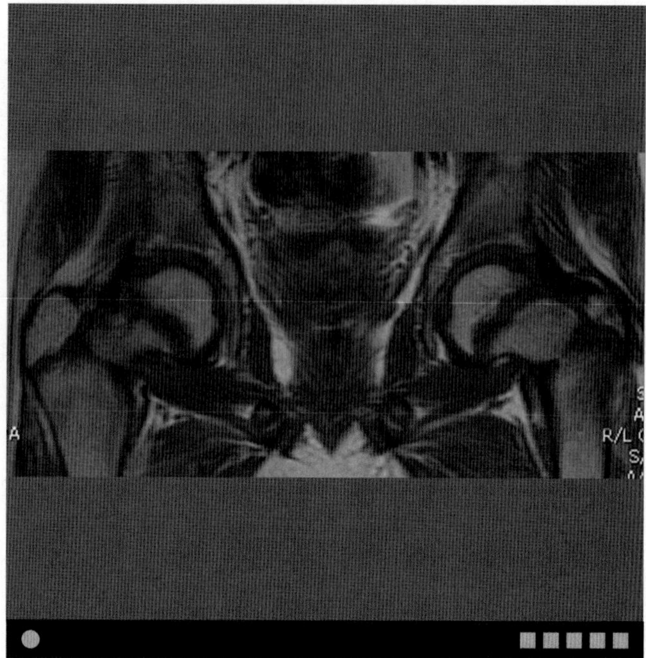

A. Rickets with SCFE: Coronal T1-weighted image of the pelvis shows widening of the physis of the head and neck junction bilaterally. Note bilateral SCFE.

COMMENTS

The patient is a 13-year-old boy with the history of generalized bone pain diagnosed with rickets. Radiographs show failure of ossification and metaphyseal widening with irregularities. Rickets is a disorder caused by deficiency of vitamin D or its active metabolite 1, 25-dihydroxy cholecalciferol leading to abnormal mineralization of bones, especially at the metaphyses of long bones. This is associated with abnormal cartilaginous growth, lacking calcium deposition and endochondral ossification. The radiographic features of rickets are most prominent at the junction of metaphyseal bone and cartilage, showing lack of ossification and physeal widening and decreased density on radiograph in the zone of provisional calcification. There is usually cupping, fraying, and brushing of metaphysis with threadlike shadows into epiphyseal cartilage in weight bearing bones. Coarse trabeculation (not ground-glass pattern as seen in scurvy) may be seen. In comparison with the normal age and sex group, the physeal cartilage is at least 50% wider. Deformities such as bowing of soft diaphysis, molding of epiphysis, and fractures are common. MRI shows the unossified cartilage as high signal intensity on T2-weighted image, which can be easily distinguished from the lower signal intensity of the epiphyseal cartilage. Also wide physis of the secondary ossification center and absence of zone of provisional center can be seen. Associated findings include SCFE and pathologic fractures with periosteal reaction and bone marrow edema.

PEARLS

- **Radiographic manifestations of rickets include widening of the physeal cartilage (at least more than 50% of the normal age and sex), secondary to lack of ossification in provisional zone of calcification.**
- **Radiographic appearances include metaphyseal cupping and fraying.**
- **Typical MR features of rickets are widened physis with increased T2 signal, absence of zone of provisional center, and similar changes at the periphery of the secondary ossification centers.**

ADDITIONAL IMAGES

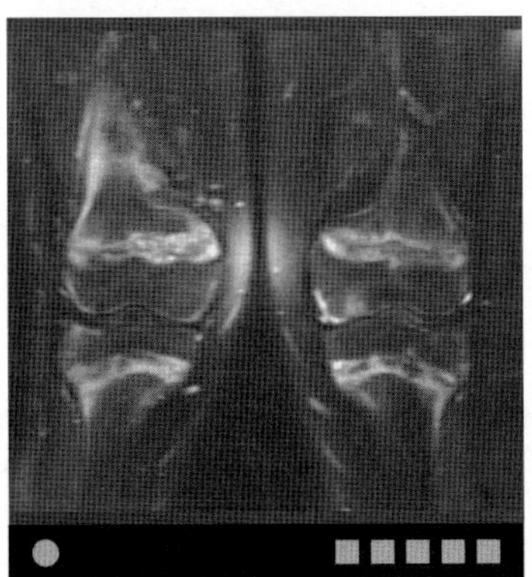

B. Rickets: Coronal T2-weighted fat-saturated image of the knees shows increased signal in the physis bilaterally. Also, note possible fracture of the right distal femur and bone marrow edema along with periosteal reaction.

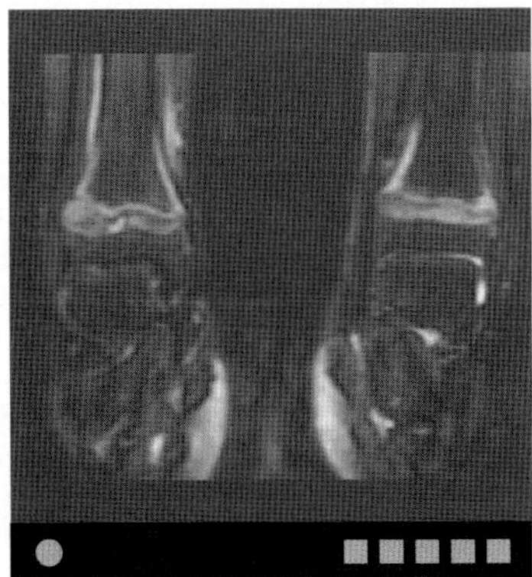

C. Rickets: Coronal T2-weighted fat-saturated image of the ankles shows bilateral increased signal intensity in the distal tibial physis.

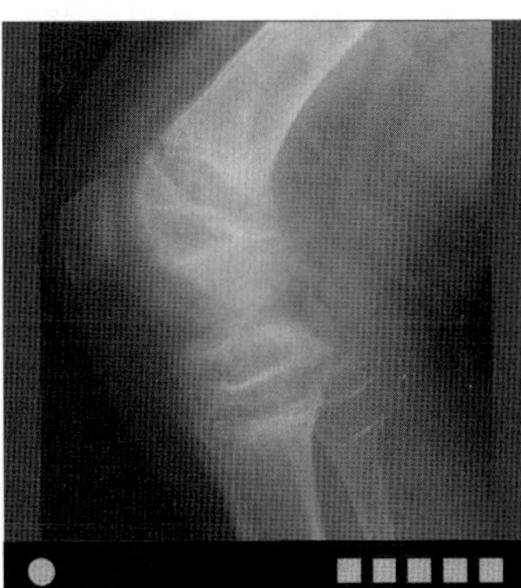

D. Rickets: Lateral knee radiograph shows demineralization of bones with widening of the physis at the distal femur and proximal tibia and fibula.

E. Rickets: AP radiograph of the right ankle shows demineralization of bones with distal physeal widening of tibia and fibula.

IMAGE KEY

Common

Rare

Typical

Unusual

DIFFERENTIAL DIAGNOSES IMAGES

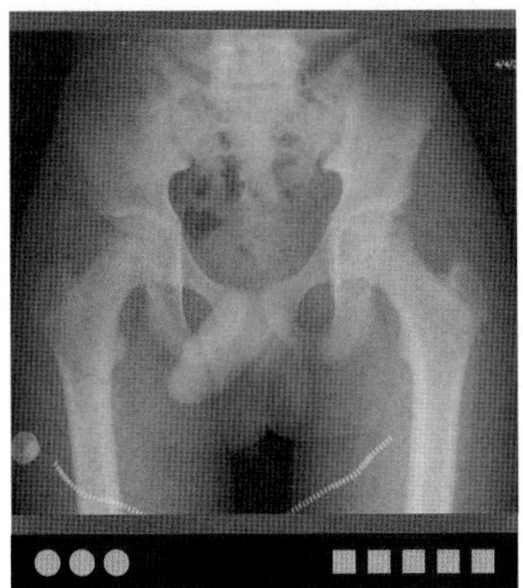

F. SCFE: AP radiograph of the pelvis demonstrates subtle widening of the right proximal femoral physis and subtle displacement of the femoral capital epiphysis caused by stress related type I Salter fracture.

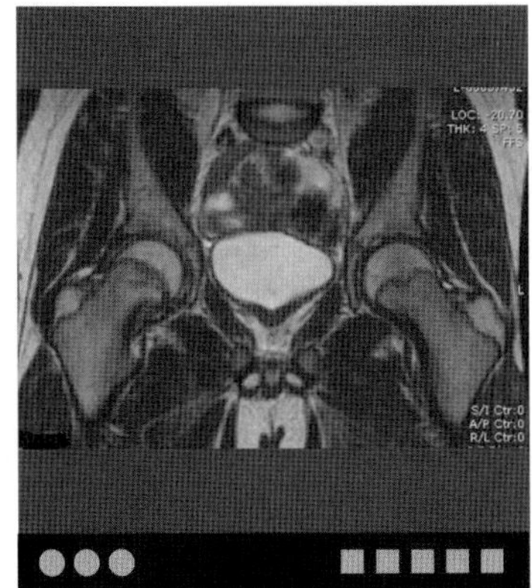

G. SCFE: Coronal T2 MR (same patient as image F) shows the widened right proximal femoral physis and the posterior and inferior slippage of the femoral capital epiphysis.

Chapter 19

Arthritis, Connective Tissue and Crystal Deposition Disorders

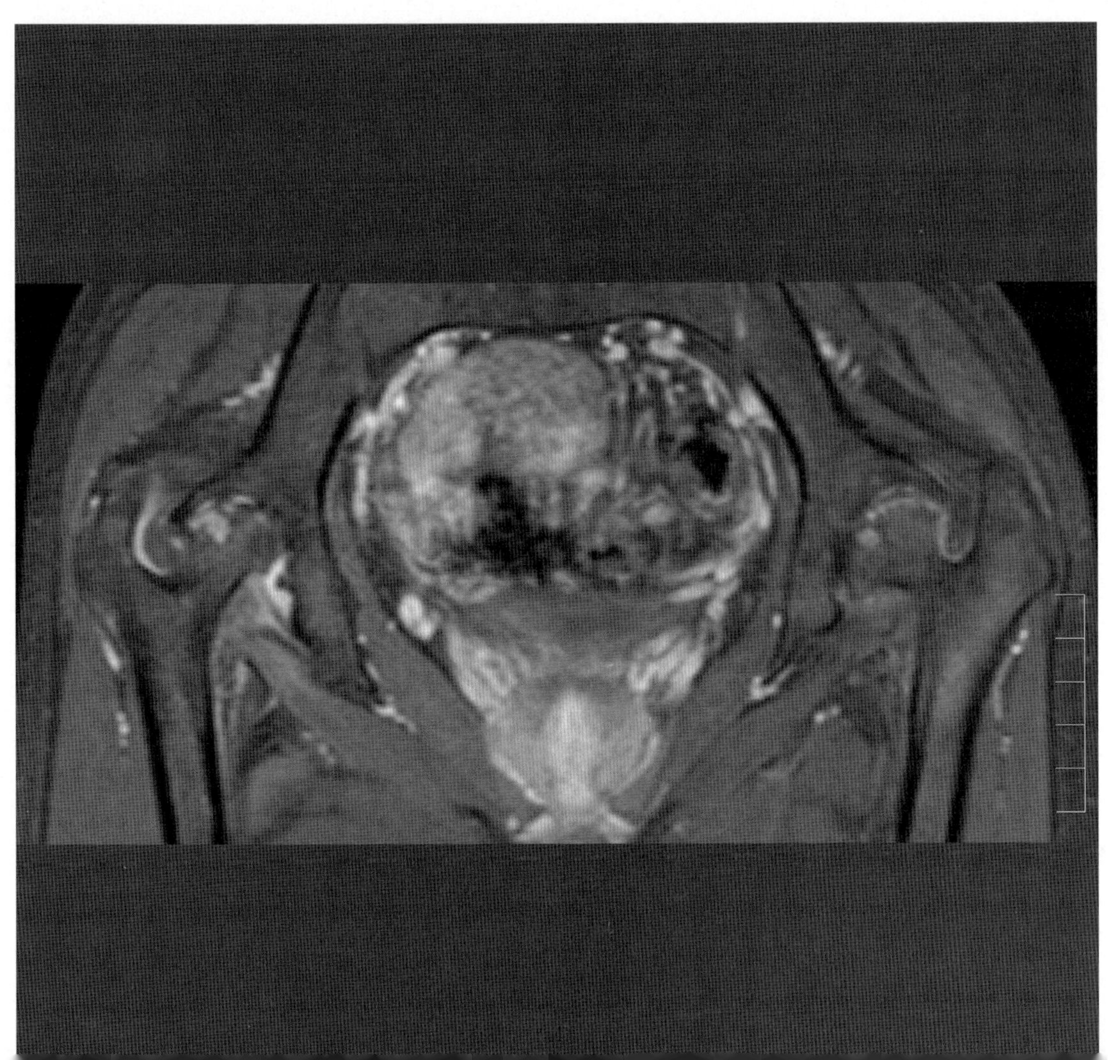

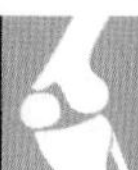

19–1 Juvenile Rheumatoid Arthritis of the Hip

Peyman Borghei and John Shin

PRESENTATION

Hip pain and stiffness

FINDINGS

MRI shows extensive erosions on both femoral head and neck with bilateral effusion. Subchondral cysts and erosions are also seen on the acetabulum.

DIFFERENTIAL DIAGNOSES

- *Hemophilic arthritis:* There may be hemosiderin deposits present, which have low signal on MRI. There is history of hemophilia.
- *Seronegative spondyloarthropathy:* Sacroiliac joint is involved and the involvement of the peripheral joints is usually asymmetric.
- *Osteoarthritis:* Superior-lateral joint narrowing is associated with osteophytes, bony sclerosis and subchondral cysts.
- *Rheumatoid arthritis:* The small joints of the hand and wrist are involved.

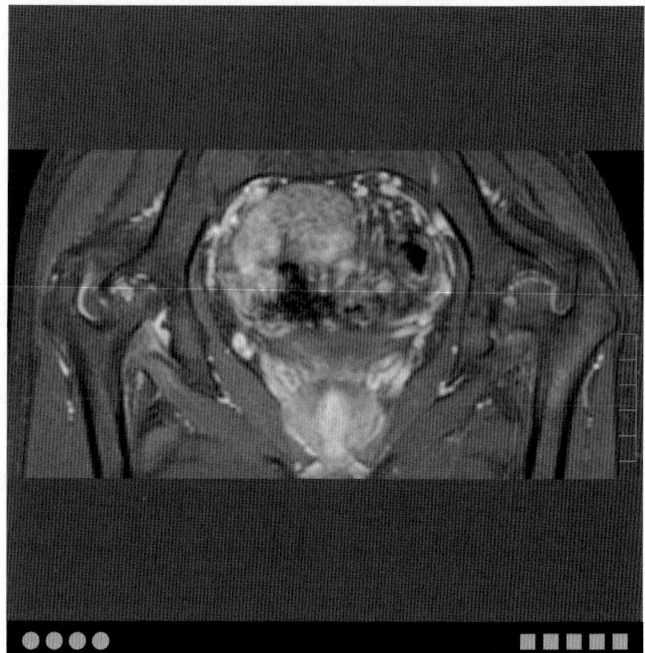

A. Juvenile rheumatoid arthritis: Coronal T1-weighted fat-saturated post contrast image shows extensive erosion of the both femoral heads and acetabula. Typical foreshortening of the femoral necks bilaterally is noted. Contrast enhancement of the inflamed synovium and pannus erosion are also seen.

COMMENTS

The patient is an 18-year-old male with the complaint of hip pain and stiffness during weight-bearing activity diagnosed with juvenile rheumatoid arthritis (JRA). JRA is the most common chronic arthritis in children and can be characterized as arthritis that causes persistent joint inflammation and stiffness for more than 6 weeks. In contrast to adult rheumatoid arthritis, JRA mainly affects the large joints such as knees, wrists, ankles, and hips rather than small joints. It is usually associated with growth disturbances. Besides pain and limited motion, other clinical symptoms of JRA in the hip joint include: thigh or posterior knee pain, limping, altered gait, and difficulty climbing stairs or standing up. JRA begins as acute synovitis that becomes chronic, eventually leading to synovial proliferation and formation of pannus. Pannus erodes the cartilage and the bone at the femoral head. Acute inflamed pannus is seen as hyperintense to the joint effusion on post contrast T1-weighted and hypointense on T2-weighted images. Contrast enhancement of pannus is rapid and prominent; however, it is slower and modest for the synovial effusion; thus, helping to differentiate these two structures. Radiological signs are similar to rheumatoid arthritis (except for involvement of large joints, late onset of bony changes, wide metaphyses, and joint fusion). Other findings may include: subchondral cysts, erosions, joint space narrowing, sclerosis, and subluxation in more extreme cases. Soft tissue manifestations include bursitis, tenosynovitis, and rupture of tendons and ligaments.

PEARLS

- **JRA, a common chronic arthritis in children, can be characterized as arthritis that causes persistent joint inflammation and stiffness for more than 6 weeks.**
- **In contrast to adult rheumatoid arthritis, JRA mainly affects the large joints such as knees, wrists, ankles, and hips rather than smaller joints.**
- **Acute inflamed pannus is seen as hyperintense to the joint effusion on post contrast T1-weighted and hypointense on T2-weighted images.**
- **Radiographic manifestations include joint effusions, marginal erosion, thinning of the cartilage, and juxta-articular osteoporosis.**

ADDITIONAL IMAGES

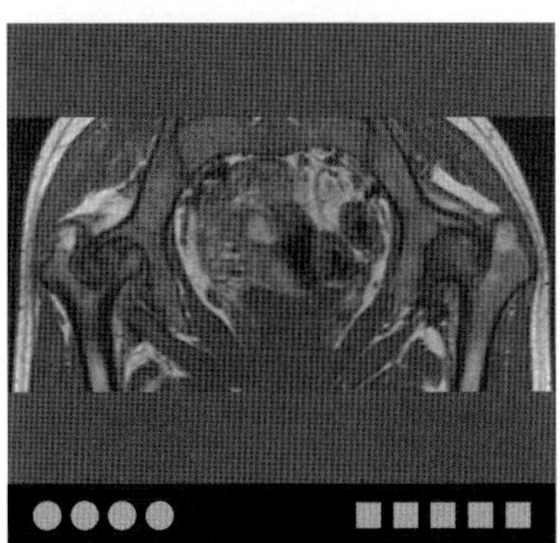

B. Juvenile rheumatoid arthritis: Coronal T1-weighted image shows foci of decreased signal intensity in the femoral head and neck due to marrow edema and bone erosion.

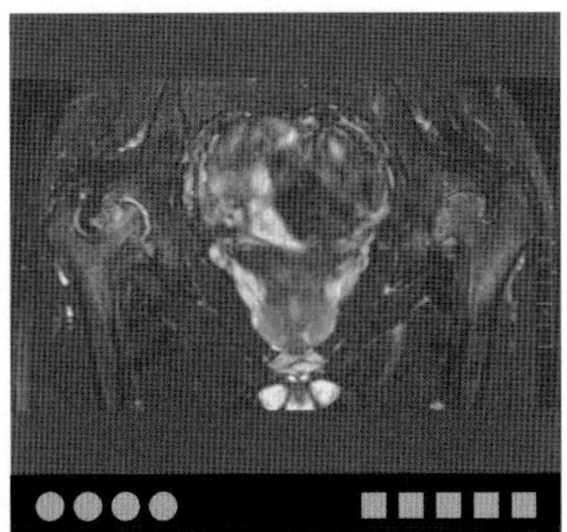

C. Juvenile rheumatoid arthritis: Coronal T2-weighted fat-saturated image shows marrow edema in both femoral head and neck. The effusion and erosions appear bright and they are more prominent on the right hip than the left.

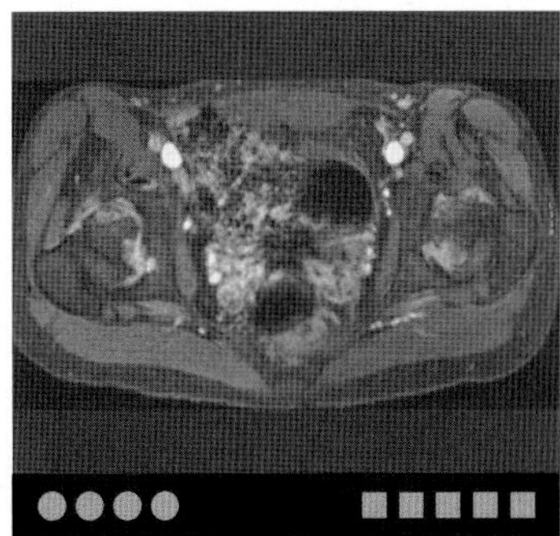

D. Juvenile rheumatoid arthritis: Axial T1-weighted fat-saturated post contrast image shows bilateral foci of contrast enhancement of the both femoral heads and acetabula representing pannus formation and erosions.

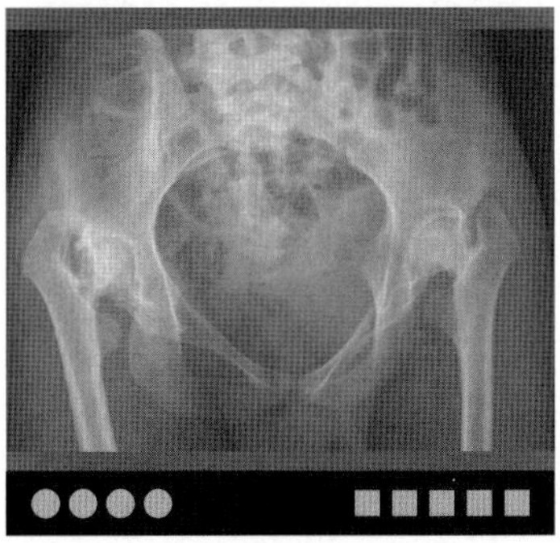

E. Juvenile rheumatoid arthritis: AP radiograph of the pelvis shows erosive changes of the both head and neck and typical foreshortening of the femoral necks bilaterally. There is also concentric narrowing of both hip joints.

DIFFERENTIAL DIAGNOSES IMAGES

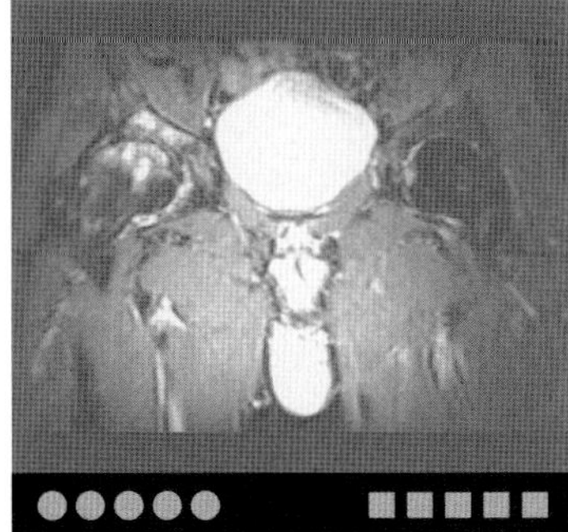

F. Osteoarthritis of hip: Coronal STIR image of the hip joints shows superior-lateral joint narrowing with fluid in the joint, bone marrow edema with subchondral cysts in the right femoral head, and acetabulum indicative of osteoarthritis.

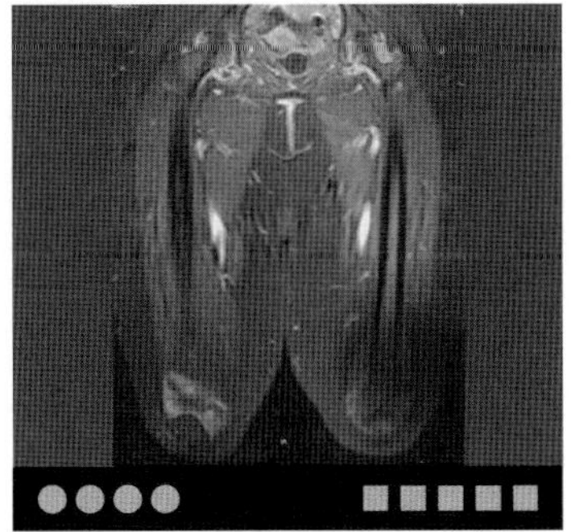

G. Adult rheumatoid arthritis: Coronal T1-weighted fat-saturated post contrast image shows narrowing of the hip joints, with synovial proliferation and bone erosion of the femoral head and neck on the left, and bone erosions in the femoral head on the right. Synovial proliferation and enhancement of the knee joints are also noted.

IMAGE KEY

Common

Rare

Typical

Unusual

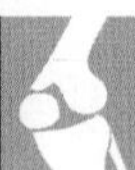

19–2 Septic Arthritis and Osteomyelitis of Symphysis Pubis

Mohammad Reza Hayeri and Jamshid Tehranzadeh

PRESENTATION

Bacteremia and abscess

FINDINGS

MRI reveals septic symphysis pubis joint with osteomyelitis and abscesses formation.

DIFFERENTIAL DIAGNOSES

- *Osteitis pubis:* This is a sterile, inflammatory often self-limited condition of symphysis pubis occurring after trauma, pregnancy, or gynecologic and urologic surgery, and is a relatively common condition in athletes.
- *Spondyloarthropathy:* Conditions such as psoriatic arthritis and ankylosing spondylitis may be associated with inflammatory changes of symphysis pubis.
- *Hyperparathyroidism:* May be associated with widening of symphysis pubis as a result of bone resorption.
- *Osteoarthritis:* Posttraumatic dislocation or subluxation of symphysis may result in osteoarthritis of this joint.

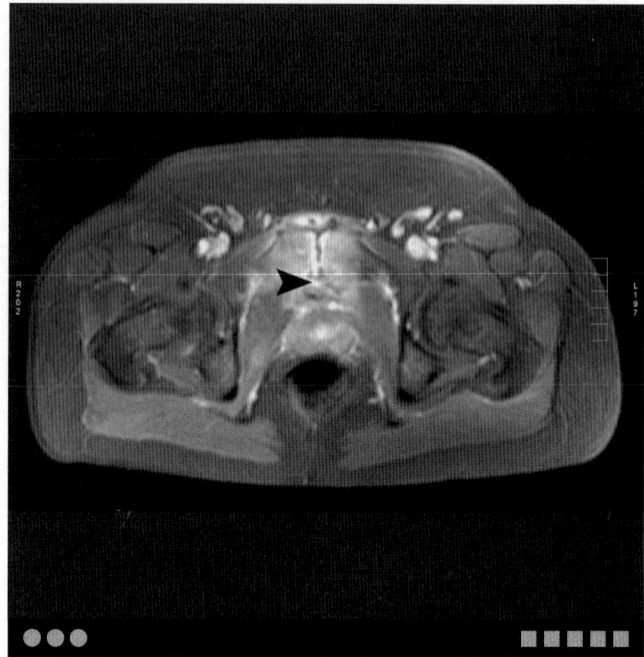

A. Septic arthritis and osteomyelitis of symphysis pubis: Axial T1-weighted, fat-saturated, postcontrast image shows enhancement of both pubic bones. The fluid is seen as dark signal at symphysis pubis with a retro pubic abscess (arrowhead).

COMMENTS

The patient is a 47-year-old man with bacteremia and several abscesses. Septic arthritis of the symphysis pubis is a rare disease and because of its insidious and low clinical suspicion is not usually diagnosed early. Septic arthritis of the symphysis pubis usually presents with pubic pain. The pain, because of the insertion of hip adductors on the pubic bones, can also localize to groin, thigh, and hip. Many cases of osteomyelitis of symphysis pubis are wrongly diagnosed as osteitis pubis, which is a sterile, inflammatory condition of the pubis occurring after trauma, pregnancy, or rheumatic disorders in athletes or gynecologic and urologic surgery. Septic arthritis of the pubis and osteitis pubis can appear in one patient at the same time. Inflammation from preexisting osteitis pubis may predispose to septic arthritis of the symphysis pubis, if transient staphylococcal bacteremia occurs. For unknown reason, intravenous drug users and patients with pelvic surgery are more prone to septic arthritis of the pubic symphysis. Delay in diagnosis and treatment may lead to pelvic instability, pubic diastasis, and even urinary bladder perforation. The radiographic features include mild to moderate subchondral bony irregularity of the symphysis pubis with resorption. A whole body bone scintigraphy will show hyperactivity at the pubis. On MRI, decreased marrow signal of the inflamed pubic bone on T1, and high signal on T2-weighted images could be seen. Fluid is detected in septic joint as a bright signal, while same fluid has dark signal on T1 and T1 fat-saturated postcontrast images.

PEARLS

- **Many cases of osteomyelitis of symphysis pubis are wrongly diagnosed as osteitis pubis, which is a sterile, inflammatory condition of the pubis.**
- **Intravenous drug users and patients with pelvic surgery are more prone to septic arthritis of the pubic symphysis.**
- **The radiographic features include mild to moderate subchondral bony irregularity of the symphysis pubis with resorption.**
- **On MRI, decreased marrow signal of the inflamed pubic bone on T1, and high signal on T2-weighted images could be seen.**

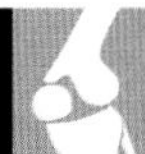

ADDITIONAL IMAGES

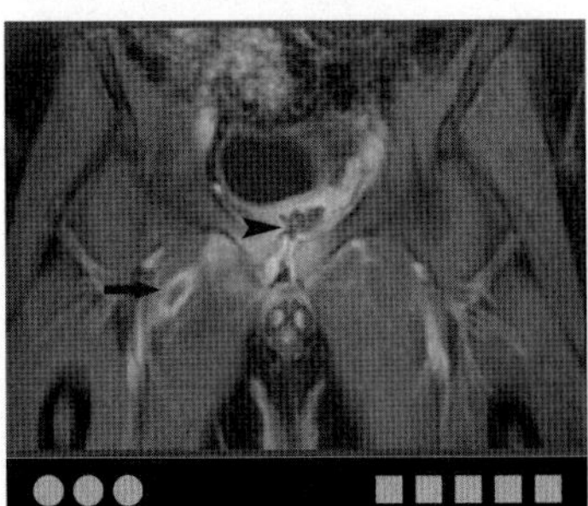

B. Septic arthritis and osteomyelitis of symphysis pubis: Coronal T1-weighted fat-saturated, postcontrast image, of the same patient as in image A, shows enhancement of both pubic bones. The fluid is seen as low signal at symphysis pubis with a retro pubic abscess (arrowhead) and as an intermediate signal in pectineus muscle with representing abscess (arrow).

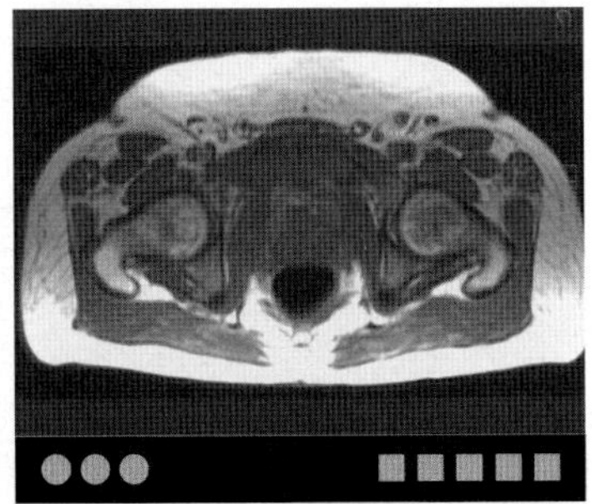

C. Septic arthritis and osteomyelitis of symphysis pubis: Axial T1-weighted image of the same patient (as in images A and B) shows decreased marrow signal of the inflamed pubic bone on both sides.

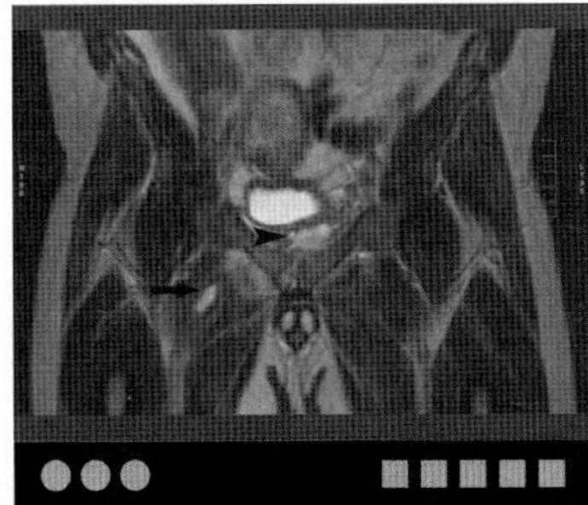

D. Septic arthritis and osteomyelitis of symphysis pubis: Coronal T2-weighted image of the same patient (as in images A to C) shows fluid in the symphysis pubis. Suprapubic (arrowhead) and pectineus abscesses (arrow) are also seen. Note erosion of the right pubic bone at the symphysis pubis

E. Septic arthritis and osteomyelitis of symphysis pubis: Coronal T2-weighted image of the same patient (as in images A to D) shows fluid in the symphysis pubis. Suprapubic (arrow) and pectineus abscesses (arrowhead) are also seen. Note erosion of the right pubic bone at the symphysis pubis

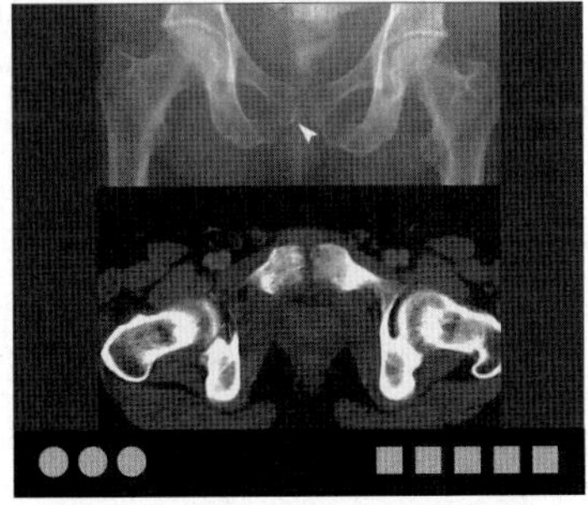

F. Septic arthritis and osteomyelitis of symphysis pubis: AP radiograph and CT examination of the same patient (as in images A to E) shows erosion of the right pubic bone at the symphysis pubis. Note sclerotic and necrotic cortex at the right pubic bone (arrowhead)

IMAGE KEY

Common

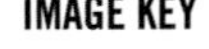

Rare

Typical

Unusual

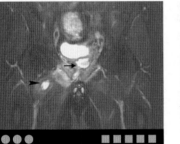

DIFFERENTIAL DIAGNOSIS IMAGE

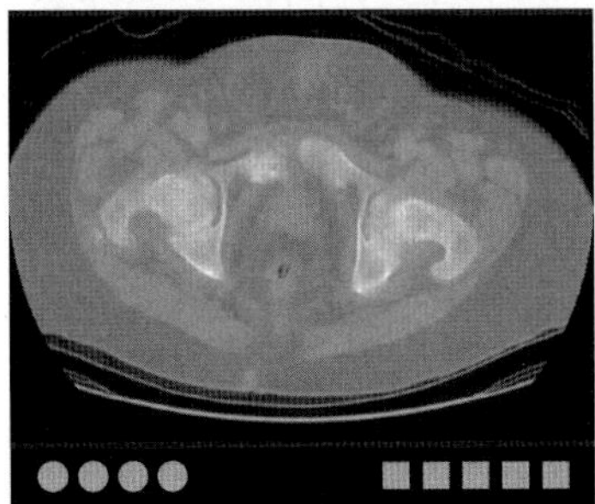

G. Hyperparathyroidism: Axial CT image demonstrates subchondral resorption, commonly seen about the symphysis pubis in hyperparathyroidism.

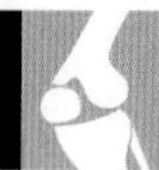

19–3 Sacroiliitis in Inflammatory Bowel Disease

Gideon Strich

PRESENTATION

Back pain

FINDINGS

MRI shows erosion and sacroiliitis of left sacroiliac joint with bone marrow edema on both sides of the sacroiliac joint.

DIFFERENTIAL DIAGNOSES

- *Ankylosing spondylitis:* Sacroiliac joint arthritis progresses to bony ankylosis. Vertebral body involvement is most common with progressive ankylosis to "bamboo" spine. The hip and shoulder are also commonly involved.
- *Septic sacroiliitis:* May be seen in patients with inflammatory bowel disease caused by salmonella or other infection. It is often unilateral and may occur spontaneously in other patients as a result of contiguous or hematogenous spread.
- *Insufficiency fracture of the sacrum:* The sacrum is a common location for insufficiency fractures in postmenopausal women, but also in athletes, particularly long distance runners.

COMMENTS

This young man with a history of Crohn's disease presented with back pain. As many as 10% to 20% of the patients with inflammatory bowel disease develop chronic arthropathy. The most common sites of involvement are the knees and ankles, followed by the joints of the arm and the small joints of the extremities. Episodes of arthritis are intermittent and may coexist or predate bowel symptoms. Permanent joint deformity is unusual however. Sacroiliac joint disease is common in patients with Crohn's disease with equal frequency in men and women. Approximately 50% of patients with Crohn's disease who develop sacroiliitis have a positive HLA-B27 antigen. In fact, the sacroiliac and spine manifestations may be indistinguishable from ankylosing spondylitis. Involvement may be unilateral initially, or bilateral, and is characterized by edema and erosions centered on the sacroiliac joint. The disease may progress to bony fusion of the sacroiliac joints. Involvement of the spine is not uncommon with marginal erosions and sclerosis, and eventually the classic bamboo spine. Infectious sacroiliitis has been reported although this may be a result of psoas abscesses, which may occur in up to 5% of patients with Crohn's disease. Spondyloarthropathies such as psoriatic arthritis, reactive arthritides, and pseudogout may present unilateral or bilateral sacroiliitis; however, they often show asymmetrical involvement.

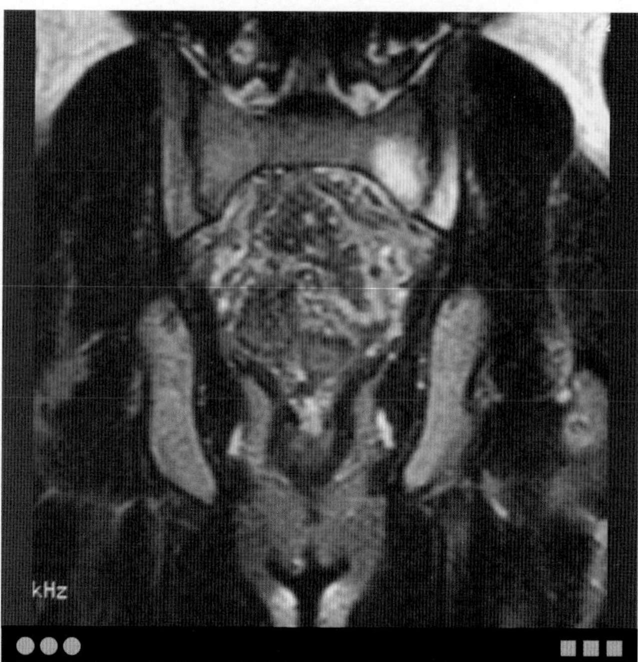

A. Inflammatory bowel disease: Coronal T2-weighted image shows sacroiliitis with erosion of the left sacroiliac joint.

PEARLS

- **Arthropathy is seen in 10% to 20% of patients with inflammatory bowel disease.**
- **The most common joints involved are the knees and ankles followed by joints of the arms. Findings may be unilateral or bilateral and are usually intermittent without permanent deformity.**
- **HLA-B27 antigen is positive in 50% of Crohn's patients with sacroiliitis. Radiographic findings may be indistinguishable from ankylosing spondylitis.**
- **Sacroiliitis may result from bacterial etiology and may be associated with psoas abscess.**

ADDITIONAL IMAGES

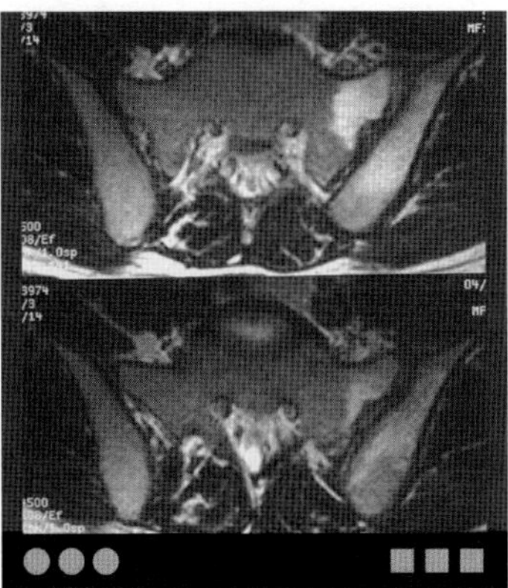

B. Inflammatory bowel disease: Axial T2-weighted fast spin echo images show unilateral sacroiliitis with edema on both sides of the joint.

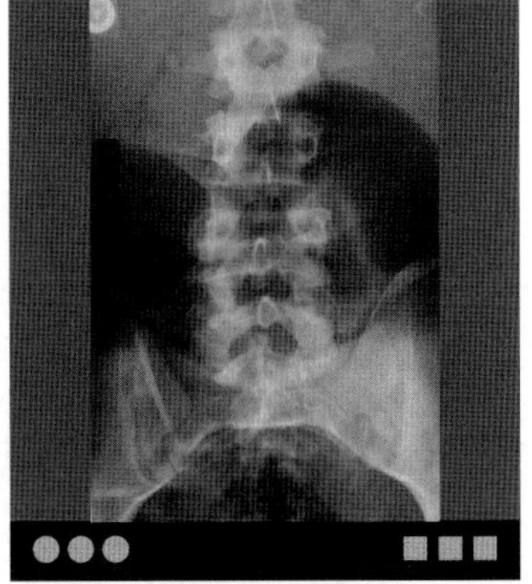

C. Inflammatory bowel disease: AP radiograph shows sclerosis and erosion of the left sacroiliac joint. Note surgical sutures in the abdomen from previous bowel resection.

DIFFERENTIAL DIAGNOSES IMAGES

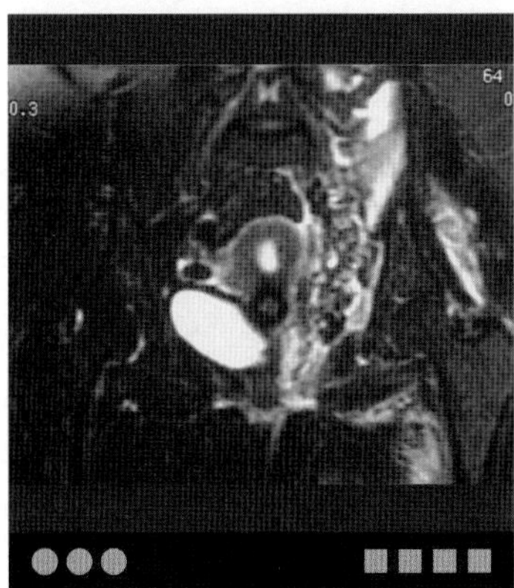

D. Infectious sacroiliitis: Coronal inversion recovery sequence demonstrates edema of the left side of the sacrum and adjacent soft tissues.

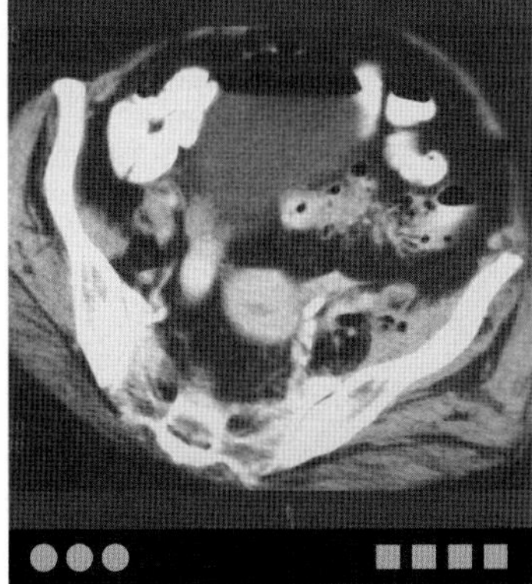

E. Infectious sacroiliitis: CT scan shows psoas abscess with fluid and air pockets adjacent to the left sacroiliac joint.

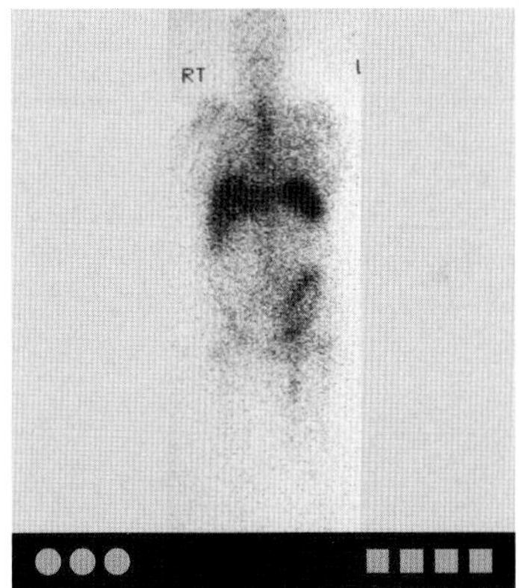

F. Infectious sacroiliitis: Radionuclide white blood cell scan shows uptake in the left sacroiliac joint and in the adjacent psoas abscess.

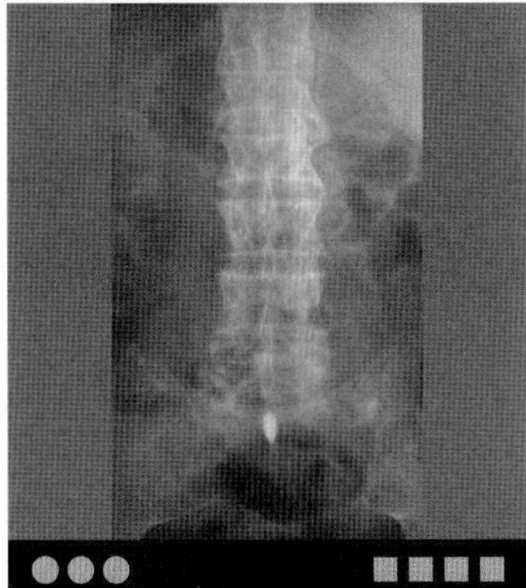

G. Ankylosing spondylitis: Late findings of ankylosing spondylitis include complete fusion of the sacroiliac joints. Note the bony ankylosis of the thoracolumbar spine.

IMAGE KEY

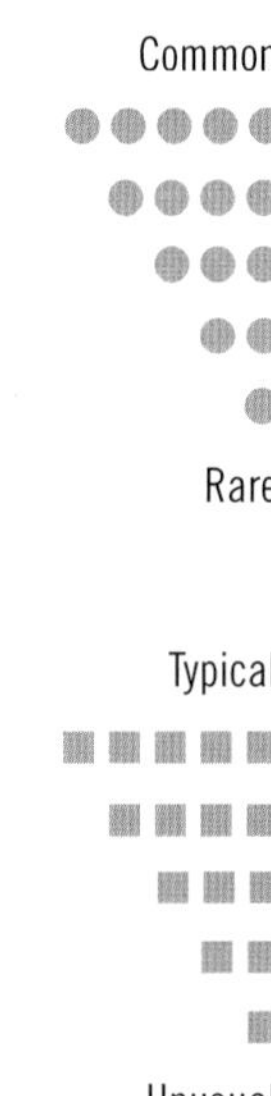

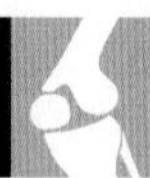

19–4 Dialysis-Related Amyloidosis

Christopher Lee and Peyman Borghei

PRESENTATION

Left hip pain

FINDINGS

MRI shows a 1.4 cm focal area of low signal intensity on T1-weighted and low to intermediate signal on T2-weighted images in the articular surface of the left femoral head and lateral acetabular margin.

DIFFERENTIAL DIAGNOSES

- *Pigmented villonodular synovitis (PVNS):* PVNS has similar MR characteristics as amyloid deposits. In contrast to dialysis-related amyloidosis (DRA), PVNS is commonly a monoarticular disease.
- *Gouty arthritis:* Gouty tophi deposition in and around the joint has similar signal intensity to amyloid.
- *Osteoarthritis:* The primary pathology is in articular cartilage, leading to joint narrowing, osteophyte formation, subchondral sclerosis, and cystic changes.
- *Brown tumor:* Patients with renal osteodystrophy on dialysis may develop intraosseous lytic changes of brown tumor; however, amyloid depositions are often at the enthesis.

COMMENTS

The patient is a 68-year-old female with end-stage renal disease on hemodialysis presenting with left hip pain of 1-month duration diagnosed with amyloidosis. DRA, a disorder characterized by tissue deposition of beta 2-microglobulin, develops in long-term dialysis patients and incidence is closely related to years of treatment. Renal clearance of beta 2-microglobulin, the light chain of the HLA class I complex, normally occurs by free glomerular filtration with subsequent reabsorption and catabolism in the proximal tubules. Because of reduced clearance in the end-stage renal disease and incomplete filtration with hemodialysis, the fibrils formed from beta 2-microglobulins undergo nonenzymatic modification to form advanced glycation end products (AGEs) and deposit preferentially in bone and tenosynovial tissue. DRA is associated with large and small joint symptoms, erosive spondyloarthropathies, bony cysts, carpal tunnel syndrome, and pathologic fractures especially involving the femoral neck. Amyloid deposits have tendency to collect at enthesis. On radiograph, early changes may be impossible to distinguish from osteoarthritis. Distinguishing features on radiograph include subchondral bone cysts, most commonly involving the acetabulum, carpal bones and distal radius and ulna. Magnetic resonance imaging may reveal diffuse synovial thickening with intra-articular deposition of amyloid. Amyloid deposits demonstrate low to intermediate signal intensity on both T1-weighted and T2-weighted sequences, although high signal intensity is often present on T2-weighted sequences with focal fluid collections. Following administration of gadolinium contrast, lesions demonstrate peripheral enhancement.

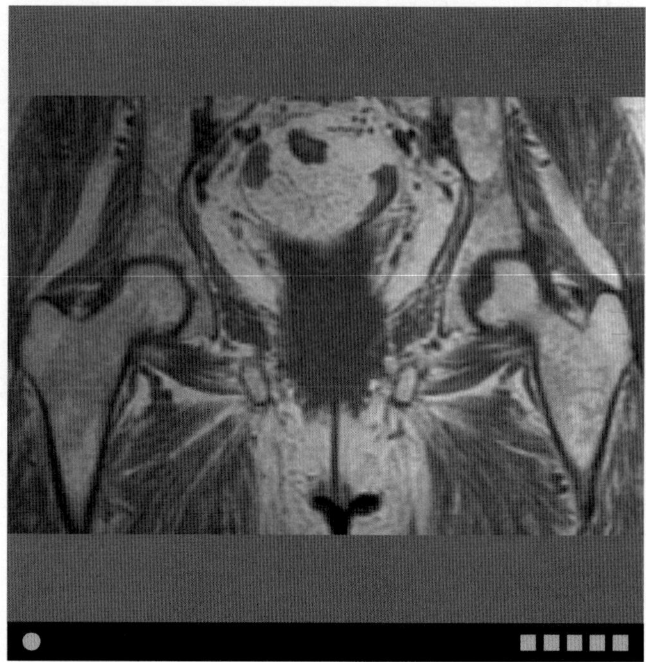

A. Dialysis-related amyloidosis: Coronal T1-weighted image shows a low signal intensity lesion in the articular surface of the left femoral head at approximately 10 o'clock position and another focus at lateral acetabular margin.

PEARLS

- **Amyloid deposits as a result of ESRD usually manifest with large and small joint disease and erosive spondyloarthropathies.**
- **Magnetic resonance imaging typically reveals low to intermediate signal intensity of amyloid deposits on both T1-weighted and T2-weighted images.**
- **High signal intensity from focal fluid collections is often present on T2 sequences.**
- **Amyloid deposits show moderate peripheral enhancement in post contrast sequences.**

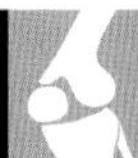

ADDITIONAL IMAGES

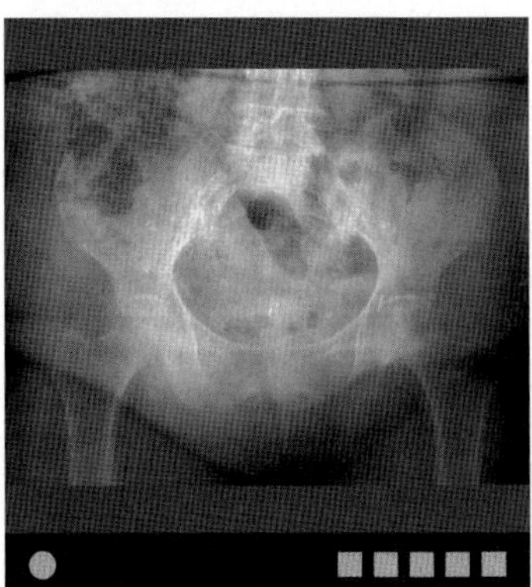

B. Dialysis-related amyloidosis: Radiograph demonstrates severe osteoporosis and vascular calcifications.

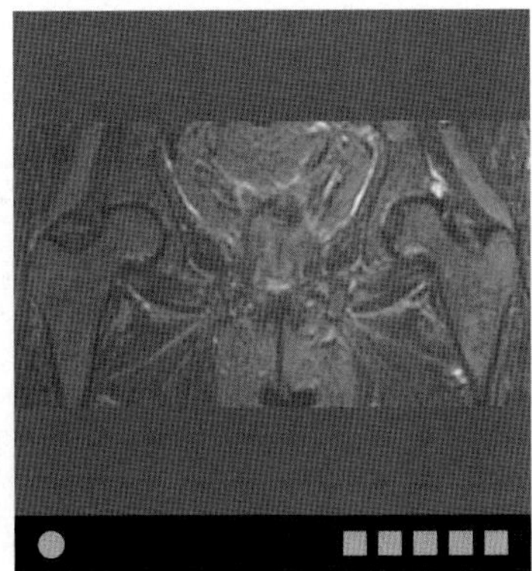

C. Dialysis-related amyloidosis: Coronal T2-weighted image shows the low signal intensity lesion in the articular surface of the left femoral head at approximately 10 o'clock position and mixed bright signal at acetabular margin related to edema with amyloid deposit.

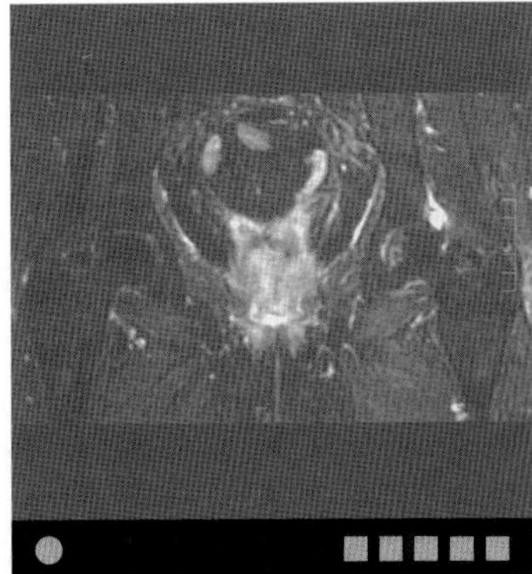

D. Dialysis-related amyloidosis: Coronal T2-weighted fat-saturated image shows an intermediate signal lesion in the articular surface of the left femoral head at approximately 10 o'clock position and a mixed bright focus at acetabular margin related to edema with amyloid deposit.

E. Dialysis-related amyloidosis: Axial T1-weighted image shows two foci of low signal in left femoral head representing amyloid deposits (arrows).

DIFFERENTIAL DIAGNOSIS IMAGES

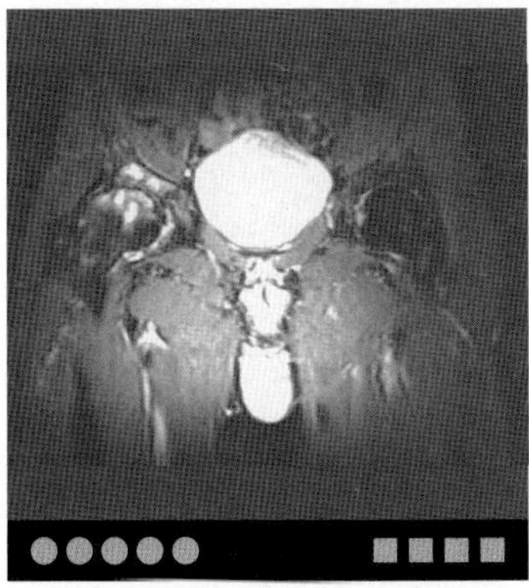

F. Osteoarthritis: STIR image of the hip shows narrowing of the right hip joint with subchondral degenerative cysts and edema of the femoral head and acetabulum.

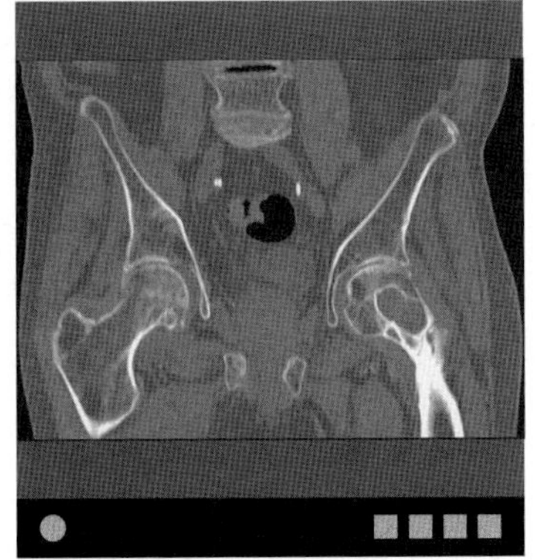

G. Brown tumor: Reformatted CT-Scan of the pelvis shows large lytic lesion at the femoral head and neck on the left side representing brown tumor in another patient with renal osteodystrophy.

IMAGE KEY

Common

Rare

Typical

Unusual

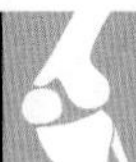

19–5 Calcinosis Cutis Universalis

Kambiz Motamedi

PRESENTATION

Difficulty sitting because of calcified buttock mass

FINDINGS

CT scan shows calcified soft tissue masses of the pelvic area.

DIFFERENTIAL DIAGNOSES

- *Scleroderma with calcinosis cutis:* Radiographs demonstrate calcium deposits along the cutaneous tissue of the fingers.
- *Tumoral calcinosis:* CT scan shows fine diffuse calcifications of the soft tissues
- *Metastatic calcifications:* Cross-sectional imaging reveals dystrophic calcifications of the soft tissues
- *Heterotopic ossification:* Calcified soft tissue mass with characteristic zonal calcification.

COMMENTS

The patient is a 10-year-old boy with difficulty sitting and palpable soft tissue masses of the trunk, pelvis, and extremities. Calcinosis cutis is a term used to describe a group of disorders in which calcium deposits form in the skin. Calcinosis cutis is classified into four major types according to etiology: dystrophic, metastatic, iatrogenic, and idiopathic. A few rare types have been variably classified as dystrophic or idiopathic. These include calcinosis cutis circumscripta, calcinosis cutis universalis (CCU), tumoral calcinosis, and transplant-associated calcinosis cutis. CCU is characterized by the deposit of calcium salts in the skin, subcutaneous tissue, tendons, and muscles. Most cases become apparent during the first decade of life. Clinical aspects may vary from arthralgia to movement limitation, with calcification of soft tissues. Deposition of calcium salts in the skin and subcutaneous tissue occurs in a variety of rheumatic diseases as well, being most commonly associated with scleroderma, CREST (calcinosis, Raynaud phenomenon, esophageal dysfunction, sclerodactyly, and telangiectasia), dermatomyositis, and overlap syndromes, but is a rare complication of systemic lupus erythematosus (SLE). Calcinosis is classified into four subsets: dystrophic, metastatic, idiopathic, or calciphylaxis/iatrogenic. Imaging reveals characteristic sheath-like calcium deposits along the fascia. In advanced cases, there are diffuse calcified soft tissue masses throughout the trunk and extremities sparing the face and skull.

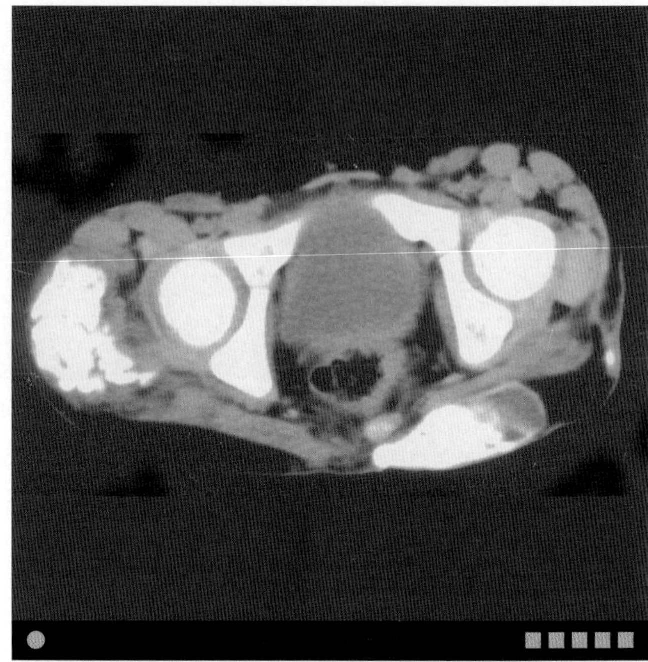

A. Calcinosis cutis universalis: Axial nonenhanced CT scan shows calcified soft tissue masses of the intramuscular and subcutaneous compartments.

PEARLS

- **Sheath-like calcifications along the fascia planes**
- **The calcification affects the extremities, trunk, and pelvis commonly sparing the face and skull**
- **May be associated with rheumatic disease, especially lupus erythematodes as in CREST syndrome.**

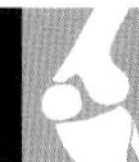

ADDITIONAL IMAGES

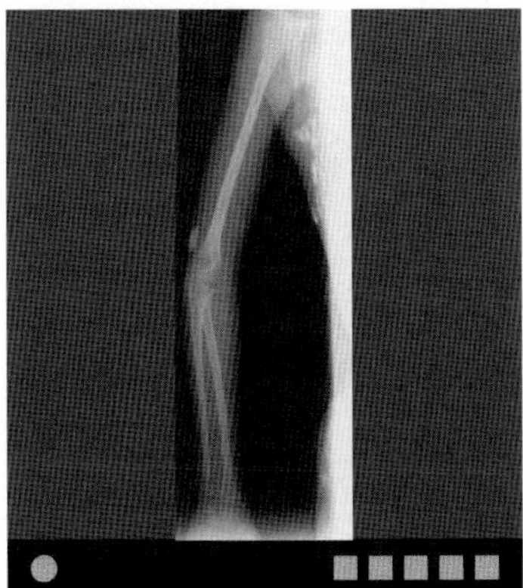

B. Calcinosis cutis universalis: AP radiograph of the upper extremity shows chunk of calcifications along the superficial fascia of the upper arm.

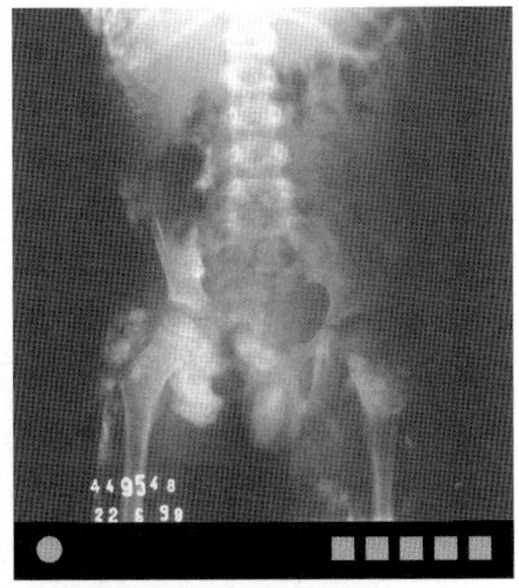

C. Calcinosis cutis universalis: AP radiograph of the trunk demonstrates the extent of the disease affecting the left chest and abdominal wall and bilateral gluteal regions and upper thighs.

DIFFERENTIAL DIAGNOSES IMAGES

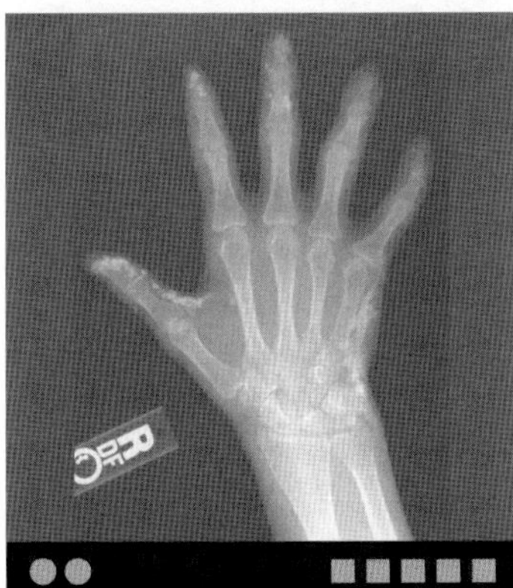

D. Scleroderma with calcinosis cutis: AP radiograph of the hand shows sheaths of calcification along the fingertips and volar aspects. Note the soft tissue wasting of the finger tips.

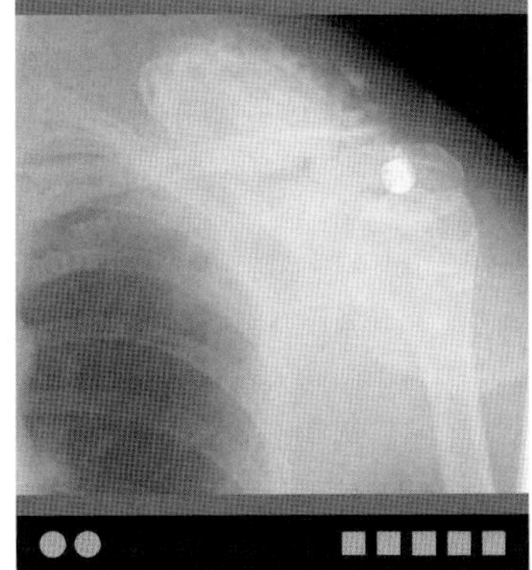

E. Tumoral calcinosis: AP view of the chest coned down to the shoulder shows a cloudy calcified mass of the shoulder.

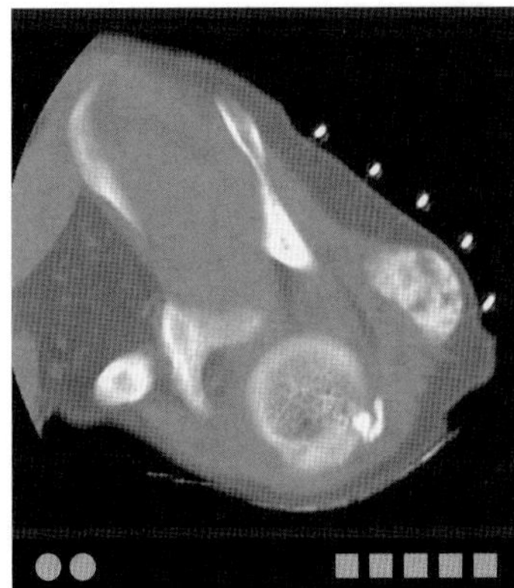

F. Metastatic calcification: Axial CT scan of the shoulder at the level of the humeral head reveals a focus of dystrophic calcification of the soft tissues in a patient with renal disease.

IMAGE KEY

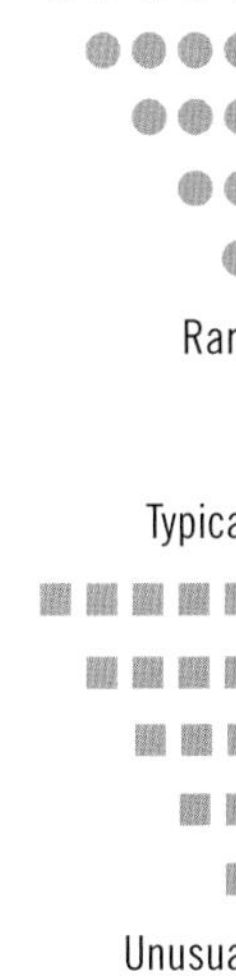

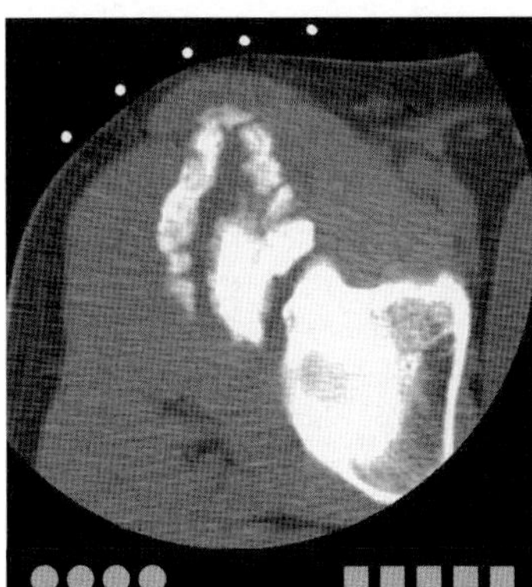

G. Heterotopic ossification: Axial CT scan reveals soft tissue mass of the rectus femoris with characteristic peripheral zonal calcification.

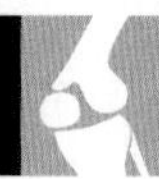

19–6 Tophaceous Calcium Pyrophosphate Deposition Disease (Tophaceous Pseudogout)

Stephen E. Ling and William R. Reinus

PRESENTATION

Asymptomatic to localized pain of acute onset, with swelling and palpable mass

FINDINGS

Cystic erosion(s) and lobulated/lobular calcified soft tissue mass or masses.

DIFFERENTIAL DIAGNOSES

- *Gout:* Negatively birefringent crystals under polarized light.
- *Chondroid tumors:* These have cartilaginous matrix with chondroid calcifications.
- *Giant cell tumor of tendon sheath*: Presents with soft tissue mass with no significant calcifications.
- *Amyloidoma:* These have similar signal changes on MRI, but may occur more at the enthesis.

COMMENTS

Tumoral calcium pyrophosphate dihydrate (CPPD) deposition disease represents a rare presentation of the condition, characterized by the presence of one or more mass-like deposits of CPPD crystals. As with the more typical types of CPPD disease, common areas for tumor-like crystal deposition are the knee, wrist, pelvis such as the pubic symphysis and SI joints, spine, shoulder, and ankle, in descending order of frequency. In addition, tophaceous CPPD disease has been reported in unusual locations such as the TMJ joint, sternoclavicular joint, craniovertebral junction, transverse ligament of C1, infratemporal fossa, facet joints, cubital tunnel, MTP joints, and great toe. The CPPD tumors are often seen near synovial tissue, but are not limited to these areas. Patients may experience sudden onset of acute paint and inflammation, in which, the disease may be confused with gout. In these cases the clinical presentation is known as pseudogout. Weakly positively birefringent rhomboid type/shaped, and rod like crystals under polarized light are characteristics for CPPD in contrast to the negatively birefringent needle shaped crystals of gout. Histopathologically, the tumoral lesions are foreign body inflammatory granulomatous masses with predominance of giant cells. Radiographs typically show one or more cystic osseous erosions and calcifications in both hyaline cartilage and fibrocartilage within the joint space. MRI shows these same erosions as well as the calcifications, which appear as low signal areas on all sequences. In addition, MRI may depict the calcium pyrophosphate based mass or masses that are associated with the erosions.

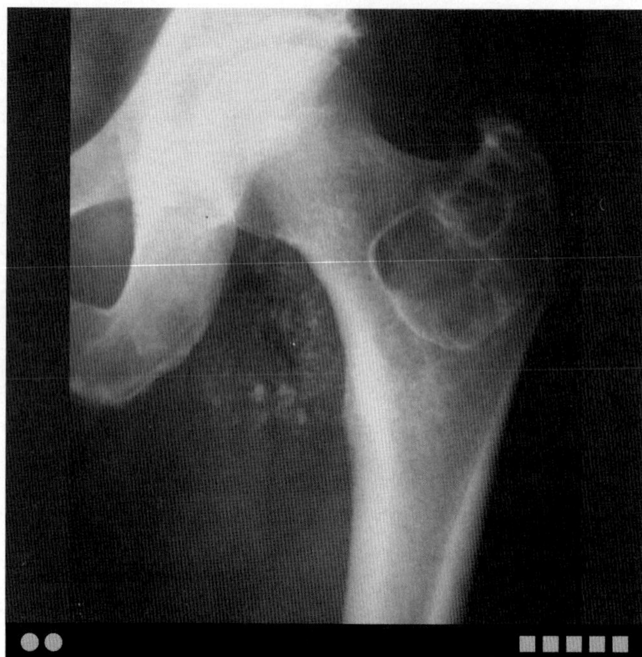

A. Tumoral CPPD deposition disease: AP radiograph of the left hip shows a lytic lesion with thin sclerotic border in the left intertrochanteric region. Note the cluster of calcifications more medially adjacent to the ischium, some of which have a somewhat "flocculent", "rings and arcs" appearance, typically seen in chondroid lesions.

PEARLS

- **Tophaceous pseudogout may be the only manifestation and a solitary, isolated presentation of CPPD disease, without clinical or radiological evidence of disease at other sites.**
- **CPPD calcifications radiographically resemble the "rings and arcs" calcified cartilaginous matrix seen in chondroid tumors such as chondrosarcoma.**
- **Tissue or synovial fluid obtained from fine needle aspiration is sufficient to make the diagnosis of tophaceous CPPD disease in most cases, obviating the need for surgical biopsy.**

ADDITIONAL IMAGES

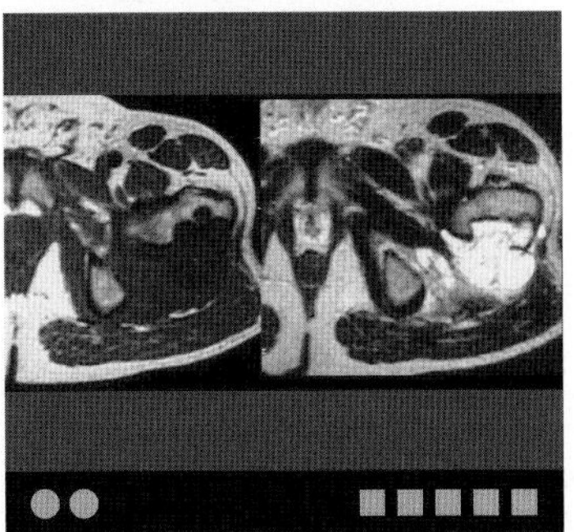

B. Tumoral CPPD deposition disease: Axial T1-weighted image and T2-weighted image show a T1 hypointense and very T2 hyperintense lobulated mass in the posterior soft tissues of the left hip with remodeling of the posterior proximal femur. Note the thin T1 and T2 hypointensity at the margin of the mass indicating sclerosis.

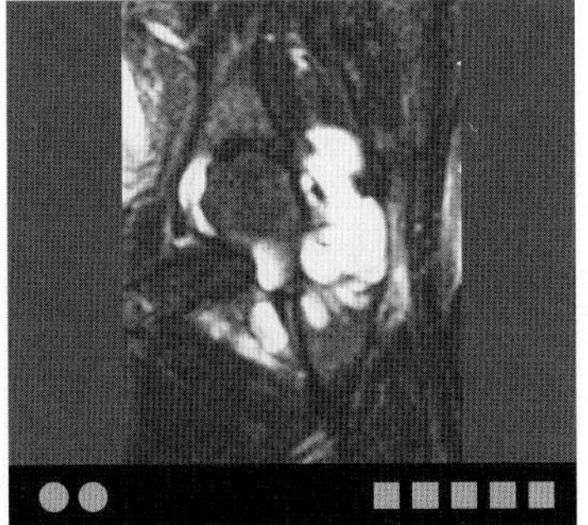

C. Tumoral CPPD deposition disease: Coronal short T1 inversion recovery (STIR) image demonstrates the extensive soft tissue and adjacent osseous involvement by the T2 hyperintense mass previously seen in images A and B.

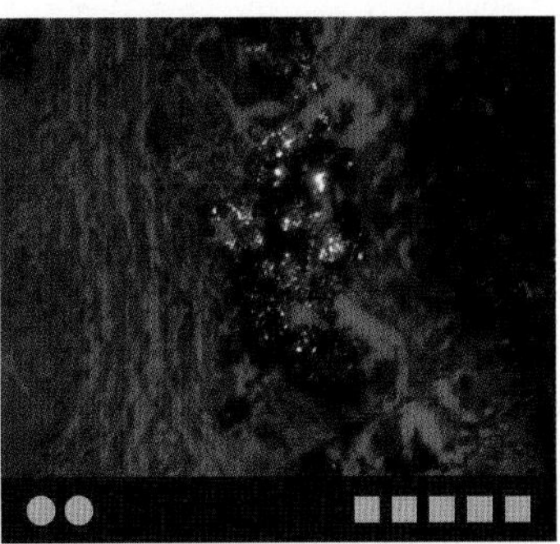

D. Tumoral CPPD deposition disease: Polarized light section demonstrates the positive birefringence of the CPPD crystals characteristic for the disease.

DIFFERENTIAL DIAGNOSES IMAGES

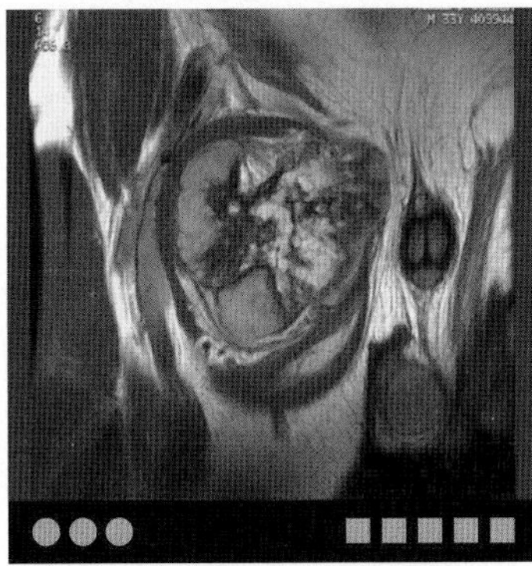

E. Chondrosarcoma: Coronal T1-weighted image shows a large, very heterogeneous mass in the anterior soft tissues of the lower right pelvis displacing the neurovascular bundle laterally.

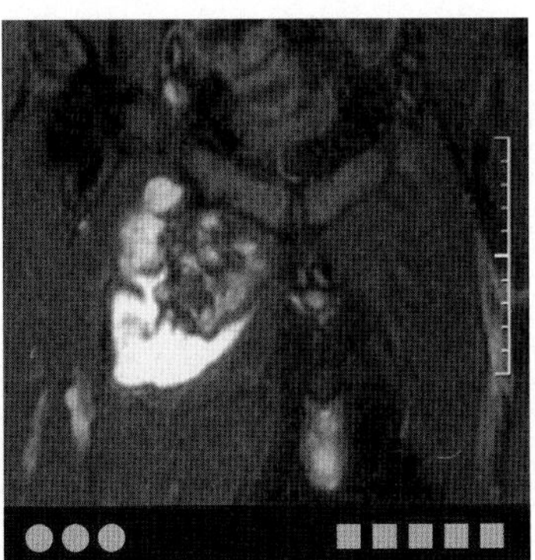

F. Chondrosarcoma: Coronal T2-weighted image at a level posterior to image E, shows the same mass to also have marked T2 heterogeneity.

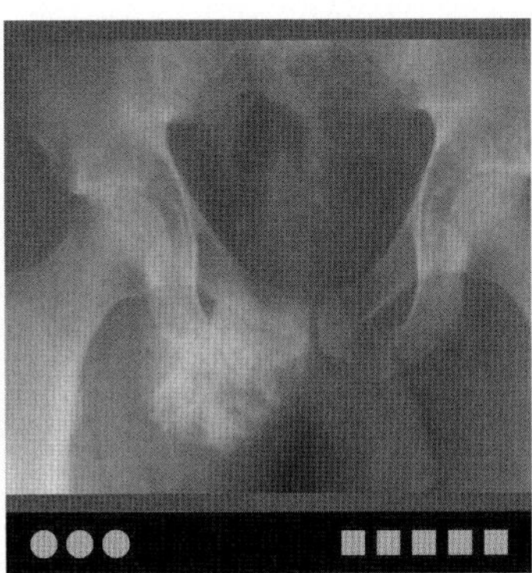

G. Chondrosarcoma: AP view of the pelvis shows a calcified mass projecting over the right ischium and pubic rami that corresponds with the mass seen in images E and F.

IMAGE KEY

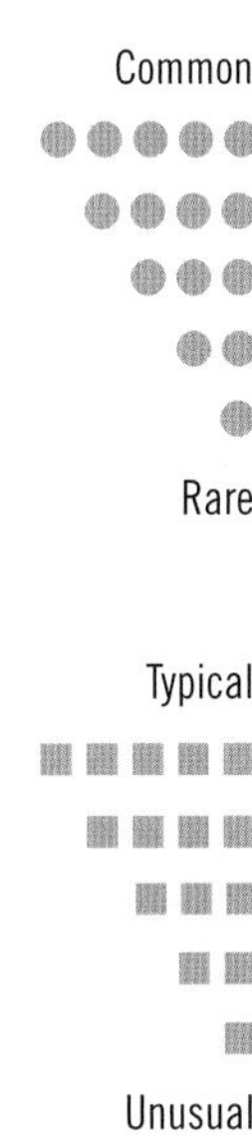

Chapter 20

Infections

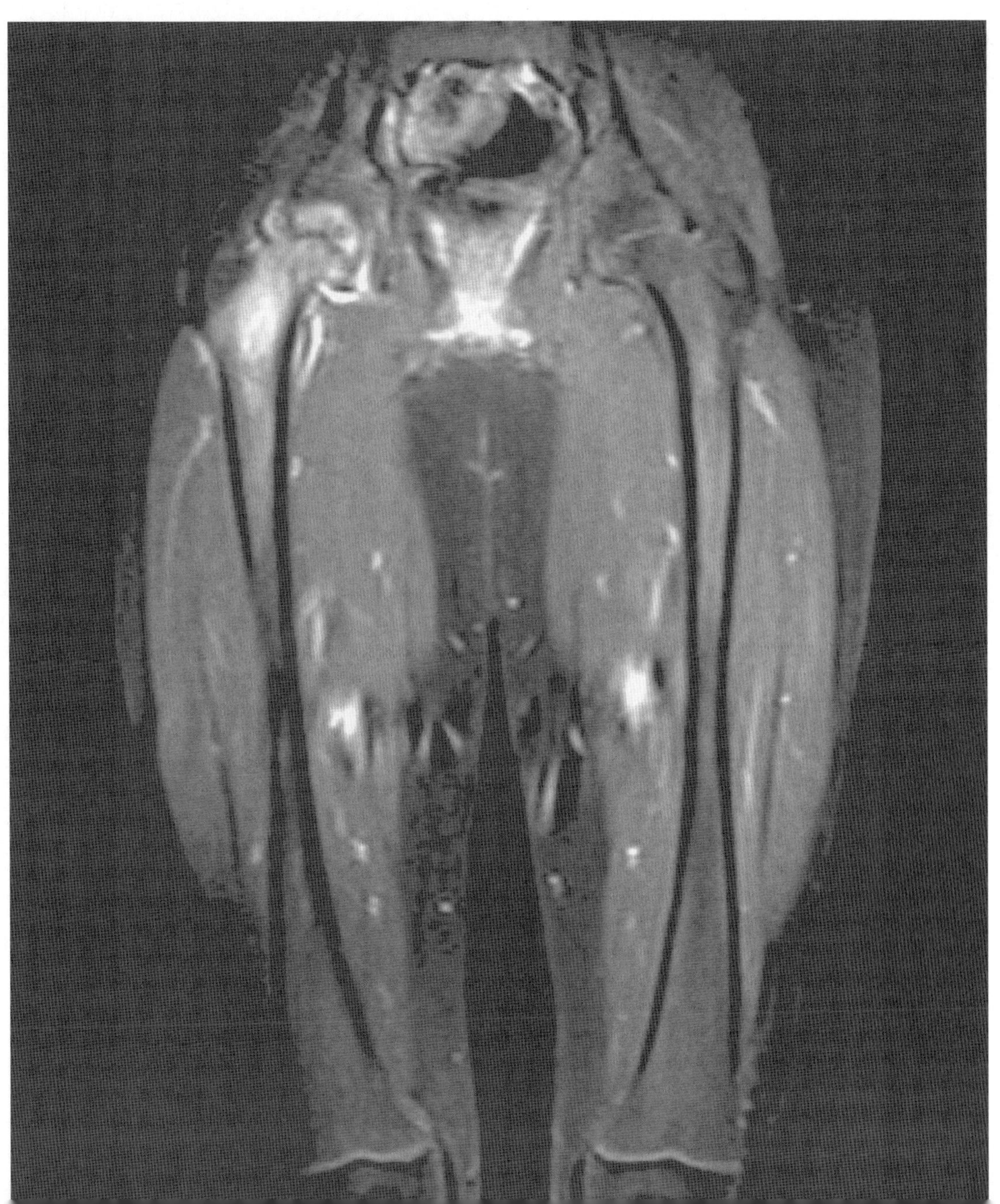

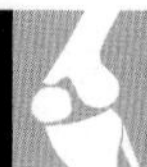

20–1 Osteomyelitis and Septic Arthritis

Eric Chen and Jamshid Tehranzadeh

PRESENTATION

Right hip pain

FINDINGS

MR images show soft tissue, synovium, and bone marrow edema of right hip with contrast enhancement.

DIFFERENTIAL DIAGNOSES

- *Septic arthritis*: Presence of fluid in the joint is associated with marrow inflammation and edema.
- *Toxic synovitis:* A condition occurring in children and masquerading as septic joint.
- *Chondrolysis*: This aseptic condition may create radiographic and MR changes similar to septic joint.
- *Transient osteoporosis:* This is associated with osteoporosis in the hip with MR changes of marrow edema.

COMMENTS

This 9-year-old boy with *Salmonella agona* osteomyelitis presents with right hip pain. Acute hematogenous osteomyelitis occurs predominately in children with the metaphysis of long bones being the most vascularized and most commonly involved. In neonates and children older than 16 years, the infection can spread to the metaphysis and adjacent joint, but in children with open physis (1–16 years), the growth plate often stops the spread of infection from the metaphysis to epiphysis and vice-versa. Subacute and chronic osteomyelitis occur in adults and develops secondary to trauma or local infection. Although radiography changes may not appear until two weeks after infection, it is commonly the initial imaging modality and findings which include soft tissue swelling, focal osteopenia, periosteal new bone formation, osteolysis, and finally sequestra. Three-phase Tc-99m methylene diphosphonate (MDP) detects changes days to weeks before appearance on radiography; however, local disturbances in vascular perfusion, clearance rate, permeability, and chemical binding (e.g., postsurgical changes, stress fractures) affect imaging. CT is superior to MRI for detection of sequestra, cloacae, and intraosseous gas. But MRI is superior for early detection and evaluating the extent of infection by delineating sinus tracts, cellulitis, and intramedullary involvement. MRI is also more specific and sensitive than the three-phase Tc-99m MDP. Edema and exudates of active infection have a low-intensity signal on T1-weighted image and high-intensity signal on T2-weighted image. Fat-saturated contrast-enhanced MR imaging is significantly more specific than nonenhanced MRI in patients with complicating clinical factors (e.g., postoperative states and conditions in which bone remodeling occurs).

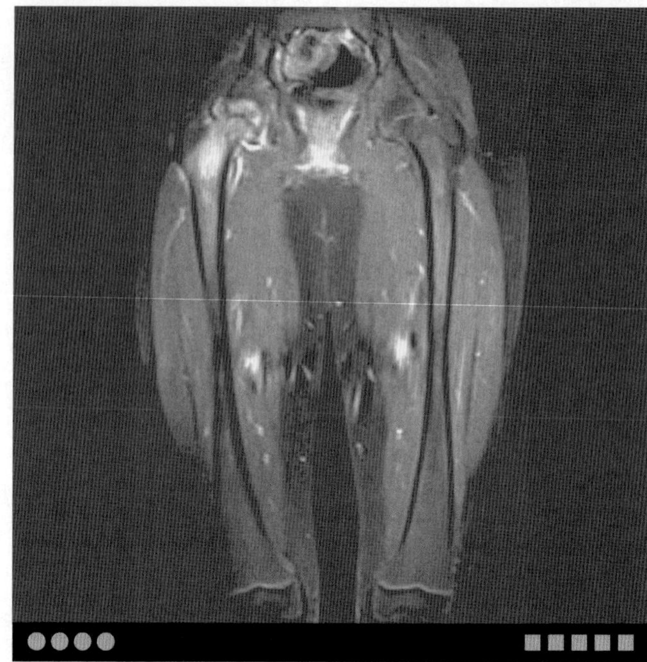

A. Osteomyelitis and septic arthritis of right hip: Coronal T1 fat-saturated postcontrast image shows bright enhancing signal of the right hip joint and right proximal femur.

PEARLS

- **Radiography findings may take 2 weeks after infection to develop and include focal osteoporosis, osteolysis, periosteal new bone formation, widening of joint, and finally sequestra**
- **Three-phase Tc-99m MDP is sensitive in early stage but is not specific in a complicated clinical setting**
- **MRI is the modality of choice in early detection and determining the extent of infection for surgical planning or in complicated clinical situations.**

ADDITIONAL IMAGES

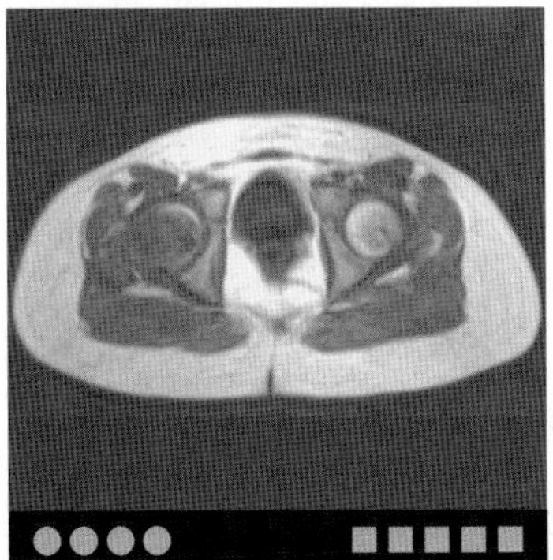

B. Osteomyelitis and septic arthritis of right hip: Axial T1-weighted image shows low signal intensity of right femoral head and neck due to marrow edema.

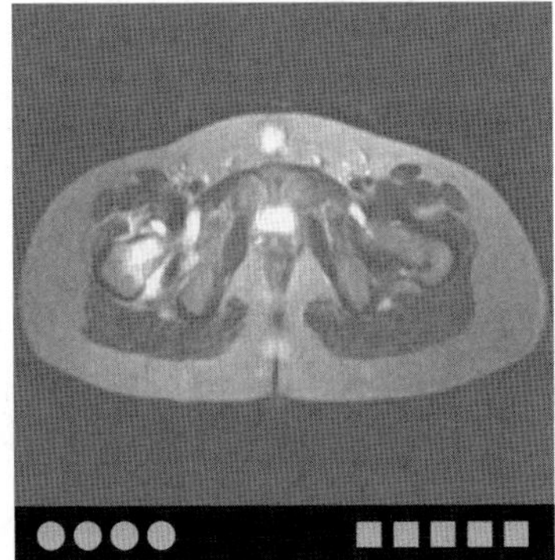

C. Osteomyelitis and septic arthritis of right hip: Axial T2-weighted image shows bright signal in the femoral neck and joint fluid on the right hip.

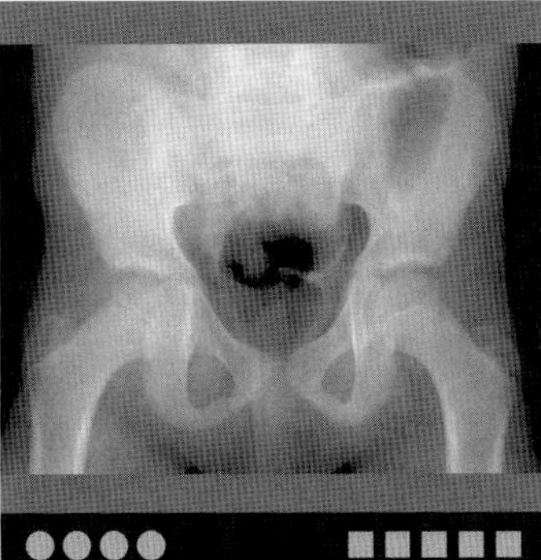

D. Osteomyelitis and septic arthritis of right hip: AP radiograph of pelvis shows focal osteopenia of right leg with obscuration of soft tissue fat lines because of soft tissue inflammation. Note osteolysis of epiphysis and metaphysis of the right femur caused by osteomyelitis.

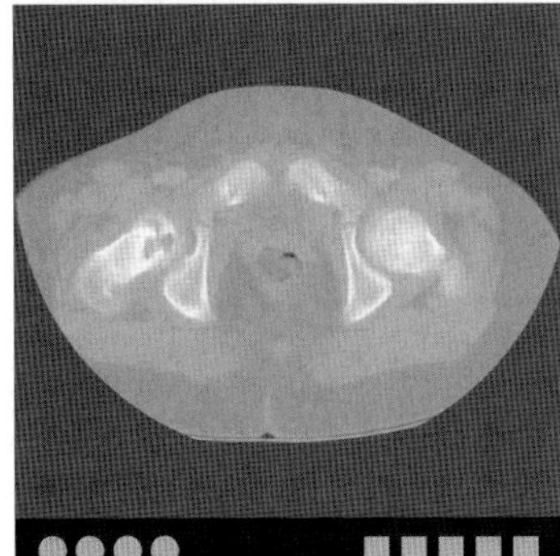

E. Osteomyelitis and septic arthritis of right hip: CT scan of hips shows widening of right hip joint occurring because of the presence of joint fluid with ostelysis of the femoral head and neck with marginal sclerosis

IMAGE KEY

Common

Rare

Typical

Unusual

DIFFERENTIAL DIAGNOSES IMAGES

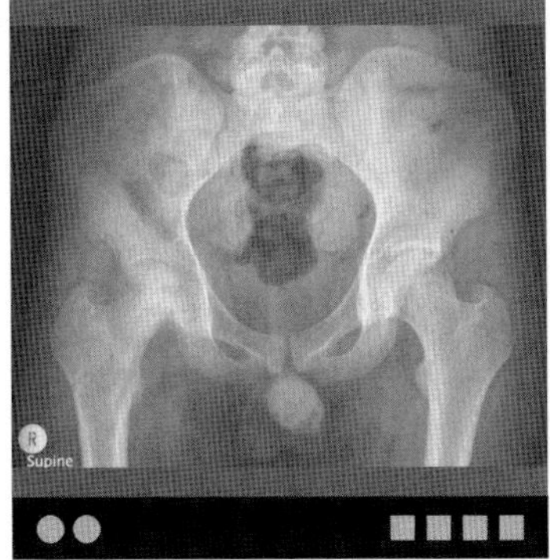

F. Ewing sarcoma: AP view of the pelvis shows a mixed lytic and sclerotic lesion of the proximal right femoral head and neck, with loss of joint space associated with an adjacent soft tissue mass. A needle track at the biopsy site is also noted.

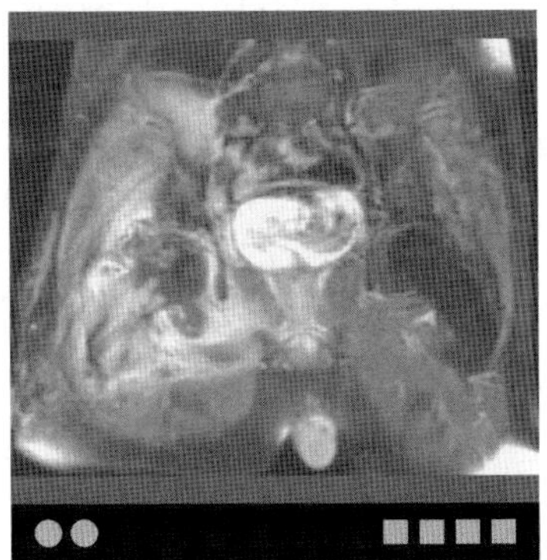

G. Ewing sarcoma: Coronal fat-saturated T1-weighted image with contrast shows marked soft tissue edema and fluid in the joint, which appears as low signal and is delineated by the enhanced peripheral synovium. Enhancement of the bone marrow indicates osseous involvement.

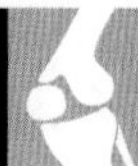

20–2 Tuberculosis of the Sacroiliac Joint

Nuttya Pattamapasong and Wilfred CG Peh

PRESENTATION

Back pain, hip pain, and sacroiliac tenderness

FINDINGS

Frontal radiograph and axial CT show irregularity of the right sacroiliac joint with adjacent subchondral sclerosis. The CT also shows juxta-articular erosion with preservation of the width of the right joint. The left sacroiliac joint is normal.

DIFFERENTIAL DIAGNOSES

- *Pyogenic arthritis:* Rapid joint space narrowing and more severe bony sclerosis. Bony ankylosis occurs more frequently.
- *Seronegative spondyloarthropathy:* Typically bilateral sacroiliac joint involvement. No para-articular abscess or associated myositis is seen.
- *Hyperparathyroidism:* Subarticular bone resorption without para-articular abscess. There would be other hyperparathyroidism-related bone changes.

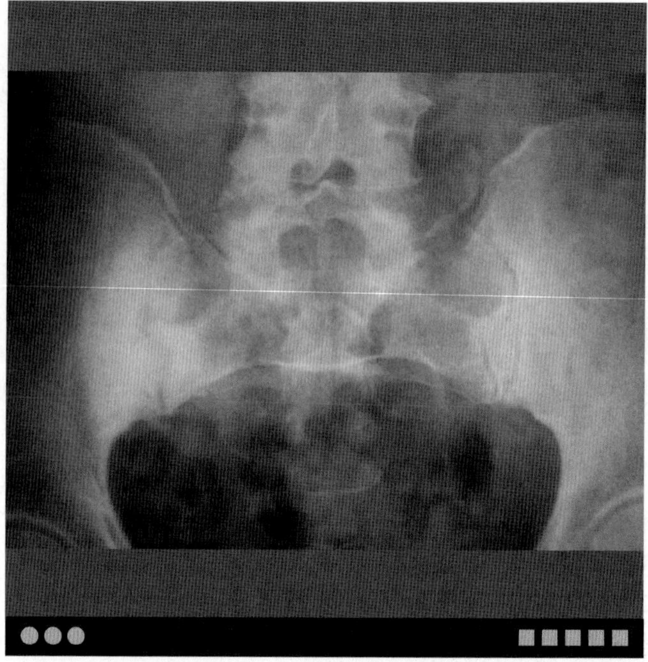

A. Tuberculous sacroiliitis: Frontal radiograph shows right sacroiliac joint irregularity and subchondral sclerosis. The left sacroiliac joint is normal.

COMMENTS

The patient is a 59-year-old man with low back pain for several years, with recent worsening. Tuberculous arthritis occurs often secondary to tuberculous osteomyelitis. *Mycobacterium tuberculosis* spreads hematogenously to one side of subchondral bone; it subsequently extends to the joint and another articular site causing subarticular bone erosions. Characteristic findings of tuberculous arthritis in the early stage are juxta-articular osteoporosis, preserved joint space, and lack of sclerosis or periostitis. Joint space narrowing is often delayed because of the lack of proteolytic enzymes in *M. tuberculosis.* The on-going process leads to the large para-articular abscesses and sinus tracts. Fistulas between the infected joint and the bowel or bladder provide the pathway for spread of the organism to adjacent visceral organs. In the late stage of disease, periostitis and bony sclerosis may be present, but these features occur more prominently in pyogenic arthritis. As any other infectious joint disease, tuberculous arthritis is usually monoarticular. CT can demonstrate both bone destruction and surrounding soft tissue extension. Associated myositis, cellulitis, and sinus track formation are better appreciated on MR imaging than on CT. Para-articular fluid aspiration and tissue biopsy is necessary for an accurate diagnosis. However, contamination of the bacteria via sinus tracts may potentially result in misinterpretation of pyogenic arthritis.

PEARLS

- **Unilateral sacroiliitis should be regarded as infection until proven otherwise. Para-articular abscess is characteristic of infectious arthritis, and this finding is helpful to distinguish infectious sacroiliitis from sacroiliitis occurring because of other causes.**
- **Sinus tracks, delayed joint space narrowing, and slow disease progression are characteristic findings of tuberculous arthritis.**
- **Infection of adjacent pelvic organs may be seen secondary to tuberculous sacroiliitis.**

ADDITIONAL IMAGE

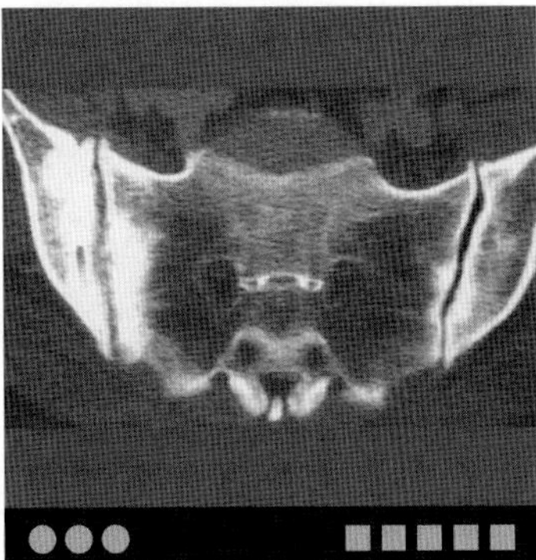

B. Tuberculous sacroiliitis: Axial CT image shows right sacroiliac joint marginal erosions and adjacent subchondral sclerosis. The surrounding prominent bony sclerosis is indicative of long-standing infection.

DIFFERENTIAL DIAGNOSES IMAGES

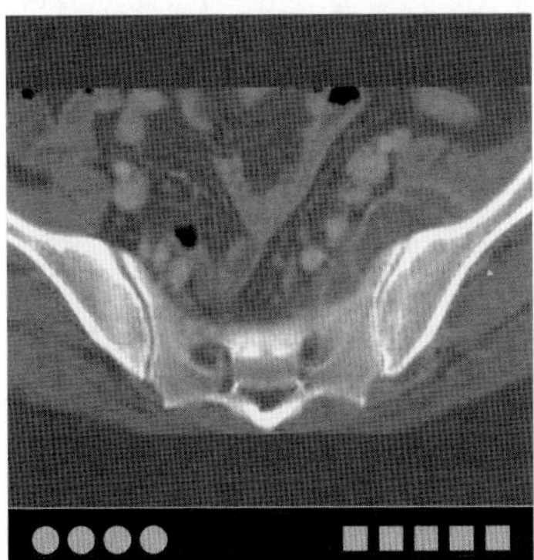

C. Pyogenic sacroiliitis: Axial CT image shows narrowing of the left sacroiliac joint, particularly the posterior aspect, and a large rim-enhancing anterior para-articular abscess.

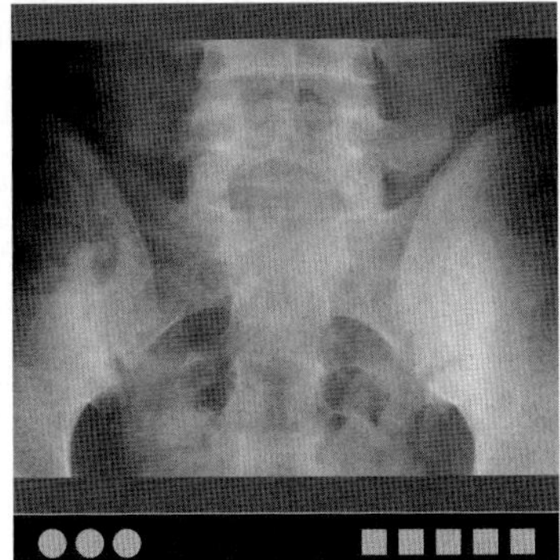

D. Ankylosing spondylitis: Frontal radiograph shows symmetrical irregularity of both sacroiliac joints with adjacent subchondral sclerosis.

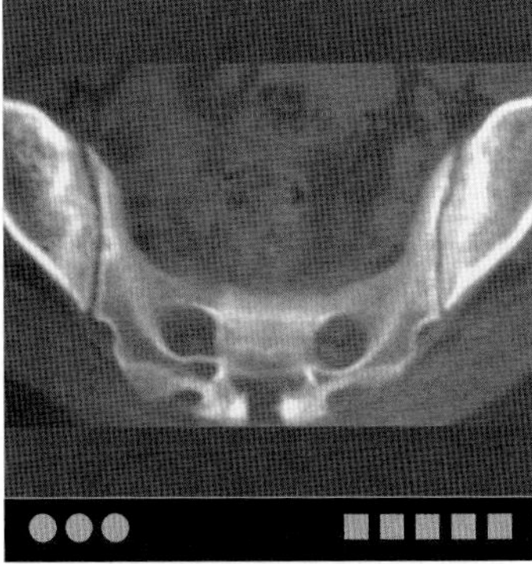

E. Ankylosing spondylitis: Axial CT image shows multiple small marginal erosions at both sacroiliac joints, with adjacent subchondral sclerosis.

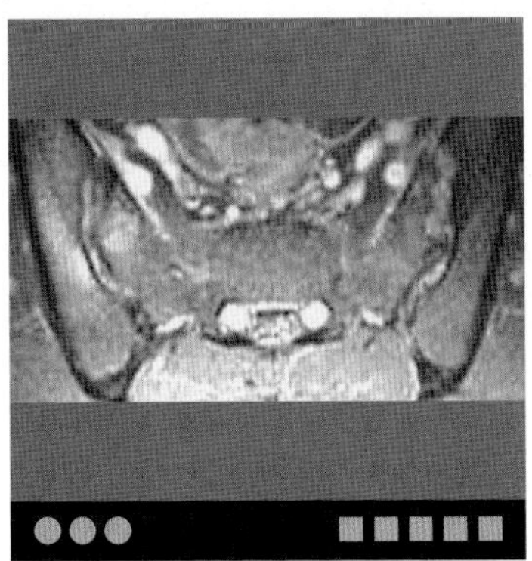

F. Ankylosing spondylitis: Axial fat-suppressed FSE T2-weighted MR image shows effusions within both sacroiliac joints, with patchy bone marrow edema adjacent to the right sacroiliac joint.

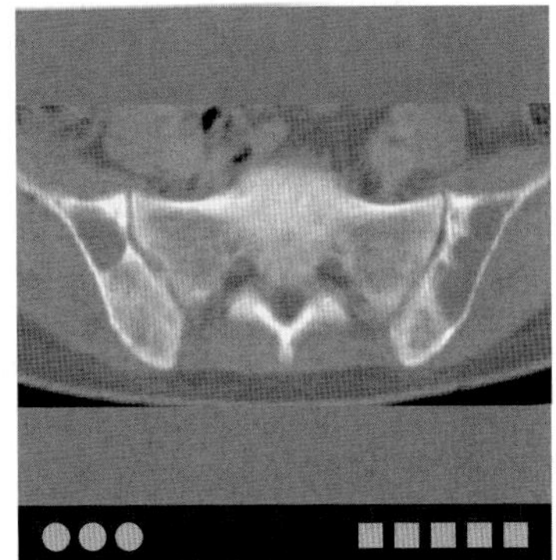

G. Hyperparathyroidism: Axial CT image shows slight erosions of the posterior aspect of the left sacroiliac joint. Multiple osteolytic lesions representing brown tumors are present.

IMAGE KEY

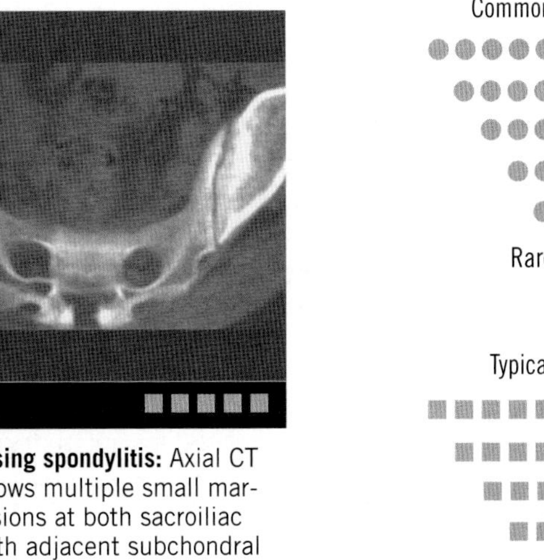

Common

Rare

Typical

Unusual

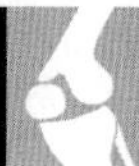

20–3 Left Iliac Bone Coccidioidomycosis

Shahla Modarresi and Daria Motamedi

PRESENTATION

Pelvic pain

FINDINGS

STIR MR image shows a bright signal lesion of the left iliac bone with no soft tissue mass.

DIFFERENTIAL DIAGNOSES

- *Chronic bacterial osteomyelitis:* CT shows sclerosis, cortical thickening, thickened disorganized trabeculae and cystic change, poorly defined areas of osteolysis, and periosteal reaction. It may contain sequestrum.
- *Prior surgery for bone graft (bone harvest):* Evidence and history of prior bone graft surgery. Bone defect is well defined on CT or radiograph.
- *Malignant primary or secondary bone lesion:* CT or radiograph shows permeative or destructive lesion with ill-defined border and soft tissue mass.
- *Benign bone tumors (e.g. Brown tumor, fibrous dysplasia):* CT shows single or multiple well-defined radiolucent bone lesions with sclerotic borders.

COMMENTS

The patient is a 35-year-old male presenting with left-sided pelvic pain and weight loss for several months. Coccidioidomycosis is caused by inhalation of spores of *Coccidioides immitis*, a dimorphic fungus, which is endemic in the soil of southwestern USA and parts of Central America, South America, and Mexico. Coccidioidomycosis is an acute pulmonary infection, which is often asymptomatic but could manifest as a flue-like illness or pneumonia. Dissemination of the disease is rare, most commonly occurring in immunosuppressed patients. Common sites of dissemination include skin, bone, joint, and meninges. The skin is the most common site of extra pulmonary disease. Coccidioidomycosis of the bone typically causes chronic osteomyelitis, often draining to soft tissue and creating fistulae. Long bones, bones of the hands, feet, pelvis, and skull may be involved. Approximately 60% are limited to a single bone, with 20% involving two bones and 10% involving three bones. Infection also affects joints, causing synovitis with knees most commonly involved. Vertebral osteomyelitis can affect any part of the vertebra, sparing the disc with increased risk of meningitis. In patients with osteomyelitis, the radiographs show lytic lesions, periosteal elevation, and bony destruction. The high-resolution CT or MRI can better delineate the extent of bone, joint, and overlying soft tissue involvement, including sinus tracts or fistulae. A bone scan may detect multiple sites of bony involvement.

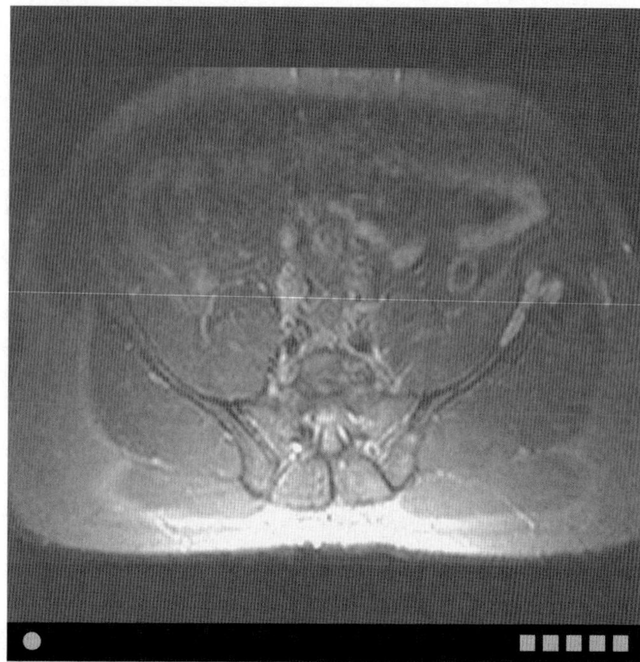

A. Coccidioidomycosis: Axial STIR image shows high signal intensity lesion of the left ileum, which is a nonspecific finding. There is no soft tissue mass.

PEARLS

- **Coccidioidomycosis is caused by inhalation of *Coccidioides immitis* spores, a fungus endemic in the soil of southwestern USA, parts of Mexico and South America.**
- **Coccidioidomycosis is an acute pulmonary infection, which in rare occasions can disseminate to skin, bone, joint, and meninges mostly in immunosuppressed patients.**
- **Coccidioidomycosis of the bone typically causes chronic osteomyelitis in long bones, hands, feet, pelvis, and skull with approximately 60% limited to a single bone.**
- **Radiographs show lytic lesions, periosteal elevation, and bony destruction. High-resolution CT or MRI can better delineate the extent of bone involvement.**

ADDITIONAL IMAGES

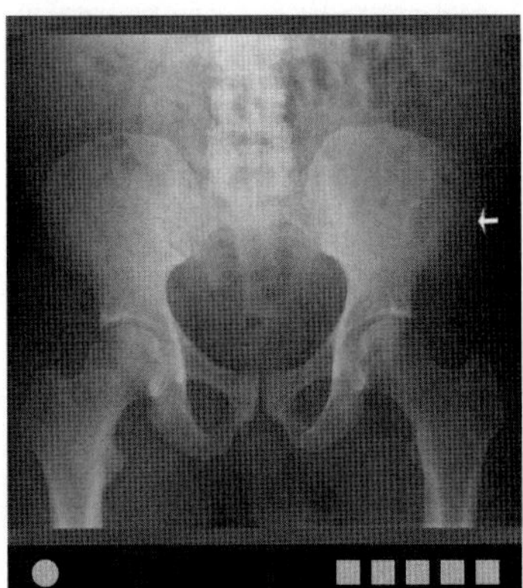

B. Coccidioidomycosis: AP radiograph shows destructive lesion of the left iliac bone with sclerotic margin suggesting slow growth process.

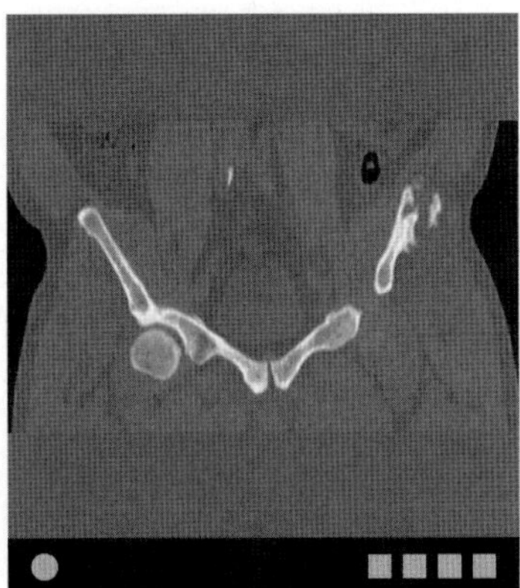

C. Coccidioidomycosis: Coronal reconstructed CT scan with bone window shows destructive lesion with sclerotic border suggesting chronic process.

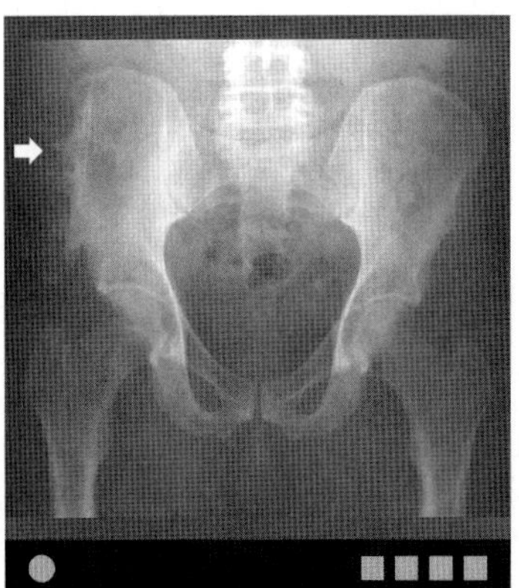

D. Coccidioidomycosis: AP radiograph of pelvis shows irregular benign appearing bony defect of the right iliac crest consistent with prior bone harvest (arrow).

DIFFERENTIAL DIAGNOSES IMAGES

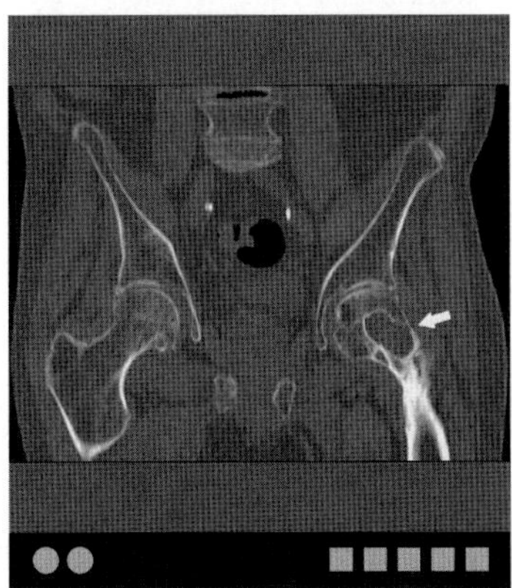

E. Brown tumor: Coronal CT scan with well-defined benign appearing lytic lesion of the left femoral neck without soft tissue mass, compatible with brown tumor (arrow).

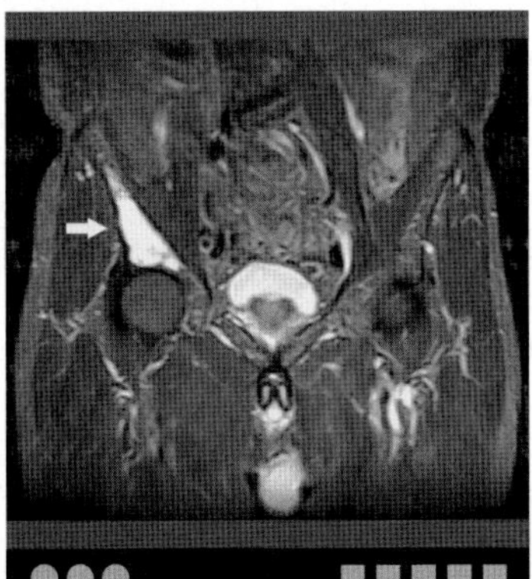

F. Fibrous dysplasia: Coronal STIR image showing bright, slightly expansile lesion of the right iliac bone (arrow), consistent with fibrous dysplasia, a nonspecific finding.

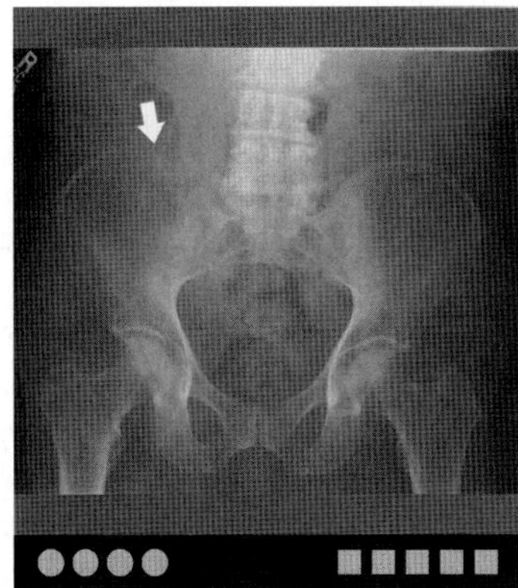

G. Metastasis: AP radiograph of the pelvis shows a lytic ill-defined malignant lesion of the right iliac bone consistent with metastasis (arrow).

IMAGE KEY

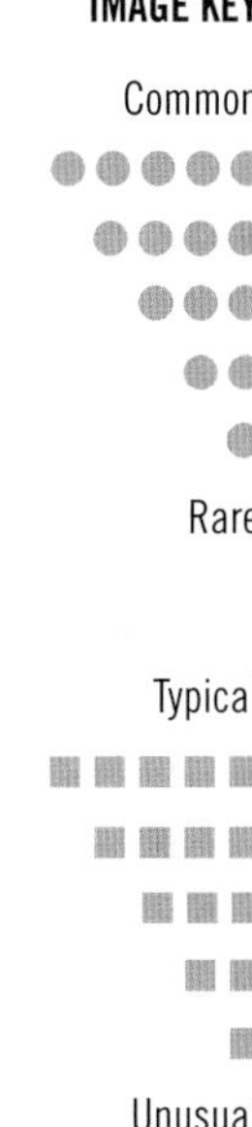

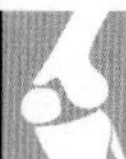

20–4 Paget Disease with Insufficiency Fractures

Kira Chow

PRESENTATION

Thigh pain

FINDINGS

Coronal inversion recovery MRI demonstrates hyperintensity along the lateral femoral shaft.

DIFFERENTIAL DIAGNOSES

- *Stress fracture:* These are divided in fatigue fractures and insufficiency fractures.
- *Looser's zones:* These typically occur in the setting of osteomalacia on the concave edge of the bone, as opposed to the insufficiency fractures of Paget disease, which occurs on the convex side.

COMMENTS

Paget disease is a disorder of abnormal osseous remodeling, common in patients older than 40 years. There are three phases of Paget disease. In the initial purely lytic phase, classic findings include osteoporosis circumscripta (focal lysis in the skull) and sharply defined edge of lucency known as the "blade of grass" or "flame." In the mixed phase, there is cortical and trabecular thickening most commonly recognized in the pelvis as prominence of the iliopectineal and ischiopubic lines, and in the spine as the "picture frame" appearance caused by thickening of vertebral body cortex. In contrast to hemangiomas, which also demonstrate vertical densities in the vertebral body, the appearance in Paget disease is coarser. CT findings are similar to those seen radiographically, but are visualized in greater detail. The MRI appearance is variable. Most often MRI demonstrates maintenance of fatty marrow, sometimes with increased fatty content. Another pattern is T1 and T2 signal heterogeneity. In the final sclerotic phase of Paget disease, there is diffuse sclerosis, and marrow is T1 and T2 hypointense owing to sclerosis on MR imaging. Complications of Paget disease are usually caused by the osseous weakening, which results from the combined abnormal activity of osteoclasts and osteoblasts. As in this case a bowing deformity occurs, initially followed by incomplete cortical fractures on the convex side. These fractures can continue through the medullary space to become complete fractures, also known as "banana fractures." Insufficiency fractures also occur commonly in the thoracolumbar spine.

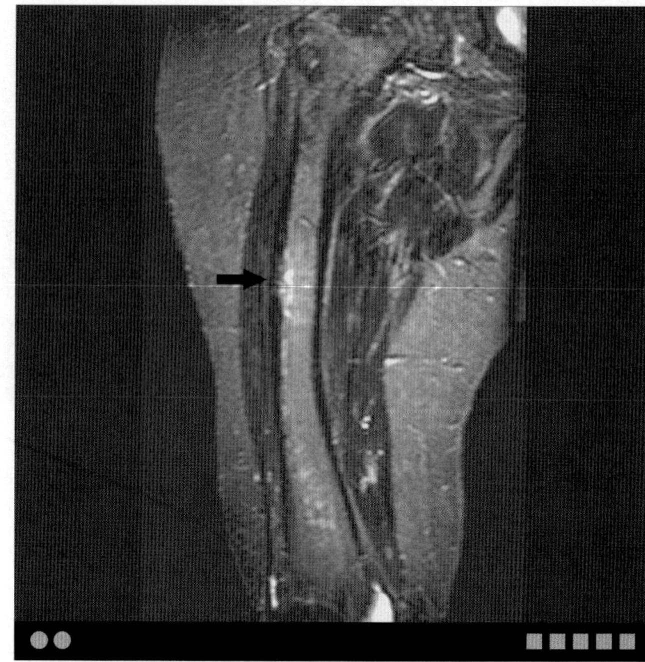

A. Paget disease with insufficiency fracture: Coronal inversion recovery MRI demonstrates hyperintensity (arrow) along the lateral femoral shaft, corresponding to the insufficiency fracture identified on radiograph (image C).

PEARLS

- **Initial phase of Paget disease is lytic, followed by mixed and finally sclerotic.**
- **Insufficiency fractures in Paget disease typically occur on the convex side of the bone.**

ADDITIONAL IMAGES

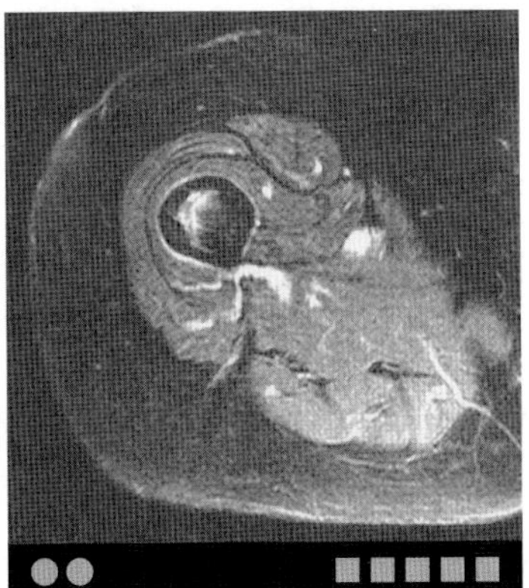

B. Paget disease with insufficiency fracture: Axial T2-weighted fat-saturated sequence at the level of interest on coronal sequence demonstrates marrow hyperintensity along the lateral femoral cortex.

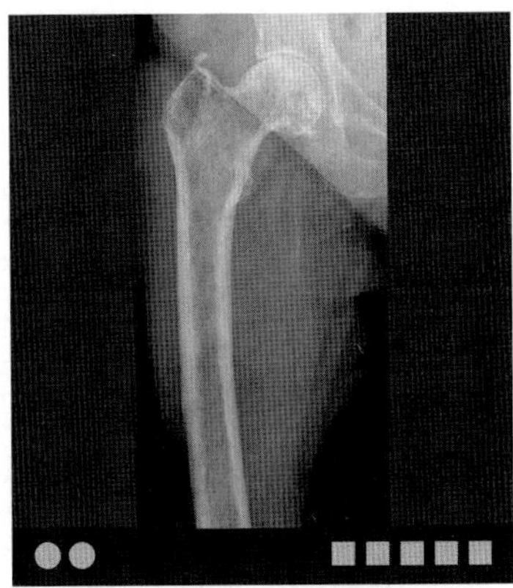

C. Paget disease with insufficiency fracture: Frontal radiograph of the right femur shows a linear horizontally oriented lucency in the lateral femoral cortex.

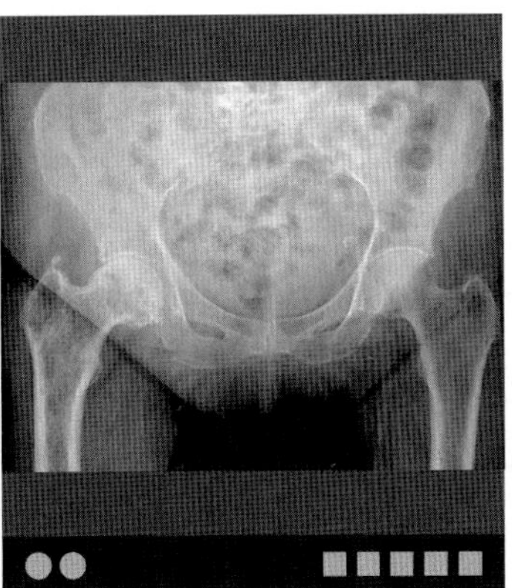

D. Paget disease with insufficiency fracture: Frontal radiograph of the pelvis demonstrates changes typical of Paget disease in the right hip. In comparison to the normal left femoral head, right femur has cortical and trabecular coarsening and thickening of the iliopectineal line.

IMAGE KEY

Common

Rare

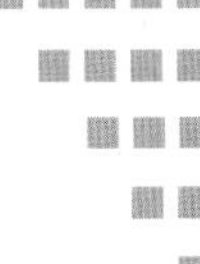

Typical

Unusual

DIFFERENTIAL DIAGNOSES IMAGES

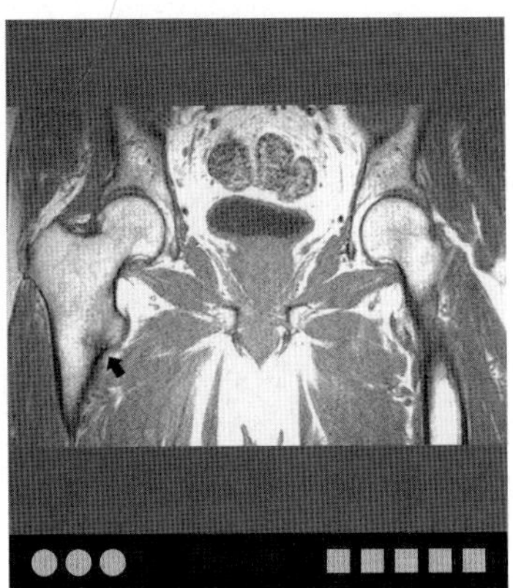

E. Fatigue fracture of the proximal femur: Coronal T1 turbo spin echo (SE) shows a dark line of fatigue fracture in the proximal right femur (arrow).

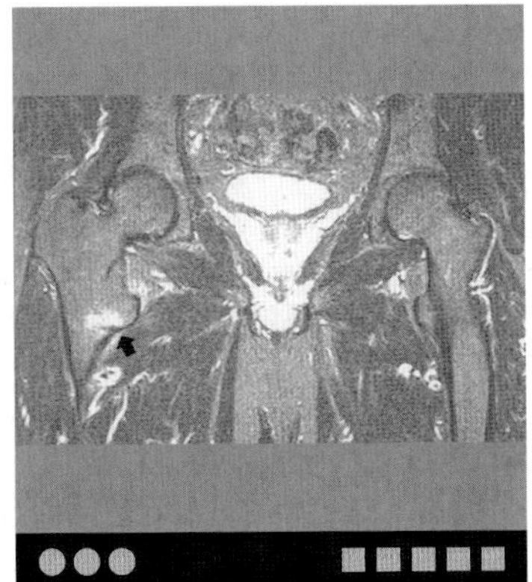

F. Fatigue fracture of the proximal femur: Coronal STIR imaging of proximal femur shows dark linear fatigue fracture surrounded by bright bone marrow edema (arrow).

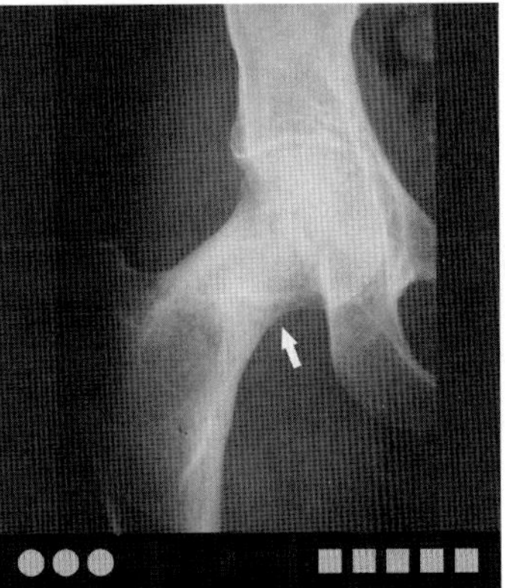

G. Fatigue fracture of the proximal femur: AP radiograph in another patient with stress fracture of femoral neck (arrow).

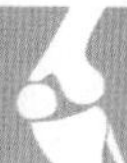

20–5 Sacral Paget Disease

Charles H. Bush

PRESENTATION

Low back pain

FINDINGS

A lateral radiograph of the lumbar spine shows subtly increased density with cortical thickening in the sacrum. MRI shows no significant abnormality.

DIFFERENTIAL DIAGNOSES

- *Blastic metastasis:* This must be considered in a patient with prostate carcinoma, but it would be unheard of for such a lesion to involve the entire sacrum as well as to be invisible on MRI.
- *Fibrous dysplasia:* The cortices and bone trabecula are not thick unlike Paget disease.

COMMENTS

A 72-year-old male with prostate carcinoma is found to have a blastic lesion in the sacrum on lumbar spine radiographs obtained for low back pain. Paget disease of bone (osteitis deformans) is a common metabolic affliction of older adults, in which bone turnover and remodeling are dramatically increased. Paget disease is of uncertain etiology, but viral, genetic, and environmental causes are all considerations. Paget disease of bone evolves through three stages: an early lytic phase, an intermediate or mixed phase, and a late phase marked by dense bone formation. The early phase of Paget disease is characterized by excessive osteoclastic resorption of bone, usually commencing at the end of the affected bone and progressing distally, with a geographic demarcation of the boundary of osteolysis. The initial appearance of reparative woven bone formation marks the intermediate phase, with thickening of both cortical and cancellous bone. The late phase is marked by a decline in the rapidity of bone turnover. Paget disease of bone has a propensity to eventually involve an entire bone. Usually, patients with Paget disease are asymptomatic, and the disease is discovered as an incidental finding on radiographs. However, the complications of Paget disease often bring the patient to medical attention. Paget disease in the skull can cause cranial nerve compression. When the long bones of the lower extremity are afflicted, bowing deformity, insufficiency fractures, and limb length discrepancy can result from weight bearing.

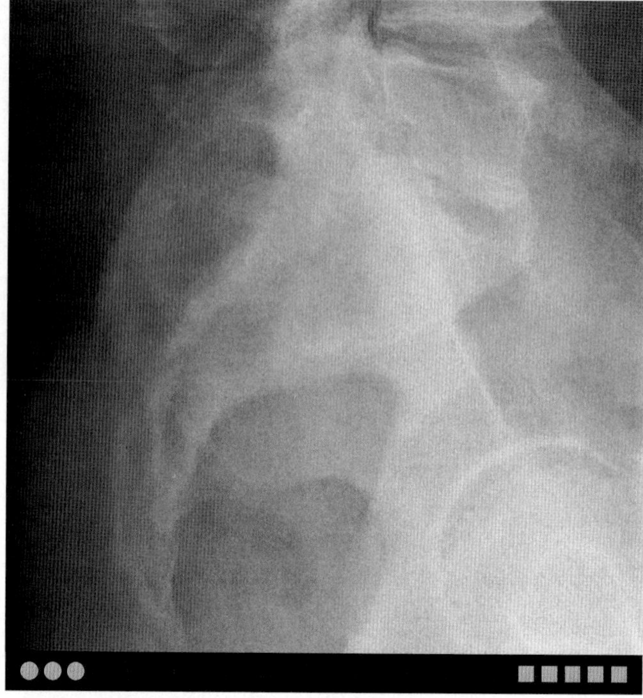

A. Paget disease: A lateral radiograph of the lower lumbar spine shows subtly increased density in the sacrum.

Secondary arthritis also commonly results from Paget disease, usually in the lower extremity. Sarcomatous degeneration is a fortunately rare complication of longstanding Paget disease, with a poor prognosis.

PEARLS

- **The radiographic appearance of the initial phase of Paget disease is characterized by the sharp demarcation between affected and normal bone, which is particularly common in the calvarium, where it is termed osteoporosis circumscripta.**
- **An oblique margin to the front of osteolysis in long bones, the so-called "blade of grass" appearance is characteristic.**
- **Radiographic finding in late-stage Paget disease are usually pathgnomonic, but MRI in confusing cases shows preservation of fatty marrow on all pulse sequences in intermediate and late phase Paget disease.**

ADDITIONAL IMAGES

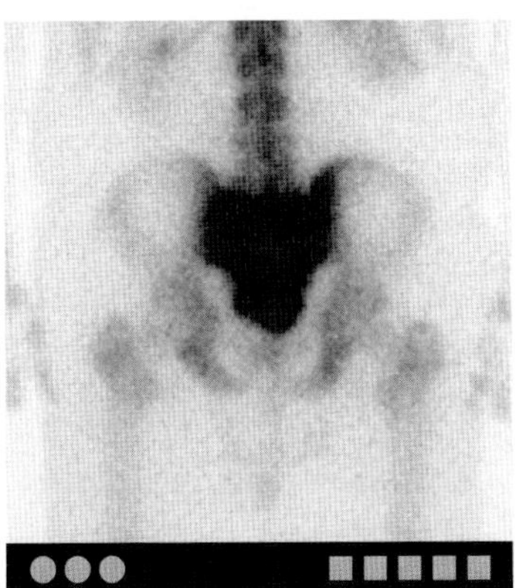

B. Paget disease: Static frontal view from radionuclide Tc-99 m MDP bone scan shows dramatically increased uptake of tracer in the entire sacrum.

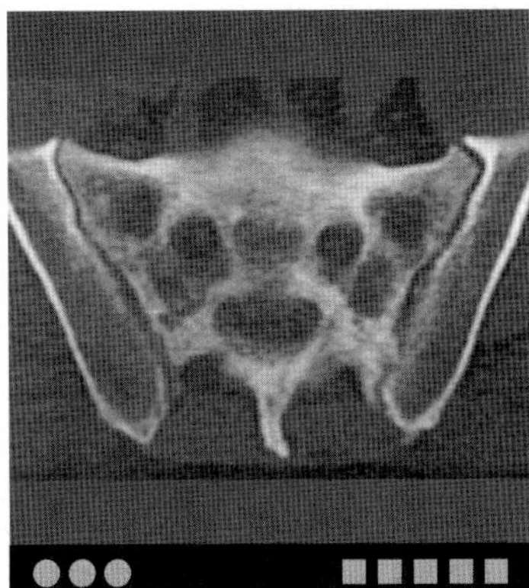

C. Paget disease: CT through the sacrum at the level of S1 shows cortical thickening and trabecular coarsening, typical for late-stage Paget disease of bone.

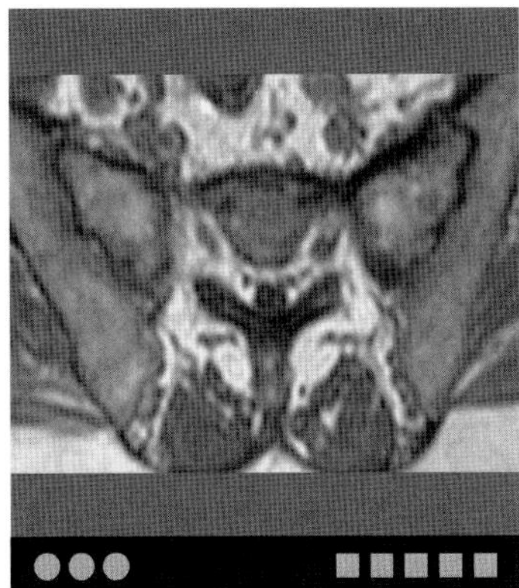

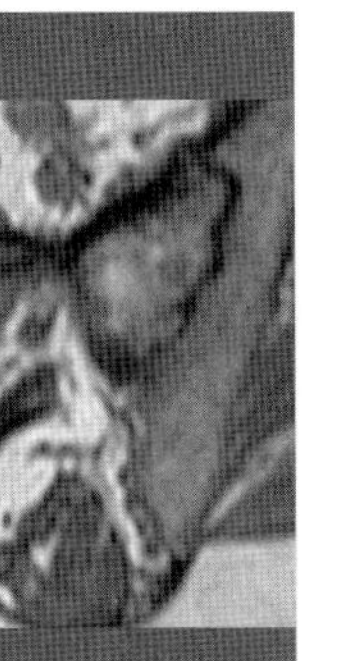

D. Paget disease: Axial T1-weighted MR image shows mostly fatty marrow signal in the sacrum, with no evidence of a space occupying lesion.

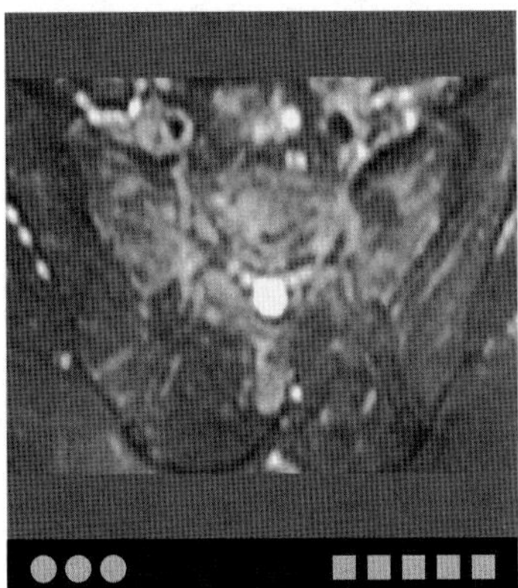

E. Paget disease: Axial T2-weighted MR image shows mostly fatty marrow signal in the sacrum, with no evidence of a space occupying lesion.

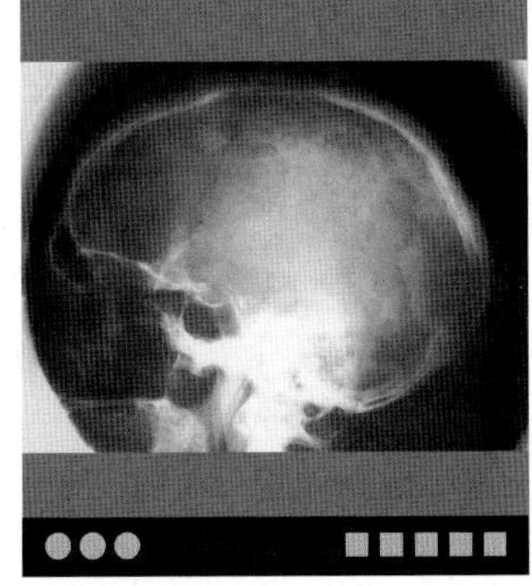

F. Paget disease: A lateral radiograph of the skull in another patient shows a well-circumscribed osteolytic lesion in the calvarium (osteoporosis circumscripta), consistent with early lytic-phase Paget disease.

IMAGE KEY

Common

Rare

Typical

Unusual

DIFFERENTIAL DIAGNOSIS IMAGE

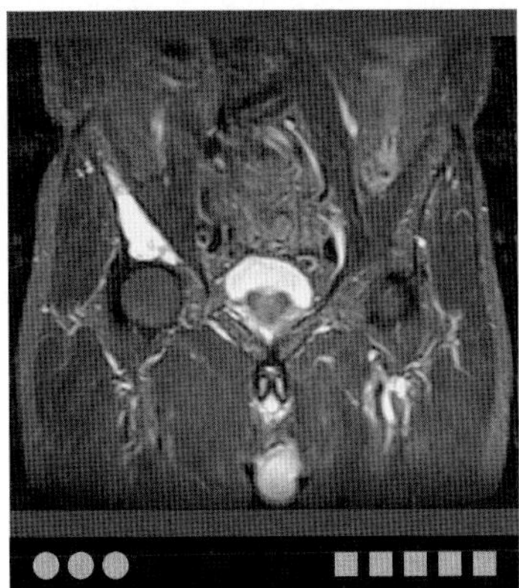

G. Fibrous dysplasia: Coronal T2-weighted FS image shows expansile lesion of the right ilium and ischium showing bright signal.

Chapter 21

Tumors and Tumor Like Lesions

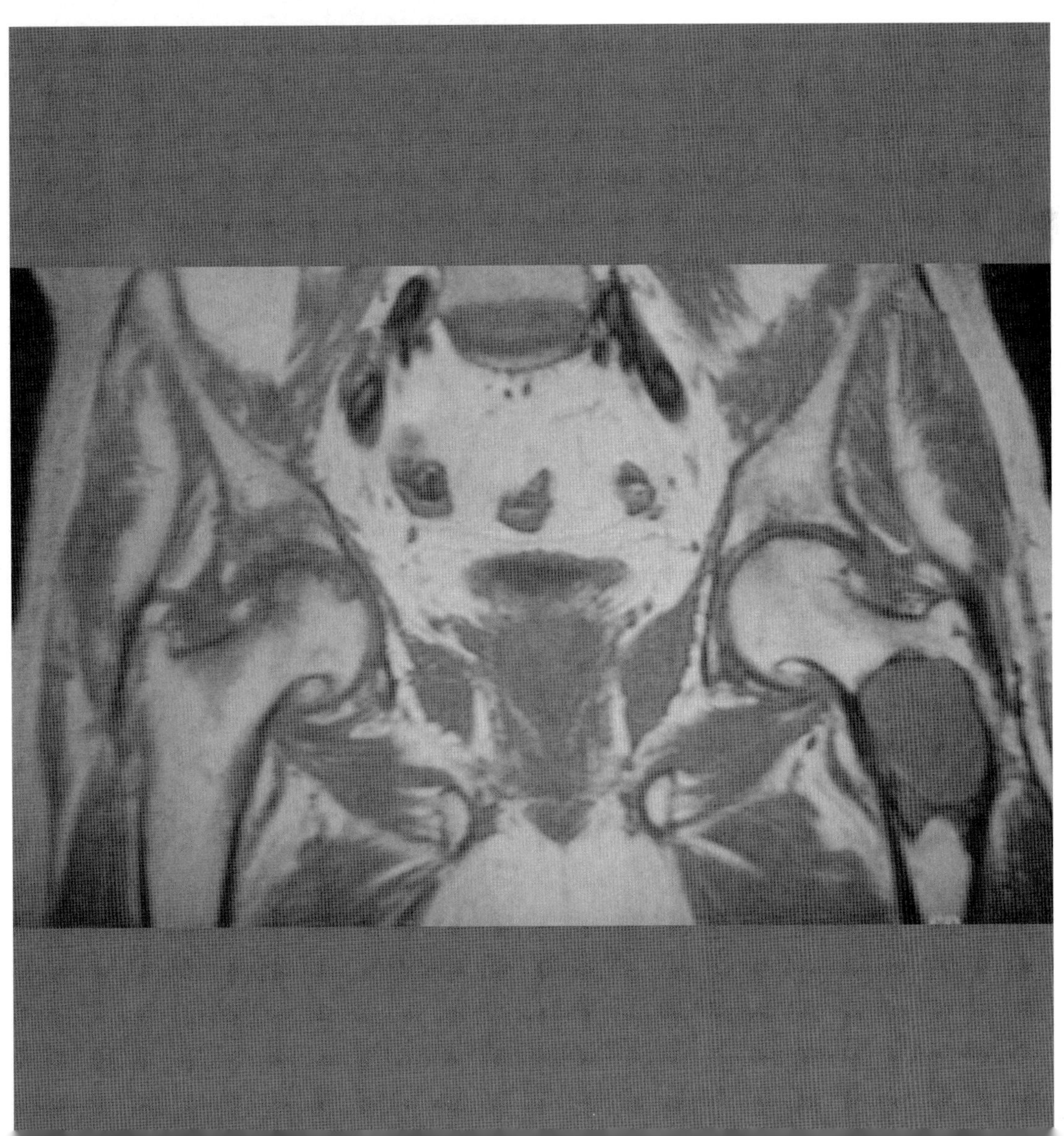

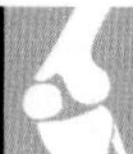

21–1 Cystic Fibrous Dysplasia

Janis Owens

PRESENTATION

Asymptomatic, pain, or enlarging mass

FINDINGS

There is a circumscribed lesion with a low signal rim that corresponds to a thick sclerotic rim on the radiograph. The internal signal of the lesion is consistent with fluid on MRI.

DIFFERENTIAL DIAGNOSES

- *Bone cysts:* The sclerotic rim is thinner than the rim in fibrous dysplasia.
- *Enchondroma:* There is no sclerotic or low signal rim. Chondroid matrix calcifications may be present.
- *Brown tumor (osteoclastoma):* There may be multiple lesions in various locations. Other signs of hyperparathyroidism are present.

COMMENTS

This is a 34-year-old male with rheumatoid arthritis who was being evaluated for hip replacement surgery. Fibrous dysplasia is a hamartomatous malformation of bone. It is seen in 1% of autopsies and is commonly seen in the proximal femur in its monostotic form. It is usually asymptomatic and diagnosed in the second or third decade as an incidental finding on radiography. The typical appearance is a geographic lesion with a bubbly "ground glass" appearance or lytic lesion with a thick sclerotic rim. MRI typically demonstrates a circumscribed lesion, which low-to-intermediate signal on the T1W sequences and intermediate to high signal on the T2W sequences. When high signal is present, it is usually lower in signal than fluid. Fibrous dysplasia may undergo cystic degeneration. When this occurs, the radiograph will retain its appearance as fibrous dysplasia and the MRI will show characteristics of a cystic fluid collection. When cystic degeneration occurs, the patient may complain of pain and the lesion may increase in size. On pathological evaluation, there is a fibrous capsule instead of the true epithelial lining seen unicameral bone cyst. The fluid in the lesion is similar to that seen in unicameral bone cyst on analysis and not blood as seen in aneurysmal bone cyst.

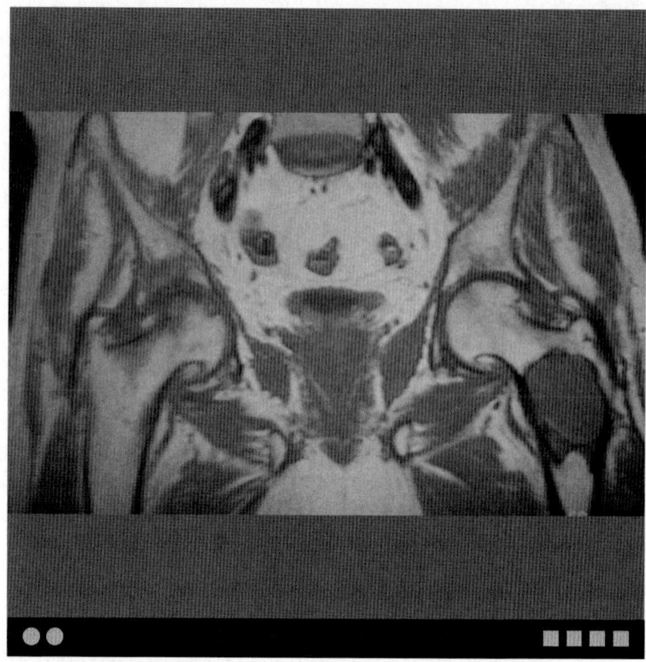

A. Cystic fibrous dysplasia: Coronal T1W sequence shows a low signal peripheral rim around an intermediate signal fluid collection in the left proximal femur.

PEARLS

- **Geographic lesion with a well-formed thick sclerotic round or oval rim.**
- **Low signal rim with internal fluid signal on MRI.**
- **Rare form of fibrous dysplasia.**

ADDITIONAL IMAGES

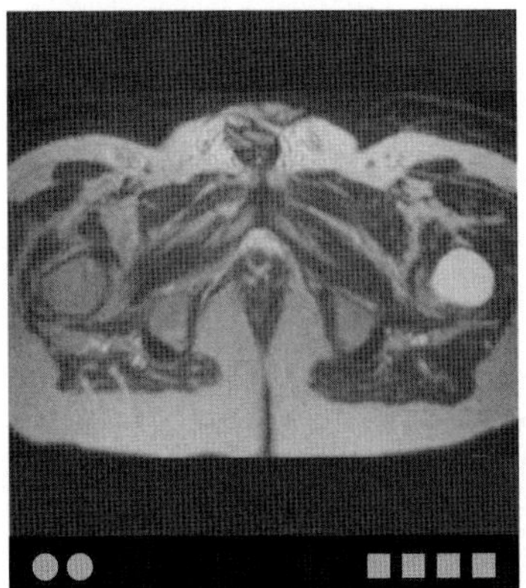

B. Cystic fibrous dysplasia: Axial T2W sequence shows the high signal fluid and the peripheral low signal rim.

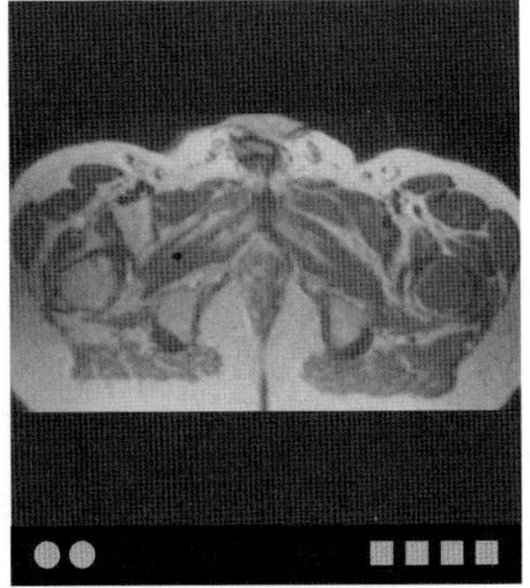

C. Cystic fibrous dysplasia: Axial T1W sequence shows the low/intermediate signal fluid and the peripheral low signal rim in the left proximal femur.

DIFFERENTIAL DIAGNOSES IMAGES

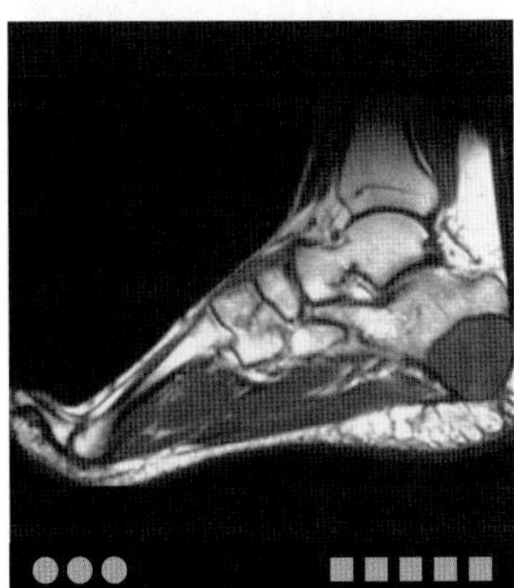

D. Bone cyst: Sagittal T1WI shows a low signal peripheral rim around an intermediate signal fluid collection in the calcaneus.

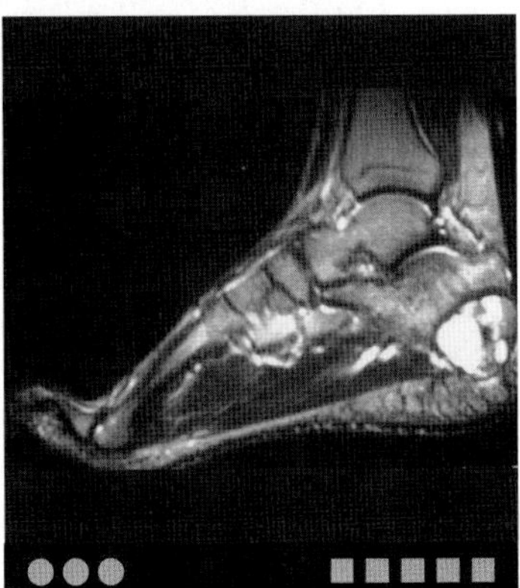

E. Bone cyst: Sagittal T2W sequence shows the high signal fluid collection and the peripheral low signal rim, which is thinner than the one in cystic fibrous dysplasia. Fluid–fluid levels are also present in this aneurysmal bone cyst.

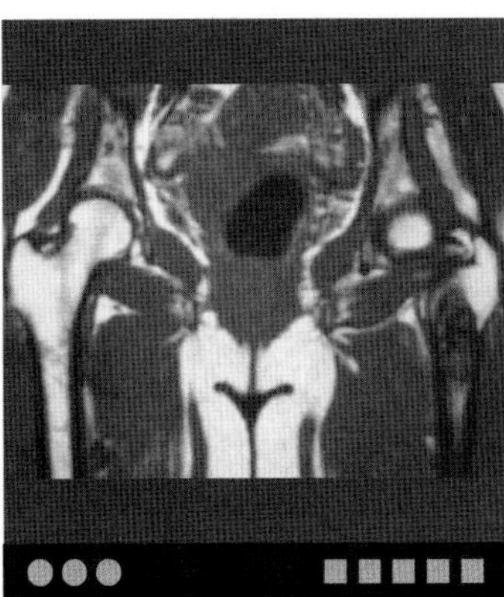

F. Enchondroma: Coronal T1WI shows an intermediate signal lesion in the left proximal femur. Internal low signal mineralization is present.

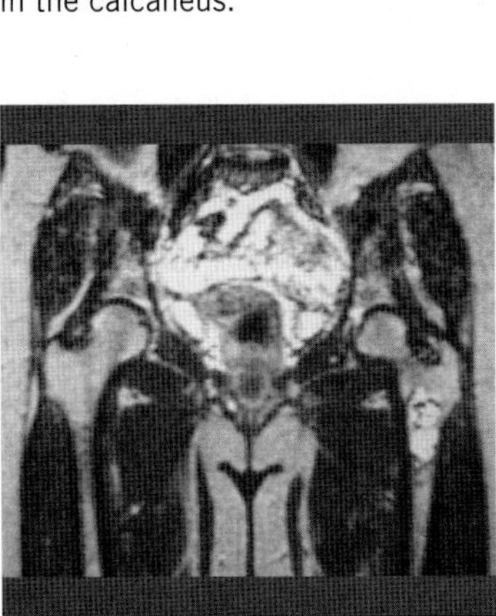

G. Enchondroma: Coronal T2WI shows the high signal lesion and no peripheral rim in the left proximal femur. Internal low signal mineralization is present.

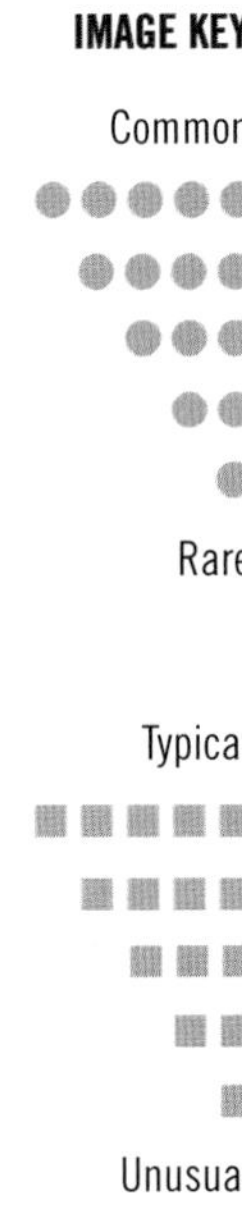

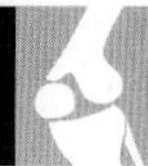

21–2 Simple Bone Cyst of the Ilium

Oganes Ashikyan and Jamshid Tehranzadeh

PRESENTATION

Pelvic pain without history of trauma

FINDINGS

CT examination of pelvis shows a cystic lesion in the ileum with narrow zone of transition and cortical microfractures.

DIFFERENTIAL DIAGNOSES

- *Langerhans cell histiocytosis:* Eosinophilic granuloma and simple bone cyst can appear similar on imaging studies. Both lesions can present with pain. Soft tissue mass with cortical erosion and histologic findings of Langerhans cells and eosinophils help differentiate eosinophilic granuloma from simple bone cyst.
- *Aneurysmal bone cyst:* This lesion has aggressive expansile "soap bubble" eccentric appearance. Fluid–fluid levels related to presence of blood in the lesion can be seen on CT or MRI.
- *Brown tumor:* Also can present as an expansile lytic well-marginated cystlike lesion. Fibrous tissue and giant cells can be seen histologically.
- *Chondromyxoid fibroma:* This lesion can occur in iliac bone and has expansile appearance with often septated matrix.
- *Osteomyelitis of iliac bone:* There is often a lytic lesion with or without sclerotic pattern.

COMMENTS

This is a 12-year-old girl who presented with pelvic pain and no history of trauma. Simple bone cyst is also known as solitary bone cyst and unicameral bone cyst. The etiology of the simple bone cyst formation is unknown and maybe related to trauma with synovial entrapment or poor interstitial drainage. Simple bone cysts usually occur during active phase of bone growth and as such are more common in the 3- to 19-year-old age group. There is a 3:1 male to female predominance. Simple bone cysts are usually asymptomatic until microfractures result in pain, which usually leads to diagnosis. Ilium is an uncommon location for the unicameral bone cyst. This lesion is usually found in the proximal humerus, proximal femur, fibula, and calcaneus. Fine sclerotic rim around the lesion and slight bone expansion can be seen. CT or MRI occasionally may reveal fluid level in bone cysts. The lesions are photopenic on bone scan, unless fractures develop. When fractured, a fallen bone fragment (fallen fragment sign) can be seen at the dependent aspect of the lesion. Biopsy demonstrates presence of clear yellowish fluid. The wall of the cyst is lined by fibrous tissue. Hemosiderin and giant cells maybe present. The cysts can spontaneously regress. When lesions are large and pathologic fracture is a concern, interventions such as curettage, bone grafting, injection of steroids, injection of autologous bone marrow, or multiple drill holes can be performed.

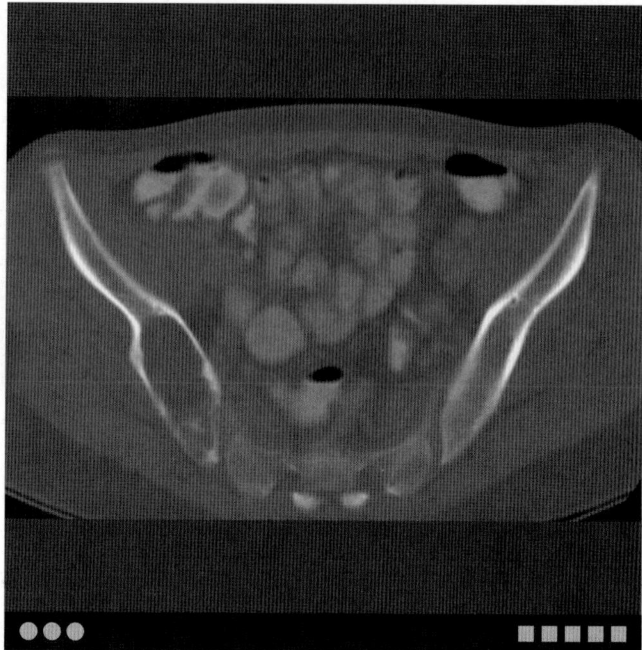

A. Simple bone cyst of ilium: Axial CT image demonstrates cystic lesion in the posterior right ilium adjacent to the right sacroiliac joint.

PEARLS

- **The etiology of the unicameral bone cyst formation is unknown and maybe related to trauma with synovial entrapment or poor interstitial drainage.**
- **This lesion is usually found in the proximal humerus, proximal femur, fibula, and calcaneus.**
- **Fine sclerotic rim around the lesion and slight bone expansion can be seen.**
- **Fallen fragment sign and fluid level in simple bone cyst have been reported.**
- **The lesions can spontaneously regress. When pathologic fracture is likely, various interventions to induce healing of the bone cyst can be performed.**

ADDITIONAL IMAGES

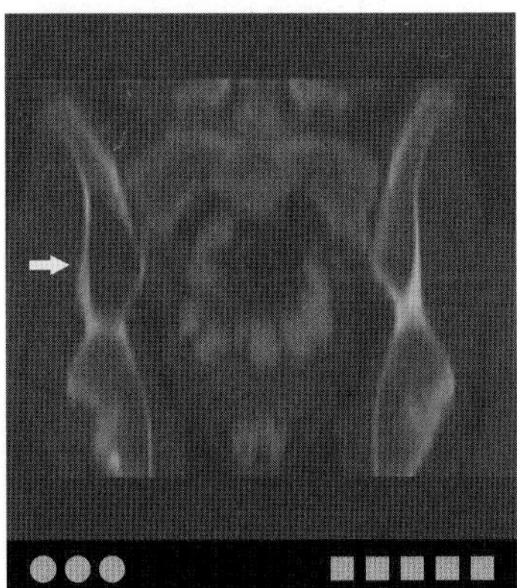

B. Simple bone cyst of ilium: Reconstructed CT image in sagittal plane demonstrates expansile cystic lesion in the posterior right ilium (arrow).

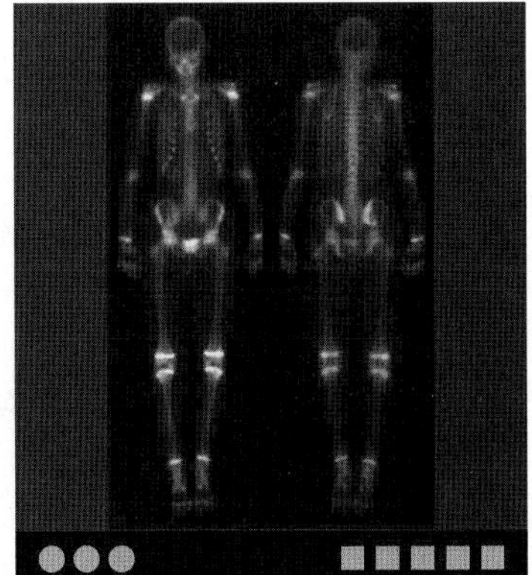

C. Simple bone cyst of ilium: Anterior and posterior projection views from the whole body bone scan obtained after administration of Tc-99m labeled MDP demonstrate mild increase in uptake of radiopharmaceutical at the borders of the lesion related to microfractures. The lesion itself remains photopenic.

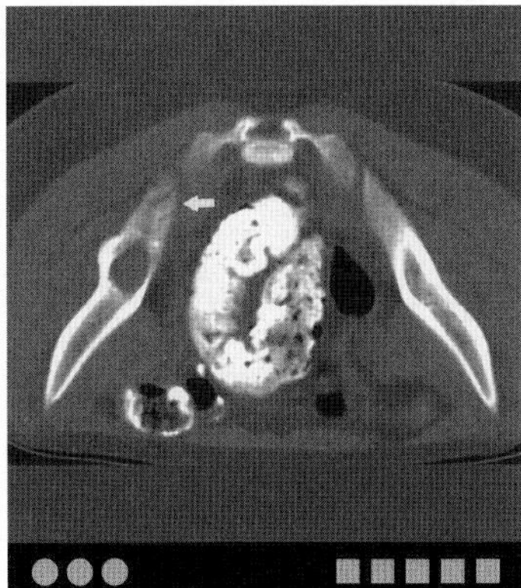

D. Simple bone cyst of ilium: Axial CT image obtained prior to CT-guided biopsy demonstrates lucent lines in the cortex of posterior right ilium adjacent to the sacroiliac joint. These lines represent microfractures, which resulted in patient's pain (arrow).

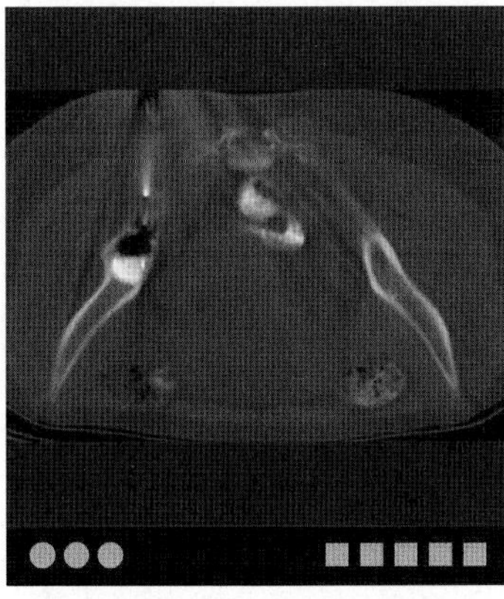

E. Simple bone cyst in the posterior right ilium: Axial CT images obtained after injection of contrast into the lesion demonstrates a single air-contrast level within the lesion.

IMAGE KEY

Common

●●●●●
●●●●
●●●
●●
●

Rare

Typical

■■■■■
■■■■
■■■
■■
■

Unusual

DIFFERENTIAL DIAGNOSES IMAGES

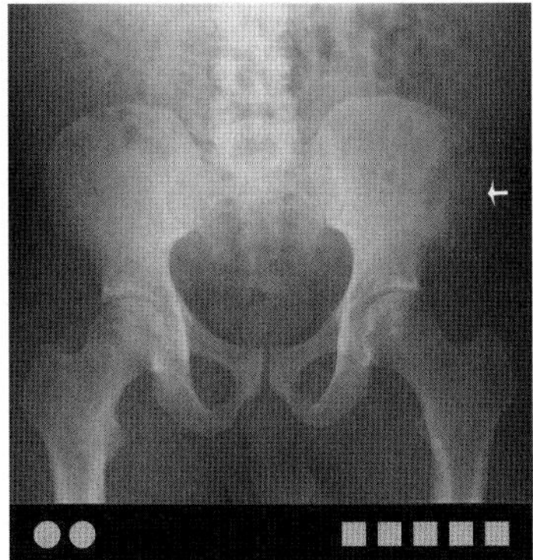

F. Coccidioidomycosis: AP radiograph shows destructive lesion of the left iliac bone with sclerotic margin (arrow) suggesting slow growth process.

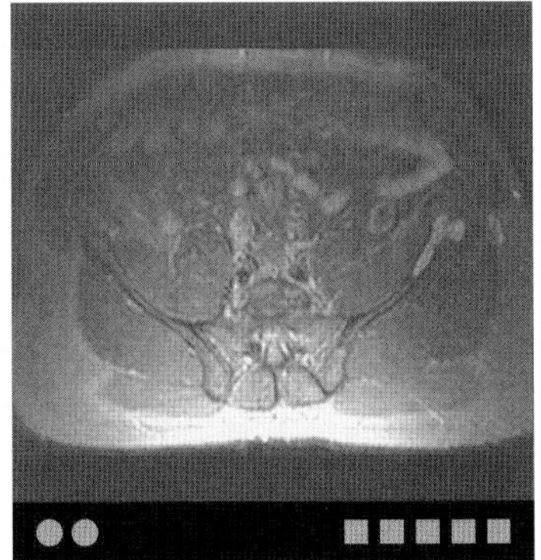

G. Coccidioidomycosis: Axial STIR image shows high signal intensity lesion of the left ileum, which is a nonspecific finding. There is no soft tissue mass.

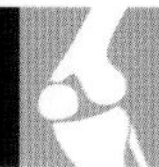

21–3 Benign Peripheral Nerve Sheath Tumor of the Sacrum

Kambiz Motamedi

PRESENTATION

Several year history of back pain

FINDINGS

CT shows widening and osteolytic changes of the right S1 sacral foramen by a solid mass.

DIFFERENTIAL DIAGNOSES

- *Tarlov cyst:* MRI may show widening of a neural foramen by a cystic mass.
- *Langerhans cell granulocytosis:* Cross sectional imaging will demonstrate a bony tumor which may invade the neural foramina. Any round cell tumor may affect the sacrum.
- *Metastatic disease:* CT may reveal a lytic or blastic rather destructive lesion of the sacrum with possible invasion of the neural foramen.

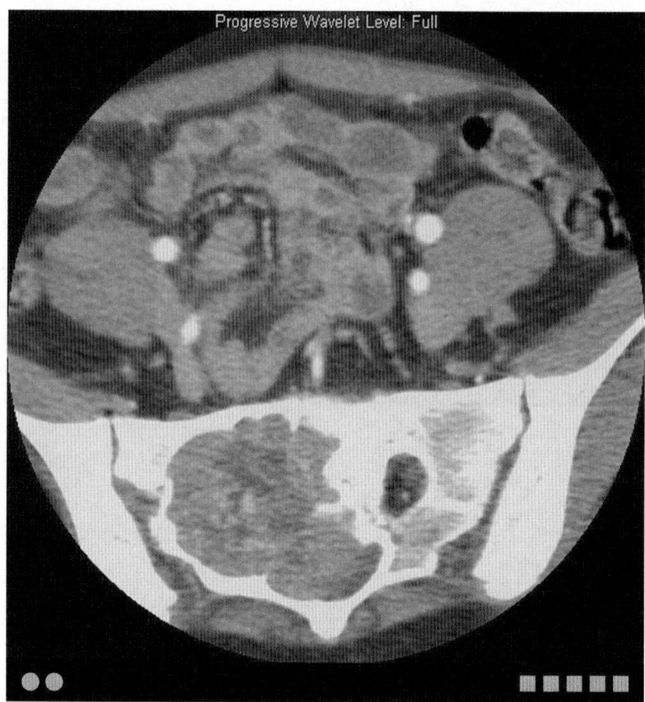

A. BPNST: The axial CT scan of the sacrum at the S1 level demonstrates a solid soft tissue mass occupying and enlarging the neural foramen.

COMMENTS

This 16-year-old patient had a 5-year history of occasional back pain and right radiculopathy. A neurilemoma is a benign, usually encapsulated neoplasm derived from Schwann cells and, along with neurofibroma, constitutes one of the two most common benign peripheral nerve sheath tumors (BPNST). The peripheral nervous system can be defined as nervous tissue outside the brain and spinal cord. It extends from the glial–schwannian junction in the cranial nerves and spinal roots to the termination of the nerve fibers in their end organ receptors and includes the posterior root ganglia and those of the autonomic nervous system. BPNSTs may affect any location in the course of the peripheral nervous system (i.e., cranial and spinal nerve roots, cranial and peripheral nerves, end organ receptors, small nerve twigs). They are common in paravertebral locations and the flexor regions of the extremities (especially near the elbow, wrist, and knee). Most BPNSTs are of the conventional (common) type, arise as solitary tumors smaller than 10 cm, and are not associated with a genetic syndrome. Neurologic symptoms tend to present late. Secondary neurologic symptoms may be present if the tumor is large. Lesions in the sciatic nerve can mimic discogenic low back pain. Commonly though symptoms can be vague, with an average interval of up to 5 years before the diagnosis is established. No racial or sex predilection is recognized with most patients between 20 and 50 years.

PEARLS

- **The sclerotic rim of the widened neural foramen reflects the nonaggressive and indolent nature of this lesion.**
- **The widened neural foramen is occupied by a solid mass.**
- **The symptoms are insidious and long standing.**

ADDITIONAL IMAGES

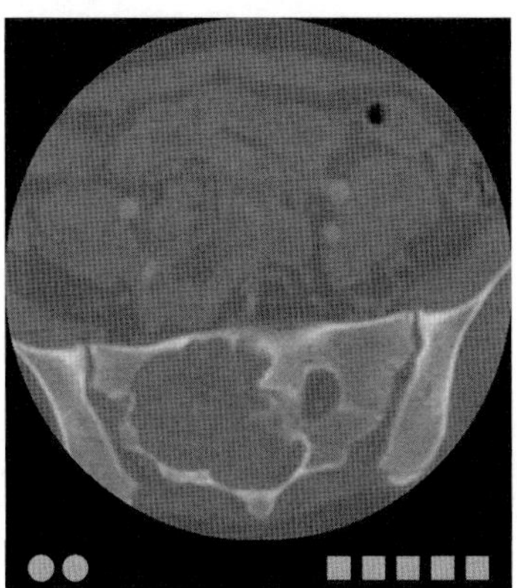

B. BPNST: Same axial CT scan in bone window shows readily the sclerotic rim of the widened neural foramen. Note cortical break at the right sacroiliac joint.

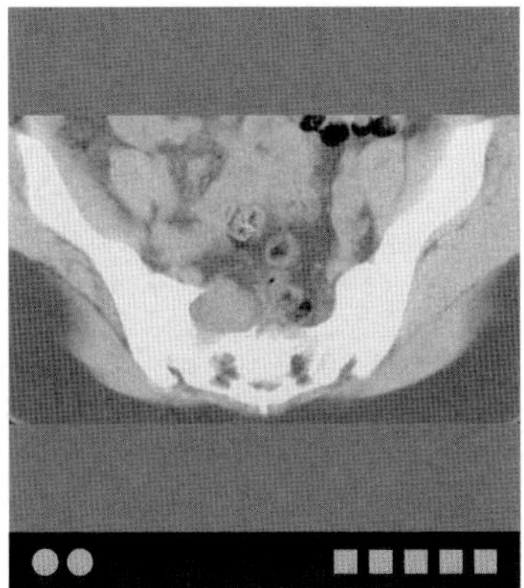

C. BPNST: An axial image at a level more superior reveals the course of the mass along the peripheral sacral nerve.

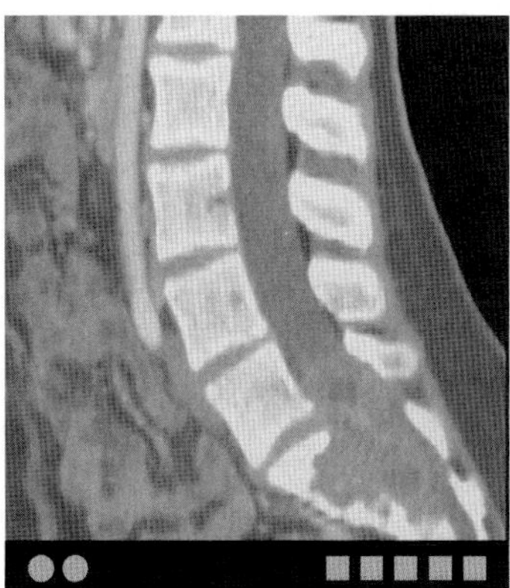

D. BPNST: The sagittal reformatted CT image shows the craniocaudal extent of the tumor and scalloping of the sacrum anteriorly.

IMAGE KEY

Common

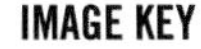

Rare

Typical

Unusual

DIFFERENTIAL DIAGNOSES IMAGES

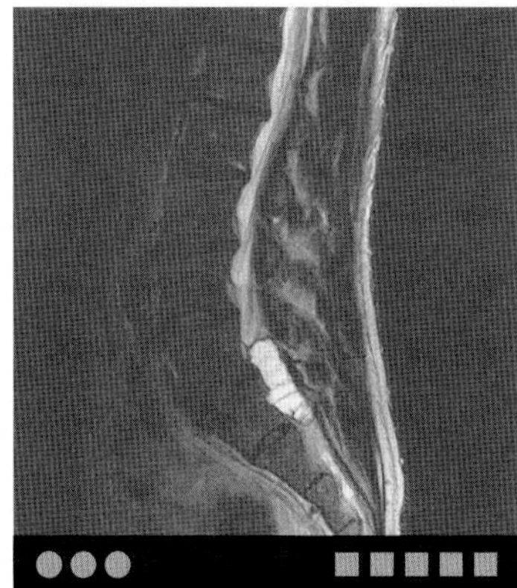

E. Tarlov Cyst: A T2W sagittal image of the lumbar spine demonstrates a cystic lesion of the spinal canal at the L5-S1 level.

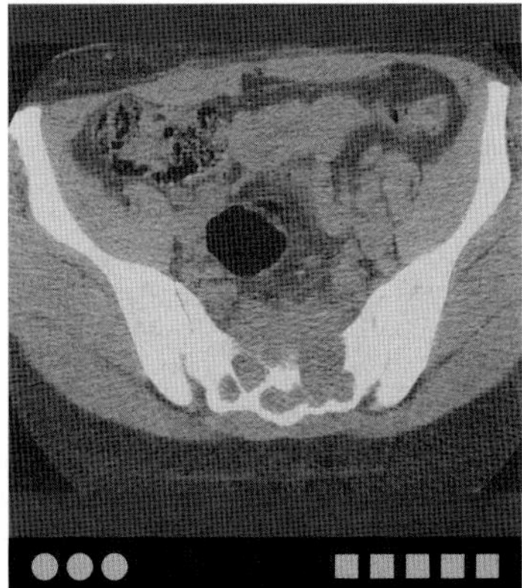

F. Langerhans cell granulocytosis: CT reveals a lytic lesion of the sacrum invading the neural foramina.

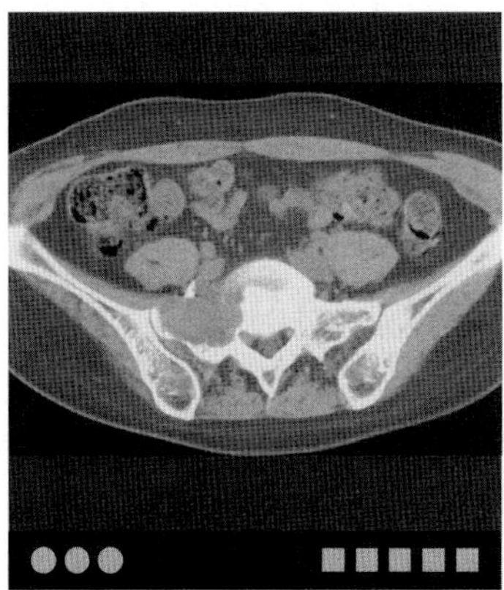

G. Metastatic disease: The axial CT scan of the sacrum at the S1 level shows a destructive presacral lesion. Incidentally this is a metastatic focus of a malignant peripheral nerve sheath tumor.

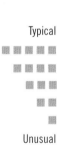

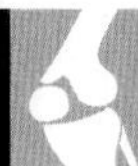

21–4 Synovial Chondromatosis of the Hip

Sulabha Masih

PRESENTATION

Pain and discomfort in the right hip

FINDINGS

Radiographs and CT show multiple intra-articular calcified loose bodies. MR images show multiple low signal intensity loose bodies on all sequences in the synovial fluid.

DIFFERENTIAL DIAGNOSES

- *Pigmented villonodular synovitis:* This condition is associated with synovial villi containing hemosiderin pigment, which appear as dark signal on all sequences. Cystic erosions of the subchondral bones are often present.
- *Synovial sarcoma:* Non-intra-articular malignant tumor, which appears as soft tissue mass with amorphous calcification on radiographs. MR shows low signal on T1W and inhomogeneous increase signal on T2WI.
- *CPPD (Calcium pyrophosphate deposition disease):* Commonly seen in patients with pseudogout, hemochromatosis, and hyperparathyroidism. Intra-articular and chondral calcifications are best seen on radiographs and CT.

COMMENTS

This is a 38-year-old male with pain and discomfort in the right hip. Synovial chondromatosis is a benign condition, always monoarticular, affecting the large joints, shows two to fourfold predilection for males compared to females and present in the third to fifth decade. Synovial chondromatosis is classified into two categories: primary or idiopathic and secondary type. Primary or idiopathic form is uncommon benign disorder due to synovial metaplasia with formation of multiple loose bodies in the joint. Initially, these loose bodies are not calcified, but later do become calcified and exhibit same size. Clinically, patients complain of tightness and swelling. Eventually these bodies imbed the synovium with cartilage erosion. Treatment includes removal of loose bodies and synovectomy. Secondary synovial chondromatosis is much more common and usually results from trauma to the cartilage with cartilage disruption and formation of loose bodies in the joint. They may or may not calcify. They vary in size and are fewer in number. Premature osteoarthritis is the end result. Treatment is removal of loose bodies and smoothening of the cartilaginous defect. On radiographs and CT multiple intra-articular calcified loose bodies are noted. MR images show multiple rounded low signal intensity loose bodies on all the sequences. Synovial fluid is low intermediate signal intensity on T1WI and high signal intensity on T2WI.

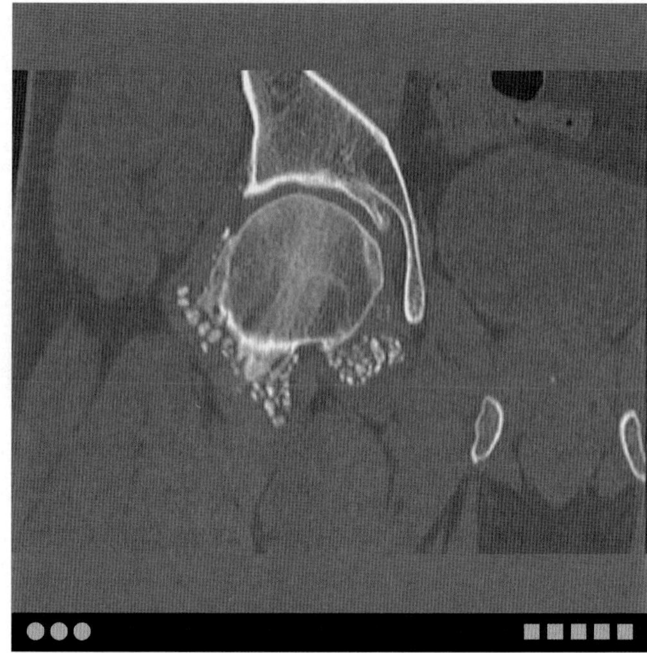

A. Synovial chondromatosis: CT scan shows multiple intra-articular loose bodies in the right hip joint well.

PEARLS

- **Primary synovial chondromatosis because of synovial metaplasia with formation of multiple same size loose bodies in the joint.**
- **Secondary synovial chondromatosis usually because of trauma to the cartilage with cartilage disruption and formation of varying size loose bodies in the joint. Premature osteoarthritis is the end result.**
- **On radiographs and CT, intra-articular calcified loose bodies are noted. MR images show multiple rounded low signal intensity loose bodies on all the sequences in the synovial fluid.**

ADDITIONAL IMAGES

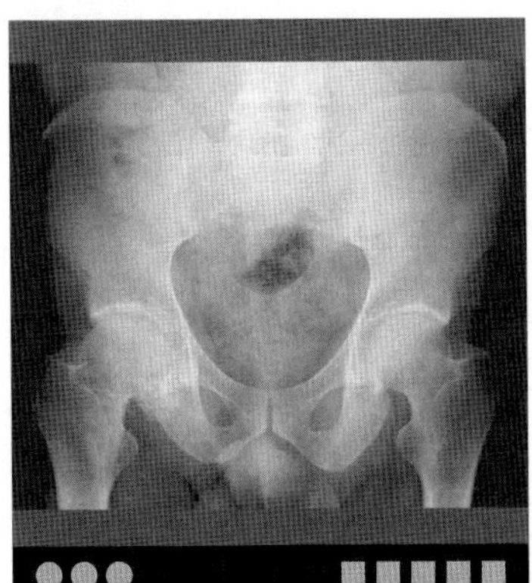

B. Synovial chondromatosis: AP pelvis radiograph demonstrates multiple calcified loose bodies in the right hip joint.

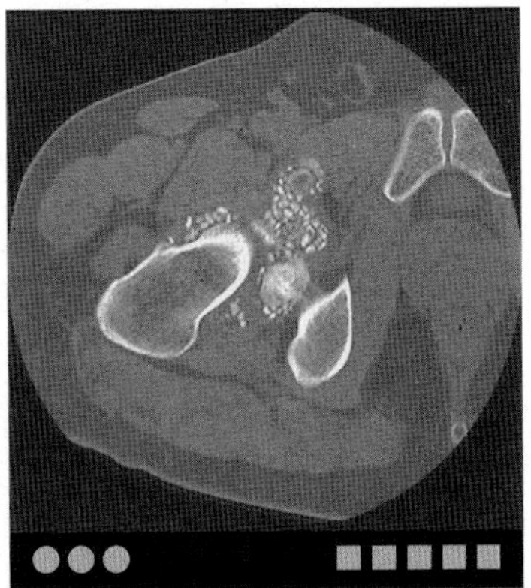

C. Synovial chondromatosis: CT scan shows intra-articular loose bodies in the right hip joint well.

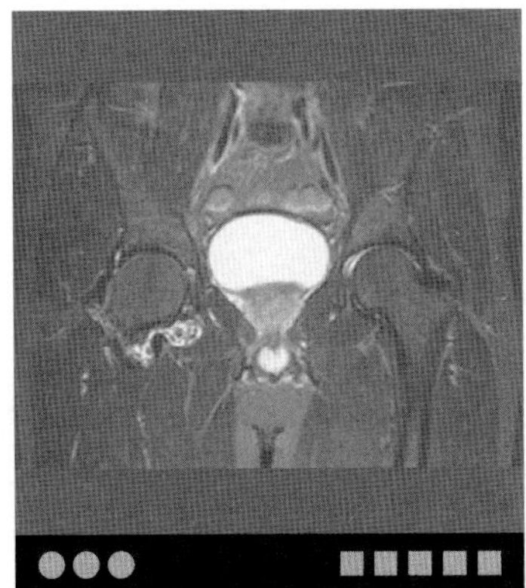

D. Synovial chondromatosis: MR coronal STIR image shows rounded low signal intensity loose bodies in the synovial fluid.

IMAGE KEY

Common

Rare

Typical

Unusual

DIFFERENTIAL DIAGNOSES IMAGES

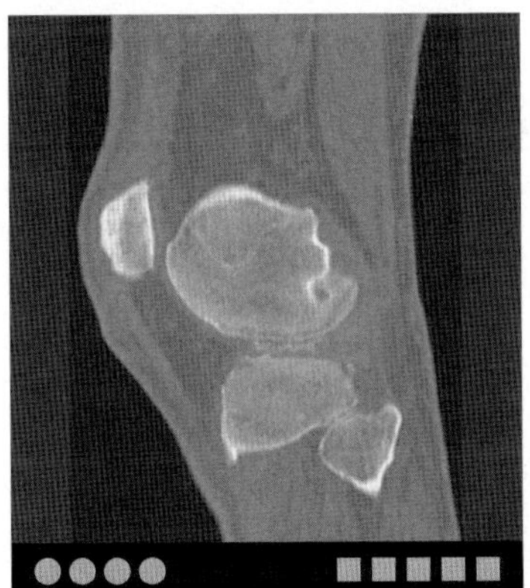

E. CPPD: Sagittal CT scan shows intra-articular chondrocalcinosis.

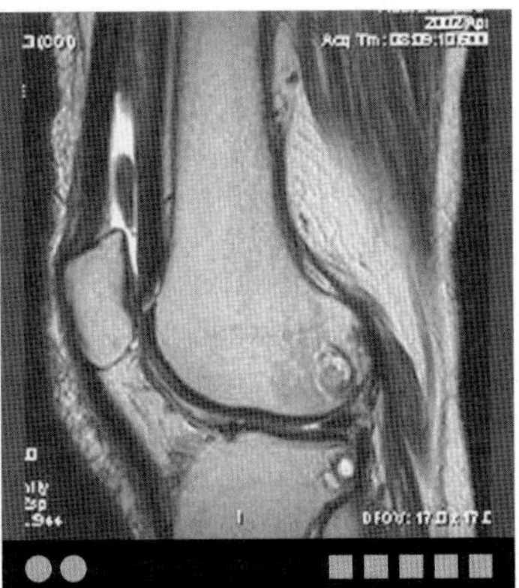

F. PVNS: Sagittal T2W images shows high signal intensity effusion &and low signal intensity hemosiderin.

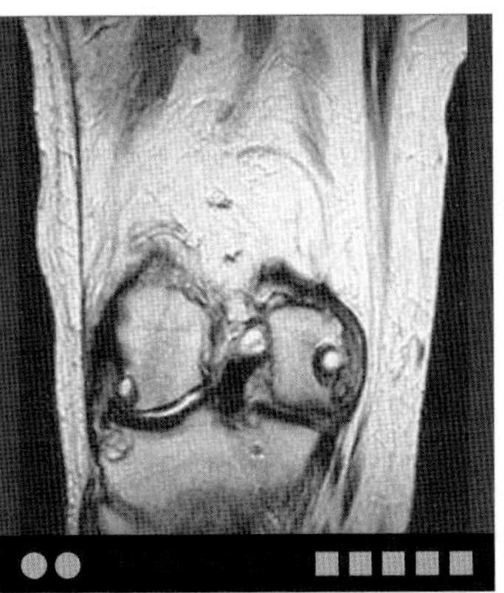

G. PVNS: Coronal T2WI shows multiple bony erosions distal femur and proximal tibia.

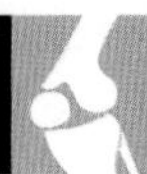

21–5 Chondroid Lipoma

George Hermann

PRESENTATION

Left upper thigh mass

FINDINGS

MRI shows a large soft tissue mass with heterogeneous signal changes.

DIFFERENTIAL DIAGNOSES

- Myxoid liposarcoma usually shows heterogeneous SI with low SI septation.
- Extraskeletal chondrosarcoma is a rare malignant tumor, which may show multinodular masses that are high SI on T2WI. Histologically, it may be difficult to differentiate between the two entities.
- MFH shows prominent lobulation and septation on T2WI. It is difficult to differentiate it from other spindle cell sarcomas.

COMMENTS

This is a 35-year-old woman with a 3-month history of an enlarging mass on the left upper thigh. She was diagnosed with chondroid lipoma. Chondroid lipoma is an uncommon benign fatty tumor containing elements of cartilage and even ossification can be observed in the lesion. The tumors are well circumscribed, usually arising in the deep subcutaneous, superficial muscular fascia, or skeletal muscle of the extremities. Occasionally, it is found in the maxillofacial region. It is more common in females. The male-to-female ratio is approximately 1:4. The age of onset ranges from the second to the eighth decade of life. The tumor is usually well defined, encapsulated and averaging in size 4 to 5 cm. Cross-sectional imaging may provide valuable information. On MRI the mass presents heterogeneously septated tissue structures. On T1WI, it shows predominantly decreased SI with scattered increased SI elements embedded inside the mass. On STIR images the lobulated low SI structures appear bright, suggesting chondroid elements. On the other hand, the bright SI area that was seen on T1 WI became suppressed on STIR images that were typical of fat.

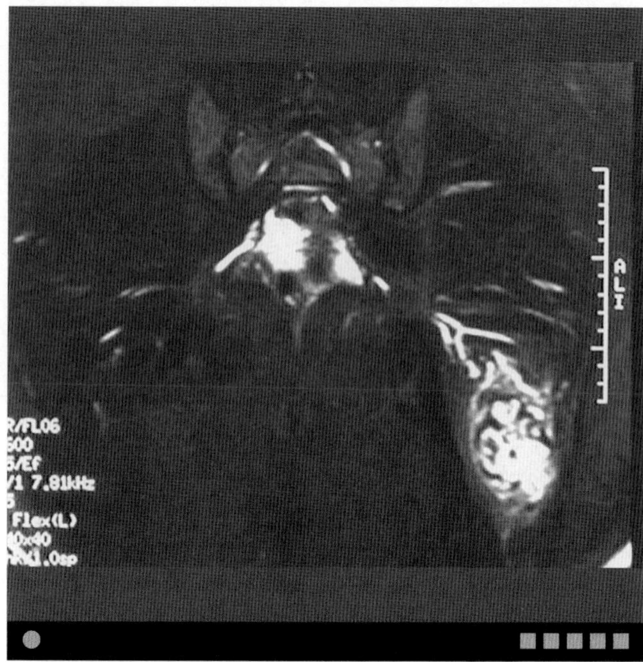

A. Chondroid lipoma: Coronal STIR image shows scattered signal void in the high SI mass.

PEARLS

- **Chondroid lipoma is a rare benign adipose tumor, which histologically resembles extraskeletal chondrosarcoma and liposarcoma.**
- **It usually involves the extremities.**
- **On MRI, the mass consisted of increased SI lobulated tissue on STIR images. The lobules are separated by low SI septae.**

ADDITIONAL IMAGES

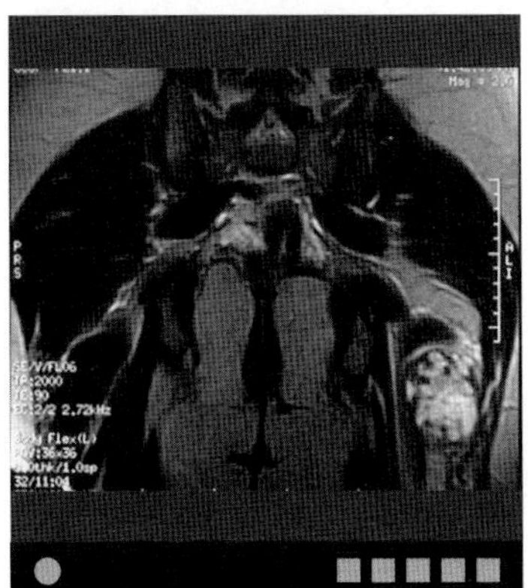

B. Chondroid lipoma: Coronal T2WI shows a well-defined mass with lobulated nodularity. Note the scattered low SI dots.

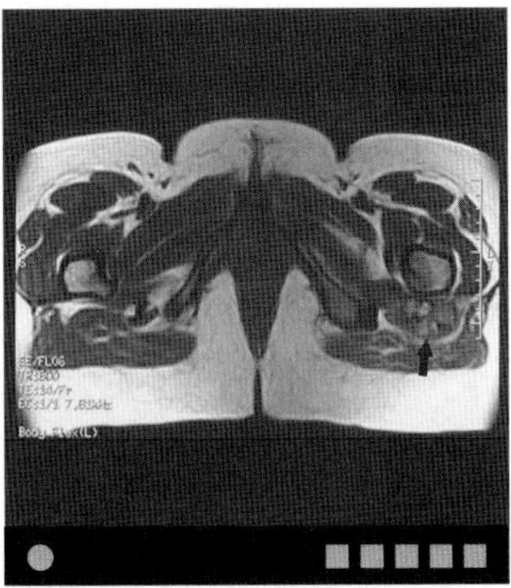

C. Chondroid lipoma: Axial T1WI demonstrates a slightly increased SI mass (arrow) behind the lesser trochanter. Note the high SI structure at the center.

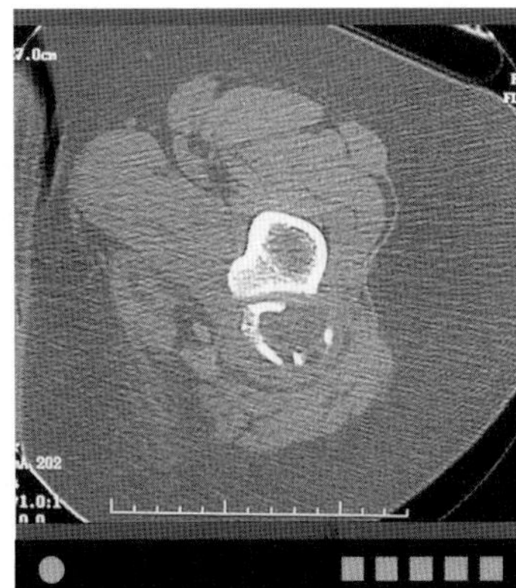

D. Chondroid lipoma: CT of the proximal thigh reveals a low attenuated soft tissue mass surrounded by a calcified rim behind the lesser trochanter.

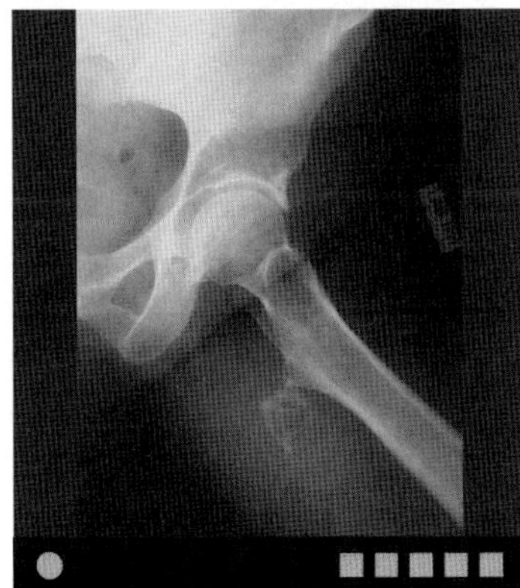

E. Chondroid lipoma: Oblique radiograph of the left hip shows an ossified mass adjacent to the lesser trochanter.

DIFFERENTIAL DIAGNOSES IMAGES

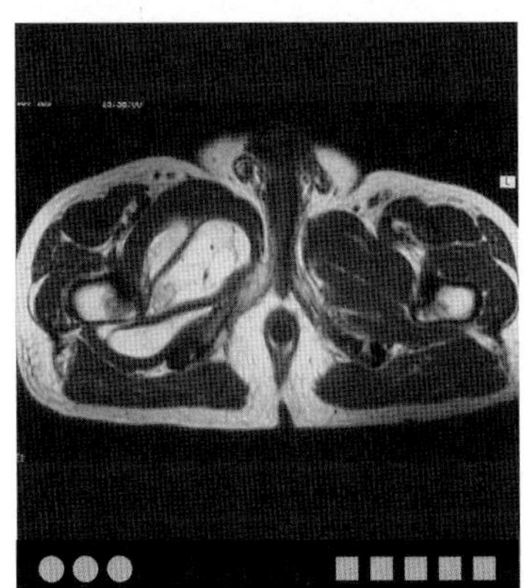

F. Liposarcoma: Axial T2WI shows scattered low SI foci in the bright mass.

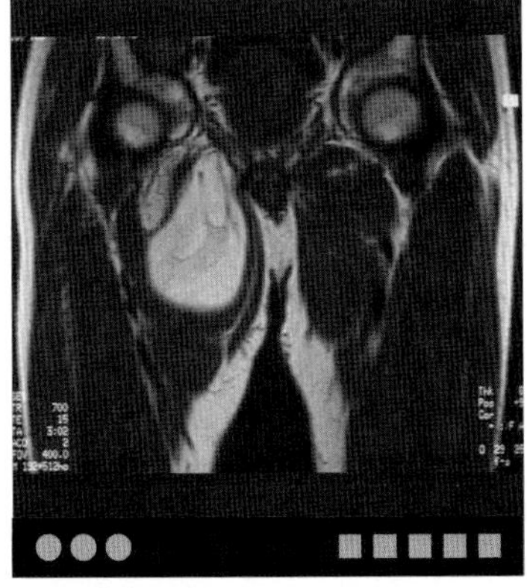

G. Liposarcoma: Coronal T1WI shows a high SI mass. Scattered low SI septae are in the mass. It is difficult to differentiate from lipoma.

IMAGE KEY

Common

Rare

Typical

Unusual

21–6 Hibernoma

James Coumas

PRESENTATION

Painless, slow-growing soft tissue mass

FINDINGS

MR images show a prominent soft tissue mass with tissue characterization similar to fat on T1 weighting with prominent septations and vessels.

DIFFERENTIAL DIAGNOSES

- *Liposarcoma:* Although variants exist, a discrete lipomatous mass with a nonlipomatous component can be seen with a well-differentiated liposarcoma.
- *Traumatized Lipoma:* Increased vascularity or bleeding within a lipoma because of trauma may produce scarring and septations.

COMMENTS

This is a 32-year-old male with a painless soft tissue mass of the thigh that has increased in size. Hibernoma is an uncommon benign slow-growing mass most commonly located in the thigh. Hibernoma is brown fat. "Hiber-" means winter, and this is the fat that warms to bring bears out of hibernation. Everybody has some, and you can recognize it (in health or as a tumor) because its cells have several vacuoles and pink mitochondria between the vacuoles. The tumor is composed of brown fat, which is thought to arise from regions of embryologic brown adipose tissue found in fetuses and newborns. Alternate sites of involvement include the soft tissues of the chest wall, axilla, and neck. Four histologic subtypes are described. Clinical presentation is most common in the third and fourth decades of life. No gender predilection has been noted. The mass is often encapsulated and extramuscular with displacement of adjacent structures. Ultrasound is not helpful in the diagnosis. MR imaging is helpful in demonstrating a lipoma-like pattern with prominent septations and vessels. To date, no malignant transformation has been reported. Treatment is marginal resection if possible. Histology is not predictive of local recurrence. Recurrence is more commonly associated with intralesional excision. Because of extensive vascularity, intralesional resection is associated with significant bleeding.

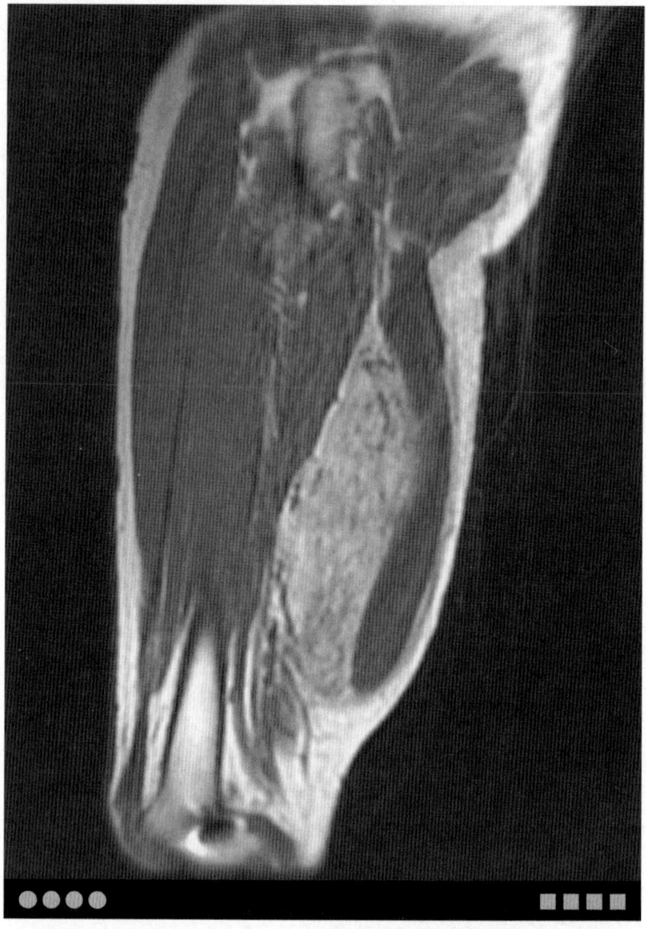

A. Hibernoma: Sagittal T1W MR image shows an intermuscular mass with fat signal and thickened septations.

PEARLS

- **Hibernoma is a lipoma-like variant on MR imaging with extensive vascularity, prominent septations, and should be entertained when a diagnosis of liposarcoma is considered.**
- **STIR MR imaging will demonstrate a relatively uniform heterogeneous increase in signal intensity throughout the mass.**

ADDITIONAL IMAGES

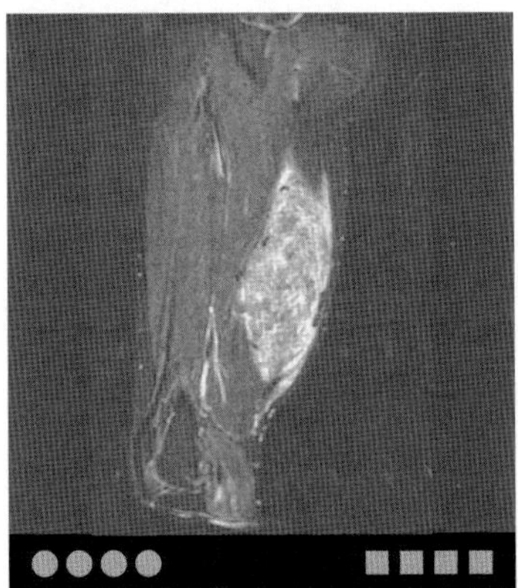

B. Hibernoma: Axial T1WI shows an intermuscular mass with fat signal and thickened septations.

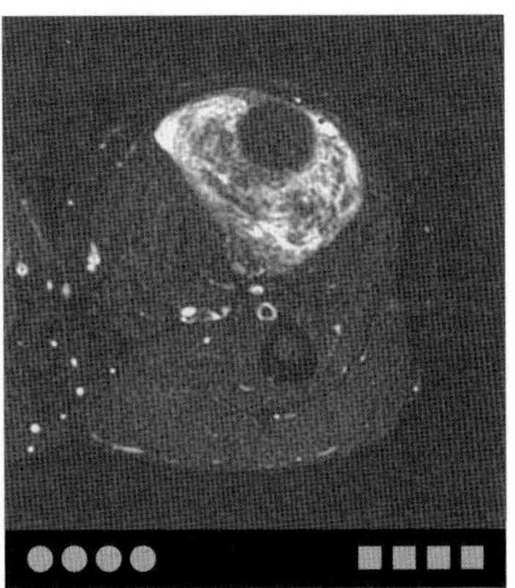

C. Hibernoma: Sagittal T2W fat-suppressed image shows uniform heterogeneous pattern with prominent peripheral vascularity.

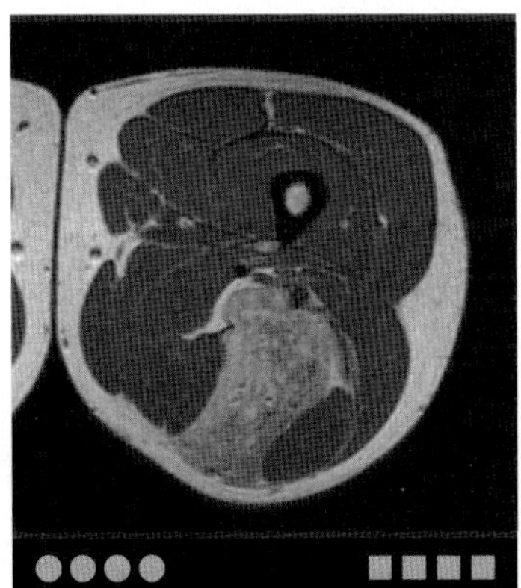

D. Hibernoma: Axial STIR image in prone position shows diffuse increased signal in mass surrounding the hamstring musculature.

DIFFERENTIAL DIAGNOSES IMAGES

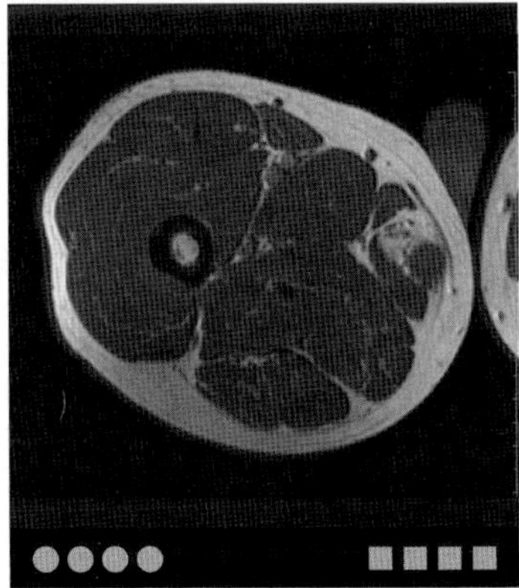

E. Liposarcoma: Axial T1WI shows a fatty component as well a focal nodular soft tissue mass isointense with muscle involving the gracilis muscle.

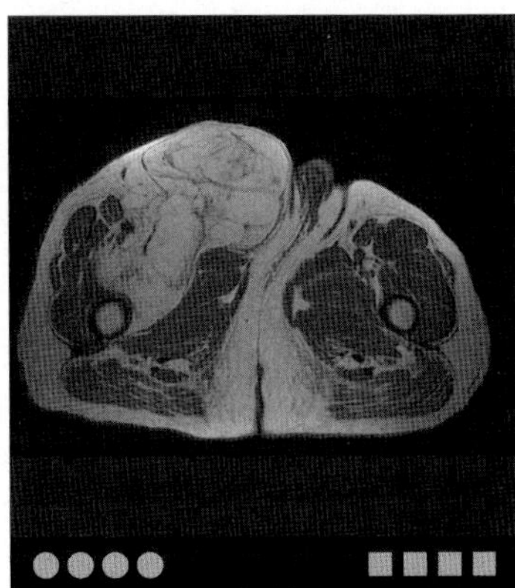

F. Liposarcoma: Axial T1WI in another patient with liposarcoma shows a large high signal mass with septations in the thigh.

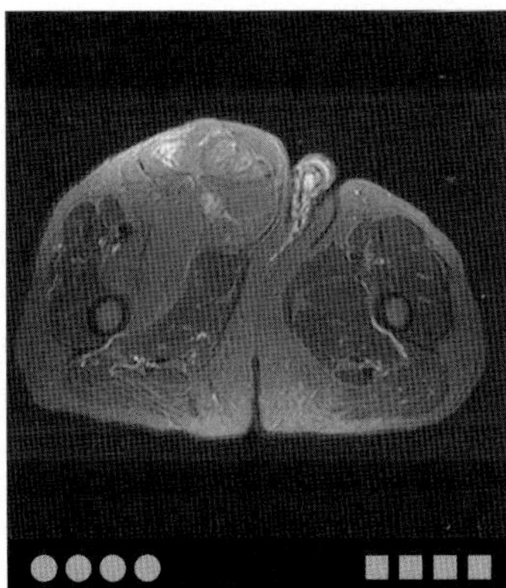

G. Liposarcoma: Axial STIR image in the same patient as image F shows a large mass with decreased signal (intermediate signal) and septations.

IMAGE KEY

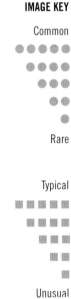

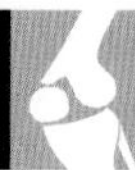

21–7 Neurofibromatosis

Ingrid B. Kjellin

PRESENTATION

Chronic hip pain and limping; multiple skin lesions

FINDINGS

MRI shows a chronic deformity of the left hip with an adjacent infiltrating mass. There are also small skin nodules.

DIFFERENTIAL DIAGNOSES

- *Angiomatous lesion:* Such is as a hemangioma. The angiomatous lesions are superficial and/or deep, often poorly marginated masses. Skin involvement is common. Occasional bone overgrowth and periosteal reaction are seen.
- In Klippel-Trenaunay-Weber syndrome, a triad of bone and soft tissue hypertrophy, varicose veins and cutaneous hemangiomas, the patients typically present with cosmetic deformity, bleeding, chronic venous insufficiency, and pain.
- *Fibromatoses:* This is a group of soft tissue lesions related to proliferation of benign fibrous tissue. They are classified as either superficial or deep. The growth pattern is often infiltrative without metastatic potential. Local recurrence is common.
- *Malignant soft tissue tumors:* Such is as malignant fibrous histiocytoma, liposarcoma, leiomyosarcoma, fibrosarcoma, and soft tissue metastasis should also be considered whenever there is a large deep soft tissue lesion in a middle-aged or elderly person.

COMMENTS

This is a 61-year-old with neurofibromatosis I, which is inherited as an autosomal dominant trait with a high penetrance. About 50% of cases result from new mutations. There are multiple criteria for diagnosis, including café-au-lait spots of a certain size, neurofibromas, axillary or inguinal freckling, optic glioma, Lisch nodules, distinct osseous lesions, and a first-degree relative with neurofibromatosis I. At least two of these findings have to be present. Skeletal abnormalities are common and are related to mesodermal dysplasia. They include kyphoscoliosis, facial, orbital and left lambdoid suture defects, pseudarthrosis, multiple nonossifying fibromas, rib deformity, posterior vertebral body scalloping, and meningoceles. Fracture healing may be defective and lead to further deformity. Anterolateral bowing of the tibia with pseudarthrosis is a deformity seen in young children with neurofibromatosis I. Focal or diffuse soft tissue hypertrophy, referred to as elephantiasis neuromatosa may coexist with bone overgrowth or underdeveloped of the adjacent bones. There are three forms of neurofibromas in neurofibromatosis I: localized, plexiform, and diffuse. The localized neurofibroma is the most frequent type, and the plexiform neurofibroma is the most characteristic lesion of neurofibromatosis I. Malignant transformation has been found to occur in about 5%, and typically involves a major nerve trunk. The patients may present with pain, neurological symptoms or rapid growth of a neurofibroma. Local recurrence and metastases are common, despite aggressive treatment.

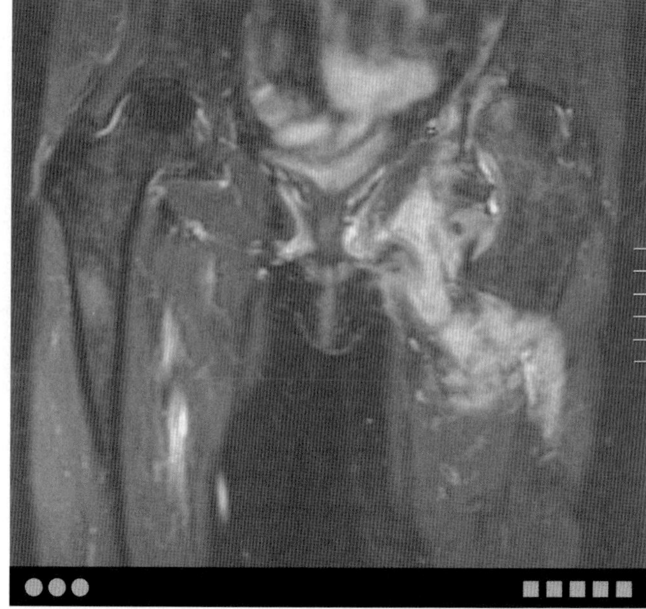

A. Neurofibromatosis: A coronal STIR image shows a poorly marginated hyperintense soft tissue mass in the left hip and thigh. There is coxa valga and cortical irregularity of the acetabulum. There are small bilateral soft tissue nodules.

PEARLS

- **Neurofibromatosis I is one of the most common genetic diseases with a frequency of 1 in 3000 births.**
- **Criteria for diagnosis include café'-au-lait spots, neurofibromas, axillary or inguinal freckling, optic glioma, Lisch nodules, distinct osseous lesions, and a first-degree relative with neurofibromatosis I.**
- **There are three types of neurofibromas in neurofibromatosis I: localized, plexiform, and diffuse.**
- **Malignant transformation has been estimated to be about 5%.**

ADDITIONAL IMAGES

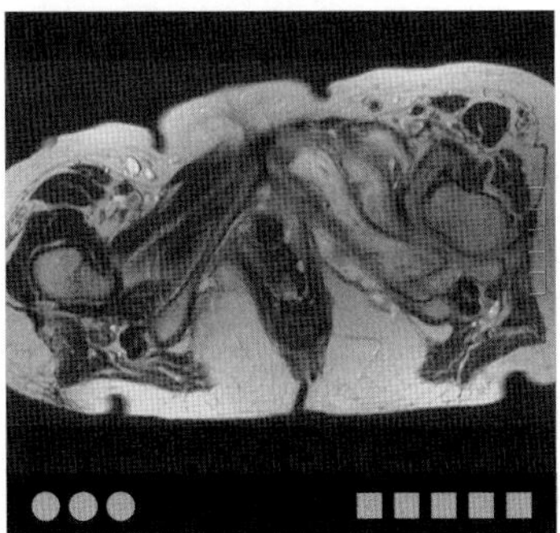

B. Neurofibromatosis: A T2W axial image without fat saturation shows a poorly defined, infiltrating mass along the left ischiopubic ramus, which is deformed. There is a small skin nodule in the anterior right thigh, consistent with molluscum fibrosum, which is a common cutaneous lesion of neurofibromatosis I.

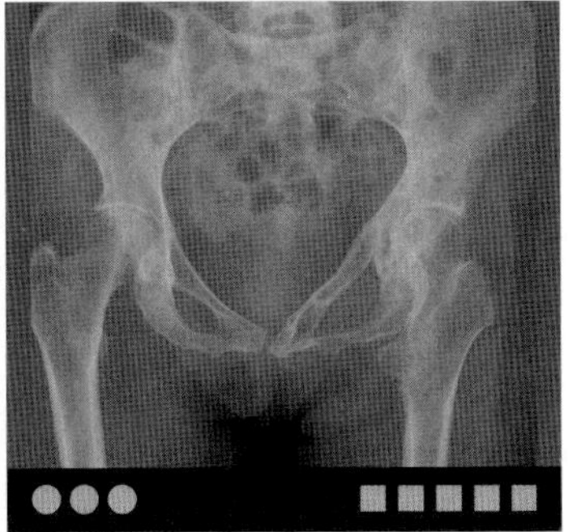

C. Neurofibromatosis: A frontal radiograph of the pelvis more clearly defines the chronic skeletal deformity, which is related to mesodermal dysplasia.

DIFFERENTIAL DIAGNOSES IMAGES

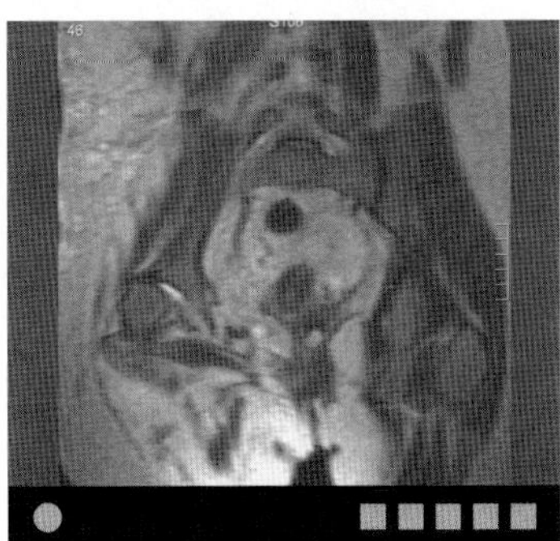

D. Klippel-Trenaunay-Weber syndrome: A coronal T2WI without fat saturation shows fatty overgrowth of the right flank with diffuse heterogeneity of the subcutaneous fat, consistent with diffuse angiomatous lesions. There is a chronic deformity of the right hip.

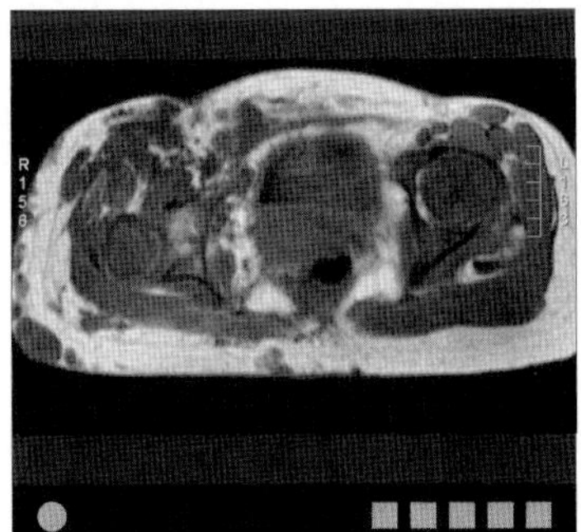

E. Klippel-Trenaunay-Weber syndrome: A T1W axial image shows extensive cutaneous lesions, consistent with angiomas, along with fatty overgrowth. The right acetabulum is dysplastic and the right femoral head is small.

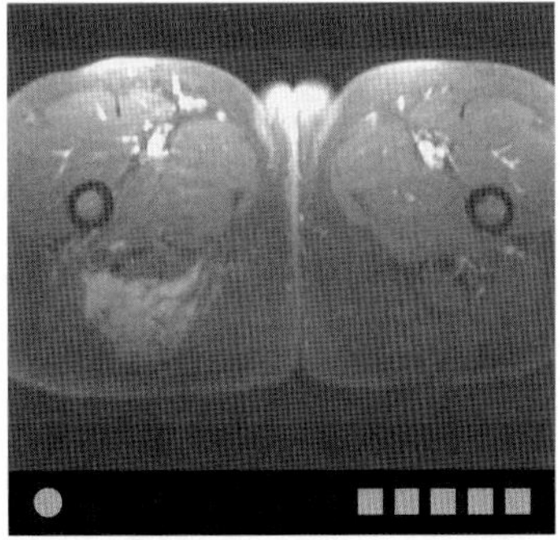

F. Fibromatosis: An axial T1W post-contrast image shows a large poorly marginated, enhancing mass in the posterior right thigh.

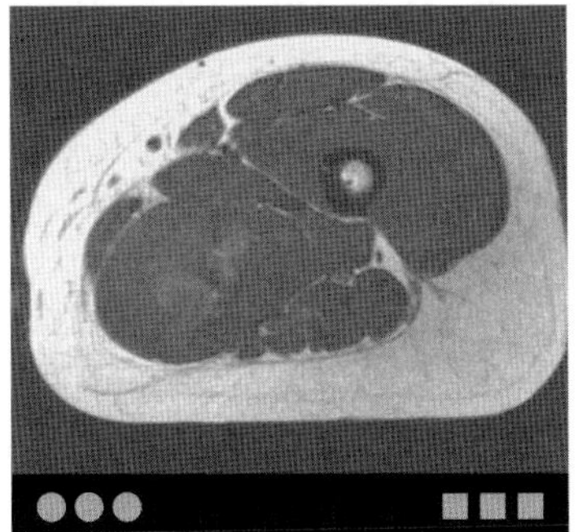

G. Liposarcoma: An axial T1WI shows a mainly isointense mass deep in the thigh. There are small regions of increased signal within the mass, consistent with fat.

IMAGE KEY

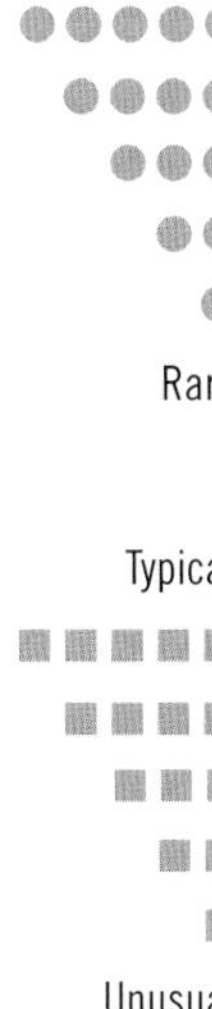

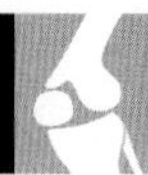

21–8 Amputation (Stump) Neuroma

Joon Kim

PRESENTATION

Small painful mass in lower extremity stump

FINDINGS

MR images show a small mass within a right lower extremity stump at an above the knee amputation.

DIFFERENTIAL DIAGNOSES

- *Peripheral nerve sheath tumor (PNST):* Both benign and malignant PNSTs tend to occur adjacent to a nerve trunk. Their MR signal characteristics are nonspecific and will vary depending on the degree of necrosis and its histology.
- *Soft tissue sarcoma:* MR signal characteristics are nonspecific; will vary depending on the degree of necrosis and its histology.
- *Hematoma:* This has a nonenhancing heterogeneous mass and variable signal characteristic depending on the age of hematoma. Thin rim of hypointense signal suggest a chronic hematoma.
- *Soft tissue lymphoma:* Imaging appearance may mimic that of soft tissue sarcomas and PNSTs.

COMMENTS

The patient is a 23-year-old man who underwent an above-the-knee amputation at the age of 11 for osteosarcoma resection. He presented to his primary care physician with a small painful mass, located within the distal right lower extremity stump. The MR images, in conjunction with the clinical presentation, were consistent with a neuroma. Amputation (stump) neuromas are benign masses that arise as a result of focal proliferation of Schwann cells, axons, and surrounding connective tissue after partial or total transection of a nerve. Amputation neuromas can potentially develop at any part of the body where a nerve is transected. These tumors tend to form 1 to 10 years after surgery. They usually do not grow larger than 2 cm in size. Most neuromas arise from peripheral sensory nerves, but neuromas from motor and nerves of the autonomic nervous system have been reported. Neuromas present as small nodules, typically proximal to the surgical incision site. These tumors are typically painful or tender and may be associated with dysesthesia. In above the knee amputations, neuromas most commonly arise from the sciatic nerve, as seen in this patient. MR imaging is useful in diagnosing amputation neuromas. Classically, these masses follow MR signal characteristics similar to a nerve; isointense to muscle on T1 and hyperintense on T2 or inversion recovery sequences. If the mass or nodule is seen connected to or adjacent to a nerve trunk, an amputation neuroma is highly suggestive.

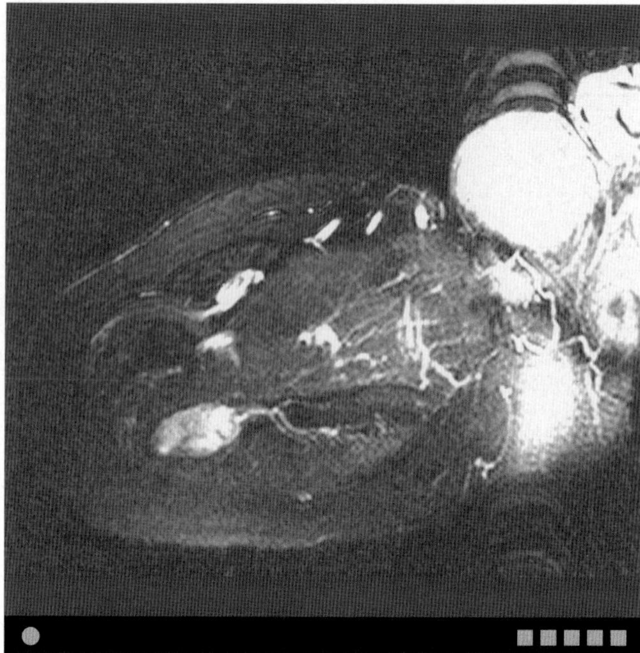

A. Amputation neuroma: Axial T2W fat-suppressed image shows a circumscribed, oval-shaped, hyperintense soft tissue mass within proximal right lower extremity stump posteriorly. The mass appears contiguous with the sciatic nerve and demonstrate signal characteristics similar to the nerve.

PEARLS

- **Amputation (stump) neuromas are benign masses composed of abnormal focal proliferation of Schwann cells, axons, and connective tissue surrounding the site of a transected nerve.**
- **Tend to develop 1 to 10 years after surgery.**
- **Neuromas typically present clinically as small painful nodules, usually proximal to a surgical incision site.**
- **MR imaging is useful in diagnosing amputation neuromas. If the mass or nodule is connected to or located adjacent to a nerve trunk, an amputation neuroma is highly suggestive.**

ADDITIONAL IMAGES

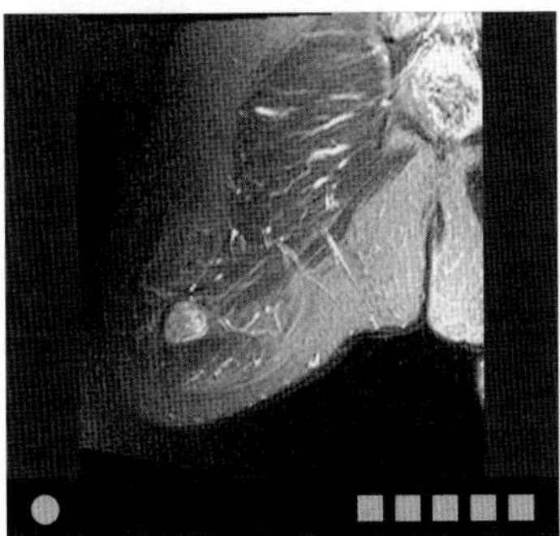

B. Amputation neuroma: Coronal inversion recovery image of the right lower extremity stump shows the mass to be close to the distal end of the stump.

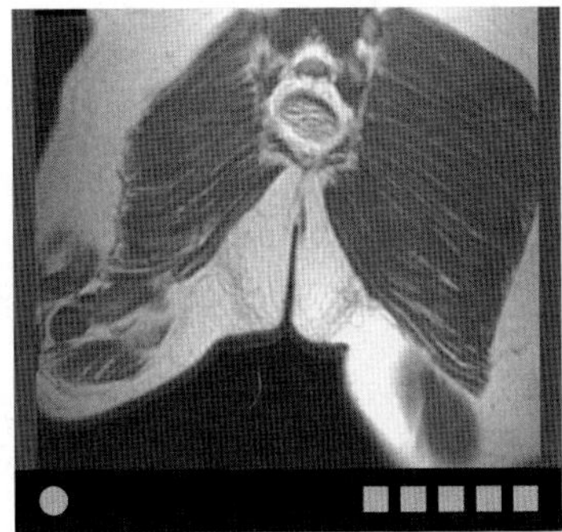

C. Amputation neuroma: Coronal T1W image shows the mass to be isointense to muscle.

DIFFERENTIAL DIAGNOSES IMAGES

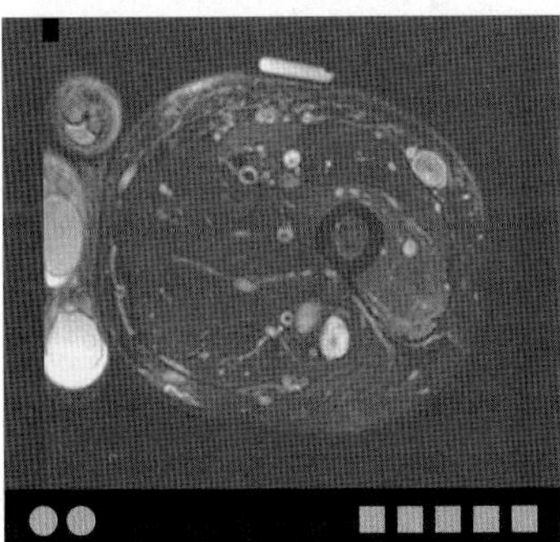

D. Peripheral nerve sheath tumors: Axial T2W fat-suppressed image shows multiple small oval or round hyperintense masses within the subcutaneous fat and musculature of the proximal left thigh in this patient with neurofibromatosis 1. Several of these masses demonstrate a "target" appearance.

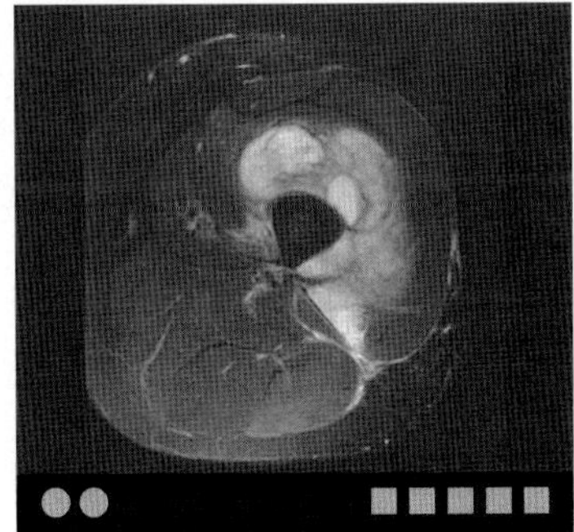

E. Intramuscular high grade sarcoma: Axial T2W fat-suppressed image shows a heterogeneous, but predominantly hyperintense mass occupying most of the vastus intermedius muscle.

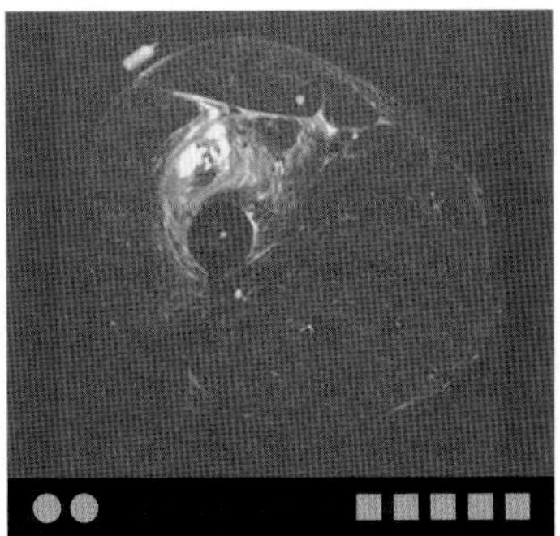

F. Intramuscular hematoma: Axial T2W fat-suppressed image shows a heterogeneous, but predominantly hyperintense mass occupying most of the vastus intermedius muscle. Fluid signal at the musculotendinous junction is consistent with a high-grade tear.

IMAGE KEY

Common

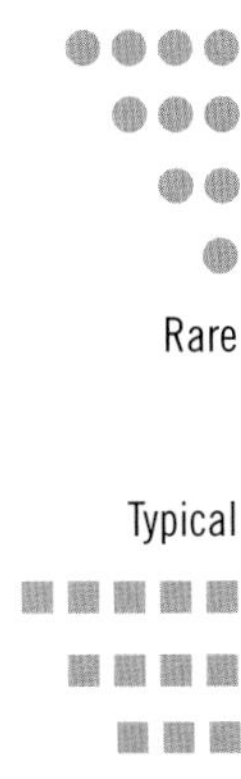

Rare

Typical

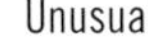

Unusual

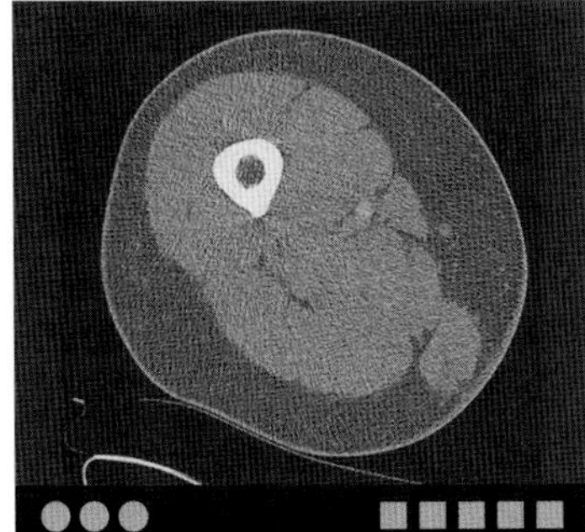

G. Subcutaneous lymphoma: Axial CT scan of the mid thigh shows a soft tissue lymphoma as a subcutaneous mass along the medial thigh in this patient with non-Hodgkins lymphoma.

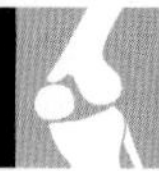

21–9 Liposarcoma of Thigh

Sulabha Masih

PRESENTATION

Slow growing right inguinal mass

FINDINGS

MR images show large inhomogeneous fatty mass in right upper thigh.

DIFFERENTIAL DIAGNOSES

- *Lipoma:* Presents as a well-defined, benign fatty tumor with homogenous high signal on T1WI.
- *Hibernoma:* A Rare, benign, slow growing, well circumscribed soft tissue mass. With serpentine vasculature and contains fat.
- *Lipoma arborescence:* Large, villous frondlike, intraarticular fat intensity mass with associated effusion.
- *Soft tissue Hemangioma:* A mass that often contains phlebolith. Postcontrast images will demonstrate "can of worm" appearance.

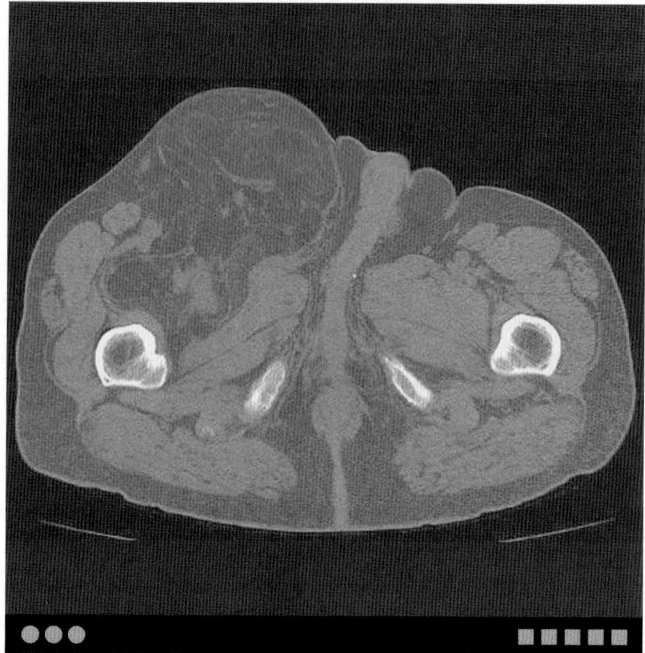

A. Liposarcoma: CT study shows a low density mass in right upper thigh.

COMMENTS

This case is a 64-year-old male with slow growing right inguinal mass for the last 2 years. Liposarcoma is the second most common soft tissue malignant tumor. Usually seen in middle aged and elderly population. It is extremely rare in children. Liposarcoma is malignant mesenchymal tumor, arising de novo from the deep-seated stroma rather than the submucosal or subcutaneous fat and does not originate from lipoma. Classification according to world health organization include well differentiated, myxoid, pleomorphic, and dedifferentiated and goes in order from low- to high-grade malignancy. Clinical symptoms are mainly the result of mass effect on the surrounding structures. The anatomical distribution is related to the histologic type. Well-differentiated liposarcoma tends to occur in deep soft tissues of the thigh, glutei, and retroperitoneum. Myxoid and pleomorphic liposarcomas have predilection to the limbs and dedifferentiated type occurs predominantly in the retroperitoneum. Metastasis to lung and liver are common with high-grade tumor and 5-year survival rate is less than 50%. Treated by wide surgical excision and radiation therapy. On radiograph, poorly defined mass of low-density fat and water density is noted. Calcification or ossification may be present in low-grade tumors. On CT, ill-defined inhomogeneous fatty and water low density mass can be seen with inhomogeneous contrast enhancement. MR imaging will show variable fat with inhomogeneous contrast enhancement. Thick septae and/or nodularity can also be noted.

PEARLS

- **Liposarcoma is distinct entity arising de novo and does not originate from lipoma. Usually located in the thigh, glutei, and retroperitoneum.**
- **Classified as well-differentiated, myxoid, pleomorphic, and dedifferentiated in order from low to high grade.**
- **Metastasis to lung and liver are common with high-grade tumor and 5-year survival rate is less than 50%.**
- **On CT, ill-defined fatty low density mass can be seen. MR imaging shows variable fat.**

ADDITIONAL IMAGES

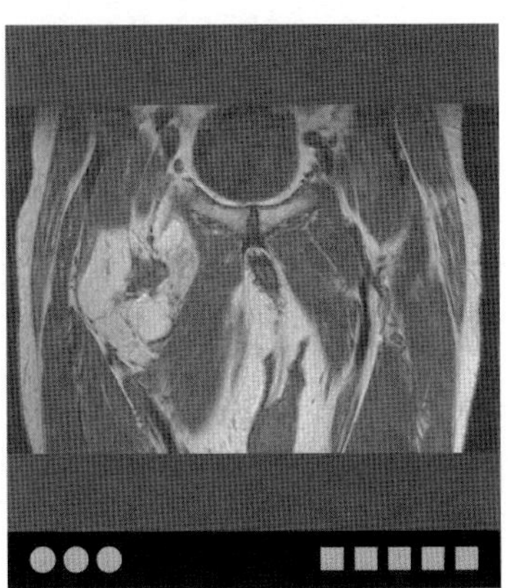

B. Liposarcoma: Coronal T1WI show an inhomogeneous fatty high signal upper thigh mass.

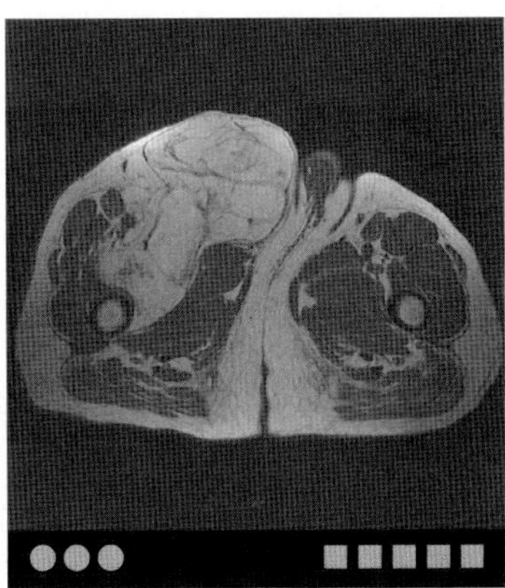

C. Liposarcoma: Axial T1WI show inhomogeneous fatty high signal upper thigh mass.

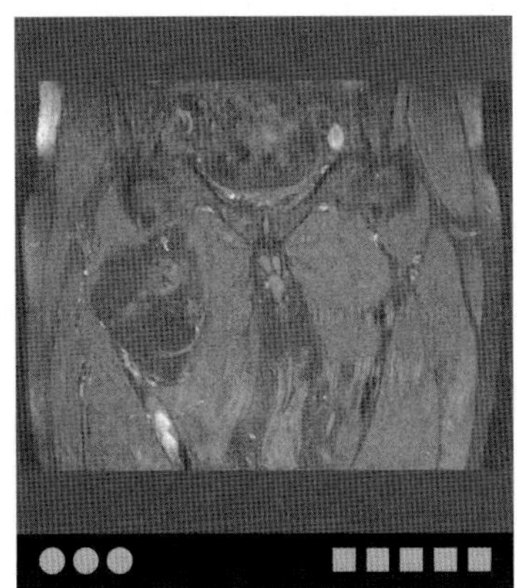

D. Liposarcoma: Coronal proton density fat-saturated image demonstrates inhomogeneous fat suppression of this mass.

DIFFERENTIAL DIAGNOSES IMAGES

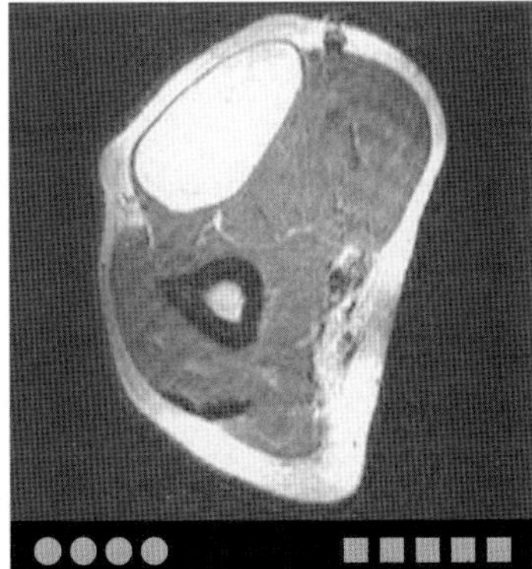

E. Lipoma: Axial T1WI shows well-defined, homogenous fatty high signal intensity mass.

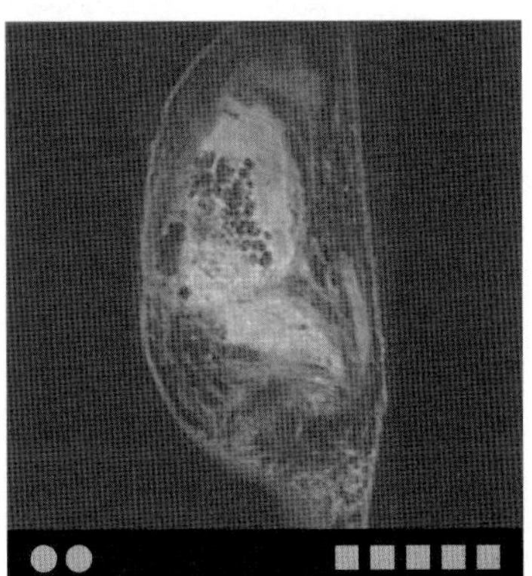

F. Lipoma arborescens: Sagittal STIR image shows low signal frond-like villous fat inside the synovial fluid.

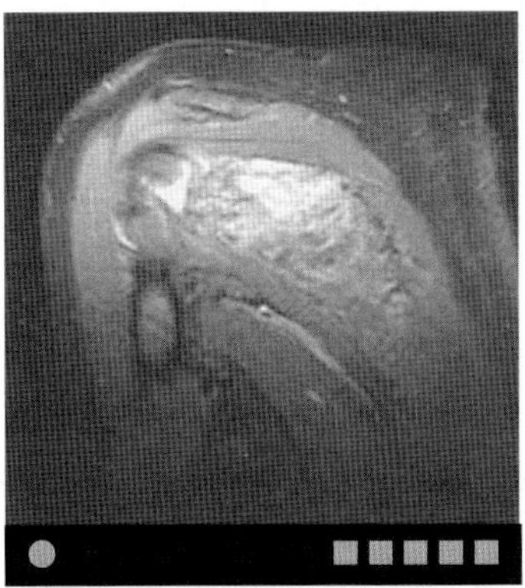

G. Hibernoma: Sagittal T2WI shows heterogeneous fatty mass with branching low signal vascular structures.

IMAGE KEY

Common

Rare

Typical

Unusual

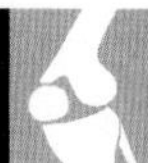

21–10 Synovial Sarcoma of Thigh

Peyman Borghei and Jamshid Tehranzadeh

PRESENTATION

Left thigh mass

FINDINGS

MRI shows lobulated cystic mass of the thigh with mixed signals.

DIFFERENTIAL DIAGNOSES

- *Liposarcoma:* MRI of liposarcoma shows a sharp mass with inhomogeneous contrast enhancement on T1W and mixed intermediate and high intensity signals on T2WI.
- *Malignant fibrous histiocytoma:* The soft tissue mass usually is associated with bony invasion and cortical destruction showing intermediate signal intensity (SI) on T1WI and high SI on T2WI.
- *Fibroblastic sarcoma:* Typically manifests as a poorly circumscribed mass with multinodular appearance and heterogenous enhancement. Extensive tendon sheath involvement is usually present.
- *Leiomyosarcoma:* Depending on tissue differentiation, this tumor may manifest different signal intensities on MR imaging.

COMMENTS

This is a 26-year-old female with a history of left thigh mass of 6-months duration diagnosed with synovial sarcoma. Synovial sarcoma, the fourth most common soft-tissue sarcoma, is a malignant mesenchymal tumor of uncertain origin. It primarily arises from the para-articular regions, usually in association with tendon sheaths, bursae, and joint capsules, with 71% invading, eroding, or touching adjacent bone. Most commonly it occurs in the lower extremities followed by upper extremities, trunk, and parapharyngeal region of the head and neck. Smaller lesions are often well circumscribed and homogenous, while larger lesions tend to be more heterogeneous. MR imaging is considered the procedure of choice for detection and staging. The characteristic MRI features include T2 inhomogeneity, areas of T1 and T2 hyperintensity reflecting hemorrhage, fluid—fluid levels, internal septations, and the triple signal intensity pattern. The triple signal intensity pattern consists of areas that are hyperintense, isointense, and hypointense relative to fat on T2WI and occurs in approximately 35% of patients. Recently differentiation between low- and high-grade synovial sarcoma by the use of CT and MRI has been proposed. Proximal distribution of the lesion, large tumor size (≥10 cm), the absence of calcification, tumor possessing cyst, the presence of hemorrhage, and the presence of the triple signal all favor high-grade tumor and poorer prognosis.

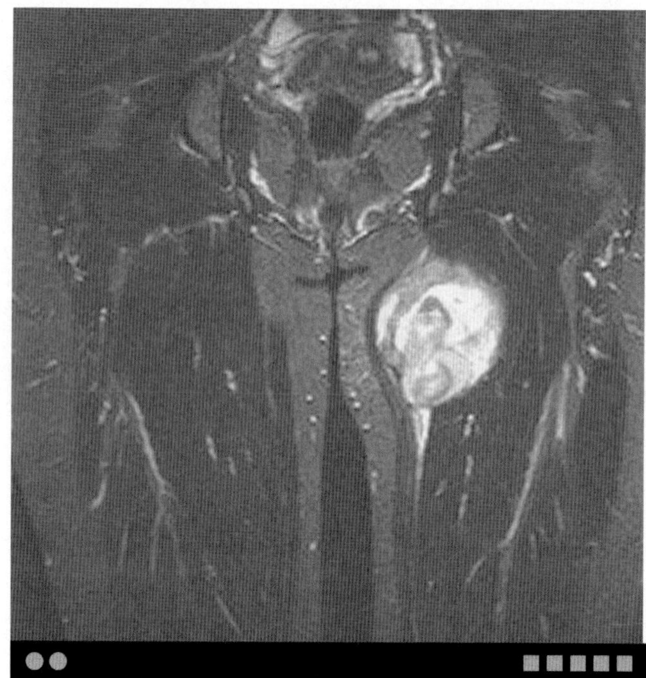

A. Synovial sarcoma: Coronal STIR image shows a large soft tissue mass with mixed intermediate and bright signals in the medial aspect of the thigh.

PEARLS

- **As the fourth most common soft tissue tumor, synovial sarcoma mostly occurs in the lower extremity.**
- **It is usually in association with tendon sheaths, bursae, and joint capsule.**
- **MRI features include inhomogeneity because of necrosis, calcification, and hemorrhage. Fluid—fluid levels, internal septation, and triple signal intensity pattern may also be seen.**
- **Large proximal lesions with cystic components and triple signal intensity pattern without calcification favors poorer prognosis.**

ADDITIONAL IMAGES

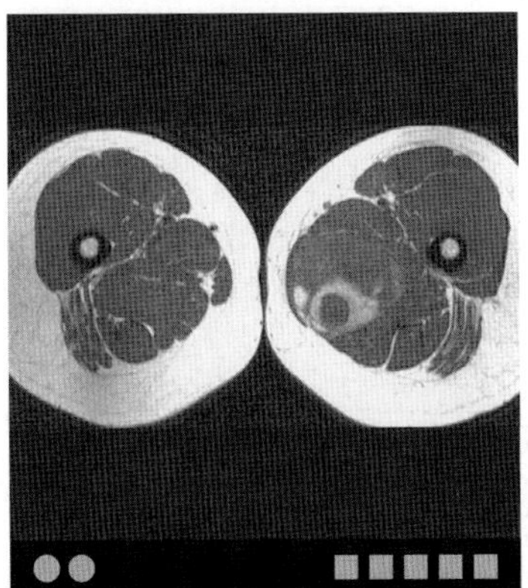

B. Synovial sarcoma: Axial T1WI shows soft tissue mass with round focus of low SI in the center and intermediate signal at the periphery of the lesion.

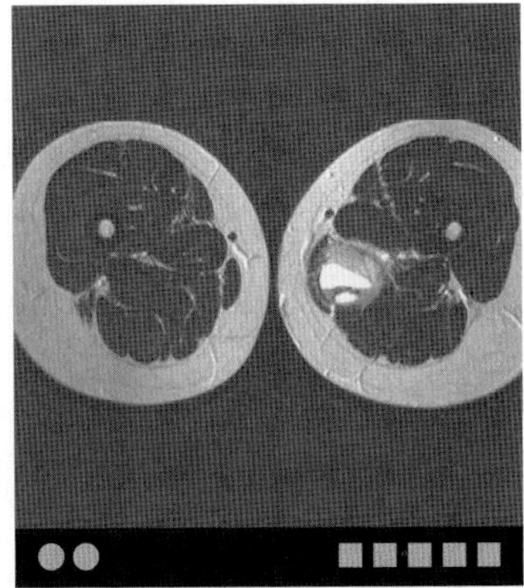

C. Synovial sarcoma: Axial fat-saturated T2WI shows cystic soft tissue mass with fluid–fluid level and triple signal pattern.

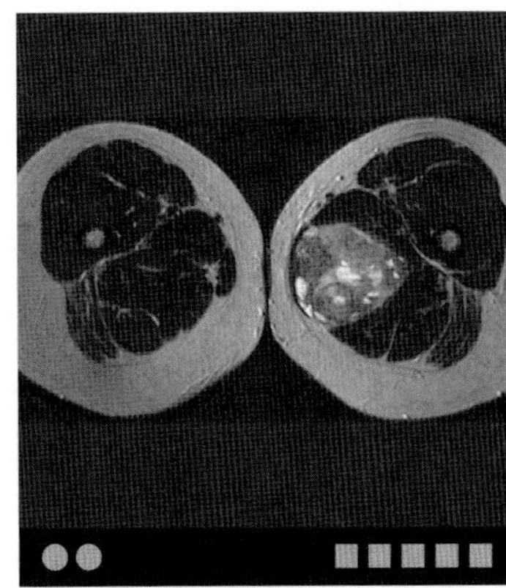

D. Synovial sarcoma: Axial fat-saturated T2WI shows lobulated soft tissue mass with dark intermediate and bright signal pattern.

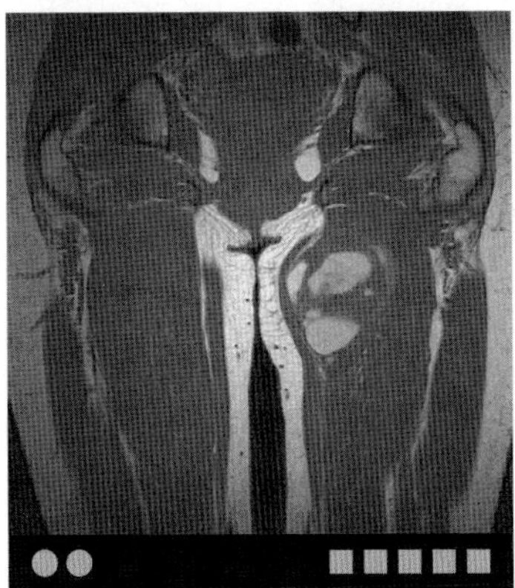

E. Synovial sarcoma: Coronal T1WI shows lobulated soft tissue mass in the medial aspect of the thigh.

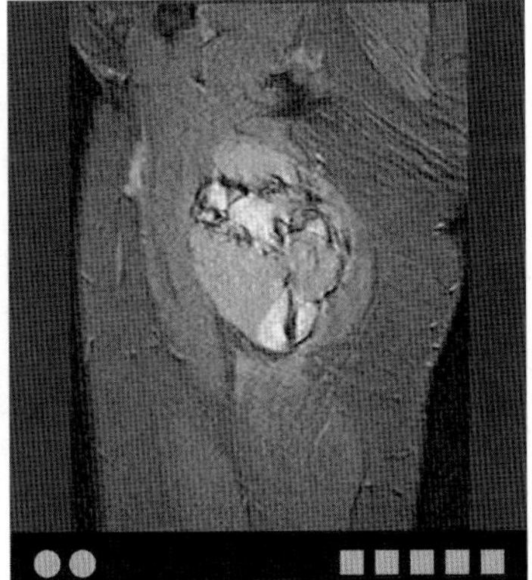

F. Synovial sarcoma: Sagittal fat-saturated T2WI shows large soft tissue mass with low, intermediate, and high SI components.

IMAGE KEY

Common

Rare

Typical

Unusual

DIFFERENTIAL DIAGNOSIS IMAGE

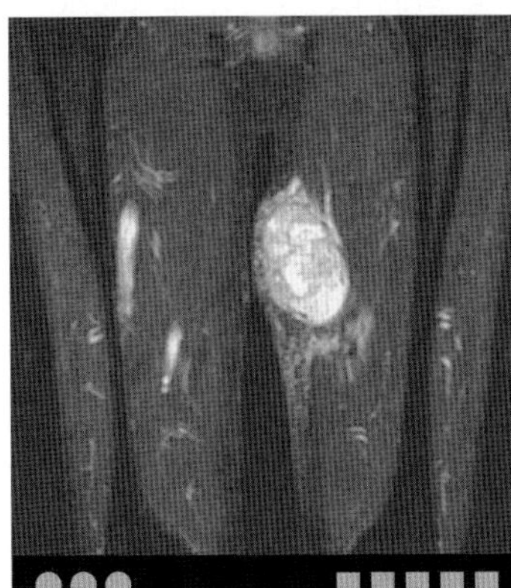

G. Liposarcoma: Coronal T2W fat-saturated MR image shows large soft tissue mass with mixed intermediate to bright signal intensity.

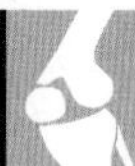

21–11 Leiomyosarcoma of Thigh

Peyman Borghei and Jamshid Tehranzadeh

PRESENTATION

Thigh mass with pathological fracture of femur

FINDINGS

There is a large heterogeneous soft tissue mass at the region of popliteal fossa with bone invasion and pathologic fracture of the distal femur. The femurs bilaterally had preexisting bone infarct.

DIFFERENTIAL DIAGNOSES

- *Malignant fibrous histiocytoma (MFH):* This tumor may occur with preexisting bone infarct.
- *Liposarcoma:* MRI of liposarcoma shows a sharp mass with inhomogeneous contrast enhancement on T1W and mixed intermediate and high-intensity signals on T2WI.
- *Synovial sarcoma:* The mass is usually isointense with muscle on T1W and inhomogenous high SI often with areas of hemorrhage and sometimes fluid—fluid levels or lobulation on T2WI.
- *Malignant schwannoma:* Usually present with neuralgia because of the compression of adjacent nerves. The mass is hypointense on T1WI, hyperintense on fat-saturated T2WI, with strong central enhancement.

COMMENTS

This is a 47-year-old man with a 2-year history of right thigh mass diagnosed with leiomyosarcoma. The mass involves the patella and also encases the neurovascular bundle in the popliteal region. Leiomyosarcoma, the third most common malignant soft tissue tumor is usually seen in adult population, with a tendency to occur in lower extremity. Leiomyosarcomas show different histological patterns such as well-differentiated, pleomorphic, myxoid, and undifferentiated. Depending the origin of the leiomyosarcoma (vessels, retroperitoneum, deep soft tissue, and cutaneous or subcutaneous tissue), the prognosis would be different. Like other soft tissue tumors, leiomyosarcoma is low-to-intermediate signal intensity (SI) on T1W and high SI on T2WI. However leiomyosarcoma is usually associated with focal cystic changes, hyalinization, hemorrhage, and necrosis. These variable features may influence the MRI findings in different cases. Cystic areas with hemorrhage are usually seen in large leiomyosarcomas, which manifest as areas of low signal intensity on T2WI because of the magnetic susceptibility effect produced by hemosiderin and increased signal on T1WI because of hemorrhage. Hyalinized areas show low signal on T2W sequences. Sometimes leiomyosarcoma is associated with metaplastic bone and cartilage formation, which on T2W sequences shows signal voids compatible with calcification.

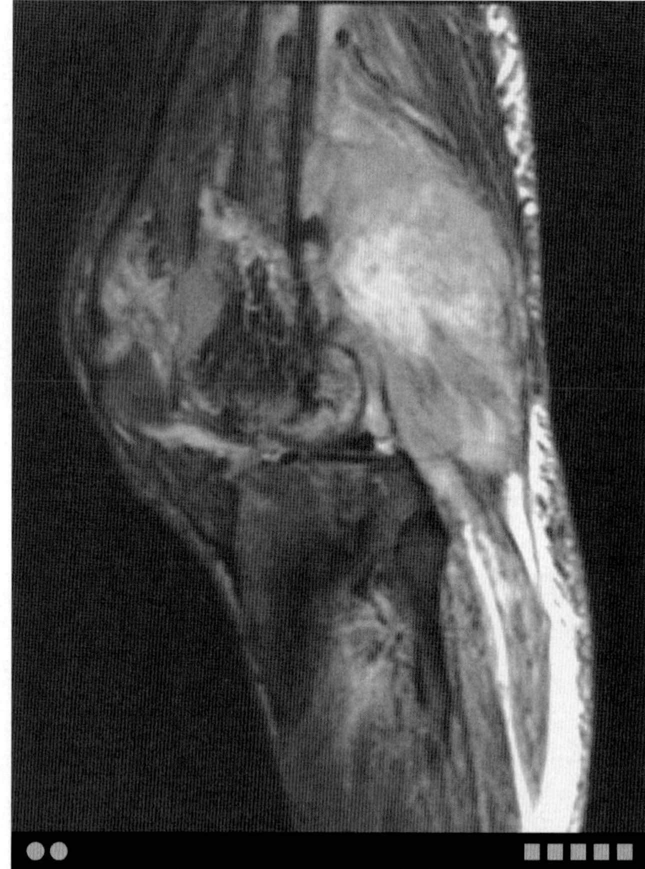

A. Leiomyosarcoma: Sagittal STIR image shows bone infarct and massive tumor of soft tissue extending into the bone anteriorly with presence of soft tissue mass posteriorly leading to pathologic fracture of femur. Note destruction of superior pole of patella.

PEARLS

- **Leiomyosarcomas are rare soft tissue sarcomas with varying MR signal characteristics and histologic components.**
- **Similar to other soft tissue tumors leiomyosarcoma has low to intermediate SI on T1W and high SI on T2WI.**
- **Low intensity signals on T2WI could results from fibrous tissue, hyalinization, or hemosiderin.**

ADDITIONAL IMAGES

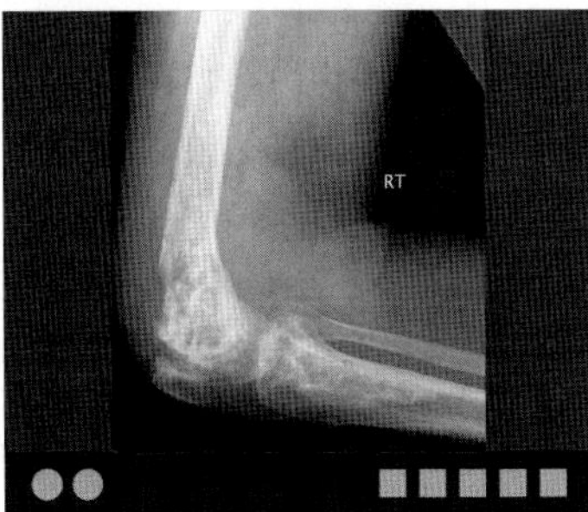

B. Leiomyosarcoma: Lateral radiograph of the knee shows evidence of bone infarct in distal femur and proximal tibia associated with permeative and destructive osteolytic changes of the distal femur with posterior and anterior soft tissue masses and loss of the anterior cortex.

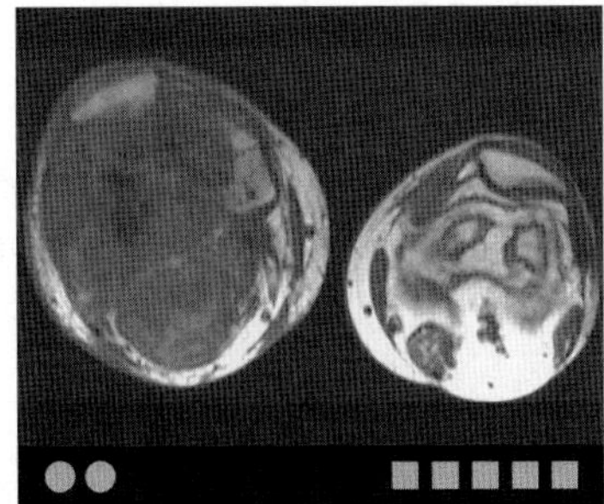

C. Leiomyosarcoma: Axial T1 SE image shows large concentric soft tissue mass with extension to distal femur on the right side. Note total loss of the cortex of the right knee. Also note presence of bone infarct on the left side.

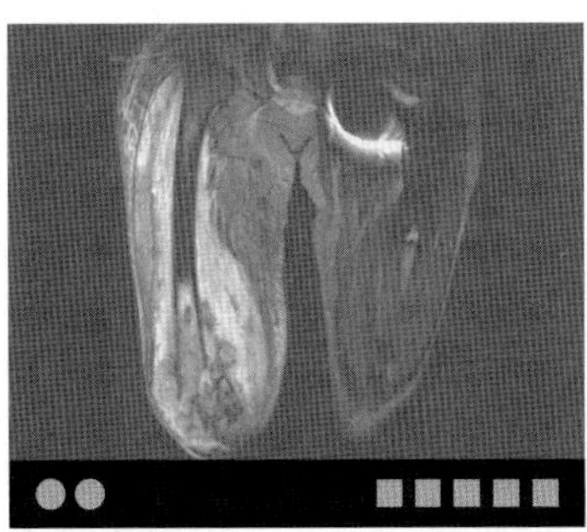

D. Leiomyosarcoma: Coronal STIR image shows pathological fracture of the distal femur surrounded by extensive soft tissue mass and edema extending up to proximal femur.

E. Leiomyosarcoma: Postcontrast T1WI of both knees shows coronal position of the left knee and sagittal position of the right knee caused by pathologic fracture and rotation. Note peripheral inhomogeneous enhancement of the soft tissue mass, while the main soft tissue tumor does not enhance significantly.

IMAGE KEY

Common

Rare

Typical

Unusual

DIFFERENTIAL DIAGNOSES IMAGES

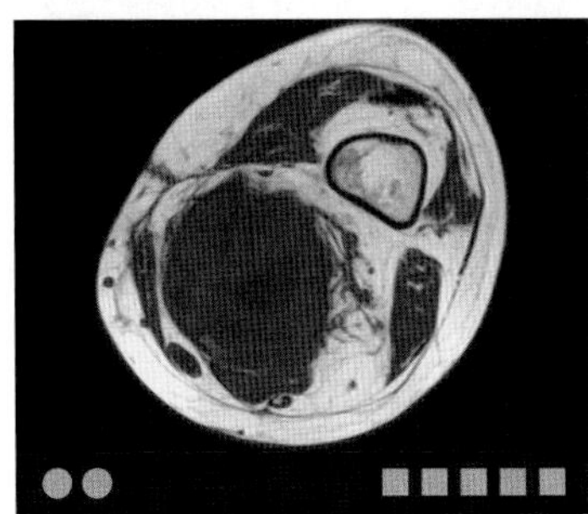

F. Synovial sarcoma: Axial T1 SE image shows large multiloculated irregular soft tissue mass in the popliteal fossa. The mass has low–intermediate signal foci.

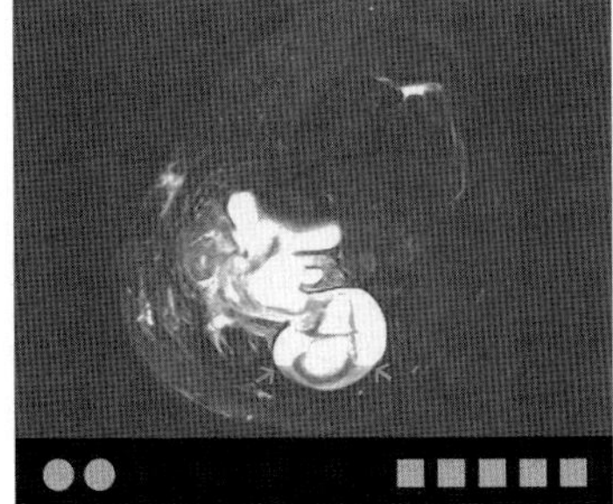

G. Synovial sarcoma: Axial fat-saturated T2WI shows the soft tissue mass in the popliteal fossa with mostly bright signal suggesting cystic tumor mass. Note fluid—fluid levels (arrows) and also areas of low signal, which may represent fibrous and necrotic tissue.

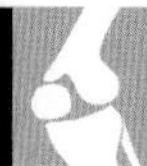

21–12 Malignant Fibrous Histiocytoma of Thigh

Peyman Borghei and Jamshid Tehranzadeh

PRESENTATION

Right thigh mass

FINDINGS

MRI shows a 9.8 × 8.7 × 8.3 cm soft tissue mass at the posteromedial aspect of the thigh with contrast enhancement at the periphery and no contrast enhancement at the center because of necrosis.

DIFFERENTIAL DIAGNOSES

- *Liposarcoma:* MRI of liposarcoma shows a sharp mass with inhomogeneous contrast enhancement on T1W and mixed intermediate- and high-intensity signals on T2WI.
- *Synovial Sarcoma:* The mass is usually isointense with muscle on T1W and inhomogenous high SI often with areas of hemorrhage and sometimes fluid—fluid levels or lobulation on T2WI.
- *Fibrosarcoma:* Typically manifests as a poorly circumscribed mass with multinodular appearance and heterogenous enhancement.
- *Dermatofibrosarcoma Protuberance:* This superficial lesion with involvement of skin and subcutaneous tissue often shows marked contrast enhancement.

COMMENTS

This is a 44-year-old female with a painful distal right thigh mass of 5-month duration and diagnosed with malignant fibrous histiocytoma (MFH). The mass displaced the sciatic nerve and branches of femoral artery. MFH is the most common soft tissue tumor in the adult population, accounting for 20% to 30% of all soft tissue sarcomas. It is mostly seen in lower extremities followed by upper extremity and trunk. Histologic appearance is usually storiform-pleomorphic, containing both fibroblastic and histiocytic elements with no surrounding capsule. The patient usually presents with pain and swelling at the region of tumor. MRI plays an important role in the assessment of preoperative extent of the tumor and the evaluation of neurovascular, bone, and joint involvement, but has no specificity for definite diagnosis of the lesion. The usual MRI findings are heterogeneous signal intensity on T2W sequences with peripheral and nodular-contrast enhancement. In large tumors, central necrosis may be seen showing nonenhancing confluent foci of low signal intensity on contrast-enhanced T1W MR images. These areas may calcify, which could also be seen on conventional radiographs.

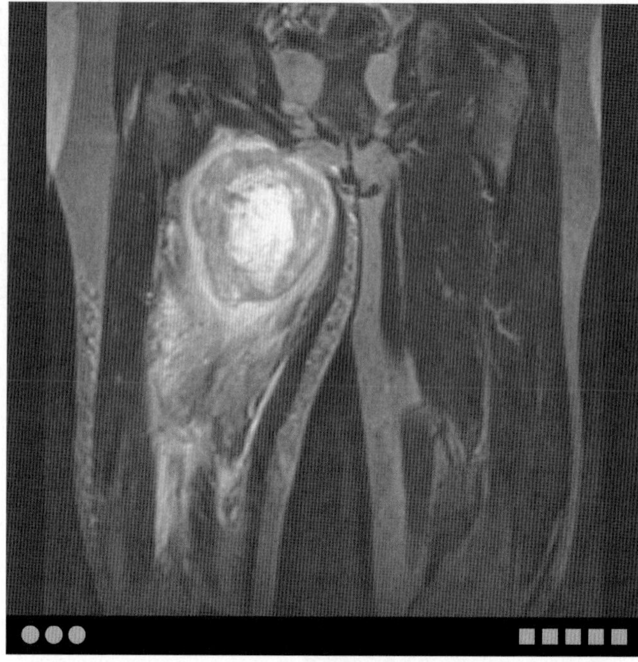

A. MFH: Coronal T2 SE image shows inhomogeneous large signal intensity mass involving the proximal medial soft tissue of the right thigh with extensive edema.

Hemorrhage within the tumor may be seen showing high signal intensity on T1WI, which may be mistaken as rapid tumor growth. An important differential feature to look for is the presence of fat seen in liposarcoma, which is absent in MFH. Treatment is en bloc resection, sometimes associated with preoperative chemotherapy and/or postresection radiotherapy. Unfortunately, prognosis is not favorable and recurrence is a common finding seen in 50% to 100% of patients.

PEARLS

- **MFH is the most common adult soft tissue sarcoma with a predilection to occur in lower extremity.**
- **The tumor lacks a surrounding capsule and so involvement of nearby structures such as neurovascular bundle, bone, and joint may occur.**
- **Patient usually presents with pain and swelling at the site of tumor.**
- **MRI is helpful in determining the tumor extension preoperatively, but is not useful for definitive diagnosis of the tumor.**
- **MRI manifestation varies upon necrosis or hemorrhage within the tumor; however, it usually shows peripheral contrast enhancement.**

ADDITIONAL IMAGES

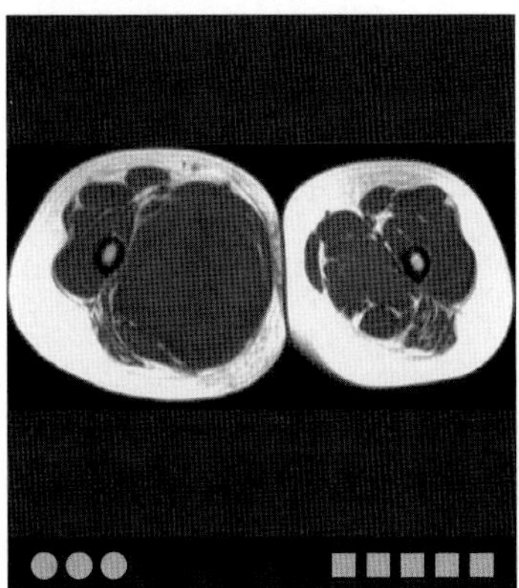

B. MFH: Axial T1WI shows a large soft tissue mass at the medial aspect of thigh, which is isointense to muscle.

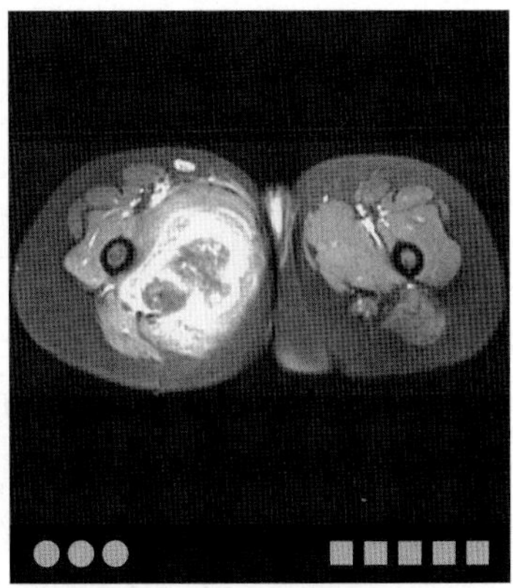

C. MFH: Axial fat-saturated postcontrast T1WI shows peripheral enhancement of this septated soft tissue mass with central necrosis.

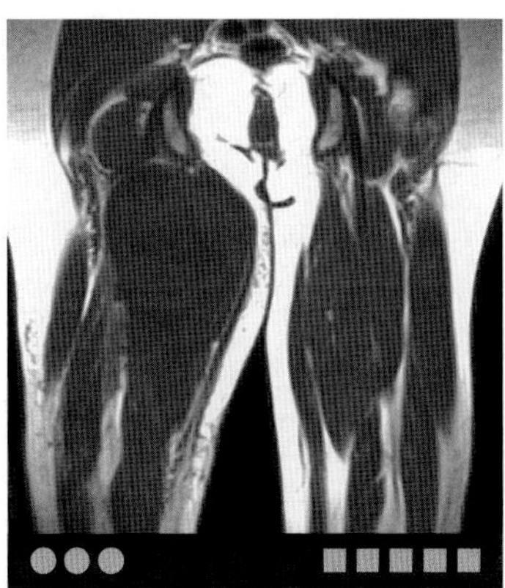

D. MFH: Coronal T1 SE image shows a soft tissue mass in the medial aspect of the thigh with isointense signal intensity to muscle.

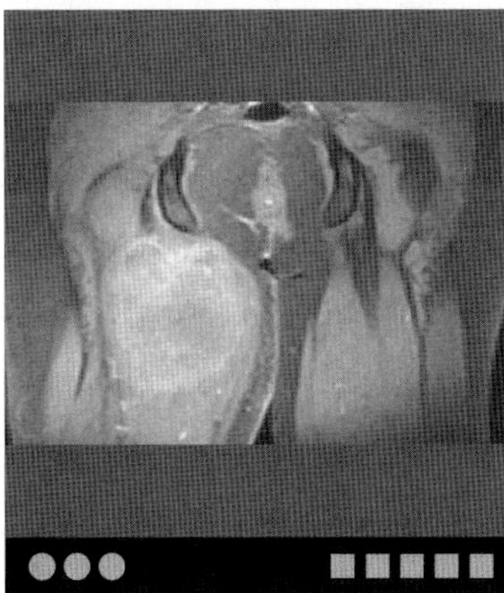

E. MFH: Coronal fat saturated post contrast T1WI shows peripheral enhancement of the tumor with several foci of central necrosis.

DIFFERENTIAL DIAGNOSES IMAGES

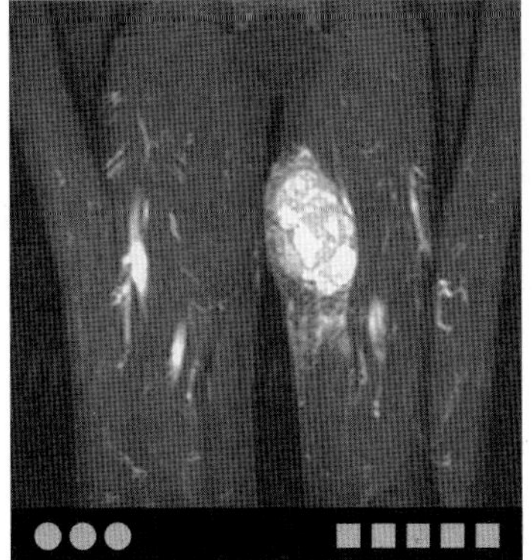

F. Liposarcoma: Coronal STIR image shows a large soft tissue mass with lobulation. Note inhomogenous, large size mass with absence of low SI which favors malignancy.

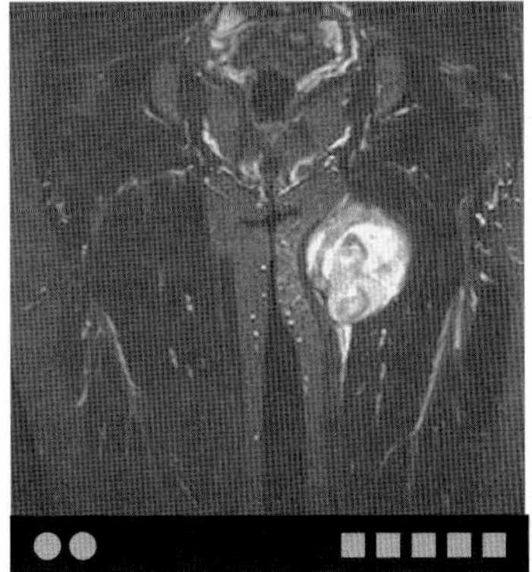

G. Synovial Sarcoma: Coronal STIR image shows a large soft tissue mass with mixed intermediate and bright signals in the medial aspect of the thigh.

IMAGE KEY

Common

Rare

Typical

Unusual

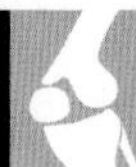

21–13 Myxoid Liposarcoma of Buttock

Janis Owens

PRESENTATION

Slow growing soft tissue mass

FINDINGS

This is a multicystic appearing mass in the right buttock with a central focus of mature fat on MRI and CT. The lesion is low/intermediate signal on T1W sequences and high signal on T2W sequences with low signal septations.

DIFFERENTIAL DIAGNOSES

- *Differentiated soft tissue sarcoma:* These may occasionally appear cystic on MRI.
- *Pleomorphic sarcoma:* These lesions may appear cystic on MRI.
- *Peripheral nerve sheath tumor:* Associated with major nerve. These may have central low signal area on T2W sequences.

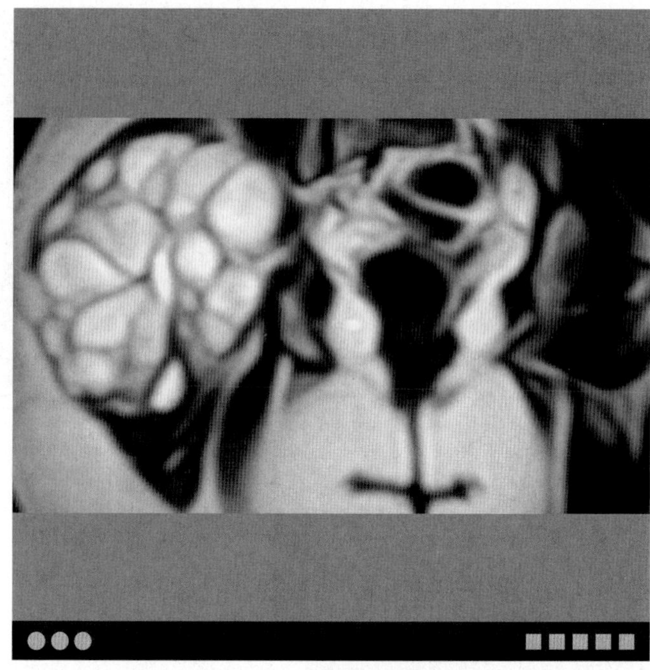

A. Myxoid liposarcoma: Coronal T2W sequence of the posterior pelvis shows the high signal mass with low signal septations.

COMMENTS

This is a 52-year-old female with a right buttock mass. Liposarcoma is the second most common soft tissue neoplasm and accounts for 20% of soft tissue sarcomas. It is usually diagnosed in the third to fifth decade with an average of diagnosis of 42 years old. Myxoid liposarcoma is an intermediate grade malignancy and accounts for 30% to 40% of liposarcomas. Myxoid liposarcoma is seen most commonly in the thigh, followed in frequency by the buttock, lower leg, and retroperitoneum. They arise from the deep intramuscular fat planes and may contain a small amount of mature fat. Twenty-two percent may appear cystic on CT or MRI. The lesions are low/intermediate signal on T1W sequences. The myxoid component is high signal on the T2W sequences. The mature fat component is identifiable on both CT and MRI. There is variable gadolinium enhancement of the lesions. Ultrasound examination confirms that there is a complex solid mass with no cystic areas and that the cyst-like areas on the other studies actually represent the myxoid component. Myxoid liposarcomas may be differentiated from other soft tissue sarcomas invading fat in that the appearance of the fat is mottled in the later condition and generally not as large as the mature fat contained in the liposarcoma.

PEARLS

- **Multicystic appearing mass with internal mature fat.**
- **Involves buttock and proximal thigh.**
- **Arises from deep fat planes.**

ADDITIONAL IMAGES

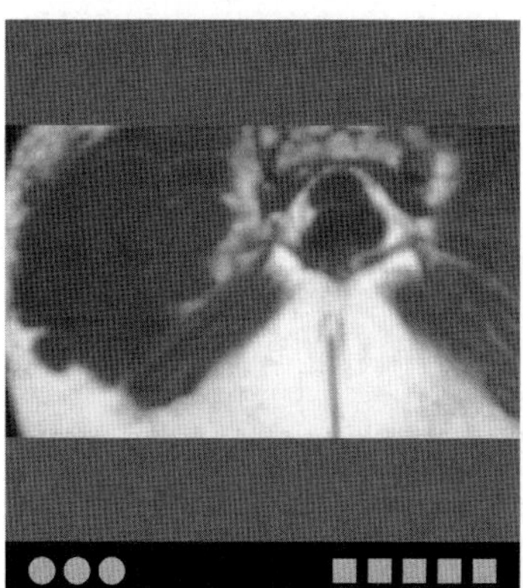

B. Myxoid liposarcoma: Coronal T1W sequence of the posterior pelvis shows a heterogeneous low/intermediate signal mass in the right buttock.

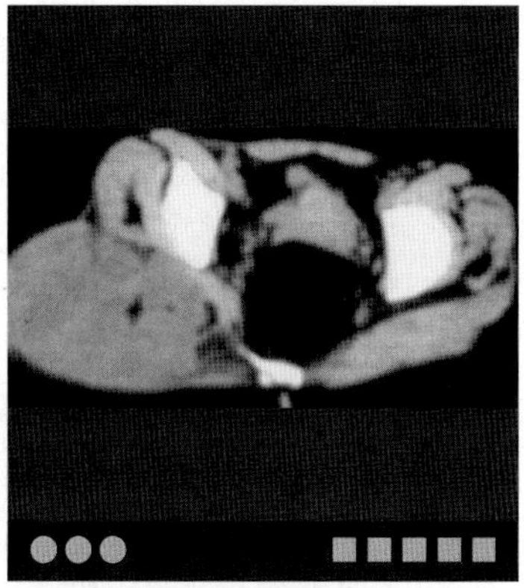

C. Myxoid liposarcoma: CT pelvis shows a multicystic appearing mass with a central fat focus.

DIFFERENTIAL DIAGNOSES IMAGES

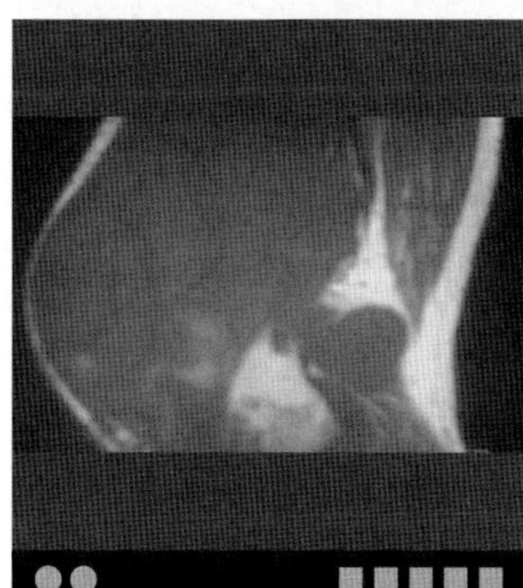

D. Synovial sarcoma: Sagittal T1W sequence of lower thigh shows a low/intermediate signal heterogenous mass in the anterior distal thigh.

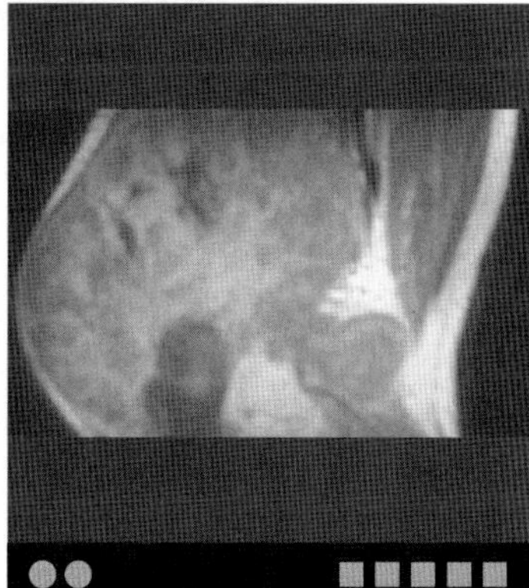

E. Synovial sarcoma: Sagittal T1W sequence post gadolinium contrast of lower thigh shows the heterogenous high signal enhancing mass with central necrosis in the anterior distal thigh.

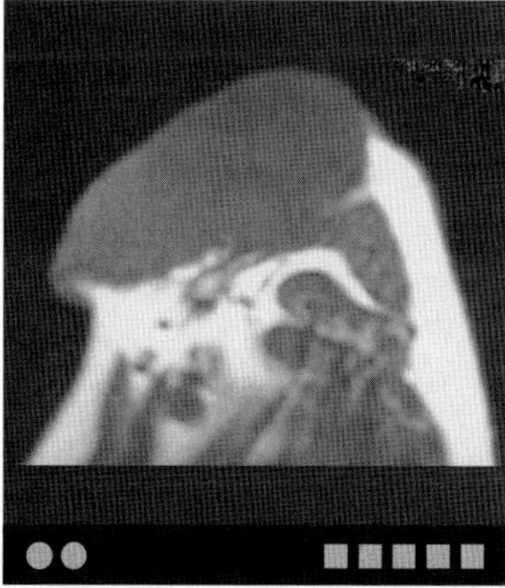

F. Malignant peripheral nerve sheath tumor: Sagittal T1W sequence of the shoulder shows the intermediate signal mass in the region of the left shoulder.

IMAGE KEY

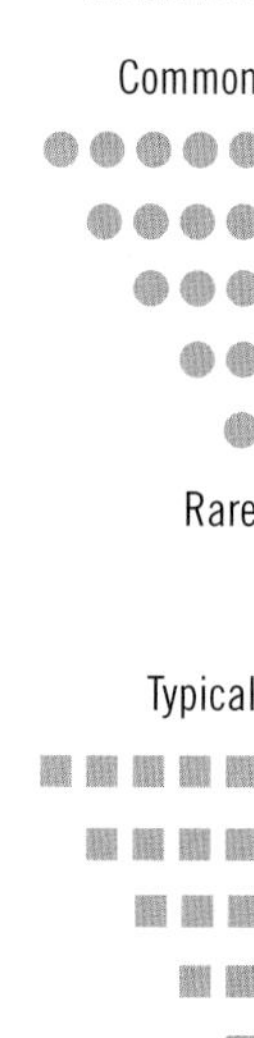

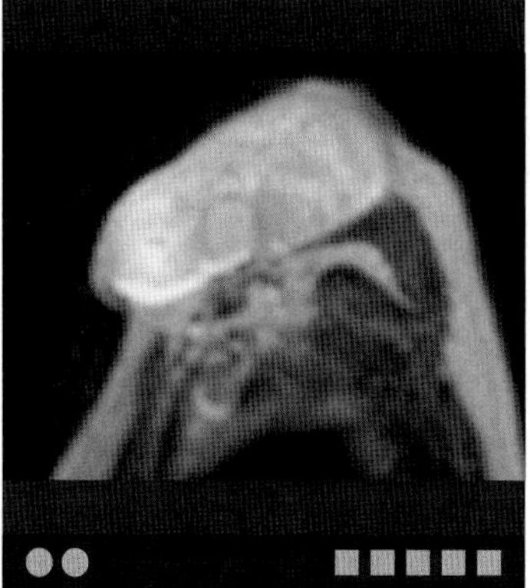

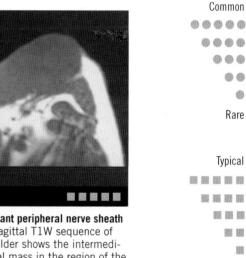

G. Malignant peripheral nerve sheath tumor: Sagittal T2W sequence of the shoulder shows the heterogenous high signal mass.

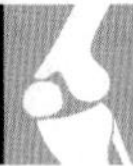

21–14 Dermatofibrosarcoma Protuberans

Carlos Molina and Rajeev K. Varma

PRESENTATION

Left buttock mass

FINDINGS

MRI shows a well-circumscribed, pedunculated, enhancing mass projecting off the left buttocks. Extension is seen to the neighboring gluteus maximus muscle.

DIFFERENTIAL DIAGNOSES

- *Fibroblastic sarcoma:* Typically manifests as a poorly circumscribed mass with multinodular appearance and heterogeneous enhancement. Extensive tendon sheath involvement is usually present.
- *Malignant fibrous histiocytoma:* The soft tissue mass usually is associated with bony invasion and cortical destruction showing intermediate signal intensity (SI) on T1W and high signal on T2WI.
- *Leiomyosarcoma:* Depending on tissue differentiation, this tumor may manifest different signal intensities on MR imaging.
- *Neurofibroma:* May present with skin pigmentations (café au lait spots), which have smooth margins.

COMMENTS

This is a 43-year-old African American man admitted to surgery–oncology for a giant left buttock mass. This patient also gave the history of injecting unknown substances into this area. Dermatofibrosarcoma protuberans (DFSP) is a rare soft tissue neoplasm that arises from the dermis, invades deeper subcutaneous tissue, and typically metastasizes by local extension. The cellular origin of DFSP is not clear at this time. Evidence exists that supports the cellular origin being fibroblastic, histiocytic, or neuroectodermal. The initial presentation is usually that of a large, indurated skin plaque with red to brown discoloration. Distant metastases are very rare, although they can occur. DFSP represents approximately 1% of all soft tissue sarcomas and usually occurs in adults from age 20 to 50. The diagnosis is usually made by skin biopsy because of the superficial nature of this lesion. MRI, CT, and PET/CT are typically used only when distant metastasis are suspected. MRI

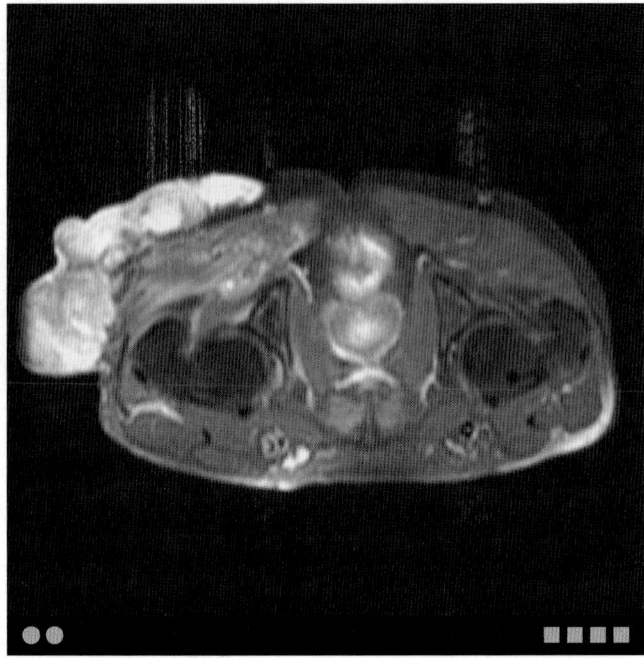

A. Dermatofibrosarcoma protuberans: Contrast-enhanced axial T1WI with fat saturation shows prominent, heterogeneous enhancement in dermal-based mass.

features include prominent, well-circumscribed lesion which is isointense to muscle T1WI, high signal on T2WI and enhances with contrast. Case reports have been sited of DFSP arising from prior injection sites. Although metastasis of DFSP is rare, all metastasis cases have been associated with local recurrence and poor prognosis. Most patients with metastatic DFSP die within 2 years.

PEARLS

- **Rare, slow growing, locally aggressive, dermal-based sarcoma.**
- **Distant metastasis is rare.**
- **MRI features include prominent, well-circumscribed lesion to muscle on T1WI, high signal on T2WI and contrast enhancement.**
- **Definitive diagnosis is usually achieved by skin biopsy.**

ADDITIONAL IMAGES

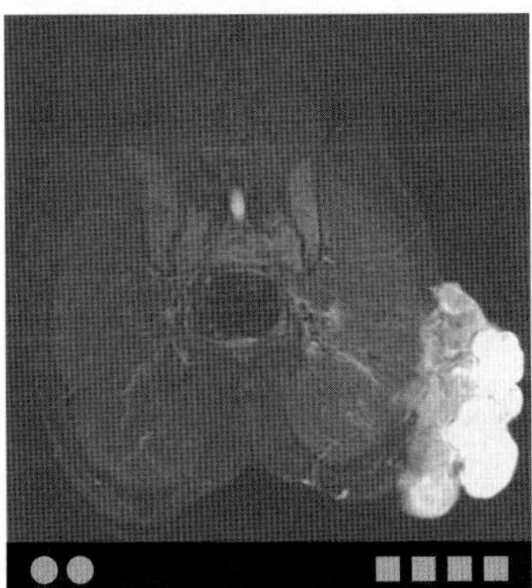

B. Dermatofibrosarcoma protuberans: Coronal STIR image shows the mass to be predominantly high signal with extension to neighboring gluteus maximus.

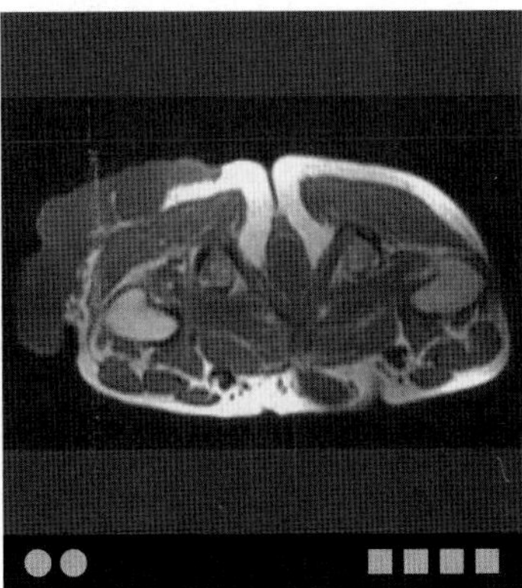

C. Dermatofibrosarcoma protuberans: Axial T1WI (prone) shows the pedunculated nature of this lesion with signal intensity isointense to muscle.

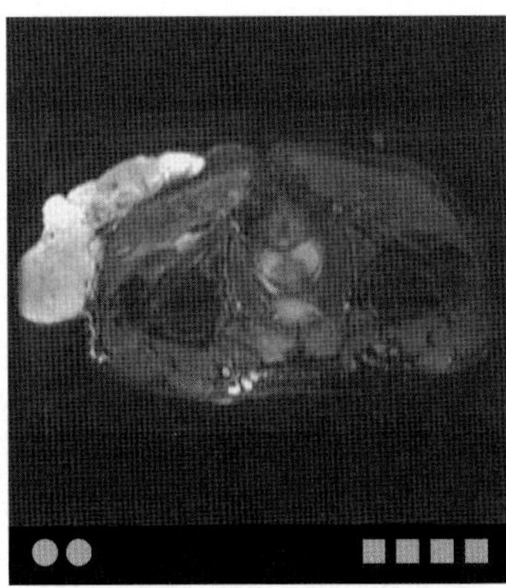

D. Dermatofibrosarcoma protuberans: Axial STIR image in prone position again shows the predominantly high signal nature of this lesion on fluid-sensitive sequences.

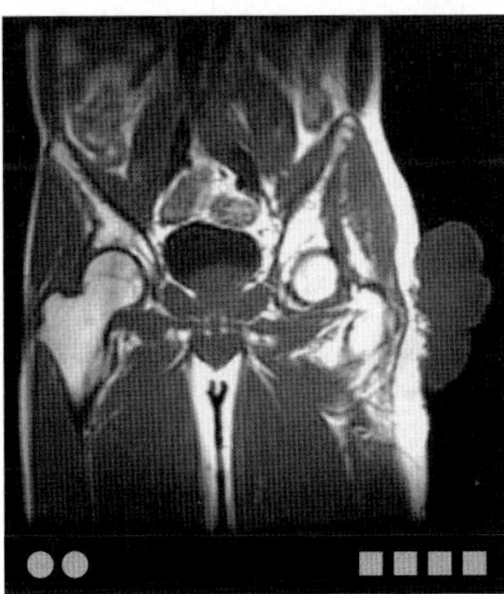

E. Dermatofibrosarcoma protuberans: Coronal T1WI shows a large, well-circumscribed, dermal-based mass with signal intensity isointense to muscle.

DIFFERENTIAL DIAGNOSES IMAGES

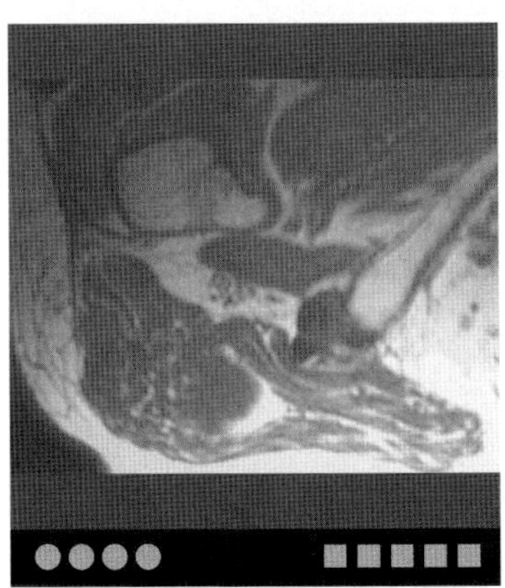

F. Neurofibroma: Axial T1WI shows low signal intensity mass in the gluteal area.

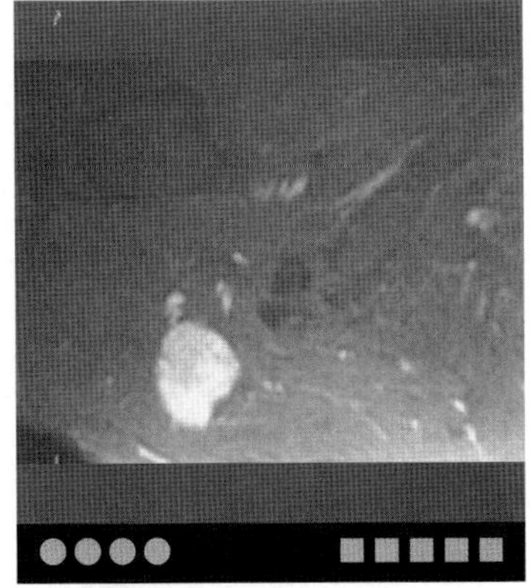

G. Neurofibroma: Axial STIR image shows bright signal intensity mass in the gluteal area.

IMAGE KEY

Common

Rare

Typical

Unusual

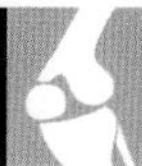

21–15 Extraskeletal Osteosarcoma of Thigh

Melitus Maryam Golshan and Jamshid Tehranzadeh

PRESENTATION

Thigh mass and pain

FINDINGS

Axial CT shows large soft tissue mass with inhomogeneous irregular, aggressive calcification, and central necrosis in the anterolateral thigh involving quadriceps muscle.

DIFFERENTIAL DIAGNOSES

- *Myositis ossificans:* Presents with ringlike ossification in soft tissue ("zonal phenomenon") best imaged by CT scan. Mature lesions have MRI signal characteristic of bone and bone marrow.
- *Ossifying fibromyxoid tumor:* May show thin and incomplete ring or shell-like ossification in radiography.
- *Synovial sarcoma:* Presents as well or poorly marginated, usually inhomogeneous mass isointense to muscle on T1 and hyperintense to subcutaneous fat on T2WI. Calcifications may be evident as area of decreased signal intensity on all pulse sequences.
- *Other soft tissue sarcomas:* Such as liposarcoma and soft tissue chondrosarcoma may show focal areas of calcification.

COMMENTS

This is a 53-year-old man with left thigh pain for several months. Extraskeletal osteosarcoma is characterized by production of osteoid or bone and/or cartilage. Soft tissue osteosarcoma is a relatively rare lesion compared with osteosarcoma of bone, and most commonly occurs in lower extremity in patients older than 40 years of age. Typically, this tumor is deep seated without attachment to the skeleton, but occasionally it presents in the subcutaneous tissue. Extraskeletal osteosarcoma is generally a high-grade sarcoma. Several predisposing factors may influence the development of extraskeletal osteosarcoma, including trauma, radiation, intramuscular injection, and diagnostic procedures with radioactive thorium dioxide. "Zonal phenomenon" refers to soft tissue mass with central calcification in extraosseous osteosarcoma, while absence of central calcification and presence of peripheral calcification indicate myositis ossificans. Radiograph shows a soft tissue mass with peripheral mineralization and irregular margin. CT is more accurate to show peripheral ossification clearly and demonstrates isolation of the lesion from adjacent bone. MR imaging is useful in the evaluation of extent of the mass. Signal intensity in MRI is inhomogeneous and varies greatly. The tumor usually shows overall low signal intensity on T1WI and a mixed high signal intensity on T2WI. Densely ossified tumors or tumor portions show low signal intensity on all pulse sequences. After intravenous gadolinium administration, contrast enhancement of the tumor is inhomogeneous and extensive. Bone scan shows intense radioactivity in the tumor.

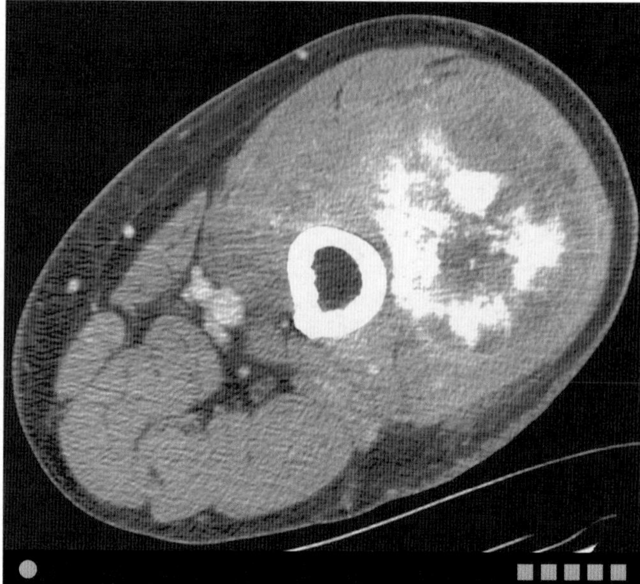

A. Osteosarcoma: Axial CT scan with soft tissue window shows large soft tissue mass with inhomogeneous, irregular and aggressive calcification with central necrosis in the anterolateral thigh involving quadriceps muscle. Note femur is not involved.

PEARLS

- **Extraskeletal osteosarcoma is a relatively rare, but aggressive neoplasm, which occurs mostly in lower extremity in patients older than 40 years of age.**
- **Radiograph shows soft tissue mass without bone involvement, but with aggressive and irregular ossification.**
- **"Zonal phenomenon" is best imaged by CT scan and refers to soft tissue mass with central calcification in extraosseous osteosarcoma, while absence of central calcification and presence of peripheral calcification indicate myositis ossificans.**
- **MR imaging shows extension of ossified soft tissue mass with contrast enhancement. It usually shows overall low signal intensity on T1WI and a mixed high signal intensity on T2WI. Ossified parts of tumor have low signal intensity on all pulse sequences**

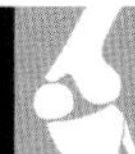

ADDITIONAL IMAGES

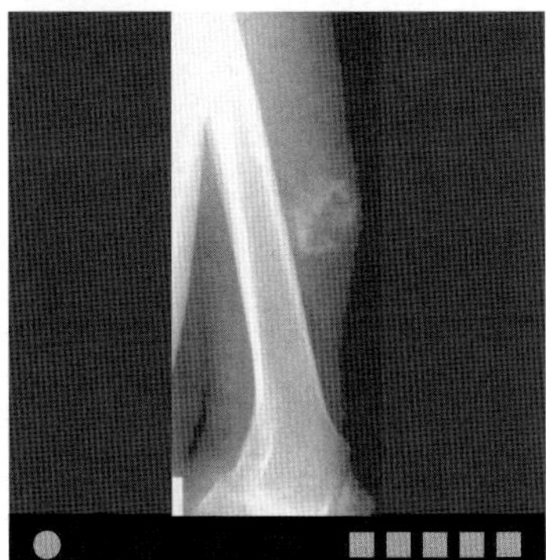

B. Osteosarcoma: Oblique radiograph of the femur shows soft tissue calcification with aggressive and irregular margin and sunburst appearance in the anterior soft tissue of the thigh.

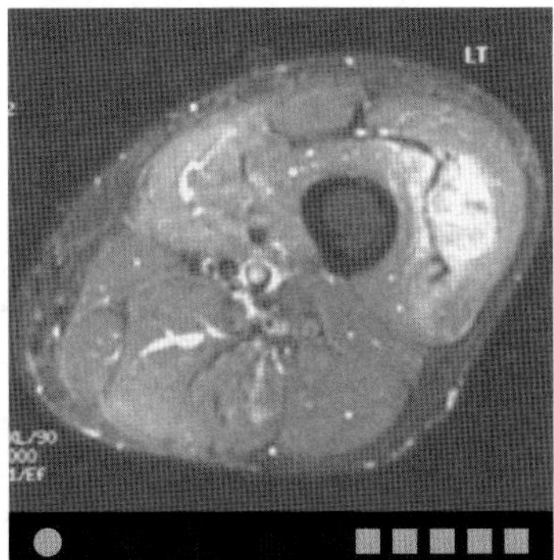

C. Osteosarcoma: Axial PD fat-saturated image shows soft tissue mass of the quadriceps muscle with internal foci of low signal irregular calcifications.

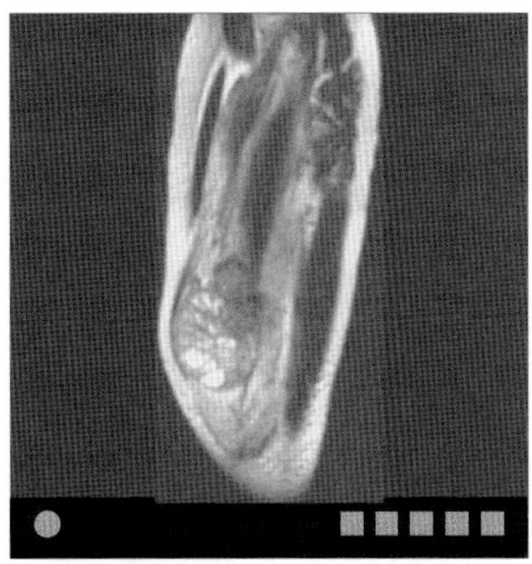

D. Osteosarcoma: Sagittal T2WI shows intermediate signal intensity mass with foci of bright signal and smaller foci of low signal in the lesion.

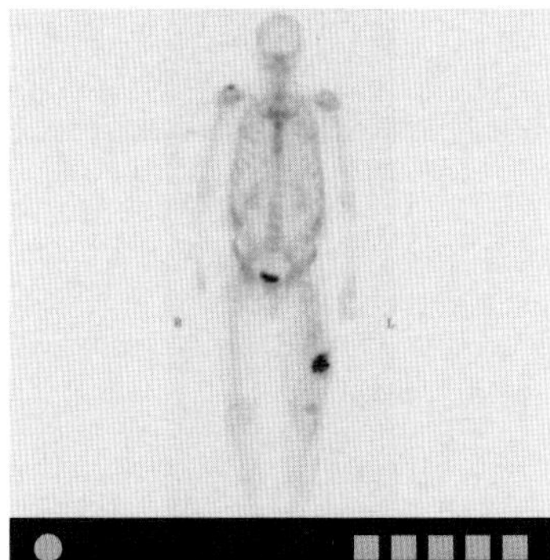

E. Osteosarcoma: Techneciuim99 methylene diphosphonate (Tc99^{99}-MDP) shows highly intense radionuclide activity in the soft tissue of the left thigh.

IMAGE KEY

Common
●●●●●
●●●●
●●●
●●
●
Rare

Typical
■■■■■
■■■■
■■■
■■
■
Unusual

DIFFERENTIAL DIAGNOSES IMAGES

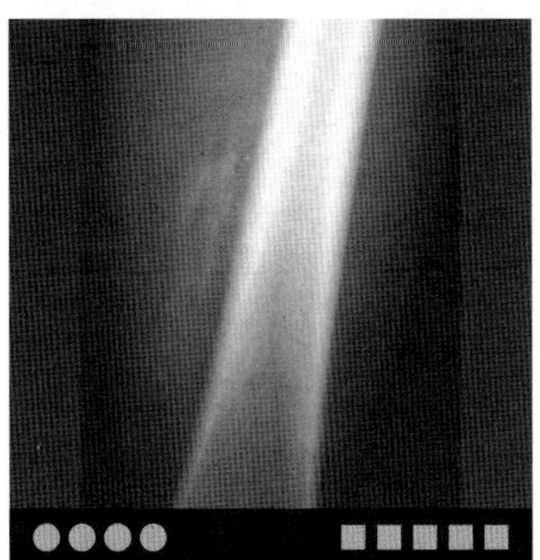

F. Myositis ossificans: AP radiograph of the femur shows a tracklike calcification in the soft tissue of the thigh. Note smooth ringlike soft tissue ossification with absence of central calcification.

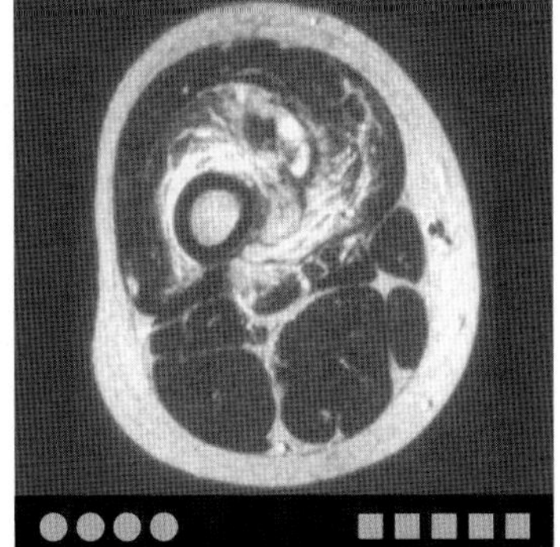

G. Myositis ossificans: MRI axial T2WI shows a mixed signal intensity lesion in the anterior soft tissue of the thigh with foci of bright signal suggesting edema or inflammation with presence of focal low signal intensity calcification.

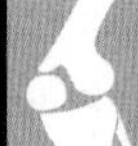

21–16 Chordoma of Sacrum

Joon Kim

PRESENTATION

Sacrococcygeal pain

FINDINGS

Conventional radiographic and CT images show a destructive mass arising from the distal sacrum.

DIFFERENTIAL DIAGNOSES

- *Chondrosarcoma/chondroma:* Differentiating these tumors from chordomas can be extremely difficult on all types of imaging. However, they tend to be less often midline in location.
- *Metastasis:* Various osteoblastic or osteolytic metastatic lesions may be seen in the sacrococcygeal region. Imaging appearance may vary depending on the type of metastasis.
- *Giant cell tumor:* Typically lytic, expansile, locally aggressive lesions without significant sclerotic margins or periosteal reaction.
- *Partial sacral resection:* Segmental resection of the sacrum, usually for locally aggressive sacral tumors or rectal carcinoma.

COMMENTS

Chordomas arise from remnant embryonic cells of the primitive notochord, explaining for its frequent midline location. They are slow-growing tumors, which are locally aggressive with high recurrence rates despite wide surgical resection. The tumors are more commonly seen in men (male-to-female ratio of 2:1). Chordomas are predominantly found in adults, with the highest prevalence occurring in patients in their 50s to 70s. It is the most common primary malignant sacrococcygeal tumor. More than half of chordomas occur in the sacrococcygeal region with the second most common location occurring within the clivus. On radiographs, chordomas are expansile lytic lesions with or without signs of local bone destruction. On CT, chordomas tend to be isodense to muscle and demonstrate heterogeneous enhancement. Calcification is found in less than half of the cases. It is frequently associated with local bone destruction and a large extraosseous soft tissue component. On MR imaging, most chordomas are isointense to hypointense on T1W sequences and hyperintense on T2W sequences. MR imaging is particularly useful in determining extraosseous involvement, particularly of the neural foramina or spinal canal, which can determine surgical planning. Differentiating chondrosarcomas or chondromas from chordomas can be very difficult in all types of imaging, but the latter have predilection for the midline.

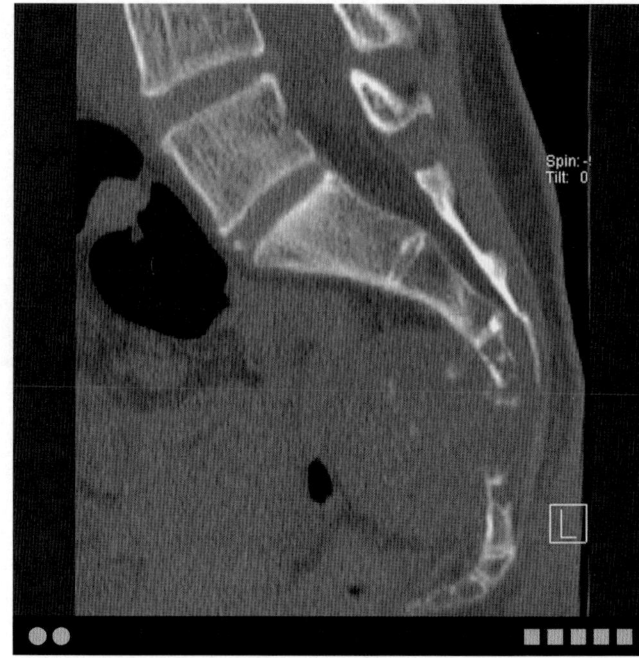

A. Sacrococcygeal chordoma: Sagittal reformatted CT scan of the sacrococcygeal region showing a destructive lesion at in the S4 vertebra, associated with a large soft tissue component anteriorly. There is tumor extension into the central canal. There are foci of high densities within the soft tissue mass, which may represent foci of calcifications or destroyed bone fragments.

PEARLS

- **Chordomas arise from remnant embryonic cells of the primitive notochord, explaining for its frequent midline location, particularly within the sacrococcygeal and clival locations.**
- **Chordomas are the most common primary malignant sacrococcygeal tumor.**
- **They are slow growing tumors, which are locally aggressive with high recurrence rates.**
- **The tumors are frequently associated with local bone destruction and a large extraosseous soft tissue component.**
- **MR imaging is useful in determining extraosseous involvement, particularly of the neural foramina or spinal canal.**

ADDITIONAL IMAGES

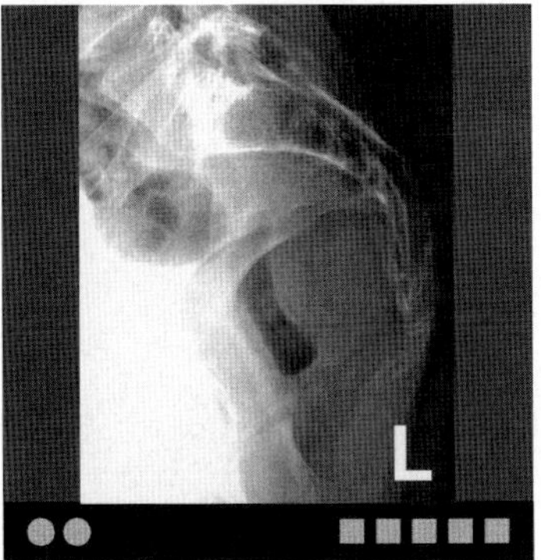

B. Sacrococcygeal chordoma: Lateral radiograph of the sacrococcygeal region show subtle loss of the anterior cortex of the distal sacrum. Note the large soft tissue mass located within the presacral space, displacing the rectum anteriorly.

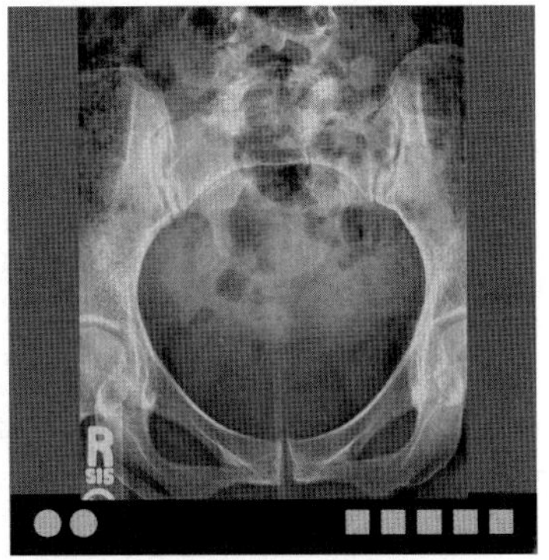

C. Sacrococcygeal chordoma: Coned-down AP radiograph of the sacrococcygeal region shows a subtle expansile lesion in the distal sacrum with loss of the normal sacral arcuate lines.

DIFFERENTIAL DIAGNOSES IMAGES

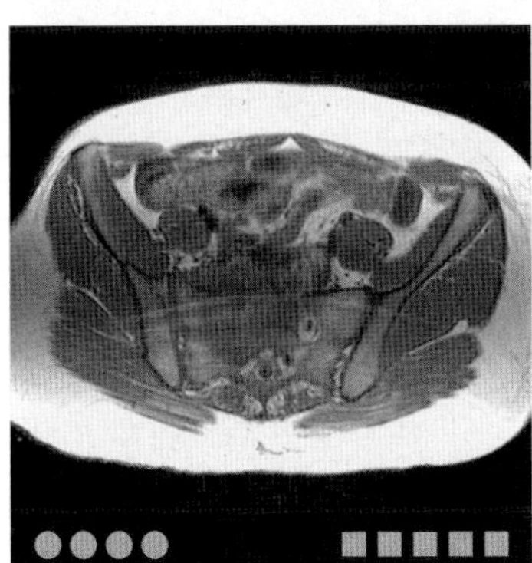

D. Metastasis: Axial T1W MR image shows a hypointense, mildly expansile, destructive lesion occupying the sacral promontory in a patient with metastatic meningioma. There is tumor extension into several of the right neural foramina.

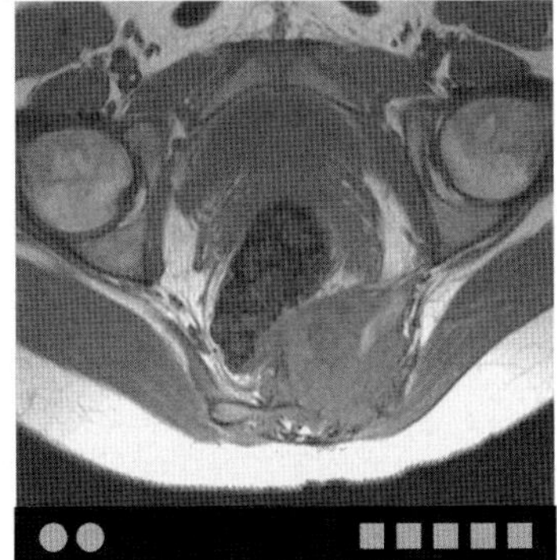

E. Ewing sarcoma: Axial T1W MR image shows a destructive mass arising from the left side of the distal sacrum/coccyx that is associated with a large heterogeneous soft tissue component anteriorly, displacing the rectum.

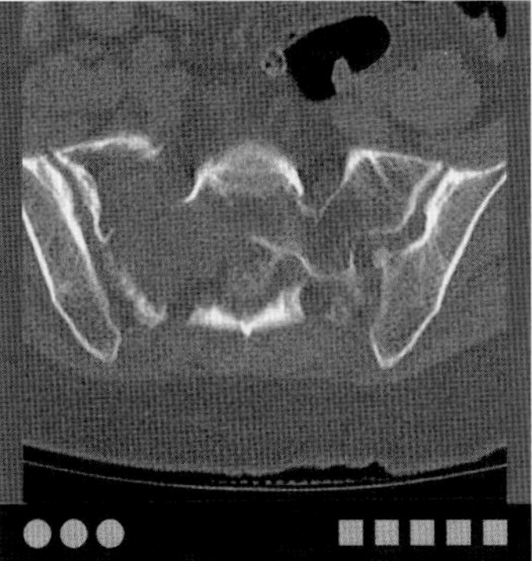

F. Giant cell tumor: Axial CT scan of the sacrum shows a mildly expansile soft tissue density lesion in the right sacrum, with involvement of the adjacent neural foramina. There is no significant sclerotic margin or periosteal reaction.

IMAGE KEY

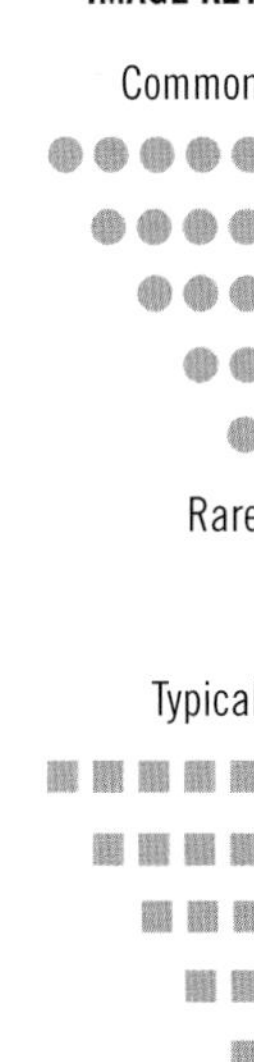

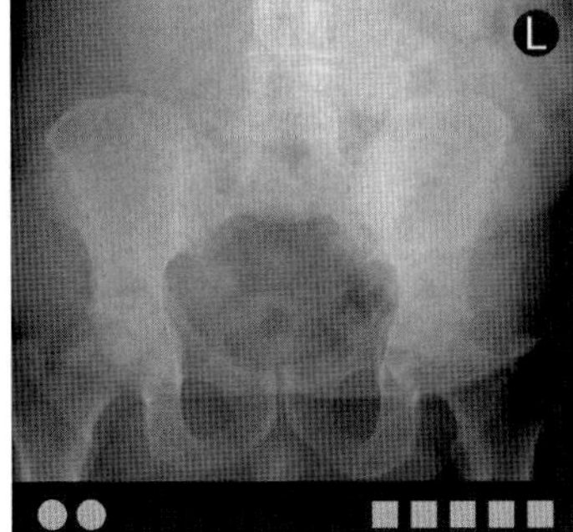

G. Partial sacral resection: AP radiograph of the pelvis shows absence of the mid to distal sacrum, consistent with partial sacral resection. The surgical margin is smooth.

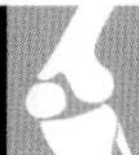

21–17 Osteoid Osteoma of Proximal Femur

John C. Hunter

PRESENTATION

Hip and groin pain

FINDINGS

MR showed nonspecific oval-shaped area of increased signal intensity in the lesser trochanter.

DIFFERENTIAL DIAGNOSES

- *Stress fracture:* The proximal medial femoral neck is a common location for stress fracture. While they may present with periosteal reaction from healing and could be confused with osteoid osteoma, seeing the fracture line on MR or CT imaging rather than a lucent nidus distinguish these entities.
- *Osteoblastoma/Osteosarcoma:* Other bone producing neoplasms must be considered. The lucent nidus, however, is characteristic. Many orthopedic tumor surgeons and MSK radiologists treat osteoid osteoma with RF ablation without biopsy if this classic appearance is present on imaging.
- *Melorheostosis:* This entity is characterized by "flowing" cortical bone and has been described as "dripping candlewax."
- *Infection (Brodie's abscess):* This focal subacute infection often resides in metaphysis and shows fuzzy sclerotic margin.

COMMENTS

This is a 13-year-old boy who presented with pain in the hip and groin, worse at night, relieved partially by salicylates. He was referred for biopsy and potential radiofrequency (RF) ablation of his lesion. Presenting radiographs were interpreted as normal. Bone scan (not shown) revealed an area of markedly increased uptake in the left lesser trochanter. CT showed a radiolucent nidus surrounded by sclerotic periosteal reaction. Osteoid osteoma is a benign osteoblastic tumor of bone mainly found in the cortex of long bones, with intra-articular and subperiosteal variants seen less frequently. The lesion is seen in the first three decades of life with a male predominance. The tumor has a central core of vascularized osteoid. The nidus is surrounded by a zone of sclerotic bone. The amount of sclerosis surrounding the nidus is less in cancellous bones and in intra-articular lesions. Approximately 70% of lesions are in long bones, with the femur and tibia dominating. Intra-articular lesions may demonstrate synovitis or periostitis regional to the lesion. Spasm and scoliosis may be seen in spinal lesions. On the radiograph and CT, the nidus is lucent with variable amounts of central calcification. On MR, the nidus demonstrates low SI on T1 and high SI on T2WI with variable enhancement postcontrast. There may be considerable surrounding soft tissue and bony edema on MR, which may cloud the diagnosis. For this reason, many prefer CT to detect the characteristic nidus. Treatment includes surgical resection or percutaneous radiofrequency ablation. There have been cases reported with spontaneous regression.

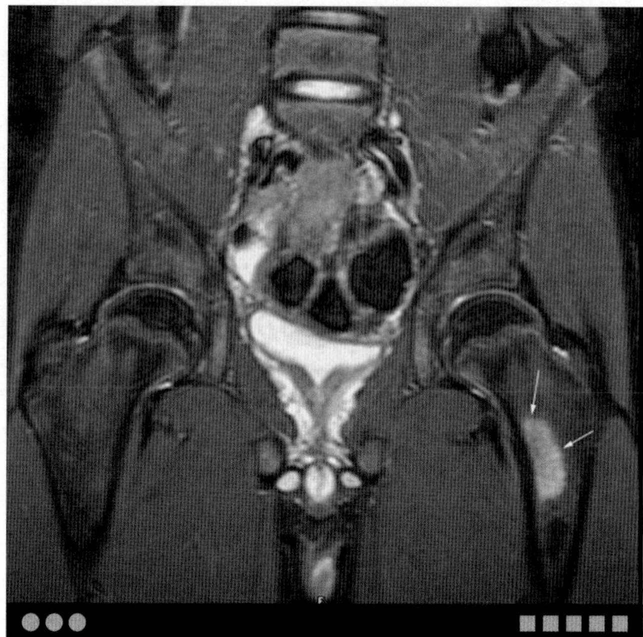

A. Osteoid osteoma: Coronal IR image shows an oval area of increased signal intensity in the region of the left lesser trochanter (arrows) in this 14 year boy with left hip pain.

PEARLS

- **Classic history of night pain relieved with salicylates is seen in the majority of patients.**
- **CT is preferred by many MSK radiologists for the detection of the nidus of osteoid osteoma. MRI often shows marked edema obscuring the characteristic findings.**
- **Lower extremity long bones are the most frequent site of osteoid osteoma.**
- **Treatment with RF ablation is becoming the therapy of choice.**

ADDITIONAL IMAGES

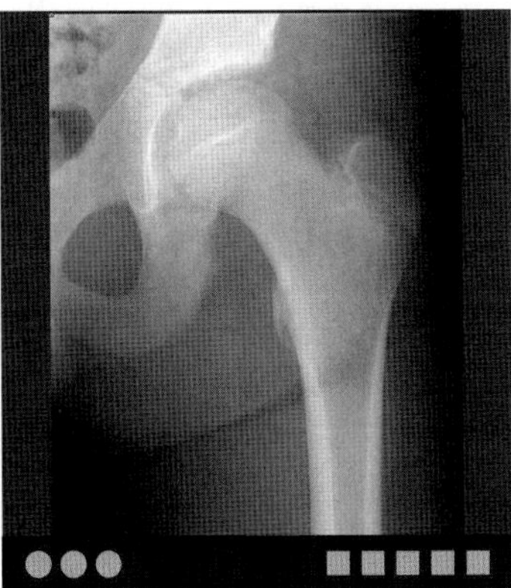

B. Osteoid osteoma: AP radiograph of hip was unremarkable.

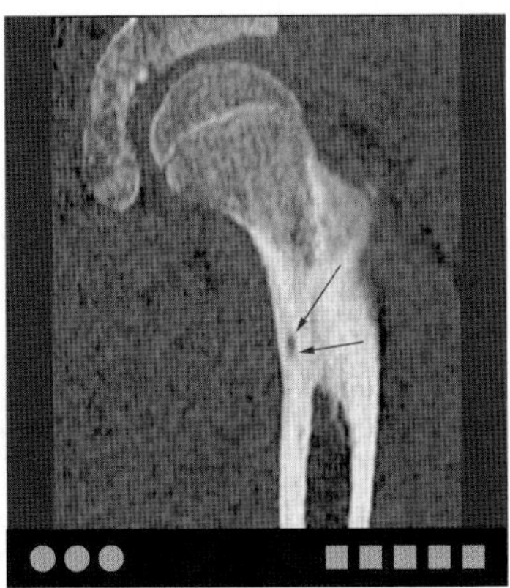

C. Osteoid osteoma: Coronal reformation from high resolution CT of the area shows sclerotic periosteal reaction surrounding a lucent nidus in the medial cortex (arrows).

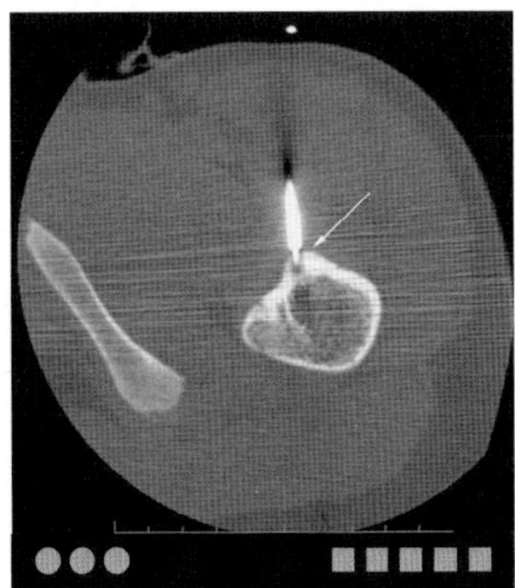

D. Osteoid osteoma: Axial CT during RF ablation procedure shows the RF probe at the nidus of the osteoid osteoma (arrow).

IMAGE KEY

Common

Rare

Typical

Unusual

DIFFERENTIAL DIAGNOSES IMAGES

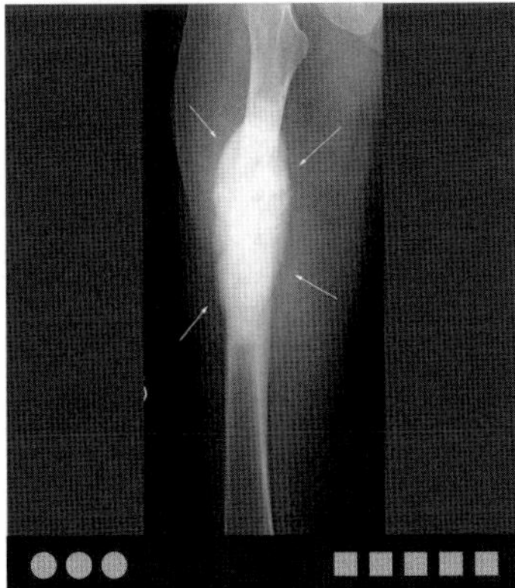

E. Osteosarcoma: Dense periosteal reaction predominates the conventional radiograph (arrows).

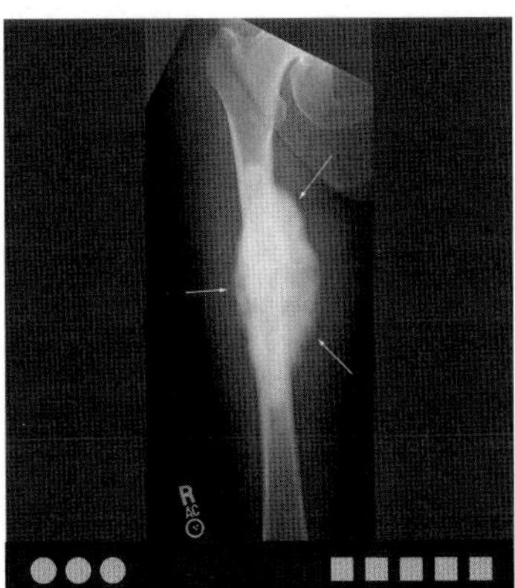

F. Osteosarcoma: Dense periosteal reaction predominates the conventional radiograph (arrows).

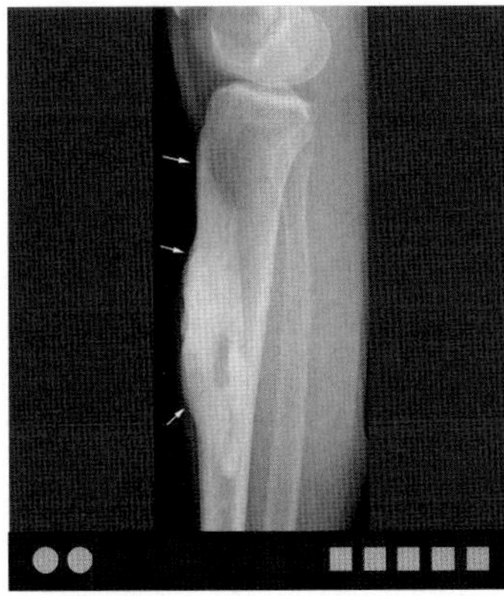

G. Melorheostosis: Dense, flowing cortical bone seen along anterior tibial cortex (arrows)

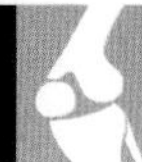

21–18 Chondroblastoma of the Greater Trochanter

Stephen E. Ling and William R. Reinus

PRESENTATION

Pain, swelling, tenderness, chronic synovitis

FINDINGS

Well-circumscribed, round, or ovoid lytic lesion in greater trochanter apophysis (epiphyseal equivalent).

DIFFERENTIAL DIAGNOSES

- *Brodie's abscess:* Clinical history, thick surrounding reactive sclerosis.
- *Eosinophilic granuloma:* Younger patient population, more common in skull and axial skeleton, and usually diaphyseal when involving a long bone.
- *Clear cell chondrosarcoma:* This can be very difficult to differentiate from chondroblastoma on imaging studies.
- *Giant cell tumor:* Older age group usually with closed physis, generally no sclerotic margins, no calcified matrix.
- *Intraosseous ganglion cyst:* Older patients.

COMMENTS

Chondroblastoma is a cartilaginous neoplasm most commonly seen in skeletally immature patients, with a peak incidence during the first through third decades (10–25 years). It affects both long and to a lesser extent flat bones, with the most common sites of involvement being the femur, proximal humerus, and proximal tibia. These locations collectively account for over 70% of cases. Most chondroblastomas are eccentric in position. The disease is invariably monostotic. The tumor originates from the physeal plate/epiphyseal cartilage plate, and typically extends into the epiphysis. Involvement of the metaphysis is less common (25%–50%). Typical radiographic features include a lytic epiphyseal lesion with a thin sclerotic border and calcifications. When present, calcifications show the "ring and arc" and "flocculent" appearance typical of cartilaginous matrix. Nonaggressive appearing periosteal bone formation may be present (30%), and it can be located remote to the lesion. Reactive joint effusion may be present. MR signal characteristics are relatively nonspecific, with low-to-intermediate signal on T1WI and hyperintensity on T2WI being most common. Although chondroblastomas usually behave in a benign fashion, they may occasionally show aggressive behavior, with local extension into soft tissues and adjacent bones. Joint seeding/intra-articular tumor, occurring most often because of spillage of tumor into the joint during surgery, can also be seen. There can even be malignant transformation with distant spread, most commonly to the lungs, but this is quite rare (1%–2%). Curettage followed by packing with either bone graft/chips or methylmethacrylate is the standard treatment for chondroblastoma. Unfortunately, there is a significant rate of local recurrence (10%–35%).

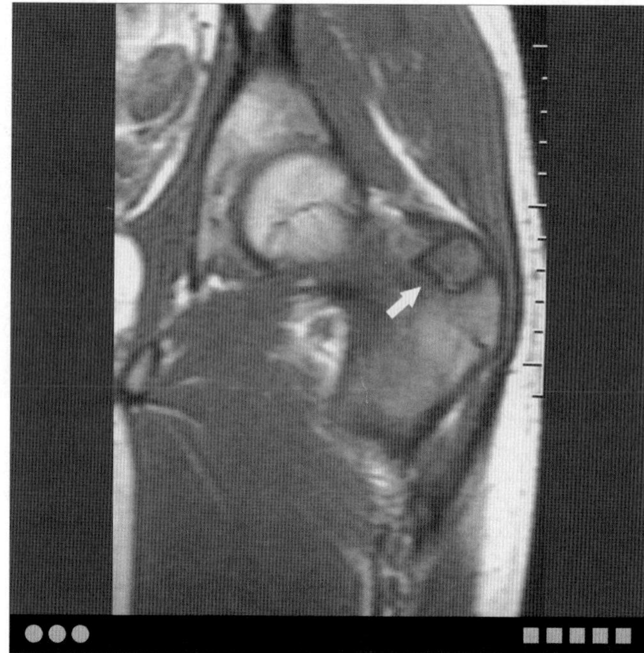

A. Chondroblastoma: Coronal T1WI shows an isointense lesion in the left greater trochanter (arrow) with a large amount of edema in the adjacent bone marrow.

PEARLS

- **Chondroblastoma is one of a number of benign lesions (i.e., osteomyelitis, osteoid osteoma, osteoblastoma, eosinophilic granuloma, and giant cell tumor) that may show quite aggressive features on MRI, such as surrounding bone marrow edema and soft tissue signal abnormalities.**
- **Chondroblastomas occur not only in epiphyses, but also in epiphyseal equivalents including apophyses. Examples include the greater and lesser trochanters, patella, calcaneus, talus, and tarsal and carpal bones.**
- **Presence or absence of calcifications is not an accurate diagnostic criterion, with only 30% to 50% of lesions having calcified matrix.**
- **Intra-articular lesions, such as those in the proximal femur, often go clinically undiagnosed for a long period of time. Patients may present with chronic synovitis.**

ADDITIONAL IMAGES

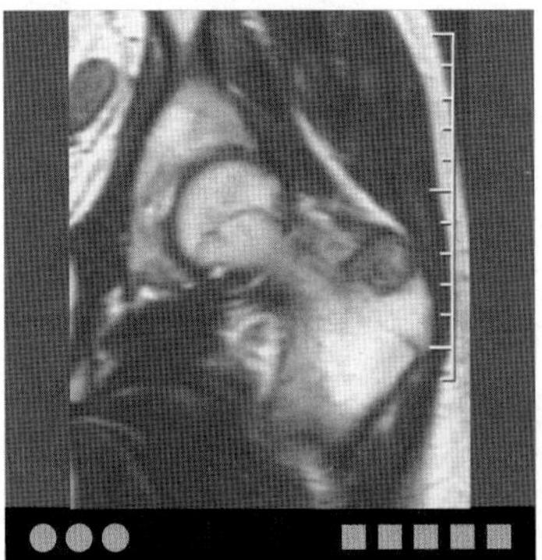

B. Chondroblastoma: Coronal T2WI shows the same lesion to be hyperintense with the extensive surrounding bone marrow edema. Note the hip joint effusion and thin T1 and T2 hypointensity at the lesion periphery indicating sclerosis.

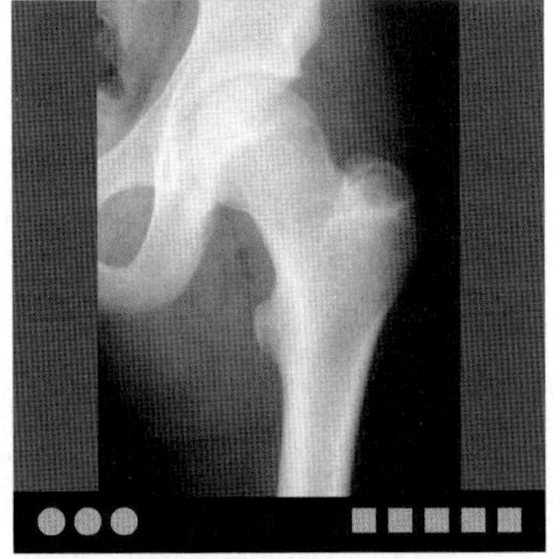

C. Chondroblastoma: AP radiograph of the left hip shows a round, well-circumscribed lytic lesion with a relatively thin sclerotic margin.

DIFFERENTIAL DIAGNOSES IMAGES

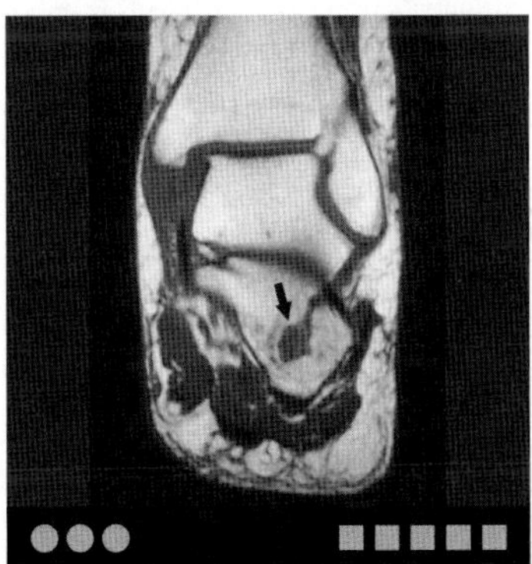

D. Brodie's abscess: Coronal T1WI shows an intraosseous fluid collection in the calcaneus (arrow) surrounded by bone marrow edema. Note the tract extending from the abscess to the surface of the calcaneus.

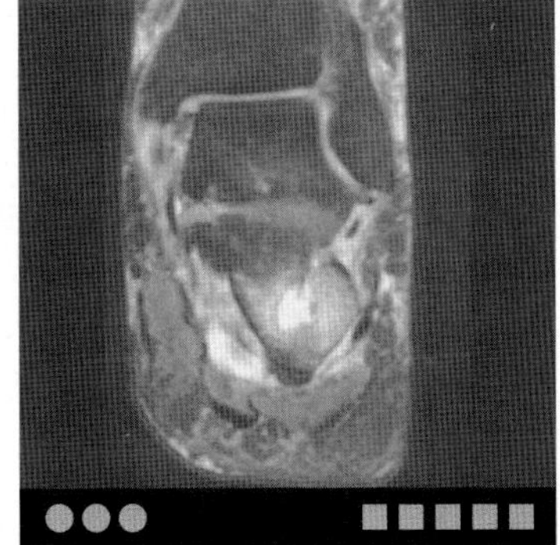

E. Brodie's abscess: Coronal fat-saturated T2WI shows an intraosseous fluid collection in the calcaneus surrounded by bone marrow edema. Note the tract extending from the abscess to the surface of the calcaneus.

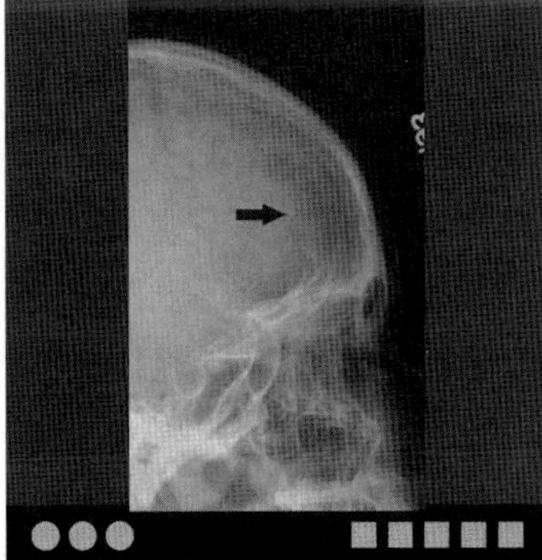

F. Eosinophilic granuloma: Lateral radiograph of the calvarium shows a lytic lesion with beveled edges in the right frontal bone (arrow).

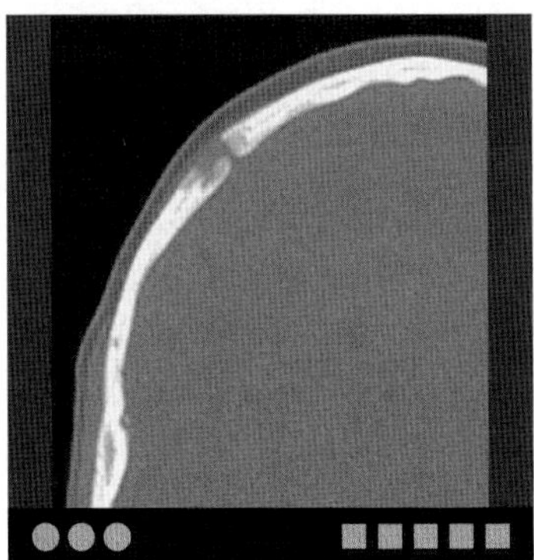

G. Eosinophilic granuloma: Axial head CT image shows a destructive lesion involving both the inner and outer tables of the right frontal bone.

IMAGE KEY

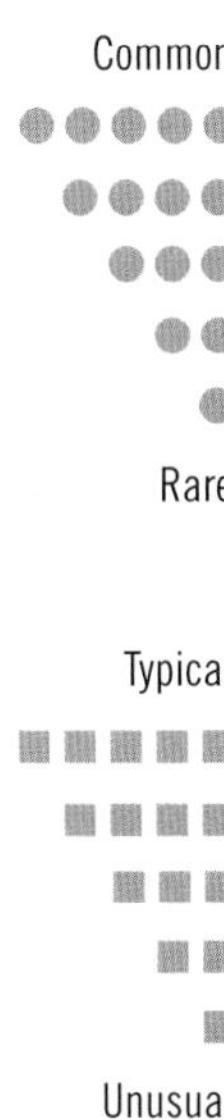

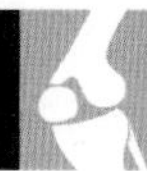

21–19 Diaphyseal Aclasis with Iliac Sarcomatous Transformation

Neerjana Doda and Wilfred CG Peh

PRESENTATION

Recent onset of pain, growing mass, neurological, or vascular symptoms

FINDINGS

Radiograph shows multiple exostoses (osteochondromas) at both femoral necks, with characteristic undertubulation deformity. A large ill-defined osteolytic lesion is present at the right ilium, with associated matrix calcification.

DIFFERENTIAL DIAGNOSES

- *Metastases:* Clinical history of known malignancy. No cartilage cap is present. Mostly osteolytic unless post-treatment or if primary is bone forming.
- *Chordoma:* Midline, destructive expansile, foci of calcification.
- *Sarcomatous transformation in Paget's disease:* Patients older than 50 years. The osteosclerotic phase is most distinctive, particularly in the axial skeleton and pelvic bone. There is bone expansion, cortical thickening, and coarse trabeculation. Sarcomatous transformation carries a poor prognosis.

COMMENTS

This is a 21-year-old woman, known to have diaphyseal aclasis (hereditary multiple exostosis), who complained of a progressively painful mass over her right upper buttock. Axial T2W MR image shows a lobulated mass arising from the right ilium. It is septated and markedly hyperintense. Diaphyseal aclasis is an autosomal dominant condition presenting with multiple osteochondromas and are associated with short stature and deformity. Malignant degeneration is more common (1%–20%) than in solitary osteochondromas. This complication occurs at a later age (fourth decade), and is more common in axial lesions than peripherally located osteochondromas. In 90% of cases, they transform to chondrosarcoma, with only 10% transforming to osteosarcoma, fibrosarcoma, or spindle cell sarcomas. Clinically, patients present with recent onset of pain and continued growth, even after skeletal maturity. Radiographic features include a cartilage cap greater than 2 cm in thickness, scattered calcific foci in soft tissue mass, focal regions of radiolucency, irregular osteochondral surface, and erosion of adjacent bone. CT is helpful to assess the cap, soft tissue mass, involvement of adjacent structures and distant metastases. MR imaging shows a lobulated mass with intermediate signal on T1- and hyperintense signal on T2WI, with interspersed areas of low signal because of calcification, septae or fibrous tissue. Intraosseous extension, cartilage cap, and the local spread are also well delineated. MR imaging is essential for local staging prior to treatment planning, especially in assessment of surgical margins. It is also helpful to detect local recurrence after surgery.

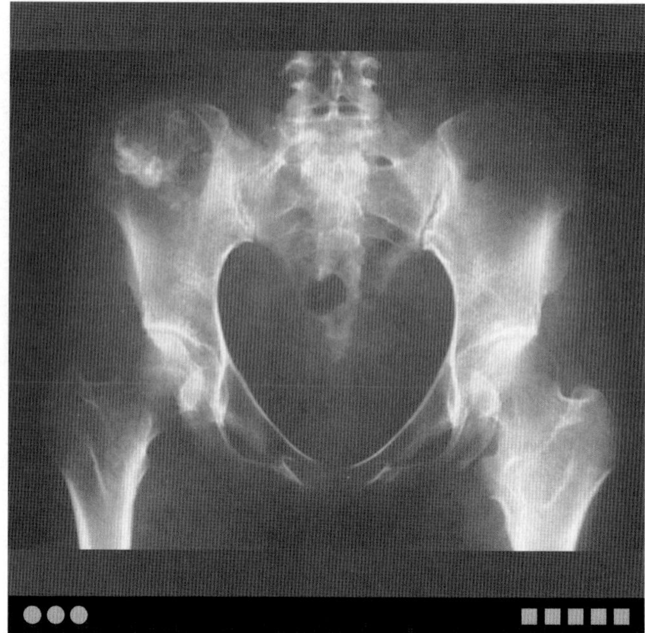

A. Chondrosarcoma developing in diaphyseal aclasia: Frontal radiograph shows a large osteolytic lesion in the right ilium, with chondroid calcifications within. Note small exostoses and remodelling of both femoral necks.

PEARLS

- **Sarcoma should be suspected when there is growth of tumour after puberty and new onset of pain.**
- **Cartilage cap thickness of more than 2 cm.**
- **Large soft tissue mass with flocculent/streaky calcification and dense radiopaque center with steaks radiating to periphery.**
- **MR imaging shows intermediate signal on T1W and hyperintense signal on T2WI.**

ADDITIONAL IMAGES

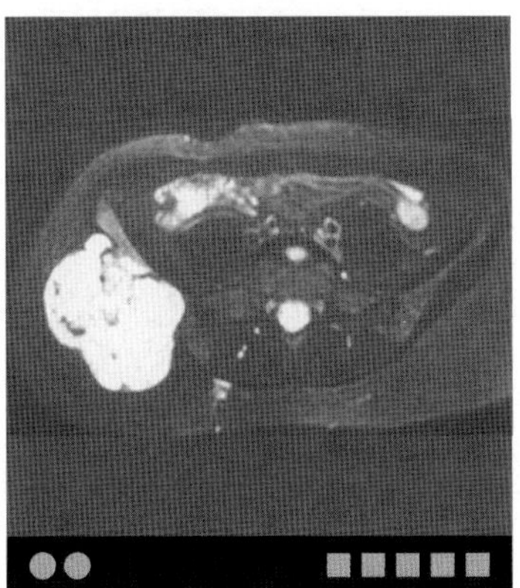

B. Chondrosarcoma developing in diaphyseal aclasia: Axial fat-suppressed FSE T2W MR image shows a large lobulated mass arising from the posterior aspect of the right ilium. The mass is markedly hyperintense and is septated.

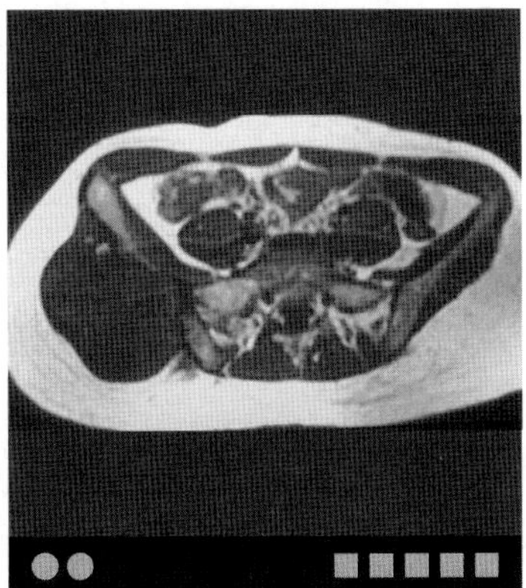

C. Chondrosarcoma developing in diaphyseal aclasia: Axial SE T1W MR image shows a large lobulated mass arising from the posterior aspect of the right ilium. The mass is isointense and invades into the adjacent gluteal muscles.

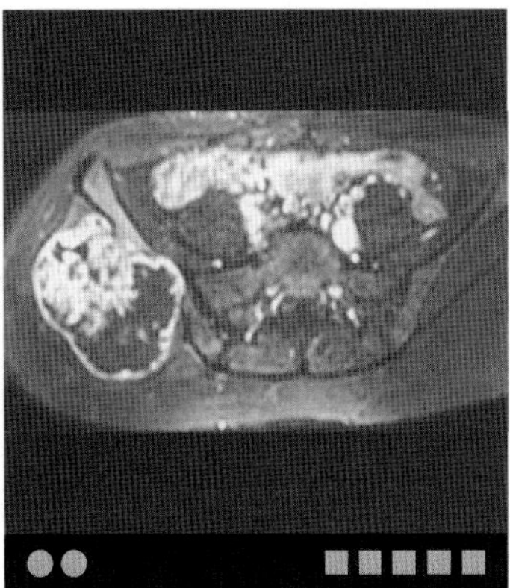

D. Chondrosarcoma developing in diaphyseal aclasia: Contrast-enhanced axial fat-suppressed SE T1W MR image shows a large lobulated mass arising from the posterior aspect of the right ilium. It shows surface and septal enhancement typical of chondroid tumors, with a large area of heterogeneous enhancement.

IMAGE KEY

Common

Rare

Typical

Unusual

DIFFERENTIAL DIAGNOSES IMAGES

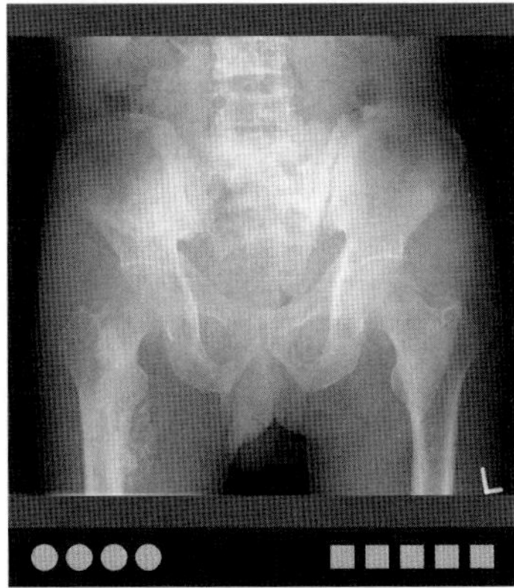

E. Bony metastases from treated bladder carcinoma: Frontal radiograph shows mixed osteolytic–sclerotic lesions in the right ilium and right femoral intertrochanteric region. There is also prominent new bone formation along the medial upper femoral shaft.

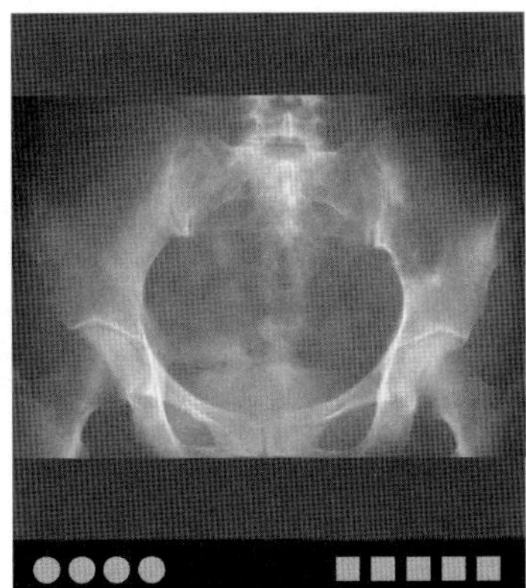

F. Bony metastases from adenocarcinoma of the lung: Frontal radiograph of the pelvis shows a large osteolytic lesion in the left medial ilium. It has ill-defined margins.

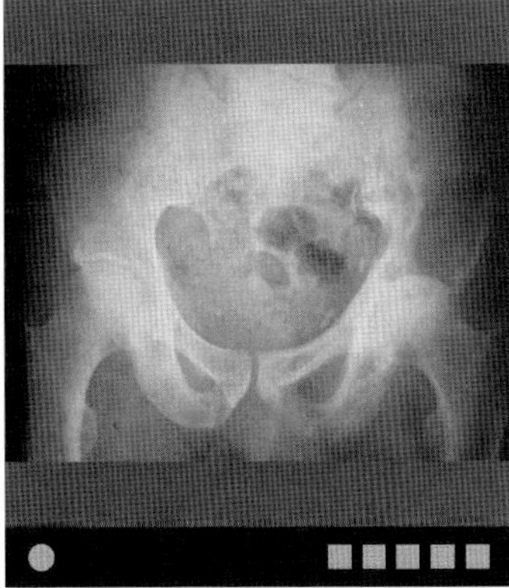

G. Osteosarcoma developing in Paget's disease: This is a 62-year-old man. Frontal radiograph shows slight expansion, sclerosis, and cortical thickening of the bones of the left hemipelvis, typical of Paget's disease. A large ill-defined osteolytic lesion is present in the supra-acetabular ilium.

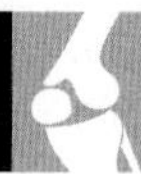

21–20 Solitary Bone Plasmacytoma

Joon Kim

PRESENTATION

Pelvic pain

FINDINGS

Conventional radiographic and CT images show a large expansile lytic lesion within the right hemipelvis.

DIFFERENTIAL DIAGNOSES

- *Lytic metastasis:* Metastases from thyroid or renal cell carcinoma are classically lytic. Differentiating a lytic metastasis from a plasmacytoma or multiple myeloma on imaging can be difficult without knowing clinical history.
- *Fibrous dysplasia:* Classically seen as a lucent lesion with ground glass or hazy density with a narrow zone of transition and sclerotic margins.
- *Ewing's sarcoma:* Usually is an aggressive appearing lesion with a large extraosseous soft tissue component. Should be considered in children, particularly during puberty.

COMMENTS

A solitary bone plasmacytoma is a lesion resulting from abnormal proliferation of monoclonal plasma cells within the bone marrow. These lesions have a predilection for the axial skeleton, but they can occur in practically every bone. Plasmacytomas are typically seen in 50 to 60 year olds, more commonly in men (male-to-female ratio of 2:1). Five percent of patients with multiple myeloma may initially present with a solitary plasmacytoma. Most patients with plasmacytomas will ultimately develop multiple myeloma; 60%to 80% at 10 years and 70% to 95% at 15 years. The most common clinical presentation is pain, particularly when a plasmacytoma is associated with a pathologic fracture. On conventional radiographs, plasmacytomas are typically described as "punched-out" lytic lesions with nonsclerotic margins and a narrow zone of transition. They are usually expansile lesions, associated with cortical thinning or endosteal scalloping. Plasmacytomas can be associated with diffuse bone destruction, especially when it is located within the pelvis or sacrum. On MR imaging, the lesions demonstrated nonspecific signal characteristics, often isointense to hypointense on T1W sequences and hyperintense on T2W sequences. A radionuclide bone scan is often not useful since the false-negative rate is high. When associated with the rare POEMS syndrome (polyneuropathy, organomegaly, endocrinopathy, M protein, and skin changes), plasmacytomas are sclerotic.

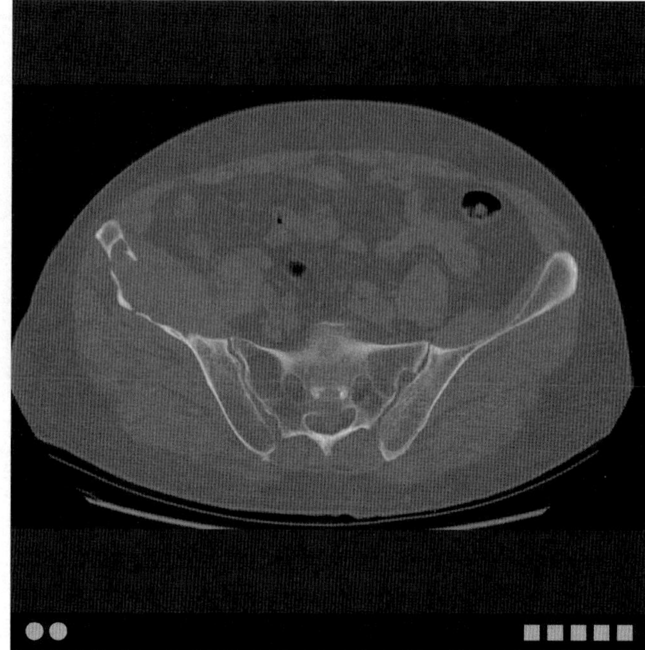

A. Plasmacytoma: Noncontrast axial CT scan of the pelvis shows large lytic lesion with cortical destruction anteromedially and the cortical thinning posterolaterally. Note the well-defined margin and the extraosseous soft tissue component.

PEARLS

- **A solitary bone plasmacytoma is a single focus of abnormal proliferation of monoclonal plasma cells.**
- **Typically seen in 50 to 60 year olds with a predilection toward males.**
- **Classically described as "punched-out" lytic lesions with nonsclerotic margins and a narrow zone of transition.**
- **On MR imaging, the lesions demonstrate nonspecific signal characteristics. Radionuclide bone scan is often not useful due to a high false-negative rate.**
- **Plasmacytomas can be associated with diffuse bone destruction resulting in pathologic fractures.**

ADDITIONAL IMAGES

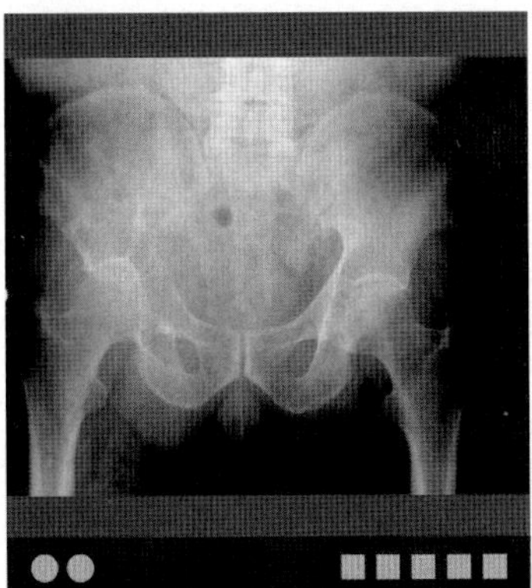

B. Plasmacytoma: AP pelvic radiograph shows a large expansile destructive lytic lesion within the right hemipelvis, involving the iliac wing, acetabulum, iliopubic eminence, and the pubic rami.

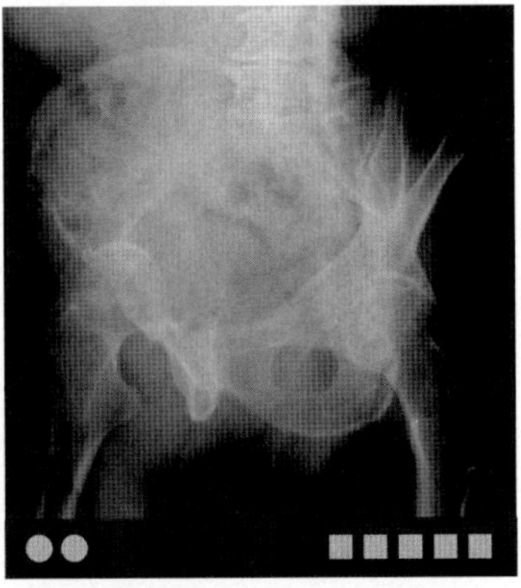

C. Plasmacytoma: External (iliac) oblique Judet view of the right hip again shows the extensive pelvic involvement. The cortical destruction along the greater sciatic notch and ischial spine is better appreciated.

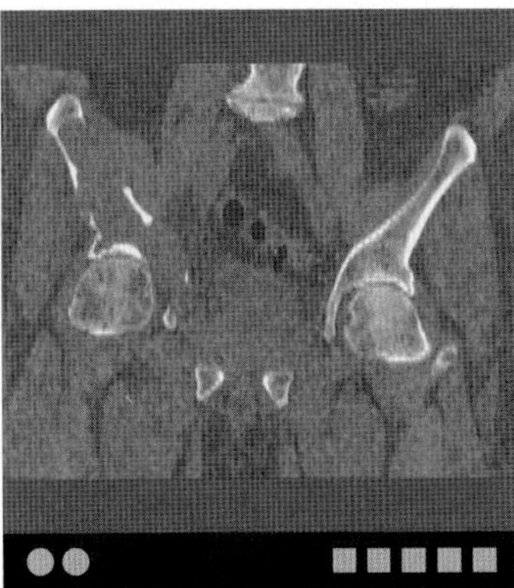

D. Plasmacytoma: Coronal reformatted CT scan of the pelvis shows involvement of the acetabulum.

DIFFERENTIAL DIAGNOSES IMAGES

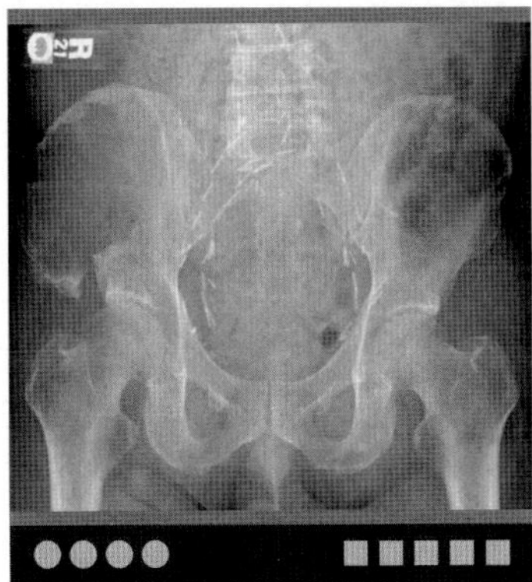

E. Metastasis: AP pelvic radiograph shows a large destructive lytic lesion involving the right iliac wing with pathologic fracture near anterior inferior iliac spine in this patient with metastatic thyroid carcinoma.

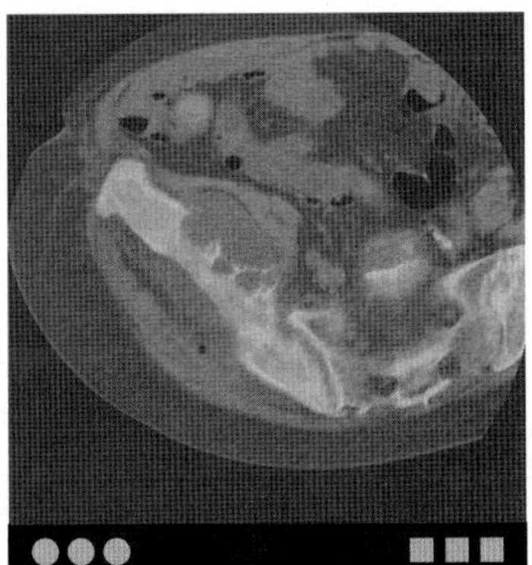

F. Fibrous dysplasia: Noncontrast CT of the pelvis during biopsy shows an expansile lesion within the right iliac wing with hazy or "ground glass" density. Extraosseous soft tissue component and cortical destruction is suggesting malignant transformation.

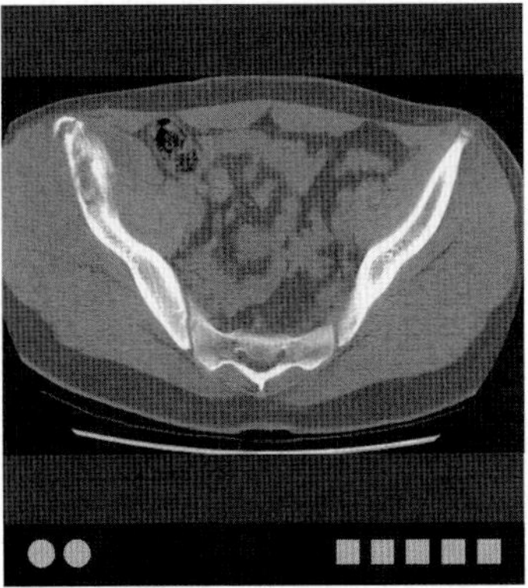

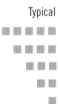

G. Ewings sarcoma: Noncontrast CT scan of the pelvis shows an aggressive mixed sclerotic and lytic lesion within the anterior right iliac wing, associated with a lamellated ("onion skin") periosteal reaction and a large extraosseous soft tissue mass.

IMAGE KEY

Common

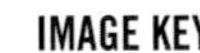

Rare

Typical

Unusual

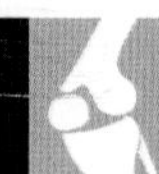

21-21 Extraskeletal Mesenchymal Chondrosarcoma (EMC)

Edward Mossop and Jamshid Tehranzadeh

PRESENTATION

Pain and swelling in groin

FINDINGS

MRI shows a large soft tissue mass in the groin with low signal on T1WI and high signal on T2WI with irregular internal dark signals representing mineralization.

DIFFERENTIAL DIAGNOSES

- *Synovial sarcoma:* The mass is usually isointense with muscle on T1WI and inhomogeneous high SI often with areas of hemorrhage and sometimes fluid–fluid levels or lobulation on T2WI.
- *MFH (malignant fibrous histiocytoma):* The soft tissue mass usually is associated with bony invasion and cortical destruction showing intermediate signal intensity (SI) on T1WI and high SI on T2WI.
- *Liposarcoma:* MRI of liposarcoma shows a sharp mass with inhomogeneous contrast enhancement on T1WI and mixed intermediate and high-intensity signals on T2WI.
- *Malignant schwannoma:* Usually presents with neuralgia because of compression of adjacent nerves. The mass is hypointense on T1WI and hyperintense on fat-saturated T2WI with strong central enhancement.

COMMENTS

This patient is a 14-year-old girl with pain and swelling in the right groin. Mesenchymal chondrosarcoma is a rare malignant tumor comprising 1% to 3% of chondrosarcoma. The peak incidence is in the second and third decades, affecting males and females equally. Extraskeletal origin of this tumor can represent 30% to 50% of all mesenchymal chondrosarcomas. The etiology of this malignancy has not been fully elucidated, but recent cytogenetic studies have found that the chromosomal translocation der (13; 21) (q10; q10) might play a causative role in its tumorigenicity. Under the microscope a mesenchymal chondrosarcoma is biphasic. There is a portion composed of small, undifferentiated round, or slightly spindled cells and a second pattern composed of islands of well-differentiated hyaline cartilage with areas of necrosis and calcification. Radiographs show a lobulated soft tissue mass containing several patterns of mineralization. Bone invasion is rare. CT more clearly depicted the intratumoral calcification and may show peripheral enhancement after contrast administration. MR imaging demonstrates a lobulated soft tissue mass, with areas of signal void corresponding to internal mineralization. T1W MR sequences often reveal a low signal intensity mass that is isointense to muscle, with high signal intensity seen on T2W and proton density MR sequences. The calcified areas show low intensity in both T1WI and T2WI. An enhancing high signal intensity mass with central foci containing low signal intensity is seen on gadolinium-enhanced T1W MR sequences. Angiography has been used to further evaluate ECM and may show neovascularization with arteriovenous shunting.

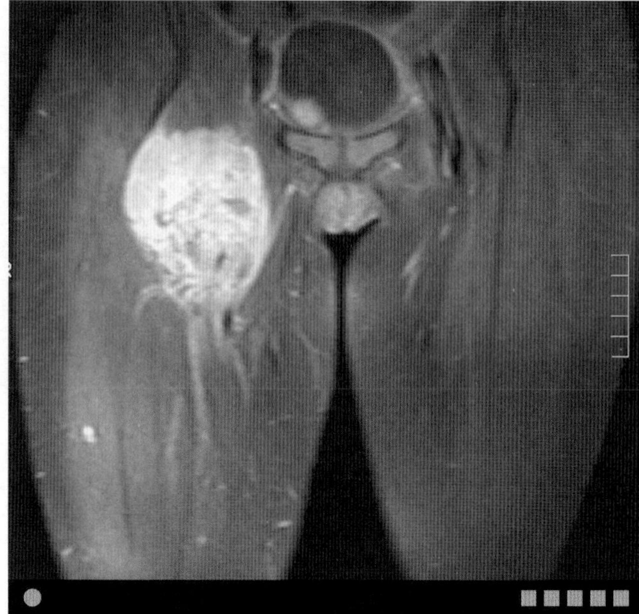

A. EMC: Coronal fat-saturated T1 postcontrast MR image shows a large enhancing soft tissue mass in the right groin with irregular internal dark signals.

PEARLS

- **Mesenchymal chondrosarcoma is a rare malignant tumor comprising about 1% to 3% of chondrosarcomas.**
- **Extraskeletal origin of this tumor represents 30% to 50% of all mesenchymal chondrosarcomas.**
- **MR imaging shows a lobulated soft tissue mass as low signal on T1 and high signal on T2 and PD-weighted images.**
- **Areas of signal void on MRI correspond to areas of calcification.**
- **After IV contrast administration the mass enhances with areas of low signal calcification.**

ADDITIONAL IMAGES

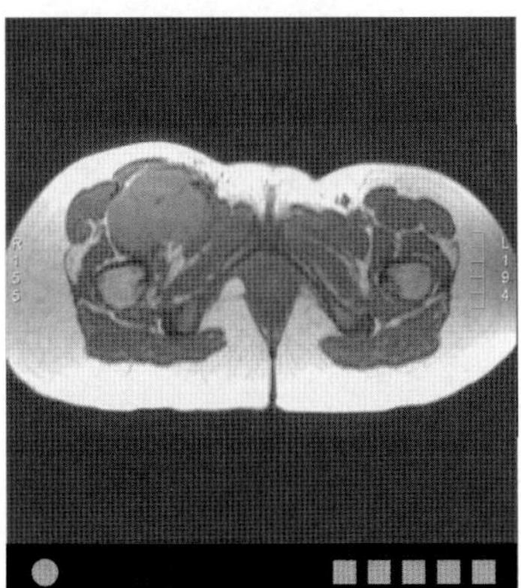

B. EMC: Axial T1W MR image shows an oval intermediate signal soft tissue mass in the right groin area.

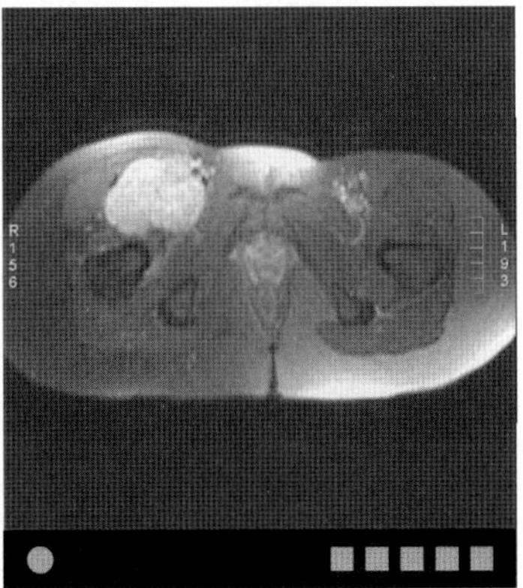

C. EMC: Axial fat-saturated T1 post-contrast MR image shows the mass is markedly enhancing in the right groin area.

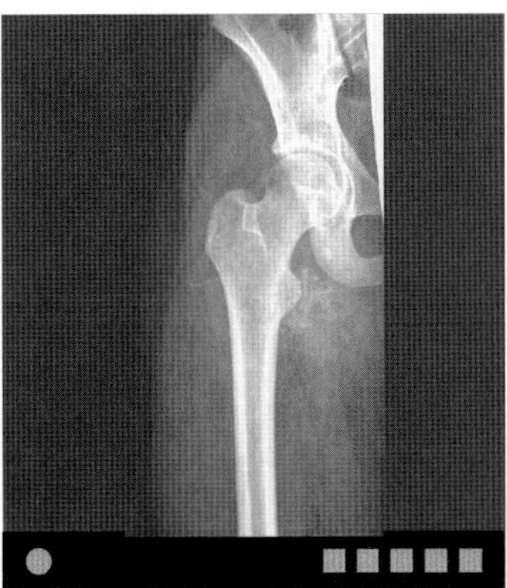

D. EMC: Plain AP radiograph of the right hip shows irregular calcifications in the soft tissue adjacent to the lesser trochanter.

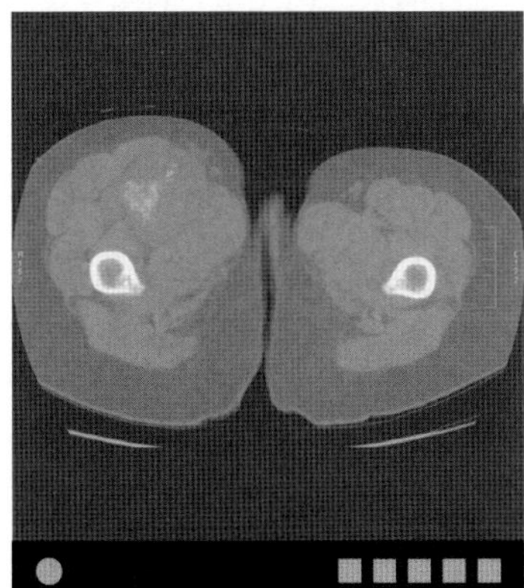

E. EMC: CT scan shows a round soft tissue mass with irregular calcifications in the right groin area.

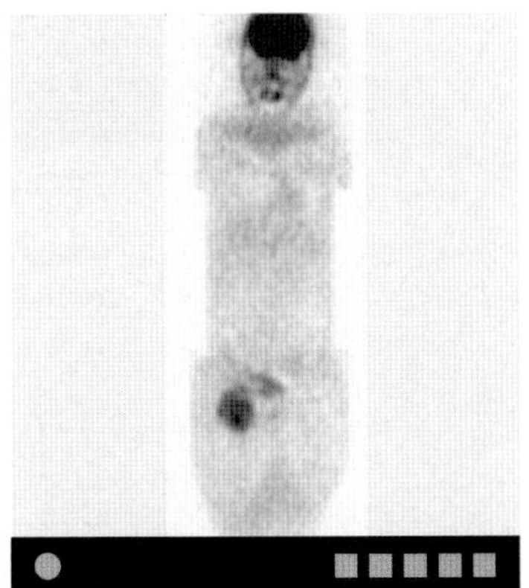

F. EMC: FDG PET scan shows avid uptake of the radionuclide by the tumor.

IMAGE KEY

Common

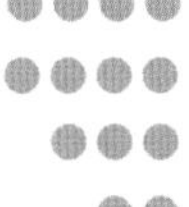

Rare

Typical

Unusual

DIFFERENTIAL DIAGNOSIS IMAGE

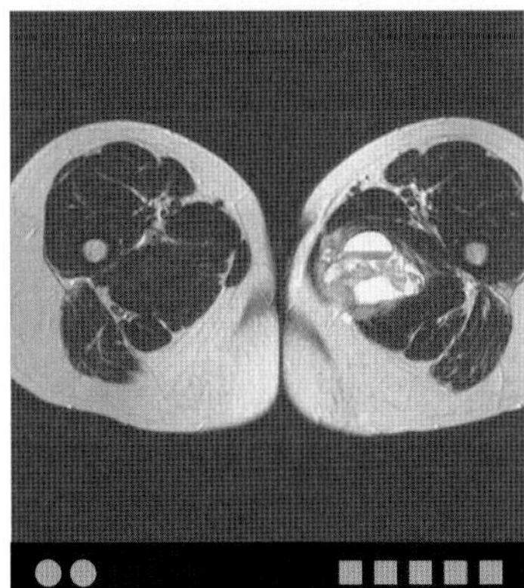

G. Synovial Sarcoma: Axial T2W MR image shows large soft tissue mass with lobulation and fluid–fluid level.

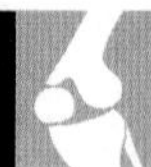

21–22 Bone Marrow Infiltration in Chronic Myelogenous Leukemia

Peyman Borghei and Jamshid Tehranzadeh

PRESENTATION

Pain and swelling of right knee

FINDINGS

MRI shows overall decreased signal intensity consistent with diffuse marrow involvement and patchy infiltration of bone marrow because of leukemic infiltration.

DIFFERENTIAL DIAGNOSES

- Marrow reconversion because of chronic anemia such as sickle cell anemia, thalassemia, spherocytosis, and HIV/AIDS marrow changes.
- Marrow infiltration and replacement like neoplastic or inflammatory processes, metastasis, lipidoses, and histiocytosis.
- Myeloid depletion as seen in chemotherapy, radiotherapy, and aplastic anemia.
- Marrow edema such as osteomyelitis and bone contusion.
- Marrow ischemia such as medullary infarct in systemic lupus erythematosus and steroid therapy.

COMMENTS

This is a 21-year-old female with a history of chronic myelogenous leukemia (CML) for 14 years, complaining of progressive pain and swelling in her right knee and left hip diagnosed with leukemic infiltration by bone marrow aspiration. CML is one of the myeloproliferative syndromes resulting from clonal expansion of hematopoietic progenitor cells usually associated with marked leukocytosis and elevated basophiles. The usual clinical presentation is anemia with constitutional symptoms and organomegaly. Packing of the marrow spaces with leukemic cells causes pressure atrophy of cancellous trabeculae and is noted radiographically as diffuse osteopenia seen in 50% of cases. Nodular collections of leukemic cells cause focal areas of medullary, cortical, or subperiosteal bone destruction. In the long bones, they are commonly seen in the metaphysis. MRI shows diffuse low signal abnormality because of the replacement of fatty marrow by hematopoietic cells. In addition, neoplastic infiltration shows low signal intensity foci on T1WI. Changes in T2WI are more variable, though an increase in signal intensity is usually present. Compared to T2WI, STIR sequences improve the visualization of leukemic process.

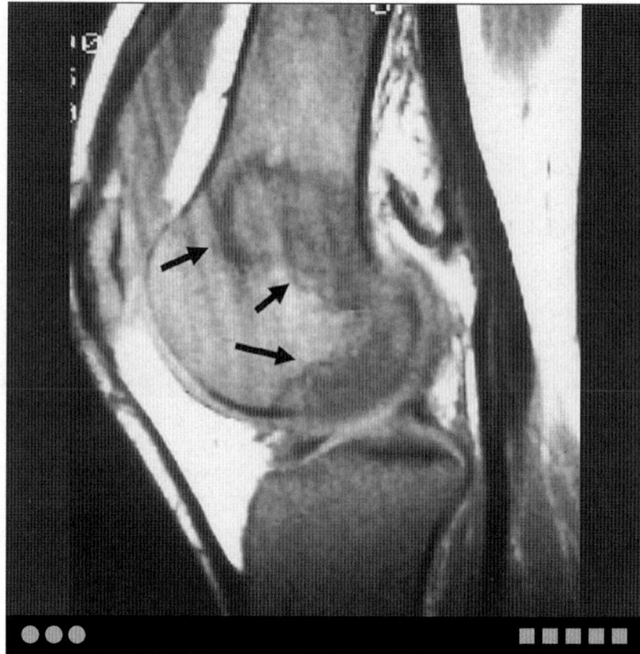

A. Bone marrow infiltration in CML: Sagittal T1WI of the knee shows diffuse decreased marrow signal because of anemia. Note patchy low signal intensity lesion in the posterior distal femur, consistent with leukemic infiltration (arrow).

PEARLS

- **CML is a myeloproliferative disorder characterized by constitutional symptoms, anemia, and organomegaly.**
- **Leukemic infiltration can involve marrow spaces and also soft tissues.**
- **Anemia associated with leukemia is responsible for diffuse low signal changes of the marrow in T1WI.**
- **MRI shows low signal intensity foci on T1WI and usually high signal intensity foci on T2WI in the areas of leukemic infiltrate.**

ADDITIONAL IMAGES

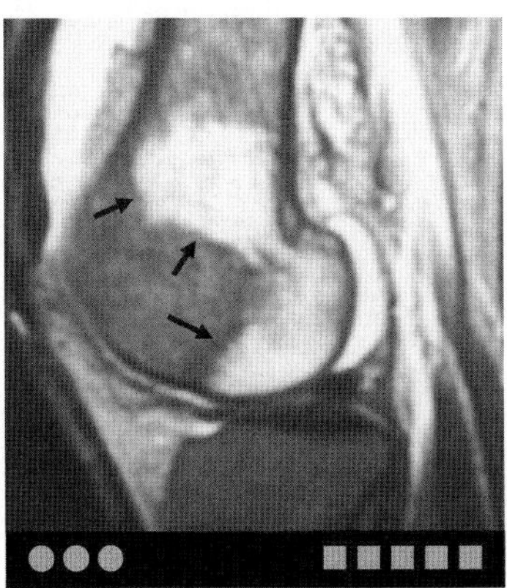

B. Bone marrow infiltration in CML: Sagittal T2WI shows a patch of leukemic infiltration showing high signal intensity focus in the distal femur (arrow).

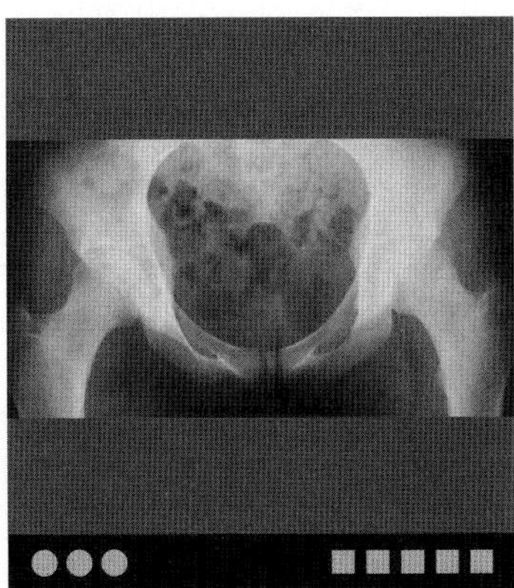

C. Bone marrow infiltration in CML: AP view of pelvis shows no definite abnormality.

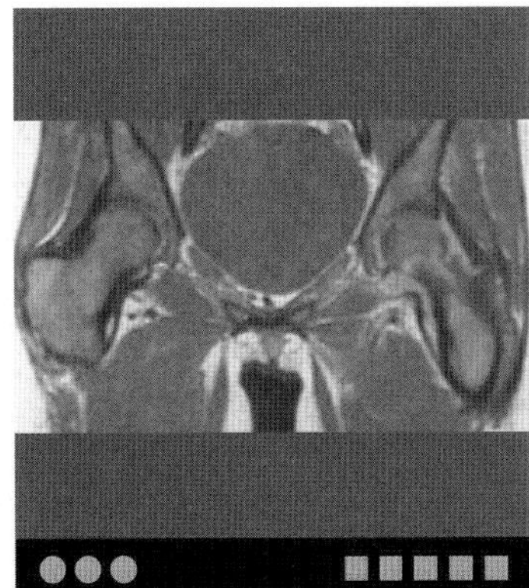

D. Bone marrow infiltration in CML: Coronal proton density of the pelvis showing diffuse low signal marrow because of anemia and foci of high signal intensity lesion on the neck of left femur because of leukemic infiltrates. Also note left hip joint effusion.

E. Bone marrow infiltration in CML: Coronal T2W MR image of the pelvis showing diffuse low signal marrow because of anemia and foci of high signal intensity lesion on the neck of left femur because of leukemic infiltrates. Also note left hip joint effusion.

IMAGE KEY

Common

Rare

Typical

Unusual

DIFFERENTIAL DIAGNOSES IMAGES

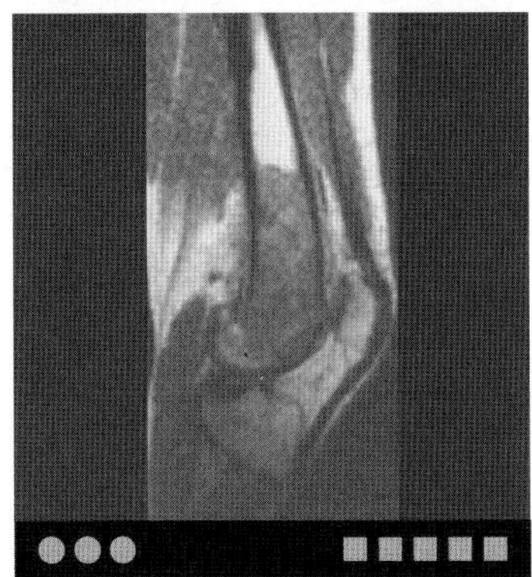

F. Osteosarcoma: Sagittal T1WI of distal femur shows osteosarcoma before chemotherapy. Low signal intensity lesion is seen at the region with osteosarcoma.

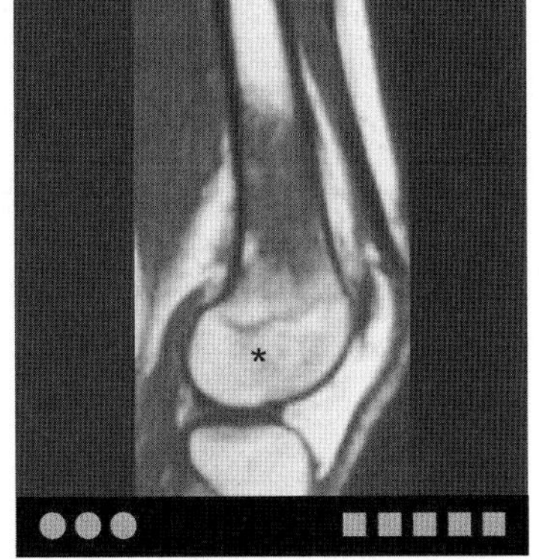

G. Osteosarcoma postchemotherapy: Sagittal T1WI of distal femur post chemotherapy. Note the return of normal fatty marrow signal in distal femur (*).

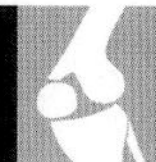

21–23 Ewing Sarcoma of Hip

Jimmy Ton and Jamshid Tehranzadeh

PRESENTATION

Right hip pain

FINDINGS

MR images show large soft tissue edema, joint effusion, and mass of the right hip.

DIFFERENTIAL DIAGNOSES

- *Tuberculous arthritis and osteomyelitis:* Patients typically present with chronic fever, tenderness, and elevated ESR. Aspiration of lesion may reveal acid-fast microorganisms.
- *Osteosarcoma:* These typically occur at the metaphysis of long bones and often present with osteoid formation.
- *Primary lymphoma:* These occur in older patients and usually involve less bone destruction.

COMMENTS

Ewing sarcoma (ES) was initially described in 1921 by James Ewing. The tumor occurs most frequently in children between 5 and 15 years of age and represents the second most common primary bone malignancy in children. Although any bone can be affected, ES usually involves the long bones of the extremities (femur, humerus, fibula, and tibia) and the pelvis. Clinically, patients with ES present with localized swelling and tenderness of several weeks to month's duration. Initially, the pain may be mild and intermittent but then rapidly intensifies. Furthermore, as the tumor grows, a palpable soft tissue mass can be appreciated on physical examination. Constitutional symptoms including fever, fatigue, weight loss, and anemia might also be present. On radiographs, ES appears as a poorly defined destructive lesion that is frequently associated with a soft tissue mass. Periosteal reaction is typically present giving an onionskin or sunburst appearance. MRI is the preferred imaging modality to evaluate accurately the extent of soft tissue and intramedullary involvement, as well as for the presence of skip lesions. The tumor exhibits low signal intensity on T1WI and appears hyperintense on T2WI. The tumor is often associated with a large soft tissue mass and it can spread throughout the marrow in the long bones. Furthermore, it may cause systemic manifestations and bone-to-bone metastasis.

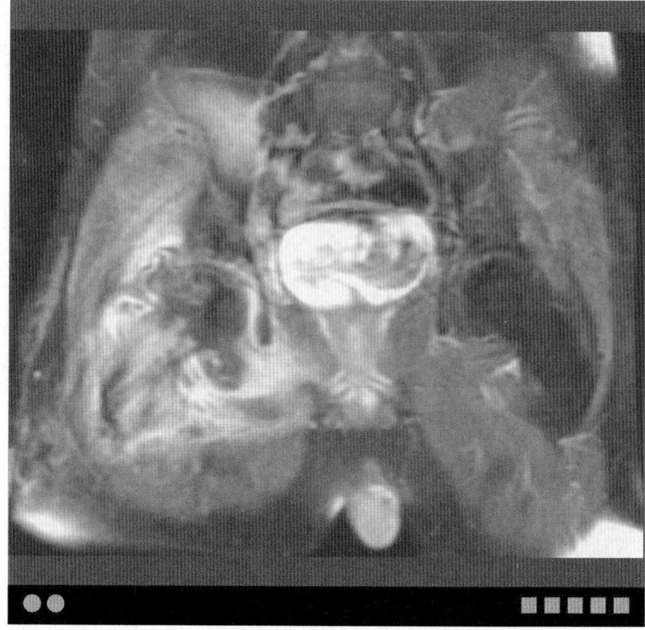

A. Ewing sarcoma: Coronal fat-saturated T1WI with contrast shows marked soft tissue edema and fluid in the joint, which appears as low signal and is delineated by the enhanced peripheral synovium. Enhancement of the bone marrow indicates osseous involvement.

PEARLS

- **ES most frequently occurs in the long bones of the extremities (femur, humerus, tibia, and fibula) and the pelvis.**
- **ES appears as a poorly defined lesion with an associated large soft tissue mass on radiographs. Periosteal reaction resulting in an onionskin or sunburst appearance might be present.**
- **MRI is useful for evaluating soft tissue involvement and typically shows low intensity on T1WI and hyperintensity on T2WI.**

ADDITIONAL IMAGES

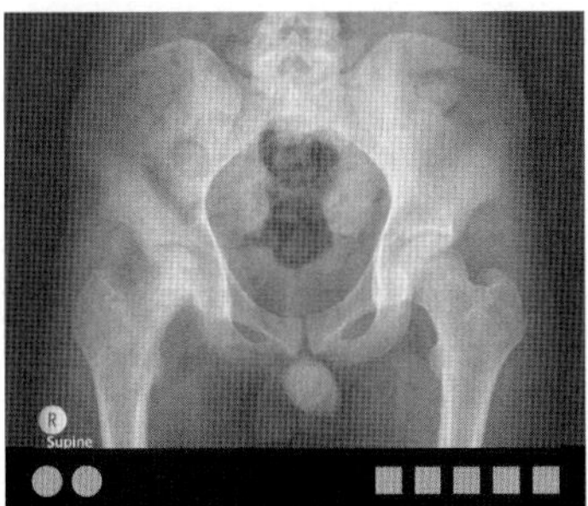

B. Ewing sarcoma: AP view of the pelvis shows a mixed lytic and sclerotic lesion of the proximal right femoral head and neck with loss of joint space associated with an adjacent soft tissue mass. A needle track at the biopsy site is also noted.

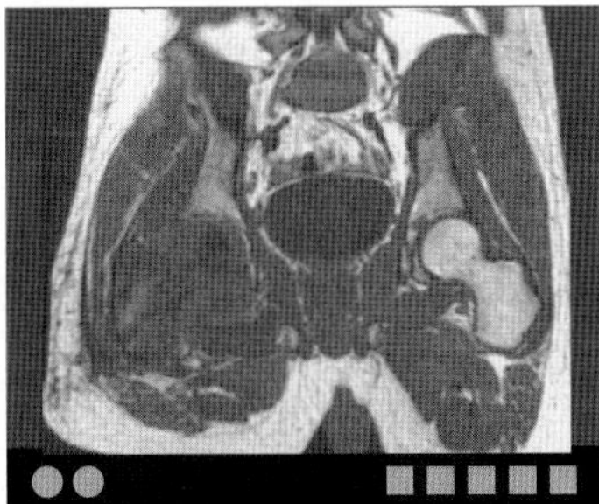

C. Ewing sarcoma: Coronal T1WI shows diffuse dark signal of the right proximal femur with adjacent soft tissue mass.

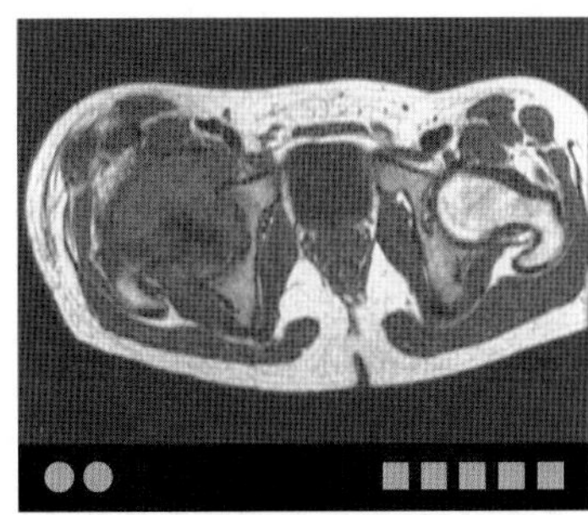

D. Ewing sarcoma: Axial spin echo T1WI shows dark signal of the right femur head and neck with surrounding soft tissue mass.

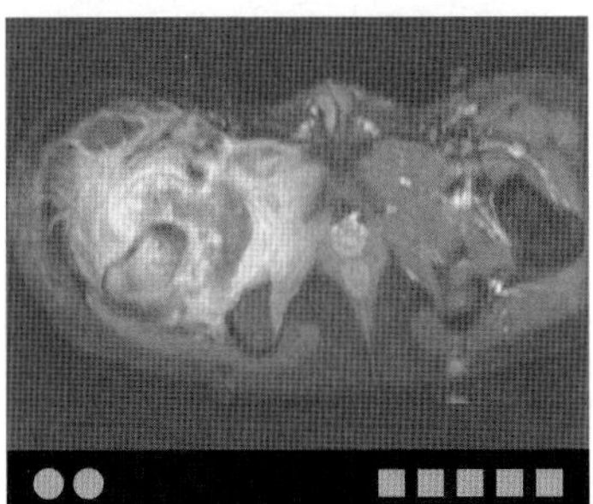

E. Ewing sarcoma: Axial fat-saturated postcontrast T1WI shows significant enhancement around the right hip and dark unenhanced joint fluid that is delineated by the peripheral contrast enhancement. Note extensive enhancement of the soft tissue mass and the right femoral neck.

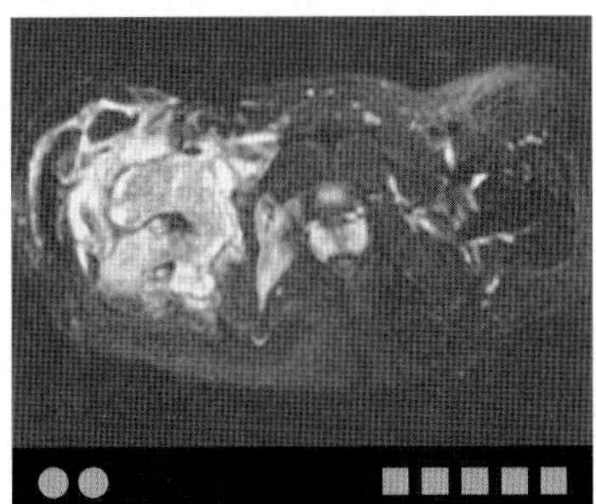

F. Ewing sarcoma: Axial fat-saturated T2WI shows soft tissue mass and fluid surrounding the right femoral head and neck. Note abnormal bright marrow signal in the right femoral head and neck.

IMAGE KEY

Common

Rare

Typical

Unusual

DIFFERENTIAL DIAGNOSIS IMAGE

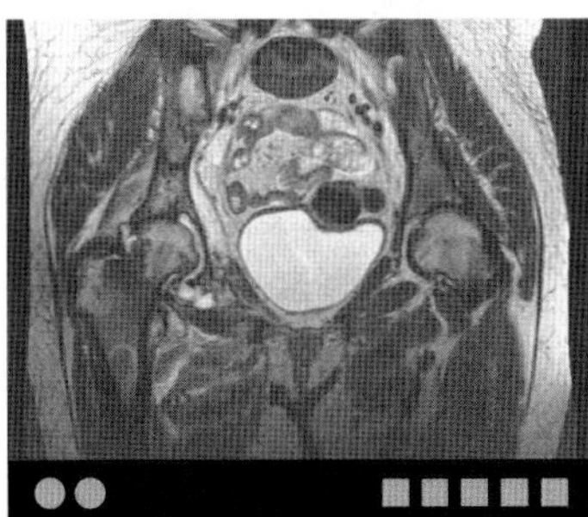

G. Tuberculous arthritis and osteomyelitis: Coronal T2WI shows loss of joint space and fluid in the right hip with abnormal bright signal in the right femoral head and the acetabulum with adjacent soft tissue edema in the medial side of the hip joint at the iliopsoas muscle insertion. There is abnormal hyperintense signal in the ilium and the proximal femoral shaft.

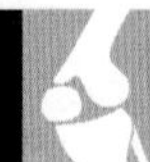

21–24 Osteosarcoma of the Femur

Michelle Chandler

PRESENTATION

Painful extremity mass

FINDINGS

MR axial SPGR postcontrast image shows an enhancing lesion involving the medullary cavity with permeation of the cortex and elevation of the periosteum of the distal femur.

DIFFERENTIAL DIAGNOSES

- *Ewing's sarcoma:* The periosteal reaction in Ewings sarcoma is lamellated as opposed to sunburst in character and the lesion is more likely to involve the metadiaphyseal region instead of the metaphysis with a permeative pattern lacking bone production.
- *Neuroblastoma metastasis:* The imaging appearance would be similar, but the lesion would likely be multiple and occur in a younger age group.
- *Osteomyelitis:* The clinical history would be helpful to make this distinction. The central cavity of any associated abscess formation may be difficult to distinguish from the necrosis that may be associated with an osteosarcoma. Osteoid formation would indicate an osteogenic tumor and would not be characteristic of an infectious process.

COMMENTS

This case involves a 6-year-old boy presenting with leg pain and a palpable mass. Osteosarcoma is the most common malignant bone tumor in the pediatric population with the typical age midteens to young adults. The typical conventional osteosarcoma is a medullary-based lesion that produces osteoid. The most common pattern of osteoid production is cloudlike. A "sunburst" pattern is another characteristic pattern. Other osteosarcoma subtypes produce chondroblastic and fibroblastic matrices and the lesion may arise from the surface of the bone. The most common location is around the knee in the distal femur and proximal tibia. Plain film radiography is the diagnostic method of choice, but MR imaging is used for surgical planning and staging. The appearance on plain film radiography is that of a destructive lytic or mixed lytic and sclerotic metaphyseal lesion. The extent of soft tissue involvement is best assessed in the setting of mineralized osteoid production. The goal of MRI is to determine extent of involvement of the medullary cavity and joint and soft

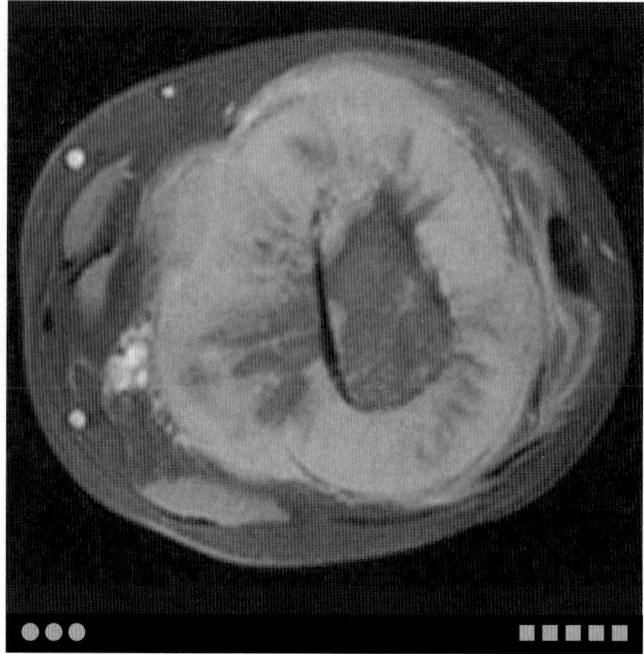

A. Osteosarcoma: Postcontrast SPGR axial MR image through the distal femur demonstrates a medullary-based lesion with diffuse enhancement of the soft tissue component. Absent enhancement centrally may indicate the presence of necrosis.

tissue structure invasion. Coronal or sagittal MR images of the entire bone involved should be obtained to evaluate for skip lesions. T1W MR images are considered the most accurate to assess the extent of medullary involvement. High-intensity fat will be replaced with low signal on T1W MR and T2W MR will better assess the extramedullary involvement along with postcontrast images. The presence of extension across the physis into the epiphysis should also be determined. Joint and vascular involvement are best assessed on post contrast images.

PEARLS

- **Osteosarcoma is the most common malignant bone tumor in the pediatric population.**
- **A lesion producing "cloudlike" osteoid or "sunburst" periosteal reaction is typical of the conventional osteosarcoma.**
- **Although MR imaging is used for staging and surgical planning, plain film radiography is considered the diagnostic modality of choice.**

ADDITIONAL IMAGES

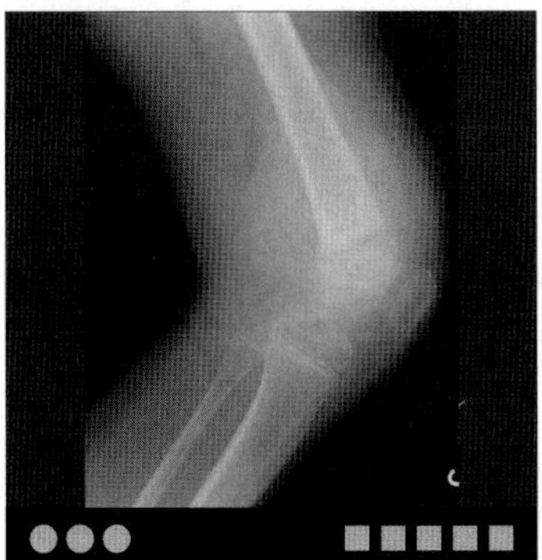

B. Osteosarcoma: Radiograph of the knee shows the "cloudlike" osteoid production most commonly found in conventional osteosarcomas.

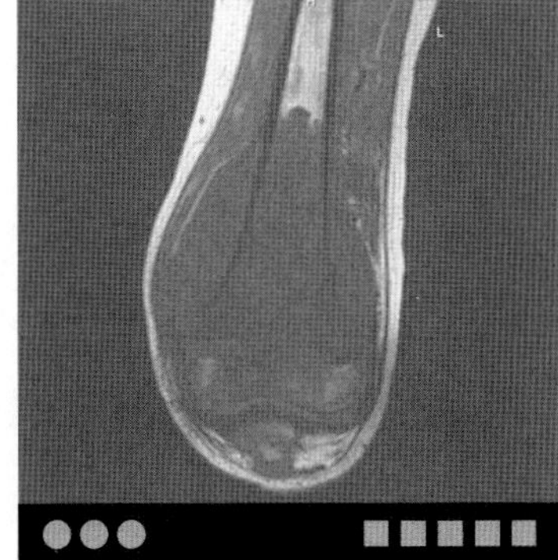

C. Osteosarcoma: Coronal T1 MR clearly demonstrates the border of the tumor with the normal medullary cavity.

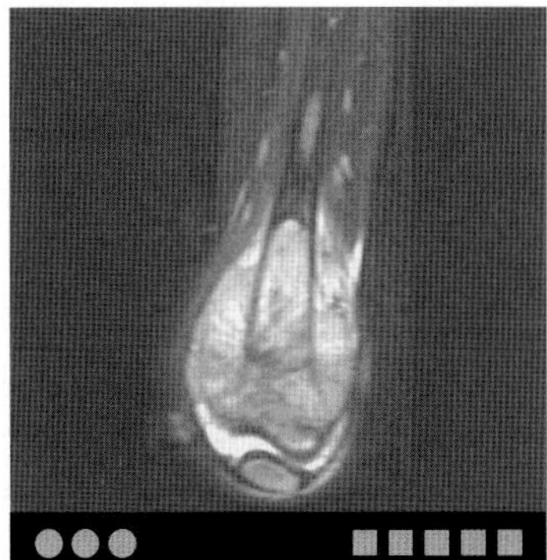

D. Osteosarcoma: Coronal T2 with fat saturation MR demonstrates the extent of soft tissue involvement including extension into the joint and associated edema in the soft tissues.

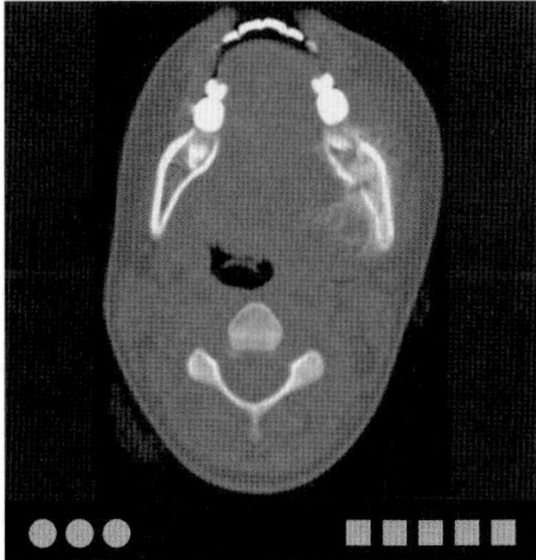

E. Osteosarcoma: CT in another patient shows the "sunburst" type of periosteal reaction seen in conventional osteosarcomas; in this case the lesion involves the jaw.

IMAGE KEY

Common

Rare

Typical

Unusual

DIFFERENTIAL DIAGNOSES IMAGES

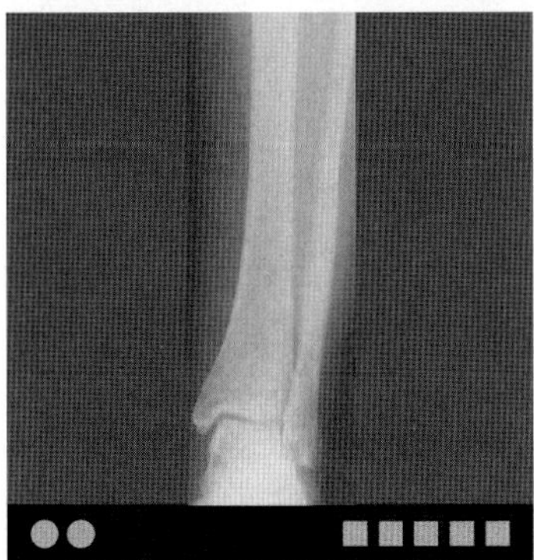

F. Ewing's sarcoma: Radiograph of the distal tibia and fibula demonstrates a permeative lesion in the distal tibia with lamellated thick periosteal reaction most characteristic of Ewing's sarcoma. Although there are typical radiographic features of Ewing's and osteosarcoma the imaging findings may often overlap placing both as high differential considerations in many cases.

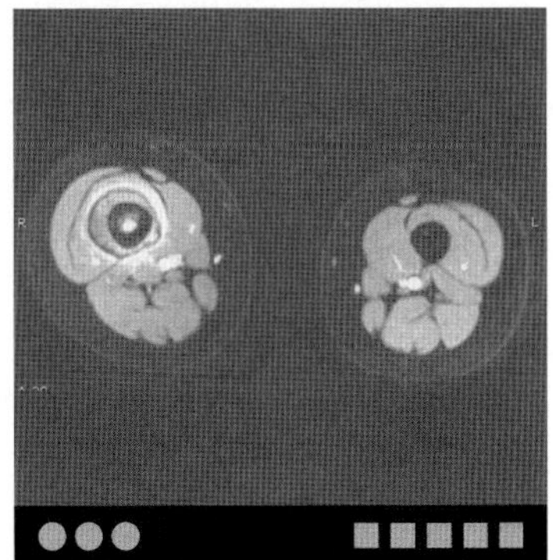

G. Metastatic neuroblastoma: Axial T1 postcontrast with fat saturation demonstrates an enhancing lesion replacing the marrow cavity and extending through the cortex with a "sunburst" appearance of the periosteal reaction in this patient with metastatic neuroblastoma. This should be considered in the differential of the younger child.

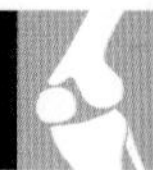

21–25 Chondrosarcoma of Acetabulum

Joon Kim

PRESENTATION

Hip pain

FINDINGS

Conventional radiographs, CT, and MR images show a destructive lesion involving the right acetabulum.

DIFFERENTIAL DIAGNOSES

- *Metastasis:* Lesions can be lytic or sclerotic depending on the origin of the metastasis. They usually lack internal chondroid matrix.
- *Lymphoma:* Tend to be associated with a large extraosseous soft tissue component.
- *Multiple myeloma/plasmacytoma:* Classic appearance is that of a circumscribed, lucent, and round "punched-out" lesion on conventional radiographs and CT.

COMMENTS

Chondrosarcomas are malignant bone tumors containing cartilaginous matrix. It is the second most common type of primary bone neoplasm, occurring most commonly in the middle aged and the elderly. They usually occur at the metaphysis of long bones and at the center of flat bones, most frequently involving the proximal femur, shoulder girdle, and the pelvis. They may develop de novo (primary chondrosarcoma), but may also arise in preexisting benign bone lesions (secondary chondrosarcoma) such as enchondromas or osteochondromas or in preexisting conditions such as multiple hereditary exostoses, Ollier's disease, and Maffucci's syndrome. On conventional radiographs and CT, chondrosarcomas tend to be lucent, expansile, and destructive lesions containing internal chondroid matrix (classically referred to having a pattern of "rings" and "arcs"). They may be associated with an extraosseous soft tissue component, which is better evaluated with cross-sectional imaging. On MR imaging, chondrosarcomas are typically lobulated, often containing internal septations. The lesions tend to be very bright on T2W sequences and hypointense/isointense on T1W sequences. There may be internal foci of signal voids, representing the calcified chondroid matrix. Differentiating chondrosarcomas from enchondromas may sometimes be difficult on imaging, but findings such as endosteal scalloping, cortical destruction, an extraosseous soft tissue component, and poorly defined borders suggest chondrosarcoma. Clinically, pain that is associated with a cartilage-based tumor is suggestive of malignancy. Prognosis of chondrosarcoma depends on its grade, ranging from grade I (90% 5-year survival rate) to grade III (Less than 50% 5-year survival rate).

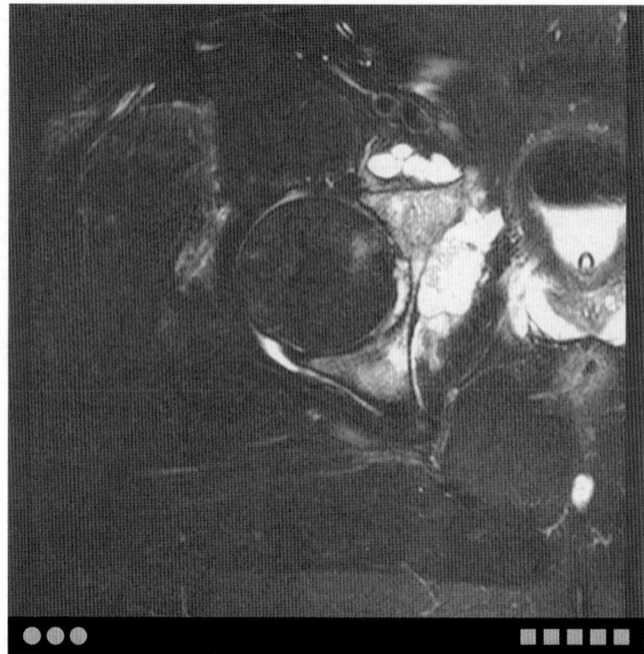

A. Chondrosarcoma: Axial T2W fat-suppressed MR image shows a hyperintense lesion in the right acetabulum with a multilobulated hyperintense extraosseous soft tissue component containing internal septations.

PEARLS

- **Chondrosarcomas are the second most common malignant primary bone tumors.**
- **Usual locations include the metaphysis of long bones and at the center of flat bones. Occurs most commonly in the middle aged and the elderly.**
- **Tend to be lucent, expansile, and destructive lesions containing internal chondroid matrix on conventional radiographs and CT.**
- **On MR imaging, they are typically hyperintense on T2W imaging, often lobulated with internal septations.**
- **Differentiating chondrosarcomas from enchondromas may sometimes be difficult, but aggressive characteristics suggest malignancy.**

ADDITIONAL IMAGES

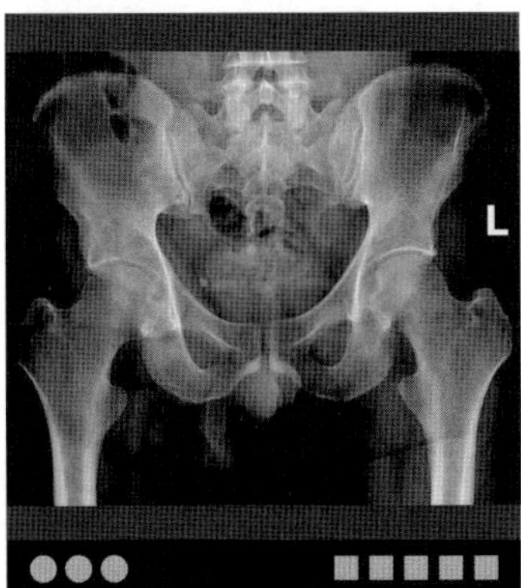

B. Chondrosarcoma: Conventional AP radiograph of the pelvis shows an expansile lucent lesion in the right acetabulum with internal chondroid matrix.

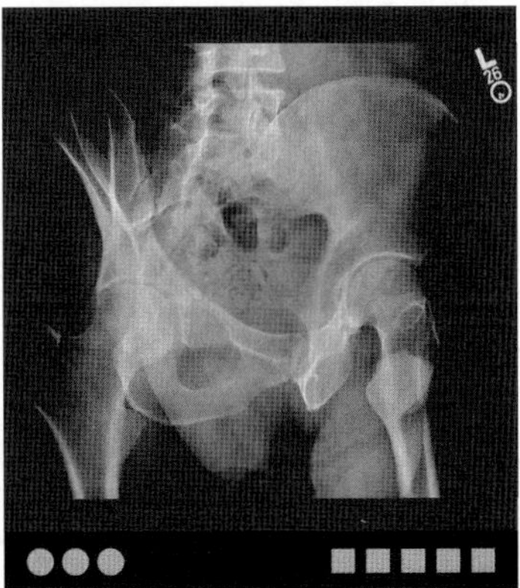

C. Chondrosarcoma: Internal oblique (Judet) view of the right hip shows that the lesion extends into the iliopubic eminence and into the superior pubic ramus, where cortical destruction is better appreciated.

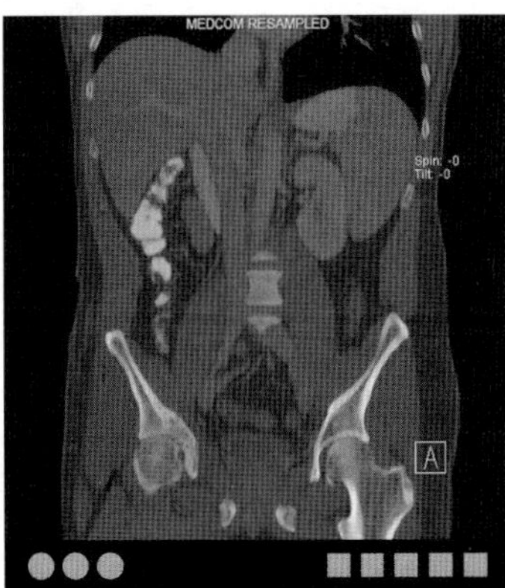

D. Chondrosarcoma: Reformatted coronal CT of the abdomen and pelvis with intravenous contrast demonstrating the destructive lesion in the right acetabulum.

IMAGE KEY

Common

Rare

Typical

Unusual

DIFFERENTIAL DIAGNOSES IMAGES

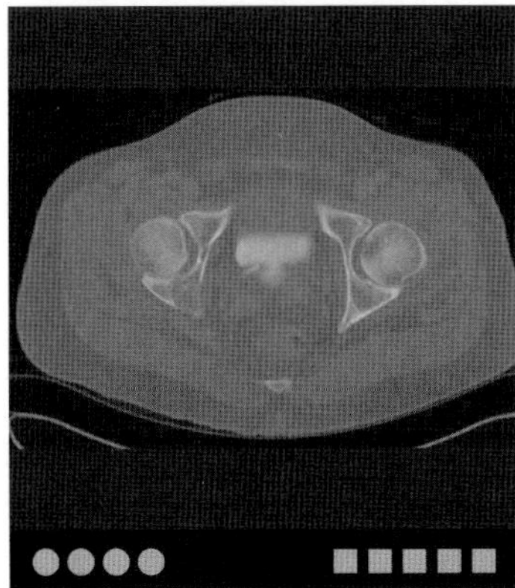

E. Metastasis; renal cell carcinoma: CT of pelvis with intravenous contrast shows a mildly destructive lesion in the posterior right acetabulum in a patient with metastatic renal cell carcinoma.

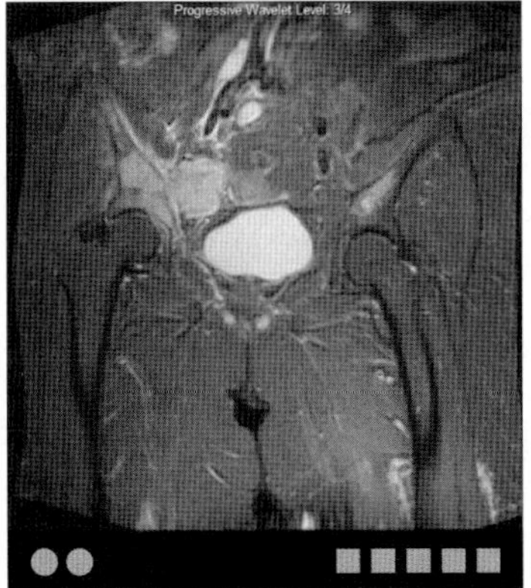

F. Lymphoma: Coronal inversion recovery image of the pelvis demonstrates a hyperintense lesion in the right acetabulum with a large intrapelvic extraosseous soft tissue component. Another lesion is in the left superior acetabulum extending into the iliac wing.

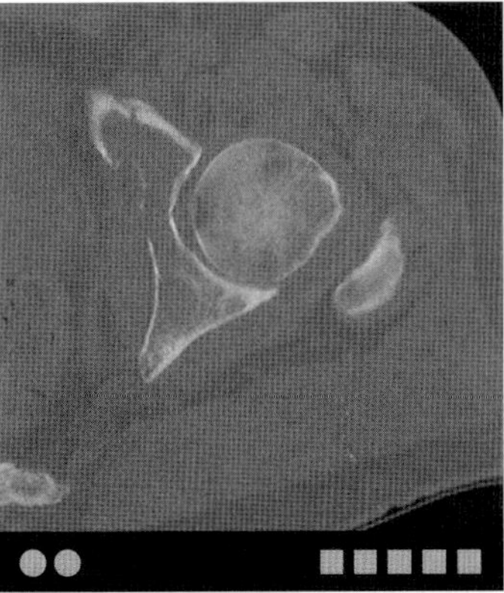

G. Plasmacytoma: Coned-down axial noncontrast CT of the left hip shows a mildly expansile lesion in the acetabulum extending into the superior pubic ramus. Note the pathologic fracture and mild cortical thickening along the anterior cortex.

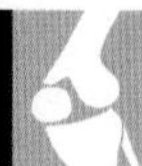

21–26 Clear Cell Chondrosarcoma

Janis Owens

PRESENTATION

Hip pain

FINDINGS

There is a circumscribed lesion in the epiphyseal–metaphyseal region of the right proximal femur, which is low/intermediate signal on T1W and high signal on T2W sequences. There is enhancement of the lesion with intravenous gadolinium contrast material with a focal area of necrosis within the lesion.

DIFFERENTIAL DIAGNOSES

- *Giant cell tumor:* There is a similar MRI appearance. More than 55% of giant cell tumors occur at the knee.
- *Chondroblastoma:* The patient age is younger. Chondroblastoma usually has associated bone marrow edema.
- *Osteonecrosis:* Variable internal signal on T1W and T2W sequences. There is a peripheral low signal rim on T1W and a low and high signal rim on T2W sequences (double line sign).

COMMENTS

This is a 28-year-old male who presented with right hip pain. Clear cell chondrosarcoma is a rare form of low-grade chondrosarcoma, which on histological evaluation contains neoplastic chondroid cells with clear cytoplasm instead of the usual neoplastic chondroid cells. Clear cell chondrosarcoma accounts for 2% of chondrosarcomas. Diagnosis is usually made in the third or fourth decade with the average age at diagnosis being 34 years. Depending on the series, 58% to 68% of clear cell chondrosarcomas occur in the proximal femur in the epiphyseal–metaphyseal location. Radiographically, clear cell chondrosarcoma is a geographic lesion, which may have focal indistinct borders Twenty percent of clear cell chondrosarcomas are lytic lesions with a thin sclerotic rim. Chondroid mineralization resembling chondroblastoma is present in 50% of the lesions; however, clear cell chondrosarcoma lacks the bone marrow edema typically seen with chondroblastoma on MRI and the age for chondroblastoma is younger than that for clear cell chondrosarcoma. The typical MRI appearance is homogeneous low/intermediate signal on T1W sequences, homogeneous high signal on T2W sequences and enhancement following gadolinium contrast injection and is similar in appearance to giant cell tumor of bone. Focal low signal areas may be seen on MRI if chondroid mineralization is present. CT scan best demonstrates areas of mineralization in the lesion.

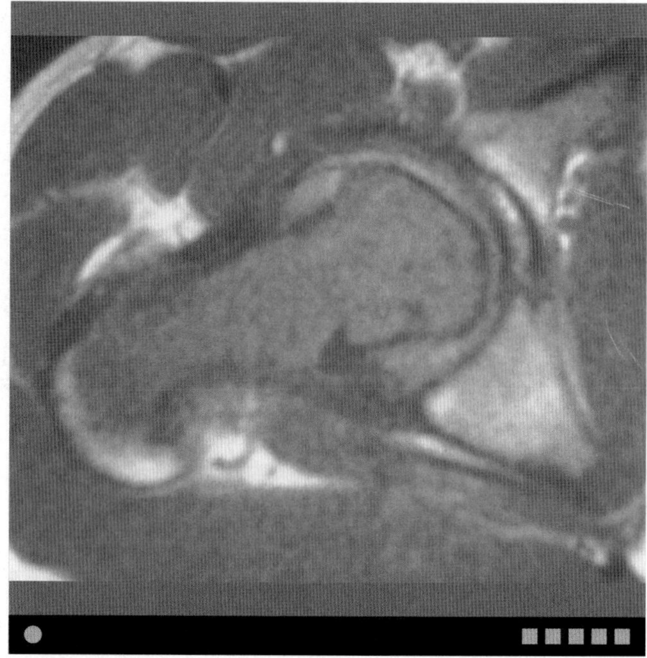

A. Clear cell chondrosarcoma: Axial T1W sequence shows a homogeneous low signal lesion in the right femoral head neck.

> **PEARLS**
>
> - **Epiphyseal–metaphyseal lesion in the proximal femur.**
> - **Geographic lesion with or without chondroid mineralization and a sclerotic rim is 20%.**
> - **Older age than chondroblastoma with no bone marrow edema on MRI.**
> - **Rare form of chondrosarcoma.**

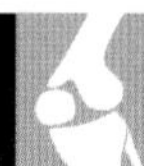

ADDITIONAL IMAGES

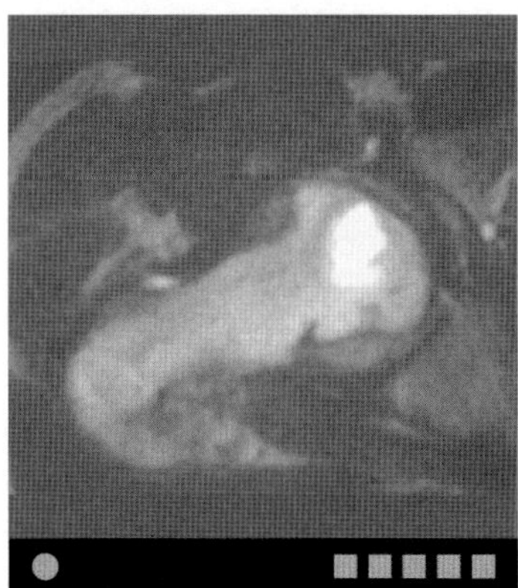

B. Clear cell chondrosarcoma: Axial T2W sequence shows a high signal lesion in the right femoral head and neck with focal cystic change or necrosis.

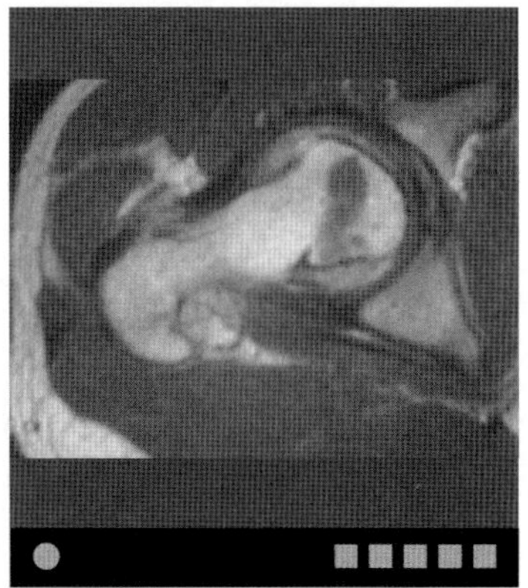

C. Clear cell chondrosarcoma: Axial T1W post-gadolinium image shows homogeneous enhancement of the lesion in the right femoral head neck with a focal area of necrosis or cystic change.

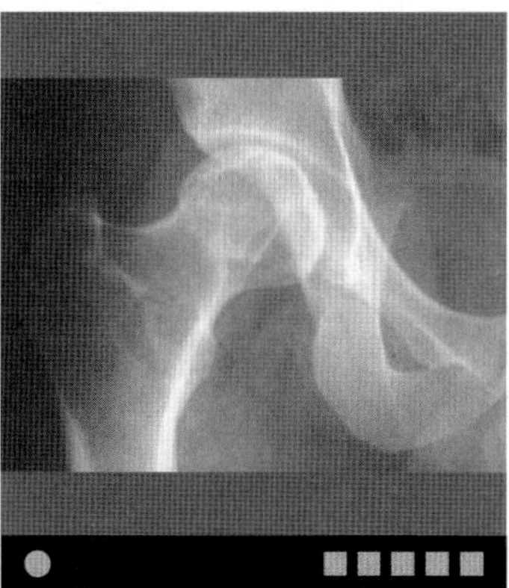

D. Clear cell chondrosarcoma: AP right hip shows a geographic lytic epiphyseal-metaphyseal lesion in the right proximal femur.

DIFFERENTIAL DIAGNOSES IMAGES

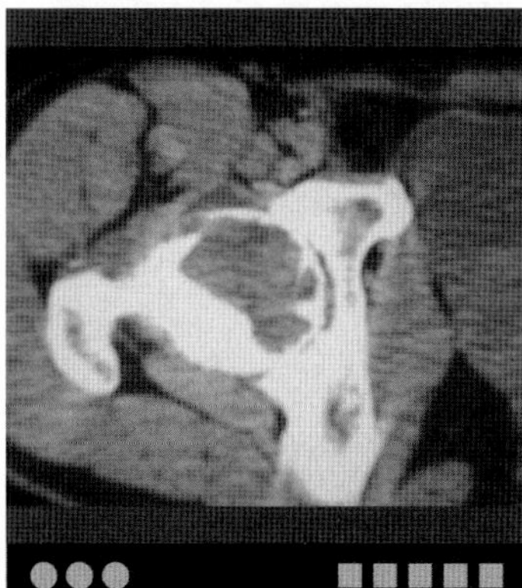

E. Giant cell tumor: Axial CT shows an isodense to muscle geographic lytic lesion in the epiphyseal-metaphyseal region with cortical break.

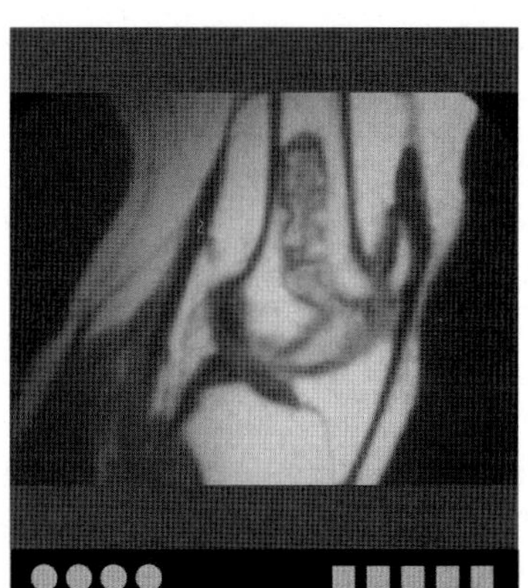

F. Osteonecrosis: Sagittal T1W sequence shows the internal high signal marrow and the peripheral low signal rim in the distal femur.

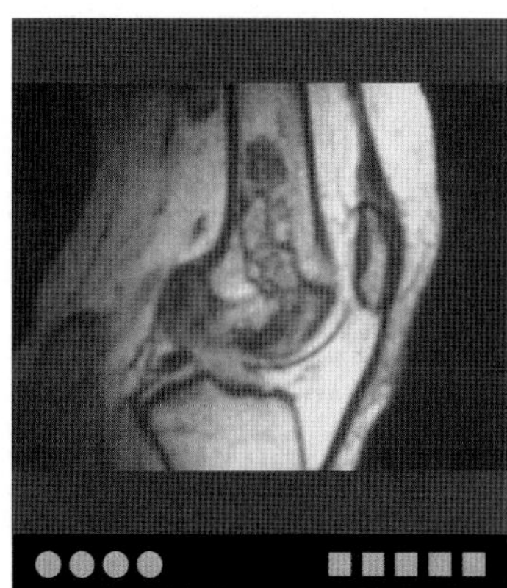

G. Osteonecrosis: Sagittal T2W sequence shows a low signal peripheral rim with internal fat signal in the epiphyseal-metaphyseal region of the distal femur.

IMAGE KEY

Common

Rare

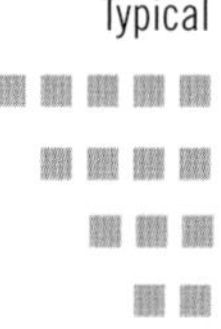

Typical

Unusual

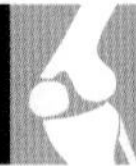

21–27 Primary Osseous Lymphoma of the Pelvis

Hakan Ilaslan

PRESENTATION

Gradually worsening leg pain and weakness

FINDINGS

There is a large marrow infiltrating lesion in left hemipelvis with a large soft tissue component. Sacral nerve roots are encased by the lesion.

DIFFERENTIAL DIAGNOSES

- *Metastatic disease:* Metastatic bone disease could present with identical imaging findings. Multiplicity of metastatic lesions usually helps although secondary lymphoma may also present with multiple sites of bony involvement.
- *Ewing's sarcoma:* The pelvic bones and femur are affected most often as the primary site of origin. The peak incidence is in second decade, although it may occur at any age. Imaging features are of an aggressive tumor with lytic, permeative bony involvement and associated large soft tissue component.
- *Osteosarcoma:* The age distribution of osteosarcoma is bimodal; it occurs most frequently in those aged 10 to 20 years and a second smaller peak is seen in patients older than 50 years, and this peak is associated with a relative increase in pelvic involvement and a decrease in involvement of extremity bones.

COMMENTS

The patient is a 35-year-old male with gradually worsening left leg pain and weakness over 1 year. Primary osseous lymphoma accounts for less than 5% of all primary bone tumors and defined as lymphoma with no evidence of systemic disease at the time of diagnosis or within 6 months of discovery of the original lesion. Secondary osseous lymphoma is systemic lymphoma with osseous involvement at the initial diagnosis or systemic disease within 6 months of osseous disease with distant nodal and/or soft tissue tumor. Primary osseous lymphoma has a predilection for the appendicular skeleton, with vertebral involvement only seen in the multifocal variant of primary osseous lymphoma, while secondary osseous lymphoma has a vertebral predilection. In recent years, PET scan gained popularity in the staging of lymphomas. The lytic-destructive pattern is the most common radiographic appearance of primary bone lymphoma, as it was reported in approximately 70% of cases and believed to result from an osteoclast-stimulating factor. Radiographically, primarily sclerotic lesions are rare in primary bone lymphoma compared to secondary lymphomatous involvement of bone. However, a mixed lytic lesion with sclerotic areas can be seen with soft tissue extension in the majority of cases. The presence of a solitary lytic-permeative, metadiaphyseal lesion in a long bone with aggressive periosteal reaction on radiographs and a soft-tissue mass on MR images, especially in an adult patient older than 30 years, is highly suggestive of lymphoma. The presence of soft-tissue mass and marrow changes associated with minimal cortical destruction favors diagnosis of primary bone lymphoma.

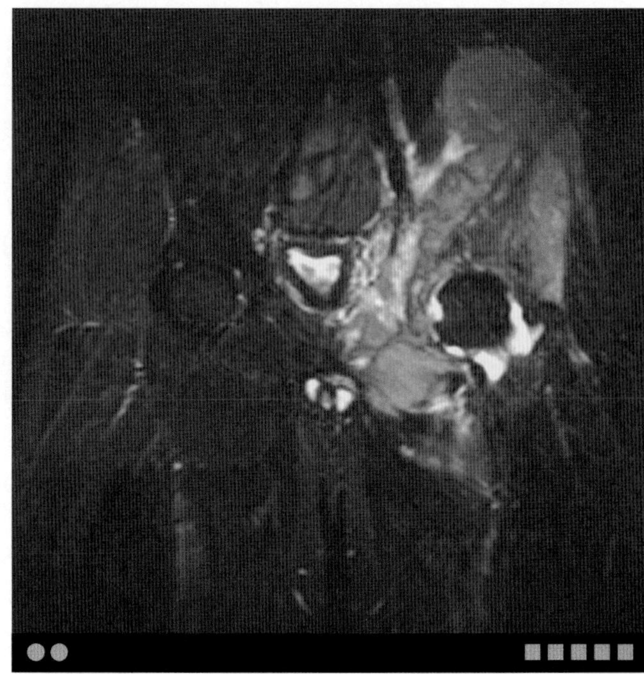

A. Primary osseous lymphoma: Coronal STIR image of the pelvis shows a large marrow infiltrating mass involving left hemipelvis with large soft tissue component.

PEARLS

- **Primary osseous lymphoma is a rare tumor accounting for less than 5% of all primary bone tumors.**
- **Typically seen in adult patients older than 30 years.**
- **Lytic pattern is the most common although mixed lytic–sclerotic lesions may be seen.**
- **On MRI, soft tissue involvement is common.**
- **A search should be made to rule out systemic lymphoma within 6 months of discovery of original osseous lymphoma lesion.**

ADDITIONAL IMAGES

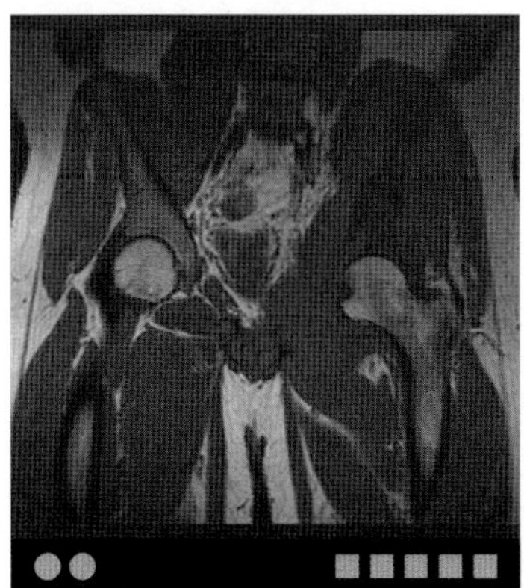

B. Primary osseous lymphoma: T1W coronal image of the same patient showing the extent of the lesion.

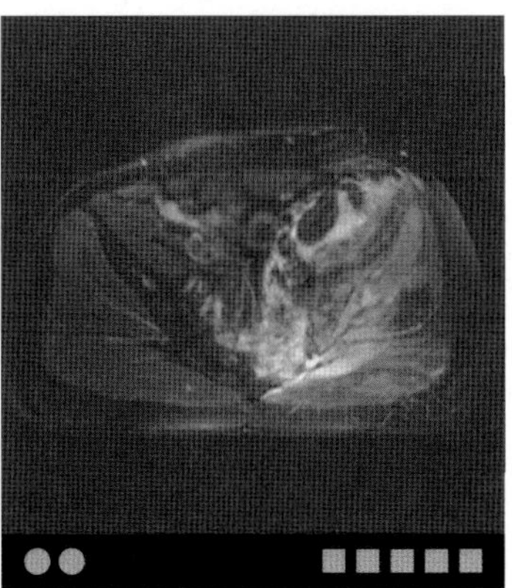

C. Primary osseous lymphoma: T2W axial image with fat suppression shows the invasion of sacral neural foramina and extension into gluteal musculature posteriorly.

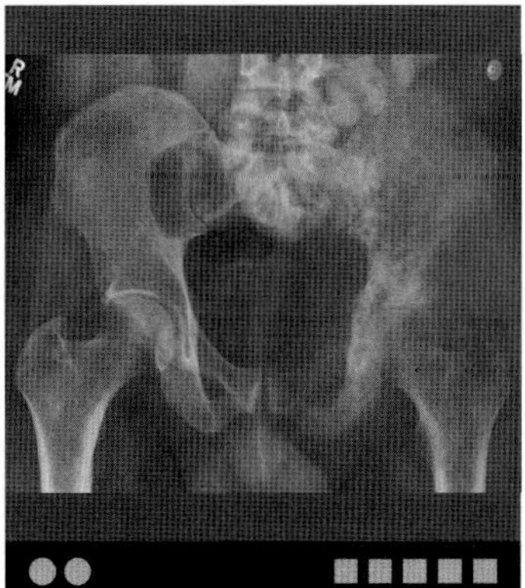

D. Primary osseous lymphoma: Radiograph of the pelvis showing the predominantly sclerotic lesion on the left side.

DIFFERENTIAL DIAGNOSES IMAGES

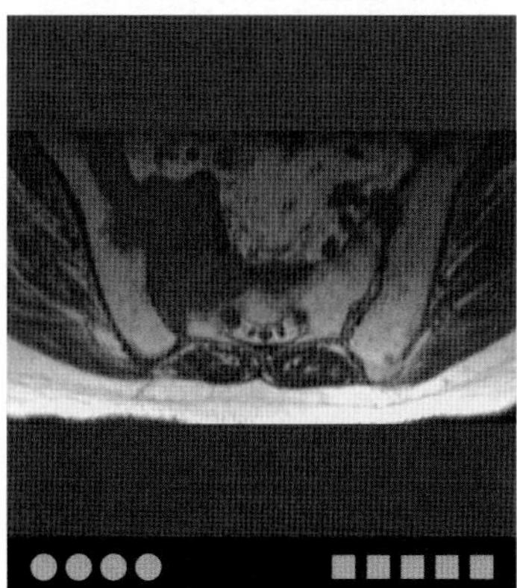

E. Metastasis: This is an 82-year-old male patient with known renal cell carcinoma. T1W axial image of the pelvis shows a large lesion with anterior soft tissue extension in left sacrum and ileum with invasion of sacroiliac join.

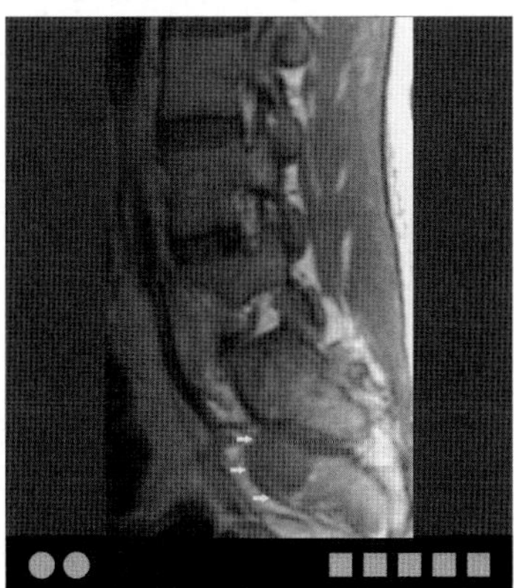

F. Ewing sarcoma: A 17-year-old male patient with Ewing sarcoma. Axial T1W post-gadolinium image shows a large, enhancing sacral mass with presacral soft tissue extension (arrows).

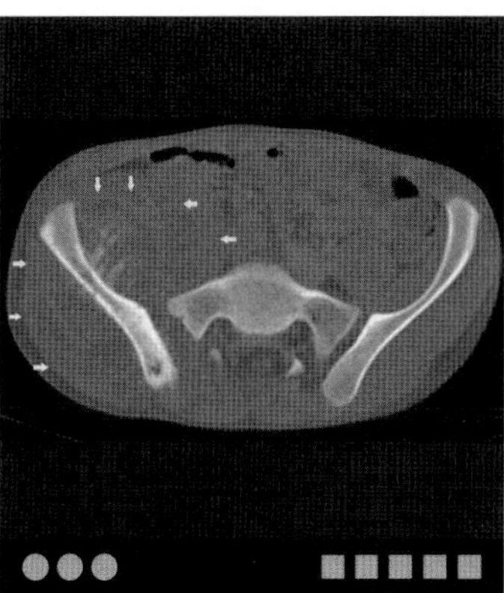

G. Osteosarcoma: This is a 9-year-old male patient with osteosarcoma. Axial pelvic CT image shows a sclerotic lesion involving right ileum extending into sacroiliac joint and large soft tissue component (arrows). Note the aggressive sunburst periostitis.

IMAGE KEY

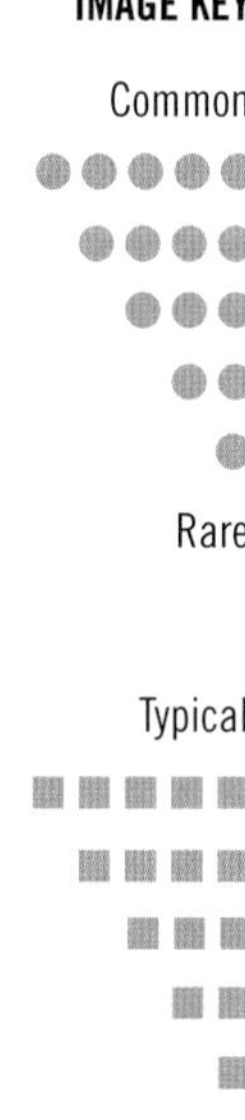

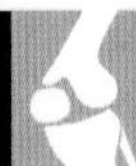

21–28 Bony Metastases of Femoral Neck

Michael A. Bruno

PRESENTATION

Localized bone pain

FINDINGS

This case demonstrates the appearance of a metastatic lesion to the proximal femur in multiple imaging modalities; this is a biopsy-proven metastatic carcinoma of the lung (non-small-cell type).

DIFFERENTIAL DIAGNOSES

- *Synovial herniation pit (Pitt's pit):* could have a similar appearance in this location.
- *An intracapsular osteoid osteoma:* A benign bony lesion could also have a similar appearance in this location.
- *Plasmacytoma or multiple myeloma:* Osteolytic or rarely sclerotic plasmacytoma or in case of multiple lesions multiple myeloma may be in differential.

COMMENTS

This is an example of an osteolytic metastatic focus, imaged in multiple modalities, including planar radiographs, CT (with coronal reconstruction), MRI and 18-F-[2-deoxy] Glucose PET. Skeletal metastasis may arise from breast, prostate, lungs, thyroid, kidneys, and gastrointestinal tract. However other processes such as melanoma, Ewing, osteosarcoma, neuroblastoma, etc., may metastasize to skeletal system. Axial skeleton including spine and pelvis are the most common site of metastasis. While renal and thyroid metastases are purely osteolytic, others such as breast and lungs could be lytic or sclerotic or mixed. Prostate metastases are mostly sclerotic but rarely may manifest as mixed lesions. In majority of the cases, bone metastasis is easy to differentiate from primary bone tumors. The key to this distinction is the multiplicity of the lesions, relative absence of large soft tissue mass and lack of significant periosteal reactions in case of skeletal metastasis. The main differential diagnosis radiologically is with multiple myeloma. However clinical and laboratory findings can help to make this distinction. Although radionuclide bone scan is often used to look for skeletal metastasis, whole body MRI, PET scan, or PET CT could be more sensitive. The most common manifestation of multiple myeloma is osteoporosis. Because of the lack of sensitivity of bone scan for small cell tumors, traditionally skeletal survey rather than bone scan was used to screen for bony metastasis in myelomas. However, the whole body MRI is more sensitive than radiograph. Rarely prostate and lung metastases to the long bones of the extremities may mimic primary bone tumors such as osteosarcoma with sunburst and laminated periosteal reactions.

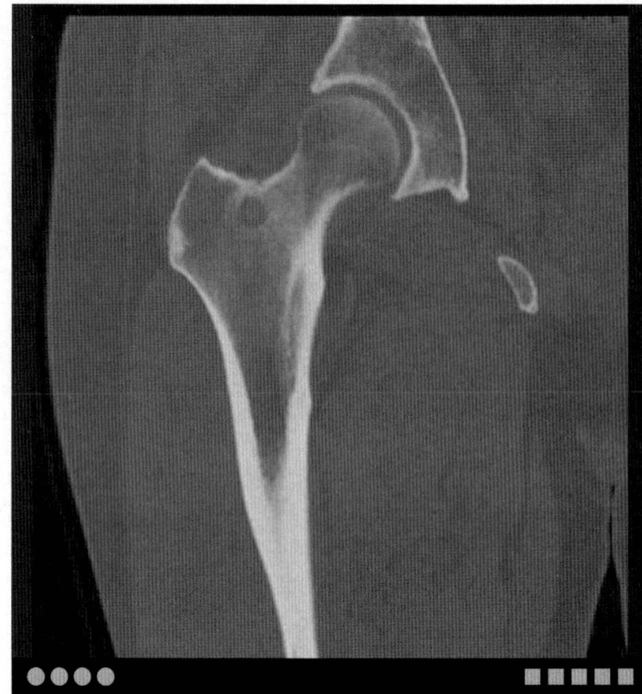

A. Bony metastases: Coronal CT scan shows a rounded, well-circumscribed lucent lesion at the base of the femoral neck, with some surrounding sclerosis. This lesion may mimic osteoid osteoma on CT.

PEARLS

- **A known antecedent primary makes multiple myeloma unlikely.**
- **In osteoid osteoma, a central nidus can be identified with CT and/or MRI; no nidus is seen in this case. Instead, MRI shows a large region of marrow edema.**
- **Osteoblastic metastases are often more readily detected on PET than on bone scan.**

ADDITIONAL IMAGES

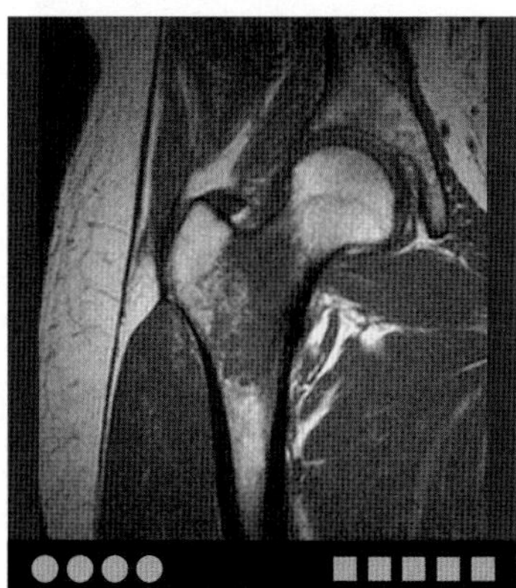

B. Bony metastases: Coronal MRI, T1W image showing extensive marrow edema (low signal) surrounding the known location of the lesion seen in image A.

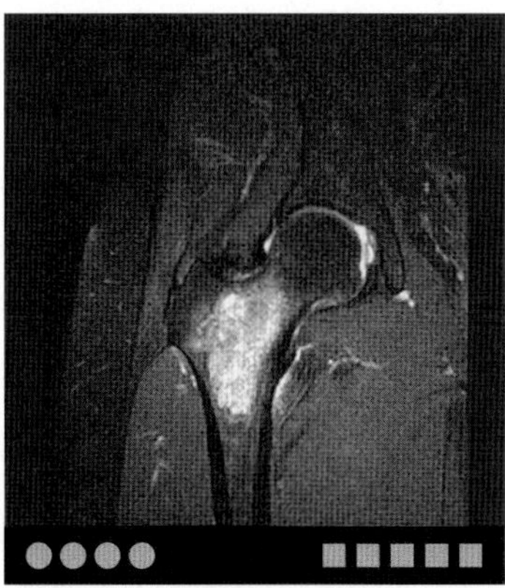

C. Bony metastases: Coronal MRI fat saturated T2W image, again showing extensive marrow edema surrounding the known location of the lesion. As in image B, the margins of the lesion are not well delineated.

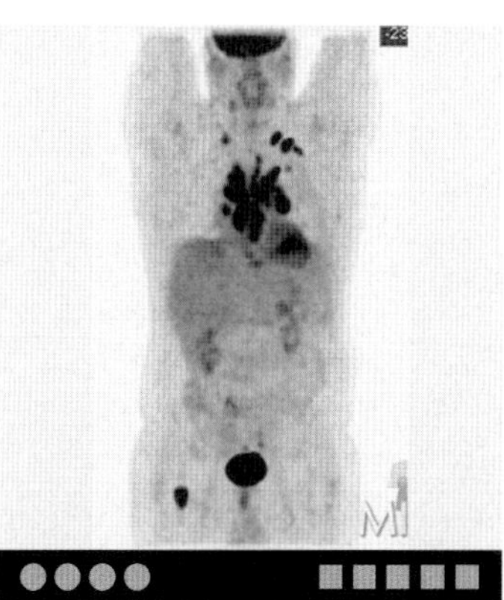

D. Bony metastases: Coronal 18FDG PET scan shows intense uptake in the lesion.

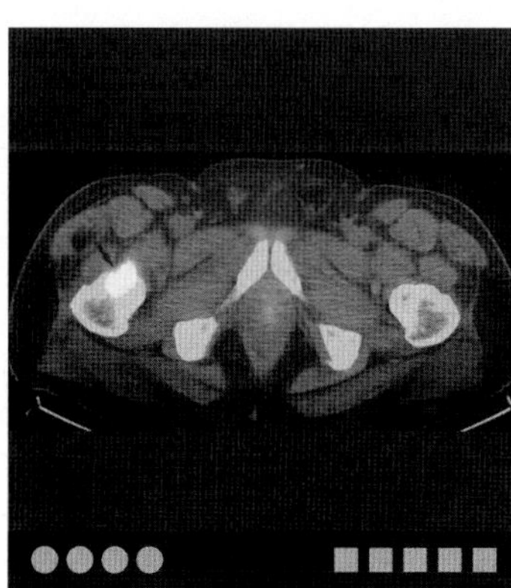

E. Bony metastases: Combined PET/CT Scan confirms location of intense FDG uptake to the base of the right femur (arrow).

DIFFERENTIAL DIAGNOSES IMAGES

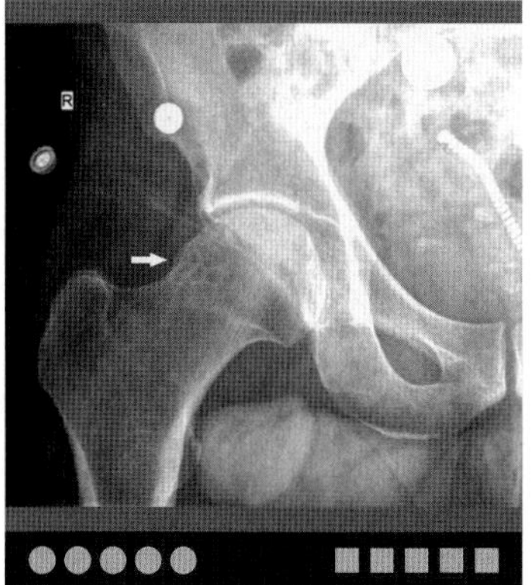

F. Synovial herniation pit (Pitt's pit) x-ray: The principal differential diagnosis, a benign synovial herniation pit, or "Pitt's pitt," as seen in this case, has a very similar appearance.

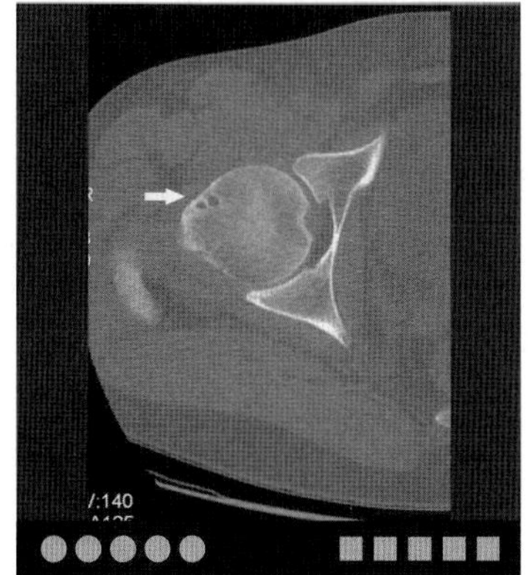

G. Synovial herniation pit (Pitt's pit) CT: CT scan (same patient as in image F). Note the similarity of appearance in this benign lesion to image A.

IMAGE KEY

Common

Rare

Typical

Unusual

Chapter 22

Miscellaneous

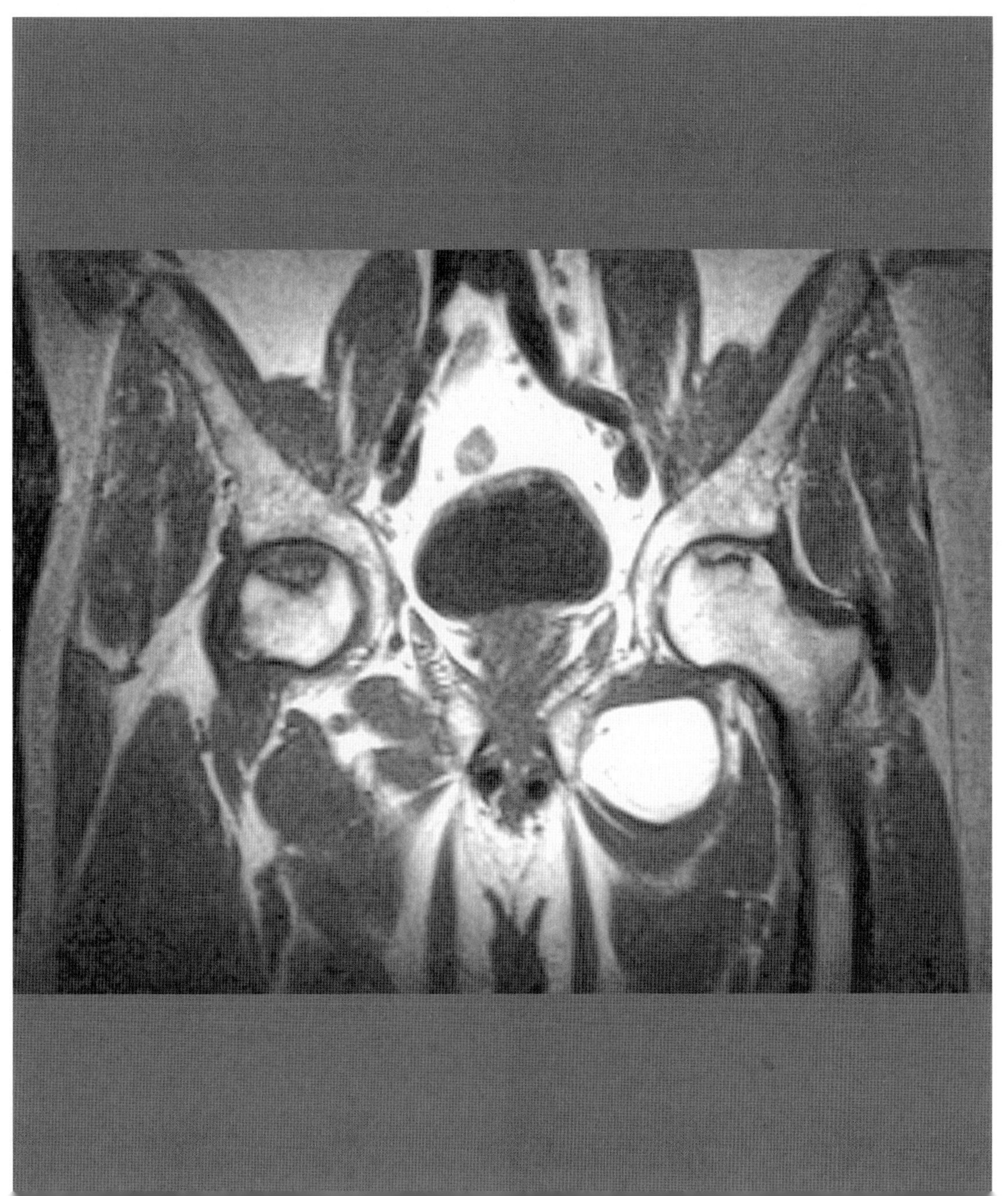

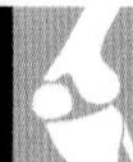

22–1 Avascular Necrosis of Femoral Head

Shahla Modarresi and Daria Motamedi

PRESENTATION

Progressive bilateral hip joint pain

FINDINGS

MR imaging shows a focus of low signal in the right femoral head surrounded by a serpiginous, peripheral, and a dark band of sclerosis. Early changes of avascular necrosis (AVN) of the left hip are also noted.

DIFFERENTIAL DIAGNOSES

- *Idiopathic transient osteoporosis of the hip:* MR imaging shows marrow edema with decreased T1 and increased T2 signal extending from femoral head to intertrochanteric region without subchondral low signal line. Similar MR appearance may noted in early AVN.
- *Fracture:* Stress or insufficiency fractures occur in femoral neck and subcapital region. MR shows low signal fracture line with surrounding low signal edema on T1-weighted and high signal in T2-weighted images.
- *Osteoarthritis of the hip joint:* MR shows severe joint space narrowing with cartilage loss, osteophytes, subchondral cysts and subarticular edema of both sides of the joint, the acetabulum, and femoral head.
- *Infection, septic joint:* MR shows monoarticular joint effusion, synovitis showing low T1, and high T2 signal with postcontrast synovial enhancement. Diffused, adjacent soft tissue and marrow edema from hyperemia or infection are noted.

COMMENTS

AVN is a common cause of musculoskeletal dysfunction creating both diagnostic and therapeutic challenge. AVN usually progresses to joint destruction requiring total hip replacement in younger individuals. Early detection and joint preservation have significant role in delaying the progression of the disease. AVN represents an inability to supply adequate oxygen to underlying bone characterized by areas of dead bone extending to the subchondral plate. The weight bearing anterolateral aspect of the femoral head is typically involved. Nontraumatic AVN is commonly bilateral occurring in a younger population. Common causes include exogenous steroids, trauma, and alcoholism. Less common causes are caisson disease, pancreatic disease, hemoglobinopathy, renal transplant, and HIV/AIDS to mention a few. A staging system using radiographic findings has been developed by Ficat and Arlet, used widely for treating AVN. This has been supplanted by the classification system of Steinberg et al, which incorporates MRI and scintigraphy findings. High magnetic field (1.5 or 3 tesla), MRI is the most sensitive imaging modality diagnosing AVN at its earliest stage. SPECT is an alternative when MRI cannot be performed or contraindicated. The coronal plane is the most important imaging plane for evaluating AVN. Coronal T1-weighted image shows low signal at ischemic area; T2-weighted and fat-suppressed sequence are obtained showing the double line sign, which is pathognomonic for AVN. STIR images may be obtained using FSE techniques to reduce imaging time.

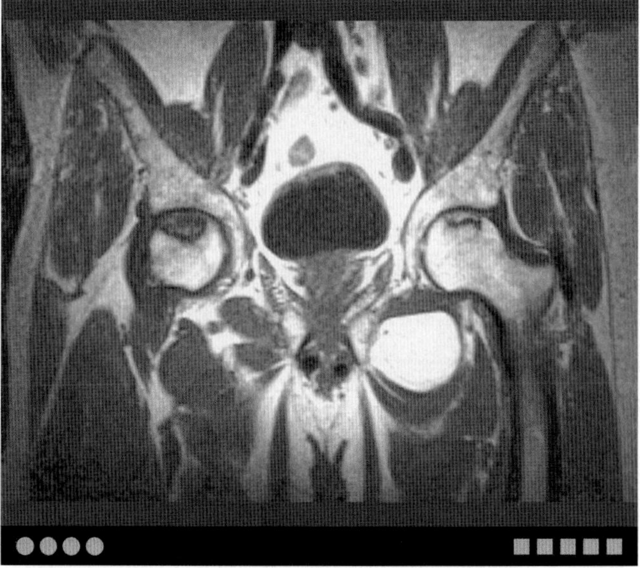

A. AVN: Coronal T1-weighted image shows a focus of low signal with peripheral, dark band of sclerosis on the right. Early changes of AVN of the left hip are also noted. Note large lipoma in left adductor muscles.

PEARLS

- **Hip AVN is a common cause of disability resulting from inadequate oxygen supply to femoral head characterized by areas of dead bone extending to the subchondral plate.**
- **Common causes include exogenous steroids, trauma, and alcoholism. Nontraumatic AVN is commonly bilateral and occurs in a younger population.**
- **High magnetic field (1.5 tesla), MRI is the most sensitive of all imaging modalities to diagnose AVN at its earliest stage.**
- **Coronal T1-weighted image shows low signal at ischemic area; T2-weighted and fat-suppressed sequence are obtained showing the double line sign, which is pathognomonic for AVN.**

ADDITIONAL IMAGES

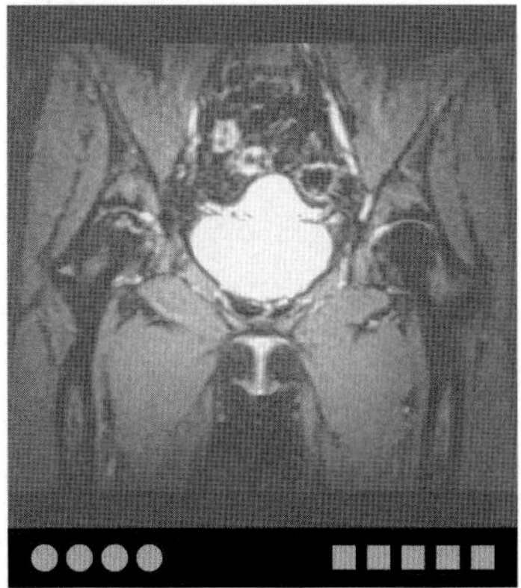

B. AVN: Coronal STIR image shows early AVN of the right femoral head with double line sign.

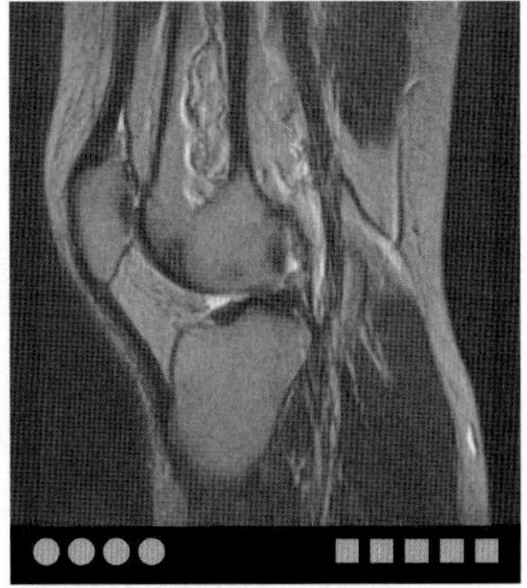

C. Medullary infarct of femoral shaft: Sagittal T2-weighted image the knee shows serpiginous double line sign of distal femoral shaft infarct/avascular necrosis.

DIFFERENTIAL DIAGNOSES IMAGES

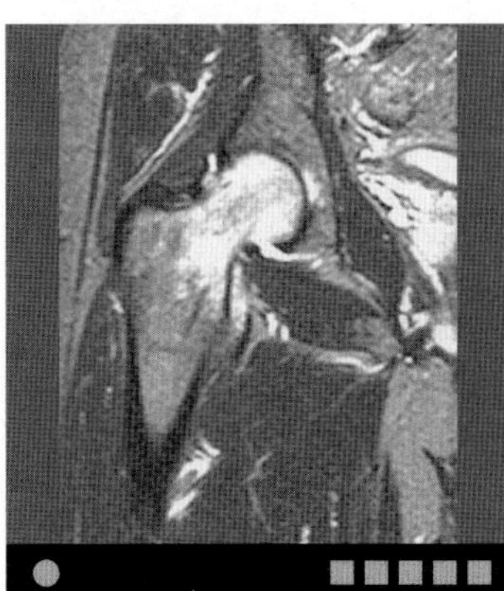

D. Idiopathic transient osteoporosis: Coronal STIR image of the hip shows bright signal in head/neck of the femur.

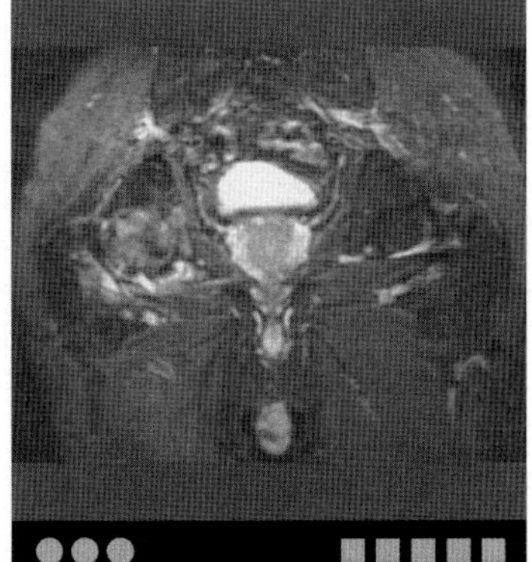

E. Insufficiency fracture: Coronal STIR image shows right, femoral subcapital insufficiency fracture with femoral head and neck marrow edema.

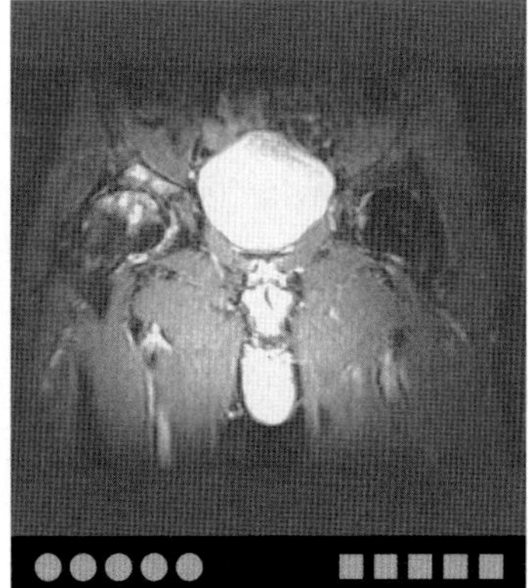

F. Osteoarthritis: Coronal STIR image shows severe osteoarthritis with joint space narrowing, subarticular marrow edema, and subchondral cysts of the acetabulum and femoral head.

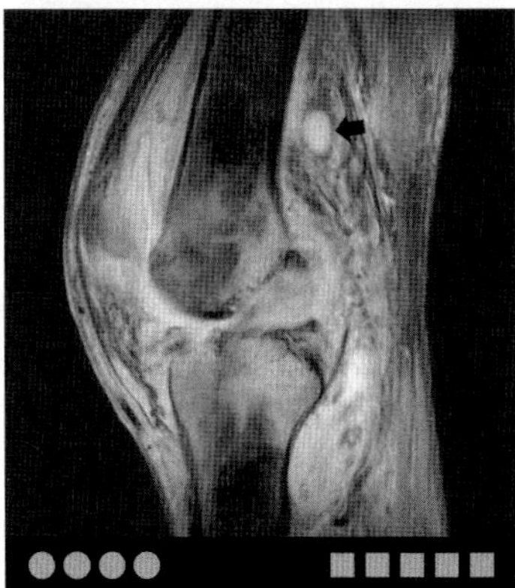

G. Osteomyelitis and septic arthritis: Sagittal STIR image of the knee shows osteomyelitis of distal femur and proximal tibia with joint effusion, diffuse soft tissue and synovial swelling, and marrow edema. Note lymph node enlargement (arrow).

IMAGE KEY

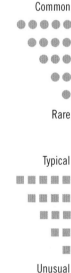

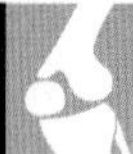

22–2 Radiation Necrosis of Pelvis

Ashkan Afshin and Jamshid Tehranzadeh

PRESENTATION

Pelvic Pain

FINDINGS

There are sclerotic changes of pelvic bone at sacrum and bilateral, iliac bone corresponding to the radiation port.

DIFFERENTIAL DIAGNOSES

- *Paget disease:* This condition presents as enlargement of the bone with cortical thickening and coarsening of the bony trabeculae.
- *Primary osseous lymphoma:* Conventional radiographs show the presence of a solitary, permeative, and metadiaphyseal lesion with a layered, periosteal reaction.
- *Osteosarcoma:* Conventional radiographs show mixed, sclerotic, and lytic lesion of the bone. Periosteal reaction may take the sunburst or onion peel appearance, and soft tissue mass shows new bone formation.
- *Fibrous dysplasia:* It is a noninherited, developmental bone disease in which normal bone marrow is replaced by fibro-osseous tissue presenting with ground glass matrix.
- *Ewings sarcoma:* Radiographs show permeative diaphyseal tumor with mottled or patchy density. Cortical involvement may produce periosteal reaction (onion skin pattern).

COMMENTS

The patient is a 71-year-old woman who presented with the cancer of cervix and radiation therapy. Generally, bones receive radiotherapy either for treatment of a painful metastatic bone lesion or for treatment of an adjacent soft tissue neoplasm. The effect of the radiation on bone depends on various factors including the dosage, quality of the x-ray beam, age of the patient, method of fractionation, duration of therapy, existence of trauma, or infection at the site. The radiation of a bone may have different effects, the most important of which are disruption of normal growth and maturation, scoliosis, osteonecrosis, and neoplasm formation. Radiation-induced sarcomas as a rare complication of the bone radiation have been shown to develop approximately 10 years after therapy. Osteonecrosis occurs in a mature skeleton and is dose-dependant. Radiation osteitis is usually observed at the lower dosage of radiation, and osteoradionecrosis is associated with higher dosage radiation. Radiation osteitis includes potentially reversible changes such as temporary cessation of growth, periostitis, bone sclerosis and increased fragility, ischemic necrosis, and infection. Radiographs will show bone, which is mottled demonstrating both osteopenia and sclerosis and areas of coarse trabeculation. The changes are observed at different time intervals depending on which bone is irradiated. Pelvis radiation can cause pelvic bone osteonecrosis, which is a rare but disabling complication. Avascular necrosis of the femoral head can be seen. In 2% of patients, fractures of the femoral head may occur. The SI joints may also be affected showing bilateral, symmetric sclerosis.

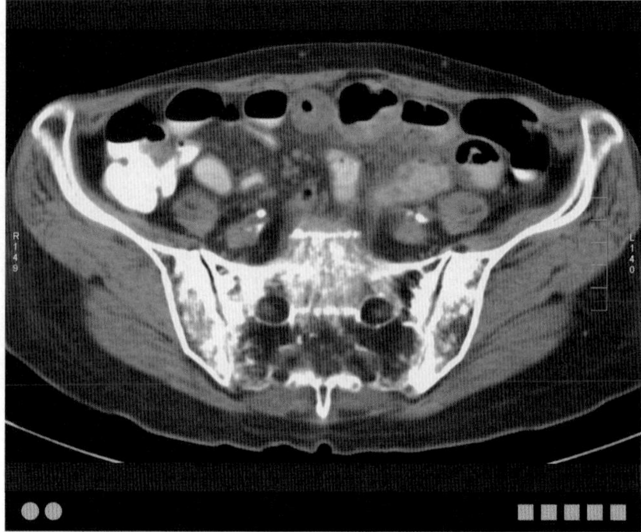

A. Radiation osteonecrosis of the pelvic bone: Axial CT scan of the pelvis shows mottled, sclerotic appearance of the sacrum and bilateral, and iliac bones.

PEARLS

- **The radiation of a bone have different effects the most important of which are disruption of normal growth and maturation, scoliosis, osteonecrosis, and neoplasm formation.**
- **Osteonecrosis occurs in a mature skeleton and is dose-dependant.**
- **Radiation osteitis is usually seen at the lower dosage of radiation, and osteoradionecrosis is associated with higher dosage radiation.**
- **Radiation osteitis includes potentially reversible changes such as temporary cessation of growth, periostitis, bone sclerosis and increased fragility, ischemic necrosis, and infection.**
- **Radiographs show bone which is mottled demonstrating both osteopenia and sclerosis and areas of coarse trabeculation.**
- **Pelvic bone osteonecrosis is a rare but disabling complication of pelvic radiation.**

ADDITIONAL IMAGE

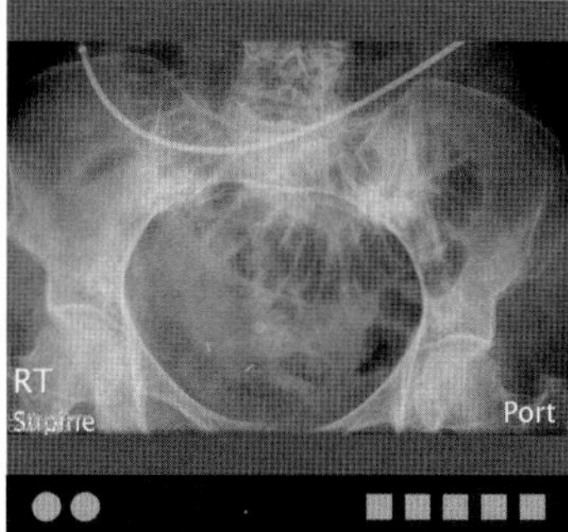

B. Radiation osteonecrosis of the pelvic bone: AP radiograph of the sacrum shows sclerotic changes of the sacrum and bilateral, iliac bones especially around the sacroiliac joints.

DIFFERENTIAL DIAGNOSES IMAGES

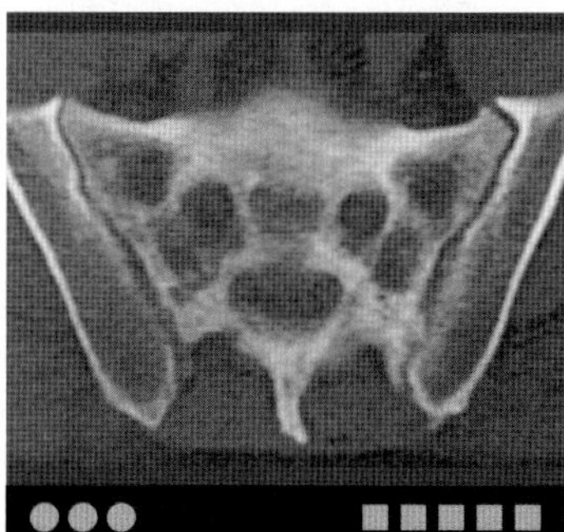

C. Paget disease of sacrum: CT scan through the sacrum at the level of S1 shows cortical thickening and trabecular coarsening, typical for late stage Paget's disease of bone.

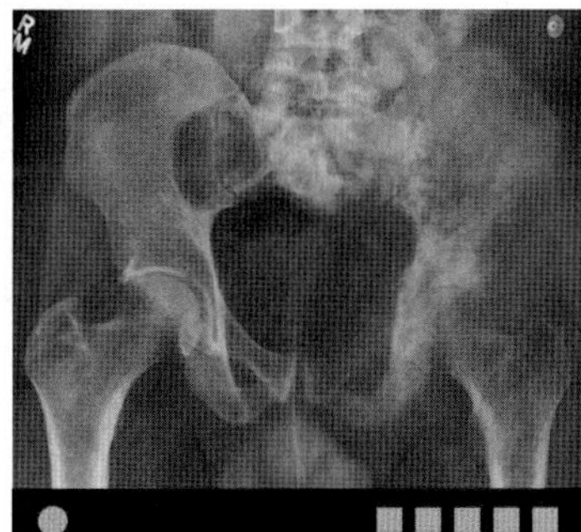

D. Primary osseous lymphoma: Radiograph of the pelvis showing the predominantly sclerotic lesion on the left side.

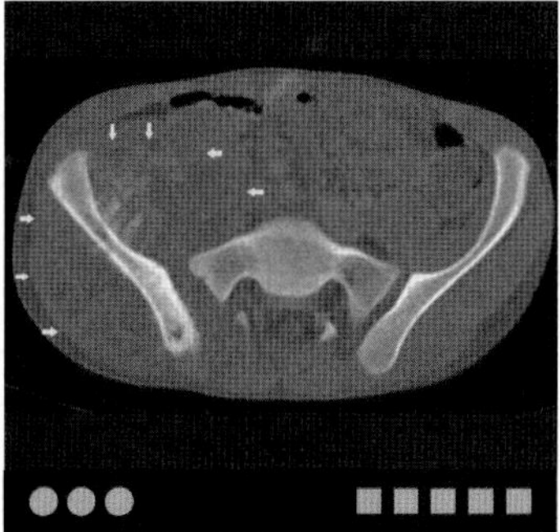

E. Osteosarcoma: This is an image of a 9-year-old boy with osteosarcoma. Axial pelvic CT scan image shows a sclerotic lesion involving right ileum extending into sacroiliac joint and large soft tissue component (arrows). Note the aggressive sunburst periostitis

IMAGE KEY

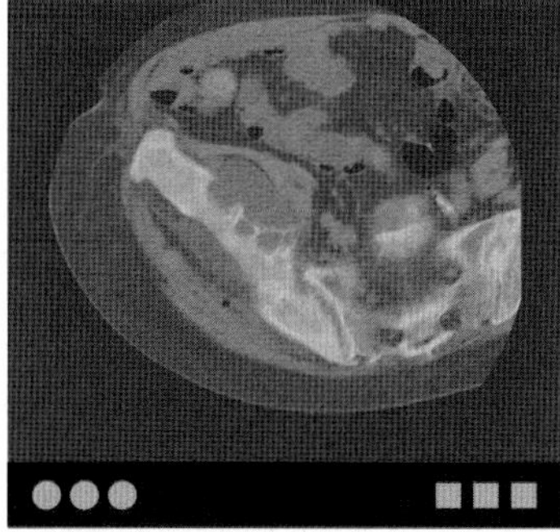

F. Fibrous dysplasia: Noncontrast CT scan of the pelvis during biopsy shows an expansile lesion within the right iliac wing with hazy or ground-glass density. Extraosseous soft tissue component and cortical destruction is suggesting malignant transformation.

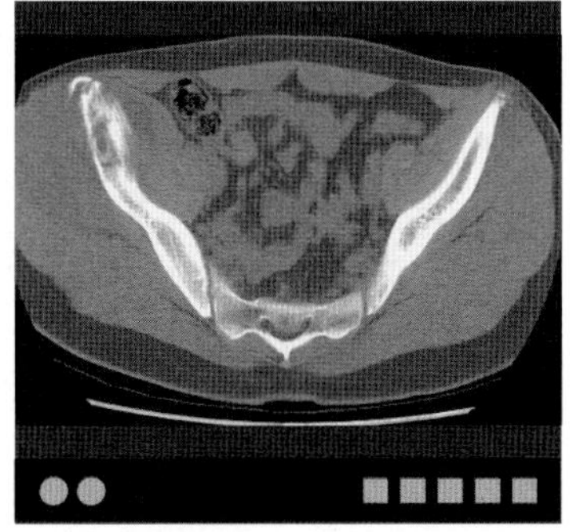

G. Ewings sarcoma: Noncontrast CT scan of the pelvis shows an aggressive, mixed sclerotic and lytic lesion within the anterior right iliac wing, associated with a lamellated (onion skin) periosteal reaction and a large extraosseous soft tissue mass.

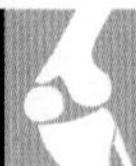

22–3 Transient Osteoporosis of the Hip

Gideon Strich

PRESENTATION

Acute onset of hip pain

FINDINGS

MRI shows unilateral hip joint effusion with diffuse bone marrow edema extending from the femoral head to the intertrochanteric area.

DIFFERENTIAL DIAGNOSES

- *Avascular necrosis:* In addition to bone marrow edema, MRI shows typical subchondral double lines on T2-weighted images, which are often bilateral.
- *Stress fracture:* Typical location is along the medial cortex of the femoral neck, which is usually unilateral.
- *Infectious or inflammatory synovitis:* Predominant finding is joint effusion although there may be reactive edema. Diagnosis is confirmed clinically or by joint aspiration.

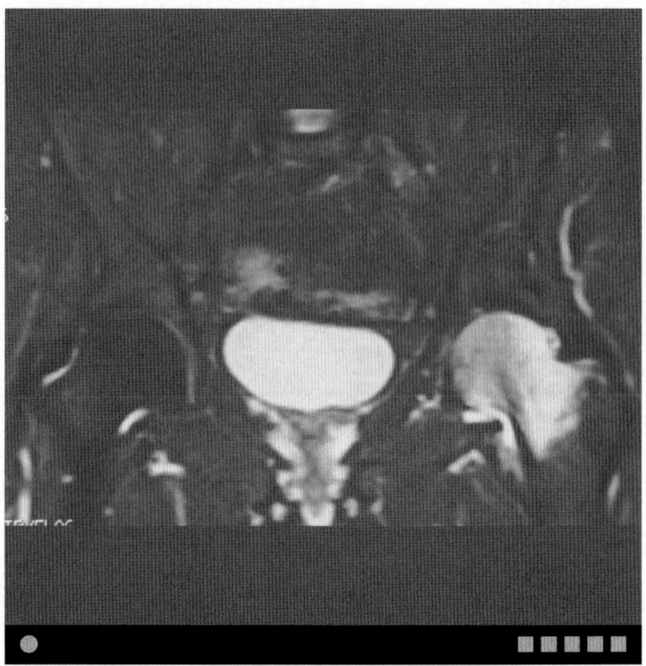

A. Transient osteoporosis of the hip (TOH): Coronal STIR image shows diffuse bone marrow edema involving the entire femoral head and neck with small effusion.

COMMENTS

This is an image of a middle-aged male who presented with a history of acute onset of unilateral hip pain. Transient osteoporosis of the hip (TOH), also known as bone marrow edema of the hip is most common in middle-aged males and also in pregnant women, more commonly in the left hip. Otherwise, there are no specific risk factors for avascular necrosis. Plain x-rays or CT scan may be normal or demonstrate regional osteoporosis involving only the femoral head and neck. MRI is more sensitive, demonstrating characteristic uniform bone marrow edema extending to the level of the trochanters. Triple phase bone scan demonstrates hyperemia as well as diffused uptake in the femoral head and neck, but cannot differentiate early avascular necrosis, insufficiency fracture, or inflammatory synovitis. MRI images should be carefully scrutinized for early signs of typical stress fracture or avascular necrosis. Transient osteoporosis of the hip may be related to regional migratory osteoporosis, a similar entity which then progresses to multiple consecutive large joints usually in the lower extremity. There may also be an association with reflex sympathetic dystrophy syndrome. The clinical course of TOH is self-limiting with resolution of symptoms usually after several months with conservative therapy only. Occasionally patients may progress to avascular necrosis. Follow-up MRI is often recommended.

PEARLS

- **TOH is most common in middle-aged men (either in hip) and in pregnant women (most often in the left hip).**
- **Typical MRI features are unilateral, diffuse bone marrow edema including the entire femoral head and neck with associated joint effusion that resolves after several months with conservative therapy.**
- **Careful observation of T1-weighted and T2-weighted images is essential to rule out treatable lesions, such as AVN or fracture.**
- **TOH may be associated with regional migratory osteoporosis or reflex sympathetic dystrophy syndromes.**

ADDITIONAL IMAGES

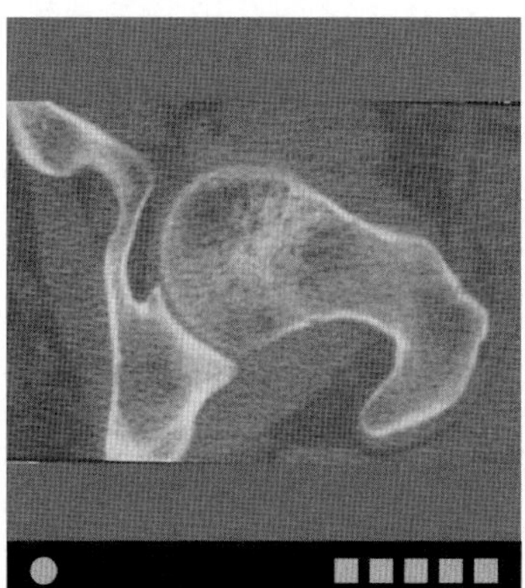

B. TOH: Axial CT scan image demonstrates osteoporosis with accentuation of primary trabecula. No fracture is seen.

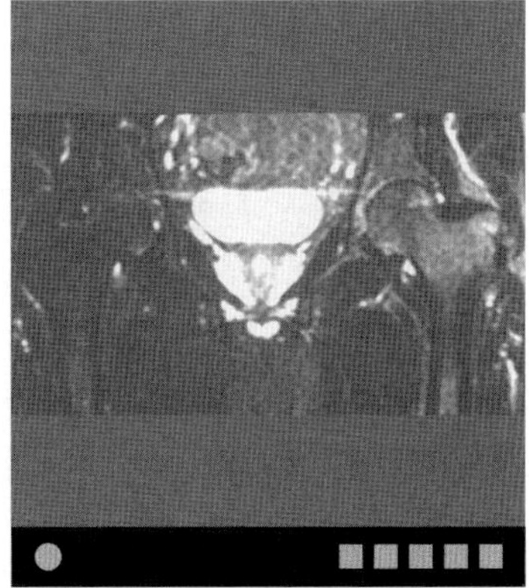

C. TOH: After 6 months, STIR images demonstrate almost complete resolution of bone marrow edema and joint effusion.

DIFFERENTIAL DIAGNOSES IMAGES

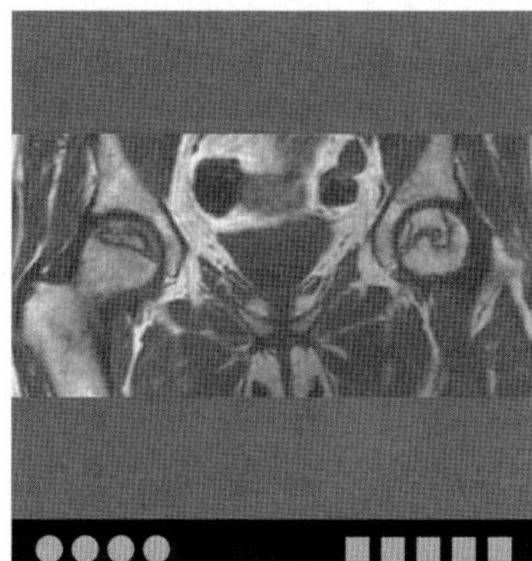

D. Avascular necrosis: Coronal T1-weighted image shows geographic low signal lesions of both femoral heads. Note slight flattening (collapse) of the femoral head on the right side consistent with stage III disease.

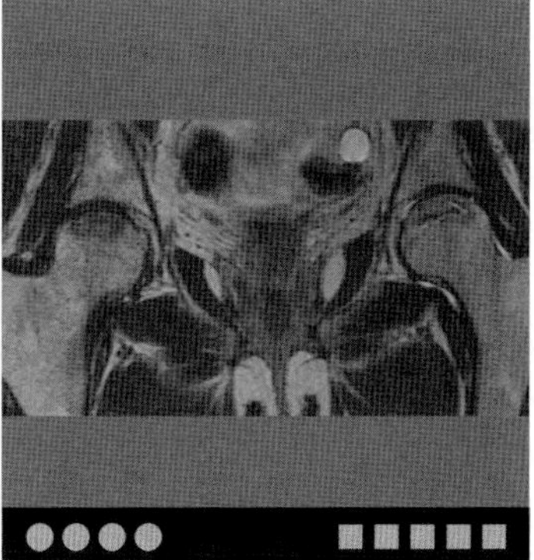

E. Avascular necrosis: Coronal T2-weighted image, showing double line sign on both femoral heads. There is no evidence of cortical collapse or compression on the left side, which is consistent with stage II disease.

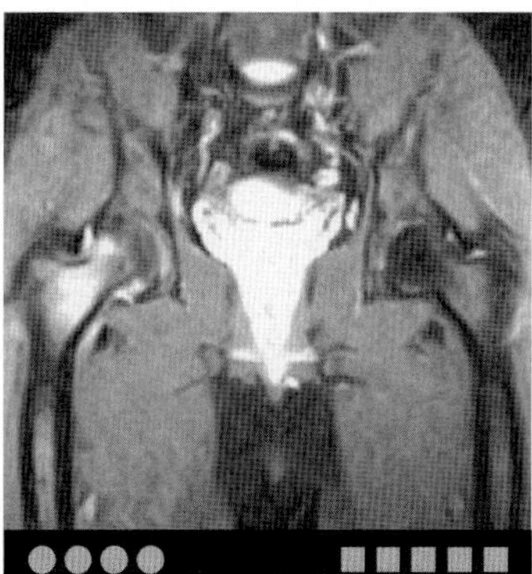

F. Stress fracture: Coronal STIR images demonstrate unilateral bone marrow edema and joint effusion.

IMAGE KEY

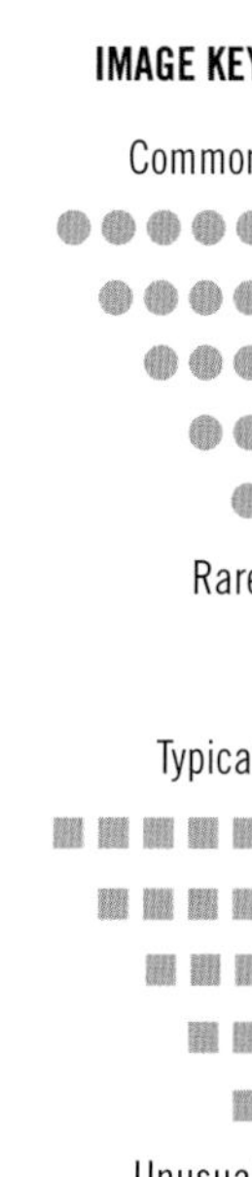

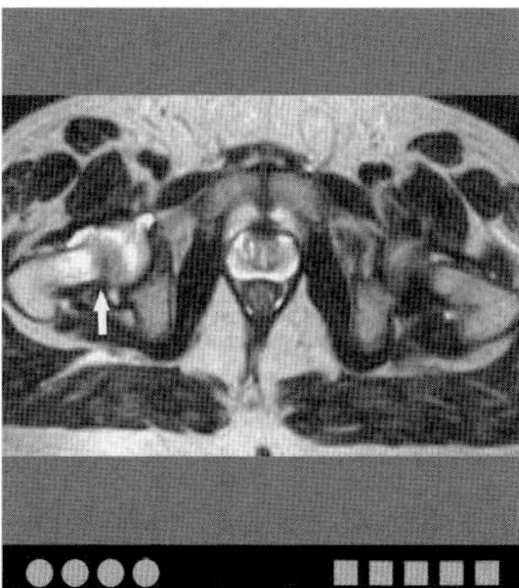

G. Stress fracture: Axial T2-weighted image shows early stress fracture at typical site in medial femoral neck (arrow).

SECTION V

KNEE

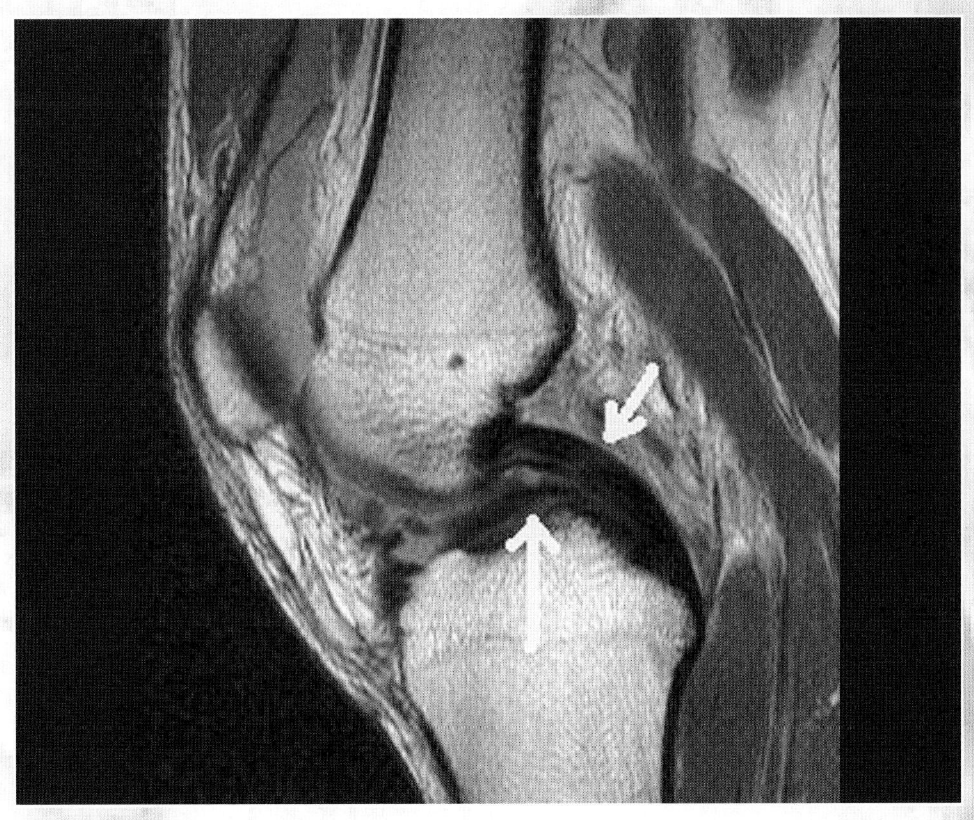

Chapter 23

Sport Medicine and Trauma

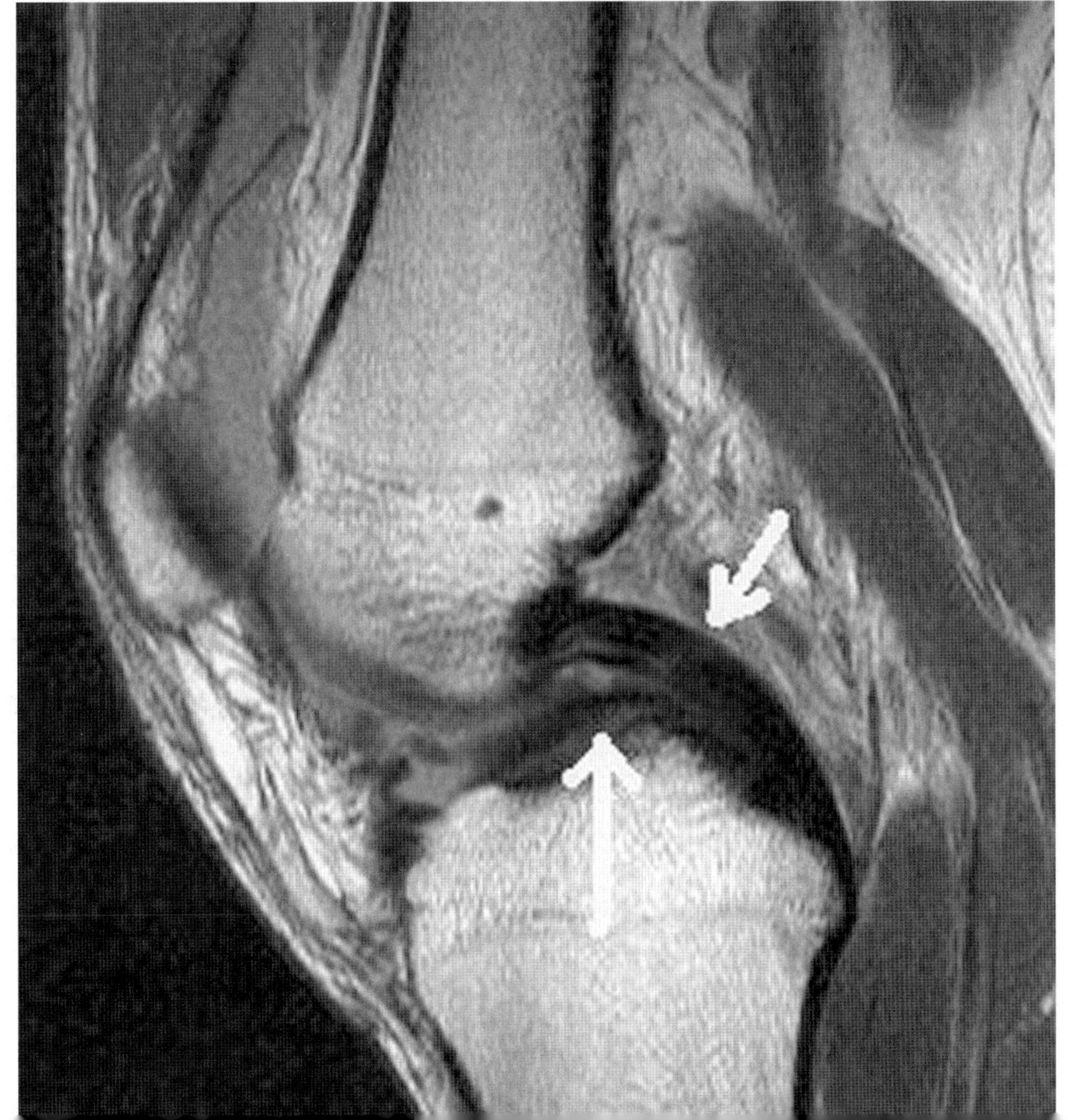

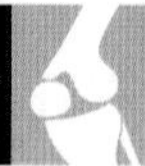

23–1 Bucket Handle Tear of the Meniscus

Arash Tehranzadeh and Sulabha Masih

PRESENTATION

Acute onset of knee pain

FINDINGS

MR images show the "double PCL sign" and "fragment in notch sign" consistent with a bucket handle tear of the medial meniscus.

DIFFERENTIAL DIAGNOSES

- *Transverse (radial tear):* The posterior and midportions of the lateral meniscus are often involved. The orientation of the tear radiates in a linear fashion from the inner margin toward the periphery of the meniscus.
- *Longitudinal tear:* In addition to the bucket handle tear, two other subtypes of longitudinal tears exist and include a horizontal cleavage tear often involving the central horizontal plane and the peripheral tear classically described as a vertical tear in the peripheral third of the meniscus.
- *Oblique tear:* These tears are composed of both vertical and horizontal components and commonly extend to the inferior surface of the meniscus. Perimeniscal cysts may be associated with horizontal tears. The center of these cysts would be at the level of the meniscus.

COMMENTS

The patient is a 24-year-old male with acute onset of knee pain, inability to straighten leg, and swelling, clicking, locking, catching, and a positive McMurray test. The bucket handle tear represents a vertical longitudinal tear of the meniscus (bucket), with displacement of the attached inner fragment (handle). The medial meniscus is commonly involved. It begins as a vertical or an oblique posterior horn tear, and propagates anteriorly and longitudinally. On physical examination a positive McMurray's test may be elicited. About 10% of meniscal tears are of a bucket handle configuration. Normal sagittal imaging of the meniscus demonstrates a bow-tie configuration of the meniscus on at least two contiguous sagittal images. If less than two bow ties are visualized at the periphery of the meniscus, then a meniscal tear should be suspected. The fragment in notch sign (coronal view) represents the displaced fragment and is seen as a band of low signal intensity in the intercondylar notch. On the sagittal plane, the double PCL sign is seen as a band of low signal intensity located between the PCL and tibial plateau and is parallel to the PCL. The peripheral remnant of the meniscus will often appear truncated. A much less common presentation is the double ACL sign where a band of low signal intensity is seen in the intercondylar notch and parallel to the ACL. However, this tear is commonly seen with lateral bucket handle meniscal tears. Another variant of the bucket handle tear involves the displacement of the torn meniscus (handle) from posterior to anterior and is called the "flipped meniscus sign."

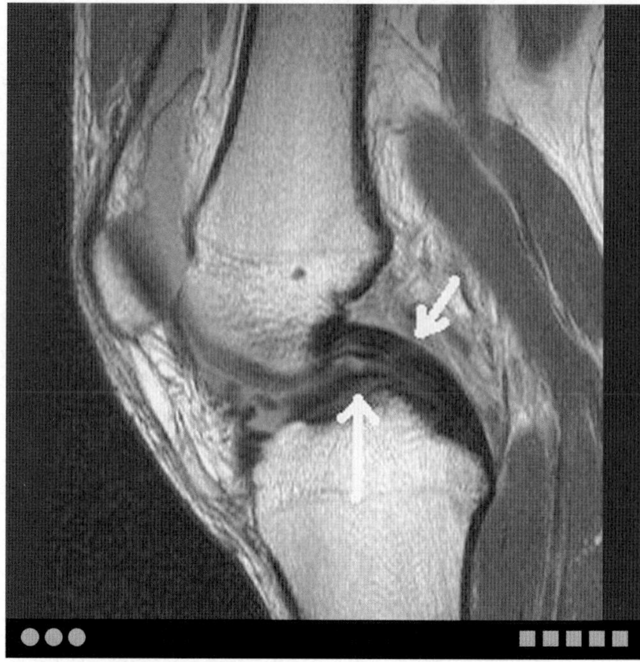

A. Bucket handle tear: Sagittal proton density turbo spin echo image identifies the normal PCL and a second arrow pointing to the double PCL sign of the bucket handle torn meniscus.

PEARLS

- **Bucket handle tear is a traumatic longitudinal vertical tear involving the medial meniscus and rarely is found in the lateral meniscus. The unstable inner fragment is displaced toward the notch.**
- **MRI shows an abnormal or blunted medial meniscus with a displaced meniscus presenting as a fragment in notch sign best appreciated on coronal views and a double PCL sign on sagittal views.**
- **Flipped meniscus sign is another manifestation of bucket handle tears.**
- **The "absent bow-tie sign" and double ACL sign have been described with bucket handle tears.**

ADDITIONAL IMAGES

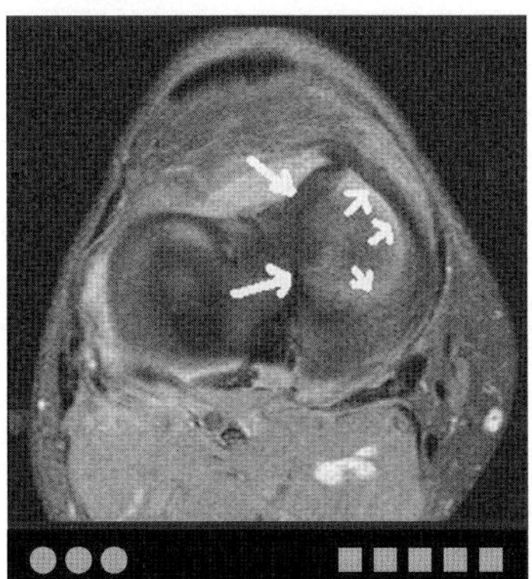

B. Bucket handle tear: Axial turbo spin echo fat-saturated image shows the bucket handle tear. The large arrows show the handle of the bucket flipped into the intercondylar notch. The small arrows mark the peripheral remnant of the torn meniscus.

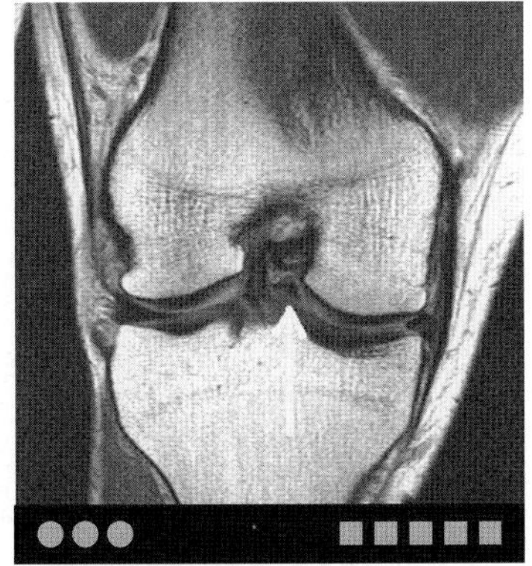

C. Bucket handle tear: Coronal proton density turbo spin echo. The arrow shows the fragment in the intercondylar notch.

DIFFERENTIAL DIAGNOSES IMAGES

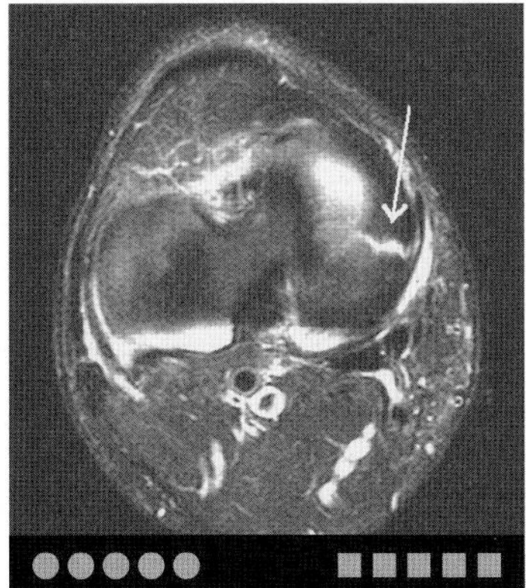

D. Radial tear: Axial turbo spin echo fat-saturated image shows radial tear of the medial meniscus marked by the white arrow.

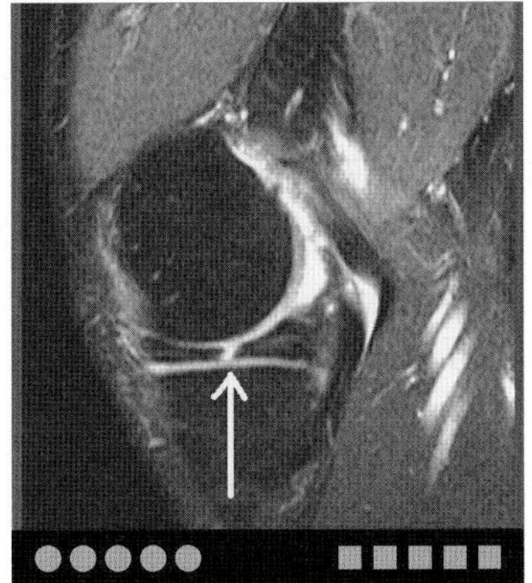

E. Radial tear: Sagittal turbo pin echo fat-saturated image demonstrates a radial tear.

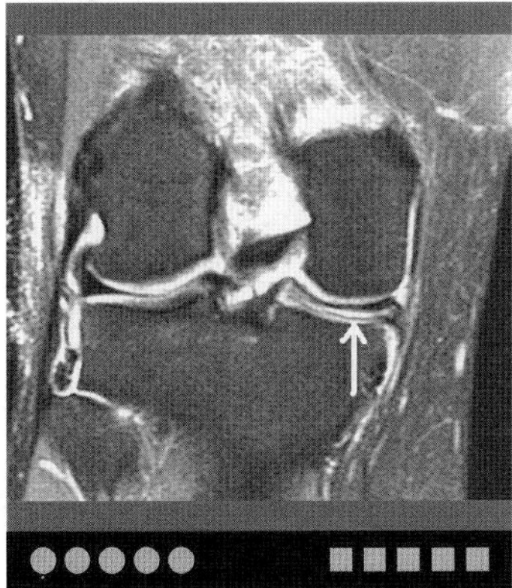

F. Horizontal tear: Coronal proton density fat-saturated image documents a horizontal tear of the medial meniscus.

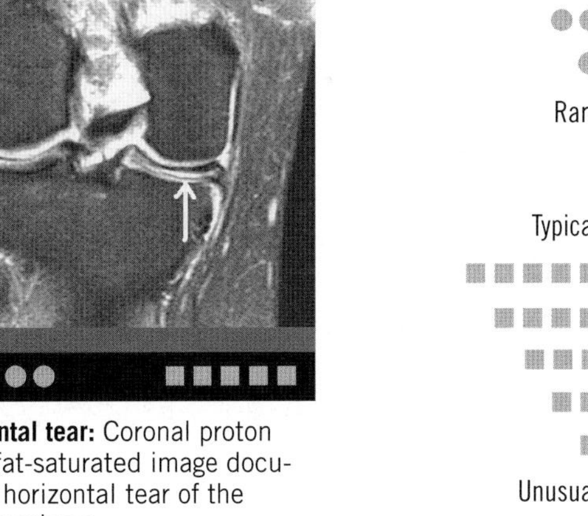

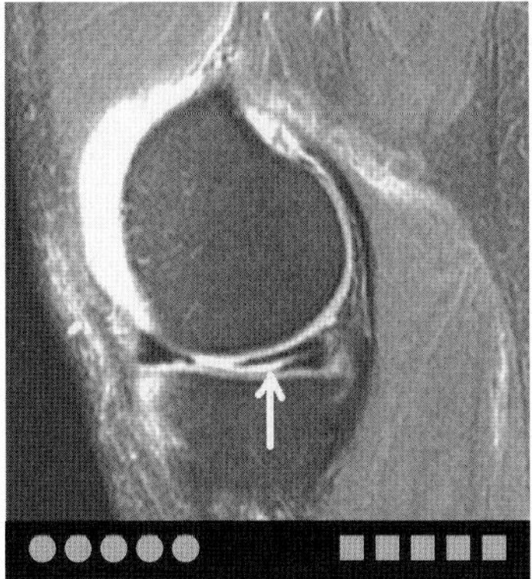

G. Oblique tear: Sagittal proton density fat-saturated image demonstrating an oblique tear violating the inferior articular surface.

IMAGE KEY

Common

Rare

Typical

Unusual

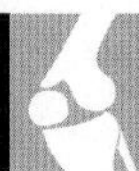

23–2 Medial Meniscus Tear in a Postoperative Patient

Joshua Farber

PRESENTATION

Knee pain after a fall and a remote history of knee surgery

FINDINGS

Multidetector computed tomography (MDCT) reformatted image (MPR) of the right knee after arthrography demonstrates contrast extending into the posterior horn of the medial meniscus. There is metal about the knee from prior surgery.

DIFFERENTIAL DIAGNOSES

- *Fracture:* The cortical margins are intact and there is no depression.
- *Ligament tear:* All ligaments, including the ACL, are intact on this exam.
- *Fixation screw loosening:* The fixation screws from prior surgery are intact with good boney purchase.
- *Osteoarthritis:* Osteoarthritis may be expected in a 69-year-old male, but osteophytes, sclerosis, and joint space narrowing are not seen on this exam.

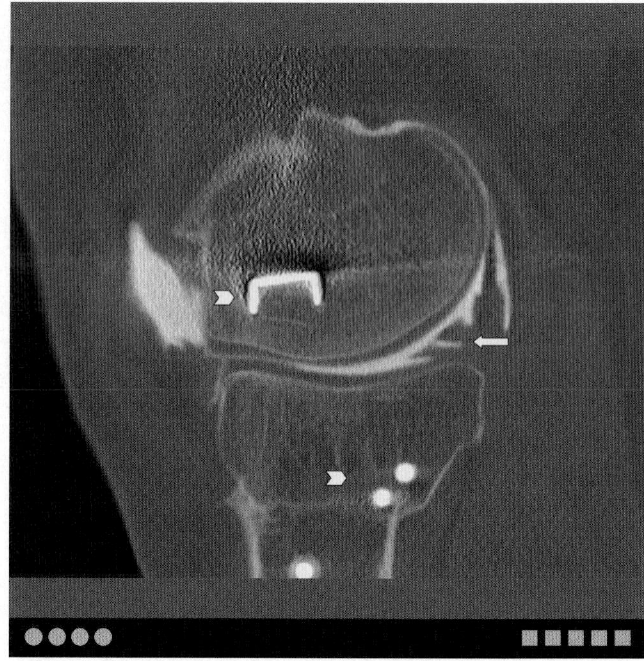

A. Tear of the posterior horn of the medial meniscus: Sagittal MPR of the right knee from an MDCT arthrogram demonstrates a tear of the posterior horn of the medial meniscus (arrow). Metal is present from prior surgery (arrow heads). Image courtesy of the Department of Radiology, Indiana University School of Medicine.

COMMENTS

The patient is a 69-year-old male with knee pain after a fall and a remote history of knee surgery. In the case presented here, this male patient had pain despite negative radiographs. Because of the fixation screws from prior surgery, MDCT arthrography was chosen to evaluate for internal derangement and occult fracture and to assess the integrity of the orthopedic screws. Axial slices of 2 mm were obtained at 1-mm intervals. The pitch was less then 1, and the mAs was 300. MPRs were obtained at 2-mm intervals. The thin slices with 50% overlap produce an essentially isotropic data set, which in turn produces robust MPRs in any plane. The low pitch and appropriate mAs allow scanning through the fixation screws without significant degradation from metallic artifact. The arthrogram was performed with full strength contrast from a retro-patellar approach under fluoroscopic control. In this case, the medial meniscus tear is seen easily as contrast extending into the meniscus from the arthrogram injection. In addition, this patient has a fissure in the articular cartilage of the lateral tibial plateau. Note that the ACL is outlined by contrast and is intact. On all the images, the fixation screws are seen nicely, and their integrity and good bony purchase is confirmed. MDCT arthrography is an excellent modality to evaluate the knee in postoperative patients who have metal in the joint that may degrade MR images and make accurate diagnosis impossible. MDCT arthrography of the knee is useful also in patients who have a contraindication to MRI.

PEARLS

- **Pain in the elderly trauma patient may be caused by various etiologies, including chronic conditions**
- **MDCT arthrography can assess the bones and evaluate for internal derangement**
- **MDCT arthrography is an excellent technique to use in patients who have a contraindication to MRI or who have a significant amount of metal in or about the knee**
- **With proper scanning technique, high-resolution MPRs may be produced and no significant metallic artifact is present.**

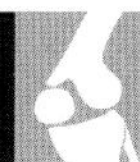

ADDITIONAL IMAGE

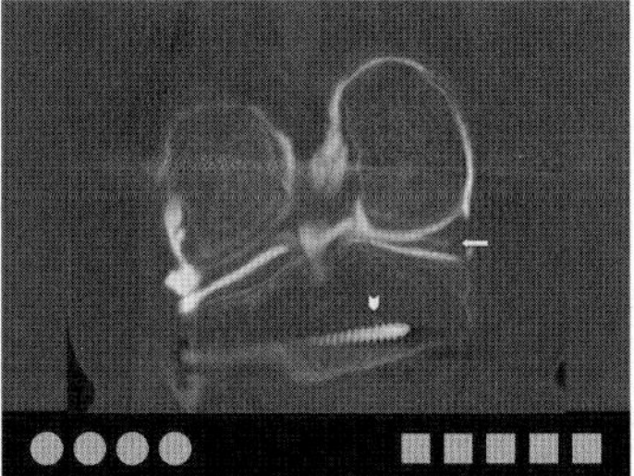

B. Tear of the posterior horn of the medial meniscus: Coronal MPR of the right knee after MDCT arthrography confirms the tear of the posterior horn of the medial meniscus (arrow). Note the lack of significant metallic artifact. Image courtesy of the Department of Radiology, Indiana University School of Medicine.

DIFFERENTIAL DIAGNOSES IMAGES

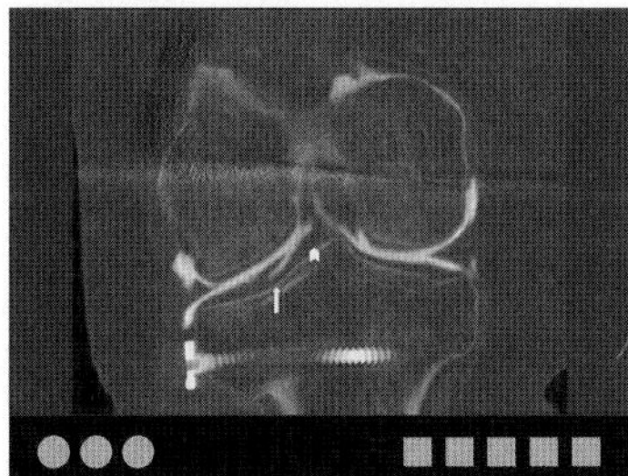

C. Fissure in the articular cartilage: Coronal MPR of the right knee after MDCT arthrography demonstrates a fissure in the articular cartilage of the lateral tibial plateau (arrow). The ACL is visualized on this image and is intact (arrow head). Image courtesy of the Department of Radiology, Indiana University School of Medicine.

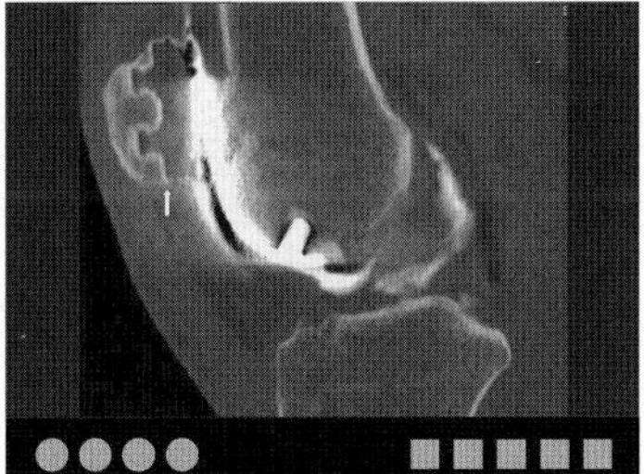

D. Status-post patellar-femoral joint resurfacing: Sagittal MPR image through the right knee after MDCT arthrography in a patient who is status-post patellar-femoral joint resurfacing and presents with pain. Despite the large orthopedic hardware metallic artifact is not significant. Image courtesy of the Department of Radiology, Indiana University School of Medicine.

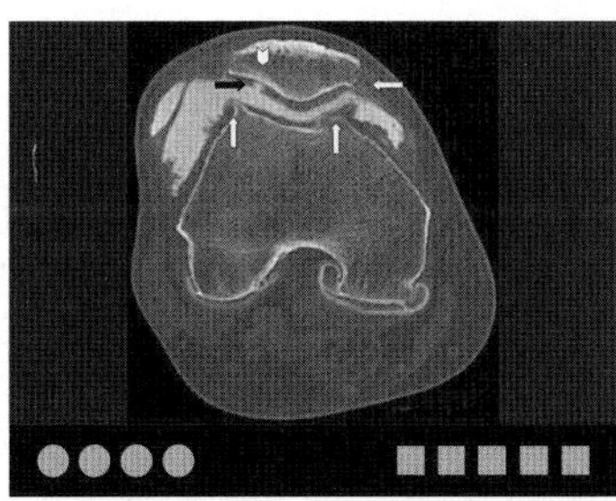

E. Osteoarthritis and a medial meniscus tear: This image is of a 75-year-old female after a fall. Axial source image from an MDCT arthrogram of the right knee shows osteophyte formation (white arrows) and sclerosis (arrow heads). There is articular cartilage fissuring as well (black arrows). Image courtesy of the Department of Radiology, Indiana University School of Medicine.

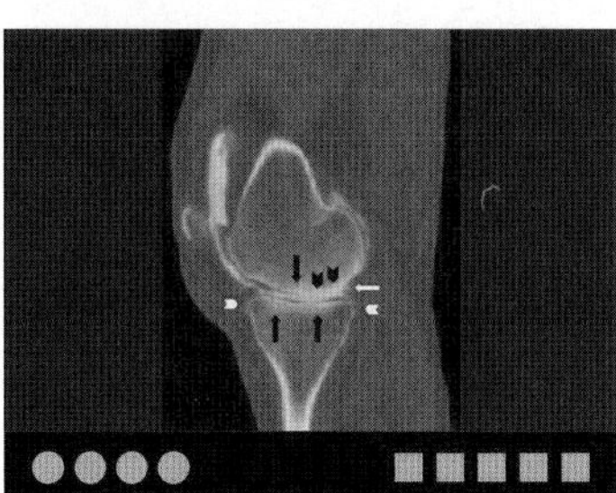

F. Osteoarthritis and a medial meniscus tear: Sagittal MPR from an MDCT arthrogram of the right knee (same patient as in image E) shows a tear of the posterior horn of the medial meniscus (white arrow) and findings of osteoarthritis: Sclerosis (black arrow), osteophytes (white arrow heads), and articular cartilage denudement (black arrow heads). Image courtesy of the Department of Radiology, Indiana University School of Medicine.

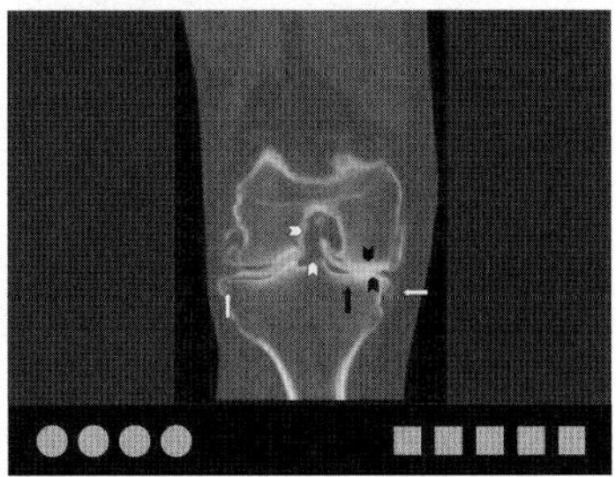

G. Osteoarthritis and a medial meniscus tear: Coronal MPR from an MDCT arthrogram of the right knee (same patient as images E and F) shows severe osteoarthritis of the medial compartment: Osteophyte formation (white arrows), articular cartilage denudement (black arrow heads), and sclerosis (black arrows). Note also that the medial compartment is narrowed and that less severe degenerative changes are seen in the lateral compartment. The ACL is intact (white arrow heads).

IMAGE KEY

Common

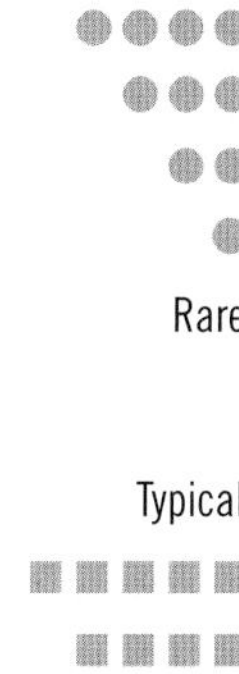

Rare

Typical

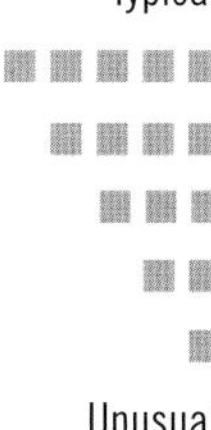

Unusual

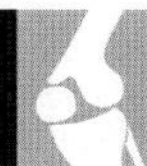

23–3 Meniscal Root Tear

Raymond Kuo and Rajeev K. Varma

PRESENTATION

Instability and pain

FINDINGS

Discontinuity of the meniscal root, fluid between the posterior cruciate ligament (PCL) attachment and posterior tibial eminence (medial root tear) and meniscal extrusion >3 mm may be associated with meniscal root tears.

DIFFERENTIAL DIAGNOSES

- *Free edge tear of posterior horn:* This meniscal tear defect does not extend to the periphery.
- *Bucket handle tear:* Less than two bowtie, double PCL sign, and flipped meniscus sign may be present.

COMMENTS

Meniscal root tears or avulsions are a newly recognized pathology and occur in 2.2% to 9.8% of patients undergoing MRI of the knee. It is important to recognize this type of tear as they may be easily missed and result in complications. There is an association of meniscal root tears with extrusion of the meniscus. Extrusion is more common with medial-side root tears. The meniscus is considered extruded when it extends beyond the margin of the tibia. Meniscal extrusions of greater than 3 mm are associated with tears of the posterior meniscal root. Because of abnormally increased contact forces across the joint, there is increased risk of accelerated osteoarthritis and also subchondral insufficiency fracture. The presence of meniscal extrusion is nonspecific and may also be associated with meniscal degeneration, complex tear, and large radial tear. When substantial meniscal extrusion is identified, there is a high likelihood that one of these lesions is present, causing loss of meniscal stability. Meniscal root tears may occur in conjunction with ACL disruptions. In this setting, lateral root tears are more prevalent than medial root tears. Meniscus extrusion that occurs with lateral root tears may be related to absence of or injury to the meniscofemoral ligament and is associated with more extensive lateral compartment bone contusions.

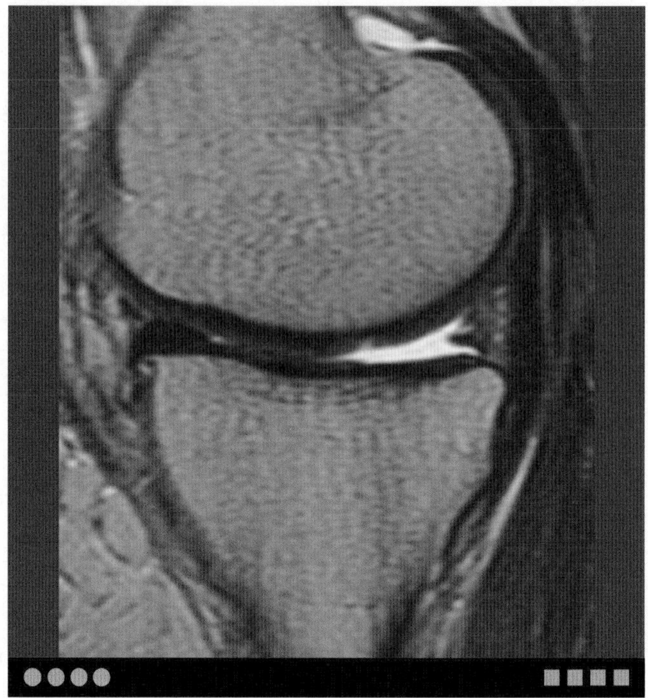

A. Meniscal root tear: Sagittal T1 image at the inner margin of the medial meniscus shows fluid in the expected location of the posterior horn, representing a tear.

PEARLS

- **The posterior meniscus should be seen on every sagittal image up to the one that shows the PCL**
- **In the coronal plane, the posterior meniscal root is horizontally oriented and extends to attach at the medial tibial eminence**
- **The differential diagnosis for medial meniscus extrusion (>3 mm) includes meniscal root tear, severe meniscal degeneration, extensive tear, complex tear, and large radial tear**

ADDITIONAL IMAGES

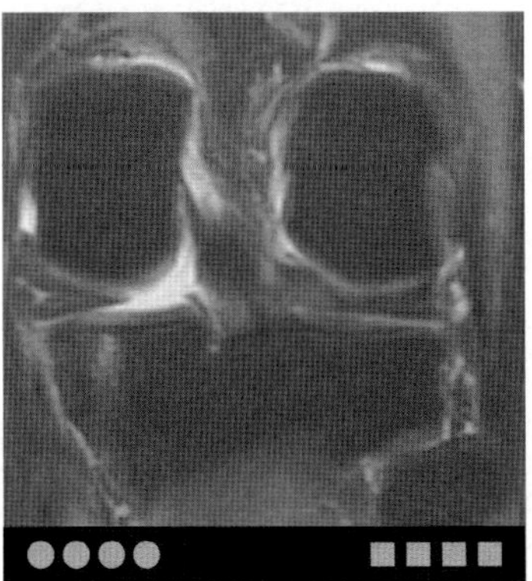

B. Meniscal root tear: Coronal T2 image showing defect of the medial meniscal root.

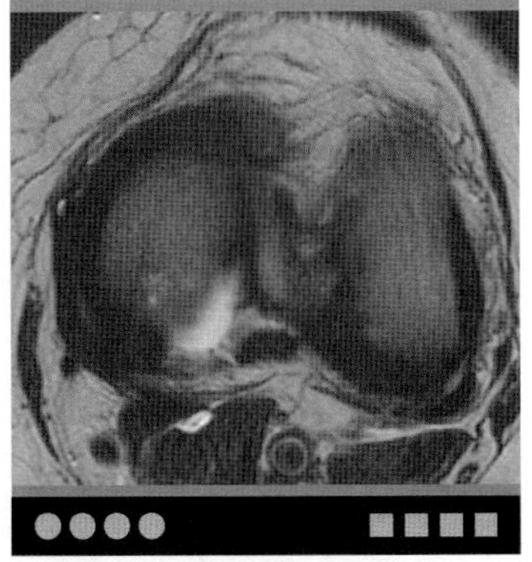

C. Meniscal root tear: Axial T2 image through the menisci nicely demonstrates the meniscal root tear as evidenced by high signal (fluid) within the defect in the posterior medial meniscus.

DIFFERENTIAL DIAGNOSES IMAGES

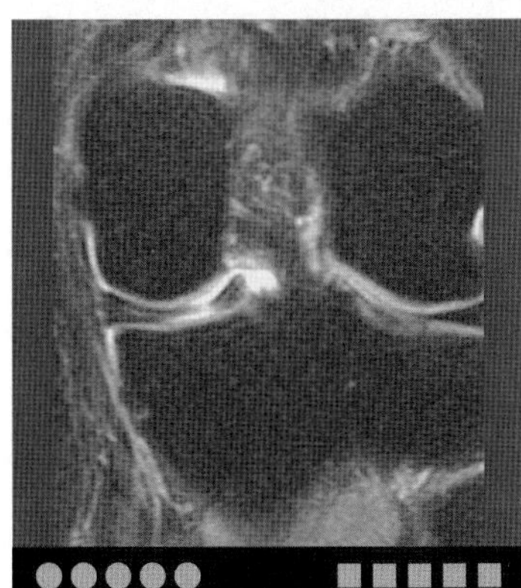

D. Free edge tear: Coronal T2 image shows focal abnormal fluid signal in the posterior horn of the medial meniscus within a tear. No significant meniscal extrusion is present.

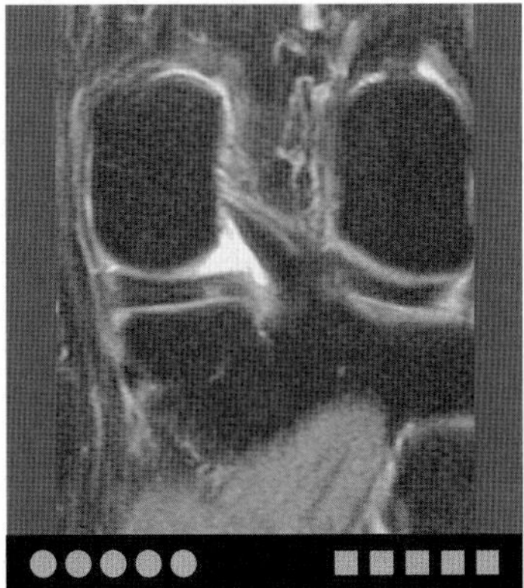

E. Free edge tear: A more posterior slice shows that the peripheral posterior meniscus remains intact, although there is slight signal abnormality representing contusion.

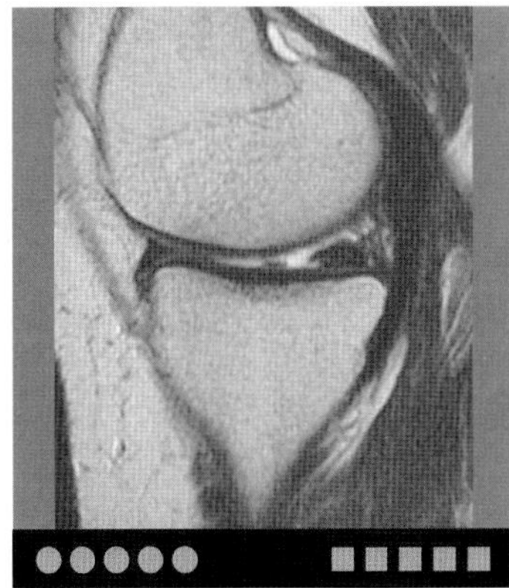

F. Free edge tear: A sagittal proton density image showing a tear at the free edge.

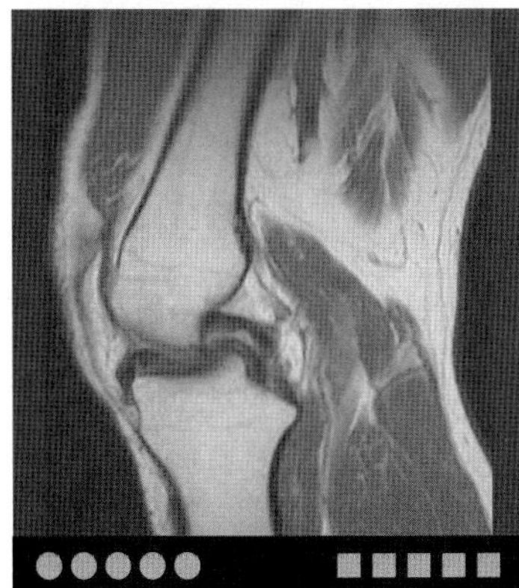

G. Bucket handle tear: Sagittal proton density image shows double posterior cruciate sign and flipped meniscus sign.

IMAGE KEY

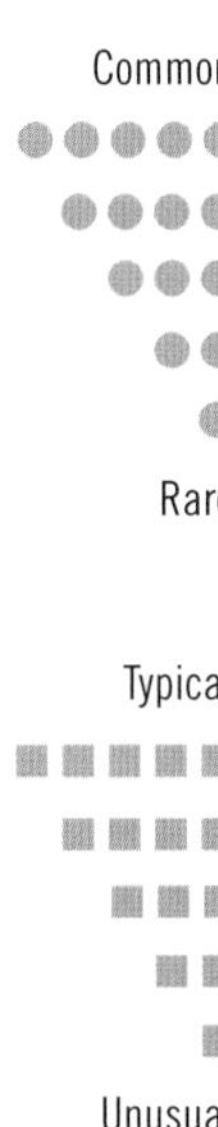

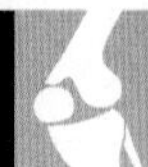

23–4 Meniscocapsular Separation

Stephen E. Ling and William R. Reinus

PRESENTATION

Joint line pain, tenderness, and instability

FINDINGS

There is fluid between the periphery of the meniscus and knee joint capsule with discontinuous or irregular heterogeneous meniscal attachments.

DIFFERENTIAL DIAGNOSES

- *Tibial collateral ligament (TCL) bursitis:* This is located peripheral to the meniscocapsular junction between the superficial and deep fibers of the medial collateral ligament (MCL).
- *Parameniscal/meniscal cyst:* This is also usually situated between the superficial and deep fibers of the MCL or within the meniscus, respectively. Meniscal tear is seen in the majority of cases.

COMMENTS

Meniscocapsular separation (MCS) is a circumferential tear of the peripheral capsular attachment of the meniscus. If the detachment is complete, the result is a meniscus that is free-floating. MCS usually arises from trauma, and thus is most commonly seen in young, active patients. It is often associated with other knee ligament injuries, particularly injury to the MCL. The medial and lateral menisci are intimately associated with the knee joint capsule. The deep fibers of the MCL (also known as the medial capsular ligament and meniscofemoral/meniscotibial ligaments) blend with the joint capsule, and together they firmly anchor the periphery of the meniscus. The lateral meniscus is anchored to the capsule throughout most of its course, but posteriorly around the popliteus tendon bursa it is anchored by the superior and inferior meniscal fascicles that give rise to the bursa. MCS is more common in the medial meniscus than the lateral meniscus, as the latter has a stronger solid attachment to the joint capsule. Overall, the meniscotibial/coronary ligament at the attachment of the posterior horn of the medial meniscus to the capsule is most frequently involved in MCS. Meniscocapsular separation often heals spontaneously because of the nearby perimeniscal capillary plexus and the adjacent "red," "vascular" zone of the meniscus. Although MRI is useful in diagnosing MCS, it is often overlooked, particularly if the T2-weighted fat-suppressed sequences are not studied carefully. Failure to make the diagnosis of meniscocapsular separation puts the patient at risk for increased meniscal mobility and instability, especially if the injury is large (>1 cm).

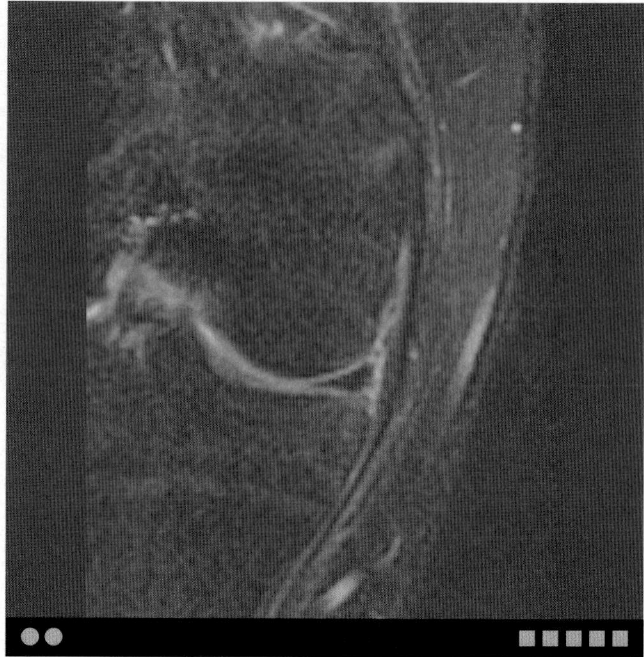

A. Meniscocapsular separation (MCS): Coronal fat saturation T2-weighted image (T2WI) shows fluid located between the peripheral aspect of the body of the medial meniscus and knee joint capsule.

PEARLS

- **The most common location for meniscocapsular separation is the meniscotibial attachment/coronary ligament of the posterior horn of the medial meniscus**
- **Coronal and sagittal images are the preferred planes in which to diagnose meniscocapsular separation (MCS)**
- **T2-weighted fat-saturated images are essential to make the diagnosis effectively**
- **Small (<1 cm) or nondisplaced tears are usually treated conservatively, as the injury tends to be able to heal on its own because of the intrinsic rich vascularity of the meniscus periphery**

ADDITIONAL IMAGE

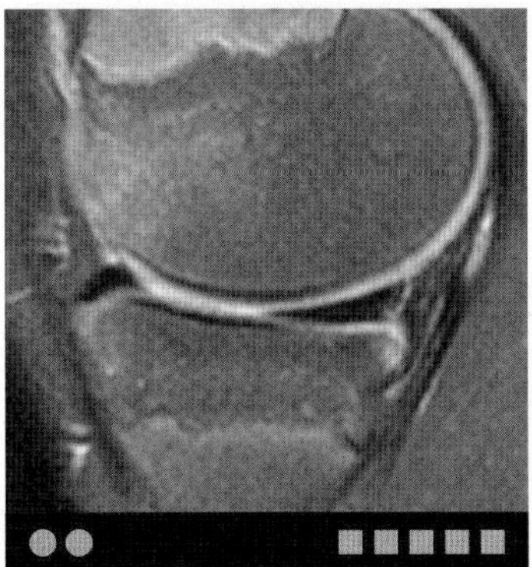

B. Meniscocapsular separation (MCS): Sagittal fat saturation T2-weighted image shows fluid interposed between the outer margin of the medial meniscus posterior horn and joint capsule.

DIFFERENTIAL DIAGNOSES IMAGES

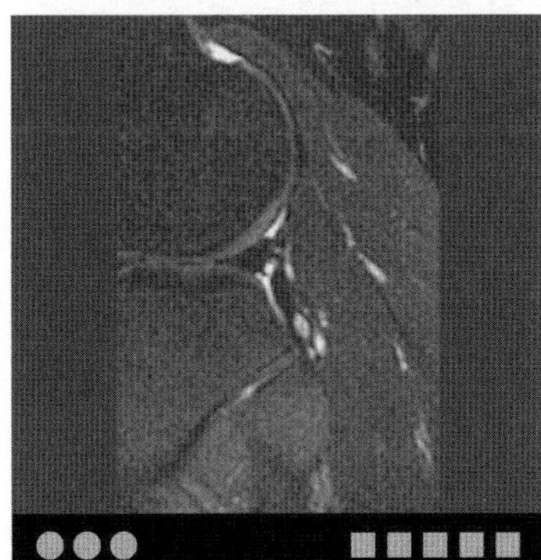

C. Popliteus hiatus: Sagittal fat saturation T2-weighted image shows fluid adjacent to the popliteus tendon and periphery of the lateral meniscus as the tendon traverses the joint capsule.

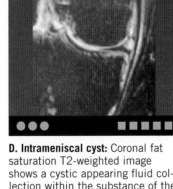

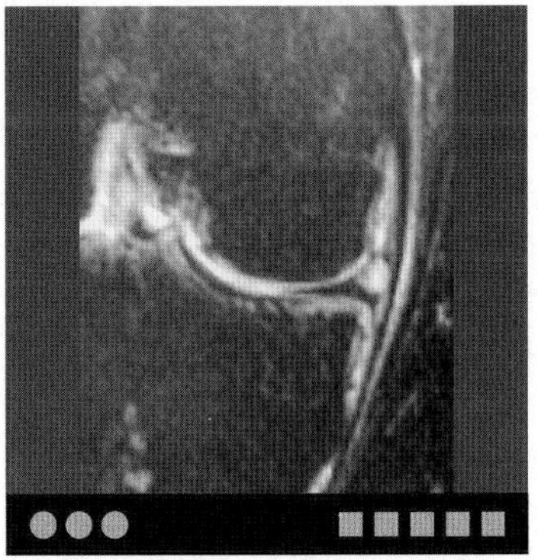

D. Intrameniscal cyst: Coronal fat saturation T2-weighted image shows a cystic appearing fluid collection within the substance of the peripheral portion of the body of the medial meniscus.

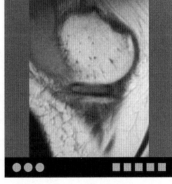

E. Intrameniscal cyst: Sagittal proton density-weighted image (PDWI) shows a cystic appearing fluid collection within the substance of the peripheral portion of the body of the medial meniscus.

F. Parameniscal cyst: Coronal fat saturation T2-weighted image shows a multilocular cystic structure deep to the lateral collateral ligament and abutting the outer edge of the lateral meniscus body. Note the horizontal tear of the meniscus.

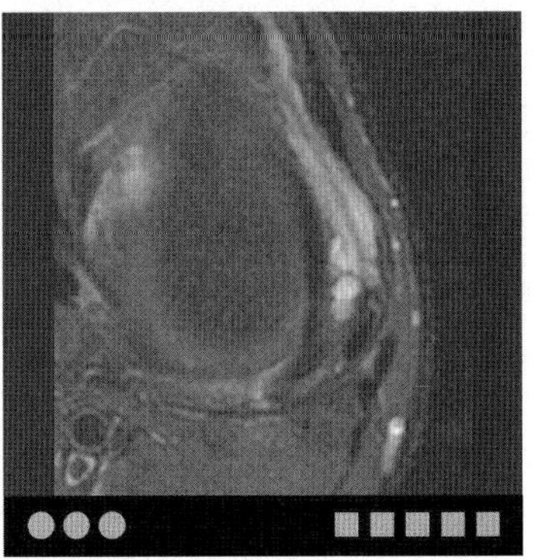

G. Parameniscal cyst: Axial fat saturation T2-weighted image shows a multilocular cystic structure deep to the lateral collateral ligament and abutting the outer edge of the lateral meniscus body.

IMAGE KEY

Common

Rare

Typical

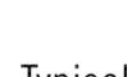

Unusual

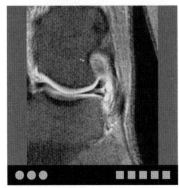

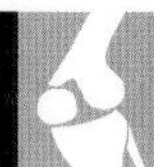

23–5 Medial Meniscal Cyst

Maria Pia Altavilla and Rajeev K. Varma

PRESENTATION

Medial joint line tenderness and palpable mass

FINDINGS

High signal intensity fluid collection on T2-weighted images along the posterior medial aspect of the tibial femoral joint.

DIFFERENTIAL DIAGNOSES

- *Pes anserine bursitis:* Fluid collection and bursitis arising at inserting tendons of sartorius, gracilis, and semitendinosus muscles.
- *Ganglion cysts:* Has a fibrous capsule instead of bursal synovial lining.
- *Medial collateral ligament bursitis:* Arise around the medial collateral ligament.

COMMENTS

The patient is a 39-year-old male who complained of medial joint tenderness and a palpable mass. Medial meniscal cysts usually present after a history or prior trauma to the knee. Most of the literature states that this cyst develops after a meniscal tear, typically a horizontal cleavage tear. This causes herniation of synovial fluid into or through the meniscal tear. The tear can act as a one-way valve mechanism causing build up of pressure, aiding cyst formation. Lateral meniscal cysts are more common than medial meniscal cyst. On MR imaging these cysts are round or oval masses of high signal intensity on T2-weighted image. On T1-weighted images the mass may be intermediate or low signal intensity, depending on the protein content of the cyst. The cyst is usually located along the lateral margin of the meniscus (parameniscal) or within meniscus. Identification of a parameniscal cyst prompts a search for a meniscal tear. Ultrasound images demonstrate a hypoechoic mass with through transmission along the periphery of the meniscus. MR imaging shows a cystic mass on the medial or lateral aspect of the knee joint, which has intermediate to low signal on T1-weighted and high signal on T2-weighted and fluid sensitive sequences. The typical cyst is associated with horizontal meniscal tear best seen on coronal images.

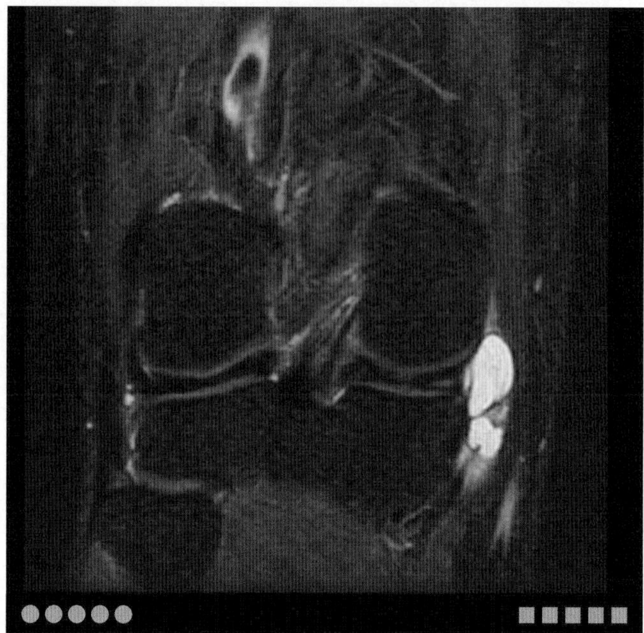

A. Medial meniscal cyst: Coronal T2 with fat saturation showing a lesion at the medial aspect of the tibial femoral joint. Note the linear high signal at the medial meniscus representing the meniscal tear.

PEARLS

- **Cyst within (intrameniscal) or adjacent to (parameniscal) the meniscus, is typically in continuity with a meniscal tear**
- **On MRI a round or oval-shaped mass with increased signal on T2-weighted images, which is intermediate to low signal in T1-weighted images**
- **Meniscal cysts can sometimes be lobulated and septated, especially if parameniscal**

ADDITIONAL IMAGES

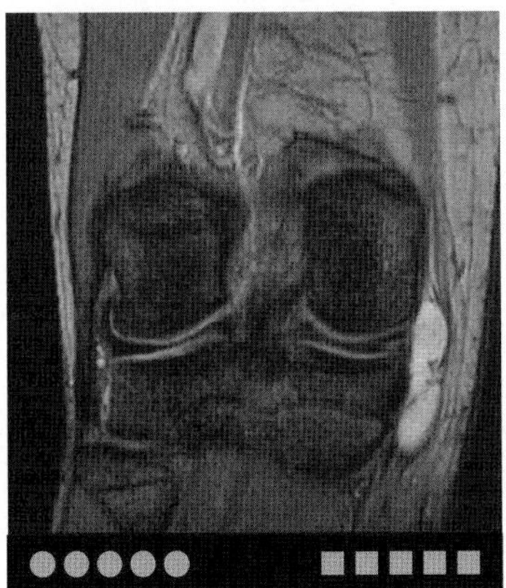

B. Medial meniscal cyst: Coronal gradient echo image showing the lesion along the medial aspect of the joint communicating with the meniscal tear.

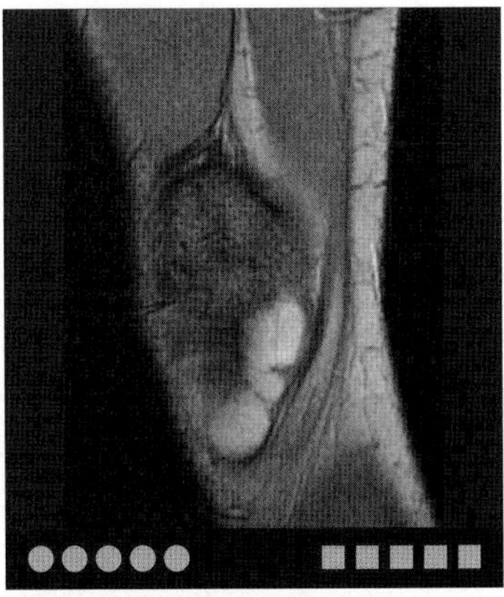

C. Medial meniscal cyst: Sagittal gradient echo image showing semi-oval mass at the medial aspect of the tibial femoral joint.

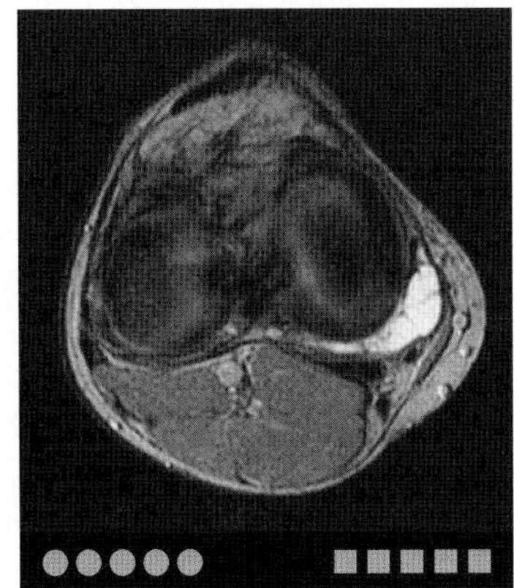

D. Medial meniscal cyst: Axial T2-weighted image with fat saturation showing a fluid collection at the posterior medial aspect of the tibial femoral joint. Note the internal septations.

DIFFERENTIAL DIAGNOSES IMAGES

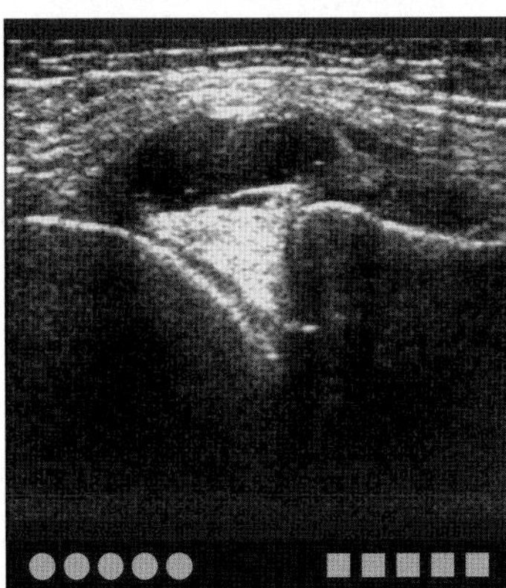

E. Medial meniscal cyst: Axial ultrasound image of the joint line of the knee demonstrating a hypo echoic lesion with through transmission consistent with a cyst.

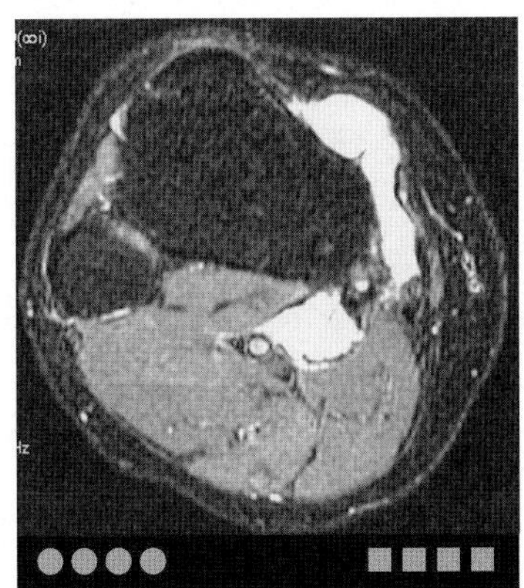

F. Pes anserine bursitis: Axial T2-weighted image with fat saturation shows a lobulated bright fluid containing bursa extending from posterior to the anterior aspect of medial tibia.

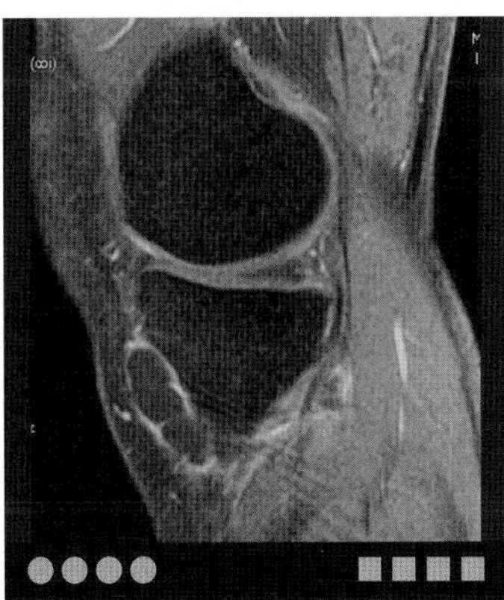

G. Pes anserine bursitis: Sagittal T1-weighted image with fat saturation post contrast shows low signal fluid containing bursa with marginal enhancement.

IMAGE KEY

Common

●●●●●
●●●●
●●●
●●
●

Rare

Typical

■■■■■
■■■■
■■■
■■
■

Unusual

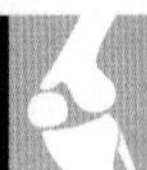

23–6 Lateral Meniscal Cyst

Gideon Strich

PRESENTATION

Lateral knee mass and peroneal neuropathy

FINDINGS

MRI shows a heterogeneous fluid-filled mass at the lateral joint line with erosion of the adjacent bone.

DIFFERENTIAL DIAGNOSES

- *Ganglion, bursa, or other fluid collection around the knee:* These are usually homogeneous with low signal on TW1 images and high signal on T2-weighted images.
- Benign synovial processes such as synovial hypertrophy, rheumatoid arthritis, gout, or pigmented villonodular synovitis are usually more diffuse and may have characteristic MR appearance depending on the entity.
- Malignant synovial or bone tumors demonstrate invasion of adjacent bone and soft tissues.
- Peroneal neuropathy may be associated with posterolateral corner injury, with a typical traumatic history and examination.

COMMENTS

The patient is a middle-aged male who presents with a history of lateral knee pain with a clinical examination demonstrating palpable mass at the lateral joint line and a mild peroneal neuropathy. Meniscal cysts, also known as parameniscal cysts, are synovial or ganglion cysts often containing joint fluid or mucinous or myxoid material. They are more common laterally than medially and are centered on the joint line. They are usually associated with tear of the adjacent meniscus. When larger, they may cause erosion of the adjacent bone and in the case of lateral meniscal cysts may produce symptoms related to the adjacent common peroneal nerve. Etiology of most meniscal cysts is thought to be related to extension of joint fluid through an adjacent horizontal cleavage tear of the meniscus. This communication may be demonstrated by intra-articular injection of gadolinium followed by MR arthrography. Treatment usually consists of surgical resection of the ganglion with resection or repair of the underlying torn meniscus. The differential diagnosis of a meniscal cyst may include any ganglion or bursa related to synovitis of joint or popliteal tendon sheath at this region. Pes anserinus and medial collateral ligament cysts are on the medial side.

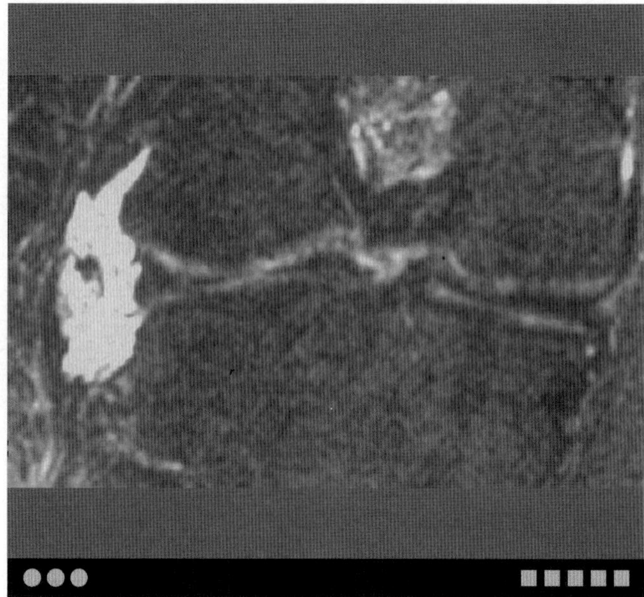

A. Meniscal cyst: Coronal STIR MRI shows a bright heterogeneous mass predominantly of fluid signal centered on the lateral joint line with an adjacent horizontal cleavage tear of the lateral meniscus.

PEARLS

- **Meniscal cysts are located at the level of the joint line and they are more common laterally than medially**
- **Most meniscal cysts are associated with adjacent meniscal tears. Treatment of symptomatic meniscal cysts usually also involves treatment of the adjacent meniscal tear.**
- **Where the appearance is unusual or diagnosis is in doubt, MR arthrography may confirm the connection with the joint**

ADDITIONAL IMAGES

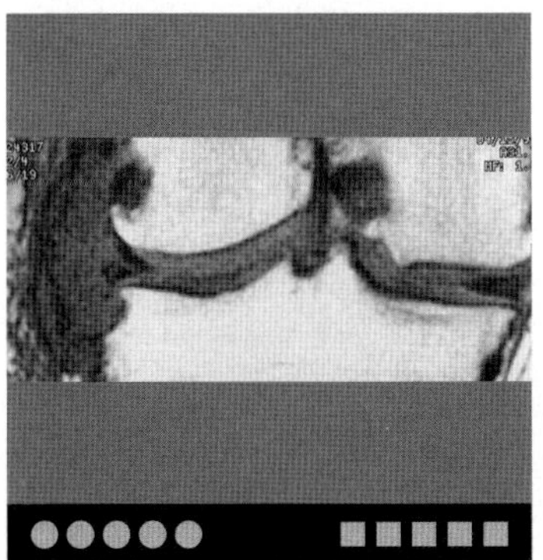

B. Meniscal cyst: T1-weighted image shows a heterogeneous mass predominantly of fluid signal centered on the lateral joint line with an adjacent horizontal cleavage tear of the lateral meniscus.

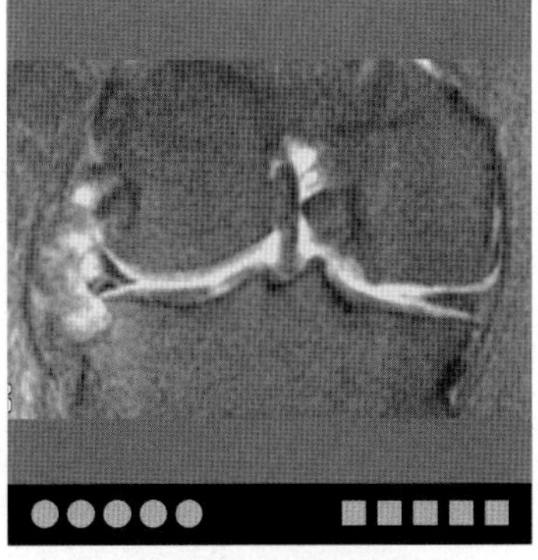

C. Meniscal cyst: MR arthrogram: T1-weighted coronal image with fat saturation shows communication of the cyst with the joint through the horizontal meniscal tear as well as filling defects in the cyst probably representing myxoid or synovial material.

DIFFERENTIAL DIAGNOSES IMAGES

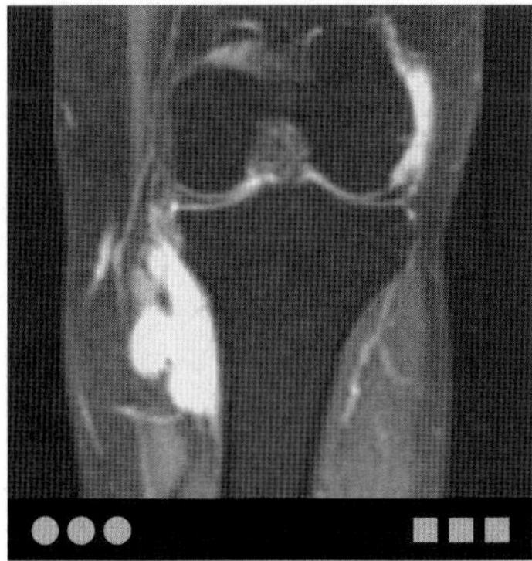

D. Pes anserinus bursa: Axial proton density image demonstrates a cystic mass just below the level of the medial joint line surrounding tendons of the pes anserinus.

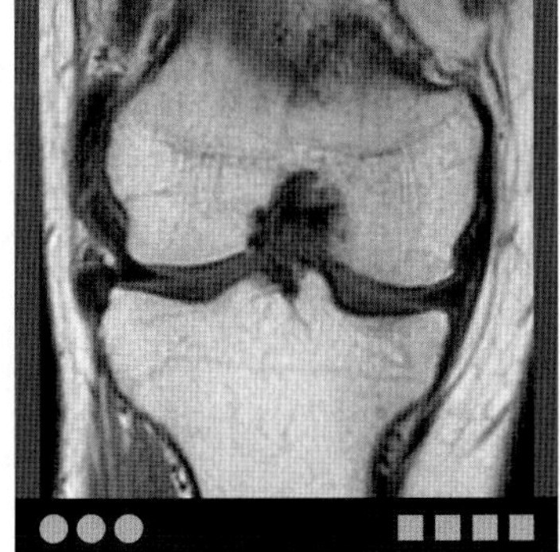

E. Pigmented villonodular synovitis: Coronal T1-weighted image demonstrates synovial mass at and above the joint line with mild erosion of underlying bone.

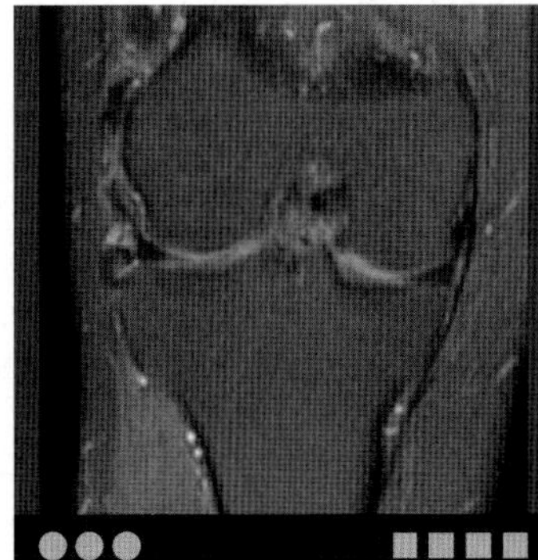

F. Pigmented villonodular synovitis: PD FSE image with fat saturation shows that although there is fluid in the joint and adjacent "mass," there is persistent low signal on all pulse sequences characteristic of PVNS.

IMAGE KEY

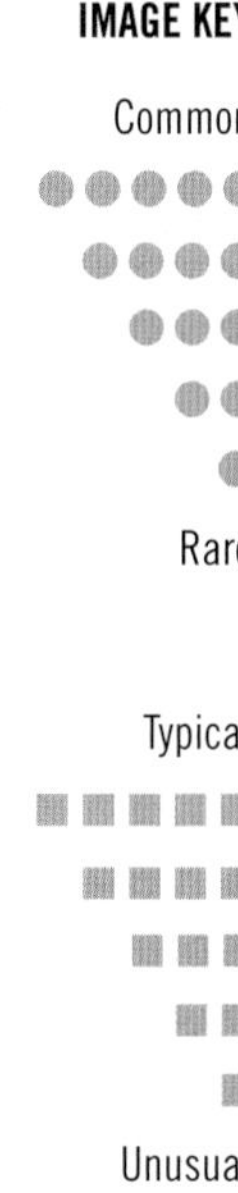

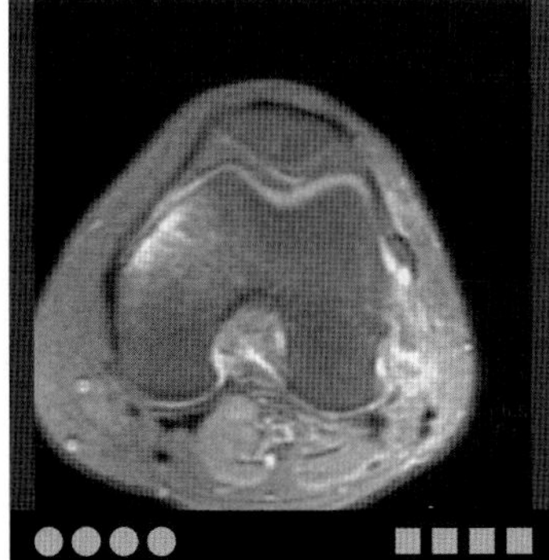

G. Posterolateral corner injury: Axial PD FSE with fat saturation shows edematous "mass" consisting of torn fibular collateral ligament. Peroneal neuropathy is secondary to stretching injury of the peroneal nerve. Note additional medial bone bruising.

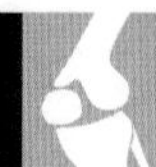

23–7 Sonographic Appearance of Meniscal Cyst

Stefano Bianchi and Ibrahim F. Abdelwahab

PRESENTATION

Soft tissue mass at the medial aspect of the knee

FINDINGS

MRI demonstrates a cystic mass located close to the medial meniscus.

DIFFERENTIAL DIAGNOSES

- *Pes anserinus ganglion:* Presents with a similar appearance but lies in a more distal location. It is not connected to the medial meniscus and the meniscus is normal. Based on the location pes anserinus ganglia and ganglia originating from the superior tibiofibular joint can be easily differentiated from meniscal cyst.
- *Pes anserinus bursitis:* Presents as a cystic lesion adjacent to bone and interdigitating with the pes anserinus tendons.
- *Soft tissue tumor:* Has a solid appearance and do not present internal fluid.

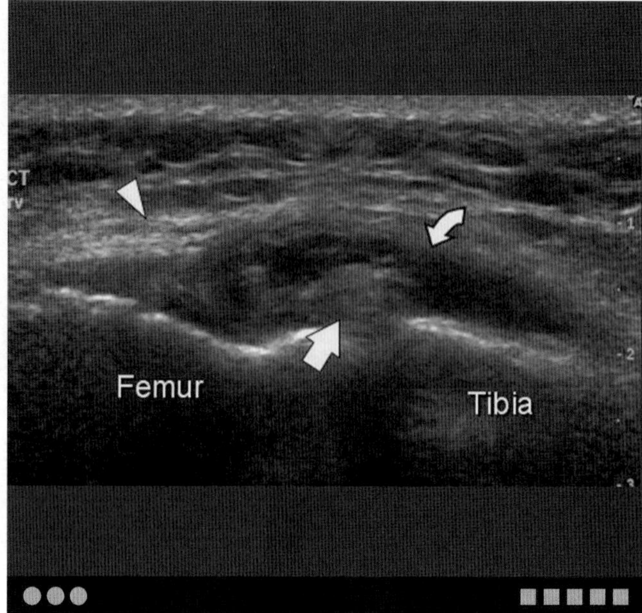

A. Meniscal cyst: Coronal US image obtained in the same patient shows the cyst (curved arrow) as a mass located close to the meniscus (arrow) and deep to the medial collateral ligament (arrowhead). The cyst presents a mixed internal structure.

COMMENTS

The patient is a 54-year-old man who developed a painless lump of the anteromedial aspect of the right knee associated with signs of internal derangement of the knee. Physical examination showed normal skin overlying an ill-defined mass that was not attached to the overlying skin. Meniscal cysts (MCs) are parameniscal lesions filled by thick, mucoid fluid that follows degenerative meniscal tears. In oblique or horizontal meniscal tear, the synovial fluid can penetrate the meniscal body and accumulate forming a small intrameniscal cyst. Being a one-way mechanism, fluid accumulates inside the meniscus and progressively thickens because of water resorption. With time, the cyst increases in size and develops within the parameniscal tissues and later inside the subcutis. Cysts arising from the medial meniscus can present a long pedicle and enlarge at considerable distance from the meniscal rupture. Clinically, MC presents with local pain and localized palpable, firm to semifluctuant swelling that can decrease in size till it disappears with different degrees of knee flexion. The cyst can present intermittent changes in size or gradually increase to cause compression on the adjacent structures. Diagnosis of MC is usually made clinically; however, MRI is frequently obtained for confirmation and to diagnose meniscal tears. Ultrasound can depict meniscal cyst by sagittal or coronal sonograms. It demonstrates cysts as expanded lesions located close to the outer meniscal surface. Their appearance varies from a unilocular hypoechoic mass to the most frequent multilocular lesion presenting internal mixed echogenicity. Color Doppler shows no internal flow signal.

PEARLS

- **Meniscal cysts are usually associated with degenerative meniscal tears**
- **The diagnosis can be suspected when a focal indolent mass is located close to the knee joint line and is associated with clinical signs of a meniscal tear**
- **Although ultrasound can easily assess meniscal cysts, only MRI can accurately evaluate the meniscus and detect associated degenerative tears**

ADDITIONAL IMAGES

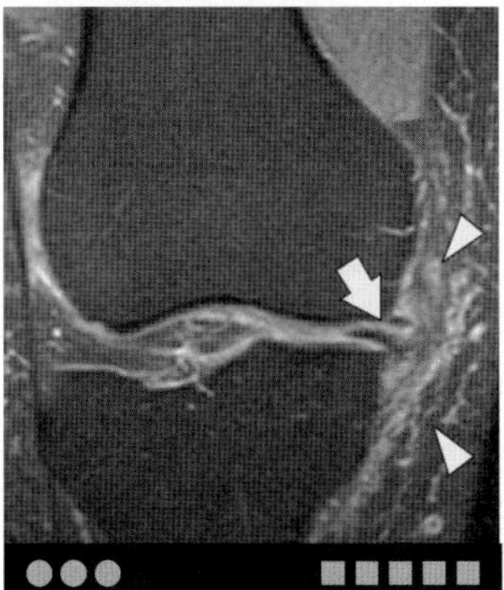

B. Meniscal cyst: Coronal proton density fat-saturated MRI image obtained at a more anterior level than image A shows a horizontal degenerative tear (arrow) of the anterior horn of the medial meniscus. Note edema of the parameniscal tissues (arrowheads).

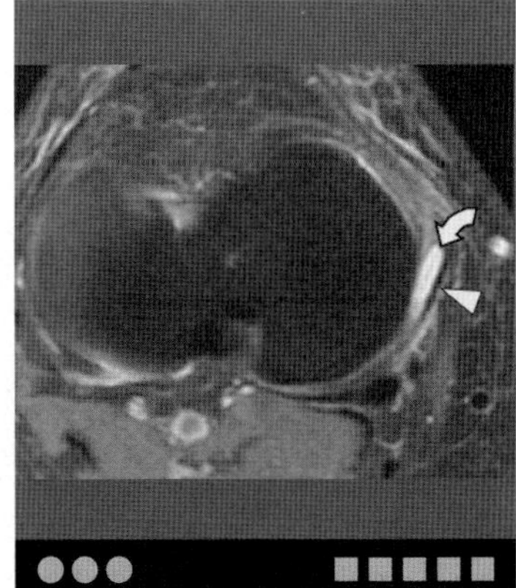

C. Meniscal cyst: Axial proton density fat-saturated MRI image obtained at the level of the tibial epiphysis shows the meniscal cyst (curved arrow) and its relation with the medial collateral ligament (arrowheads).

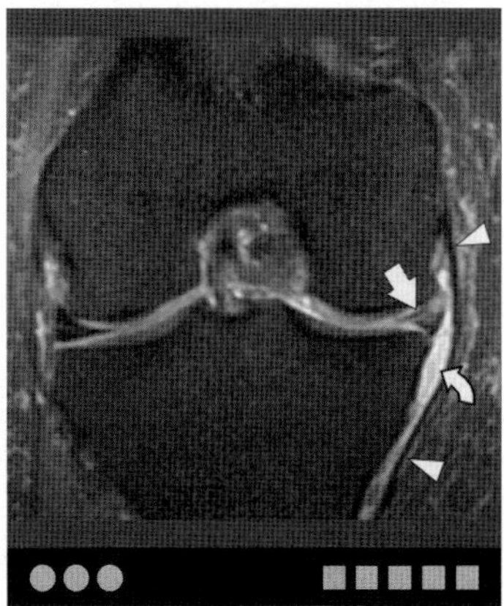

D. Meniscal cyst: Coronal proton density fat-saturated MRI image obtained at the level of intercondylar notch shows the meniscal cyst (curved arrow) appearing as a hyperintense mass located deep at the medial collateral ligament (arrowheads). Note the irregular medial meniscus (arrow).

IMAGE KEY

Common

Rare

Typical

Unusual

DIFFERENTIAL DIAGNOSES IMAGES

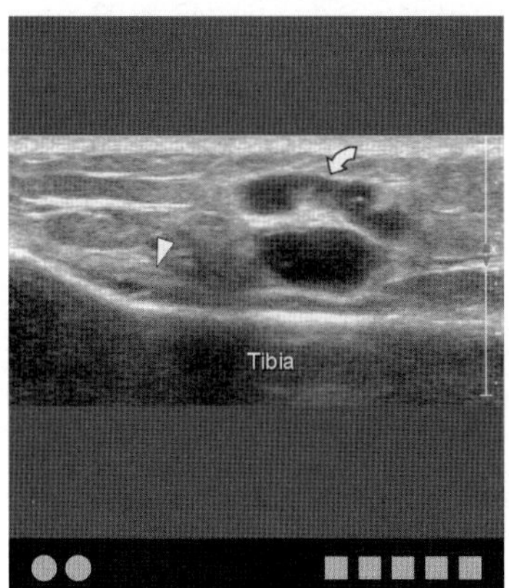

E. Pes anserinus ganglion: Coronal US image obtained over the pes anserinus region shows a mass (curved arrow) with well-marginated border arising from the tendon sheath of the pes anserinus tendons (arrowhead). The internal structure is made by alternating anechoic areas, corresponding to mucoid fluid, and hyperechoic septa giving the ganglion a multiloculated appearance.

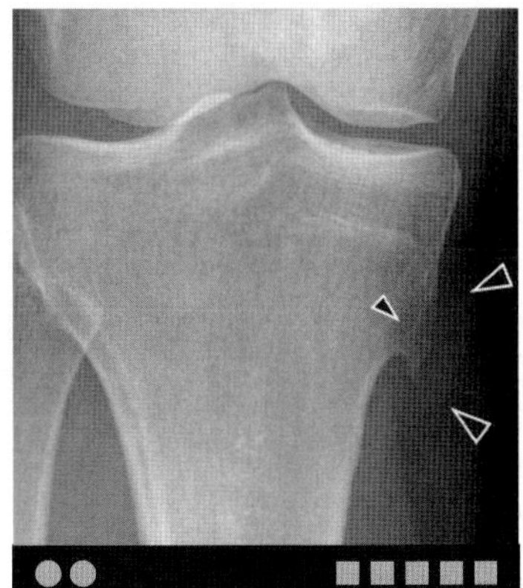

F. Pes anserinus bursitis and bursa exostotica: AP radiograph shows a metaphyseal exostosis (black arrowhead) of the tibia and an adjacent ill-defined soft tissue mass (open arrowheads). The knee joint is normal.

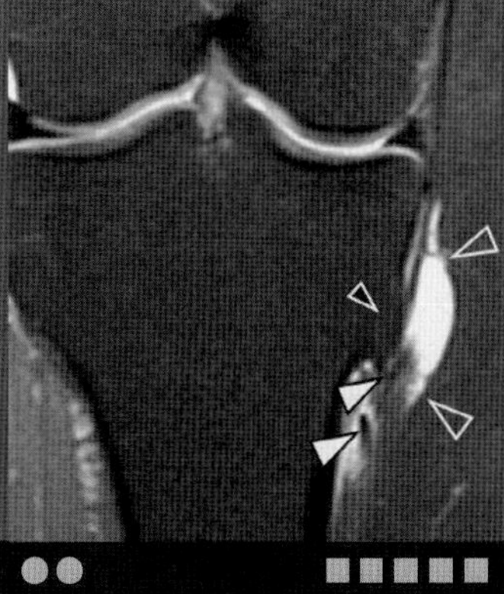

G. Pes anserinus bursitis and bursa exostotica: Coronal proton density fat-saturated MRI image shows the exostosis (black arrowhead) and an adjacent fluid collection consistent with bursa exostotica (open arrowheads). The pes anserinus tendons (white arrowheads) are normal.

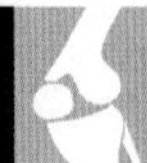

23–8 Discoid Lateral Meniscus

Peyman Borghei and Jamshid Tehranzadeh

PRESENTATION

Knee pain

FINDINGS

Coronal image shows a rectangular-shaped lateral meniscus.

DIFFERENTIAL DIAGNOSES

- *Bucket handle tear:* MRI findings include less than two contiguous bowties or absence of a bowtie, presence of double posterior cruciate ligament sign, double anterior horn sign, flipped meniscus sign, disproportional posterior horn sign, and fragment within the intercondylar region.
- *Normal meniscus:* Two bowties should be present at the periphery of medial or lateral menisci.

COMMENTS

The patient is a 14-year-old girl with the complaint of knee pain diagnosed with discoid lateral meniscus. Discoid meniscus is enlarged and disc shaped rather than normal semilunar. Lateral discoid menisci are 10 times more common than the medial ones, and also bilateral involvement of lateral discoid meniscus is not uncommon. The disc-shaped meniscus results in greater tibial surface coverage, which leads to abnormal shearing force across the knee joint. They are usually asymptomatic unless complicated by tears, degeneration, and cystic formation. The diagnosis of a discoid meniscus is strongly suggested by the patient's history, with symptoms that include knee pain, snapping, and locking in a child or adolescent. Three subgroups of discoid meniscus have been explained: **Complete,** in which the lateral discoid meniscus (LDM) completely covers the lateral tibial plateau and attaches to it. **Incomplete,** in which the LDM attaches to the lateral tibial plateau but does not cover it completely, **Wrisberg,** in which the LDM covers the lateral tibial plateau completely with attachments only to posterior meniscofemoral ligament and not to tibial plateau. On MRI the bowtie appearance of the meniscal body is seen on more than three contiguous 5-mm thick sagittal images. Also the transverse width at the mid-portion of the meniscal body usually exceeds 14 mm, the normal central tapering is absent and the height of the meniscus is increased by at least 2 mm when compared with the opposite normal side.

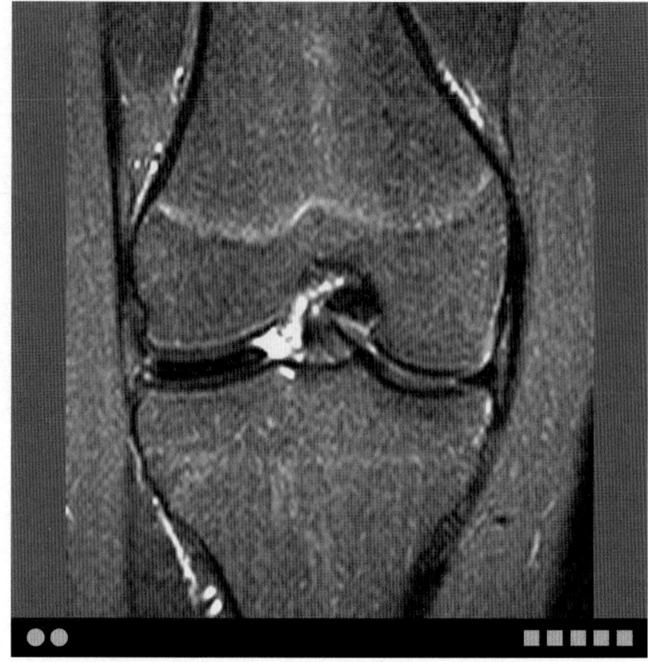

A. Discoid lateral meniscus: Coronal STIR image of the right knee shows a rectangular-shaped and thickened lateral meniscus. Note that the mesial portion of the meniscus does not taper as normal meniscus does.

PEARLS

- **The discoid lateral meniscus is an abnormally thick and disc-shaped meniscus that widely covers the articular surface of the tibial plateau, and is prone to complications like tear**
- **It is more common in the lateral side**
- **The three types of DLM include: Complete, Incomplete, and Wrisberg**
- **MRI manifestations include: Three or more bowties seen on sagittal images; midportion transverse width is more than 14 mm; the involved meniscus is 2 mm taller than the normal other side**

ADDITIONAL IMAGES

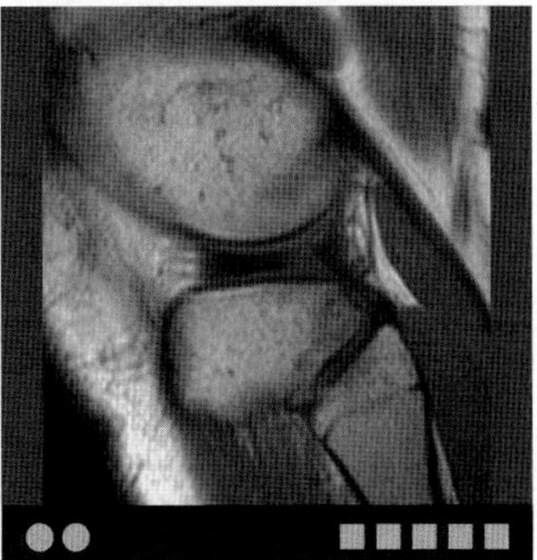

B. Discoid lateral meniscus: The first of the three consecutive 5 mm sagittal PD image shows a complete bowtie appearance.

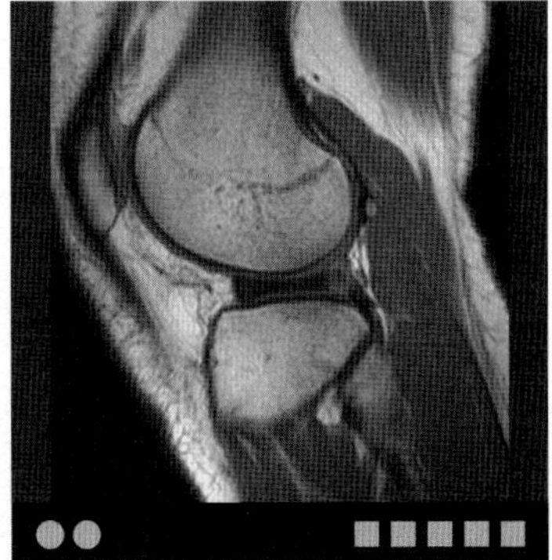

C. Discoid lateral meniscus: The second of the three consecutive 5 mm sagittal PD image shows continuity of bowtie appearance.

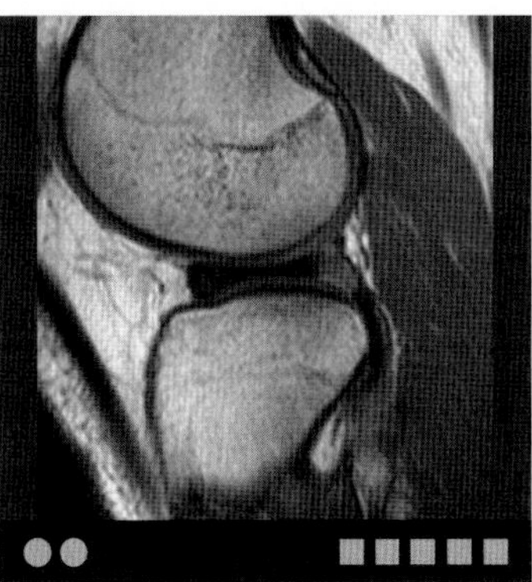

D. Discoid lateral meniscus: The third of the three consecutive 5-mm thick sagittal PD image shows a complete bowtie appearance.

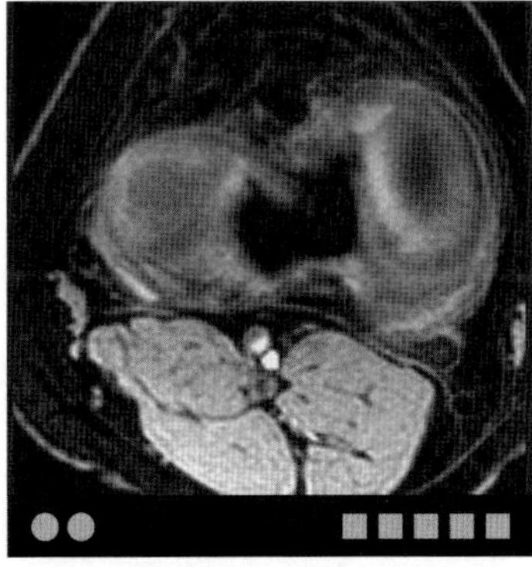

E. Discoid lateral meniscus: Axial fat-saturated T2-weighted image shows disc-shaped lateral meniscus. Note increased transverse width at the midportion of the meniscal body which is more than 14 mm.

DIFFERENTIAL DIAGNOSES IMAGES

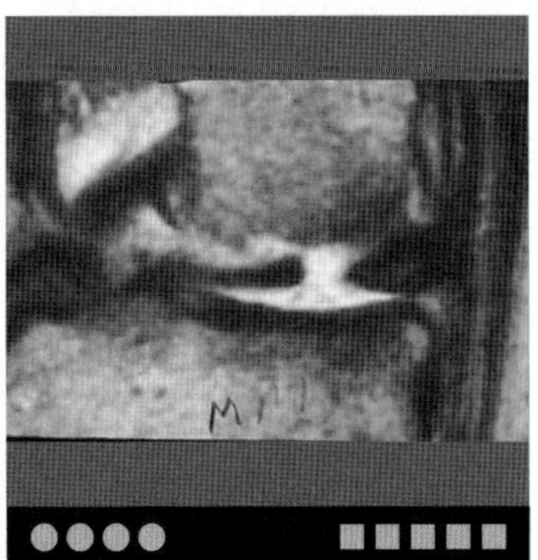

F. Bucket handle tear: Coronal T2-weighted image shows a wide gap between two pieces of medial meniscus representing a bucket handle tear. Adjacent osteochondral defect of the femoral condyle is also noted.

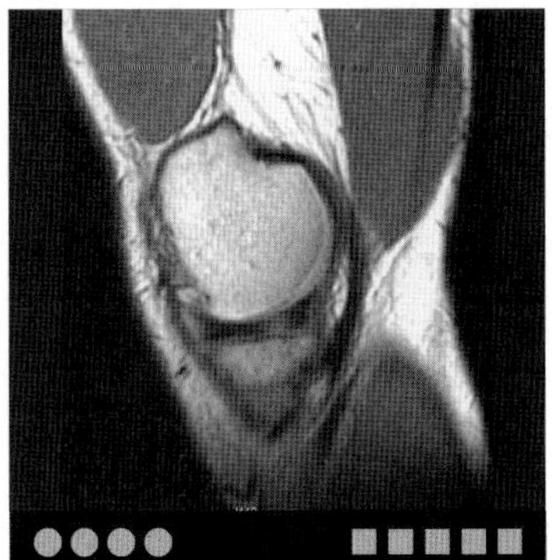

G. Bucket handle tear: Sagittal PD image of another patient shows even the first slice of the peripheral aspect of the meniscus does not show a complete bowtie showing a vertical bucket handle tear.

IMAGE KEY

Common

Rare

Typical

Unusual

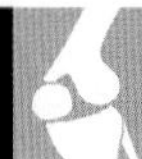

23–9 Meniscus Ossicle

Ayodale S. Odulate and Piran Aliabadi

PRESENTATION

Knee pain and swelling

FINDINGS

Smooth rounded lesion inside the meniscus that follows marrow signal on all MR sequences.

DIFFERENTIAL DIAGNOSES

- *Meniscus tear/degeneration:* Varied appearance from intrasubstance degeneration to complex tears extending to the articular surface.
- *Meniscus calcification:* This is a condition with diffuse calcification of the meniscus associated with calcium pyrophosphate dehydrate crystal deposition disease (CPPD), which is best appreciated on plain radiographs. MR signal intensity varies from hypo- to hyperintense linear signal intensity.
- *Popliteus tendon avulsion:* A posterolateral corner injury of the knee. Rarely an isolated injury commonly associated with lateral meniscal and ACL injuries. Radiographs may demonstrate an avulsion fracture of the lateral femoral condyle.

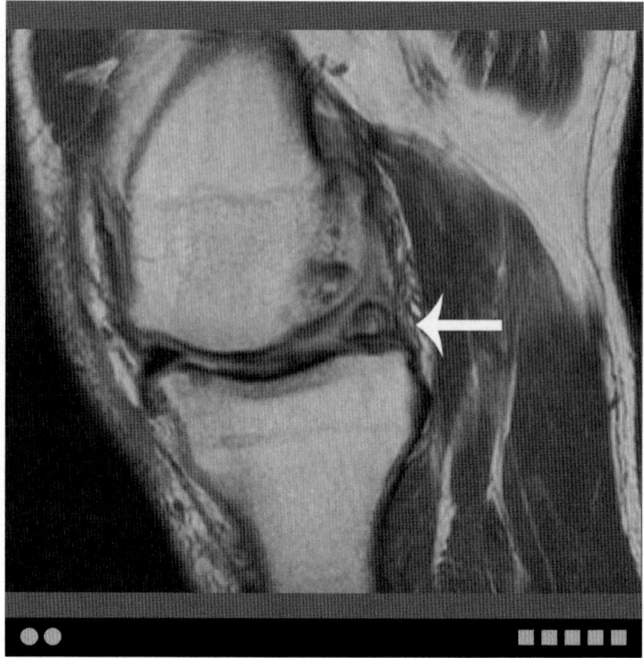

A. Meniscus ossicle: Sagittal T1-weighted image demonstrates a meniscal ossicle (arrow) in the posterior horn of the medial meniscus.

COMMENTS

The patient is a 27-year-old male with knee pain without history of trauma. A meniscal ossicle is a rare diagnosis by MRI or arthroscopy. The ossicle is often found within the posterior horn of the medial meniscus. They are diagnosed in young males with chronic knee pain and/or swelling. Often a history of trauma can be elicited and the ossicle is believed to have developed within the meniscus as a result of the reparative process following a tear. If there is no history of trauma, and the patient is asymptomatic, the ossicle may be a developmental variant from rest of mesenchymal cells within the meniscus. No therapy is indicated in asymptomatic patients; however, symptomatic patients may need arthroscopy for resection and debridement of the meniscus. On radiograph, the ossicle appears as a well-circumscribed corticated smooth rounded or triangular calcification that may be mistaken for an intra-articular loose body within the joint. The MR imaging characteristics are pathognomonic. A smooth lesion within the meniscus with a hypointense rim representing cortical bone and internal signal intensity that follows marrow signal on all sequences. On T1-weighed image, the ossicle has increased signal, similar to that of fatty marrow. Chondrocalcinosis on the other hand usually has punctate linear signal abnormalities without the well-defined cortical border. Intra-articular bodies may be the result of osteochondritis dissecans, osteoarthritic osteophytes, or fracture. The MR imaging characteristics are similar to meniscal ossicles; however, they will lie within the joint capsule.

PEARLS

- **Meniscal ossicle is a rare entity in young males; often misdiagnosed as intra-articular loose bodies on radiograph and it may be asymptomatic**
- **Round smooth signal abnormality in the meniscus that follows marrow signal on all MRI sequences**

ADDITIONAL IMAGES

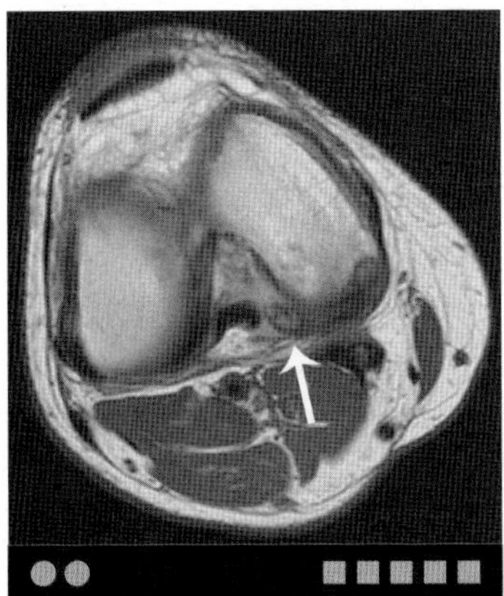

B. Meniscus ossicle: Axial proton density images show a round corticated ossicle (arrow) within the posteromedial horn of the medial meniscus.

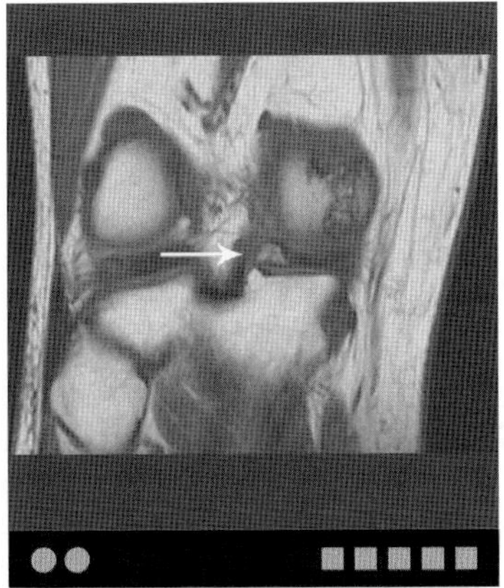

C. Meniscus ossicle: Coronal T1-weighted image demonstrates the ossicle (arrow) in the posterior medial meniscus.

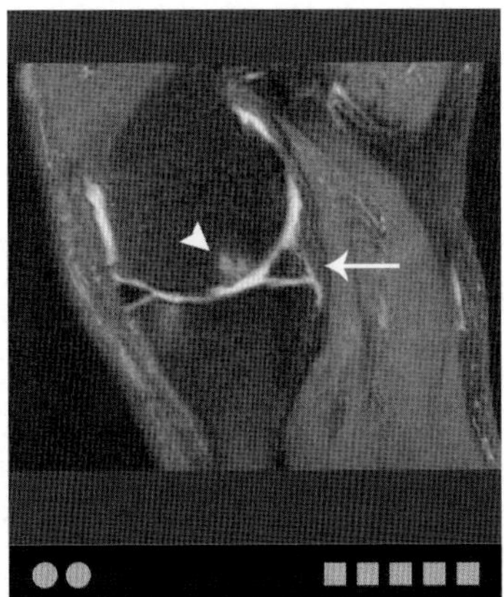

D. Meniscus ossicle: Sagittal proton density fat-saturated image shows abnormal signal within the medial femoral condyle (arrowhead). Note that the signal intensity of the ossicle (arrow) follows that of marrow on all sequences.

DIFFERENTIAL DIAGNOSES IMAGES

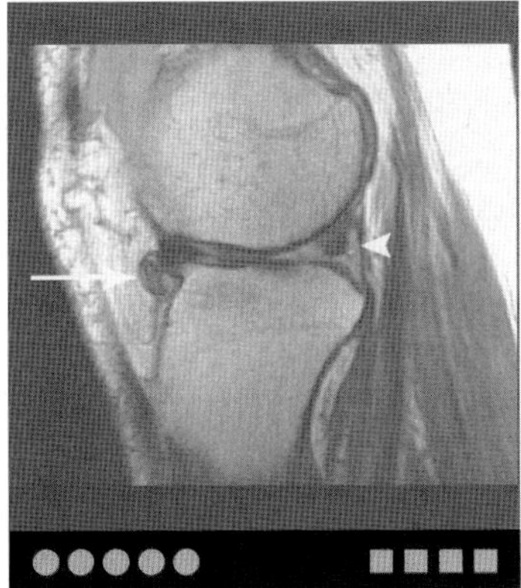

E. *Intra-articular loose bodies:* Sagittal proton density image shows a corticated loose body (arrow) in the anterior joint. A tear of the posterior horn of the meniscus is also seen (arrowhead).

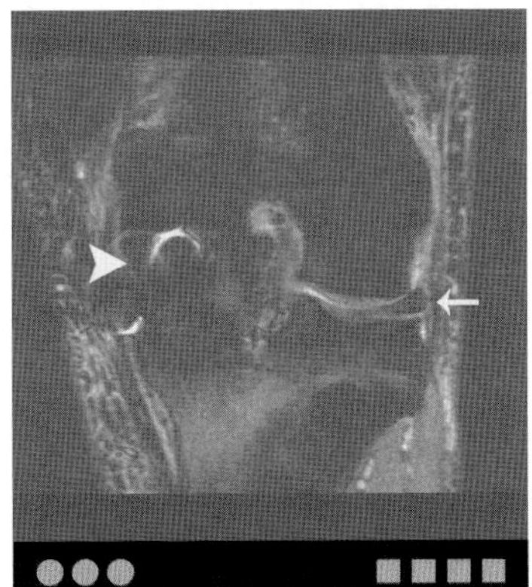

F. *Meniscus calcification:* Coronal STIR image shows subtle increased signal intensity in the lateral meniscus (arrow). Metal artifact from the unicondylar prosthesis is seen (arrowhead).

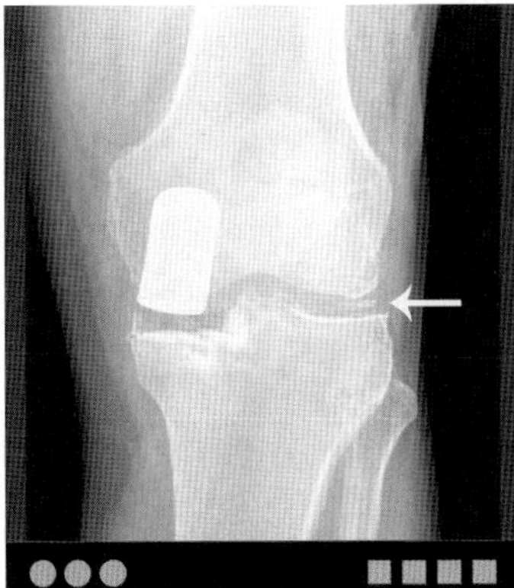

G. *Meniscus calcification:* Frontal radiograph of the knee from the same patient shows calcifications of the lateral meniscus (arrow). A medial unicondylar prosthesis is seen.

IMAGE KEY

Common

Rare

Typical

Unusual

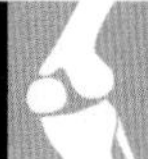

23–10 Ruptured Dissecting Bakers Cyst

Shahla Modarresi and Daria Motamedi

PRESENTATION

Pain and swelling of the calf

FINDINGS

Sagittal proton density (PD) MR image shows mass with mixed low and high signal compressing gastrocnemius muscle.

DIFFERENTIAL DIAGNOSES

- *Hematoma:* MR image shows confined mass-like collection of blood with no muscle fiber coursing through the mass, showing age-dependent signal of blood on T1 and T2-weighted images.
- *Gastrocnemius muscle tear:* MR image shows intraparenchymal bleeding, high signal on T2-weighted image with muscle fibers coursing through the abnormal area. Muscle may be enlarged.
- *Soft tissue/synovial sarcoma:* MR image usually shows low signal on T1-weighted and high signal on T2-weighted image showing contrast enhancement. It can occasionally mimic the fluid and be very intense on T2-weighted sequence.

COMMENTS

The patient is a 50-year-old man with pain and tightness behind the knee with swelling of the calf. Baker's cyst, also termed popliteal cyst, is a synovial cyst located posterior to the medial femoral condyle between the medial head of the gastrocnemius muscle and semimembranosus tendon. This usually communicates with the joint via a slit-like opening at the posteromedial aspect of the knee capsule just superior to the joint line. A Baker's cyst is lined by a true synovium, as it is an extension of the knee joint. The common underlying conditions are osteoarthritis and Charcot joint. A popliteal mass is the most common presenting complaint or symptom. Baker's cyst can rupture or dissect down the posterior calf causing acute pain behind knee. More common medical conditions associated with popliteal cysts, in descending order of frequency are (1) *arthritides*: osteoarthritis (most common), RA, juvenile RA, gout, reiter syndrome, psoriasis, systemic lupus erythematosus; (2) *internal derangement*: meniscal tears, anterior cruciate ligament tears, osteochondral fractures; (3) *infection*: septic arthritis, tuberculosis. Although prevalence of Baker's cyst in patients with inflammatory arthritis is higher than in patients with osteoarthritis, osteoarthritis is much more common than inflammatory arthritis. The incidence of popliteal cysts detected on knee MRI varies (5–18%), depending on the patient population. MR detection revealed that 84% of Baker's cysts had meniscal tears, mostly in the posterior horn of the medial meniscus. MR shows a low T1, high T2 cystic mass in typical location at the popliteal fossa.

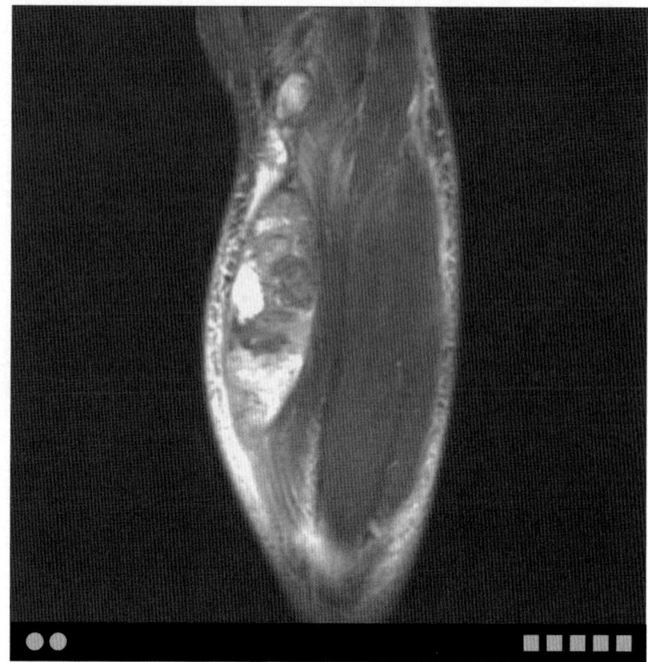

A. Ruptured dissecting Baker's cyst: Sagittal PD image showing mass with low and high signal fluid compressing gastrocnemius muscle.

PEARLS

- **Baker's cyst is a synovial cyst between the medial head of the gastrocnemius muscle and semimembranosus tendon**
- **Baker's cyst can rupture or dissect in the soft tissues of posterior calf causing acute pain and mass behind the knee joint**
- **First diagnostic step is ultrasound to rule out DVT**
- **Most common medical condition associated with Baker's cyst is osteoarthritis**

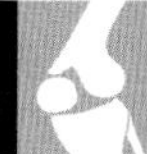

ADDITIONAL IMAGES

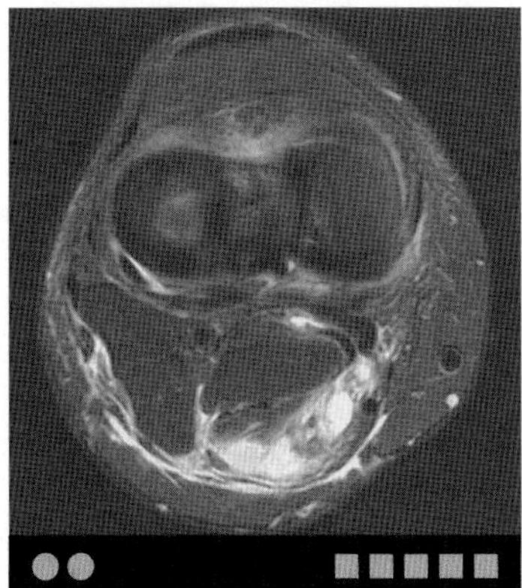

B. Ruptured dissecting Baker's cyst: Axial STIR image shows high signal fluid and blood of ruptured dissecting Baker's cyst compressing medial head of gastrocnemius muscle.

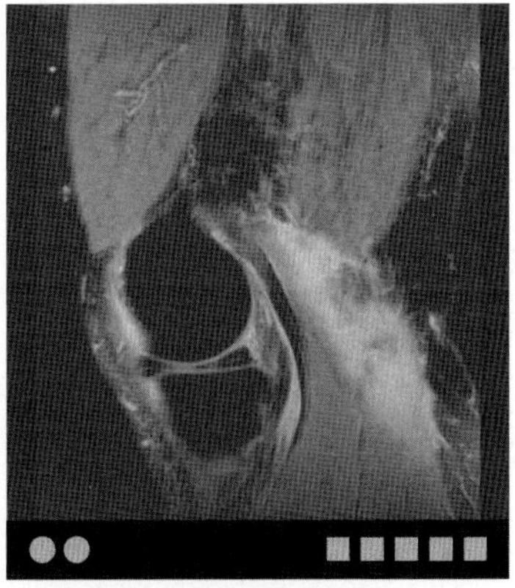

C. Ruptured dissecting Baker's cyst: Sagittal STIR image shows mixed signal fluid ruptured dissecting Baker's cyst between gastrocnemius muscle and semimembranous tendon.

DIFFERENTIAL DIAGNOSES IMAGES

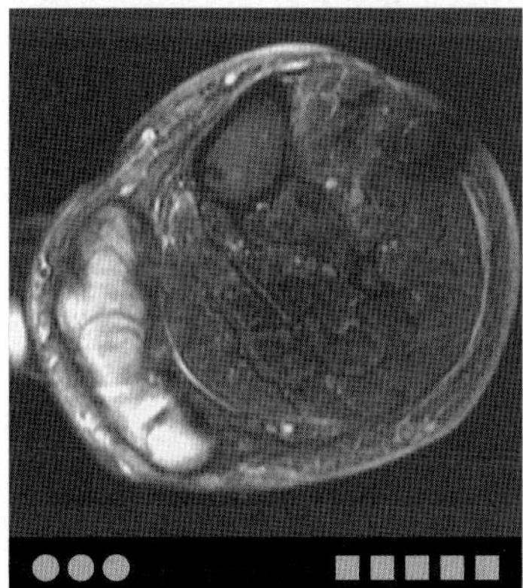

D. Hematoma: Axial STIR image shows high signal organized subacute hematoma compressing the gastrocnemius muscle.

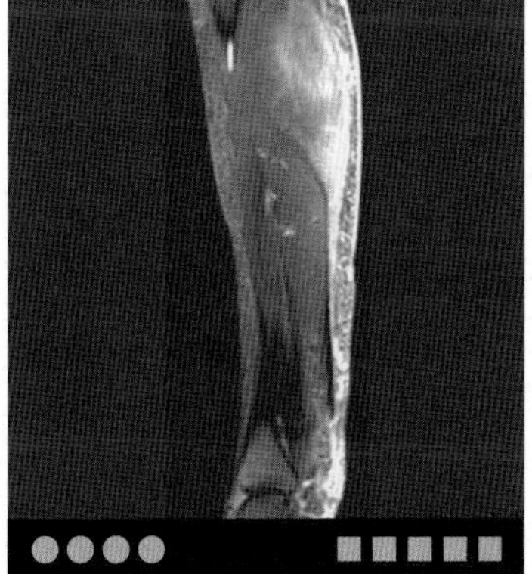

E. Intramuscular hemorrhage: Sagittal T2-weighted image shows high signal intraparenchymal bleeding with muscle fibers coursing through the abnormal area. Note muscle is enlarged.

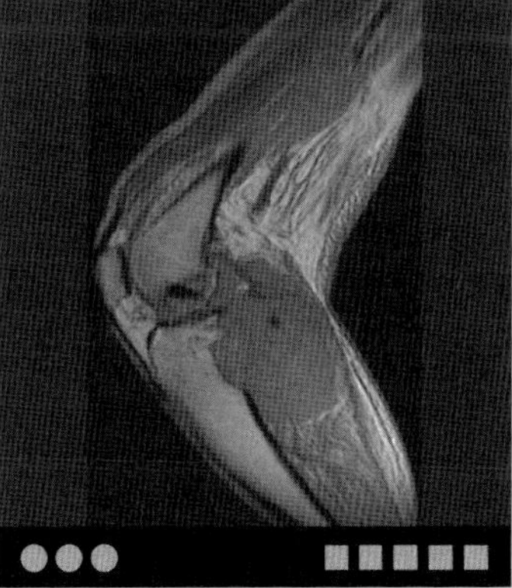

F. Synovial sarcoma: Sagittal PD image shows soft tissue mass with intermediate signal posterior to proximal tibia with bony erosion extending to the joint consistent with synovial sarcoma.

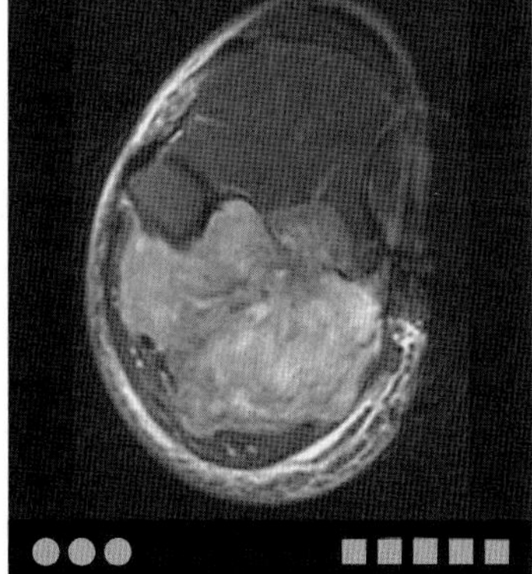

G. Synovial sarcoma: Axial STIR image shows high signal soft tissue mass posterior to proximal tibia with bony erosion extending to the joint consistent with synovial sarcoma.

IMAGE KEY

Common

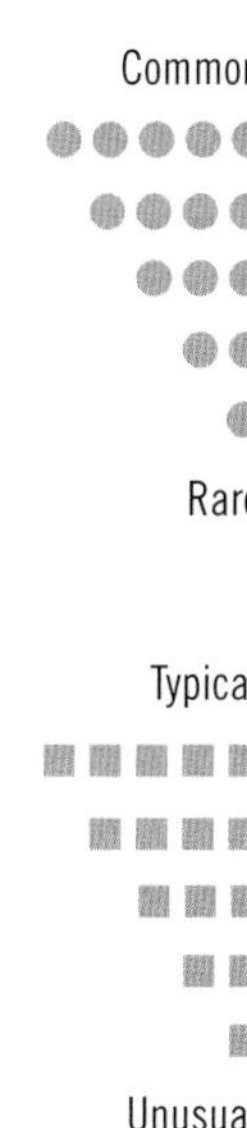

Rare

Typical

Unusual

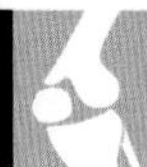

23–11 Sonographic Appearance of Ruptured Baker's Cyst

Stefano Bianchi and Ibrahim F. Abdelwahab

PRESENTATION

Acute pain in the calf

FINDINGS

Ultrasound image shows an anechoic structure taking origin from the semimembranosus-medial gastrocnemius head synovial bursa (SMHSB) and extending distally in the calf.

DIFFERENTIAL DIAGNOSES

- *Thrombosis of the popliteal vein:* The clinical picture is very similar to a ruptured Baker's cyst. US study allows direct demonstration of the hypoechoic thrombus filling the uncompressible vein. In doubtful cases, color Doppler allows a definite diagnosis. Posterior medial knee scanning reveals a normal SMHSB.
- *Soft tissue tumors:* They appear as hypoechoic solid masses that are not related to the SM-MH bursa.
- *Intramuscular myxoma:* Can present with a similar US appearance. It does not communicate with the knee joint, and is uncommon in the leg.
- *Tennis leg:* The term refers to tears of the distal myotendineous junction of the medial gastrocnemius. They are traumatic in nature. US easily shows the disruption of the distal internal architecture of the muscle as well as presence of secondary hematomas.

COMMENTS

The SMHSB is located between the external semimembranosus tendon and the internally located medial head of the gastrocnemius muscle. The bursa has a synovial lining and contains a small amount of synovial fluid that facilitates sliding among the adjacent tendons and posterior joint structures. Contrary to what is observed in children, the bursa in most adults communicates with the knee cavity. Baker's cysts are pathological enlargement of the semimembranosus-medial head synovial bursa. Standard radiographs and CT are most helpful when the bursa contains calcific loose bodies. Ultrasound can accurately evaluate the size of Baker's cysts, their proximal and distal extensions, wall and internal synovial vegetations, as well as their relation with adjacent vessels and nerves. Nevertheless, US cannot assess the vast majority of internal disorders causing the cysts. MRI is the method of choice in evaluating internal knee disorders associated with Baker's cyst. It is also an extremely accurate tool in evaluating the size, location, and internal structure of the cysts.

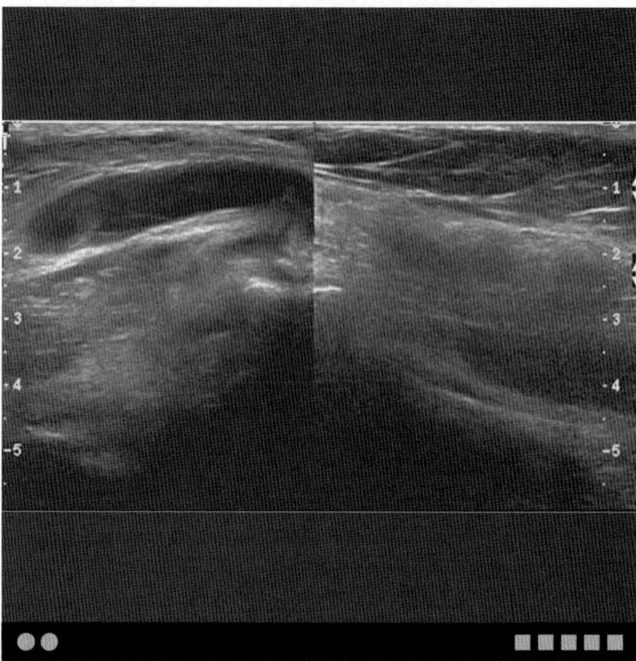

A. Ruptured Baker's cyst: Sagittal split-off US image obtained over the proximal calf shows rupture of the cyst and extension of fluid distally in the proximal part of the soleus muscle.

When subject to excessive internal pressure, Baker's cyst can rupture releasing their contents into the adjacent soft tissues. Patient experiences calf pain and local swelling mimicking thrombophlebitis. US is the method of choice in assessing cyst ruptures since it can detect the cyst and the extravasated fluid and it can evaluate popliteal and calf veins.

PEARLS

- **In adults the SMHSB almost invariably communicates with the knee joint. Knee effusions can cause distension of the bursa and therefore allowing the formation of Baker's cysts.**
- **A ruptured Baker's cyst causes diffusion of the fluid within the soft tissues of the calf producing local swelling and pain**
- **US study detects fluid inside the distal soft tissues secondary to cyst rupture. It also allows an accurate assessment of the popliteal vein**
- **The connection of the cyst with the SMHSB is the major criterion for differentiating Baker's cysts from intramuscular myxoma and other nerve sheath tumors.**

ADDITIONAL IMAGES

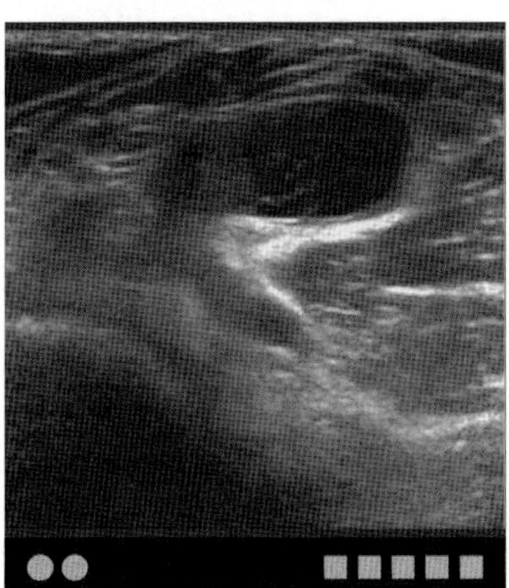

B. Ruptured Baker's cyst: Axial US image obtained over the popliteal space shows the cyst located between the medial head and semimembranosus tendon.

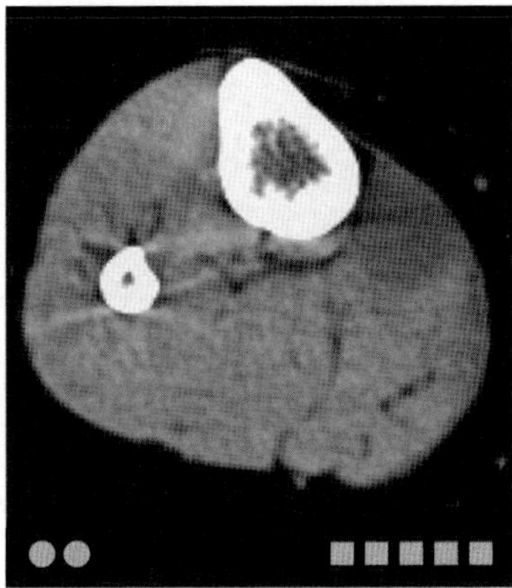

C. Ruptured Baker's cyst: Axial CT shows distal accumulation of fluid as an area of hypodensity located inside the soleus muscle.

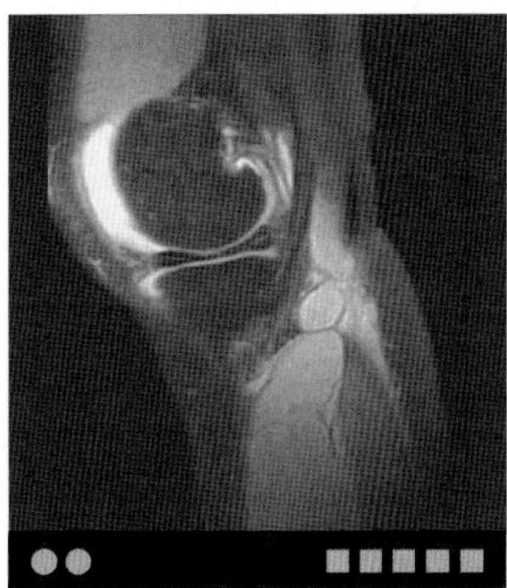

D. Ruptured Baker's cyst: Sagittal T2-weighted image shows the cyst, its distal tear, and presence of intra-articular knee fluid.

DIFFERENTIAL DIAGNOSES IMAGES

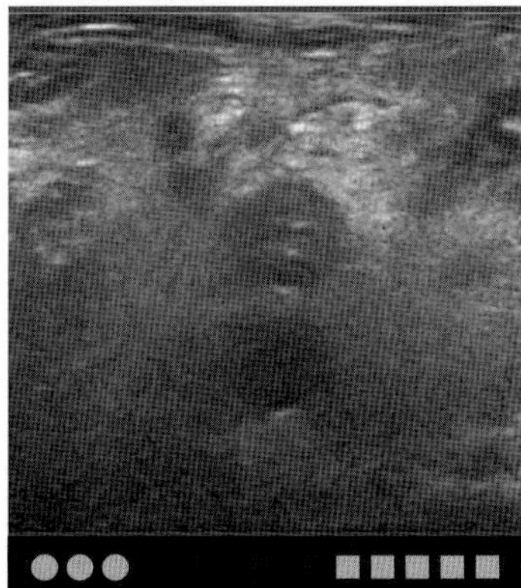

E. Popliteal vein thrombosis: Transverse US image shows an enlarged popliteal vein presenting a thickened wall and internal hypoechoic content corresponding to thrombus. The anterior popliteal artery appears normal.

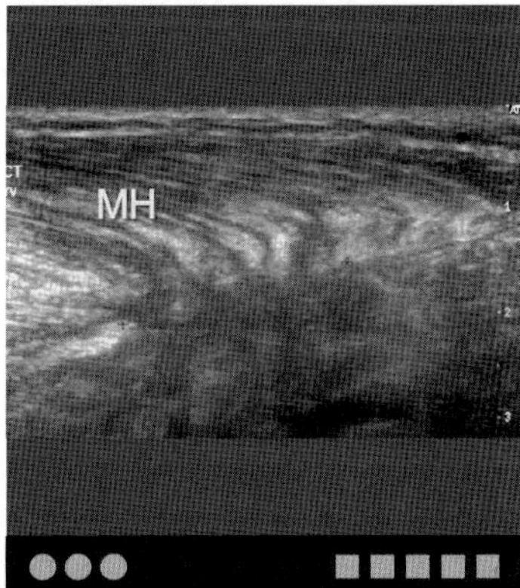

F. Tennis leg: Sagittal US image shows disruption (callipers) of the distal myotendineous junction of the gastrocnemius medial head (MH).

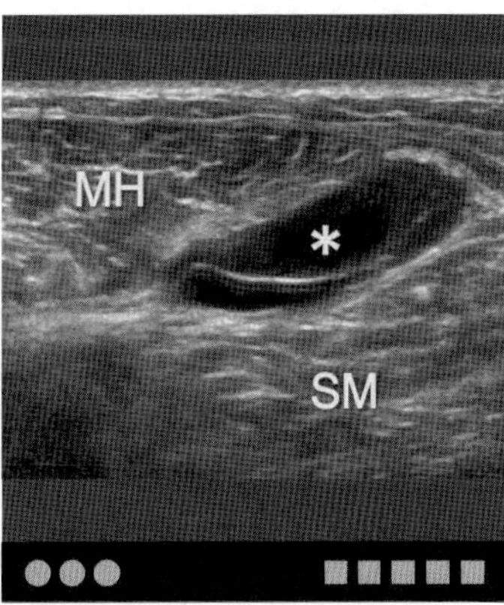

G. Tennis leg: Transverse US image obtained in a different patient shows a hematoma (asterisk) located between the disrupted medial head (MH) and the soleus muscle (SM).

IMAGE KEY

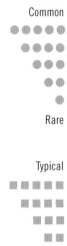

Common

Rare

Typical

Unusual

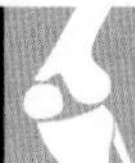

23–12 Lipohemarthrosis of Knee

Sulabha Masih

PRESENTATION

Knee pain, after a fall

FINDINGS

MR images show joint effusion with three layers. Superior is the fatty layer with high signal intensity on T1-weighted and low signal intensity on fat-suppressed images. The middle layer is high signal intensity on T2-weighted and STIR images. The most inferior layer shows low signal intensity on all the sequences.

DIFFERENTIAL DIAGNOSES

- *Pigmented villonodular synovitis (PVNS):* Hemarthrosis may result from synovial inflammation and hemosiderin deposition, with mixed signal intensity.
- *Hemophilia:* Bleeding disorder causing hypertrophic synovial membrane with pannus formation and cartilage erosion.
- *Synovial hemangioma:* It is a rare tumor, common in young females and involves mostly knee. It is an intra-articular mass with villonodular pattern. Usually it is associated with cutaneous and soft tissue hemangiomas.
- *Lipoma arborescens:* Presents as large, villous, frond-like intra-articular fat intensity mass with effusion on MR images.

COMMENTS

The patient is a 54-year-old male, who slipped and fell down causing pain in the knee. Lipohemarthrosis is simply a mixture of fat and blood in the joint cavity following trauma. Lipohemarthrosis of the knee was first described in 1929. Osteochondral defect at the articular surface after trauma causes fat and blood to escape from the marrow space into the joint. Fat is lighter than blood and floats on the blood surface. Nondisplaced fractures of the knee can be sometimes very difficult to diagnose. Lipohemarthrosis can be detected with several different imaging modalities. On lateral radiograph, horizontal beam technique allows the detection of fat fluid level, and on CT, transaxial images provide the diagnosis because of differences in attenuation between the blood and fat. MR imaging is very sensitive in the diagnosis of subtle occult fractures. Sagittal proton density and sagittal and axial fat-suppressed proton density images demonstrate joint effusion with three layers of fluid within the joint. The most superior layer has signal characteristic of fat, which is high in signal intensity on T1-weighted and is low signal intensity on fat-suppressed images. The middle layer is high signal intensity on T2-weighted and STIR images because of serum content. The most inferior layer shows low signal intensity on all the sequences because of hemosiderin. On MR imaging, subtle fracture lines are diagnosed as linear low signal intensity on all the sequences. T2-weighted and STIR images may show bright signal bone marrow edema surrounding the subtle fracture.

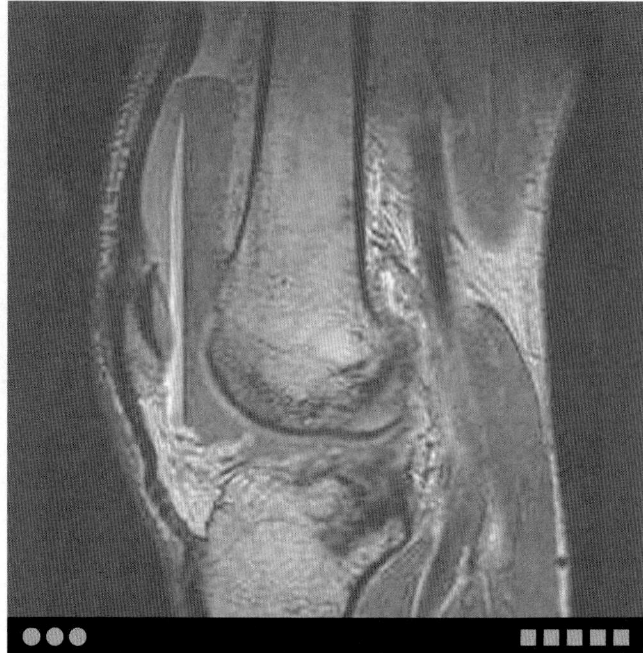

A. Lipohemarthrosis: Sagittal fat-saturated proton density image shows Lipohemarthrosis.

PEARLS

- **Lipohemarthrosis is a mixture of fat and blood in the joint cavity following trauma**
- **On horizontal beam lateral radiograph & transaxial CT, fat fluid level is detected in the joint because of differences in attenuation of fat and fluid**
- **On MR imaging, detection of lipohemarthrosis is very helpful in diagnosing occult intra-articular fractures and subtle fracture lines. T2-weighted and STIR images may demonstrate bright signal bone marrow edema surrounding the fracture.**

ADDITIONAL IMAGES

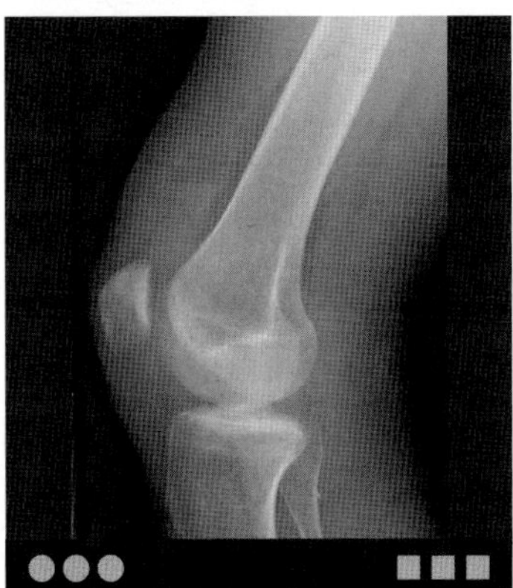

B. Lipohemarthrosis: Lateral standing radiograph demonstrates fat fluid level at suprapatellar region.

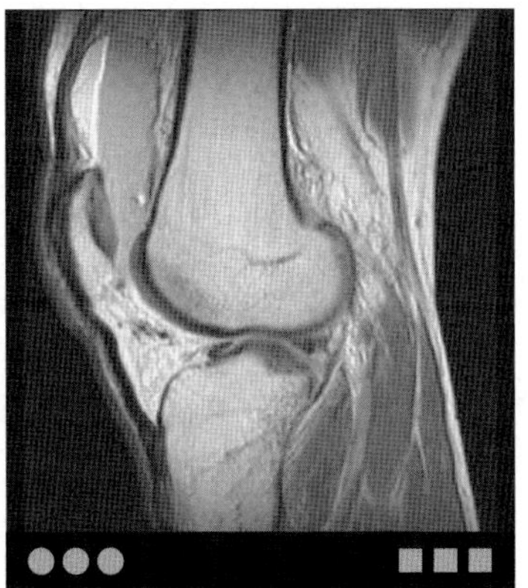

C. Lipohemarthrosis: Sagittal proton density image shows high signal intensity fat and isointense fluid signal.

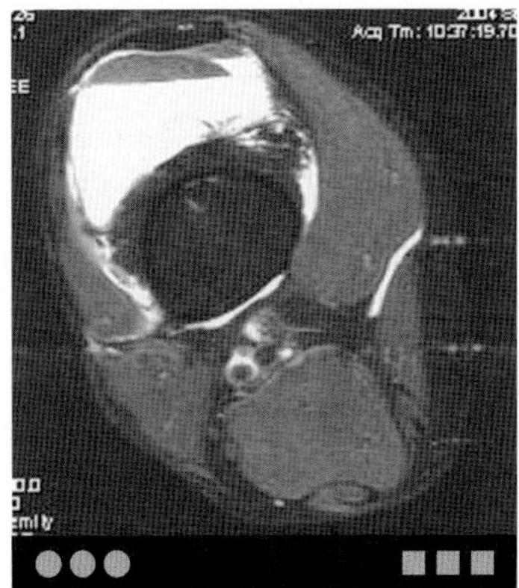

D. Lipohemarthrosis: Axial STIR image demonstrates fat fluid level.

DIFFERENTIAL DIAGNOSES IMAGES

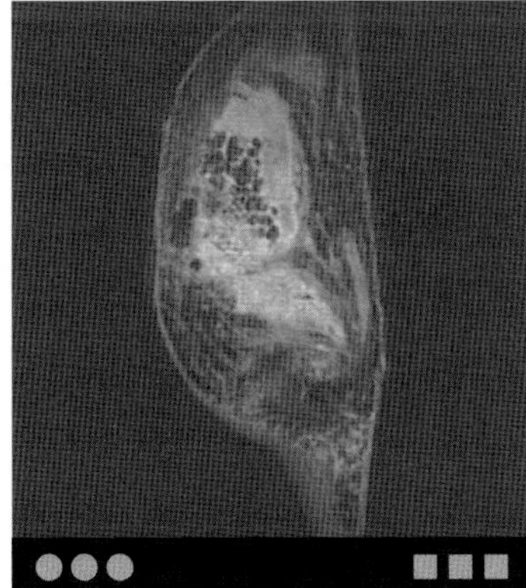

E. Lipoma arborescens: Sagittal STIR image shows low signal frond-like villous fat inside the synovial fluid.

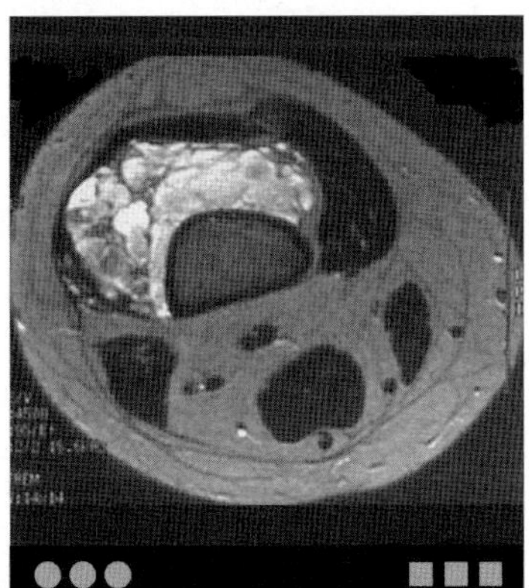

F. Synovial hemangioma: Axial T2-weighted image shows inhomogeneous intra-articular high signal intensity lesion.

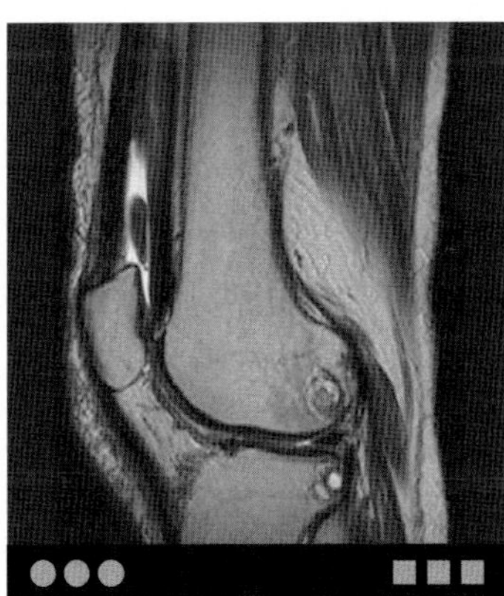

G. PVNS: Sagittal T2-weighted image shows hemarthrosis with intra-articular low signal intensity hemosiderine and bone erosion.

IMAGE KEY

Common

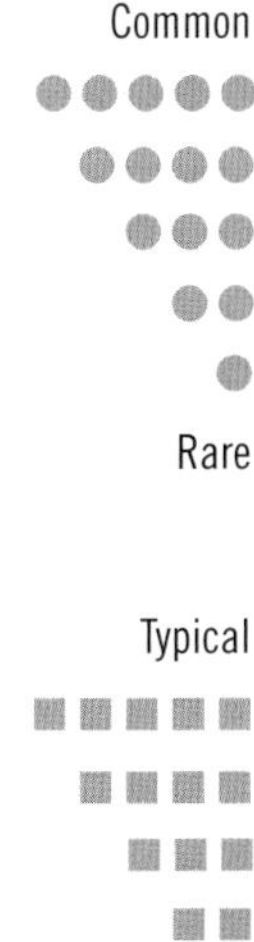

Rare

Typical

Unusual

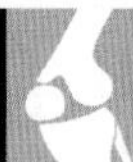

23–13 Anterior Cruciate Ligament Tear with Deep Sulcus Sign

Charles H. Bush

PRESENTATION

Knee pain after twisting injury

FINDINGS

A lateral radiograph of the right knee shows a joint effusion with subtle central depression of the articular cortex of the lateral femoral condyle.

DIFFERENTIAL DIAGNOSES

- *Lateral femoral impaction and contusion:* This impaction may be the result of direct impaction and is isolated. However in osteochondral impaction fracture of the lateral femoral condyle, the deep sulcus sign, resulting from a twisting injury to the knee the anterior cruciate ligament (ACL) tear is noted.
- *Segond fracture:* This avulsion injury of the lateral tibial condyle could be associated with ACL tear and medial meniscal tear.
- *Avulsion of anterior tibial spine:* Detection of this fracture should alert the physician of ACL avulsion.

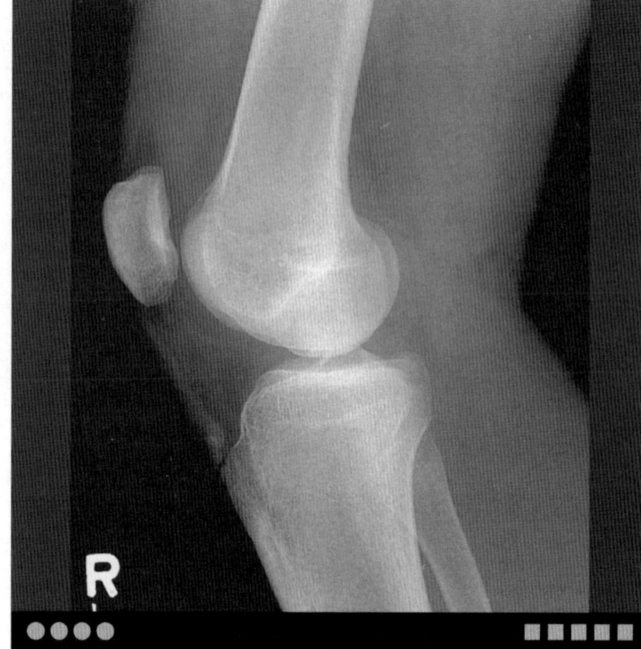

A. ACL tear: Lateral radiograph of the right knee showing the deep sulcus sign of a pivot shift injury to the knee. Note the joint effusion in the suprapatellar recess.

COMMENTS

The patient is a 20-year-old male who injured his right knee after being tackled in a football game. The injury that occurred was a valgus stress to the knee of a planted, fixed lower extremity, with the knee in flexion with external rotation of the tibia or internal rotation of the femur. This is a common mechanism for tears of the anterior cruciate ligament (ACL), which is termed a "pivot shift" injury. The resultant instability allows the tibia to sublux anteriorly with respect to the femur, causing impaction of the lateral femoral condyle on the posterior margin of the lateral tibial condyle. The contusion pattern that results has a high specificity for ACL tears, and is prominently seen on T2-weighted sagittal MR images. Extension of the contusion into the posterior margin of the medial tibial condyle can also be seen, which results from contrecoup forces in the medial compartment occurring after the valgus force has dissipated. Sometimes, the force of the injury is sufficient to cause an osteochondral impaction fracture of the lateral femoral condyle, which can be seen on radiographs as the "deep sulcus" sign. Other sports that can result in a pivot shift injury of the ACL and a deep sulcus sign include skiing, basketball, and gymnastics. The deep sulcus sign should be distinguishable from the shallower, normal lateral condylopatellar sulcus, which is similar in depth on lateral radiograph.

PEARLS

- **Deep sulcus sign is caused by osteochondral impaction fracture of the lateral femoral condyle resulting from a twisting injury to the knee. This is a common mechanism for tears of the anterior cruciate ligament (ACL), which is termed a "pivot shift" injury.**
- **Other signs associated with ACL tear that may be visible on conventional radiographs are a lateral tibial margin fracture (Segond fracture), avulsion of the lateral tibial eminence, and avulsion fracture of the styloid process of the fibular head. The latter, the arcuate sign, also has a high correlation with posterolateral corner injuries.**
- **Meniscal tears (both medial and lateral) occur in 50% to 60% of acute ACL tears.**

ADDITIONAL IMAGES

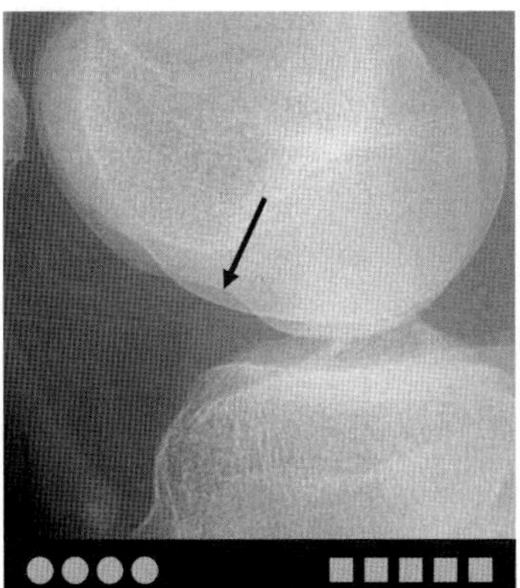

B. ACL tear: Close up lateral radiograph of the knee shows the deep sulcus (arrow).

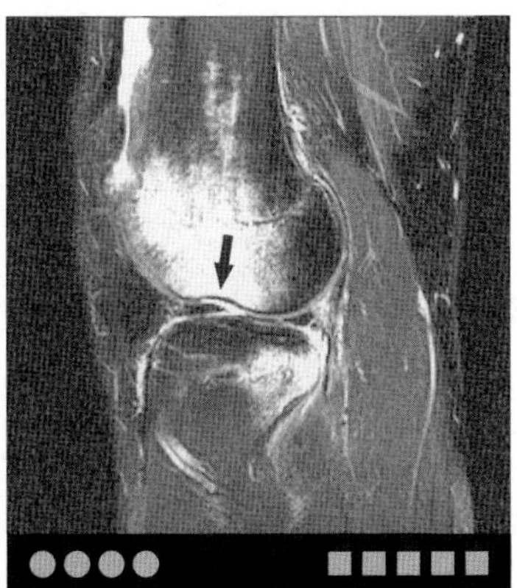

C. ACL tear: A T2-weighted sagittal image with fat suppression shows the deep sulcus (arrow) corresponds to an osteochondral fracture of the lateral condyle, with extensive marrow edema.

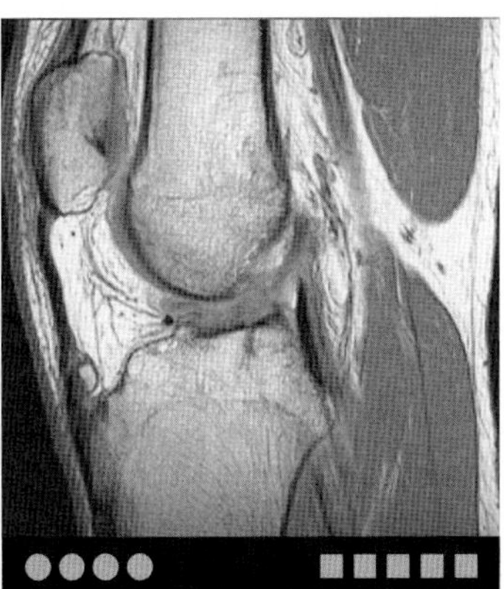

D. ACL tear: A proton density sagittal image more medially shows the disrupted anterior cruciate ligament.

DIFFERENTIAL DIAGNOSES IMAGES

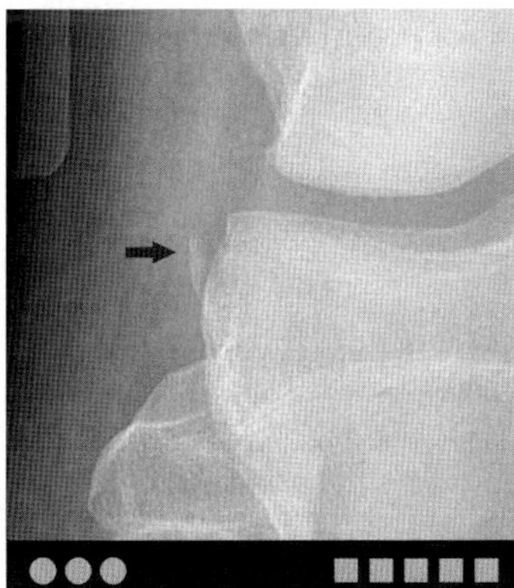

E. Segond fracture: An AP radiograph of the right knee of another patient shows a Segond fracture (arrow).

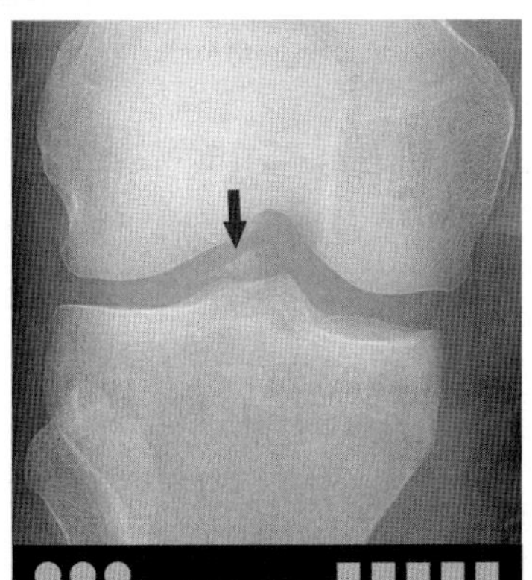

F. Avulsion of anterior tibial spine: An AP radiograph of the right knee of another patient shows an avulsion fracture of the lateral tibial eminence by the anterior cruciate ligament.

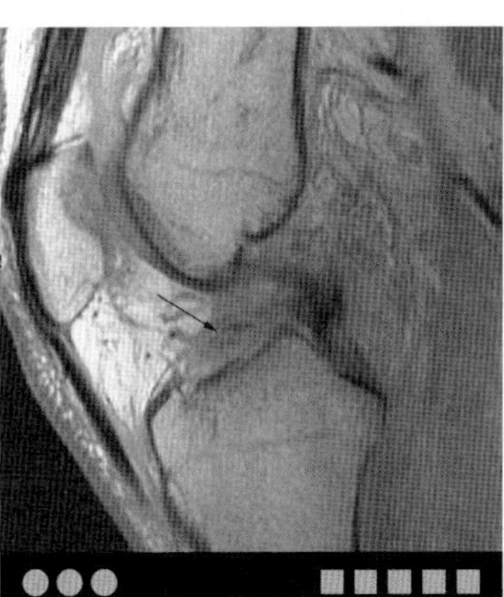

G. Avulsion of anterior tibial spine: Sagittal MRI of the same patient as image F, showing the avulsion fracture (arrow).

IMAGE KEY

Common

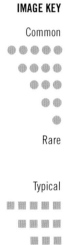

Rare

Typical

Unusual

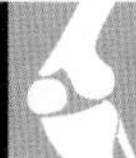

23–14 Cyclops Lesion

Kira Chow

PRESENTATION

Decreased range of motion

FINDINGS

Coronal proton density sequence demonstrates an oval mass in the anterior knee, resembling an eye.

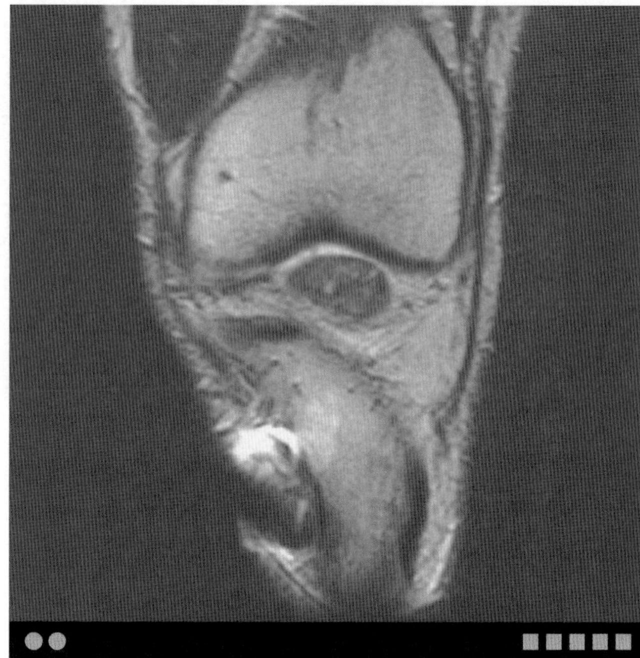

A. Cyclops lesion: Coronal proton density sequence demonstrates an oval mass in the anterior joint space, demonstrating intermediate signal intensity. In this plane, the lesion resembles an eye, thus the name cyclops.

DIFFERENTIAL DIAGNOSES

- *Pigmented villonodular synovitis (PVNS):* Hemosiderin-rich synovial masses most commonly involve the knee. PVNS is characterized by predominantly low signal intensity on all sequences, although T2-weighted sequences can demonstrate variable signal intensity.
- *Synovial osteochondromatosis:* Osseous intra-articular bodies can occur anterior to the anterior cruciate ligament. These usually demonstrate signal intensity similar to marrow with hypointense rim. However, some bodies can be diffusely hypointense similar to osseous cortex.
- *Meniscal cyst:* Meniscal cysts follow the signal characteristics of fluid and are associated with horizontal meniscal tears.

COMMENTS

Anterior cruciate ligament (ACL) reconstruction can be complicated by inflammation and synovial hyperplasia around the ACL graft, leading to formation of fibrosis which may be diffusely present anterior and posterior to the graft. A focal nodule of fibrosis may form, known as a cyclops lesion. This occurs along the anterior aspect of the ACL graft just above the entry site into the tibial tunnel posterior to the Hoffa fat pad. This complication occurs in up to 10% of patients after ACL reconstruction. No association with intercondylar notch width or ACL graft impingement has been documented. One study has shown MRI to be 85% sensitive for these lesions. On MRI, cyclops lesions demonstrate hypointensity on T1-weighted sequences and intermediate or variable signal on proton density and T2-weighted sequences; margin is hypointense. Although these lesions are fibrotic, they can show intermediate signal probably related to inflammation. Cyclops lesions can occur in patients with an ACL tear even without ACL reconstruction. Patients with cyclops lesions present with decreased range of motion, especially loss of extension; typical treatment is arthroscopy for resection of the focal mass. At arthroscopy, the cyclops lesion looks like an "eye," a round fibrous mass with discolored regions of red and blue.

PEARLS

- **Cyclops lesion is a common cause of loss of extension after anterior cruciate ligament reconstruction**
- **Arthroscopic resection is the treatment of choice**
- **Unlike T1/T2 hypointensity typical of fibrous lesions, cyclops lesions show intermediate and variable signal which is thought to be caused by inflammation**

ADDITIONAL IMAGES

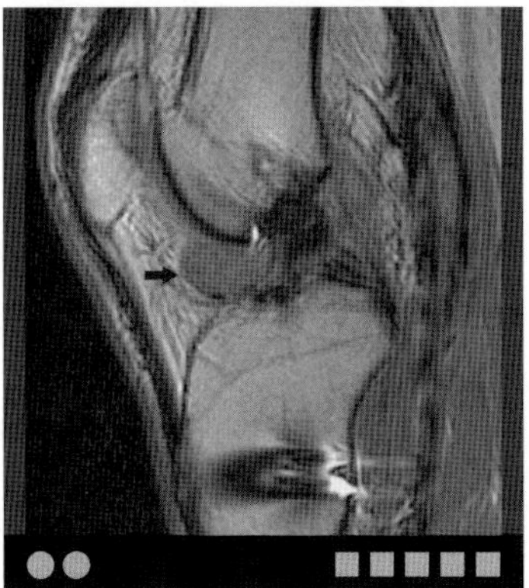

B. Cyclops lesion: Sagittal proton density sequence demonstrates the intermediate signal oval mass along the anterior aspect of the ACL graft, just proximal to the entry site into the tibial plateau (arrow).

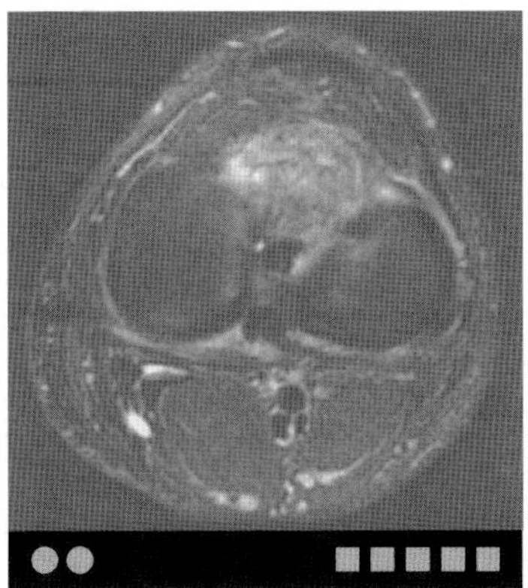

C. Cyclops lesion: Axial T2-weighted sequence shows an intermediate signal rounded focus posterior to the Hoffa fat pad.

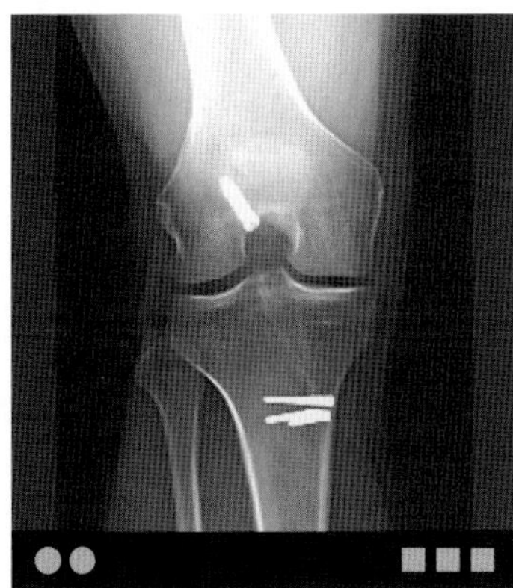

D. Cyclops lesion: Frontal radiograph of the knee shows the typical interference screws of ACL reconstruction.

DIFFERENTIAL DIAGNOSES IMAGES

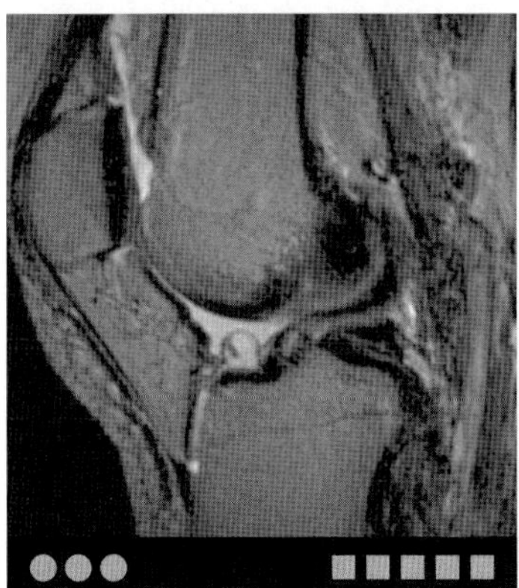

E. Meniscal cyst: T2-weighted sagittal MRI shows a T2 hyperintense round lesion in the anterior joint space.

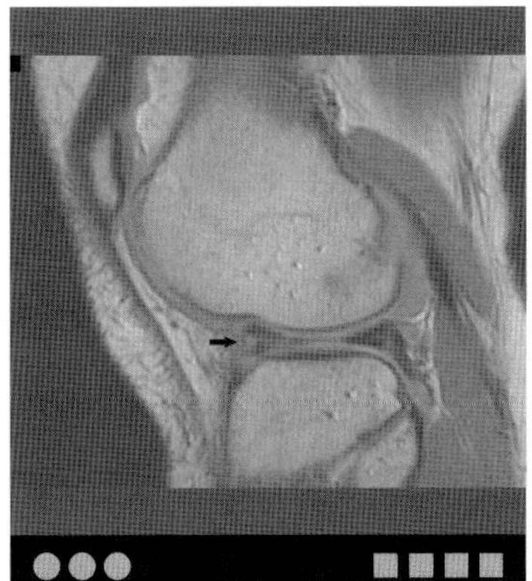

F. Meniscal cyst: Proton density sagittal MRI in the same patient as Figure E demonstrates an anterior horn lateral meniscus horizontal tear communicating with the anterior meniscal cyst (arrow).

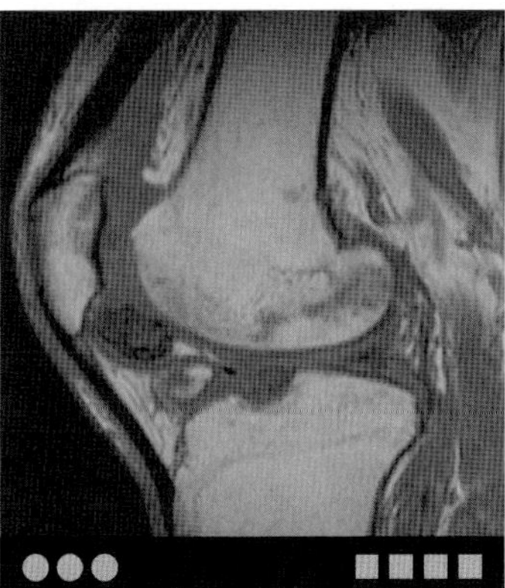

G. Synovial osteochondromatosis: Osteochondral body in the anterior joint space demonstrates internal marrow signal with hypointense periphery representing cortication.

IMAGE KEY

Common

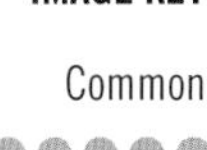

Rare

Typical

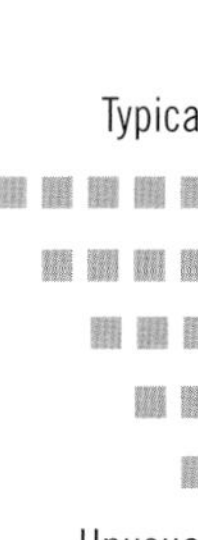

Unusual

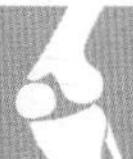

23–15 Anterior Cruciate Ligament Reconstruction Graft Tear

Eli J. Bendavid

PRESENTATION

Instability, status-post anterior cruciate ligament (ACL) reconstruction

FINDINGS

MRI demonstrates a previous ACL reconstruction. Low to intermediate signal intensity ACL graft is not identified.

DIFFERENTIAL DIAGNOSES

- *Normal ACL reconstruction:* Normal low to intermediate signal intensity ACL reconstruction graft is identified within the intercondylar notch.
- *ACL ganglion cyst:* A cystic lesion is often noted adjacent to ACL.
- *PCL ganglion cyst:* A cystic lesion is seen adjacent to posterior cruciate ligament (PCL).
- *PCL tear:* Discontinuity of the PCL is noted.

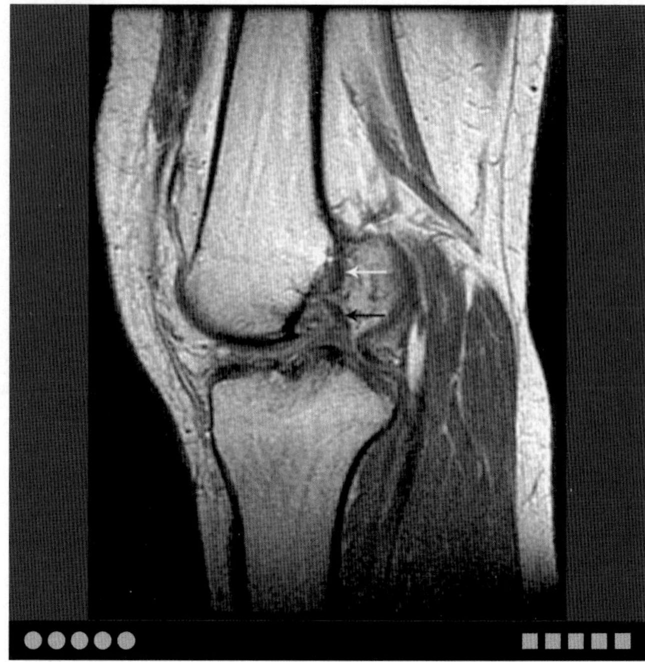

A. ACL reconstruction graft tear: Sagittal proton density image shows a short proximal remnant of the torn ACL reconstruction graft (white arrow). The intact PCL is partially visualized (black arrow).

COMMENTS

The patient is a 36-year-old female with a history of instability, following a previous anterior cruciate ligament (ACL) reconstruction. Distal femoral and proximal tibial interference screw artifact is noted. Expected low to intermediate signal intensity ACL reconstruction graft is only identified at the end of the femoral interference screw, indicative of a graft tear. Common sources for an ACL graft include patellar tendon autograft, semi-tendinosis tendon autograft, or allograft. The most common underlying cause of ACL graft failure is improper tunnel and screw placement, which may lead to graft impingement and instability. Improper screw placement may be readily noted radiographically prior to the occurrence of a tear. Other technical causes predisposing to tear include fixation failure, intrinsic graft failure secondary to improper selection, or improper graft tensioning. Associated injury to the remaining ligaments of the knee may occur in conjunction with the initial ACL injury. Laxity or tear of these ligaments may predispose to graft failure. Acute trauma may be an independent factor for tear, or contribute to the mechanisms listed above. Graft tears most commonly occur at either end of their attachment. Failed ACL reconstructions are typically re-treated surgically, with residual fiber removal, scar debridement, possible re-drilling and graft placement, and treatment of concomitant ligament injuries. Short of a tear, other causes for reconstruction failure include biological factors (infection or allograft rejection) or arthrofibrosis. Postoperative arthrofibrosis consists of scar extension to Hoffa's fat pad, and results in decreased range of motion.

PEARLS

- **Absence of low to intermediate signal intensity graft fibers within the intercondylar notch**
- **Instability frequently noted on physical examination**
- **Improper reconstruction screw placement or graft impingement may be noted prior to a graft tear**
- **Arthrofibrosis may be an associated finding**
- **Sagittal imaging plane is most sensitive for diagnosis**

ADDITIONAL IMAGES

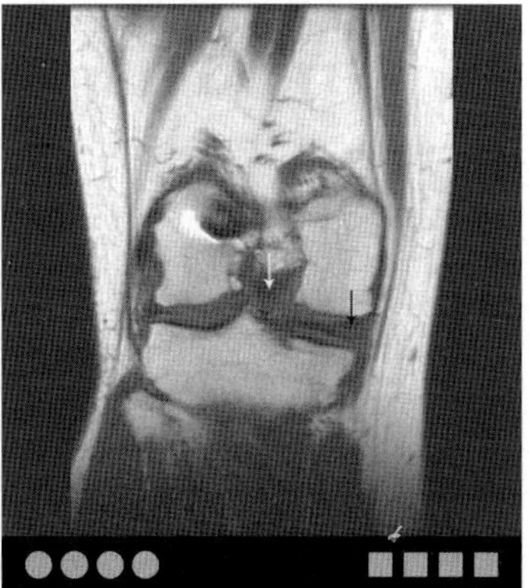

B. ACL reconstruction graft tear: Coronal T1 image demonstrates absence of the reconstruction graft within the intercondylar notch (white arrow). A medial meniscus tear is partially visualized (black).

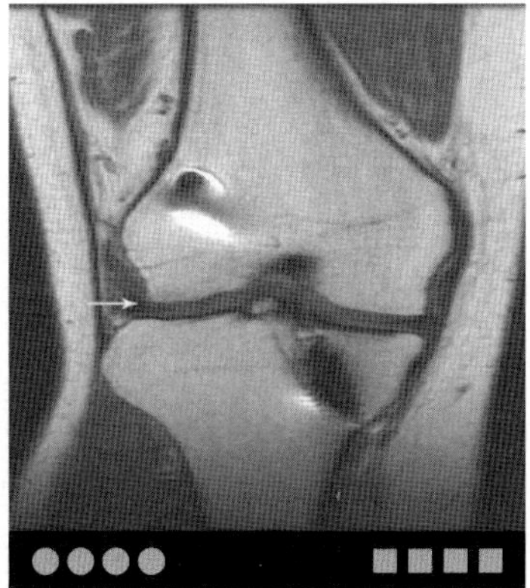

C. ACL reconstruction graft tear: Coronal T1 image shows the distal femoral and proximal tibial interference screw artifacts. A lateral meniscus tear is partially visualized (arrow).

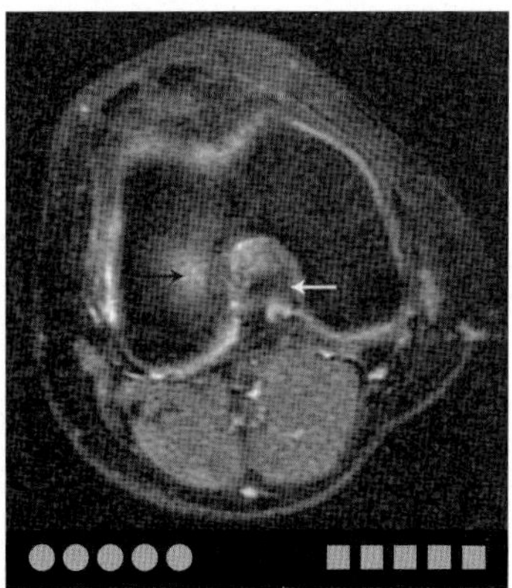

D. ACL reconstruction graft tear: Axial fat-saturated proton density image demonstrates absence of reconstruction graft within the intercondylar notch. The PCL (white arrow) and artifact from the femoral interference screw (black arrow) are partially visualized.

DIFFERENTIAL DIAGNOSES IMAGES

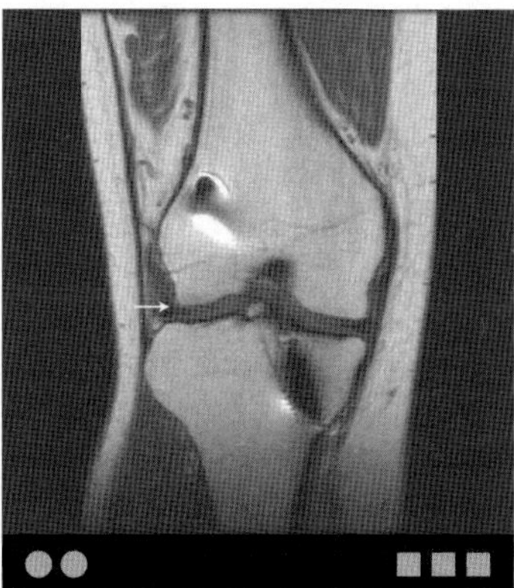

E. Anterior cruciate ligament ganglia: Coronal T2-weighted image shows septated ganglion at femoral insertion (arrow).

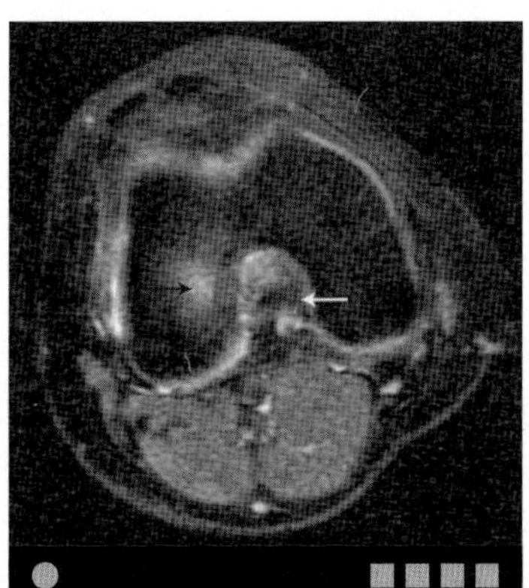

F. Ganglion of the posterior cruciate ligament: Axial fat saturation PD MR image shows the CLG as a well-delimited septated cystic lesion located inside the femoral notch.

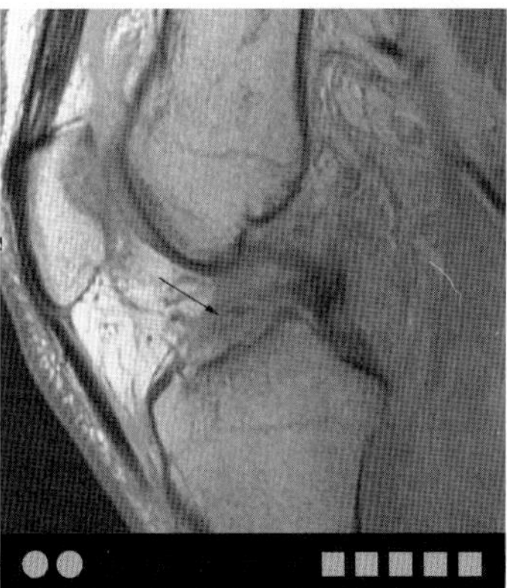

G. Posterior cruciate ligament tear: Sagittal proton density FSE image demonstrates a complete rupture (arrow) of the posterior cruciate ligament.

IMAGE KEY

Common

Rare

Typical

Unusual

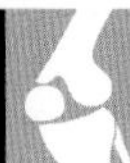

23–16 Posterior Cruciate Ligament Tear

Ayodale Odulate and Piran Aliabadi

PRESENTATION

Knee pain following fall on bended knee

FINDINGS

MRI shows a truncated, wavy, and thickened ligament with abnormal signal intensity.

DIFFERENTIAL DIAGNOSES

- *Magic angle phenomenon:* An imaging artifact when the ligament lies at 55 degrees to the main magnetic field. This can be eliminated by viewing the ligament with alternative planes of imaging.
- *Posterior cruciate ligament (PCL) avulsion fracture:* This ligament rarely avulses removing a piece of bone from the insertion site at posterior tibia.
- *Bucket handle tear of the medial meniscus:* The entirety of the PCL is intact with normal morphology and signal intensity with absence of the medial portion of the medial meniscus.
- *Eosinophilic degeneration:* Often in elderly patients with abnormal signal intensity on T1-weighted images that have normal signal intensity on T2-weighted imaging sequences.

COMMENTS

The patient is a 25-year-old male who sustained an injury to the knee. Hyperflexion injuries such as falling on bended knees or motor vehicle accidents are common causes of posterior cruciate ligament (PCL) injuries. An isolated injury of the PCL is uncommon and associated major knee injuries often involve the ACL, medial meniscus, meniscofemoral ligaments, and collateral ligaments. Physical examination demonstrates a positive posterior Drawer test. Isolated PCL injuries are treated conservatively with immobilization and antisteroidal medications. Chronic untreated PCL rupture may lead to patellofemoral arthrosis because of posterior dislocation of the tibia with abnormal tracking of the patella. MRI is the imaging modality of choice and demonstrates abnormally thickened ligament with disrupted fibers and increased signal intensity on fluid sensitive sequences in the acute stage. A normal ligament has hypointense signal on all imaging sequences. The transverse diameter of a normal PCL is 13 mm, slightly larger than the ACL. The PCL is composed of two bands, the larger stronger anterolateral and posteromedial bands. Grade I sprain represents microtears or stretching with preservation of the outer ligament. Grade II sprain represents partial tear possibly involving one margin with intact fibers. Grade III tear represents a complete tear with both margins of the ligament showing abnormal signal intensity. Plain radiographs may show posterior subluxation of the tibia on the lateral view. Additionally, avulsion fractures of the femur and tibia may be seen.

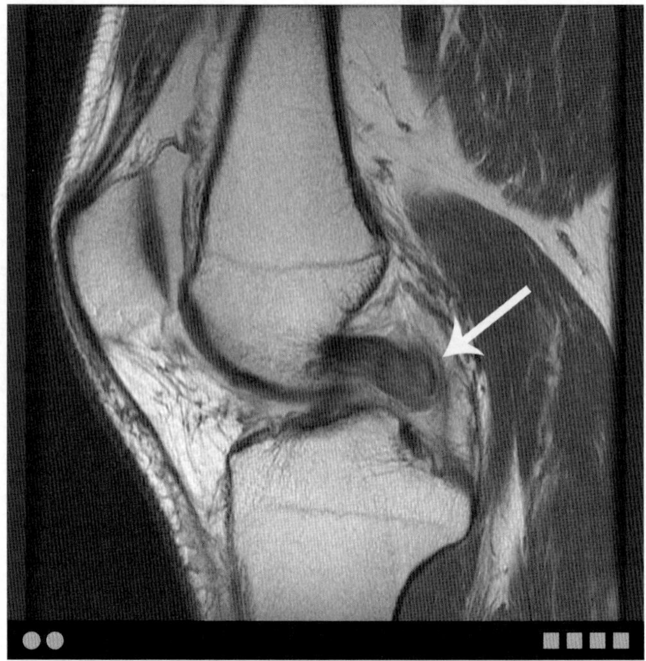

A. PCL tear: Sagittal proton density FSE image demonstrates a complete rupture (arrow) of the posterior cruciate ligament.

PEARLS

- **High association with other injuries such as ACL, medial meniscus, and collateral ligament injuries in dashboard injuries**
- **Can be an isolated injury in hyperflexion injuries such as fall on bended knees**
- **MRI demonstrates abnormally thickened ligament with abnormally increased signal**
- **Suspect PCL injury with posterior subluxation of the femur on plain radiographs**

ADDITIONAL IMAGES

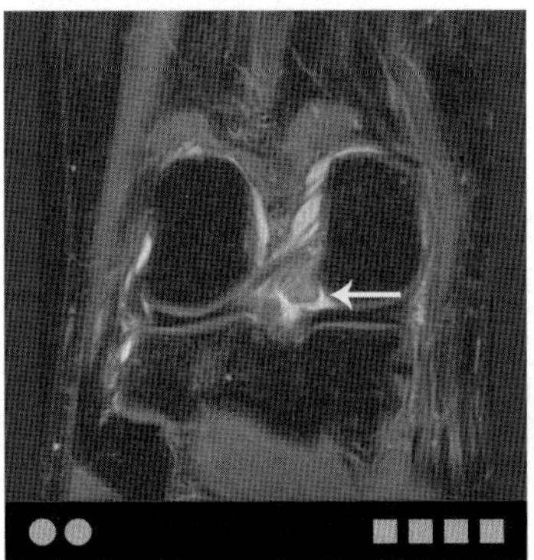

B. PCL tear: Coronal STIR image shows truncation, bulbous enlargement, and abnormal increased signal intensity of the PCL (arrow).

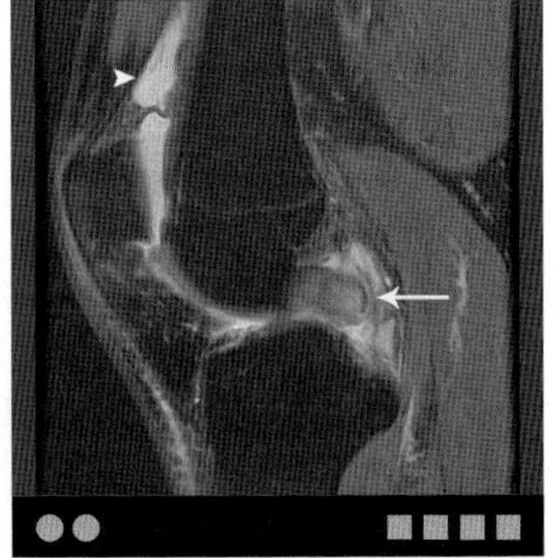

C. PCL tear: Sagittal proton density fat-saturated image shows increased signal intensity of the PCL with a bulbous appearance of the margin (arrow) and absence of the origin. A joint effusion is also seen (arrowhead).

DIFFERENTIAL DIAGNOSES IMAGES

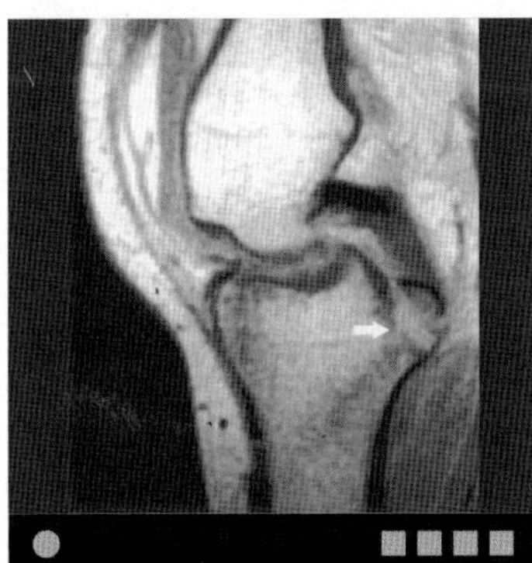

D. Avulsion fracture of PCL: Sagittal spin echo T2-weighted image shows avulsion fracture of PCL from attachment site of posterior tibia (arrow).

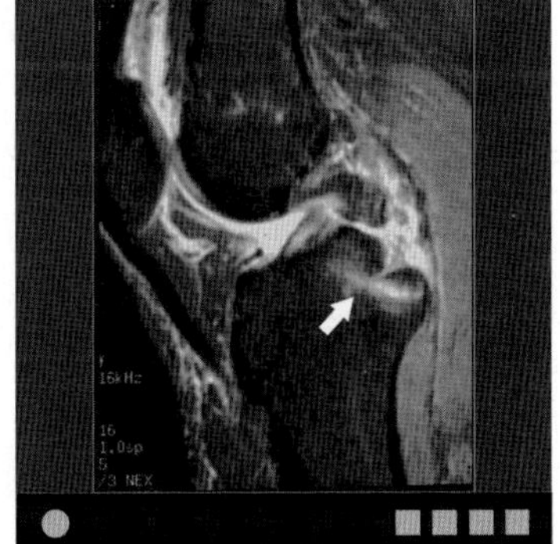

E. Avulsion fracture of PCL: Sagittal STIR image in another patient shows avulsion fracture of PCL from attachment site of posterior tibia (arrow).

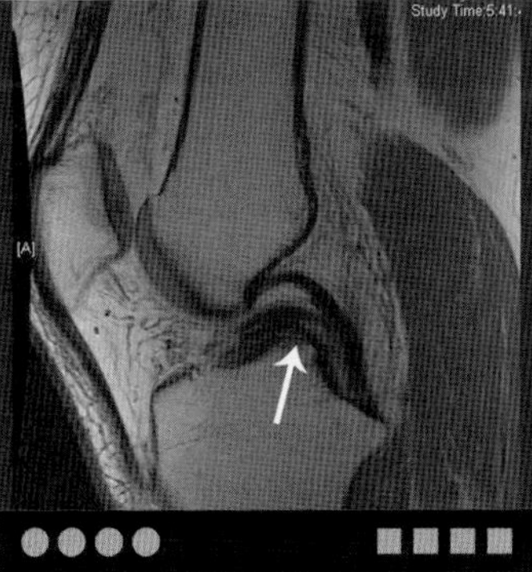

F. Bucket handle tear: Sagittal proton density fat-saturated image, a normal intact PCL is posterior to the flipped medial meniscal fragment (arrow). This may be confused for a tear of the PCL.

IMAGE KEY

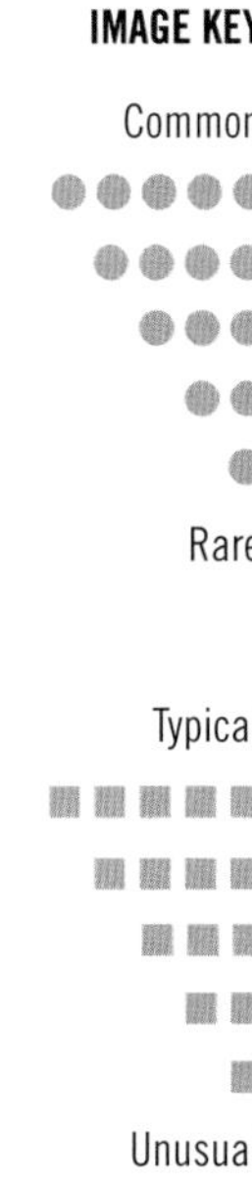

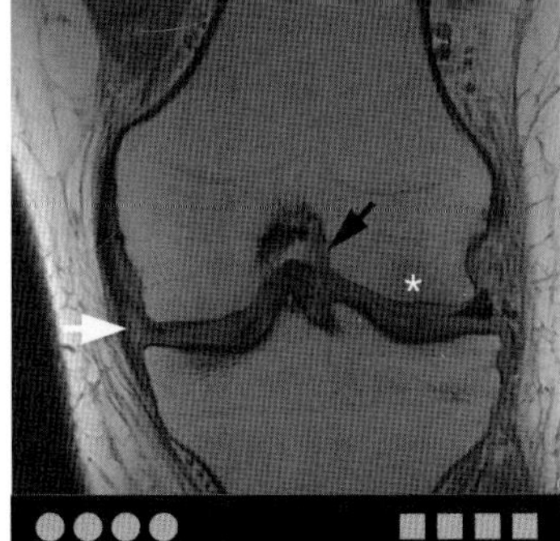

G. Bucket handle tear: Coronal T1-weighted image shows absence of the medial meniscus (white arrow) with the meniscal fragment in the intercondylar notch (black arrow). Edema of the lateral femoral condyle represents a bone contusion (asterisk).

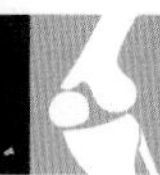

23–17 Complete Medial Collateral Ligament Tear

Peyman Borghei and John Shin

PRESENTATION

Left knee pain

FINDINGS

Coronal image shows complete disruption of superficial a deep layers of MCL.

DIFFERENTIAL DIAGNOSES

- *Medial collateral ligament strain:* A slight irregularity or thickening may be evident, often associated with edema but there is no discontinuity.
- *Partial medical collateral ligament tear:* In partial tears discontinuity of some ligamentous fibers or separation of fibers from adjacent cortical bone may be evident.
- *Medial collateral ligament bursitis:* It is an inflammation of the bursa between the superficial and the deep fibers of the medial collateral ligament.

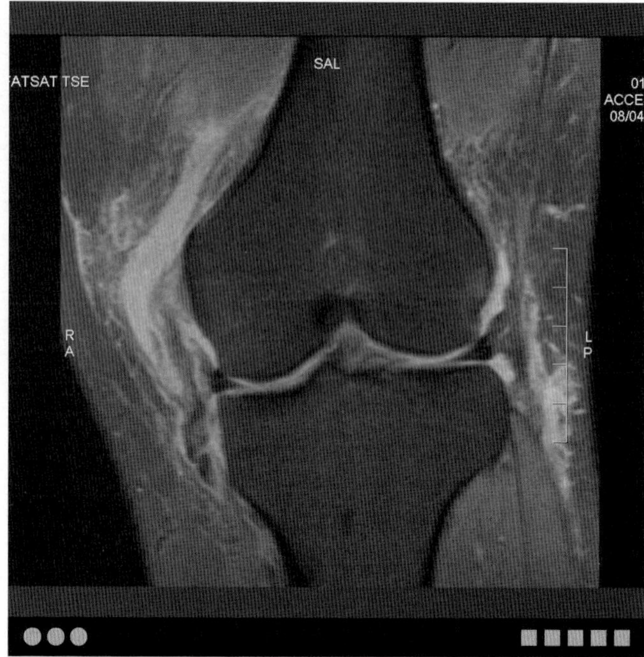

A. Complete MCL tear: Coronal PD FS image of the left knee shows marked irregularity and edema of MCL. The MCL is wavy and completely disrupted.

COMMENTS

The patient is a 19-year-old male with medial collateral ligament (MCL) tear of the left knee after being struck by a car in an auto versus pedestrian accident. He also suffered a tear of his anterior cruciate ligament (ACL). The MCL is composed of superficial and deep fibers; the superficial extends from the medial femoral condyle to the medial aspect of the tibia. The deep fibers reinforce the knee joint capsule beneath the superficial portion that attaches to medial meniscus. The biomechanic of MCL injury is usually valgus stress with external rotation. There is a bursa between the superficial and deep fibers of MCL, which can be seen on coronal MRI views at the level of joint and should not be mistaken with small tears in the ligament. Complete MCL tear is usually associated with tears in ACL and medial meniscus (O' Donahue's triad) and contusion of the lateral femoral condyle and tibial plateau. MCL tears may be associated with extensive joint effusion. On MRI, a ruptured MCL appears thickened or completely disrupted and surrounded by edema (intermediate signal on T1-weighted and high signal on T2-weighted images). In the complete tears of MCL the superficial fibers are always completely torn; however, the deep fibers may be normal. The primary signs of an acutely torn ACL on MRI include poor or nonvisualization, focal or diffuse increased signal intensity within the ligament, abrupt angulation, and wavy contour of this ligament.

PEARLS

- **Medial collateral ligament is consisted of superficial and deep fibers that are separated by a bursa at the level of knee joint. Care should be taken not to mistake this bursa with small tears.**
- **A ruptured MCL on MRI appears thickened or completely disrupted, which is surrounded by edema (intermediate signal on T1-weighted and high signal on T2-weighted images).**
- **The primary signs of a torn ACL on MRI include poor or nonvisualization, focal or diffuse increased signal intensity within the ligament, abrupt angulation, and wavy contour of the ligament.**

ADDITIONAL IMAGES

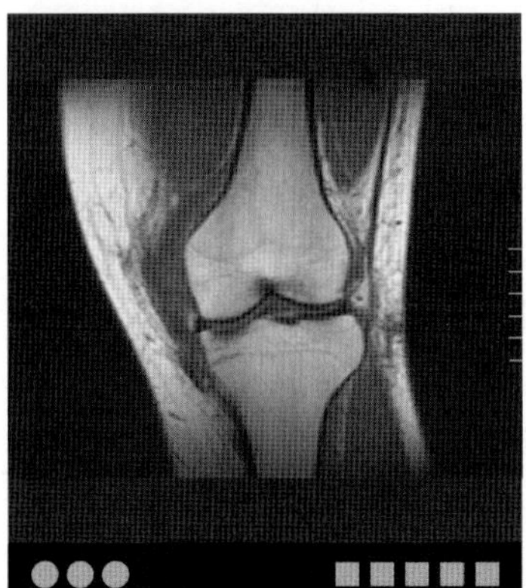

B. Complete MCL tear: Coronal T1-weighted image of the knee shows a wide area of low signal intensity at the region of MCL, which is consistent with edema and hemorrhage caused by complete tear.

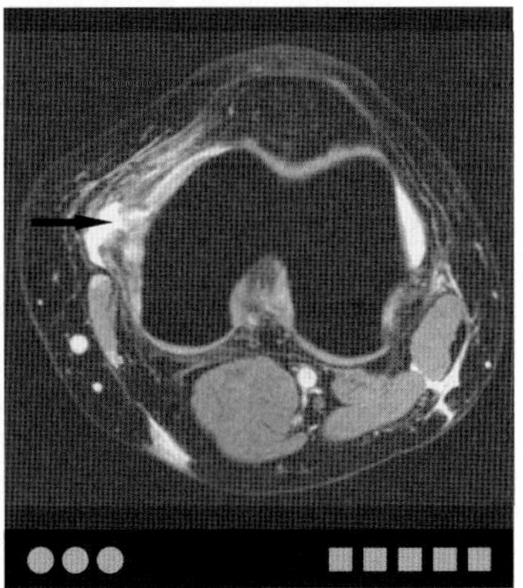

C. Complete MCL tear: Axial T2-weighted image of the left knee shows fluid signal around the MCL because of complete rupture. Note disrupted fragment of MCL in the blood pool (arrow).

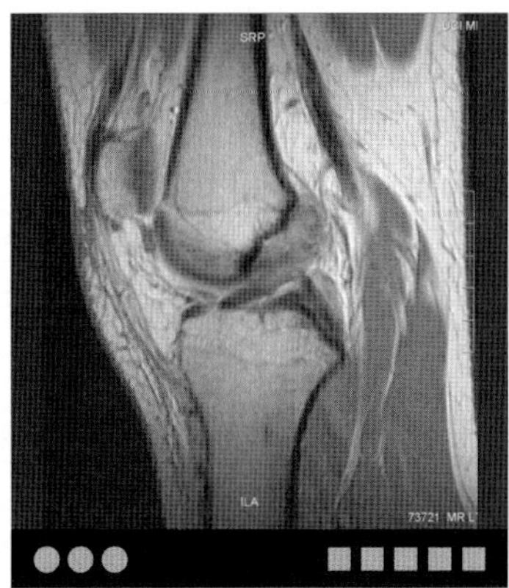

D. Complete MCL tear: Sagittal proton density image shows associated tear of the ACL.

DIFFERENTIAL DIAGNOSES IMAGES

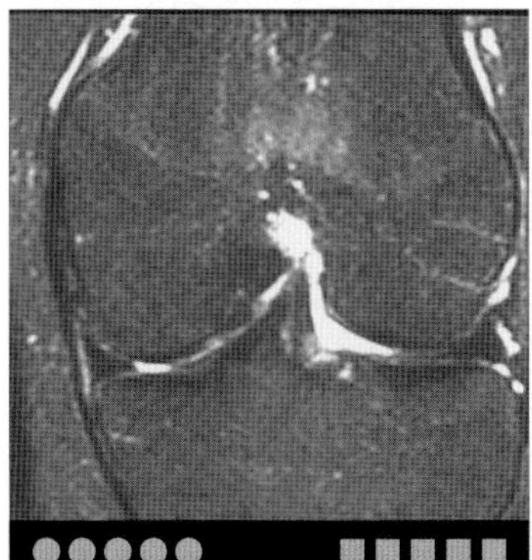

E. Normal MCL: Coronal T2-weighted FS image of the knee for comparison shows normal MCL.

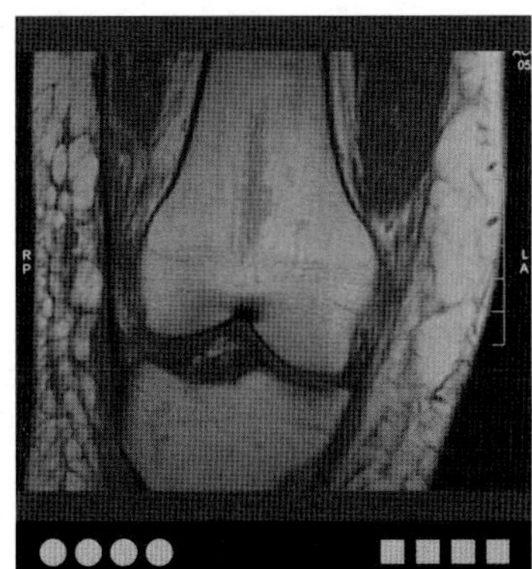

F. Partial MCL tear: Coronal T1-weighted image shows partial tear of the deep fibers of MCL.

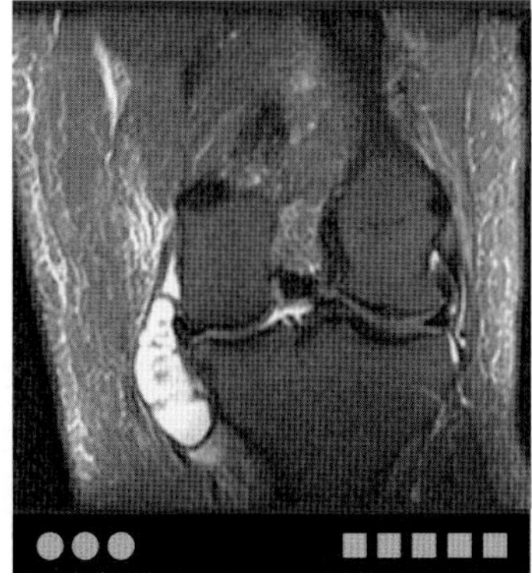

G. MCL bursitis: Coronal T2-weighted FS image shows enlargement of MCL bursa containing fluid.

IMAGE KEY

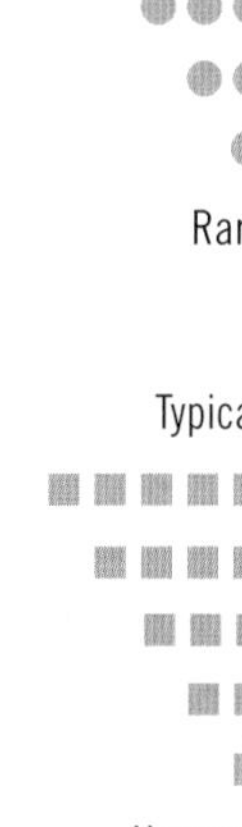

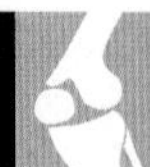

23–18 Sonographic Appearance of Medial Collateral Ligament

Mélanie Morel, Nathalie Boutry, and Anne Cotten

PRESENTATION

Knee injury, medial knee pain, and swelling

FINDINGS

Sonography shows a hypoechoic thickening of the proximal medial collateral ligament (grade 2).

DIFFERENTIAL DIAGNOSES

- *Medial collateral ligament bursitis:* The fluid collection is deep to the medial collateral ligament, extending above and below the medial joint line.
- *Medial capsulomeniscal separation:* This is diagnosed when fluid is completely interposed between the meniscus and the capsule.
- *Medial parameniscal cyst:* MRI often shows a connection between the fluid parameniscal collection and a horizontal tear of the posterior horn of the medial meniscus.
- *Pes anserinus bursitis:* Imaging shows a fluid collection located medially, just inferior to the joint line, beneath the pes anserine tendons (sartorius, gracilis, and semitendinosus tendons) against the distal portion of the tibial collateral ligament and the medial tibial condyle.
- *Medial retinaculum injury:* This may be associated with MCL sprain. In this case, the femoral attachment of the retinaculum is hypoechoic, and of high signal intensity on T2-weighted images.

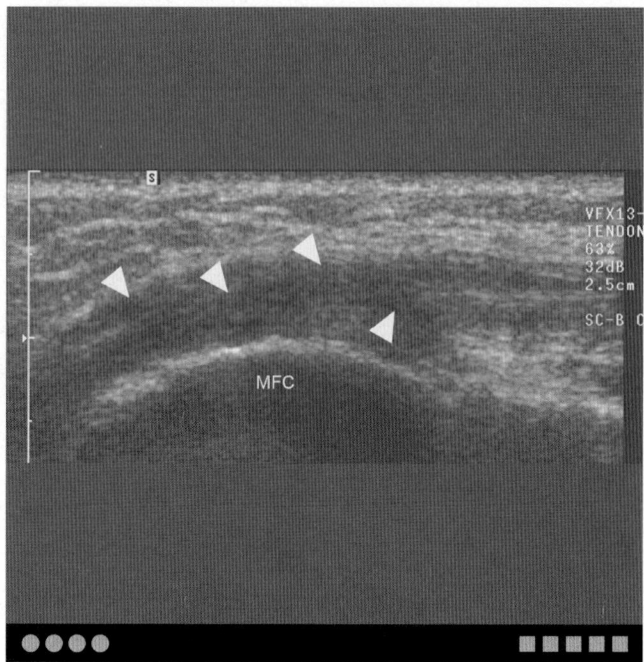

A. Partial tear of the MCL (grade 2): Longitudinal sonogram demonstrates focal hypoechoic areas (arrows) at the proximal insertion of the MCL (MFC, medial femoral condyle). The proximal ligament is thickened and some fibers remain intact.

COMMENTS

This is the case of a 30-year-old man with a history of acute pain along the medial side of the knee while going sledging, diagnosed as a partial tear of the medial collateral ligament (MCL). Injury to the MCL occurs with a valgus stress to a flexed knee. It may be associated with other injuries in the knee, especially tears of anterior cruciate ligament and posterior horn of the medial meniscus. Proximal MCL tear is more frequent than distal MCL lesion. Grade 1 tear (sprain) is defined by subcutaneous edema. Sonogram exhibits an ill-defined hypoechoic subcutaneous area. MRI shows increased signal intensity in the soft-tissue adjacent to the MCL, with a normal appearing ligament. Grade 2 (partial tear) is present when there is partial ligament disruption, and/or internal increased signal intensity on T2-weighted images. Sonography shows a thickened ligament with hypoechoic areas because of partial rupture, but with some intact fibers. Grade 3 represents a complete ligament tear. Bone edema can be detected in the femoral condyles and tibial plateaus on MR images. Pellegrini–Stieda syndrome is a sequela of MCL sprain and is demonstrated on a knee radiograph: a layer of ossification or calcification is seen along the proximal attachment of the ligament. US study can also detect this lesion.

PEARLS

- **MCL injuries are caused by valgus stress to a flexed knee.**
- **Other injuries (anterior cruciate ligament, posterior horn of the medial meniscus) can be associated.**
- **3 grades (sprain, partial tear, complete tear) can be described on US and MRI studies.**

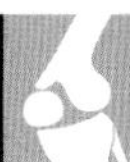

ADDITIONAL IMAGES

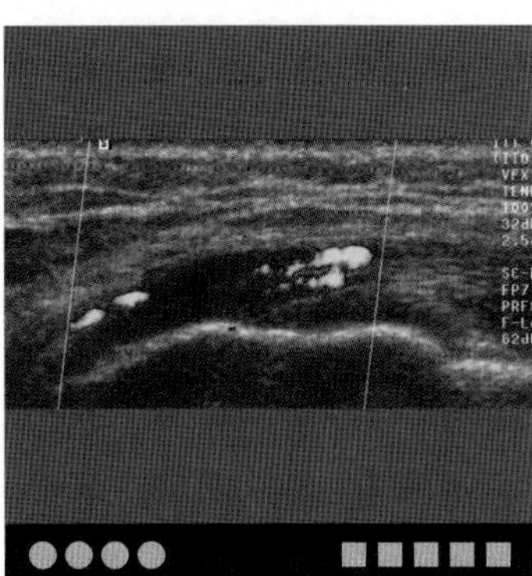

B. Partial tear of the MCL (grade 2): Doppler ultrasound exhibits hyperemia at the proximal insertion of the thickened MCL.

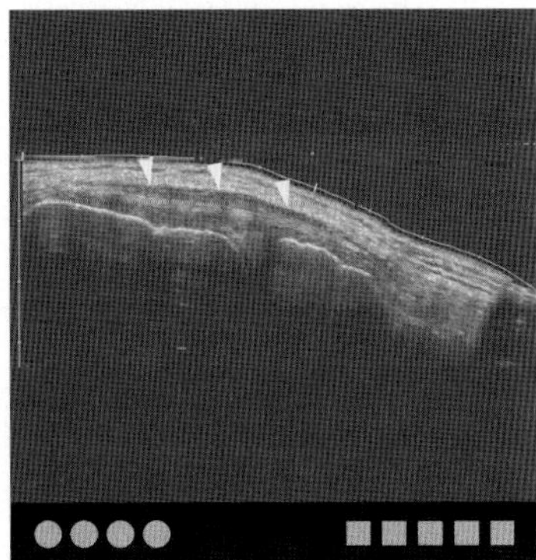

C. Sprain of the MCL (grade 1): Longitudinal sonogram shows hypoechoic soft-tissue edema (arrowheads) along the MCL, without any hypoechoic area within the ligament.

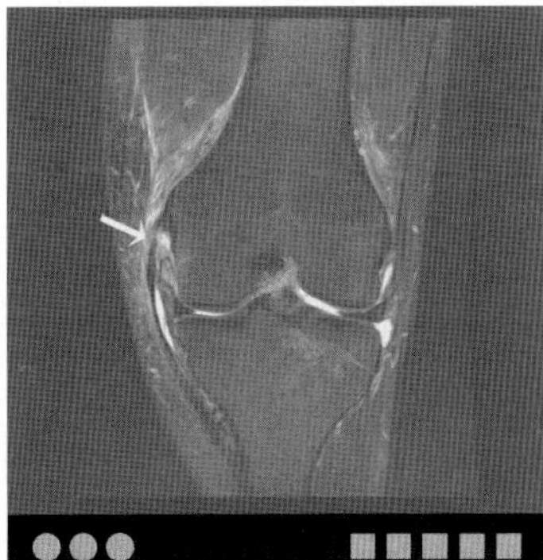

D. Complete tear of the MCL (grade 3): Coronal T2-weighted fat-saturated MR image shows complete fiber discontinuity of the MCL (arrow) next to its proximal insertion.

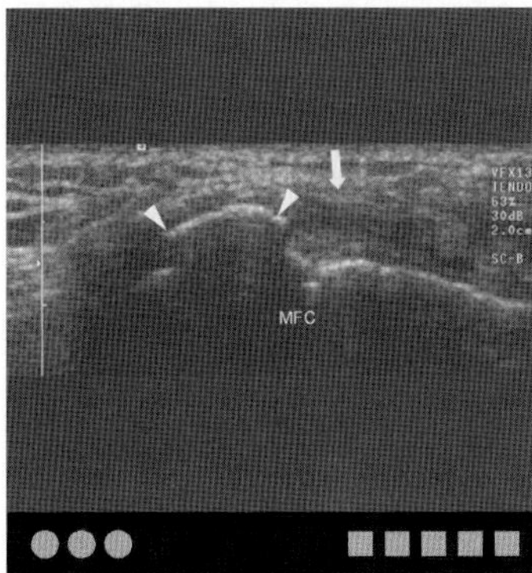

E. Pellegrini–Stieda syndrome: Hyperechoic calcification with posterior attenuation (arrowheads) is found at the insertion of the MCL (arrow) on the medial femoral condyle (MFC).

IMAGE KEY

Common

Rare

Typical

Unusual

DIFFERENTIAL DIAGNOSES IMAGES

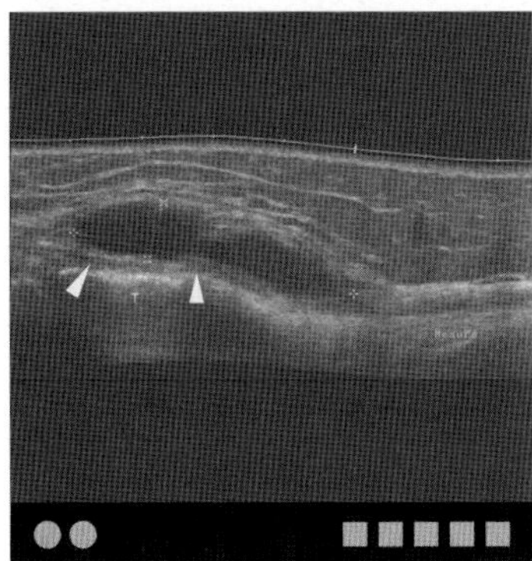

F. Medial collateral ligament bursitis: Longitudinal sonogram reveals a cystic lobulated lesion adjacent to the MCL (arrowheads).

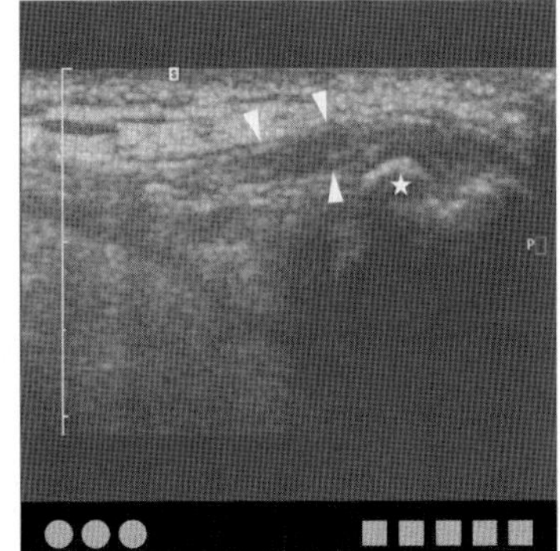

G. Medial retinaculum injury: Axial sonogram shows a hypoechoic thickening of the patellar insertion of the medial retinaculum (arrowheads). Note the bone avulsion of the medial aspect of the patella (star; P).

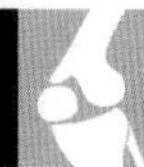

23–19 Pellegrini Stieda Disease

Eli J. Bendavid

PRESENTATION

Chronic pain

FINDINGS

MRI demonstrates clustered signal voids along the expected course of the proximal medial collateral ligament.

DIFFERENTIAL DIAGNOSES

- *Loose body:* Ossified loose bodies have low T1 and T2 signals, but are located within the joint space.
- *Pigmented villonodular synovitis (PVNS):* Hemosiderin deposition results in foci of decreased T1 and T2 signal intensity. As the name indicates, findings are found along the synovium of the joint. Presentation along the tendon sheaths of the large joints is rare.
- *Complete tear of MCL:* There is total disruption of this ligament, which is replaced by fluid.
- *Partial tear of MCL:* Interruption of the fibers is not complete. Some fibers are torn and the rest are intact.
- *Pes anserine bursitis:* Localized fluid collection is noted deep to the common "goose foot" junction of the gracilis, sartorius, and semitendinous tendons.

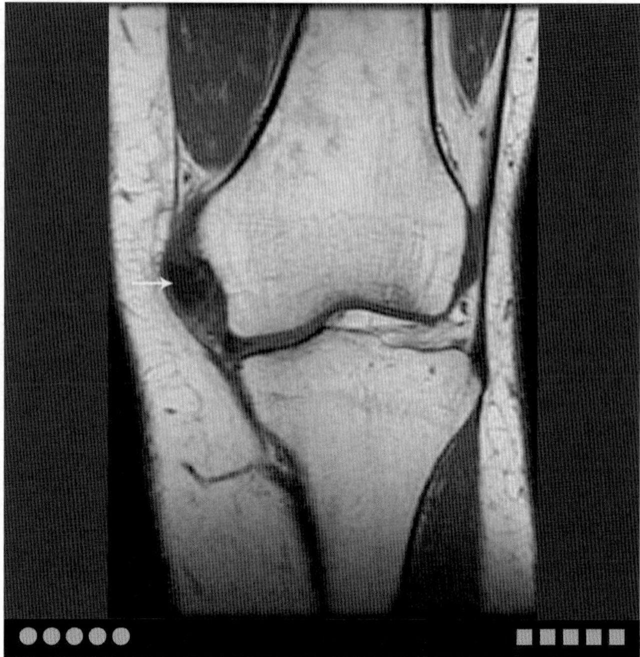

A. Pellegrini Stieda disease: Coronal T1 image shows signal voids, corresponding to ossifications, along the proximal fibers of the torn superficial MCL (arrow).

COMMENTS

The patient is a 56-year-old female with a history of chronic medial knee pain. Focal areas of signal void along the proximal medial collateral ligament (MCL) correspond to ossification foci. The MCL is thickened and demonstrates intermediate signal intensity, indicative of chronic tear. Ossification of the chronically injured MCL is known by the eponym, Pellegrini Stieda disease. Valgus trauma most commonly occurs with a direct blow to the lateral aspect of the knee, resulting in stretch and tear of the superficial and/or deep layers of the MCL. The ossification within the MCL is thought to represent the sequela of localized hemorrhage, following initial trauma and tear. Routine frontal radiographs of the knee can reliably demonstrate and confirm the presence of MCL ossification. In some cases, T1 sequence MR may demonstrate foci of increased signal intensity, corresponding to bone marrow, within the signal voids, confirming the presence of bony ossification. In addition to indicating the extent of superficial and/or deep layer MCL disruption, MRI indicates whether other structures commonly associated with MCL tears, namely the medial meniscus or anterior cruciate ligament, are torn. Tears of all three of these structures are known as O' Donohue's unhappy triad. Examination findings of an MCL tear may include pain, swelling, valgus instability, or limited range of motion. In addition, the ossified portion of the MCL may be palpable. Failing conservative therapy, surgical removal of the ossifications and/or MCL reconstruction may be contemplated.

PEARLS

- **Chronic, posttraumatic ossification (low T1 and T2) of the proximal MCL**
- **Frontal radiograph may confirm findings**
- **Tear of deep MCL fibers or medial meniscus may be noted**
- **Coronal imaging plane is most sensitive for diagnosis**

ADDITIONAL IMAGES

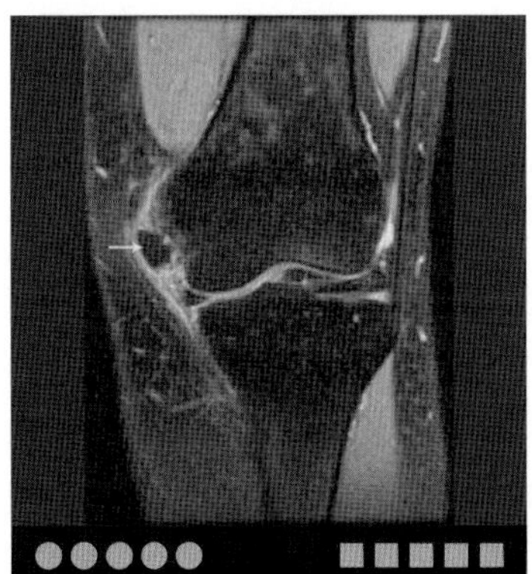

B. Pellegrini Stieda disease: Coronal fat-saturated proton density image redemonstrates ossification along the torn proximal, superficial MCL (arrow).

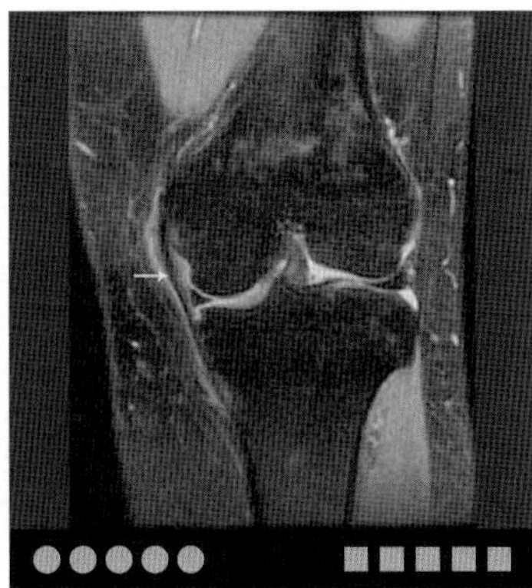

C. Pellegrini Stieda disease: Coronal fat-saturated proton density image, posterior to the image from image B, shows intact deep fibers of the MCL (arrow).

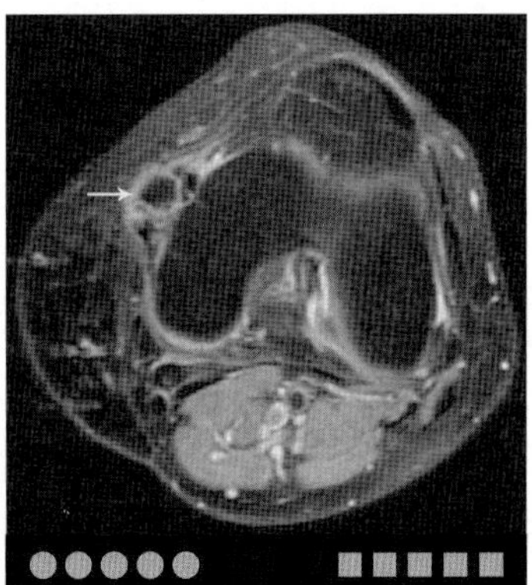

D. Pellegrini Stieda disease: Axial fat-saturated proton density image demonstrates multiple ossifications along the disrupted course of the MCL (arrow).

DIFFERENTIAL DIAGNOSES IMAGES

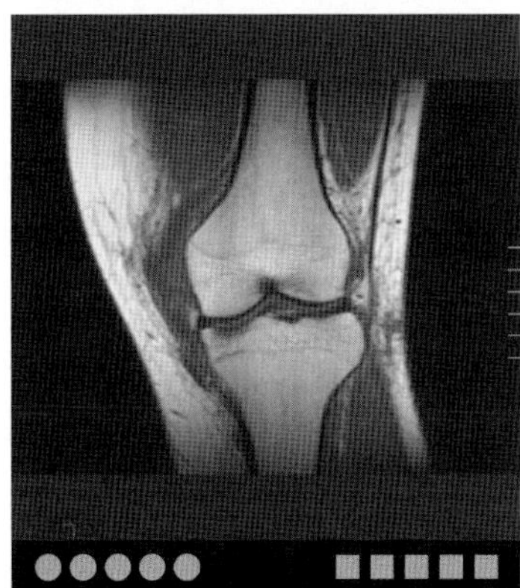

E. Complete MCL tear: Coronal T1-weighted image of the knee shows a wide area of low signal intensity at the region of MCL, which is consistent with edema and hemorrhage caused by complete tear.

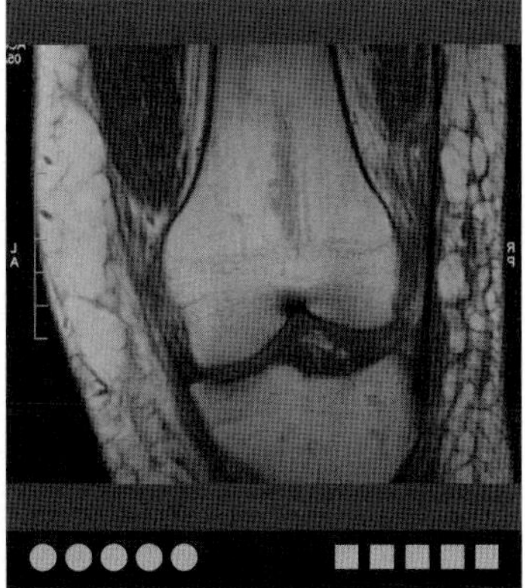

F. Partial MCL tear: Coronal T1-weighted image shows partial tear of the deep fibers of MCL.

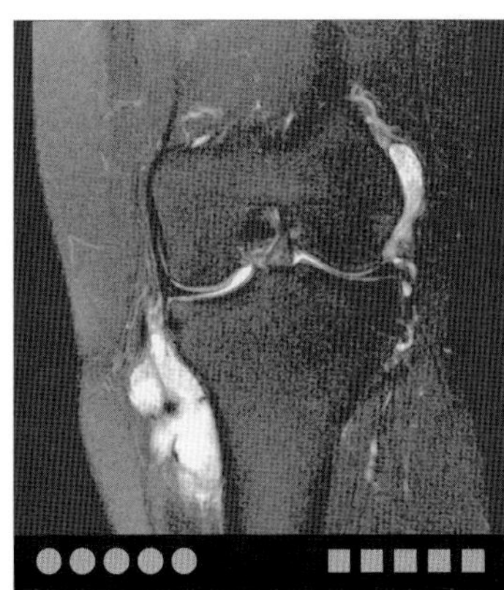

G. Pes anserinus bursitis: Coronal fat-saturated T1-weighted spin echo post contrast image shows a lobulated cystic lesion in the medial aspect of the proximal left tibia. Note rice bodies in the joint representing synovitis.

IMAGE KEY

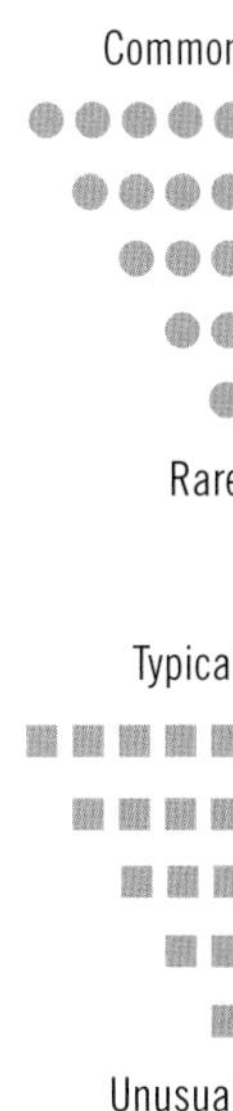

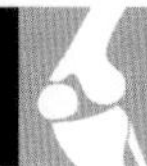

23–20 Posterolateral Corner Injury

Stephen E. Ling and William R. Reinus

PRESENTATION

Pain, swelling, and posterolateral instability

FINDINGS

Traumatic injury involving the soft tissues and/or osseous structures of the posterolateral complex (PLC) of the knee.

DIFFERENTIAL DIAGNOSES

- *Segond fracture:* Cortical avulsion of the lateral tibial condyle that can be associated with anterior cruciate ligament (ACL), medial meniscus and lateral joint capsule tear. This also could present in association with posterior lateral corner injury.
- *Iliotibial band syndrome:* This is associated with edema and fluid around the iliotibial band that inserts anteriorly on Gerdy's tubercle.

COMMENTS

The posterolateral complex (PLC) of the knee has several components: (1) lateral collateral ligament, (2) popliteus tendon, (3) popliteofibular ligament, (4) fabellofibular ligament, (5) arcuate ligament, (6) posterolateral joint capsule, and (7) the lateral head of the gastrocnemius muscle. Injury to the posterolateral corner (PLCI) occurs via several mechanisms – valgus stress with external femoral rotation, varus stress, and direct blow to the tibia, hyperextension, and rotational, twisting injury. Although PLCI may occur in isolation, it is frequently associated with cruciate ligament injuries. Radiographs are usually normal, but may show a fibular head avulsion fracture (Arcuate sign) or lateral joint space widening. Other radiographic findings arise from coexisting injury to a cruciate ligament. ACL injury may be associated with a Segond fracture (lateral tibial rim avulsion at the insertion of the lateral capsular ligament), tibial intercondylar eminence avulsion (ACL footprint), depression of the lateral condylopatellar sulcus (>1.5 mm) secondary to tibial impaction ("lateral notch sign"), or impaction fracture of the posterolateral tibial plateau. Avulsion fracture of the posterior tibia (PCL footprint) may be present with PCL injury. MR is sensitive for PLCI, in part because of its excellent contrast resolution. Beyond the associated bone contusions and fractures, MR findings are similar to those seen with all myotendinous, ligamentous, and capsular injuries. Since 1.5T MRI does not routinely image the smaller structures in PLCI, care should be taken to look for popliteus muscle or tendon tears, proximal fibular edema and anatomic disorganization in this region. Failure to recognize and repair a PLCI associated with an ACL tear virtually condemns the ACL reconstruction to failure.

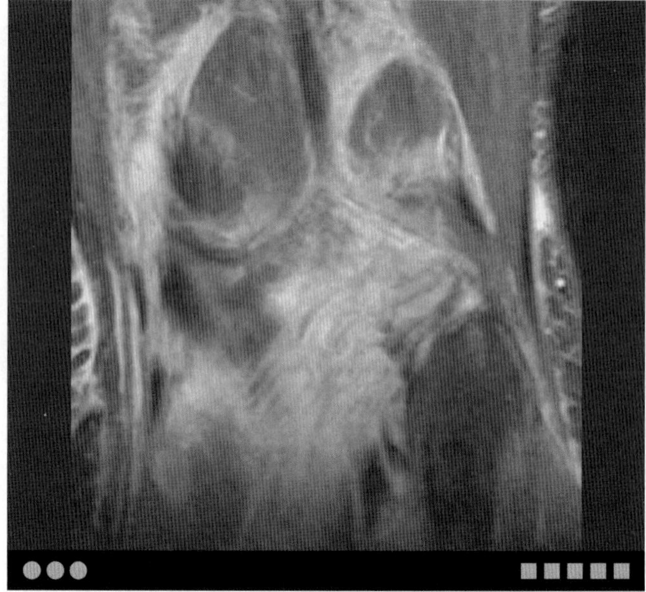

A. Posterolateral corner injury (PLCI)—Popliteus: Coronal T2-weighted image with fat saturation shows diffuse edema in the popliteus including its myotendinous junction with irregularity of muscle fibers and loss of normal muscle architecture, consistent with strain and posterolateral corner injury (PLCI).

PEARLS

- **Avulsion fracture of the fibular head (arcuate sign) is essentially pathognomic for injury to the posterolateral corner (PLC).**
- **In the setting of ACL tear, it is very important to diagnose any concomitant posterolateral complex injury, as failure to surgically address this abnormality significantly increases the incidence of graft rupture/failure following ACL reconstruction.**
- **Posterolateral complex injuries may be treated with repair, augmentation, or reconstruction, with acute cases having better results than longer standing ones, including those treated as soon as 4 to 5 days following the traumatic event.**
- **Some of the smaller soft tissue structures of the posterolateral corner are currently not well demonstrated by conventional MR imaging, but they may potentially be better visualized on a routine basis in the future utilizing 3T MR.**
- **Avulsion fractures of the Segond type can be subtle and are often overlooked on MRI because of the relative paucity of bone marrow edema. CT better evaluates these small fractures.**

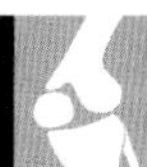

ADDITIONAL IMAGES

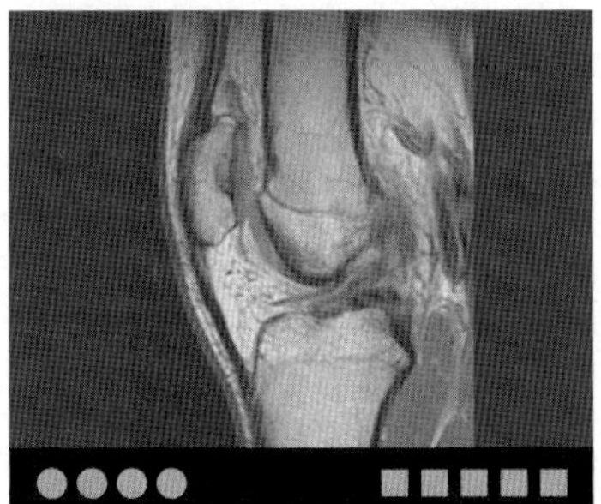

B. ACL injury: Sagittal proton density weighted image (PDWI) in another patient with posterolateral corner injury (shown in image C) shows a complete tear of the ACL in its proximal third.

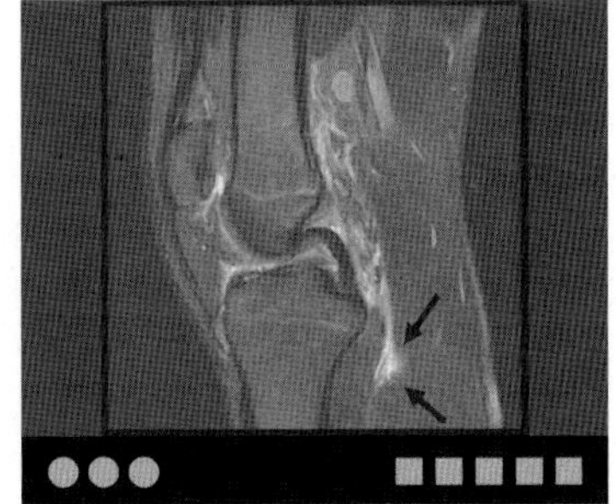

C. Posterolateral corner injury (PLCI)—Popliteus: Sagittal T2-weighted image with fat saturation from the same study as image B shows mild fluid and edema around the popliteus at the myotendinous junction posteriorly (arrows) indicating concomitant posterolateral complex injury.

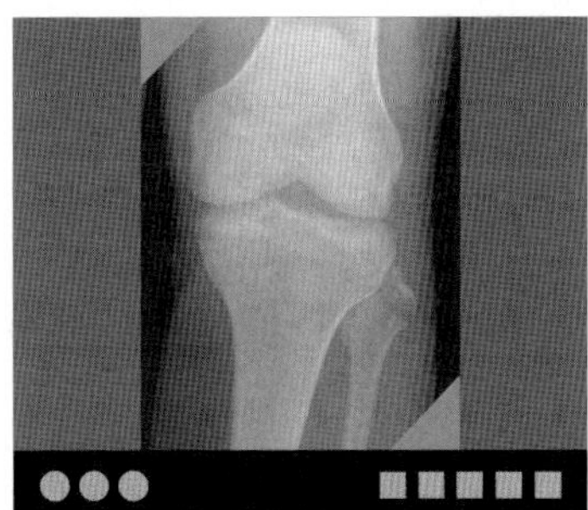

D. Posterolateral corner injury (PLCI)—-Fibular head: AP radiograph of the knee in a third case shows a large avulsion fracture off the fibular head (arcuate sign) diagnostic of posterolateral corner injury.

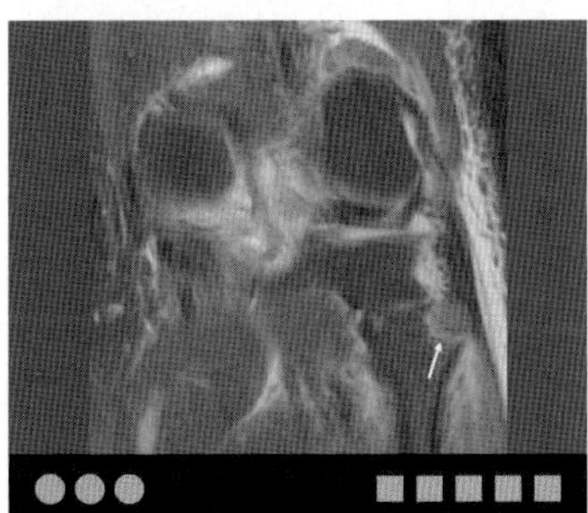

E. Posterolateral corner injury (PLCI)—-Fibular head: Coronal T2-weighted image with fat saturation shows a fibular head avulsion fracture (arrow) at the conjoined biceps femoris tendon–lateral collateral ligament insertion corresponding with the arcuate sign seen in image D. Note the paucity of bone marrow edema in the fibula proper despite the relatively large size of the avulsion fracture.

IMAGE KEY

Common

Rare

Typical

Unusual

DIFFERENTIAL DIAGNOSES IMAGES

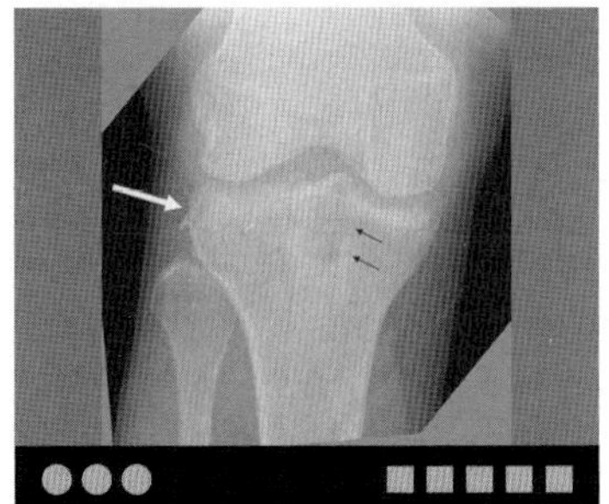

F. Segond fracture: AP radiograph of the knee in another patient shows a small fragment of cortical bone consistent with an avulsion fracture (white arrow) off the lateral tibial rim (Segond fracture), the attachment site of the lateral capsular ligament. Note also the evidence of prior ACL reconstruction (small black arrows).

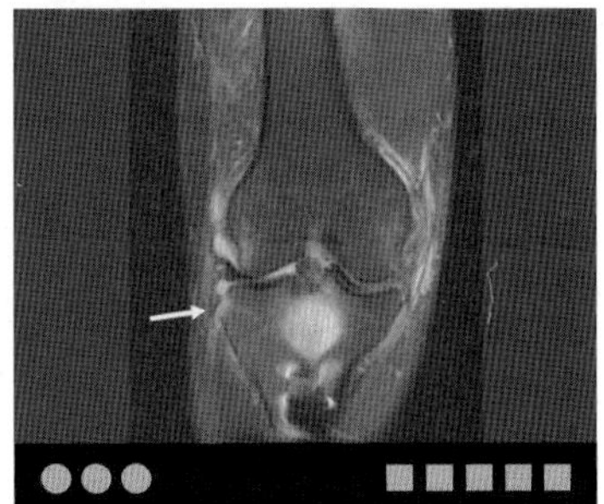

G. Segond fracture: Coronal T2-weighted image with fat saturation in the same patient as image F shows an avulsion fracture off the lateral tibial rim (arrow).

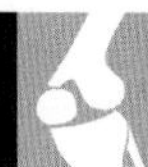

23–21 Anterior Cruciate Ligament Mucoid Degeneration

Ayodale S. Odulate and Piran Aliabadi

PRESENTATION

Knee pain, stiffness, and locking

FINDINGS

Abnormally thickened anterior cruciate ligament (ACL) with abnormal increased signal on MRI sequences.

DIFFERENTIAL DIAGNOSES

- *ACL tear:* The ligament will appear thickened with increased signal intensity on fluid sensitive sequences. Discontinuity of the fibers may be seen in complete rupture.
- *ACL ganglion:* Discrete fluid signal cystic structure within interspersed intact ligament fibers on MR.
- *ACL graft tear:* There is history of knee surgery. Intraosseous tunnel and interference screws indicate ACL graft.

COMMENTS

The patient is a 47-year-old male with no known history of trauma and left knee pain and swelling for 4 months. ACL mucoid degeneration is often found in middle-aged patients without a history of trauma. Patients may present with knee pain and stiffness. Treatment can include nonsteroidal anti-inflammatory medications, arthroscopy with dissection of the mucoid material from the intact ACL fibers and notchplasty. Mucoid degeneration of ACL is believed to represent less than 1% of all finding on MR imaging of the knee. The ACL originates from the lateral femoral condyle and inserts onto the anteromedial tibia and measures approximately 1 cm in transverse diameter. The ligament is enlarged, intact, and homogeneous in increased signal intensity with a described "celery stalk" appearance on all imaging sequences. The MR appearance may sometimes be confused for an ACL tear. A tear will have disruption of fibers, thickened tendon at the site of tear, and edema in the remaining tendon in the acute stage. Mucoid degeneration is thought to lie along the spectrum of disease termed ACL synovial inflammatory pseudomass or ASIP. Homogeneous increased signal intensity suggests mucoid degeneration. If discrete foci of fluid are seen around or in the abnormally thickened ligament, an ACL ganglion may be the diagnosis. ACL ganglia may even insinuate into the joint and surrounding bone. Occasionally, ASIP may be confused for a neoplasm.

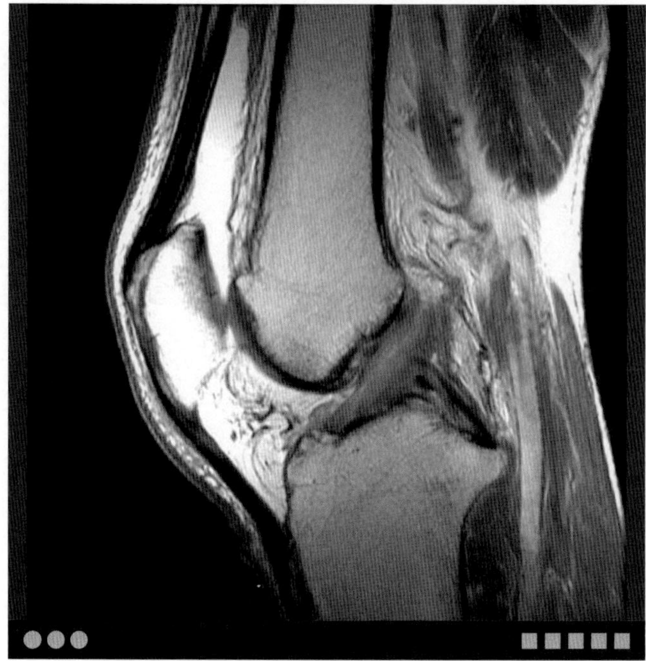

A. ACL mucoid degeneration: Sagittal proton density image demonstrates homogeneous increased signal intensity in the ACL (arrows).

PEARLS

- **Mucoid degeneration presents as "Celery stalk" homogeneous appearance of an enlarged ACL**
- **ACL mucoid degeneration presents as an intact ligament with increased girth and increased signal intensity often in middle-aged patients without a history of trauma**
- **Treatment may be notchplasty and debridement of the mucinous material**

ADDITIONAL IMAGE

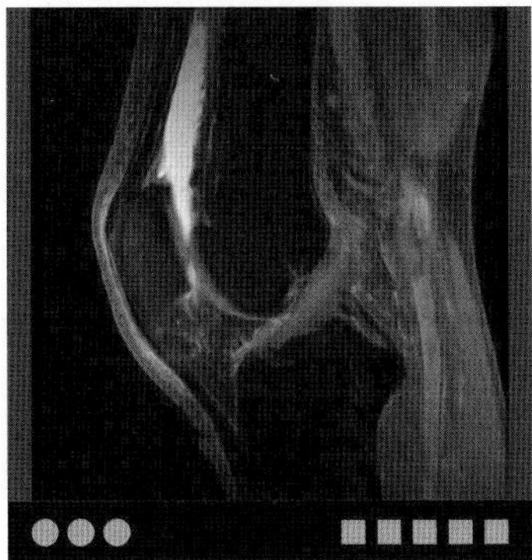

B. ACL mucoid degeneration: Sagittal fat-saturated proton density image demonstrates enlargement of the ACL and joint effusion (arrowheads). Strands of fibers are interspersed between the mucinous tissues giving a "celery stalk" appearance (arrow).

DIFFERENTIAL DIAGNOSES IMAGES

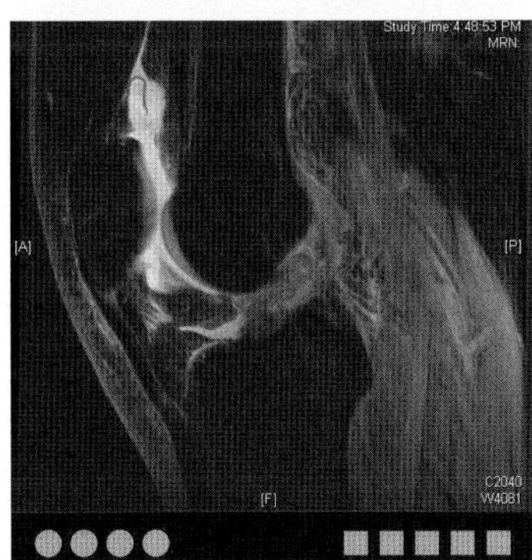

C. ACL tear: Sagittal fat-saturated T2-weighted image shows heterogeneous increased signal intensity of the ACL representing a complete rupture (arrow). A joint effusion (arrowhead) is also seen. Slight anterior subluxation of the tibia is seen.

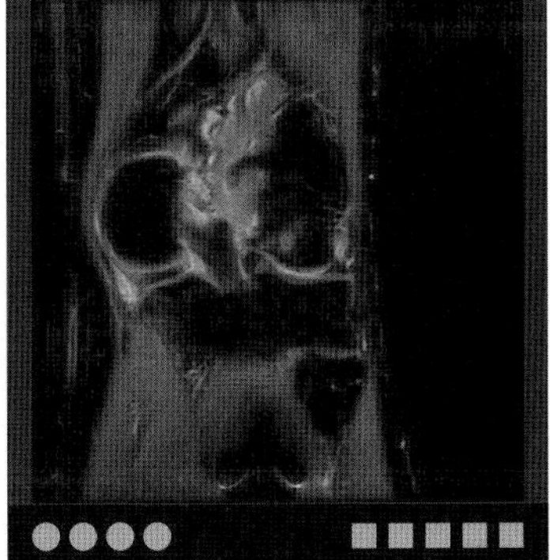

D. ACL tear: Coronal T1-weighted image demonstrates bulbous heterogeneity of the ACL origin on the lateral femoral condyle (arrow). The ligament is diffusely enlarged.

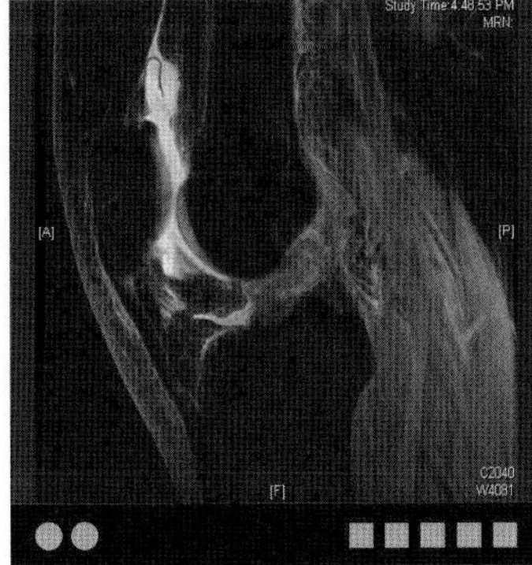

E. ACL ganglion: Sagittal STIR image from a different patient shows a discrete hyperintense signal collection (arrow) oriented along the long axis of the ACL.

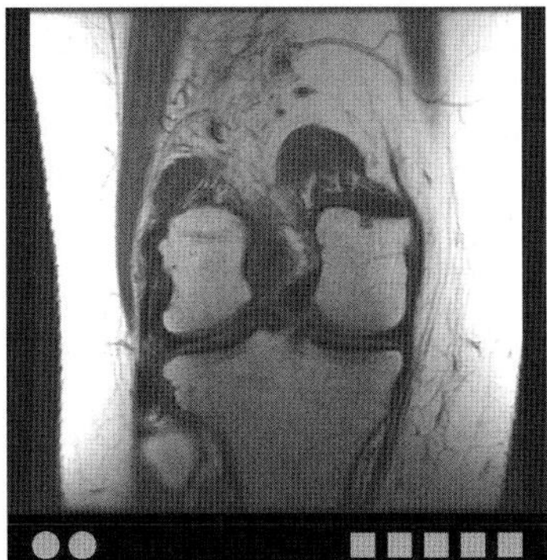

F. ACL ganglion: Coronal STIR image demonstrates the ganglion (arrow) at the origin of the ACL along the lateral femoral condyle.

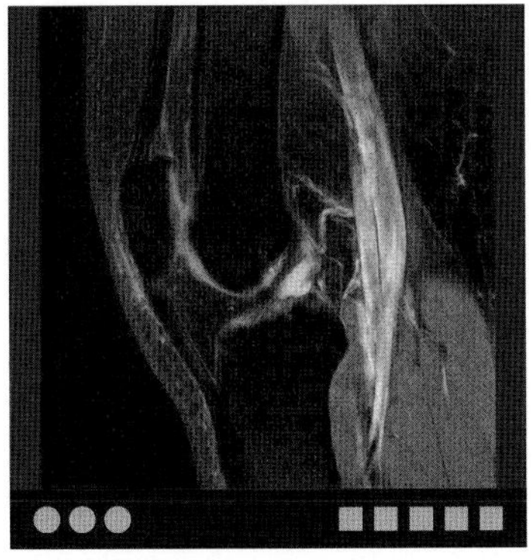

G. ACL graft tear: Sagittal T2-weighted image shows ACL graft tear. Note anterior drawer sign.

IMAGE KEY

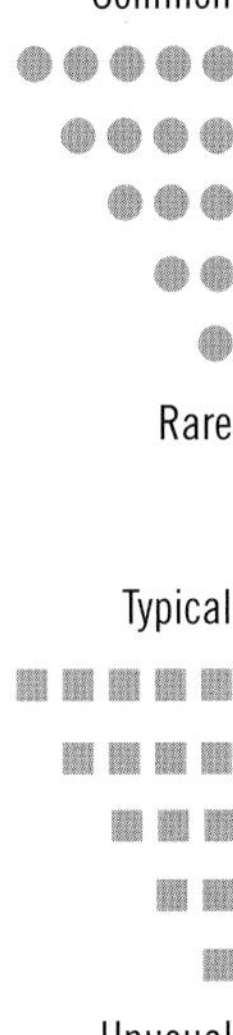

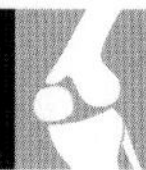

23–22 ACL Ganglia and Mucoid Degeneration

Marcia F. Blacksin

PRESENTATION

Chronic knee pain, no trauma

FINDINGS

Thickened anterior cruciate ligament (ACL) with an increased signal intensity and cruciate cysts at tibial and femoral insertion sites is seen.

DIFFERENTIAL DIAGNOSIS

- *High-grade partial ACL tear*: Noted in young patients who are active in sports. Increased signal in ACL with thickening.
- *Full-thickness ACL tear*: Increased signal in ACL with discontinuity of fibers. Bone marrow edema at posterolateral tibia and lateral, femoral condyle.

COMMENTS

Intra-articular ganglia of the cruciate ligaments have a variable presentation. They can be incidental findings, or a cause of "fullness" and pain at the knee joint. The cause of these cysts has not been fully delineated. Recent literature now shows an association between mucoid degeneration of the ACL and these cysts. The mean age of this patient population is 45 years. The patients do not demonstrate knee instability. Mucoid degeneration will cause a thickened ACL with an increased signal intensity. Cysts were identified across both the proximal and distal halves of the ACL and some of them involved the entire ACL. These cysts may be septated and multilobulated. In one study of 74 patients, 35% of patients had both ganglia and mucoid degeneration. Other incidental findings were intraosseous ganglia, seen in 66% of patients with cruciate ganglia. The bone findings may be secondary to pressure erosion of the intrasubstance ligament ganglia into the articular surfaces of the knee joint. Differential diagnosis includes ACL tears. A history of trauma is usually present, and the secondary signs of ACL injury can be searched for on MR. These include bone marrow edema in the posterolateral aspect of the tibial plateau, bone marrow edema in the weight bearing surface of the lateral femoral condyle, or a deep, lateral sulcus sign. Other signs include tears in Hoffa's fat pad, buckling of the PCL, and posterior translation of the femur on the tibia.

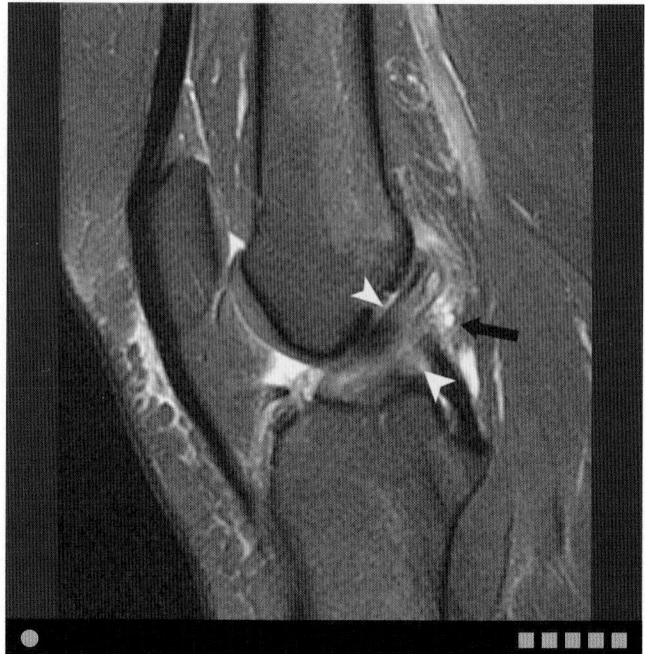

A. ACL ganglia: Sagittal T2-weighted image shows thickened ACL with an increased signal (arrowhead). Note ACL ganglion at insertion (arrow).

PEARLS

- **There is an association between cruciate ganglia and mucoid degeneration of the ACL.**
- **Full-thickness ACL tears often demonstrate secondary MR findings.**
- **Cruciate cysts or ganglia may be seen as an incidental finding on MR images.**

ADDITIONAL IMAGES

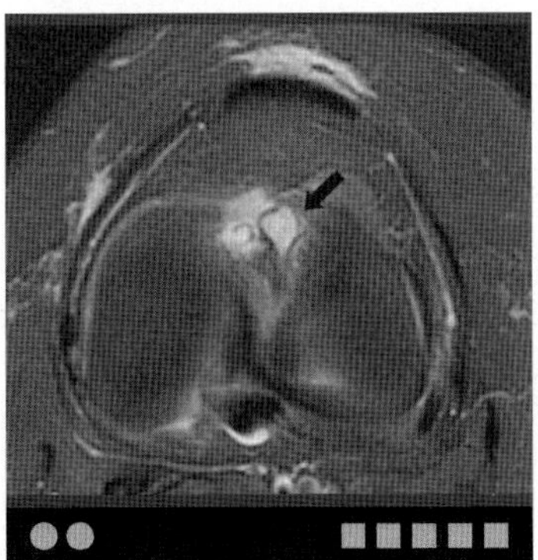

B. ACL ganglia: Axial T2-weighted image shows ganglion at tibial insertion of ACL (arrow).

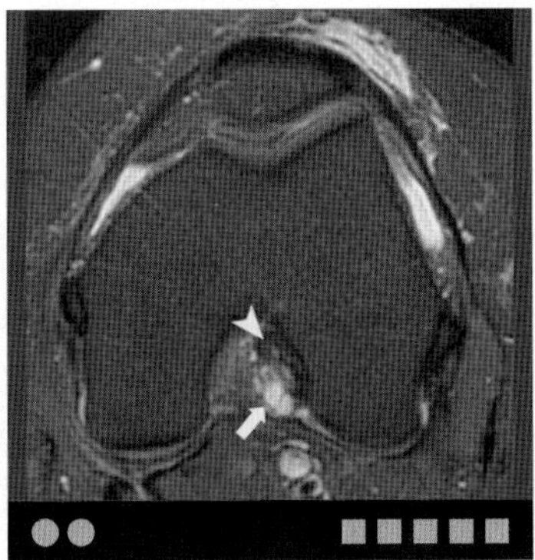

C. ACL ganglia: Axial T2-weighted image shows ganglion at femoral ACL insertion (arrow). Note increased interstitial signal in ACL (arrowhead).

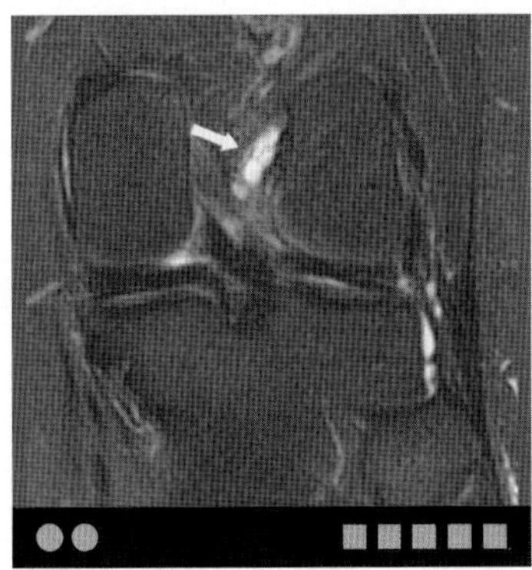

D. ACL ganglia: Coronal T2-weighted image shows septated ganglion at femoral insertion (arrow).

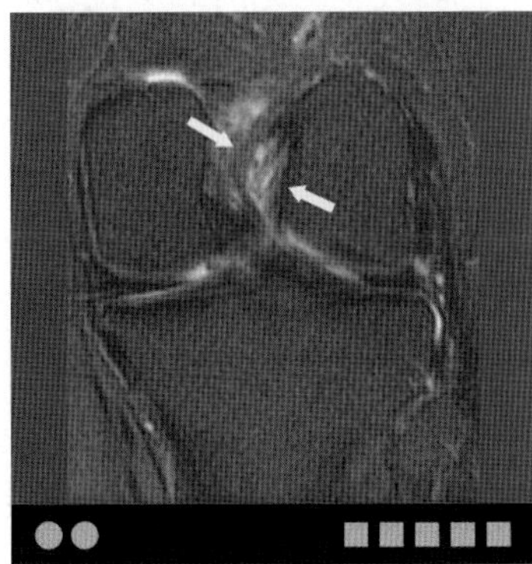

E. ACL ganglia: Coronal T2-weighted image with an increased signal in ACL (arrows)

DIFFERENTIAL DIAGNOSES IMAGES

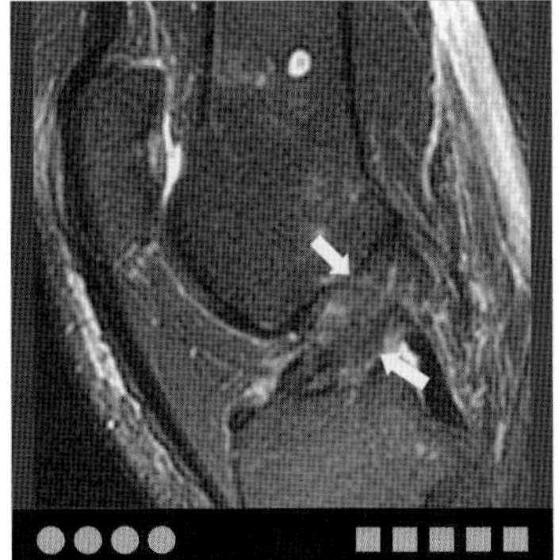

F. ACL tear: Sagittal T2-weighted image shows increased signal, thickening, and discontinuity in ACL (arrows).

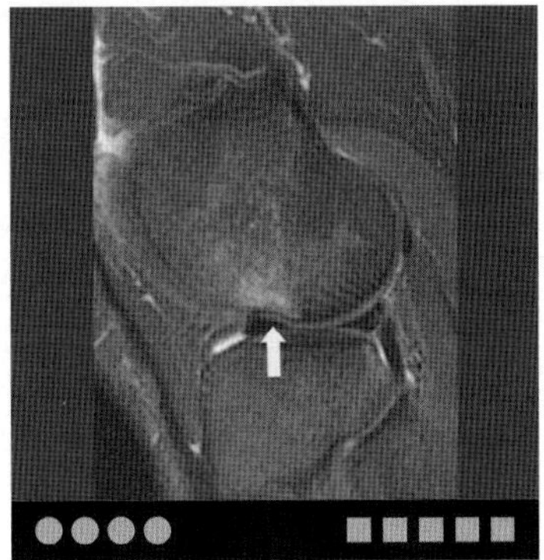

G. ACL tear: Sagittal image in same patient with lateral, femoral condyle bone marrow edema and deep, lateral sulcus sign (arrow).

IMAGE KEY

Common

Rare

Typical

Unusual

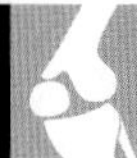

23–23 Ganglion of the Posterior Cruciate Ligament

Stefano Bianchi and Ibrahim F. Abdelwahab

PRESENTATION

Painless limitation in knee flexion

FINDINGS

MRI shows a well-circumscribed, cystic mass located inside the intercondylar notch.

DIFFERENTIAL DIAGNOSES

- *Meniscal cysts:* Parameniscal cysts are usually connected with a degenerative tear of the meniscus.
- *Pigmented villonodular synovitis (PVNS):* Solid mass presenting internal hypointense areas both in T1 and T2-weighted images corresponding to hemosiderin deposition.
- *Synovial hemangioma:* Rare vascular tumors that may demonstrate phleboliths.

COMMENTS

The patient is a 48-year-old female who presented with progressive limitation of the flexion of the left knee associated with a slight pain. Ganglia are cysts with a fibrous wall and a viscous content that result from mucoid degeneration of the para-articular connective tissue. The most common ganglia of the knee region are meniscal cysts (MC). More rarely are cruciate ligaments ganglia (CLG). They may be located inside the femoral notch. The etiology is still unknown. Since the advent of MRI, they became more commonly recognized. CLG may lie anterior, between, posterior, or inside the ligaments. Intraligamentous cysts appear as fusiform cysts extending along the course of the ligaments. CLG can be asymptomatic or present with unspecific pain and locking of the knee. MRI is the preferred method to assess CLG. Gadolinium injection is necessary to differentiate them from pigmented villonodular synovitis, synovial hemangioma, and synovial sarcoma. MRI is also helpful to appreciate their size, location, and relation with the adjacent structures. They appear as well-defined, multiloculated masses with intermediate signal intensity on T1-weighted and increased signal on T2-weighted images with a relatively hypointense wall. Typically only the wall and internal septa enhance following IV gadopentetate. Imaging guided needle puncture or arthroscopy is necessary in the rare cases in which MRI appearance is nonspecific.

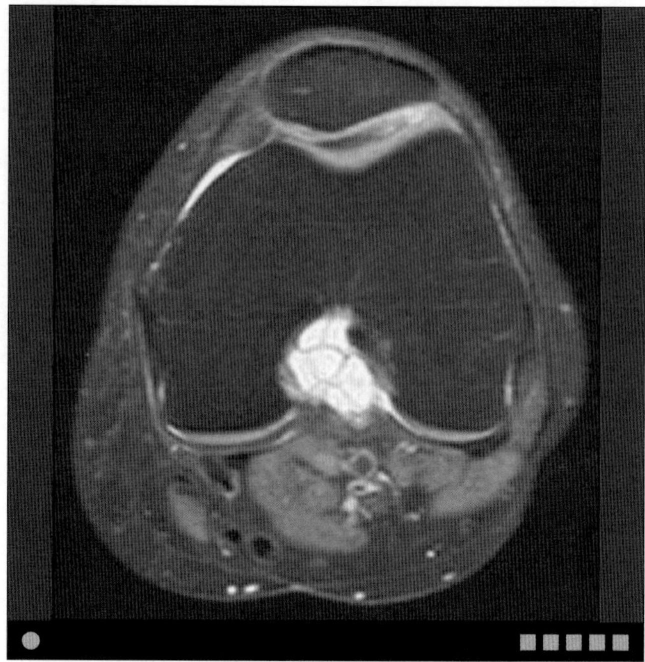

A. Ganglion of the posterior cruciate ligament: Axial fat saturation PD MR image shows the CLG as a well-delimited septated cystic lesion located inside the femoral notch.

PEARLS

- **CLG are cystic lesions containing mucoid fluid located inside or adjacent to the cruciate ligaments. They may be asymptomatic or cause a painless limitation of knee extension or flexion.**
- **MRI is the preferred method to assess CLG. Gadolinium injection is necessary to differentiate them from pigmented villonodular synovitis, synovial hemangioma, and synovial sarcoma.**
- **Imaging guided needle puncture or arthroscopy is necessary in the rare cases in which MRI appearance is nonspecific.**

ADDITIONAL IMAGES

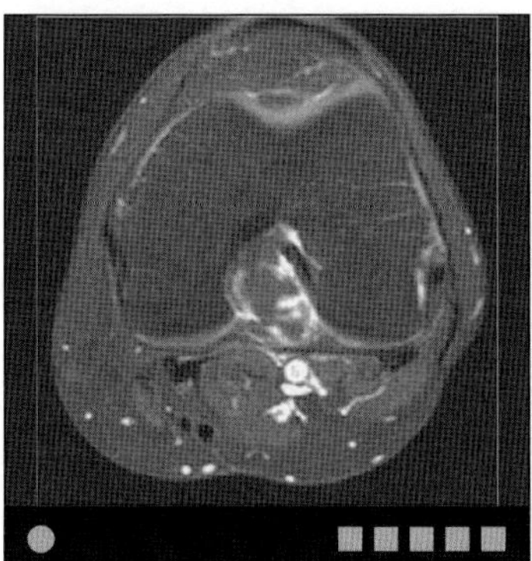

B. Ganglion of the posterior cruciate ligament: Post contrast fat saturation axial T1-weighted MRI image showing enhancement of the peripheral wall and septa after gadolinium injection.

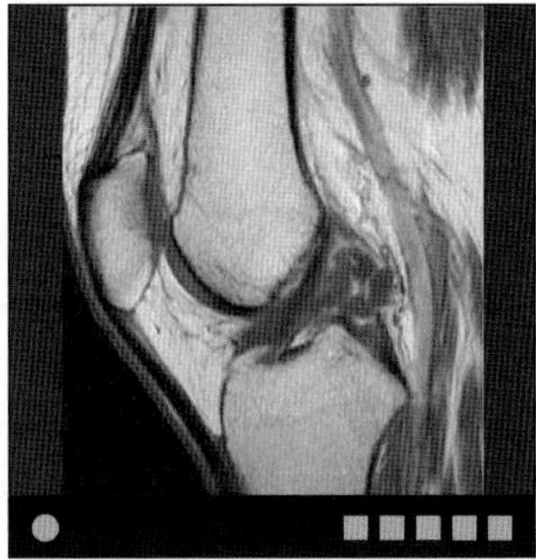

C. Ganglion of the posterior cruciate ligament: Post contrast fat saturation sagittal T1-weighted MRI demonstrates that the ganglion is located behind the normal ACL.

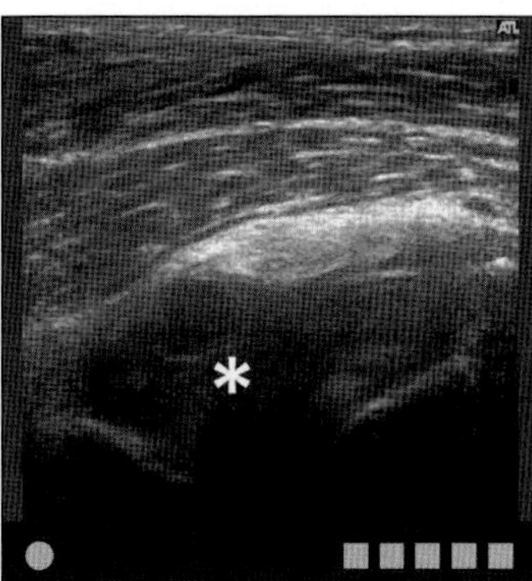

D. Ganglion of the posterior cruciate ligament: Sagittal US image shows the ganglion (asterisk) as an unechoic cystic lesion with internal septa.

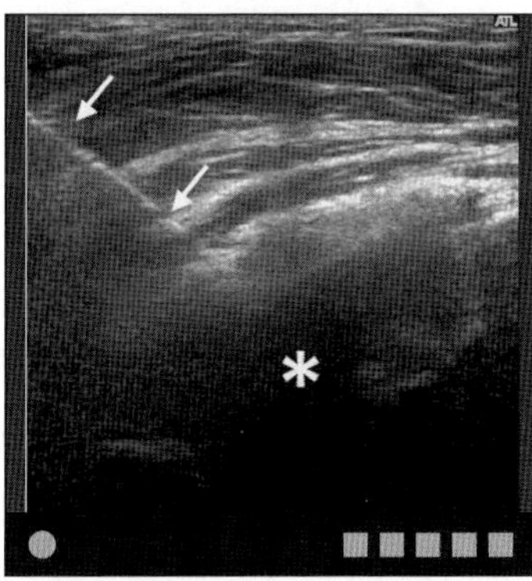

E. Ganglion of the posterior cruciate ligament: US-guided needle puncture. Note the needle (arrows) advancing under US guidance toward the ganglion (asterisk).

IMAGE KEY

Common

●●●●●
●●●●
●●●
●●
●

Rare

Typical

■■■■■
■■■■
■■■
■■
■

Unusual

DIFFERENTIAL DIAGNOSES IMAGES

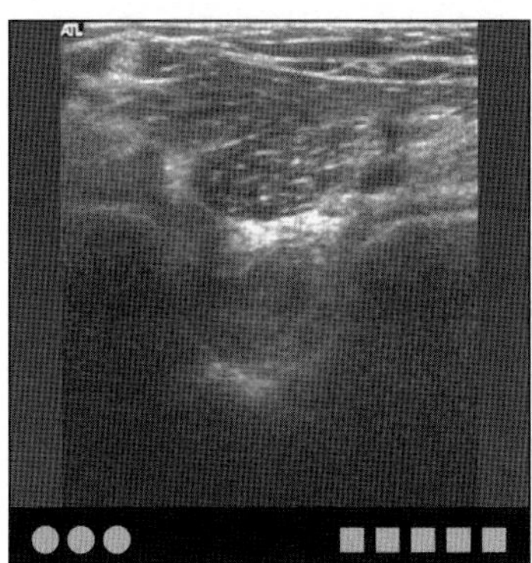

F. PVNS: Axial posterior sonogram obtained at the level of the intercondylar notch shows a hypoechoic mass located between the two condyles.

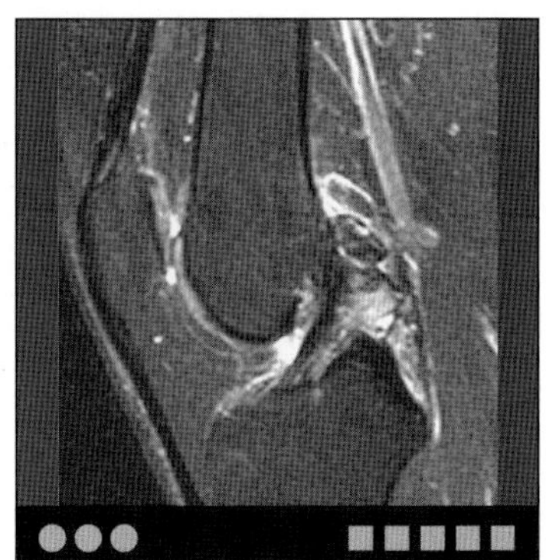

G. PVNS: Sagittal T2-weighted MRI image shows a solid mass located posterior to the ACL. Please note the hypointense signals inside the superior part of the mass, consisting with PVNS.

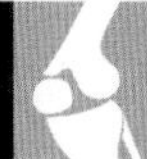

23–24 Jumper's Knee

Stefano Bianchi and Ibrahim F. Abdelwahab

PRESENTATION

Pain localized in the patellar region

FINDINGS

US demonstrated a swollen irregular proximal portion of the patellar tendon. MRI shows thickened patellar tendon with partial tear.

DIFFERENTIAL DIAGNOSES

- *Tear of the patellar or trochlear cartilages:* Presents with partial or full-thickness fissures or ulcers of the patellofemoral articular cartilages. The patellar tendon and the Hoffa fat pad are normal.
- *Patellar tendon–lateral femoral condyle friction syndrome:* It follows impingement of the superolateral aspect of the fat pad located between the patellar tendon and femoral condyle. It manifests as increased signal on T2-weighted fat-saturated images noted in the superolateral aspect of the Hoffa fat pad.

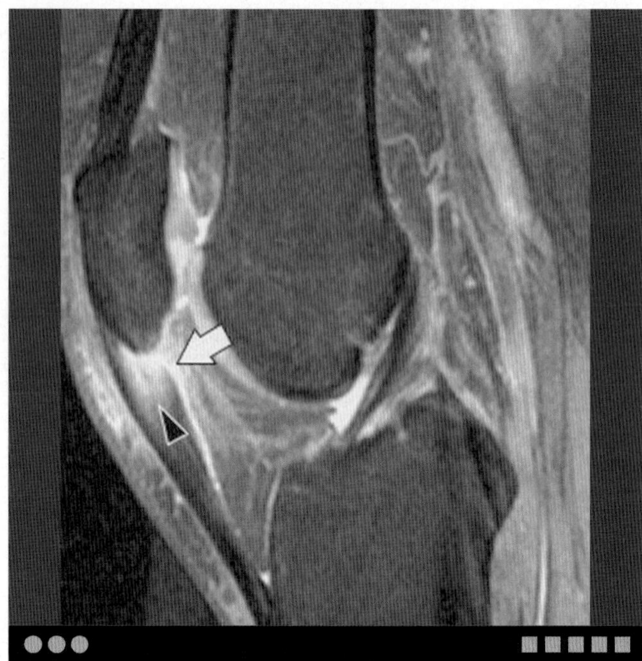

A. Jumper's knee: Sagittal fat-saturated proton density MRI image shows thickening (arrow) of the proximal patellar tendon, associated with internal hyperintensity (arrowhead) reflecting edema.

COMMENTS

A 25-year-old sportsman developed a sharp pain on the patellar region. Physical examination showed absence of joint effusion and tenderness over the lower pole of the patella. Tendinopathy of the patellar tendon mostly affects the proximal tendon and is secondary to repetitive overuse. The condition mainly affects young active subjects involved in sports or recreational activities that require powerful contraction of the QM such as kicking, running, or jumping. The pathogenesis is focal tearing of collagen fibers followed by mucoid degeneration possibly secondary to the local poor vascularity. The clinical appearance of jumper's knee is quite typical to allow a confident diagnosis. US typically shows an anechoic, fusiform area affecting the posterior part of the middle third of the tendon. In axial images the posterior border of the tendon shows a central bulging caused by the presence of the rounded degenerative nodule. The medial and lateral third are typically unaffected and present a normal hyperechoic appearance. Frequently, the most superficial part of the tendon appears normal. The nodule appears hypoechoic with possible focal internal hyperechoic spots and posterior shadowing caused by calcifications. Color Doppler shows increased vascularity in acute cases. Both MRI and US can accurately assess jumper's knee. MRI may be limited only to the exceptional cases in which uncertainty exists in US. Although control examinations are frequently asked by the clinician in an effort to follow the evolution and mostly to decide if the athlete can return to agonistic activity, US has a limited value in such evaluation.

PEARLS

- **Jumper's knee is an acute tendinopathy affecting the proximal portion of the patellar tendon**
- **It affects young subjects involved in sports in which powerful contraction of the quadriceps muscle is required**
- **Jumper's knee can be easily diagnosed by US. If US is negative MRI must be performed to accurately evaluate the cartilage of the patellofemoral articulation and the Hoffa fat pad**

ADDITIONAL IMAGE

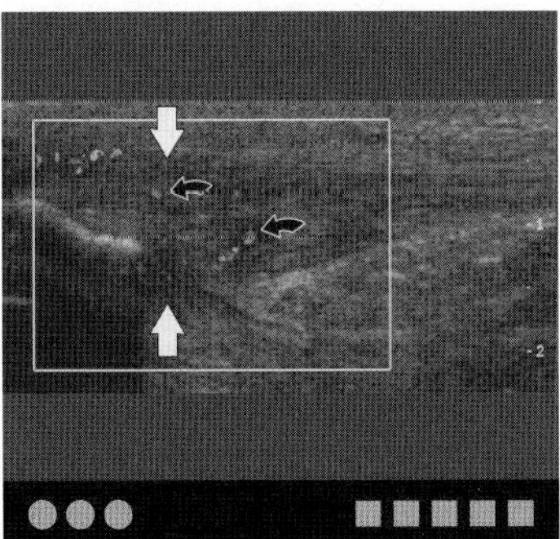

B. Jumper's knee: Sagittal color Doppler US image over the anterior aspect of the lower pole of the patella shows thickening (arrows) of the proximal patellar tendon, associated with hypoechoic area and internal flow signals (curved arrows).

DIFFERENTIAL DIAGNOSES IMAGES

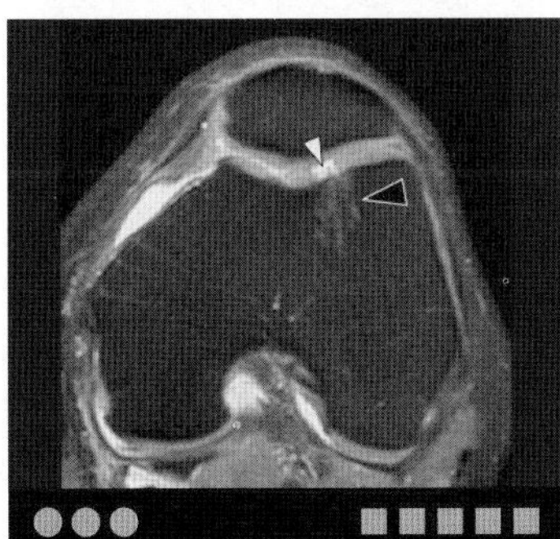

C. Tear of the trochlear cartilage: Axial fat-saturated proton density MRI image shows a full-thickness tear of the trochlear cartilage (white arrowhead) associated with local bone marrow edema (black arrowhead).

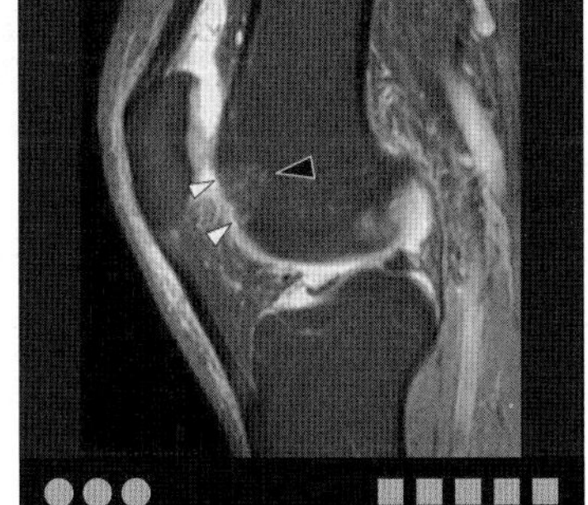

D. Tear of the trochlear cartilage: Sagittal fat-saturated proton density MRI image obtained in the same patient confirms a full-thickness tear of the trochlear cartilage (white arrowheads) and bone marrow edema (black arrowhead). Note the normal patellar articular cartilage and the joint effusion.

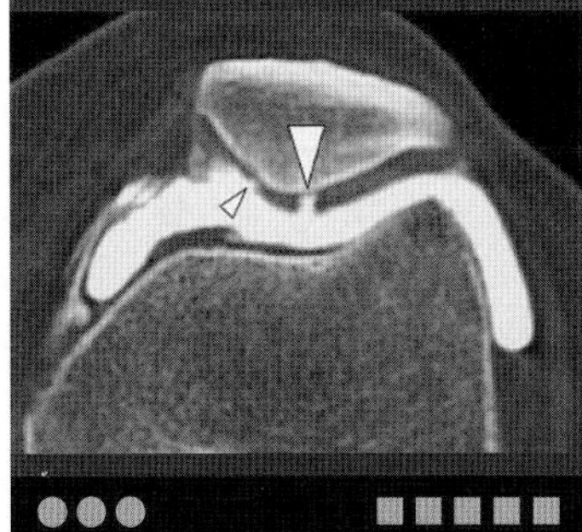

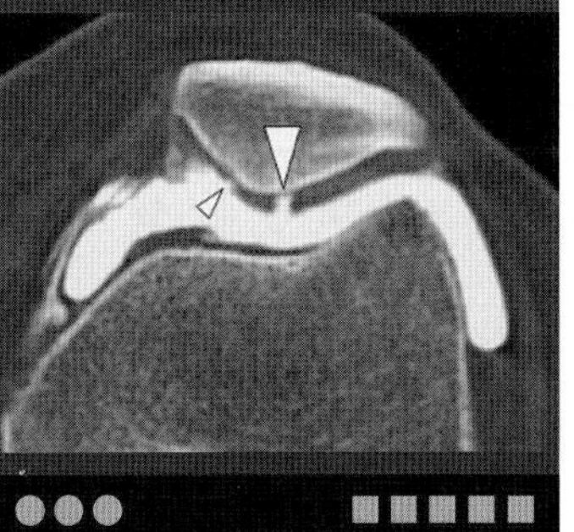

E. Tear of the patellar cartilages: Axial CT-arthrography image obtained at the level of the patella shows a full-thickness tear of the patellar cartilage (large arrowhead) of the lateral facet. A smaller partial-thickness tear is evident in the medial facet (small arrowhead). Both tears are filled with contrast.

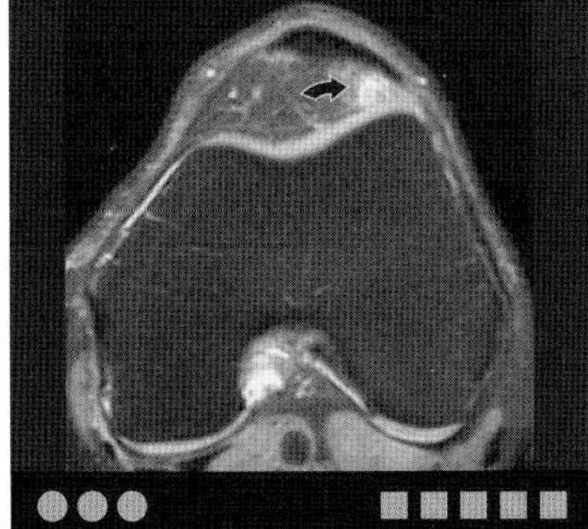

F. Patellar tendon–lateral femoral condyle friction syndrome: Axial fat-saturated proton density MRI image obtained at the level of the proximal patellar tendon shows focal hyperintensity of the superolateral part of the Hoffa fat pad (curved arrow). Note the normal patellar tendon and trochlear cartilage.

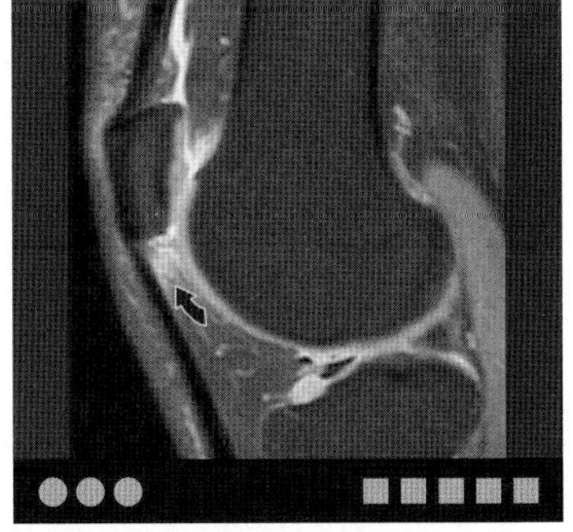

G. Patellar tendon–lateral femoral condyle friction syndrome: Sagittal fat-saturated proton density MRI image obtained in the same patient confirms focal edema localized at the superolateral part of the Hoffa fat pad (curved arrow).

IMAGE KEY

Common

Rare

Typical

Unusual

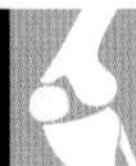

23–25 Sonographic Appearance of Patellar Tendinosis

Mélanie Morel, Nathalie Boutry, and Anne Cotten

PRESENTATION

Anterior knee pain

FINDINGS

Sonography reveals hypoechoic areas in the thickened proximal patellar tendon with intratendinous calcifications.

DIFFERENTIAL DIAGNOSES

- *Inflammatory patellar enthesopathy:* In inflammatory disorders (psoriatic arthritis), enthesophytes and erosions can be seen at the inferior pole of the patella. Hyperemia on Doppler sonography would be specifically located at the bone-enthesis junction rather than at the inner face of the proximal patellar tendon.
- *Sinding–Larsen–Johansson disease:* It occurs in younger patients (adolescents between 10 and 14 years). The sonographic appearance is quite similar to patellar tendinosis. On radiographs, the lower end of the patella is usually fragmented. Edema of the lower pole of the patella can be detected on MR images.
- *Enthesopathy of the distal patellar tendon:* Its US and MRI appearance is similar to patellar tendinosis, but the location is different.
- *Complete rupture of the patellar tendon:* The clinical diagnosis is usually obvious, with discontinuity and retraction of the tendon.
- *Deep infrapatellar bursitis:* Ultrasound shows an anechoic area between the anterior aspect of the tibia and the inferior patellar tendon, with peripheral hyperemia on Doppler study. Its content is fluid on T2-weighted images and its walls enhance after intravenous contrast injection.

COMMENTS

The patient is a 27-year-old man complaining of chronic anterior knee pain at the lower end of the patella, diagnosed as proximal patellar tendon enthesopathy. "Patellar tendinosis" is a frequent syndrome affecting individuals involved in sports requiring violent contraction of the quadriceps muscle (volleyball, running, etc.). Chronic recurrent anterior knee pain is associated with tenderness of the proximal patellar tendon next to its patellar insertion. It is a mechanical enthesopathy with mucoid degeneration near the bone attachment. Ultrasonography shows a hypoechoic thickening of the central deep portion the patellar tendon adjacent to the lower pole of the patella.

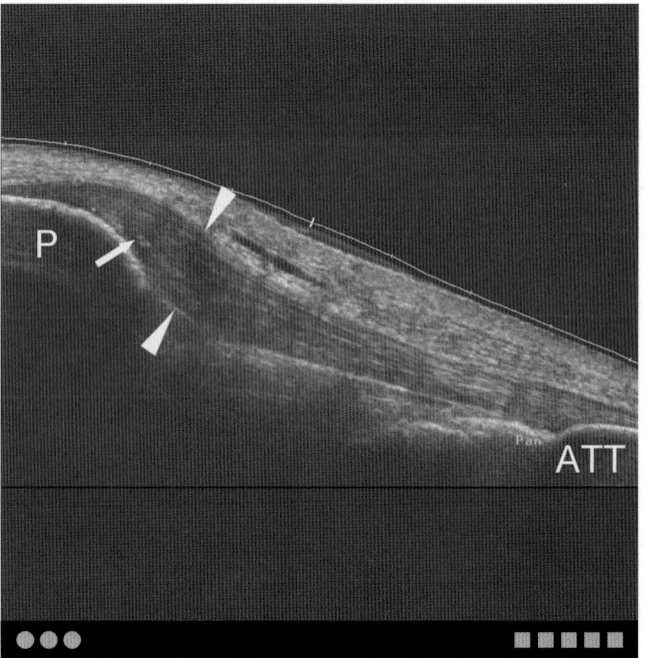

A. Patellar tendinosis: Longitudinal sonography shows thickening of the proximal patellar tendon (arrowheads) with intratendinous calcifications (arrow) (P: patella; ATT: anterior tibial tuberosity).

This area is nodular on axial planes and spindle-shaped on sagittal sections. Hyperemia may be found around it with power Doppler. In case of chronic enthesopathy, hyperechoic intratendinous calcifications and irregularities of the lower part of the patella can be observed. A thickened area of increased signal-intensity corresponding to partial tears can be seen at the posterior portion of the tendon at its junction with the patella on T1 and T2-weighted MR images. Abnormal signal intensity extends also to the paratendinous fat deep to the tendon. STIR images sometimes reveal high signal in the lower end of the patella.

PEARLS

- **Patellar tendinosis is a mechanical enthesopathy of the proximal patellar tendon**
- **It is commonly encountered in "jumping" athletes**
- **Sonography shows enlarged proximal enthesis, with hypoechoic foci**
- **Doppler study exhibits intra-tendinous and adjacent Hoffa's fat hyperemia**
- **T2-weighted MR images demonstrate high signal intensity zone at the inner face of the proximal tendon**

ADDITIONAL IMAGES

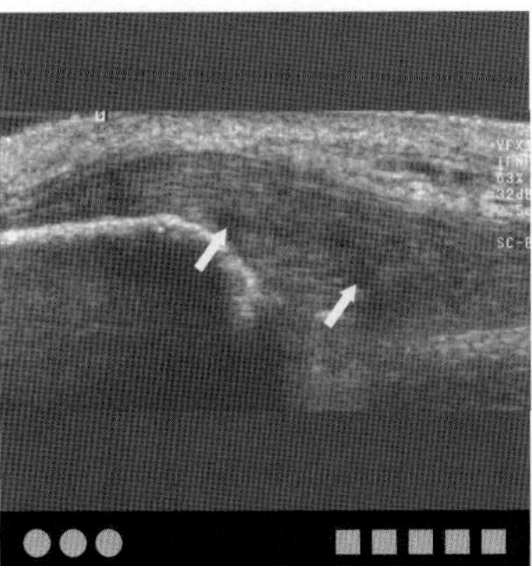

B. Patellar tendinosis: Longitudinal sonogram exhibits intratendinous focal hypoechoic areas (arrows).

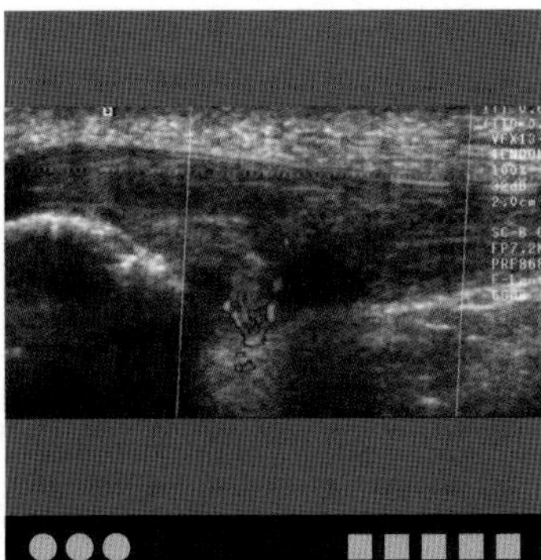

C. Patellar tendinosis: Doppler study reveals hyperemia located at the inner face of the proximal patellar tendon and in the infrapatellar fat-pad.

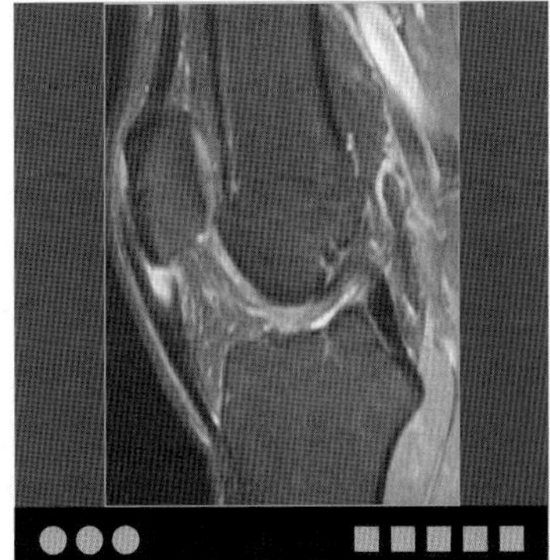

D. Patellar tendinosis: T2-weighted sagittal image demonstrates a partial tear with high signal intensity at the proximal end of the patellar tendon.

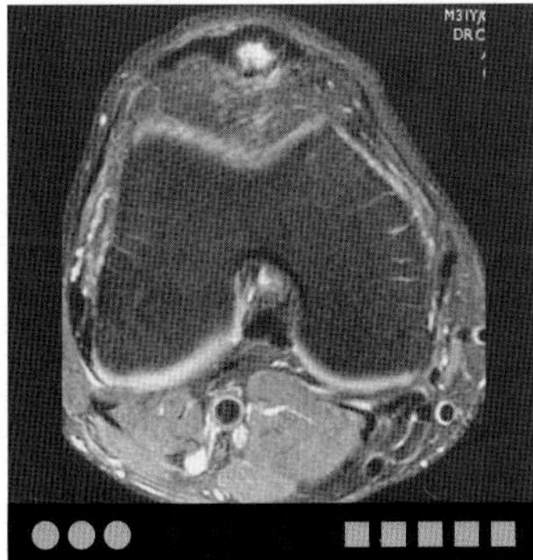

E. Patellar tendinosis: T2-weighted axial image shows a high signal intensity nodule located at the middle part of the inner face of the proximal patellar tendon.

DIFFERENTIAL DIAGNOSES IMAGES

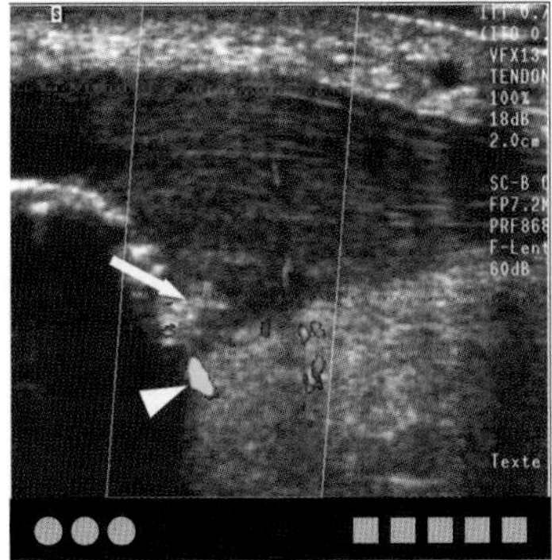

F. Inflammatory patellar enthesopathy in psoriatic arthritis: Proximal enthesis of the patellar tendon is thickened. Irregularities of the patellar bone and enthesophyte (arrow) are obvious. Doppler study reveals hyperemia at the bone–enthesis junction (arrowhead), in addition to intratendinous and fat-pad hyperemia.

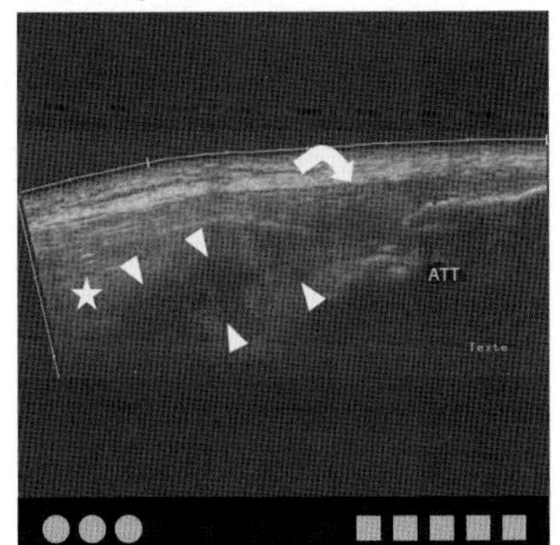

G. Infrapatellar bursitis: Longitudinal sonogram exhibits an anechoic collection (arrowheads) in the infrapatellar fat-pad (star), next to the inner face of the distal patellar tendon (curved arrow) and the anterior tibial tuberosity (ATT).

IMAGE KEY

Common

●●●●●
●●●●
●●●
●●
●

Rare

Typical

■■■■■
■■■■
■■■
■■
■

Unusual

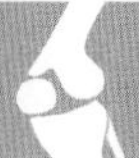

23–26 Prepatellar Bursitis

Sulabha Masih

PRESENTATION

Pain, swelling in front of the knee cap

FINDINGS

MR images show fluid collection superficial to the patella.

DIFFERENTIAL DIAGNOSES

- *Tumor in the prepatellar soft tissue:* Shows as variable signal intensity with contrast enhancement.
- *Trauma to the prepatellar soft tissue:* Variable signal intensity depending on the degradation of blood products.
- *Patellar tendon tear:* Blood from patellar tendon tear may extend in the prepatellar bursa with variable signal intensity.
- *Pretibial bursitis:* Is inflammation of pretibial bursa with fluid collection.

COMMENTS

The patient is a 42-year-old male carpet layer with history of pain and swelling around the anterior of the knee cap. Bursa is a fluid filled sac, which acts as a cushion between tendons, bones, and skin. Prepatellar bursa is a potential space, which is located between the front of the kneecap (patella) near the attachment of the patellar tendon and overlying skin. Prepatellar bursitis, also known as Housemaid's knee, is an irritation and inflammation of a bursa causing pain and swelling above the knee cap with limited range of motion at the joint. Bursitis can result from overuse, a direct blow to the area, and chronic friction from frequent kneeling. Plumbers, carpet layers, gardeners, housemaids, football and basketball athletes, and patients with motor vehicle injuries are at risk of developing prepatellar bursitis. Crystal deposition diseases, such as gout and pseudogout can also contribute toward development of prepatellar bursitis. Incidence of prepatellar bursitis is higher in males than females. Radiographs show soft tissue swelling anterior to the patella. On MR imaging, fluid collection is seen superficial to the patella, which is low signal intensity on T1-weighted images and high signal intensity on T_2-weighted images. Treatment consists of avoidance of aggravating activity, drainage or excision, anti-inflammatory drugs and antibiotics if it gets infected.

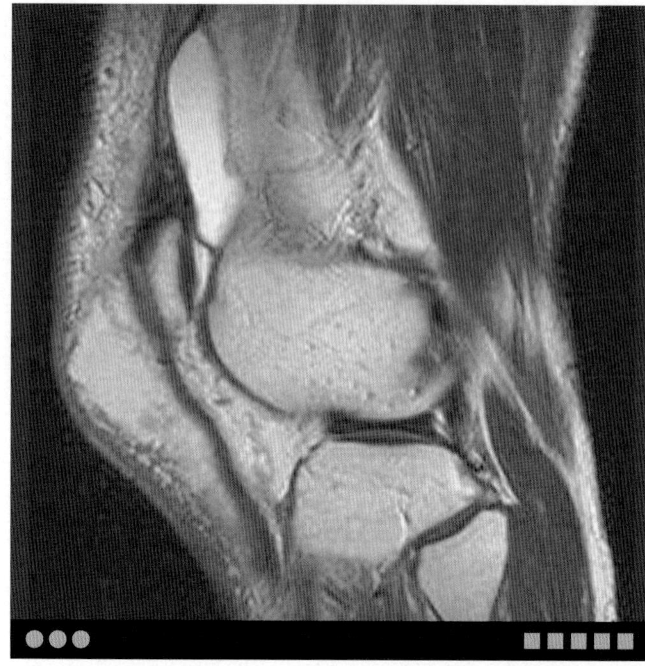

A. Prepatellar bursitis: Sagittal T2-weighted image demonstrates bright fluid signal prepatellar bursa.

PEARLS

- **Prepatellar bursitis is inflammation of a bursa, located in front of patella, near the attachment of the patellar tendon and overlying skin.**
- **Plumbers, carpet layers, gardeners, housemaids, football and basketball players, and patients involved with motor vehicle injuries are at higher risk of developing prepatellar bursitis.**
- **MR imaging shows fluid collection superficial to the patella.**

ADDITIONAL IMAGES

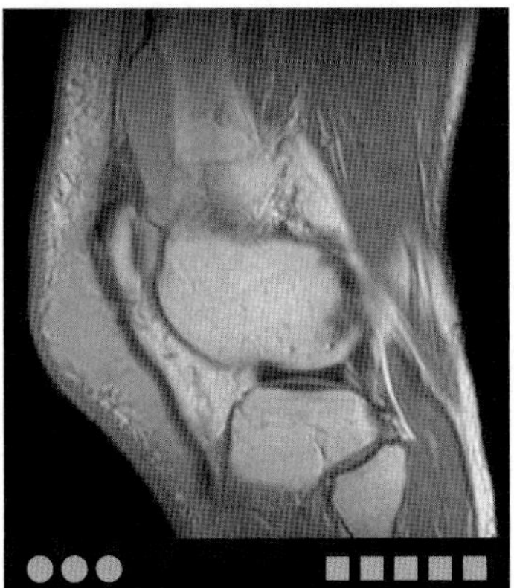

B. Prepatellar bursitis: Sagittal T1-weighted image shows intermediate signal intensity fluid collection prepatellar bursa.

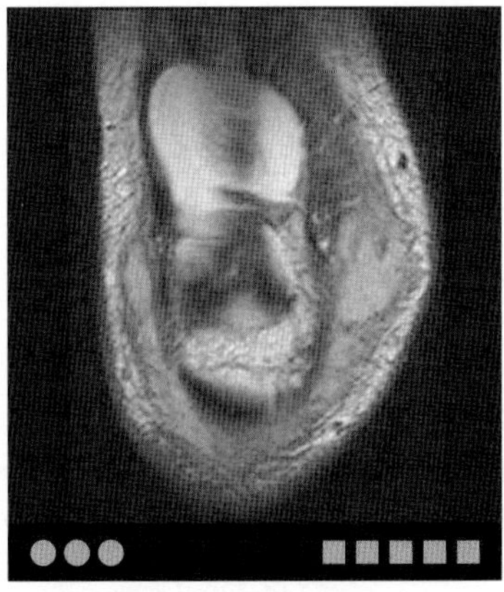

C. Prepatellar bursitis: Coronal T2-weighted image shows high signal intensity fluid in prepatellar bursa.

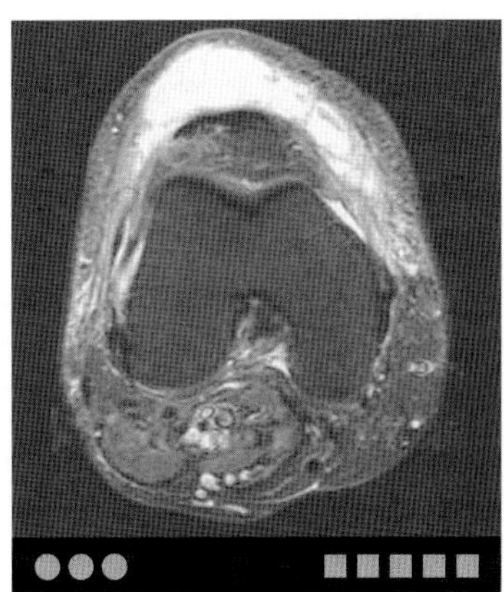

D. Prepatellar bursitis: Axial STIR weighted image shows fluid-filled structure prepatellar bursa.

IMAGE KEY

Common

Rare

Typical

Unusual

DIFFERENTIAL DIAGNOSES IMAGES

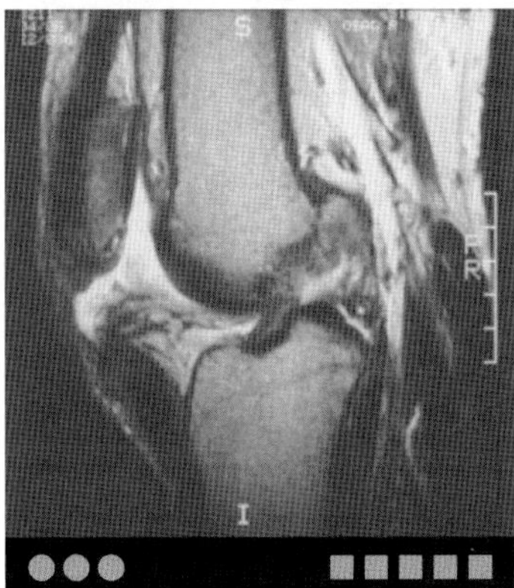

E. Patellar tendon tear: Sagittal T2-weighted image shows blood from patellar tendon tear extending in the prepatellar bursa with high signal intensity.

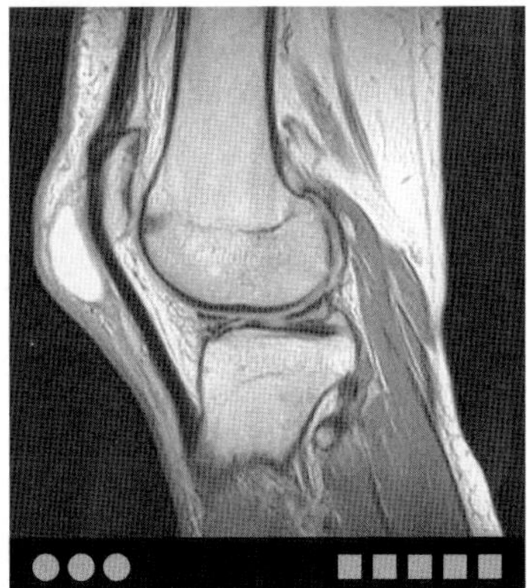

F. Trauma to the prepatellar soft tissue: Sagittal T1-weighted image shows high signal intensity subacute blood.

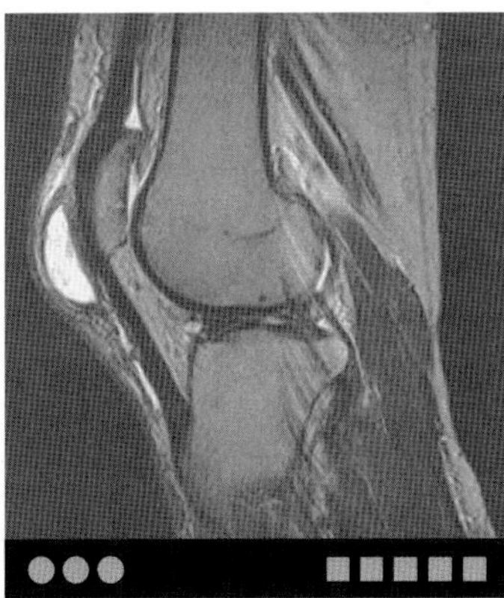

G. Trauma to the prepatellar soft tissue: Sagittal T2-weighted image shows high signal intensity blood in prepatellar bursa.

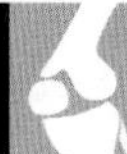

23-27 Pes Anserinus Bursitis

Melitus Maryam Golshan and Jamshid Tehranzadeh

PRESENTATION

Pain, tenderness, and soft tissue mass

FINDINGS

MR images show fluid in the pes anserine bursa in medial aspect of the knee joint.

DIFFERENTIAL DIAGNOSES

- *Atypical synovial cyst:* Extension to the joint could be traced in different planes.
- *Meniscal or perimeniscal cyst:* The center of these cysts would be at the level of the meniscus.
- *Medial collateral ligament bursitis:* This would be along the medial collateral ligament.
- *Soft tissue tumors of medial knee joint:* These would often enhance with IV Gad. Contrast agent.

COMMENTS

The patient is a 49-year-old woman with arthritis, pain, and tenderness in the medial side of the knee. Pes anserinus is the anatomic term used to identify the insertion of the conjoined tendons into the anteromedial proximal tibia. From anterior to posterior, pes anserinus is made up of the tendons of the sartorius, gracilis, and semitendinosus muscles. The term literally means "goose's foot," describing the webbed foot-like structure. The conjoined tendon lies superficial to the tibial insertion of the medial collateral ligament (MCL) of the knee. Theoretically, bursitis results from stress to this area (e.g., stress may result when an obese individual with anatomic deformity from arthritis ascends or descends stairs). Acute cases are the results of overuse especially in runners. Pathological studies do not indicate whether symptoms are attributable predominantly to true bursitis, tendonitis, or fascistic at this site. Ultrasound can aid the physician when diagnosing pes anserine bursitis. Large cystic bursal swellings have been evidenced by ultrasound and computed tomography (CT) scans. MRI is the preferred imaging technique to help the clinician confirm the diagnosis. A collection of fluid with low signal intensity is observed on T1-weighted images, and a homogenous increase in signal intensity is observed on T2-weighted images. Early images post contrast will outline the bursal margin. However, leakage of contrast agent into the cyst will follow soon, which will enhance the cyst in its entirety.

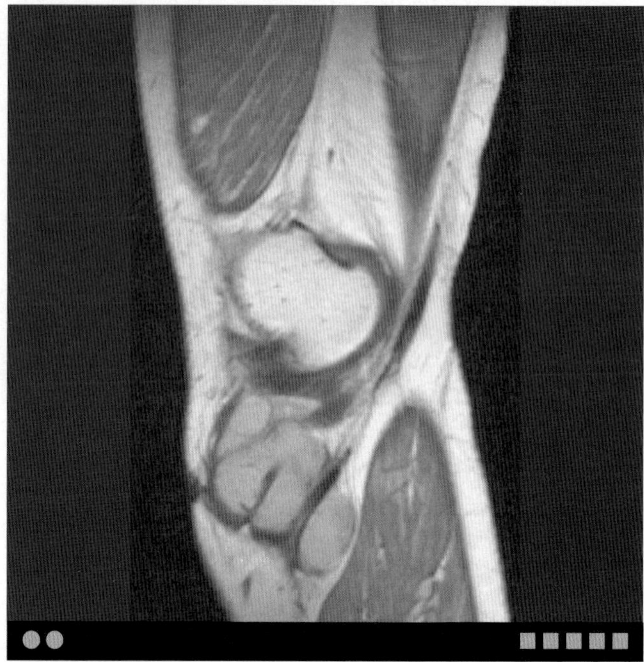

A. Pes anserinus bursitis: Sagittal proton density MR image shows a trident lobular digit-like cystic lesion in the medial aspect of the proximal tibia, representing pes anserinus bursitis.

PEARLS

- **Pes anserinus bursitis involves the three conjoined tendons in the medial aspect of the knee including sartorius, gracilis, and semitendinosus muscles.**
- **This bursitis has the appearance of webbed foot of a goose and best detected by MRI. US could also be useful.**
- **MRI shows a low signal mass on T1-weighted image in the medial aspect of the tibia with peripheral enhancement with contrast and homogenous bright signal on T2-weighted image.**

ADDITIONAL IMAGES

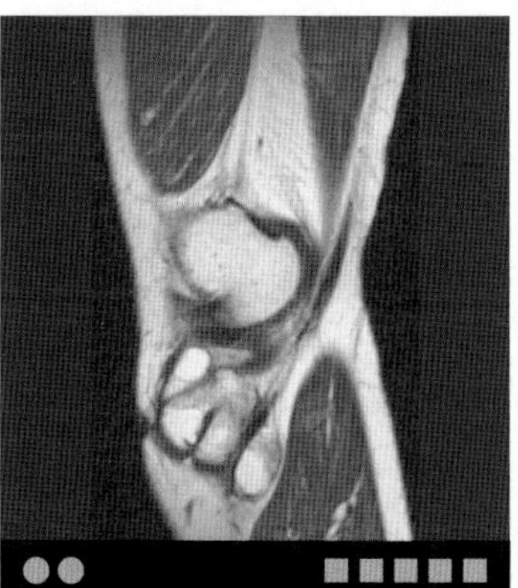

B. Pes anserinus bursitis: Sagittal T2-weighted image shows a trident lobular digit-like cystic lesion in the medial aspect of the proximal tibia, representing pes anserinus bursitis.

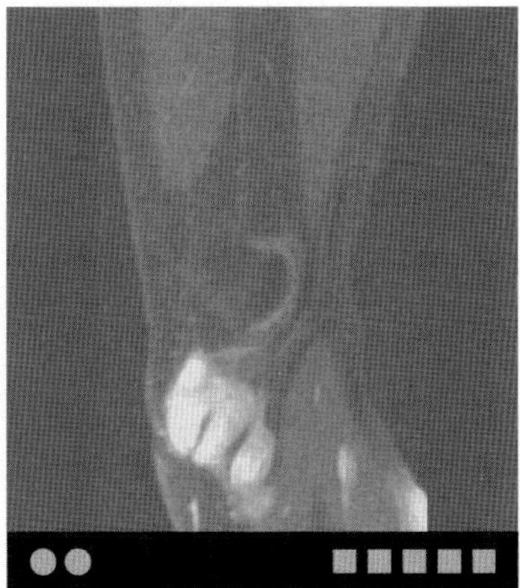

C. Pes anserinus bursitis: Sagittal fat-saturated T1-weighted post contrast image shows trident-shaped pes anserinus bursa with bright signal.

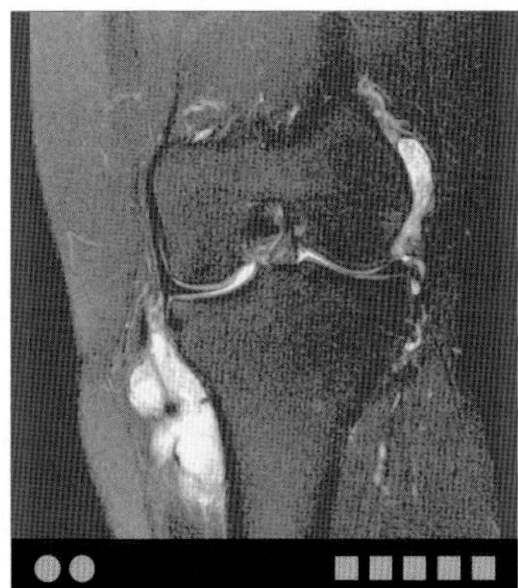

D. Pes anserinus bursitis: Coronal fat-saturated T1-weighted spin echo post contrast image shows a lobulated cystic lesion in the medial aspect of the proximal left tibia. Note rice bodies in the joint representing synovitis.

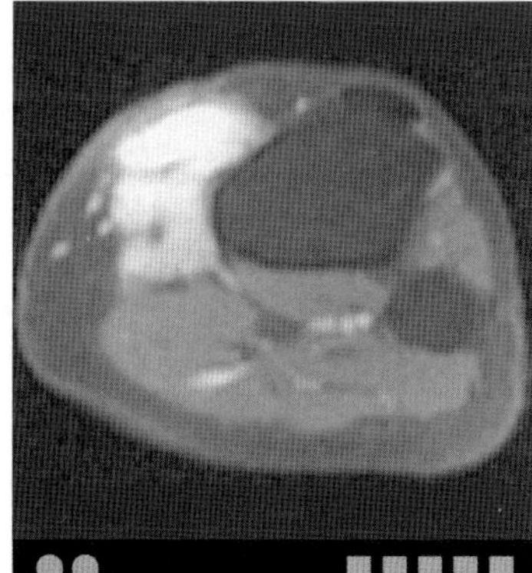

E. Pes anserinus bursitis: Axial fat-saturated post contrast T1-weighted image shows the bursa on the medial side of the left knee.

IMAGE KEY

Common

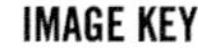

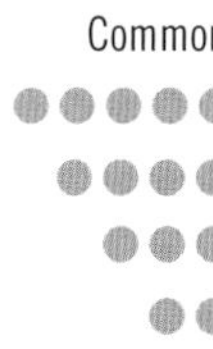

Rare

Typical

Unusual

DIFFERENTIAL DIAGNOSES IMAGES

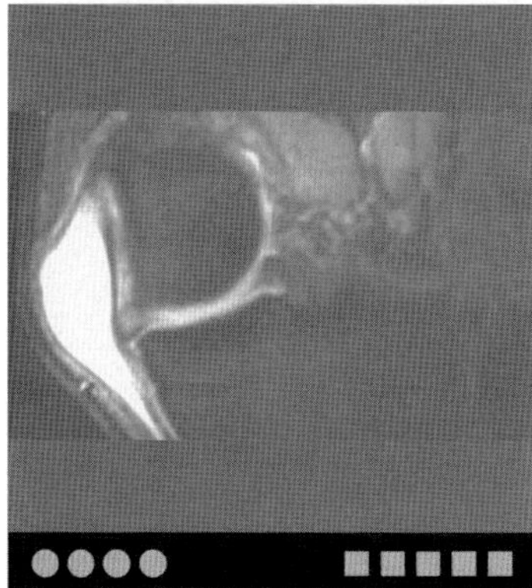

F. Perimeniscal cyst associated with bucket handle meniscal tear: Note the center of the cyst is at the level of the meniscus.

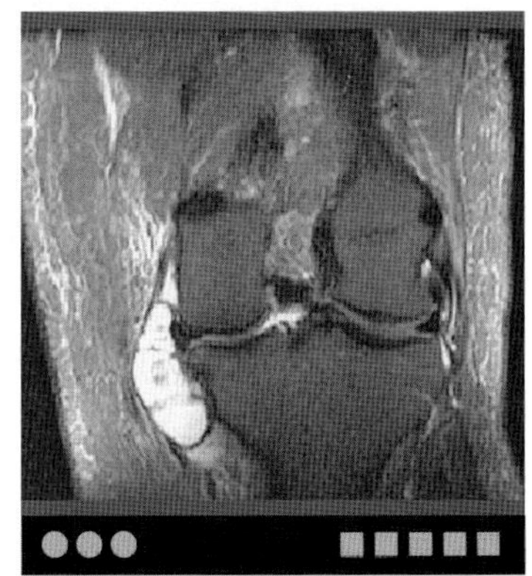

G. Medial collateral ligament bursitis: Coronal fat-saturated T2-weighted image shows fluid-containing cyst in the medial aspect of the knee joint.

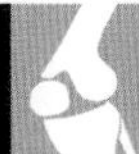

23–28 Tennis Leg

Kambiz Motamedi

PRESENTATION

Calf pain following sports activity

FINDINGS

MRI shows fluid within the compartment between the medial gastrocnemius and soleus muscles.

DIFFERENTIAL DIAGNOSES

- *Lymphoma/Leukemia:* MRI reveals an infiltrative mass of the musculature with spindle-shaped growth. The signal properties are nonspecific.
- *Necrotizing fasciitis:* MRI commonly shows microabscesses and enhancing edema along the deep fascial planes. Scattered muscle edema may also be encountered.
- *Soft tissue sarcoma:* MRI usually reveals a soft tissue mass of varying appearance. The mass may be homogenous with high fluid signal or heterogeneous after internal bleeding.

COMMENTS

This 54-year-old male patient experienced intense calf pain following a tennis match. Tennis leg is a common clinical condition that affects both young athletes and sedentary people. The classic presentation is that of acute pain in the middle portion of the calf after relatively innocuous activity like walking up stairs or pivoting to get to the ball while playing tennis or some other sport. Affected individuals often report a "pop" or "tearing sensation" at the onset of symptoms; however, the event is often not painful enough to prevent them from doing whatever activity they were doing immediately. In fact, the greatest pain develops over the next 24 to 48 hours and is associated with significant tenderness and regional swelling that can take on a purplish skin discoloration from hemorrhage. The role of the plantaris muscle tendon in this type of injury has been questioned on several reports. In patients with symptoms consistent with tennis leg, MRI and/or ultrasound proven rupture of the plantaris tendon was observed in only 1.4% of affected individuals. In the majority of the cases (88%), there was a tear in the medial head of the gastrocnemius muscle (66.7%) or a fluid collection between the aponeurosis of the medial gastrocnemius and soleus. MR images through the calves often show a collection of fluid between the soleus and the gastrocnemius that can take on a tubular configuration. A torn or retracted tendon helps with the diagnosis. The follow-up imaging shows decrease and eventual resolution of the fluid collection.

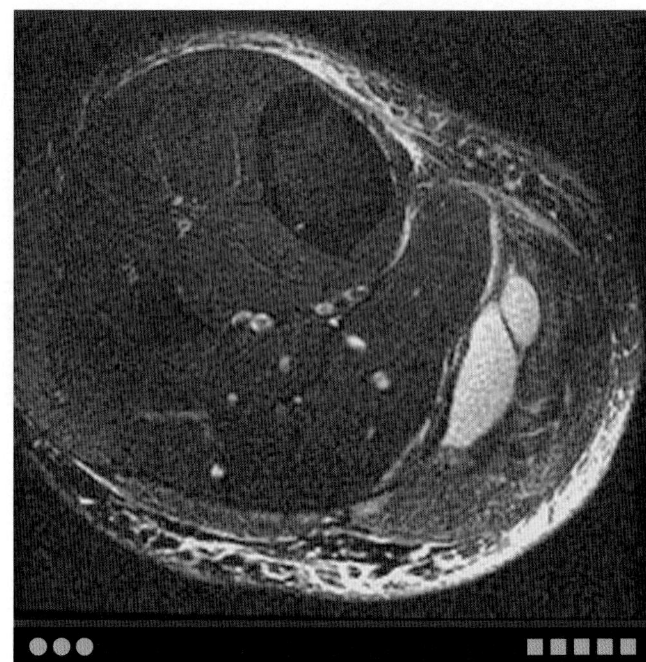

A. Tennis leg: Axial fat-saturated T2-weighted image shows fluid collection along the aponeurosis of the medial gastrocnemius muscle and edema of the muscle itself.

PEARLS

- **The fluid collection with or without edema of the medial gastrocnemius muscle are the hallmarks of this entity.**
- **Follow-up imaging may be indicted in equivocal cases to ensure resolution and exclude a soft tissue mass.**
- **Follow-up may be performed with ultrasound.**

ADDITIONAL IMAGES

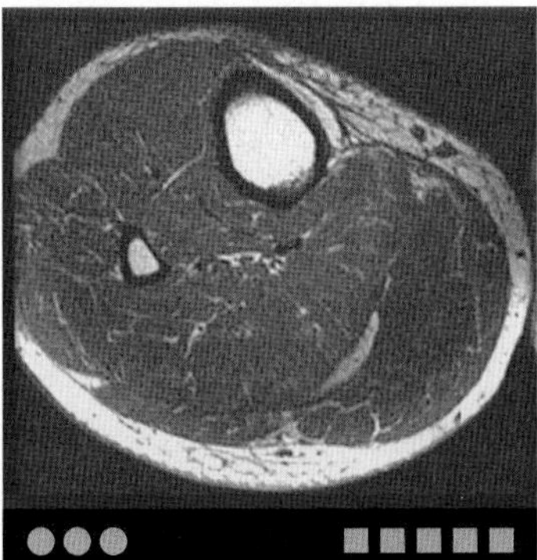

B. Tennis leg: Axial T1-weighted image reveals a low signal fluid collection indicating chronic hematoma. Note the obliteration of the fatty marbling of the medial gastrocnemius muscle consistent with edema.

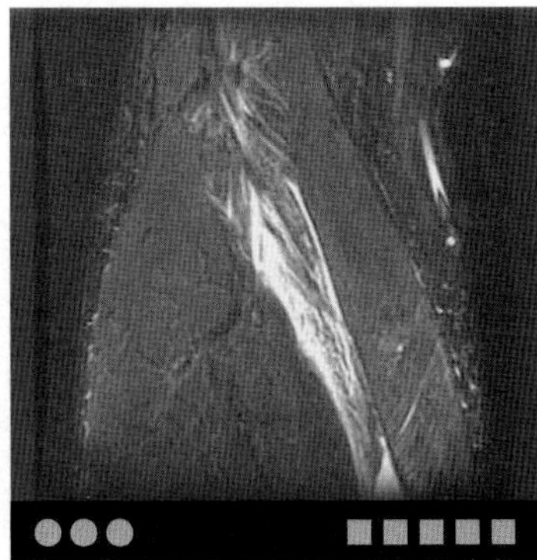

C. Tennis leg: Coronal inversion recovery image confirms the elongated hematoma collection along the course of the plantaris tendon.

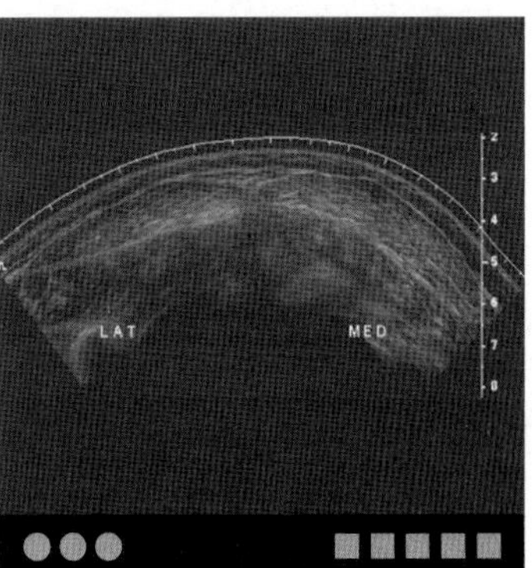

D. Tennis leg: Follow-up panorama sonographic image demonstrates the normal symmetric echo texture and morphology of the contralateral gastrocnemius muscle.

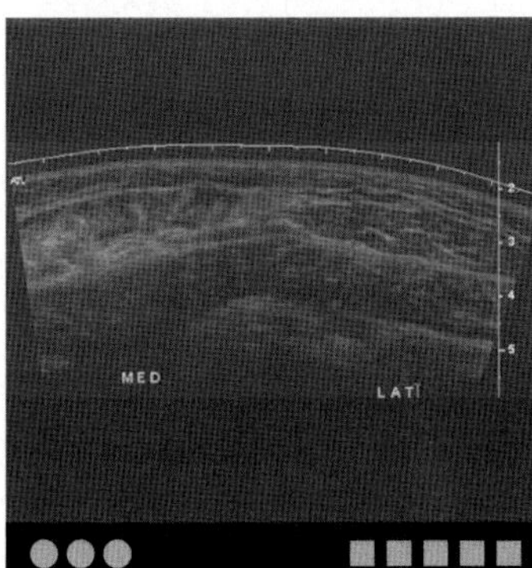

E. Tennis leg: Follow-up panorama sonographic image reveals the architectural distortion of the medial gastrocnemius muscle compartment indicating edema. This becomes most conspicuous in comparison to the contralateral aspect.

IMAGE KEY

Common

Rare

Typical

Unusual

DIFFERENTIAL DIAGNOSES IMAGES

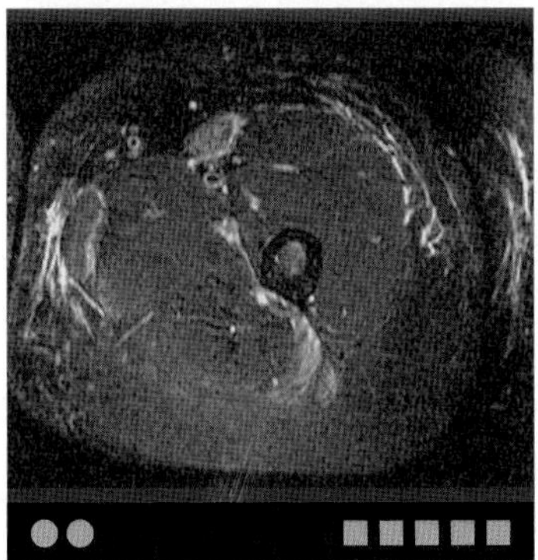

F. Leukemic infiltrates: Axial fat-saturated MR image demonstrates the enhancing fascial edema with patchy edema of the rectus femoris and subcutaneous compartments.

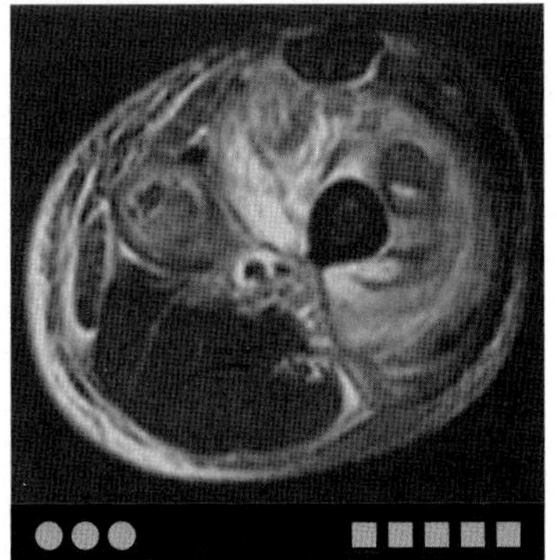

G. Necrotizing fasciitis: Axial fat-saturated MR image shows microabscesses along with deep fascial and muscular edema.

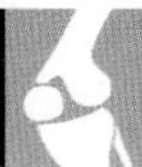

23–29 Sonographic Presentation of Tennis Leg

Mélanie Morel, Nathalie Boutry, and Anne Cotten

PRESENTATION

Acute, sports-related, medial calf pain

FINDINGS

Sonography shows a fusiform heterogenous collection between the medial head of the gastrocnemius muscle and the aponeurosis of the soleus muscle.

DIFFERENTIAL DIAGNOSES

- *Rupture of the plantaris tendon:* Discontinuity of the plantaris tendon can be seen on longitudinal sonograms. The muscle belly is retracted proximally between the popliteus tendon and the lateral head of the gastrocnemius muscle. An intermuscular fluid collection can be seen between the soleus and the medial head of the gastrocnemius muscles, typically proximal to the collection found in tennis leg.
- *Intramuscular contusion/rupture of the soleus muscle:* Sonogram shows heterogeneous hypoechoic hematoma within the muscle, and distortion of the normal architecture. MRI is more convenient than sonography to study these deep lesions.
- *Rupture of the calcaneal tendon:* In case of complete tear, sonography shows a cleft in the tendon and a hematoma between the separated tendon ends. Partial rupture is defined by the presence of intact fibers within an enlarged tendon and hypoechoic or anechoic areas corresponding to the tear.
- *Ruptured Baker's cyst:* Sonography shows fluid superficial to the medial head of the gastrocnemius muscle, distal to a popliteal cyst with irregularities at its distal aspect.
- *Deep venous thrombosis:* Sonography shows a loss of compressibility of the vein, intraluminal thrombi, and color defect on Doppler sonogram.
- *Soft tissue calf mass:* MRI is the gold standard if a solid or hypervascular soft tissue mass is found with ultrasound examination.

COMMENTS

The patient is a 42-year-old man complaining of acute pain in the calf while skiing, associated with a snapping sensation, followed by local edema and functional impairment. Tennis leg usually occurs in a middle-aged person during active plantar flexion of the foot and simultaneous extension of the knee. The sudden pain in the calf arises from the detachment of the medial head of the gastrocnemius muscle from its peripheral aponeurosis next to its distal musculo-tendinous junction. Sonography is useful for assessing the severity of the tear. A partial tear is defined by focal disruption of muscle fibers at the musculo-aponeurotic junction. The distal portion of the medial head of gastrocnemius muscle has a heterogeneous appearance (with hyper or/and hypoechoic areas) instead of its normal regular fibrillar appearance. Longitudinal sonogram shows a blunting of the triangular configuration of this distal portion. A complete tear is diagnosed when the entire medial head of the gastrocnemius muscle is involved, with proximal retraction of muscle fibers. A hypoechoic or anechoic fluid collection is commonly found between the medial head of the gastrocnemius muscle and the aponeurosis of the soleus muscle. US guided drainage of the fluid collection may produce a rapid relief of symptoms, but is often followed by recurrence of the collection when calf compression is not performed. Hemorrhagic collection in the fascial plane separating the soleus and the medial head of gastrocnemius muscles is clearly depicted.

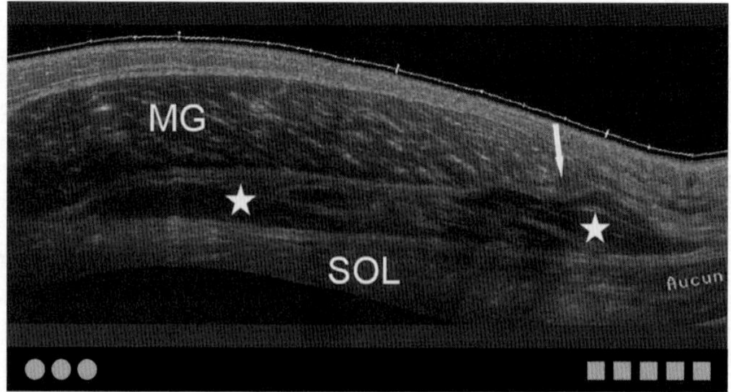

A. Tennis leg (complete tear): Longitudinal sonogram of the anteromedial calf shows a loss of triangular pattern of the distal portion of the retracted medial head of the gastrocnemius muscle (MG), with hypoechoic areas (arrow). Heterogeneous blood collection (stars) is seen between the gastrocnemius muscle aponeurosis and the soleus muscle aponeurosis (SOL).

PEARLS

- **This is one of the most common sports-related injury in middle-aged persons, but it may also result from daily activities.**
- **The distal fibers of the medial head of the gastrocnemius muscle detach from its peripheral aponeurosis.**
- **US image typically shows disruption of the medial head of the gastrocnemius muscle, and a fluid collection separating the medial head and the soleus muscle.**
- **US enables to appreciate the size of the tear and to follow-up the healing.**
- **MRI is not needed for diagnosis, but is useful for assessing the severity of the injury.**

ADDITIONAL IMAGES

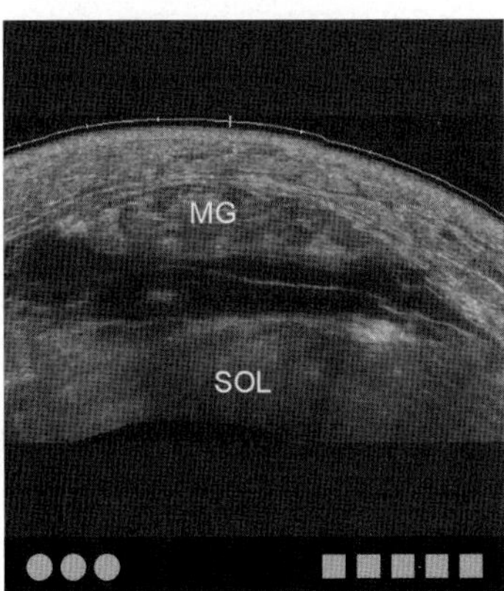

B. Tennis leg (complete tear): Axial sonogram depicts the entire medial head of the gastrocnemius muscle (MG) and shows it is a complete tear (SOL: soleus muscle).

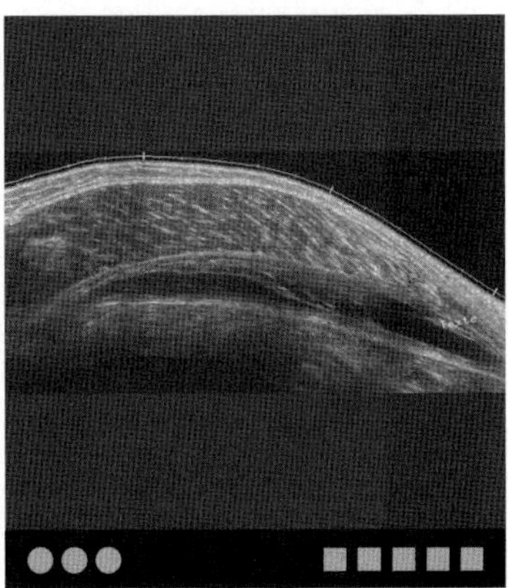

C. Tennis leg: The 1-month follow-up after blood collection evacuation shows recurrence of hematoma which is less echoic.

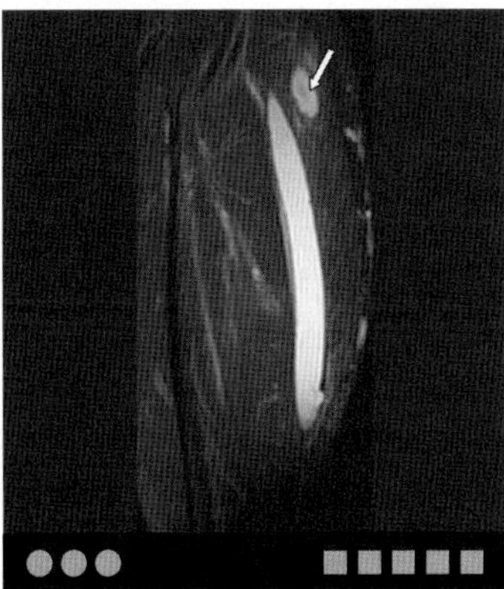

D. Tennis leg (complete tear): Sagittal T2-weighted fat-saturated image shows the blood collection between the retracted medial head of the gastrocnemius muscle and the soleus muscle. Venous thrombosis is associated in this patient (arrow).

DIFFERENTIAL DIAGNOSES IMAGES

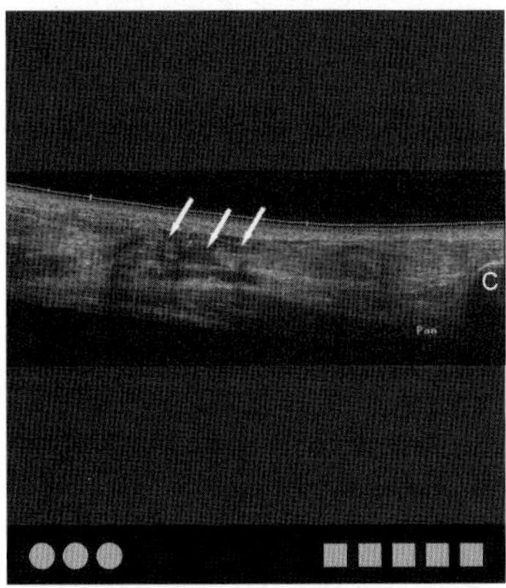

E. Complete rupture of the calcaneal tendon: Longitudinal sonogram shows a complete disruption of the calcaneal tendon fibers (arrows), with a retracted upper fragment (C: calcaneus).

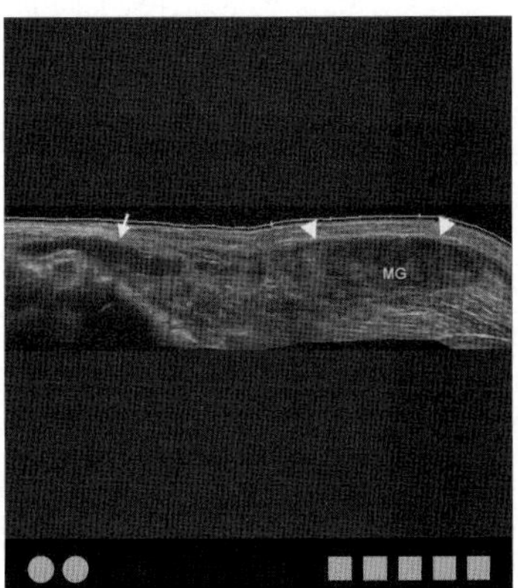

F. Ruptured Baker's cyst: A fluid collection (arrowheads) can be seen superficial to the medial gastrocnemius muscle (MG), distally to the popliteal cyst (arrow).

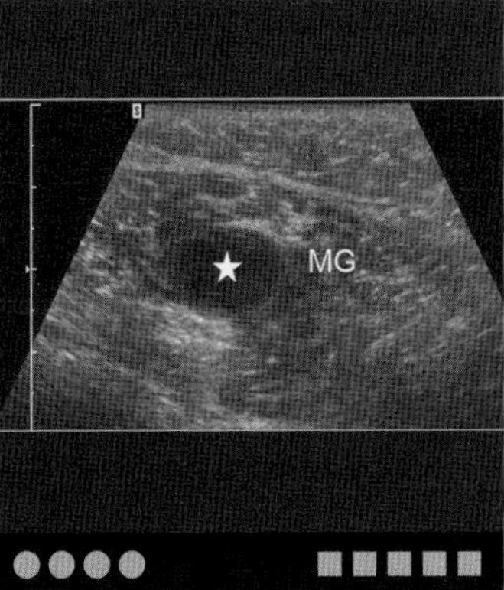

G. Venous thrombosis: Axial sonogram of the posterior medial calf exhibits a loss of compressibility of the vein (MG: medial head of the gastrocnemius muscle) and intraluminal thrombi (star).

IMAGE KEY

Common

Rare

Typical

Unusual

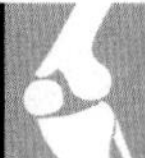

23–30 Transient Patellar Dislocation

Hakan Ilaslan

PRESENTATION

Persistent knee pain and swelling after football injury

FINDINGS

MRI shows bone marrow contusions of medial patellar facet and lateral femoral condyle. Interruption of medial patellar retinaculum fibers with associated edema and fluid-like signal consistent with partial thickness tear.

DIFFERENTIAL DIAGNOSES

- *MCL injury:* Although MCL and medial patellar retinaculum are intimately related, careful evaluation demonstrate the abnormality within and surrounding MCL fibers. Bone marrow contusion pattern of transient patellar dislocation (TPD) is typically absent.
- *Post-traumatic bone marrow contusions:* This finding may be isolated or associated with ligamentous injuries. However, location of bone marrow contusions of TPD is classic.

COMMENTS

Transient patellar dislocation (TPD) is a common cause of acute traumatic hemarthrosis in young active patients. TPD is thought to occur either as a result of a noncontact injury with internal rotation of the femur and valgus position of the knee while on a planted foot (most common), or direct blow to the medial aspect of the patella. When the patella spontaneously relocates after dislocation, bone marrow contusions of the medial patellar facet and lateral femoral condyle occur owing to impaction injury. In addition, chondral or osteochondral fractures may also be seen in one or both of these locations. Injury to the medial patellar retinaculum is typically seen after TPD. The medial patellar retinacular complex is the medial restraint of the patella and is composed of three layers. The most superficial layer (Layer I) invests both the sartorius and gastrocnemius muscles. Layer II is deep to Layer I and contains the major ligaments including medial patellofemoral ligament, the superficial portion of MCL and patellotibial ligament. Layer III is the deepest layer and is composed of deep MCL fibers and joint capsule. Osteochondral fractures most frequently occur on the inferomedial patella and may be difficult to see on radiographs. MRI is the modality of choice for the diagnosis of TPD. Typically, bone marrow contusions of medial patellar facet and lateral femoral condyle are present (kissing contusions). Medial patellar retinacular complex is best evaluated on the axial plane, and frequently demonstrates thickened and irregular fibers with associated edema and fluid-like signal.

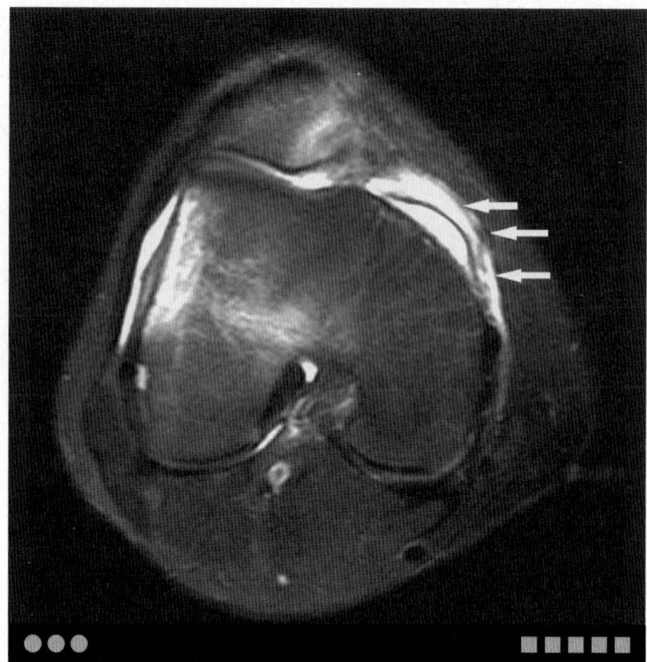

A. Transient patellar dislocation: Axial T2-weighted image of the right knee demonstrates bone marrow contusions of medial patellar facet and lateral femoral condyle. There is also interruption of medial patellar retinaculum fibers with associated edema and fluid-like signal consistent with partial thickness tear (arrows).

PEARLS

- **On MRI, the classic triad of this entity includes bone marrow contusions of medial patellar facet and lateral femoral condyle with associated medial retinacular injury.**
- **Chondral or osteochondral fractures may be seen, typically at the inferomedial patella.**
- **Effusions or hemarthrosis are common.**
- **Clinically, TPD may not be suspected at the initial presentation.**

ADDITIONAL IMAGES

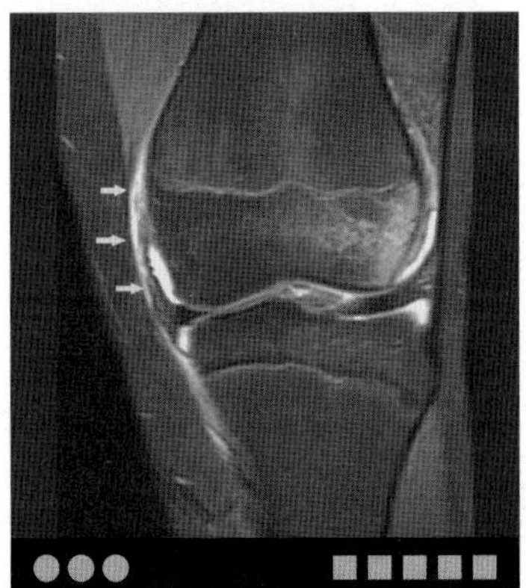

B. Transient patellar dislocation: Coronal T2-weighted image of the right knee demonstrates bone marrow contusion of lateral femoral condyle and edema-like signal about the medial patellar retinaculum (arrows).

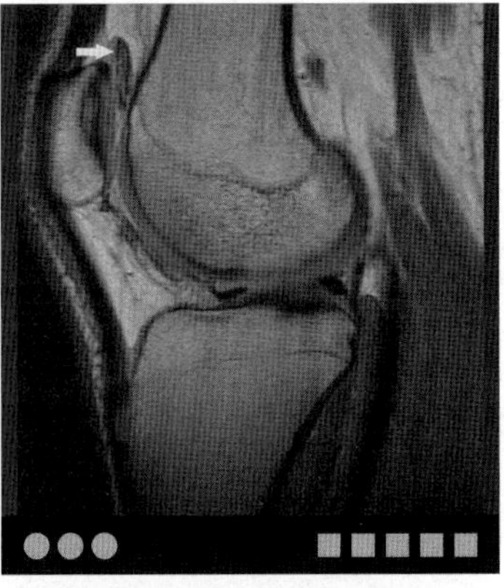

C. Transient patellar dislocation: Sagittal PD image of the left knee after TPD shows osteochondral free fragment (arrows).

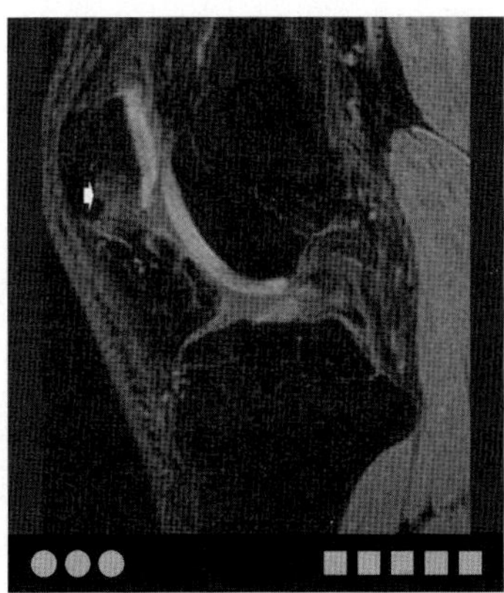

D. Transient patellar dislocation: Sagittal gradient echo 3D image of the left knee demonstrates the donor site in the inferomedial patella (short arrow).

IMAGE KEY

Common

●●●●●
●●●●
●●●
●●
●

Rare

Typical

■■■■■
■■■■
■■■
■■
■

Unusual

DIFFERENTIAL DIAGNOSES IMAGES

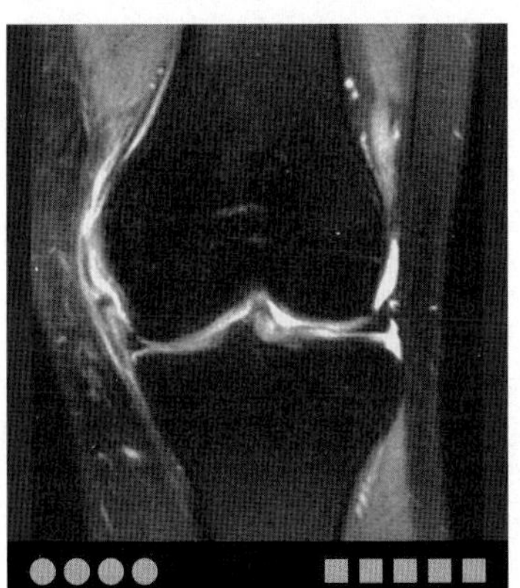

E. Medial collateral ligament sprain: Coronal proton density weighted FS image shows irregular MCL fibers with surrounding fluid and edema-like signal consistent with MCL sprain.

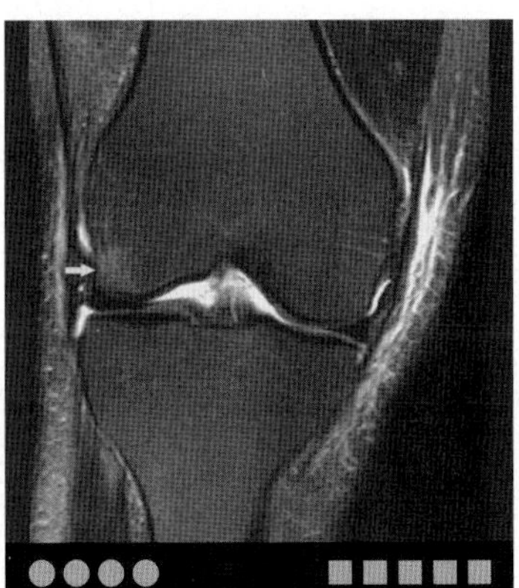

F. Bone marrow contusion in ACL tear: Coronal T2-weighted image of the right knee demonstrates bone marrow contusion of lateral femoral condyle (arrow) in a patient with ACL tear. Also note the mild MCL sprain medially.

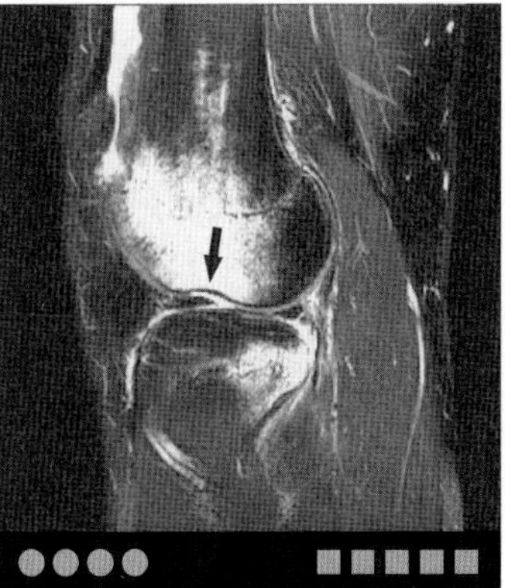

G. Osteochondral impaction and contusion of lateral condyle in ACL tear: Sagittal T2-weighted image with fat suppression in another patient shows the deep sulcus (arrow) corresponds to an osteochondral fracture of the lateral condyle, with extensive marrow edema.

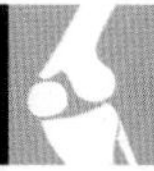

23–31 Partial Tear of Quadriceps Tendon

Shahla Modarresi and Daria Motamedi

PRESENTATION

Knee pain, swelling, and function loss after trauma

FINDINGS

MR images show partial thickness tear of quadriceps tendon.

DIFFERENTIAL DIAGNOSES

- *Myxoid degeneration/tendinosis:* Occurs with aging and chronic overuse. MR imaging shows normal size or thickened tendon with increased internal signal in T1-weighted and T2-weighted images.
- *Arthritis:* Pannus or tophi may involve the tendon resembling partial tear. MR imaging shows thickened tendon, low T1, intermediate to high T2 signal in rheumatoid arthritis; intermediate T1, intermediate to low T2 signal in gout.
- *Xanthoma of the tendon:* Occurs in patients with familial hyperlipidemia, most common in Achilles tendon. MR imaging shows thickened tendon with internal low and high signal. It may not be distinguishable from partial tear.
- *Giant cell tumor of the tendon sheet (PVNS):* It presents as a nonpainful, soft tissue mass. MR imaging shows intermediate or low signal in both T1 and T2-weighted images. It may resemble partial tear.

COMMENTS

The quadriceps muscle is formed of four muscle groups: the vastus intermedius, vastus medialis, vastus lateralis, and rectus femoris. The quadriceps tendon is multilayered formed by the convergence of all four muscles just proximal to the superior patella. The rectus femoris tendon is the most superficial layer inserting on the patella with some of its fibers continued over the anterior patellar surface to join distally to the patellar tendon. Myxoid degeneration of tendons occurs with aging or chronic overuse, which weakens the tendon leading to partial or full thickness tear as the most common cause. Quadriceps tendon rupture is infrequent, unilateral, occurring in those older than over 40, about 2 cm above the patella. It could be bilateral with systemic diseases including hyperparathyroidism, chronic renal failure, gout, obesity, RA, diabetes, steroid abuse, and tumors. Patellar tendon ruptures are less common occurring in younger patients. Jumper's knee involves the patellar tendon but can involve the quadriceps in 25% of cases. Complete tendon rupture requires early diagnosis and surgery for best results. Surgery of complete tear up to one year following injury is

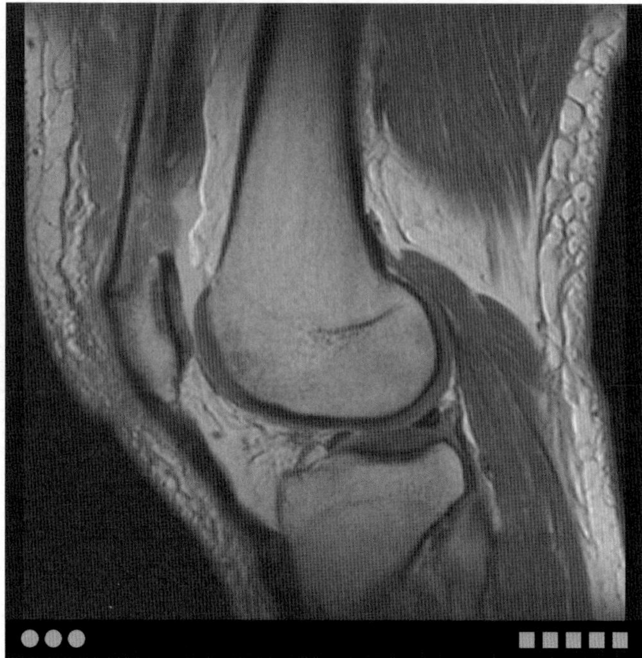

A. Partial quadriceps tendon tear: Sagittal proton density (PD) image shows partial thickness tear of the quadriceps tendon.

indicated. Partial tears are treated conservatively unless they remain refractory to conservative management. MRI is the imaging modality of choice. Complete ruptures show transection of all tendon layers. Incomplete ruptures show discontinuities of individual layers, with the remaining layers being intact and showing high T2 signal.

PEARLS

- **The quadriceps tendon is formed by convergence of four muscles: the vastus intermedius, vastus medialis, vastus lateralis, and rectus femoris inserting on the patella.**
- **Myxoid degeneration of tendons occurs with aging or chronic overuse, which weakens the tendon leading to partial or full thickness tear as the most common cause.**
- **Many systemic diseases such as hyperparathyroidism, chronic renal failure, gout, obesity, RA, diabetes, steroid abuse, tumors predispose the tendon to bilateral tear.**
- **Patellar tendon ruptures are less common occurring in younger patients. Jumper's knee involves the patellar tendon but can involve the quadriceps in 25% of cases.**
- **MRI is the imaging modality of choice. Complete transection of all tendon layers or incomplete discontinuity of some tendon layers is demonstrated.**

ADDITIONAL IMAGE

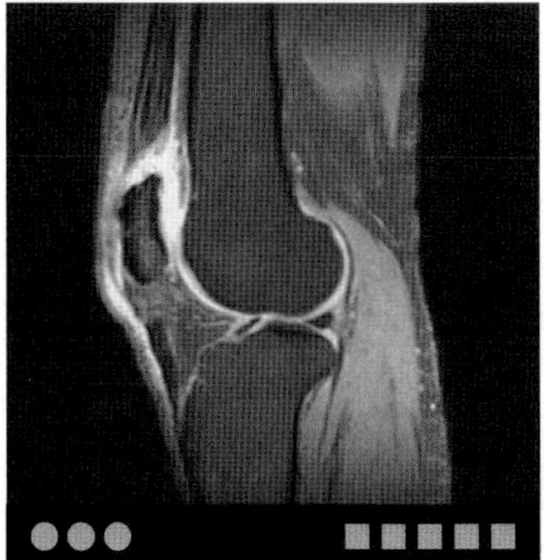

B. Partial quadriceps tendon tear: Sagittal STIR image in another patient shows partial thickness tear of quadriceps tendon and patellar tendon.

DIFFERENTIAL DIAGNOSES IMAGES

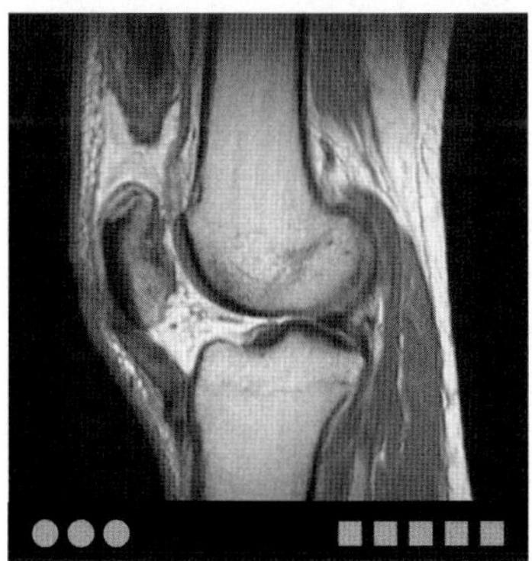

C. Complete quadriceps tendon tear in patient with gout: Sagittal PD image shows complete tear and retraction of the quadriceps tendon. Note partial thickness tear of patellar tendon.

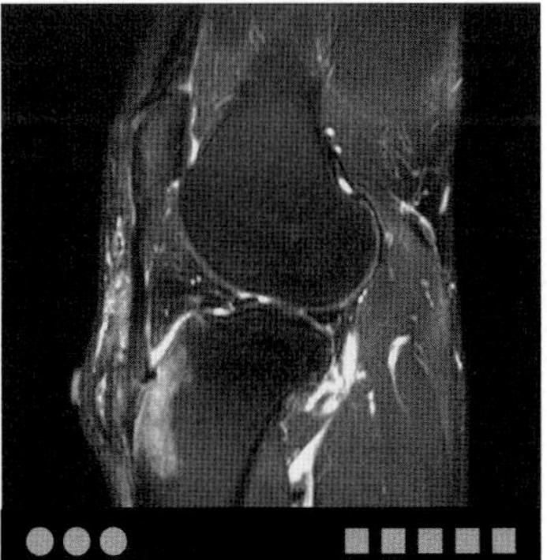

D. Pattelar tendinosis: Sagittal STIR image shows tendinosis vs. partial thickness tear of distal patellar tendon with bone marrow edema/contusion of tibial tubercle.

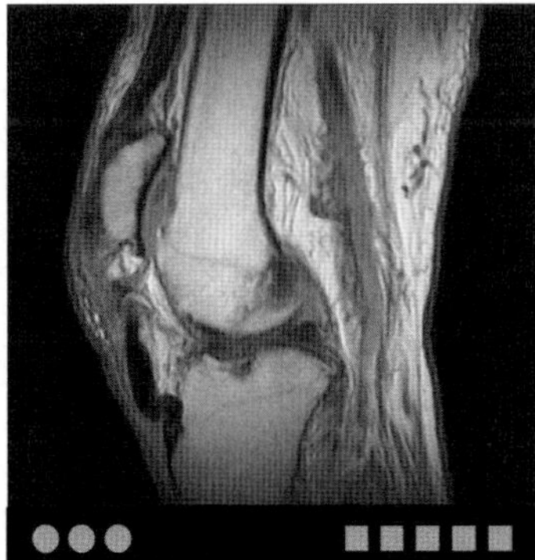

E. Complete patellar tendon tear: Sagittal PD image shows full thickness tear of patellar tendon and prepatellar hematoma. Note retraction of quadriceps tendon and patella.

IMAGE KEY

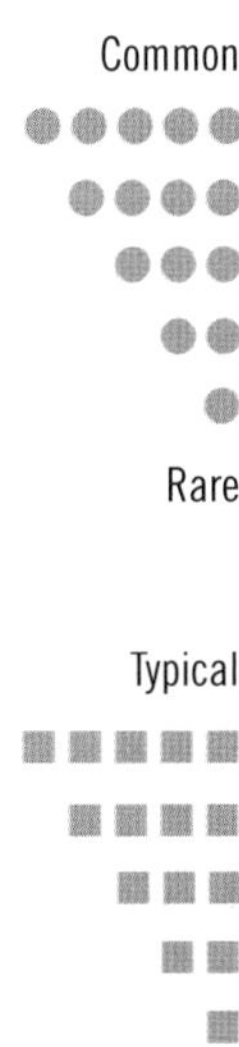

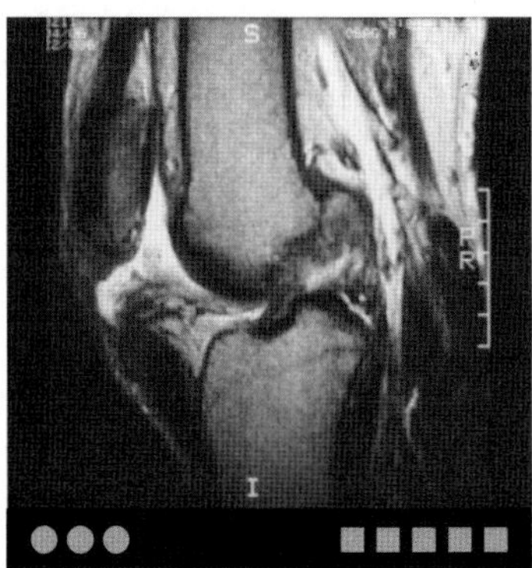

F. Complete patellar tendon tear: Sagittal T2-weighted image in another patient shows complete tear of proximal patellar tendon tear. Note retraction of quadriceps tendon and patella.

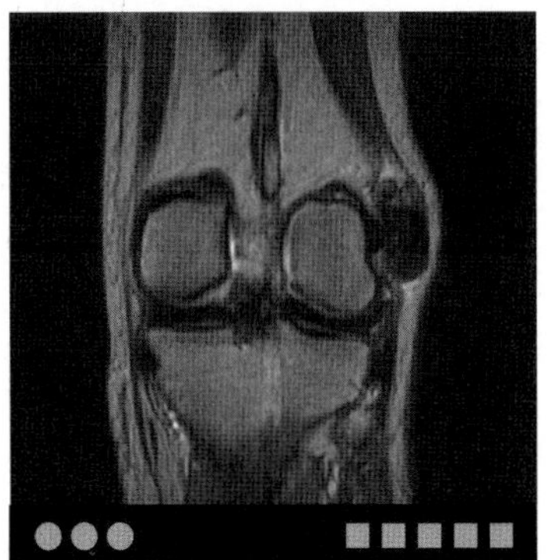

G. Giant cell tumor of tendon sheet: Coronal T2-weighted image shows intermediate to low signal mass of biceps femoris tendon consistent with giant cell tumors that may resemble tendon tear.

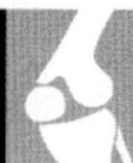

23–32 Tibial Plateau Fracture/Bumper Fracture

Edward Mossop and Jamshid Tehranzadeh

PRESENTATION

Knee pain after trauma

FINDINGS

MRI shows fracture of the lateral tibial plateau with bone contusion extending to the midline and partial tear of the lateral collateral ligament.

DIFFERENTIAL DIAGNOSES

- *Segond fracture:* A cortical avulsion fracture of lateral tibial condyle that could be associated with anterior cruciate ligament (ACL), medial meniscus, and lateral joint capsule tear.
- *Moderate to severe contusion of the lateral tibial condyle without fracture:* Occasionally bone contusions may mask tibial plateau fractures.
- Tear of the lateral collateral ligament may occur without fracture.
- Avulsion fracture of the fibula with tear of lateral collateral ligament is responsible for posterolateral knee instability and is called arcuate sign.

COMMENTS

Tibial plateau fractures were originally termed bumper fractures because of their association with automobile impacts to the knee. Only 25% are related to automobile trauma, the remaining are caused by a fall in which the knee is forced into valgus or varus. Tibial plateau fractures are most common in adults between 50 and 60 years of age because of the increasing osteoporosis, but may occur in adults of any age. Force is directed from the femoral condyles onto the medial and lateral portions of the tibial plateau, resulting in fracture. Fractures of the lateral plateau occur more frequently (75% to 80%) and can be accompanied by disruption of the ACL and medial collateral ligament. Medial plateau injuries are usually more severe with damage to the posterior cruciate ligament (PCL) and popliteal artery. Soft tissue injuries occur in approximately 10% of patients. Patients may present with pain, stiffness, deformity, and knee effusion. Fractures can be missed on conventional radiograph. MRI shows a well-defined linear area of low signal intensity in the epiphysis on T1-weighted images that would be surrounded by an area of bright bone edema on T2-weighted images or STIR imaging. In acute fracture, with associated fluid or hemorrhage, MRI with contrast may be useful in displaying fracture morphology. MRI is also an excellent modality for showing ligamentous and meniscal injuries.

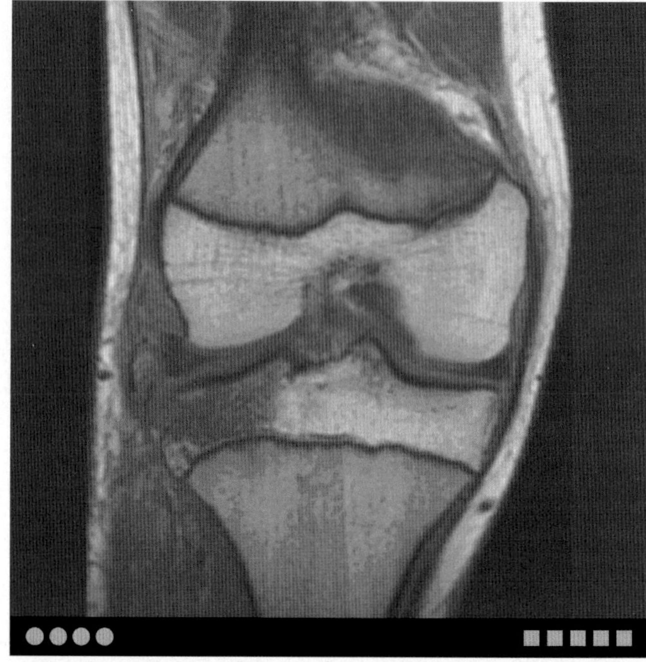

A. Bumper fracture: Coronal T1-weighted image shows large area of low signal in the medial aspect of the tibial plateau from bumper fracture.

PEARLS

- **75% of tibial plateau fractures occur after a fall with axial loading.**
- **75% to 80% of fractures involve the lateral tibial plateau.**
- **Soft tissue injuries occur in 10% of this fracture and include damage to the cruciate and collateral ligaments.**
- **MRI shows fracture as a low signal intensity line on T1-weighted images, which would be surrounded by an area of bright bone contusion on T2-weighted or STIR imaging.**
- **MRI is necessary for evaluation of ligamentous injuries accompanying this fracture.**

ADDITIONAL IMAGES

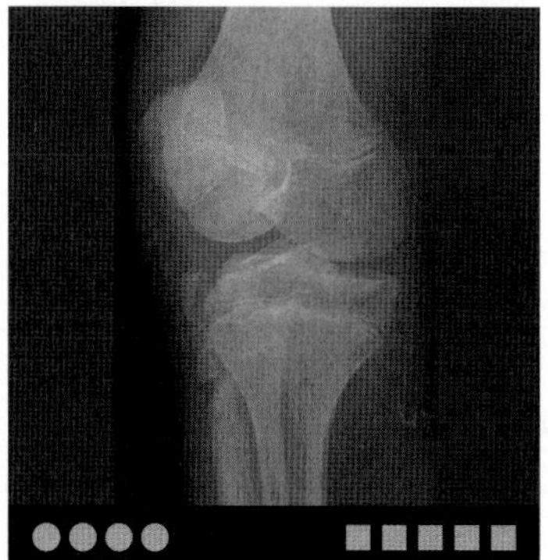

B. Bumper fracture: Oblique radiograph shows bumper fracture of the lateral tibial plateau.

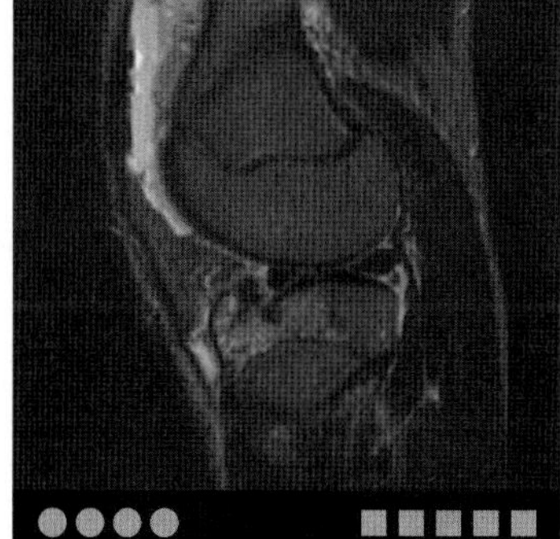

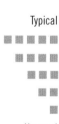

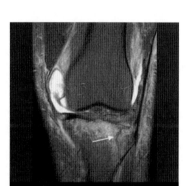

C. Bumper fracture: Sagittal T2-weighted image shows large area of high signal involving the lateral aspect of the tibial plateau consistent with bone contusion from bumper fracture. Note fluid levels or serum cellular separation within suprapatellar bursa.

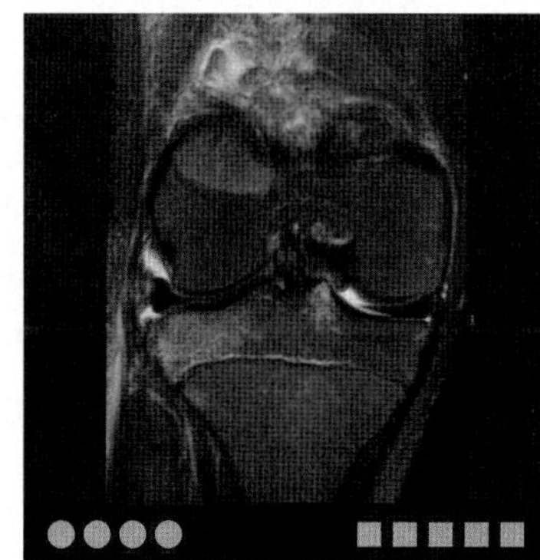

D. Bumper fracture: Coronal T2-weighted image shows increased signal in the lateral aspect of the tibial plateau consistent with bone contusion from bumper fracture.

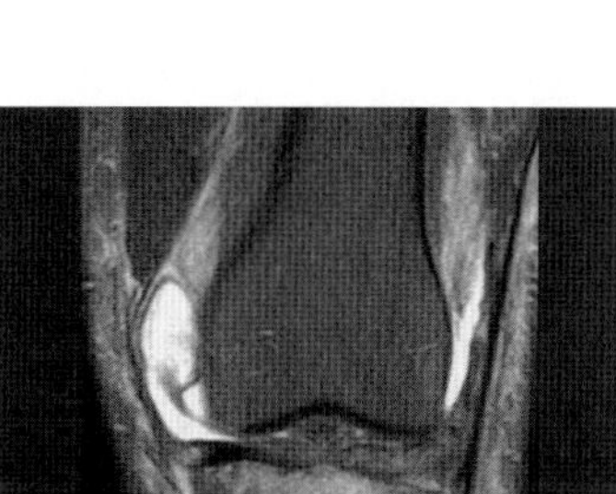

E. Bumper fracture: Coronal T2 fat-saturated image shows fracture line (arrow) with tibial plateau edema.

IMAGE KEY

Common

Rare

Typical

Unusual

DIFFERENTIAL DIAGNOSES IMAGES

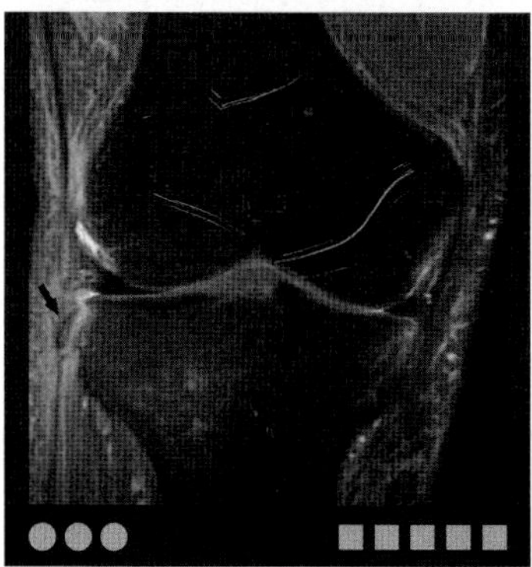

F. Segond fracture: Coronal proton density fat-saturated MRI sequence shows the tiny avulsed elliptical osseous fragment (arrow) from the proximal lateral tibia.

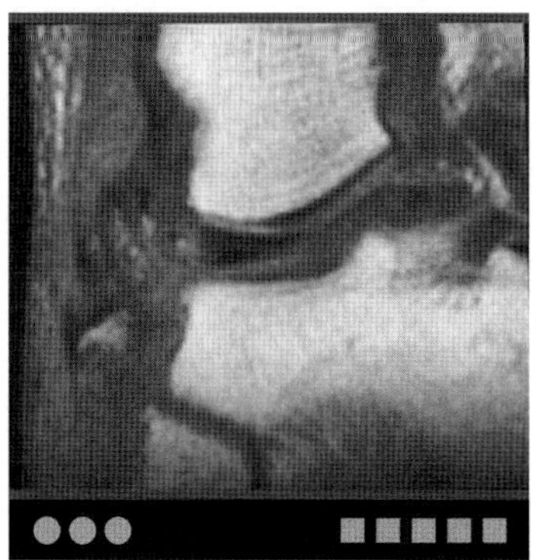

G. Avulsion fracture of proximal tibia: T1-weighted image shows avulsion fracture of the proximal fibula with tear of the lateral collateral ligament.

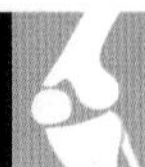

23–33 Segond Fracture

Kira Chow

PRESENTATION

Pain after fall

FINDINGS

Frontal knee radiograph demonstrates tiny elliptical fragment just distal to the lateral tibial articular surface.

DIFFERENTIAL DIAGNOSES

- *Lateral tibial plateau fracture (bumper fracture):* A far lateral sagittally oriented tibial condyle fracture extending to the tibial plateau could mimic a Segond fracture.
- *Avulsion of the Gerdy tubercle:* In contrast to the Segond fracture with directly lateral fracture fragment, the Gerdy tubercle avulsion fragment is anterolateral.

COMMENTS

The Segond fracture, first described by Paul Segond in 1879, remains controversial in many ways. The mechanism is not completely defined, but the injury is thought to be secondary to excessive internal rotation and varus stress. The anatomy of the lateral soft tissue structures is not totally understood. Most investigators agree upon divisions of the lateral structures into superficial, middle, and deep layers as well as anterior, middle, and posterior portions. The region involved in the Segond fracture is the lateral capsular ligament, which is the middle third of the deep layer. The classic radiographic appearance of the Segond fracture is a tibial avulsion fracture just distal to the articular surface of the lateral plateau, at the attachment site of the lateral capsular ligament. The small elliptical avulsion fragment is constant in size, is separated from the parent bone by a sagittally oriented fracture line, and is best seen on AP radiographs of the knee. This seemingly minimal radiograph finding has importance because of the high incidence of associated injuries, such as anterior cruciate ligament (ACL) tears, meniscal tears, avulsion fractures, and posterolateral corner injury. The Gerdy tubercle avulsion is adjacent to the Segond fracture, but these are distinguished by the direct lateral position of the Segond fracture fragment in contrast to the anterolateral position of the Gerdy tubercle avulsion. Therefore, a straight AP will demonstrate the Segond fracture but not the Gerdy tubercle avulsion.

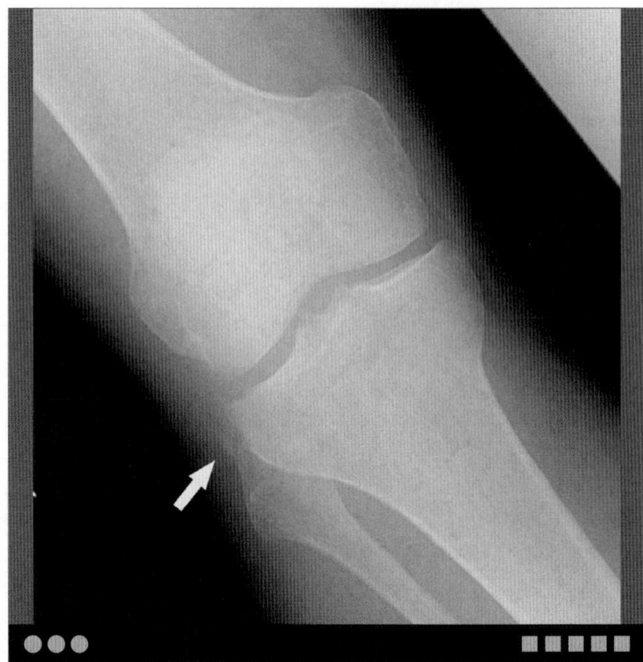

A. Segond fracture: Frontal radiograph of the knee demonstrates a tiny elliptical fracture fragment (arrow) just distal to the articular surface of the lateral tibial plateau, separated from parent bone by sagittally oriented fracture line.

PEARLS

- **Best view for visualization of Segond fracture is a straight AP view.**
- **The Segond fracture is an avulsion of the lateral capsular ligament attachment.**
- **The Segond fracture is associated with internal derangement, most commonly ACL tears and meniscal tears.**

ADDITIONAL IMAGES

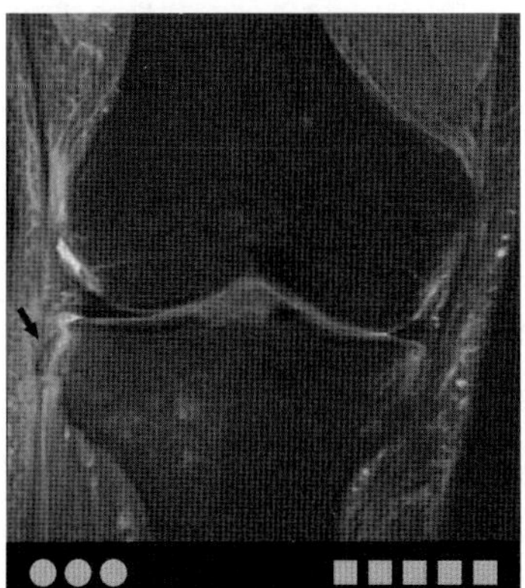

B. Segond fracture: Coronal proton density fat-saturated MRI sequence shows the tiny avulsed elliptical osseous fragment (arrow) from the proximal lateral tibia.

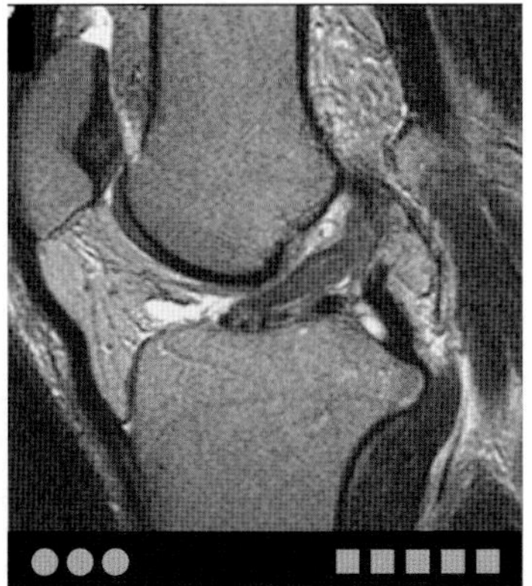

C. Segond fracture: Sagittal T2-weighted MRI sequence shows an associated ACL tear and joint effusion.

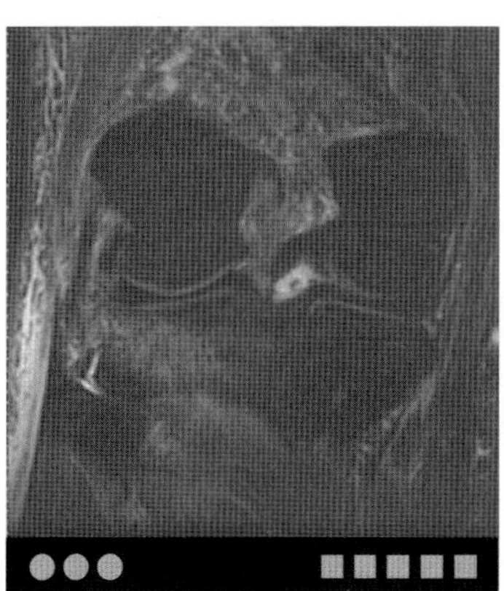

D. Segond fracture: Coronal T2-weighted fat-saturated MRI shows marrow edema in the lateral tibial plateau.

DIFFERENTIAL DIAGNOSES IMAGES

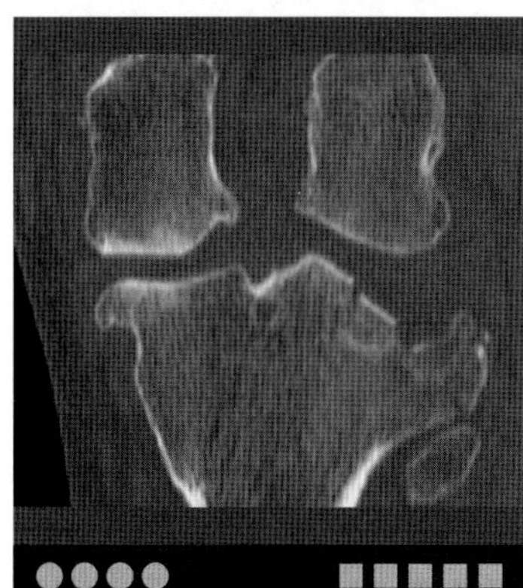

E. Lateral tibial plateau fracture (bumper fracture): Reformatted CT image in the coronal plane shows a sagittally oriented fracture through the lateral tibial plateau. In contrast to a Segond fracture, this is involving the articular lateral tibial plateau surface.

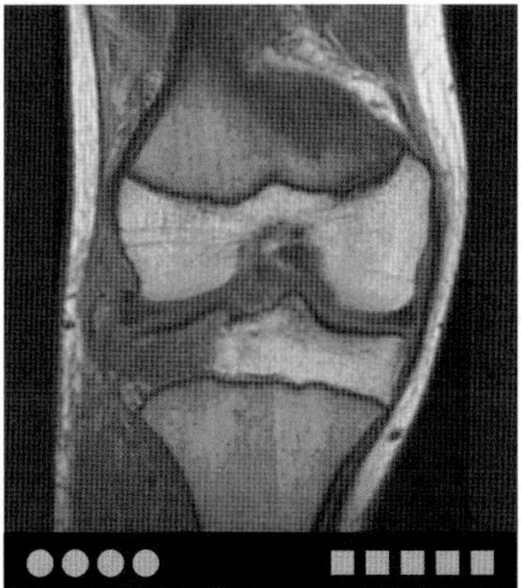

F. Bumper fracture of tibia: Coronal T1-weighted image in another patient shows large area of low signal in the medial aspect of the tibial plateau from bumper fracture.

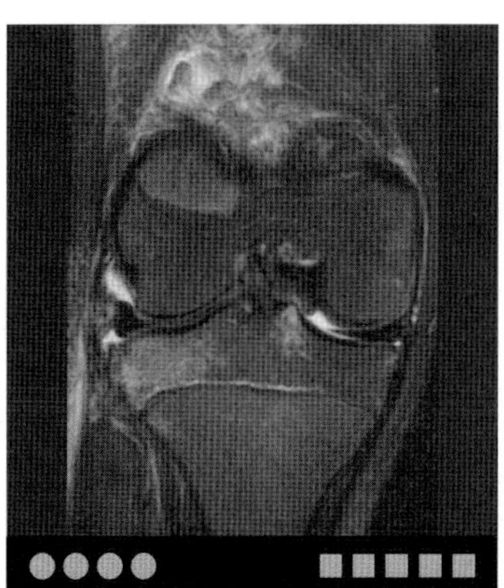

G. Bumper fracture of tibia: Coronal T2-weighted image shows increased signal in the lateral aspect of the tibial plateau consistent with bone contusion from bumper fracture.

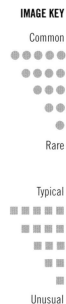

IMAGE KEY

Common

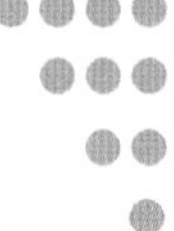

Rare

Typical

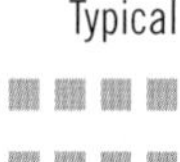

Unusual

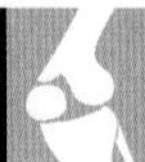

23–34 Stress Fracture of the Tibia

Sailaja Yadavalli

PRESENTATION

Athlete with recent onset of left leg pain

FINDINGS

MRI shows linear transverse low signal with periosteal reaction, early callus formation, and adjacent bone marrow and soft tissue edema.

DIFFERENTIAL DIAGNOSES

- *Stress reaction:* Early changes of stress may include cortical thickening, periosteal changes, and surrounding soft tissue edema. Areas of microfractures may exist.
- *Shin splints:* Believed to occur because of periostitis that results from rupture of Sharpey's fibers, which extend from muscle into cortical bone. No fracture line is seen on MRI.
- *Infection:* Bone marrow and soft tissue edema with periostitis are characteristic of osteomyelitis. Cortical erosive changes and soft tissue abscess may also be present.

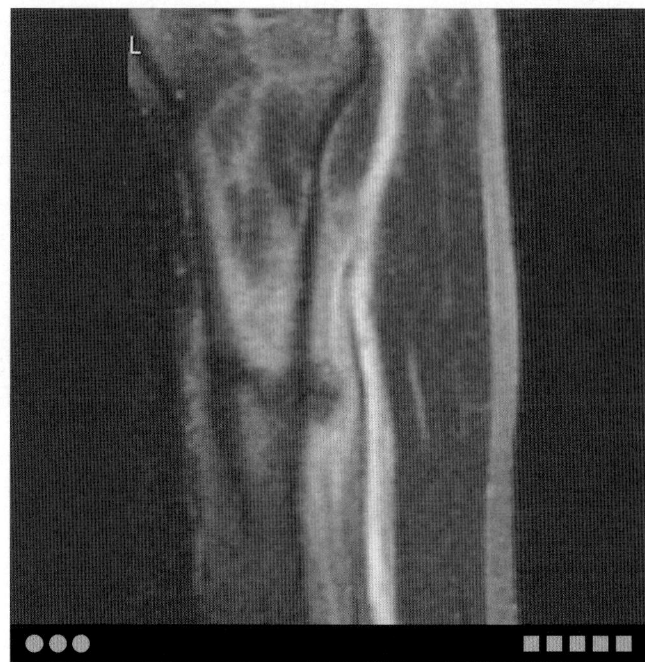

A. Stress fracture: Sagittal T2-weighted fat-saturated image shows fracture line, callus formation, associated bone marrow and soft tissue edema.

COMMENTS

Proximal tibial stress fractures often occur in athletes who perform jumping or leaping activities as with basketball or volleyball. Mid and distal shaft fractures are seen with long-distance running. Distal tibial stress fractures may be seen in patients who begin weight bearing with a healing proximal traumatic fracture or after ankle or subtalar arthrodesis. Proximal stress fractures are more often seen in the posteromedial aspect of the cortex than the anterolateral aspect. The anterior stress fractures should be differentiated from shin splints. Repetitive submaximal loading causes accelerated bone remodelling, which may lead to a stress fracture with continued activity. The fracture begins as a cortical break that progresses with continued stress. In tubular bones, stress fractures are often transverse, but can be longitudinal or oblique, especially in the tibia. Patients have pain associated with the activity, which is relieved with rest. Clinical findings may include focal soft tissue swelling and tenderness. Primary treatment involves pain relief and rest. On MRI linear low signal intensity is seen on both T1-weighted and fluid-sensitive sequences with adjacent areas of bone marrow edema. Associated periosteal changes and edema in the surrounding soft tissues are also present. Periosteal and endosteal callus formation may also be seen. Early radiographs often show mild cortical thickening. As the stress changes progress a linear cortical radiolucency with associated periosteal and endosteal changes may develop. Multiple radiolucent striations may be seen within the cortex. However, CT is more sensitive in detection of these findings.

PEARLS

- **Stress fractures are classified as fatigue fractures or insufficiency fractures.**
- **Location of tibial stress fracture depends on the activity.**
- **Anterior tibial stress fractures should be differentiated from shin splints.**
- **MRI typically shows linear low signal on T1-weighted and fluid-sensitive sequences surrounded by an area of bone marrow edema.**
- **Recognition of early cortical changes on radiographs or CT and periosteal and endosteal changes on MRI is important.**

ADDITIONAL IMAGES

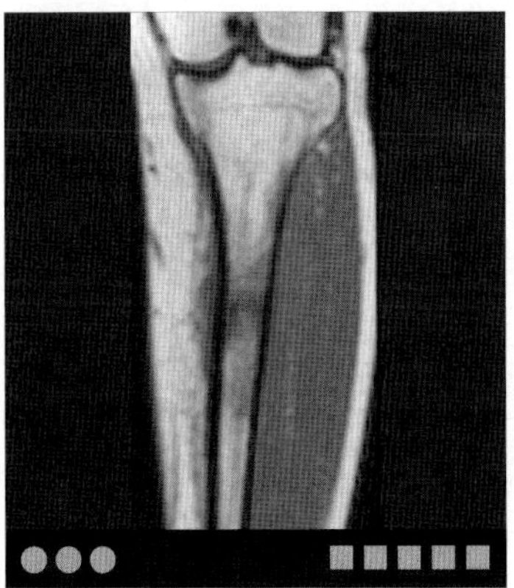

B. Stress fracture: Coronal T1-weighted image shows linear low signal in the proximal diaphysis of the tibia with callus formation.

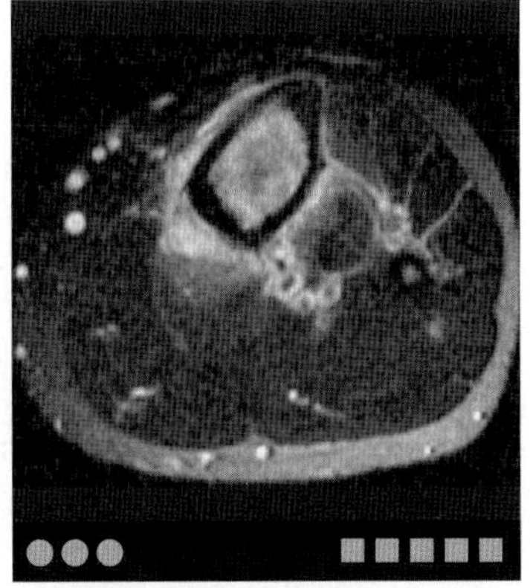

C. Stress fracture: Axial T2-weighted fat-saturated image shows bone marrow edema, periosteal and endosteal changes along the anteromedial cortex, and extensive soft tissue edema.

DIFFERENTIAL DIAGNOSES IMAGES

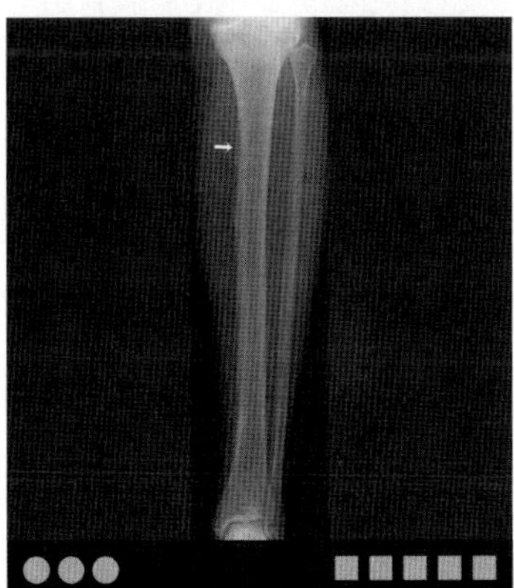

D. Early stress changes (DDX): AP radiograph of the tibia shows subtle periosteal and endosteal changes.

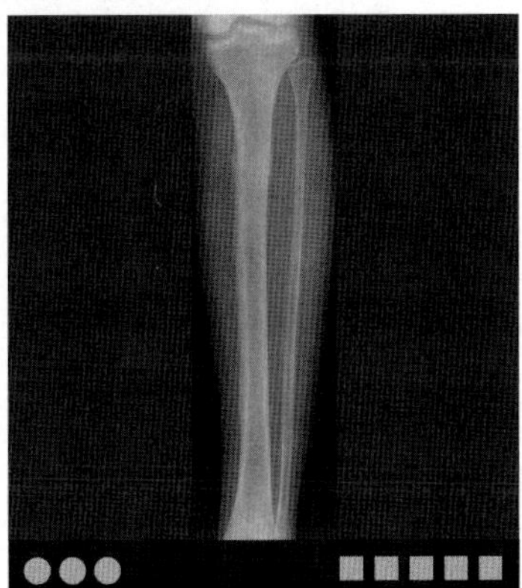

E. Progression to stress fracture: AP radiograph one month later shows a proximal tibial stress fracture with callus formation.

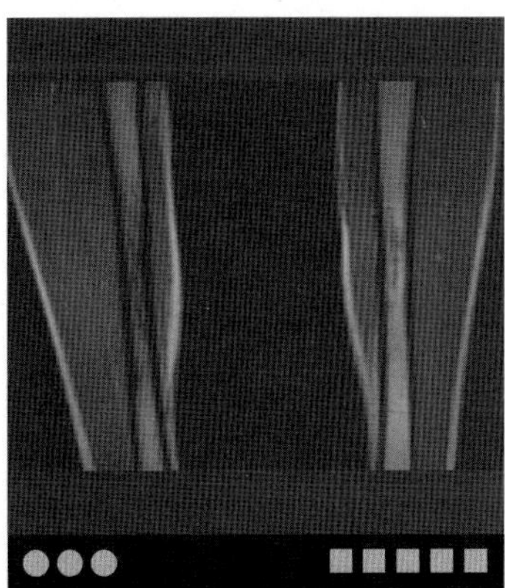

F. Early stress changes (DDX): Coronal T1-weighted image shows longitudinal low signal in the diaphysis of both tibia with no evidence of cortical break.

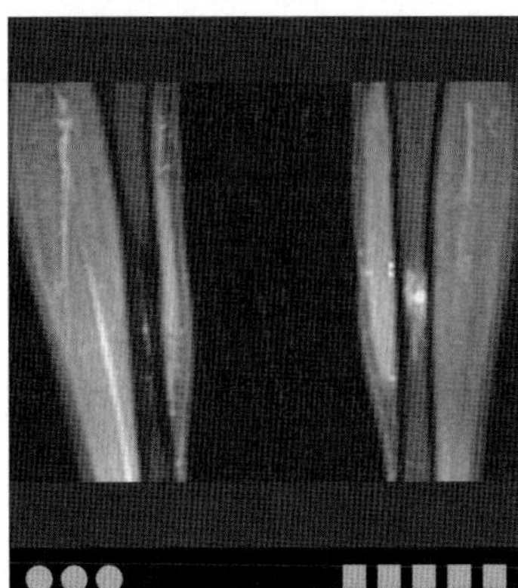

G. Early stress changes (DDX): Coronal STIR image shows mild bone marrow and soft tissue edema in both legs of this runner.

IMAGE KEY

Common

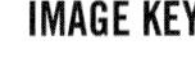

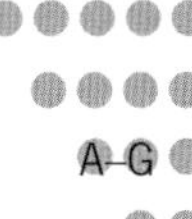

Rare

Typical

Unusual

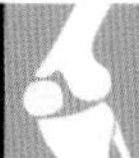

23-35 Semimembranous–Tibial Collateral Bursa

Ayodale S. Odulate and Piran Aliabadi

PRESENTATION

Medial joint pain after playing basketball

FINDINGS

Comma-shaped fluid collection deep to the semimembranosus–tibia collateral ligament.

DIFFERENTIAL DIAGNOSES

- *Pes anserinus:* Fluid collection that will extend inferior to the joint line with a characteristic "goose foot" appearance of the bursa.
- *Baker's cyst:* Fluid collection in the posterior knee that can often be seen communicating with the joint.
- *Meniscal cyst:* Intra-articular cyst associated with meniscal injury.

COMMENTS

The patient is a 28-year-old male with chronic medial knee pain. There are many causes of medial joint pain including meniscal injury, bursitis, and tendonitis. A semimembranosus-tibial collateral bursa develops after continuous repetitive trauma, and the bursa can enlarge and be a cause of medial and sometimes posterior knee pain. This bursa lies between the semimembranosus muscle and medial head of the gastrocnemius. It is important to differentiate the semimbraneous-tibial collateral bursa from other fluid collections in the medial knee that cause pain such as a Baker's cyst or pes anserinus. Treatment is conservative, rest and nonsteroidal anti-inflammatory medications. Rarely, surgical resection is indicated. Semimembranosus-tibial collateral bursa is found on approximately 5% of MR knee examinations. The MRI findings are well described as a comma-shaped homogeneous fluid collection on coronal images at the level of the joint posterior and medial to the semimembranosus muscle and tendon. The margins of the bursa are smooth and well circumscribed. The bursa can become inflamed and rupture and may have the appearance of a mass. The lining of the bursa may enhance; however, the internal homogeneous fluid should not enhance. A Baker's cyst, also known a popliteal cyst, communicates with the joint and is extra-articular. Pes anserinus is a fluid collection that can easily be confused; however, lies inferior to the joint at the level of the head of the fibula and has a characteristic "goose foot" appearance. A meniscal cyst is a smooth well-circumscribed intra-articular fluid collection at the joint line adjacent to the meniscus.

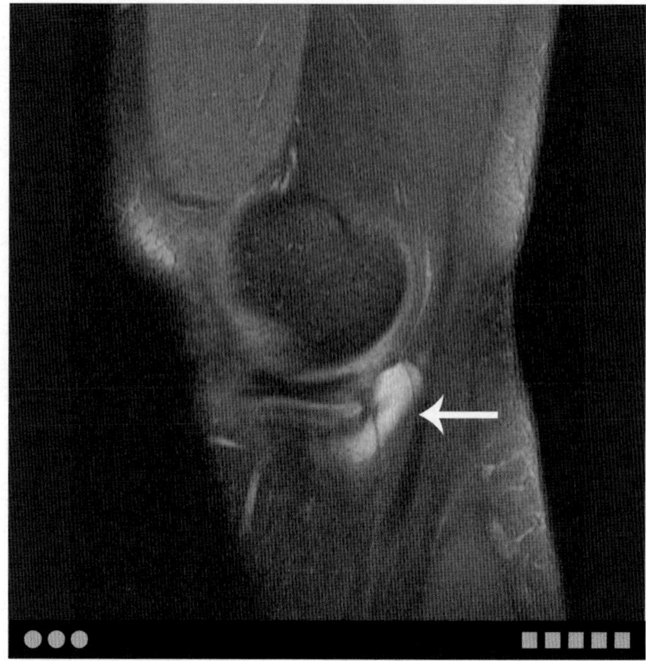

A. Semimembranosus–tibial collateral bursa: Sagittal fat-saturated proton density image shows a discrete comma-shaped (arrow) smooth fluid collection.

PEARLS

- **Comma-shaped bursa located at the level of the medial knee joint does not communicate with the joint.**
- **Can enlarge and extend into the posterior knee.**

ADDITIONAL IMAGES

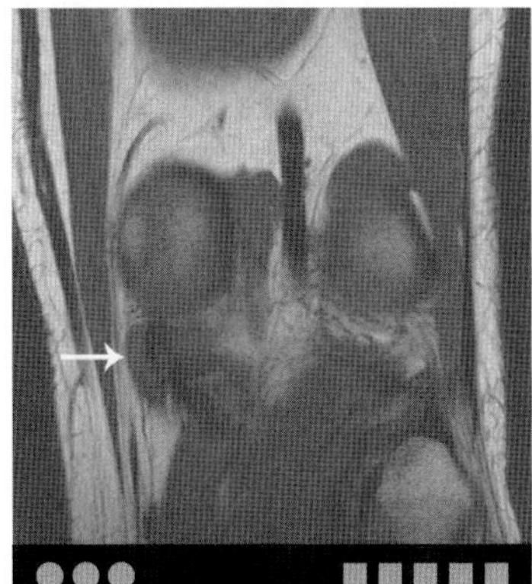

B. Semimembranosus–tibial collateral bursa: Coronal T1-weighted image shows a smooth comma-shaped hypointense signal lesion (arrow) outside of the medial joint capsule.

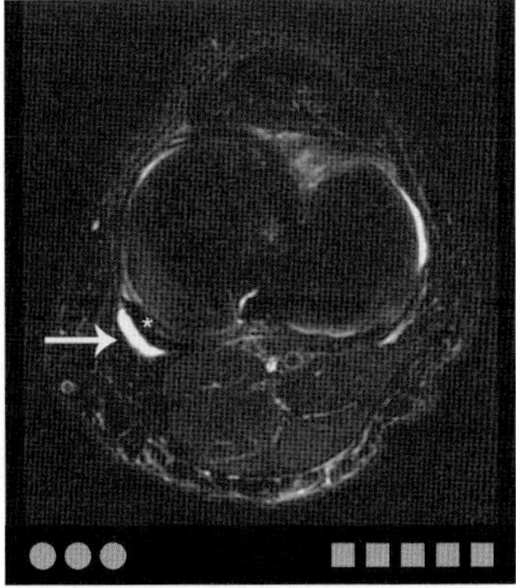

C. Semimembranosus–tibial collateral bursa: Axial T2 fat-saturated image again shows the medial fluid collection (arrow) medial to the semimembranous muscle (asterisk) outside of the joint capsule.

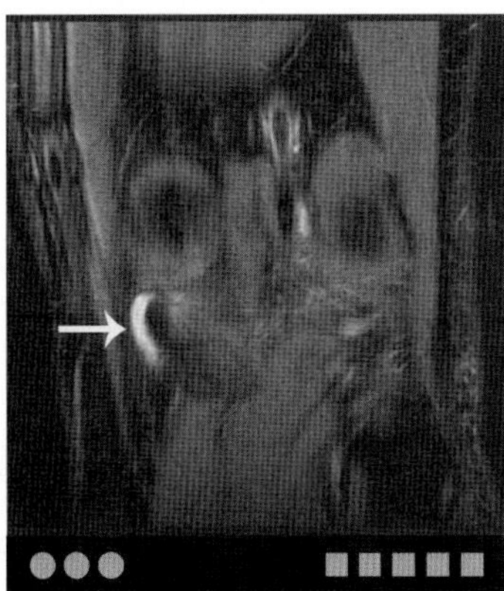

D. Semimembranosus–tibial collateral bursa: Coronal STIR image demonstrates the comma-shaped semimembranous–tibial collateral bursa (arrow).

DIFFERENTIAL DIAGNOSES IMAGES

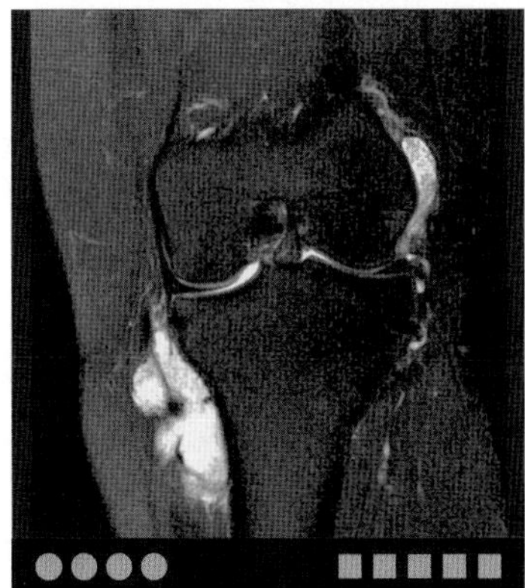

E. Pes anserinus bursitis: Coronal fat-saturated proton density MR image shows a trident lobular digit-like cystic lesion in the medial aspect of the proximal tibia, representing pes anserinus bursitis.

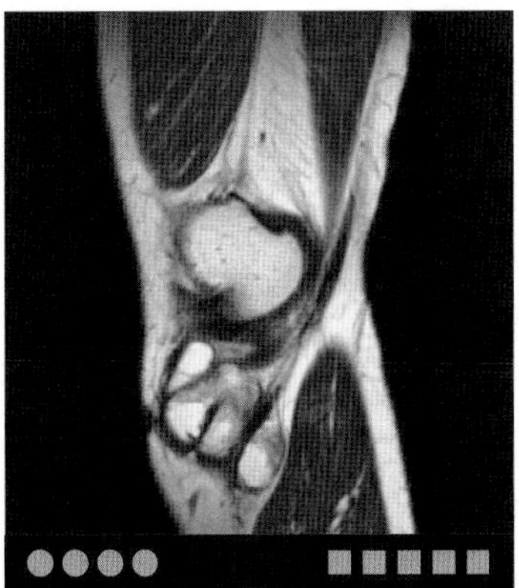

F. Pes anserinus bursitis: Sagittal T2-weighted image shows a trident lobular digit-like cystic lesion in the medial aspect of the proximal tibia, representing pes anserinus bursitis.

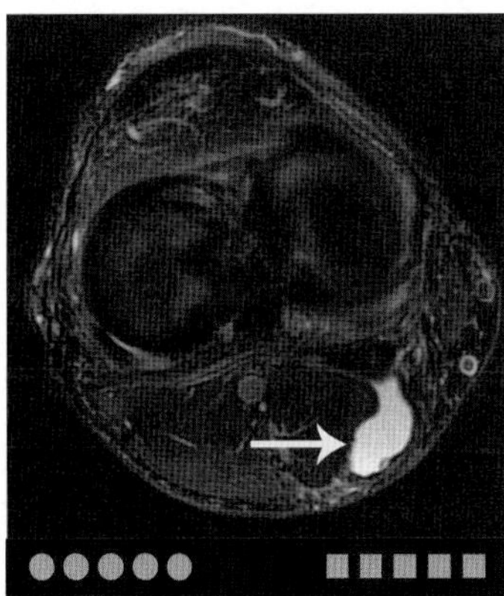

G. Baker's cyst: Axial fat-saturated T2-weighted image shows a Baker's cyst (arrow) at the level of the joint line. The tail of the cyst points toward the joint capsule.

IMAGE KEY

Common

●●●●●

●●●●

●●●

●●

●

Rare

Typical

■■■■■

■■■■

■■■

■■

■

Unusual

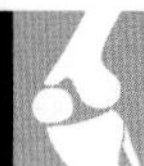

23–36 Chondromalacia of Patella

Eric Chen and Jamshid Tehranzadeh

PRESENTATION

Anterior knee pain and swelling

FINDINGS

MRI shows focal loss of articular cartilage of medial facet of patella (Grade IV), with edema, and subchondral cystic changes.

DIFFERENTIAL DIAGNOSES

- Chondromalacia patella Grade III: shallow dent in cartilage
- Normal patellar cartilage
- Patellofemoral osteoarthritis
- Pseudogout with involvement of the femoral–patellar joint
- Inflammatory arthritis such as rheumatoid arthritis

COMMENTS

The patient is a 62-year-old woman with anterior knee pain and swelling. Chondromalacia of patella typically is characterized by anterior knee pain, abnormal cartilage softening, swelling, and edema. Literally, chondromalacia means "soft cartilage," and historically anterior knee pain was thought to be caused by abnormally soft patellar cartilage. Current theory suggests multiple etiologies for anterior knee pain not limited to cartilage softening. Cartilage lesions most commonly develop along the posterior medial patella and develop from the basal layers. Histologically, it is attributed to a decrease in sulfated mucopolysaccharides in the ground substance. Conventional radiographs are insensitive for detection of cartilage damage and MRI is the preferred imaging modality. Spoiled gradient echo technique or gradient echo images with magnetization transfer provide the best contrast between subchondral bone, cartilage, and joint fluid. Chondromalacia is classified into one of five grades:

- Grade 0 corresponds to normal cartilage.
- Grade I changes are minimal with localized softening or swelling and little or no break in the cartilage surface.
- Grade II changes include fragmentation or fissuring up to 1.3 cm in diameter.
- Grade III changes show articular cartilage surface irregularities and definite fibrillation with fissuring extending greater than 1.3 cm; classically described as "crab meat appearance" in arthroscopic picture.
- Grade IV represents cartilage loss down to subchondral bone.

Grades I and II are not detected with regular MRI techniques.

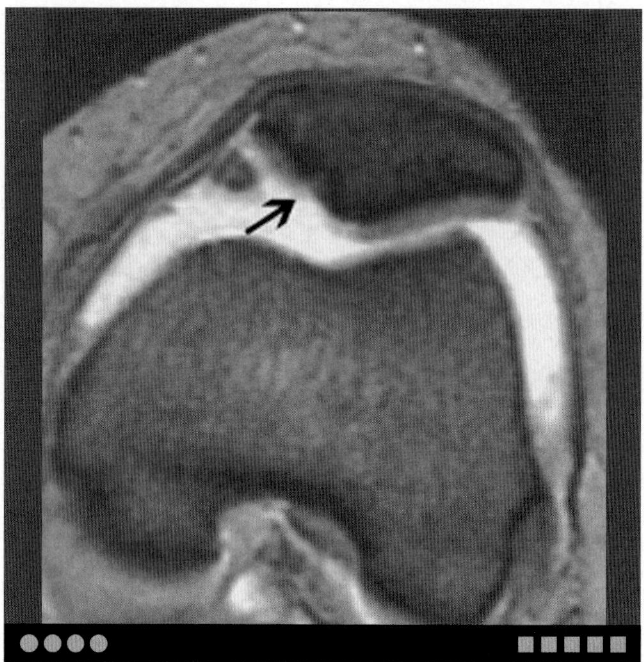

A. Grade IV chondromalacia: Axial gradient echo image showing large defect (arrow) in the medial dorsal patellar cartilage exposing underlying bone indicating grade IV defect.

PEARLS

- **Chondromalacia patella is typically characterized by anterior knee pain, abnormal cartilage softening, swelling, and edema.**
- **Grade III indicates focal and superficial cartilage defect and grade IV is complete loss of cartilage with exposure of underlying bone.**
- **Presentation is usually in young female patients.**
- **Spoiled gradient echo technique or gradient echo images with magnetization transfer and proton density images provide the best contrast between subchondral bone, cartilage, and joint fluid.**

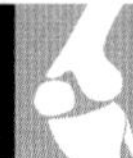

ADDITIONAL IMAGES

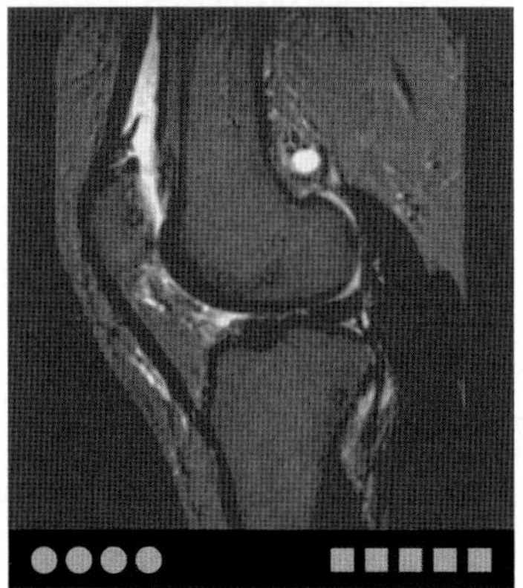

B. Grade IV chondromalacia: Sagittal fat-saturated T2-weighted image shows joint effusion and irregular dorsal patellar cartilage.

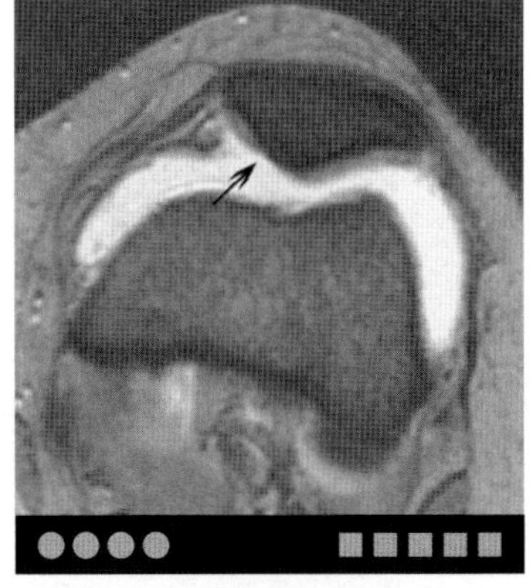

C. Grade IV chondromalacia: Axial gradient echo image showing large defect (arrow) in the medial dorsal patellar cartilage exposing underlying bone indicating grade IV defect.

DIFFERENTIAL DIAGNOSES IMAGES

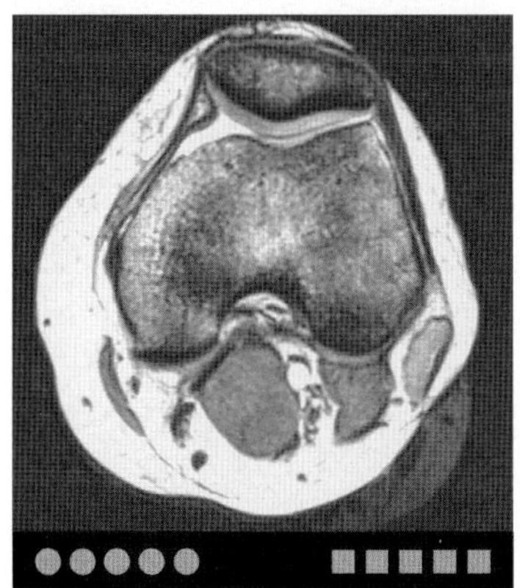

D. Normal patellar cartilage: Axial gradient echo image with magnetization transfer is showing normal patellar cartilage.

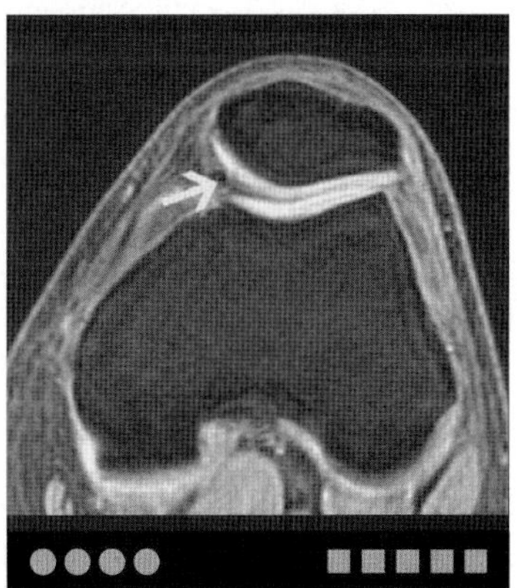

E. Mild Grade III chondromalacia: Axial gradient echo shows a small dent in the medial dorsal cartilage of patella (arrow).

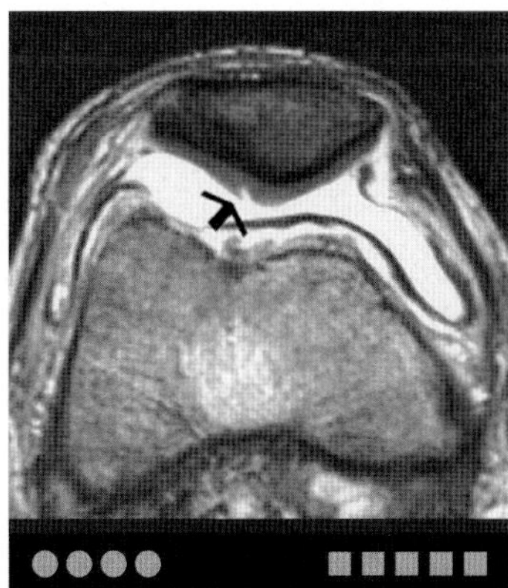

F. Severe Grade III chondromalacia: Axial gradient echo with magnetization transfer shows a large dent in the lateral patellar cartilage (arrow) indicating grade III chondromalacia.

G. Severe Grade IV chondromalacia: Axial gradient echo shows total loss of medial articular cartilage of patella (arrow).

IMAGE KEY

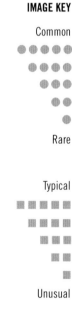

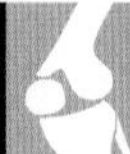

23–37 Iliotibial Band Bursitis

Lynne Steinbach and Jeffrey N. Masi

PRESENTATION

Anterolateral knee pain

FINDINGS

High-intensity signal is seen between iliotibial band (ITB) and lateral femoral condyle on T2-weighted images.

DIFFERENTIAL DIAGNOSES

- *Effusion in suprapatellar bursa:* Fluid separate from iliotibial adventitial bursa, may be associated with trauma, osteoarthritis, and synovitis.
- *Lateral collateral ligament (LCL) tear:* Prior trauma, T2 hyperintensity lateral or within LCL complex.
- *Lateral meniscus tear:* Meniscal abnormalities.
- *Infra-patellar bursitis:* Fluid in infrapatellar bursa.

COMMENTS

The patient presents with anterolateral knee pain. This condition is common in runners and is unilateral in 80% of the cases. When the tightly stretched iliotibial band fibers repeatedly traverse the lateral femoral epicondyle, as in running, reactive changes may ensue resulting in the classic findings of ITB syndrome. Typically, there is a complaint of pain with recent increase in distance of running or hill running. Unilateral presentation is most common; however, 20% of the runners have symptoms bilaterally. Physical exam may reveal crepitus with flexion and extension as well as point pain and tenderness laterally. Normally appearing as a dark band on MR, the iliotibial band is best seen on coronal images. Thickening of the ligament may be seen with regions of increased signal intensity medially in an adventitial bursa on T2-weighted images. The more posterior aspect of the iliotibial band is involved. Tears of the band may be associated with LCL damage. Although LCL injuries are relatively uncommon, suspicion should be raised if the mechanism of injury involved varus stress with the knee flexed and the tibia internally rotated. In lateral meniscus tears, the classical presentation is of a catch or snapping sound when changing direction along with a physical exam finding of joint line tenderness. T1-weighted and proton density weighted images show increased signal intensity in the lesion. Vertical tears usually have traumatic etiology while horizontal tears are typically the result of a degenerative process.

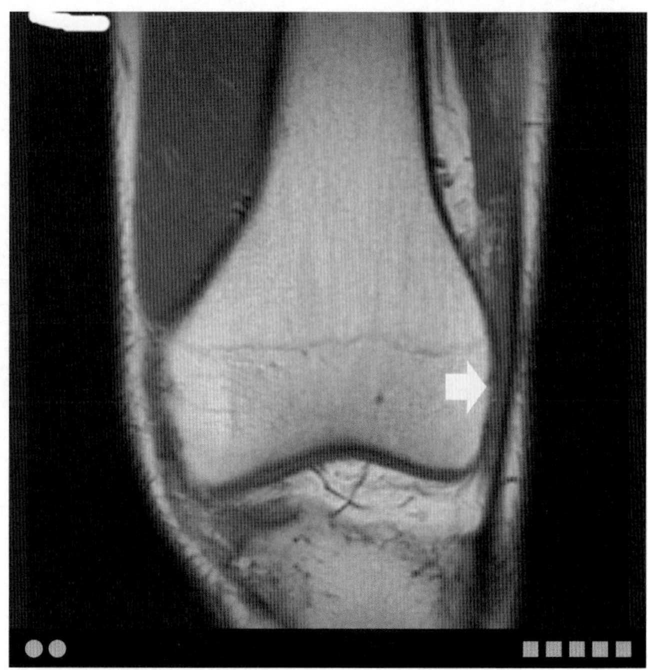

A. Iliotibial band friction syndrome: T1-weighted coronal MR image of a knee demonstrates low signal intensity fluid mesial to the iliotibial band (arrow) in this runner who had lateral knee pain.

PEARLS

- **The current view is that posterior ITB fibers run tighter against the lateral femoral epicondyle than the anterior fibers of the ITB, and it is under this area where abnormal signal often predominates.**
- **Lateral gluteal weakness, running downhill and running repeatedly in the same direction around the track have been cited as factors that increase the risk of ITB bursitis.**
- **Although joint fluid is often seen in the lateral knee recess of asymptomatic patients, joint fluid in the bursa is uncommon in asymptomatic individuals.**
- **Look for this problem in athletes who have an otherwise normal knee MRI.**

ADDITIONAL IMAGES

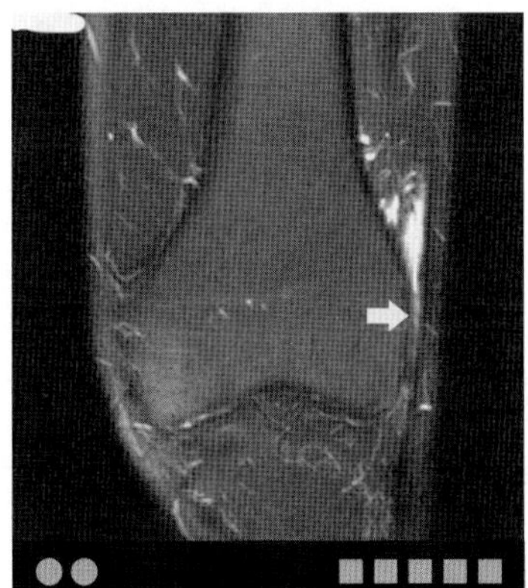

B. Iliotibial band friction syndrome: The fluid increases in signal intensity on the T2-weighted fat-suppressed coronal MR image of the same patient as in image A (arrow).

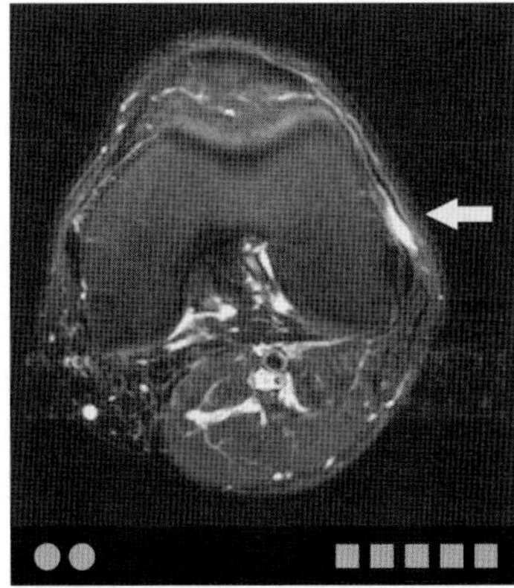

C. Iliotibial band friction syndrome: There is high signal intensity fluid within an adventitial bursa mesial to the iliotibial band on this axial fat-suppressed T2-weighted coronal MR image of the same patient as in images A and B (arrow).

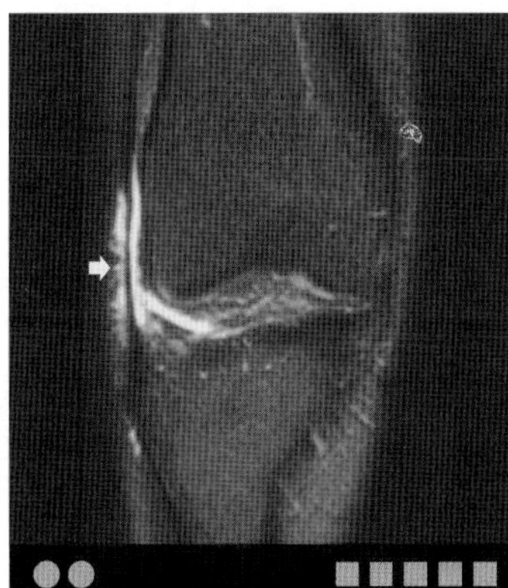

D. Iliotibial band friction syndrome: In this runner, the T2 hyperintensity on this fat-suppressed T2-weighted coronal MR image is noted not only in the bursa but lateral to the iliotibial band (arrow).

DIFFERENTIAL DIAGNOSES IMAGES

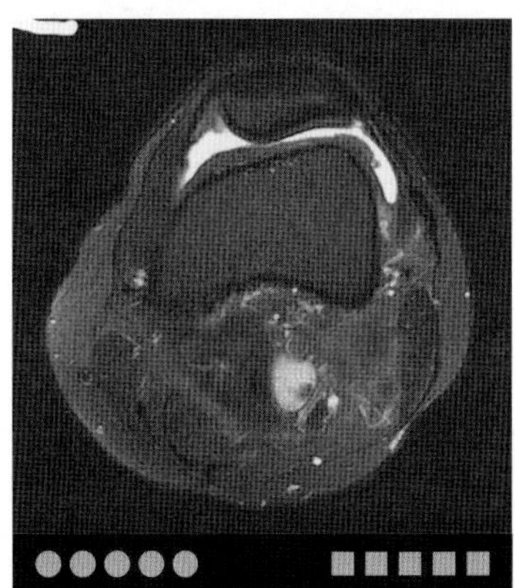

E. Normal suprapatellar effusion: The fluid in the suprapatellar bursa saddlebags around the femur anteriorly, unlike an adventitial bursa of ITBFS on this axial fat-suppressed FSE T2-weighted MR image of the patellofemoral region.

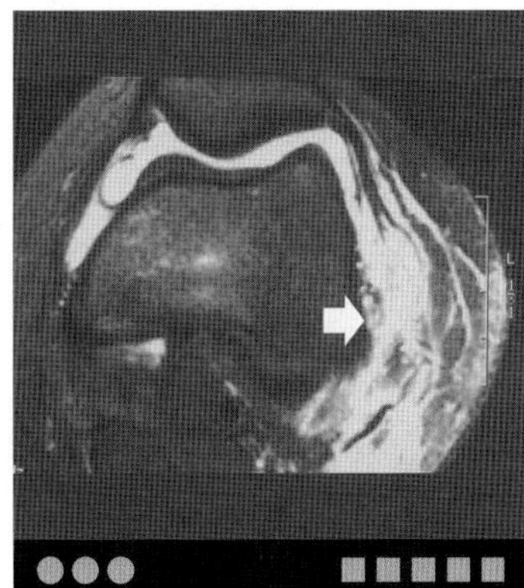

F. Lateral collateral ligament and patellofemoral ligament complex tears: Demonstrate complete disruption of the ligamentous structures on this fat-suppressed T2-weighted axial MR image (arrow).

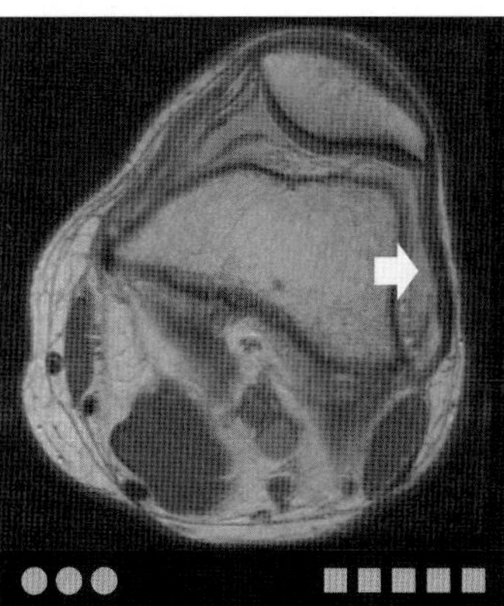

G. Thickened lateral patellofemoral ligament from chronic patellofemoral tracking disorder: An axial PD image of the patellofemoral joint reveals thickening of the lateral patellofemoral ligament (arrow). There is also injury to the medial patellofemoral ligament. This ligament is anterior to the iliotibial band.

IMAGE KEY

Common

●●●●●
●●●●
●●●
●●
●

Rare

Typical

■■■■■
■■■■
■■■
■■
■

Unusual

Chapter 24

Congenital, Systemic and Metabolic Disorders

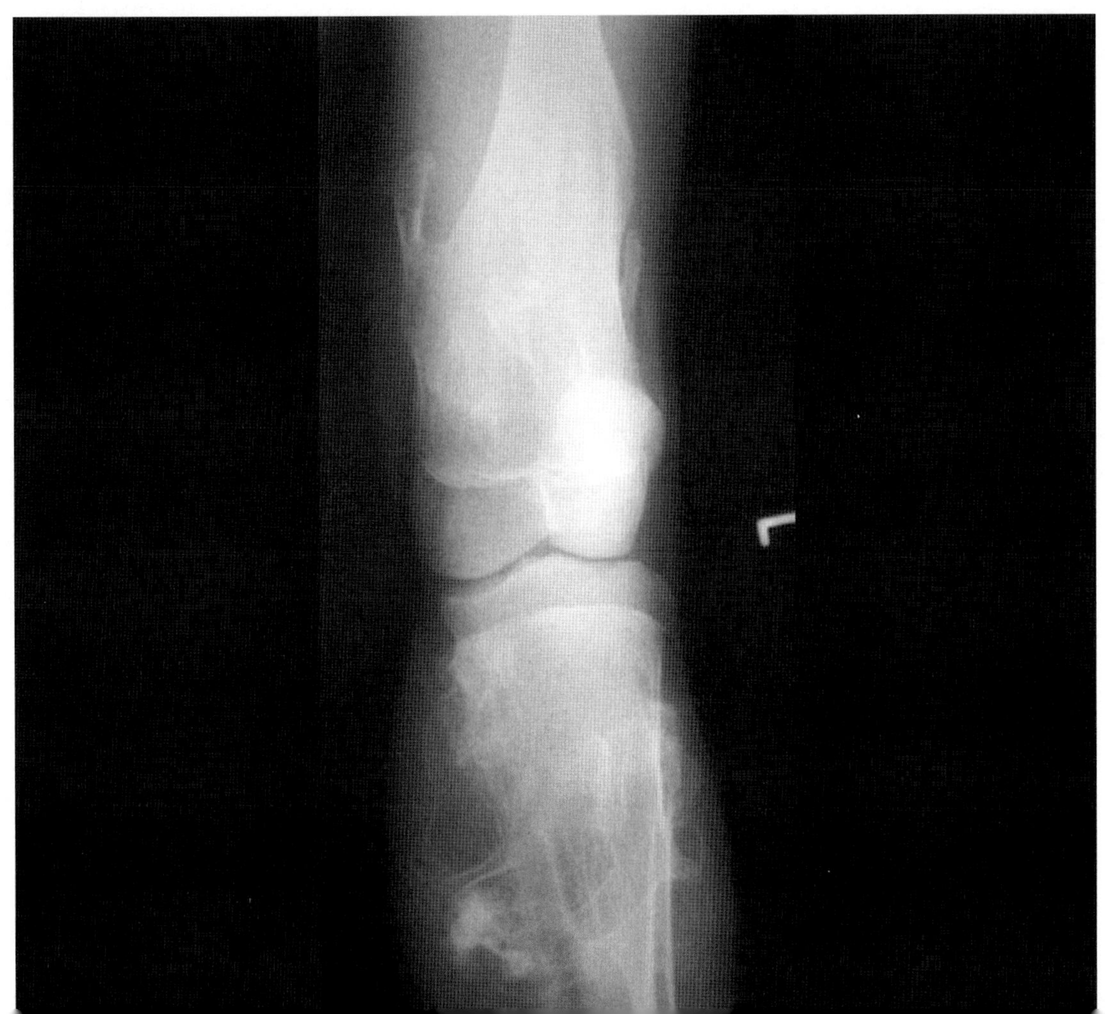

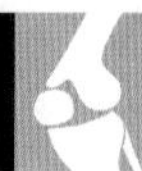

24–1 Hereditary Multiple Exostoses (Diaphyseal Aclasis)

Neerjana Doda and Wilfred CG Peh

PRESENTATION

Deformity, mass, fracture, pain, neurological, or vascular compromise

FINDINGS

Radiographs and CT scan show multiple bony protuberances arising from the metaphyses of the distal femur, proximal tibia, and proximal fibula bilaterally. These lesions are well-defined and point away from the joint.

DIFFERENTIAL DIAGNOSES

- *Solitary exostosis (or osteochondroma):* This common benign bone tumor occurs in 1% to 2% of the population. This lesion shows a growth pattern similar to hereditary multiple exostoses.
- *Supracondylar process of the humerus:* This bony overgrowth points toward the joint in contrast osteochondromas which points away from nearest joint.
- *Spur:* This normal variant may result from a variety of causes such as prominent muscular attachments and accessory ossification centers.

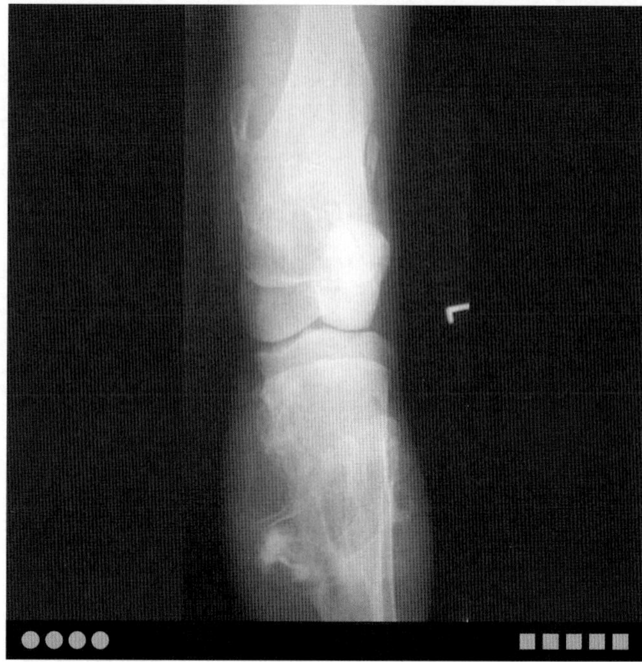

A. Hereditary multiple exostoses: Frontal radiograph of the left knee shows multiple bony protuberances arising from the metaphysis of the distal femur, and proximal tibia and fibula. Note that the tips of the exostoses point away from the knee joint.

COMMENTS

The patient is a 12-year-old girl who felt multiple bony lumps. She had previous excision of an exostosis from her left elbow. In these lesions, the characteristic continuity of cortical and cancellous bone from the host bone to the lesion is seen. There is no associated destruction or soft tissue mass. Also known as multiple osteochondromas and diaphyseal aclasis, hereditary multiple exostoses are autosomal dominant conditions in which asymmetric lesions are associated with short stature and deformities. These lesions are mostly diagnosed in the first decade, and there is a male predominance. Patients may present with deformity, pain, mass, or fracture. Bony outgrowths are located close to the metaphysis, and may be sessile or pedunculated. A characteristic feature is cortex and medullary continuity of the lesion with parent bone. Exostoses possess equivalent of a growth plate that ossifies and closes with onset of skeletal maturity. The knee is a common site of occurrence, with approximately 70% of affected individuals having a clinically apparent exostoses around the knee. Neurological or vascular complications may occur. Risk of malignant degeneration is 1% to 20% and is much more common than in solitary exostosis. Hereditary multiple exostoses of the long bones are easily diagnosed on radiographs. CT scan is useful in detecting and assessing lesions of pelvis, shoulder, and spine. Ultrasonography aids in evaluating the cartilaginous cap and detection of vascular complications. MR imaging best demonstrates continuity of medulla and cortex with parent bone and is particularly useful in assessing cartilage cap thickness and associated soft tissue complications.

PEARLS

- **Hereditary multiple exostoses of the long bones have a characteristic appearance and are easily diagnosed on radiographs.**
- **Lesions show cortical and medullary continuity with parent bone. Well appreciated on CT scan and MR imaging.**
- **The risk of malignant degeneration should always be kept in mind, with clinical and radiological assessment during follow-up being useful.**

ADDITIONAL IMAGES

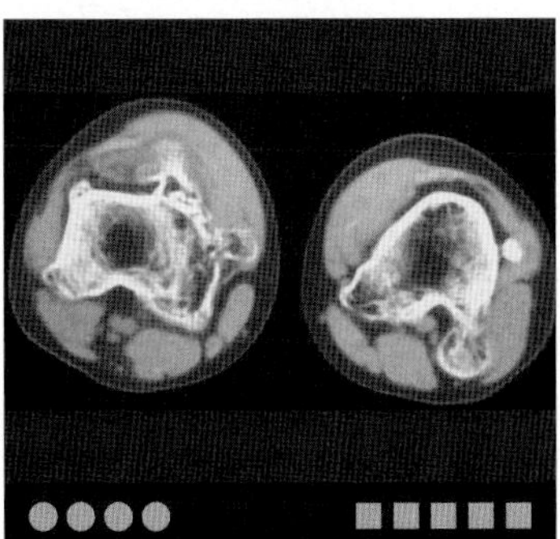

B. Hereditary multiple exostoses: Axial CT scan image of both distal femurs shows multiple well-corticated exostoses arising from both femurs. There is no associated soft tissue mass. Note cortico-medullary continuity between the exostoses and parent bone.

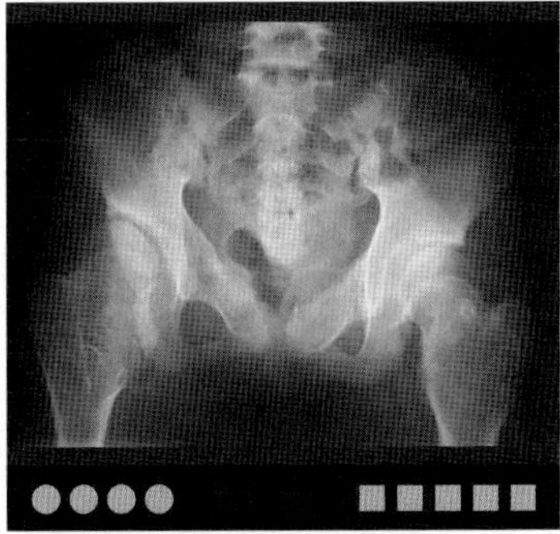

C. Hereditary multiple exostoses: Frontal radiograph of the pelvis shows several small exostoses in the iliac bones and pubic rami, as well as both femoral necks. Remodelling deformities of both proximal femurs are noted.

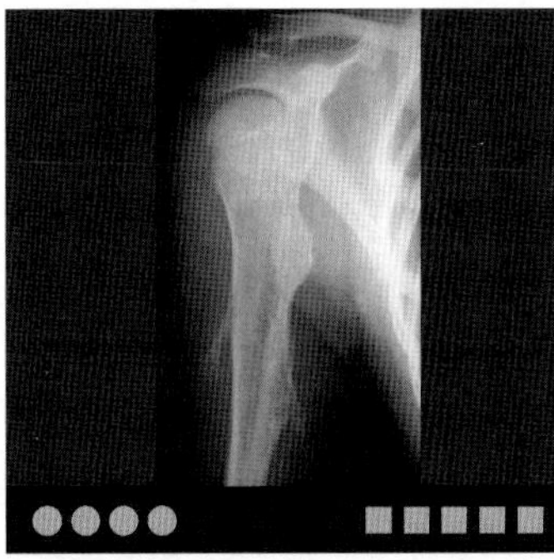

D. Hereditary multiple exostoses: Frontal radiograph of the right humerus shows multiple exostoses of the upper humeral shaft.

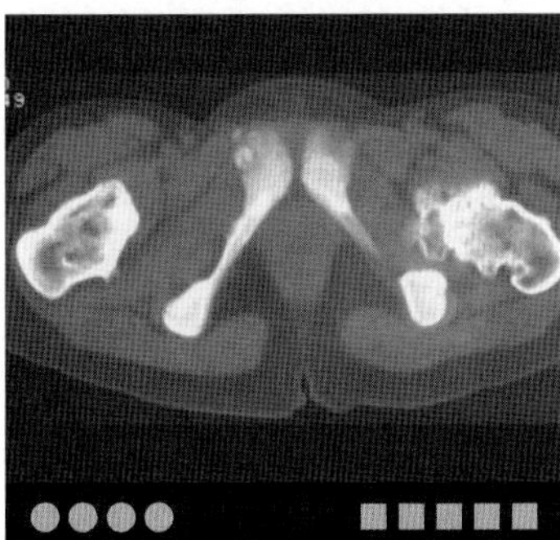

E. Hereditary multiple exostoses: This is an image of a 14-year-old girl. Axial CT scan image of the hips shows exostoses arising from both femoral necks. There is cortico-medullary continuity between lesion and parent bone and no associated soft tissue mass. Both proximal femurs show remodelling.

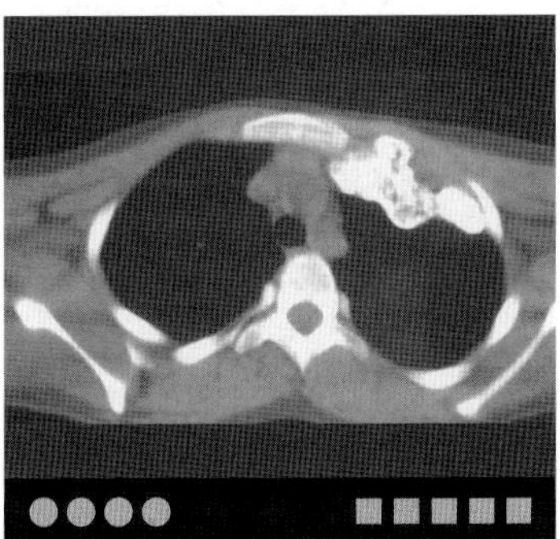

F. Hereditary multiple exostoses: This is an image of a 14-year-old girl. Axial CT scan image of the upper chest wall shows a large exostosis arising from the left upper rib. A calcified cartilage cap is noted.

IMAGE KEY

Common

Rare

Typical

Unusual

DIFFERENTIAL DIAGNOSIS IMAGE

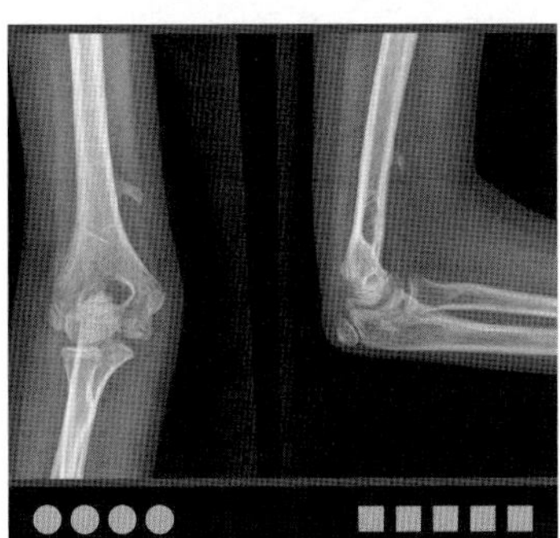

G. Supracondylar process of distal humerus: AP and lateral radiograph of the elbow shows supracondylar process of humerus. Note unlike osteochondromas, this bony excrescence is pointing toward the joint.

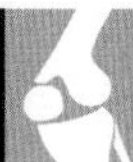

24–2 Hypertrophic Pulmonary Osteoarthropathy

Stephen E. Ling and William R. Reinus

PRESENTATION

Pain, swelling/clubbing, and arthritis/synovitis

FINDINGS

The images show nonaggressive appearing well-formed, symmetrical, and solid periosteal bone formation.

DIFFERENTIAL DIAGNOSES

- *Chronic venous insufficiency/stasis:* Phleboliths, usually only involves lower extremities, typically bilateral.
- *Cellulitis:* Typically unilateral and accompanied by obvious signs of superficial infection of the soft tissues.
- *Congestive heart failure:* Periosteal new bone associated with long-standing heart disease.
- *Pachydermoperiostosis (primary hypertrophic osteoarthropathy):* Rare disease. Genetic disorder with thickened skin and epiphyseal involvement, irregular periostitis seen primarily in blacks.
- *Thyroid acropachy:* Thyroid dysfunction, predilection for small bones of the hands and feet, and typically seen in patients with a known history of thyroid disease—usually treated as Graves disease.

COMMENTS

Hypertrophic pulmonary osteoarthropathy (HPOA) is a radiologically benign appearing manifestation of significant underlying systemic disease. Tubular bones, both large and small and of both the upper and lower extremities, are frequently involved with thick, periosteal new bone formation. Typically, this periosteal new bone extends from proximal metaphysis to distal metaphysis, sparing the epiphyses. Flat bones such as the ribs, scapula, mandible, and maxilla are less commonly affected. HPOA is often seen in patients with one of various lung tumors, especially primary lung cancer (accounts for 80%–90% of cases), but also with malignant mesothelioma, lymphoma, metastases, and benign fibrous tumor of the pleura. Chronic diseases such as pulmonary interstitial fibrosis, bronchiectasis, COPD, cyanotic congenital heart disease, liver dysfunction from cirrhosis and hepatitis, and GI tract diseases such as inflammatory bowel disease can also cause this entity. In fact, the first case of HPOA was described with a peritoneal malignant mesothelioma. Chemical irritant/toxic substances, parasympathetic neurogenic dysfunction, and hypervascularity have all been proposed as the causes of this disorder. The leading candidate at the current time appears to be a vagally mediated neuralgic reflex. Radiographs and radionuclide bone scan have a very high sensitivity for detection of this disorder. The high association of HPOA with pulmonary disease mandates that a chest radiograph be performed in patients in whom HPOA is discovered. When caused by a neoplasm, clinical and radiographic findings may regress/disappear or reappear in concert with tumor treatment and recurrence of tumor, respectively. Thoracotomy can cause remission of the periosteal reaction and limb pain even in the case of nonresectable tumor.

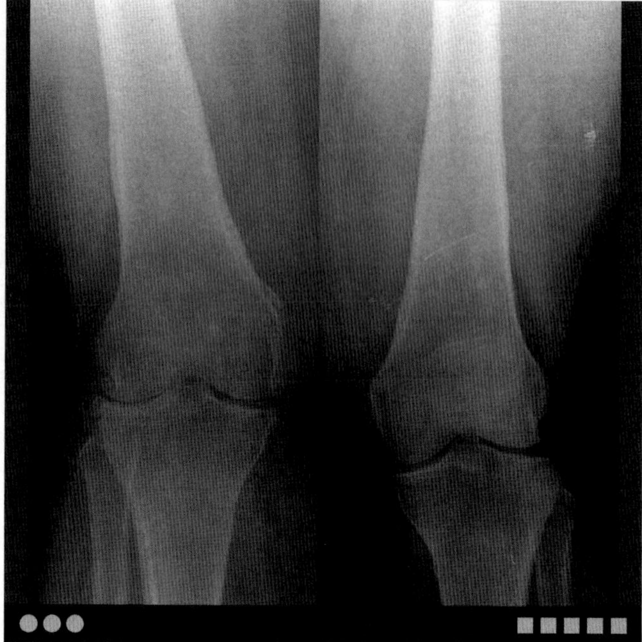

A. Hypertrophic pulmonary osteoarthropathy (HPOA): AP radiographs of both knees show thick, solid, and symmetrical periosteal reaction along the metadiaphysis of distal femurs, proximal tibia, and proximal fibula.

PEARLS

- **The clinical findings of HPOA can mimic inflammatory arthritis with swelling and arthralgia. As a result, HPOA is often first discovered on bone radiographs.**
- **If a patient shows periosteal bone formation on radiographs or increased uptake on bone scan typical of HPOA and has no known clinical history to explain the imaging finding, the clinician should be advised to obtain a chest x-ray.**
- **Secondary HPOA can be distinguished from other causes of symmetric periosteal reaction such as pachydermoperiostitis, thyroid acropachy, and chronic venous stasis on the basis of clinical history and physical examination.**

ADDITIONAL IMAGES

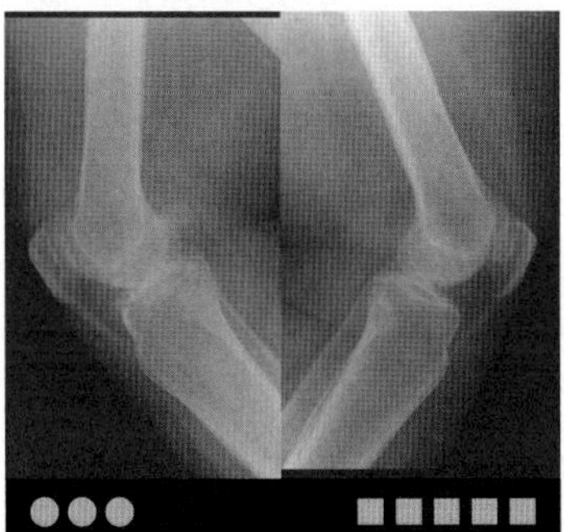

B. Hypertrophic pulmonary osteoarthropathy (HPOA): Corresponding lateral radiographs of both knees show findings similar to those seen in image A.

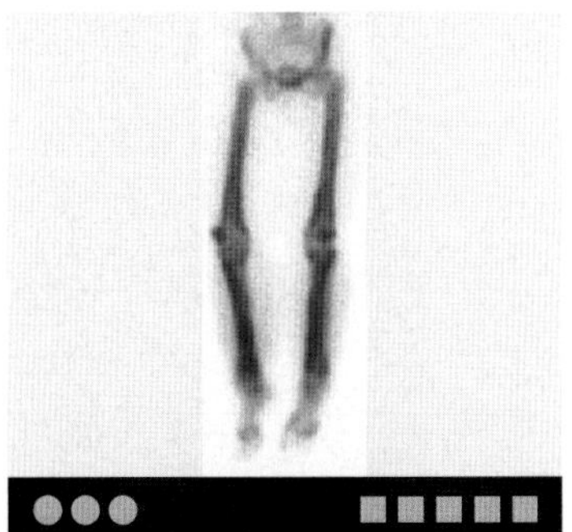

C. Hypertrophic pulmonary osteoarthropathy (HPOA): Delayed static images from a radionuclide bone scan demonstrate linear, longitudinally oriented increased uptake by both tibia and femora superficially.

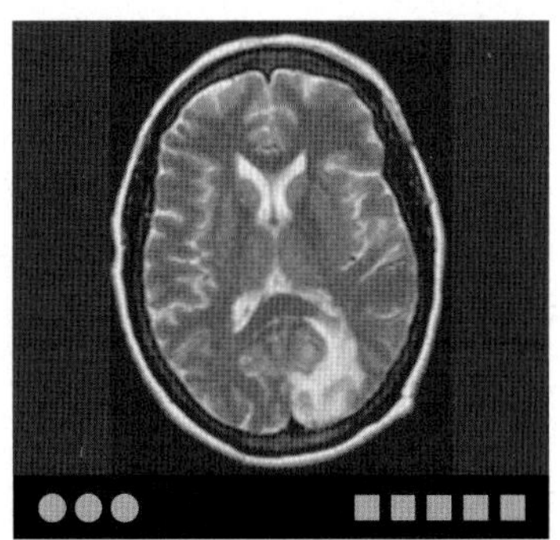

D. Hypertrophic pulmonary osteoarthropathy (HPOA): Axial T2-weighted image at the level of the third ventricle demonstrates hyperintense vasogenic edema in the white matter of the left parietal occipital region.

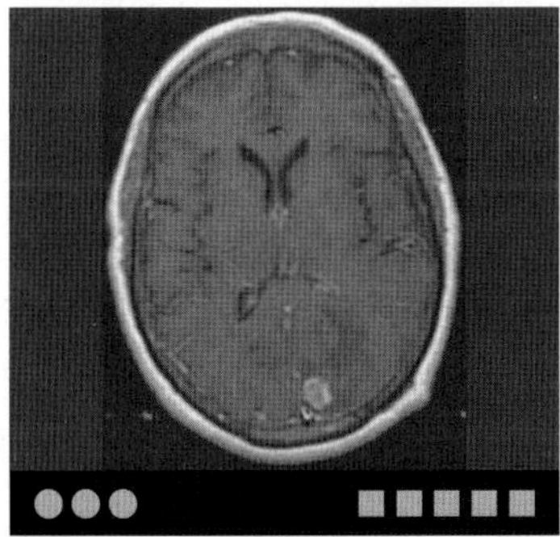

E. Hypertrophic pulmonary osteoarthropathy (HPOA): Postcontrast axial T1-weighted image (at the same level as image D) shows a rim enhancing mass surrounded by low signal vasogenic edema in the left parietal occipital region, consistent with a metastasis from lung cancer.

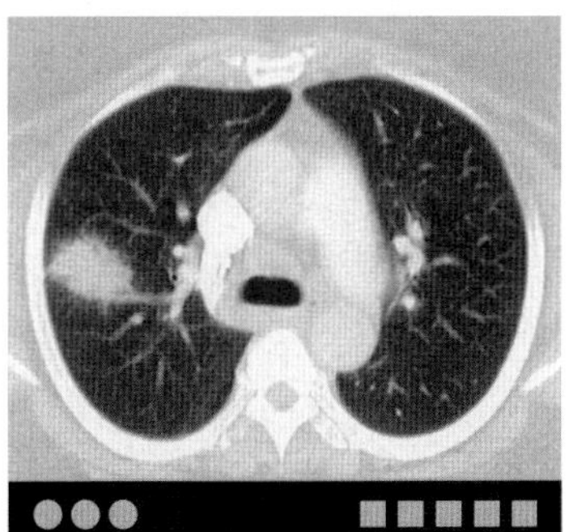

F. Hypertrophic pulmonary osteoarthropathy (HPOA): Axial CT scan image demonstrates a spiculated mass in the right upper lobe representing the patient's primary lung cancer.

DIFFERENTIAL DIAGNOSIS IMAGE

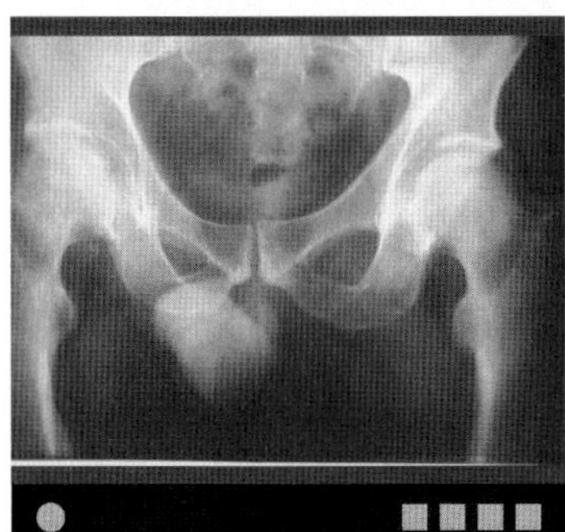

G. Pachydermoperiostitis: AP view of the pelvis shows well formed, nonaggressive appearing and bilateral, periosteal bone formation at both proximal femurs.

IMAGE KEY

Common

Rare

Typical

Unusual

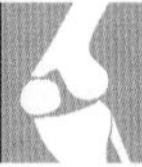

24–3 Sickle Cell Anemia

Gideon Strich

PRESENTATION

Knee pain

FINDINGS

MRI shows patchy, cellular bone marrow replacement throughout the long bones with focal areas of bone infarct.

DIFFERENTIAL

- *Avascular necrosis:* Bone infarcts of sickle cell anemia are more commonly metaphyseal and also commonly occur in the small bones of the hands and feet (hand-foot syndrome) as well as in the diaphysis of larger tubular bones. AVN of other etiologies is more common in the hip and shoulder.
- *Osteomyelitis:* With osteomyelitis, the metaphyseal lesion is heterogeneous and bright on T2-weighted images rather than showing a serpiginous low signal pattern of bone infarct. Periosteal reaction and septic arthritis are also associated.
- *Gaucher disease and other storage diseases:* Results in remodeling of the metaphysis (Erlenmeyer flask deformity) as well as bone infarcts and vertebral abnormalities similar to those in sickle cell disease.

COMMENTS

The patient is a young black male who presented with multiple episodes of bone pain predominantly involving the knees, but also the hands, feet, and shoulders. Sickle cell disease is a congenital anemia resulting from an abnormal form of hemoglobin (Hb S). The trait may be homozygous, causing sickle cell disease, occurring in approximately 1% of American blacks, or may be combined with other anemias (i.e., sickle cell thalassemia). The less severe sickle cell trait (Hb AS) occurs in approximately 7% of the American black population and is not associated with such severe symptoms. The disease is characterized by microvascular occlusion because of the abnormal shape and clumping of the sickle cells resulting in bone marrow ischemia manifesting as dactylitis in the hands and feet, metaphyseal bone infarcts in the large tubular bones, and typical central compression fractures in the vertebrae. MR images of the extremities show the typical serpiginous pattern of hypointensity in the metaphyses of the long bones because of bone infarcts, corresponding to sclerosis on radiographs. Other manifestations include marrow hypercellularity with diffusely decreased signal on T1-weighted MR images.

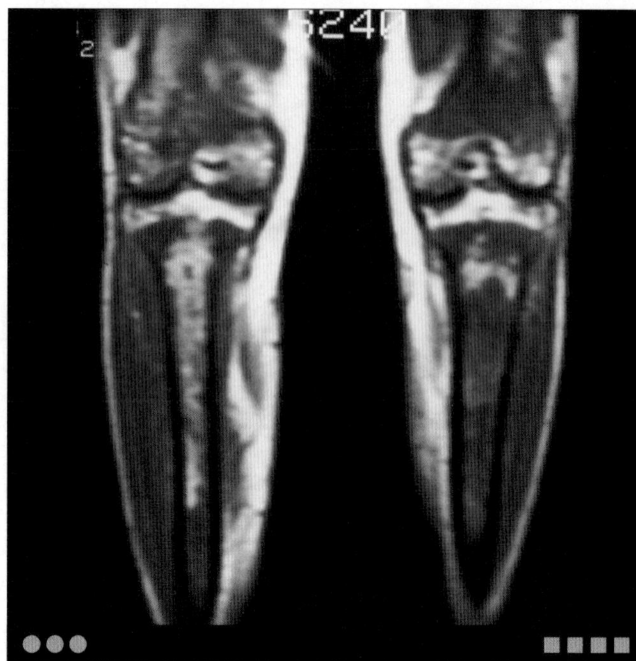

A. Sickle cell disease: Coronal T1-weighted image of the knees demonstrates diffused bone marrow replacement with multiple bone infarcts predominantly involving the metaphyses.

Osteomyelitis and septic arthritis are more common in patients with sickle cell anemia. Although staphylococcus is the most common organism, there is a much larger proportion of salmonella infections than in the general population. Osteomyelitis has a more aggressive lytic appearance than typical bone infarct, and it is commonly associated with septic arthritis. Although radionuclide white cell scans are usually strongly positive in septic arthritis and osteomyelitis, abnormal uptake may also be seen in bone infarcts. MRI may help differentiate infarct from osteomyelitis, and may be useful in guiding bone biopsy if necessary.

PEARLS

- **Sickle cell disease is a congenital anemia resulting from abnormal hemoglobin (Hb S) and affects 1% to 2% of the American black population.**
- **Most bone manifestations of sickle cell disease result from ischemia secondary to microvascular occlusion by abnormal sickle cells as well as diffused cellular marrow conversion because of anemia.**
- **Multiple bone infarcts in the metaphyses of the large bones and dactylitis in the small bones of the hands and feet are common.**
- **Osteomyelitis and septic arthritis are common complications of sickle cell disease and must be differentiated from acute bone infarcts.**

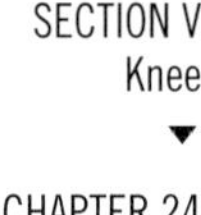

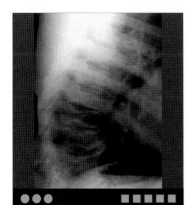

ADDITIONAL IMAGES

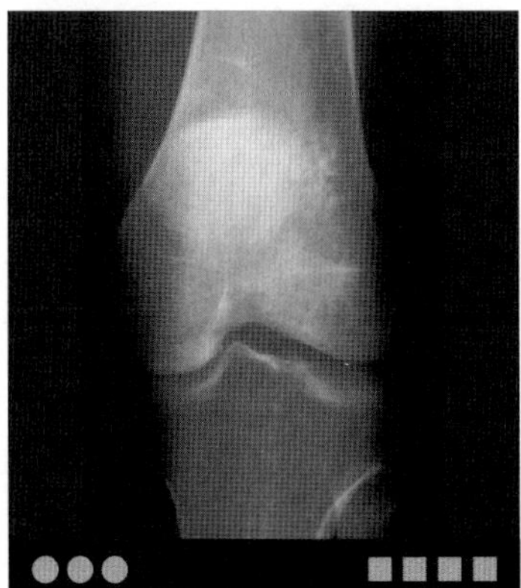

B. Sickle cell disease: AP radiograph shows typical sclerotic metaphyseal bone infarct is seen in the distal femur.

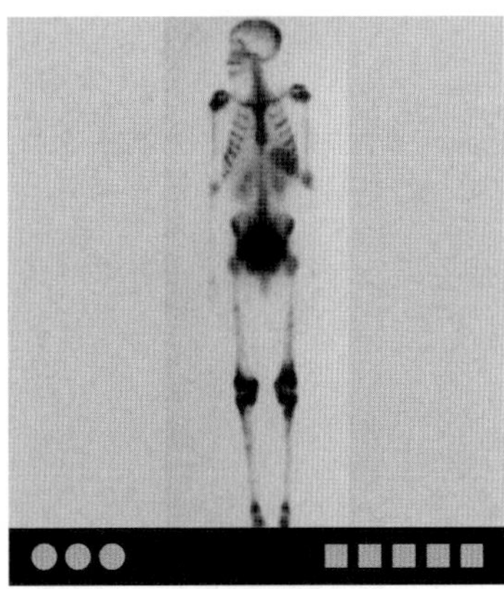

C. Sickle cell disease: Radionuclide bone scan shows multiple areas of abnormal uptake because of infarcts on the long bones. Uptake in the spleen is typical in sickle cell disease towing to splenic infarct.

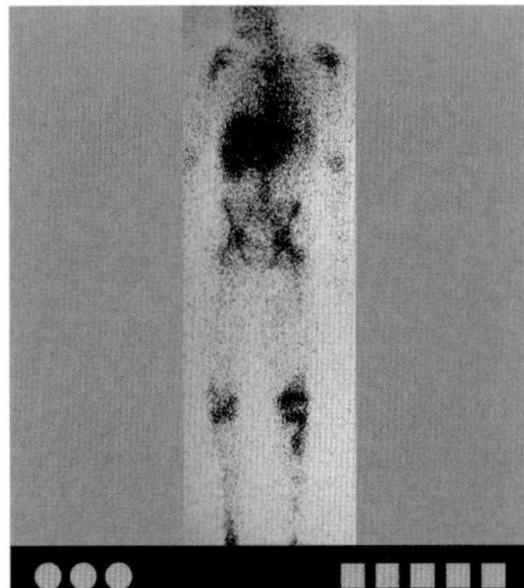

D. Sickle cell disease: White blood cell scan demonstrates expansion of the bone marrow as well as abnormal white cell uptake in acute bone infarcts adjacent to the knee. Note the absence of white cell activity in the spleen owing to autosplenectomy.

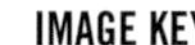

E. Sickle cell disease: Radiograph shows diffused sclerosis of the ribs and "H-shaped" vertebral bodies because of microvascular infarction.

IMAGE KEY

Common

Rare

Typical

Unusual

DIFFERENTIAL DIAGNOSES IMAGES

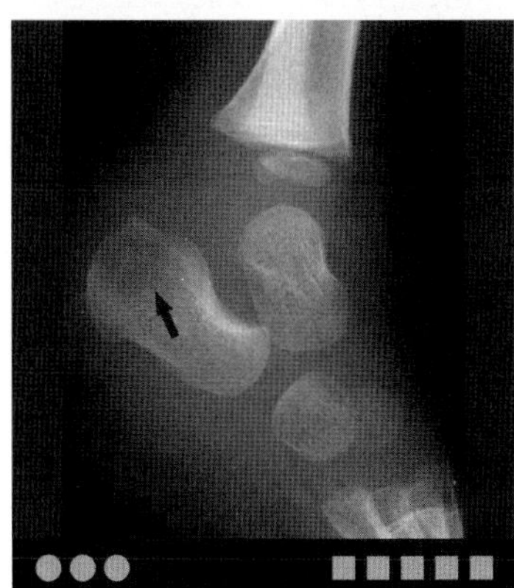

F. Osteomyelitis: Lateral radiograph of the ankle shows joint effusion and subtle bone destruction in calcaneus (arrow).

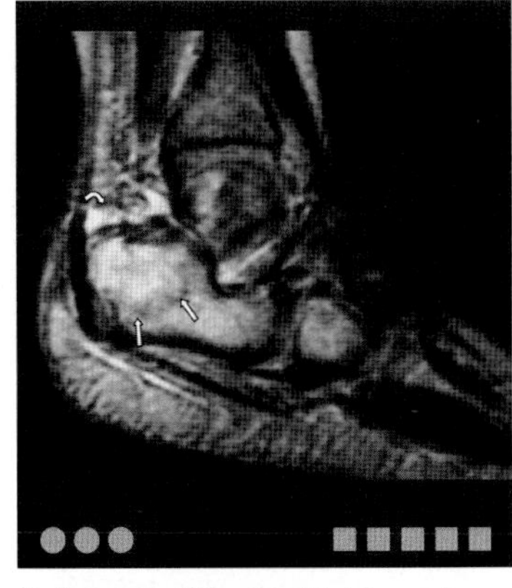

G. Osteomyelitis: Sagittal inversion recovery image shows osteomyelitis of calcaneus (arrows) and joint effusion (curved arrow.)

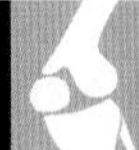

24–4 Erdheim-Chester Disease

Kambiz Motamedi

PRESENTATION

Knee pain

FINDINGS

MRI shows geographic lesions of the distal femurs and proximal tibias with mixed signal. There is no soft tissue mass.

DIFFERENTIAL DIAGNOSES

- *Langerhans cell granulocytosis (LCG):* Very similar MRI appearance with a different age distribution. LCG is a disease of childhood.
- *Medullary bone infarcts:* MRI reveals predominantly metaphyseal lesions without extension into the diaphysis. Depending on the stage of bone infarct, the appearance varies from signal properties corresponding to central edema to necrosis and return of yellow marrow.
- *Enchondroma:* Usually monostotic with lobular appearance and metaphyseal location. The cartilaginous lesions follow on MRI, and the signal intensity of simple fluid is caused by their high water content.

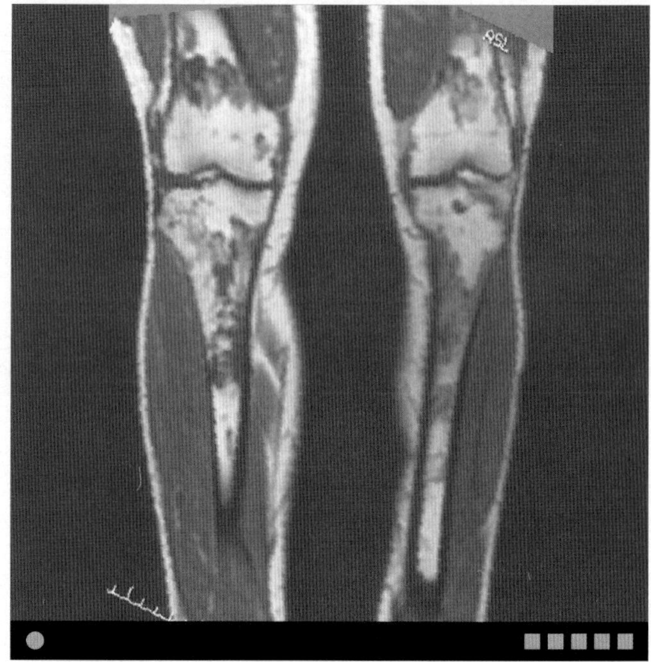

A. ECD: Coronal T1-weighted image shows the geographic lesions of bilateral, tibial diametaphyses. There are lesions of the distal femoral metaphysis with a single epiphyseal focus (radiographically usual sparing of the epiphyses is a common feature).

COMMENTS

The patient is a 40-year-old patient who presented with a 7-month history of lower extremity and knee pain. Bone pain is a common first presentation of Erdheim-Chester disease (ECD). ECD is rare and very similar to LCG in its histopathology and distribution and was thought to represent the same disease process. The main difference is the age distribution. ECD is a disease of the adult with a median age of 53 years. The ECD lesions do not share the same immunohistology and electron microscopy properties: The LCG lesions stain positive for S-100 antigen and demonstrate Birbeck granules on electron microscopy. The ECD bone lesions are often symmetric, sclerotic, and involve the metadiaphyses of long bones, whereas the LCG lesions are typically lytic and are found commonly in the axial skeleton. The MRI appearance corresponds well to the typical scintigraphic findings of symmetric streaks of radionuclide uptake and radiographic findings of sclerosis in the diametaphyseal regions of the long bones sparing the epiphyses. The sclerotic foci are of low MR signal interspersed with signal properties corresponding to normal marrow and edema. The nonosseous disease affects commonly the central nervous system with predominance of hypothalamic and pituitary involvement resulting in diabetes insipidus. Renal, cutaneous, and pulmonary involvements have all been described as well.

PEARLS

- **Polyostotic symmetric appearance is the hallmark of this disease.**
- **It is a rare disease with only 80 cases reported in the literature.**
- **Diametaphyseal infarct-like lesions of the long bones on MRI may prompt further investigation.**

ADDITIONAL IMAGES

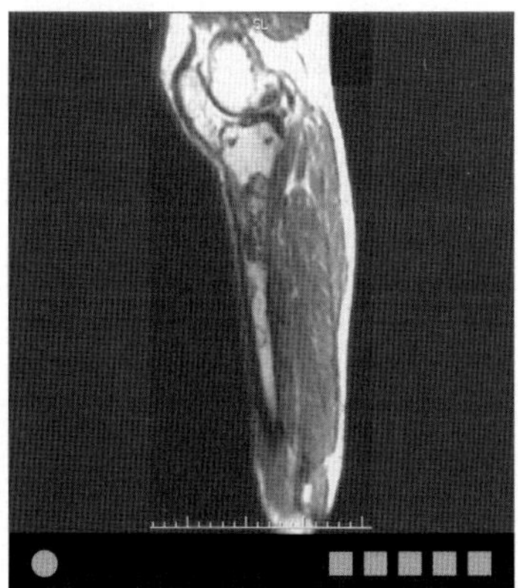

B. ECD: Sagittal T1-weighted image of the proximal tibia and distal femur demonstrates the geographic low signal lesion of both bones.

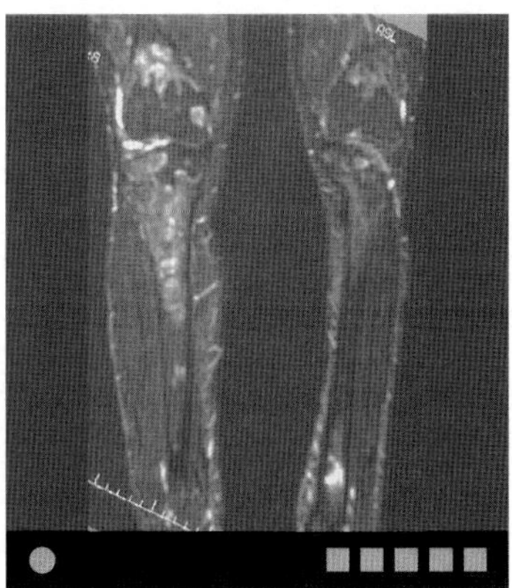

C. ECD: Coronal STIR images show the mixed signal properties of these lesions.

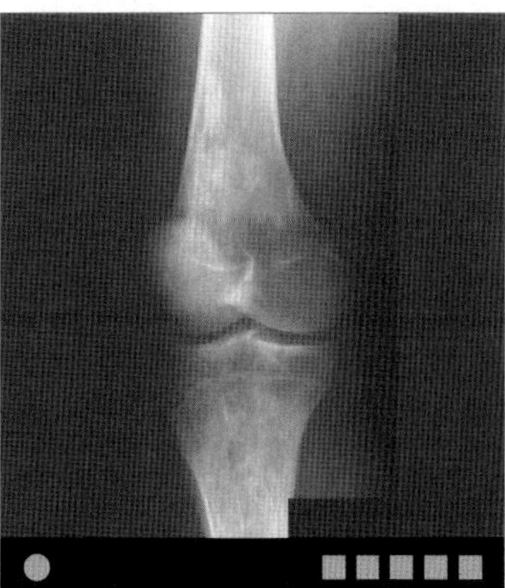

D. ECD: The AP radiograph of the knee demonstrates the characteristic streaky, sclerotic lesions of the distal femur and proximal tibia.

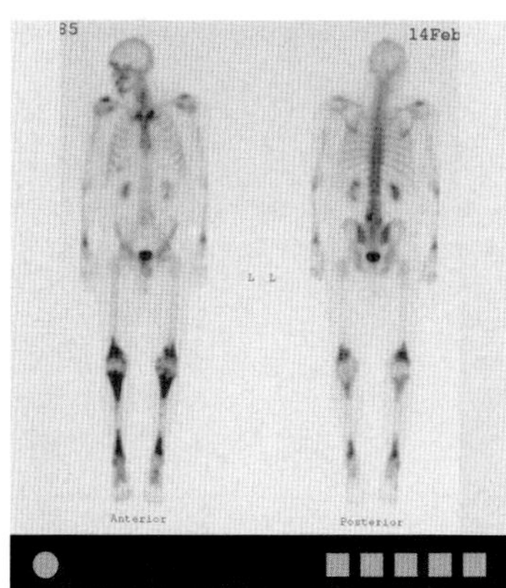

E. ECD: The bone scintigram displays the symmetric radionuclide uptake in the long bones.

IMAGE KEY

Common

Rare

Typical

Unusual

DIFFERENTIAL DIAGNOSES IMAGES

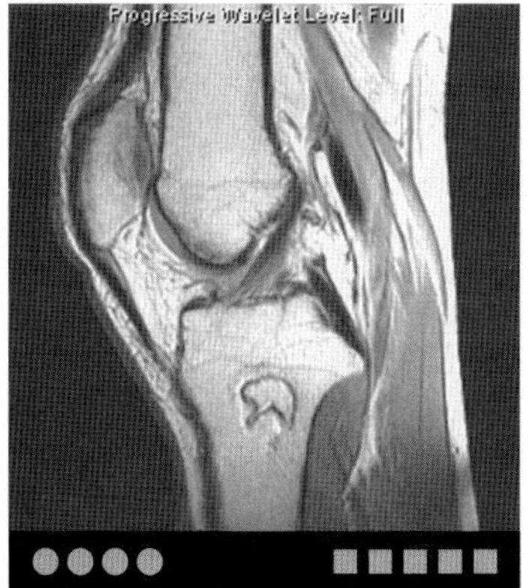

F. Bone infarct: The sagittal PD image of the knee shows a focus of bone infract in the proximal tibia.

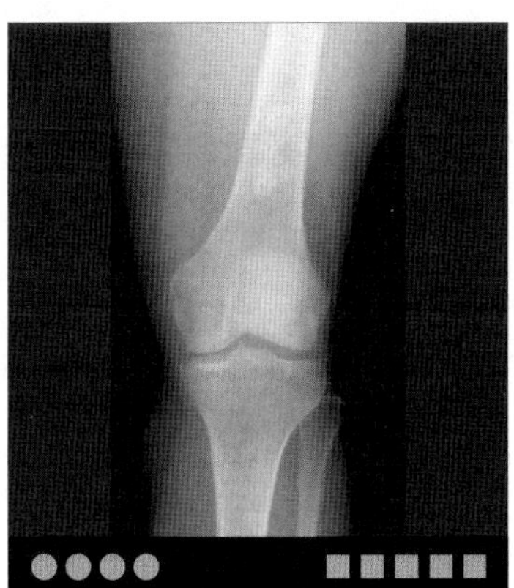

G. Encondroma: The AP radiograph of the knee reveals a medullary, mineralized low grade cartilage lesion, such as an enchondroma.

Chapter 25

Arthritis, Connective Tissue and Crystal Deposition Disorders

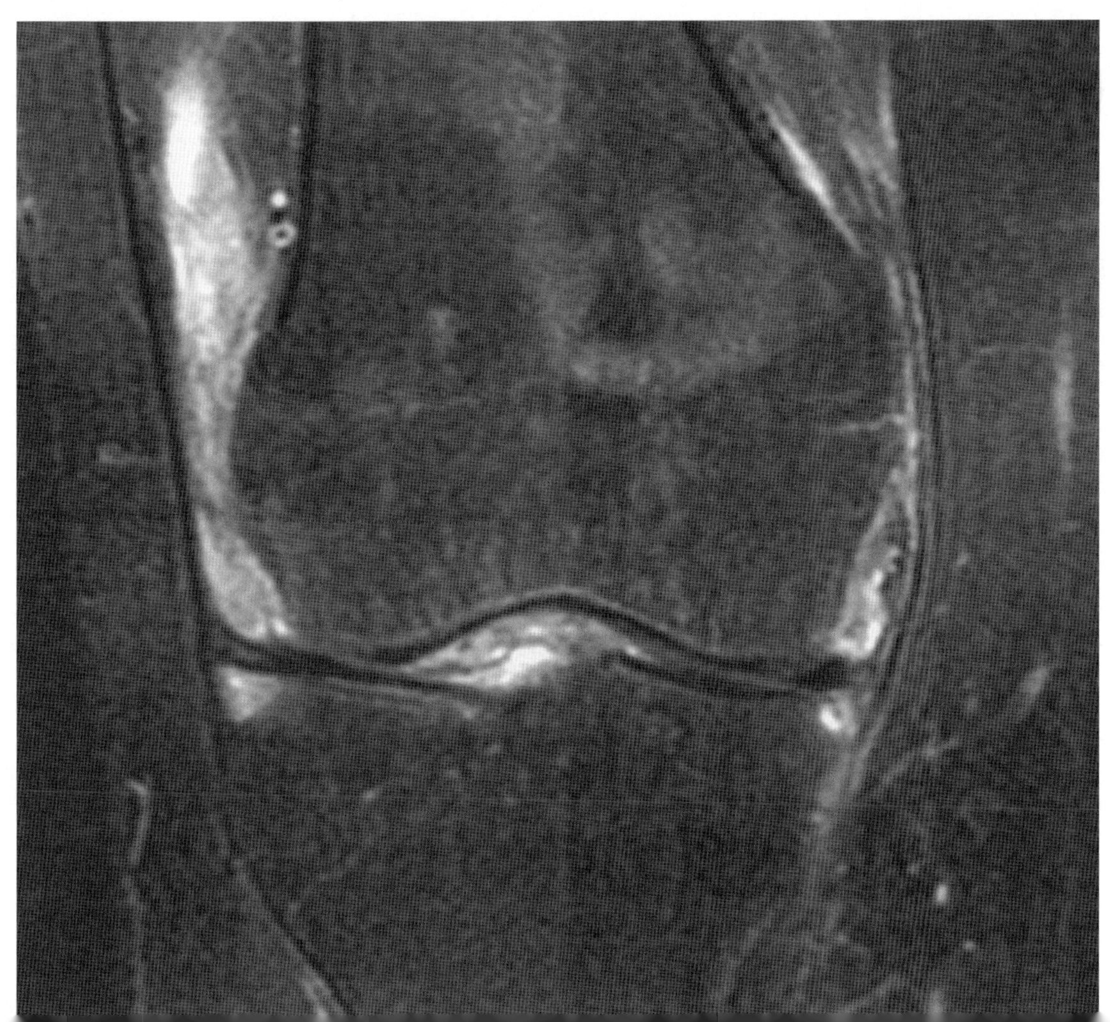

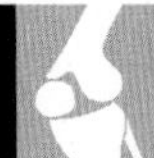

25–1 Rheumatoid Arthritis of the Knee

Edward Mossop and Jamshid Tehranzadeh

PRESENTATION

Knee pain and swelling.

FINDINGS

MRI shows marked synovial proliferation with rice bodies, joint effusion, and bone marrow edema.

DIFFERENTIAL DIAGNOSES

- *Psoriatic arthritis:* Erosions are more asymmetrical and central. They can be associated with enthesopathy, periostitis, and new bone formation. Patients often have the cutaneous or nail changes of psoriasis.
- *Septic arthritis and osteomyelitis: Staphylococcus aureus* is the most common cause. The course of the disease is much more acute and rapidly progressive and patients often exhibit systemic upset.
- *Reiter's arthritis:* Occurs more commonly in young men with urethritis and uveitis and is associated with enthesopathy and erosions that have indistinct margins and are surrounded by periosteal new bone formation.
- Other inflammatory arthritides may simulate rheumatoid arthritis (RA) changes.

COMMENTS

The patient is a 26-year-old female with known (RA). RA is a chronic systemic inflammatory disease of undetermined etiology involving primarily the synovial membranes and secondarily the articular structures of multiple joints. The disease is often progressive and results in pain, stiffness, and swelling. Prevalence is approximately 1% in the United States and affects women three times more than men between the age of 25 and 50 years. Chronic inflammation induces hypertrophy and villous thickening of the synovium into folds known as pannus. This invades the joint causing destruction of cartilage and bone. Multiple joints are affected and 80% of patients have bilateral, symmetrical knee involvement. On T1-weighted images, the synovial proliferation exhibits low signal, which enhances markedly after IV contrast. Small fibrinated areas of pannus known as rice bodies may be visualized within the joint fluid. Synovial proliferations present as low to intermediate signal rice bodies in bright synovial fluid on T2-weighted images. Marginal erosions of the bone and cartilage appear as areas of low signal foci on T1-weighted images and as regions of heterogeneous or bright signal on T2-weighted images. Cyst-like bone erosions are viewed as low signal on T1-weighted images and high signal on T2-weighted images and may enhance after contrast. Other signs can include: osteonecrosis, loss of joint space, and an irregular fat pad.

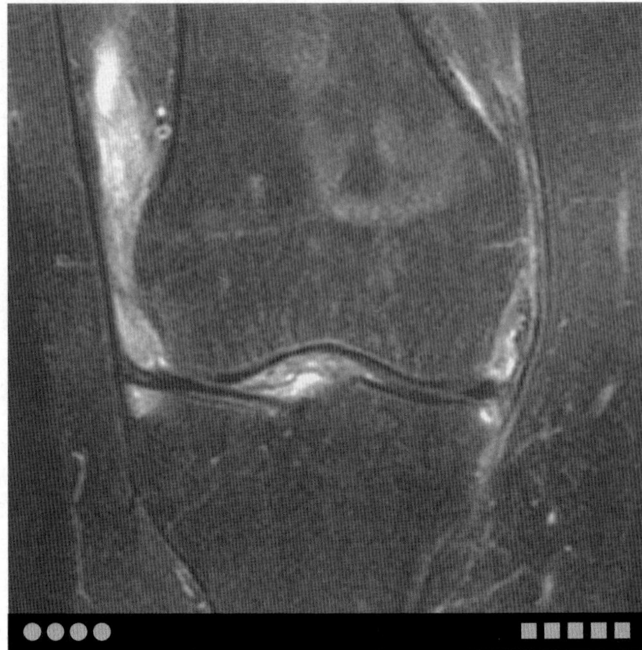

A. Rheumatoid Arthritis: Coronal T2 fat-saturated image shows joint fluid with intermediate rice body signals because of synovial proliferation and mild edema of the distal femur caused by RA.

PEARLS

- **RA is a chronic systemic inflammatory disease of undetermined etiology involving primarily the synovial membranes and secondarily the articular cartilages and bones of multiple joints.**
- **On T1-weighted images the synovial proliferation exhibits low signal, which enhances markedly after IV contrast. Synovial proliferation presents as low signal rice bodies within bright joint fluid on T2-weighted images.**
- **Marginal erosions of the bone and cartilage appear as areas of low signal foci on T1-weighted images, which enhance with contrast and present as regions of high signal on T2-weighted images.**
- **Other changes include cyst-like changes, joint effusions, osteonecrosis, and an irregular fat pad.**

ADDITIONAL IMAGES

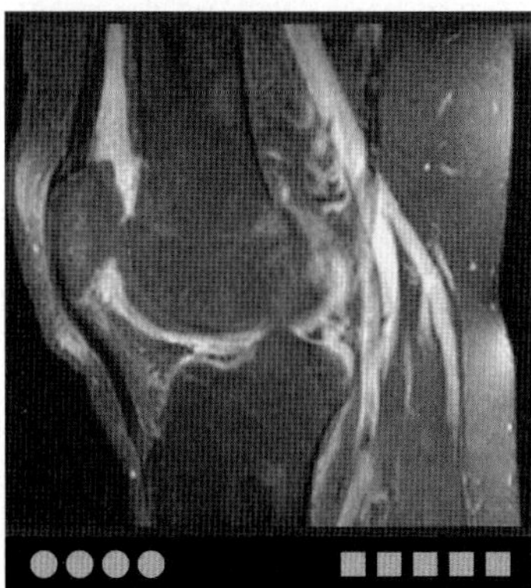

B. RA: Sagittal T1 fat-saturated postcontrast image shows joint fluid with intermediate signal rice bodies in the joint. Note erosion of the dorsal articular cartilage in the lower pole of the patella. Note edema in both the prepatellar area and bone marrow.

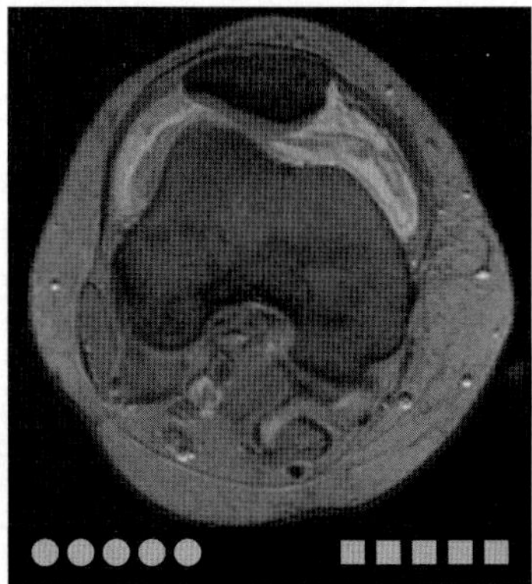

C. RA: Axial GRE image shows low to intermediate signal synovial proliferation in the suprapatellar bursa. Note dorsal articular cartilage erosion of the medial patella.

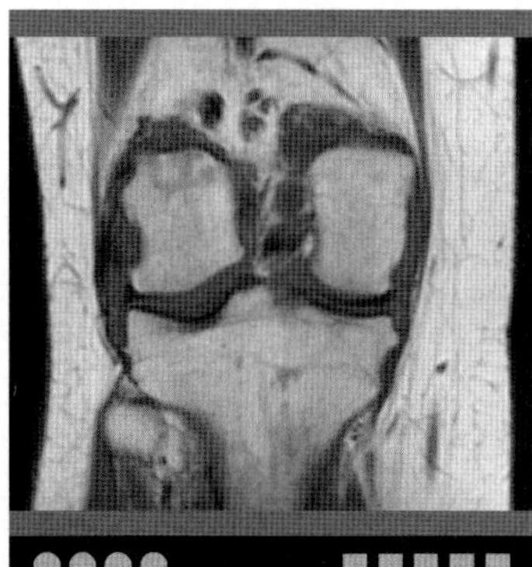

D. RA: Coronal T1-weighted image shows joint fluid and synovial proliferation.

E. RA: Axial T1 fat-saturated post-contrast image shows synovial enhancement surrounding low signal fluid. Note dorsal patella cartilage erosion on the medial side (arrow).

IMAGE KEY

Common

Rare

Typical

Unusual

DIFFERENTIAL DIAGNOSES IMAGES

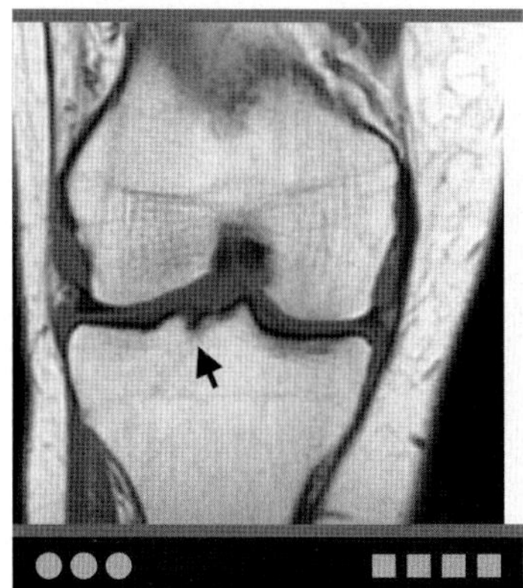

F. Psoriatic Arthritis: Coronal T1-weighted image of psoriatic arthritis shows central erosion (arrow) with fluid and synovial proliferation in the joint.

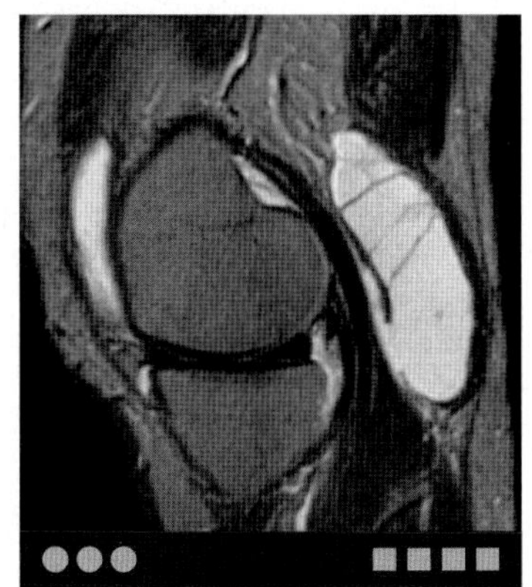

G. Psoriatic Arthritis: Sagittal T2 fat-saturated image of psoriatic arthritis shows joint fluid and synovial thickening in the Bakers cyst.

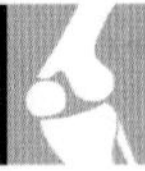

25–2 Dissecting Suprapatellar Bursa in Rheumatoid Arthritis

Shahla Modarresi and Daria Motamedi

PRESENTATION

Chronic knee joint pain and swelling.

FINDINGS

MR images show large, heterogeneous, low signal proliferative synovium in the dissecting suprapatellar bursa.

DIFFERENTIAL DIAGNOSES

- *Deposition diseases, e.g., gouty tophus:* On MR study, tophaceous mass reveals heterogeneously low to intermediate signal intensity with erosive changes of adjacent bone or joints.
- *Synovial proliferation, PVNS:* On MRI, the mass contains some loss of signal intensity on T2-weighted images representing combination of fibrosis and scattered hemosiderin deposit.
- *Lipoma arborescens:* MRI shows proliferation of synovial tissue and fingerlike fatty masses in the joint.
- *Synovial sarcoma:* Nonspecific MR signal showing high signal on T2-weighted and STIR images. Calcification may be seen as low signal foci within the lesion.
- *Infectious granulomatous disease (TB and Coccidiomycosis):* Hypertrophied synovium with nonspecific low to intermediate T1, PD, high T2, and STIR signal intensities.

COMMENTS

Rheumatoid arthritis (RA) is a chronic inflammatory, likely autoimmune systemic disease characterized by multiple joint involvement with pain, swelling, redness, morning stiffness, synovial proliferation, and eventual deformity. The most common joints involved are the fingers, wrists, elbows, shoulders, jaw, hips, knees, and toes. The prevalence of RA increases with age with a peak incidence in 40 to 60 years. The disease is three times more common in females than males and affects 1 in every 100 Americans. A patient has RA if he or she has at least four of seven following symptoms: morning stiffness for at least 1 hour, arthritis of three or more joint areas, symmetric arthritis, and arthritis of the hands, rheumatoid nodules, serum RF, and radiographic changes. RF is found in the serum of approximately 90% of patients with RA. Following osteoarthritis, the other two most commonly seen arthropathies are RA and calcium pyrophosphate dihydrate (CPPD) deposition disease. The characteristic radiographic features of RA include soft tissue swelling, periarticular osteoporosis, joint space narrowing, and articular and marginal erosions. RA rarely shows any productive bone formation such as periostitis, enthesopathy, and osteophyte unless there is secondary osteoarthritis present. MR imaging findings of RA of knee joints include: joint effusion, erosion of the articular cartilage, meniscus, ligaments, synovial membrane proliferation (pannus) in the forms of popliteal cyst or enlarged (dissecting) suprapatellar bursa, and eventual erosive and destructive changes in osseous structure.

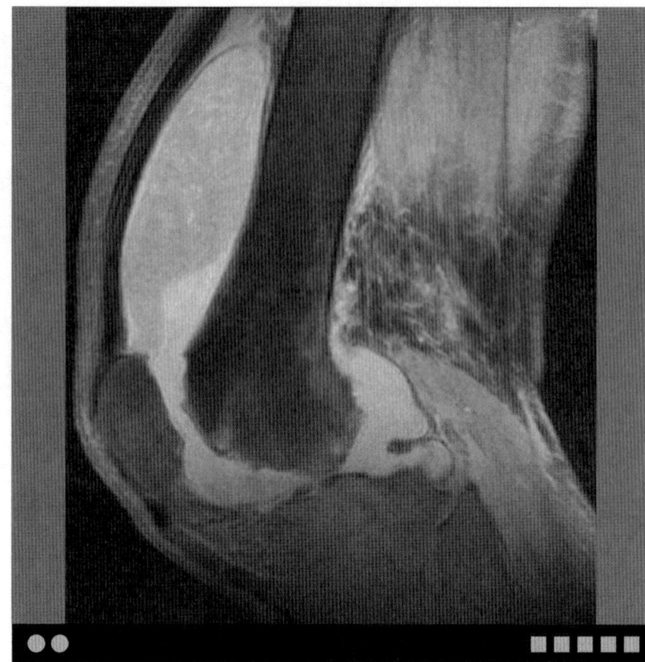

A. Dissecting suprapatellar bursa in RA: Sagittal postcontrast fat-saturated T1-weighted image shows diffusely enhancing synovial pannus in a dissecting suprapatellar bursa.

PEARLS

- **RA is a chronic inflammatory disease characterized by multiple joint involvement with pain, swelling, synovial proliferation, and eventual deformity.**
- **Following osteoarthritis, two most commonly seen arthropathies are RA and CPPD deposition.**
- **The characteristic radiographic features of RA include: soft tissue swelling, periarticular osteoporosis, joint space narrowing, and articular and marginal erosions.**
- **MR imaging findings of RA of knee joints include: joint effusion, erosion of the articular cartilage, meniscus, ligaments, synovial membrane proliferation (pannus) in the forms of popliteal cyst or enlarged (dissecting) suprapatellar bursa, and eventual erosive and destructive changes in osseous structure.**

ADDITIONAL IMAGES

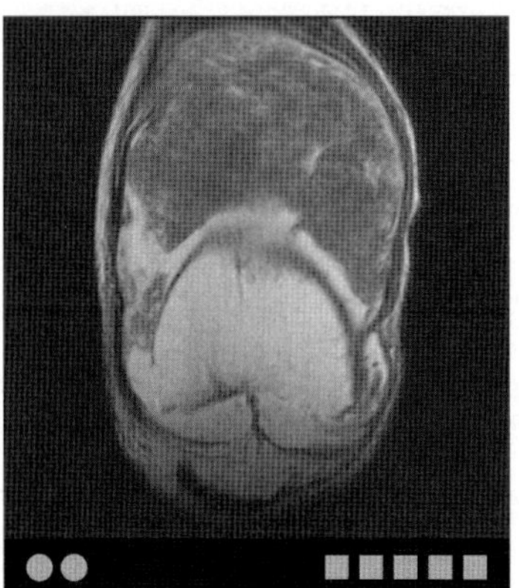

B. Dissecting suprapatellar bursa in RA: Axial PD image shows large, heterogeneous, low signal proliferative synovium in suprapatellar bursa.

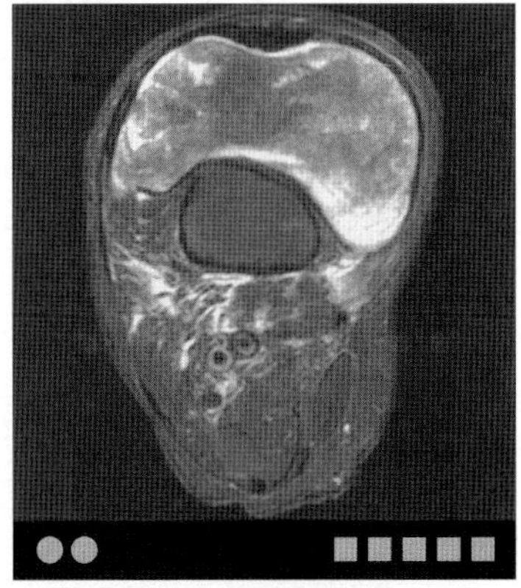

C. Dissecting suprapatellar bursa in RA: Axial T2-weighted fat-saturated image shows synovial proliferation in hyperextended fluid-filled suprapatellar bursa.

DIFFERENTIAL DIAGNOSES IMAGES

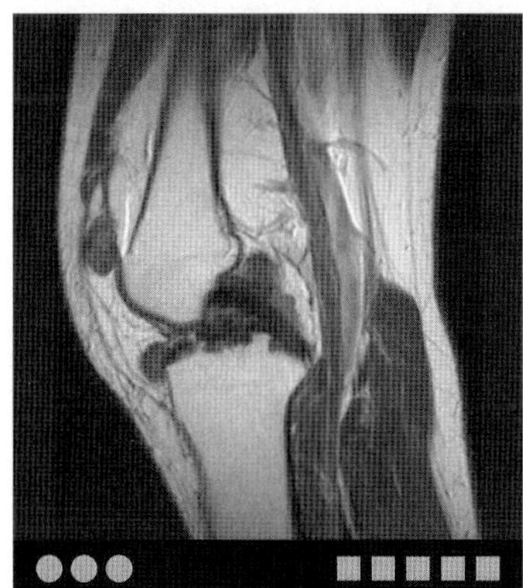

D. Gout: Sagittal T2-weighted image shows multiple low signal gouty tophi in the joint space with bony erosions.

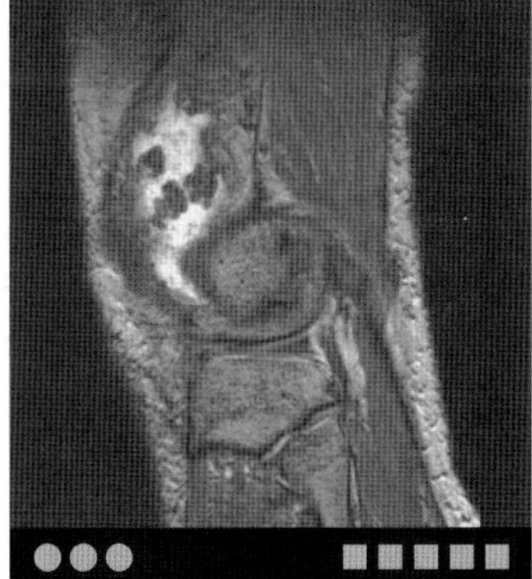

E. Synovial osteochondromatosis: Sagittal STIR image shows multiple low signal loose bodies within joint space with joint effusion consistent with synovial osteochondromatosis.

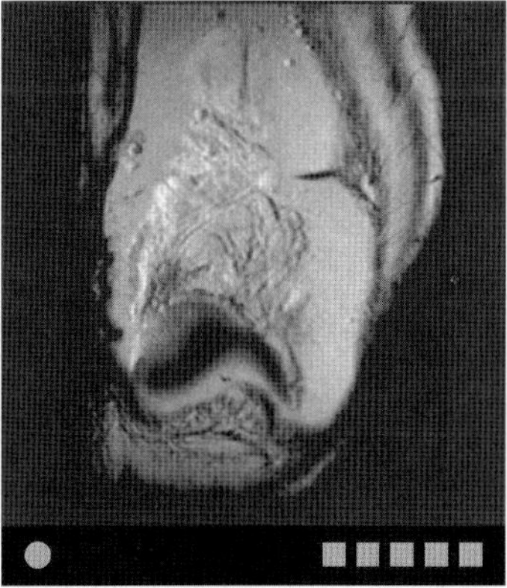

F. Lipoma arborescens: Coronal T2-weighted image shows fatty synovial proliferation and fingerlike fatty masses in the joint with large effusion, consistent with lipoma arborescence.

IMAGE KEY

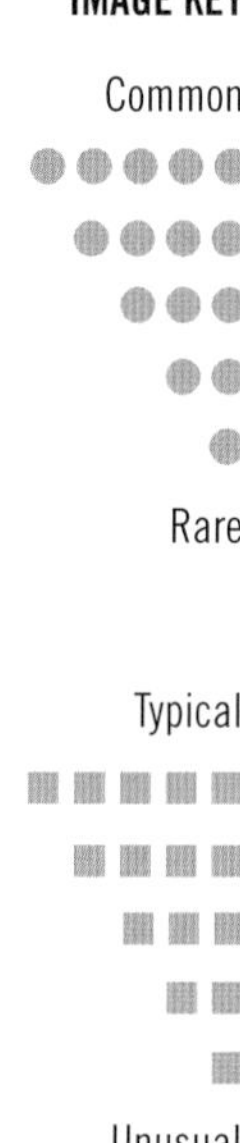

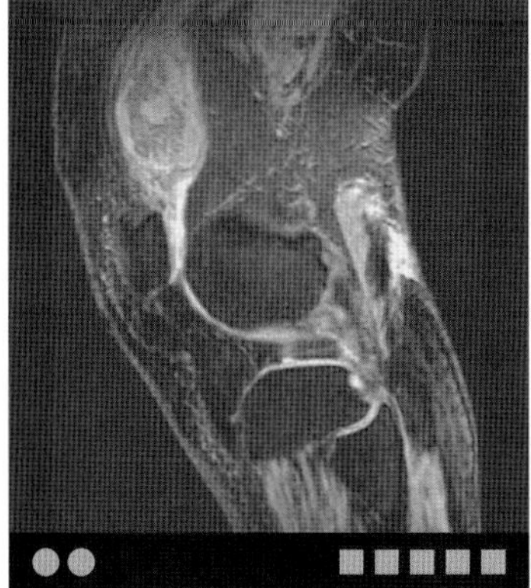

G. PVNS: Sagittal STIR image shows low signal mass surrounded by fluid in the suprapatellar pouch representing hemosiderin deposits in pigmented villonodular synovitis.

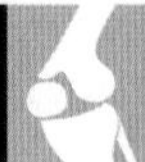

25–3 Hemophilic Arthritis of Knee

Rosemary J. Klecker

PRESENTATION

Chronic knee pain and decreased range of motion.

FINDINGS

MR image shows thickening of the synovium, severe cartilage loss with joint space narrowing, synovitis, and large subchondral cysts.

DIFFERENTIAL DIAGNOSES

- *Rheumatoid arthritis (RA):* Hemarthrosis and epiphyseal overgrowth are not seen in RA. Large subchondral cysts and severe joint destruction are characteristics more frequently seen in hemophilic arthropathy. Severe joint destruction is inconsistently seen in late stage of RA.
- *Juvenile rheumatoid arthritis (JRA):* Differentiated from hemophilic arthropathy by lack of joint destruction, large subchondral cysts, and hemarthrosis.
- *Pigmented villonodular synovitis (PVNS):* It is usually monoarticular and is characterized by synovial proliferation with hemosiderin deposition. The localized form is most commonly seen in the hands and feet whereas diffuse synovitis is often seen in the knee. Erosions are present approximately 50% of the time.

COMMENTS

The patient is a 38-year-old male with chronic knee pain and decreased range of motion. Hemarthrosis occurs in approximately 75% to 90% of patients with hemophilia. Severity of joint degeneration depends on frequency and the age of initial occurrence of the hemarthrosis. The most commonly affected joints in descending order of frequency are the knee, elbow, ankle, hip, and glenohumeral joint. With repeated episodes of bleeding, the synovial lining becomes thickened secondary to synovial absorption of hemosiderin. On MR imaging, this presents as a thickened, irregular synovial lining that is low signal intensity on all sequences. Repeated hemarthrosis also results in periarticular osteopenia, and cartilage and subchondral bone destruction resulting in an irregular contour of the articular surfaces resulting in symmetric joint destruction. The intercondylar notch of the femur is often widened as a result of repeated hemorrhage around the cruciate ligaments. Squaring of the inferior pole of the patella has been associated with hemophilia. This finding, however, is not specific to hemophilia and has also been described as associated with JRA, and thinning and elongation of the patella may

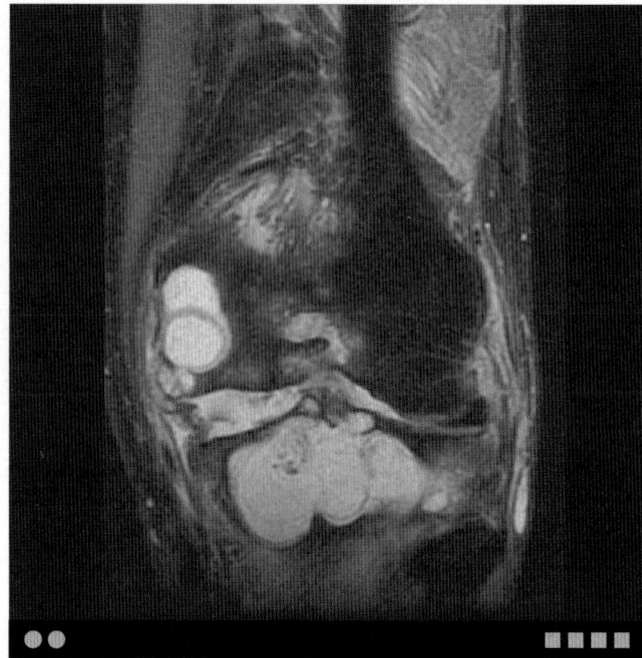

A. Hemophilic arthritis: Coronal STIR-weighted image of the knee shows synovitis with large central cysts and marginal erosions, and cysts with edema of the surrounding soft tissues. There is complete cartilage loss of the medial compartment.

also be seen. Epiphyseal overgrowth is a manifestation of chronic synovitis and hemarthrosis. Osseous cystic lesions are prominent in this disease and are often multiple of varying size, occurring marginally and centrally, and often communicating with the articular surface. Trabecular thinning and resorption gives rise to enlarging marrow spaces, which may appear cystic and intraosseous or periosteal hemorrhage creates neoplastic-like lesions known as hemophilic pseudotumors.

PEARLS

- **Classic radiographic findings include diffuse joint narrowing with marginal erosions and subchondral cysts, periarticular osteopenia, epiphyseal overgrowth, dense effusions, synovial thickening, widened intercondylar notch, and abnormal patellar morphology.**
- **On MR, the synovial lining may appear thick and low signal intensity on all sequences secondary to presence of hemosiderin.**
- **May be distinguished from inflammatory arthropathies early in the disease process by presence of subchondral cysts and erosions with joint space preservation.**

ADDITIONAL IMAGE

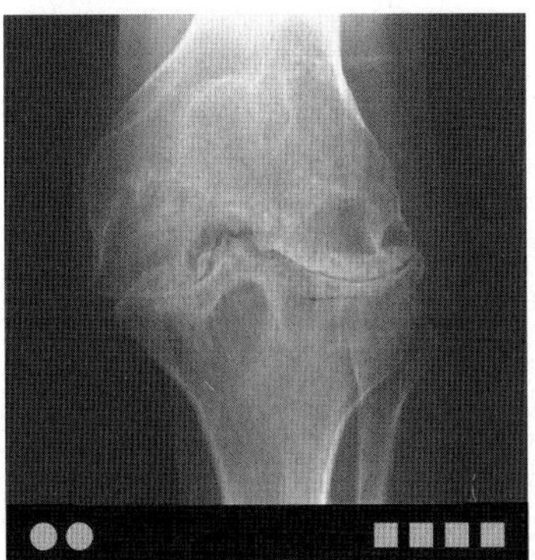

B. Hemophilic arthritis: Radiograph of the same patient demonstrates the irregularity of the articular surfaces secondary to bone resorption. There is widening of the intercondylar notch.

DIFFERENTIAL DIAGNOSES IMAGES

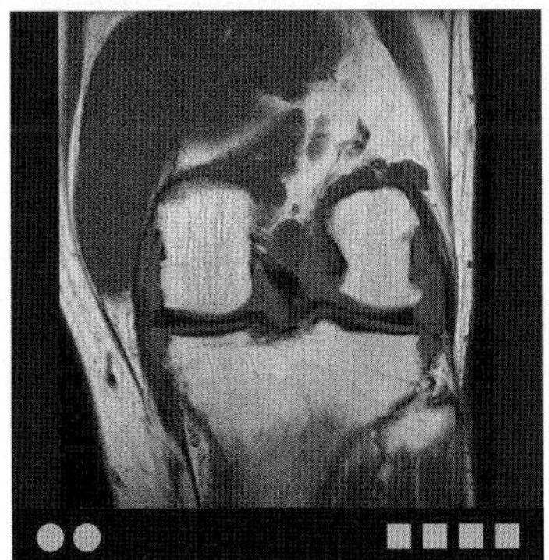

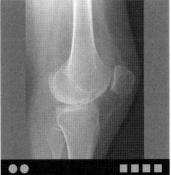

C. Rheumatoid arthritis: Coronal T1-weighted MR image of the knee demonstrates a large joint effusion and marginal erosions.

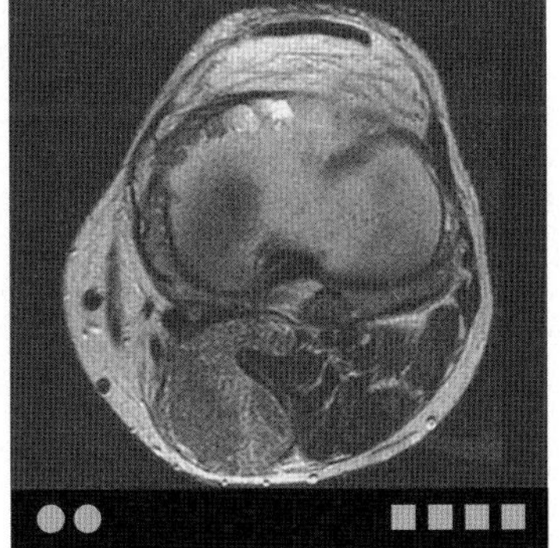

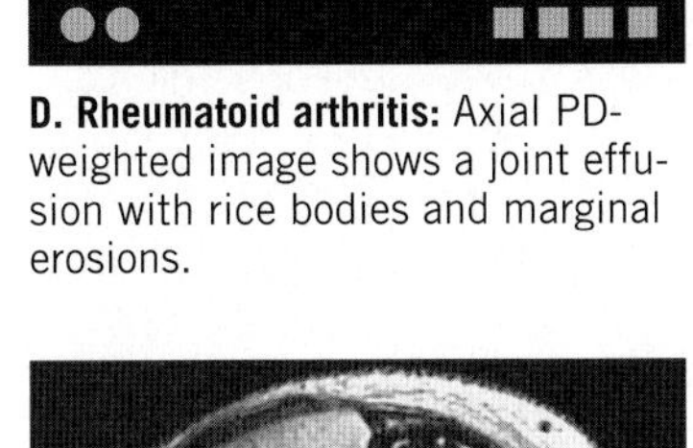

D. Rheumatoid arthritis: Axial PD-weighted image shows a joint effusion with rice bodies and marginal erosions.

E. Juvenile rheumatoid arthritis: Radiograph demonstrates joint effusion, overgrowth of the epiphysis, and squaring of the patella. The chondral surfaces are intact.

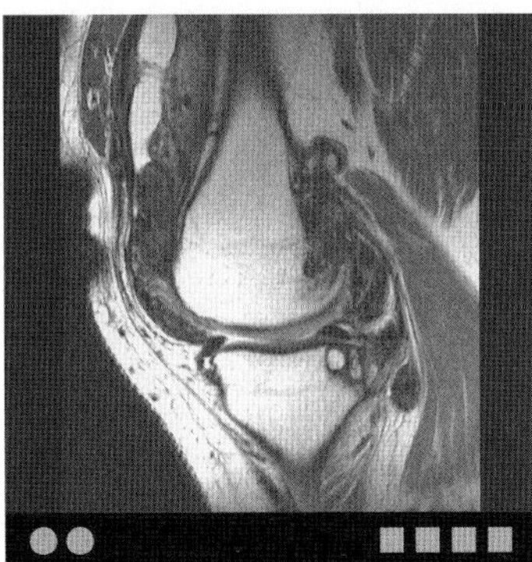

F. Pigmented villonodular synovitis: Sagittal PD-weighted image shows intra-articular nodular masses of low signal intensity in the joint. Hemosiderin deposition accounts for the characteristic low signal intensity of the masses. There are marginal erosions with preservation of the joint space.

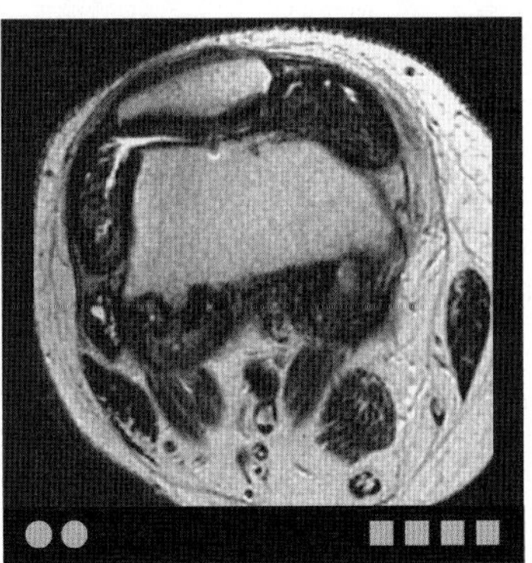

G. Pigmented villonodular synovitis: Axial T2-weighted image shows intra-articular nodular masses of low signal intensity in the joint. Hemosiderin deposition accounts for the characteristic low signal intensity of the masses. There are marginal erosions with preservation of the joint space.

IMAGE KEY

Common

Rare

Typical

Unusual

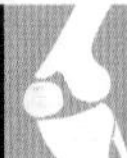

25–4 Osteoarthrosis of the Knee with Meniscal Subluxation

Edward Mossop and Jamshid Tehranzadeh

PRESENTATION

Left knee pain and reduced range of movement.

FINDINGS

Severe osteoarthrosis (OA) of the left knee with narrowing of the medial femorotibial compartment, osteophytes, subchondral sclerosis with cyst formation, muscle atrophy, and subluxation of the anterior horn of the medial meniscus.

DIFFERENTIAL DIAGNOSES

- *Rheumatoid arthritis (RA):* Inflammation and proliferation of synovial tissue causes joint effusions, loss of cartilage, and subchondral erosions. Acute inflamed pannus is hypointense on T1-weighted images and enhances with contrast.
- Calcium pyrophosphate deposition diseases such as pseudogout, hyperparathyroidism, and hemochromatosis are associated with chondrocalcinosis and premature degenerative changes in the joint.
- *Psoriatic arthritis:* Erosions are more central in the joint and can be associated with enthesopathy and new bone formation. Patients often have the cutaneous or nail changes of psoriasis.
- *Reiter's arthritis:* Occurs more commonly in young men with urethritis and uveitis and is associated with enthesopathy and erosions that have indistinct margins, and are surrounded by periosteal new bone.

COMMENTS

The patient is a 59-year-old female with confirmed OA. OA is defined as a "heterogeneous group of conditions that leads to joint symptoms and signs, which are associated with defective integrity of articular cartilage, in addition to related changes in the underlying bone at the joint margins." Its prevalence after the age of 65 years is 60% in men and 70% in women. The etiology of OA is multifactorial with inflammatory, metabolic, and mechanical causes. A number of risk factors such as obesity, occupation, and trauma may be involved. OA indicates the degeneration of articular cartilage with changes in subchondral bone and mild intra-articular inflammation. In the knee, the menisci function as buffers by distributing axial load and protecting the articular cartilage. Degeneration/subluxation of menisci occurs more often in association with OA. MRI shows thinning of the articular cartilage as inhomogeneous decreased signal intensity on T2/T1-weighted images and the presence of osteophytes. Areas of subchondral sclerosis are foci of low signal intensity on MR sequences, which are surrounded by low signal on T1-weighted and high signal on T2-weighted images representing bone marrow edema. Subchondral cysts appear as high signal fluid containing foci surrounded by thin low signal borders. Meniscal subluxation resembles the filling of an oreo cookie pushed out and resting beyond the margin of the joint ("Oreo Cookie sign").

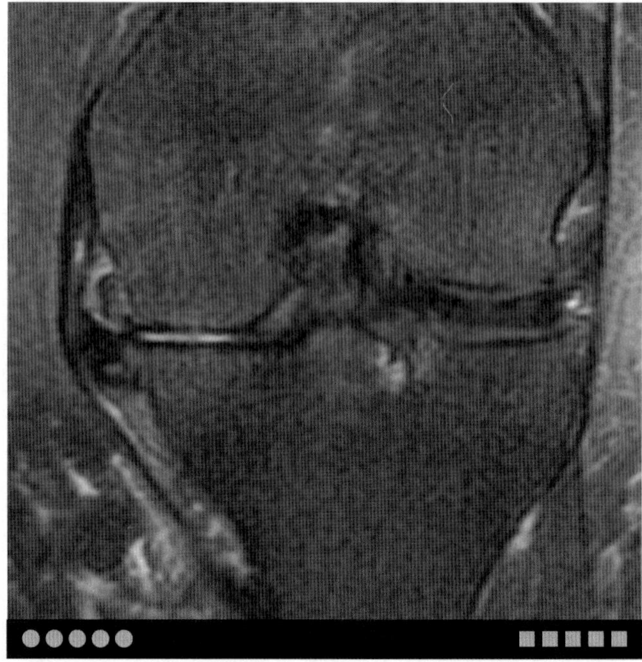

A. Osteoarthrosis: Coronal T2 fat-saturated image shows OA of the knee joint with loss of articular cartilage from the medial joint. Note subluxation of the medial meniscus (Oreo Cookie sign).

PEARLS

- **OA is a degenerative disease of articular cartilage and is the most common type of arthritis.**
- **The prevalence of OA after the age of 65 years is about 60% in men and 70% in women.**
- **Subluxation of menisci occurs more often in association with OA.**
- **This resembles the filling of an oreo cookie pushed out under force ("Oreo Cookie sign").**
- **Coronal MR images characteristically show subluxation of menisci beyond the margins of the joint.**

ADDITIONAL IMAGES

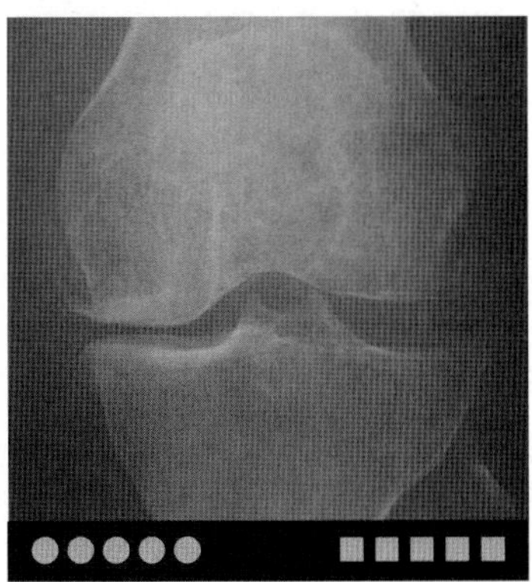

B. OA: AP radiograph of the left knee shows medial joint space narrowing, osteophytes and subchondral sclerosis consistent with OA.

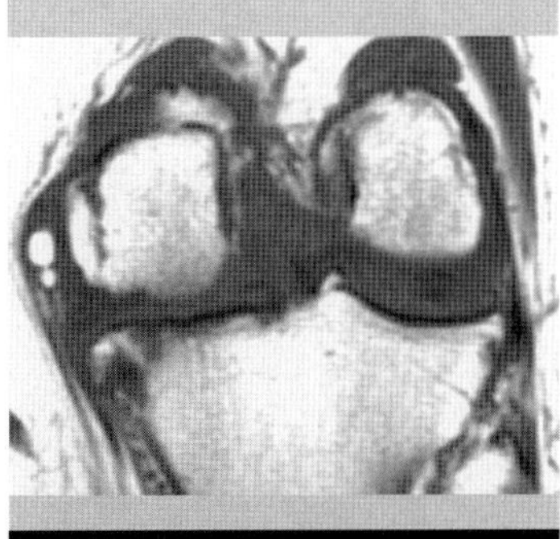

C. OA: Coronal T1-weighted image shows OA of the knee joint. Note hypertrophic osteophytes of the femoral and tibial condyles, asymmetrical medial joint narrowing, and subchondral sclerosis with subluxation of the medial meniscus.

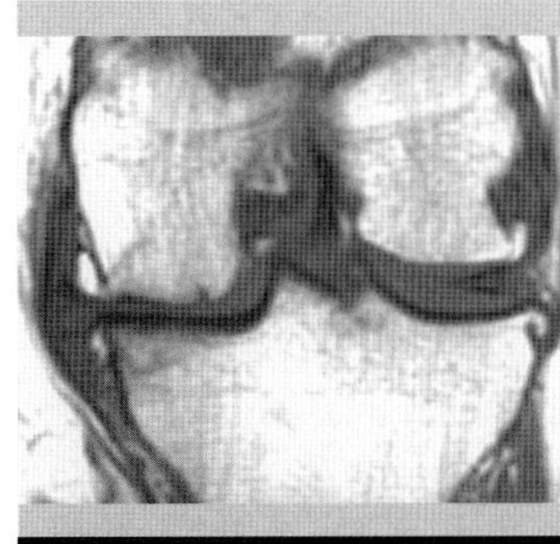

D. OA: Coronal T1-weighted image shows OA of the knee joint. Note hypertrophic osteophytes of the femoral and tibial condyles, asymmetrical medial joint narrowing, and subchondral sclerosis with subluxation of the medial meniscus.

E. OA: Sagittal proton density image shows osteophytes and subchondral focus of low signal of the femoral condyle.

DIFFERENTIAL DIAGNOSES IMAGES

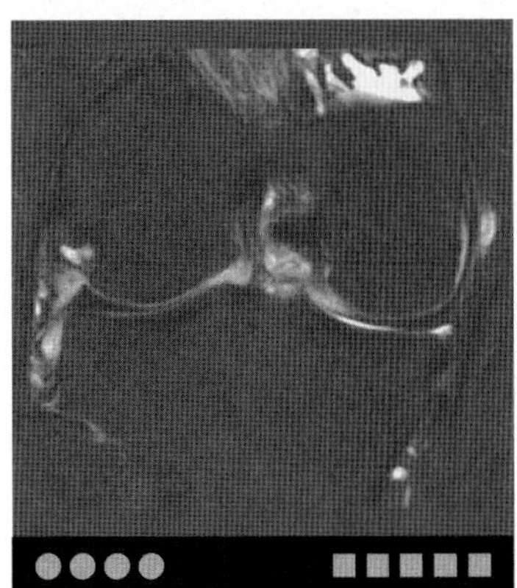

F. RA: Coronal T2 fat-saturated image shows RA of the knee with symmetrical loss of joint space and fluid within the joint. Note the presence of rice bodies within the joint representing synovial proliferation.

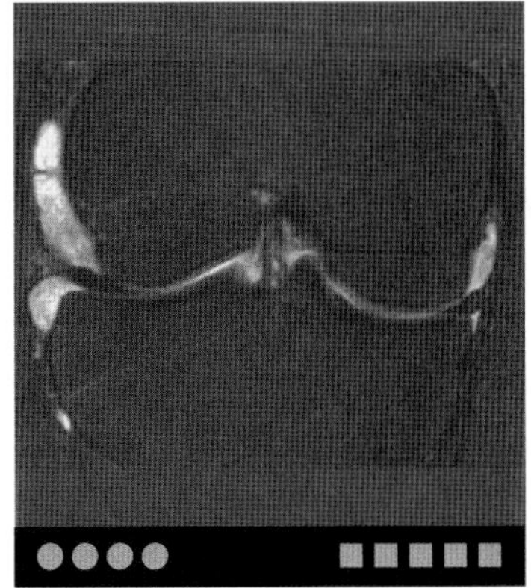

G. RA: Coronal T2 fat-saturated focused image shows RA of the knee with symmetrical loss of joint space and fluid within the joint. Note the presence of rice bodies within the joint representing synovial proliferation.

IMAGE KEY

Common

Rare

Typical

Unusual

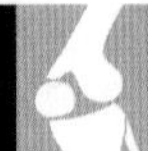

25–5 Gout of Patella

Melitus Maryam Golshan and Jamshid Tehranzadeh

PRESENTATION

Knee pain.

FINDINGS

Radiograph and CT show osteolytic lesion in posterior aspect of patella. MR images show erosion of patella with low signal intensity on T1-weighted image and contrast enhancement.

DIFFERENTIAL DIAGNOSES

- *Chondroblastoma:* Lobulated MRI margins are typical of cartilaginous lesions; it is isointense to muscle in T1-weighted image and intermediate heterogeneous to high signal intensity in T2-weighted image, and often presents with cartilaginous matrix calcification.
- Boride's abscess and other infections such as tuberculosis. They usually have soft tissue involvement as well.
- Synovial erosion in rheumatoid arthritis and degenerative cyst of osteoarthrosis.
- Other benign tumors such as giant cell tumor and osteoid osteoma may occur in patella.

COMMENTS

This is the case of a 67-year-old man with a history of knee pain for five months. Gout is a common inflammatory arthritis, especially in men. Diagnosis is typically established by clinical and laboratory assessment. These include detection of urate crystals in joint aspirate and elevated serum uric acid. The knee is the third most commonly affected site in gout after the foot and ankle. Gouty tophi may produce bony erosions and cystic changes of the adjacent bone resulting in chronic deforming arthritis. Gout has tendency to involve extensor tendons of the joints such as olecranon attachment of triceps, Achilles tendon, and patellar tendon. However, isolated involvement of patella is rare, when present typically is accompanied by changes in the femur and tibia. Gout tends to involve primarily superior lateral aspect of patella. Atypical presentation of gout does occur, which may relate to intra-articular tophaceous deposits in which, further imaging evaluation is necessary. Such deposits present as masses on MR images. Gouty tophi are mostly of low or intermediate signal intensity of T1-weighted image and reveal a characteristic increase in signal intensity after intravenous administration of gadolinium. The imaging findings of tophi on T2-weighted image are variable, but usually contain low signal regions. These features relate primarily to internal calcifications, which are most evident on CT images.

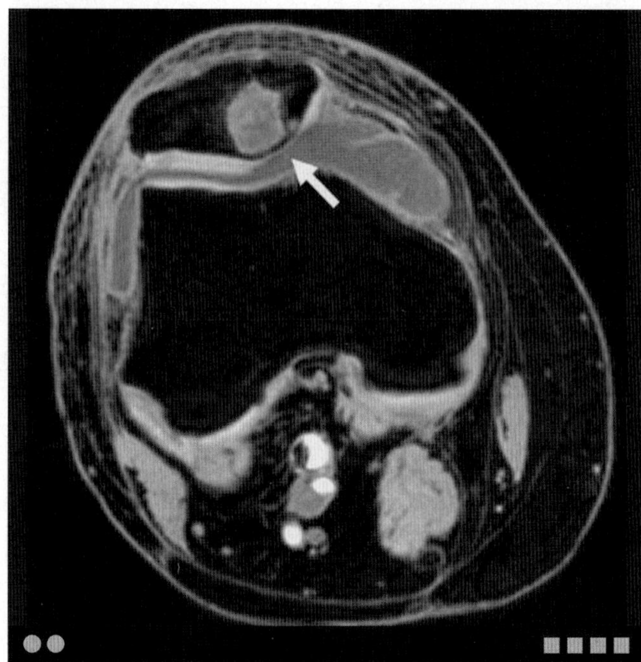

A. Gout: 3D spoiled gradient echo axial image of the knee shows intermediate signal lesion in the patella. Note adjacent cartilage erosion (arrow) and joint effusion.

PEARLS

- **Gout is an important cause of arthralgia in middle age male group.**
- **Intra-articular tophi of the knee may appear in patients with either chronic gout or atypical presentation, which imaging studies needed for accurate diagnosis.**
- **Gout has a tendency to occur at extensor tendon insertion sites and in patella, superior lateral part is primarily affected.**
- **MRI shows low to intermediate signal intensity on T1-weighted image, which enhances with contrast agent. T2-weighted images are more variable and it may have nonhomogeneous, mostly, low or foci of high signal intensity.**
- **CT scanning often allows accurate diagnosis of stippled calcifications in intraosseous tophi.**

ADDITIONAL IMAGES

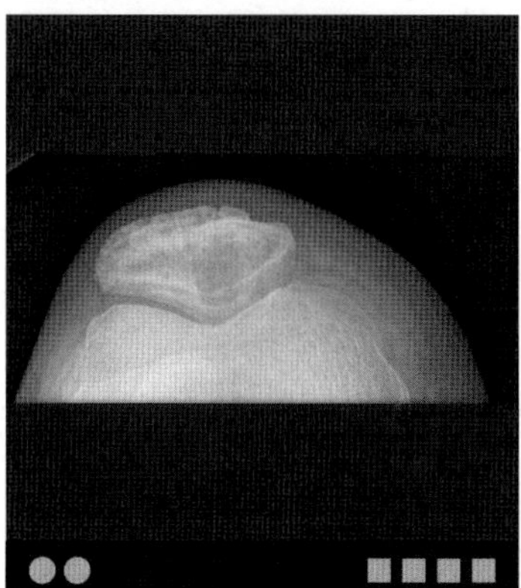

B. Gout: Sunrise radiographic view of the knee shows cystic lesion in the patella close to posterior surface.

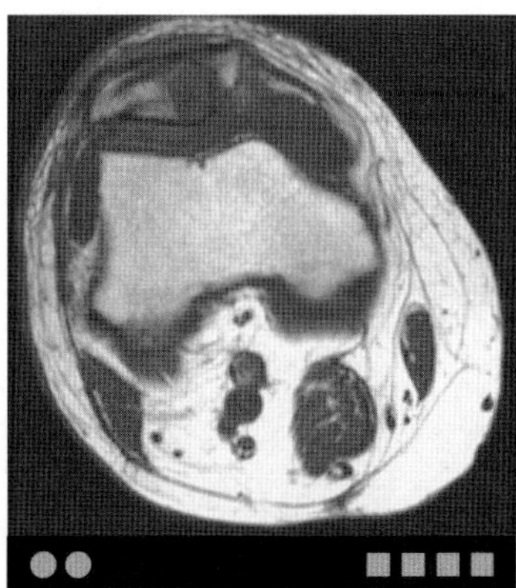

C. Gout: Axial T1-weighted image of knee shows a focus of low signal lesion in the patella with cortical disruption.

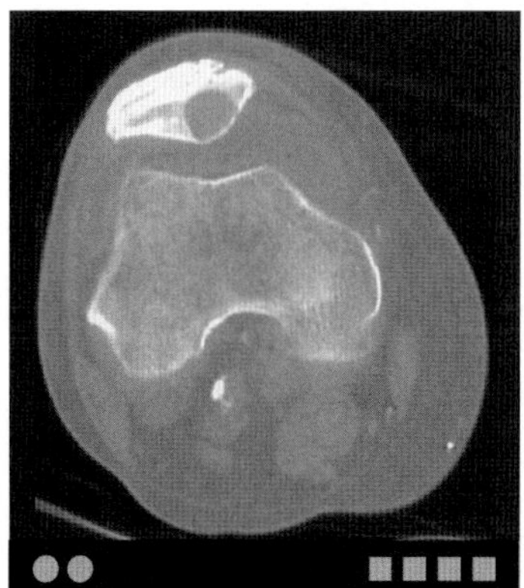

D. Gout: Axial CT of the knee shows osteolytic lesion in posterior part of patella.

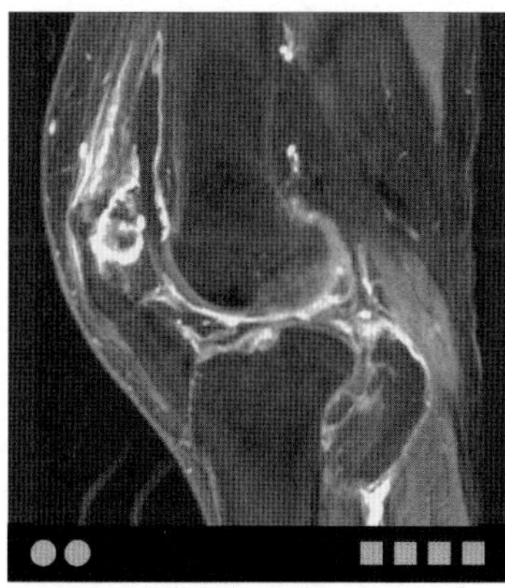

E. Gout: Sagittal T1-weighted fat-saturated postcontrast image shows nonhomogenous and marginal enhancement around and in the patellar erosion. Note also synovial enhancement.

IMAGE KEY

Common

Rare

Typical

Unusual

DIFFERENTIAL DIAGNOSES IMAGES

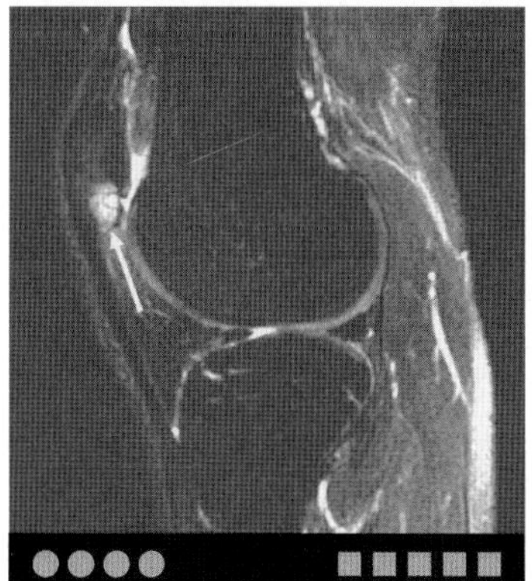

F. RA: Sagittal T2 fast spin echo fat saturated image shows bright focal erosion in inferior lateral pole of patella (arrow) in a 45-year-old female with RA.

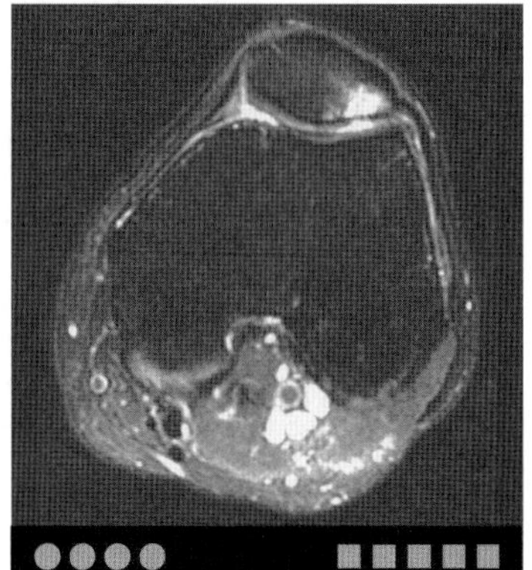

G. RA: Axial T2 fast spin echo fat-saturated image shows bright focal erosion of patella with adjacent dorsal articular cartilage defect in a 45-year-old female with RA.

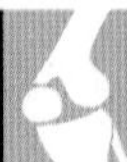

25–6 Amyloidosis of the Knee

George Hermann

PRESENTATION

Knee pain.

FINDINGS

MRI shows a low signal mass in the knee joint eroding the endplate of the tibia.

DIFFERENTIAL DIAGNOSES

- *Synovial chondromatosis:* This usually presents with extensive erosion of the joint with soft tissue mass.
- *Osteoarthritis:* This is characterized by joint space narrowing with subarticular sclerosis, cyst formation, and proliferative changes around the joint.
- *Pigmented villonodular synovitis:* This may present with soft tissue mass, bony erosions, and presence of hemosiderin.
- *Gouty arthritis:* This is associated with elevated serum uric acid.

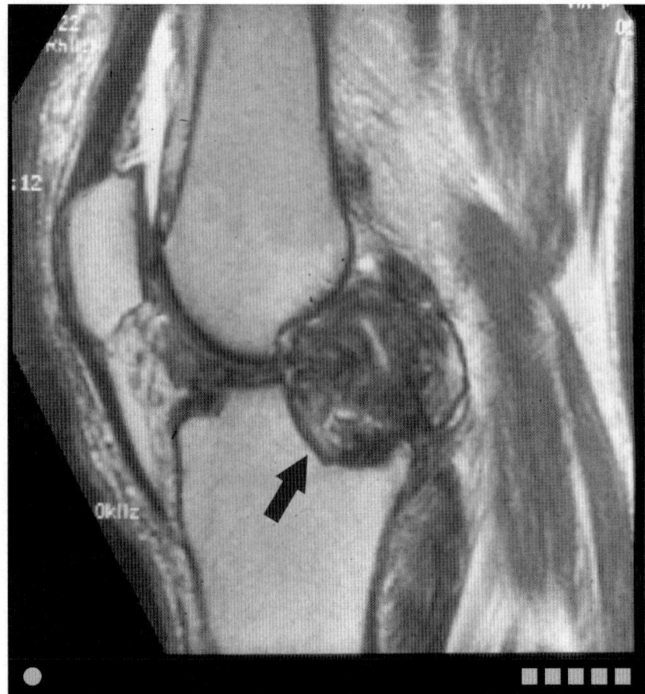

A. Amyloidosis: Sagittal T2-weighted image of the knee reveals moderately decreased signal intensity mass of the central portion of the joint. Note the bony erosion of posterior tibial plateau (arrow).

COMMENTS

The patient is a 51-year-old male treated with hemodialysis for 21 years. He was diagnosed with amyloidosis involving multiple sites. Amyloidosis, in general, may be classified as primary, idiopathic, or secondary to some other condition or familial. Chronic hemodialysis related amyloid (AB_2-microglobulin) derived from B_2–microglobulin, which is found in the serum of normal individuals. The B_2-m protein is normally filtered by the glomerulus and reabsorbed by the proximal tubules in the kidney. Conventional dialysis membranes do not remove it from the bloodstream. As a result, the serum levels become elevated and deposit in the various tissues. Periarticular soft tissue masses, cystic lesions in tubular bones, flat and irregular bones are common. Amyloid deposition may lead to spondyloarthropathy or carpal tunnel syndrome. MRI is very useful in evaluating intra-articular involvement and also subchondral deposition of amyloid. While the MR appearance may be variable, depending on the tissue constituents, the low signal intensity on T1 and T2-weighted image is common and related to the presence of fibrous tissue. Similar low signal lesions with erosions are seen in patients with pigmented villonodular synovitis (PVNS), gout, and synovial chondromatosis. Clinical correlation and laboratory data and examination of other joints help in differential diagnosis. Synovial chondromatosis and PVNS are usually monoarticular.

PEARLS

- **Amyloid deposition in the musculoskeletal system may occur in up to 80% of patients on long-term hemodialysis (10 years or more).**
- **Joint erosion surrounded with soft tissue mass favors the diagnosis of amyloidosis in patients on long-term hemodialysis.**
- **Decreased signal intensity on T1 and T2-weighted image is highly suggestive of amyloid deposition.**

ADDITIONAL IMAGES

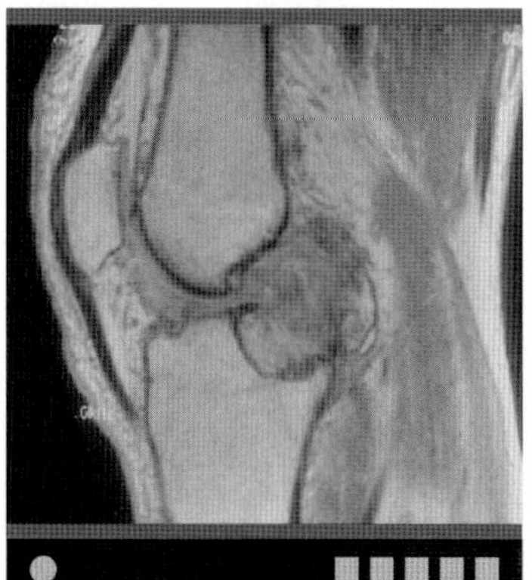

B. Amyloidosis: Sagittal T1-weighted image reveals decreased signal intensity with bony erosion.

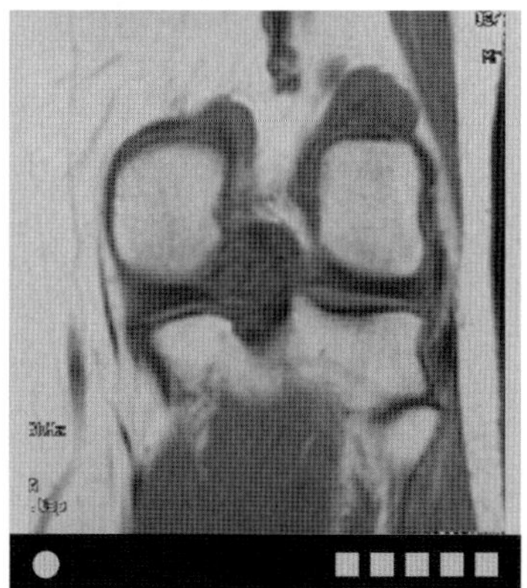

C. Amyloidosis: Coronal T1-weighted image shows a decreased signal intensity at the center of the tibial plateau.

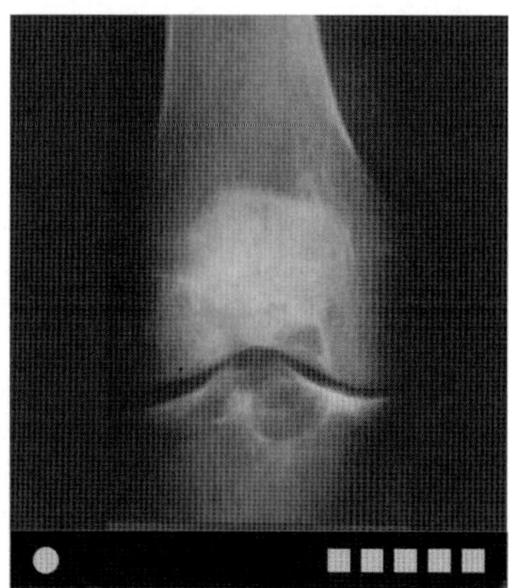

D. Amyloidosis: AP radiograph shows subarticular lytic lesions around the joint.

DIFFERENTIAL DIAGNOSES IMAGES

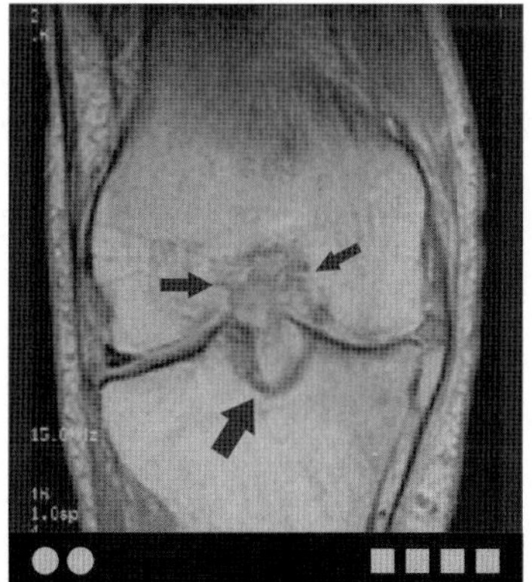

E. Pigmented villonodular synovitis: Coronal T1-weighted image shows decreased signal intensity mass at the intercondyle notch and bony erosions (arrows).

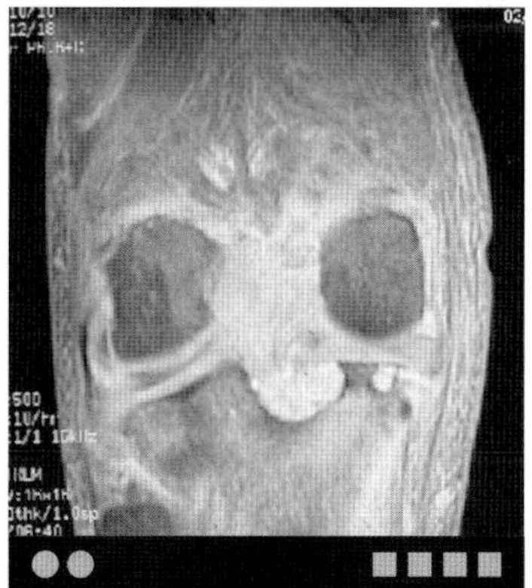

F. Pigmented villonodular synovitis: Coronal T2-weighted image shows relatively decreased signal intensity and bony erosions at the same areas as figure E.

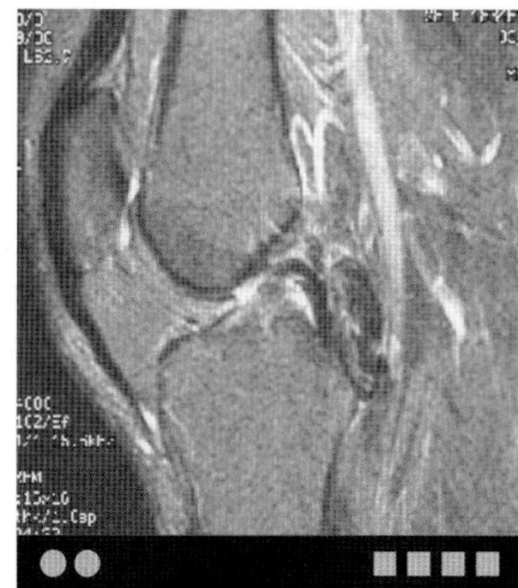

G. Pigmented villonodular synovitis: Sagittal STIR image shows an oval mass of low signal with minimal marginal increased signal intensity behind the knee joint.

IMAGE KEY

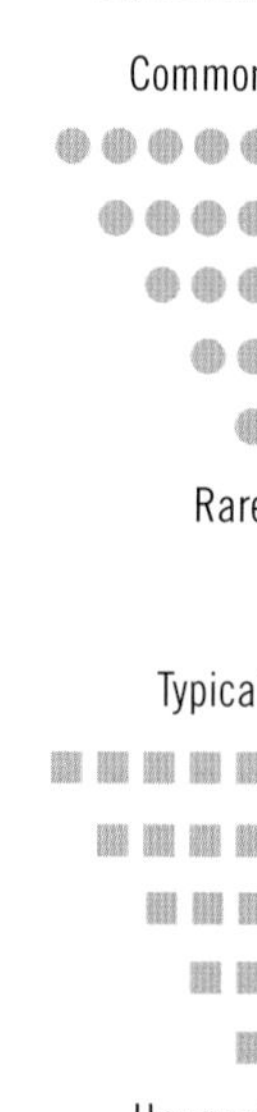

Chapter 26

Infections

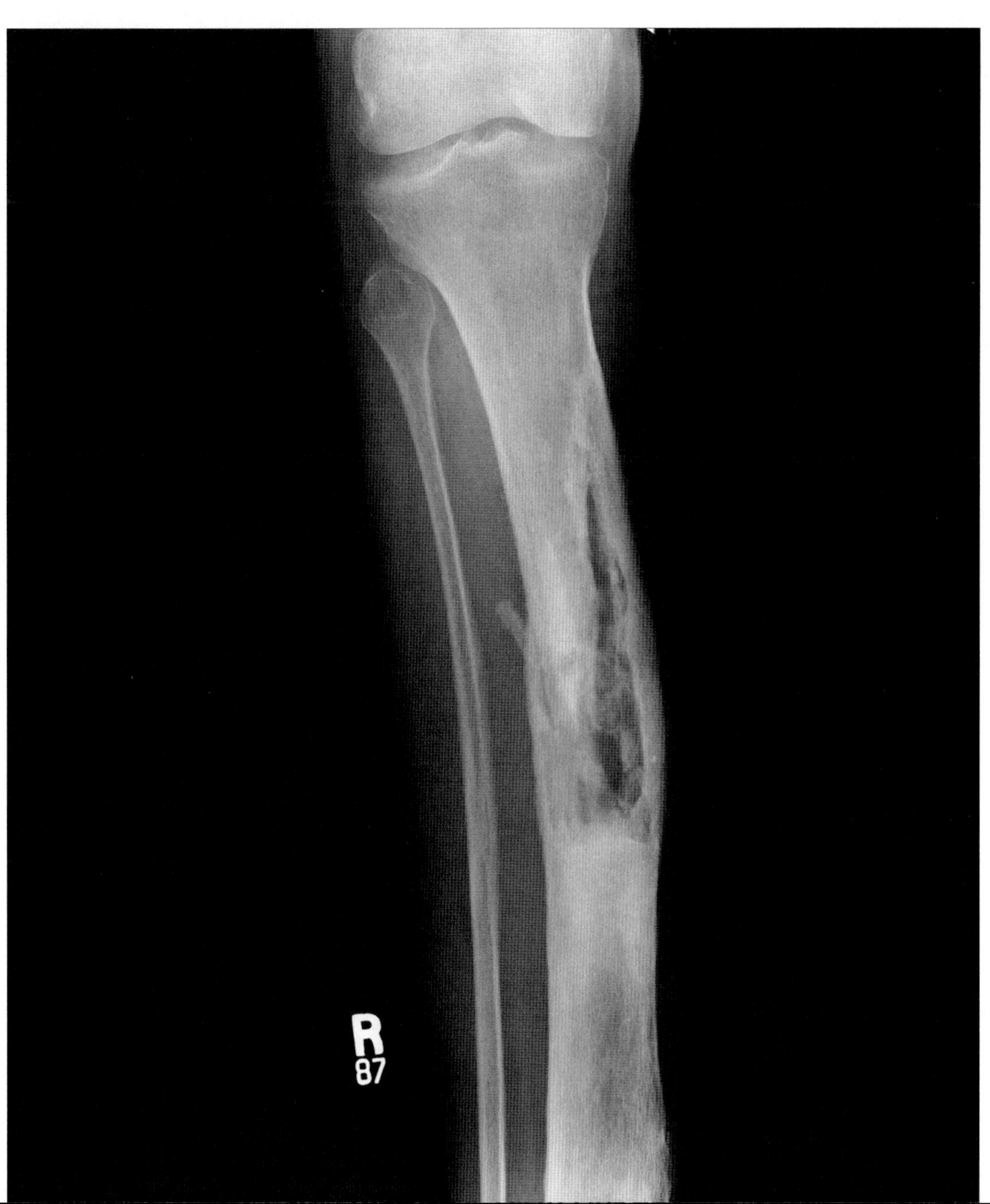

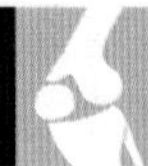

26–1 Chronic Osteomyellitis of Tibia

Michael A. Bruno

PRESENTATION

Long-standing, mild pain, and purulent drainage

FINDINGS

Radiographs show a well-circumscribed, expansile medullary lucency with irregular inclusions and some "onionskin" bony remodeling. CT scan shows characteristic draining sinus and involucrum. Nuclear bone scan and labeled WBC study are both positive, confirming the diagnosis.

DIFFERENTIAL DIAGNOSES

- *Eosinophilic granuloma:* This is a common cause of osteolytic lesion in children. The diagnosis is especially strong if multiple sites are noted.
- *Chondrosarcoma:* This can sometimes mimic, chronic osteomyelitis especially if occurs in the long bones.
- *Ewing sarcoma:* Aggressive, multilayered, and periosteal new bone and adjacent soft tissue mass can masquerade osteomyelitis.

COMMENTS

This patient presented with chronic pain and purulent drainage. Initial radiographs were highly suggestive of chronic osteomyelitis, with an expansile onion skin pattern of bony remodeling. CT scan was confirmatory of this diagnosis, with visualization of a draining sinus from the medullary cavity to the skin surface, and CT scan also reveals a circumferential bony involucrum within the medullary cavity. A three-phase nuclear bone scan was then performed in conjunction with a nuclear radiolabeled WBC scan. Since these utilize different radioisotope tracers, it is possible to simultaneously acquire both images simultaneously, and coregister or "map" the WBC images onto the bone scan images. In this case, the bone scan and the WBC scan were both positive, indicating active infection. The WBC activity primarily maps to the medullary space, where the active infection lies, and the bone scan primarily maps to the cortical periphery, where most of the bony remodeling is taking place. Within the most commonly used classification (Roberts), this case would be a type IV (in the Roberts classification, six subtypes of chronic osteomyelitis are described: Type I is solitary and can mimic eosinophilic granuloma, type II is metaphyseal and can mimic osteogenic sarcoma, type III is diaphyseal and periosteal and can mimic osteoid osteoma, type IV is diaphyseal and can demonstrate onion-skinning bony remodeling, mimicking Ewing sarcoma, type V occur in the epiphysis and can show concentric radioloucency, and type VI occur in the vertebral body).

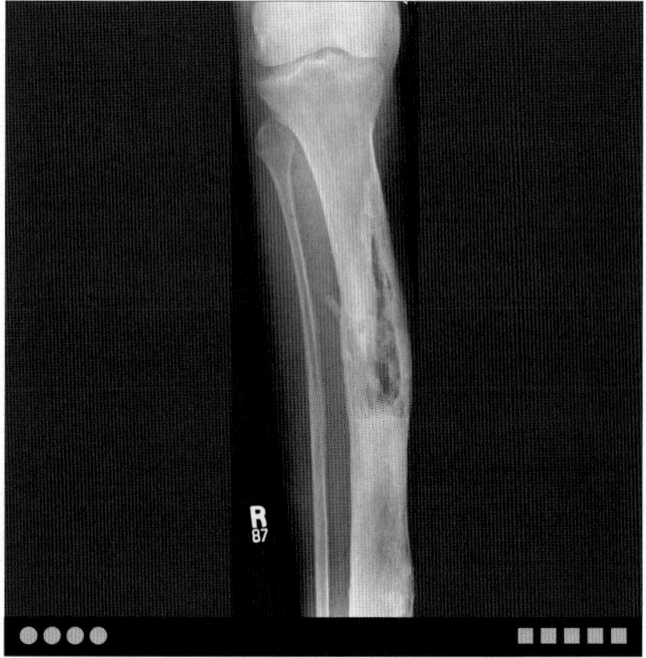

A. Chronic osteomyelitis: AP radiograph of tibia/fibula showing large, expansile, and diaphyseal lesion with onionskin bony remodeling and an irregular central lucency.

PEARLS

- **Low-grade pyogenic abscess of bone.**
- **Subacute or chronic infection.**
- **Usually the infectious agent is *Staphylococcus aureus* (60% of cases). Also *Streptococcus*, *Pseudomonas aeruginosa* (especially in IV drug-abusing patients), and *Haemophilus influenzae*.**
- **Bones with chronic osteomyelitis may contain involucrum (periosteal new bone), sequestrum (dead necrotic bone), and cloaca (fistulous tract).**

ADDITIONAL IMAGES

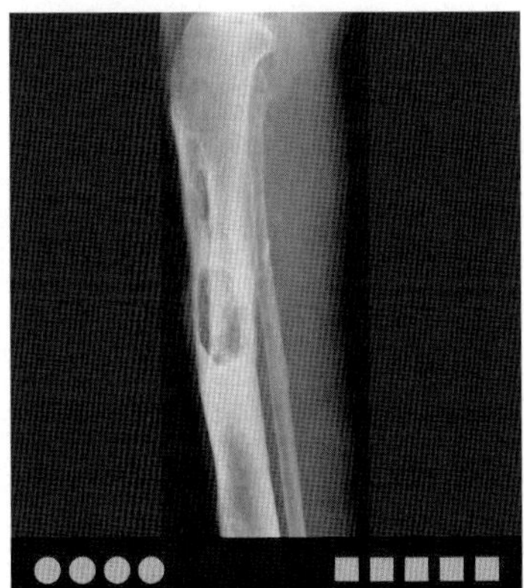

B. Chronic osteomyelitis: Lateral radiograph seen in the same patient.

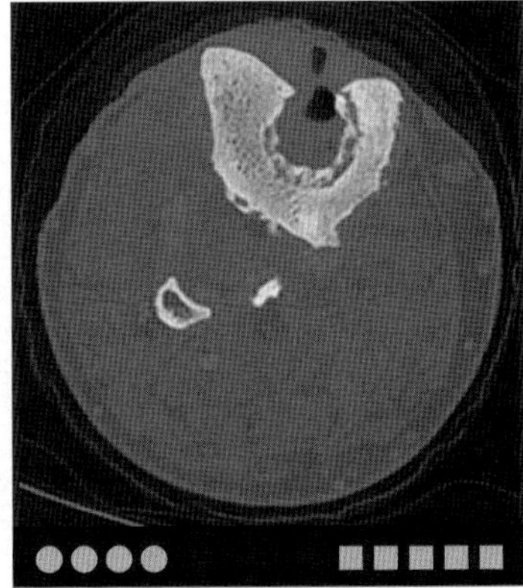

C. Chronic osteomyelitis: CT scan of same patient through the lesion showing open drainage pathway (wide mouthed sinus) from the medullary space.

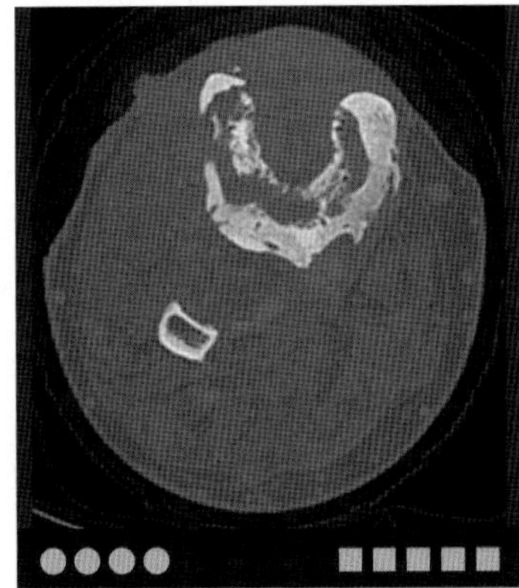

D. Chronic osteomyelitis: Another axial CT scan showing the bony involucrum within the medullary cavity.

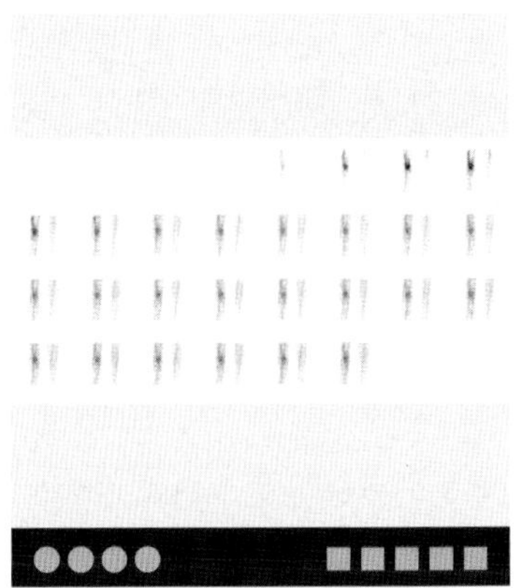

E. Chronic osteomyelitis: Nuclear bone scan, flow images, with positive early uptake of tracer in the region of the abscess.

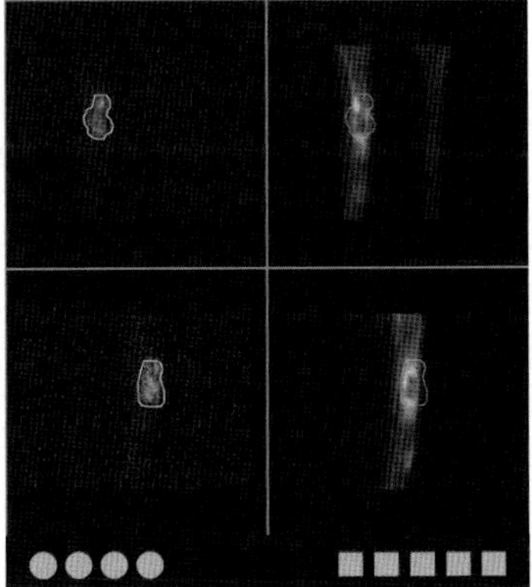

F. Chronic osteomyelitis: Coregistration of delayed images of nuclear bone scan and WBC images, as discussed in the comments section.

IMAGE KEY

Common

Rare

Typical

Unusual

DIFFERENTIAL DIAGNOSIS IMAGE

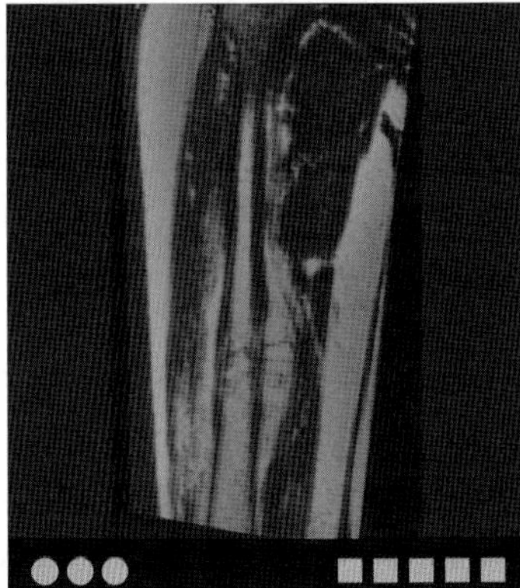

G. Ewing sarcoma: Coronal T2-weighted image shows midshaft femoral lesion with periosteal new bone and bright soft tissue mass.

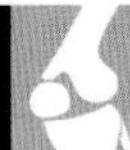

26–2 Lyme Arthritis

Sandra Leigh Moore

PRESENTATION

Knee pain and swelling

FINDINGS

MRI demonstrates joint effusion, synovial thickening, early erosions, and posterolateral synovial involvement.

DIFFERENTIAL DIAGNOSES

- *Rheumatoid arthritis(RA):* Presents with synovial thickening and inflammation and results in symmetrical joint narrowing and finally bone erosion. Small joints of hand and wrist are often involved.
- *Septic arthritis:* Rapid course of joint inflammation which leads to irregular joint destruction.
- *Tuberculous arthritis:* Chronic pain leading to osteoporosis, erosion in nonweight bearing margins of the joint, and finally kissing sequestra may appear.

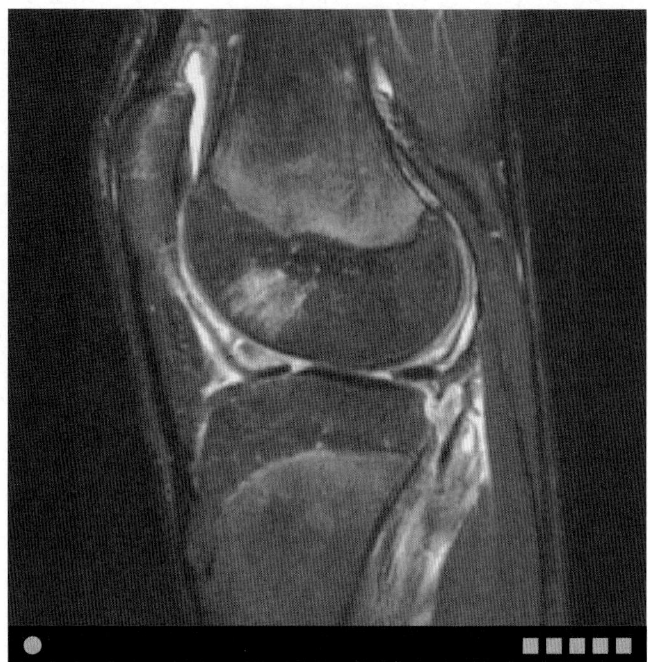

A. Lyme arthritis: Adolescent male; with a history of tick bite. Sagittal intermediate density fat-saturated image shows joint effusion, synovial thickening, early trochlea erosion, and posterolateral involvement of subpopliteus bursa and popliteus tendon sheath.

COMMENTS

This is an image of a adolescent male who presented with knee pain and swelling, and a history of a tick bite. Ticks can transmit bacterial, viral, and/or protozoal infections to humans. Lyme disease is the most frequent tick transmitted illness, and the most frequent vector disease in the United States. Lyme borreliosis, caused by the spirochete Borrelia burgdorferi is transmitted to humans in the saliva of the *ixodes scapularis* tick. The clinical manifestations include rash, chills, fever, constitutional and neurological signs, large joint swelling, and arthritis. Large joint inflammatory oligoarthritis (knee most common) in endemic areas should arouse suspicion of Lyme disease. Diagnosis is based on known exposure and characteristic clinical features, but outside endemic areas may be overlooked. Often the clinical presumption is of juvenile rheumatoid arthritis, or less likely pyogenic arthritis. Serologic tests (ELISA and Western Blot) do not always confirm or exclude Lyme disease. MRI may be ordered to evaluate response to treatment or in clinically challenging cases. MRI of Lyme arthritis demonstrates findings in common with rheumatoid arthritis and pyogenic septic arthritis including bare area erosions, marrow edema, and synovial proliferation. No large MR series of patients with Lyme arthritis have been performed, but in small comparative series, septic arthritis characteristically shows more subcutaneous edema than Lyme disease on MRI. Striking popliteus fossa lymphadenopathy and posterior lateral synovial involvement may be helpful in distinguishing Lyme from rheumatoid arthritis.

PEARLS

- **Large joint inflammatory oligoarthritis in endemic areas should raise consideration of Lyme disease.**
- **Although there are no pathognomonic imaging findings, on MR images: a paucity of subcutaneous edema, the presence of prominent popliteal fossa nodes, and posterolateral synovial involvement are suggestive of Lyme arthritis.**

ADDITIONAL IMAGES

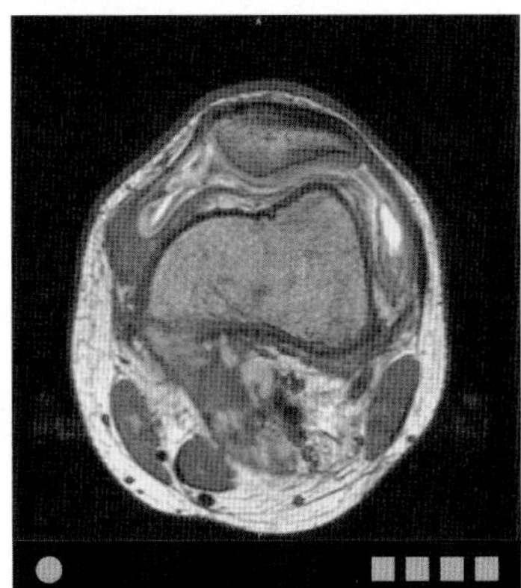

B. Lyme arthritis: Adolescent male; living in endemic area; serology positive. Axial T1-weighted image shows synovial thickening.

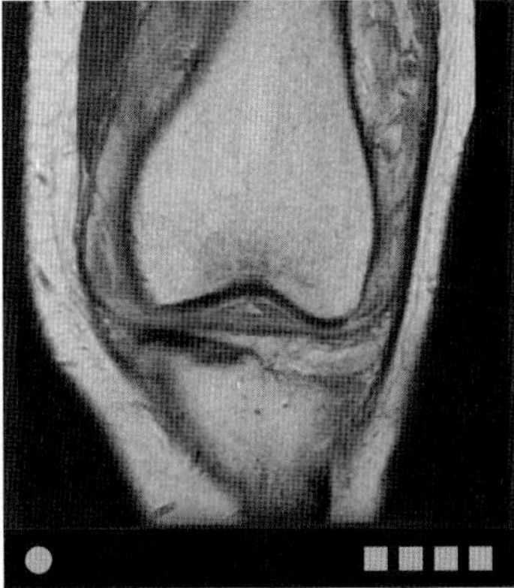

C. Lyme arthritis: Adolescent female; living in endemic area; a history of tick bites. Coronal T1-weighted image shows synovitis, joint effusion, and myriad rice bodies.

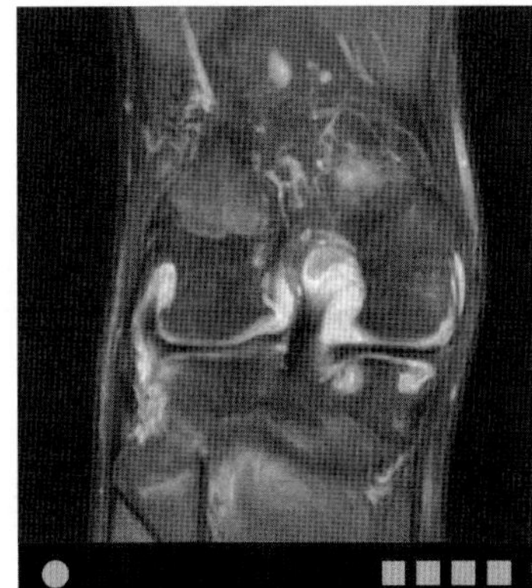

D. Lyme arthritis: Adolescent male living in endemic area; a history of tick bite: Coronal intermediate density fat-saturated image shows a joint effusion, synovial thickening, and marginal erosions.

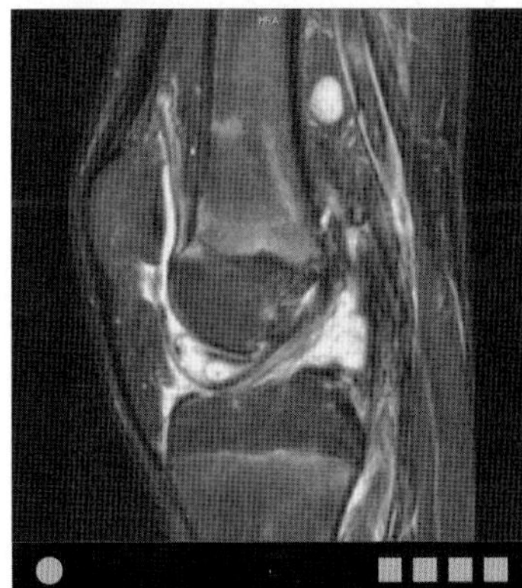

E. Lyme arthritis: Adolescent male living in endemic area with positive serology. Sagittal intermediate density fat-saturated image shows synovitis and popliteal fossa node.

IMAGE KEY

Common

Rare

Typical

Unusual

DIFFERENTIAL DIAGNOSES IMAGES

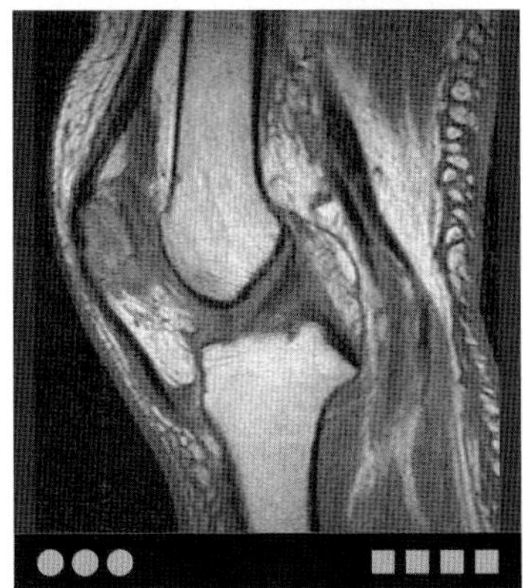

F. Tuberculous arthritis: Middle-aged female with atypical mycobacterium infection: Osteomyelitis of the patella. Subcutaneous edema is a differentiating point from Lyme arthritis.

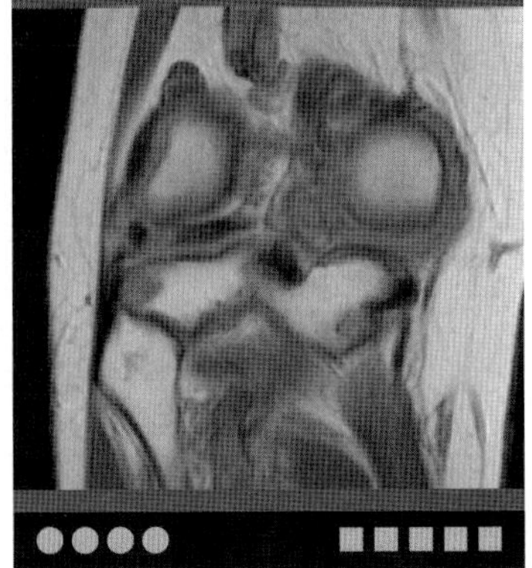

G. Rheumatoid arthritis: Middle-aged female with RA: Synovitis and marginal erosions are common to Lyme arthritis and RA.

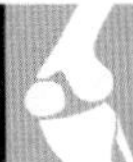

26–3 Prepatellar Abscess

Melitus Maryam Golshan and Jamshid Tehranzadeh

PRESENTATION

Knee pain, swelling, and fever

FINDINGS

MR imaging shows well-defined cystic lesions in prepatellar area with low signal intensity on T1 and high signal intensity on T2-weighted images. Note marked enhancement of the abscess wall.

DIFFERENTIAL DIAGNOSES

- *Prepatellar bursitis:* Shows bright fluid collection on T2-weighted image in the prepatellar bursa without a thick wall.
- *Hematoma:* Subacute hematoma: shows a bright signal in both T1- and T2-weighted images because of high level of methemoglobin. Old hematoma shows low signal on T2 images because of the presence of hemosiderin and ferritin.
- *Soft tissue infections (cellulitis, phlegmon, and fasciitis):* These lesions are not well-defined and do not have an enhancing capsule.

COMMENTS

The patient is a 3-year-old girl who presented with a history of knee pain, swelling, tenderness, and low-grade fever after falling on the gravel and developing skin ulcer 3 days later. Most bacterial infections (predominantly Staphylococcus aureus) in the soft tissues remain localized and commence as cellulitis. These infections can extend and develop into an abscess depending on the immunologic status of the patient. Common causes of soft tissue abscesses include penetrating trauma, iatrogenic interventions, spreading from contagious infection, and septic emboli. The radiographic findings are similar to cellulitis with soft tissue swelling and loss of fascial planes. Abscess formation cannot always be diagnosed clinically and ultrasound (US) may be useful. US typically demonstrates a focal anechoic mass within a region of cellulits. However, the fluid may appear hyper or isoechoic within the surrounding inflamed area. CT scan or MRI with intravenous contrast enhancement may also be used to demonstrate the extent of the lesion and differentiate between cellulitis and abscess. An abscess is seen as a necrotic center with ring enhancement and surrounding edema. The finding of gas (on any imaging modality) within a mass suspected of being infective is characteristic of an abscess. MR imaging will show a well-demarcated fluid collection that is hypointense on T1-weighted image and hyperintense on T2-weighted image. The abscess is surrounded by a low signal intensity pseudocapsule in all sequences, and demonstrates a peripheral rim enhancement after intravenous administration of Gadolinium contrast. These features are useful in differentiating abscesses from cellulitis or fasciitis.

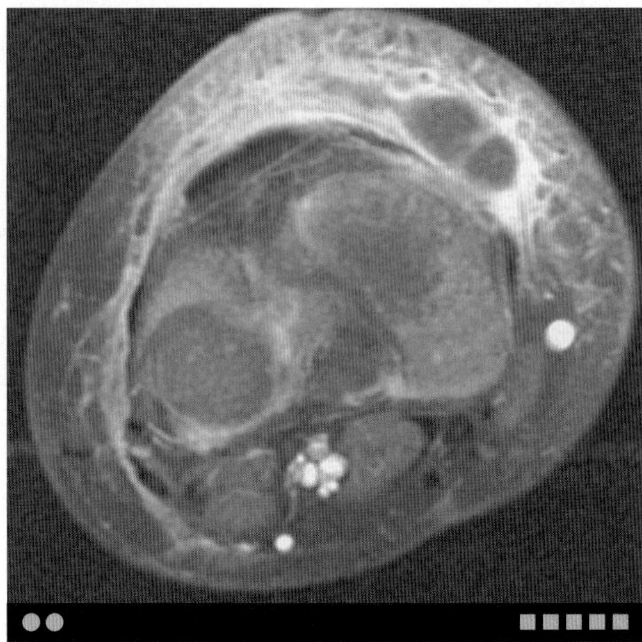

A. Prepatellar abscess: Axial postcontrast fat-saturated T1-weighted image shows loculated abscess with peripheral wall enhancement and adjacent cellulitis.

PEARLS

- **Most bacterial infections of soft tissue are localized as cellulitis, but they may progress to abscess which presents as unspecific soft tissue swelling in radiography and hypoechoic mass within region of cellulitis in US.**
- **CT scan and MRI with intravenous contrast show peripheral ring enhancement in abscesses and demonstrate peripheral cellulitis.**
- **Soft tissue abscess is hypointense on T1 and hyperintense on T2-weighted images with peripheral low signal fibrous capsule in all sequences, which enhances after contrast administration.**

ADDITIONAL IMAGES

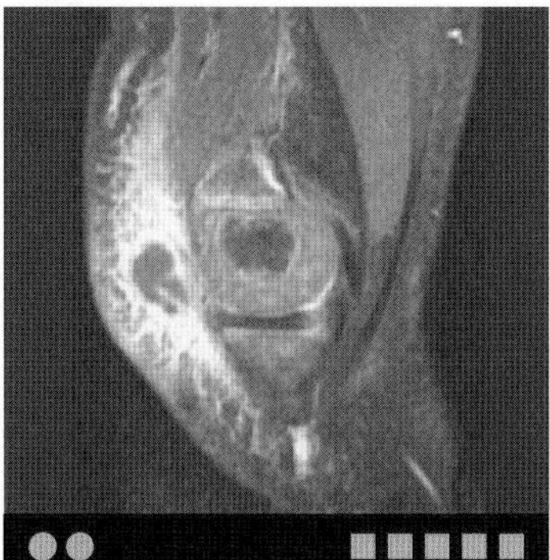

B. Prepatellar abscess: Sagittal postcontrast fat-saturated T1-weighted image shows lobulated low signal intensity abscess in prepatellar region with peripheral rim enhancement. Note soft tissue enhancement and edema surrounding the abscess.

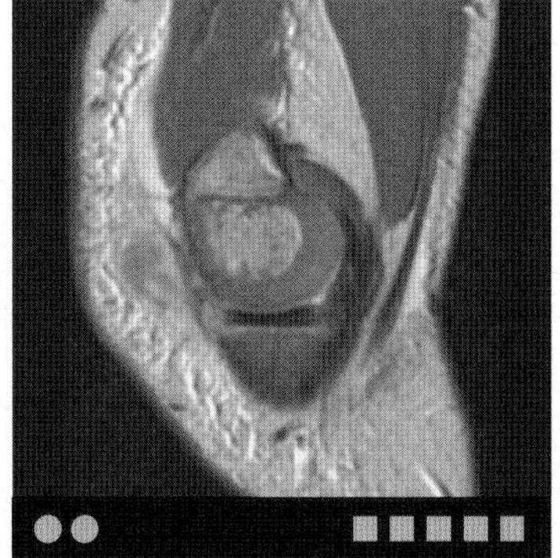

C. Prepatellar abscess: Sagittal proton density MR image shows the loculated abscess with central intermediate signal intensity (SI). Note peripheral soft tissue edema with high SI and swelling in prepatellar area.

DIFFERENTIAL DIAGNOSES IMAGES

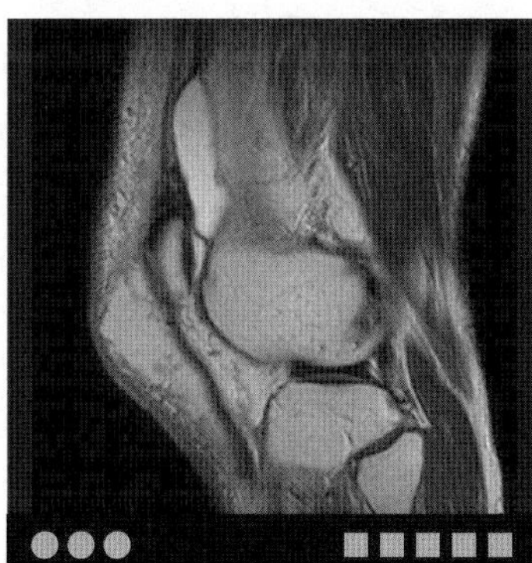

D. Prepatellar bursitis: Sagittal T2-weighted image shows an oval shape collection of fluid in front of patellar tendon representing bursitis.

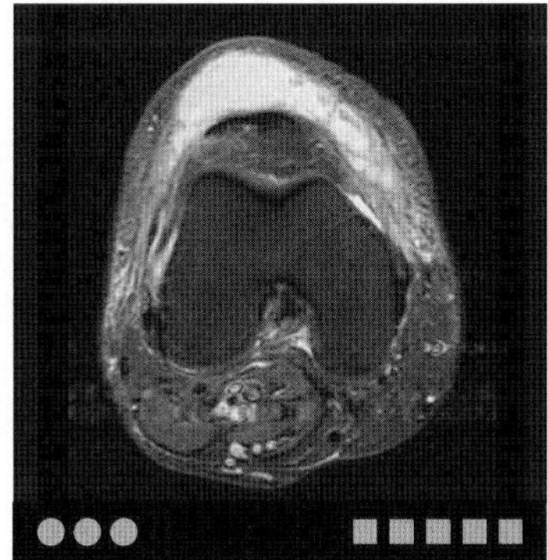

E. Prepatellar bursitis: Axial fat-saturated T2-weighted image shows fluid-filled bursa in prepatellar region.

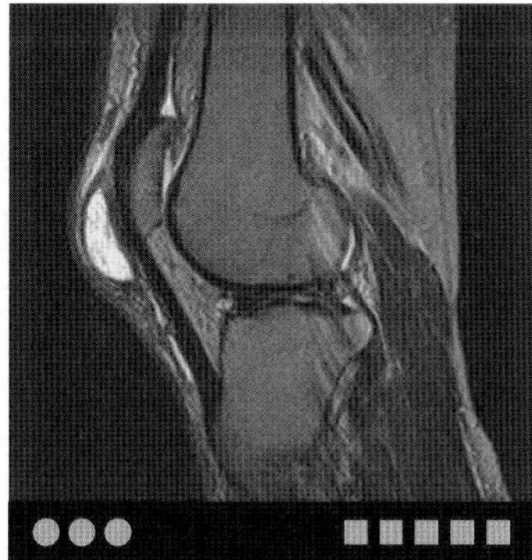

F. Prepatellar subacute hematoma: Sagittal proton density image shows a well-defined, oval shape high SI collection in prepatellar region.

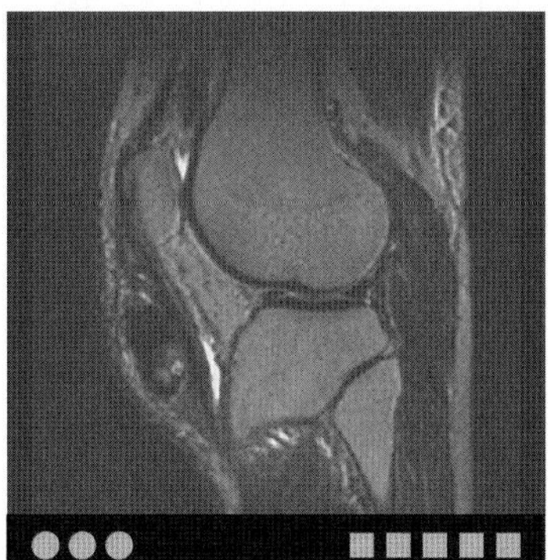

G. Prepatellar old hematoma: Sagittal proton density image shows a low SI oval mass with some foci of bright signals in it in prepatellar region representing an old hematoma in a 25-year-old man with hemophilia.

IMAGE KEY

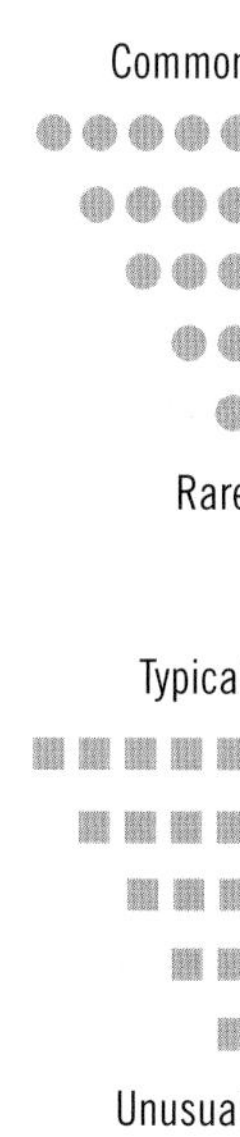

Chapter 27

Tumors and Tumor Like Lesions

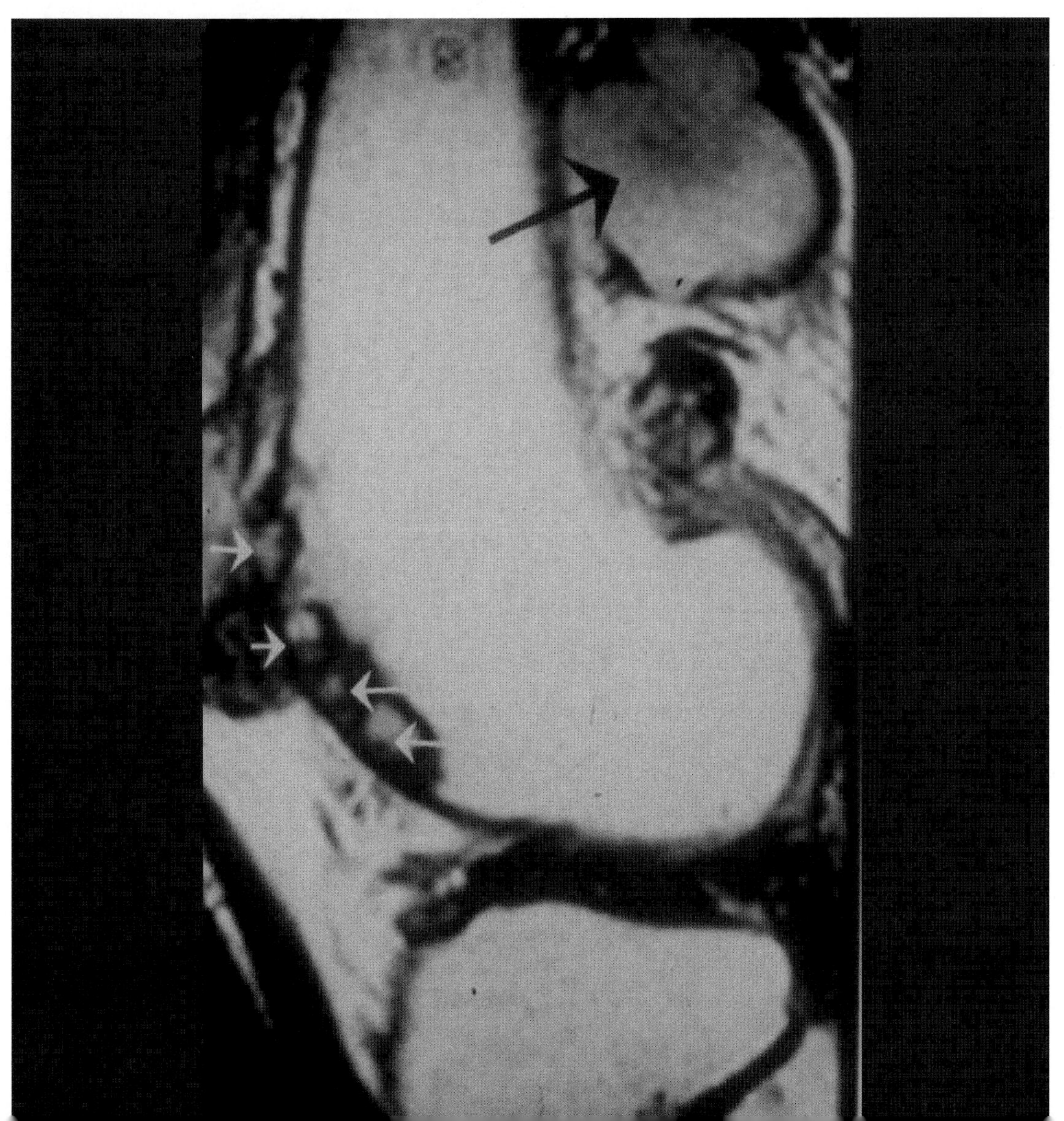

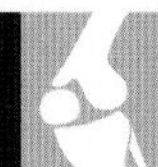

27–1 Soft Tissue Amyloidoma of the Knee

George Hermann

PRESENTATION

Knee pain

FINDINGS

MRI shows a large soft tissue mass (large arrow) above the popliteal fossa; erosions of femoral condyle and patella are noted (small arrows).

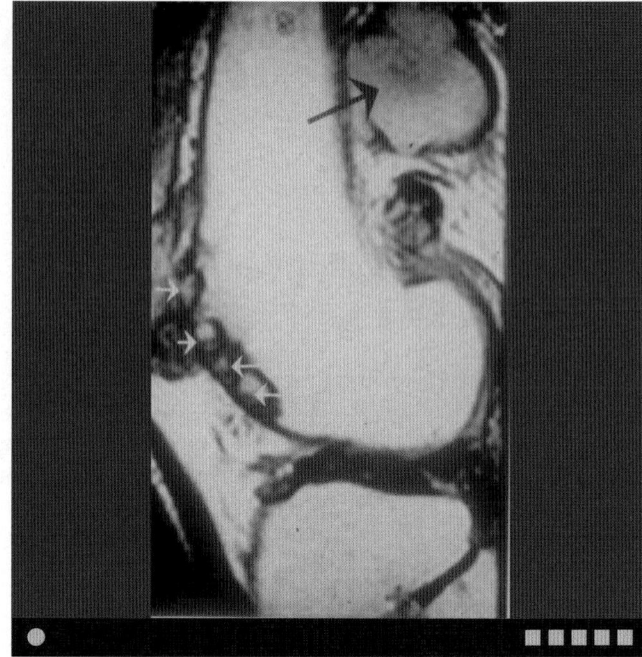

A. Soft tissue amyloidoma: Sagittal T1-weighted image demonstrates a well-defined mass behind the distal femur (large arrow). Note erosion of the femoral condyle and the patella (small arrows).

DIFFERENTIAL DIAGNOSES

- *Lipoma:* This shows increased SI on T1-weighted image isointense to subcutaneous fat.
- *Liposarcoma:* This shows scattered decreased SI on T1-weighted image and appears heterogeneous. Occasionally, it is difficult to differentiate from lipoma.
- *Malignant fibrous histiocytoma (MFH):* This tumor usually presents as a high SI lobulated mass on T2-weighted image with low SI septae separating the lobules.
- *Neurofibroma:* This tumor shows high signal on T2-weighted image with a low SI central area known as the "target sign."

COMMENTS

The patient is a 53-year-old woman diagnosed with amyloidoma of the right distal thigh. She had been treated with hemodialysis for 16 years. Deposition of dialysis-related amyloid in joints and soft tissue is a known complication of long-term hemodialysis. B_2 microglobulin amyloidosis (AB_2 m) is dialysis related and occurs exclusively in patients undergoing long-term hemodialysis (5–10 years or longer). B_2 microglobulin is a protein that normally is present in the blood, filtered by the glomerulus and reabsorbed by the proximal tubules. The blood level is increased 40 to 50 times in renal failure. Amyloidosis predominantly involves the musculoskeletal system. The clinical manifestations include carpal tunnel syndrome, arthropathy as a result of the deposition of amyloid in the synovial membrane, and bone around the joints. Amyloidoma may occur in the brain, nasopharynx, spleen, or adrenal glands in primary amyloidosis. Amyloid deposits in hemodialysis patients are usually concentrated in joints, most often in the knee. In these instances it may be the result of chronic inflammation of the synovium. MRI usually shows decreased SI on both T1 and T2-weighted image. There is no clear explanation of the reason for signal loss on T2-weighted image. Decreased proton density as a result of unusual protein configuration may contribute to the T2 signal loss. It might be that the densely packed B structure excludes water.

PEARLS

- **Amyloid deposition in the soft tissue is a relatively uncommon complication of chronic hemodialysis**
- **Bony erosions are common manifestation of amyloidosis**
- **Soft tissue mass usually surrounds the involved joint**
- **MRI demonstrates decreased SI both on T1- and T2-weighted images**

ADDITIONAL IMAGES

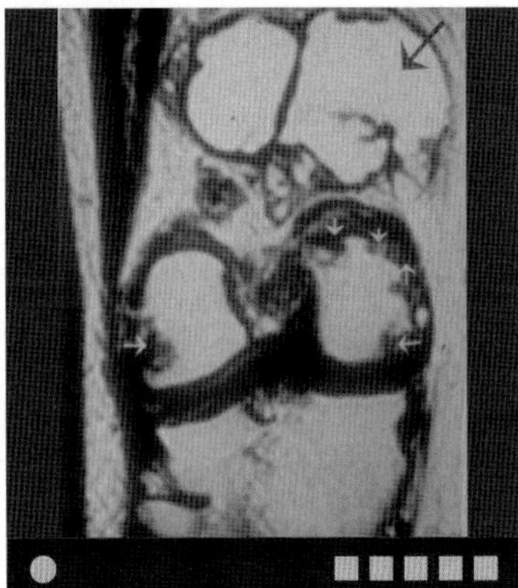

B. Soft tissue amyloidoma: Coronal T2-weighted image shows slightly increased SI (large arrow). Note femoral condyle erosions (small arrows).

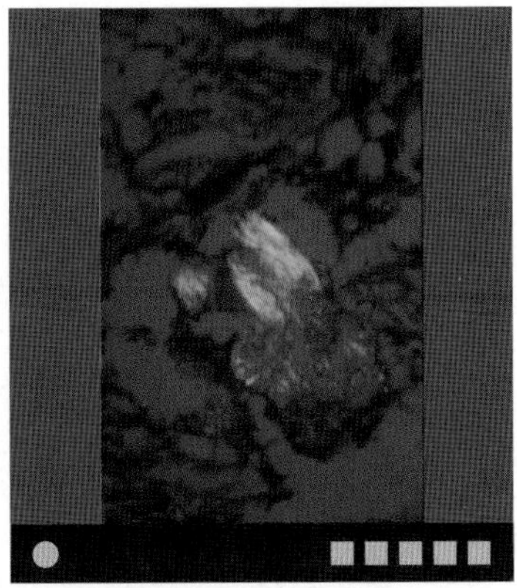

C. Soft tissue amyloidoma: Congo red stain of the tumor shows apple-green birefringence, which is diagnostic of amyloid crystals.

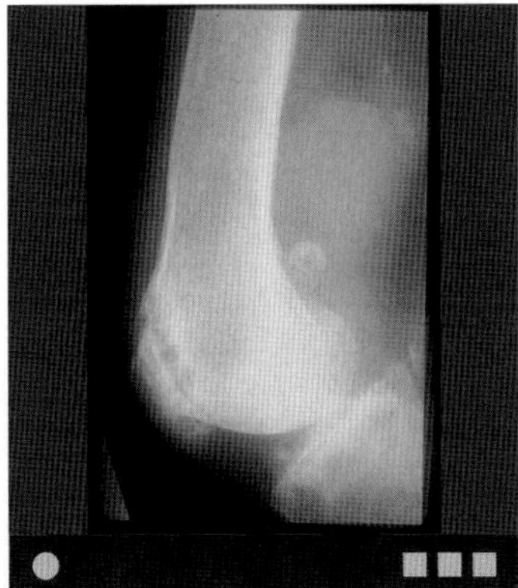

D. Soft tissue amyloidoma: Lateral radiograph of the knee reveals a large soft tissue mass above the popliteal fossa with femoropatellar erosions.

IMAGE KEY

Common

Rare

Typical

Unusual

DIFFERENTIAL DIAGNOSES IMAGES

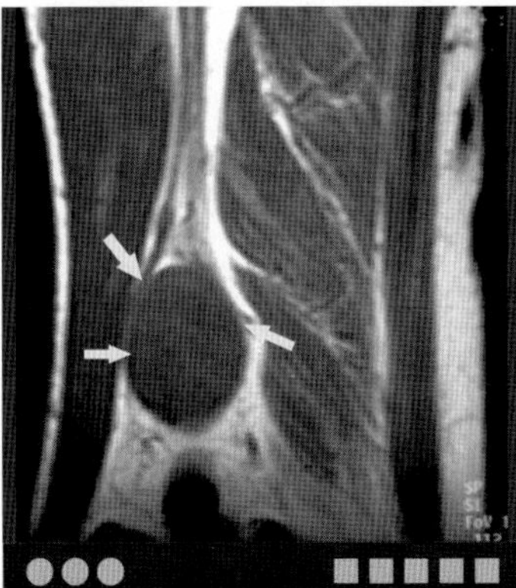

E. Neurofibroma: Sagittal T1-weighted image reveals a decreased SI mass (arrows) behind the distal femur.

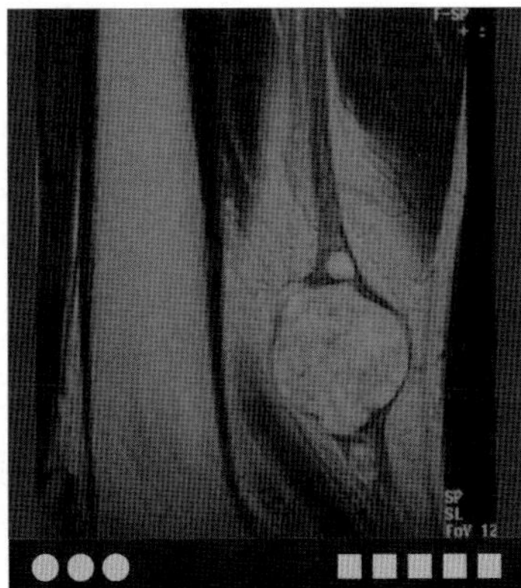

F. Neurofibroma: Sagittal T2-weighted image reveals a relatively low SI at the central region surrounded by a high signal periphery. Note that the mass is connected with the nerve root.

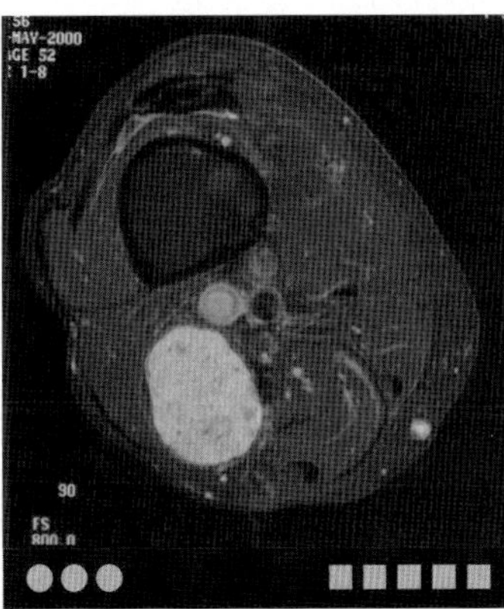

G. Neurofibroma: Axial STIR images reveal the "target sign." The center of the mass shows decreased SI surrounded with a bright SI rim.

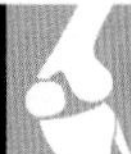

27–2 Lipoma Arborescens of Knee

Sulabha Masih

PRESENTATION

Right knee pain

FINDINGS

MR imaging shows a large, villous, frond-like intra-articular fat intensity mass associated with joint effusion.

DIIFERENTIAL DIAGNOSES

- *Pigmented villonodular synovitis (PVNS):* On MRI, this lesion shows mass-like lesions of synovial proliferation with foci of low signal intensity hemosiderin on T1- and T2-weighted images.
- *Synovial hemangioma:* Intra-articular vascular mass with villonodular filling defects. It is commonly associated with cutaneous and deep soft tissue hemangiomas.
- *Synovial lipoma:* Occurs exclusively in the knee with round to oval masses of fat in the joint.
- *Lipohemarthrosis:* This is usually secondary to trauma with fat–fluid level on CT and MRI.

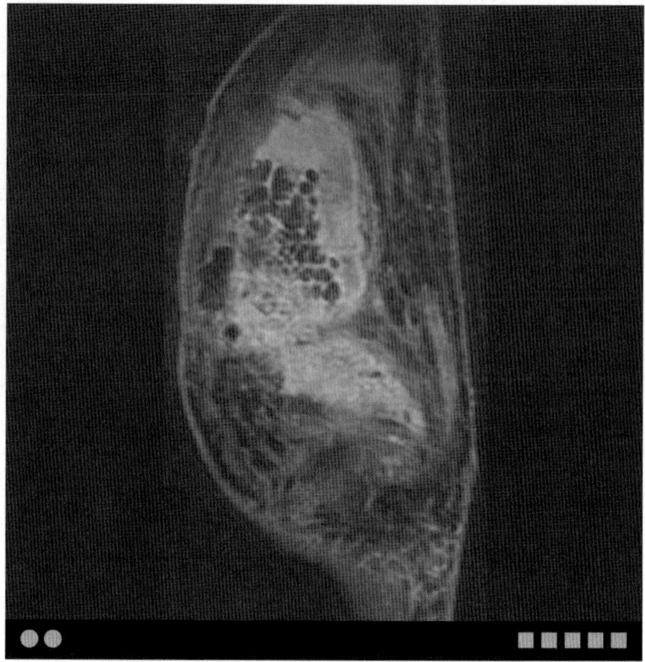

A. Lipoma arborescens: Sagittal STIR image demonstrates fat-suppressed low signal frond-like villous fat inside the synovial fluid.

COMMENTS

The patient is a 70-year-old man with right knee pain. Lipoma arborescence is a benign, rare, intra-articular lesion, characterized by replacement of synovial tissues by fatty proliferation. Frond-like villous arborization of the fat, appropriately names this entity, as lipoma arboresence. Lipoma arborescence may be painless, but is often symptomatic with pain and joint effusion. Clinical course often shows intermittent exacerbations with extensive effusion lasting for several days because of trapped hypertrophic villi between the joint surfaces. Even though, the most common location is knee, shoulder and hips are occasionally involved. Hypertrophic synovial villi are distended with fat. Even though the etiology is unknown, it usually is a reaction to the chronic synovitis. It is frequently associated with prior trauma, chronic rheumatoid arthritis and degenerative joint disease. It can arise independent of an underlying arthritis. The laboratory findings are usually unremarkable. Radiographs are nonspecific or may demonstrate radiolucency within an effusion. Multiple well-defined defects are noted on arthrography. On CT, low attenuation mass that is consistent with fat is noted outlining the synovial fronds. The lesion is not enhanced after the intravenous contrast injection and helps to differentiate from pigmented villonodular synovitis, which shows contrast enhancement and is of high attenuation. The appearance of lipoma arborescence on magnetic resonance imaging is pathognomonic. On MR imaging, definite frond-like, villous, arborizing pattern of fat with high signal intensity on T1-weighted and low signal intensity on fat-suppressed images is noted within the hypertrophied high signal intensity synovial fluid on T2 and STIR weighted images.

PEARLS

- **Hypertrophied synovium is distended with frond-like villous fat**
- **Frequently associated with prior trauma, chronic rheumatoid arthritis, and degenerative joint disease**
- **On MR, high signal intensity synoval fluid on T2-weighted and STIR weighted images, with intra-articular frond-like villi of fat with high signal intensity on T1-weighted image and low signal intensity on fat-suppressed images is characteristic findings.**

ADDITIONAL IMAGES

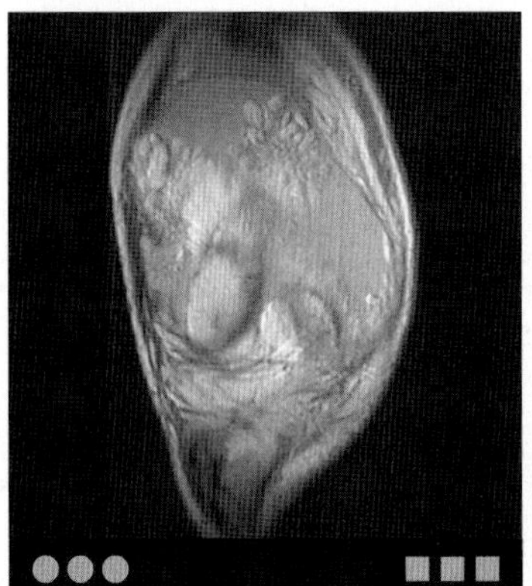

B. Lipoma arborescens: Coronal T1-weighted image shows high signal intensity arborizing fat.

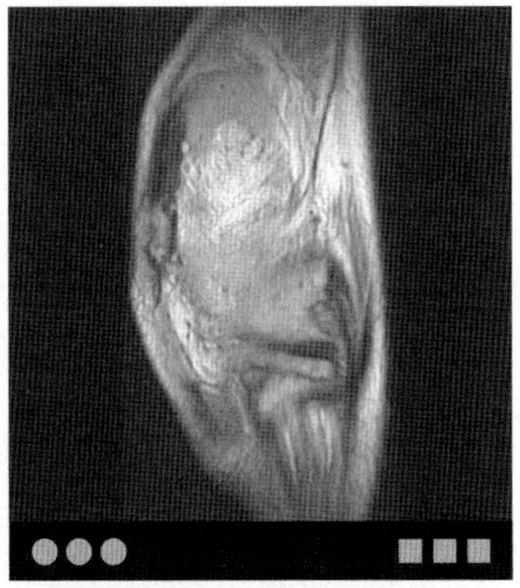

C. Lipoma arborescens: Sagittal proton density image of the knee shows frond-like intra-articular fat intensity mass.

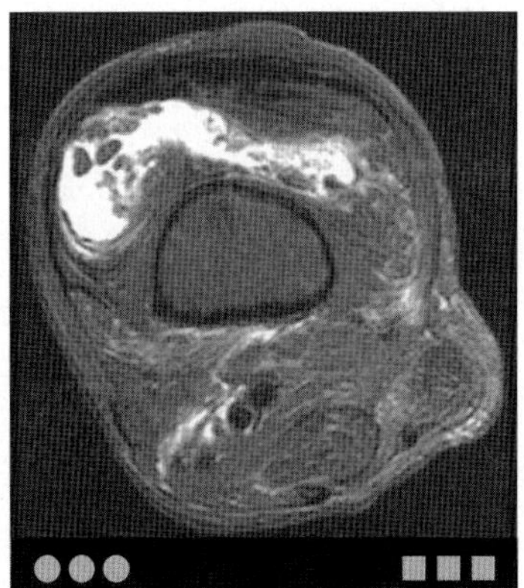

D. Lipoma arborescens: Axial STIR shows multiple fat-suppressed low signal intensities inside the high signal synovial fluid.

DIFFERENTIAL DIAGNOSES IMAGES

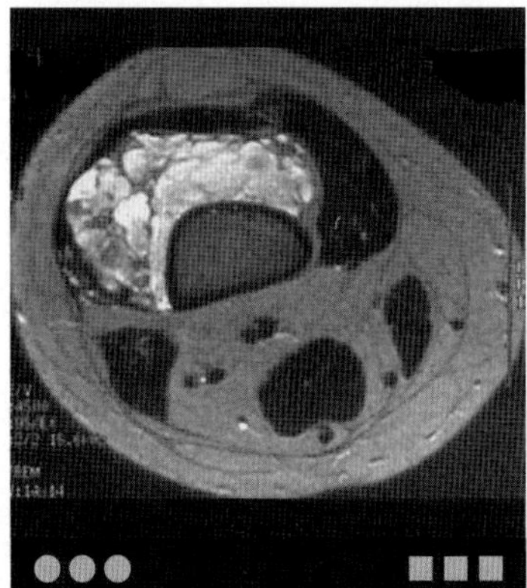

E. Synovial hemangioma: Axial T2-weighted image shows inhomogeneous intra-articular high signal intensity lesion.

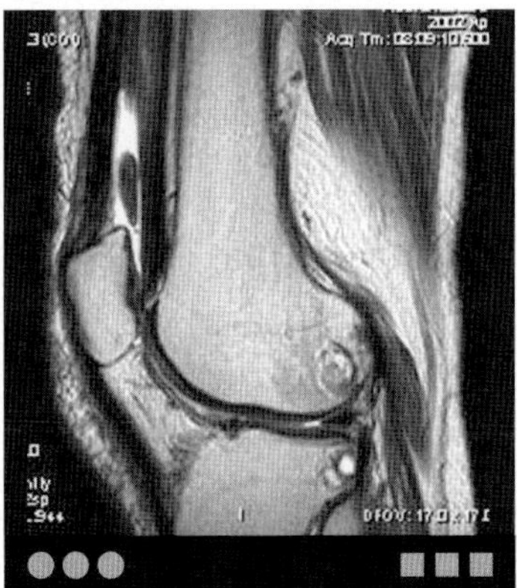

F. PVNS: Sagittal T2-weighted image shows low signal intensity hemosiderine inside the joint fluid.

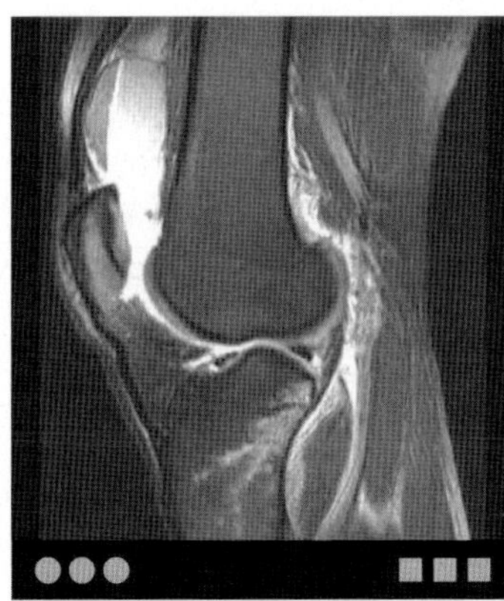

G. Lipohemarthrosis: Sagittal fat-saturated proton density image shows fat-fluid level.

IMAGE KEY

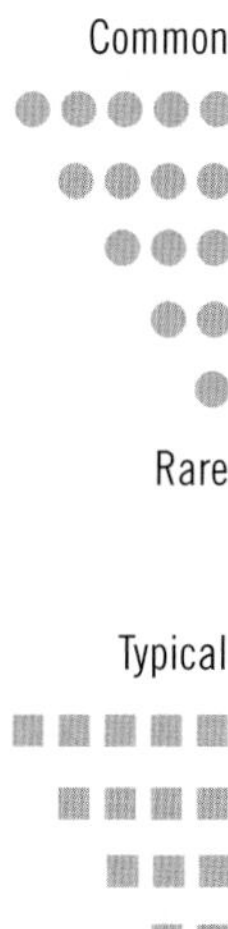

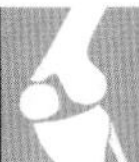

27–3 Angiolipoma of the Calf

Alya Sheikh and Rajeev K. Varma

PRESENTATION

Enlarging calf mass

FINDINGS

MRI reveals a mass within the left soleus with considerable fat as well as curvilinear and serpigenous soft tissue structures.

DIFFERENTIAL DIAGNOSES

- *Well-differentiated liposarcoma:* It is difficult to differentiate it from the lipoma variants. It may contain thickened septae (>2 mm), nonlipomatous soft tissue component foci of increased T2-weighted signal, and enhancement.
- *Cavernous hemangioma:* This can be associated with reactive fat overgrowth and fat with serpentine vessels. MRI demonstrates marked increase in T1/T2-weighted signal and enhancement. Angiogram shows tortuous feeding vessels and early draining vein.
- *Lymphangioma:* These are multiloculated cystic lesions with septations that can have fat, but unlikely to have obvious vessels. MRI shows increased T1-weighted and decreased T2-weighted signal, without enhancement.

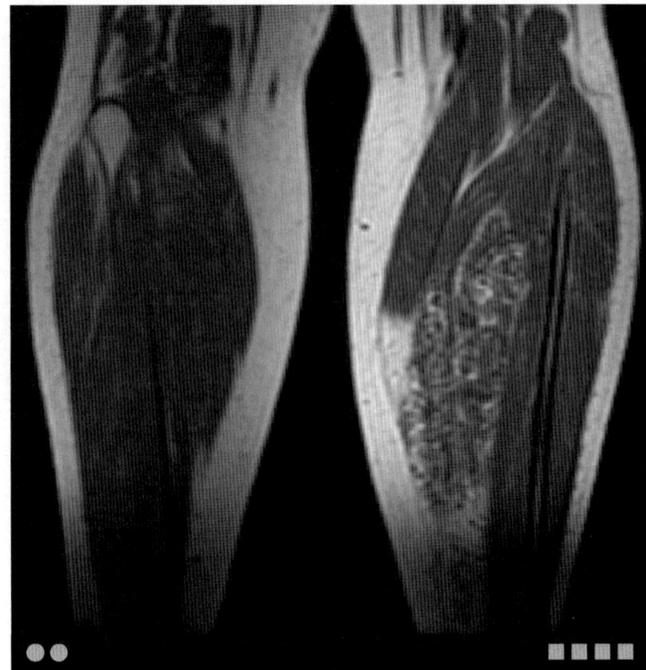

A. Angiomyolipoma: Coronal T1-weighted image shows mass within the left calf with considerable fat as well as curvilinear or serpigenous soft tissue structures likely representing vessels with flood void.

COMMENTS

The patient is a 20-year-old female with a 3 year history of enlarging mass diagnosed as an angiolipoma predominantly of the left soleus muscle. Angiolipoma is also known as hemangiolipoma, angiomyolipoma, vascular lipoma, and fibromyolipoma. This is a rare subset of lipoma variants, which includes entities such as chondroid lipoma, osteolipoma, and hibernoma among others. Histologically, this entity is an encapsulated lipoma with vascular channels which contain intravascular fibrin thrombi. This benign subcutaneous lesion typically occurs in young healthy males in the second and third decades. Usual presentation is that of a subcutaneous mass that is tender on palpation. The most common sites are the extremities, trunk, and neck. Multiple lesions are seen in approximately 70% of the cases. Angiolipomas classically were divided into noninfiltrating and infiltrating types. The former is more common, and is described above. The infiltrating angiolipoma is rare, occurs usually in the extremities, and may infiltrate into bone, muscle, and nerves; however, this is now being considered by the World Health Organization as an intravascular hemangioma. Typically, the noninfiltrating angiolipoma is hyperintense and inhomogeneous on T1-weighted images; the degree of central hypointensity on the T1-weighted study may be reflective of vascularity. There is marked enhancement on the fat-suppressed T1-weighted images. The T2-weighted signal is variable though usually hyperintensity is noted. Surgery is considered curative. Dedifferentiation and local recurrence do not usually occur.

PEARLS

- **It is a rare benign subset of lipoma variants that occurs in young healthy males**
- **It usually is located in extremities, trunk, and neck**
- **Important characteristics include encapsulation, intravascular thrombus, septations, and multiplicity.**
- **Areas of low T1-weighted signal corresponding to regions of increased T2-weighted signal likely represent vascularity.**

ADDITIONAL IMAGES

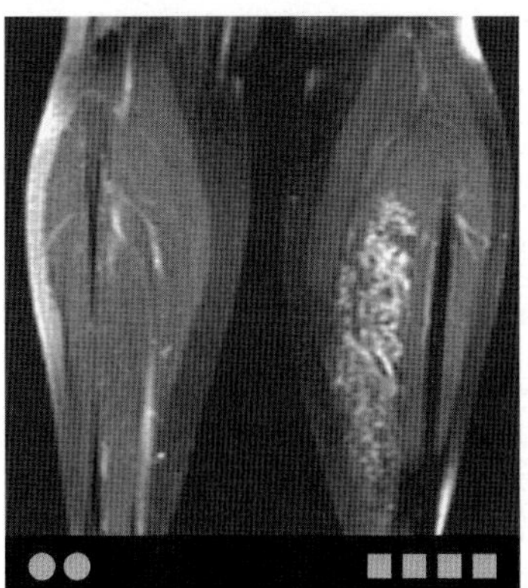

B. Angiomyolipoma: Coronal STIR sequence shows serpigenous increased signal within the mass.

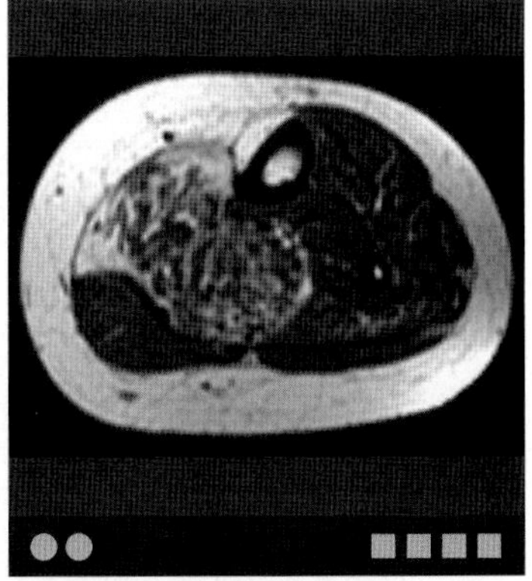

C. Angiomyolipoma: Axial T1-weighted image shows serpigenous increased signal within the mass.

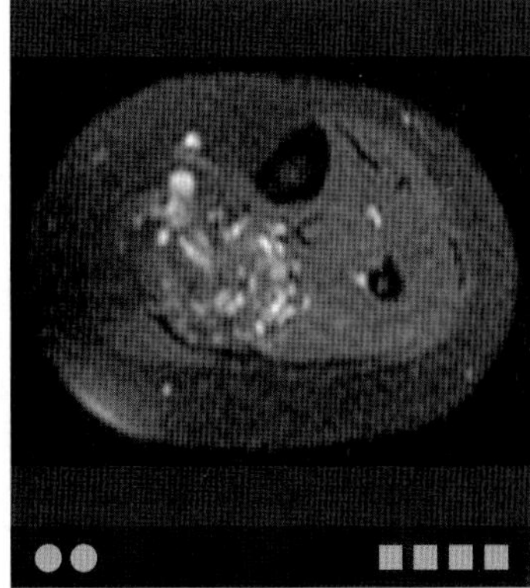

D. Angiomyolipoma: Axial STIR image with increased signal mixed with low signal fat.

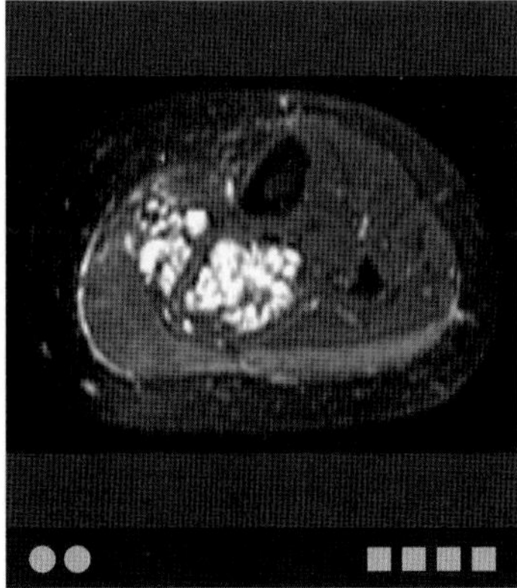

E. Angiomyolipoma: Axial contrast-enhanced T1-weighted image with fat suppression shows increased uptake in the mass with hypointense areas likely representing septations, phleboliths, or vascular components.

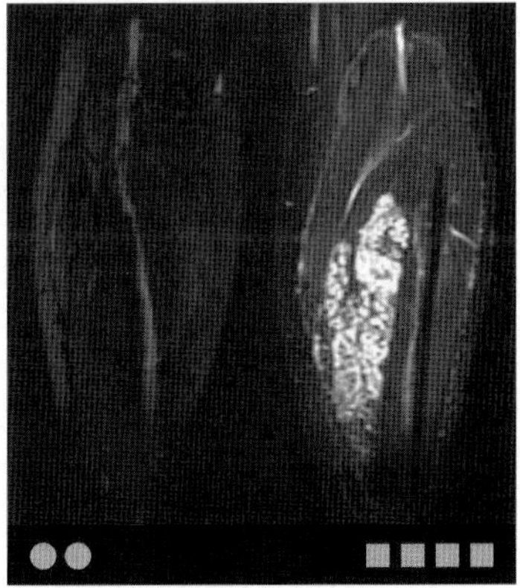

F. Angiomyolipoma: Coronal contrast-enhanced T1-weighted image with fat suppression shows increased uptake in the mass with hypointense areas likely representing septations, phleboliths, or vascular components.

IMAGE KEY

Common

Rare

Typical

Unusual

DIFFERENTIAL DIAGNOSIS IMAGE

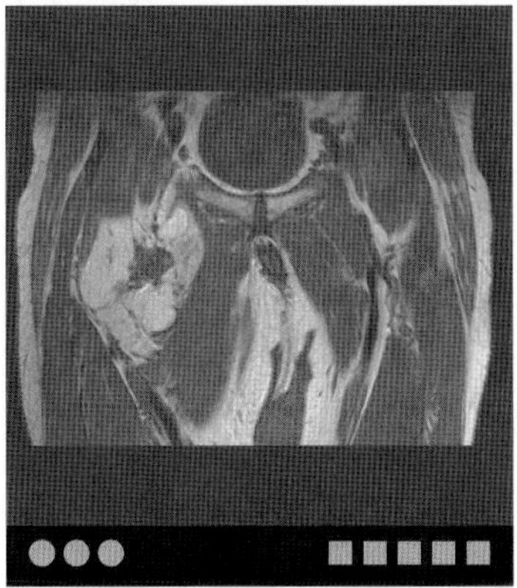

G. Liposarcoma: Coronal T1-weighted image shows a large inhomogeneous fatty mass in the proximal thigh with septations and no defined capsule.

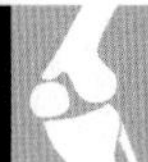

27–4 Periosteal Hemangioma of the Tibia

Kambiz Motamedi

PRESENTATION

Long-standing leg pain

FINDINGS

Radiographs showed a surface lesion of the periosteum with increased thickening. The MRI demonstrates an eccentric lesion of the tibial diaphysis with soft tissue component and high signal tubular channels on fluid-sensitive sequences.

DIFFERENTIAL DIAGNOSES

- *Periostitis ossificans:* CT usually shows mature bone formation along the cortex commonly with mature medullary cavity
- *Surface chondroma:* Cross-sectional imaging shows a chondroid lesion arising from the cortex. CT may reveal a chondroid matrix, whereas MRI would show a lobular high signal (fluid-sensitive sequences) lesion.
- *Surface osteosarcoma:* Radiographs and cross-sectional imaging show a surface lesion with usually osteoid mineralization

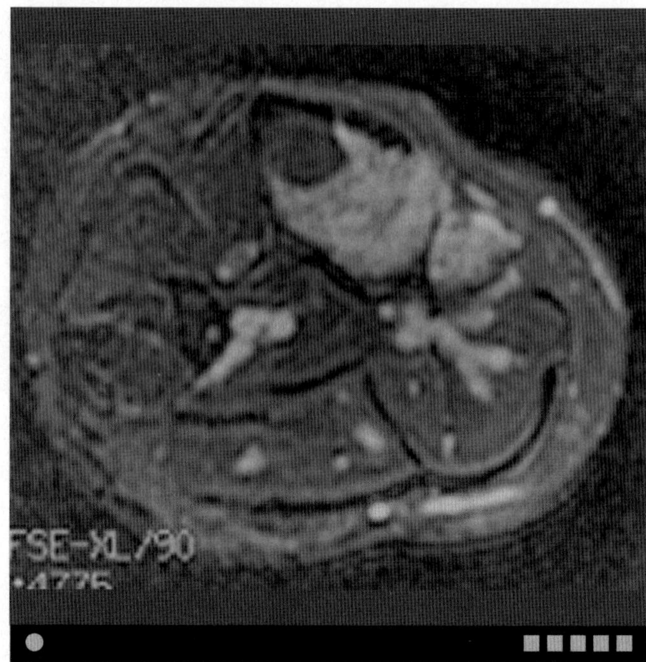

A. Periosteal hemangioma: Axial fat-saturated T2-weighted image shows a cortically based high-signal lesion with a soft tissue component.

COMMENTS

The patient is a 54-year-old female, who presented with a 4-year history of leg pain and palpable tibial mass. Bone hemangiomas are benign, and malformed vascular lesions which overall constituting less than 1% of all primary bone neoplasms. They occur most frequently in the vertebral column and skull (up to 70%), whereas involvement of other sites (including the long bones, short tubular bones, and ribs) is extremely rare. Bone hemangiomas are usually asymptomatic lesions discovered incidentally on imaging or postmortem examination and mostly encountered in the middle aged. The symptoms are largely nonspecific and depend on the site, size, and aggressiveness of the tumors. Bone hemangiomas usually occur in the medullary cavity but uncommonly, surface-based hemangiomas are encountered in the cortex, periosteum, and subperiosteal regions. Radiographic patterns may be nonspecific, necessitating further imaging or histology to achieve diagnosis. Radiographs may not suffice and the diagnosis may remain equivocal. CT is especially helpful to access changes in bone trabeculae, such as increased sclerosis and periosteal thickening. CT in general supports the radiographic findings but provide greater detail. The superior soft tissue and bone marrow contrast resolution of MRI allows for better evaluation of extra osseous extension and depiction of the characteristic fatty content in bone hemangiomas. The multiplanar capabilities of MRI are also crucial in defining the extent of the bone involvement and planning therapeutic interventions.

PEARLS

- **Hemangiomas of the appendicular skeleton are rare**
- **Radiographs and CT may show increased sclerosis with vascular channels**
- **MRI demonstrates the soft tissue component along with the fatty contents and tubular structures**

ADDITIONAL IMAGES

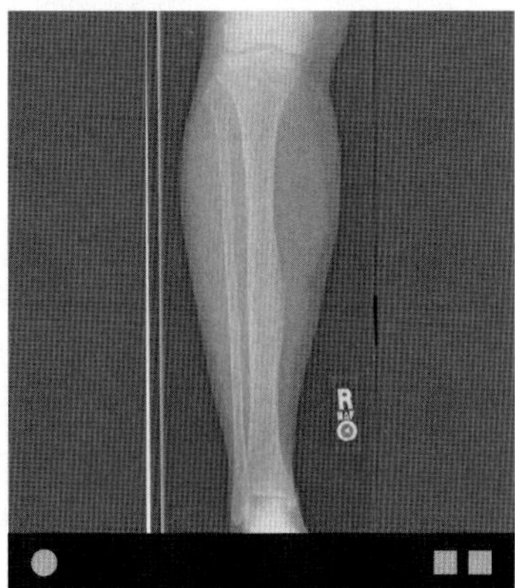

B. Periosteal hemangioma: AP radiograph shows medial cortical thickening of the mid-tibial shaft with increased sclerosis.

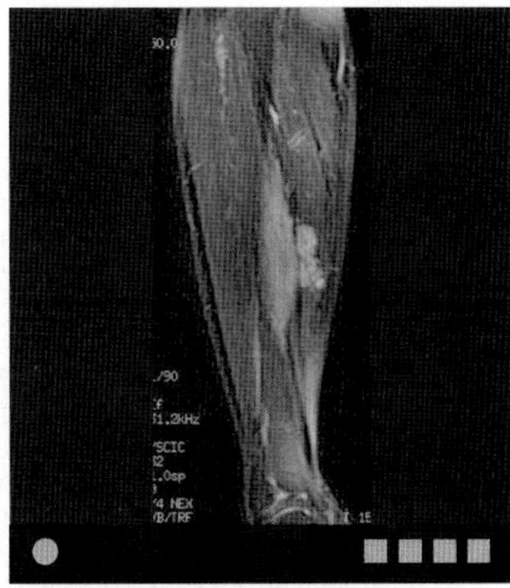

C. Periosteal hemangioma: Coronal fat-saturated T2-weighted image reveals the area of mid-shaft cortical thickening as a high signal soft tissue mass with a soft tissue component composed of tubular structures.

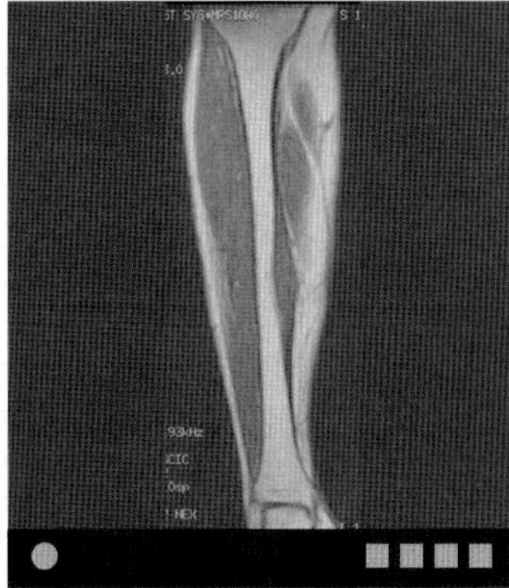

D. Periosteal hemangioma: Coronal T1-weighted image reveals the cortically based lesion to be of low to intermediate signal.

E. Periosteal hemangioma: Contrast-enhanced fat-saturated axial T1-weighted image demonstrates heterogeneous enhancement of the lesion.

IMAGE KEY

Common

Rare

Typical

Unusual

DIFFERENTIAL DIAGNOSES IMAGES

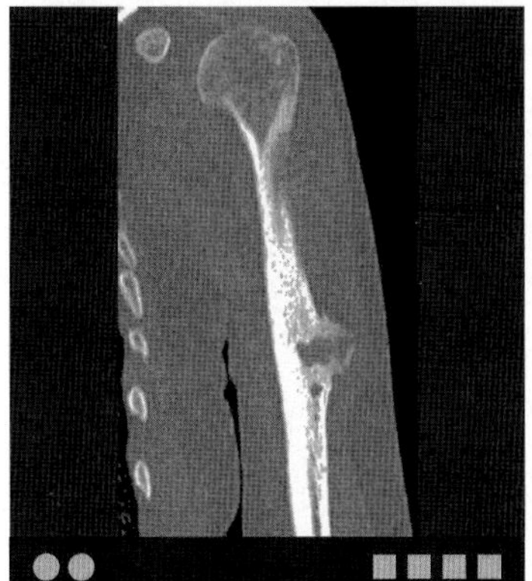

F. Surface chondroma: Coronal reformatted CT scan of the humerus in bone algorithm demonstrates a partially lytic lesion of the lateral cortex.

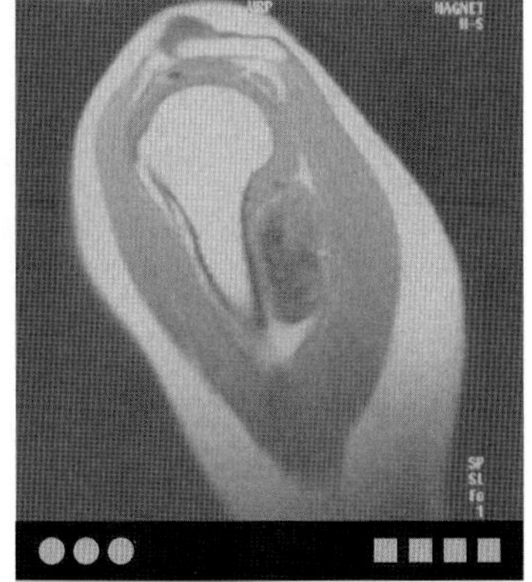

G. Parosteal osteosarcoma: Sagittal T1-weighted image shows a surface lesion of the proximal humerus with low-to-intermediate signal.

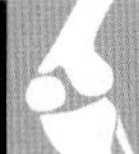

27–5 Synovial Osteochondromatosis of the Knee

Maria Pia Altvilla and Rajeev K. Varma

PRESENTATION

Joint pain and swelling of the knee

FINDINGS

Calcified intra-articular loose bodies on radiograph are a signature finding. T2-weighted MR Image shows multiple low signal loose bodies within the knee joint.

DIFFERENTIAL DIAGNOSES

- *Pigmented villonodular synovitis (PVNS) (localized form):* Owing to hemosiderin content, this aggressive but benign villonodular synovial lesion often presents with dark signal on most MR sequences.
- Amyloidosis often presents with similar MR signal appearance with more homogenous enhancement.
- Gouty tophi often show intra-articular masses that are low signal intensity on T1-weighted image which enhance after contrast administration.
- Loose bodies secondary to osteoarthritis usually vary in size and are few in number.

COMMENTS

The patient is a 49-year-old male, who complained of intermittent pain and swelling, and occasional locking of his knee for several years. Synovial osteochondromatosis (SOC) usually affects men two to four times more than women, and typically in the third to fifth decade of life. The disease is a synovial proliferation and metaplasia that manifests in cartilaginous or osteocartilaginous intra-articular bodies. These bodies may be loose within the joint or adherent to the synovium. They range in size from 1 to 3 cm, and tend to be uniform in size.

This benign entity most frequently occurs in the knee. Other common locations include the hip, shoulder, and elbow. SOC usually is monoarticular and frequently seen in conjunction with a joint effusion. The bodies may cause erosions within the joint and subsequent secondary osteoarthritis.

For the more classic presentation, MR T2-weighted and proton density images will demonstrate multiple low signal intensity bodies within synovial fluid. MRI plays an important role for the diagnosis when the loose bodies are not calcified on radiograph. On T2-weighted images, a soft tissue mass of predominantly high signal intensity can be seen within the joint and may have low signal foci secondary to the calcium deposits. The mass can be low or intermediate signal intensity on T1-weighted images. Bony erosions can be appreciated on both radiograph and MR from these loose bodies. Early osteoarthrosis may result in chronic cases.

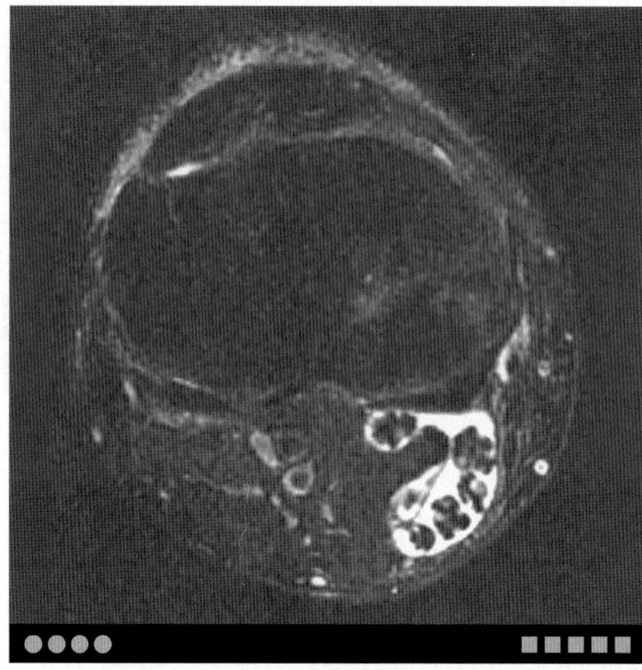

A. Synovial osteochondromatosis: STIR axial sequence shows hypointense loose bodies in the popliteal cyst.

PEARLS

- **Typically diagnosed on radiograph as multiple intra-articular calcified loose bodies**
- **Loose bodies are usually the same size, ranging from 1 to 3 cm**
- **MRI is the key to the diagnosis when the loose bodies are not calcified and the diagnosis is not obvious on radiograph**
- **Bony erosions can be appreciated on both radiograph and MR from these loose bodies. Early osteoarthrosis may result in chronic cases**

ADDITIONAL IMAGES

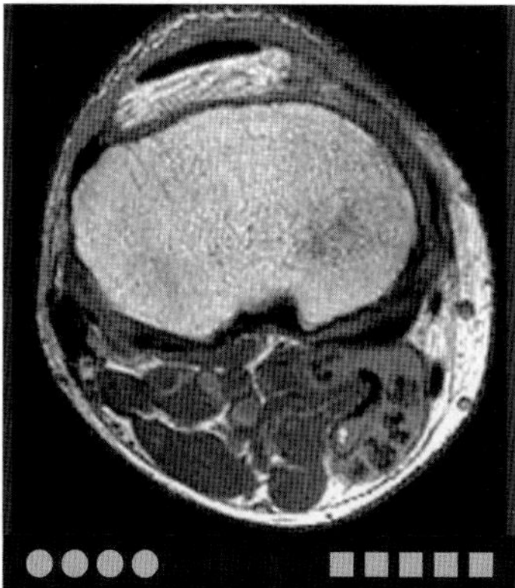

B. Synovial osteochondromatosis: Proton density (PD) axial image shows mixed signal loose bodies in the popliteal cyst.

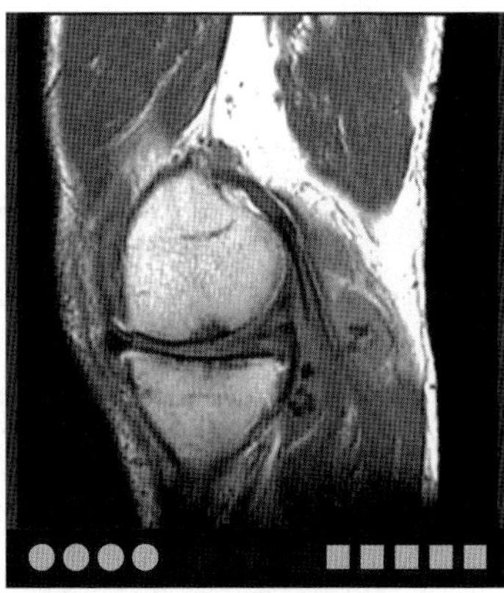

C. Synovial osteochondromatosis: Sagittal PD image shows loose bodies within the knee joint capsule as well as popliteal cyst.

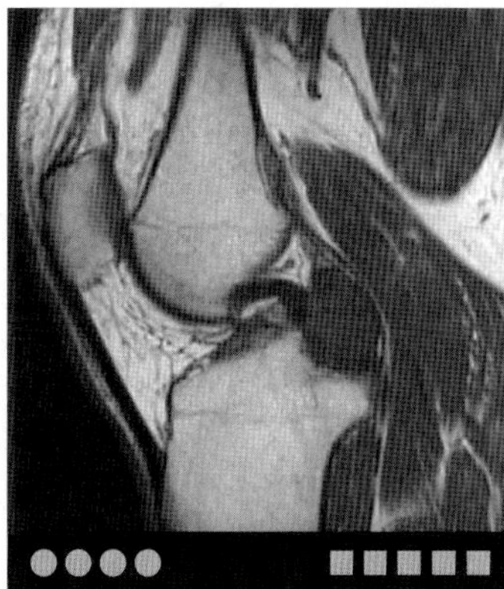

D. Synovial osteochondromatosis: A different patient with an isolated rather large osteochondromatous loose body seen as hypointense mass posterior to PCL on this T1-weighted sagittal image.

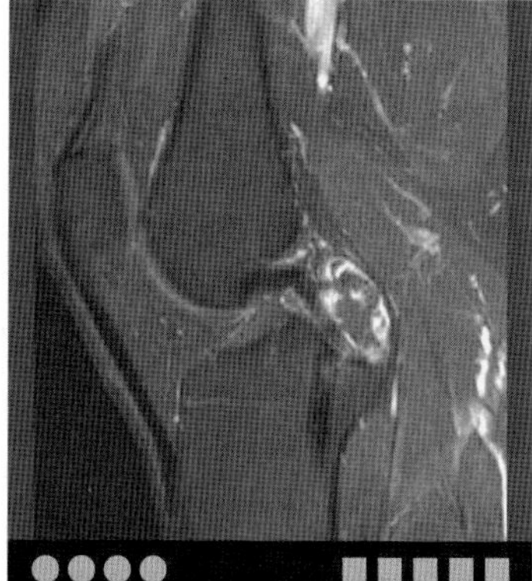

E. Synovial osteochondromatosis: Contrast-enhanced T1-weighted image with fat suppression (same patient as in Figure D) shows the osteochondromatous lesion.

IMAGE KEY

Common

Rare

Typical

Unusual

DIFFERENTIAL DIAGNOSES IMAGES

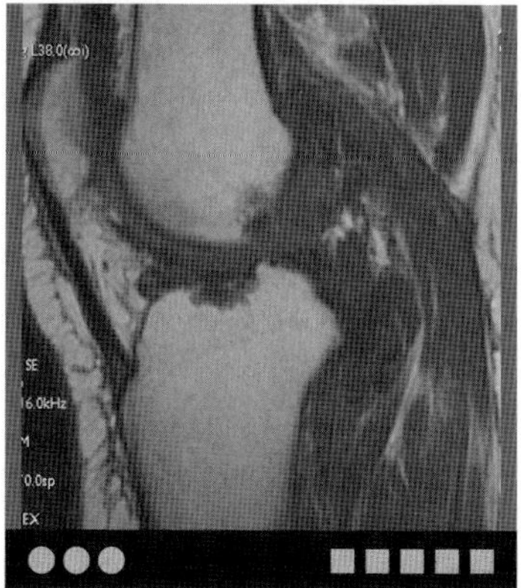

F. PVNS: multiple nodules with signal almost isointense to muscle are seen in the knee joint on this T1-weighted sagittal image.

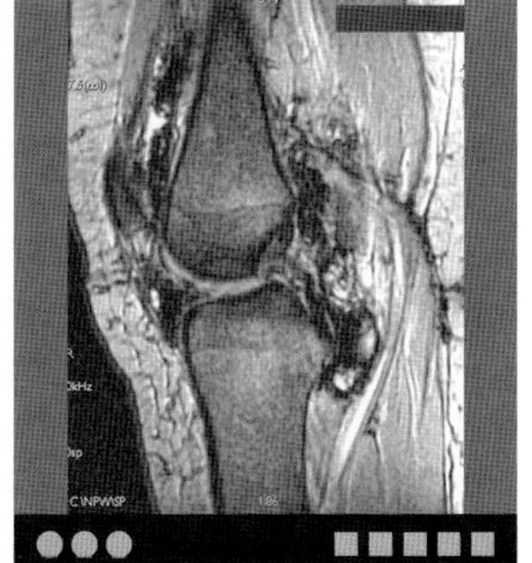

G. PVNS: T2*-weighted image in the sagittal plane shows blooming artifacts characteristic of PVNS related hemoglobin by-products.

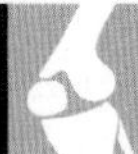

27–6 Neurofibromas of the Knee

Janice Ancheta and Rajeev K. Varma

PRESENTATION

Soft tissue mass

FINDINGS

MRI shows a chain of nodular soft tissue masses in the popliteal fossa of the knee with low signal on T1-weighted and bright signal on T2-weighted and STIR images.

DIFFERENTIAL DIAGNOSES

- *Neurofibrosarcoma:* Inhogenous signal on T2-weighted images and inhomogeneous contrast uptake which might be because of areas of necrosis. They are treated as any soft tissue sarcoma.
- *Schwannoma:* The target sign on T2-weighted images is usually absent. But MR cannot reliably distinguish between Schwannoma and neurofibroma. Prognosis is better for surgical removal of a Schwannoma since it does not infiltrate along the nerve bundles.

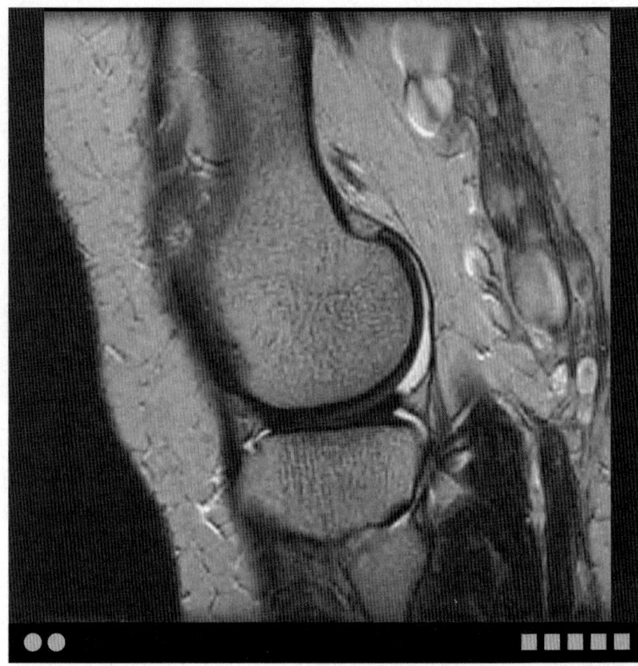

A. Neurofibroma: Sagittal T2-weighted image shows a chain of multiple round and oval densities with increased signal representing neurofibromas. The target sign is not evident though.

COMMENTS

Neurofibromas account for approximately 5% of all benign soft tissue tumors and can form in peripheral nerves, bone, soft tissue, or skin. On T2-weighted images, neurofibromas are bright and usually have an inhomogeneous hypointense center, giving them a characteristic "target" appearance. It is the larger neurofibromas that tend to lose this target appearance. On T1-weighted images, neurofibromas are isointense to muscle. They tend to be well-circumscribed but not encapsulated and do enhance with contrast. When arising from a peripheral nerve, neurofibromas are more fusiform in shape than other nerve sheath tumors. Solitary neurofibromas are smaller and much more common than those associated with neurofibromatosis-1. When associated with NF-1, neurofibromas can be localized, diffuse, or plexiform. Plexiform neurofibromas appear as multiple tortuous masses that develop along the course of a major nerve. They have a characteristic "bag of worms" appearance and are diagnostic of NF-1.

Malignant transformation of solitary neurofibromas is exceedingly rare while the rate of malignant degeneration is 4% in nonplexiform neurofibromas associated with NF-1 and 10% in plexiform neurofibromas. Malignant degeneration of a neurofibroma into a neurofibrosarcoma is difficult to discern on MRI. However, experts observe that neurofibromas that display the characteristic target appearance tend to be benign. Other leg findings in NF-1 including bowing of the tibia and fibula, pseudarthrosis, and focal gigantism with unilateral overgrowth of limbs, are better evaluated on radiograph.

PEARLS

- **Neurofibromas characteristically display a "target" appearance—bright on T1-weighted images with an inhomogeneous hypointense center**
- **Neurofibromas associated with NF-1 are generally larger and much less common than solitary neurofibromas**
- **Plexiform neurofibromas appear as multiple tortuous masses along the course of a major nerve, like a "bag of worms"**
- **Malignant transformation is most common in plexiform neurofibromas, less common in other neurofibromas associated with NF-1, and very uncommon in solitary neurofibromas**

ADDITIONAL IMAGES

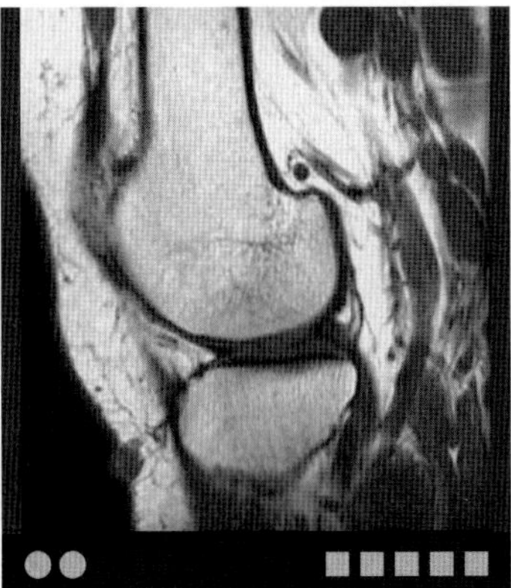

B. Neurofibroma: Sagittal T1-weighted image shows multiple round and oval hypointense structures in the subcutaneous tissue around the knee.

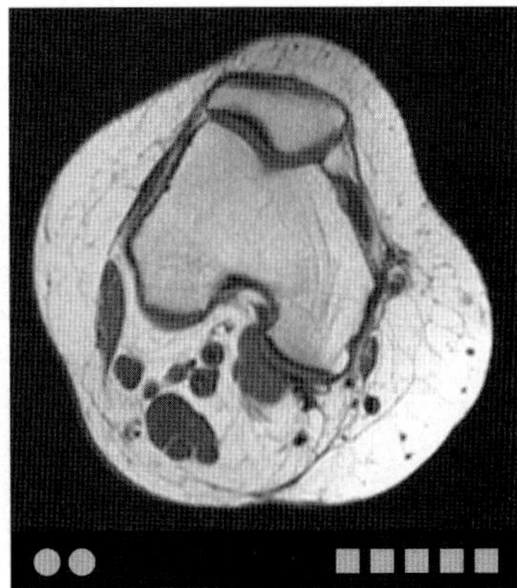

C. Neurofibroma: Axial T1-weighted images show the hypointense lesions in the nerves around the knee.

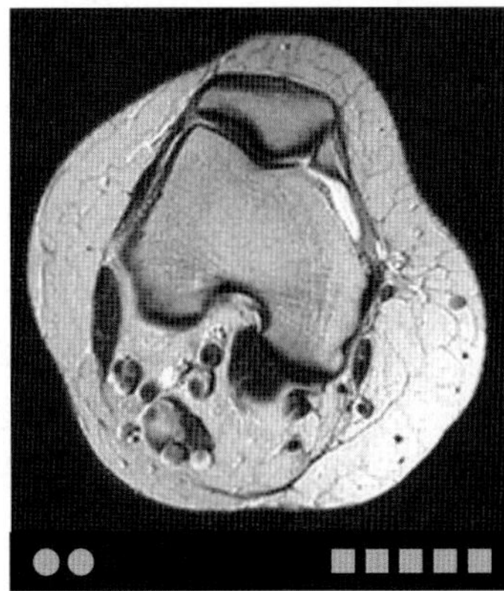

D. Neurofibroma: Axial T2-weighted images show the hyperintense lesions in the nerves around the knee.

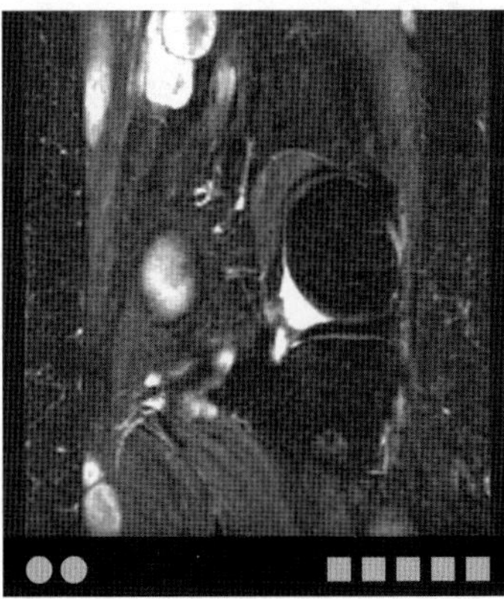

E. Neurofibroma: Coronal STIR image shows the neurofibromas as hyperintense signal lesions.

DIFFERENTIAL DIAGNOSES IMAGES

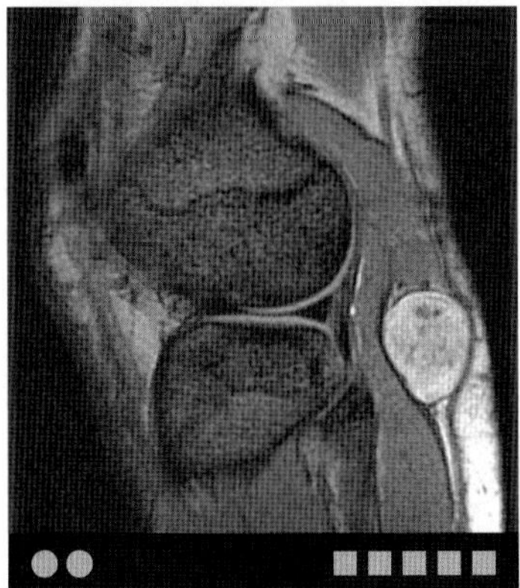

F. Nerve sheath tumor: Sagittal T2* GRE image shows a tumor of the common peroneal nerve, the patient had presented with foot drop.

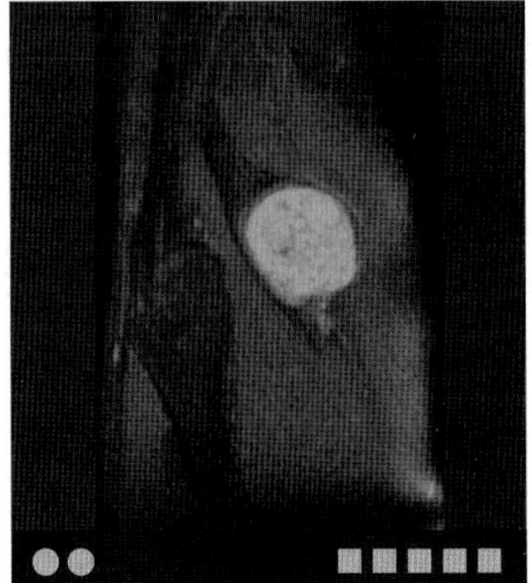

G. Schwannoma of the common peroneal nerve: Sagittal T1-weighted contrast-enhanced image with fat suppression (same patient as Figure F) illustrâtes contrast enhancement.

IMAGE KEY

Common

Rare

Typical

Unusual

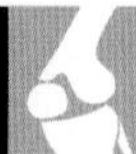

27–7 Nonossifying Fibroma

Amilcare Gentili

PRESENTATION

Knee pain

FINDINGS

MR images show a lesion abutting the posterior femoral cortex with mixed signal intensity.

DIFFERENTIAL DIAGNOSES

- *Osteosarcoma:* Most common & aggressive sarcoma.
- *Giant cell tumor:* Subchondral osteolytic lesion.
- *Metastases:* Osteolytic or blastic which is often multiple.

COMMENTS

The patient is a 20-year-old man with knee pain. Nonossifying fibroma and fibrous cortical defects have the same histology and differ only in size with fibrous cortical defects being smaller than 3 cm. They are also called fibroxanthomas as they contain spindle-shaped fibroblasts and xanthoma (foam) cells. They are the most common benign lesions of bone and have been reported in 30% of normal children. They are a non-neoplastic developmental aberration. Most are asymptomatic and disappear spontaneously. There is a male predominance with a 1.5 to 1 male-to-female ratio. Their peak incidence is around 10 years of age. These defects are usually localized to the metaphysis of a long bone and are most frequent about the knee (distal femur and proximal tibia). They are infrequent in the upper extremities. Their radiographic appearance is often pathognomonic, and no additional studies are usually necessary. They are frequently seen as incidental findings on MR examinations of the knee and can have a variable MR appearance. In their early stages, when the lesion is completely lytic on radiographs, the lesion may have high signal on T1-weighted images becuae of an abundance of xanthoma (foam) cells containing fat. Linear structures with low signal are often present and represent fibrous septa or osseous pseudosepta. When the lesion starts healing it has low signal intensity on both T1 and T2-weighted images because of increased fibrous collagen, mineralization, and possibly hemosiderin deposits. The lesions are always well defined, and are never surrounded by bone marrow edema.

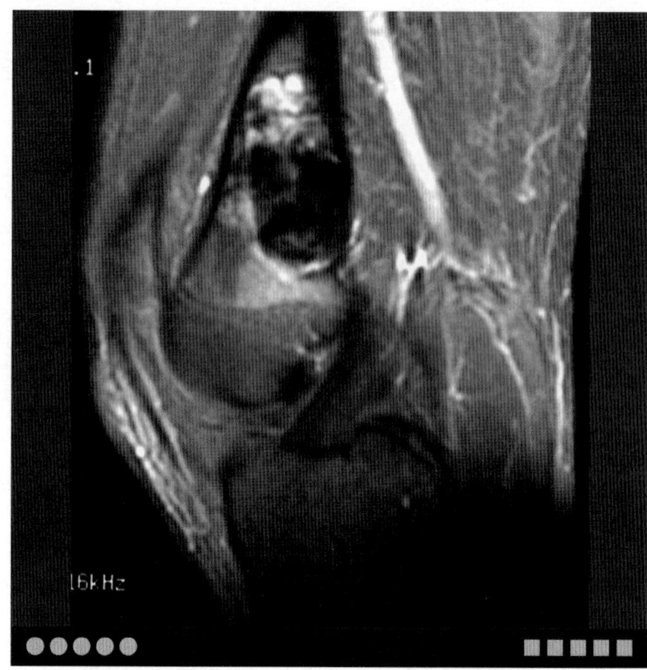

A. Nonossifying fibroma: Sagittal T2-weighted fat-suppressed image shows large lesion in the distal femur extending from the metaphysis into the diaphysis. Part of the lesion has high signal while the rest has low signal.

PEARLS

- **Nonossifying fibromas and fibrous cortical defects are the same lesion histologically**
- **They are always cortically based**
- **They are usually asymptomatic unless large enough to cause weakening of the bone**
- **They spontaneously heal with sclerosis on radiograph**

ADDITIONAL IMAGES

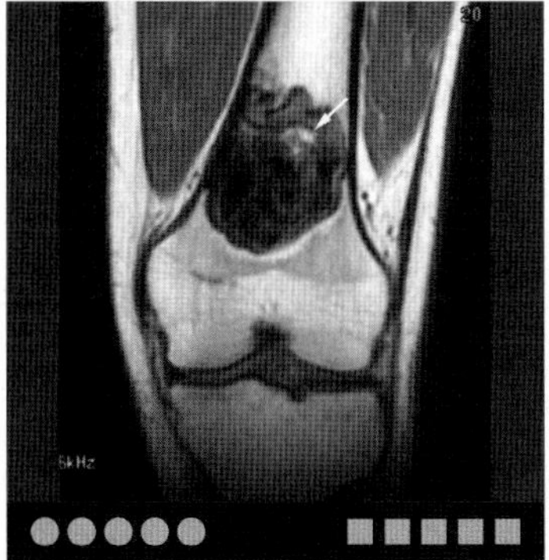

B. Nonossifying fibroma: Coronal T1-weighted image shows large lesion in the distal femur. Most of the lesion has low signal intensity, the area with high signal (arrow) most likely represent an area reach with xanthoma cells.

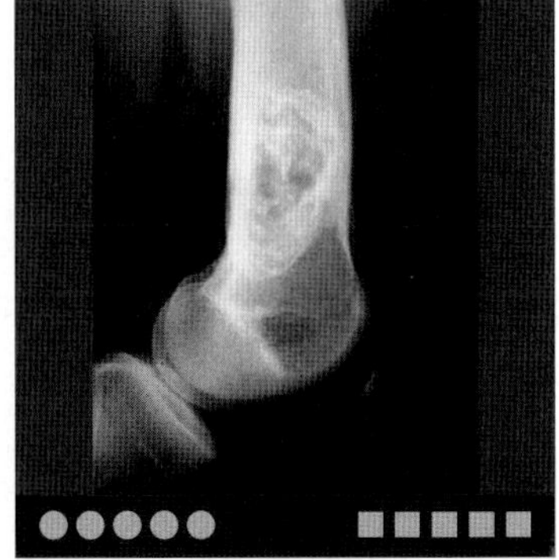

C. Nonossifying fibroma: Lateral radiograph of the knee shows osteolytic lesion with a thick sclerotic border in the distal femur.

DIFFERENTIAL DIAGNOSES IMAGES

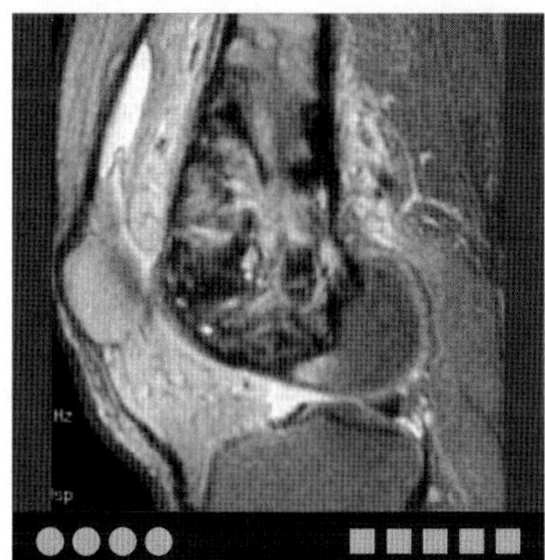

D. Giant cell tumor: Sagittal T2-weighted image with fat saturation shows a lesion extending from the diaphysis of the distal femur to the epiphysis. The lesion extends to the subchondral bone of the knee joint. The lesion has heterogeneous signal intensity with areas of low signal caused by hemosiderin deposits.

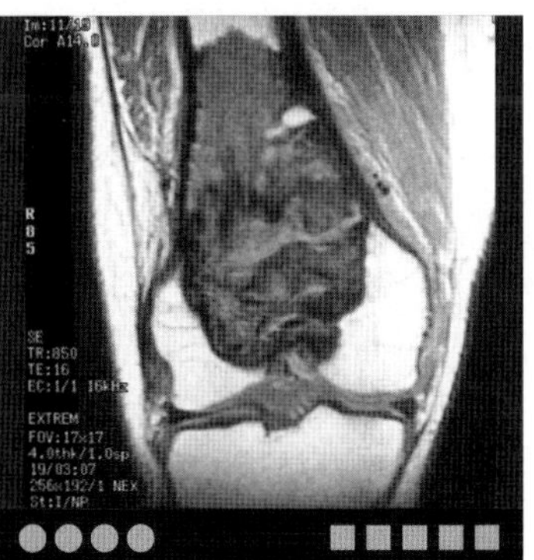

E. Giant cell tumor: Coronal T1-weighted image shows the lesion to have low to intermediate signal intensity.

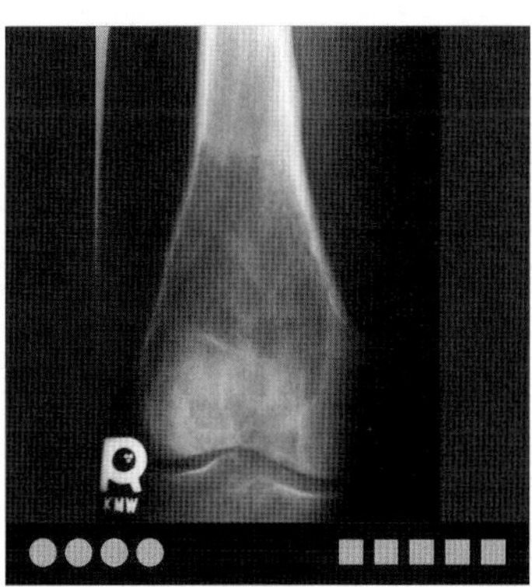

F. Giant cell tumor: AP radiograph shows a well-defined lytic lesion without sclerotic borders.

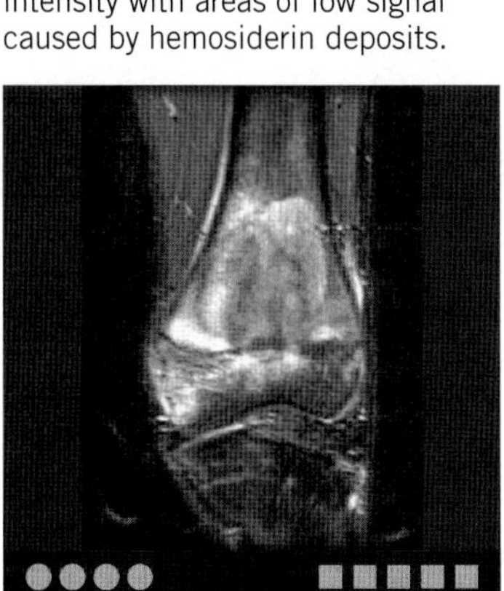

G. Osteosarcoma: Coronal T2-weighted with fat saturation shows a lesion extending from the diaphysis of the distal femur into the epiphyses.

IMAGE KEY

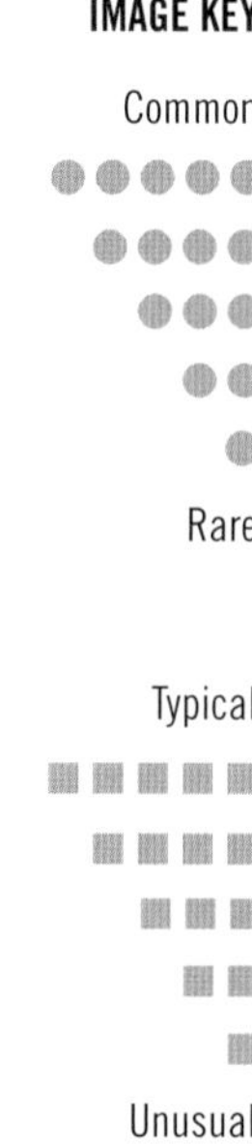

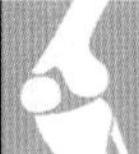

27–8 Soft Tissue Chondroma of the Hoffa Fat Pad

Kambiz Motamedi

PRESENTATION

Palpable mass below the patella

FINDINGS

MRI demonstrates a cartilaginous mass of the Hoffa fat pad.

DIFFERENTIAL DIAGNOSES

- *Focal nodular synovitis:* MRI may show a low signal to intermediate soft tissue mass of the Hoffa fat pad.
- *Cyst of the Hoffa fat pad:* A ganglion cyst or meniscal cyst arising from the internal knee structures would demonstrate signal properties consistent with simple fluid on MRI.
- *Heterotopic ossification:* Cross-sectional imaging of a mature focus reveals a well-corticated bony mass with fatty marrow.

COMMENTS

The patient is a 64-year-old patient, who noticed an enlarging lump of the anterior aspect of her knee over a period of 4 months. The Hoffa fat pad is the fatty tissue anterior and inferior to the knee joint and deep to the patellar tendon. This is an extra-synovial space without synovial lining. However, joint-related lesions may extend into this space and create a palpable mass with or without discomfort. Examples of joint-related entities are a meniscal cyst from a meniscal tear, a synovial cyst from inflammatory arthritis, or focal nodular synovitis, formerly known as pigmented villonodular synovitis (PVNS). Alternatively a ganglion cyst, without synovial lining may cause a mass effect in this space. Inflammation of the deep infrapatellar bursa may cause fluid accumulation in this bursa with superior extension into this space. Soft tissue masses are usually rare. The most common one is a soft tissue chondroma. Occasionally a soft tissue sarcoma, such as synovial cell sarcoma, may occur in this space. The soft tissue chondromas are rare benign tumors. In one study they comprised only 1.5% of all soft tissue chondromas. They are usually embedded in the soft tissues of the extremities such as between the metatarsals or the metacarpal bones. These masses are usually painless and mobile on palpation. The surgical excision is often the treatment of choice with a negligible recurrence rate.

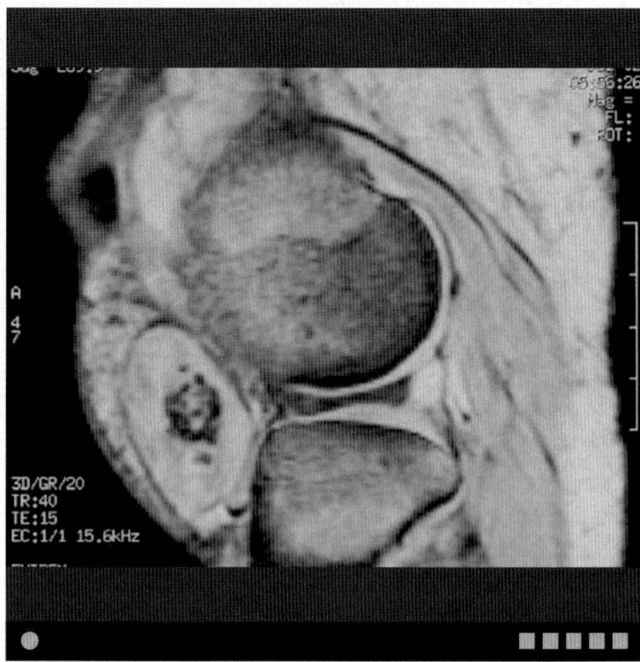

A. Hoffa fat pad chondroma: The sagittal gradient echo MR image shows the cartilage lesion of the Hoffa fat pad.

PEARLS

- **The location of a lesion deep to the patellar tendon and surrounded by fat locates this lesion within the Hoffa fat pad**
- **There is commonly a chondroid mineralization**
- **Cartilage sensitive sequences will readily demonstrate the chondroid matrix of these lesions**

ADDITIONAL IMAGES

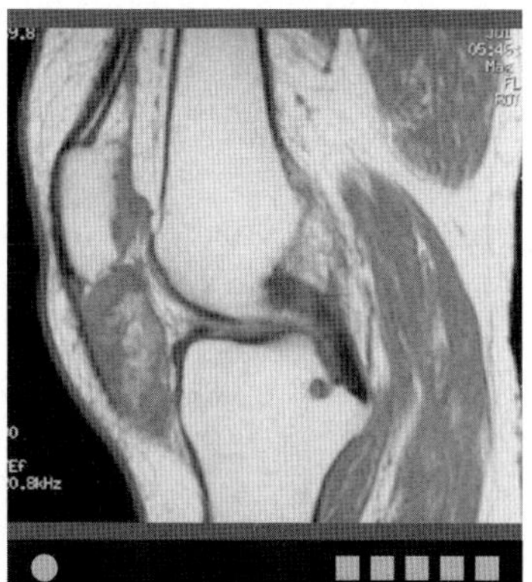

B. Hoffa fat pad chondroma: The sagittal T1-weighted MR image demonstrates the location of the mass within the Hoffa fat pad.

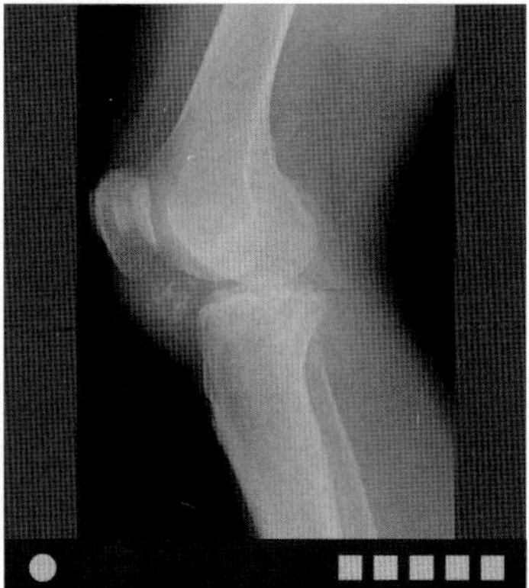

C. Hoffa fat pad chondroma: The lateral radiograph of the knee reveals a partially mineralized mass anterior to the knee joint and deep to the patellar tendon.

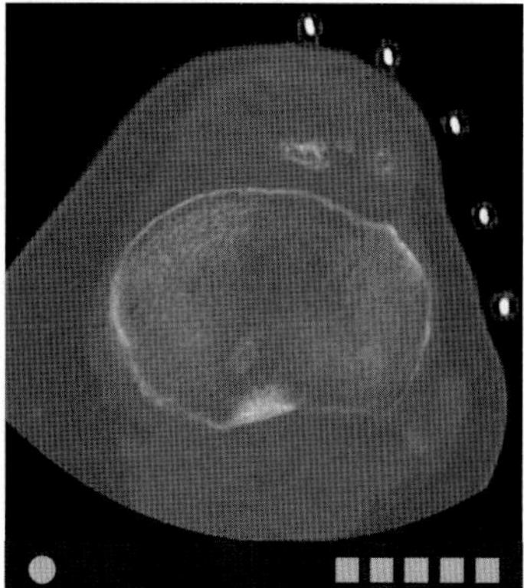

D. Hoffa fat pad chondroma: The axial CT scan for biopsy planning with bone window shows the anatomic location of the lesion and readily shows the mineralized chondroid matrix of the lesion.

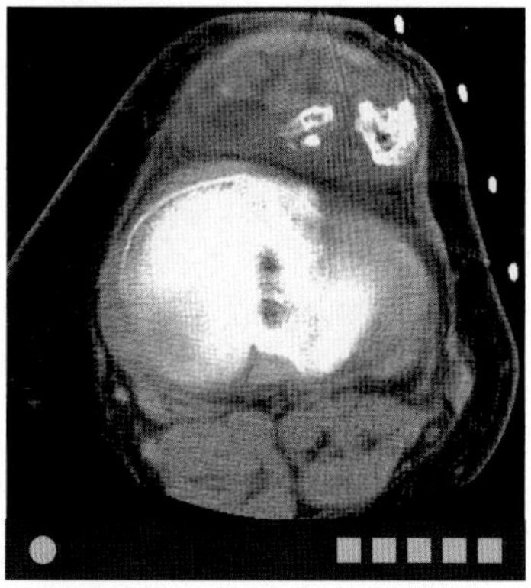

E. Hoffa fat pad chondroma: The axial CT scan in a plane higher than the prior figure within soft tissue window reveals the partially low density matrix of this lesion suggestive of cartilaginous or myxoid matrix.

IMAGE KEY

Common

Rare

Typical

Unusual

DIFFERENTIAL DIAGNOSES IMAGES

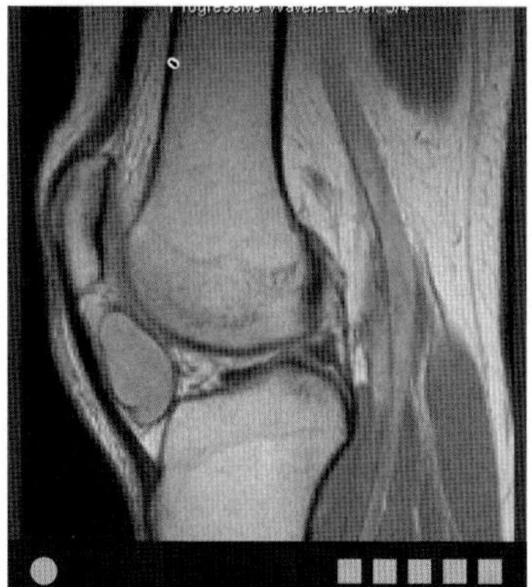

F. Ganglion cyst: Proton density MR image demonstrated a well-marginated homogenous oval lesion of the Hoffa fat pad.

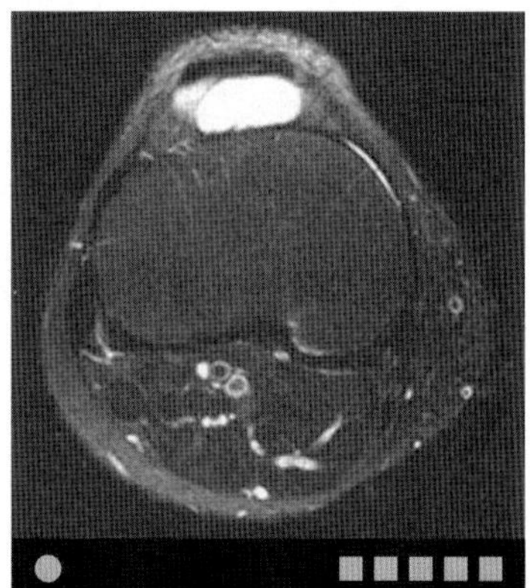

G. Ganglion cyst: The axial MR image reveals the homogenous high signal of this lesion suggestive of simple fluid.

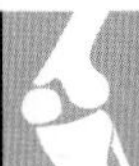

27–9 Squamous Cell Carcinoma of Soft Tissue of Tibia

Shahla Modarresi and Daria Motamedi

PRESENTATION

Large ulcer of soft tissue of tibia

FINDINGS

MRI shows superficial cutaneous ulcerating mass with high STIR signal and showing contrast enhancement.

DIFFERENTIAL DIAGNOSES

- *T-cell lymphoma (mycosis fungoides):* CT scan or MR imaging might be necessary to determine the extent of the disease. Signal characteristic is nonspecific. Cortical destruction, periostitis, and soft tissue swelling are common.
- *Infection, osteomyelitis:* MR imaging shows superficial or deep skin ulceration with low T1, high T2, and STIR signal with contrast enhancement. Bone marrow increased T2 signal and contrast enhancement seen with osteomyelitis.
- *Malignant melanoma:* MR imaging shows well-defined intensely enhancing superficial lesion, likely high T1 and very low T2 signal that is rather specific for tumor containing melanocytes.
- *Kaposi's sarcoma:* Usually there are many lesions of various sizes. It occurs more frequently in patients with acquired immunodeficiency syndrome. MR imaging and CT are useful for staging of the disease.

COMMENTS

The patient is a 65-year-old male with chronic leukemia and large ulcer of soft tissue of tibia. Skin cancer causes significant morbidity and mortality in US. Each year approximately 500,000 new cases and 2000 deaths from nonmelanoma skin cancer are reported. Sun exposure is the most common cause and fair skinned individuals are more susceptible. Basal cell and squamous cell carcinomas (SCC) make up about 90% of skin cancers with basal cell carcinoma (BCC) being the most common. Squamous cell carcinoma of skin exhibits shallow ulcers that are frequently elevated. Like basal cell carcinomas, they can be locally aggressive with twice the rates of recurrence. Lesion size and depth of invasion influence the prognosis. There is small but definite risk of metastasis. Lesions usually arising within burns, prior radiation, trauma, and chemical exposure worsen the prognosis. These patients have 30% increase incidence of other malignancies. Cure rate for local lesions is high. Advanced skin cancer, defined as tumors >2 cm, invasion of bone, muscle, nerve, lymph node, and metastasis require more extensive therapy. Large extensive skin malignant lesions may require imaging examination such as MRI or CT to evaluate the extent of the lesion. CT can be used to assess bony involvement and MRI is best to accurately depict the anatomic extent and identify tissue of origin, depth of invasion, and relation to adjacent structures. BCC has similar MR appearance to SCC with less local invasion.

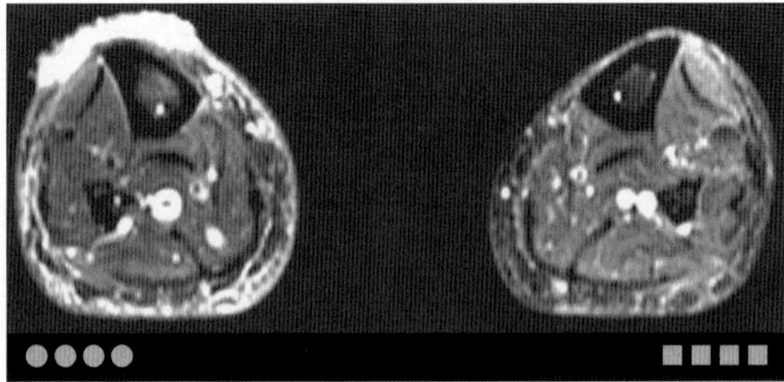

A. Squamous cell carcinoma: Axial STIR image shows high signal lesion of soft tissue of the right tibia.

PEARLS

- **Skin cancer causes significant morbidity and mortality in US with 500,000 new cases and 2000 deaths from nonmelanoma skin cancer being reported each year**
- **Sun exposure is the most common cause and fair-skinned individuals are more susceptible**
- **Basal cell and squamous cell carcinomas make up about 90% of skin cancers with basal cell being the most common**
- **Large extensive skin malignant lesions may require imaging examination such as MRI or CT to evaluate the extent of the lesion**
- **CT can assess bony involvement, and MRI accurately depicts the anatomic extent, depth of invasion, and relation to adjacent structures, such as muscles and bones.**

ADDITIONAL IMAGES

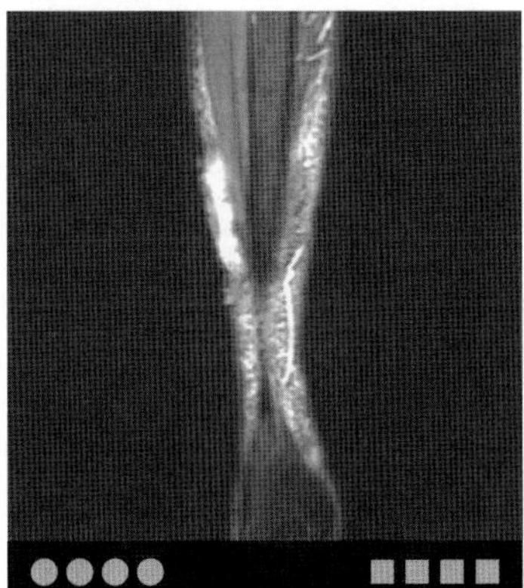

B. Squamous cell carcinoma: Sagittal STIR MR image shows high STIR signal lesion of soft tissue of the right tibia.

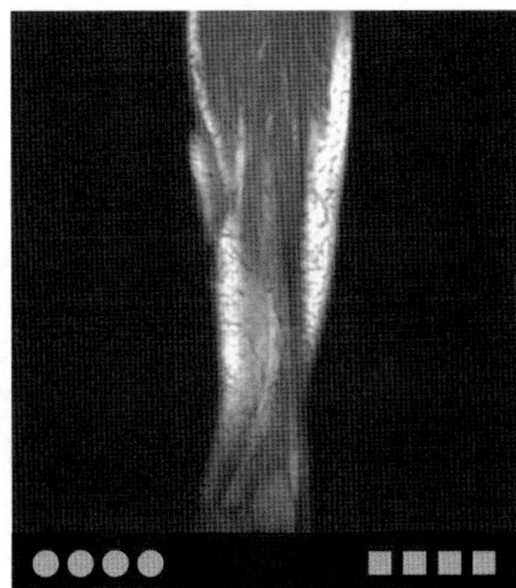

C. Squamous cell carcinoma: Sagittal PD image shows intermediate signal lesion of soft tissue of the right tibia.

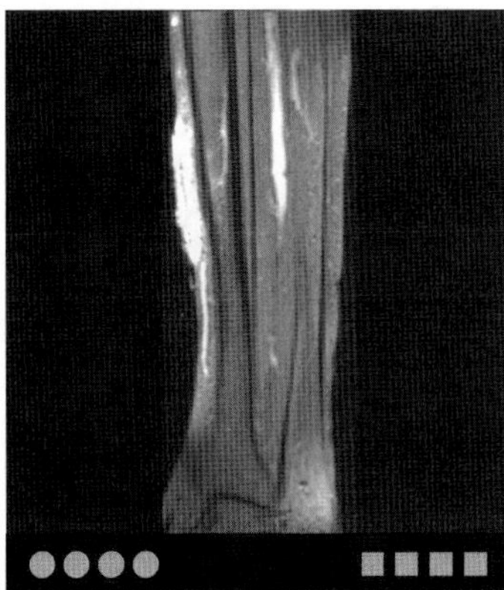

D. Squamous cell carcinoma: Sagittal post contrast fat-saturated T1-weighted image shows lesion enhancement and focal marrow enhancement.

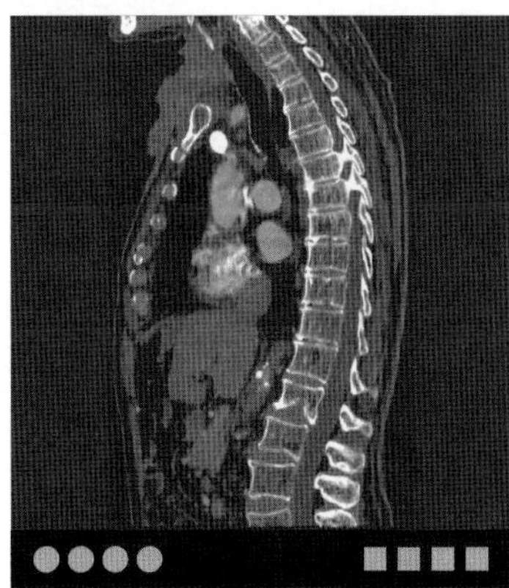

E. Squamous cell carcinoma: Sagittal reconstructed CT scan of different patients with squamous cell carcinoma of chest wall showing some enhancement.

IMAGE KEY

Common

●●●●●
●●●●
●●●
●●
●

Rare

Typical

■■■■■
■■■■
■■■
■■
■

Unusual

DIFFERENTIAL DIAGNOSES IMAGES

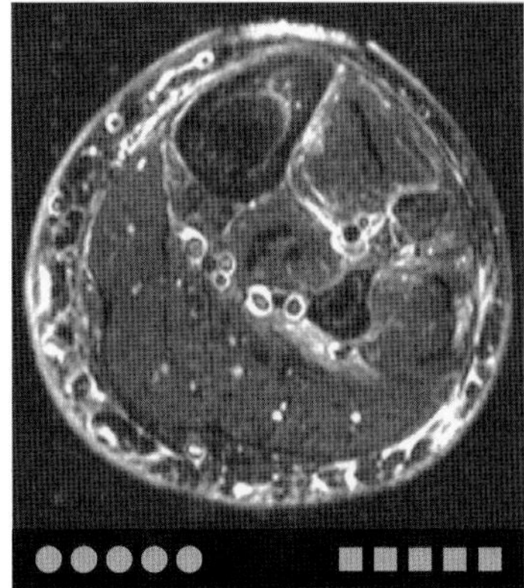

F. Osteomyelitis: Axial post contrast fat-saturated T1-weighted image shows enhancing skin ulceration with osteomyelitis.

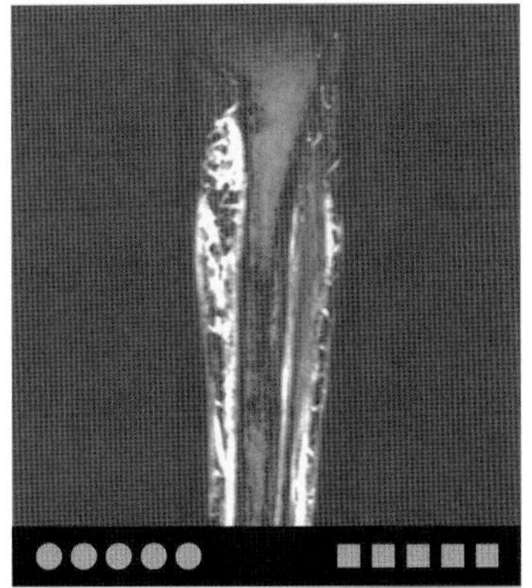

G. Infection: Coronal STIR image of diabetic patient with skin infection and ulceration of soft tissue of tibia.

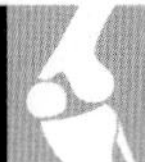

27–10 Dermatofibrosarcoma Protuberance of the Popliteal Fossa

Peyman Borghei and Jamshid Tehranzadeh

PRESENTATION

Popliteal mass

FINDINGS

MRI shows an enhancing 3 × 3.7 × 11 cm soft tissue tumor arising from popliteal fossa with an infiltrative component, which involves the subcutaneous soft tissue and a small portion of medial head of the gastrocnemius.

DIFFERENTIAL DIAGNOSES

- *Malignant fibrous histiocytoma:* The soft tissue mass may be associated with bony invasion and cortical destruction showing intermediate signal intensity (SI) on T1-weighted and high SI on T2-weighted images.
- *Liposarcoma:* MRI of liposarcoma shows a sharply marginated mass with inhomogeneous contrast enhancement on T1-weighted and mixed intermediate and high intensity signals on T2-weighted images.
- *Synovial sarcoma:* The mass is usually isointense with muscle on T1-weighted and inhomogeneous high SI often with areas of hemorrhage and sometimes fluid–fluid levels or lobulation on T2-weighted images.
- *Leiomyosarcoma:* Based on tissue differentiation this tumor may manifest different signal intensities on MR imaging.

COMMENTS

The patient is a 72-year-old man with 2 months history of popliteal mass and reddish skin changes over the mass, with tissue diagnosis of dermatofibrosarcoma protuberance (DFSP). Dermatofibrosarcoma, an intermediate grade spindle cell tumor, typically arises from the dermis as a multinodular mass, which then spreads into the subcutaneous tissues and muscle. The tumor usually is seen in second to fifth decades, with men and women affected equally. It is most commonly seen in trunk followed by proximal extremities and head and neck. The tumor growth is slow and often ignored by the patient till they become quite large. Metastatic disease is extremely rare. Treatment is surgical resection of the lesion. There is poor correlation between the size of the tumor and recurrence rate; however, obtaining inadequate margins while resecting the lesion leads to high recurrence rate. MR imaging is useful to assess the true extent and location of the tumor preoperatively and for evaluation of recurrence postoperatively. The lesion is usually well defined with lower signal intensity than subcutaneous fat on T1-weighted imaging. However, it could be isointense, hypointense, or hyperintense, compared to skeletal muscle on T1-weighted sequences. On T2-weighted images the lesion shows intermediate to high signal intensity. However, it is always high signal-like water or blood vessels in STIR imaging with marked contrast enhancement.

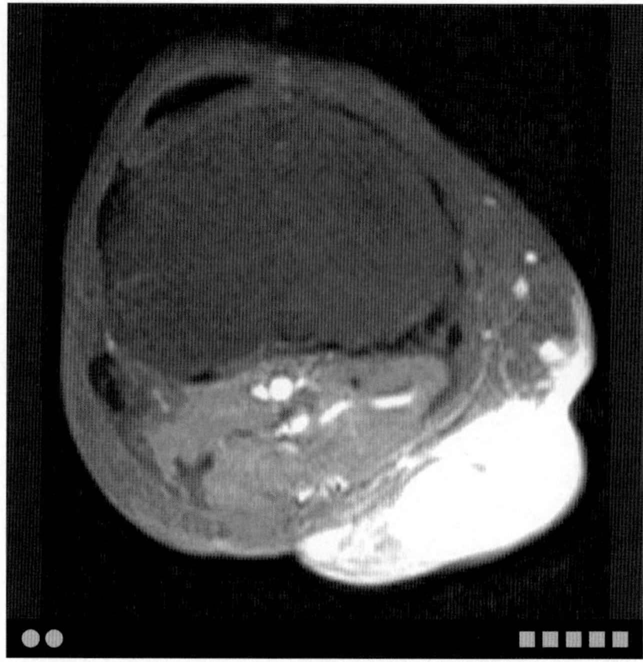

A. DFSP: Axial fat-saturated postcontrast T1-weighted image shows a large soft tissue mass with strong enhancement arising in the posterior aspect of the knee involving the skin and the subcutaneous tissue and also medial head of the gastrocnemius muscle.

PEARLS

- **DFSP is a spindle cell soft tissue tumor with intermediate malignancy**
- **DFSP usually is a slow growing, well-defined tumor with high local recurrence rate and rare distant metastasis**
- **Recurrence is mostly affected by the adequate distant excised margins, and not by the tumor size**
- **MRI is useful for localization of the tumor preoperatively and evaluation of recurrence postoperatively**
- **The classic MRI feature is low signal intensity on T1-weighted images which will strongly enhance with contrast and has intermediate to high signal intensity on T2-weighted images.**

ADDITIONAL IMAGES

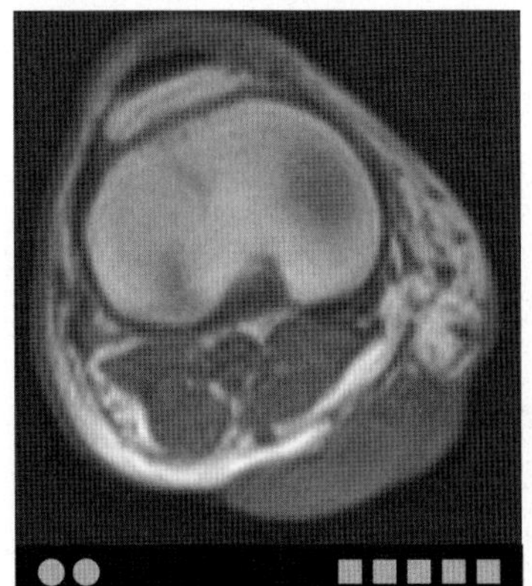

B. DFSP: Axial T1 SE image shows low–intermediate signal in the soft tissue mass.

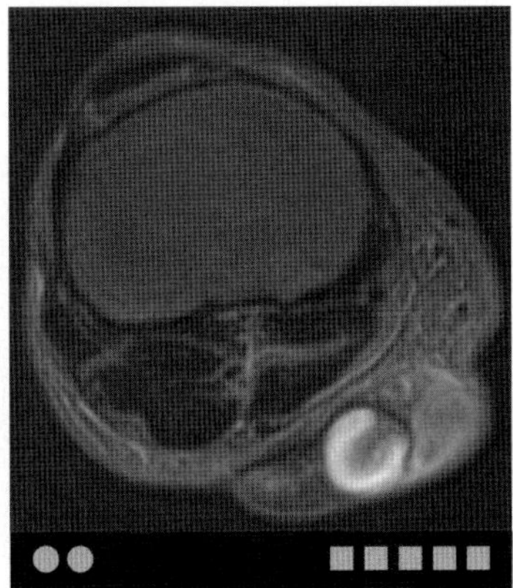

C. DFSP: Axial fat-saturated T2-weighted image shows most of the mass to be intermediate signal except for the center, which has a horseshoe-shaped hallow of bright signal.

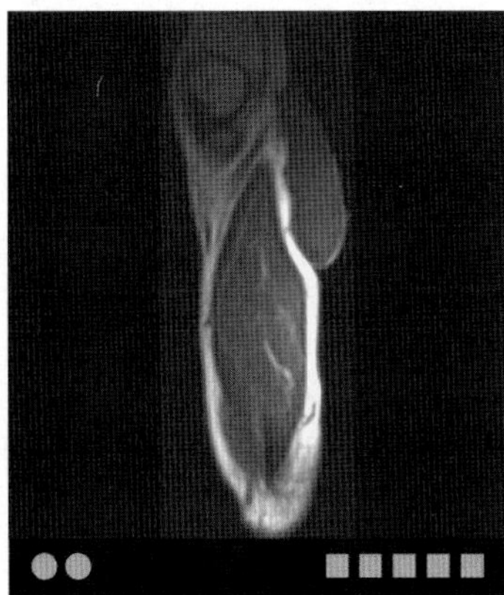

D. DFSP: Sagittal T1 SE image shows oval-shaped low to intermediate signal mass arising from the popliteal fossa.

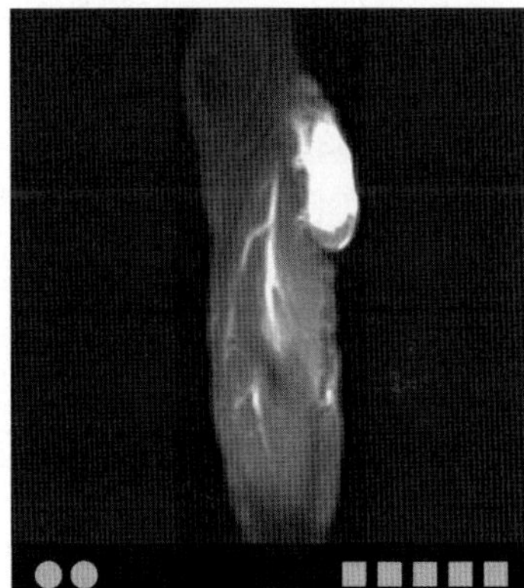

E. DFSP: Sagittal fat-saturated post contrast T1-weighted image shows marked enhancement of the soft tissue mass.

IMAGE KEY

Common

Rare

Typical

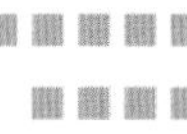

Unusual

DIFFERENTIAL DIAGNOSES IMAGES

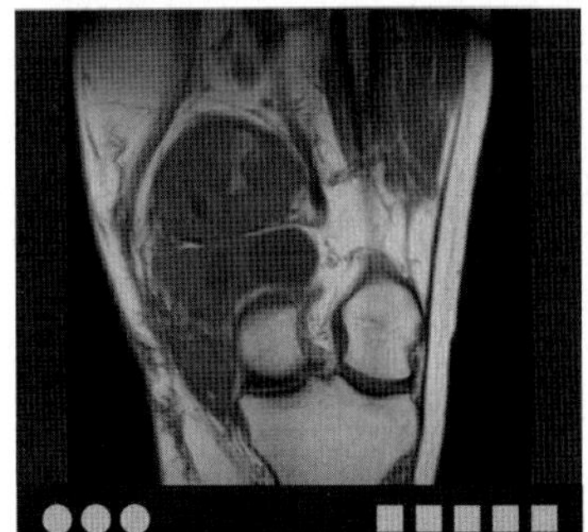

F. Synovial sarcoma: Coronal T1 SE image shows soft tissue mass with inhomogeneous intermediate and low signal intensity in the popliteal fossa extending into the medial side of the knee.

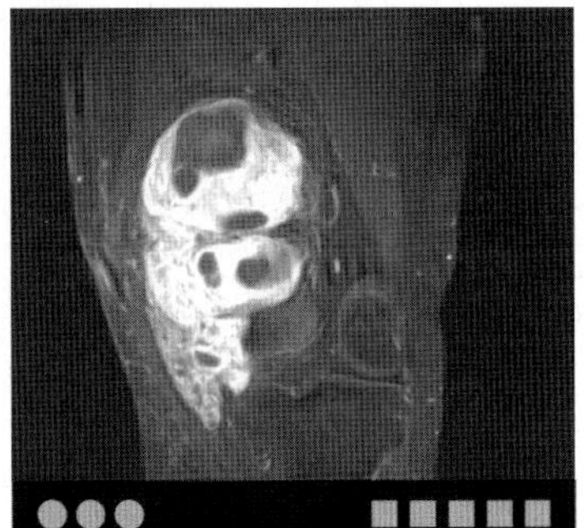

G. Synovial sarcoma: Coronal fat-saturated post contrast T1-weighted image shows large enhancing soft tissue mass with nonenhancing low signal areas of cystic change and necrosis.

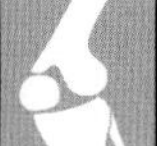

27–11 Giant Cell Tumor

Kira Chow

PRESENTATION

Pain after a fall

FINDINGS

CT scan demonstrates epiphyseal tibial lesion without matrix. There is a pathologic fracture of medial metaphysis.

DIFFERENTIAL DIAGNOSES

- *Chondroblastoma:* This is a lucent epiphyseal lesion with internal cartilaginous matrix about one third of the time. Surrounding sclerosis is more commonly seen with chondroblastoma and is unusual in giant cell tumor. Chondroblastomas are typically small, less than 4 cm.
- *Aneurysmal bone cyst*: These lytic expansile lesions usually occur in younger patients, 5 to 20 years old. Although they start in the metaphysis, after physeal fusion, they can grow into the epiphysis.
- *Sarcoma:* Osteosarcoma can occur with paucity of osteoid matrix resulting in lytic appearance. These tumors have more aggressive characteristics such as osseous destruction and extraosseous soft tissue component.
- *Other differential possibilities:* Chondromyxoid fibroma, Brown tumor, clear cell chondrosarcoma, and plasmacytoma.

COMMENTS

Giant cell tumor is a tumor consisting predominantly of multinucleated giant cells. The classic radiographic appearance is an eccentric epiphyseal lesion, which is purely lytic without internal matrix and without surrounding sclerosis. Bone is often expanded and thinned and as a result, pathologic fracture can occur. Periosteal reaction is unusual. Around 50% of giant cell tumors occur around the knee with the remainder occurring in the distal radius, proximal humerus, fibula, and sacrum. The lesion occurs most commonly in patients 20 to 40 years of age, after the physis is fused. In rare cases occurring in skeletally immature patients, the location is metaphyseal. CT scan can detect small nondisplaced fractures that often occur in the setting of pathologically thinned cortex. CT internal Hounsfield units are 20 to 70. On MRI, giant cell tumors are T2 hyperintense and may have signal intensity suggesting blood products as a result of intratumoral hemorrhage. There may also be fluid–fluid levels, which may be caused by aneurismal bone cyst components, common in giant cell tumors. Giant cell tumors often recur after curettage, usually between 1 and 3 years and rarely after 5 years. Giant cell tumors that are histologically benign can behave aggressively, underscoring the important fact that histology does not predict prognosis. Aggressive tumors can spread to the lungs or recur, typically 1 to 3 years after curettage and rarely after 5 years. Histologically, malignant giant cell tumors are extremely rare.

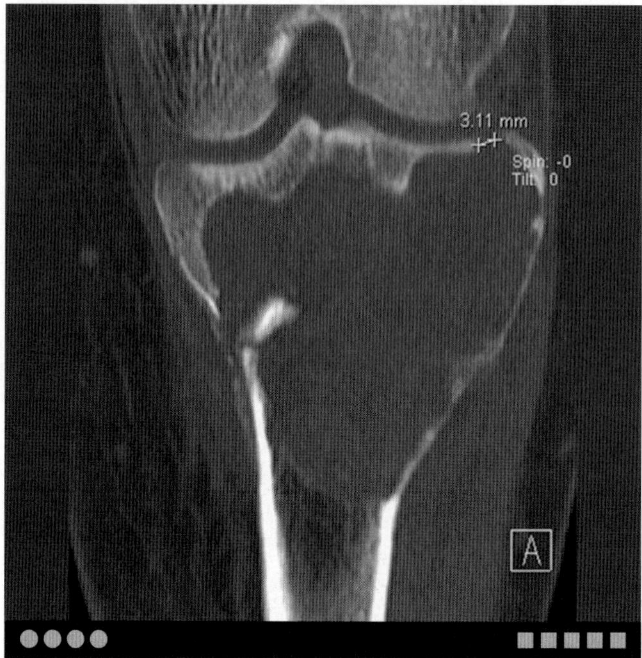

A. Giant cell tumor: Coronal CT image demonstrates a slightly expansile eccentric epiphyseal lesion with no internal matrix. There is cortical thinning along the lateral tibia. Pathologic fracture is noted along the medial metaphysis.

PEARLS

- **Epiphyseal location with purely lytic appearance is classic. Giant cell tumor can be differentiated from chondroblastoma by lack of internal chondroid matrix and lack of surrounding sclerosis.**
- **Giant cell tumor occurs in patients aging between 20 and 40 years.**
- **Benign giant cell tumor can disseminate to the lungs. Histological appearance does not predict prognosis.**
- **Recurrence usually occurs 1 to 3 years after curettage.**

ADDITIONAL IMAGES

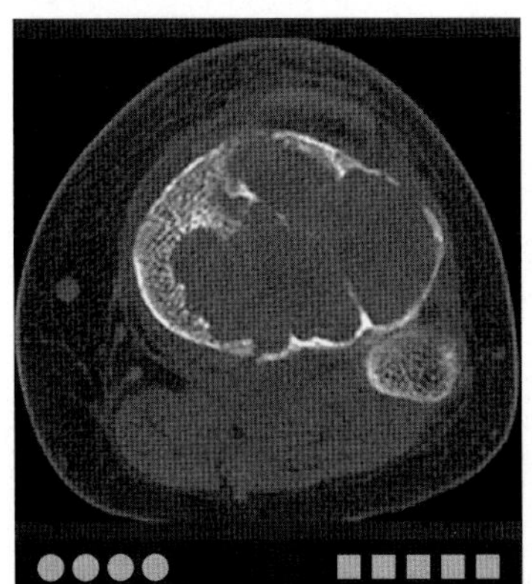

B. Giant cell tumor: Axial CT image demonstrates cortical thinning and multiple focal areas of complete cortical loss. The endosteal scalloping seen is thought to explain the radiographic appearance of pseudotrabeculation.

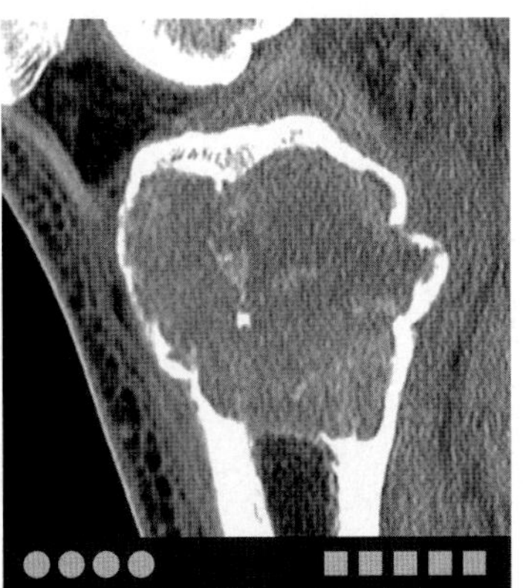

C. Giant cell tumor: Sagittal CT image in soft tissue window demonstrates density difference between normal fatty marrow and soft tissue density within the tumor.

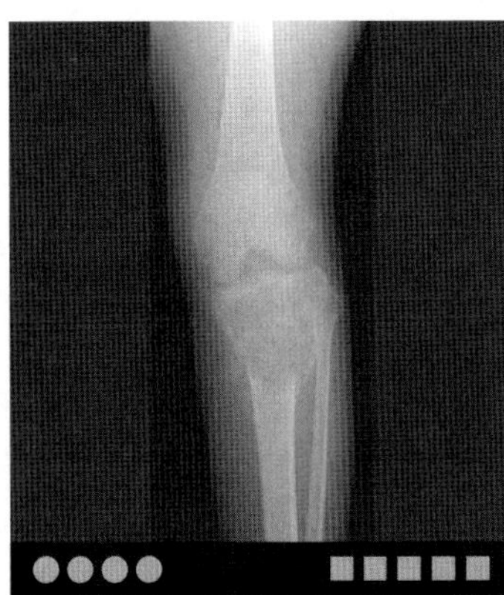

D. Giant cell tumor: Frontal radiograph of the knee demonstrates the epiphyseal lucent lesion with mild osseous expansion.

IMAGE KEY

Common

Rare

Typical

Unusual

DIFFERENTIAL DIAGNOSES IMAGES

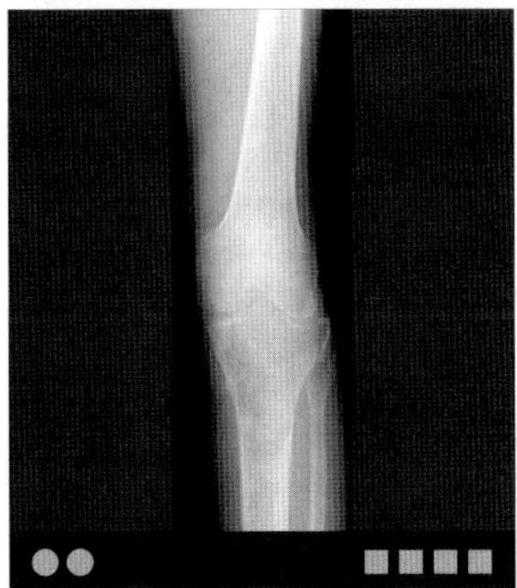

E. Spindle cell sarcoma: Frontal radiograph of the tibia demonstrates an aggressive epiphyseal lytic lesion demonstrating an ill-defined zone of transition and cortical destruction.

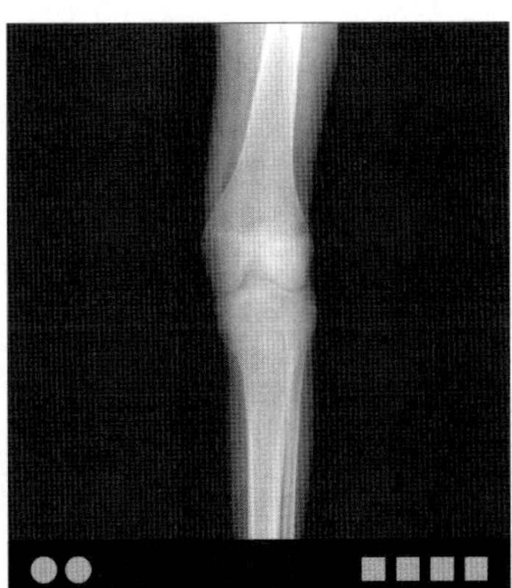

F. Chondroblastoma: Frontal radiograph of the knee demonstrates a small lesion in the epiphysis with surrounding sclerosis.

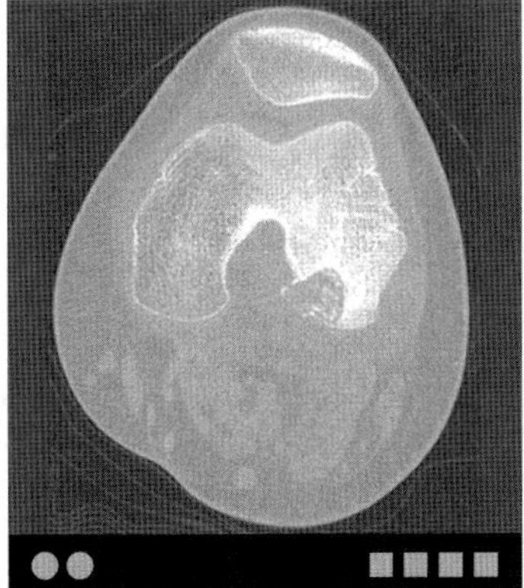

G. Chondroblastoma: CT scan in the same patient as in image F demonstrates chondroid matrix within the lesion and surrounding sclerosis.

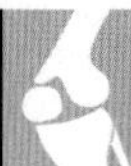

27–12 Aneurysmal Bone Cyst of the Proximal Tibia

Marcia F. Blacksin and Gideon Strich

PRESENTATION

Lower leg pain

FINDINGS

Expansile lesion of proximal tibial diametaphysis showing multi-loculated appearance with regions of high and low signal intensity on T1-weighted and fluid–fluid levels on T2-weighted images.

DIFFERENTIAL DIAGNOSES

- *Giant cell tumor:* These lesions occur most commonly in a 20- to 40-year-old age group and usually extend to subchondral bone.
- *Chondroblastoma:* These are benign lesions of epiphysis showing cartilaginous calcification in up to 50% of the cases. They are also seen in regions of the bones considered epiphyseal equivalents. Age range is first through third decades.
- *Unicameral (simple) bone cyst:* These most commonly occur in proximal humeral and femoral metaphysis of children and may extend to diaphysis.
- *Telangiectatic osteosarcoma:* These have aggressive pattern on radiograph and solid components on MR.

COMMENTS

The patient is a 5-year-old boy with leg pain. ABC is a locally aggressive expansile benign bone lesion that usually occurs in patients younger than 20 years old. It is composed of cystic cavities containing blood. Vertebra, femur, and tibia are common foci with a metaphyseal location seen in the tubular bones. The neoplasm may extend to the articular surface, once the physes close. Periosteal new bone and cortical destruction can be seen and should not be misinterpreted as an indication of malignancy. The neoplasm is usually eccentric, expansile, and trabeculated. ABC may coexist with other benign and malignant tumors such as chondroblastoma, giant cell tumor, fibrous dysplasia, and osteosarcoma. Therefore, a search for any solid components should be made on MR before diagnosis of ABC is offered. Rapid growth, bone destruction, and soft tissue extension can be seen. Recurrence is common at approximately 10% to 20%. In addition to aneurysmal bone cyst (ABC), many benign lesions can contain fluid–fluid levels. These lesions can also appear similar on radiography. They include unicameral bone cyst, giant cell tumor, chondroblastoma, and fibrous dysplasia. Malignant lesions include telangiectatic osteosarcoma. Unicameral bone cyst is usually a central lesion and may show a "fallen fragment" sign. Giant cell tumor is rare in patients who are skeletally immature (<10%) and hemosiderin may be seen on MR imaging. Fibrous dysplasia is best diagnosed on radiography and CT where the appearance is easily recognizable. Telangiectatic osteosarcoma will show solid components within the tumor on MR.

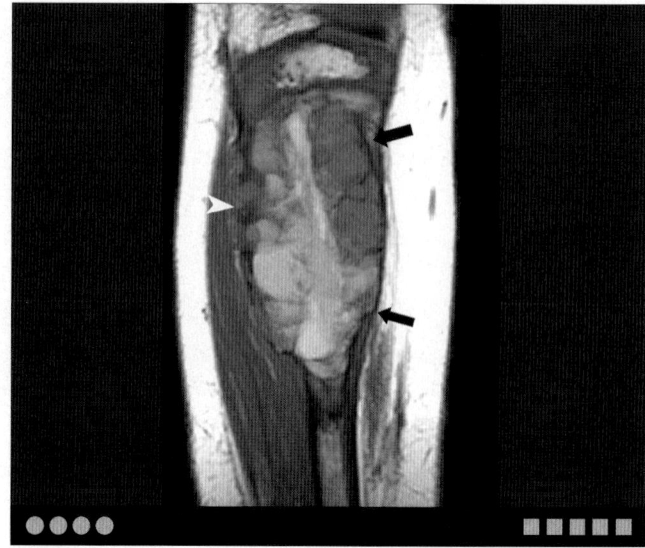

A. Aneurysmal bone cyst of proximal tibia: T1-weighted coronal image shows multiloculated, expansile lesion (arrows) with both high and low signal. Lesion is extending through lateral cortex (arrowhead).

PEARLS

- **ABC is a locally aggressive expansile benign bone lesion that usually occurs in patients younger than 20 years old.**
- **A variety of bone lesions can display fluid–fluid levels, and correlation with radiography and patient age can narrow the differential diagnosis.**
- **Bone neoplasms cannot be adequately characterized on MR without radiographic examination of matrix, lesion borders, and periostitis.**
- **If radiography is not definitive, CT may be added to characterize any increased sclerosis in bone such as cartilaginous matrix calcification or neoplastic bone.**

ADDITIONAL IMAGES

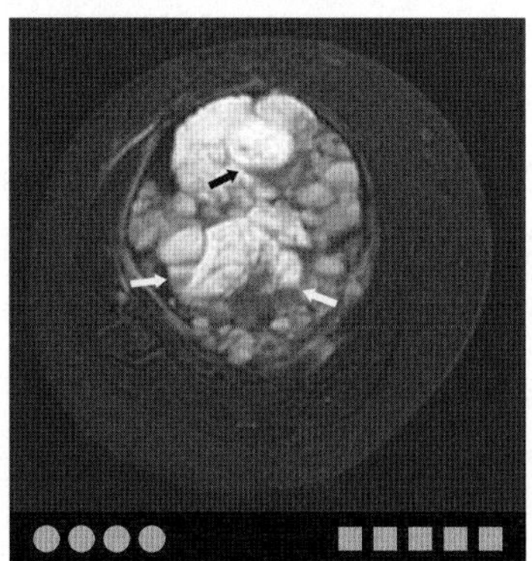

B. Aneurysmal bone cyst of proximal tibia: Axial T2-weighted image shows numerous fluid–fluid levels filling lesion (arrows).

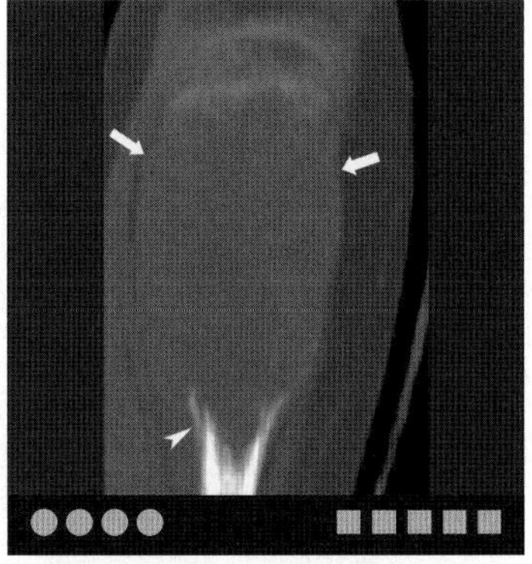

C. Aneurysmal bone cyst of proximal tibia: Coronal CT reconstruction of ABC shows almost complete osteolysis of cortical bone (arrows) and periostitis (arrowhead).

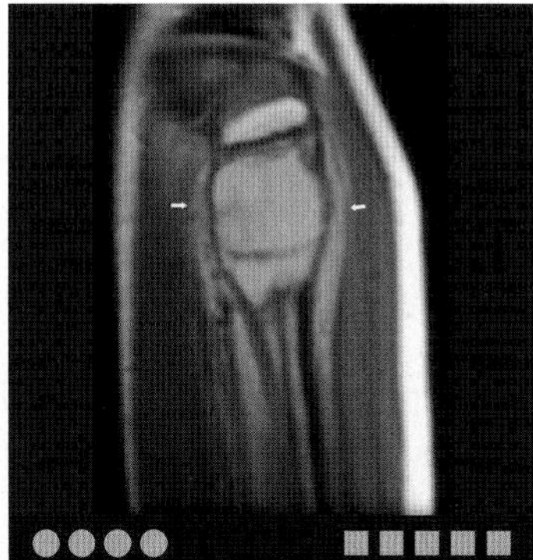

D. Aneurysmal bone cyst of proximal fibula: Sagittal proton density image in another patient with ABC of the proximal fibula shows a mixed bright signal expansile mass extending to, but not involving the epiphysis, with periosteal reaction (arrows).

E. Aneurysmal bone cyst of proximal fibula: Axial T2 fat saturation image in same patient as Figure D shows a multicystic lesion with multiple fluid–fluid levels. A thin rim of cortex is seen around the lesion. There is significant soft tissue edema related to the periosteal reaction.

IMAGE KEY

Common

Rare

Typical

Unusual

DIFFERENTIAL DIAGNOSES IMAGES

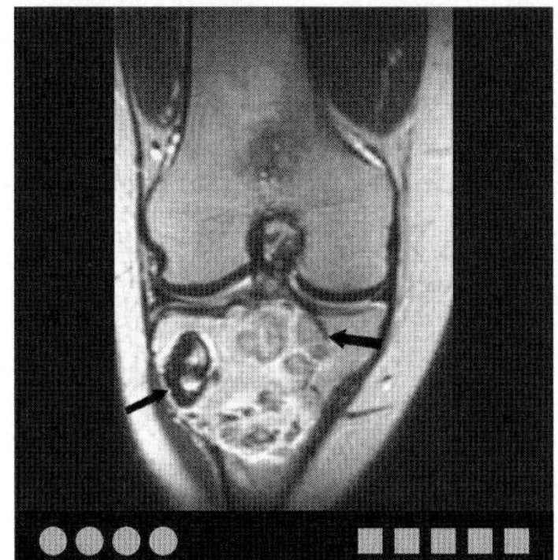

F. Giant cell tumor: Coronal T2-weighted image shows low signal intensity hemosiderin deposition (arrows) often seen in giant cell tumors.

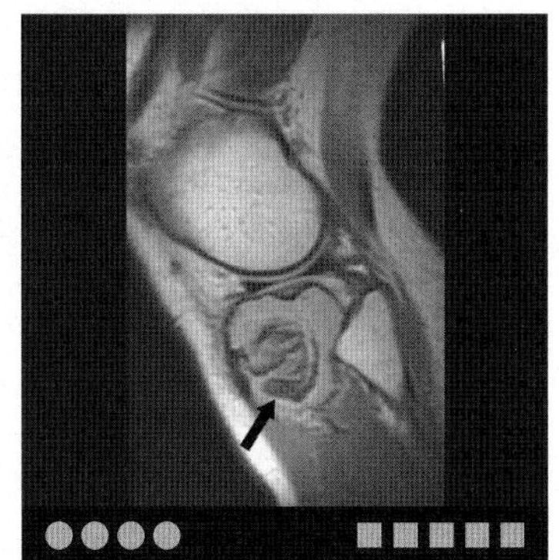

G. Giant cell tumor: Sagittal proton density MR shows hemosiderin deposition (arrow) and lesion extending proximally to articular surface.

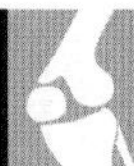

27–13 Chondromyxofibroma of Tibia

Albert Quan

PRESENTATION

Left leg pain

FINDINGS

Conventional radiography and computed tomography demonstrate a well-marginated, lobulated, lytic/lucent lesion with internal calcifications. MRI shows a heterogeneous, ovoid lesion located at the lateral aspect of the middiaphysis of the tibia.

DIFFERENTIAL DIAGNOSES

- *Aneurysmal bone cyst:* Fluid–fluid levels in an expansile lytic lesion. Periosteal bone formation may be present. However, no matrix mineralization is usually identified.
- *Adamantinoma:* Patients are more commonly elderly. Cortical destruction is evident. Periosteal reaction is not uncommon.
- *Fibroxanthoma:* There is no cortical protrusion or destruction. Periosteal reaction is rare unless there is a cortical fracture.
- *Giant cell tumor:* Eccentric and extending to the subchondral bone, this expansile lytic lesion does not typically demonstrate a matrix.

COMMENTS

The patient is a 37-year-old woman with left leg pain. As the least common benign cartilaginous lesion, chondromyxofibroma (CMF) comprises less than 1% of all primary bone tumors. Usually diagnosed by the age of 30 years (60%–75%), the clinical presentation includes focal swelling and pain, if symptomatic at all. There is a male predilection of up to 2:1 ratio in relation to females. Malignant transformation of CMF to chondrosarcoma is rare. Most commonly arising in the long bones (58%), CMF frequently is identified in the tibia, femur, and fibula and 40% to 55% occurs about the knee joint. CMF is geographic, eccentrically expansile, and usually located at the cortex. Although CMF is primarily metaphyseal, it may arise from the epiphysis or diaphysis. Matrix mineralization is rare. Pathological fractures occur at 2% to 5% of the time. Periosteal reaction occurs when there is either cortical "breakthrough" and/or pathological fracture. Conventional radiography and computed tomography classically demonstrate an ovoid, elongated, radiolucent, macrolobulated,

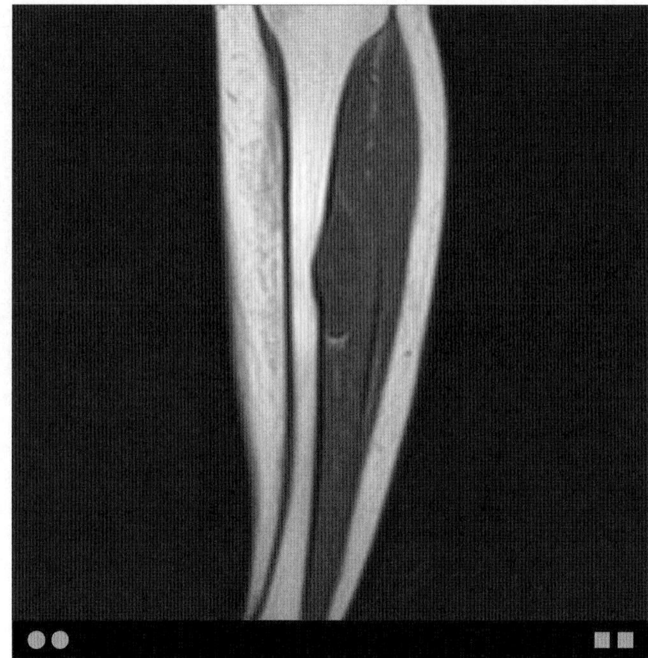

A. Chondromyxoid fibroma: Coronal T1-weighted image shows low–intermediate signal characteristics of this expansile lesion.

well-marginated lesion with a rim of sclerosis. Uncommonly, there may be complete cortical erosion/destruction and breakthrough of the cortex. Magnetic resonance imaging of CMF demonstrates signal intensity similar to or slightly lower than muscle on T1-weighted images; on T2-weighted images, the lesion is of high signal intensity.

PEARLS

- **CMF comprises 0.5% of all primary bone tumors; 2% of all benign bone tumors**
- **60% to 75% is identified by less than 30 years of age**
- **If symptomatic, presentation includes local swelling and pain**
- **It is a benign tumor; malignant transformation is rare**
- **Metaphysis (95%) of lower extremity, proximal tibia (30%)**
- **Eccentric, expansile, lucent lesion**
- **Matrix calcification is absent or very unusual**

ADDITIONAL IMAGES

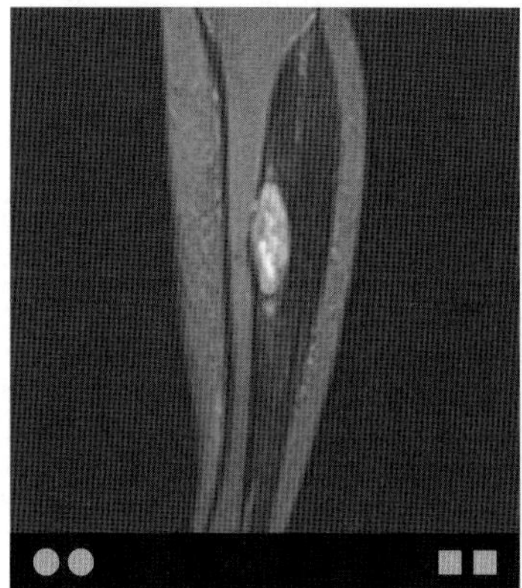

B. CMF: Coronal T2-weighted image shows the lesion is of intermediate–high signal.

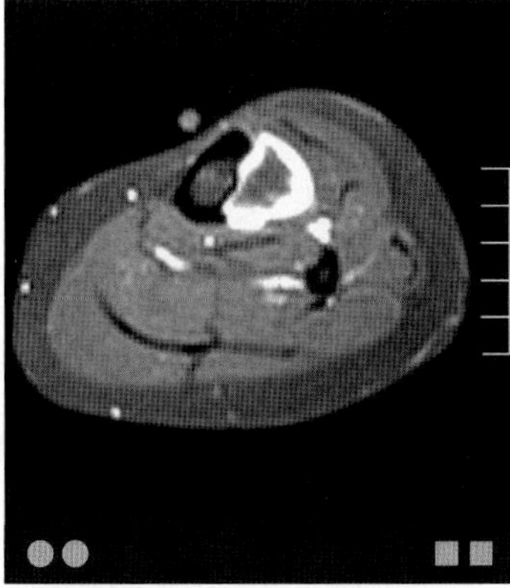

C. CMF: Axial contrast-enhanced T1-weighted fat-saturated image demonstrates peripheral enhancement as well as its erosive changes of the adjacent cortex.

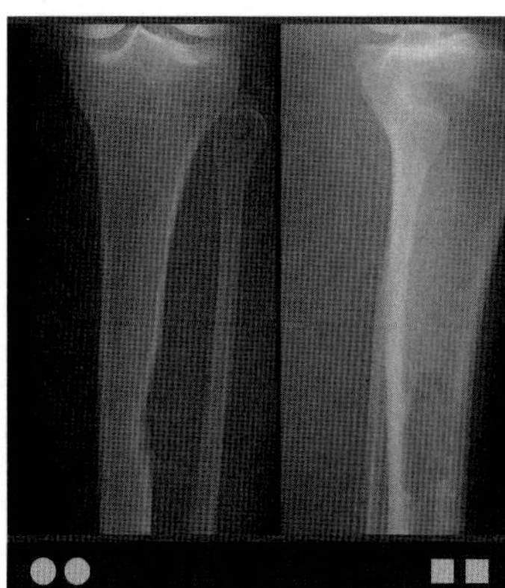

D. CMF: AP and lateral radiographs demonstrate a well-marginated, expansile, lytic lesion of the mid-shaft of the tibia.

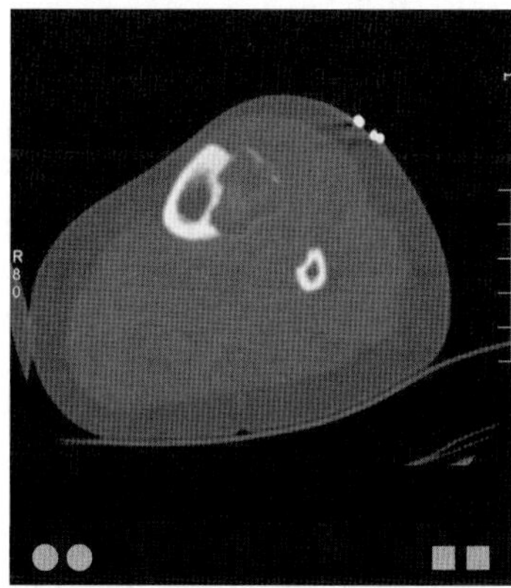

E. CMF: Axial computed tomography shows the lytic changes of the cortex as well as the expansile periosteal new bone formation.

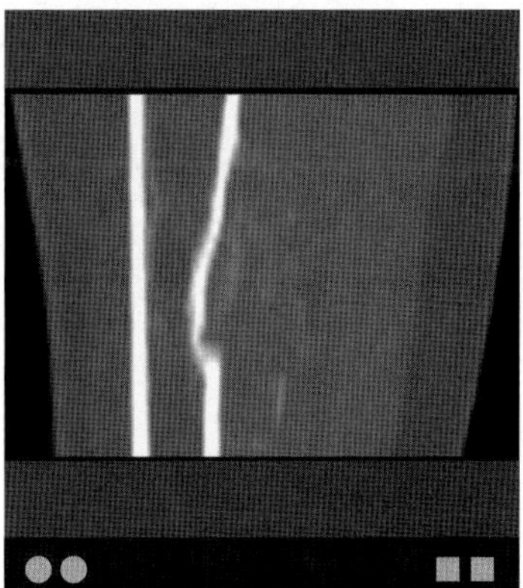

F. CMF: Coronal reformatted CT image demonstrates the lytic lesion of the tibial shaft with adjacent periosteal calcification.

IMAGE KEY

Common

Rare

Typical

Unusual

DIFFERENTIAL DIAGNOSIS IMAGE

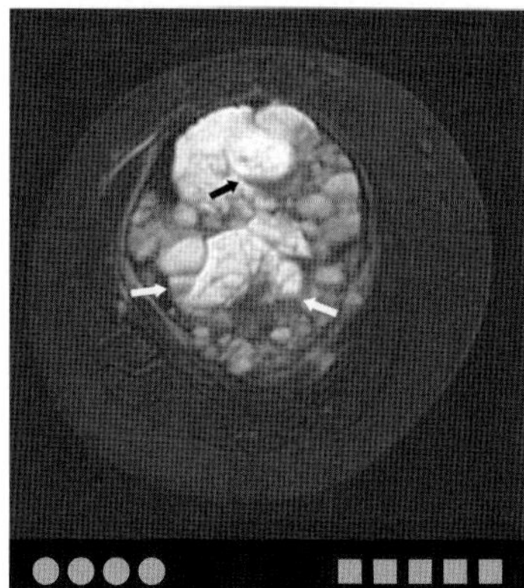

G. Aneurysmal bone cyst of tibia: Axial T2-weighted image shows numerous fluid–fluid levels filling lesion (arrows).

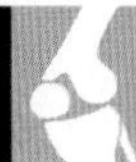

27–14 Pigmented Villonodular Synovitis of Knee

Ayodale S. Odulate and Piran Aliabadi

PRESENTATION

Episodic knee pain

FINDINGS

Extra- and intracapsular pigmented villonodular synovitis (PVNS) insinuating into the soft tissues and ligaments.

DIFFERENTIAL DIAGNOSES

- *Rheumatoid arthritis:* Polyarticular, erosions, cartilage space narrowing and soft tissue swelling.
- *Synovial chondromatosis:* Multiple small calcified bodies in the joint with thickened synovium.
- *Hemophilia:* Episodic spontaneous hemarthrosis that over time can lead to degenerative changes of the joint. A squared appearance of the patella and overgrowth of the epiphysis resulting from hyperemia is seen.
- *Tuberculosis arthritis:* Monoarticular, involving mainly large and medium sized joints. Usually diagnosis is made by synovial biopsy and culture.

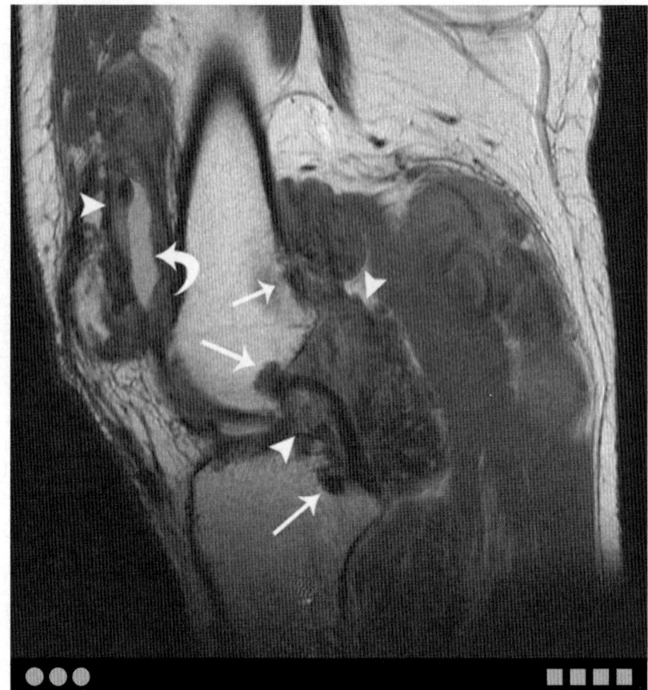

A. PVNS: Sagittal proton density image demonstrates hypertrophied synovium (arrowheads), joint effusion (curved arrow), and bone erosions (arrows), in this case of diffuse PVNS.

COMMENTS

The patient is a 29-year-old male with chronic episodic knee pain. Pigmented villonodular synovitis (PVNS) is a benign tumor of the synovium that can become locally aggressive most common in the knee, shoulder, and ankle. Two types of PVNS are described, diffuse and nodular. The diffuse form is much more common and associated with cystic changes of the joint and periarticular erosions. The nodular form of PVNS usually does not cause local destruction to the joint and diagnosis is difficult as a hemarthrosis may be the only finding. The etiology is unknown with an age range of 20 to 50 years. Patients often present clinically with swelling and pain of the joint. Early MRI findings include a synovial mass with hypointense T1–T2-weighted and proton density signal intensity with a joint effusion. The hypointense signal on T1-weighted imaging is felt to be as a result of hemosiderin deposition from multiple bouts of hemarthrosis. Isointense to hyperintense T2-weight signal intensity can also be seen secondary to the localized synovitis. During the early presentation of the disease, no cartilage space narrowing or destructive changes are present. Later in the course of the disease, cartilage space narrowing and pressure erosions in the bones from the hypertrophied synovium develop. The synovial mass can become locally aggressive and insinuate into surrounding tendons and ligaments. Imaging plays a crucial role in the diagnosis and direction of surgical management as the treatment is total synovectomy. If the mass is not completely resected, recurrence is likely. Synovectomy with curettage of the osseous component is required in diffuse form of PVNS.

PEARLS

- **Hyperplastic synovium in PVNS, large effusions, and bone erosions are characteristic**
- **Episodic haemarthrosis is characteristic in PVNS**

ADDITIONAL IMAGES

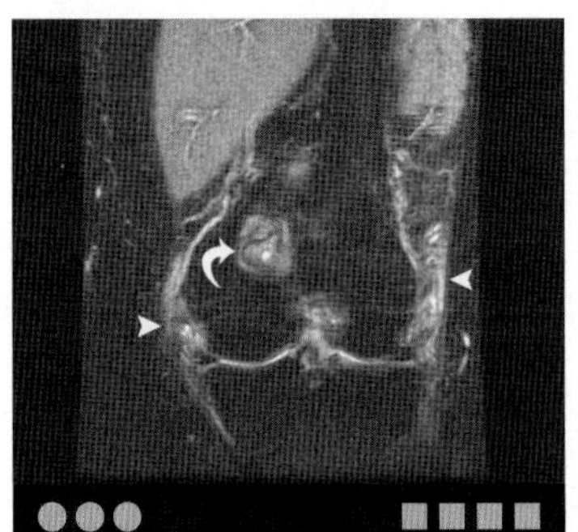

B. PVNS: Coronal STIR images demonstrate diffuse PVNS with soft tissue within erosions in the medial femoral condyle (curved arrow). Edema along the collateral ligaments (arrow) is seen.

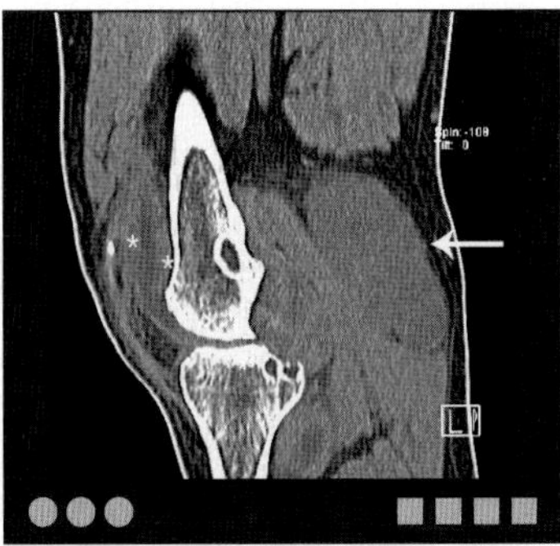

C. PVNS: Sagittal computed tomography (CT) from the same patient shows diffuse soft tissue masses in the posterior knee (arrow). Note the thickened synovium (asterisks).

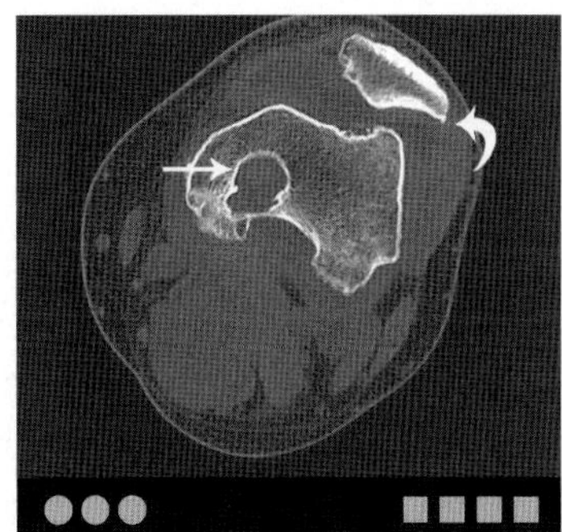

D. PVNS: Axial CT image with bone algorithm demonstrates the smooth erosion with a thin cortical margin (arrow) in the medial femoral condyle. Lateral subluxation of the patella (curved arrow) is noted.

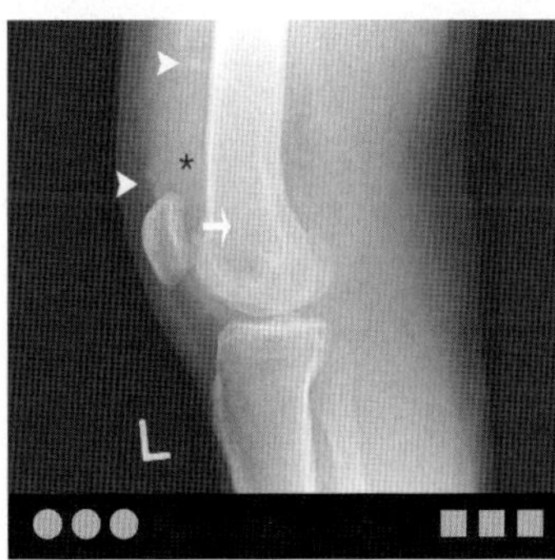

E. PVNS: Lateral radiograph from the same patient demonstrates a benign appearing lytic lesion in the distal femur (arrow) and joint effusion (asterisk). The calcifications (arrowheads) are not within the joint.

IMAGE KEY

Common

Rare

Typical

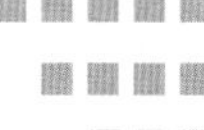

Unusual

DIFFERENTIAL DIAGNOSES IMAGES

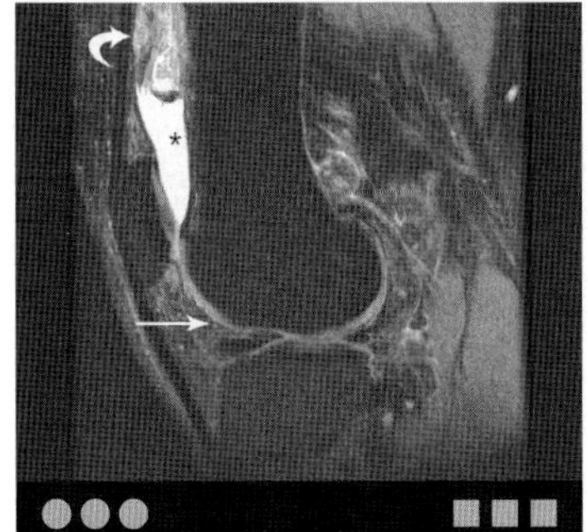

F. Rheumatoid knee: Sagittal STIR image demonstrates cartilage thinning (arrow), a joint effusion (asterisk), and synovial hypertrophy (curved arrow).

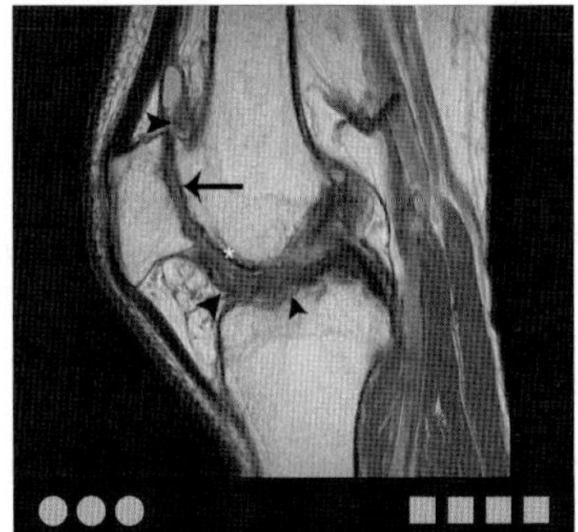

G. Hemophilic arthritis: Sagittal proton density image shows a squared patella (arrow), cartilage narrowing (asterisk), and hypointense thickened synovium (arrowheads).

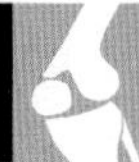

27–15 Osteochondroma of the Tibia

Hakan Ilaslan

PRESENTATION

Firm mass behind the knee and intermittent claudication

FINDINGS

Ossified mass originating from proximal tibia posteriorly noted showing corticomedullary continuity with underlying bone and overlying thin cartilage cap consistent with a sessile osteochondroma.

DIFFERENTIAL DIAGNOSES

- *Posttraumatic ossification:* Usually history of significant trauma is elicited. These lesions typically do not demonstrate corticomedullary continuity with underlying bone.
- *Parosteal osteosarcoma:* Although some of these tumors may demonstrate mature ossific matrix, absence of cartilage corticomedullary continuity and cartilage cap usually allows the differentiation.
- *Periosteal chondroma:* These lesions may simulate sessile osteochondroma in rare cases and frequently causes a saucer-like eroded area of the cortex, with a band of reactive sclerosis and a buttress of periosteal new bone. The lesion is demarcated from the medullary cavity by the intervening cortex of the bone, unlike an osteochondroma.

COMMENTS

The patient is a 17-year-old male presented with a firm mass behind the knee and intermittent claudication for approximately 1-year duration. Osteochondroma is by far the most common benign tumor of the bone. They are characterized by bony growths that project from the surface of the affected bone with overlying cartilage cap. These lesions could be solitary or multiple (multiple hereditary osteochondromatosis). The individual lesions of solitary and multiple osteochondromas are identical radiographically and pathologically. The tumors may be sessile or pedunculated. The exostosis or bony portion is produced by a progressive enchondral ossification of this growing cartilaginous cap. The cartilaginous portion of the osteochondroma acts as an enchondral plate for this abnormal growth and persists as long as there is growth activity. In the long bones, radiographs frequently provide satisfactory diagnostic information. Lesions in flat bones or complex anatomical locations such as scapula or pelvis may require confirmation with cross-sectional imaging, particularly MRI because of its ability to demonstrate cartilage cap and neurovascular structures. The growth usually stops when the growth plates are closed. Osteochondromas can be complicated by mechanical irritation, bursa formation, compression, injury of adjacent structures (i.e., nerves, vascular structures), fracture, malignant transformation, and recurrence after incomplete resection. Malignant transformation is the most worrisome complication that occurs in approximately 1% of solitary and 5% to 25% of multiple osteochondromas. Cartilage cap thicker than 2 cm, bony destruction, and associated soft tissue mass should raise the suspicion for malignant degeneration in a known osteochondroma.

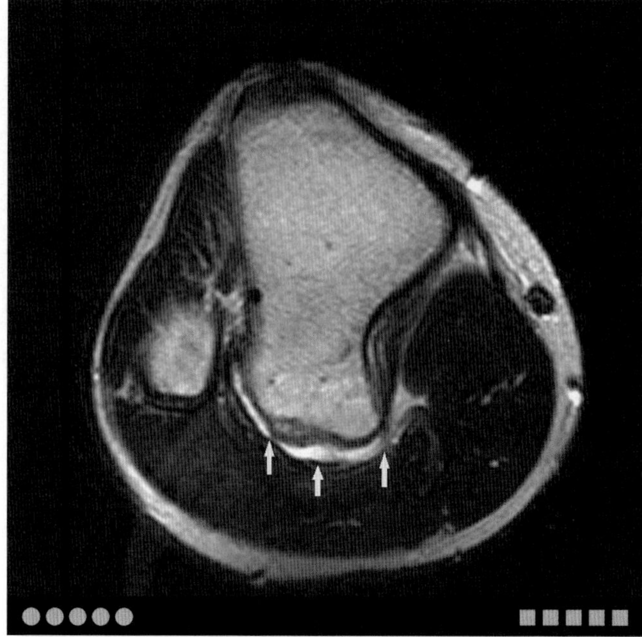

A. Osteochondroma of tibia: Axial T2-weighted image of the right knee demonstrates an ossific lesion with corticomedullary continuity and overlying thin, hyperintense rim of cartilage (arrows).

PEARLS

- **An ossified mass showing corticomedullary continuity with underlying bone is the typical imaging finding**
- **Radiographs are usually diagnostic for uncomplicated long bone lesions**
- **MRI is the preferred method to evaluate the lesions in the flat bones and diagnose complications**
- **Complications include mechanical irritation, bursa formation, compression, or injury of adjacent nerves and vascular structures, fracture, malignant transformation, and recurrence.**

ADDITIONAL IMAGES

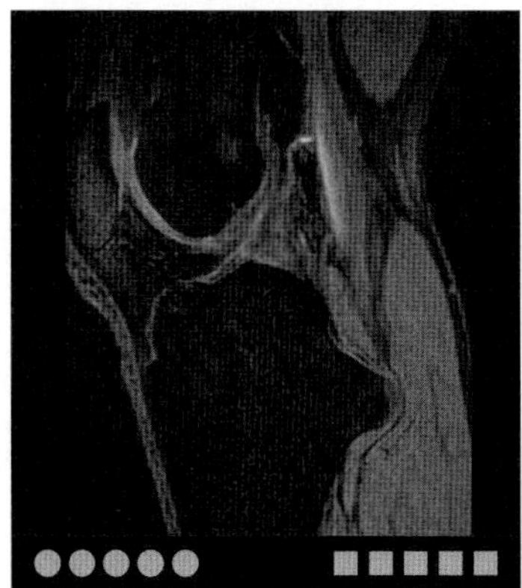

B. Osteochondroma of tibia: Sagittal gradient echo 3D image shows the extent of the lesion.

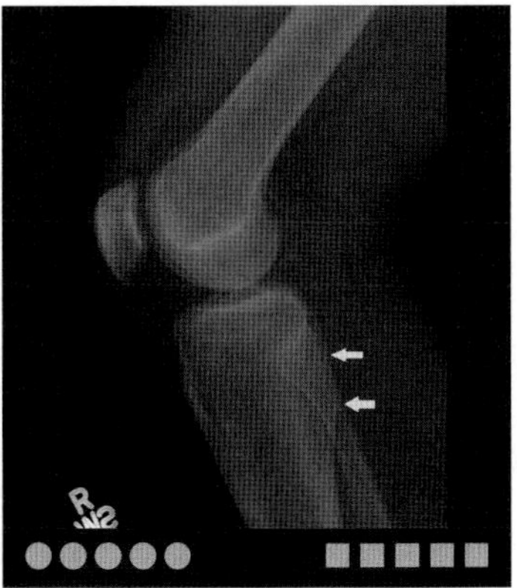

C. Osteochondroma of tibia: Lateral radiograph demonstrates the sessile osteochondroma posteriorly.

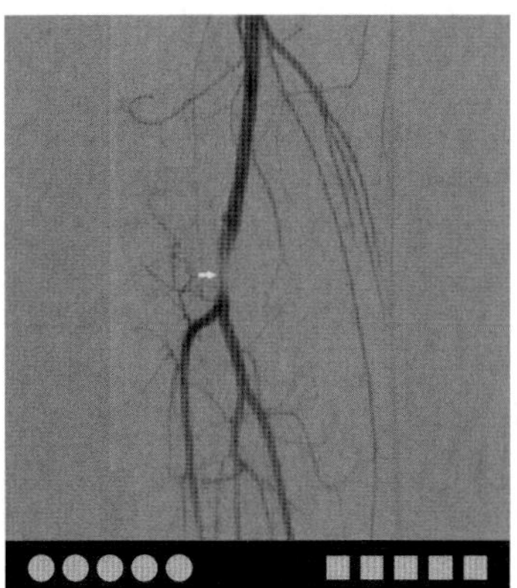

D. Osteochondroma of tibia: AP view of the knee with subtraction during an arteriogram demonstrates the compression of popliteal artery by the lesion proximal to the trifurcation (arrow).

IMAGE KEY

Common

Rare

Typical

Unusual

DIFFERENTIAL DIAGNOSES IMAGES

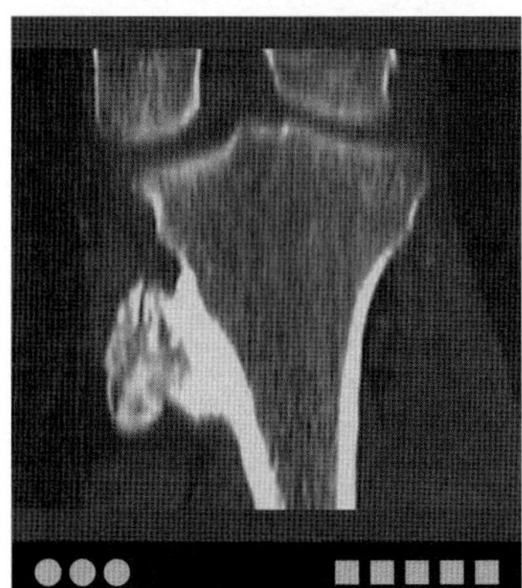

E. Parosteal osteosarcoma: Coronal reconstruction CT image of the knee shows an ossified surface tumor without corticomedullary continuity, typical of a parosteal osteosarcoma.

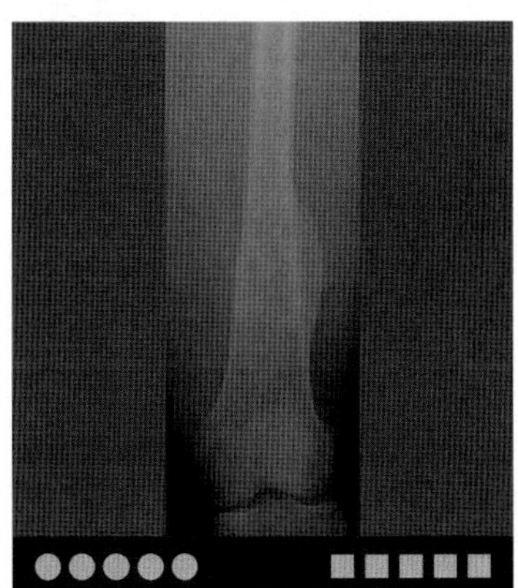

F. Posttraumatic subperiosteal heterotopic ossification: AP radiograph of the left knee shows an ossified mass associated with distal femur posteriorly.

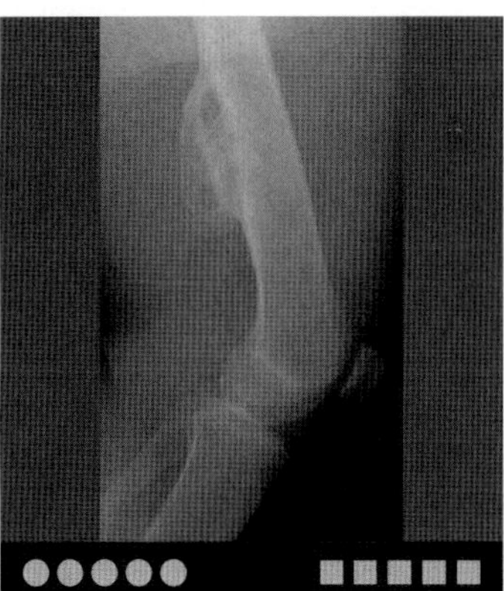

G. Posttraumatic subperiosteal heterotopic ossification: Lateral radiograph shows an ossified mass with smooth margin in the posterior distal femoral cortex. Bone scan (not shown) demonstrated only minimal uptake.

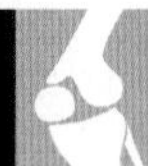

27–16 Bursitis Secondary to Osteochondroma

Marcia F. Blacksin

PRESENTATION

Palpable thigh mass and pain

FINDINGS

Osteochondroma originating from posterior femur, surrounded by a fluid-filled bursa.

DIFFERENTIAL DIAGNOSES

- *Myositis ossificans:* Also called heterotopic ossification, is a condition with new bone formation after trauma, paraplegia, or periods of immobilization. New bone begins to mineralize after a few weeks and lesions may adhere to adjacent bone.
- *Chondrosarcoma from osteochondroma:* Incidence of malignant degeneration of the cartilage cap is less than 1% with a single osteochondroma, but increases to approximately 20% with multiple hereditary exostoses.

COMMENTS

The diagnosis of osteochondroma can be made on radiography. The lesion usually grows perpendicular to the parent bone, with a continuous cortex and marrow cavity. The most common causes of pain are fracture through the neck of the osteochondroma, bursitis, or compression of a neurovascular bundle by the osteochondroma. Growth of the osteochondroma after skeletal maturity or a cartilage cap larger than 1.5 cm in thickness is associated with malignant degeneration into a chondrosarcoma or osteosarcoma. Comparison with prior radiographs can be useful in documenting a change in the pattern of matrix calcification in the cartilage cap. Cartilaginous matrix is characterized by a ring or broken ring pattern of calcification. The width of the cartilage cap can be easily measured on MR using proton density (PD) fat saturation (Fat Sat) fast spin echo (FSE) images, where the cartilage is intermediate in signal intensity, or gradient echo images where the cap is very bright in signal. Heterotopic ossification can be seen in patients with no history of trauma, and usually presents as a tender, painful soft tissue mass. Usually a zoning phenomenon is seen and the lesion ossifies from the periphery to the center. Imaging is best done with radiography or CT, where this phenomenon can be seen. MR can demonstrate aggressive signal characteristics, depending on the stage of maturation. Unless radiography is done, the lesion can be mistaken for a sarcoma.

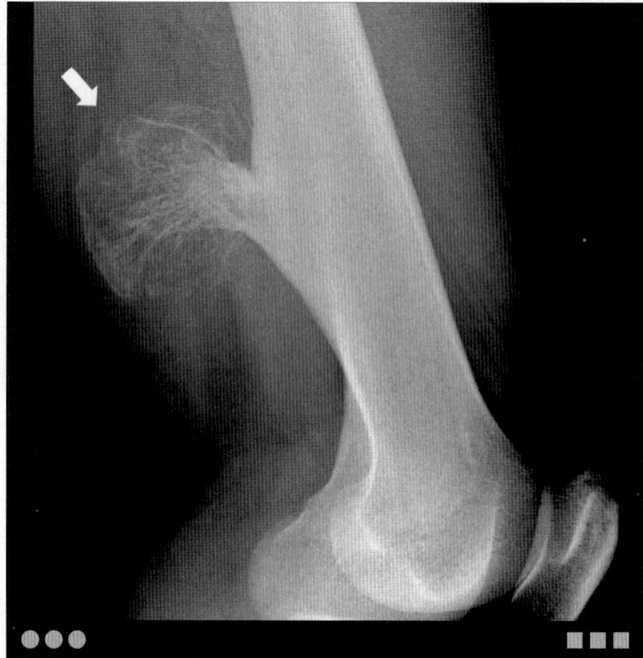

A. Bursitis secondary to osteochondroma: Sagittal radiograph of distal femur shows osteochondroma on posterior cortex, with no fractures (arrow).

PEARLS

- **Osteochondroma is a benign bone lesion that may have a cartilage cap. Pain can be caused by fracture, bursitis, or compression of surrounding structures.**
- **Malignant degeneration of a single osteochondroma is rare.**
- **Heterotopic ossification is new bone formation that may be adherent to the adjacent bone, and secondary to trauma, paraplegia, and periods of immobilization.**

ADDITIONAL IMAGES

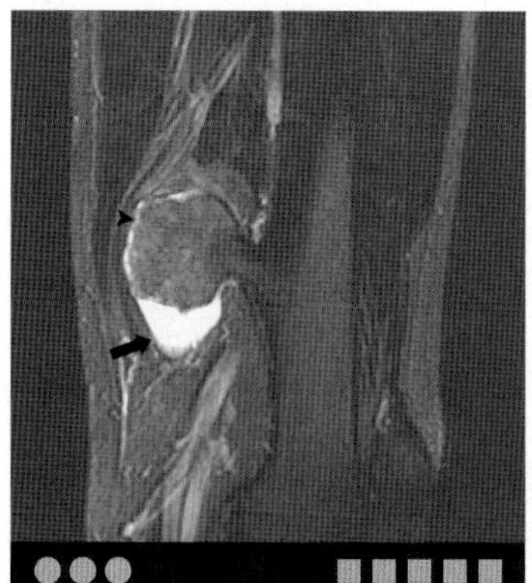

B. Bursitis secondary to osteochondroma: Sagittal fat-saturated T2-weighted MR shows osteochondroma surrounded by fluid-filled bursa (arrow). Thin intermediate signal cartilage cap (arrowhead) seen.

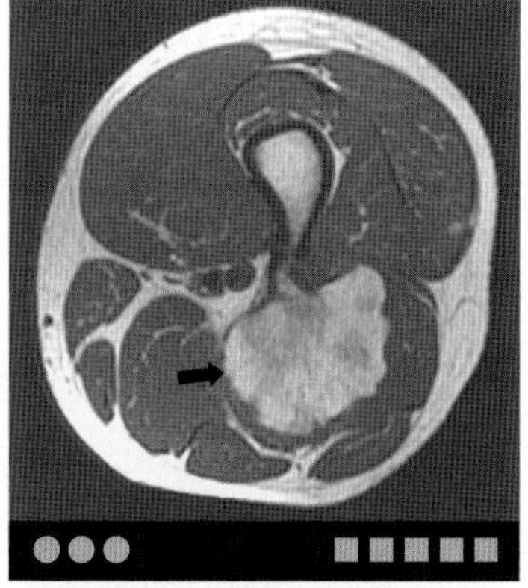

C. Bursitis secondary to osteochondroma: Axial T1-weighted MR shows osteochondroma (arrow) with signal intensity matching femoral marrow.

DIFFERENTIAL DIAGNOSES IMAGES

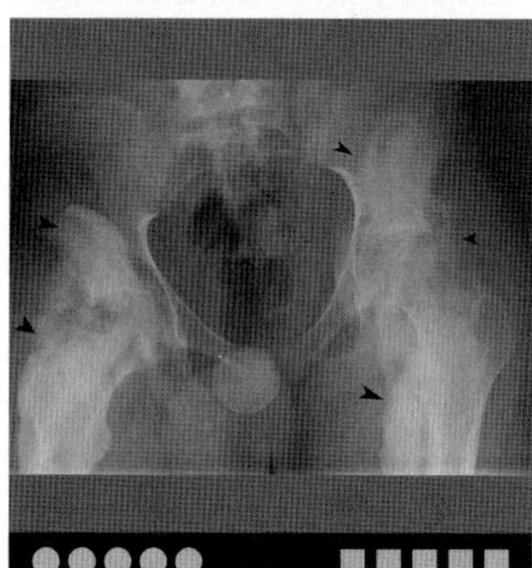

D. Heterotopic ossification: Pelvis radiograph of paraplegic with heterotopic ossification bridging both hips (arrowheads).

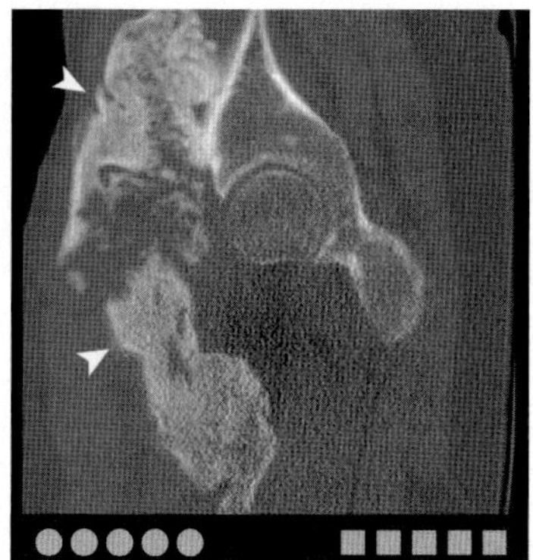

E. Heterotopic ossification: Sagittal CT reconstruction shows mature bone (arrowheads) bridging hip joint.

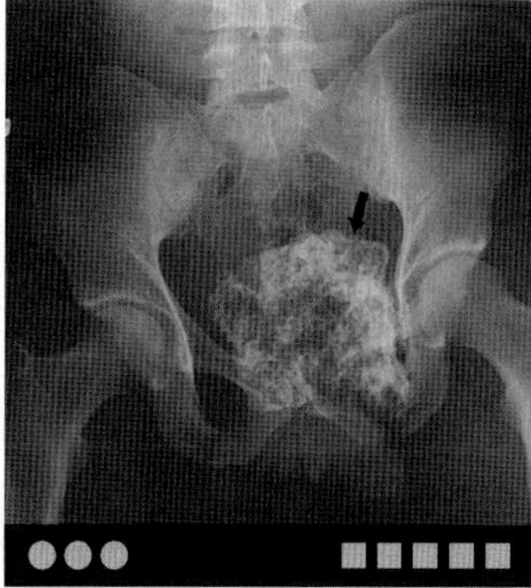

F. Osteochondroma with malignant degeneration: Radiograph of large osteochondroma (arrow) in pelvis. Recent change in lesion size is seen.

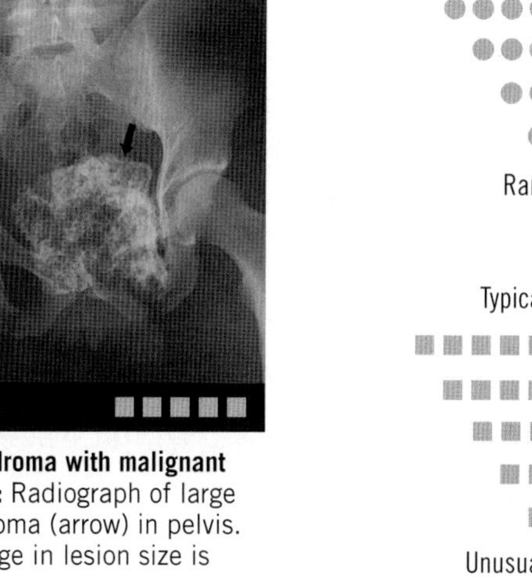

IMAGE KEY

Common

Rare

Typical

Unusual

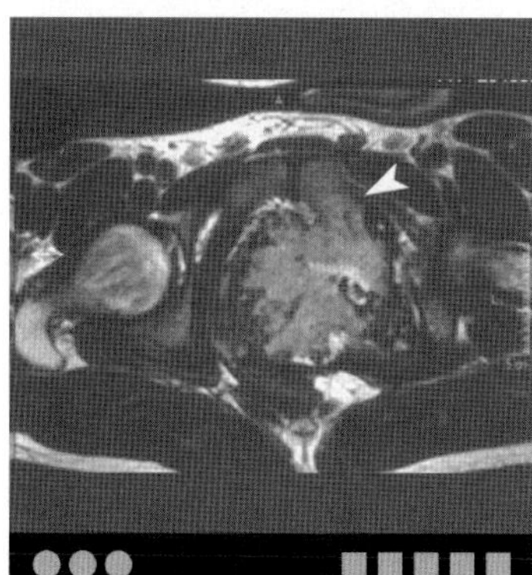

G. Osteochondroma with malignant degeneration: Axial T2-weighted MR of pelvis shows site of origination from posterior left pubic bone (arrow).

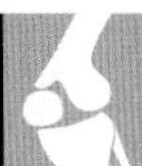

27–17 Chondroblastoma of the Knee

George Herman

PRESENTATION

Knee pain

FINDINGS

MRI shows abnormal signal changes at the medial aspect of the femoral condyle surrounded with inflammation.

DIFFERENTIAL DIAGNOSES

- *Giant cell tumor:* It may originate at the epiphysis of the mature skeleton.
- *Infection:* This usually occurs in the metaphysis but it may be situated in the epiphysis of the young child.
- *Clear cell chondrosarcoma:* It may contain cartilaginous tissue and also giant cells similar to chondroblastoma.
- *Osteoid osteoma or osteoblastoma:* These are relatively rare tumors at the epiphysis. In this case it shows decreased SI both on T1- and T2-weighted images.

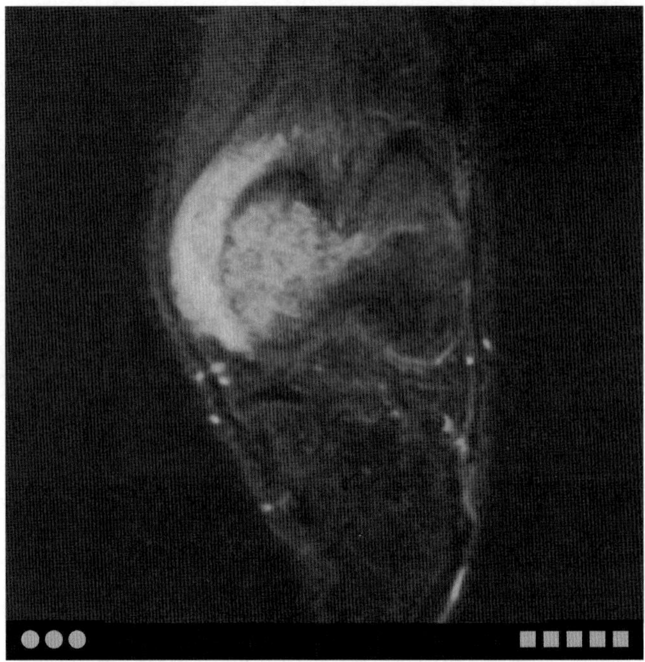

A. Chondroblastoma: MRI on coronal STIR image shows bright SI, which involves the medial aspect of the distal femoral condyle. Note the edema around the condyle.

COMMENTS

The patient is a 16-year-old boy complaining of chronic pain and swelling of the left knee. He was diagnosed with chondroblastoma. Chondrobastoma is a rare benign cartilaginous tumor that includes approximately 1% of all bone tumors. The most common location is the epiphysis of the long bones such as the knee, followed by the proximal humerus, tibia, in decreasing frequency. It may involve the hands, feet, and rarely the axial skeleton. In the majority of cases chondroblastoma occurs in the second decade of life; however, it may be seen in patients younger than 5 years of age and also over 60 years of age. The male/female ratio is approximately 2:1. On radiograph chondroblastoma characteristically appears as an osteolytic lesion located at the epiphysis. The lesion is generally round and measures less than 5 cm in diameter. It is surrounded with a thin sclerotic rim. The tumor is usually confined to the epiphysis but it may extend to the subarticular bone and/or the metaphysis (25–35%); metaphyseal origin is extremely rare. In less than half of the cases calcification may be detected within the lesion. Periosteal reaction in the adjacent metaphysis may be observed in 40% to 50% of the cases. Radiograph may show lytic lesion at the epiphysis. MRI on T1-weighted image demonstrates low SI. On T2-weighted image the SI is generally decreased owing to the presence of cellular stroma. Occasionally, however, the SI is high on T2-weighted image as a result of the inflammatory process that occurs around chondroblastoma.

PEARLS

- **Chondroblastoma typically involves the epiphysis.**
- **Periosteal reaction is unusual in tumorous processes of the epiphysis. It occurs in up to 50% of the cases of chondroblastoma.**
- **MRI usually shows decreased SI on T1-weighted image. On T2-weighted image it may show decreased SI depending on the amount of cellular stroma.**

ADDITIONAL IMAGES

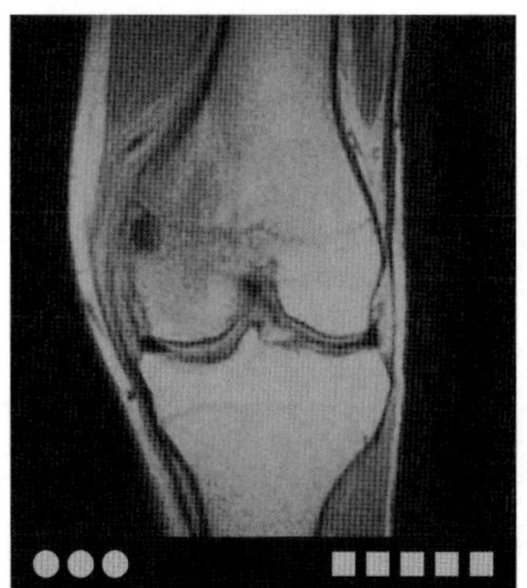

B. Chondroblastoma: MRI on coronal T1-weighted image. There is a decreased SI lesion confined to the medial femoral condyle.

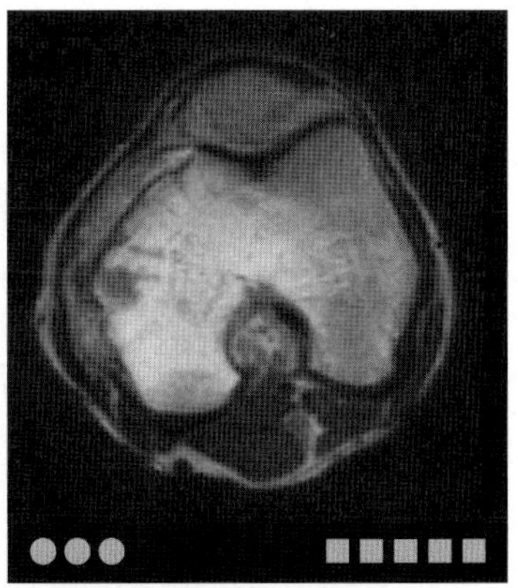

C. Chondroblastoma: Axial STIR image shows well-defined decreased SI at the medial condyle.

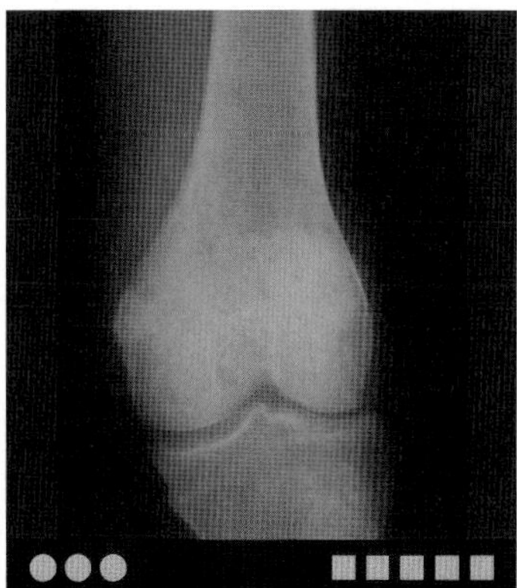

D. Chondroblastoma: AP radiograph of the knee reveals a small lesion at the medial femoral condyle. Note the reactive periosteal reaction extending to the metaphysis.

IMAGE KEY

Common

Rare

Typical

Unusual

DIFFERENTIAL DIAGNOSES IMAGES

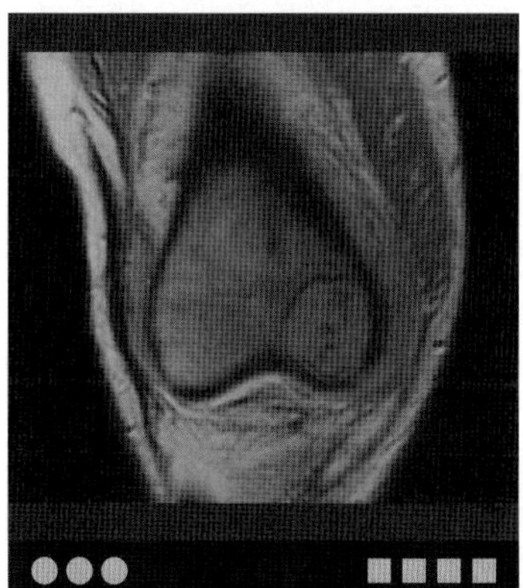

E. Osteoid osteoma: Coronal T1-weighted image reveals decreased SI at the medial condyle.

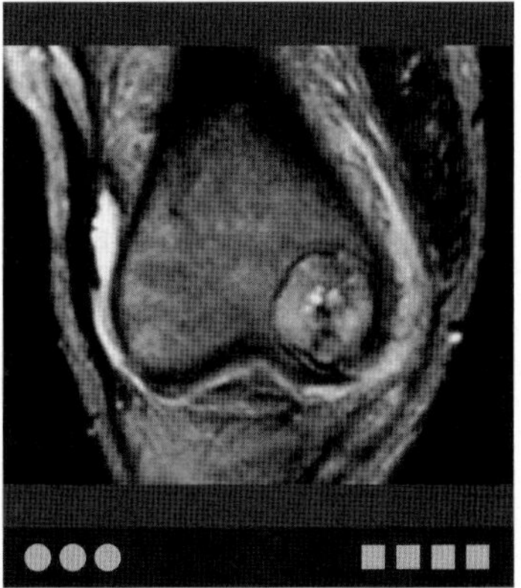

F. Osteoid osteoma: Coronal T2-weighted image reveals increased SI at the medial condyle with central calcification.

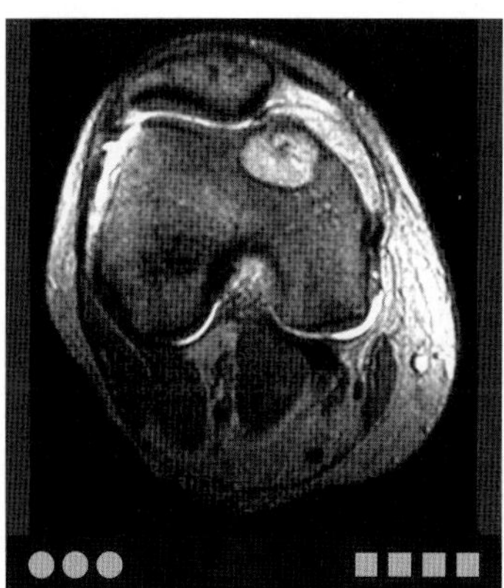

G. Osteoid osteoma: Axial T2-weighted image shows increased SI at the medial condyle with central calcification.

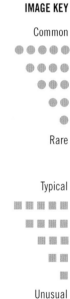

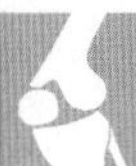

27–18 Osteoid Osteoma of Tibia

Jimmy Ton and Jamshid Tehranzadeh

PRESENTATION

Chronic leg pain and muscle wasting

FINDINGS

MR images show edema with periosteal elevation and a round target shaped lesion in the cortical defect of medial proximal tibia.

DIFFERENTIAL DIAGNOSES

- *Osteomyelitis:* Focal subacute osteomyelitis (Brodie's abscess) may present similar picture. However, the sclerotic margin in infection has a fuzzy border on radiograph.
- *Stress fracture:* Periosteal new bone formation and sclerosis in stress fracture are associated with a line of low signal intensity surrounded by bone edema.
- *Osteoblastoma:* These lesions are histologically very similar to osteoid osteoma; however, they are larger than 1.5 cm in size.
- *Ewing sarcoma:* Has larger soft tissue mass, larger bony lesion, and more aggressive periosteal reaction.

COMMENTS

Osteoid osteoma is a benign skeletal neoplasm that accounts for approximately 12% of all benign bone tumors. The tumor occurs most frequently in patients between 10 and 30 years of age and is twice as prevalent in males as in females. Although the tumor can occur in any bone, it frequently involves the metaphysis or diaphysis of long bones (e.g., proximal tibia and femoral neck) and of the spine. Approximately 80% of the tumor involves cortical bone with the remaining being intramedullary. Clinically, patients with osteoid osteoma present with severe focal skeletal pain that is exacerbated with exertion or at night. This pain has been attributed to prostaglandin secretion by the tumor and can be relieved by aspirin because of antiprostaglandin effect. Spine involvement can result in painful scoliosis. On CT, osteoid osteoma appears as a radiolucent circular or ovoid lesion with a sclerotic center. Lesions that are cortical or subperiosteal in location exhibit more surrounding sclerosis than those that are intramedullary. The nidus typically enhances with IV contrast. On MR imaging, the nidus appears as an area of high signal intensity on T2-weighted images. The surrounding sclerosis is of low signal intensity on both T1- and T2-weighted images. Soft tissue and bone marrow edema and periosteal reaction are also frequently seen. Moreover, patients with intra-articular involvement might exhibit joint effusions on MR and are prone to develop early osteoarthrosis.

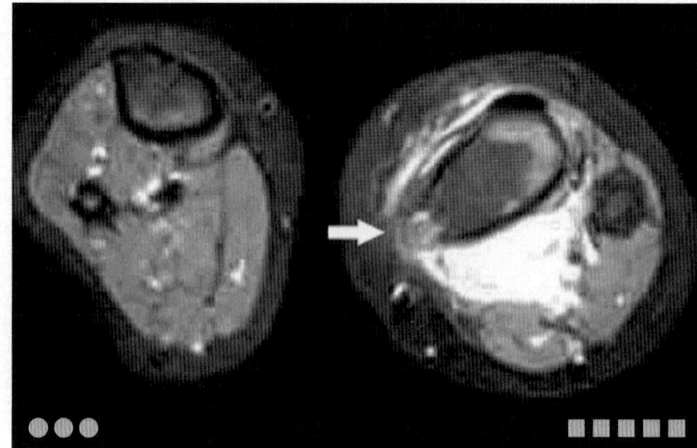

A. Osteoid osteoma of the proximal tibia: Axial fat-saturated proton density image shows marked edema of the soft tissue surrounding the left tibia, more posteriorly. There is a focal area of cortical defect with intermediate signal intensity and a target appearance in the medial cortex of the proximal tibia (arrow) suggesting osteoid osteoma. Note periosteal elevation of the anterior tibial cortex.

PEARLS

- **Osteoid osteoma is a benign osteoid tumor of the bone involving patients between the ages of 10 and 30 years. It is two times more common among the male patients.**
- **Osteoid osteoma frequently involves the cortical portion of the metaphysis or diaphysis of long bones.**
- **Cortical or periosteal osteoid osteoma exhibits more surrounding sclerosis, while cancellous locations often lack bone density.**
- **MR shows a nidus of high signal intensity on T2-weighted image with sclerosis that is of low signal intensity on both T1- and T2-weighted images.**

ADDITIONAL IMAGES

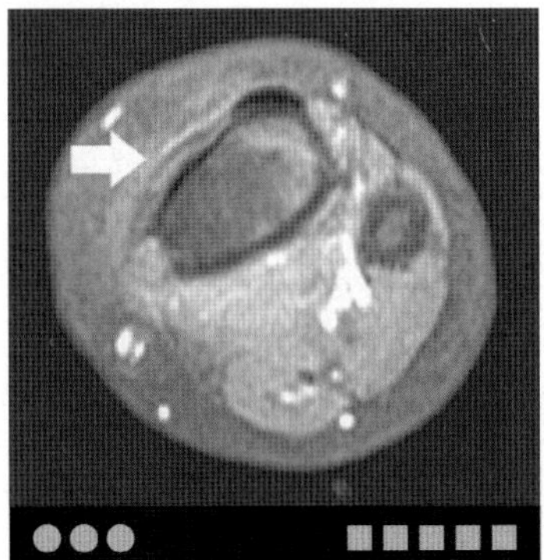

B. Osteoid osteoma of the proximal tibia: Axial spin-echo fat-saturated T1 image shows there is cortical break in the medial aspect of the tibia with a black line of periosteal elevation (arrow).

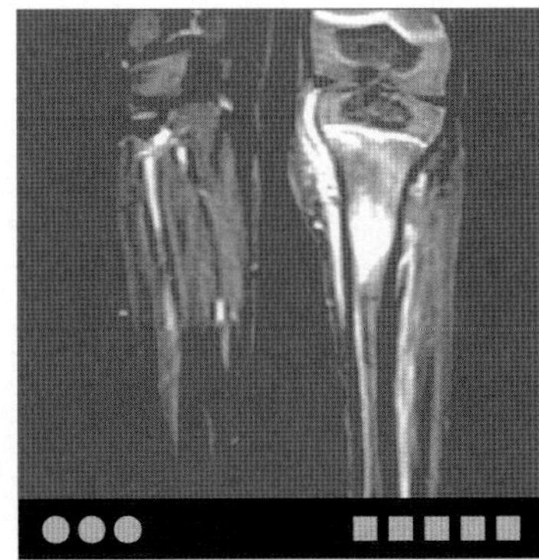

C. Osteoid osteoma of the proximal tibia: Coronal T1 fat-saturated post-contrast image shows periosteal enhancement of the medial aspect of the tibia and proximal diaphysis.

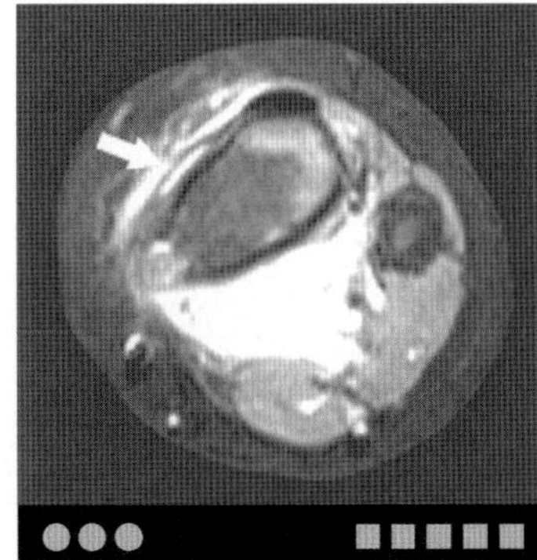

D. Osteoid osteoma of the proximal tibia: Axial fat-saturated proton density image, which is a close up of image A, shows periosteal elevation (arrow) as a black line in the center of anterior soft tissue edema.

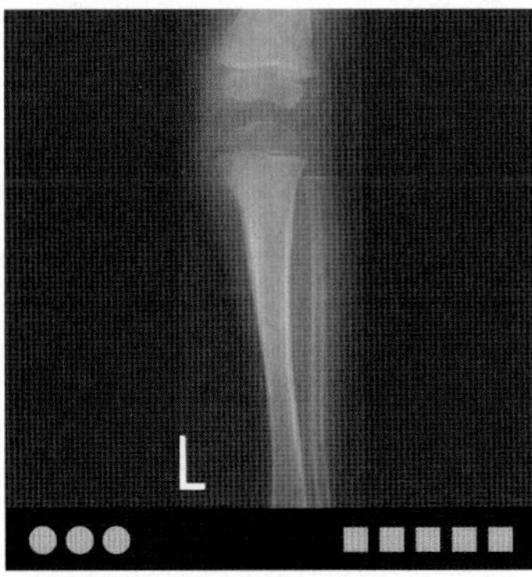

E. Osteoid osteoma of the proximal tibia: AP radiograph of the tibia shows cortical irregularity of the proximal medial tibia with adjacent sclerosis.

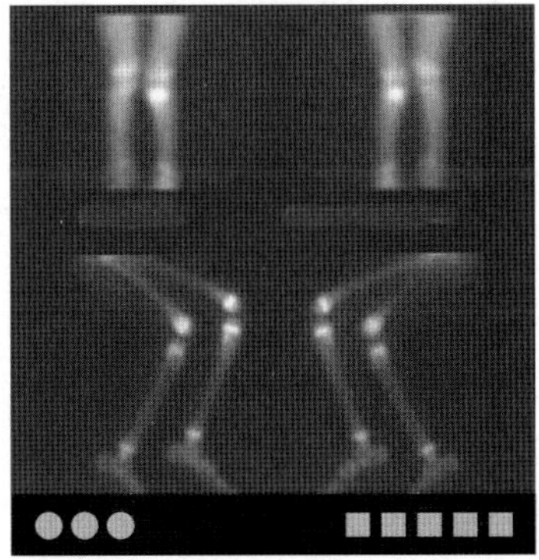

F. Osteoid osteoma of the proximal tibia: Technitium99m methylenediphosphonate bone scan shows increased radionuclide uptake in the left proximal tibia.

DIFFERENTIAL DIAGNOSIS IMAGE

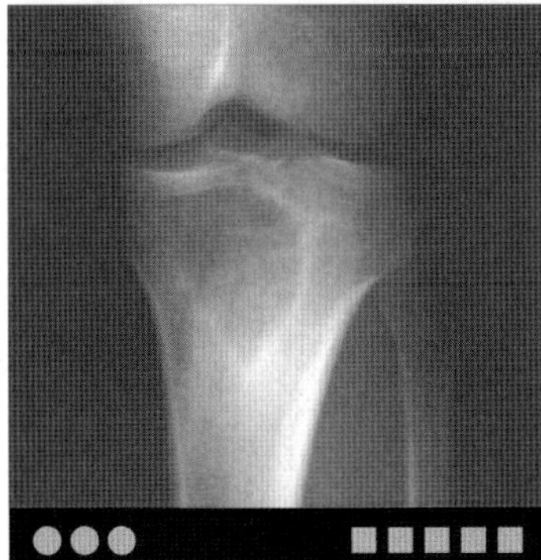

G. Brodie's abscess of the proximal tibia: AP radiograph of the proximal tibia shows osteolytic lesion with marginal sclerosis. Note that the fuzziness of the sclerosis surrounding the lesion fades away into the normal bone.

IMAGE KEY

Common

Rare

Typical

Unusual

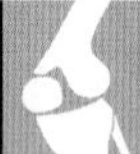

27–19 Medullary Osteoid Osteoma

Janis Owen

PRESENTATION

Pain

FINDINGS

There is a circumscribed lesion in the right distal femur metaphysis posteriorly. The lesion is low/intermediate signal on the T1-weighted, high/intermediate signal on the T2-weighted, and high signal on the gradient echo images with a central low signal area on all sequences.

DIFFERENTIAL DIAGNOSES

- *Osteoblastoma:* There is a similar appearance radiographically and pathologically with the osteoblastoma being larger in size than the osteoid osteoma.
- *Osteomyelitis:* There is low signal on T1-weighted and a high signal on T2-weighted sequences consistent with fluid and no mass present. Sequestra in the area may simulate calcifications.
- *Intraosseous lipoma:* The lesion is radiolucent radiographically with a thin sclerotic rim. A central calcification or ossified nidus is common.

COMMENTS

The patient is a 30-year-old female, who presented with right knee pain. Osteoid osteoma is a benign tumor of bone that generally involves the cortex. It may also be subperiosteal, intra-articular, or medullary (cancellous) in location. The subperiosteal and medullary locations do not cause the reactive sclerosis seen in the cortical form. Diagnosis occurs in the first through third decades. The lesion is three times more common in males than females. The usual history is pain that is worst at night and ameliorated by salicylates. The occurrence of osteoid osteomas in the long tubular bones is 71% and at the knee it is 50% to 60%. Radiographically, osteoid osteoma is a lytic nidus surrounded by reactive bone sclerosis. The nidus may or may not contain calcifications. In the medullary and subperiosteal forms, the reactive bone formation if present is often away from the nidus. The cortical form is diaphyseal, while the subperiosteal and medullary forms are metaphyseal in location. When osteoid osteoma is intra-articular, it will produce synovitis and effusion. The lesions show uptake on nuclear bone scan and the nidus will show uptake on gallium scan. CT is beneficial in demonstrating the lesions and nidus calcifications and is the modality of choice. MRI shows an intermediate signal mass with internal low signal areas when calcifications are present. Osteoid osteomas enhance following the administration of gadolinium contrast material.

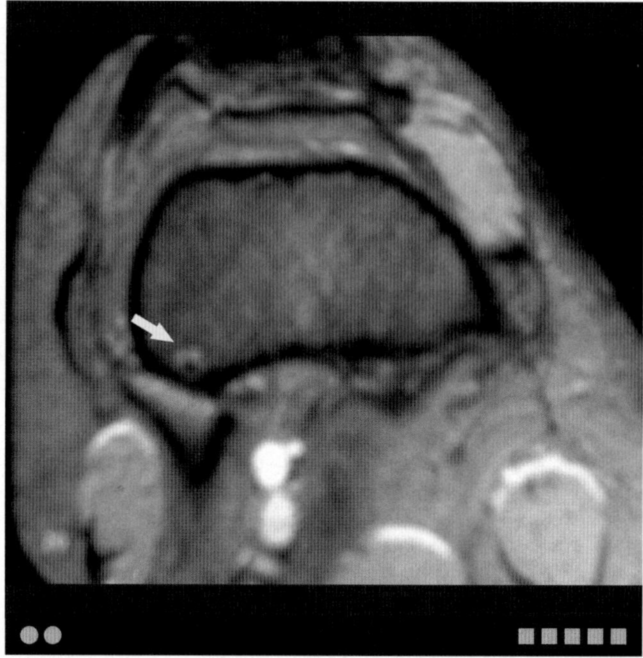

A. Medullary osteoid osteoma: Axial gradient echo sequence shows a high/intermediate signal lesion with a central low signal (arrow).

PEARLS

- **Medullary osteoid osteoma is metaphyseal lesion in tubular bones.**
- **Reactive sclerosis is absent in medullary type.**
- **Low/intermediate signal on T1, intermediate/high signal on T2-weighted images are noted.**
- **Central calcification is seen.**

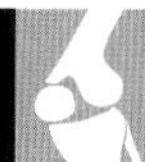

ADDITIONAL IMAGES

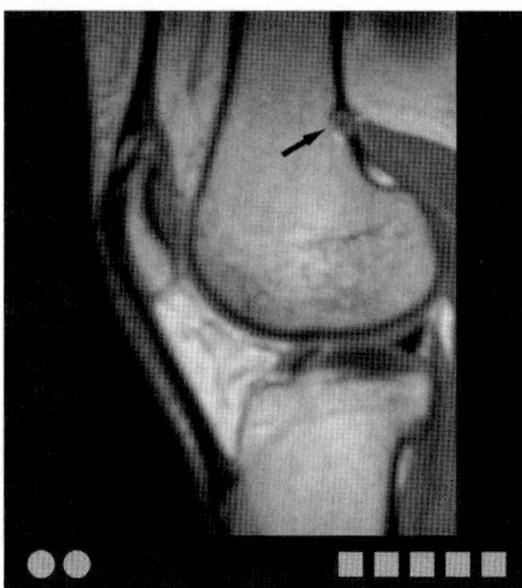

B. Medullary osteoid osteoma: Sagittal T2-weighted sequence shows a high/intermediate signal lesion with a low signal calcification (arrow).

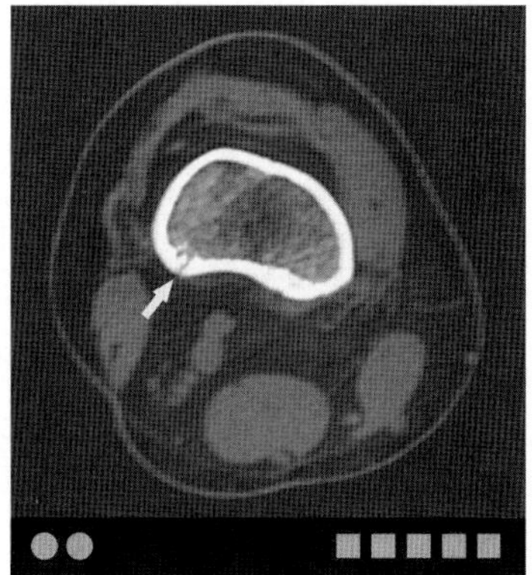

C. Medullary osteoid osteoma: Axial CT shows the lesion with central calcification and absent reactive sclerosis (arrow).

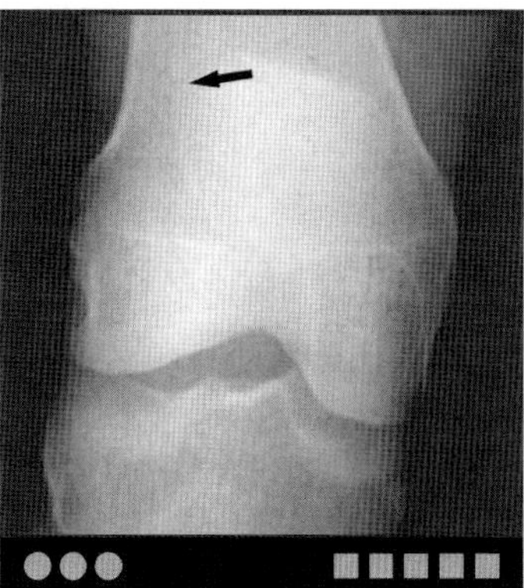

D. Medullary osteoid osteoma: AP right knee shows a geographic lytic lesion with a central calcification (arrow).

DIFFERENTIAL DIAGNOSES IMAGES

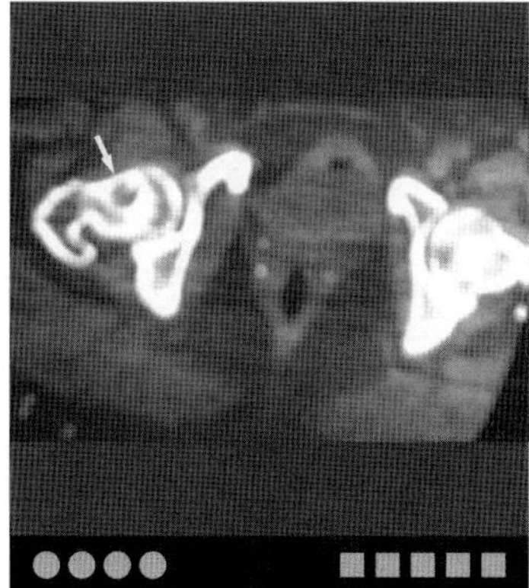

E. Osteoblastoma: CT shows a low density geographic lesion in the femur neck with internal mineralization (arrow).

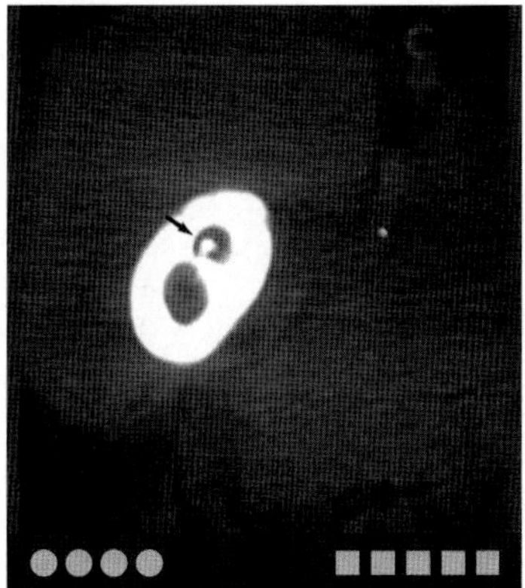

F. Chronic osteomyelitis: Axial CT of the right proximal femur shows a sequestrum (arrow) and involucrum.

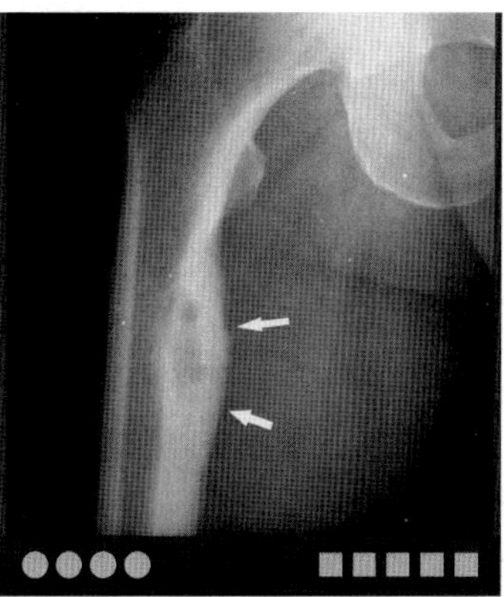

G. Chronic osteomyelitis: AP right femur shows an irregular lytic lesion with surrounding cortical periosteal reactions (arrows).

IMAGE KEY

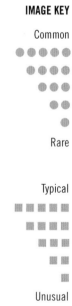

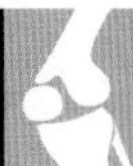

27–20 Cortical Desmoid (Cortical Avulsive Injury)

Raymond Kuo and Rajeev K. Varma

PRESENTATION

Asymptomatic or aching pain

FINDING

Cortical erosion of 1 to 3 cm, irregularity, and periostitis are noted at the posteromedial femoral metaphysis.

DIFFERENTIAL DIAGNOSES

- *Osteoid osteoma:* Cortical-based sclerotic lesion with cortical thickening and possible visible nidus are noted.
- *Parosteal osteosarcoma:* Originates at distal femur or proximal tibia. A dense bony mass separated from the cortex by a thin gap, attached at a stalk or base.
- *Osteosarcoma/other malignancy:* Often but not always with a more destructive appearance with soft tissue mass.

COMMENTS

Previously known as cortical desmoid, this entity is now more accurately referred to as cortical avulsive injury or cortical irregularity syndrome. The lesion most commonly occurs in older children, adolescents at the posteromedial femoral metaphysis, likely secondary to repetitive trauma at the attachment of the adductor magnus muscle or medial head of the gastrocnemius. Other sites include the proximal tibia, medial aspect of the proximal humerus, and distal radius. This lesion is most notable for simulating an aggressive tumor, both radiologically and histopathologically. Unfortunately its deceptive features mimicking malignancy have resulted in amputation; high T2 signal may incorrectly raise the concern for malignancy. The location of the lesion is the key discriminating sign. The diagnosis is preferentially made on conventional radiographs or CT. On radiograph, the lesion measures 1 to 3 cm in size and is irregular with areas of lucency and sclerosis. CT demonstrates a complex lesion surrounded by a mild sclerotic reaction. There may be areas of cortical thinning and thickening, with possible small cystic areas. Bone scintigraphy is generally normal; however, there may be uptake during the early reactive stages. MRI demonstrates low signal intensity on T1 and high signal on T2-weighted images and occasional low signal rim. Ages of involvement range from 3 to 20 years, and are most common in the early teen years. Most commonly the patients are male, with female patients increasingly common, especially those involved in sports.

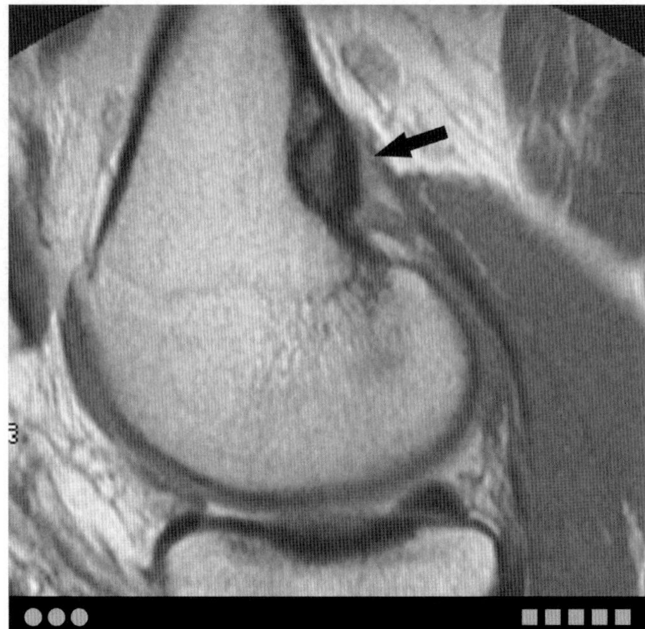

A. Cortical avulsive injury: Sagittal T1-weighted images of a cortical desmoid in the characteristic location in the posterior distal femur (arrow) shows a low signal area of sclerosis with irregular margins at the attachment site of the medial gastrocnemius muscle.

PEARLS

- **Best diagnosed on conventional radiograph**
- **Location of the lesion is the key to correct diagnosis**
- **A "leave alone" lesion as biopsy may lead to the erroneous histologic diagnosis of osteosarcoma.**

ADDITIONAL IMAGES

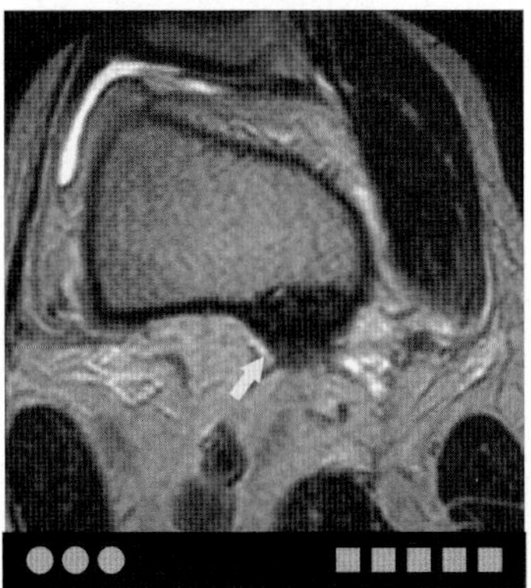

B. Cortical avulsive injury: Axial T2-weighted image shows cortical desmoid (arrow).

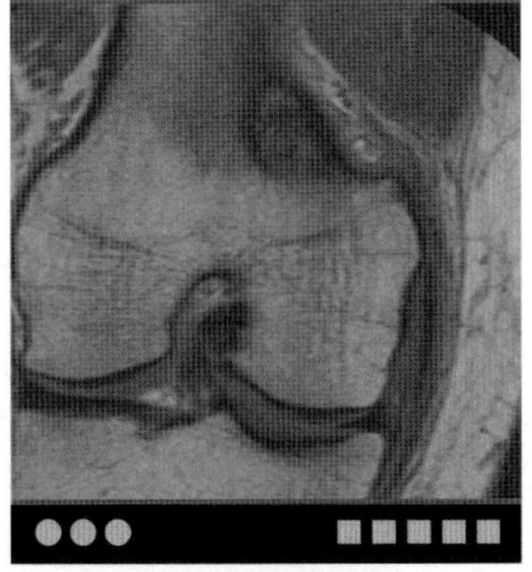

C. Cortical avulsive injury: Coronal T1-weighted image shows cortical desmoid.

DIFFERENTIAL DIAGNOSES IMAGES

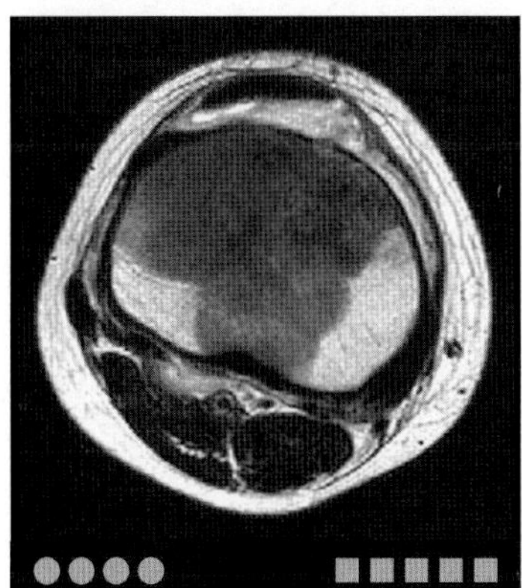

D. Osteosarcoma: Axial T1-weighted image of an osteosarcoma demonstrates an infiltrative low signal lesion involving the majority of the tibial plateau.

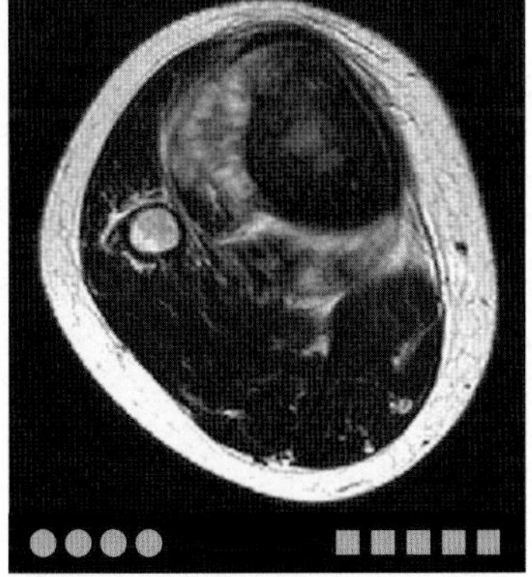

E. Osteosarcoma: Axial T2-weighted image at a more inferior level shows abnormal low signal throughout the replaced tibial marrow. The thick high-signal rim posterolaterally represents an invasive soft tissue mass. Note the radial sunburst pattern within the soft tissue extension.

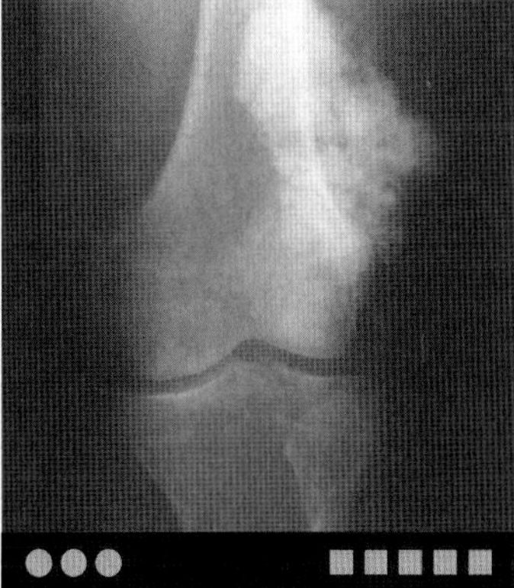

F. Parosteal osteosarcoma: AP radiograph of the knee shows a large irregular sclerotic mass at the distal femur.

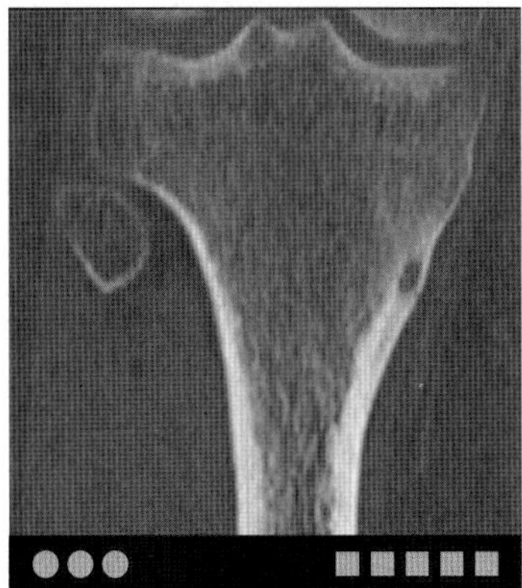

G. Osteoid osteoma: Coronal CT shows a focal radiolucent lesion (nidus) in the medial proximal tibial cortex with central calcification and adjacent reactive sclerosis.

IMAGE KEY

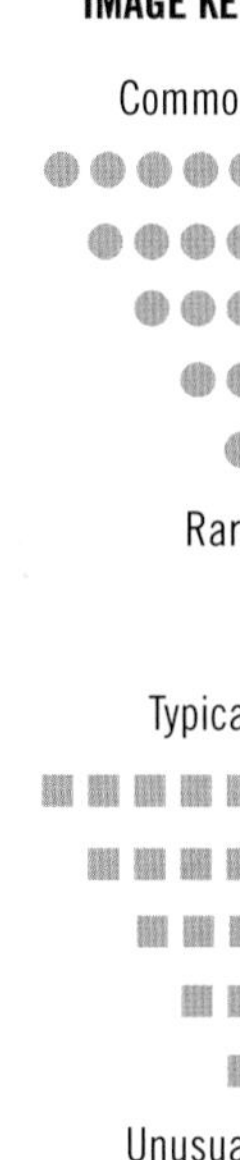

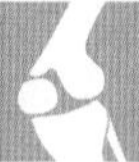

27–21 Fibrous Cortical Defect/Nonossifying Fibroma of the Tibia

Michelle Chandler

PRESENTATION

Incidental finding or pain and swelling

FINDINGS

Radiograph evaluation of the proximal tibia demonstrates a focal area of cortical lucency and expansion in the proximal tibial metaphysis.

DIFFERENTIAL DIAGNOSES

- *Simple bone cyst:* The "fallen fragment sign" indicating a fragment of bone loose within the central fluid-filled cavity of this lesion is typically noted when this lesion is discovered after pathologic fracture.
- *Aneurysmal bone cyst:* This lesion is actually composed of multiple eccentric expansile locules that may be associated with periosteal reaction or pathologic fracture.
- *Fibrous dysplasia:* This expansile lesion is typically medullary in location as opposed to a cortically based lesion.

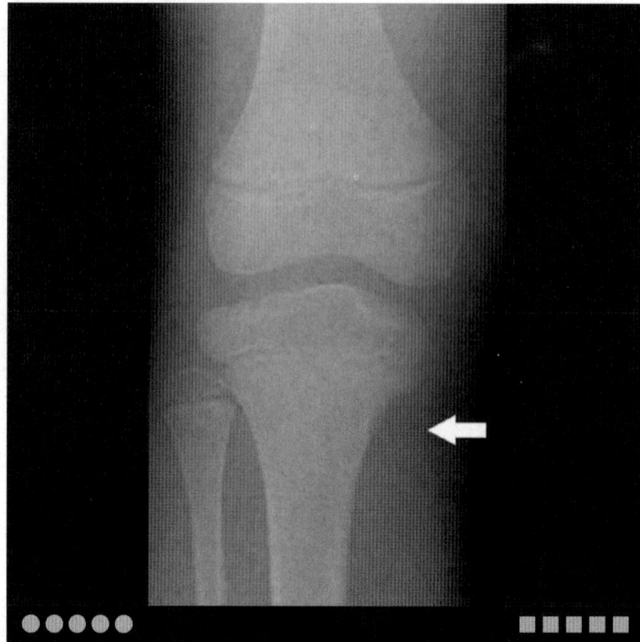

A. Fibrous cortical defect: AP radiograph of the proximal tibia shows a lucent cortically based expansile lesion in the metaphysis (arrow). Note the medial cortex is markedly thinned and difficult to visualize by radiograph.

COMMENTS

This is a preteen pediatric patient presenting with leg pain. The fibrous cortical defect is considered on a continuum with the nonossifying fibroma. This is a benign lesion and is composed of cellular stromal tissue. It is considered a normal developmental variant, found in approximately one-third of pediatric patients and is slightly more common in males. It is rarely identified before 18 months of age and the average age at presentation is 5 to 6 years. The typical course is spontaneous resolution by progressive ossification. Size is the distinguishing feature. A fibrous cortical defect is typically less than 2 cm in size without extension into the medullary cavity. The nonossifying fibroma is larger, extending into the medullary cavity, and may be symptomatic. The diagnosis of fibrous cortical defect can be readily made by radiography and is considered a "do not touch" lesion. The typical location is around the knee in the posterior metaphyseal cortex. A sclerotic finely lobulated border surrounding a lucent center is characteristic. With maturation the lesion may move away from the metaphysis. Fine septations may be present in larger lesions. The larger nonossifying fibroma may require additional imaging particularly if the patient is symptomatic. On MR the lesion is typically hypointense on both T1 and T2 and it typically enhances. The nonossifying fibroma may be surrounded by edema on MR and larger lesions may fracture. Multiple nonossifying fibroma in conjunction with café au lait skin spots, mental retardation, hypogonadism, cryptorchidism and ocular and cardiovascular malformation are known as Jaffe-Campanacci syndrome.

PEARLS

- **The typical cortically based expansile posterior metaphyseal fibrous cortical defect can be readily diagnosed by radiography and should be considered a "do not touch" lesion.**
- **The most common location is about the knee, but with maturation the lesions will ossify and eventually disappear.**
- **The lesions tend to migrate away from the physis with growth and can become larger with growth.**
- **Size is the distinguishing feature between these benign lesions felt to represent a continuum, but the occasional symptomatic patient may warrant additional imaging that will demonstrate a hypointense enhancing lesion on MR evaluation.**

ADDITIONAL IMAGES

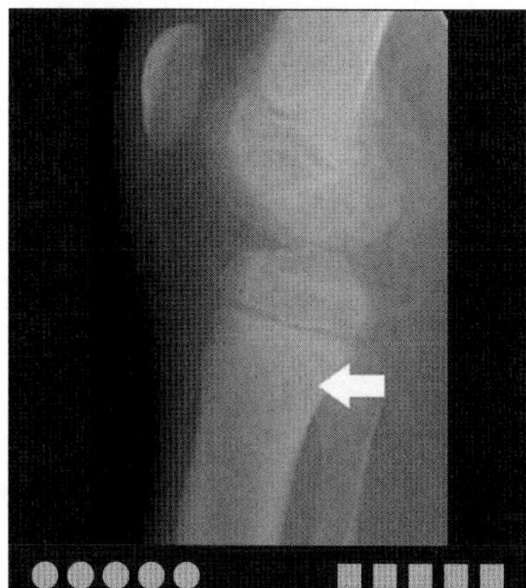

B. Fibrous cortical defect: Lateral radiograph of the proximal tibia shows the typical posterior location of the lesion (arrow).

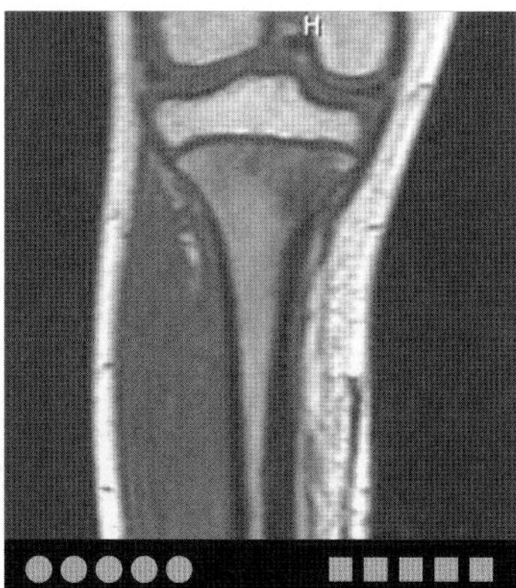

C. Fibrous cortical defect: Coronal T1 image demonstrates the hypointense appearance of the lesion and the well-defined sclerotic border that was difficult to demonstrate by radiograph.

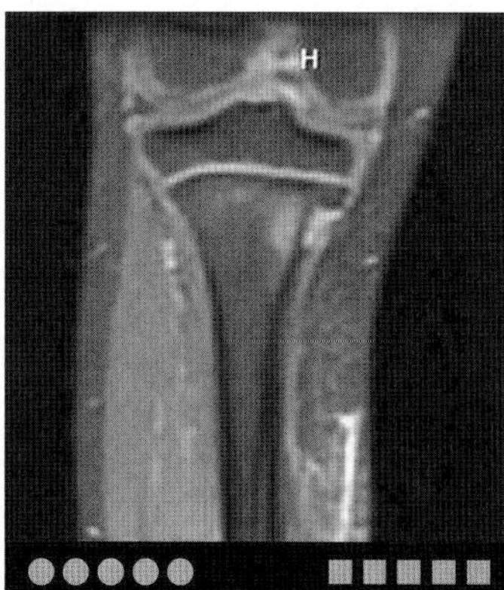

D. Fibrous cortical defect: Coronal SPGR post-gadolinium image shows diffuse homogeneous enhancement. Other characteristic patterns of enhancement include peripheral enhancement and septal enhancement.

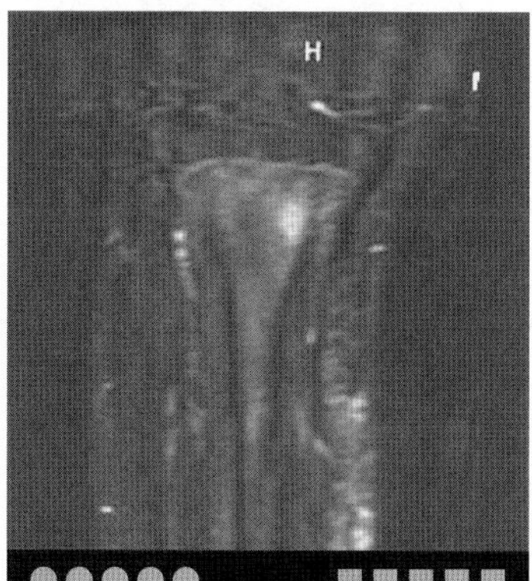

E. Fibrous cortical defect: Coronal T2 with fat saturation image shows edema associated with the lesion along the lateral aspect. This finding may account for the pain symptoms noted in this patient.

DIFFERENTIAL DIAGNOSES IMAGES

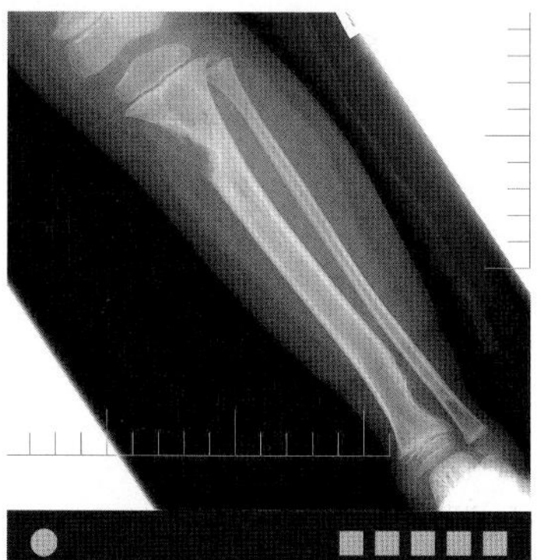

F. Jaffe-Campanacci syndrome: AP radiograph of tibia and fibula in a patient who has multiple nonossifying fibromas associated with café' au lait spots. In the setting of multiplicity of lesions this diagnosis needs to be considered.

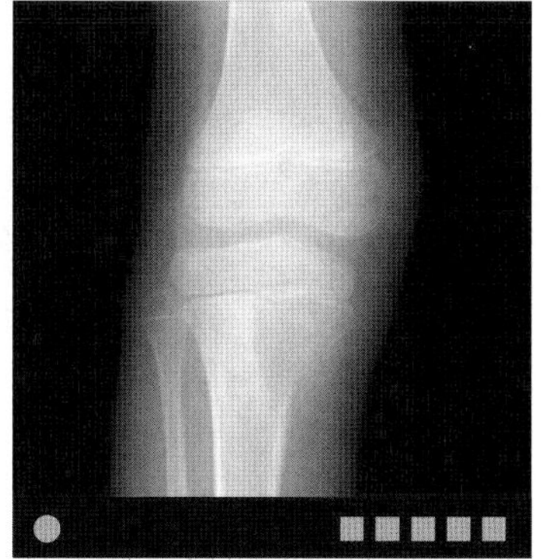

G. Aneurysmal bone cyst: Radiograph of the proximal tibia shows an expansile cortically based lucent defect representing a small aneurysmal bone cyst.

IMAGE KEY

Common

Rare

Typical

Unusual

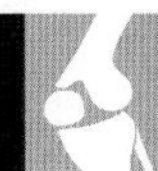

27–22 Malignant Fibrous Histiocytoma Arising in a Bone Infarct

Charles H. Bush

PRESENTATION

Painless left knee mass

FINDINGS

A lateral radiograph of the left knee shows a soft tissue mass posterior to the distal femur. MRI shows posterior cortical destruction of the distal femur, with a soft tissue mass.

DIFFERENTIAL DIAGNOSES

- *Osteomyelitis:* This is a common problem in patients with both homozygous sickle cell disease and Hgb-SC disease. Bone destruction in osteomyelitis is not usually associated with a large soft tissue mass.
- *Acute infarction:* Periosteal elevation can occur, but a soft tissue mass is not seen in osteonecrosis.

COMMENTS

A painless left knee mass arose slowly in a 51-year-old woman with known sickle-C (Hgb-SC) disease. The erythrocyte sickling occurring in Hgb-S disease and Hgb-SC disease causes bone infarction, which presents acutely as bone pain, the crisis. The diaphyses of the long bones, various epiphyses, and the spine and flat bones are commonly affected in adults. Such patients often also present with fever, swelling, and leukocytosis, and must be distinguished from osteomyelitis. Possibly because of their more normal lifespan and milder clinical manifestations, osteonecrosis may be more common in Hgb-SC disease than homozygous Hgb-S disease. Besides infarctions, patients with Hgb-SC disease can have marrow hyperplasia on MRI, but the conventional radiographic alterations are usually more subtle than in Hgb-S disease. In distinction to Hgb-S disease, patients with Hgb-SC disease usually have splenomegaly.

Patients with chronic intramedullary bone infarction are usually asymptomatic, but long-standing infarctions occasionally undergo sarcomatous degeneration. Such tumors occur usually in adults over the age of 40 years, occur usually in an infarct in the shaft of a long bone, and are histologically most often malignant fibrous histiocytoma (MFH) or fibrosarcomas, which are commonly high-grade. Prognosis of these tumors is usually dismal. On cross-sectional imaging, an aggressive, destructive bony lesion usually having a soft tissue mass arising from a site of infarction is apparent. Such patients not infrequently present with pulmonary metastases as well.

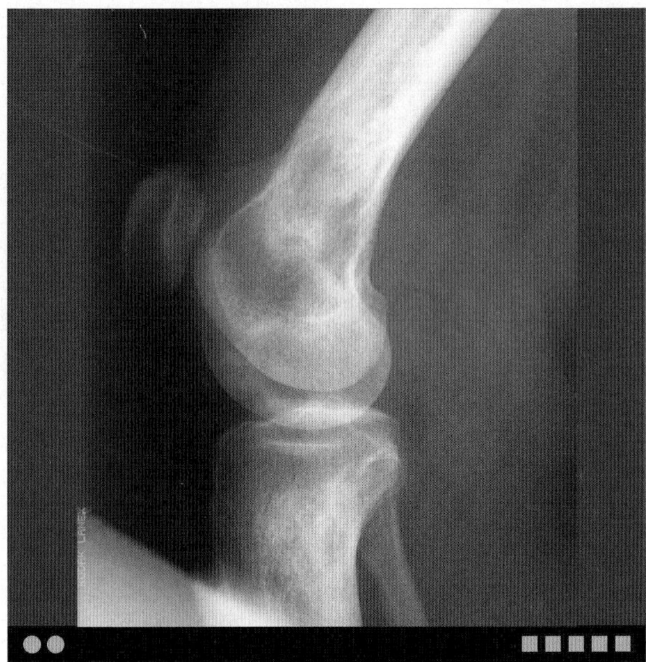

A. MFH arising in bone infarct: A lateral radiograph of the left knee shows a soft tissue mass posterior to the distal femur. The cortex of the femur shows thickening and subtle central radiolucency secondary to Hgb-SC disease. Note distal femur and proximal tibia bone infarct.

PEARLS

- **Besides old infarcts, irradiated bone and Paget disease occasionally undergo late sarcomatous degeneration.**
- **Malignant fibrous histiocytoma is the most common tumor seen in such patients, but osteosarcoma has also been reported.**

ADDITIONAL IMAGES

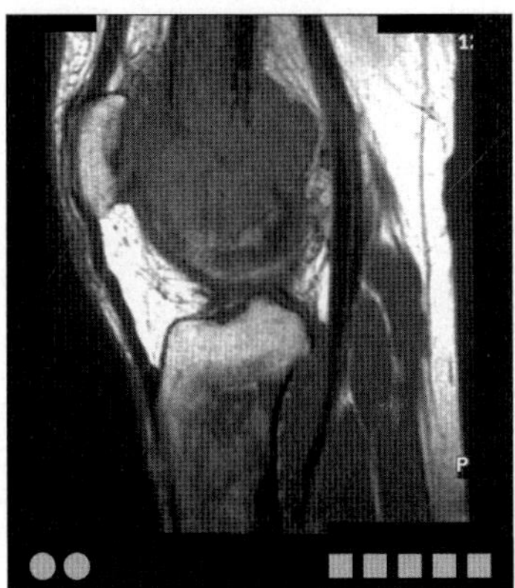

B. MFH arising in bone infarct: MR with sagittal T1-weighted image shows an aggressive bony mass of the distal femur causing posterior cortical destruction, with a large soft tissue component. Note the intramedullary infarct in the proximal tibia.

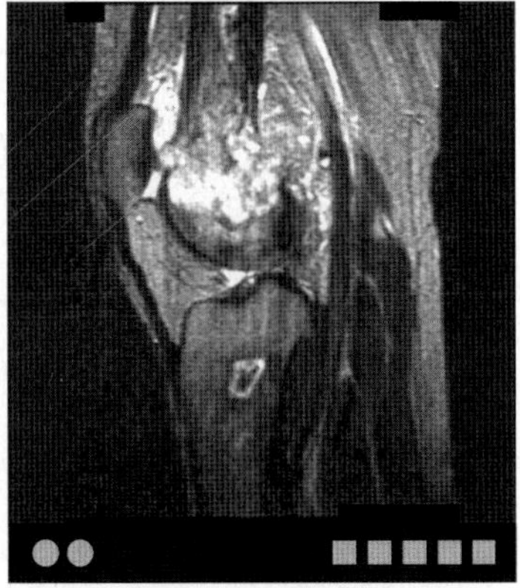

C. MFH arising in bone infarct: MR with sagittal T2-weighted image shows an aggressive bony mass of the distal femur causing posterior cortical destruction, with a large soft tissue component. Note the intramedullary infarct in the proximal tibia.

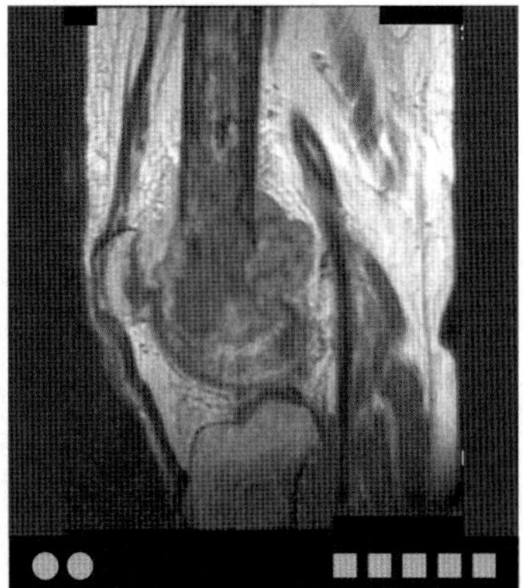

D. MFH arising in bone infarct: MR with sagittal T1-weighted image with intravenous paramagnetic contrast shows an aggressive bony mass of the distal femur causing posterior cortical destruction, with a large enhancing soft tissue component.

IMAGE KEY

Common

Rare

Typical

Unusual

DIFFERENTIAL DIAGNOSES IMAGES

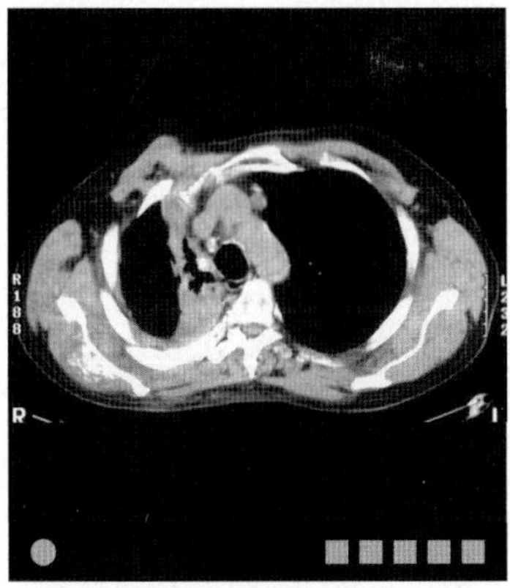

E. Radiation-induced osteosarcoma: This patient was irradiated for small cell carcinoma of the right hilum 11 years ago presents with swelling about the right scapula. CT of the chest shows a destructive mineralizing mass arising from the right scapula, a radiation-induced osteosarcoma. Note the linear fibrosis and bronchiectasis in the right hemithorax from the treatment of the primary lung tumor.

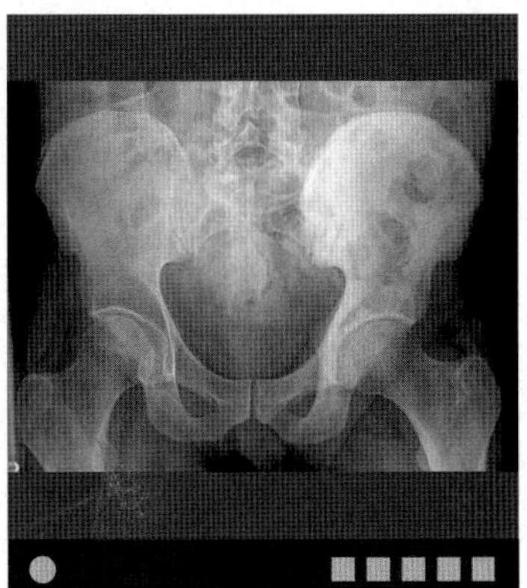

F. MFH arising in Paget disease: An AP radiograph of the pelvis shows changes of late-stage Paget disease of bone of the left hemipelvis.

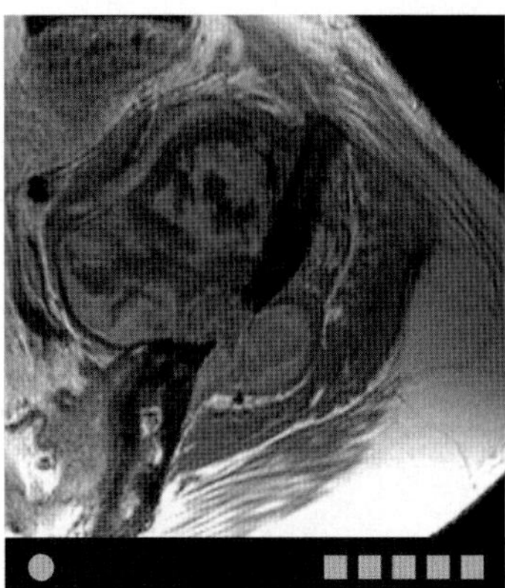

G. MFH arising in Paget disease: T1-weighted post-contrast coronal image from an MR examination of the same patient (as in image F) shows a destructive bony mass with a large soft tissue component arising from the left ilium: a secondary malignant fibrous histiocytoma arising in long-standing Paget disease.

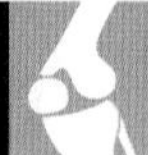

27–23 Adamantinoma of Tibia

Gideon Strich

PRESENTATION

Tibial pain

FINDINGS

MRI shows an eccentric mass originating in the cortex of the tibial diaphysis with invasion of the adjacent soft tissue.

DIFFERENTIAL DIAGNOSES

- *Ossifying fibroma (osteofibrous dysplasia)* in the tubular bones is most commonly seen in the first two decades and presents with multiloculated or "bubbly" well-marginated lucent lesions originating in the tibial cortex, and may be associated with bowing of the tibia.
- *Fibrous dysplasia:* May involve multiple bones with expansion of the medullary cavity and deformity of the long bones. Typical ground glass appearance on radiograph. In younger patients, may be associated with bowing and pseudoarthrosis.
- *Intracortical and periosteal osteosarcoma:* Rare forms of osteosarcoma primarily involve the cortex of a tubular bone with secondary invasion of the soft tissues and the medullary bone. Usually have typical soft tissue calcification.
- *Benign inflammatory process such as osteomyelitis or stress fracture:* Early osteolytic process followed by sclerotic repair.

COMMENTS

The patient is a middle-aged male with tibial pain and palpable mass. Adamantinoma of the tubular bones is a relatively rare lesion that arises in the proximal tibial diaphysis in approximately 90% of cases. It is eccentric and predominantly arises from the cortex with early invasion of the soft tissues. It is usually lytic and poorly marginated and may invade the medullary cavity. Lesions may be multifocal within the same bone, similar to fibrous dysplasia. Adamantinoma contains epithelial cells similar to ameloblastoma of the mandible. It is relatively slow growing but is locally aggressive and will recur following inadequate resection. Up to 20% of lesions will metastasize. Adamantinoma, when it invades the medullary bone may be difficult to differentiate from ossifying fibroma and the local form of fibrous dysplasia radiographically, and these three entities are thought to be part of a spectrum of disease. Ossifying fibroma and fibrous dysplasia are usually seen in younger patients and more often show tibial bowing. Cortical erosion and soft tissue invasion are commonly seen with adamantinoma. Presentation in the first two decades and bowing of the tibia is more common with ossifying fibroma and fibrous dysplasia. Ground glass appearance and pseudoarthrosis are characteristic of fibrous dysplasia.

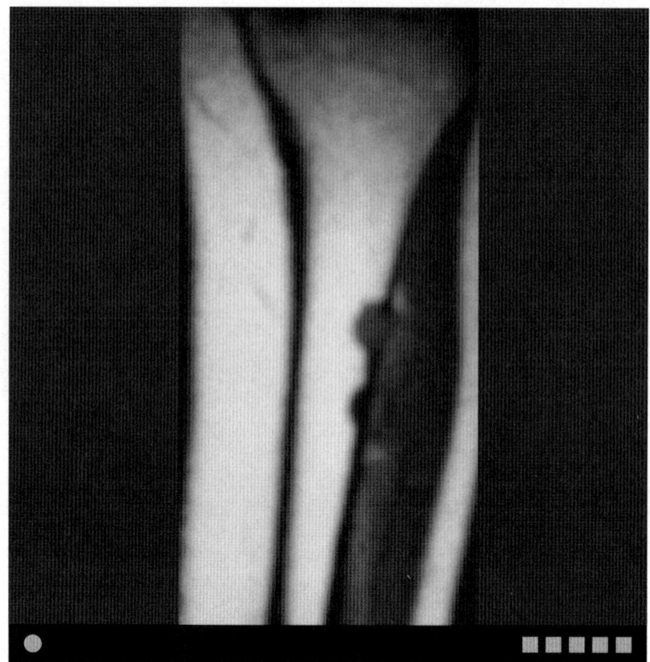

A. Adamantinoma: Coronal T1-weighted image shows cortical origin and early soft tissue invasion.

PEARLS

- **Adamantinoma of the tubular bones is a rare lesion of epithelial origin.**
- **90% arise in the cortex of the proximal tibial diaphysis.**
- **Although they are slow growing locally, they are aggressive and commonly recur or metastasize if inadequately resected.**

ADDITIONAL IMAGES

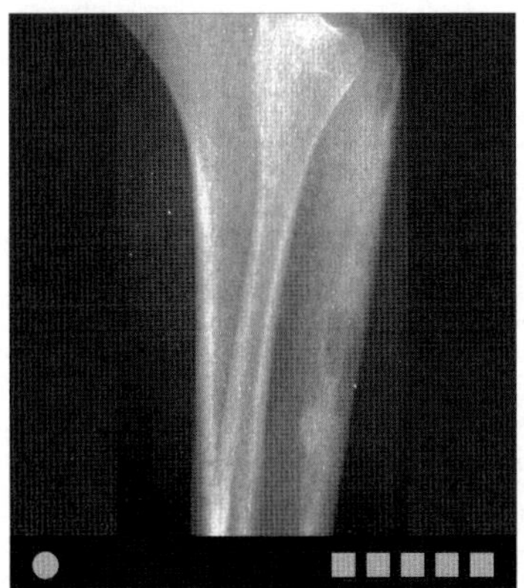

B. Adamantinoma: Oblique radiograph shows ill-defined lytic lesion of the anterior tibial cortex without apparent sclerosis or periosteal reaction.

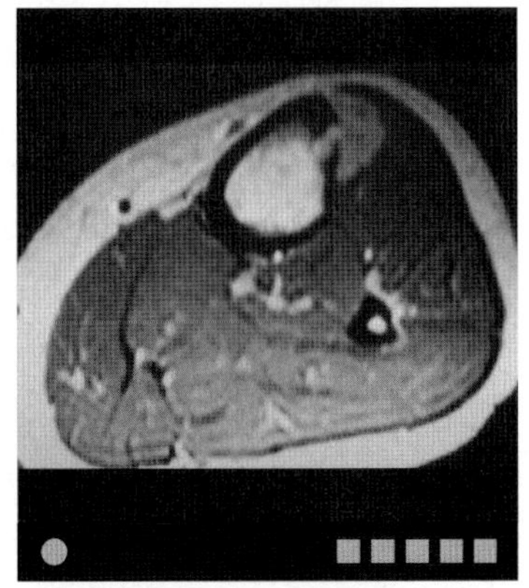

C. Adamantinoma: Axial proton density-weighted image demonstrates more soft tissue invasion than would be expected from the appearance on the radiograph.

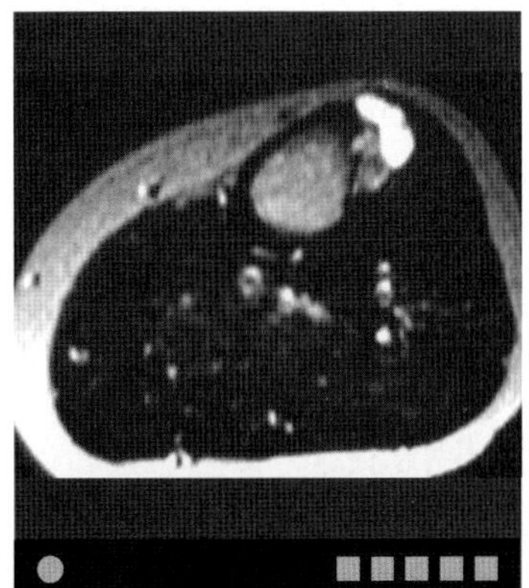

D. Adamantinoma: Axial T2-weighted image demonstrates the soft tissue has relatively bright signal on T2-weighted images.

IMAGE KEY

Common

Rare

Typical

Unusual

DIFFERENTIAL DIAGNOSES IMAGES

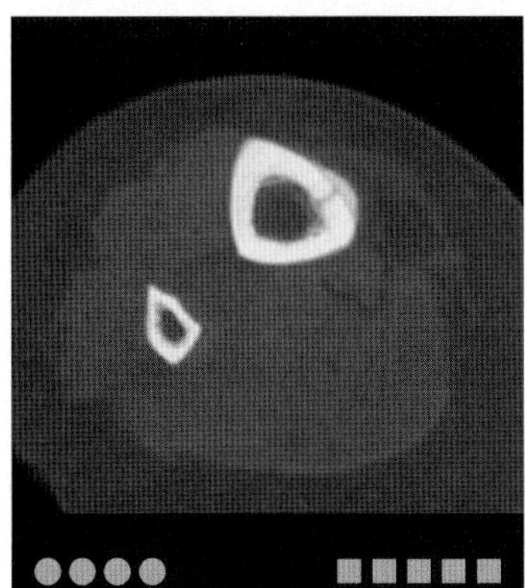

E. Tibial stress fracture: Axial CT shows cortical stress fracture and periosteal new bone.

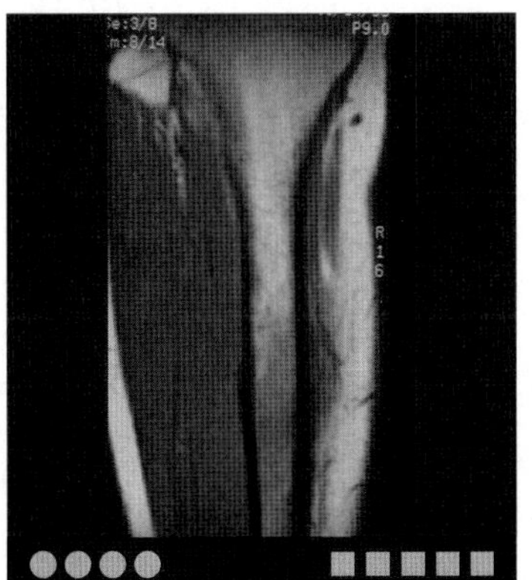

F. Tibial stress fracture: Coronal T1-weighted image shows cortical thickening and edema of bone marrow and adjacent soft tissues.

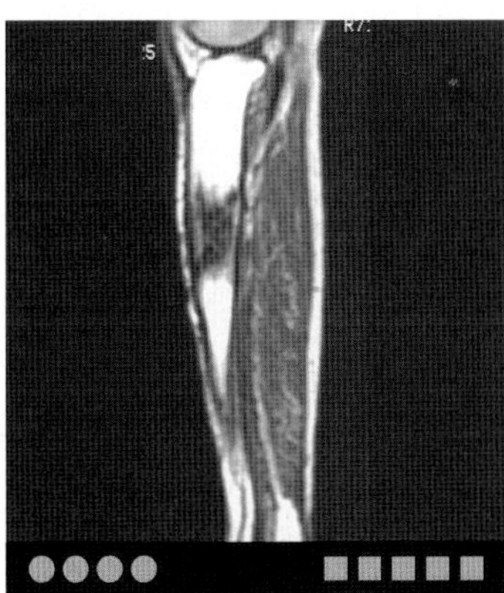

G. Osteomyelitis: Sagittal T1 image shows periosteal reaction and sclerosis surrounding sequestrum.

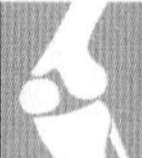

27–24 Lymphoma of the Knee

Amilcare Gentili

PRESENTATION

Knee pain

FINDINGS

Abnormal marrow signal in the medial femoral condyle and medial tibial plateau is noted.

DIFFERENTIAL DIAGNOSES

- *Metastases:* Much more common than lymphoma, even when lymphoma of bone is present it is most often metastatic lymphoma and not primary lymphoma of bone.
- *Giant cell tumor:* Usually no or minimal soft tissue extension.
- *Ewing sarcoma:* This may present with minimal cortical destruction in the presence of extensive soft-tissue extension as lymphoma, it is more common in children.
- *Spontaneous osteonecrosis of the knee (SONK):* This process which is caused by subchondral insufficiency fracture is usually seen in patients with prior meniscectomy.

COMMENTS

The patient is a 67-year-old man presenting with a history of increasing knee pain over several months. The pain was attributed to osteoarthrosis and an MRI was obtained to evaluate the menisci and ligaments. Detection of lymphoma was an unexpected finding. Primary lymphoma of bone is rare accounting for less than 5% of malignant bone tumors. Systemic lymphoma with bone involvement is much more common. Primary lymphoma of bone can be seen in any age group, but has a preference for the sixth and seventh decade of life. It affects men more frequently than women with a male-to-female ratio of 1.5 to 1. Involvement of the long bones is more common in primary lymphoma than in secondary lymphoma. In secondary bone lymphoma the axial skeleton is more frequently involved. In multifocal primary osseous lymphoma most lesions occur around the knee. Most primary lymphomas of bone are non-Hodgkin lymphomas. Radiographic appearance is very variable, lymphoma may present with either lytic or blastic lesions, or can present with normal or near-normal radiographs as in our case. On T1-weighted MR images lymphoma appears as areas of low signal intensity in the bone marrow. On T2-weighted MR images the signal intensity is variable from high signal to low signal depending on the amount of fibrosis in the lesion. One MR imaging characteristic suggestive of lymphoma is the presence of extensive bone marrow replacement, with normal or near-normal radiographs. Another feature of lymphoma is minimal cortical destruction in the presence of extensive soft-tissue and marrow involvement.

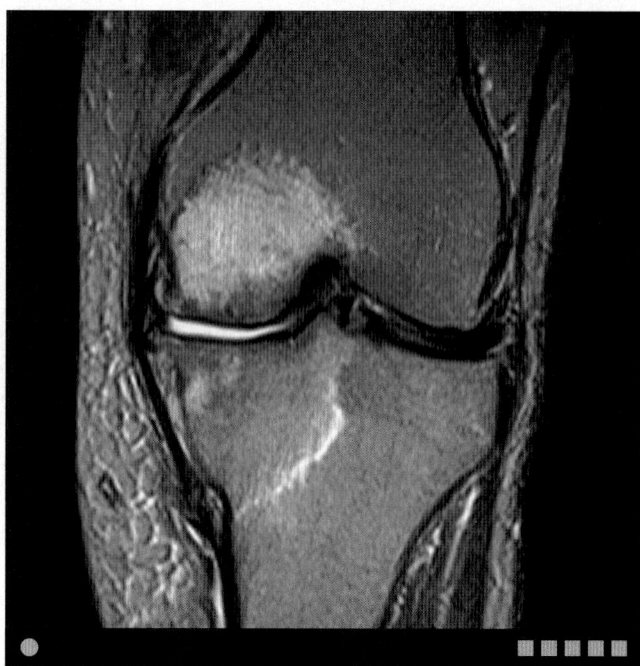

A. Lymphoma. Coronal T2-weighted MR image of the knee demonstrates bone marrow signal abnormalities in both the medial femoral condyle and medial tibial plateau, the femoral lesion has increased signal intensity while the tibial lesion has almost the same signal intensity as normal marrow.

PEARLS

- **Primary lymphoma of bone is rare accounting for less than 5% of malignant bone tumor.**
- **Radiographs and even CT may have normal or near-normal appearance and lesion may only be detected on MRI or skeletal scintigraphy.**
- **Often associated with large soft-tissue mass.**

ADDITIONAL IMAGES

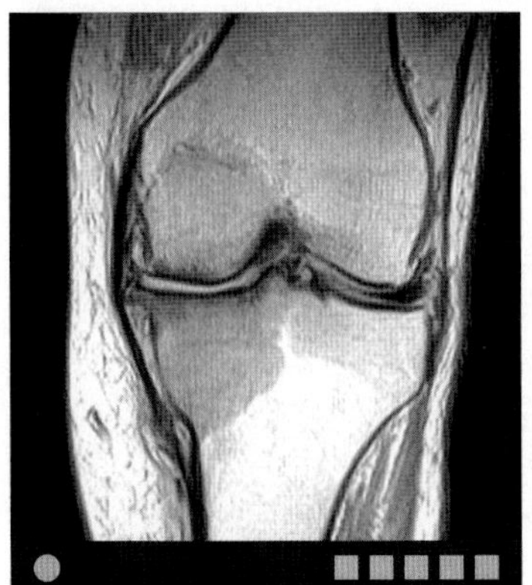

B. Lymphoma: Coronal proton density MR image of the knee demonstrates bone marrow signal abnormalities in the medial femoral condyle and medial tibial plateau; both lesions have decreased signal intensity when compared to normal marrow

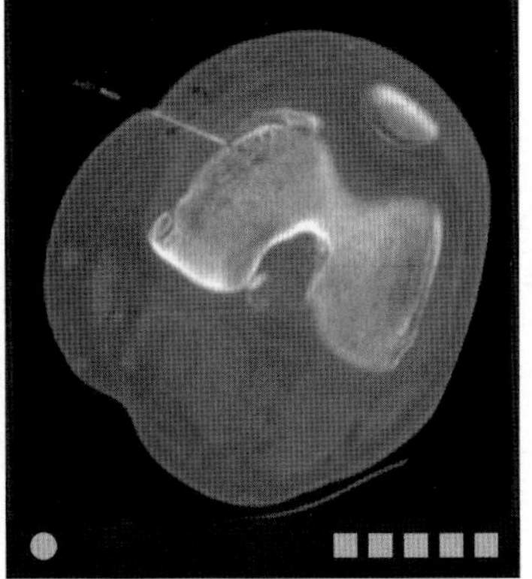

C. Lymphoma: Axial CT image obtained during CT-guided biopsy shows normal appearing bone in an area of histologically proven lymphoma.

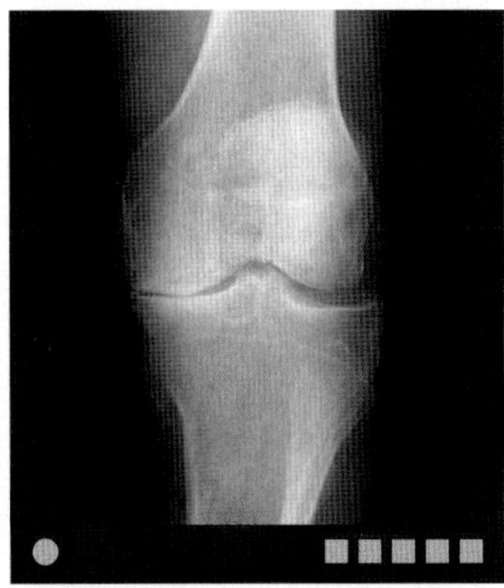

D. Lymphoma: AP radiograph of the knee demonstrates osteoarthrosis of the medial compartment, but was otherwise unremarkable.

IMAGE KEY

Common

Rare

Typical

Unusual

DIFFERENTIAL DIAGNOSES IMAGES

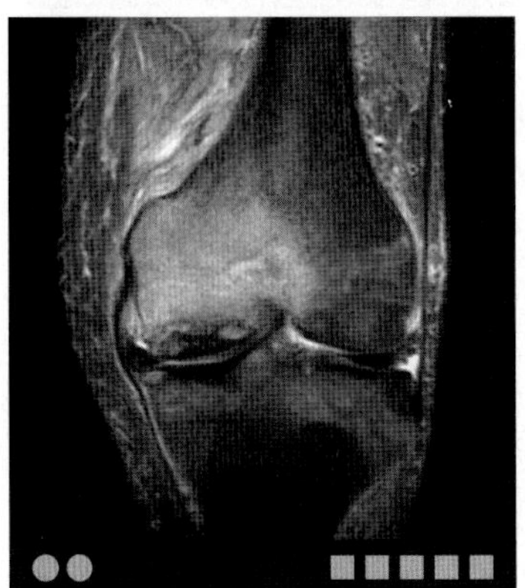

E. SONK (Insufficiency fracture): Coronal T2-weighted MR image of the knee demonstrates a subchondral fracture of the medial femoral condyle surrounded by extensive bone marrow edema.

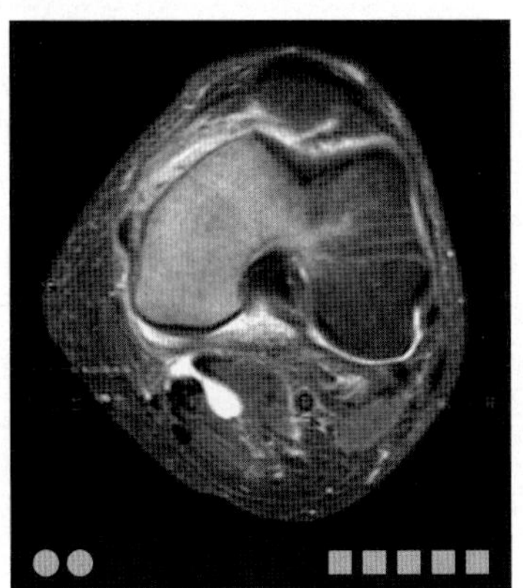

F. SONK (Insufficiency fracture): Axial T2-weighted MR image of the knee demonstrates bone marrow edema in the medial femoral condyle. Note a small joint effusion and Baker cyst.

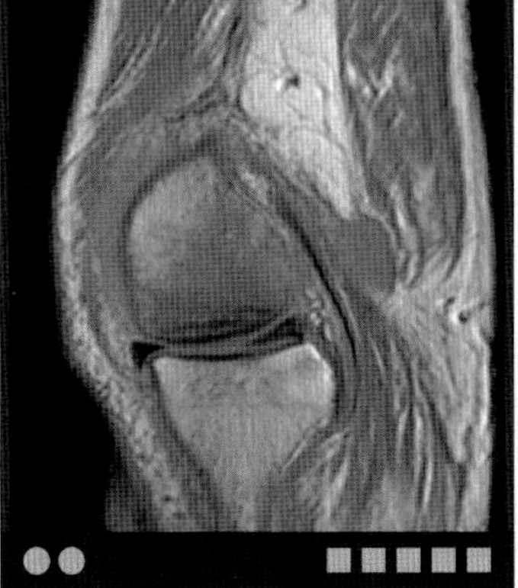

G. SONK (Insufficiency fracture): Sagittal proton density T2-weighted MR image of the knee demonstrates a subchondral fracture of the medial femoral condyle surrounded by extensive bone marrow edema.

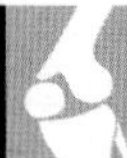

27–25 Periosteal Lymphoma of the Distal Femur

Ibrahim F. Abdelwahab and Stefano Bianchi

PRESENTATION

Soft tissue tender mass

FINDINGS

MR imaging demonstrates a subperiosteal soft tissue mass causing a superficial erosion of the lateral cortex of the distal femur. The medulla of the distal femur has normal signal intensity.

DIFFERENTIAL DIAGNOSES

- *Periosteal Ewing sarcoma:* The age of our patient is far older than the mean age of periosteal Ewing sarcoma (14 years).
- *Periosteal chondroma or chondrosarcoma:* This is often associated with intralesional calcifications.
- *Periosteal osteosarcoma:* Osteoid ossification present in this lesion is helpful to diagnose this lesion.
- *Periosteal ganglion:* Enhancement after gadolinium injection limited to the peripheral capsule and presence of mucoid fluid contained within the ganglion with no central enhancement are helpful.

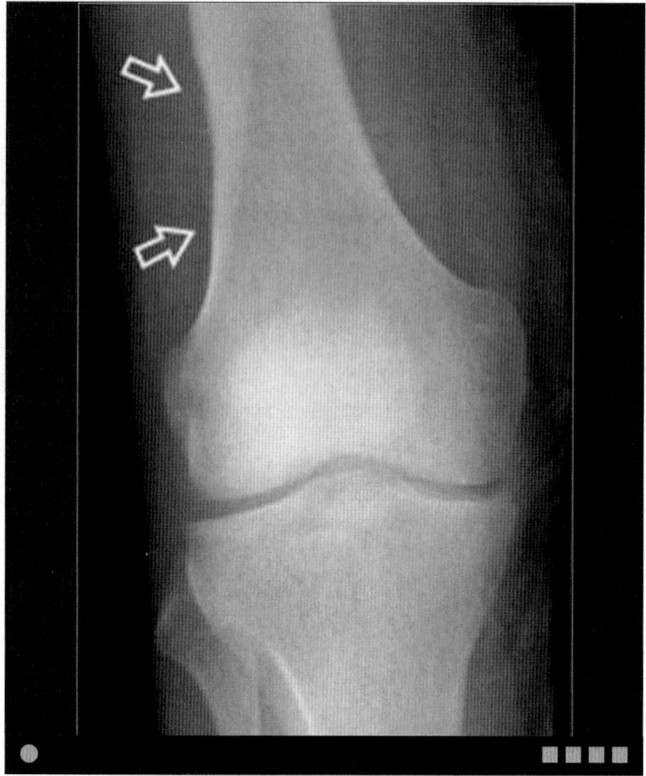

A. Periosteal lymphoma: AP radiograph of the right knee reveals focal superficial erosion in the lateral cortical margin of the metadiaphysis of the right femur (arrows). Note the ill-defined periosteal reaction.

COMMENTS

The patient is a 27-year-old man with a history of pain and swelling in the superior lateral side of the knee for 9 months. The pathologic study revealed periosteal large cell lymphoma, B-cell type. Periosteal lymphoma is very rare and can be easily confused with surface lesions not exhibiting mineralization. This lesion is arising primarily within the periosteum, without any marrow infiltration. It usually has soft tissue mass surrounding the involved bone. The primary site of primary bone lymphoma is the appendicular skeleton, mainly the lower extremity with peak incidence in the fifth decade. The typical symptoms are pain, local tenderness, and occasionally swelling in the region of the tumor, usually without any systemic symptoms. The intermediate to low signal on MR images are similar to primary intramedullary lymphoma of bone. The cortical scalloping represents cytokine-induced increased osteoclastic activity causing a "tunnel" presenting as a small linear foci of high T2 signal in the cortex of the bone. Bone scan usually shows increased uptake at the site of the cortical erosion. In addition, the fleshy, tan appearance of the gross specimen, and the diffuse large B-cell histologic appearance also simulate intramedullary bone lymphoma. Lymphoma would need to be considered in the differential diagnosis of aggressive periosteal lesions without a discernible matrix and a soft tissue mass.

PEARLS

- **Periosteal lymphoma is very rare and can be easily confused with surface lesions not exhibiting mineralization. Lymphoma would need to be considered in the differential diagnosis of aggressive periosteal lesions without a discernible matrix and a soft tissue mass.**
- **The main site of primary bone lymphoma is the appendicular skeleton, mainly the lower extremity with peak incidence in the fifth decade. This lesion is arising primarily within the periosteum, without any marrow infiltration.**
- **Periosteal lymphoma shows low to intermediate signal intensity mass within the periosteum in T1 and bright cortical tunnel lesion on T2 MR sequences without any marrow infiltration.**

ADDITIONAL IMAGES

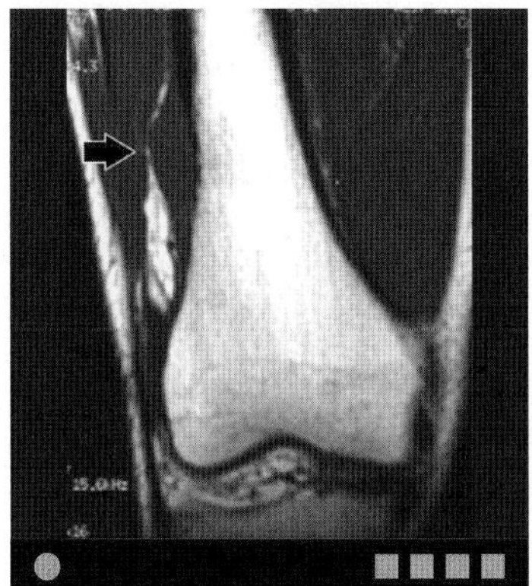

B. Periosteal lymphoma: Coronal T1-weighted image of the distal femur demonstrates a sharply defined elliptical soft tissue periosteal mass (arrow), well outlined by the displaced fat. The mass is abutting the cortical saucerization and has an isointense signal with muscles.

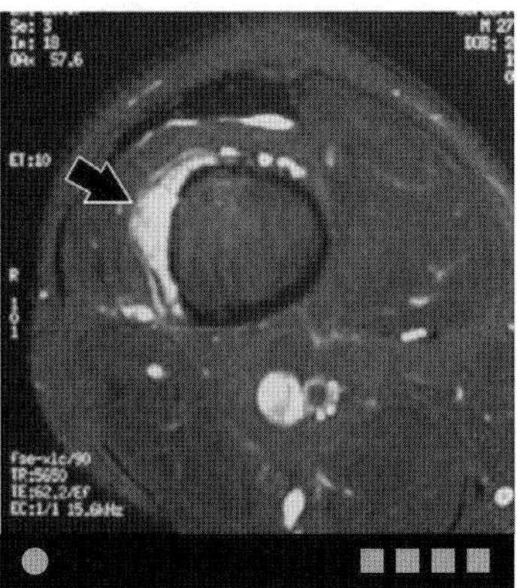

C. Periosteal lymphoma: An axial FSE fat-suppressed T2-weighted image reveals a sharply defined crescent-like periosteal soft tissue mass (arrow) abutting the cortical excavation. The mass has a homogeneous high intensity signal. The medulla has normal intensity signal.

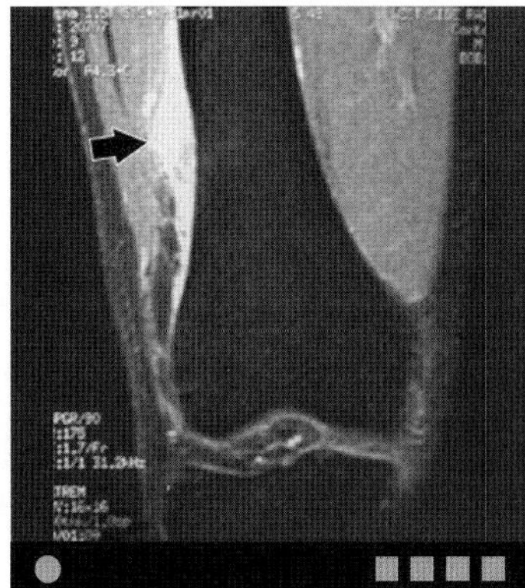

D. Periosteal lymphoma: Enhanced fat-suppressed T1-weighted image shows enhancement of the periosteal mass (arrow) with intralesional multiple, tiny areas of non-enhancement most likely representing infiltrating periosteal fibrous tissue. The medulla is not enhanced.

IMAGE KEY

Common

Rare

Typical

Unusual

DIFFERENTIAL DIAGNOSES IMAGES

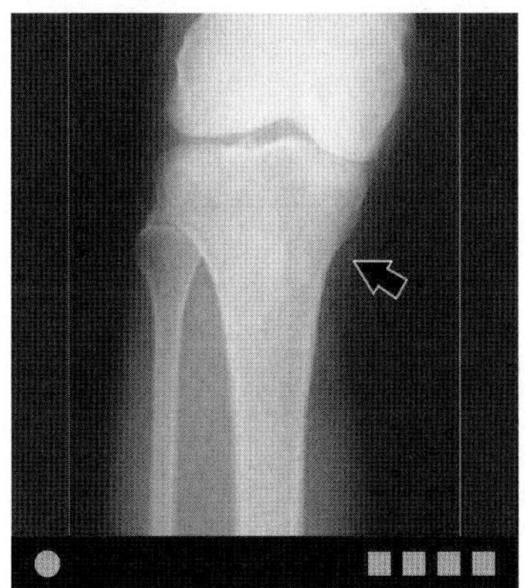

E. Periosteal ganglion: AP roentgenogram of the right knee reveals focal superficial erosion in the medial cortical margin of the metaphysis of the right tibia (arrow).

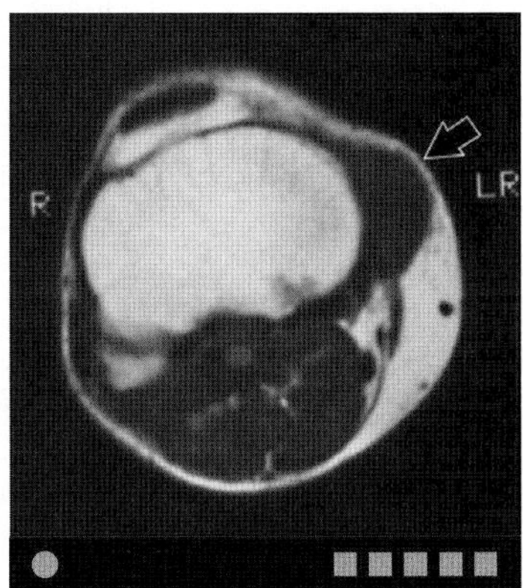

F. Periosteal ganglion: Axial T1-weighted image of the proximal tibia demonstrates a sharply defined soft tissue periosteal mass (arrow). The mass has a homogeneous low intensity signal.

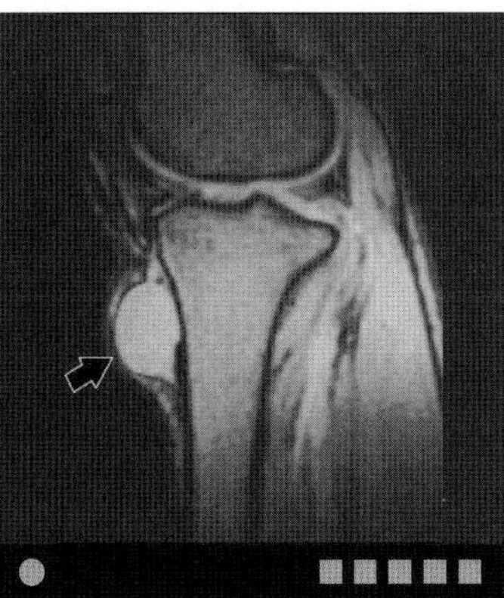

G. Periosteal ganglion: Sagittal FSE fat-suppressed T2-weighted image reveals a sharply defined periosteal soft tissue mass (arrow). The mass has a homogeneous high intensity signal.

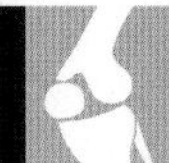

27–26 Dedifferentiated Chondrosarcoma of Femur

George Hermann

PRESENTATION

Right thigh pain

FINDINGS

MRI shows a large lesion in the medullary cavity of the distal femoral shaft. The inner aspect of the cortex is destroyed.

DIFFERENTIAL DIAGNOSES

- *Metastasis:* It may be difficult to differentiate but usually lacks calcification.
- *Central chondrosarcoma:* Well-organized ring-like calcification in the matrix may indicate low-grade chondrosarcoma.
- *Malignant lymphoma:* It may be difficult to differentiate. Matrix calcification is uncommon. It commonly presents with a large soft tissue mass on MRI.
- *Ewing sarcoma:* MRI shows increased SI on T2-weighted image surrounded with large soft tissue mass.

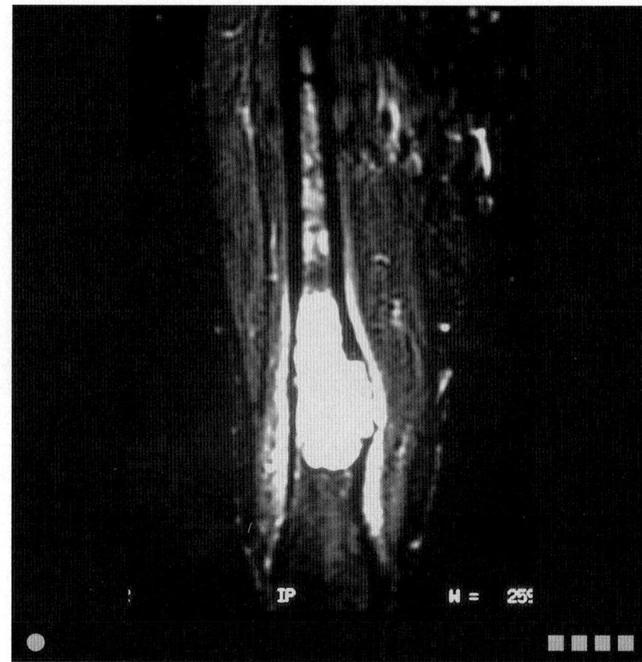

A. Dedifferentiated chondrosarcoma: Coronal STIR image shows a bright SI lesion in the medullary cavity. The cortex is destroyed. Note the bright SI along the cortices.

COMMENTS

The patient is a 44-year-old woman, who presented with a 10-month history of gradually increasing pain of the right thigh. She was diagnosed with dedifferentiated low-grade chondrosarcoma. Chondrosarcoma is usually a low- or intermediate-grade malignant hyaline cartilage tumor that generally follows an indolent course. Dedifferentiated chondrosarcoma represents 10% to 11% of all reported cases of chondrosarcoma. It is a form of chondrosarcoma composed of two distinct components: a low-grade chondrosarcoma or even an enchondroma juxtaposed to a high-grade nonchondrogenous sarcoma. The dedifferentiated component of the tumor is a more aggressive malignant lesion that eventually may destroy the primary cartilaginous tumor. The histologic features of the dedifferentiated component are usually represented by osteosarcoma (17%), fibrosarcoma (24%), or MFH (77%). The age of the patient varies. In the majority of cases the tumor involves the lower extremity. MRI is extremely useful in visualizing the intraosseal and extraosseal extent of the tumor. On T2-weighted spin-echo and STIR images the tumor may show two different features. The component of the low-grade chondrosarcoma appears hyperintense with hypointense internal septae. The high grade tumor, on the other hand, remains relatively lower in SI. The tumor may show a biphasic pattern such as lobulated high SI on T2-weighted image accompanied with an area of low SI component.

PEARLS

- **Dedifferentiated chondrosarcoma usually involves the long tubular bones, predominantly the femur.**
- **The primary tumor may be low grade or benign cartilaginous lesion, the dedifferentiated component, however, usually consists of a high-grade sarcoma.**
- **MRI of dedifferentiated chondrosarcoma shows a biphasic pattern. The high-grade component on T2-weighted image appears relatively low in SI.**
- **Low-grade dedifferentiated chondrosarcoma is extremely rare.**

ADDITIONAL IMAGES

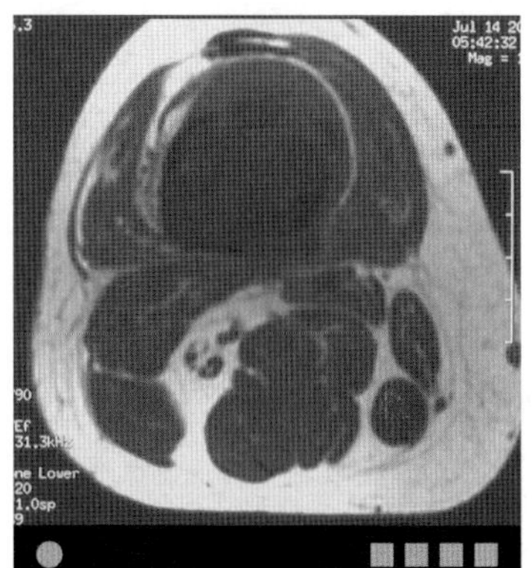

B. Dedifferentiated chondrosarcoma: Axial T1-weighted image shows a uniformly low SI in the medullary cavity. The cortex is destroyed; the tumor extends to the soft tissue.

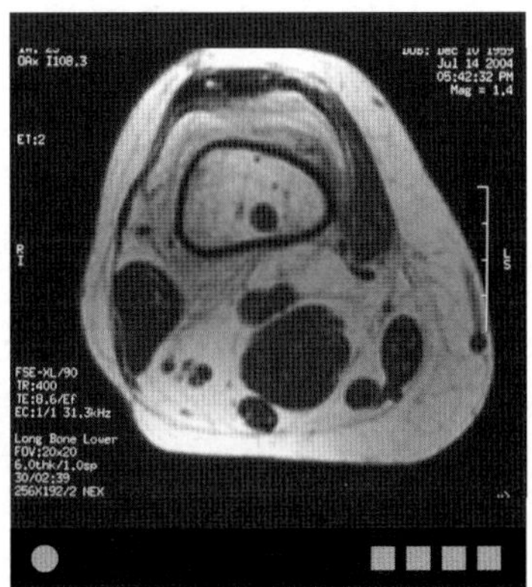

C. Dedifferentiated chondrosarcoma: Axial T1-weighted image shows a small separate ring-like lesion (dedifferentiated component) distally to the mass.

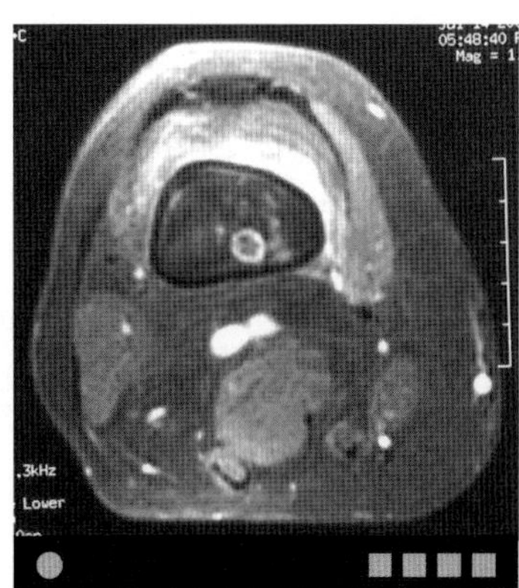

D. Dedifferentiated chondrosarcoma: Axial T1-weighted image post contrast shows unenhanced marrow. The periosseal soft tissue is enhanced.

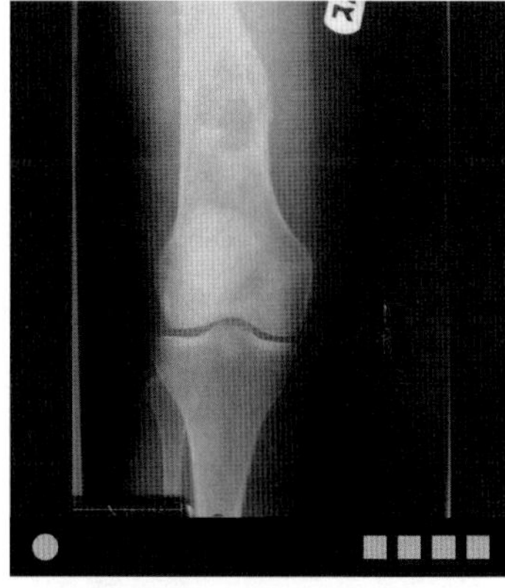

E. Dedifferentiated chondrosarcoma: Frontal radiograph of the distal femoral shaft shows a lytic lesion with a small calcification at the lower part of the lesion. The inner cortex is destroyed and periosteal reaction is present.

DIFFERENTIAL DIAGNOSES IMAGES

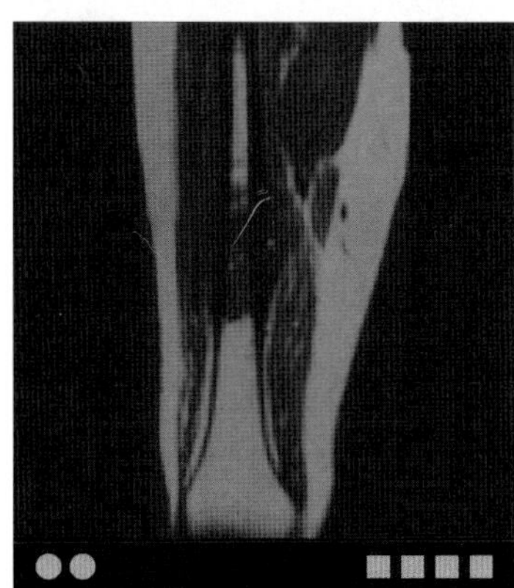

F. Ewing sarcoma: Coronal T1-weighted image shows decreased SI in the medullary cavity.

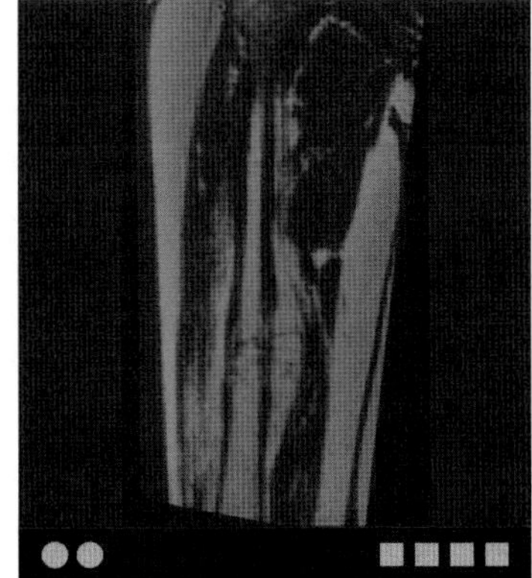

G. Ewing sarcoma: Coronal T2-weighted image shows the presence of large periosteal soft tissue mass.

IMAGE KEY

Common

Rare

Typical

Unusual

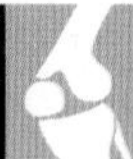

27–27 Telangiectatic Osteosarcoma of Femur

George Hermann

PRESENTATION

Knee pain

FINDINGS

MRI shows an eccentric lesion of the distal femoral metaphysis. The periosteum is elevated and fluid–fluid levels are noted.

DIFFERENTIAL DIAGNOSES

- *Giant cell tumor:* This usually involves the epiphysis following closure of the growth plate.
- *Hemangioendothelioma:* This is a rare tumor, most often occurring in the fourth to fifth decade of life. The lesion may localize to the cortex, causing osseous expansion. Frequently it is multifocal.
- *Metastasis:* Primaries such as hypernephroma, usually occurs in the older age group.
- *Aneurysmal bone cyst:* It is an expansile lesion usually eccentric, with multiple fluid levels. It may be difficult to differentiate from telangiectatic osteosarcoma.

COMMENTS

The patient is a 14-year-old girl, who presented with gradually increasing knee pain during the past 4 months. She was diagnosed with telangiectatic osteosarcoma. Osteosarcoma is the most common primary bone tumor in children and the second in frequency following plasma cell myeloma in all ages. It is characterized histologically by producing osteoid or immature bone. The tumor may be classified according to the site—central, intracortical, surface, periosteal, or parosteal. Histologically it may be osteoblastic, chondroblastic, fibroblastic, small cell, or telangiectatic. The degree of cellular differentiation may be high or low grade. Osteosarcoma in general is seen in the second to third decade of life. The male/female ratio is 2:1. Cases involving the appendicular skeleton is 80%, two-thirds of all cases occur around the knee. In some osteosarcomas the tumor includes large cystic cavities filled with blood considered a distinct variety that is called telangiectatic osteosarcoma (TOS). TOS represents approximately 10% of all osteosarcoma cases. It arises at the metaphysis of the femur, tibia, and humerus in decreasing frequency. Pathologic fracture

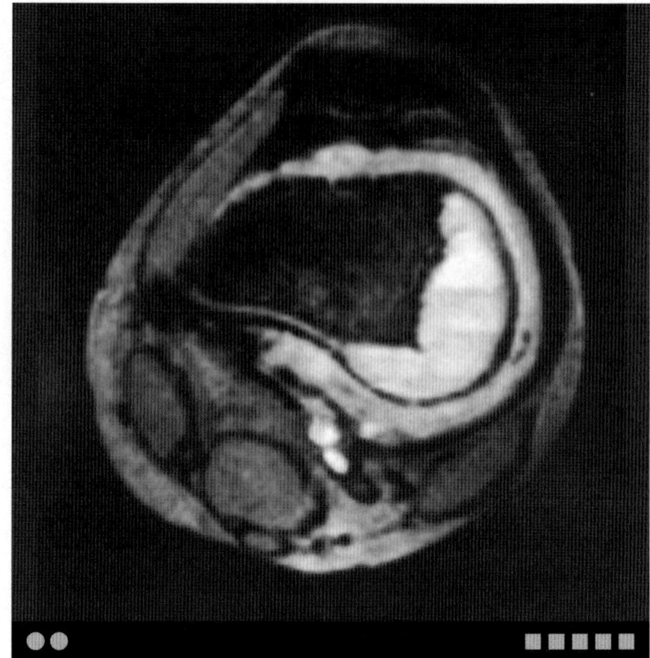

A. Telangiectatic osteosarcoma: Axial T2-weighted MR image reveals a high SI mass of the distal femoral condyle situated under the periosteum. Note the multiple fluid levels.

occurs in up to 30% of TOS cases. MRI is helpful in evaluating the content and extent of the lesion. On T1-weighted image, localized increased SI represents the bloody content. Fluid levels are similar to those seen in aneurysmal bone cyst.

PEARLS

- **Osteosarcoma is the most common primary bone tumor in children.**
- **TOS represents approximately 10% of all osteosarcoma cases.**
- **TOS arises at the metaphysis of the femur, tibia, and humerus in decreasing frequency.**
- **Pathologic fracture occurs in up to 30% of TOS cases.**
- **Fluid levels are similar to those seen in aneurysmal bone cyst.**

ADDITIONAL IMAGES

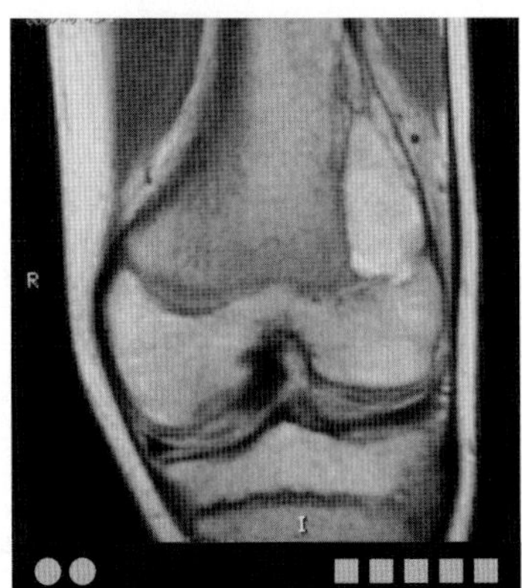

B. Telangiectatic osteosarcoma: Coronal proton density MR image reveals a quite well-defined, homogeneously higher SI lesion at the lateral aspect of the femoral metaphysis. The periosteum is elevated.

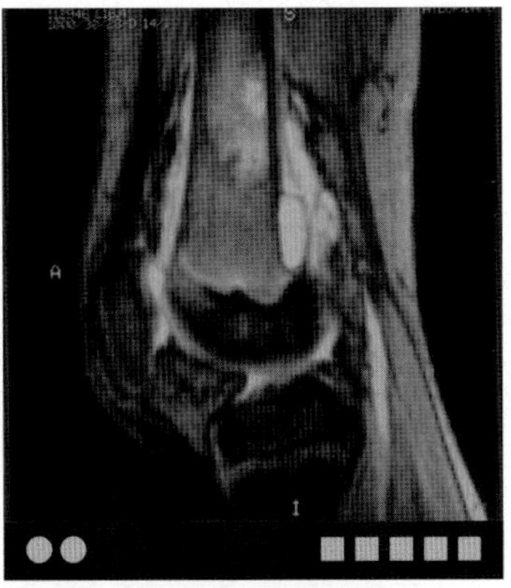

C. Telangiectatic osteosarcoma: Sagittal T2-weighted MR image reveals a destruction of the medullary cavity. Note the elevated periosteum posteriorly and presence of the soft tissue mass.

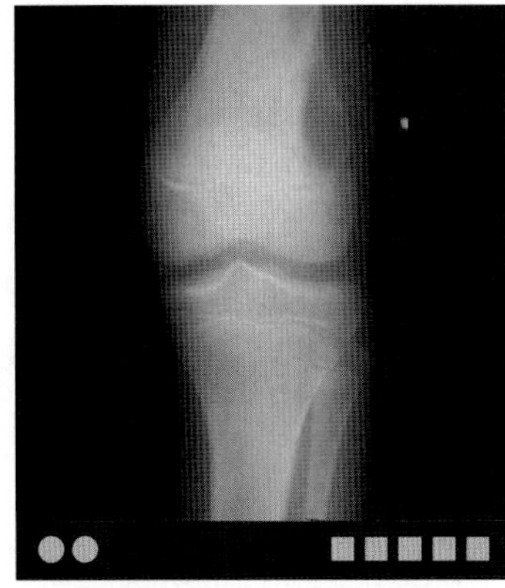

D. Telangiectatic osteosarcoma: Frontal radiograph of the knee reveals an expansile lytic lesion on the lateral aspect of the metaphysis of the distal femur. Note the thin periosteal reaction.

IMAGE KEY

Common

Rare

Typical

Unusual

DIFFERENTIAL DIAGNOSES IMAGES

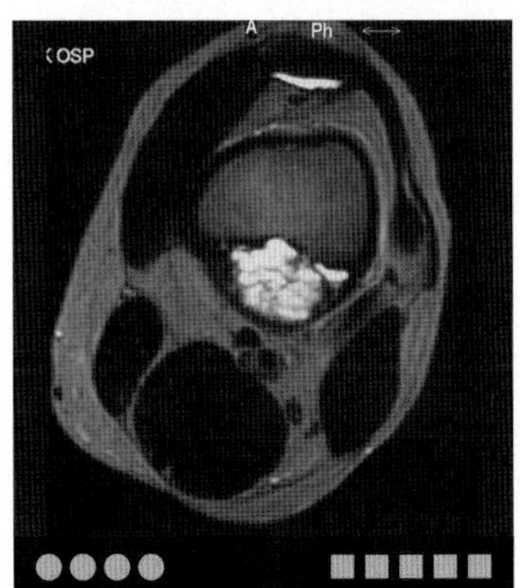

E. Aneurysmal bone cyst: Axial STIR image reveals high signal intensity mass at the posterior aspect of the distal femur. Note the fluid levels.

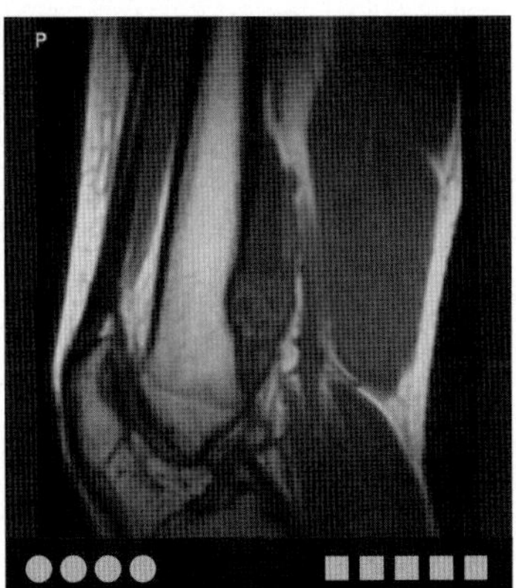

F. Aneurysmal bone cyst: Sagittal T1-weighted MR image reveals a large decreased SI mass along the posterior aspect of the distal femur.

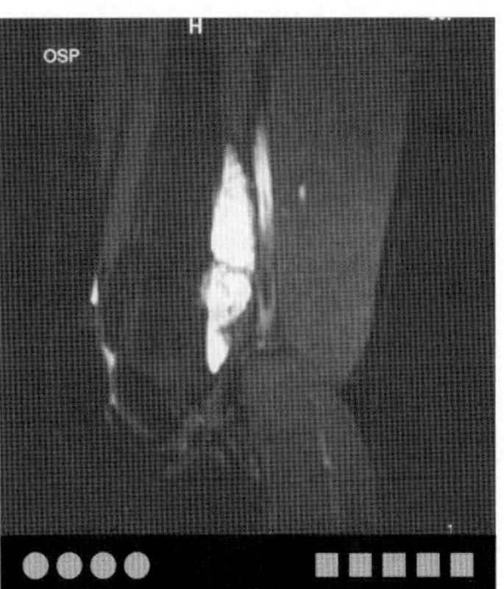

G. Aneurysmal bone cyst: Sagittal T2-weighted MR image shows the mass becomes bright.

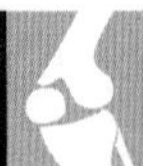

27–28 Parosteal Osteosarcoma of Distal Femur

Michael A. Bruno

PRESENTATION

Recent leg pain and swelling

FINDINGS

Radiographs of the knee and thigh show a large, dense mass extending from the posterolateral femoral margin forming a broad base. MRI shows no evidence of extension into the medullary space.

DIFFERENTIAL DIAGNOSES

- *Myositis ossificans:* This is usually posttraumatic, the ossific densities in this benign condition demonstrate three distinct zones—the central, undifferentiated zone; a surrounding zone of immature osteoid formation; and a peripheral zone with more mature bone. The characteristic zone pattern may be apparent within 10 days after the onset of symptoms. Also, myositis ossificans does not invade surrounding soft tissues nor does it invade the marrow space.
- *Periosteal osteosarcoma:* This tumor is differentiated by the presence of a region of densely thickened cortex with evidence of extrinsic pressure-type erosion along the margin of the broad-based surface soft-tissue mass. Typically, there is also significant periosteal reaction, usually oriented perpendicularly to the long bone shaft, and extending into the soft-tissue component. As with parosteal osteosarcoma, marrow invasion is rare.
- *Fibrous dysplasia:* This lesion can be considered in any dense, irregular mass.

COMMENTS

The patient is a 51-year-old man with a relatively brief history of pain but a longer and uncertain history of swelling that belies the slow, indolent progression of this tumor. The tumor exhibits a somewhat cloud-like calcification and appears to encircle the femur partially. Angiography shows the lesion to be relatively hypovascular. This is a very common location for parosteal osteosarcoma, with 50% of lesions found in this region. Lesions found at an earlier stage may interface with the cortex in a small focal region, i.e., a narrow stalk of attachment, whereas lesions found at a later stage, such as this one, demonstrate a broader base against the cortex. Medullary involvement is rare, and it changes the prognosis. The role of MRI is limited to the evaluation of the tumor extension. Angiography is no longer commonly performed as it contributes little to the diagnosis or management of these tumors. Parosteal osteosarcoma is a relatively low-grade tumor histologically. The prognosis is relatively good after wide excision, unless cortical invasion or extension of the tumor into the medullary space indicate the presence of dedifferentiation into a higher-grade tumor. This tumor should be differentiated from posttraumatic myositis ossificans. The presence of cleavage plane between heterotopic bone and host bone and well-demarcated cortical margin confirms myositis ossificans.

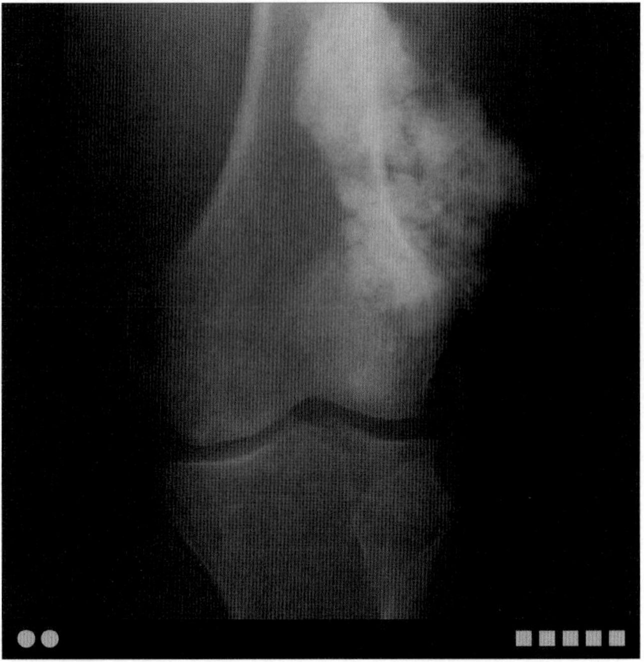

A. Parosteal osteosarcoma: AP radiograph of the distal thigh and knee demonstrating the dense mass appearing to encircle the posterolateral aspect of the distal femur. Note irregular tumor margin.

PEARLS

- **Parosteal osteosarcoma most often occurs in the distal femur and proximal humerus, growing along the bone surface and often encircling the shaft.**
- **It is a low-grade tumor with a favorable prognosis.**
- **The patient's symptoms are mild and the progression is indolent.**
- **Extension to the medullary space (best detected by MRI) is a poor prognostic sign, usually indicating dedifferentiation to a more aggressive, higher-grade malignancy.**

ADDITIONAL IMAGES

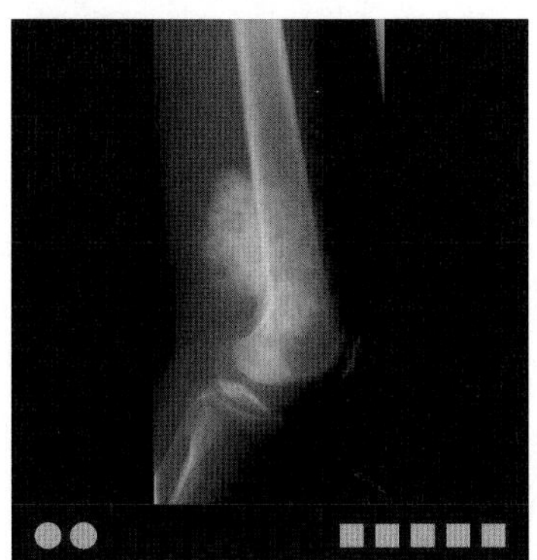

B. Parosteal osteosarcoma: Lateral view of the same patient. There is a broad base stalk and irregular margin of the mass.

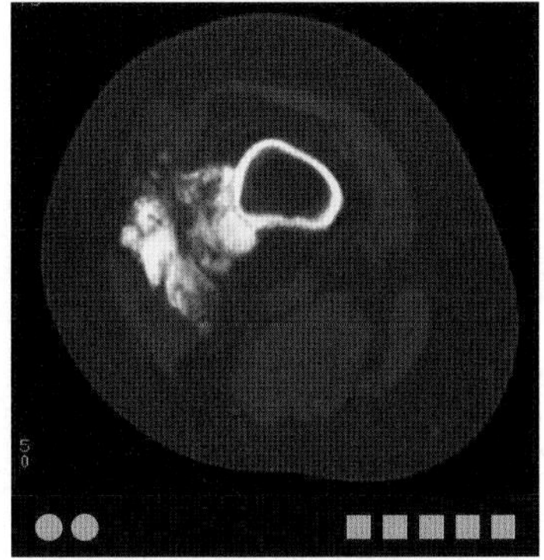

C. Parosteal osteosarcoma: Axial CT scan of the mass shows the margins of the tumors to be markedly irregular.

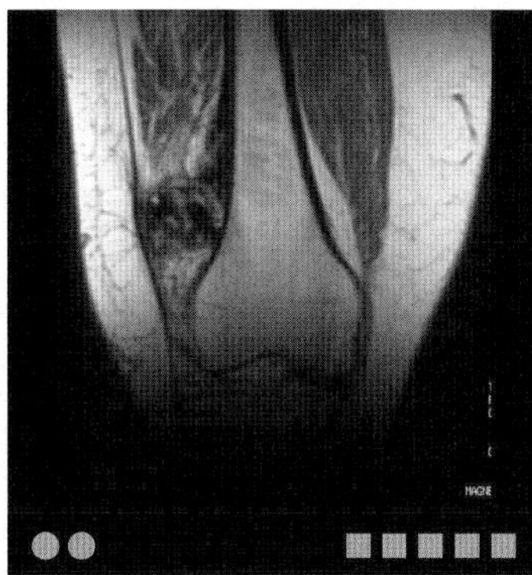

D. Parosteal osteosarcoma: Coronal T1-weighted spin-echo MR image shows the extent of the lateral soft-tissue extension of the tumor and absence of medullary involvement.

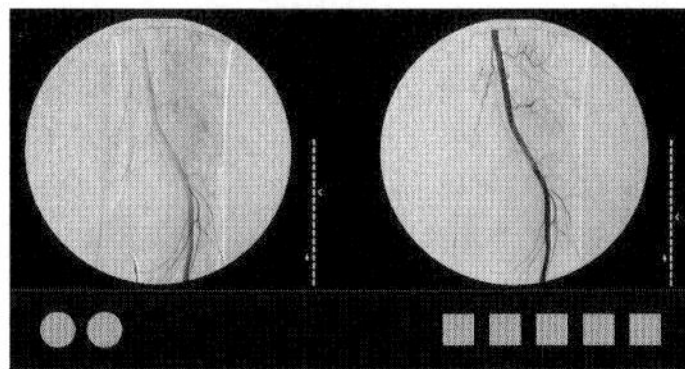

E. Parosteal osteosarcoma: Subtraction images from conventional contrast angiography. The tumor is shown to be relatively hypovascular, but shows some central early "tumor blush" and pooling of contrast.

IMAGE KEY

Common

Rare

Typical

Unusual

DIFFERENTIAL DIAGNOSES IMAGES

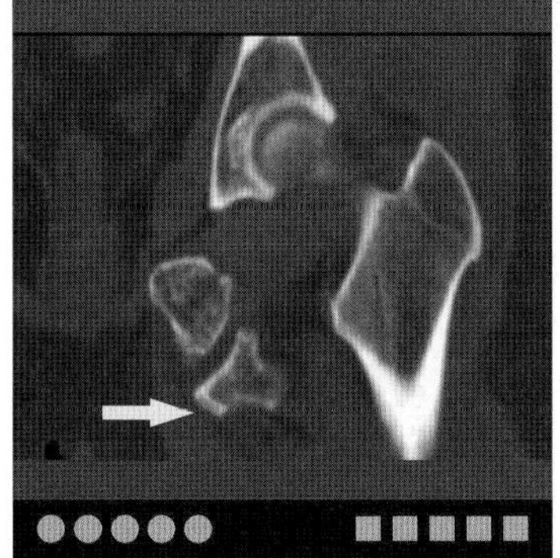

F. Posttraumatic heterotopic ossification: This is a patient with football injury several years earlier, who has pain in the leg and hip. Coronal reformatted CT shows heterotopic ossification at quadratus femoris muscle (arrow). Note there is a cleavage plane between the ischial tuberosity and this benign ossification.

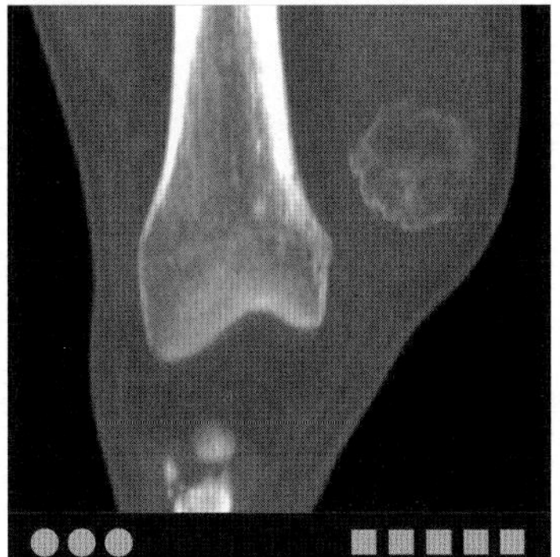

G. Myositis ossificans: AP radiograph of the knee in a different patient with a myositis ossificans lesion near the knee joint. Note the margin of this lesion is calcified and the center is relatively lucent.

27–29 Chondroblastic Osteosarcoma of Tibia

Peyman Borghei and Jamshid Tehranzadeh

PRESENTATION

Leg pain

FINDINGS

MRI shows a heterogeneous lesion in the right proximal tibia with cortical breakthrough. There is also a central area of low signal intensity with marginal enhancement on post-contrast image compatible with an area of necrosis.

DIFFERENTIAL DIAGNOSES

- *Ewing sarcoma:* This is usually seen in the shaft of long bones with large soft-tissue mass. Necrosis and hemorrhage are frequently present.
- *Telangiectatic osteosarcoma:* Presents with mostly osteolytic appearance and multiple fluid–fluid levels on CT or MRI.
- *Chondrosarcoma:* Cartilaginous matrix and typical calcification is seen.
- *Fibrosarcoma:* Fibrosarcoma and malignant fibrous histiocytoma in bone may rarely simulate osteolytic osteosarcoma.
- *Tuberculous pseudotumor:* This mixed osteolytic and osteosclerotic lesion with irregular periosteal reaction may mimic sarcomas.

COMMENTS

The patient is a 17-year-old girl with a history of leg pain diagnosed with chondroblastic osteosarcoma. High-grade intramedullary osteosarcoma or conventional osteosarcoma arises from undifferentiated mesenchymal tissue (cartilaginous, fibrous, osseous matrix) and produces osteoid or immature bone. There are three histologic types: osteoblastic (50–80%), chondroblastic (5–25%), and fibroblastic–fibrohistiocytic (7–25%). The age of the patients is usually 10 to 25 or >60 years. Patients usually present with painful swelling of 1 to 2 months duration and fever. It is most commonly seen in the metaphysis of the long bones, while the lesion is about the knee in 50% to 55% of cases. At the time of diagnosis the lesion is usually about 5 to 6 cm. The tumor can be purely osteolytic or purely osteoblastic but the mixed pattern is the most typical. Periosteal reaction can be interrupted in the form of Codman triangle, perpendicular as seen in sunburst (hair on end) or laminated (onion skin) appearance. Cortical destruction and soft tissue mass usually accompany the lesion. MRI shows an inhomogeneous

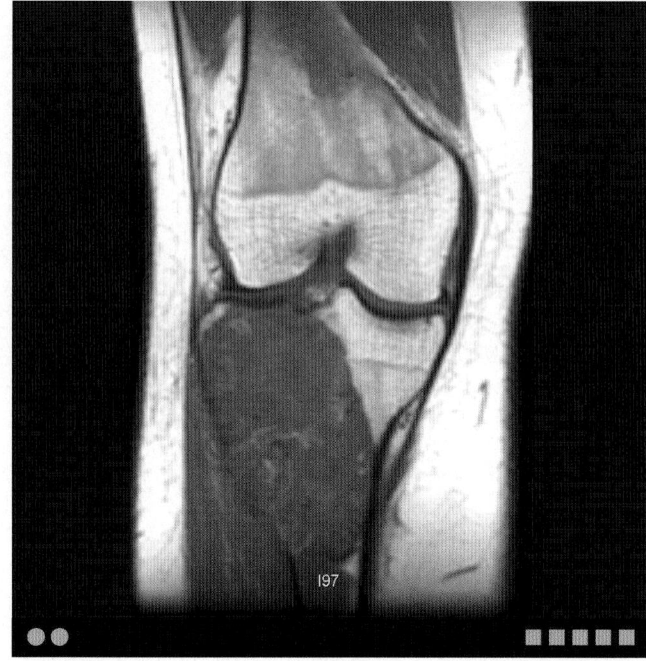

A. Osteosarcoma: Coronal T1-weighted image shows an inhomogeneous low signal mass with lateral cortical break measuring 7.7 × 4.4 × 4.7 cm in the proximal tibia extending into the tibial plateau but not into the joint.

lesion with low to intermediate signal intensity on T1-weighted and high signal intensity on T2-weighted image, which inhomogeneously enhances with the contrast. Subacute hemorrhage within the tumor is seen as high signal intensity on both T1-weighted and T2-weighted images. Necrosis and cystic changes within the tumor is seen as hypointense on T1-weighted and hyper intense on T2-weighted images. MRI also helps to evaluate the extent of soft tissue and neurovascular involvement and invasion of epiphysis and joints.

PEARLS

- **Osteosarcoma originates from the undifferentiated cartilaginous, fibrous, or osseous mesenchymal tissue.**
- **The common site of involvement is the metaphysis of the long bones, especially the distal femur and proximal tibia.**
- **MRI shows an inhomogeneous lesion with low to intermediate signal intensity on T1-weighted and high signal intensity on T2-weighted images with an inhomogeneous contrast enhancement.**
- **Peritumoral edema appears as high signal intensity on T2-weighted image, which enhances more homogeneously.**

ADDITIONAL IMAGES

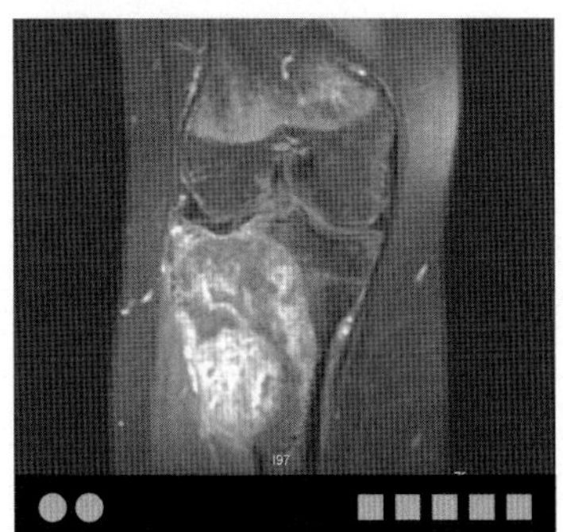

B. Osteosarcoma: Coronal fat-saturated post-contrast T1-weighted image shows an inhomogeneously enhanced lesion with cortical disruption. The small necrotic core of the tumor has little or no enhancement.

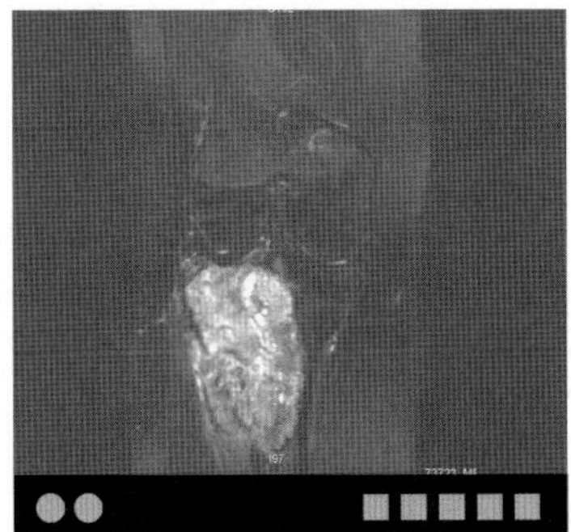

C. Osteosarcoma: Coronal fat-saturated T2-weighted image shows an inhomogeneous high signal intensity lesion with cortical disruption and soft tissue invasion by the tumor in the lateral side of proximal tibia.

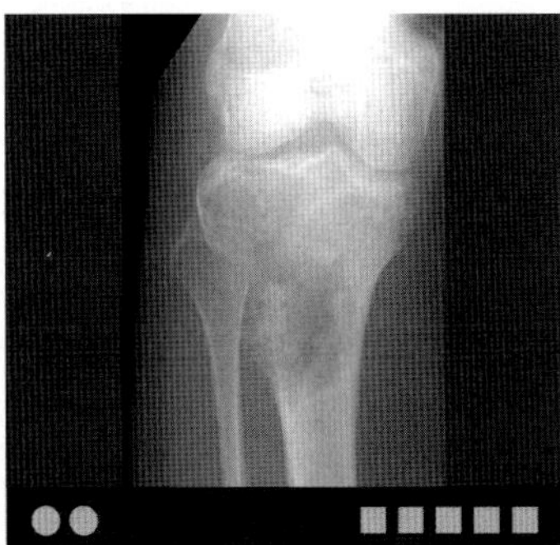

D. Osteosarcoma: Radiograph shows a large lytic lesion with a wide zone of transition at the proximal right tibial metaphysis and epiphysis with loss of cortex on the lateral side. Note a focal area of sclerotic bone near the lateral cortex.

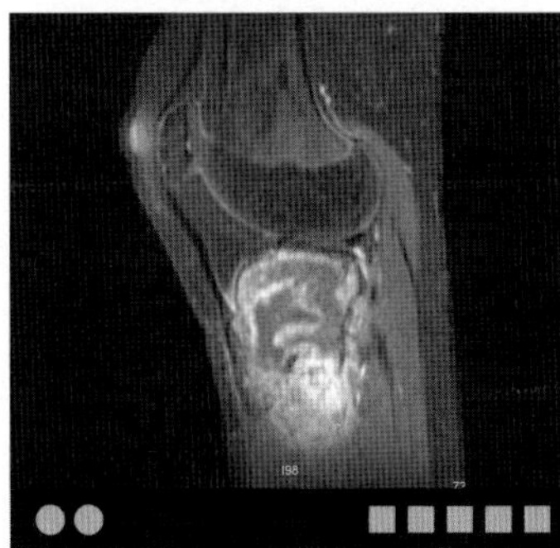

E. Osteosarcoma: Sagittal fat-saturated post-contrast T1-weighted image shows a heterogeneous lesion in the right proximal tibia with cortical breakthrough. There is also a central area of low signal intensity with marginal enhancement compatible with an area of necrosis.

IMAGE KEY

Common

Rare

Typical

Unusual

DIFFERENTIAL DIAGNOSES IMAGES

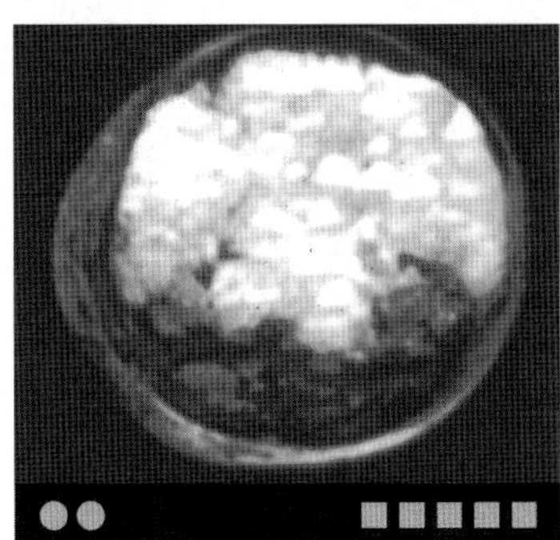

F. Telangiectatic osteosarcoma: Axial CT scan shows a large and expansile osteolytic lesion with multiple fluid–fluid levels.

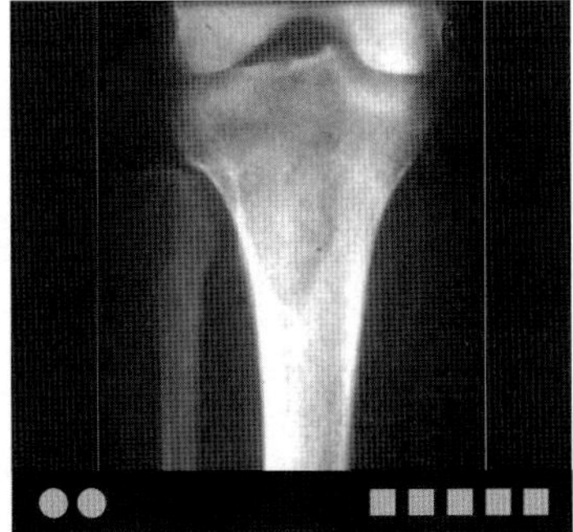

G. Tuberculous pseudotumor: AP view of the right knee shows mixed lytic and sclerotic lesion with compact endosteal bone reaction on the lateral margin of the lesion and intact articular margin. Note irregular periosteal reaction. (Courtesy of I.F. Abdelwahab)

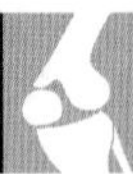

27–30 Angiosarcoma of Distal Femur

Shahla Modarresi and Daria Motamedi

PRESENTATION

Progressive hip and leg pain

FINDINGS

STIR MR imaging shows cortical destruction and slightly expansile lesion of the left femoral diametaphyses and increased signal at bone marrow and soft tissues.

DIFFERENTIAL DIAGNOSES

- *Metastasis:* Osteolytic metastasis such as lung or breast cancer. MR imaging shows multiple small or large low T1 signal lesions that become higher signal than surrounding marrow on T2-weighted sequence.
- *Osteomyelitis:* MR imaging shows permeative or mouth-eaten bone destruction, obliterating medullary fat by marrow edema causing low to intermediate on T1-weighted and high signal on T2-weighted and STIR images.
- *Plasmocytoma:* MR imaging signal is indistinguishable from metastasis. MR imaging usually shows equal or lower signal than muscle in T1-weighted image, low or high signal intensity in T2-weighted images.
- *Fibrous bone lesions:* Fibrous dysplasia shows decreased signal on T1-weighted image because of fibrous nature, heterogeneous signal on T2-weighted image which may be high, low, or mixed. It has benign appearance without soft tissue mass.

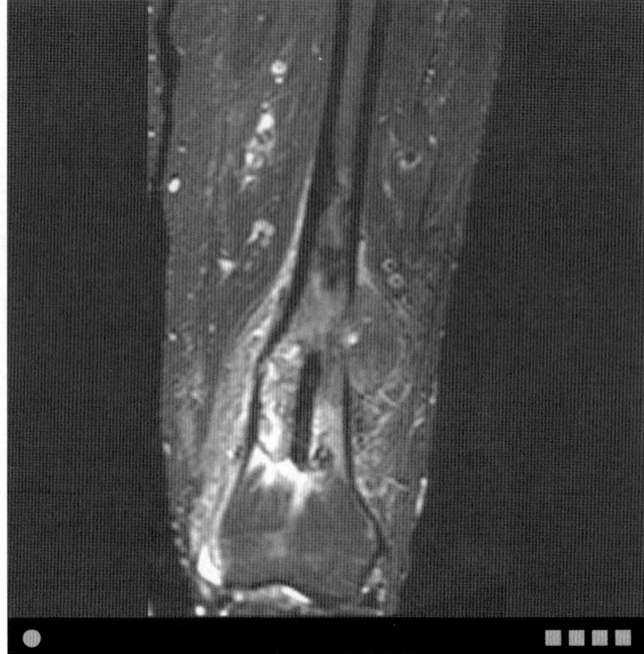

A. Angiosarcoma: Coronal STIR image shows left distal femoral cortical destruction, soft tissue mass with increased bone marrow and surrounding soft tissue signal intensity.

COMMENTS

The patient is a 70-year-old man with progressive hip and leg pain. Angiosarcoma is a high-grade malignant tumor of the blood vessel cells. Hemangioendothelioma and hemangiopericytoma are lower-grade tumors with better prognosis. Soft tissue sarcomas (1–2%) are vascular in origin. Angiosarcomas are found in the skin, soft tissue, breast, liver, and bone, and are more common in men between the ages of 40 and 70 years. High-grade skeletal angiosarcoma has two distinct clinical presentations: (1) multiple lesions in a single bone, two or more adjacent bones, having slow course and good prognosis; (2) single or multiple rapidly progressive lesions that metastasize to other bones or to the lung with very poor prognosis. Typical lesions of high-grade angiosarcoma are eccentric, lytic, metaphyseal, and diaphyseal, with focal cortical destruction and no visible calcification. They appear very aggressive with soft tissue extension and no periosteal reaction. Treatment involves a wide excision with adjuvant therapy depending on the grade and stage of the tumor at presentation. Small association with bone infarct may exist. The site and extent of the lesion is clearly seen on MRI or CT scan. MR imaging shows mixed signal intensity lesion with low T1 and high T2 signal. Focal cortical disruption with soft tissue extension may exist. MR imaging is used for staging rather than specific diagnosis of bone lesions, which are much more accurately determined with conventional radiographs.

PEARLS

- **Angiosarcoma is a high-grade malignant tumor of the blood vessel cells. Hemangioendothelioma and hemangiopericytoma are lower-grade tumors with better prognosis.**
- **High-grade skeletal angiosarcoma can appear as multiple slow growing lesions with good prognosis or rapidly progressive lesions that metastasize with very poor prognosis.**
- **The lesions of high-grade angiosarcoma are eccentric, lytic, metaphyseal, and diaphyseal, with focal cortical disruption, small calcification, and little soft tissue extension.**
- **The extent of the lesion is clearly seen on MRI or CT. MRI shows mixed signal intensity lesion with low T1 and high T2 signal characteristics.**

ADDITIONAL IMAGES

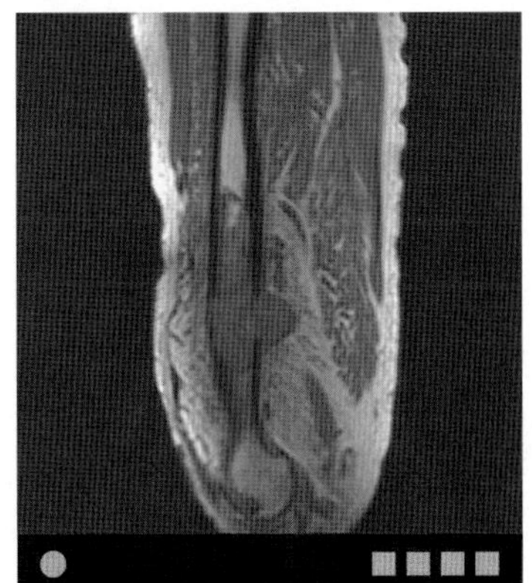

B. Angiosarcoma: Sagittal T1-weighted image shows left femoral low signal intensity lesion with cortical disruption and soft tissue mass.

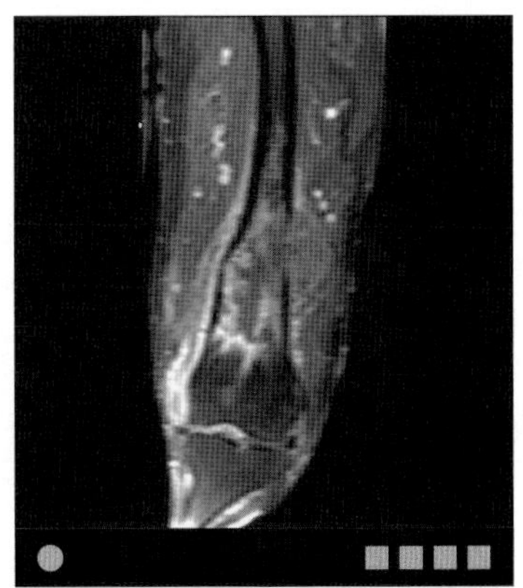

C. Angiosarcoma: Coronal postcontrast fat-saturated T1-weighted image shows diffuse bone marrow and adjacent soft tissue enhancement.

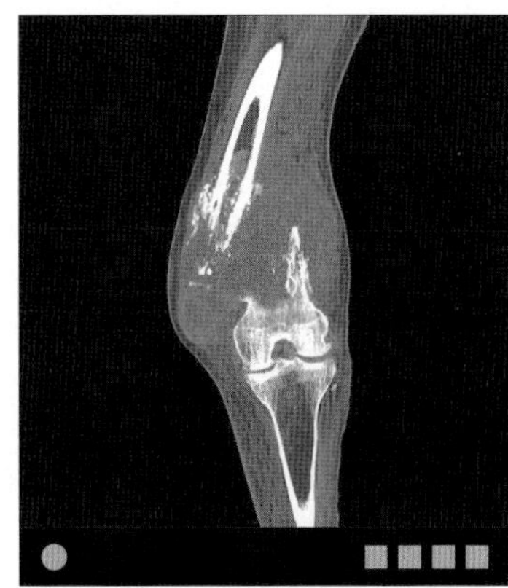

D. Angiosarcoma: Coronal reconstruction CT scan of femur showing advanced destructive angiosarcoma with displaced pathologic fracture, large soft tissue mass and calcification.

IMAGE KEY

Common

Rare

Typical

Unusual

DIFFERENTIAL DIAGNOSES IMAGES

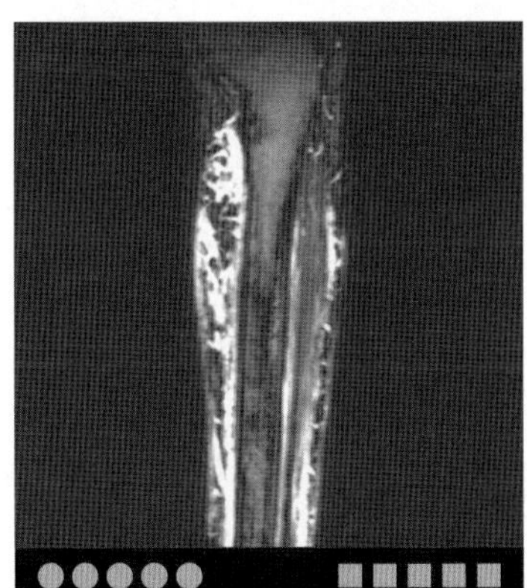

E. Osteomyelitis: Sagittal T2-weighted with fat saturation image shows permeative bone destruction and marked soft tissue edema showing increased T2 signal consistent with osteomyelitis.

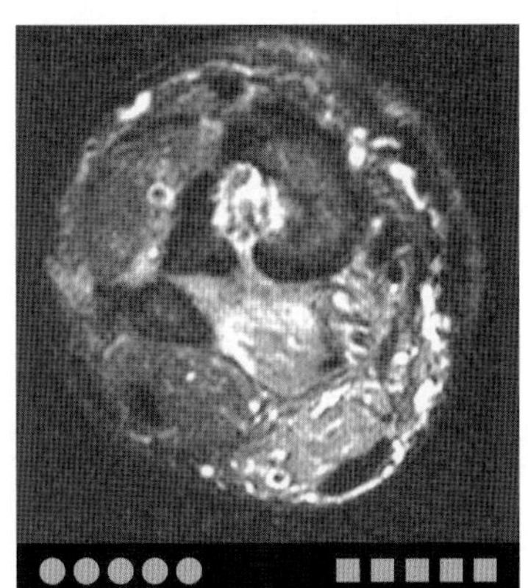

F. Osteomyelitis: Axial STIR image showing abnormal increased mar row signal in patient with chronic active osteomyelitis.

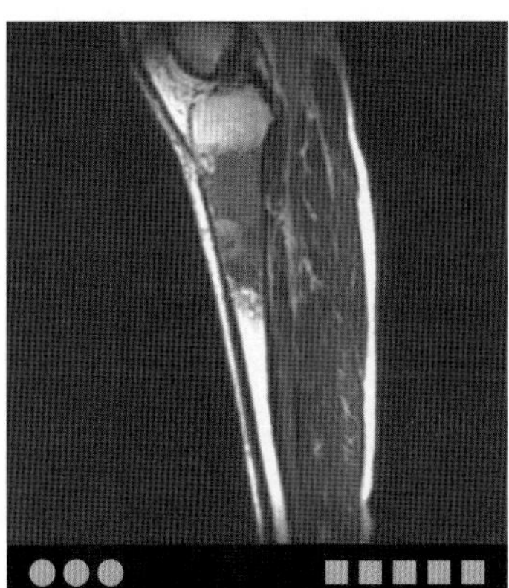

G. Fibrous dysplasia: Sagittal T1-weighted image shows low signal lesion of proximal tibia because of fibrous nature consistent with fibrous dysplasia. It has benign appearance without soft tissue mass.

Chapter 28

Miscellaneous

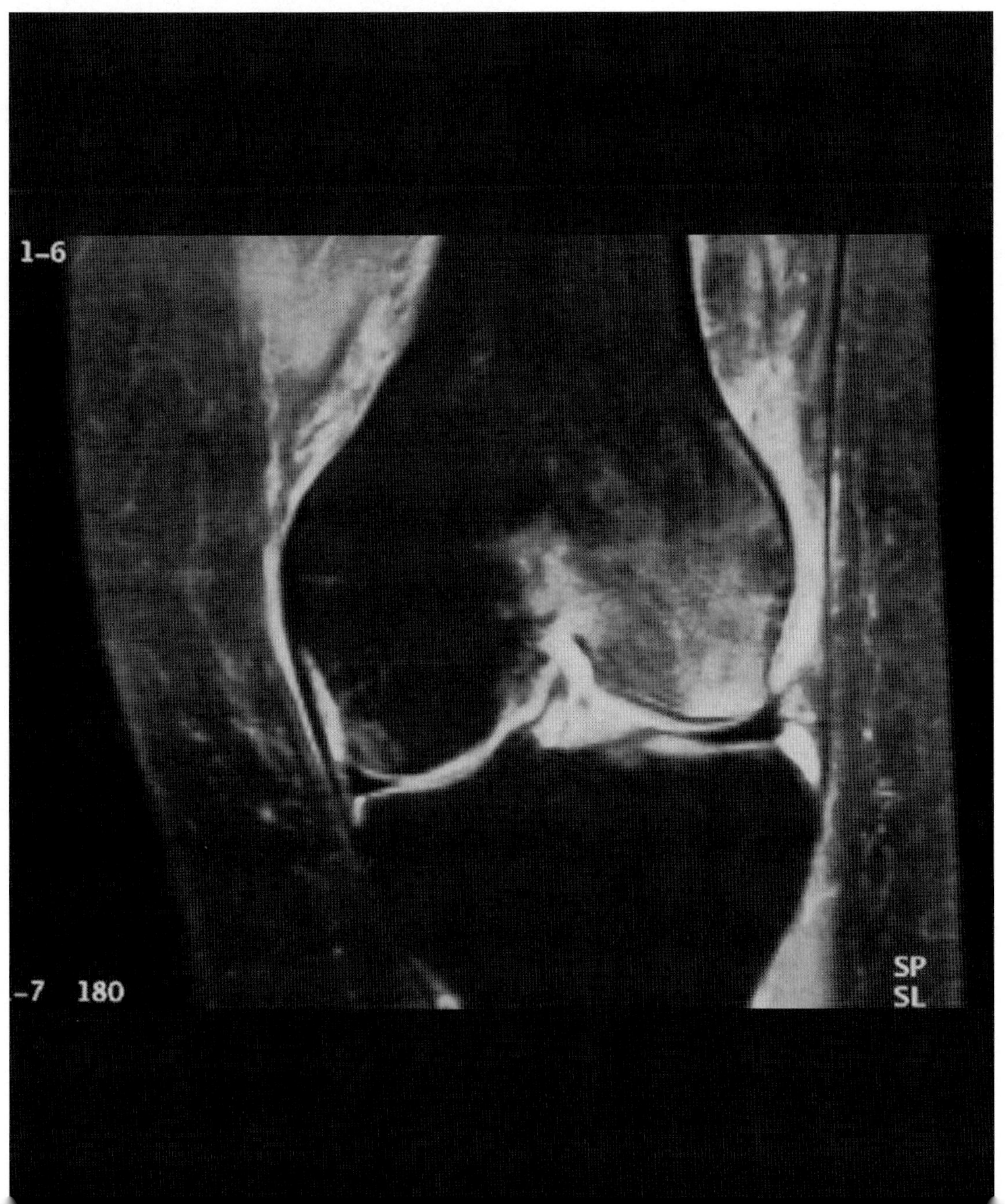

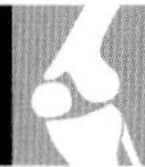

28–1 Transient Osteoporosis of the Knee

George Hermann

PRESENTATION

Knee pain

FINDINGS

MRI shows diffused edema of the lateral condyle of the left femur.

DIFFERENTIAL DIAGNOSES

- *Reflex sympathetic dystrophy:* Usually preceded by trauma; commonly, involves the upper extremity. The long-term prognosis is poor. Contracture and local circulatory changes may develop.
- *Subchondral fracture or contusion:* Usually followed by trauma or knee injury.
- *Transient edema:* Radiograph shows no osteoporosis.
- *Spontaneous osteonecrosis of the knee (sonk or sponk):* Often seen in knees with previous meniscectomy, and they represent subchondral insufficiency fractures.

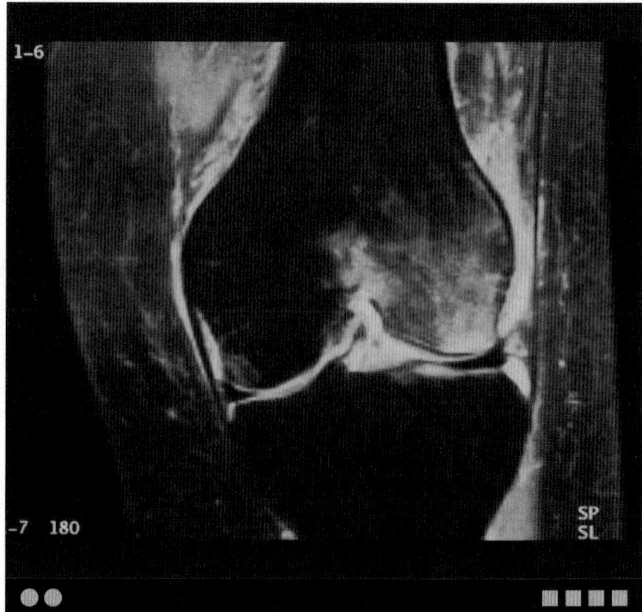

A. Transient osteoporosis of the knee: Coronal T2 images show bright SI of the lateral condyle. Note the prominent bright SI around the knee, and more on the lateral side.

COMMENTS

This is an image of a 53-year-old woman complaining of a gradual onset of left knee pain. She was diagnosed with transient osteoporosis of the left lateral femoral condyle. Transient osteoporosis is an uncommon, self-limiting condition that is characterized by pain around the involved joint and osteopenia on radiography. The condition was first described in 1959 in young women who developed transient demineralization of the hip at the third trimester of pregnancy. It is known today that the disorder is not uncommon in middle-aged men as well. Apart from the hips, it may involve the knee and ankle but rarely the upper extremity. Clinically, the patient presents with a gradual or sudden onset of pain around the joint. Typically, there is no history of trauma. At the time of presentation, there is a local tenderness, erythema, and limitation of motion. The symptoms resolve spontaneously over a period of 6 to 8 months. The condition may recur in the same joint or it may migrate and appear in a different joint. The etiology of transient osteoporosis is unknown. It should be differentiated from bone marrow edema, reflex sympathetic dystrophy. On MRI, the involved joint shows diffuse, decreased signal intensity (SI) on T1-weighted image and increased SI on T2-weighted image or fast inversion recovery, because of the marked marrow edema. While the recovery is complete in both disorders, in transient osteoporosis, and osteopenia will develop within 6 to 8 weeks intervals.

PEARLS

- **Transient osteoporosis is an uncommon disorder. Usually involves the hip, knee, occasionally the ankle, and rarely the upper extremity.**
- **On MRI, it presents with marrow edema—decreased SI on T1-weighted image and increased SI on T2-weighted image.**
- **Radiograph—initially is normal. The patient usually develops osteoporosis and joint effusion within a few weeks.**
- **Radionuclide bone scan demonstrates increased uptake.**

ADDITIONAL IMAGES

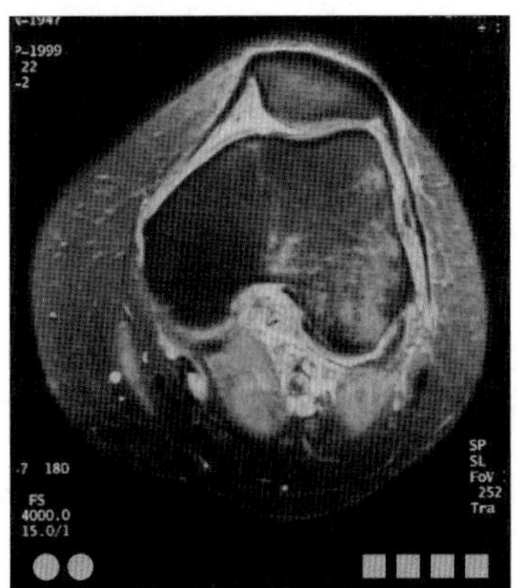

B. Transient osteoporosis of the knee: Axial STIR images show increased SI of the lateral condyle.

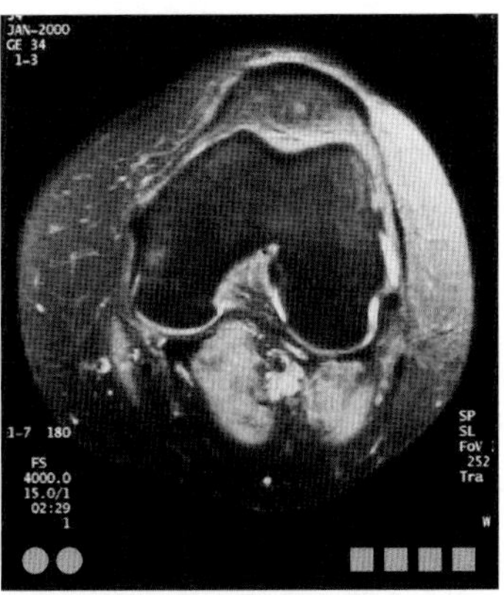

C. Transient osteoporosis of the knee: Axial STIR image 4 months later demonstrates no significant signal alteration.

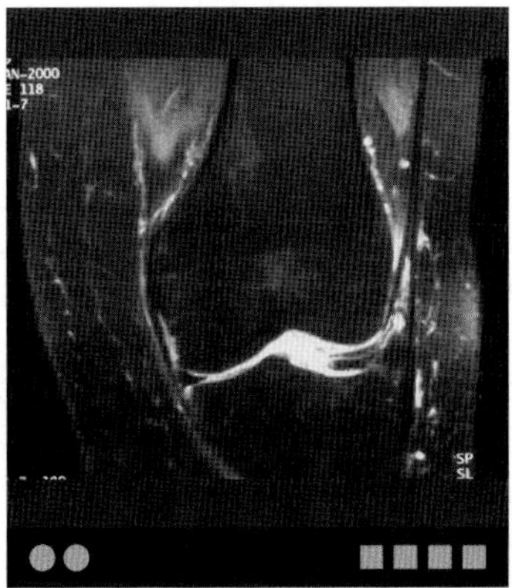

D. Transient osteoporosis of the knee: Coronal T2 image 4 months later. The lateral femoral condyle appears normal. The articular surface is intact.

IMAGE KEY

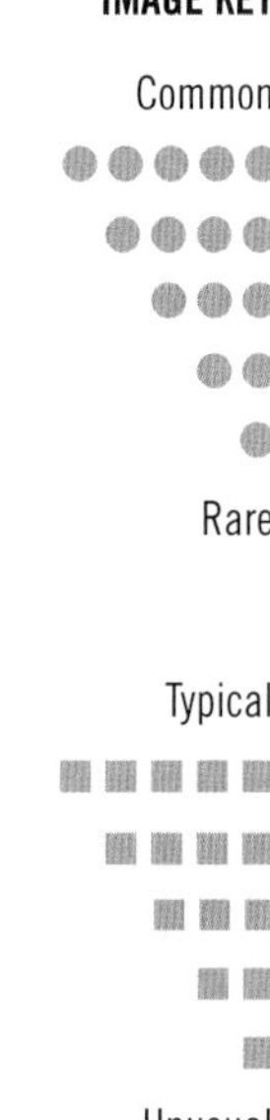

DIFFERENTIAL DIAGNOSES IMAGES

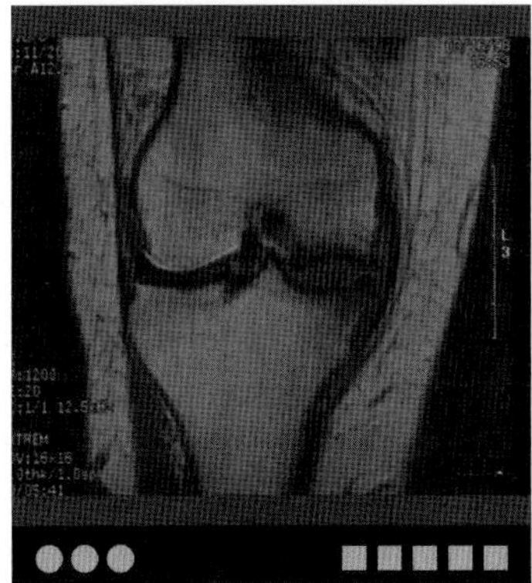

E. Osteonecrosis of femoral condyle: T1-weighted iamge shows decreased SI at the subchondral part of the medial femoral condyle. The articular surface is indistinct.

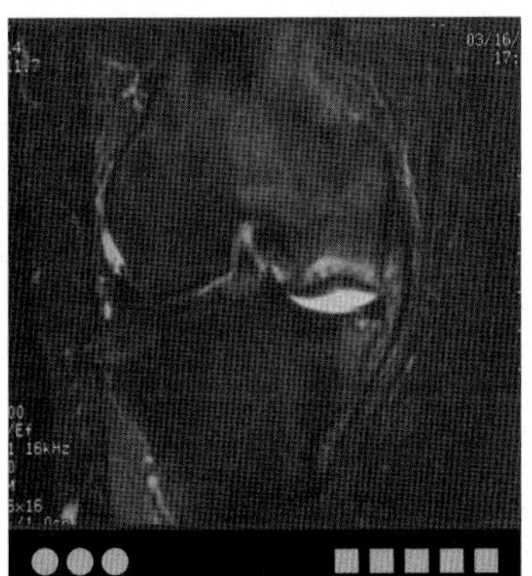

F. Osteonecrosis of femoral condyle: T2-weighted image shows increased SI at the subchondral part of the condyle.

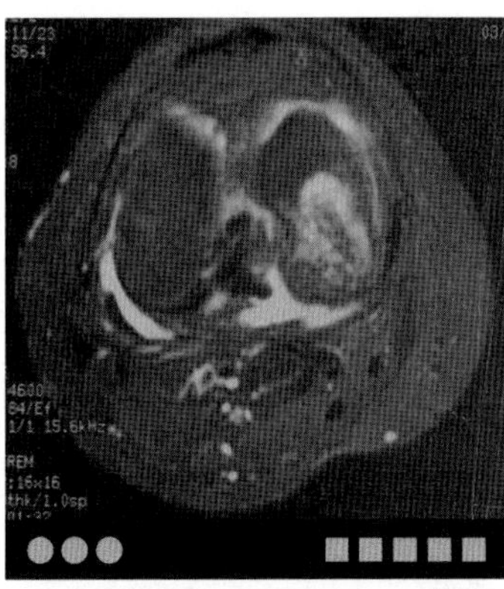

G. Osteonecrosis of femoral condyle: Axial STIR image shows mostly a high SI area at the medial condyle.

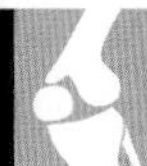

28–2 Myonecrosis

Sailaja Yadavalli

PRESENTATION

Leg swelling and pain with foot drop

FINDINGS

Postcontrast MR image shows areas of low signal intensity within the muscles of the anterior and lateral compartments of the leg with peripheral nodular enhancement. No focal fluid collection is seen.

DIFFERENTIAL DIAGNOSES

- *Abscess:* Mass with central nonenhancing fluid with peripheral rim of enhancement. Patients have clinical findings of infection.
- *Tumor:* Ill-defined, central, and nonenhancing necrotic areas with peripheral areas of enhancement may have appearance similar to myonecrosis. Patients do not have a history of sudden onset of symptoms.
- *Myositis:* Focal, nodular myositis may have the appearance of an enhancing mass. It is typically not as painful as myonecrosis.

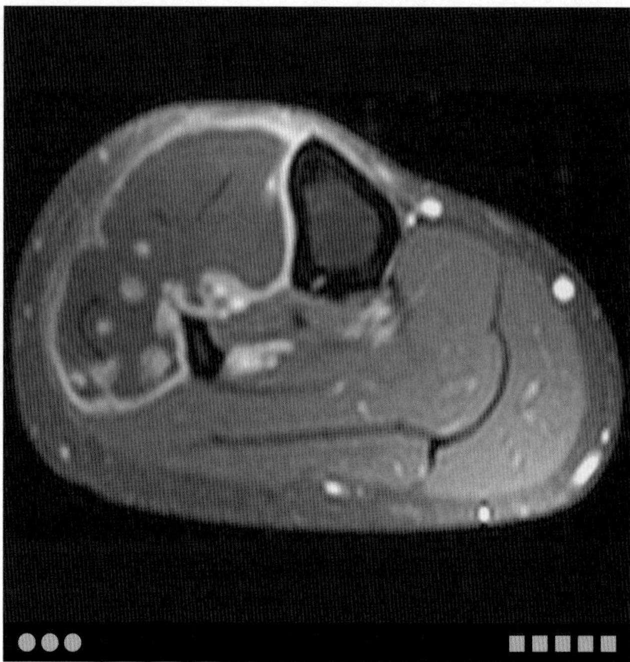

A. Myonecrosis: Axial TI-weighted contrast-enhanced fat-saturated image shows central region of low signal with peripheral enhancement and areas of nodular enhancement within.

COMMENTS

This is an image of a 33-year-old female who presented with a history of fall, leg swelling, and pain; 1 month ago presented with foot drop and pain. Myonecrosis may be idiopathic in patients with diabetes or alcohol abuse. No fever or erythema is seen. Multiple etiologies have been associated with myonecrosis. These include trauma, ischemia, infection, or neoplasm. Myonecrosis has also been described in diabetics and with alcoholism. Patients present with acute symptoms of pain, swelling, and weakness. Diagnosis of myonecrosis may be difficult in cases where there is no obvious cause as patients may not have associated erythema or fever. Patients complain of extreme pain that is typically out of proportion to the clinical signs and extent of injury. With subacute presentation creatinine kinase levels may not be high. Elevated creatinine kinase with subsequent exponential drop within a few days has been reported in patients presenting with acute symptoms. On T1-weighted MR images, the areas of myonecrosis are isointense to muscle. Swelling with loss of fascial planes may be seen in the involved muscles. On fluid sensitive sequences no intramuscular focal fluid collections are seen. Instead diffuse or patchy muscle edema is noted with perifascial fluid and subcutaneous edema. Postintravenous contrast injection central regions of low signal are seen with irregular and almost nodular areas of peripheral enhancement. Foci or streaks of enhancement may be seen within the central low signal intensity regions. These may represent viable or inflammatory tissue. Involvement of the adjacent bone depends on the etiology of the muscle necrosis.

PEARLS

- **Myonecrosis may be related to trauma, infection, neoplasm, and vascular abnormalities or may be idiopathic typically in patients with diabetes or alcoholism.**
- **Degree of pain is usually disproportionately high compared to other clinical findings.**
- **Pattern of peripheral enhancement with central area of low signal and areas of nodular and linear enhancement within the central area is typical.**
- **Area of necrosis is usually isointense to muscle on T1-weighted images.**
- **No associated focal fluid collections are seen in the muscle.**

ADDITIONAL IMAGES

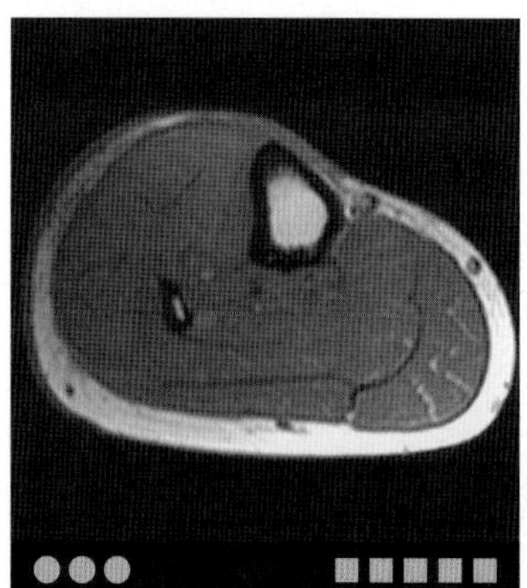

B. Myonecrosis: Axial T1-weighted nonfat-saturated image shows mild ill definition of muscle planes along the anterolateral aspect of the leg with the involved muscles slightly swollen but isointense to other muscles.

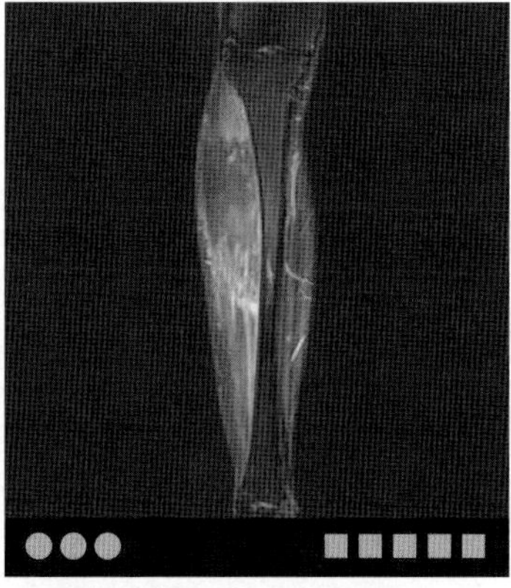

C. Myonecrosis: Coronal STIR image shows patchy muscle edema without a focal fluid collection.

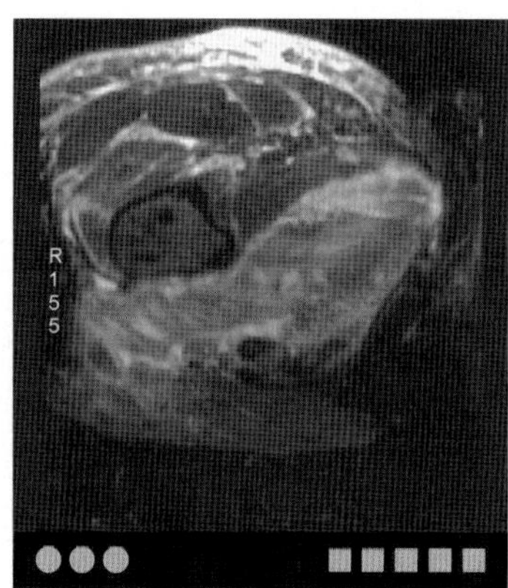

D. Myonecrosis: Axial STIR image shows patchy, increased signal in multiple muscles around the right hip in this diabetic patient with idiopathic myonecrosis.

DIFFERENTIAL DIAGNOSES IMAGES

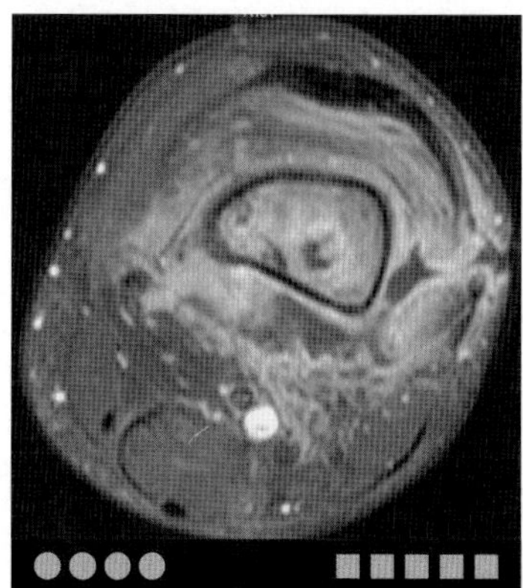

E. Abscess: Axial postcontrast T1-weighted image shows a low signal area with peripheral enhancement extending to the skin. There is also extensive enhancement of muscle and bone marrow in this patient with osteomyelitis and draining abscess.

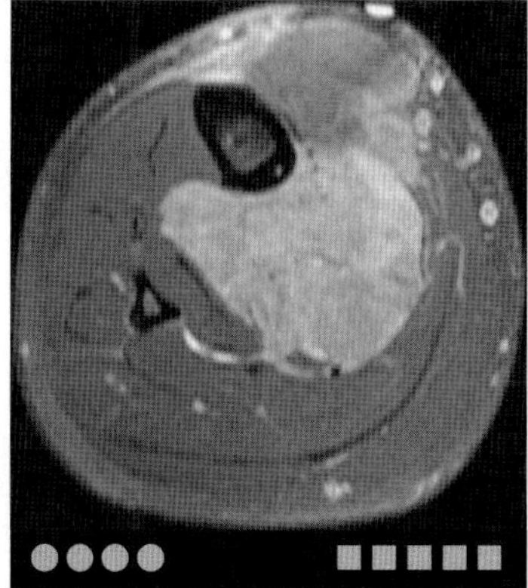

F. Tumor: Axial postcontrast T1-weighted image shows a large enhancing mass with anterior nonenhancing necrotic region in a patient with proven Ewing's Sarcoma.

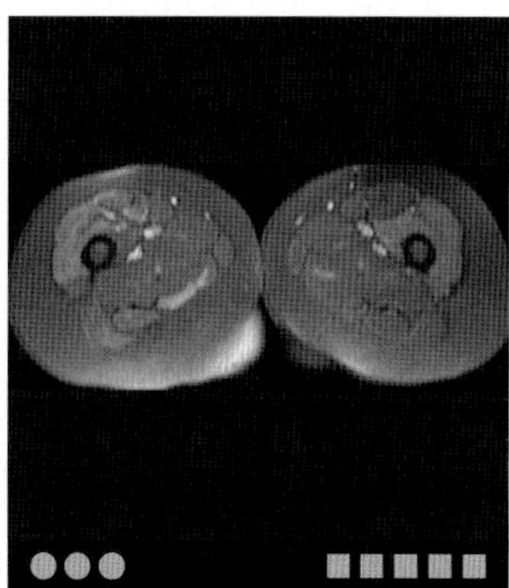

G. Myositis: Axial postcontrast T1-weighted FS image shows enhancement of multiple muscles in both thighs in a patient with polymyositis.

IMAGE KEY

Common

Rare

Typical

Unusual

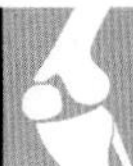

28–3 Bone Infarct in Systemic Lupus

Marcia F. Blacksin

PRESENTATION

Gradually worsening knee pain

FINDINGS

Bone infarcts in proximal tibial and distal femoral shafts extending to articular surfaces are noted.

DIFFERENTIAL DIAGNOSES

- *Sickle cell anemia:* Multiple foci of marrow infarction on radiography and MR, red marrow hyperplasia are seen.
- *Spontaneous osteonecrosis medial femoral condyle:* Usually only site of marrow edema, with low signal line running parallel to subchondral bone.

COMMENTS

Early osteonecrosis can manifest as bone marrow edema. As the area of infarction matures, the classical finding of a "double line sign' would appear. This is a band of high signal intensity on T2-weighted images that runs parallel to a line of decreased signal in the medullary canal, often with a serpentine border. On T1-weighted sequences, the low signal intensity rim is easily identified. Systemic lupus is one of several diseases that can cause marrow infarction. Osteonecrosis may be secondary to the vasculitis seen with this disease or secondary to steroids used to treat the disease. Other diseases that are associated with marrow infarction include sickle cell disease, and Gaucher's disease. MR findings seen with sickle cell disease include marrow infarction as well as red marrow hyperplasia. In these patients, red marrow will often cross the growth plate and infiltrate both the normally fatty epiphyseal and apophyseal regions of the bone. Rheumatoid arthritis and HIV disease may demonstrate bone infarcts as a complication of medications administered to treat these conditions. Differential diagnosis for this imaging study also includes "SPONK" or spontaneous osteonecrosis of the medial condyle. Though originally felt to be osteonecrosis adjacent to the medial femoral condyle subchondral plate, this process is now felt to be a stress fracture of the condyle. It occurs in older patients, and is often associated with a meniscal tear. Cases have been seen in the lateral condyle. No other foci of marrow infarction are seen in this patient population.

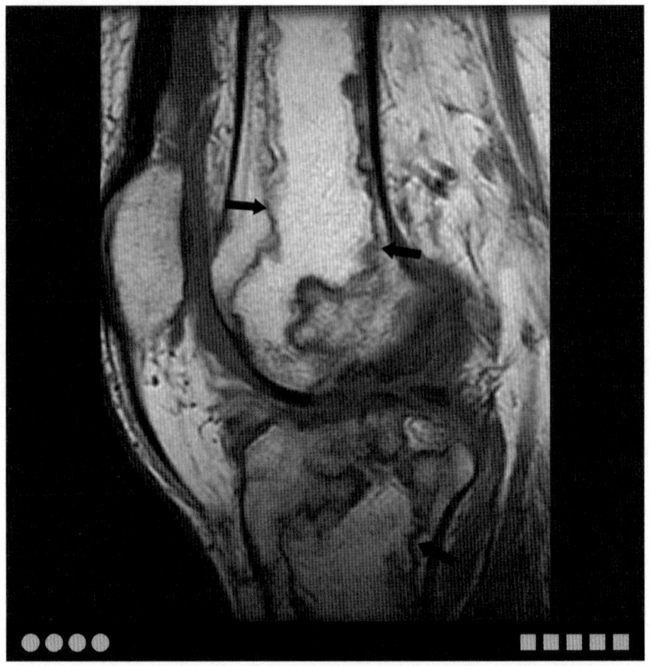

A. Systemic lupus with marrow infarction: Sagittal T1-weighted image with zones of infarction demarcated by low signal serpiginous border (arrows).

PEARLS

- **The double line sign is pathognomonic for osteonecrosis on MR images.**
- **Sickle cell anemia can demonstrate bone infarcts and red marrow hyperplasia on MR studies.**
- **Spontaneous osteonecrosis of the medial femoral condyle is a stress fracture, and associated with meniscal tear.**

ADDITIONAL IMAGE

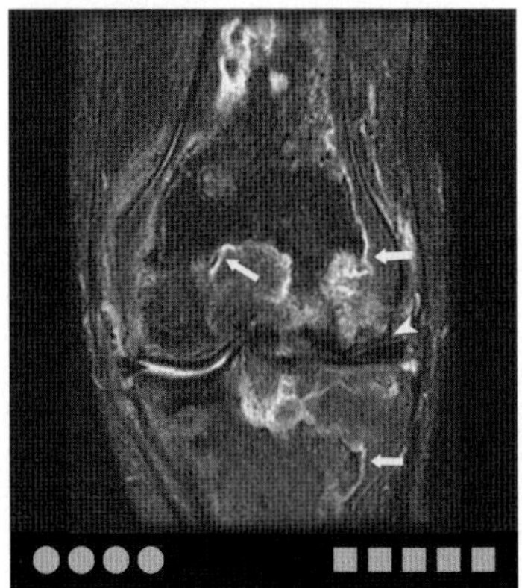

B. Systemic lupus with marrow infarction: Coronal T2-weighted image with double line sign in distal femur and proximal tibia (arrows). Note subchondral collapse of lateral femoral condyle (arrowhead).

DIFFERENTIAL DIAGNOSES IMAGES

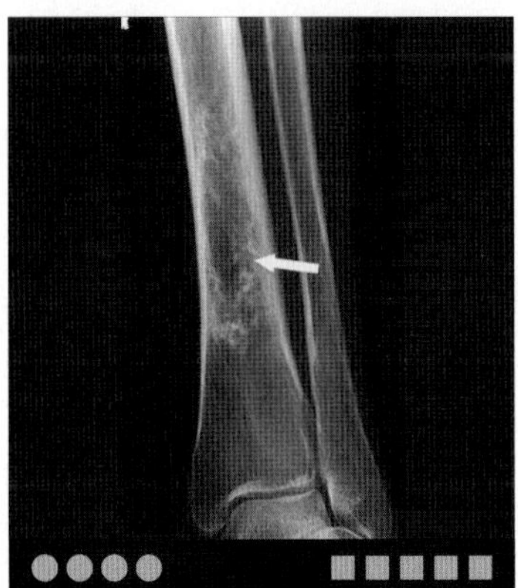

C. Sickle cell anemia: Frontal radiograph of distal tibia demonstrates typical bone infarct with serpiginous sclerotic border (arrow).

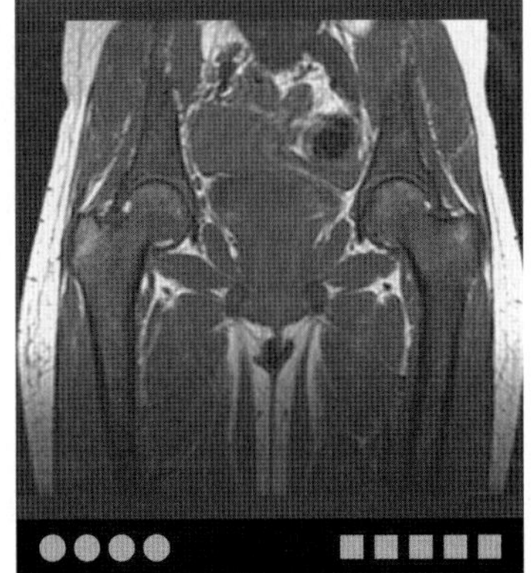

D. Sickle cell anemia: Coronal T1-weighted MR of the hips shows low signal intensity red marrow hyperplasia in all bony structures.

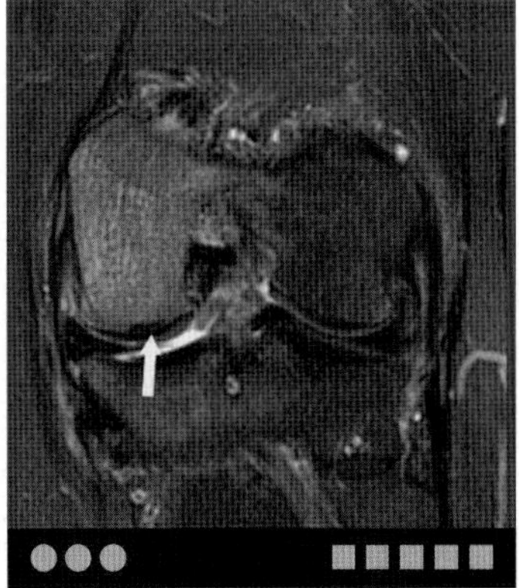

E. SPONK: Coronal Fat Sat T2-weighted MR shows diffused bone marrow edema in medial femoral condyle with low signal linear focus adjacent to subchondral plate (arrow).

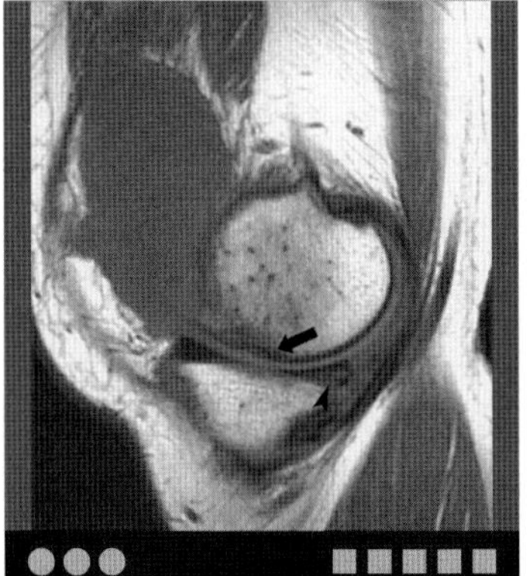

F. SPONK: Sagittal T1-weighted image shows low signal linear focus felt to be a stress fracture (arrow), and subchondral flattening. Meniscal tear (arrowhead).

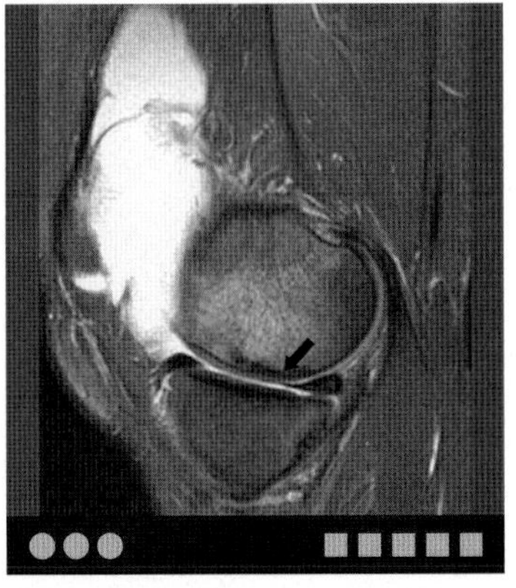

G. SPONK: Sagittal Fat Sat T2-weighted image shows stress fracture (arrow) and marrow edema.

IMAGE KEY

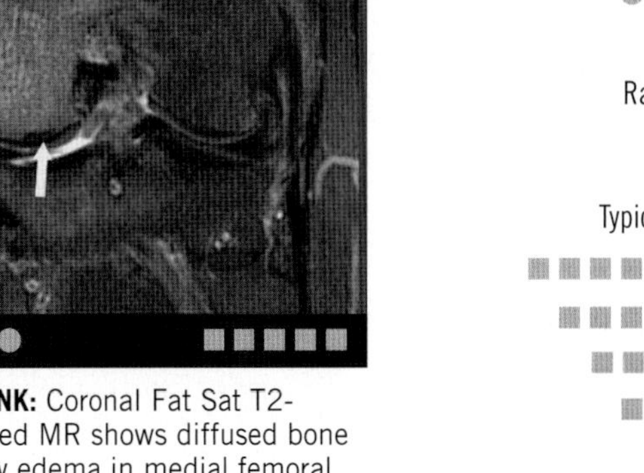

Common

Rare

Typical

Unusual

SECTION VI

ANKLE AND FOOT

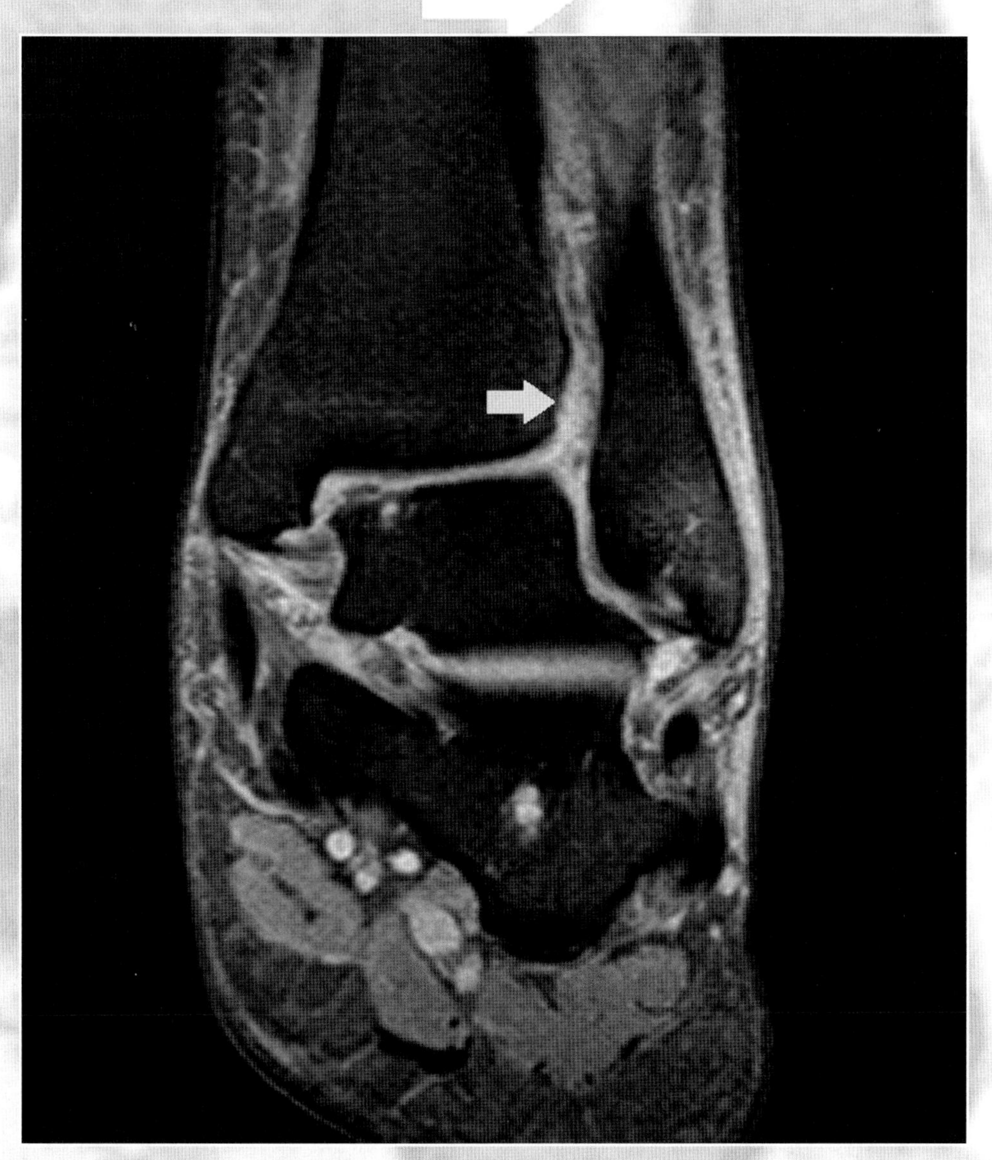

Chapter 29

Sport Medicine and Trauma

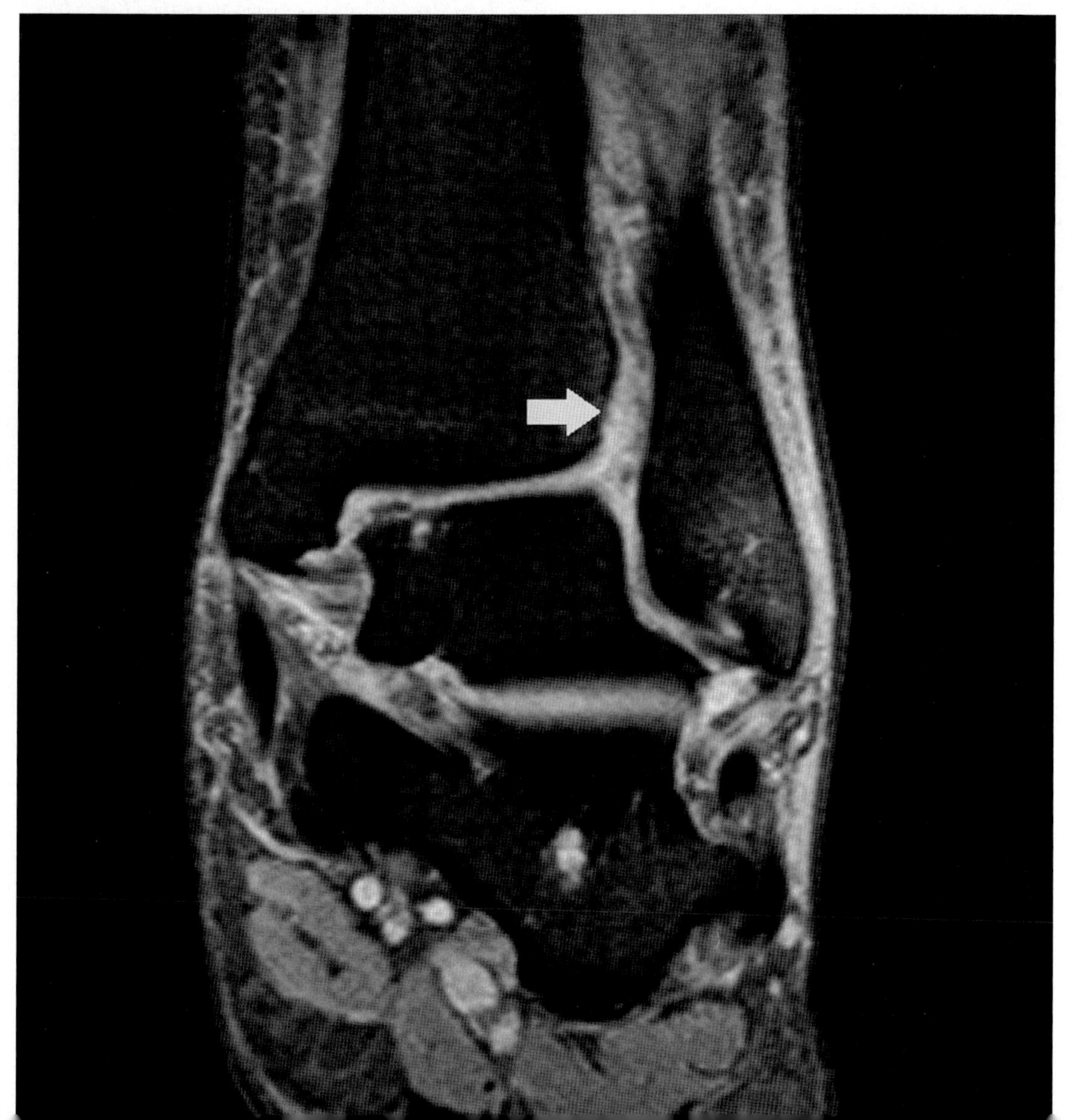

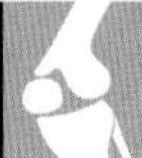

29–1 Syndesmotic Ligament Injury

Ashkan Afshin and Jamshid Tehranzadeh

PRESENTATION

Leg pain

FINDINGS

Radiographs show widening of distal tibiofibular joint. MR images demonstrate disruption of the ligaments and increased signal in distal tibia–fibular joint. Ankle arthrogram shows extravasation of contrast agent into distal tibiofibular syndesmosis and articulation.

DIFFERENTIAL DIAGNOSES

- *Fibula stress fracture:* Stress fractures are seen as a result of repetitive injury to the bone often manifested as hair-line or occult fracture not visualized on original radiograph but best seen on MRI or bone scan.
- *Juvenile tillaux fracture:* The juvenile fracture of Tillaux is an ankle joint avulsion fracture of the anterior distal tibial tubercle in adolescents, produced by external rotation force applied to the foot.
- *Osteochondral fracture (osteochondritis disseccans):* This condition is a defect in the subchondral region with partial or complete separation of the bone fragment.

COMMENTS

Syndesmosis is made up of anterior inferior tibiofibular ligament (AITF), posterior inferior tibiofibular ligament (PITF), transverse tibiofibular ligament, and interosseous membrane. Syndesmotic injury of the ankle, also called "high" ankle sprain, occurs in 10% to 20% of ankle sprains. These injuries may occur in isolation or in association with fractures such as high fibular fracture. Injuries without fractures usually result from external rotation, abduction, and dorsiflexion of the ankle or leg. The loss of ligament support and alteration in the stability of the mortise have been postulated to lead to an increase in joint reactive forces and traumatic arthritis. The patients usually complain of pain in anterolateral of the leg. In the absence of fracture, physical examination reveals swelling of the leg or ankle, tenderness over the anterior aspect of the syndesmosis and a positive squeeze or external rotation test. These patients may be unable to bear their weight. Conventional radiographs show widening of tibiofibular clear space (more than 6 mm), decreased tibiofibular overlap, and increased medial clear space (more than 4 mm). Since syndesmotic injury may not be observed radiographically, routine stress testing is necessary for detecting syndesmotic instability. MRI is the best diagnostic tool to identify syndesmotic ligament injuries. MR findings show thickening and disruption of the ligaments. Fluid hyperintensity and diastasis of syndesmotic ligaments (AITF, PITF) are also observed on MR images.

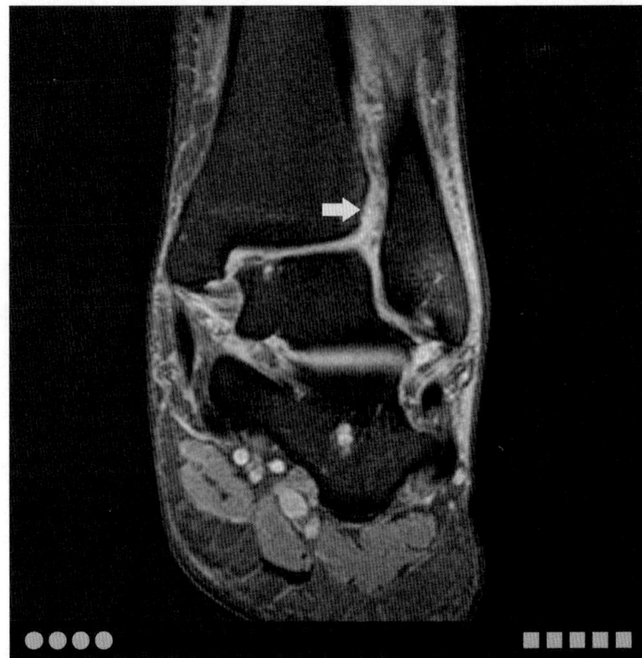

A. Syndesmotic ligament injury: Coronal proton density weighted image shows edema and fluid-like signal in the region of distal intraosseous membrane (arrow) consistent with syndesmotic injury. Also note the osteochondral injury in the medial talar dome.

PEARLS

- **Results from external rotation, abduction, and dorsiflexion injuries or is associated with factures.**
- **Sever pain on external rotation, tenderness over the anterior syndesmosis, and a positive squeeze test are common clinical findings.**
- **Increased tibiofibular clear space, decreased tibiofibular overlap, and increased medial clear space on roentgenogram.**
- **Thickening, disruption of the ligaments, fluid hyperintensity, and diastasis of AITF and PITF are on MR images.**

ADDITIONAL IMAGES

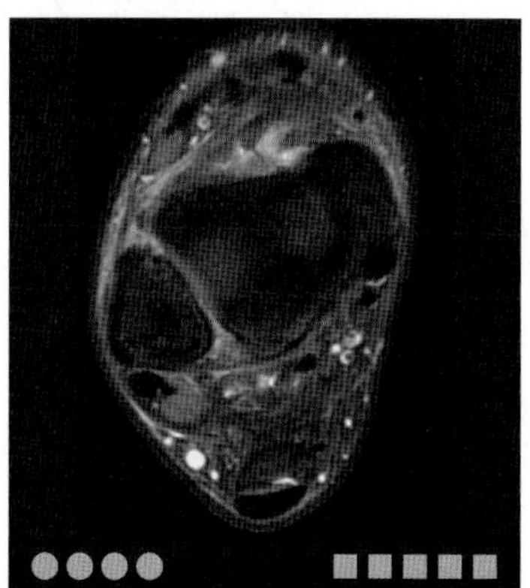

B. Syndesmotic ligament injury: Axial T2-weighted image shows complete tear of anteroinferior tibiofibular ligament tear consistent with syndesmotic injury.

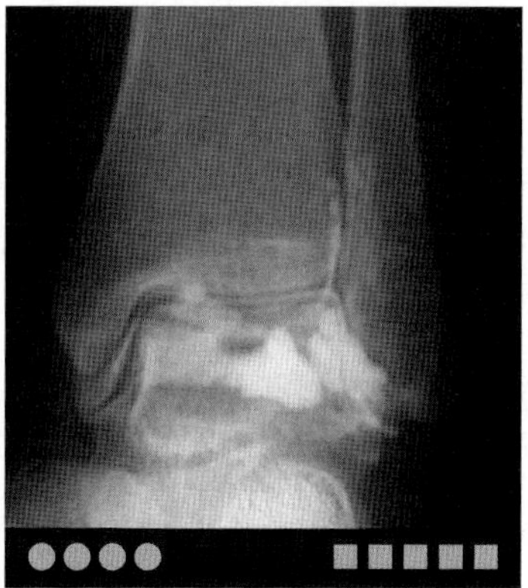

C. Syndesmotic ligament injury: Ankle arthrogram shows the contrast injected into the ankle mortise joint has extravasated between tibia and fibula at the distal tibiofibular joint indicating tear of syndesmosis.

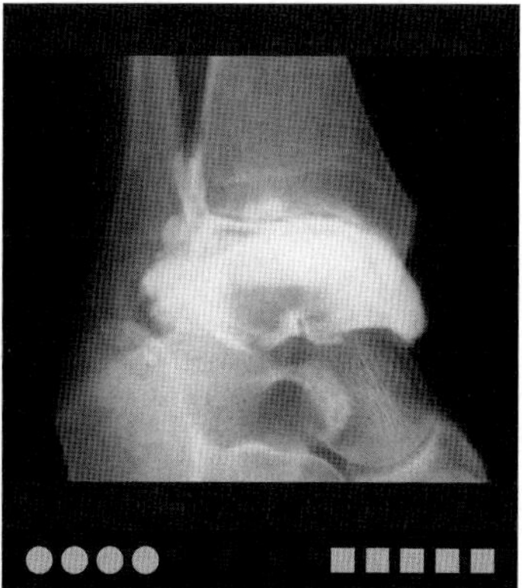

D. Syndesmotic ligament injury: Ankle arthrogram in another patient shows the contrast injected into the ankle mortise joint has extravasated between tibia and fibula at the distal tibiofibular joint indicating tear of syndesmosis.

IMAGE KEY

Common

Rare

Typical

Unusual

DIFFERENTIAL DIAGNOSES IMAGES

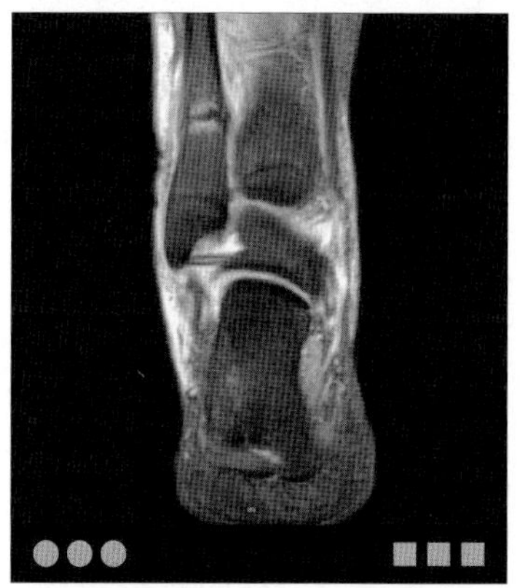

E. Fibula stress fracture: Coronal gradient echo fat-saturated fluid-sensitive image shows linear low signal surrounded by marrow edema corresponding to the fracture. Mild periosteal changes are seen.

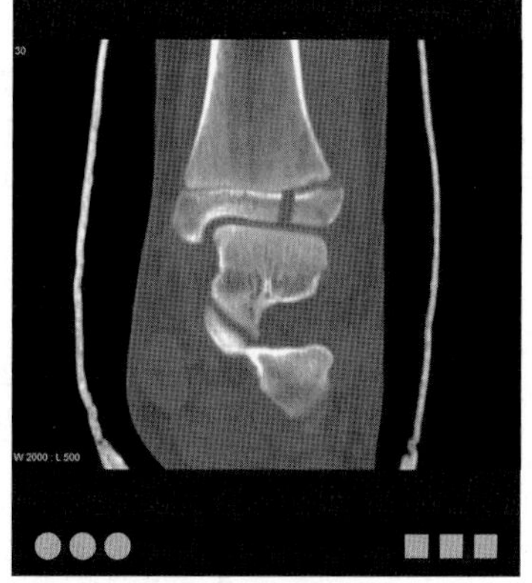

F. Juvenile tillaux fracture: Coronal CT demonstrates the vertical (Salter–Harris III) fracture through the epiphysis with intra-articular extension.

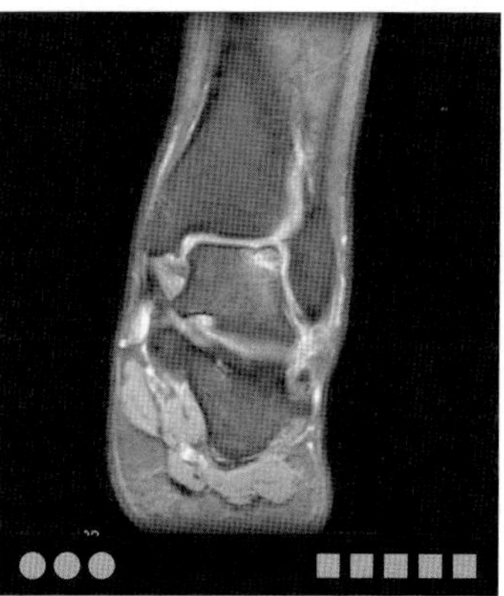

G. Osteochondral fracture (osteochondritis disseccans): Coronal MR image shows the osteochondral lesion with associated edema.

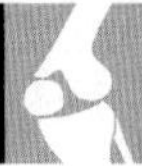

29–2 Anterior Ankle Impingement Syndrome

Mohammad Reza Hayeri and Jamshid Tehranzadeh

PRESENTATION

Pain

FINDINGS

MR imaging shows osseous spurs and synovial thickening extending over the anterior aspect of the joint. There are osteophytes of anterior tibial plafond and talus associated with osseous fragment.

DIFFERENTIAL DIAGNOSES

- *Anterolateral impingement:* This is produced by entrapment of abnormal soft tissue in the anterolateral gutter of the ankle, a space bounded by the anterolateral talus, anteromedial distal fibula, and anterolateral distal tibia.
- *Anteromedial impingement:* This condition is a rare complication of repeated supination injury with perhaps a rotational component that leads to capsular thickening and synovitis.
- *Posterior impingement:* This is the compression of the tibiotalar capsule, posterior talofibular, intermalleolar, and tibiofibular ligaments between the posterior process of the calcaneus and the tibia.
- *Posteromedial impingement:* This is because of compression of the posteromedial tibiotalar capsule and posterior fibers of the tibiotalar ligament between the talus and medial malleolus during supination injuries.

COMMENTS

Anterior ankle impingement, sometimes termed "footballer's ankle" (kicker's foot), is defined as painful mechanical limitation of full ankle movement secondary to osseous abnormality and soft-tissue thickening within the ankle joint. The underlying mechanism of injury is repeated supination injury which causes damage at the anteromedial margins of the articular cartilage. Damage of the anterior articular cartilage rim also occurs during forced dorsiflexion injuries which are especially common in soccer and ballet. Anterior tibiotalar spurs that are thought to be caused by chronic traction on the anterior capsule are a significant component of the anterior impinging. It is thought that additional capsular abnormality rather than the spurs alone are critical for producing the clinical syndrome because a significant proportion of asymptomatic athletes also have these spurs. Anterior ankle impingement presents with pain with a subjective feeling of blocking on dorsiflexion. There is a limited range of motion on dorsiflexion with occasional soft-tissue swelling and palpable mass. The typical positions of tibiotalar spurs are at the anterior and medial articular cartilage margins, which can be seen on radiographs. MR imaging can demonstrate osseous spurs and synovial thickening extending over the anterior aspect of the joint. Synovial thickening usually has low signal intensity on T1-weighted images and low to intermediate signal intensity on T2-weighted images; with an irregular contour or stranding evident if an effusion is present. Like anterolateral impingement and unlike posterior impingement, these abnormalities rarely show striking soft tissue or osseous edema.

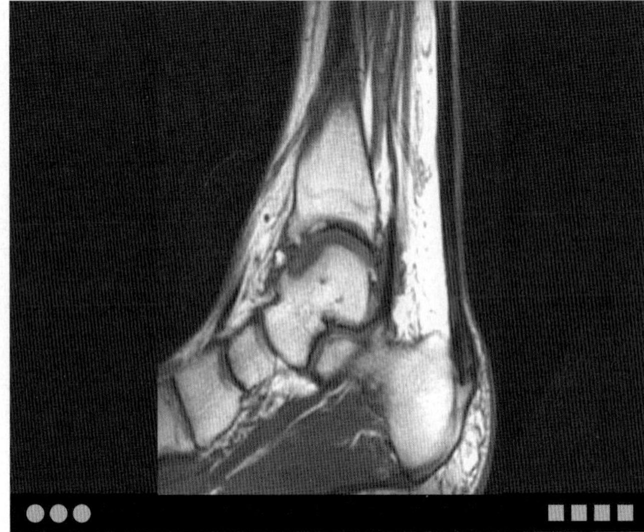

A. Anterior impingement: Sagittal T1-weighted image shows large anterior tibial plafond osteophyte associated with anterior talar traction osteophyte with osseous body in between causing anterior impingement and limitation of the ankle dorsiflexion (kicker's foot) (Courtesy of Mark Schweitzer).

PEARLS

- **Ankle impingement is defined as a painful mechanical limitation of full ankle movement, secondary to osseous abnormality and soft-tissue thickening within the ankle joint.**
- **Although tibiotalar spurs are an important part of this condition, the development of additional capsular abnormality is critical for producing the clinical syndrome.**
- **MR imaging can demonstrate osseous spurs and synovial thickening extending over the anterior aspect of the joint.**
- **Synovial thickening usually has low signal intensity on T1-weighted images and low to intermediate signal intensity on T2-weighted images; with an irregular contour or stranding evident if an effusion is present.**

ADDITIONAL IMAGE

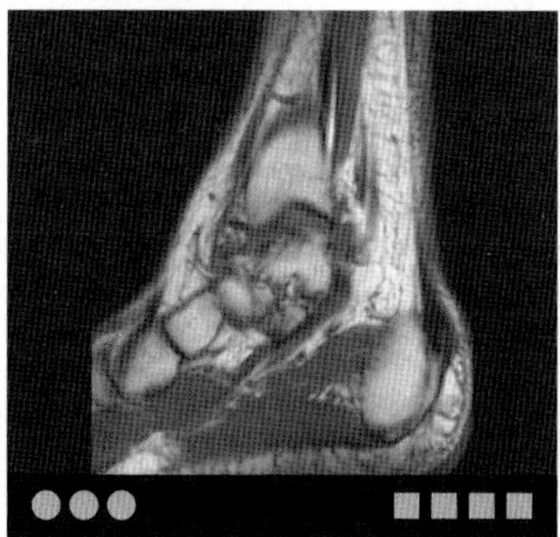

B. Anterior impingement: Sagittal T1-weighted image shows bony fragment between anterior tibial plafond and traction osteophyte of talus causing limitation of dorsiflexion (kicker's foot) (Courtesy of Mark Schweitzer).

DIFFERENTIAL DIAGNOSES IMAGES

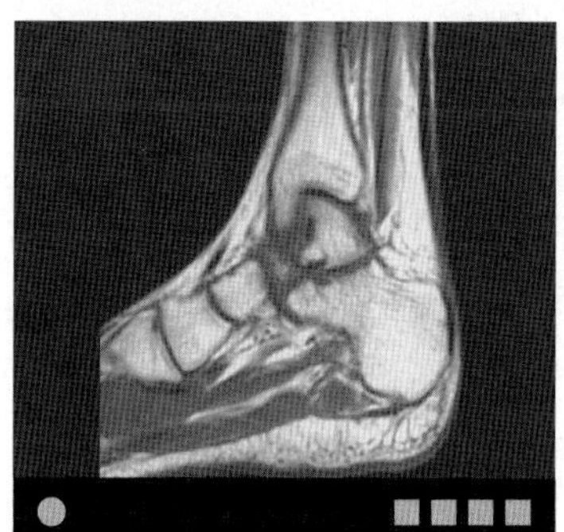

C. Anteromedial impingement: Sagittal T1-weighted image shows elongated medial malleolus causing impingement and bone marrow edema of the talus (Courtesy of Mark Schweitzer).

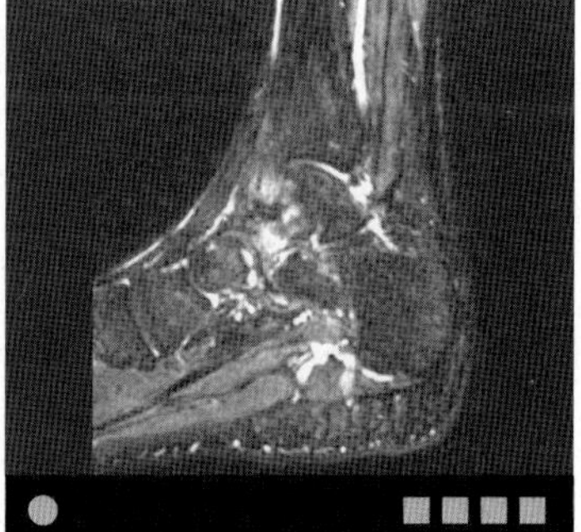

D. Anteromedial impingement: Sagittal gradient echo T2*-weighted image shows elongated medial malleolus causing impingement and bone marrow edema of the talus and medial malleolus (Courtesy of Mark Schweitzer).

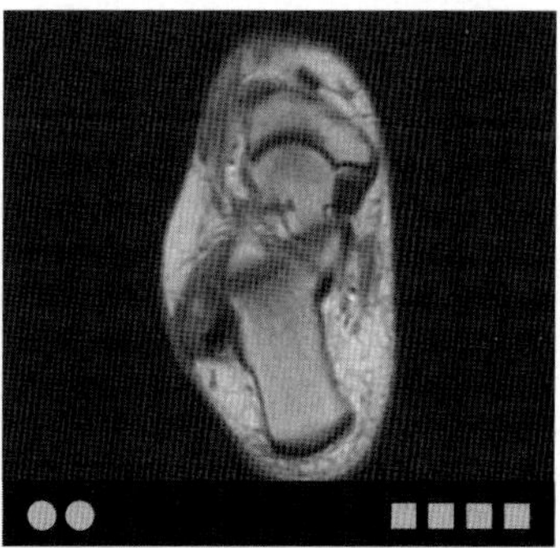

E. Lateral impingement: Axial T1-weighted image shows soft tissue mass as a result of synovial thickening in the anterior aspect of proneal tendon, which is the cause of lateral impingement (Courtesy of Mark Schweitzer).

IMAGE KEY

Common

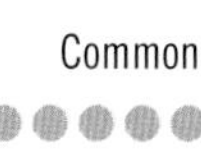

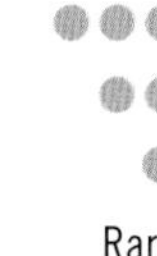

Rare

Typical

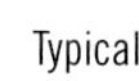

Unusual

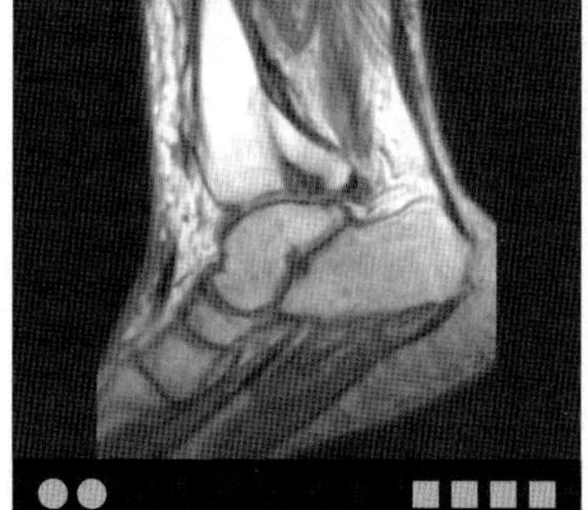

F. Posterior impingement: Sagittal T1-weighted image shows fracture of posterior malleolus extending to the tibial plafond causing impingement of posterior joint capsule (Courtesy of Mark Schweitzer).

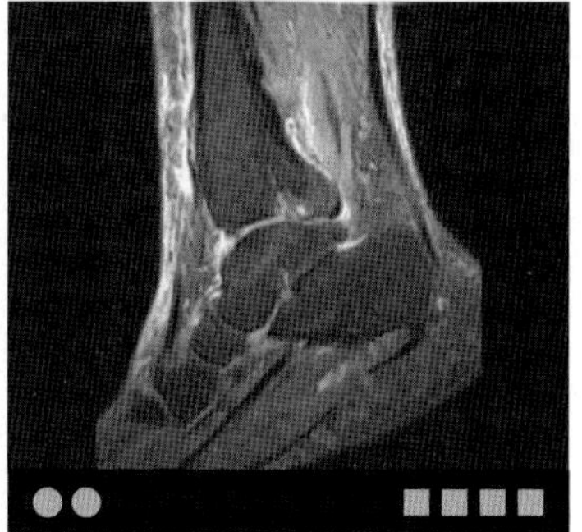

G. Posterior impingement: Sagittal fat-saturated T2-weighted image shows fracture of posterior malleolus extending to the tibial plafond causing impingement of posterior joint capsule (Courtesy of Mark Schweitzer).

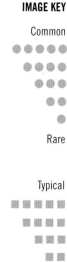

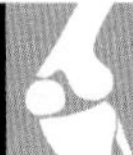

29–3 Deltoid Ligament Complex Tear

Rosemary J. Klecker

PRESENTATION

Ankle inversion injury and continued pain

FINDINGS

MR image shows abnormal laxity of the deltoid ligaments and osseous masses medial to the talus.

DIFFERENTIAL DIAGNOSES

- *Posterior tibial tendon (PTT) tear:* The PTT is posterior and medial to the medial malleolus and is superficial to the tibiospring ligament.
- *Spring ligament tear:* The spring ligament runs from the tibiospring ligament of the deltoid complex and the sustentaculum talus to the navicular bone.
- *Tendinosis of posterior tibial tendon:* Thickening of the tendon is associated with intrasubstance intermediate signal on T2-weighted images.

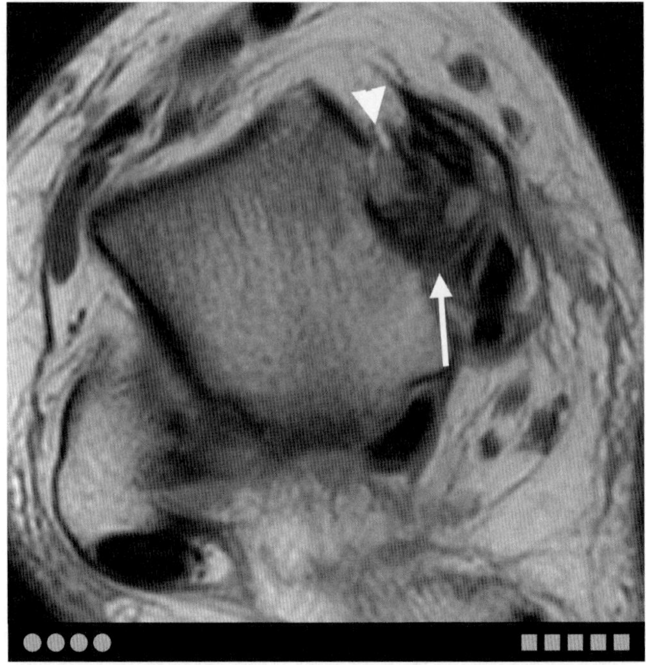

A. Deltoid ligament complex tear: Axial proton density weighted image shows laxity and decreased signal intensity in the deep deltoid ligaments (arrow) compatible with tear. There is an avulsion injury from the talar insertion (arrowhead).

COMMENTS

The patient is a 30-year-old woman with inversion injury of the ankle with continued ankle pain. The deltoid ligament complex on the medial aspect of the ankle is composed of deep and superficial ligaments. The anterior and posterior tibiotalar ligaments are the deep component. The superficial component consists of the tibionavicular, tibiospring, and tibiocalcaneal ligaments. The anterior tibiotalar ligament is inconsistently seen on MR imaging, which may reflect congenital absence or ligament tear. The posterior tibiotalar ligament is the strongest of the deltoid ligaments and is rarely torn. When torn, there is often an associated tear of one or more of the superficial deltoid ligaments. The Lauge–Hansen classification of ankle injuries considers both the mechanism of injury and the associated ligamentous disruptions. According to this classification, tears or avulsion injuries of the deltoid ligament occur secondary to pressure from the medially directed talus from a supination–adduction ankle injury. Likewise, pronation of the foot places tension on the deltoid ligaments, which are then prone to tear when the pronated foot is subjected to forceful external rotation or abduction of the talus. On MRI the posterior tibiotalar ligament is seen as a low signal intensity thick band with or without identifiable individual fibers that extends from the medial talus to the posterior colliculus of the tibia. When torn, the ligament loses its normal linear contour and may be partially obscured by edema and hemorrhage in the surrounding soft tissues. Tears of the ligament may be associated with avulsion injuries of the talus or tibia.

PEARLS

- **The deltoid ligament is composed of two deep ligaments: the anterior and posterior ligaments, and three superficial ligaments: the tibionavicular, tibiospring, and tibiocalcaneal ligaments.**
- **Deltoid ligament sprains or tears are associated with supination–adduction, pronation–external rotation, and pronation–adduction injuries of the ankle.**
- **Tears of the deltoid ligaments manifest as abnormal "wavy" contour of the ligament with edema signal in the ligament and surrounding soft tissues. It may be associated with an osseous avulsion injury.**
- **Tears of the deltoid ligaments are much less common than tears of the lateral ankle ligaments and may indicate a more severe injury.**

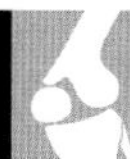

ADDITIONAL IMAGES

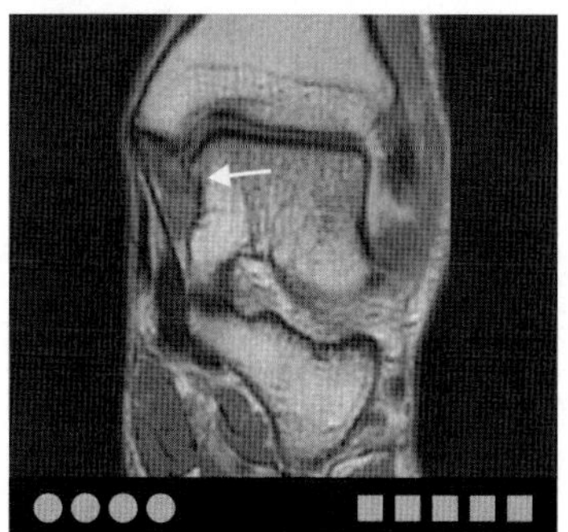

B. Deltoid ligament complex tear: Coronal T1-weighted image shows loss of normal linear morphology of deep deltoid ligaments compatible with tear from the talar insertion (arrow).

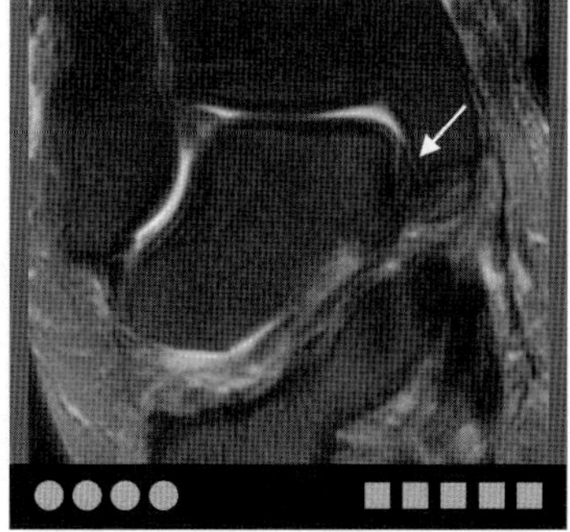

C. Deltoid ligament complex tear: Coronal T2-weighted image with fat saturation shows a tear of the deep deltoid ligaments and an osseous body (arrows) from an avulsion injury interposed between the talus and the medial malleolus of the tibia.

DIFFERENTIAL DIAGNOSES IMAGES

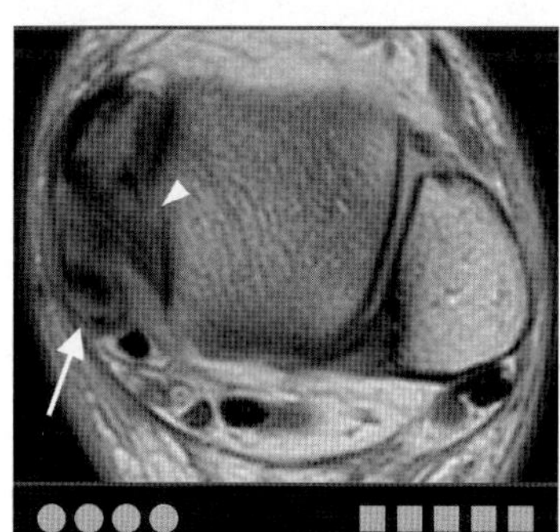

D. Posterior tibial tendon tear: Axial proton density weighted image shows a type I tear of the posterior tibial tendon (arrow). The posterior tibiotalar ligament (arrowhead) is intact.

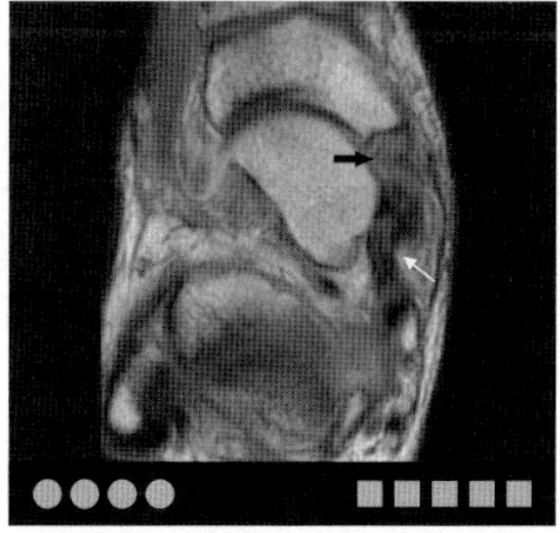

E. Sprain of spring ligament and tear of posterior tibial tendon: Axial oblique proton density weighted image shows a sprain of the spring ligament (white arrow) and a grade 1 tear of the posterior tibial tendon (black arrow).

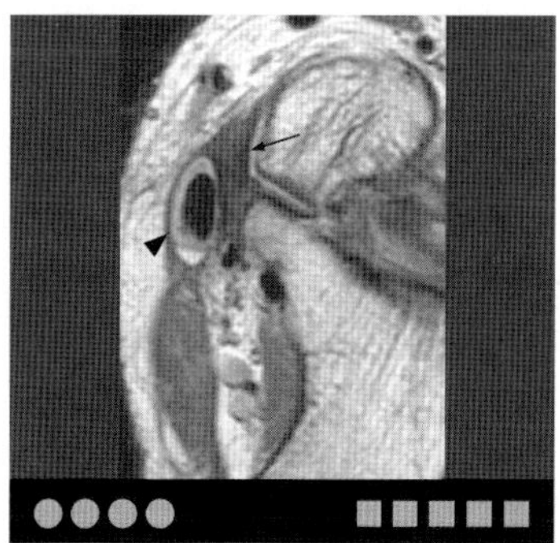

F. Sprain of spring ligament and tear of posterior tibial tendon: Axial oblique proton density weighted image shows a sprain of the spring ligament (arrow) and a grade 1 tear and fluid around the posterior tibial tendon (arrowhead).

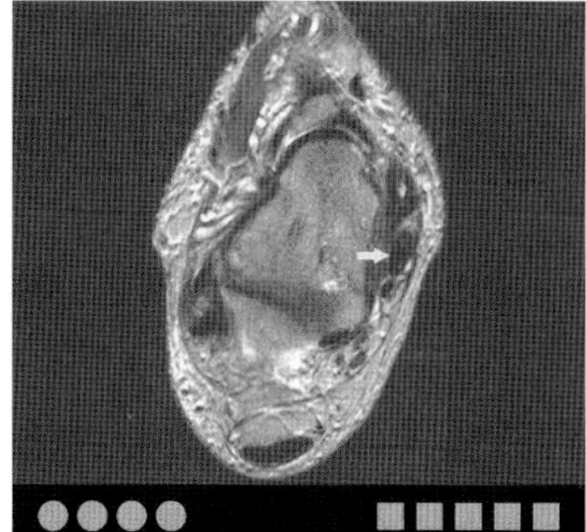

G. Tendinosis of posterior tibialis tendon: Axial T2-weighted image of the hindfoot shows intermediate signal in an enlarged posterior tibial tendon (arrow).

IMAGE KEY

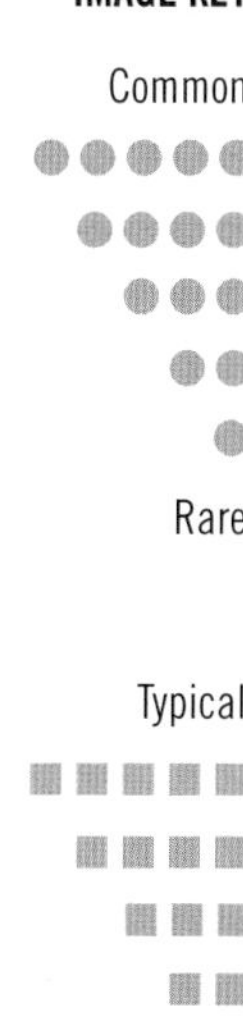

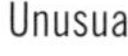

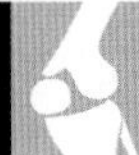

29–4 Anterior Talofibular Ligament Tear

Hakan Ilaslan

PRESENTATION

Swelling and pain following an inversion injury

FINDINGS

MRI shows interruption of fibers of anterior talofibular ligament (ATFL) with surrounding edema and extension of joint fluid into adjacent subcutaneous tissues.

DIFFERENTIAL DIAGNOSES

- *Tibiofibular ligament tear (syndesmotic injury):* There might be tibiofibular joint widening, joint incongruity, and an increased height of the tibiofibular recess. Syndesmotic injuries are typically caused by external forces that produce sudden ankle dorsiflexion or plantar flexion in combination with external rotation of the foot.
- *Calcaneofibular ligament tear:* CFL tears are associated with localized edema, peroneal retinacular thickening, tenosynovitis, and tendon subluxation. The injured ligament is frequently thickened and heterogeneous, and the surrounding fat planes are often obliterated. Interruption of ligament fibers may also be seen with acute injuries.
- *Posterior talofibular ligament tear:* This is a much thicker ligament compared to ATFL and is rarely injured, except in association with a complete dislocation of the talus.

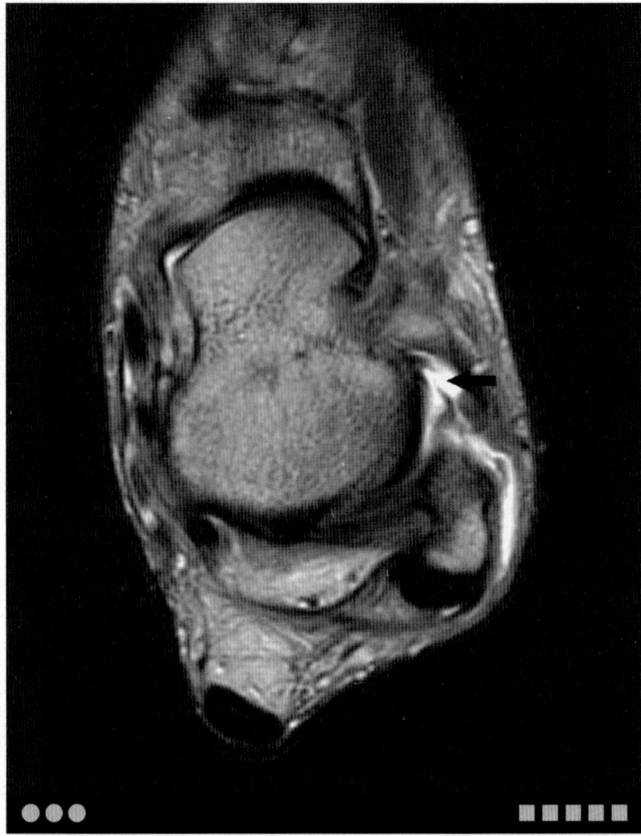

A. ATFL tear: Axial T2-weighted image shows complete tear of ATFL (arrow).

COMMENTS

The patient is an 18-year-old male, who presented with ankle pain and swelling after an inversion ankle injury. The ATFL is an intracapsular ligament and attaches anteriorly to the anterior border of the distal fibula and laterally to the neck of the talus. On MRI, ATFL is best evaluated on axial plane, typically seen at the level of distal fibular tip. Inversion injuries of the ankle are common accounting for approximately 40% of all athletic injuries. The ATFL is the weakest ligament and therefore the most frequently torn. The ATFL and the calcaneofibular ligament are sequentially injured when a plantar-flexed foot is forcefully inverted. On MRI, acute tears of ATFL present with either partial or complete ligament fiber disruption, ligament laxity, or complete absence of the ligament associated with a capsular rupture and leak of joint fluid into the anterolateral subcutaneous tissues. Associated findings such as soft tissue edema and bone bruise are frequently seen with acute injuries. There may be osteochondral lesions as well. Chronic tear often manifests as thickening, thinning, elongation, and wavy or irregular contour of the ligament. Anterolateral impingement of the ankle has been described as a complication of lateral ligamentous injuries of ankle with subsequent fibrosis and synovial scarring from hemorrhage. There are three grades of ATFL injury: Grade I sprain: When the ligament is stretched but not torn. Grade II sprain: Moderate sprain which usually results in partial tears of the ligaments. Grade III sprain: Indicates complete rupture of the ligament.

PEARLS

- **ATFL is the most commonly torn ankle ligament.**
- **Mechanism of injury usually involves forceful inversion of a plantar-flexed foot.**
- **Associated findings with acute ATFL injuries include soft tissue edema and bone bruise.**
- **If ATFL tear is present, calcaneofibular ligament should be carefully evaluated for injuries.**

ADDITIONAL IMAGES

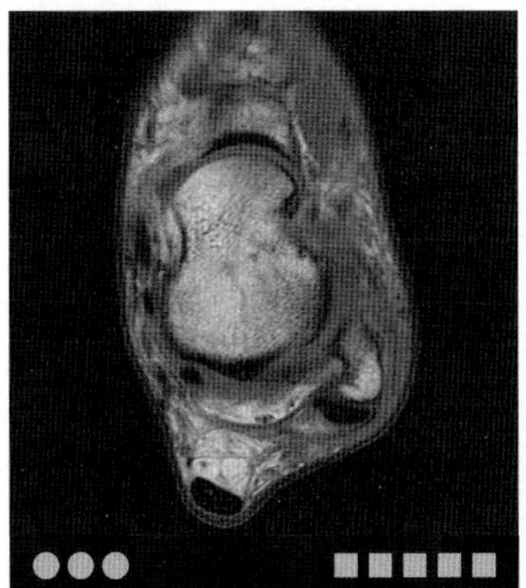

B. ATFL tear: Axial T1-weighted image shows complete tear of ATFL.

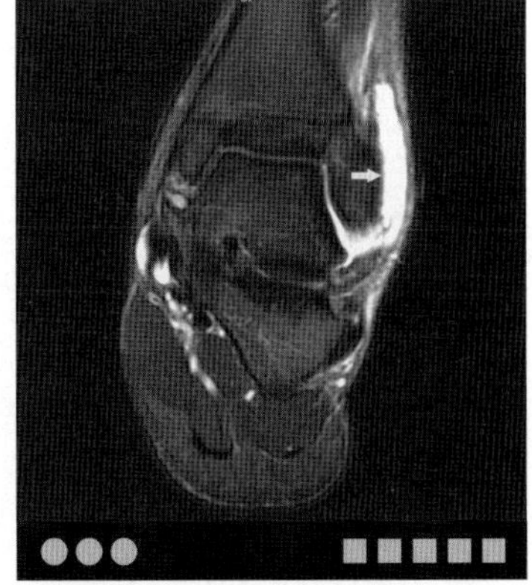

C. ATFL tear: Coronal T2-weighted fat-saturated image shows absence of ATFL consistent with tear. Note the extension of joint fluid into anterolateral subcutaneous tissues (arrow).

DIFFERENTIAL DIAGNOSES IMAGES

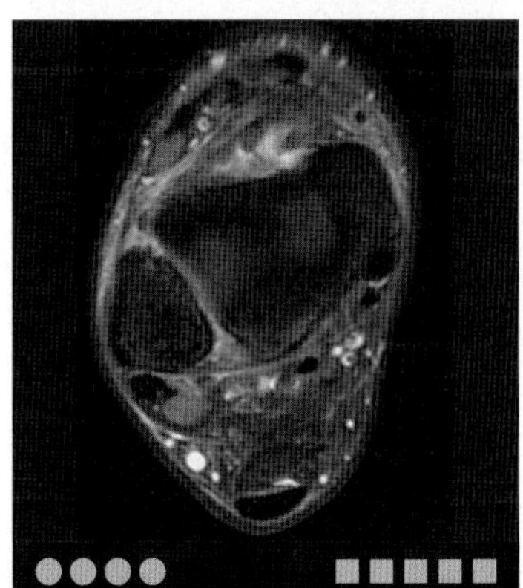

D. Syndesmotic injury: Axial T2-weighted image shows complete tear of anteroinferior tibiofibular ligament tear consistent with syndesmotic injury.

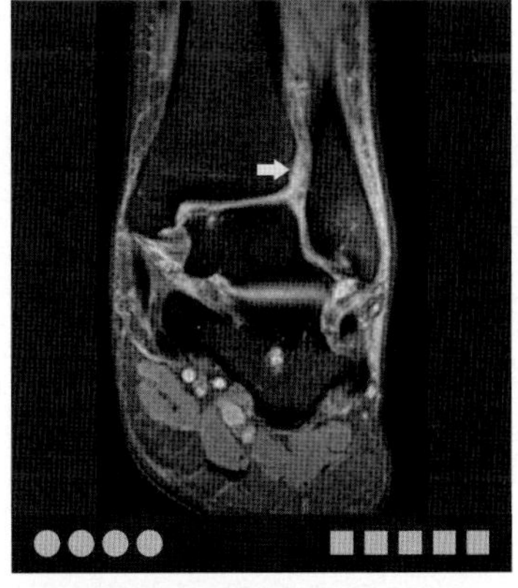

E. Syndesmotic injury: Coronal proton density weighted image shows edema and fluid-like signal in the region of distal intraosseous membrane (arrow) consistent with syndesmotic injury. Also note the osteochondral injury in the medial talar dome.

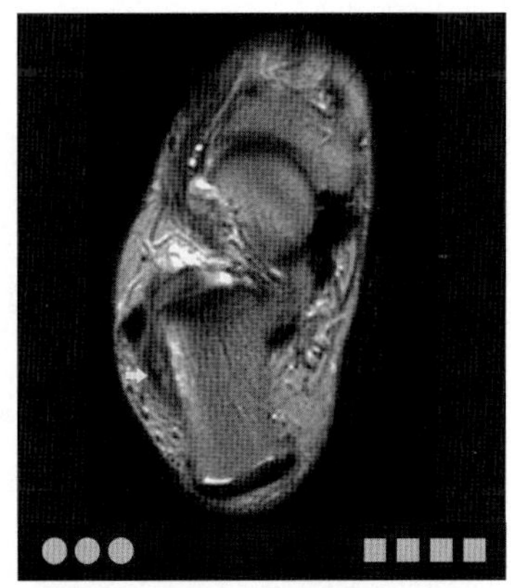

F. Calcaneofibular ligament tear: Axial T2-weighted image shows ill-defined abnormal signal in the expected location of CFL (arrow).

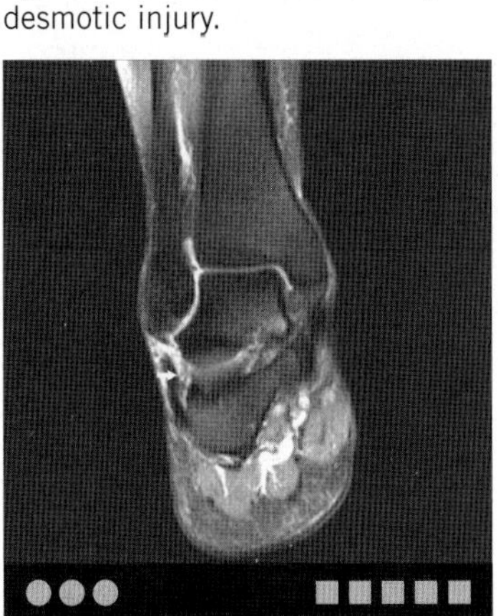

G. Calcaneofibular ligament tear: Coronal proton density weighted image shows tear of CFL (arrow) with surrounding edema-like signal deep to peroneal tendons.

IMAGE KEY

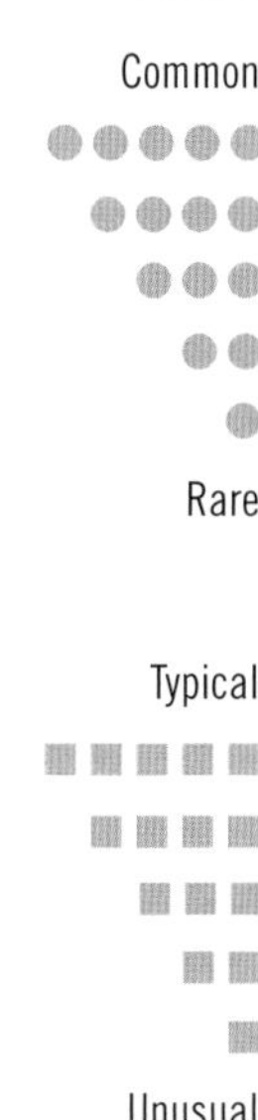

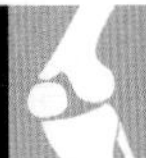

29–5 Anterior Tibial Tendon Tear

Amilcare Gentili

PRESENTATION

Anterior ankle mass and pain

FINDINGS

MR images show a thickened anterior tibial tendon above and below the region of the tear.

DIFFERENTIAL DIAGNOSES

- *Ganglion cyst:* It can occur around the ankle, it may displace the tendons, but the tendon is normal.
- *Synovial cyst:* A connection with a joint is usually present.
- *Schwannoma:* May have similar location, but a normal anterior tibial tendon is noted on MRI.

COMMENTS

The patient is a 73-year-old male, who presented with increasing ankle pain and swelling. The anterior tibial muscle originates from the lateral condyle of tibia, proximal half to two-third of the lateral surface of tibia, interosseous membrane, deep fascia and lateral intermuscular septum, and inserts on the plantar surface of the base of first metatarsal and medial plantar surface of first cuneiform. The anterior tibial tendon extends and inverts the foot at the ankle and holds up medial longitudinal arch of foot. Although the anterior tibial tendon is responsible for 80% of dorsiflexion power of the foot, compensation by the extensor hallucis longus and extensor digitorum longus muscles for the loss of function may make the diagnosis of anterior tibial tendon tear difficult. Rupture of the tibialis anterior tendon is uncommon. It can occur either after direct or indirect trauma or spontaneously. Most tears are caused by underlying chronic tendinosis and are seen in patients between ages of 60 and 70 years. The location of tear is fairly consistent. The anterior tibialis tendon usually ruptures 0.5 to 3 cm proximal to its bony insertion, where the tendon passes under the inferior extensor retinaculum. Diabetes mellitus, gout, rheumatoid diseases, hyperparathyroidism, systemic lupus erythematosus, obesity, and oral or local steroid therapy are associated with rupture of the tibialis anterior tendon. Typical clinical findings are a palpable defect between the extensor retinaculum and the anterior tibial tendon insertion site, a mass which represents the retracted tendon stump anteromedial to the ankle joint and a lack of active inversion and dorsiflexion of the ankle.

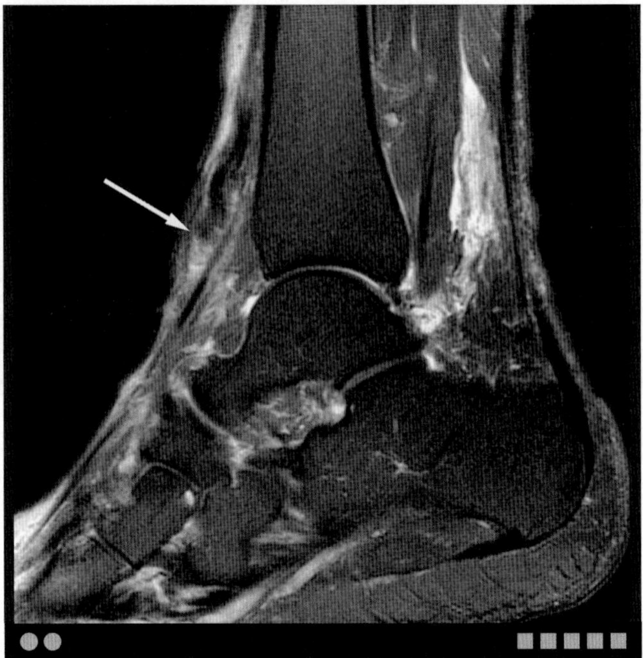

A. Anterior tibial tendon tear: Sagittal T2-weighted fat-saturated fast spin echo MR image shows complete disruption of anterior tibial tendon anterior to tibiotalar joint (arrow) and retraction of proximal stump.

PEARLS

- **A common presentation of anterior tibial tendon tear is an anterior ankle mass.**
- **Anterior tibial tendon tear are much less common than posterior tibial tendon tears.**
- **Most tear occurs without trauma, and are caused by tendon degeneration.**

ADDITIONAL IMAGES

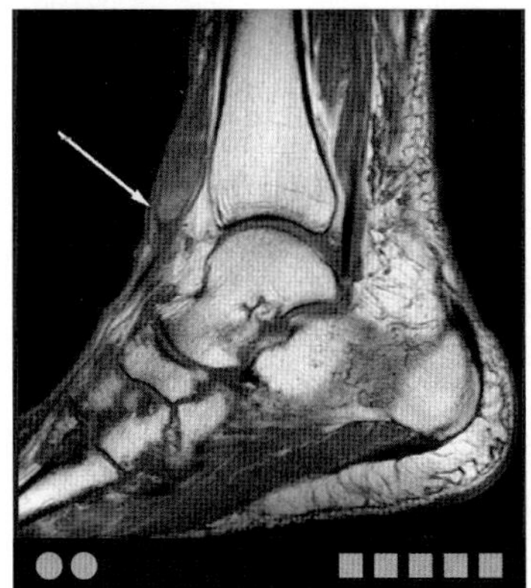

B. Anterior tibial tendon tear: Sagittal T1-weighted MR image shows complete disruption of anterior tibial tendon anterior to tibiotalar joint (arrow) and retraction of proximal stump.

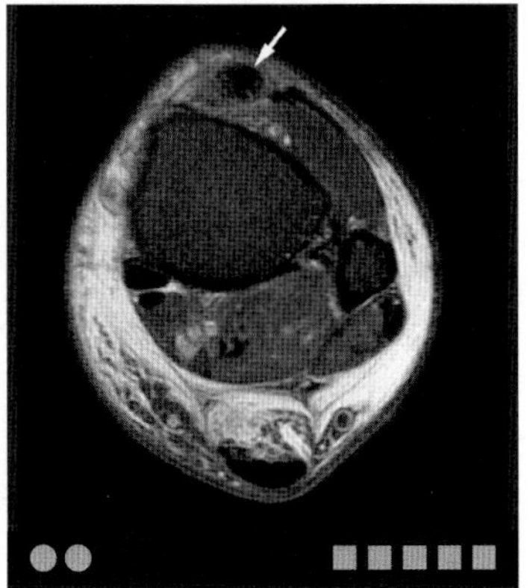

C. Anterior tibial tendon tear: Axial T2-weighted fat-saturated fast spin echo MR image shows a thickened anterior tibial tendon (arrow) just above the site of tear.

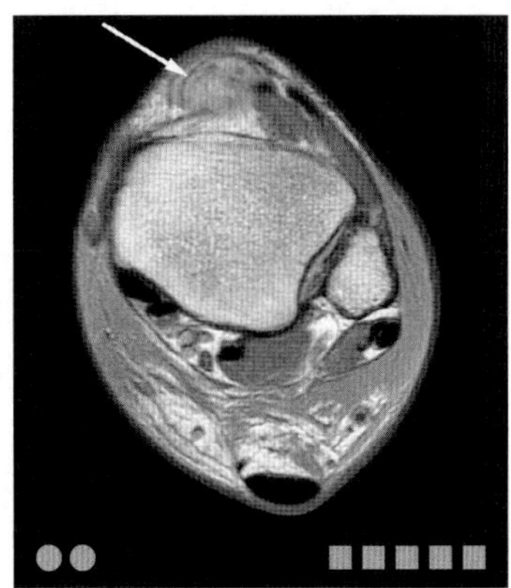

D. Anterior tibial tendon tear: Axial proton density fast spin echo MR image shows torn anterior tibial tendon (arrow).

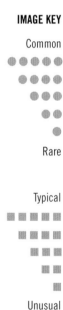

IMAGE KEY

Common

Rare

Typical

Unusual

DIFFERENTIAL DIAGNOSES IMAGES

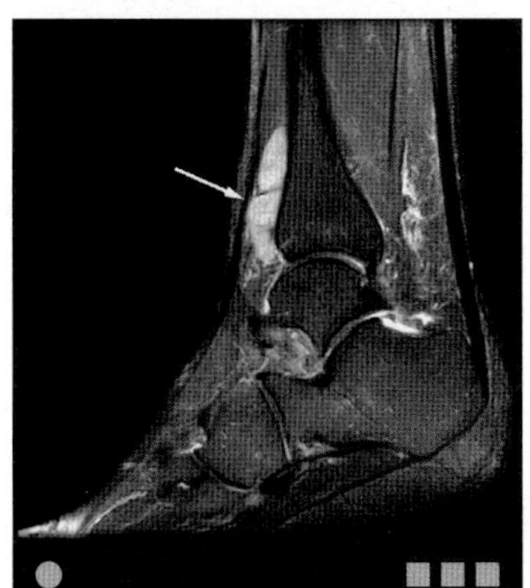

E. Schwannoma: Sagittal T2-weighted fat-saturated fast spin echo MR image shows a high signal mass anterior to the ankle.

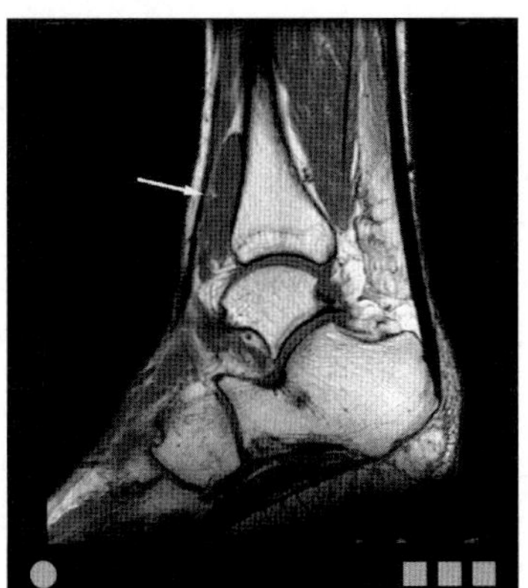

F. Schwannoma: Sagittal T1-weighted spin echo MR image shows low signal intensity mass anterior to the ankle.

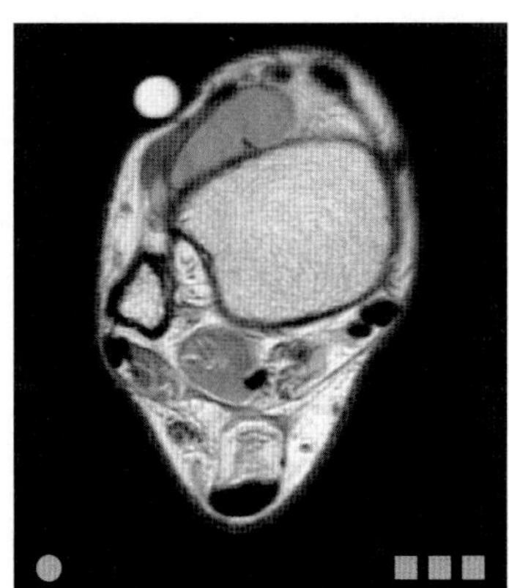

G. Schwannoma: Axial proton density fast spin echo MR image shows a mass displacing anteriorly the extensor digitorum longus muscle and tendons, but the tendons are intact.

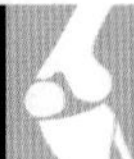

29–6 Complete Tear of Posterior Tibial Tendon

Mélanie Morel, Nathalie Boutry, and Anne Cotten

PRESENTATION

Pain and swelling of the ankle

FINDINGS

MR imaging demonstrates complete discontinuity of the posterior tibial tendon.

DIFFERENTIAL DIAGNOSES

- *Tenosynovitis of the posterior tibial tendon:* It is mainly caused by mechanical irritation of the tendon sheath (sometimes associated with a tendinopathy), but other causes including inflammatory (rheumatoid arthritis), metabolic (gout), or infectious disorders may also be encountered.
- *Dislocation of the posterior tibial tendon:* May occur as a result of severe dorsiflexion. On axial MR images, the tendon (with sometimes a partial tear) is seen medial or anterior to the medial malleolus. An avulsed or stripped flexor retinaculum can be found.
- *Deltoid ligament sprain (tibiotalar component):* MR imaging shows loss of striated appearance, and high signal intensity on T1 and T2-weighted images.

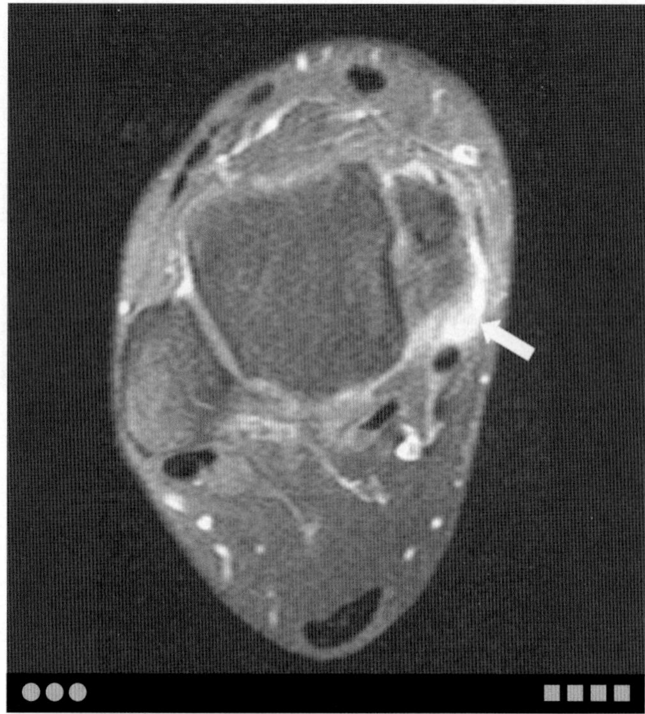

A. Complete tear of posterior tibial tendon: Axial T2-weighted fat-saturated image at the level of medial malleolus shows hyperintense fluid (arrow) anterior to the flexor digitorum longus tendon, instead of posterior tibial tendon.

COMMENTS

The patient is a 68-year-old woman complaining of pain and tenderness below and behind the medial malleolus of the ankle with change in foot shape, diagnosed as complete tear of the posterior tibial tendon. Lesions of the posterior tibial tendon are rarely caused by acute trauma. Most of them are linked to degenerative causes. Middle-aged or older women are mostly affected. Rheumatoid arthritis and accessory navicular are other common risk factors. Most tears occur at the level of or just distal to medial malleolus. Partial tear causes tendon hypertrophy with vertical split (type 1), or decrease in the dimension of the tendon (type 2). Intratendinous high signal intensity foci on T1 and T2-weighted images, and contrast-enhancement of the tendon are also encountered. Complete rupture (type 3) is diagnosed when tendon discontinuity with fluid-filled gap (low or intermediate signal intensity on T1- and high signal intensity on T2-weighted images) is found. A spur of periosteal reaction can sometimes be seen at the posteromedial aspect of the medial malleolus. Progressive flat-foot deformity is also encountered. Tears are sometimes associated with sinus tarsi syndrome and degenerative changes of the posterior subtalar joint. In case of tenosynovitis, sonography shows a widened tendon sheath with an anechoic collection of synovial fluid. Hyperemia of the sheath can be seen with power Doppler. MR T2-weighted images reveal high signal around the tendon. The tendon demonstrates normal signal intensity and morphologic characteristics if no tendinopathy is associated.

PEARLS

- **Posterior tibial tendon tear usually results from chronic degenerative tendinopathy.**
- **Middle-aged or older women are mostly affected.**
- **Pain, swelling, and flattening of medial longitudinal arch are clinically found.**
- **MR imaging demonstrates a change in tendon size and/or intrasubstance high signal intensity in case of partial tear.**
- **Complete discontinuity of the tendon with fluid-filled gap is synonymous with type 3 tear.**

ADDITIONAL IMAGES

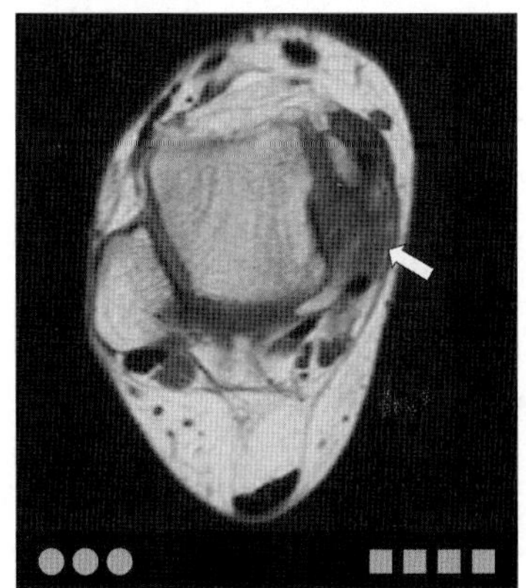

B. Complete tear of posterior tibial tendon: On axial T1-weighted image, the gap is filled with intermediate signal intensity fluid (arrow).

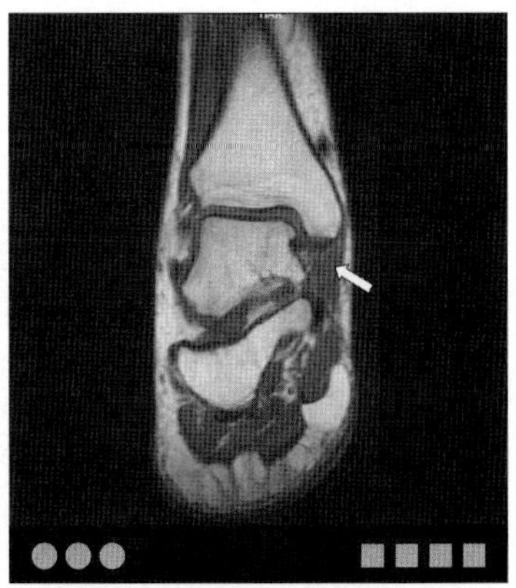

C. Complete tear of posterior tibial tendon: Coronal T1-weighted images exhibits the absence of posterior tibial tendon (arrow) just below the medial malleolus.

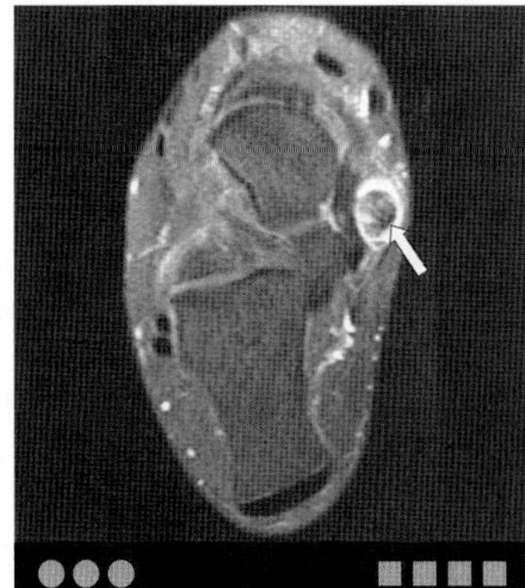

D. Complete tear of posterior tibial tendon: Axial T2-weighted fat-saturated image below the tear site demonstrates enlargement of the distal end of the posterior tibial tendon (arrow) with intrasubstance high signal (tendinopathy), surrounded by hyperintense fluid (tenosynovitis).

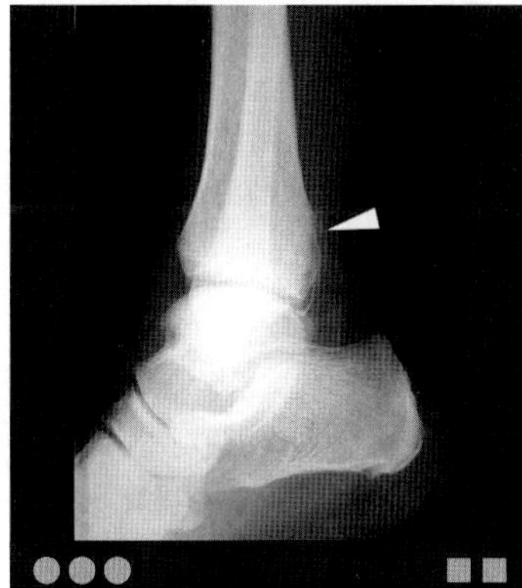

E. Complete tear of posterior tibial tendon: Ankle radiograph reveals periosteal reaction (arrowhead) along the posterior aspect of the medial malleolus.

IMAGE KEY

Common

Rare

Typical

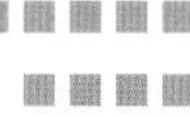

Unusual

DIFFERENTIAL DIAGNOSES IMAGES

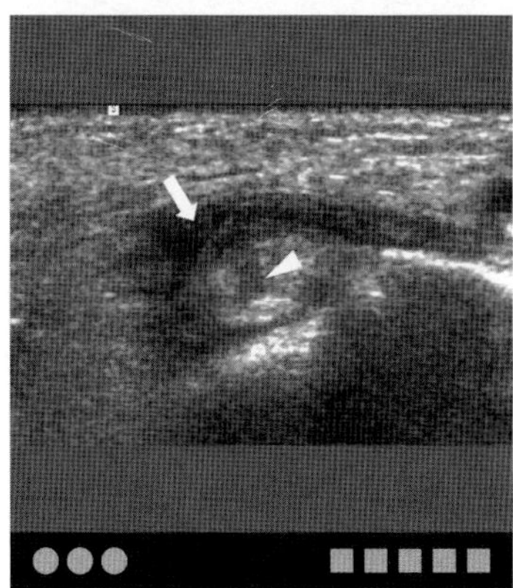

F. Tenosynovitis and tendinopathy of posterior tibial tendon: Sonogram demonstrates anechoic fluid in the tendon sheath (arrow) and hypoechoic area inside the tendon indicating tendinopathy (arrowhead) and intrasubstance tear.

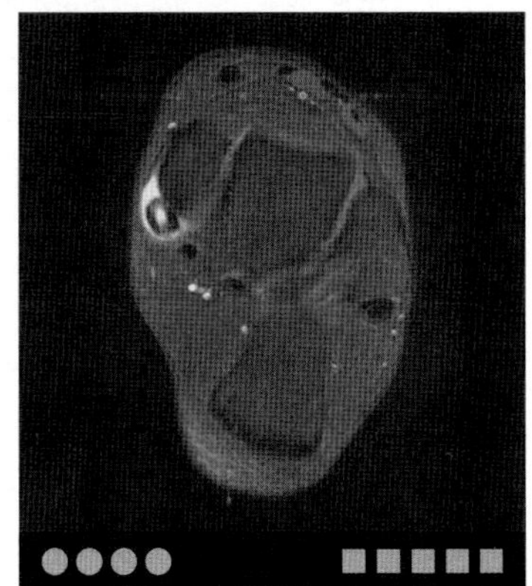

G. Tenosynovitis and tendinopathy of posterior tibial tendon: Axial MR T2-weighted fat-saturated image (same patient as in image F) exhibits hyperintense fluid in the tendon sheath. Intratendinous high signal focal corresponds to tendinopathy and intrasubstance tear.

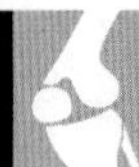

29–7 Sonographic Appearance of Tibialis Posterior Tendon

Stefano Bianchi and Ibrahim F. Abdelwahab

PRESENTATION

Pain at the posteromedial aspect of the ankle associated with flat foot.

FINDINGS

Sagittal sonogram shows a complete tear and the swollen hypoechoic and irregular proximal tibialis posterior tendon (TPT).

DIFFERENTIAL DIAGNOSES

- *TPT partial tear:* It affects only a portion of the tendon and is not associated with retraction of the tendon stump.
- *TPT tenosynovitis:* The tendon is continuous and surrounded by fluid and/or hypertrophy of the synovial membrane.
- *TPT dislocation:* The continuous tendon is dislocated anteriorly. Tenosynovitis can be an associated finding.

COMMENTS

The patient is a 67-year-old female complaining of pain at the posteromedial aspect of the left ankle. The TPT is the strongest tendon of the posteromedial group. It runs first behind the medial malleolus, reflects under it, and then inserts into the tubercle of the navicular and first two cuneiforms. It supports the longitudinal medial arch of the foot and prevents flat foot. It is postulated that there is a continuum in changes of TPT following local over use. The first stage is tenosynovitis in which fluid and synovial hypertrophy are found. In the following stage the tendon itself is affected and may present partial tears in the form of local thinning or thickening associated with internal fissures. Finally, the tendon completely tears. Complete tears are commonly seen in elderly women and are followed by increase in the angle of the longitudinal arch with resultant flat foot and valgus deformity. The best modalities to investigate TPT pathology are ultrasound and MRI. Ultrasound is inexpensive, ready, noninvasive, and allows dynamic tendon assessment. In addition to tendons, MRI can also assess the adjacent ligaments, joints, and bones. Color Doppler ultrasound and injection of gadolinium allows accurate assessment of local inflammatory changes.

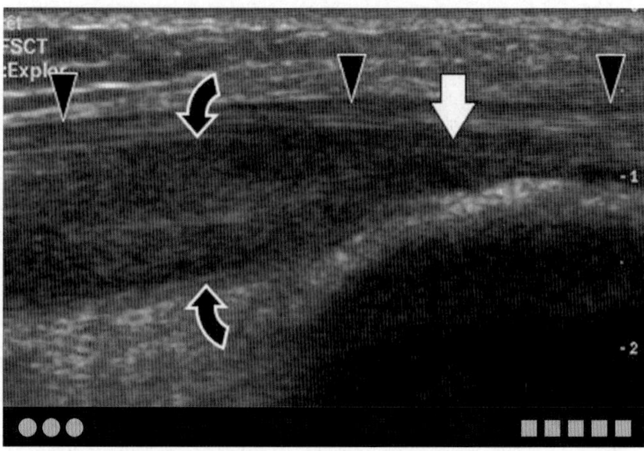

A. Complete tear of the tibialis posterior tendon: Sagittal sonogram obtained over the supramalleolar portion of the TPT shows a complete tear (arrow) and the swollen hypoechoic and irregular proximal tendon (curved arrows). Note the normal flexor digitorum tendon (arrowheads).

PEARLS

- **TPT is an essential structure in preventing flat foot and valgus of the hind foot.**
- **Secondary to local overuse the TPT shows progressive changes ranging from tenosynovitis to partial and finally complete tear.**
- **Both ultrasound and MRI are effective in following TPT changes. Color Doppler and Gd injection are essential in judging the local inflammatory changes.**
- **Ultrasound is cheaper, faster, and dynamic. MRI allows optimal assessment of tendon changes as well as the adjacent anatomic structures.**

ADDITIONAL IMAGES

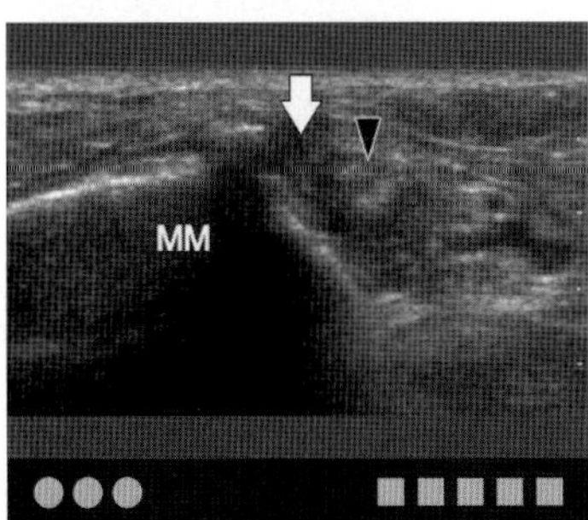

B. Complete tear of the tibialis posterior tendon: Axial sonogram obtained over the supramalleolar portion of the TPT shows absence of the tendon (arrow) and the normal flexor digitorum tendon (arrowhead). MM = medial malleolus.

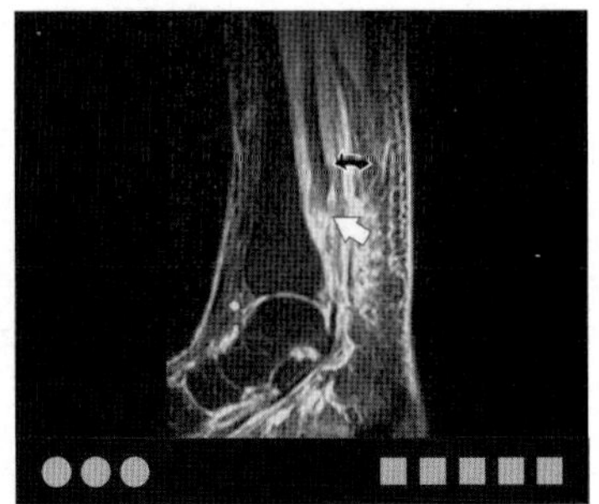

C. Complete tear of the tibialis posterior tendon: Sagittal STIR MR image shows a complete tear (arrow) of the TPT and proximal retraction of the swollen, irregular proximal tendon (curved arrow).

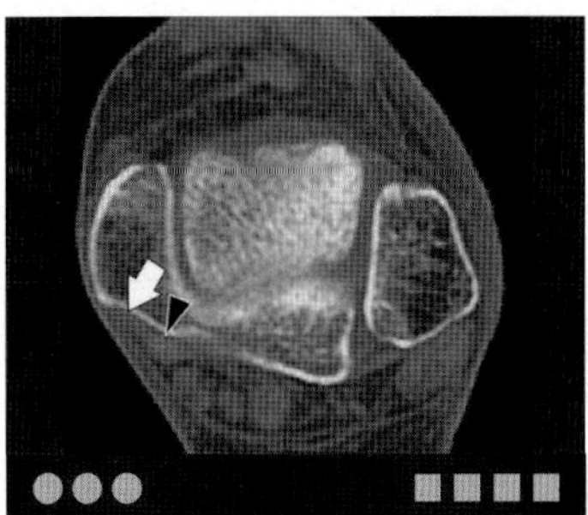

D. Complete tear of the tibialis posterior tendon: Axial CT obtained at the level of the medial malleolus shows absence of the TPT (arrow) and demonstrates the normal flexor digitorum tendon (arrowhead).

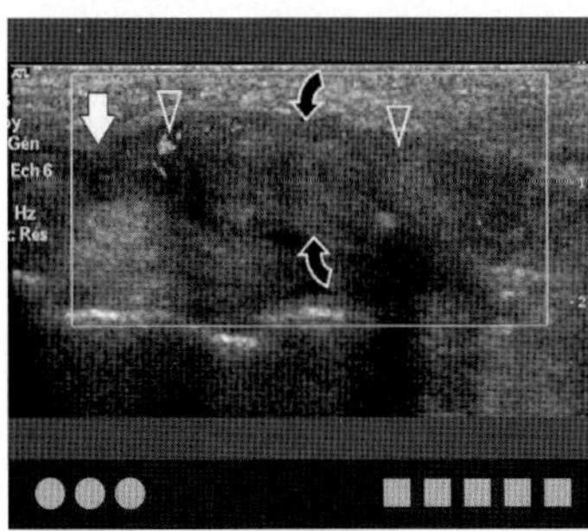

E. Complete tear of the tibialis posterior tendon: Axial oblique color Doppler sonogram obtained over the inframalleolar portion of the TPT shows the complete tear (arrow) and the swollen hypoechoic and irregular distal tendon (curved arrows). Note the flow signals corresponding to local inflammation of the parietal synovium (arrowheads).

IMAGE KEY

Common

Rare

Typical

Unusual

DIFFERENTIAL DIAGNOSES IMAGES

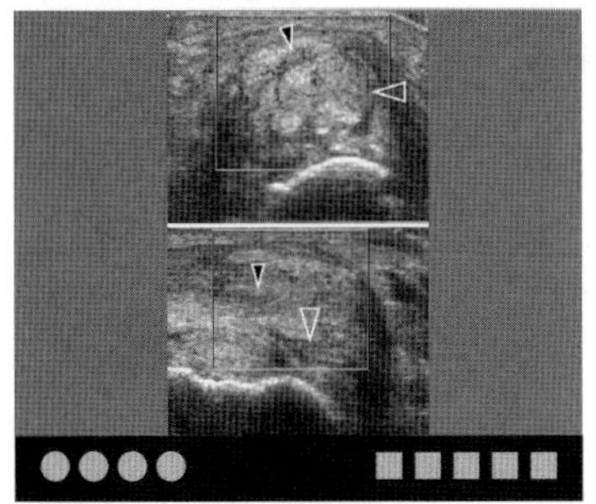

F. Partial tear and Tenosynovitis of the tibialis posterior tendon: Axial oblique color Doppler sonogram obtained over the (a) supramalleolar portion and (b) inframalleolar portion of the TPT show local inflammatory changes of the parietal synovium (void arrowheads) and internal fissures (black arrowheads) related to partial tears.

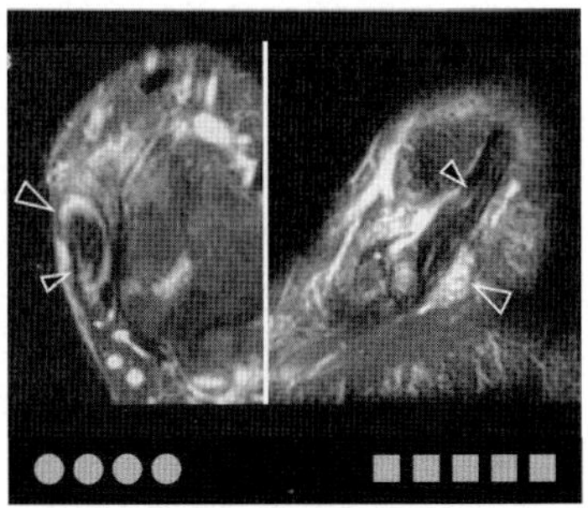

G. Partial tear and tenosynovitis of the tibialis posterior tendon: (a) axial oblique and (b) sagittal gadolinium-enhanced T1-weighted fat-saturated MR images in the same patient show contrast enhancement of the synovium (void arrowheads) and internal tendon fissures (black arrowheads).

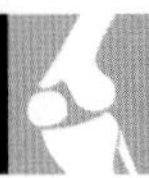

29–8 Complete Tear of Peroneus Longus Tendon

Shahla Modarresi and Jamshid Tehranzadeh

PRESENTATION

Progressive pain, swelling and tenderness

FINDINGS

MR study shows discontinuity of peroneus longus tendon. The torn distal fragment is seen in a pool of fluid near the calcaneocuboid joint. The axial view shows missing tendon is replaced by fluid in the tendon sheath.

DIFFERENTIAL DIAGNOSES

- *Tenosynovitis:* MR shows fluid collection within tendon sheath. Enlarged tendon with internal intermediate signal is noted.
- *Tendinosis:* MR shows an enlarged tendon with intermediate signal within the tendon substance.
- *Synovitis of the tendon sheath:* MR shows fluid collection within tendon sheath with otherwise normal appearing tendon.

COMMENTS

Peroneal tendons lie on the posterolateral aspect of the ankle passing through the fibular groove of the lateral malleolus superficial to calcaneofibular ligament. Peroneus brevis lies medial and anterior to the longus crossing over the cuboid to insert on the fifth metatarsal styloid. Peroneal longus tendon turns beneath the cuboid in a tunnel formed by the long plantar ligament and the groove of the cuboid. It then courses to insert onto the first metatarsal and medial cuneiform. In 20% of the population, an os peroneum may be present within the longus tendon as it turns under the cuboid bone. In 0.1%, os vesalianum is found at the insertion of the peroneus brevis tendon. The peroneal tendon is the major foot everter designed to stabilize the foot and ankle and protect them from sprains. Injuries to the peroneal tendons are not always clinically significant. Function can be severely compromised by tendon tear or for unknown reason it can be asymptomatic. Acute injuries include tendinosis, laceration, tear, rupture, and subluxation resulting from either: (1) inversion injury which is often associated with anterior talofibular ligament and/or calcaneofibular ligament disruption or (2) a powerful contraction of the peroneal muscles from forcefully dorsiflexed foot.

Chronic injuries include longitudinal tears and recurrent subluxation of the peroneus brevis tendon usually from ankle or subtalar arthritis and ankle instability. MR is an excellent modality to visualize the tendon and identify tendinosis, partial or complete tears. Tendon enlargement with internal fluid signal within the tendon sheath is a typical finding. Tendon discontinuity and fluid at ruptured site is seen in complete tendon tear.

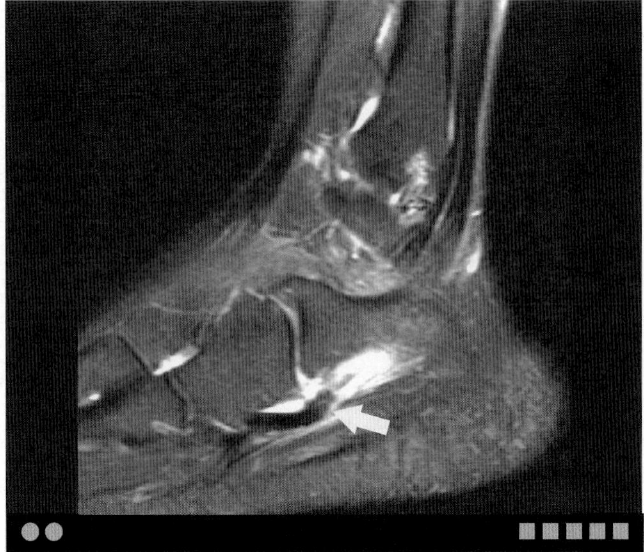

A. Complete tear of peroneus tendon tear: Sagittal fat-saturated T2-weighted image shows discontinuity of peroneus longus tendon. The torn distal tendon fragment is buckled (arrow) in a pool of fluid.

PEARLS

- **Peroneal tendons pass through the retromalleolar groove. The brevis crosses over cuboid to insert on fifth metatarsal and the longus turns beneath the cuboid to insert onto first metatarsal and medial cuneiform.**
- **Peroneal tendons are the major foot everters designed to stabilize the foot and ankle and protect them from sprains.**
- **Peroneal tendons acute injuries include tendinosis, laceration, tear, rupture, and subluxation resulting from inversion injury or forcefully dorsiflexed foot.**
- **Peroneal tendons chronic injuries include longitudinal tears and recurrent subluxation of the peroneus brevis tendon usually from ankle or subtalar arthritis and ankle instability.**
- **MRI shows enlarged tendon with increased T2-weighted internal signal in partial thickness tear and split in full thickness tear. Tendon discontinuity and fluid at ruptured site are seen in complete tendon tear.**

ADDITIONAL IMAGES

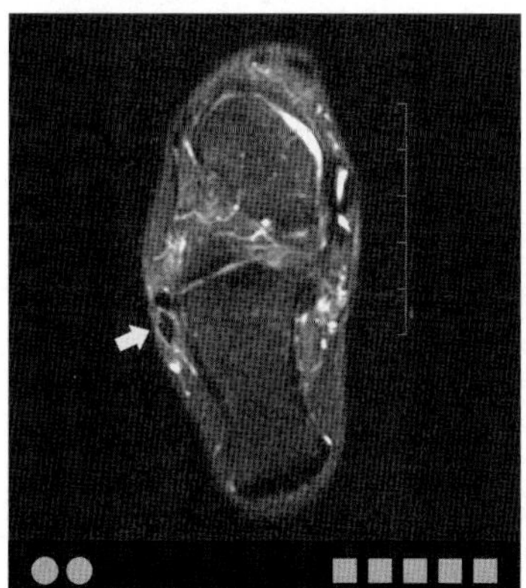

B. Complete tear of peroneus tendon tear: Axial T2-weighted fat-saturated image shows normal peroneus brevis tendon on the top and proximal segment (arrow) of torn peroneus longus on the bottom. On this section peroneus longus appears normal. However, the next section (image C) shows empty torn tendon sheath.

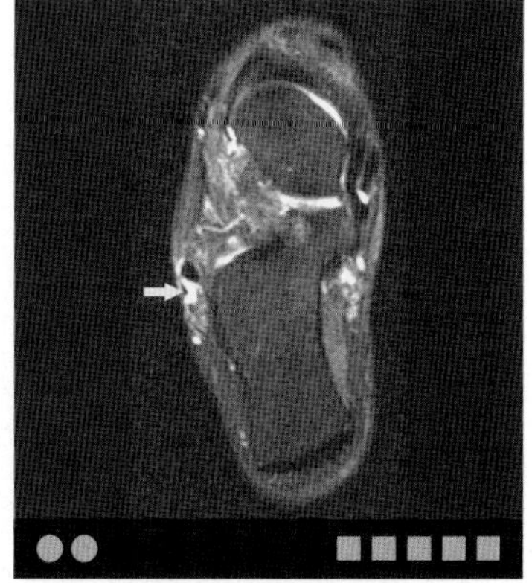

C. Complete tear of peroneus tendon tear: Axial T2-weighted fat-saturated image (next distal section to image B) shows normal peroneus brevis tendon on the top. Empty tendon sheath of peroneus longus is filled with fluid (arrow) indicating missing torn tendon.

IMAGE KEY

Common

Rare

Typical

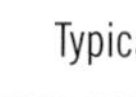

Unusual

DIFFERENTIAL DIAGNOSES IMAGES

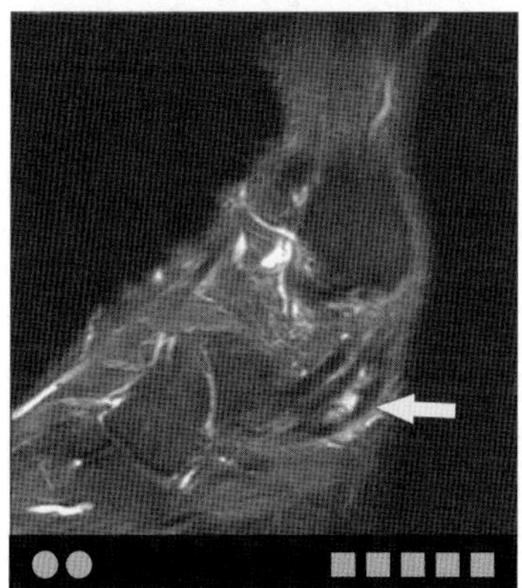

D. Split tear of peroneus longus tendon: Sagittal STIR image in another patient shows split tear of peroneus longus tendon (arrow).

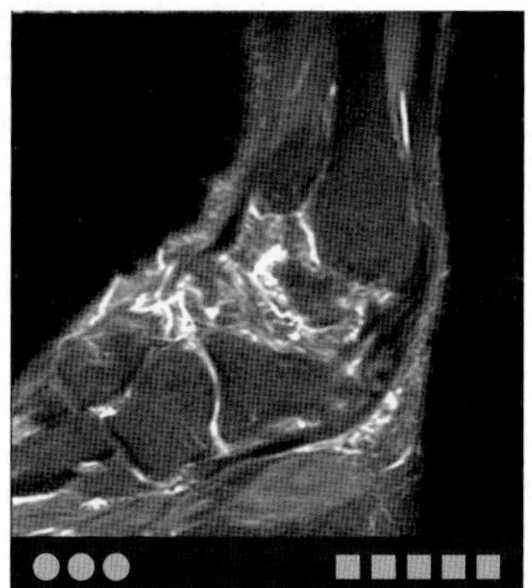

E. Partial tear of peroneus longus tendon: Sagittal STIR image shows partial tear of peroneal tendon.

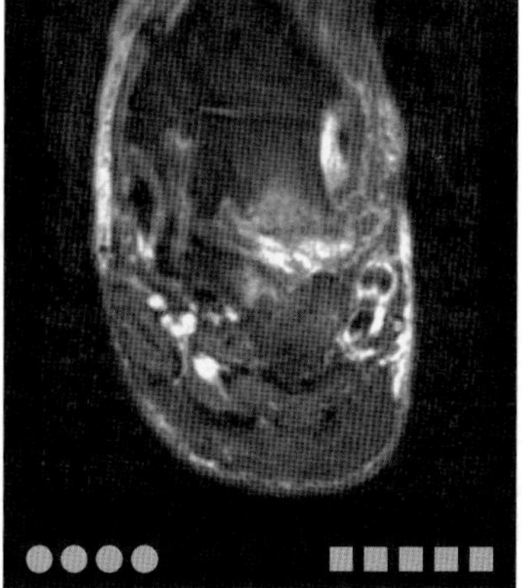

F. Tenosynovitis of peroneal tendon: Coronal STIR image of the ankle shows fluid surrounding the peroneal tendon with internal signal consistent with tenosynovitis vs. partial tear.

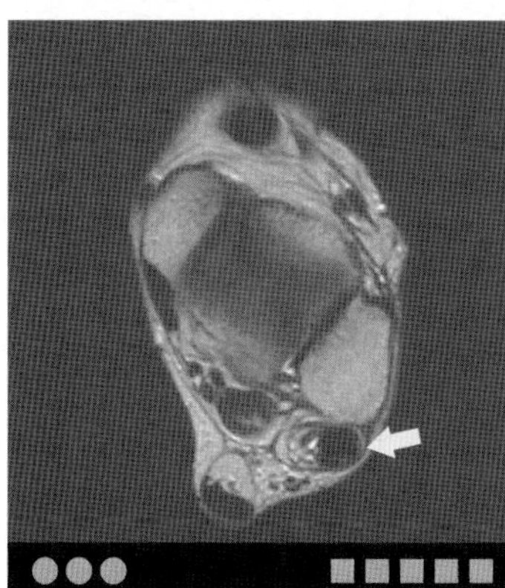

G. Peroneal tendon tendinosis: Proton density axial image of the ankle shows enlarged peroneal tendon with internal signal consistent with tendinosis (arrow).

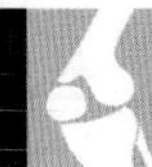

29–9 Split Tear of Peroneus Brevis Tendon

Ashkan Afshin and Jamshid Tehranzadeh

PRESENTATION

Ankle pain

FINDINGS

MR images show increased signal longitudinally along the substance of the tendon. Normal flat appearance of brevis tendon changes to an inverted U-shape appearance (boomerang appearance). Two separate tendons with only one muscle body may also be demonstrated on MR images.

DIFFERENTIAL DIAGNOSES

- *Complete tear of peroneus longus tendon:* MR findings show incontinuity of peroneus longus and empty tendon sheath of peroneus longus, which is filled with fluid.
- *Tendinosis of peroneus brevis*: Tendinosis is diagnosed when the tendon has intermediate signal on T1-weighted image and normal to intermediate signal is seen in T2-weighted sequence.
- *Complete tear of peroneus tendon:* Discontinuity of tendon is seen with fluid signal at the disrupted site.

COMMENTS

Peroneus brevis originate from distal two-third of the lateral surface of the body of fibula and the adjacent intermuscular septa and inserts to tuberosity on lateral side of proximal end of fifth metatarsal. Longitudinal tear of the brevis tendon is called peroneus brevis split tear. Certain conditions, such as a shallow retromalleolar groove, torn peroneal retinaculum, low lying brevis muscle belly, and the presence of a peroneus quartus muscle predispose this tendon to split. Pain and swelling along the peroneal tendon sheath are common complaints in peroneus brevis tendon tear. Chronic lateral ankle instability can also be associated with peroneus brevis tendon splits. MR imaging is useful in establishing the diagnosis of split tears of the peroneus brevis tendon as well as associated soft tissue findings. In MR images, the peroneus brevis tendon is usually anterior to the peroneus longus tendon and at the retromalleolar groove these two tendons often cannot be appreciated as separate structures. Both tendons are normally low signal on T1-weighted images and separate from each other at peroneal tubercle of Calcaneus. Brevis is anterior to the tubercle and longus is posterior. Splits can be seen as increased signal longitudinally along the substance of this tendon. Brevis splits are most commonly seen on axial images where normal flat appearance of brevis tendon changes to an inverted U-shape appearance (boomerang appearance). It may also be shown on sagittal images where two separate tendons and only one muscle body are demonstrated.

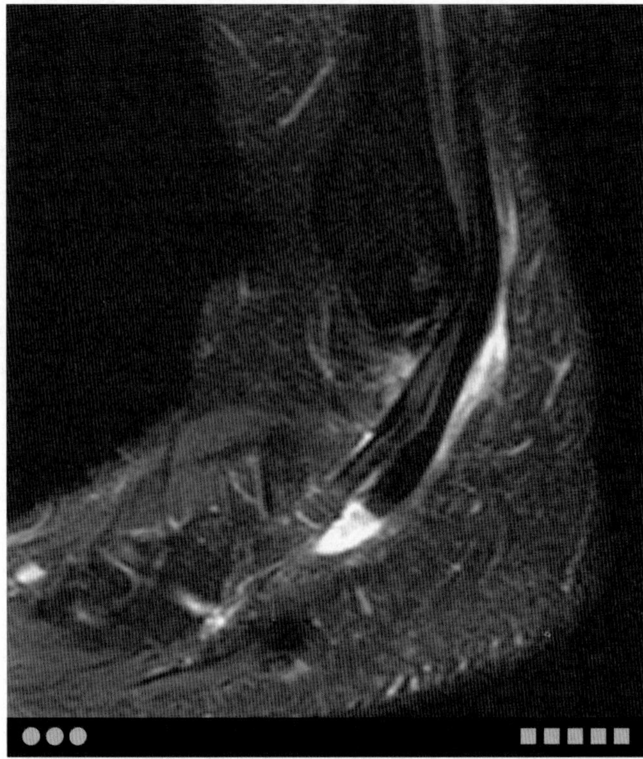

A. Split tear of peroneus brevis Tendon: Sagittal fat-saturated T2-weighted image on the lateral side of the ankle shows a line of bright signal seen along the course of peroneus brevis tendon indicating split tear of this tendon.

PEARLS

- **Peroneus brevis originates from distal of body of fibula and inserts to proximal end of fifth metatarsal bone.**
- **Shallow retromalleolar groove, torn peroneal retinaculum, low lying brevis muscle belly, and the presence of a peroneus quartus muscle predispose the tendon to split.**
- **Pain and swelling along the peroneal tendon sheath are common complaints. It may also be associated with chronic lateral ankle instability.**
- **MR imaging shows increased signal longitudinally along the substance of this tendon. Normal flat appearance of brevis tendon changes to an inverted U-shape or boomerang appearance.**

ADDITIONAL IMAGES

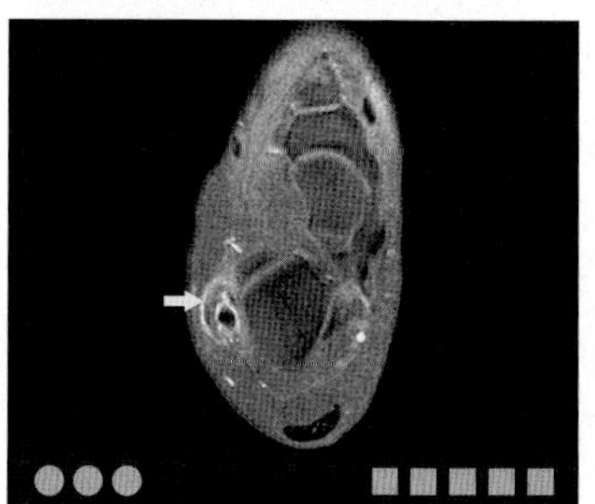

B. Split tear of peroneus brevis Tendon: Axial fat-saturated T2-weighted image shows fluid in the tendon sheaths around peroneus brevis and longus tendons. The peroneus brevis tendon which is located on the top (anterior) to peroneus longus has an inverted U-shape appearance (boomerang appearance) indicating split tear (arrow).

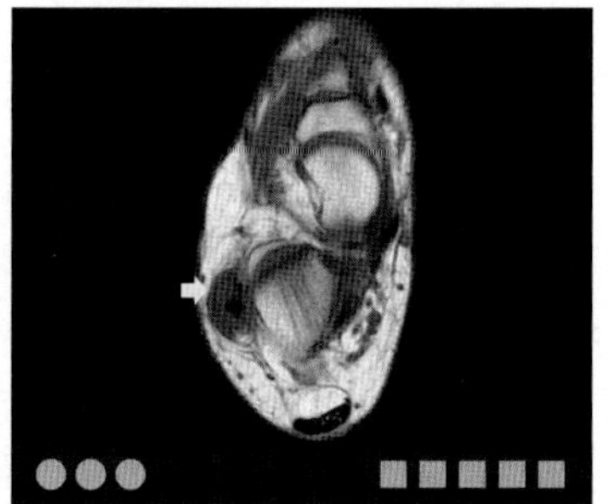

C. Split tear of peroneus brevis Tendon: Axial T1-weighted image shows fluid in the tendon sheaths around peroneus brevis and longus tendons. The peroneus brevis tendon which is located on the top (anterior) to peroneus longus has an inverted U-shaped appearance (boomerang appearance) indicating split tear (arrow).

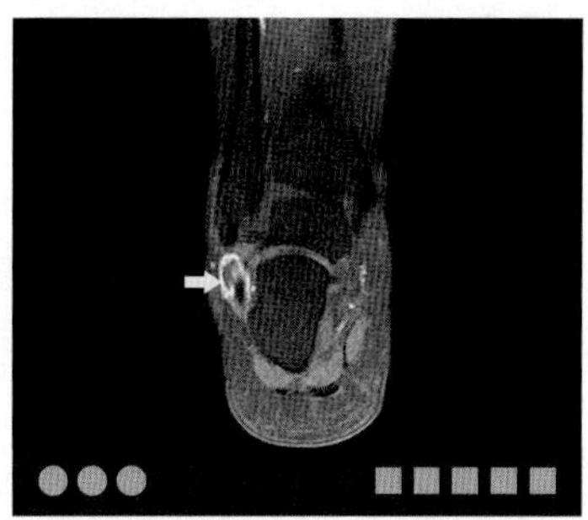

D. Split tear of peroneus brevis Tendon: Coronal fat-saturated T2-weighted image shows fluid in the tendon sheath around peroneal tendons. Peroneus longus tendon has normal dark signal. The peroneus brevis tendon has intermediate to bright signal indicating tear of the tendon (arrow).

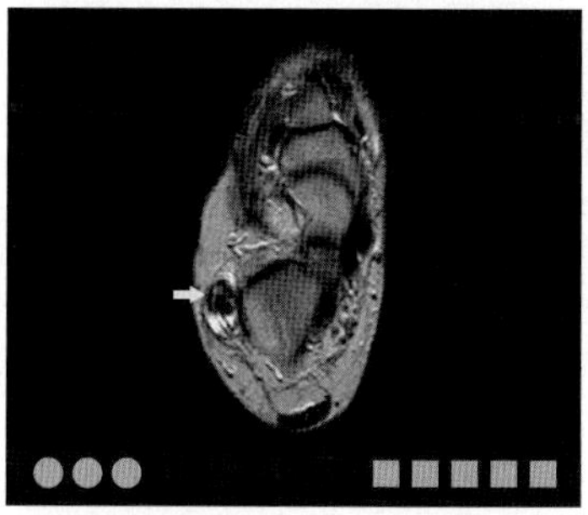

E. Split tear of peroneus brevis Tendon: Axial T2-weighted image shows fluid in the tendon sheaths around peroneus brevis and longus tendons. The peroneus brevis tendon which is located on the top (anterior) to peroneus longus has an inverted U-shaped appearance (boomerang appearance) indicating split tear (arrow).

IMAGE KEY

Common

Rare

Typical

Unusual

DIFFERENTIAL DIAGNOSES IMAGES

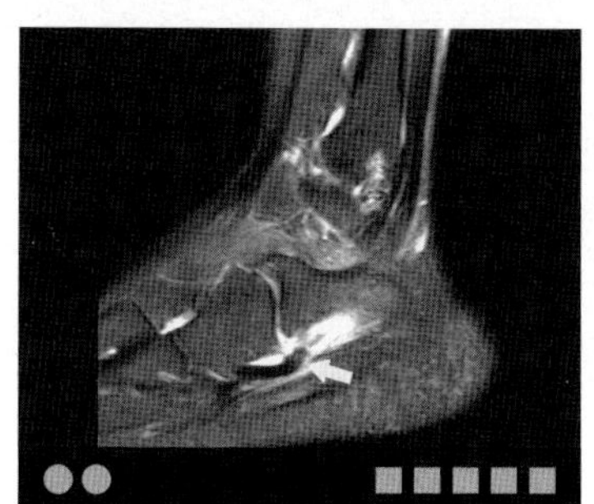

F. Complete tear of peroneus longus tendon: Sagittal fat-saturated T2-weighted image shows discontinuity of peroneus longus tendon. The torn distal tendon fragment is buckled (arrow) in a pool of fluid.

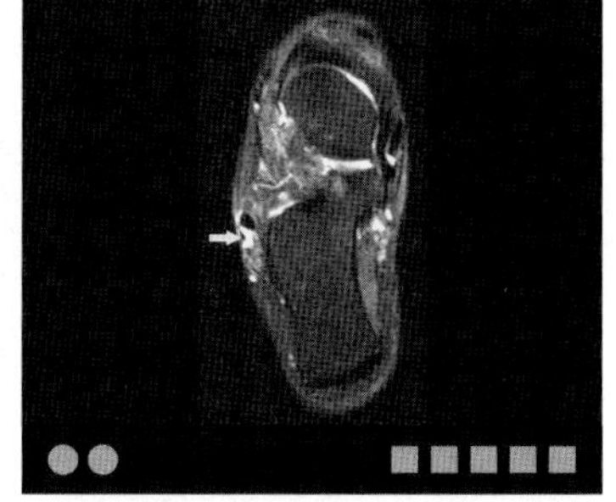

G. Complete tear of peroneus longus tendon: Axial T2-weighted fat-saturated image shows normal peroneus brevis tendon on the top. Empty tendon sheath of peroneus longus is filed with fluid (arrow) indicating missing torn tendon.

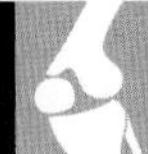

29–10 Plantar Fasciitis

Kira Chow

PRESENTATION

Heel pain

FINDINGS

Sagittal inversion recovery MRI shows edema along the plantar fascia near the calcaneal origin site.

DIFFERENTIAL DIAGNOSES

- *Plantar fibromatosis:* Nodular or irregular regions of thickening along the plantar fascia, often with infiltrative margins. In contrast to fasciitis, fibromatosis does not necessarily involve the calcaneal attachment site.
- *Plantar fascia rupture:* Discontinuity of the plantar fascia, often with surrounding edema.
- *Cellulitis, osteomyelitis:* Edema is present along the plantar fascia with marrow edema in the bone, which may represent osteomyelitis or reactive marrow edema.

COMMENTS

The plantar fascia is a fibrous aponeurosis originating from the calcaneal tuberosity and inserting onto the deep short transverse ligaments of the metatarsal heads. Of the medial, lateral, and central components, the central component is the strongest, largest, and most typically involved by plantar fasciitis. Plantar fasciitis is a chronic degeneration and inflammation that occurs in response to micro tears in the fascia. Etiology is most commonly repetitive trauma as in athletes and less commonly inflammatory arthritides such as ankylosing spondylitis, Reiters syndrome, and psoriasis. Other possible risk factors include obesity, hard walking surfaces, and age over 40. The site usually involved is the calcaneal origin but plantar fasciitis can also occur more distally. Diagnosis is more often clinical, but MRI does demonstrate abnormalities in the plantar fascia. On proton density and T1-weighted images, there is intermediate signal within the plantar fascia with fusiform thickening measuring $<$6 mm as opposed to the $<$4 mm thickness normally associated with this structure. There may also be marrow edema in the adjacent calcaneus or muscle edema in the flexor digitorum brevis muscles. Presence of muscle edema is associated with more severe pain. The relationship of heel spurs to plantar fasciitis is controversial. However, recent literature suggests that heel spurs occur independently and are not indicative of plantar fasciitis. Treatment is usually conservative, consisting of NSAIDS (nonsteroidal anti-inflammatory agents), steroid injections and behavioral modifications such as use of orthotics.

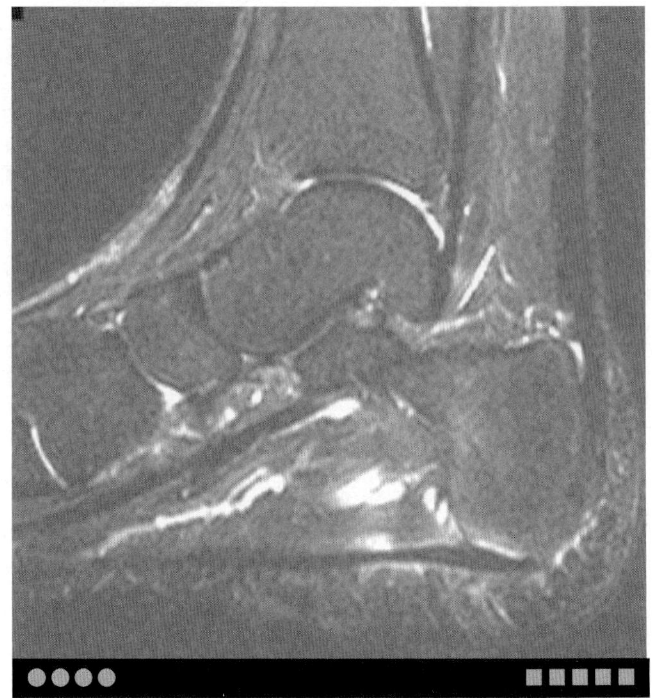

A. Plantar fasciitis: Sagittal inversion recovery MRI shows edema along the plantar fascia near the calcaneal origin site.

PEARLS

- **Classic finding is fusiform thickening ($>$6 mm) of the calcaneal origin of the plantar fascia with intermediate signal intensity.**
- **Etiology can be stress related or inflammatory arthritis.**
- **Heel spurs are not an associated radiographic finding in plantar fasciitis.**

ADDITIONAL IMAGES

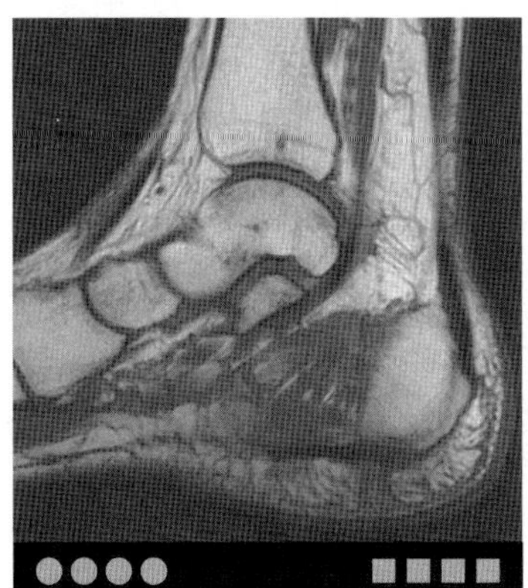

B. Plantar fasciitis: T1-weighted sagittal MRI shows intermediate signal and thickening of the calcaneal origin of the plantar fascia.

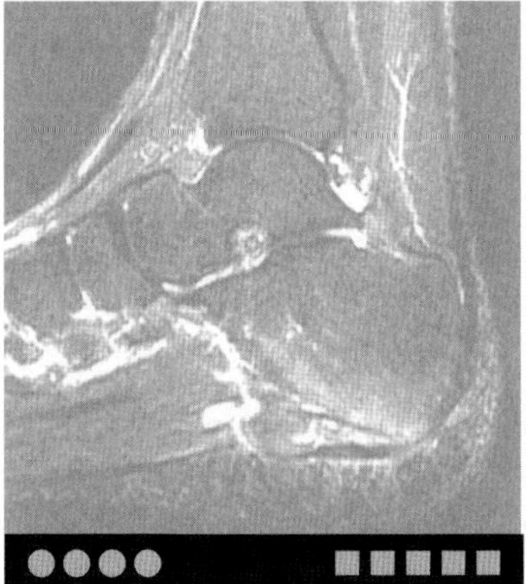

C. Plantar fasciitis: Sagittal inversion recovery MRI shows hyperintense signal representing marrow edema in the calcaneus at the plantar fascial origin site.

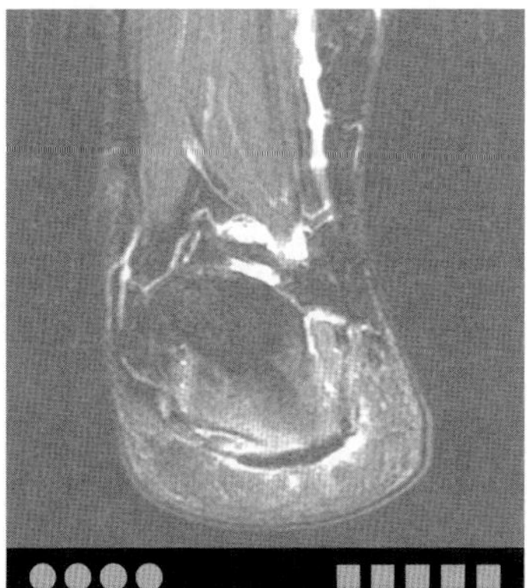

D. Plantar fasciitis: Coronal T2-weighted fat-saturated MRI demonstrates the plantar fascia with edema on its plantar and dorsal aspects.

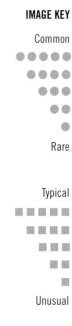

IMAGE KEY

Common

Rare

Typical

Unusual

DIFFERENTIAL DIAGNOSES IMAGES

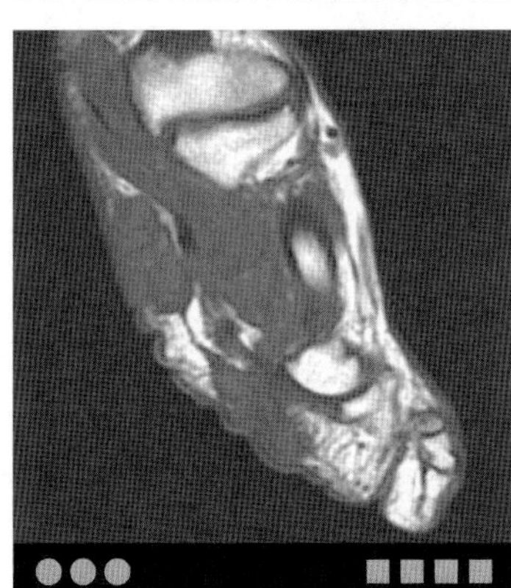

E. Plantar fibromatosis: T1-weighted sagittal MRI demonstrates two T1 hypointense nodules along the plantar aspect of the foot, involving a more distal part of the plantar fascia than is involved by plantar fasciitis.

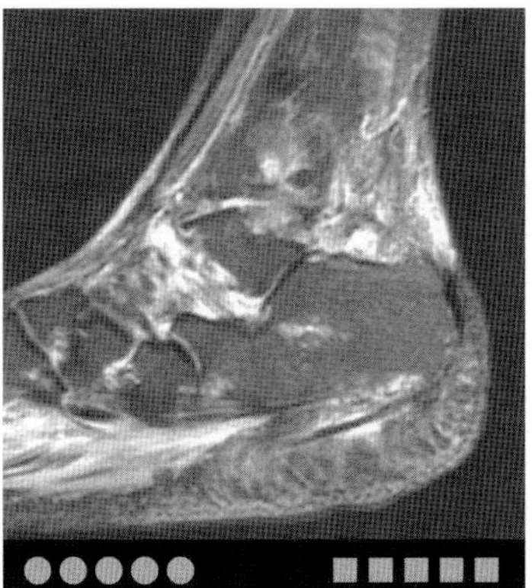

F. Cellulitis, osteomyelitis: Sagittal inversion recovery MRI demonstrates edema along the proximal plantar fascia as well as in the plantar muscle compartment. Small region of signal abnormality in the inferior calcaneus at the plantar fascial origin represents osteomyelitis.

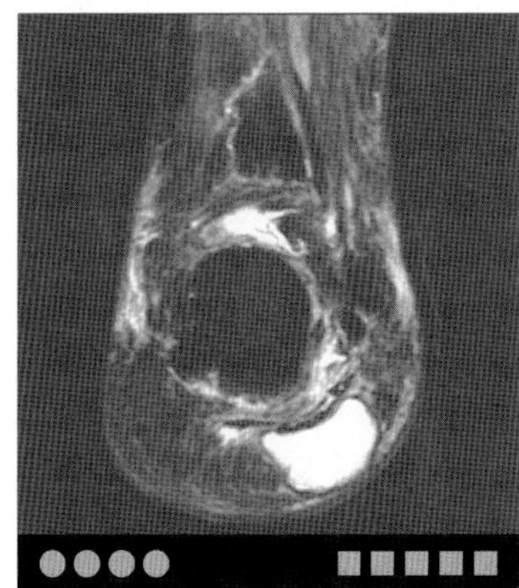

G. Heel abscess: Coronal T2-weighted fat-saturated MRI in the patient in Figure F demonstrates a hyperintense fluid collection representing an abscess.

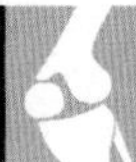

29–11 Sonographic Appearance of Plantar Fasciitis

Mélanie Morel, Nathalie Boutry, and Anne Cotten

PRESENTATION

Subcalcaneal heel pain

FINDINGS

Sonography shows hypoechoic thickening of the body of the plantar fascia with perifascial fluid. MRI also exhibits perifascial edema.

DIFFERENTIAL DIAGNOSES

- *Plantar fascia rupture:* Sonography shows a slightly undulated and thinned fascia. MRI exhibits disruption and increased signal intensity at the site of a recent rupture on T1-weighted images, and perifascial edema on T2 MR images. In case of chronic rupture, the plantar fascia is focally thickened with intrafascial intermediate to low signal intensity on all sequences (scar).
- *Plantar fascia inflammatory enthesopathy in spondylarthropathies:* Sonography shows hypoechoic thickening of the plantar fascia enthesis, erosions, and enthesophytes at the adjacent calcaneus. Bone marrow edema can be seen within the subcortical region of the medial calcaneal tuberosity. It is often bilateral and associated with Achilles tendon enthesitis and retrocalcaneal bursitis.
- *Plantar fascia mechanical enthesopathy:* Sonographic features are quite similar to the former but other enthesopathies and retrocalcaneal bursitis are usually not seen, and patients are older and frequently demonstrate overweight.

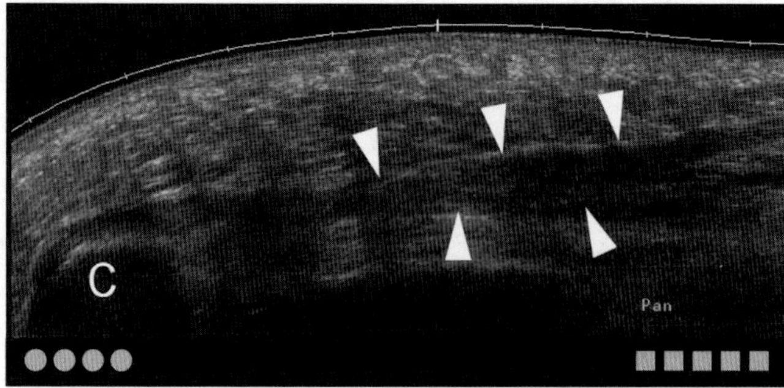

A. Plantar fasciitis: Longitudinal sonogram shows hypoechoic thickening of the proximal plantar fascia (arrowheads), located between 2 and 4 cm from its calcaneal (C) insertion.

COMMENTS

The patient is a 36-year-old woman suffering from chronic bilateral heel pain, diagnosed as plantar fasciitis. Plantar fasciitis is the most common cause of inferior heel pain, particularly (but not only) in the athlete running and jumping. It may also be associated with various foot deformities, obesity, degenerative or systemic factors. Repetitive tractions produce fibers micro-tears of the plantar fascia and perifascial inflammatory changes. The patient complains of heel pain arising in the morning and worsening with intense activity. Sagittal heel sonogram shows a thickened proximal plantar fascia (compared with the contralateral foot), focal or diffuse hypoechoic changes within it. These changes are found distant to the attachment of the plantar fascia on the calcaneus. Hyperemia of plantar fascia and surrounding soft tissues with or without perifascial fluid may also be found. MR imaging typically demonstrates fascial thickening with adjacent soft-tissue edema. Treatment of plantar fasciitis is primarily conservative. Steroid injections and surgery are reserved to chronic recalcitrant cases. Other differential diagnoses include plantar fibromatosis which usually involves distal portion of the plantar fascia, with single or multiple nodular areas of thickening of its inferior margin. The nodules are hypoechoic and blend with the fascia proximally and distally. They have low to intermediate signal intensity on T1-weighted images. Signal intensity on T2-weighted images decreases with time. Other causes of inferior heel pain include subcalcaneal bursitis, calcaneal stress fracture, calcaneal osteomyelitis, and tarsal tunnel syndrome.

PEARLS

- **Plantar fasciitis is the most common cause of inferior heel pain.**
- **It is caused by micro-tears of plantar fascia fibers, with perifascial inflammatory changes.**
- **Imaging abnormalities are proximal, but distinct from the attachment of the fascia on the calcaneus.**
- **US shows hypoechoic thickening of the plantar fascia.**
- **MRI shows fascial thickening with perifascial edema. High signal intensity of the plantar fascia on T2-weighted images is often found.**

ADDITIONAL IMAGES

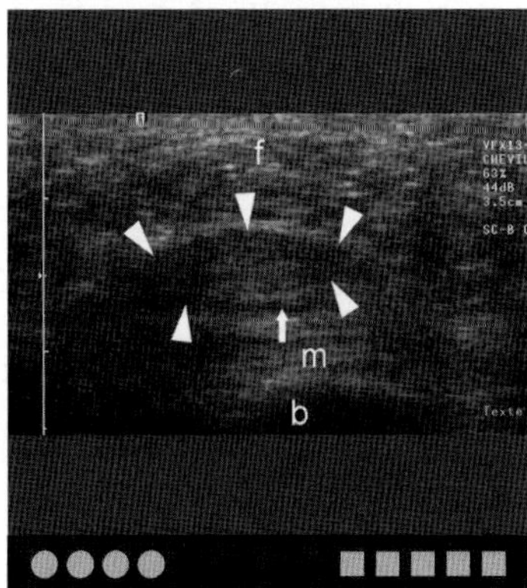

B. Plantar fasciitis: Transverse sonogram exhibits fusiform thickening of the plantar fascia (arrowheads), with perifascial fluid (arrow) (f: fat pad; b: tarsal bone; m: flexor digitorum brevis muscle).

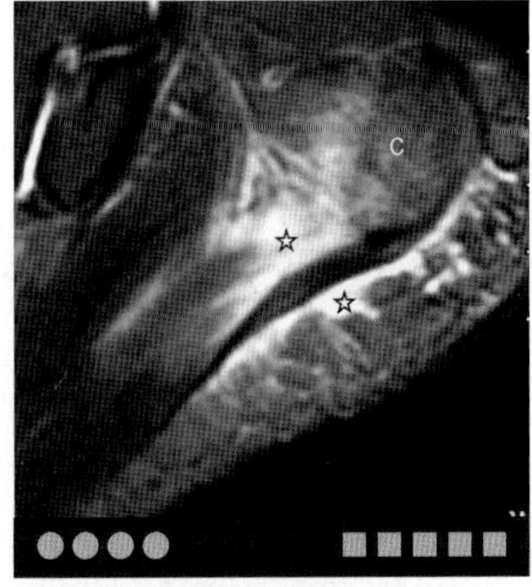

C. Plantar fasciitis: STIR sagittal MR image demonstrates high signal intensity perifascial edema (stars) on both sides of the thickened plantar fascia.

IMAGE KEY

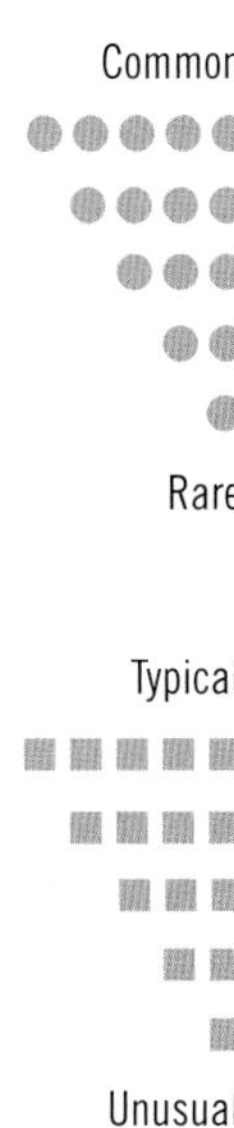

DIFFERENTIAL DIAGNOSES IMAGES

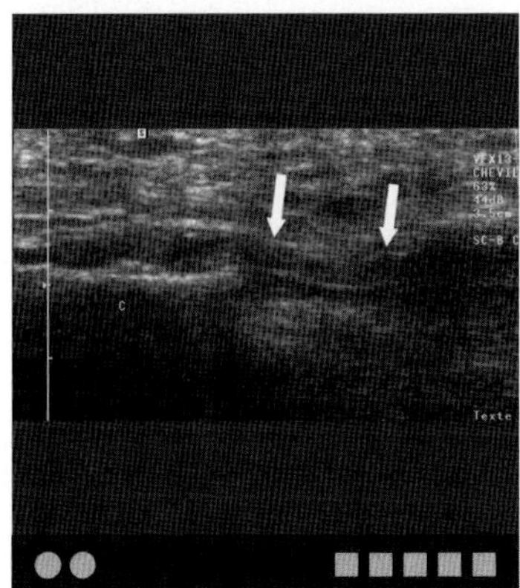

D. Plantar fascia rupture: Longitudinal sonogram reveals a slightly undulated, thinned fascia (between the arrows).

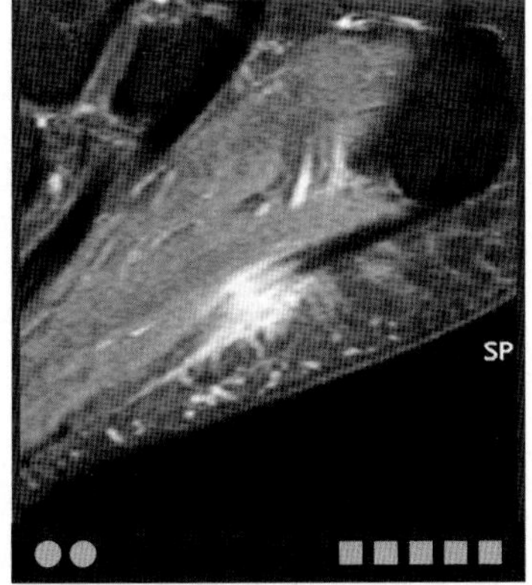

E. Plantar fascia rupture: STIR sagittal MR image shows discontinuity of the fibers of the plantar fascia, with perifascial edema.

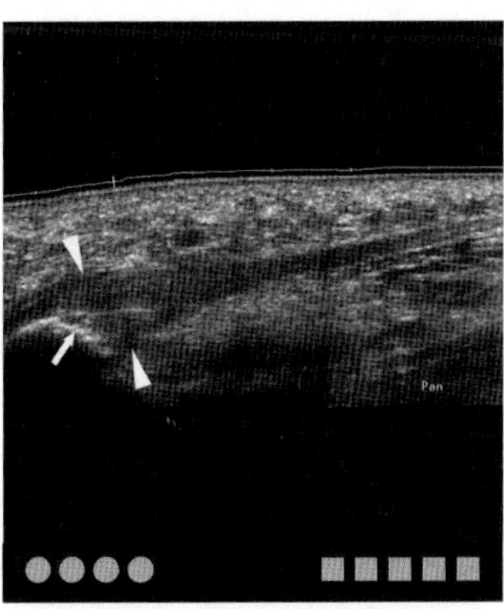

F. Plantar fascia inflammatory enthesopathy: Longitudinal sonogram exhibits thickening of the calcaneal insertion of the plantar fascia (arrowheads), calcaneal erosions (arrow), and enthesophyte.

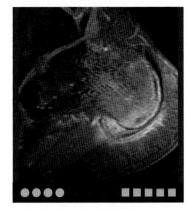

G. Plantar fascia inflammatory enthesopathy: STIR sagittal MR image demonstrates a thickened calcaneal enthesis, with perifascial and calcaneal bone edema.

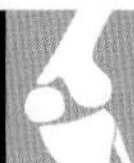

29–12 Plantar Plate Disruption (Turf Toe)

Rosemary J. Klecker

PRESENTATION

Acute first metatarsalgia

FINDINGS

MR images show disruption of the plantar plate between the sesamoid bone and the base of the proximal phalanx of the first toe.

DIFFERENTIAL DIAGNOSES

- *Intermetarsal bursitis:* Presents on MR imaging as a well-defined fluid collection at or above the intermetatarsal ligaments.
- *Flexor tendon disruption:* The disruption is of the flexor tendon which is larger than and located plantar to the plantar plate.
- *Sesamoiditis:* MR imaging findings include increased signal of the marrow of the sesamoids on T2 and STIR-weighted images and variably decreased marrow signal on T1-weighted images.

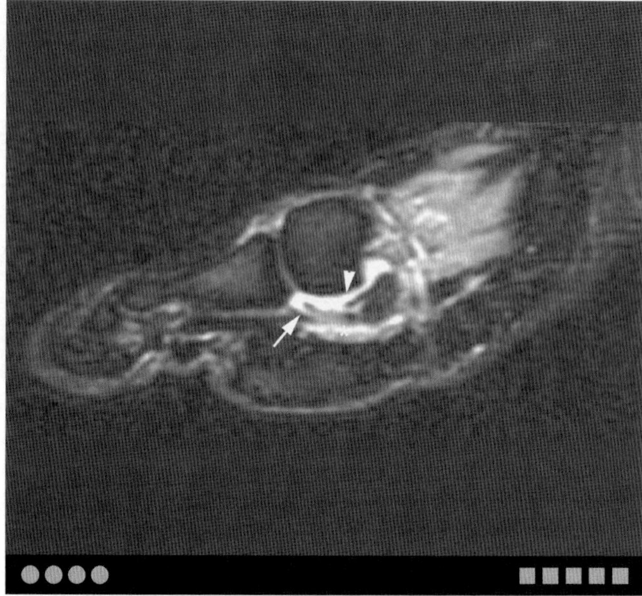

A. Plantar plate disruption: Sagittal STIR image of the forefoot: The distal insertion of the plantar plate is torn and retracted plantar to the MTP joint (arrow). The proximal insertion is interposed between the head of the first metatarsal and the sesamoid (arrowhead). Note the joint effusion, displacement of the sesamoid and the edema of the soft tissues deep to the flexor tendon (asterix).

COMMENTS

The patient is a 32-year-old male with acute first metatarsalgia. Plantar plate disruption is associated with hyperextension injury (chronic or acute) at the metatarsophalangeal (MTP) joint. Plantar plate disruption of the second through fifth MTP joints is more frequently seen in women secondary to the increased weight-bearing load and hyperextension forces placed on the joints by high-heeled shoes. The plantar plate is a fibrocartilaginous structure that reinforces the MTP capsule and extends from the volar aspect of the metatarsal necks to the proximal phalanges of the toes. On MR imaging, the plantar plate is thin along the volar aspect of the MPT joint and is of low signal intensity on all sequences. It is best visualized on the sagittal and coronal images through the forefoot. Disruption of the plantar plate is diagnosed on MR imaging as increased signal intensity in the plantar plate on T2-wighted images. Other MR imaging findings which are variably present include MTP synovitis, flexor tenosynovitis, and persistent flexion of the MTP. Plantar plate disruption of the first MTP joint is often referred to as "turf toe" and is more prevalent in football or soccer players. The name refers to the fact that this often occurs as a result of playing on artificial turf and hard surfaces while wearing lightweight, flexible shoes predisposing the MTP joints to hyperextension injuries.

PEARLS

- **Plantar plate disruption of the second through fifth digits is more common in women who wear high-heeled shoes.**
- **The second MTP joint is most commonly affected.**
- **MRI shows disruption of the fibrocartilaginous plantar plate between the metatarsal neck and the proximal phalanges of the toes.**
- **Associated MR imaging findings include flexor tendon tenosynovitis, MTP synovitis, and persistent hyperextension of the proximal phalanx.**

ADDITIONAL IMAGES

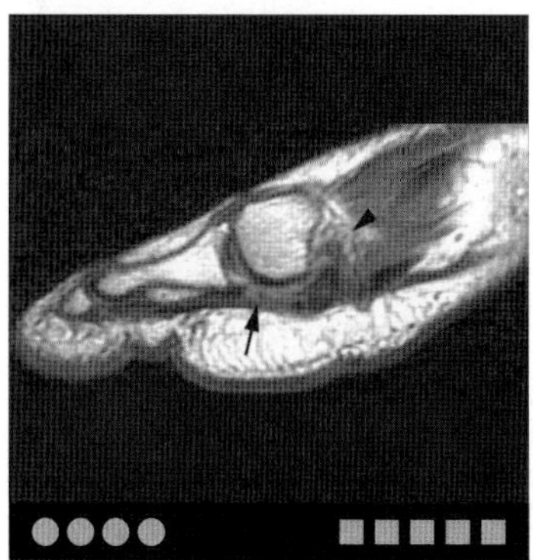

B. Plantar plate disruption: Sagittal proton density-weighted image of the forefoot shows disruption of the plantar plate (arrow) and laxity/partial tear of the joint capsule (arrowhead).

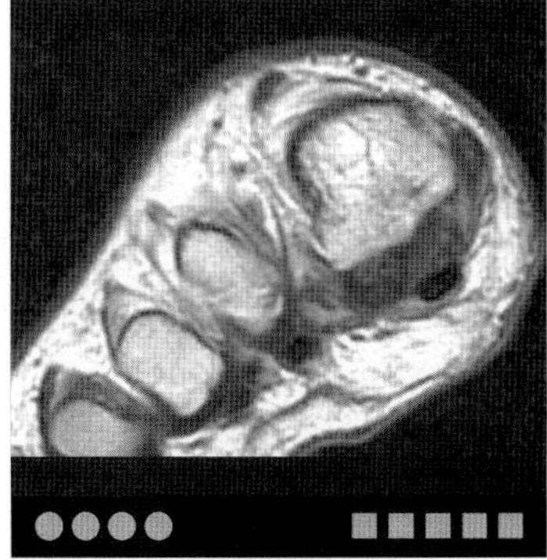

C. Plantar plate disruption: Coronal proton density-weighted image shows edema at the expected location of the planar plate. The plantar plate is not seen at the first MTP.

DIFFERENTIAL DIAGNOSES IMAGES

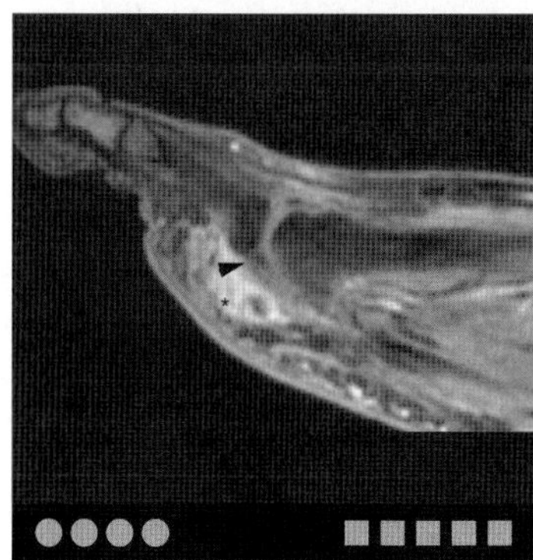

D. Intermetatarsal bursitis: Sagittal T1-weighted fat saturation with gadolinium shows enhancement of the bursa (asterix) in the soft tissues deep to the plantar plate of the third MTP joint (arrowhead).

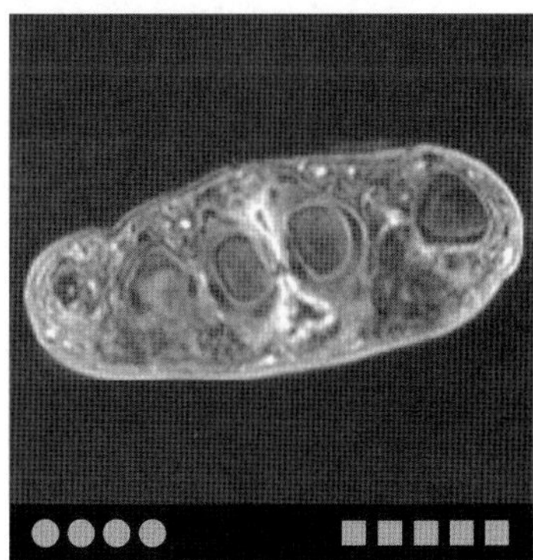

E. Intermetatarsal bursitis: Coronal T1-weighted fat saturation with gadolinium image the intermetatarsal bursa extending above and below the intermetatarsal ligament between the second and third rays.

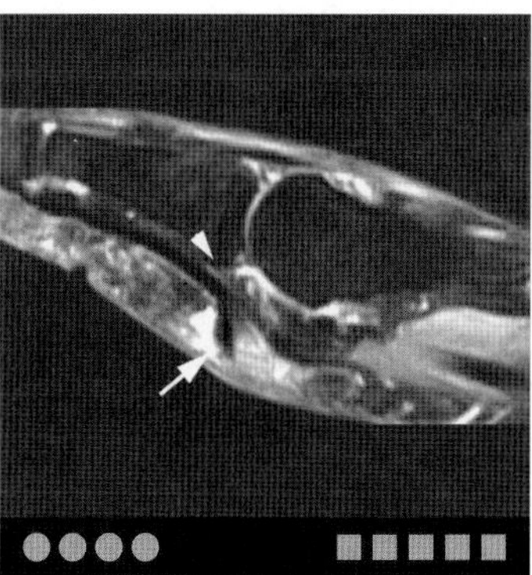

F. Tear of the flexor tendon: Sagittal STIR-weighted image of the second MTP joint shows near-complete rupture of the flexor digitorum longus tendon (arrow). The plantar plate is intact (arrowhead).

IMAGE KEY

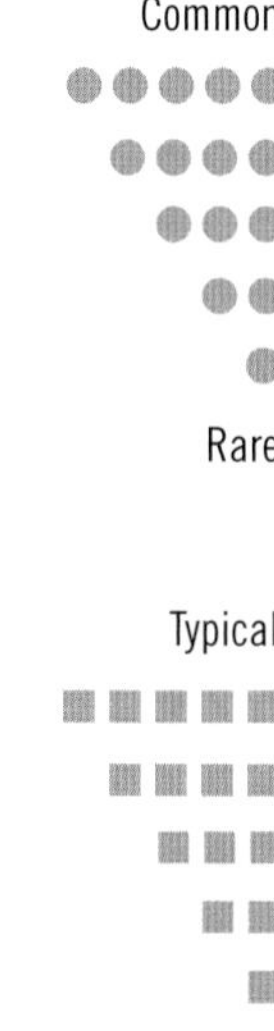

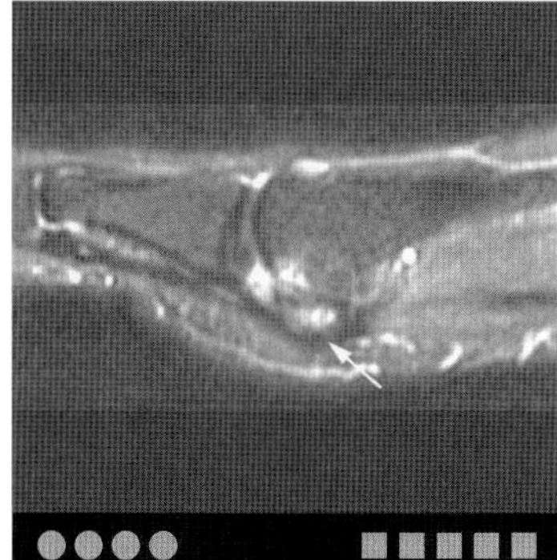

G. Sesamoiditis: Coronal T2-weighted image with fat saturation shows edema in the medial (tibial) sesamoid (arrow), MTP synovitis, and mild subchondral edema of the first metatarsal head.

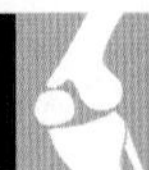

29–13 Ruptured Distal Plantaris Tendon

Marcia F. Blacksin

PRESENTATION

Sudden posterior ankle pain

FINDINGS

Increased signal intensity in tendinous structure adjacent to medial Achilles tendon with discontinuity.

DIFFERENTIAL DIAGNOSES

- *Achilles tendon tear:* Discontinuity, retraction of Achilles is associated with edema of Kagers fat pad.
- *Xanthoma of Achilles tendon:* This infiltrating deposit in Achilles tendon results in degeneration and tear of Achilles and presents as large lobulating mass.

COMMENTS

The plantaris muscle arises from the lateral femoral condyle and continues distally in the calf, deep to the lateral gastrocnemius muscle. Distally, several insertions have been reported. The tendon can blend into the medial aspect of the Achilles tendon, with a small cleft between the two tendons. The tendon can also insert into the medial aspect of the calcaneal tuberosity or 1 cm anterior and medial to the Achilles insertion on the calcaneus. This tendon has been used to repair Achilles tendon injury. Rupture of the plantaris tendon in the calf has been called "tennis leg." Sudden dorsiflexion of the ankle with the knee in extension is thought to be the mechanism of injury. The patient can experience sudden calf pain or a "pop." The injury needs to be differentiated from both Achilles tendon rupture and gastrocnemius injury. This injury is treated conservatively with rest and medications to reduce inflammation. MRI is helpful for diagnosis of tendon and ligamentous injury. Discontinuity, retraction and irregularity of the margins of this tendon are manifested by presence of low signal intensity fluid on T1-weighted images which change to increase signal and edema in T2-weighted and STIR sequences. Kagers fat pad edema is often noted with plantaris and Achilles tendon injuries.

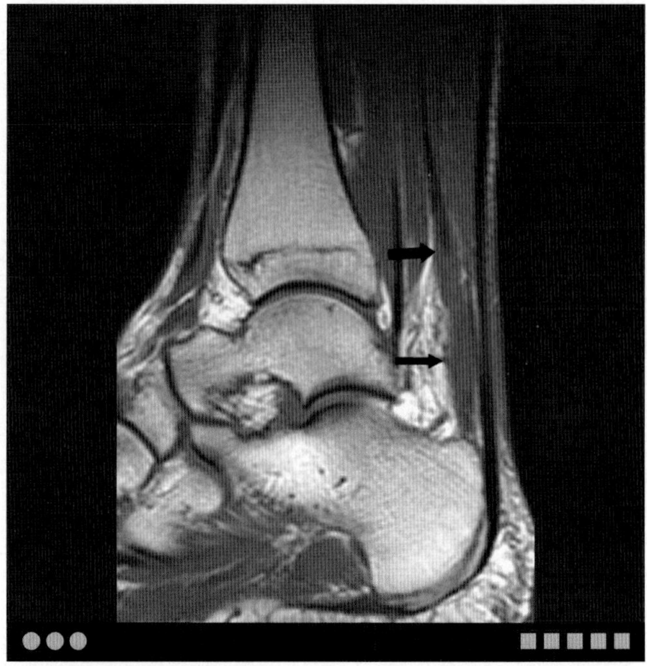

A. Plantaris tendon rupture: Sagittal T1-weighted image shows retracted tendon and distal discontinuity (arrows).

PEARLS

- **The plantaris tendon arises from the lateral femoral condyle and can blend with the medial margin of the Achilles tendon.**
- **Injuries to this tendon can mimic Achilles tendon or gastrocnemius injury.**

ADDITIONAL IMAGES

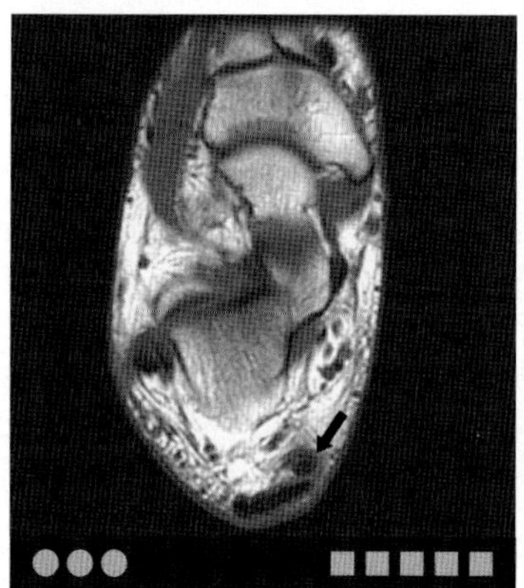

B. Plantaris tendon rupture: Axial T1-weighted image shows increased signal in tendon seen anterior and medial to Achilles (arrow).

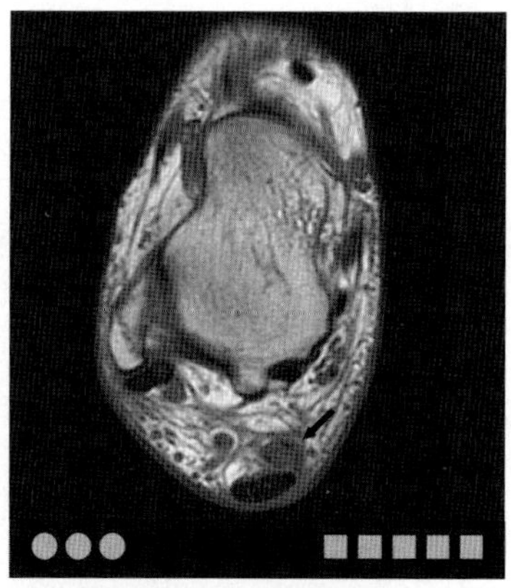

C. Plantaris tendon rupture: Axial T1-weighted image slightly distal shows tendon discontinuity (arrow).

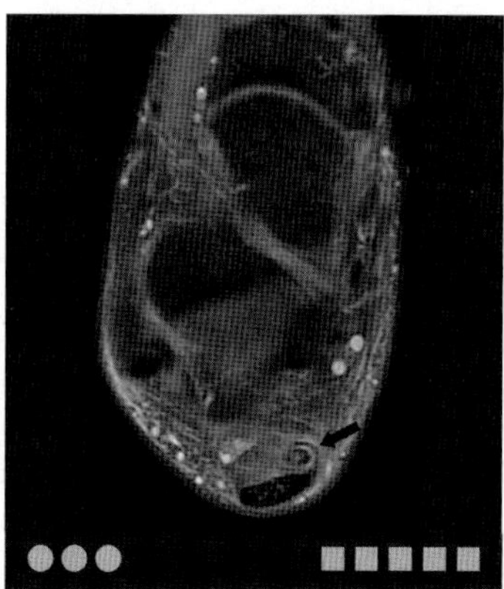

D. Plantaris tendon rupture: Axial T2-weighted image shows increased signal in plantaris tendon (arrow).

DIFFERENTIAL DIAGNOSES IMAGES

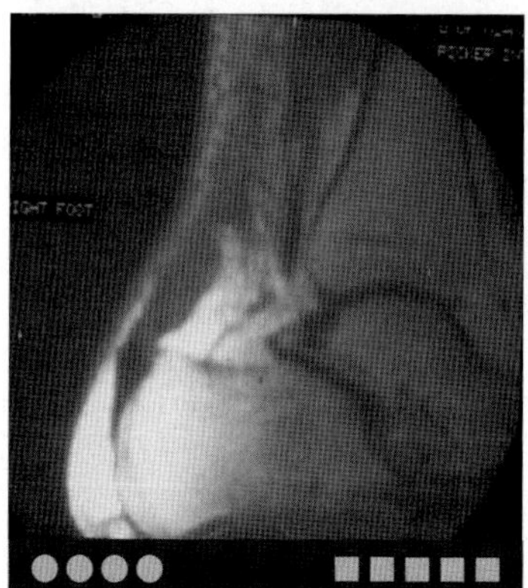

E. Achilles tendon tear: Sagittal T1-weighted image of the ankle shows tear of Achilles tendon with retraction of proximal part.

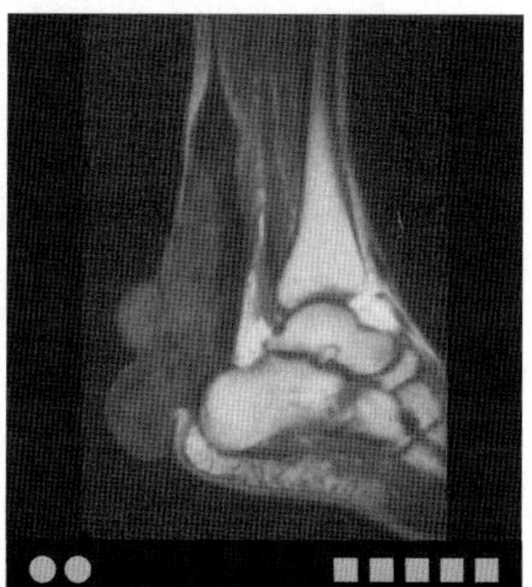

F. Xanthoma of Achilles tendon: Sagittal T1-weighted image of the ankle shows intermediate signal lobulating mass is infiltrating distal and posterior Achilles tendon in a patient with hypercholesterolemia.

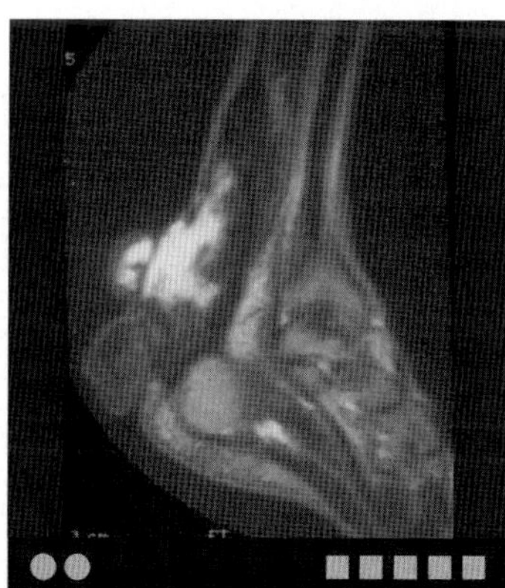

G. Xanthoma of Achilles tendon: Sagittal T2-weighted image of the ankle shows this lobulating mass has mixed signal.

IMAGE KEY

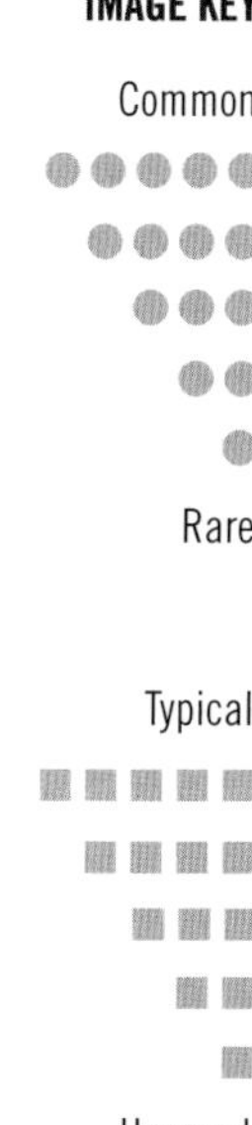

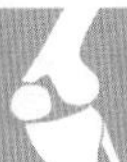

29–14 Complete Rupture of Achilles Tendon

Melitus Maryam Golshan and Jamshid Tehranzadeh

PRESENTATION

Acute posterior ankle pain

FINDINGS

MRI shows complete disruption of Achilles tendon.

DIFFERENTIAL DIAGNOSES

- *Partial Achilles tendon tear:* MRI shows either focal intra-substance increased signal or partial discontinuity of Achilles tendon, where some tendon fibers are preserved and no tendinous gap or retraction is detected.
- *Achilles tendinosis:* MRI shows thickened tendon with or without intra-substance intermediate signal in T2-weighted image.
- *Achilles tendinosis with partial tear:* Thickening of Achilles tendon is associated with bright signal in the tendon with or without partial disruption of it.
- *Plantaris tendon tear* may mimic Achilles tendon tear in medial sagittal images, but axial cuts can differentiate them especially in fat-saturated proton density fast spin echo sequences.

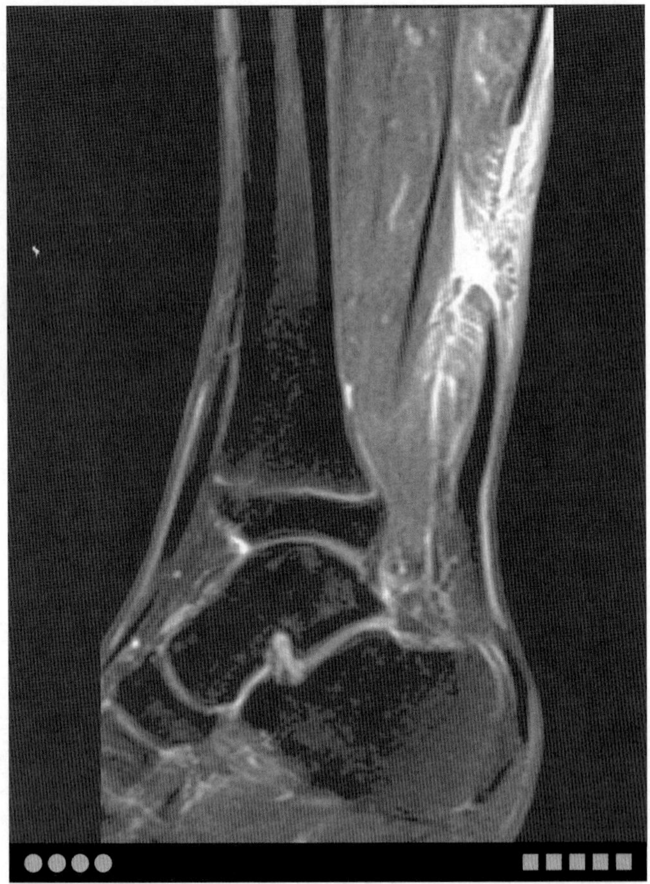

A. Achilles tendon rupture: Sagittal post-contrast T1-weighted image with fat saturation shows discontinuity of Achilles tendon with retraction of proximal fragment. Note the gap between two ends of torn fibers.

COMMENTS

The patient is a 14-year-old boy with difficulty in walking and ankle pain after trauma. Achilles tendon is the only tendon of the foot and ankle whose disorders have male predominance. Ruptures of the Achilles tendon may occur as the result of direct trauma or as the end result following Achilles peritendinosis with or without tendinosis. Patient usually identifies the exact instant, e.g., if someone kicked. It classically occurs with forced dorsiflexion of the planted foot. Abnormal stretching of the degenerated tendon leads to partial or complete macro tears. Classically it occurs 3 to 5 cm proximal to the calcaneal insertion site because this is a relatively hypovascular watershed region.

MRI is more sensitive in detecting incomplete tendon ruptures, chronic degenerative changes and fluid. There is good correlation between MRI and the surgical grading of tendon rupture. In addition, MRI is able to discern peritendinosis, bursitis, tendon thickening, and rupture and can be used to monitor tendon healing. MRI clearly demonstrates partial or full-thickness discontinuity of tendon. Within the gap between the torn fibers, the signal represents a combination of edema and hemorrhage. Edema is seen as a low or intermediate signal intensity area on T1-weighted or proton density sequences and as a hyperintense area on the T2-weighted image. With full-thickness tears, MRI can quantify the degree of tendon retraction.

PEARLS

- **Achilles tendon disorders have male predominance.**
- **Achilles tendon rupture classically occurs with forced dorsiflexion of the planted foot or after trauma.**
- **MRI clearly identifies hyperintense fluid-filled edematous gap in T2-weighted image and disruption of tendon with discontinuity with or with out wavy retracted Achilles tendon in T1 and T2-weighted sequences.**

ADDITIONAL IMAGES

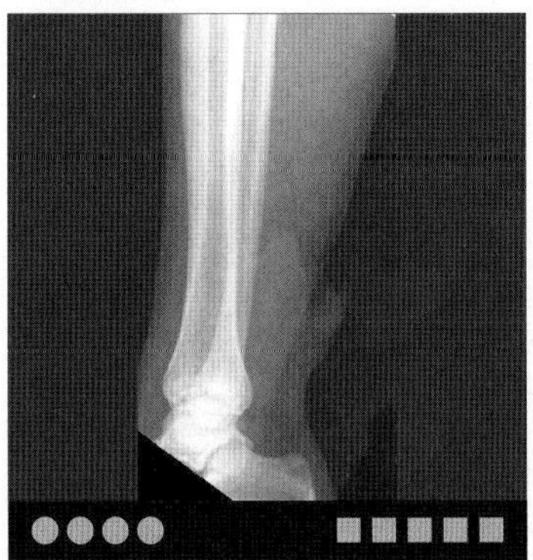

B. Achilles tendon rupture: Lateral radiograph of ankle shows soft tissue swelling and laceration of posterior calf. Note disruption of Achilles tendon.

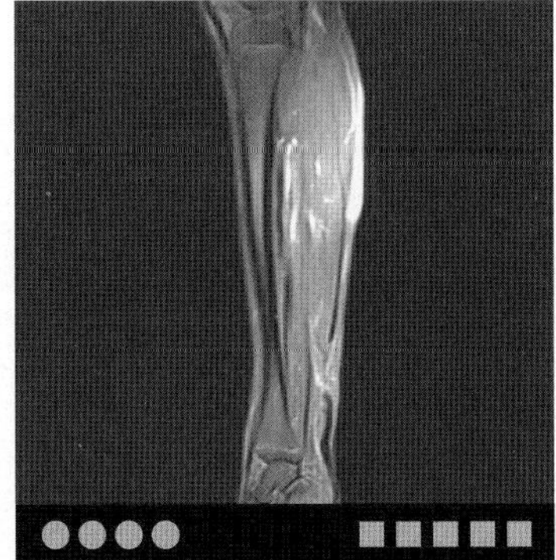

C. Achilles tendon rupture: Sagittal post-contrast T1 fast spin echo image with fat saturation of lower leg shows complete tear of Achilles tendon with retraction. Note high signal in the soft tissue gap between two ends of tendon indicating enhancement at the rupture site.

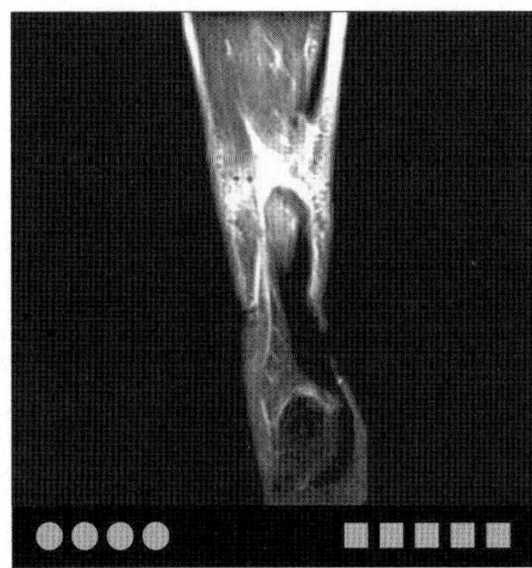

D. Achilles tendon rupture: Coronal T1-weighted fat-saturated post-contrast image shows complete tear of Achilles tendon with hyper intense signal in the gap between torn fibers indicating enhancement at the rupture site.

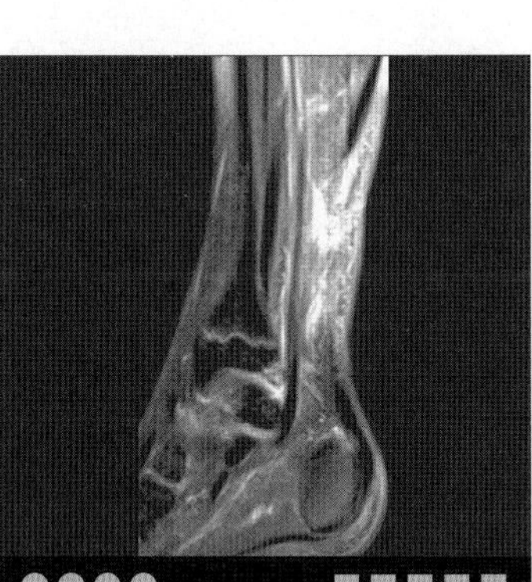

E. Achilles tendon rupture: Sagittal post-contrast T1-weighted image with fat saturation shows complete tear of Achilles tendon with hyperintense signal in the gap between torn fibers indicating enhancement at the rupture site.

IMAGE KEY

Common

Rare

Typical

Unusual

DIFFERENTIAL DIAGNOSES IMAGES

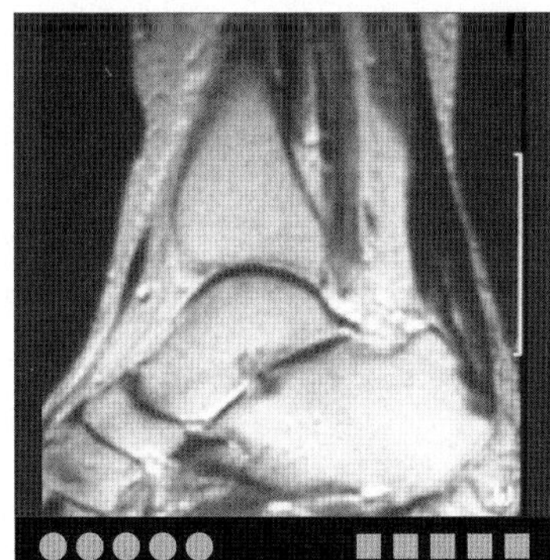

F. Chronic Achilles tendinosis with intrasubstance tear: Sagittal T2-weighted image show thickened Achilles tendon with intrasubstance high signal indicating chronic Achilles tendinosis with partial intrasubstance tear.

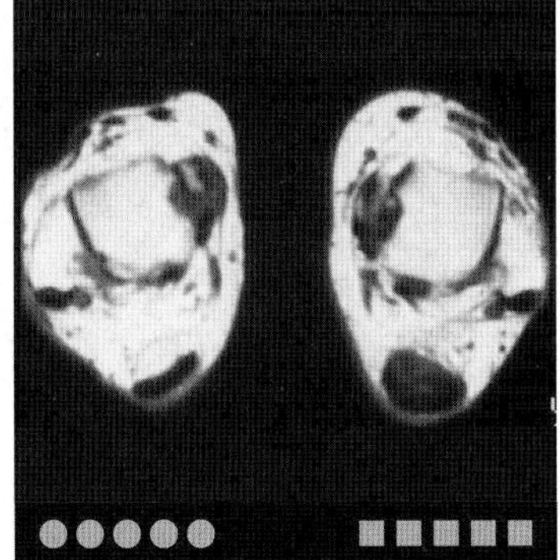

G. Chronic Achilles tendinosis with intrasubstance tear: Axial T2-weighted image show thickened Achilles tendon with intrasubstance high signal indicating chronic Achilles tendinosis with partial intrasubstance tear.

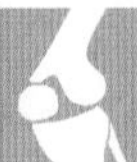

29–15 Partial Tear of Achilles Tendon

Amilcare Gentili

PRESENTATION

Pain after being struck in the Achilles tendon

FINDINGS

MR images show thickened Achilles tendon with areas of abnormal increased signal consistent with a partial tear.

DIFFERENTIAL DIAGNOSES

- *Complete tear of Achilles tendon:* the entire tendon is disrupted, no intact fiber is seen crossing the tear.
- *Chronic tendinosis:* There is thickening of the tendon but the signal is normal on fluid-sensitive sequences.
- *Stress fracture of calcaneus:* Abnormal signal is present in the calcaneus; the Achilles tendon has normal appearance.
- *"Tennis leg":* It is usually a tear of the medial head of the gastrocnemius at the musculotendineous junction, often with an associated hematoma.

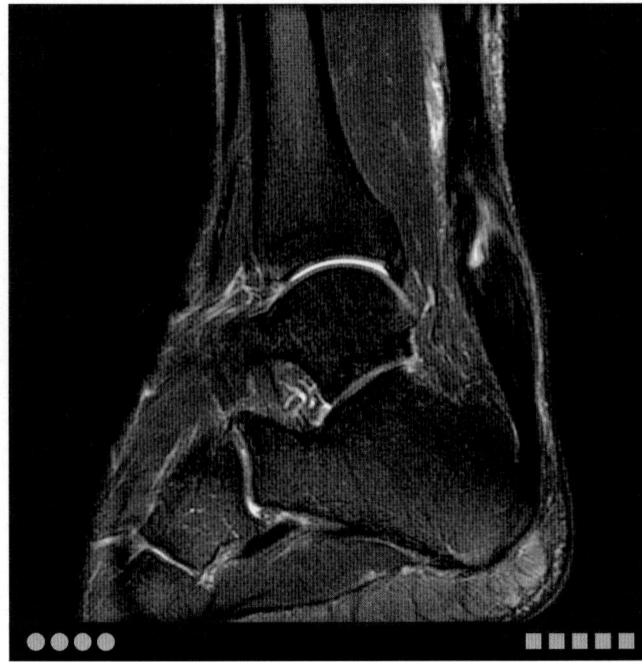

A. Partial tear of Achilles tendon: Sagittal T2-weighted fat-suppressed image shows an area of abnormal increased signal in the Achilles tendon. Note marked thickening of the Achilles tendon.

COMMENTS

The patient is a 34-year-old male, who presented with ankle pain after being struck in the Achilles tendon while playing basketball. The incidence of Achilles tendon rupture appears to be rising over the last half-century and the most likely explanation is the increased number of middle-aged persons participating in recreational sports. The mean age of rupture is approximately 35 years, with the mechanism of injury usually related to sports requiring sudden acceleration or jumping (sprinting, basketball, and tennis). Steroid and fluoroquinolone therapy have been associated with Achilles tendon rupture. The spectrum of Achilles tendon tears ranges from microtears to interstitial, partial, and complete tears. All types of tears show abnormally increased signal intensity on fluid-sensitive sequences. As normal tendons do not tear, most tendons with partial tear are thick as a result of the underlying chronic tendinosis, which predisposes to tear. The most common site of tendon tear is 3 to 4 cm proximal to the calcaneus, but tear can occasionally be seen at the musculotendineous junction and at the insertion on the calcaneus. MRI findings of partial tear include a thick tendon with discontinuity of some of its fibers, but still with some intact fibers. It is important to distinguish partial from complete tear as most partial tears are treated conservatively, while complete tear may require surgical intervention. A complete tear without retraction may be difficult to distinguish from a partial tear, and a normal plantaris tendon can be confused with remaining intact fibers of the Achilles tendon.

PEARLS

- **Partial tear is associated with tendinosis; the Achilles tendon is thicker than normal and has a convex anterior surface.**
- **The area of tear is usually 3 to 4 cm above insertion on the calcaneus.**
- **The tear has high signal intensity on fluid-sensitive sequences.**

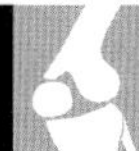

ADDITIONAL IMAGES

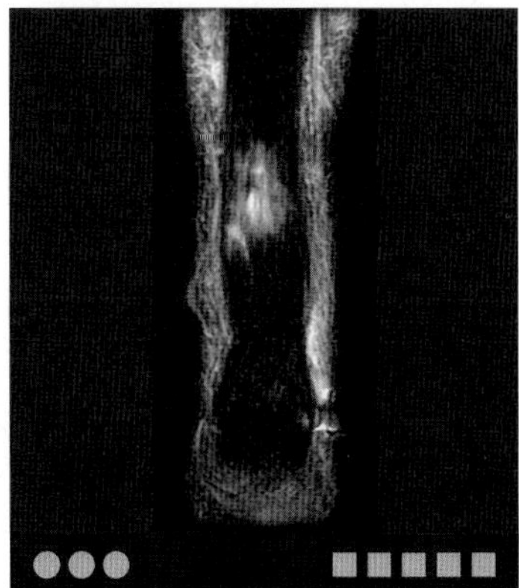

B. Partial tear of Achilles tendon: Coronal T2-weighted fat-suppressed image shows an area of abnormal increased signal in the Achilles tendon. Note intact fiber in the lateral aspect of the Achilles tendon.

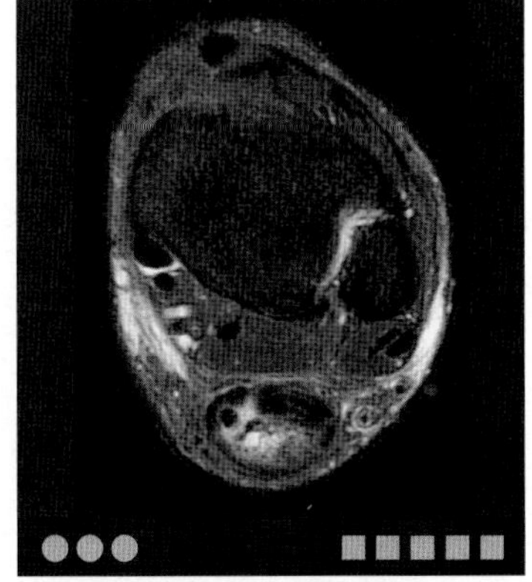

C. Partial tear of Achilles tendon: Axial T2-weighted fat-saturated image shows an enlarged Achilles tendon with intermediate signal intensity.

DIFFERENTIAL DIAGNOSES IMAGES

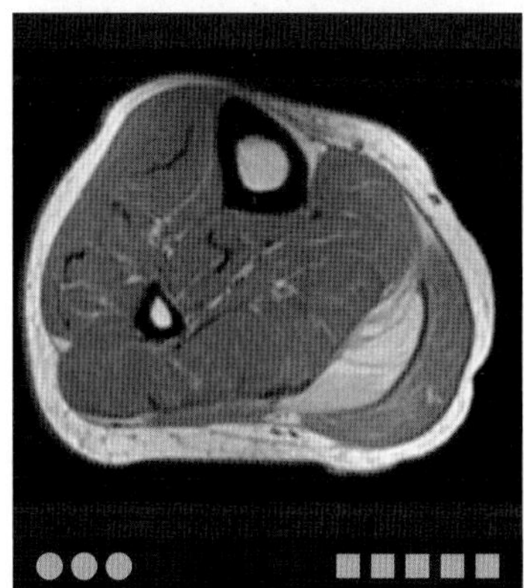

D. Tennis leg: Axial proton density image shows a fluid collection with intermediate signal between the medial head of the gastrocnemius muscle and the soleus.

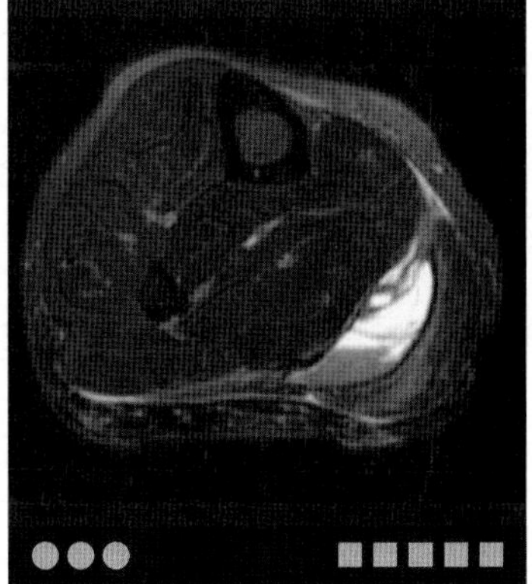

E. Tennis leg: Axial T2 fat-suppressed image shows a fluid collection with high signal between the medial head of the gastrocnemius muscle and the soleus. Note area of low signal with a fluid–fluid level within the fluid collection consistent with sedimentation of blood products in a hematoma.

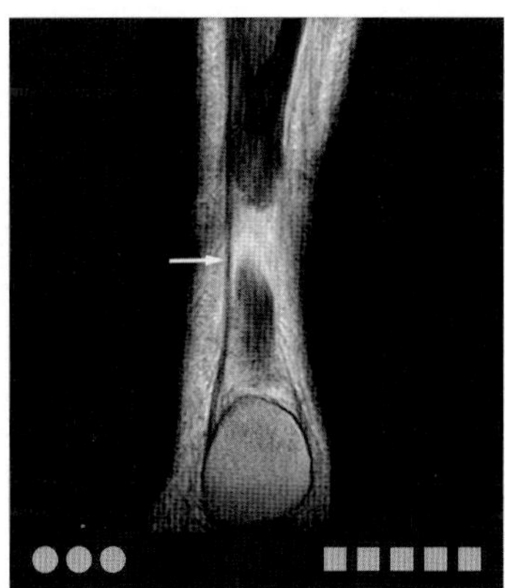

F. Complete tear of Achilles tendon: Coronal T2-weighted spin echo MR image of a complete tear of the Achilles tendon. The plantaris tendon (arrow) should not be confused with the Achilles tendon.

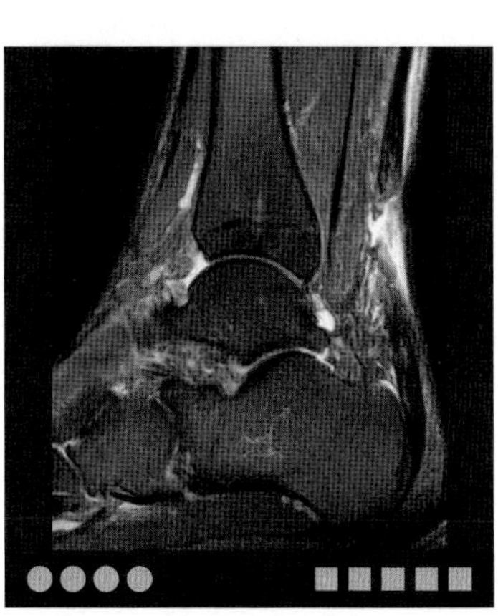

G. Complete tear of Achilles tendon: Sagittal T2-weighted spin echo fat-suppressed MR image shows a complete tear of the Achilles tendon.

IMAGE KEY

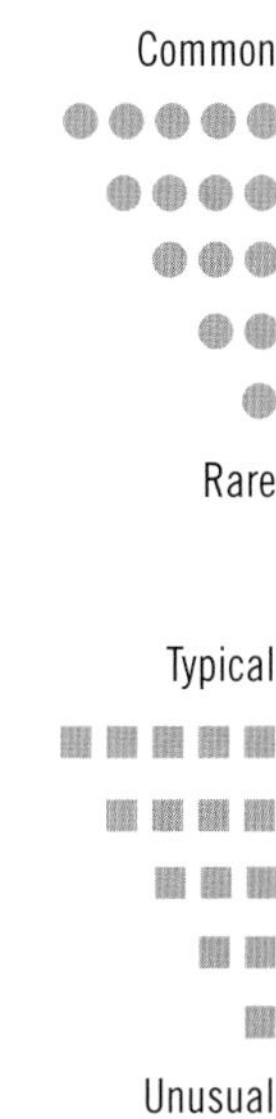

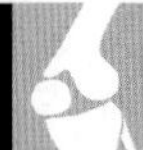

29–16 Achilles Tendinosis

Amilcare Gentili

PRESENTATION

Ankle pain

FINDINGS

MR images show extensive thickening of the Achilles tendon with loss of normal concave anterior margin. The signal intensity is normal on fluid-sensitive sequences.

DIFFERENTIAL DIAGNOSES

- *Complete tear Achilles tendon:* The entire tendon is disrupted; no intact fibers are seen crossing the tear.
- *Partial tear Achilles tendon:* Only a portion of the tendon is disrupted, intact fibers are seen crossing the tear.
- *Stress fracture of calcaneus:* Abnormal signal is present in the calcaneus; the Achilles tendon has normal appearance.
- *Haglund disease:* There is enlargement of the calcaneal tuberosity with fluid in the retrocalcaneal bursa and in the retro Achilles bursa.
- *"Tennis leg":* It is usually a tear of the medial head of the gastrocnemius at the musculotendineous junction, often with an associated hematoma.

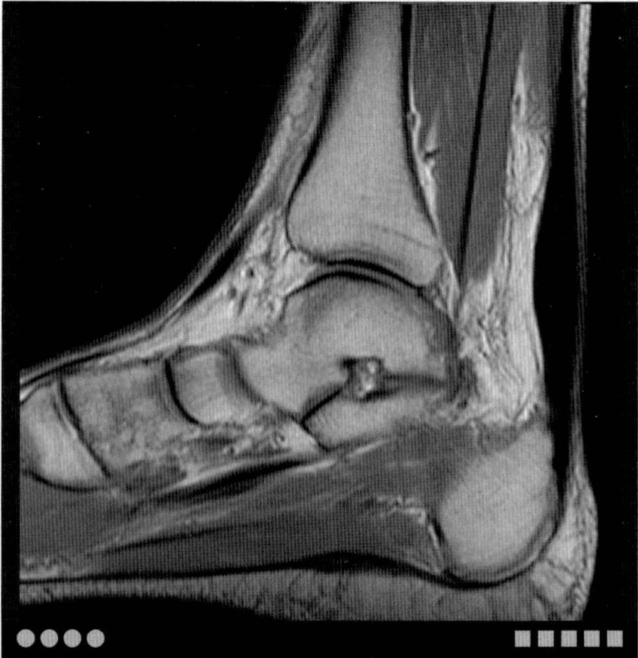

A. Achilles tendinosis: Sagittal T1-weighted image shows fusiform thickening of the Achilles tendon 3 to 6 cm above its insertion on the calcaneus. The tendon and Kager fat pad have normal signal intensity.

COMMENTS

The patient is 56-year-old male, who presented with posterior ankle pain and was diagnosed with Achilles tendon tendinosis. The Achilles tendon is the combined tendon of the gastrocnemius and soleus muscles. The tendon is surrounded by a paratenon, as opposed to a synovial sheath. The paratenon is continuous with the fascia of the gastrocnemius and soleus muscles and the periosteum of the calcaneus. The term Achilles tendinosis is preferred to Achilles tendonitis as there is tendon degeneration without inflammatory changes. The most common type of tendon degeneration is fibromatous degeneration also called "hypoxic degenerative tendinopathy." These hypoxic changes usually occur in the critical zone of the Achilles tendon (2–7 cm from the insertion on the calcaneus) and cause thickening of the tendon without signal alteration on MRI. Patients with this type of degeneration are often symptomatic and present with an enlarged and slightly tender tendon. Chronic tendinosis predisposes to Achilles tendon tear. It is rare to find a torn Achilles tendon without underlying changes of tendinosis. Tendinosis is more common in men than women. It is usually seen in middle-aged men that start exercising or in younger athletes that increase the level of their training. MRI is useful in distinguishing tendinosis from peritendinitis (inflammation of the soft tissues around the Achilles tendon and paratendinitis (inflammation of the paratenon). In paratendinitis and peritendinitis, the size of the Achilles tendon is normal while with tendinosis the Achilles tendon is thickened.

PEARLS

- **Tendinosis causes the Achilles tendon to be thicker and rounder than normal.**
- **The area of abnormality is usually 3 to 7 cm above insertion on the calcaneus.**
- **The signal intensity of the tendon is usually normal on fluid-sensitive sequences.**

ADDITIONAL IMAGES

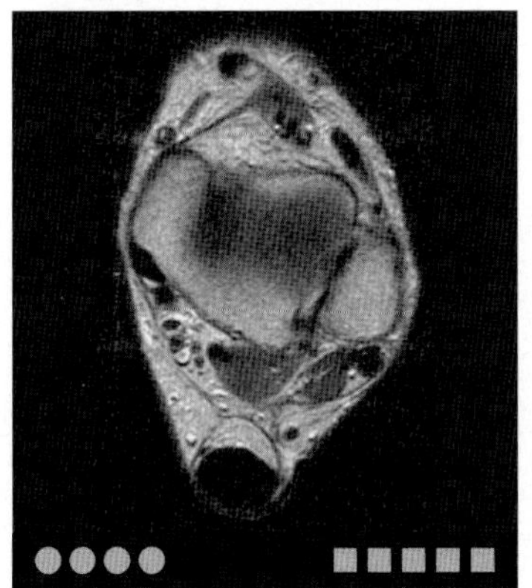

B. Achilles tendinosis: Axial T2-weighted image shows a thickened Achilles tendon with a convex anterior surface and normal signal intensity.

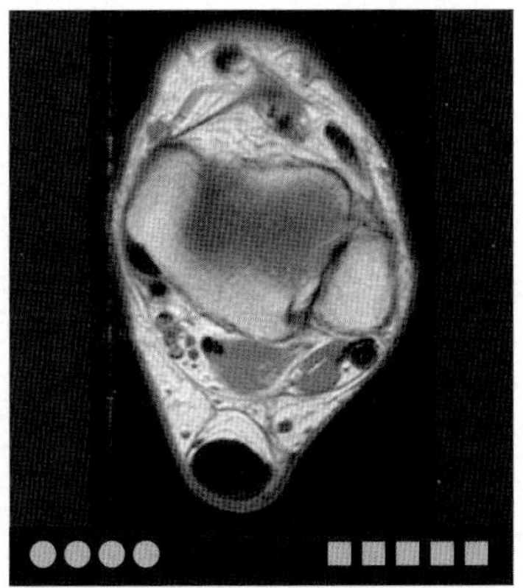

C. Achilles tendinosis: Axial proton density image shows a thickened Achilles tendon with a convex anterior surface.

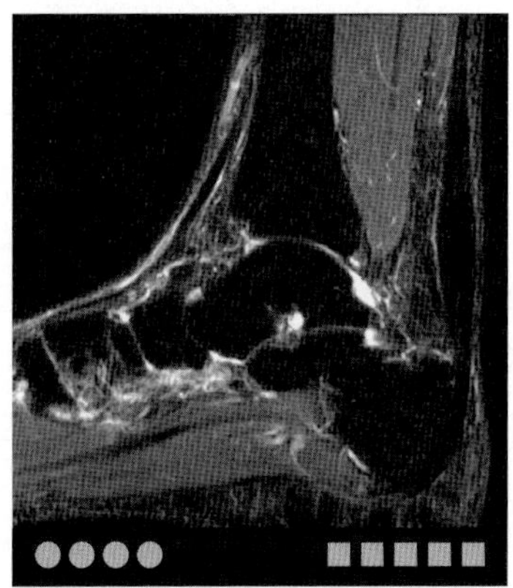

D. Achilles tendinosis: Sagittal STIR image shows fusiform thickening of the Achilles tendon 3 to 6 cm above its insertion on the calcaneus. The tendon and Kager fat pad have normal signal intensity.

IMAGE KEY

Common

Rare

Typical

Unusual

DIFFERENTIAL DIAGNOSES IMAGES

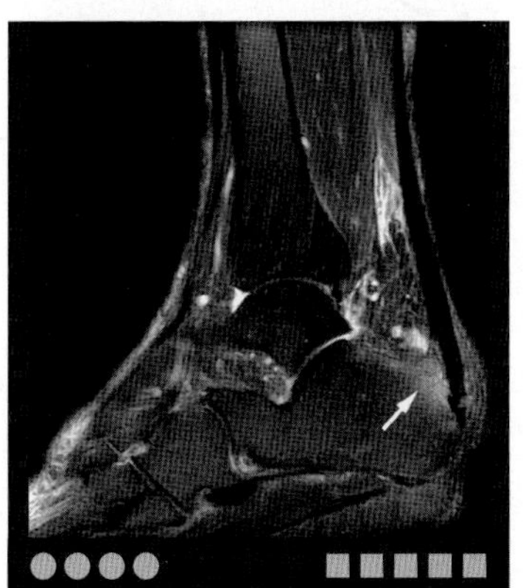

E. Haglund disease: Sagittal STIR image shows prominent posterior–superior aspect of the calcaneus and edema in the posterior aspect of the calcaneus (arrow).

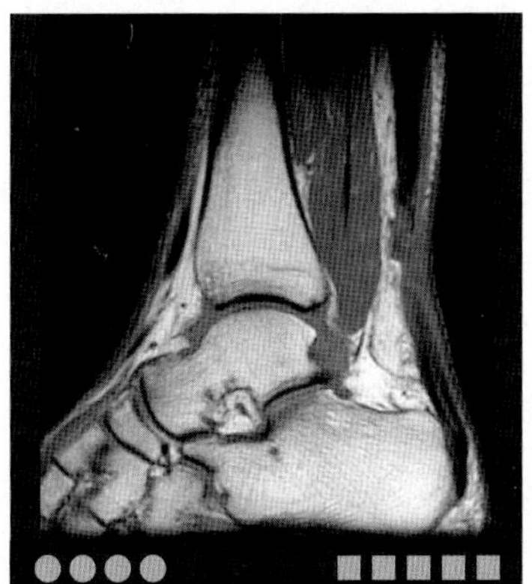

F. Achilles tendon tear: Sagittal T1-weighted spin echo MR image shows intermediate signal intensity replacing the normal low signal of the Achilles tendon.

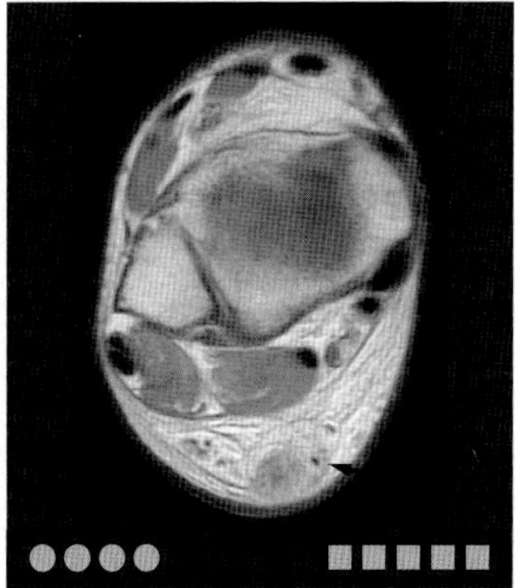

G. Achilles tendon tear: Axial proton density fast spin echo MR image, at the level of the tear, shows absence of normal fibers of the Achilles tendon. The only normal low signal fibers (arrow) represent an intact plantaris tendon.

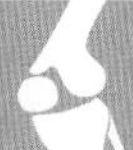

29–17 Haglund Deformity

Ayodale S. Odulate and Piran Aliabadi

PRESENTATION

Posterior heel pain and swelling

FINDINGS

Pre- and post-Achilles bursitis, Achilles insertion tendinosis, and prominent posterior calcaneal tuberosity.

DIFFERENTIAL DIAGNOSES

- *Achilles tendonopathy:* Edema within the tendon sheath or tendon, often superior to Achilles tendon insertion. This may be associated with a tear.
- *Spondyloarthropathy:* Retrocalcaneal bursitis and bone erosions. There may be additional findings such as soft tissue swelling.
- *Calcaneal stress fracture:* Discrete fracture line on MR imaging with preservation of the signal intensity of the Achilles tendon and bursae.

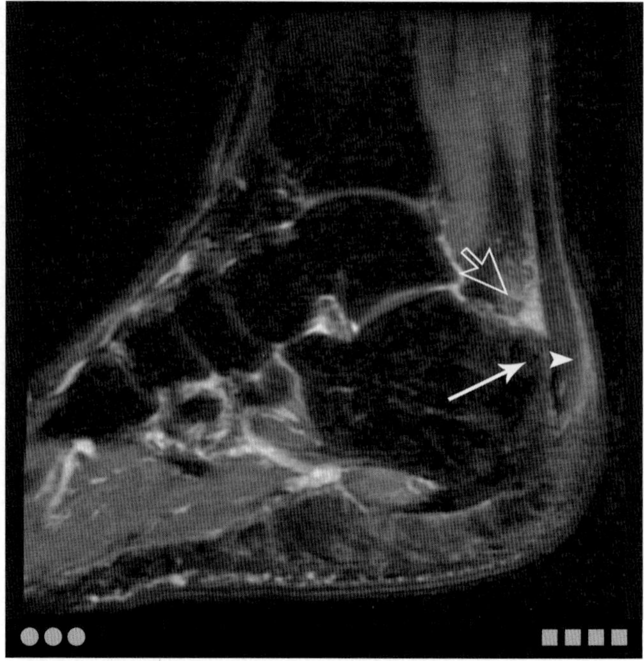

A. Haglund deformity: Sagittal STIR image shows edema in the retrocalcaneal bursa (open arrow), retro-Achilles bursa (arrowhead), and bone edema in the posterior calcaneal tuberosity (arrow).

COMMENTS

The patient is a 58-year-old male with discrete pinpoint tenderness and swelling on the heel. Clinical presentation consists of discretely painful prominent soft tissue swelling at the posterior aspect of the calcaneus near the Achilles tendon insertion. Haglund's deformity is associated with constant rubbing of the posterior aspect of the calcaneus by stiff heel cups of shoes coinciding with a prominent calcaneal tuberosity. This can be seen in any age population with varying patterns of activity, although highly associated with women wearing high-heeled shoes. The treatment is conservative and includes adding heel lifts, wearing open-backed shoes, limiting activity, and heel cord stretching. Nonsteroidal anti-inflammatory medications are often prescribed in conjunction with conservative therapy. Steroids are not routinely prescribed, as there is a slight increased risk of Achilles tendon rupture. Occasionally, surgical excision of the calcaneal tuberosity is indicated. Plain film findings include obliteration of the pre-Achilles fat pad by retrocalcaneal bursitis and prominent posterior calcaneal tuberosity. Prominent focal soft tissue swelling and thickening of the Achilles tendon at the level of the insertion are seen, so called "pump bump." Often a posterior calcaneal spur is present. MRI findings include increased signal intensity of the retrocalcaneal and retro-Achilles bursae on fluid-sensitive sequences. Abnormal fluid signal intensity of the posterior calcaneal tuberosity, tendinosis of the Achilles tendon insertion, and superficial soft tissue edema at the level of the Achilles insertion can also bee seen.

PEARLS

- **Painful thickened soft tissue near Achilles tendon insertion (pump bump).**
- **Triad of retrocalcaneal and retro-Achilles bursitis, thickened Achilles tendon insertion, and prominent posterior calcaneal tuberosity.**
- **No bone erosions; if present suggest spondyloarthropathy, commonly Reiter's syndrome or rheumatoid arthropathy.**

ADDITIONAL IMAGES

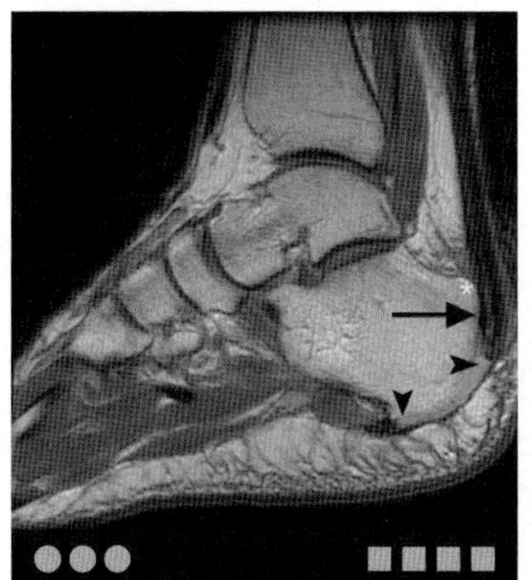

B. Haglund deformity: Sagittal proton density image of the foot reveals the prominent retrocalcaneal tuberosity (asterisk), plantar and calcaneal spurs (arrowheads), and abnormal convexity of the Achilles tendon insertion (arrow).

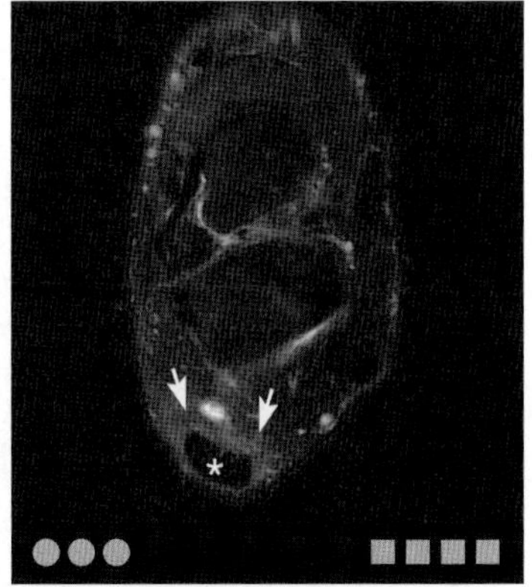

C. Haglund deformity: Axial STIR image shows abnormal convexity (asterisk) of the Achilles tendon with surrounding edema in the pre-Achilles fat pad (arrows).

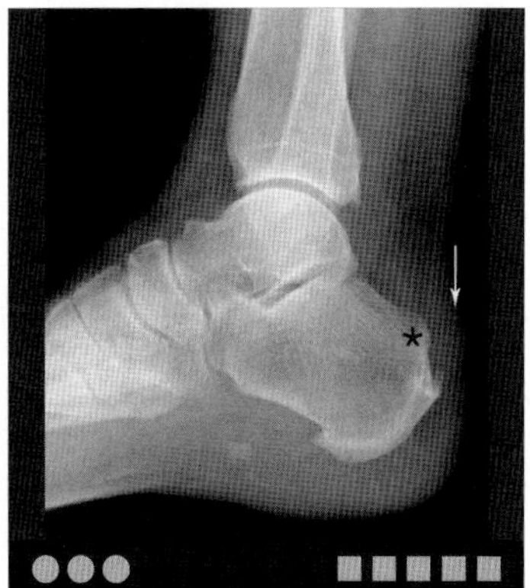

D. Haglund deformity: Lateral plain film of the foot shows enthesopathy of Achilles tendon insertion, prominent posterior calcaneal tuberosity (asterisk), and abnormal convexity of posterior soft tissues (arrow).

IMAGE KEY

Common

Rare

Typical

Unusual

DIFFERENTIAL DIAGNOSES IMAGES

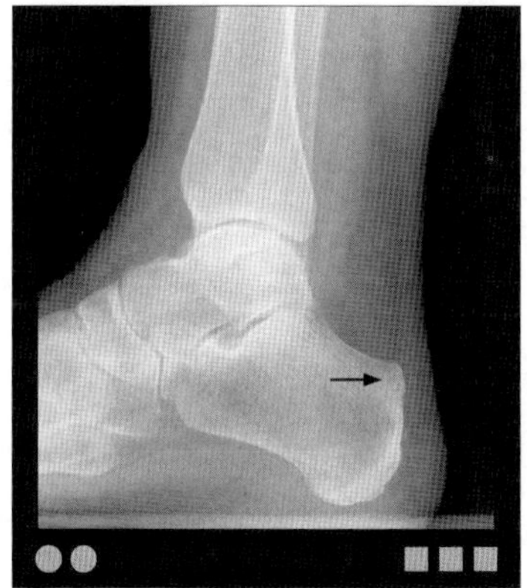

E. Spondyloarthropathy: Unlike Haglund deformity, cortical erosions of the posterior calcaneus (arrow) are often seen with inflammatory spondyloarthropathy such as in this plain film.

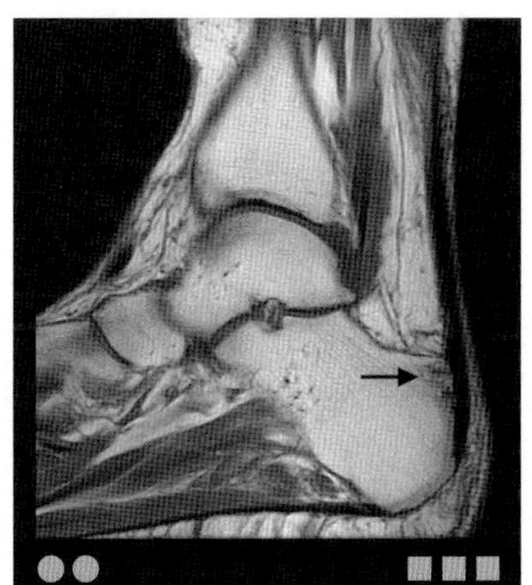

F. Spondyloarthropathy: Sagittal T1-weighted image from the same patient demonstrates abnormal hypointensity (arrow) of the calcaneus from erosions.

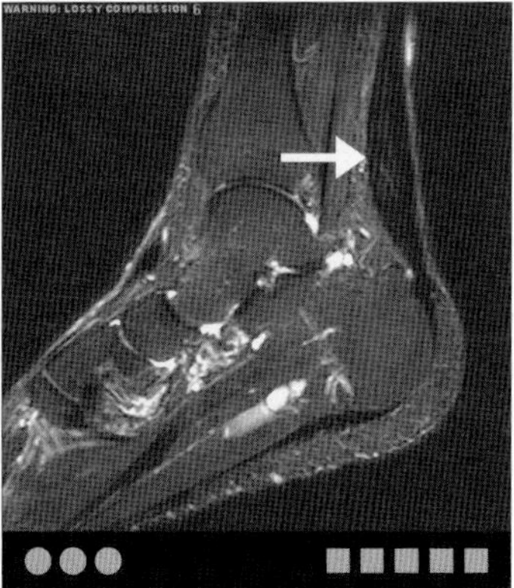

G. Achilles tendinosis & intrasubstance tear: Sagittal STIR image demonstrates an abnormal thickened Achilles tendon above the level of the tendon insertion. Linear increased signal intensity within the Achilles tendon represents an intrasubstance tear.

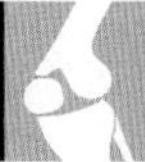

29–18 Sonographic Appearance of Tendinosis of the Achilles Tendon

Mélanie Morel, Nathalie Boutry, and Anne Cotten

PRESENTATION

Chronic pain in Achilles tendon

FINDINGS

Sonography shows fusiform hypoechoic enlargement of the Achilles tendon.

DIFFERENTIAL DIAGNOSES

- *Complete rupture of the Achilles tendon:* Sonogram shows a complete disruption of the tendon fibers with a retracted upper fragment and echogenic debris in-between. Fat herniation in the gap and posterior acoustic shadowing at the frayed tendon ends are also in favor of a full-thickness tear. By contrast, the plantaris tendon is better seen and should not be mistaken for intact Achilles tendon fibers. On T2-weighted images, high signal through the entire anteroposterior dimension of the mid-Achilles tendon can be seen.
- *Peritendinitis:* May be associated with tendinosis of the Achilles tendon. It is defined by thickening of the paratenon on axial images, and increased signal intensity of the paratenon and Kager fat pad on STIR images.
- *Xanthoma of the Achilles tendon:* Often bilateral, Achilles tendon is thickened and hypoechoic on sonogram. It contains intermediate to high signal intensity striations on T1- and T2-weighted sagittal images. Axial sequences reveal a stippled pattern of high and low signal intensities.

COMMENTS

The patient is a 44-year-old woman suffering from chronic posterior ankle pain, diagnosed as chronic tendinosis of Achilles tendon. Achilles tendon is a commonly injured tendon. Sonogram examination diagnoses tendinosis when the anteroposterior diameter of the tendon is increased, with a fusiform or nodular shape of the tendon and convex anterior margin. Homogeneous hypoechogenicity or focal intratendinous hypoechoic zones can be demonstrated. Neovascularization in the ventral side of the tendon may be seen with power Doppler. In addition to the above, other differentials include Achilles tendon inflammatory enthesopathy in rheumatoid arthritis and spondylarthropathies. In this condition, sonography shows thickening of the Achilles tendon at its calcaneal attachment, with focal hypoechoic areas. Intratendinous calcifications, calcaneal enthesophytes, and retrocalcaneal bursitis can be observed. Hyperemia with Doppler sonography is typically located at the bone–enthesis junction. MRI is also of great value. Accessory soleus muscle can be included as a differential. This is located medial to the Achilles tendon, adjacent to the posterior tibial nerve. Its tendon inserts either into the Achilles tendon or to the top of posterior calcaneus. Haglund syndrome is an impingement syndrome between an abnormal prominence of the posterior superior border of the calcaneus and the shoe. It leads to tendinosis of the Achilles tendon and retrocalcaneal bursitis. Achilles tendon thickening and anterior intratendinous hypoechoic areas are found just above its calcaneal insertion. On T2-weighted images, high-signal-intensity foci are seen in the distal Achilles tendon, the retrocalcaneal and retro-Achilles bursae, and the calcaneal tuberosity.

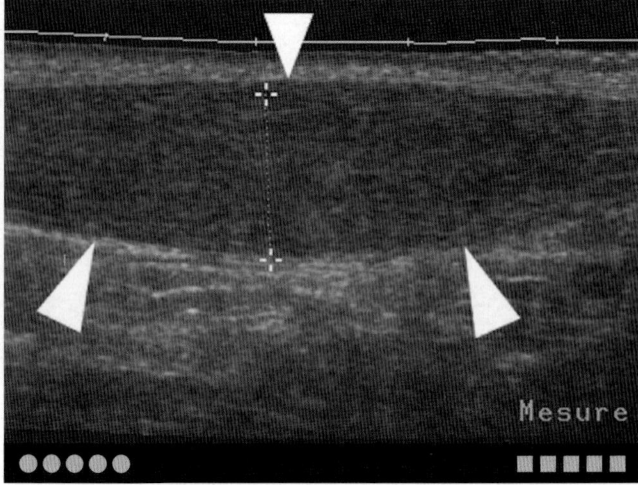

A. Tendinosis of the Achilles tendon: Sagittal sonogram reveals fusiform thickening of the Achilles tendon (arrowheads).

PEARLS

- **Achilles tendon is the most common site of tendinosis at the ankle.**
- **Sonographic pattern of tendinosis is an enlarged tendon with fusiform or nodular shape and homogeneous or focal low echogenicity.**
- **Sonogram represents an easy, cheap, and valuable method for the diagnosis of this lesion.**

ADDITIONAL IMAGES

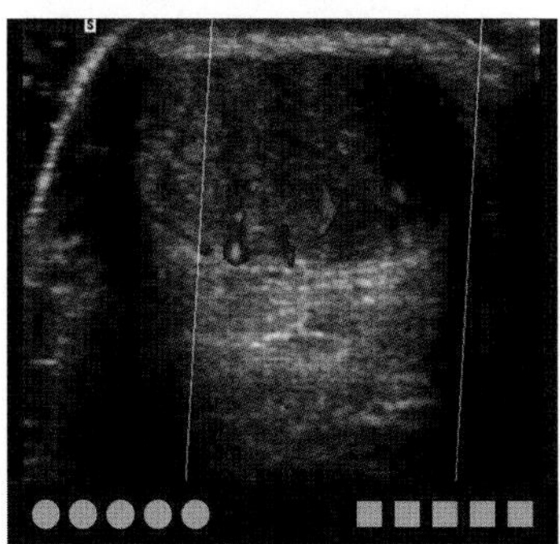

B. Tendinosis of the Achilles tendon: Axial Doppler sonography demonstrates intratendinous hyperemia at the ventral aspect of the enlarged Achilles tendon.

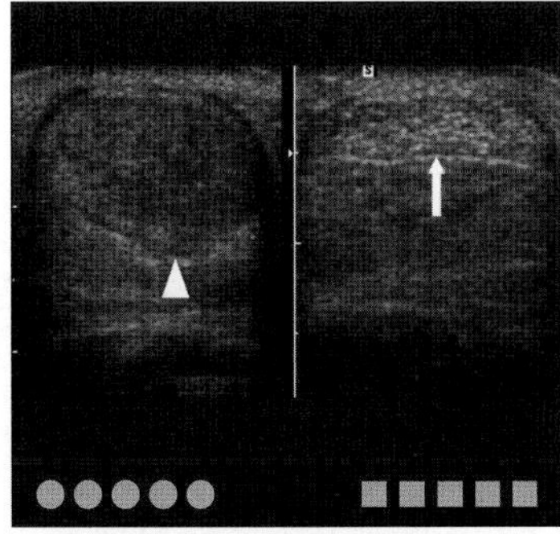

C. Tendinosis of the Achilles tendon: Axial comparative study of the Achilles tendon exhibits hypoechoic swelling (arrowhead) of the ventral side of the painful Achilles tendon (on the left), contrasting with the concave anterior margin of the normal contralateral tendon (arrow).

DIFFERENTIAL DIAGNOSES IMAGES

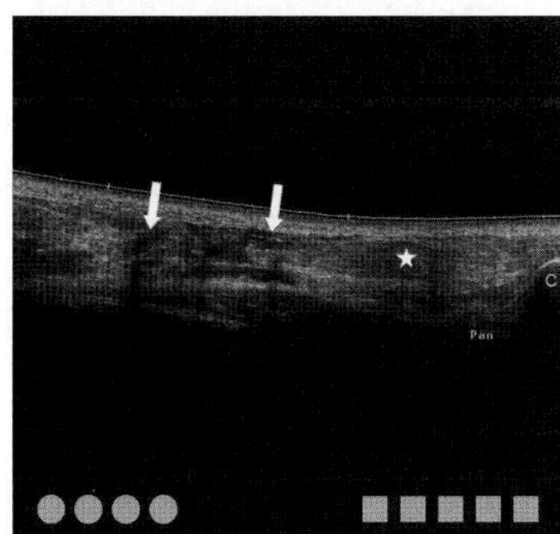

D. Complete rupture of the Achilles tendon and tendinosis: Sagittal sonography shows a complete disruption of the tendon fibers (arrows) with posterior acoustic shadows. Thickened tendon with hypoechoic areas indicate associated tendinosis of the distal Achilles tendon (star).

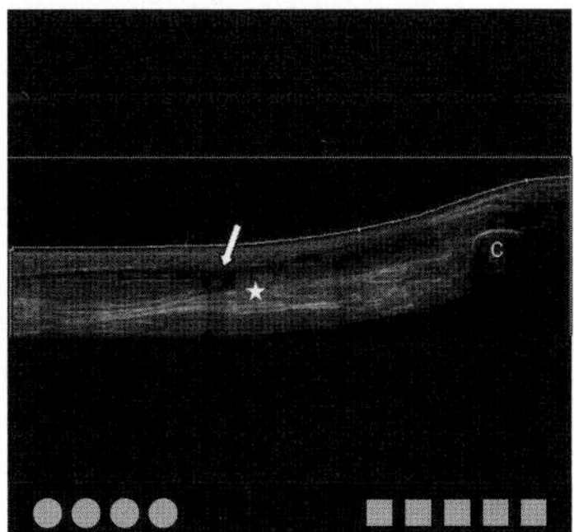

E. Complete rupture of the Achilles tendon: Sagittal sonography demonstrates the anechoic gap (arrow) between the ends of the tendon and fat herniation (star) in the rupture (C: calcaneus).

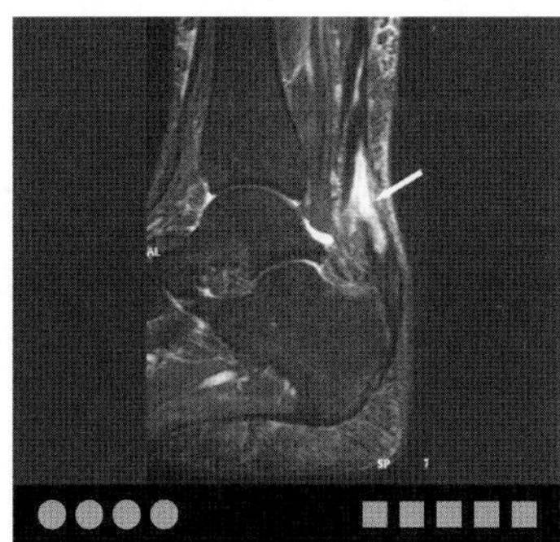

F. Complete rupture of the Achilles tendon: Sagittal T2-weighted image exhibits the complete discontinuity of the Achilles tendon (arrow) filled with a high signal intensity zone.

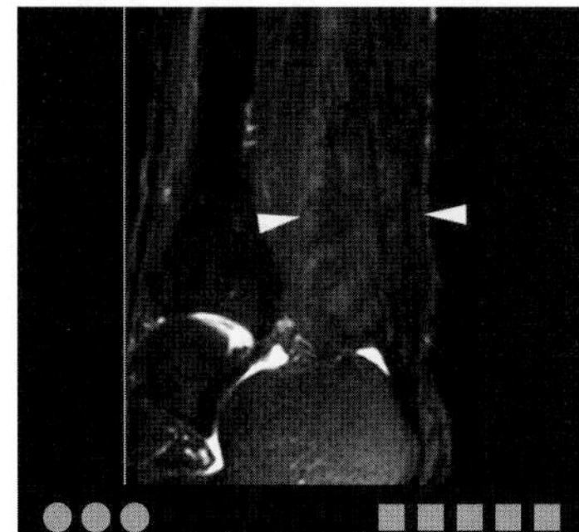

G. Xanthoma of the Achilles tendon: Sagittal T2-weighted image shows a thickened Achilles tendon (arrowheads) with intermediate signal intensity areas infiltration. No fiber discontinuity is found.

IMAGE KEY

Common

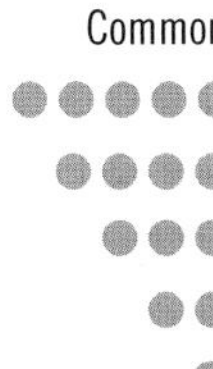

Rare

Typical

Unusual

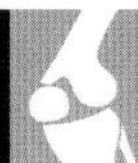

29–19 Tarsal Tunnel Ganglion

Ayodale S. Odulate and Piran Aliabadi

PRESENTATION

Medial hind foot swelling and palpable painful lump.

FINDINGS

Hyperintense nodule along the flexor digitorum longus tendon within the tarsal tunnel.

DIFFERENTIAL DIAGNOSIS

- *Plantar fasciitis:* Medial pinpoint pain along the sole of the foot.
- *Calcaneal fracture:* Linear stress fracture can cause hind foot swelling.
- *Inflammatory arthritides:* Swelling of the hind foot can be caused by inflammatory erosions of the calcaneus.
- *Nerve sheath tumor:* Heterogeneous hyperintense signal intensity on T2-weighted images with heterogeneous enhancement.

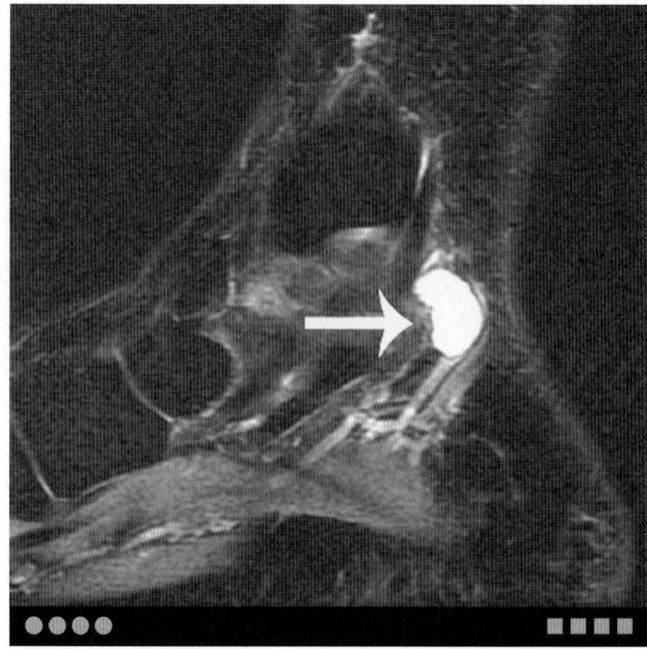

A. Tarsal tunnel ganglion: Sagittal STIR image shows a lobulated hyperintense homogeneous nodule (arrow) in the tarsal tunnel.

COMMENT

The patient is a 38-year-old male with medial hind foot swelling and radiating pain. Tarsal tunnel syndrome is caused by compression of the posterior tibial nerve by a space-occupying lesion along its course through the tarsal tunnel. Patients classically present with burning hind foot pain and paresthesia that may radiate distally that are worse with weight bearing. Ganglia are benign cystic nodules that develop along tendon sheaths and around joints. The ganglia are pathologic when they develop in sensitive areas and compress local structures. The first line of treatment is conservative. If the symptoms do not resolve, steroid injections can be tried followed by surgical decompression. Investigating the cause of tarsal tunnel syndrome can be made by various imaging modalities such as ultrasound, computed tomography, and magnetic resonance (MR). Radiograph can exclude bony etiologies such as an exostosis, pes planus, osteophytes, or coalition. MR imaging characteristics of ganglia in the foot are the same as ganglia in any other part of the body; discrete homogeneous hyperintense nodule on T2-weighted images associated with a tendon sheath does not enhance after intravenous gadolinium injection. Peripheral nerve sheath tumors will have a slightly inhomogeneous iso- to hyperintense signal compared to muscle on T1-weighted images, proton density images, and hyperintense signal intensity on T2-weighted images. A majority of nerve sheath tumors will enhance heterogeneously after administration of gadolinium. Other entities that might be diagnosed by MR include varicose veins, accessory or hypertrophied muscles, lipoma, or inflammatory masses such as a pannus associated with rheumatoid arthritis.

PEARLS

- **Ganglions are benign cystic lesions that may cause pressure on the posterior tibial nerve and cause tarsal tunnel syndrome.**
- **The cause of tarsal tunnel syndrome is often benign.**

ADDITIONAL IMAGES

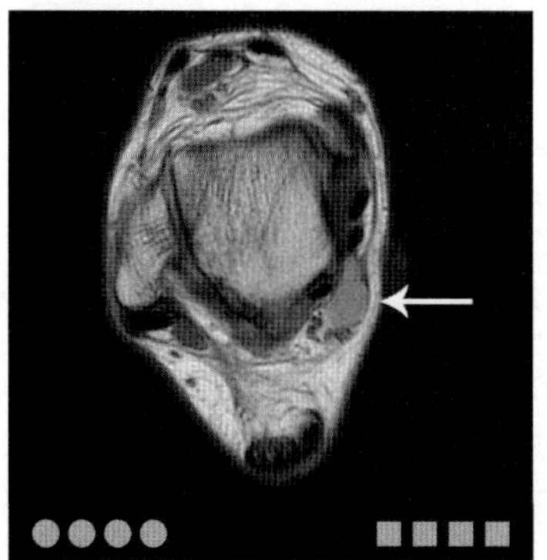

B. Tarsal tunnel ganglion: Axial proton density image again shows the ganglion (arrow) posterior to the flexor digitorum longus tendon. Note the smooth thin border and homogenous signal intensity.

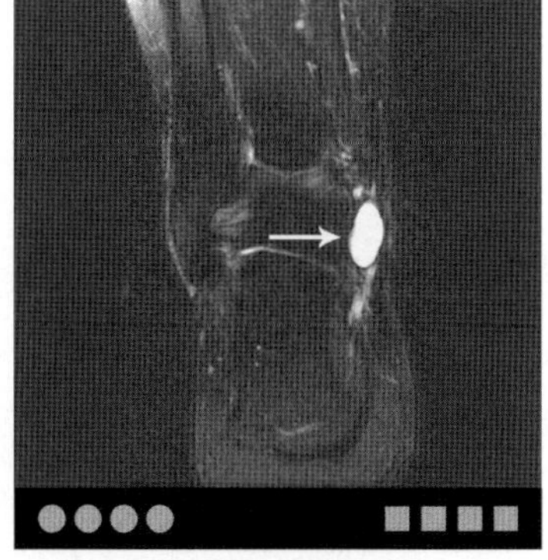

C. Tarsal tunnel ganglion: Coronal fat-saturated T2-weighted image shows the ganglion (arrow).

DIFFERENTIAL DIAGNOSES IMAGES

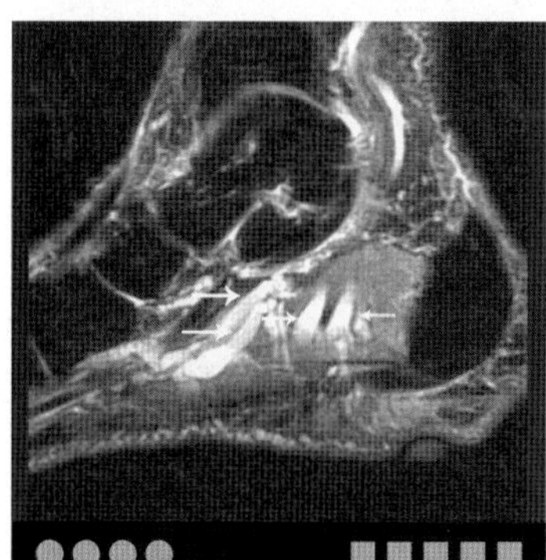

D. Varicose vein: Sagittal STIR image demonstrates numerous vessels (arrows) in the tarsal tunnel. This space-occupying lesion can cause compression on the posterior tibial nerve, thus causing tarsal tunnel syndrome.

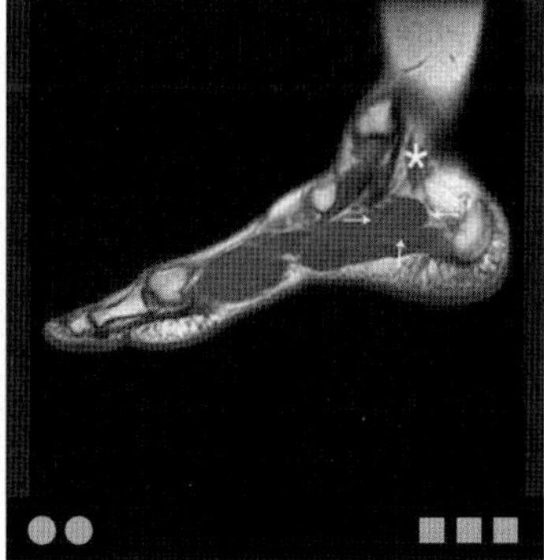

E. Schwannoma: Sagittal T1-weighted image at the level of the tarsal tunnel (asterisk) shows a homogeneous round lesion (arrows) isointense to muscle.

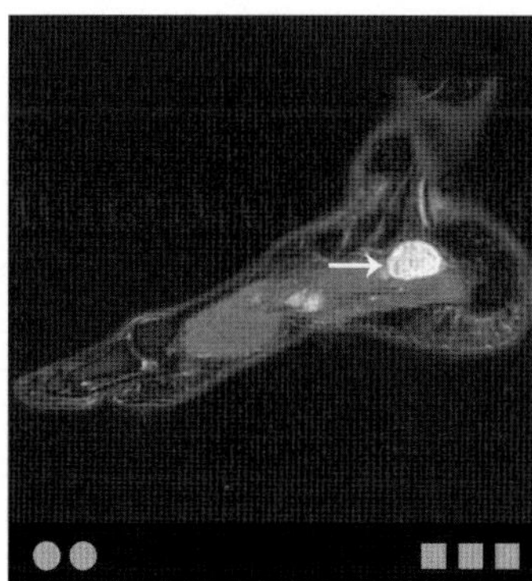

F. Schwannoma: Sagittal STIR image shows a lesion with heterogeneous hyperintense signal intensity (arrow) in the tarsal tunnel.

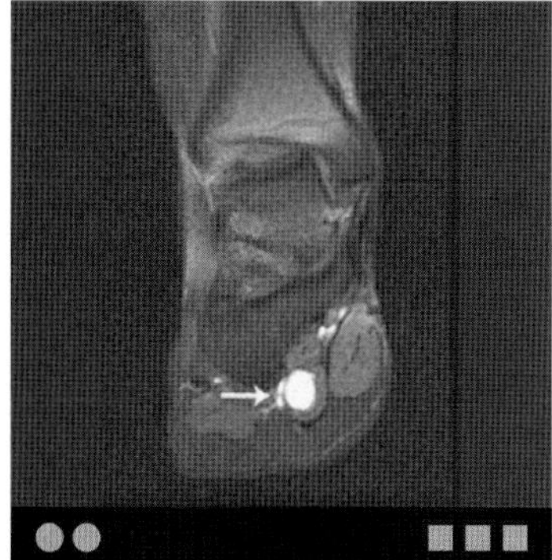

G. Schwannoma: Coronal fat-saturated T1-weighted image shows a different enhancing hyperintense intramuscular nodule (arrow) in this patient with multiple schwannomata.

IMAGE KEY

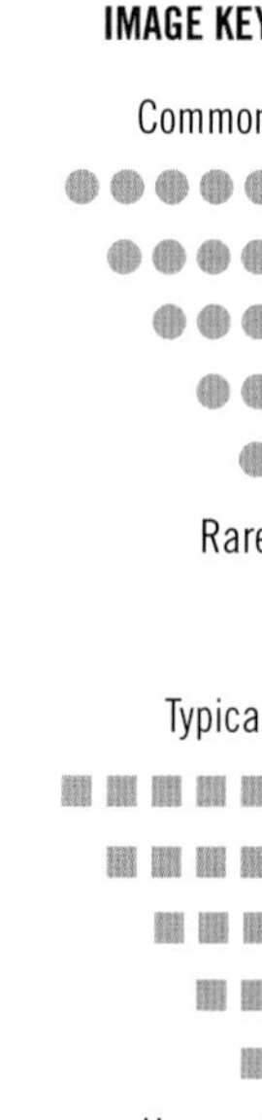

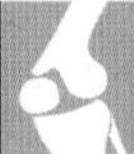

29–20 Sinus Tarsi Syndrome

Ashkan Afshin and Joshua Farber

PRESENTATION

Ankle pain

FINDINGS

Edema is seen in sinus tarsi area of subtalar joint with fat obliteration at this area.

DIFFERENTIAL DIAGNOSES

- *Tarsal tunnel ganglion cyst:* MR images show a cystic hyperintense mass in the region of tarsal tunnel.
- *Varicose veins in medial soft tissue of the ankle:* Varicosities in the soft tissue of medial ankle create increased signal in fluid-sensitive sequences. These varicose veins in tarsal tunnel may cause tarsal tunnel syndrome.

COMMENTS

The patient is a 55-year-old female with ankle pain. She is suffering from sinus tarsi syndrome secondary to mid-subtalar coalition and in addition she has chronic Achilles tendinosis. The sinus tarsi is a cone-shaped anatomical space which is bounded by the calcaneus and talus anteriorly and posterior facet of the subtalar joint posteriorly and continuous with the tarsal canal medially. This space contains interosseous talocalcaneal ligament, cervical ligament, medial, inferior, and lateral roots of the inferior extensor retinaculum and artery of the tarsal canal. Sinus tarsi syndrome results from ankle sprain in 70% of the cases. It can be associated with the lateral collateral ligament and tibialis posterior tendon injuries. Patients with sinus tarsi syndrome usually complain of localized pain on the lateral part of the foot, which is aggravated by weight-bearing activity and alleviated with rest. They may also experience the feeling of instability of the hindfoot especially while walking on uneven surfaces. Physical examination of these patients reveals tenderness on the sinus tarsi with aggravation of the pain on foot inversion or eversion. MRI is probably the best diagnostic test to show changes in the tissues of the sinus tarsi. MR images show obliteration of fat in the sinus tarsi space. The space itself may be replaced by either fluid or scar tissue, and the disruption of the ligaments may be observed. Ankle arthroscopy may also be beneficial to directly evaluate the sinus for damaged tissue.

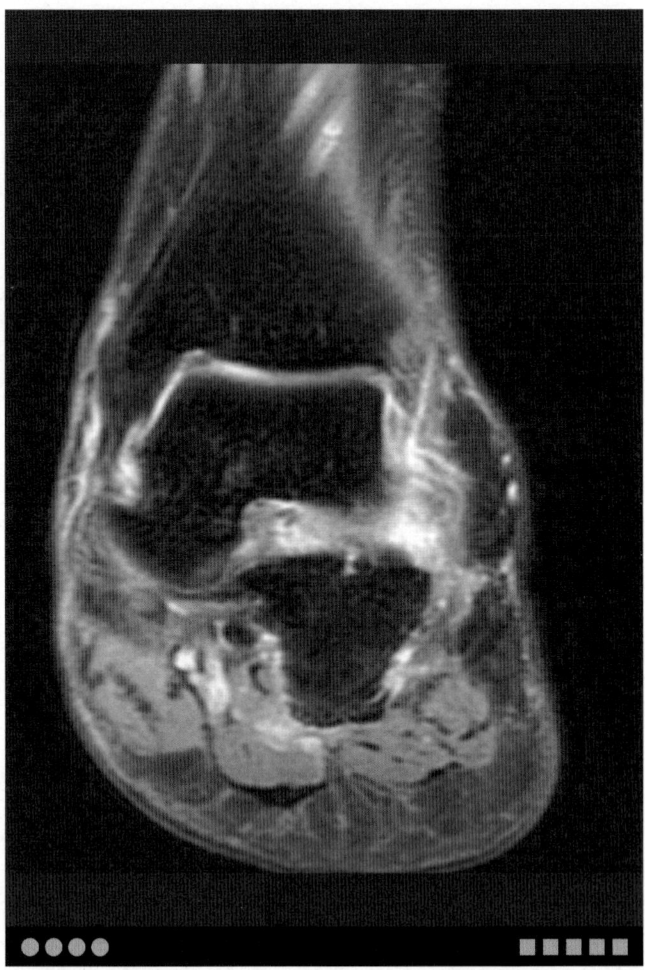

A. Sinus tarsi syndrome: Coronal fat-saturated proton density image shows fat obliteration and increased signal in the subtalar joint at the region of sinus tarsi.

PEARLS

- **Painful condition usually caused by ankle sprain**
- **Association with lateral collateral ligament and tibialis posterior tendon injuries**
- **Localized pain on the lateral part of the foot and tenderness on the sinus tarsi**
- **Obliteration of fat and presence of edema in the sinus tarsi space on MR images**

ADDITIONAL IMAGES

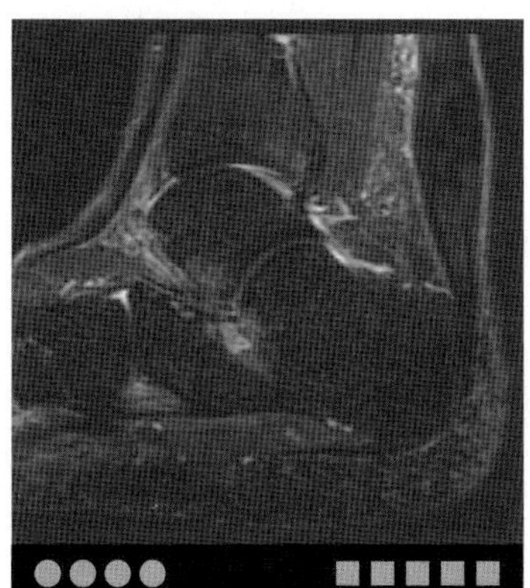

B. Sinus tarsi syndrome: Sagittal fat-saturated T2-weighted image shows increased signal in the subtalar joint and some bone marrow edema in adjacent subchondral bones of talus and calcaneus. Note thickening of Achilles tendon related to chronic tendinosis.

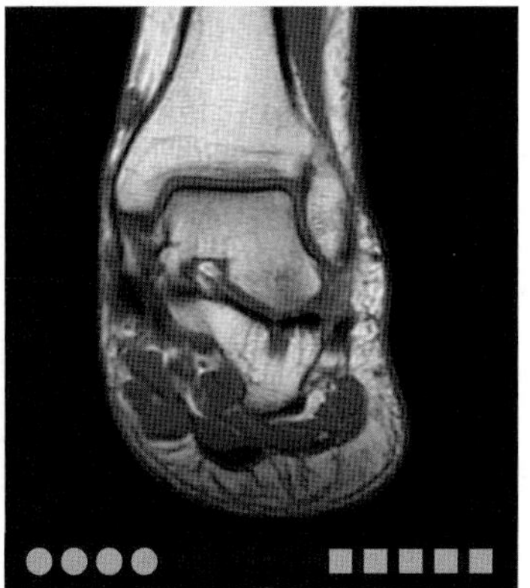

C. Sinus tarsi syndrome: Coronal T1-weighted image shows obliteration of the sustentaculum tali joint indicating mid-subtalar coalition.

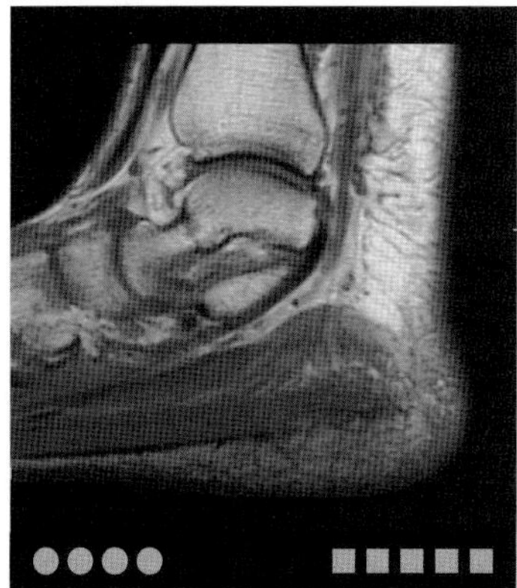

D. Sinus tarsi syndrome: Sagittal T1-weighted image in the medial aspect of the ankle joint shows obliteration of the sustentaculum tali joint and low signal representing edema in sinus tarsi in the region of mid-subtalar joint.

IMAGE KEY

Common

Rare

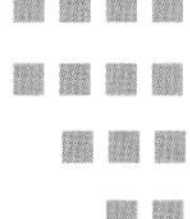

Typical

Unusual

DIFFERENTIAL DIAGNOSES IMAGES

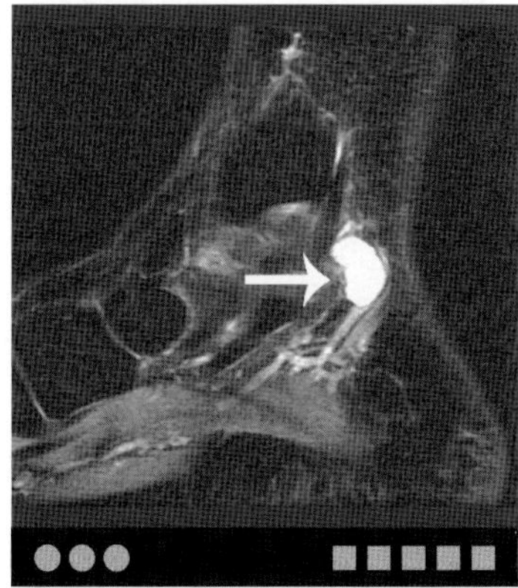

E. Tarsal tunnel ganglion: Sagittal STIR image shows a lobulated hyperintense homogeneous nodule (arrow) in the tarsal tunnel.

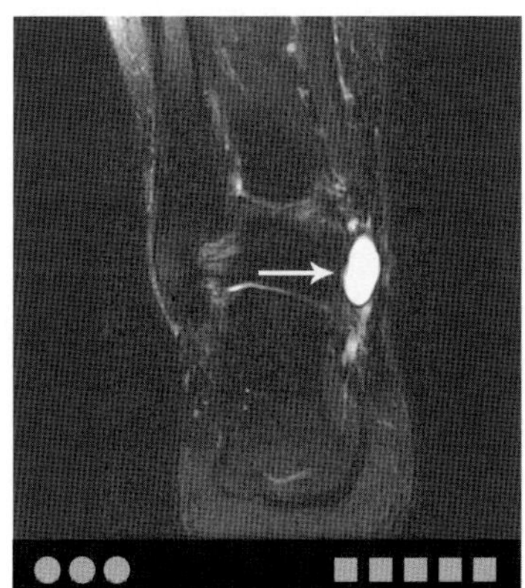

F. Tarsal tunnel ganglion: Coronal fat-saturated T2-weighted image shows the ganglion (arrow).

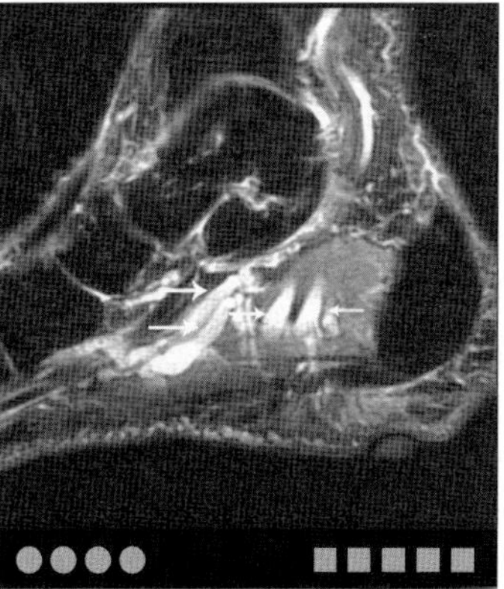

G. Varicose vein: Sagittal STIR image demonstrates numerous vessels (arrows) in the tarsal tunnel. This space-occupying lesion can cause compression on the posterior tibial nerve, thus causing tarsal tunnel syndrome.

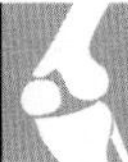

29–21 Sonographic Appearance of Ganglion Cyst in the Tarsal Tunnel

Mélanie Morel, Nathalie Boutry, and Anne Cotten

PRESENTATION

Burning and paresthesias of the foot

FINDINGS

Sonography and MRI show a cystic lobulated mass adjacent to the posterior tibial nerve in the tarsal tunnel.

DIFFERENTIAL DIAGNOSES

- *Nerve sheath tumor:* Sonography shows a fusiform hypoechoic soft-tissue mass in continuity with the posterior tibial nerve or its branches. T2-weighted image exhibits a hyperintense lesion in the space occupied by the posterior tibial nerve. T1-weighted post-contrast image demonstrates enhancement of the mass.
- *Hemangioma:* The mass may be well- or ill-defined. Doppler study identifies feeding and draining vessels. Phleboliths may be identified within the lesions. T2-weighted image shows hyperintense tortuous vessels in the tarsal tunnel.
- *Tenosynovitis of a flexor tendon:* Sonography shows a thickened tendon sheath with an anechoic collection of synovial fluid. Hyperemia of the sheath can be encountered with power Doppler. T2-weighted image reveals high signal around the tendon.
- *Varicosities:* Sonography reveals anechoic masses obliterating under probe compression. Doppler study demonstrates their venous nature.
- Other causes of tarsal tunnel syndrome include bone deformity after calcaneal fracture, synovial hypertrophy (pannus, giant cell sheath tumor, etc.), and hypertrophied abductor hallucis muscle: MRI enables to determine whether the treatment is conservative or surgical.

COMMENTS

The patient is a 36-year-old man complaining of burning and paresthesias along the sole of the foot and to the toes, diagnosed as tarsal tunnel syndrome caused by a ganglion cyst. Tarsal tunnel syndrome occurs when posterior tibial nerve or its branches are compressed in the tarsal tunnel. Posterior tibial nerve lies between the posterior tibial muscle in the proximal region of the leg and then passes to lie between the flexor digitorum longus and flexor hallucis longus muscle in the distal region of the leg. The main divisions of posterior tibial nerve are calcaneal, medial plantar, and lateral plantar nerves. Tarsal tunnel extends craniocaudally from the medial malleolus to the navicular. It is limited laterally by talus and calcaneus, and medially by flexor retinaculum and abductor hallucis muscle. Ganglion cyst is a fibrous walled mass containing clear mucinous fluid. It may communicate with an adjacent articular cavity. In case of soft-tissue ganglion cyst, sonography shows an anechoic or hypoechoic uni or multilobulated lesion without any visible wall, but with posterior intensification. CT imaging reveals a mass of fluid density (0–20 UH). On MR imaging, the signal-intensity of the mass is low on T1- and high on T2-weighted images. The cyst wall is depicted as a thin low-signal-intensity border which may enhance after intravenous contrast injection. Communication with an adjacent joint can sometimes be seen.

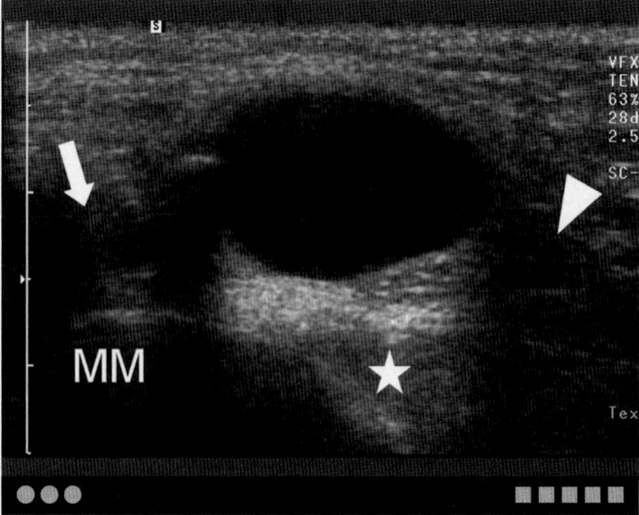

A. Ganglion cyst: Axial sonogram of the medial side of the ankle shows a cystic anechoic fluid collection next to the posterior tibial nerve (arrowhead) (MM: medial malleolus; arrow: posterior tibial tendon; star: flexor digitorum longus tendon).

PEARLS

- **Ganglion cyst is a fibrous walled mass containing clear mucinous fluid.**
- **Sonography shows an anechoic lobulated lesion.**
- **MR imaging demonstrates a fluid-filled mass.**
- **Hyperemia of the walls can be revealed on Doppler sonography and post-contrast MR images.**

ADDITIONAL IMAGES

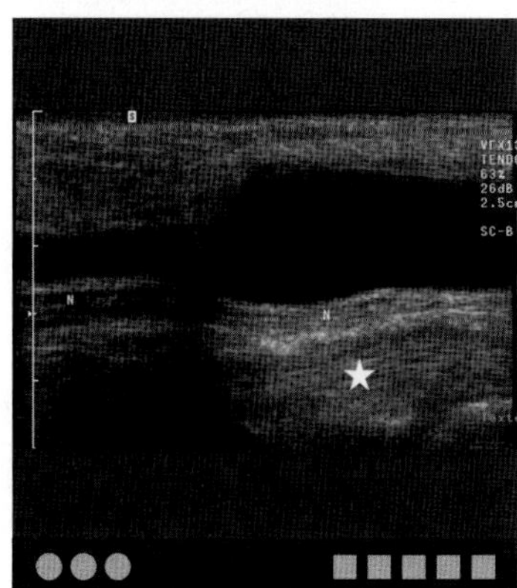

B. Ganglion cyst: Sagittal sonogram demonstrates the mass effect of the cyst on the posterior tibial nerve (N) (star: flexor digitorum longus tendon).

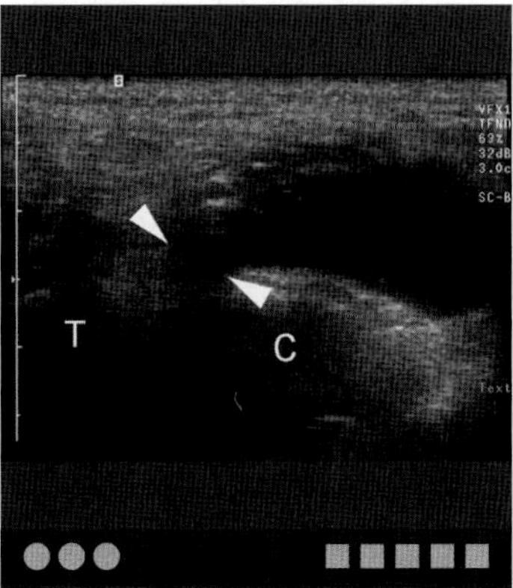

C. Ganglion cyst: Coronal view enables to suspect a communication (arrowheads) between the cystic lesion and the talocalcaneal joint (T: talus; C: calcaneus).

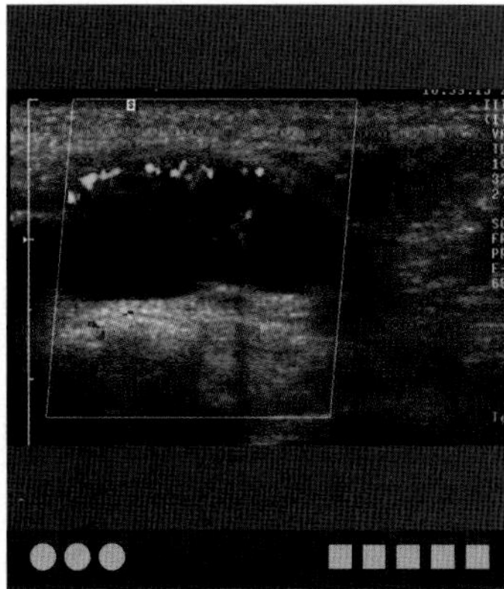

D. Ganglion cyst: Doppler sonography exhibits hyperemia of the walls of the lesion. Note also its lobulated shape.

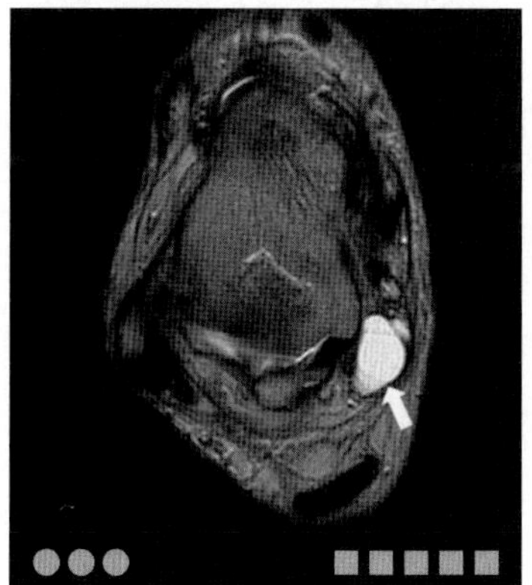

E. Ganglion cyst: In the same patient, axial T2-weighted image shows a hyperintense lobulated mass (arrow) in the space normally occupied by the posterior tibial nerve, artery, and vein.

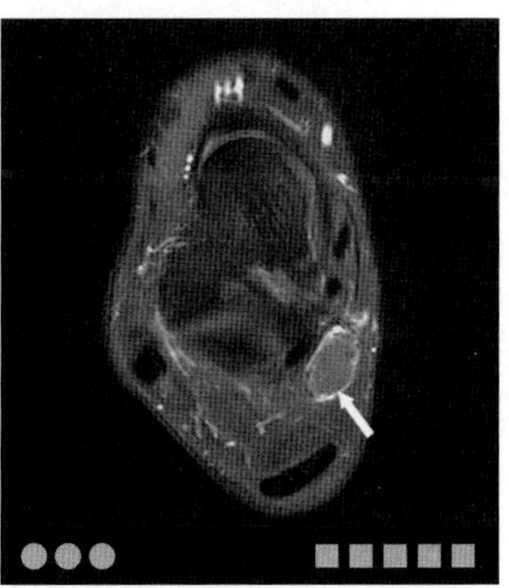

F. Ganglion cyst: Axial T1-weighted fat-saturated post-contrast image demonstrates peripheral enhancement of the mass in the tarsal tunnel.

IMAGE KEY

Common

Rare

Typical

Unusual

DIFFERENTIAL DIAGNOSIS IMAGE

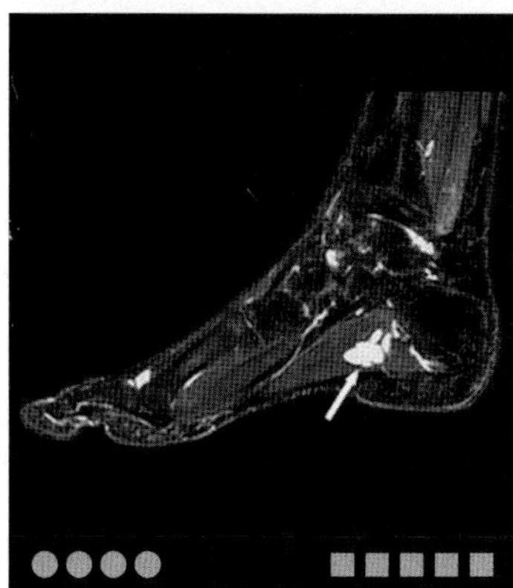

G. Venous malformation: STIR sagittal image shows increased-signal tortuous structures next to the medial plantar vessels in the tarsal tunnel.

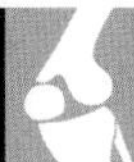

29–22 Intramuscular Ganglion

Ibrahim F. Abdelwahab and Stefano Bianchi

PRESENTATION

Pain at proximal anterolateral leg compartment radiating distally

FINDINGS

US shows a multilocular cystic mass located inside the peroneus longus muscle.

DIFFERENTIAL DIAGNOSES

- *Intramuscular myxoma:* Resembles intramuscular ganglia but are not attached to the superior tibiofibular joint. They are uncommon in the leg.
- *Nerve tumor:* Presents with similar clinical findings. It is often spindle shaped and is located in close proximity with a nerve trunk.
- *Peroneal nerve ganglia:* Hard to distinguish from IMG, although they tend to dissect proximally. Histologically, they are within the nerve sheath.
- *Hematoma:* History of previous trauma or blood dyscrasia. No communication to superior tibiofibular joint.

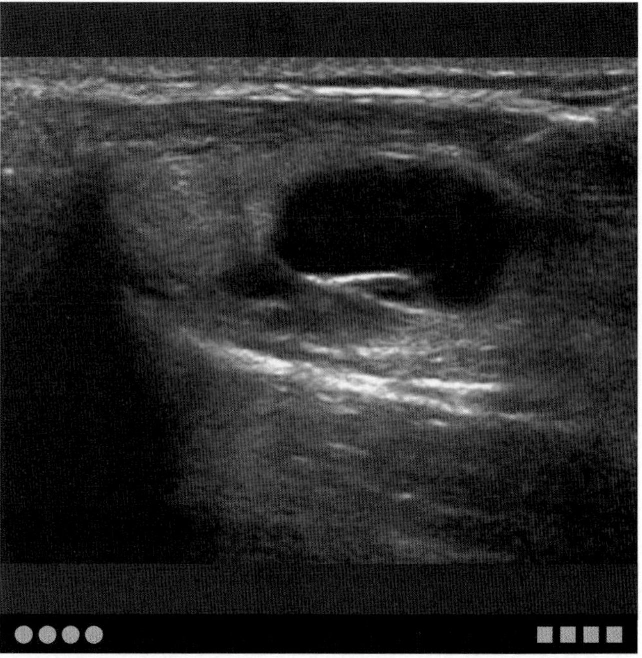

A. Intramuscular ganglion: Sagittal US image obtained over proximal aspect of the anterolateral leg compartment shows a well-circumscribed hypoechoic intramuscular ganglion.

COMMENTS

The patient is a 29-year-old man, who presented with pain over the superior part of the peroneus longus muscle radiating over the anterolateral leg secondary to an intramuscular ganglion (IMG). Intramuscular ganglia are rare lesions arising from the superior tibiofibular joint (STFJ) and mainly dissecting into the peroneus longus and the tibialis anterior muscle. They may result from repeated microtrauma to the STFJ and can cause pain radiating distally because of compression of the peroneal nerves. Physical examination reveals an ill-defined, firm muscular swelling. Because of their deep location, IMGs are seldom diagnosed clinically and require an imaging study. Standard radiographs are usually normal. In large lesions pressure erosions of the adjacent bone cortex can be seen and typically present sclerotic borders. US study shows a cystic mass generally presenting thick wall with internal septa. Its intramuscular location as well as its relations with the peroneal nerves can be accurately assessed. CT depicts the cyst as a hypodense mass. MRI shows a well-delineated expansible lesion presenting high signal on T2-weighted images and contrast enhancement of the wall and internal septa after gadolinium injection. Treatment includes needle aspiration and intralesional steroid injection that, although temporarily, can reduce patients symptoms. Surgical removal is curative. Local recurrence may be seen if the attachment of the ganglion to the joint is not excised.

PEARLS

- **Intramuscular ganglia are cystic lesions usually located in the anterolateral compartment of the leg. They communicate with the superior tibiofibular joint with a stalk.**
- **Because of their anatomic location they can cause pressure on the peroneal nerves and pain radiating down the leg.**
- **Both MRI and US studies are effective in confirming the diagnosis and demonstrating the stalk and the relation with the peroneal nerves. US can guide a needle aspiration. MRI allows exquisite assessment of the adjacent joints and bone.**

ADDITIONAL IMAGES

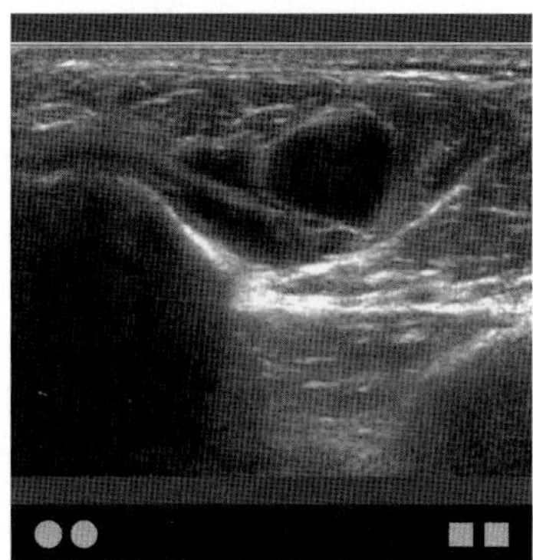

B. Intramuscular ganglion: Axial US image shows that the ganglion is located inside the peroneus longus muscle. Note the thick wall and internal septa.

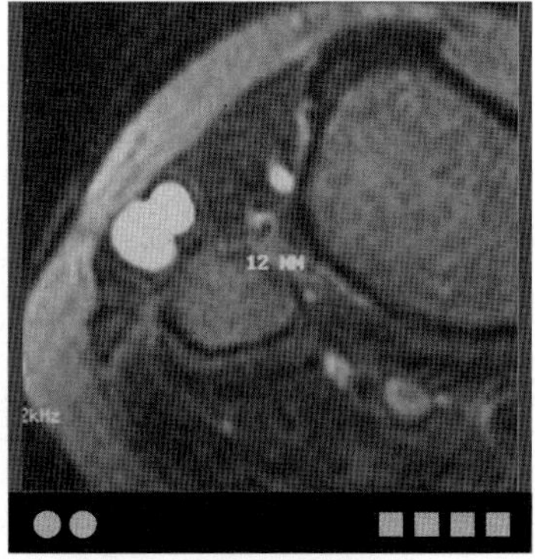

C. Intramuscular ganglion: Axial T2-weighted MRI image showing a sharply defined hyperintense mass located within the peroneus longus muscle.

DIFFERENTIAL DIAGNOSES IMAGES

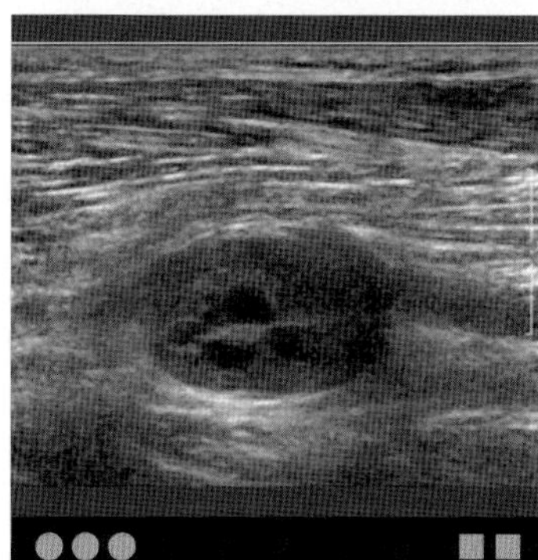

D. Schwannoma: Sagittal US image obtained over proximal aspect of the anterolateral leg compartment show an ovoid mass presenting a hypoechoic appearance with small internal cystic areas. The mass is located deep to the deep peroneal nerve.

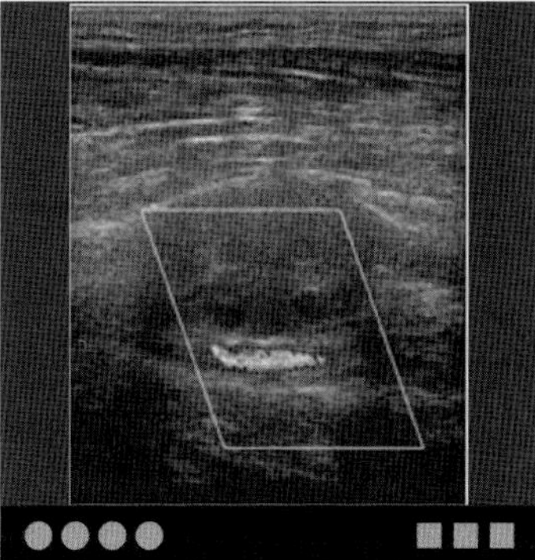

E. Schwannoma: Sagittal color Doppler US image shows that the mass is located between the deep peroneal nerve and the anterior tibial artery.

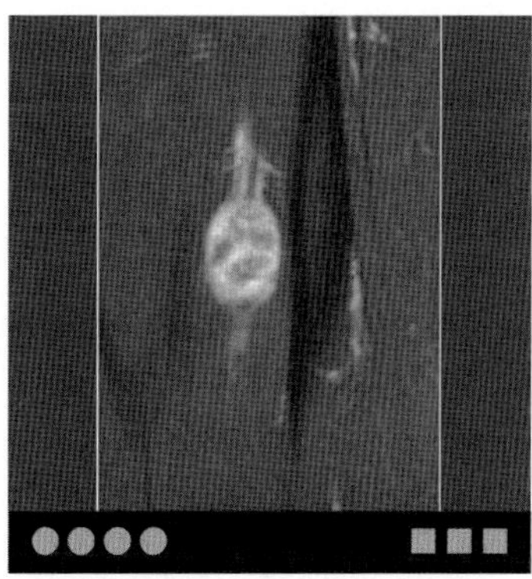

F. Schwannoma: Coronal fat saturation post Gd-T1-weighted MRI image confirms presence of a neurogenic tumor.

IMAGE KEY

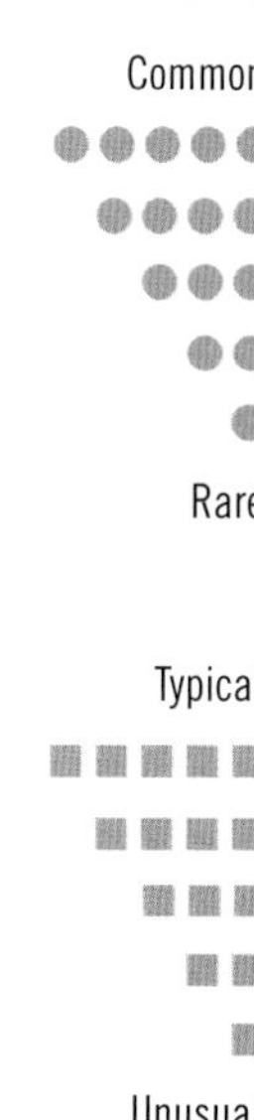

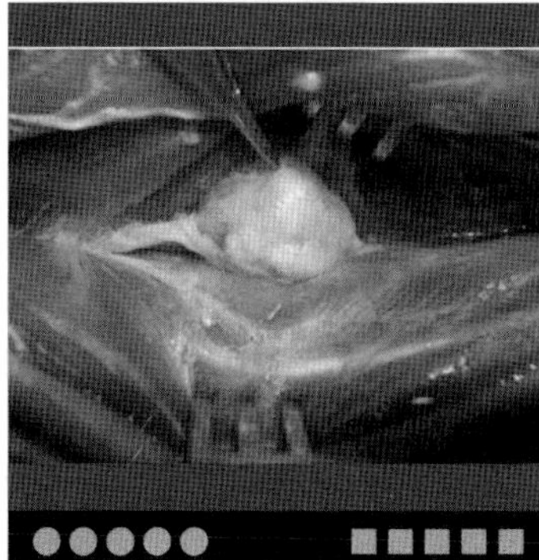

G. Schwannoma: Surgical appearance shows a spindle-shaped mass attached to the nerve trunk.

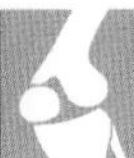

29–23 Osteochondritis Dissecans of the Ankle

John Shin and Peyman Borghei

PRESENTATION

Ankle pain

FINDINGS

MRI shows kissing osteochondral defect at the tibial plafond and dome of talus, which has low signal intensity on T1-weighted image. A line of hyperintense fluid on T2-weighted image separates the normal bone from the lesion.

DIFFERENTIAL DIAGNOSIS

- *Stress fracture:* Fractures present with dark line on T1-weighted image which are surrounded by bone edema best seen in fluid-sensitive sequences.
- *Osteonecrosis:* MRI shows fatty marrow changes caused by fat cell necrosis presenting as low signal foci on T1-weighted image, mixed signal, or double line sign on T2-weighted image and sclerosis on radiograph.

COMMENTS

The patient is a 12-year-old male with a history of right ankle pain diagnosed with osteochondritis dissecans (OCD). OCD is often as a result of a localized fracture within a segment of subchondral bone. Although it may be caused by trauma, ischemia, or genetic factors, inversion injuries of the ankle are the most common cause of ankle OCD. The usual sites of OCD of the talar dome are the posteromedial and the anterolateral aspect of the talus; such mirror-like lesions suggest trauma as the etiology. Occasionally, the articular surfaces of the tibia, fibula, or both are also involved. The severity of the lesion can range from an incomplete fracture with intact cartilage to a complete fracture with loss of cartilage integrity leading to fragment displacement. On radiographs, osteochondral lesions may appear normal or as lucencies in the articular epiphysis. Loss of the sharp cortical line of the articular surface represents more advanced lesion. On STIR or T2-weighted MRI, diffuse high signal intensity throughout the bone may signify bone marrow edema, a possible early indicator of an osteochondral lesion (stage I). Subchondral cyst or incomplete separation of the osteochondral fragment represent stage II. Fluid around an undetached, undisplaced osteochondral fragment is consistent with stage III. A complete and displaced osteochondral fragment, seen as a high signal fluid encircling the defect on T2-weighted image, represents stage IV.

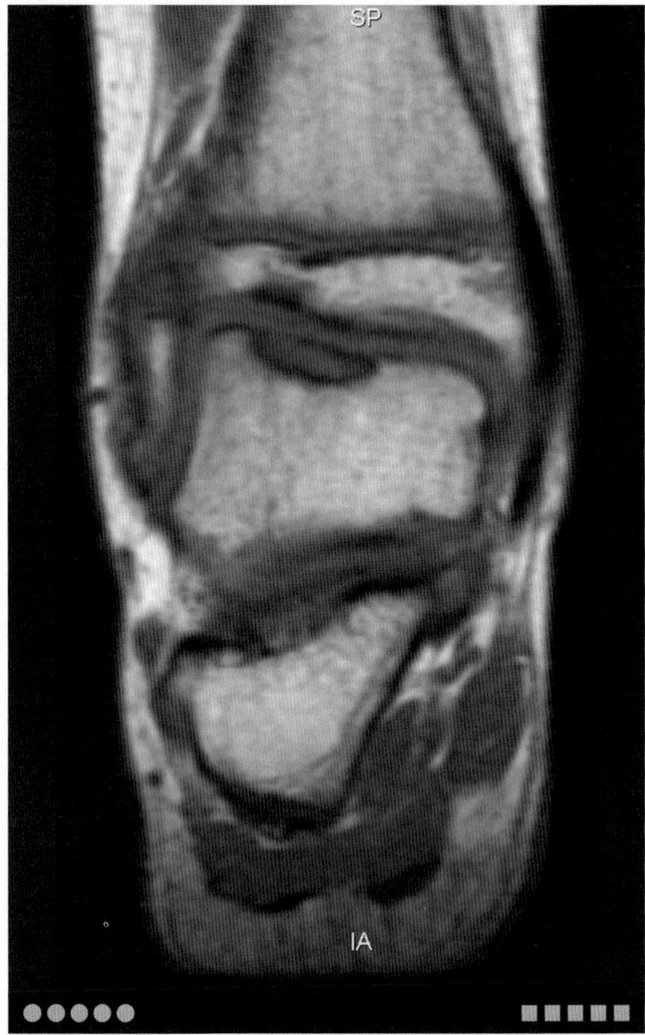

A. OCD: Coronal T1-weighted image shows kissing lesions with low signal intensity of subchondral bones of talar dome and tibial plafond.

PEARLS

- **The majority of OCD lesions involving the ankle joint typically occur on the articular surface of the talar dome, the semicircular part of the talus right beneath the tibia.**
- **Initial evaluation of patients should include conventional radiography. If the lesion appears stable and nondisplaced, MRI should be obtained to evaluate the integrity of the overlying cartilage.**
- **If the lesion appears displaced on conventional radiography, a CT scan should be obtained to more accurately assess the size and location of the lesion.**

ADDITIONAL IMAGES

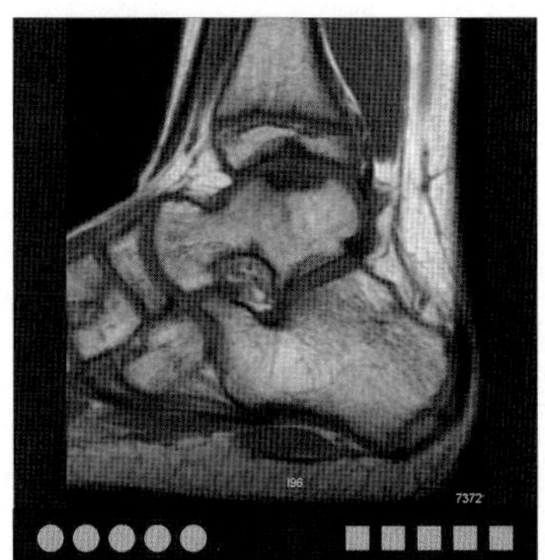

B. OCD: Sagittal T1-weighted image of the ankle shows kissing low signal intensity foci at the talar dome and tibial plafond.

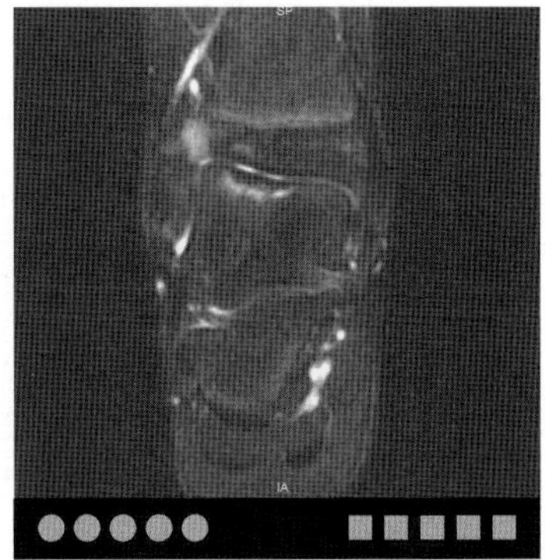

C. OCD: Coronal T2-weighted fat-saturated image shows kissing osteochondral defect. Note the fluid signal underlying the subchondral lesions of tibial plafond and talar dome consistent with stage III.

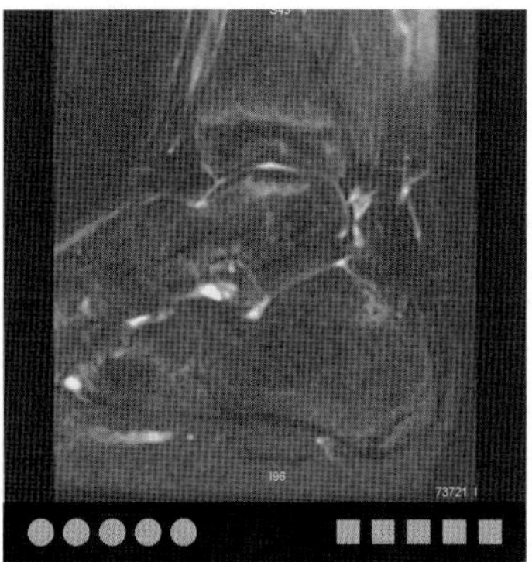

D. OCD: Sagittal T2-weighted fat-saturated image shows kissing OCD with the fluid signal underlying the subchondral lesions consistent with stage III.

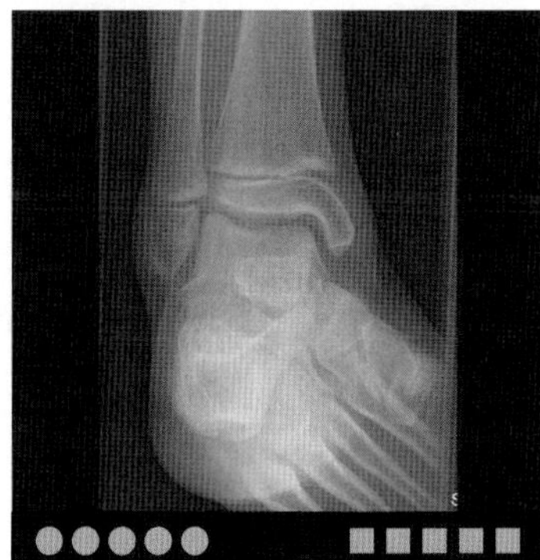

E. OCD: Internal oblique radiograph of the ankle shows osteochondral defect of the dome of the mid-talus close to the lateral side with subtle subchondral sclerosis.

DIFFERENTIAL DIAGNOSES IMAGES

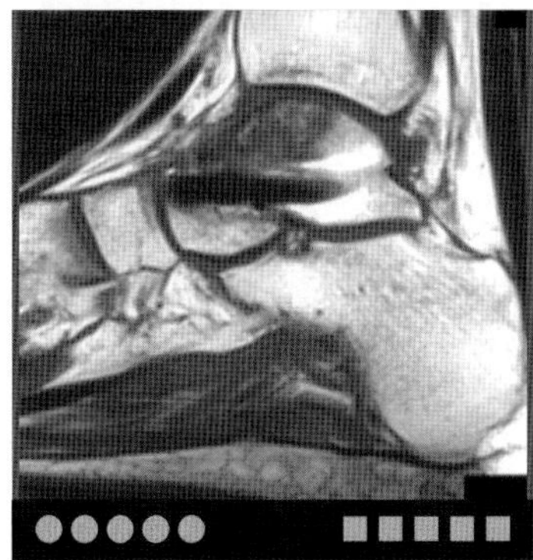

F. Osteonecrosis medial talar dome: Sagittal T1-weighted image of medial talar dome shows ischemic changes and avascular necrosis on medial anterior talar dome in a 19-year-old man, who sustained nondisplaced talar fracture. Note magnetization artifact from cancellous screws.

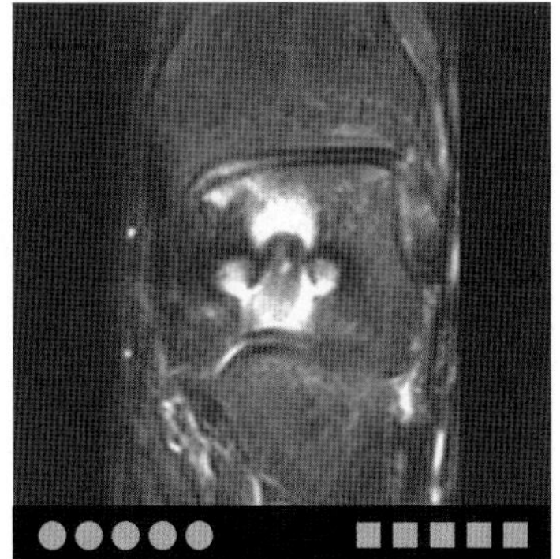

G. Osteonecrosis medial talar dome: Coronal fat-saturated T2-weighted image of ankle shows early phase of ischemia as bone marrow edema in medial dome of the talus in the same patient as Figure F.

IMAGE KEY

Common

●●●●●

●●●●

●●●

●●

●

Rare

Typical

■■■■■

■■■■

■■■

■■

■

Unusual

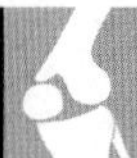

29–24 Fibular Stress Fracture

Sailaja Yadavalli

PRESENTATION

Persistent ankle pain

FINDINGS

Linear low signal on MRI with associated bone marrow and soft tissue edema shows distal fibular insufficiency fracture.

DIFFERENTIAL DIAGNOSES

- *Chronic overuse syndrome:* Diffuse patchy bone marrow edema is seen on MRI in the distal tibia and fibula, the tarsal and metatarsal bones in active children and young adults.
- *Infection:* Bone marrow and soft tissue edema with periostitis are characteristic of osteomyelitis. Cortical erosive changes and soft tissue abscess may also be present.
- *Iatrogenic:* Post-operative changes of ligament repair or screw tracts.

COMMENTS

The patient is a 61-year-old female with persistent ankle pain. Fatigue fractures occur when abnormal and repeated stress is applied to normal bone. Insufficiency fractures result when normal stress is applied to abnormal bone in conditions such as osteoporosis or rheumatoid arthritis. Typically distal fibular fatigue fractures occur with running, and proximal fractures are caused by activities that involve jumping. Proximal fibular stress fractures have been described in paratroopers. Ballet dancing may lead to stress fractures in children and adolescents. Distal fibular stress fractures may also be seen with rheumatoid arthritis, ankle or subtalar arthrodesis, and in postmenopausal females. These may occur in conjunction with distal tibial stress fractures. Repetitive sub-maximal loading causes accelerated bone remodeling, which may lead to a stress fracture with continued activity. The fracture begins as a cortical break which progresses with continued stress. In tubular bones, stress fractures are often transverse, but can be longitudinal or oblique, especially in the tibia. Patients have pain associated with the activity, which is relieved with rest. Clinical findings may include focal soft tissue swelling and tenderness. Primary treatment involves pain relief and rest. On MR imaging linear low signal intensity is seen on both T1-weighted and fluid-sensitive sequences with adjacent areas of bone marrow edema. Associated periosteal changes and edema in the surrounding soft tissues are usually present.

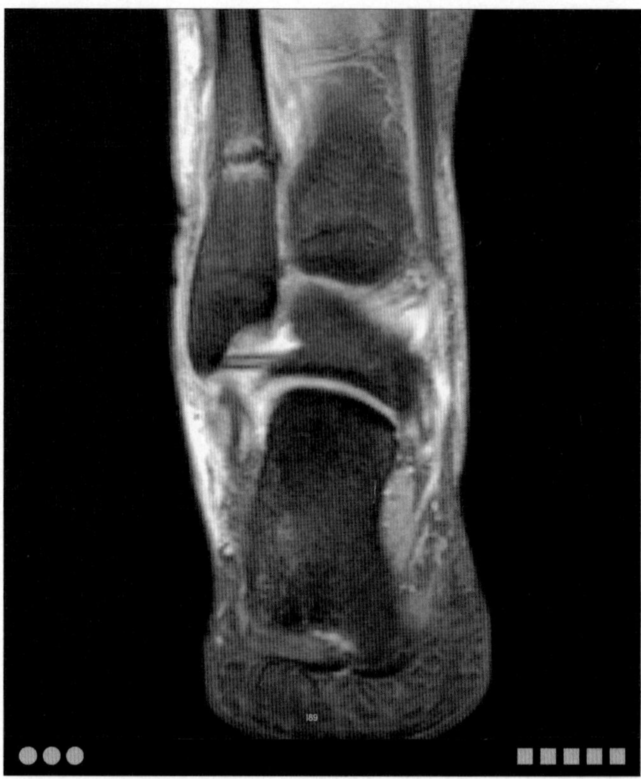

A. Stress fracture: Coronal gradient echo fat-saturated fluid-sensitive image shows linear low signal corresponding to the fracture. Mild periosteal changes are seen.

Periosteal and endosteal callus formation may also be seen. Early radiographs may often be normal or show minimal periosteal and endosteal changes. Later radiographs show a transverse sclerotic fracture line. Fibular stress fractures may easily be overlooked on ankle radiographs in a patient complaining of ankle pain.

PEARLS

- **Stress fractures are classified as fatigue fractures or insufficiency fractures.**
- **Distal fibular stress fractures are associated with long-distance running, rheumatoid arthritis, and ankle or hind foot arthrodesis.**
- **Proximal fibular stress fractures are associated with jumping activities.**
- **MRI typically shows linear low signal on T1-weighted and fluid-sensitive sequences surrounded by an area of bone marrow and soft tissue edema.**
- **May easily be overlooked on ankle radiographs.**

ADDITIONAL IMAGES

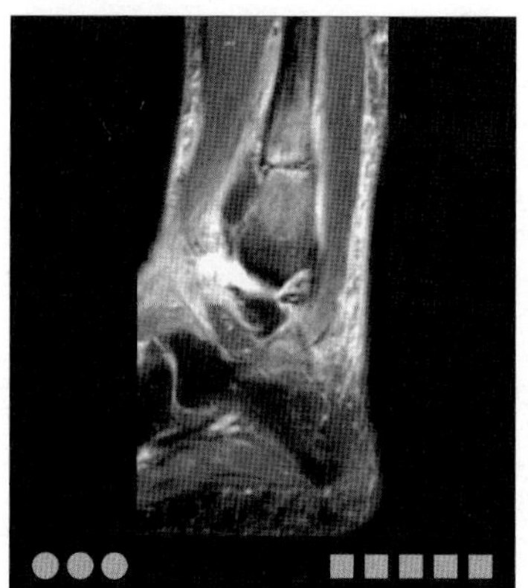

B. Stress fracture: Sagittal STIR image shows low signal fracture line with extensive bone marrow and soft tissue edema and periosteal changes.

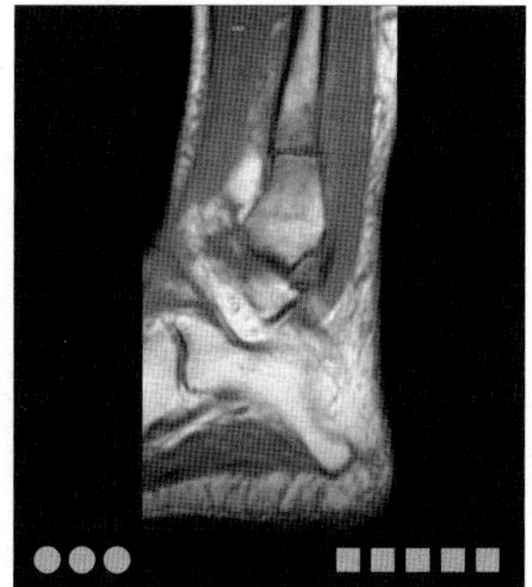

C. Stress fracture: Sagittal T1-weighted image shows linear fracture line, bone marrow changes, and periosteal changes along the posterior aspect.

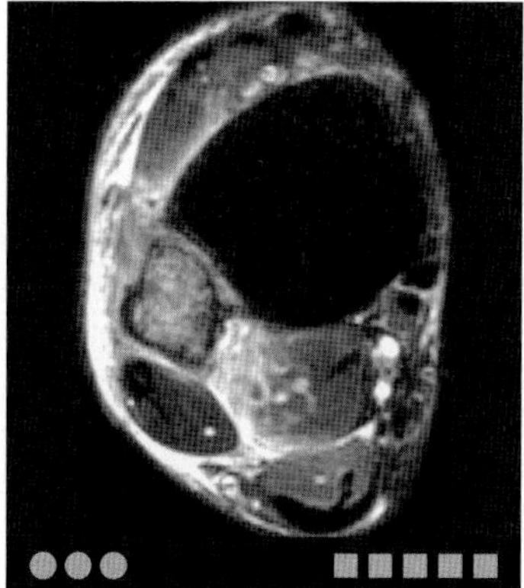

D. Stress fracture: Axial fluid-sensitive fat-saturated image shows bone marrow edema in the distal fibula with surrounding soft tissue edema. The fracture can easily be overlooked on the axial images.

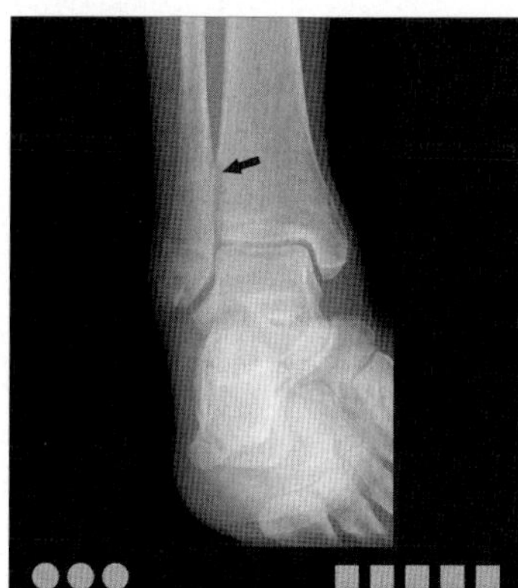

E. Stress fracture: Radiograph of the ankle shows a transverse sclerotic line across the distal fibula compatible with a stress fracture (arrow).

IMAGE KEY

Common

Rare

Typical

Unusual

DIFFERENTIAL DIAGNOSES IMAGES

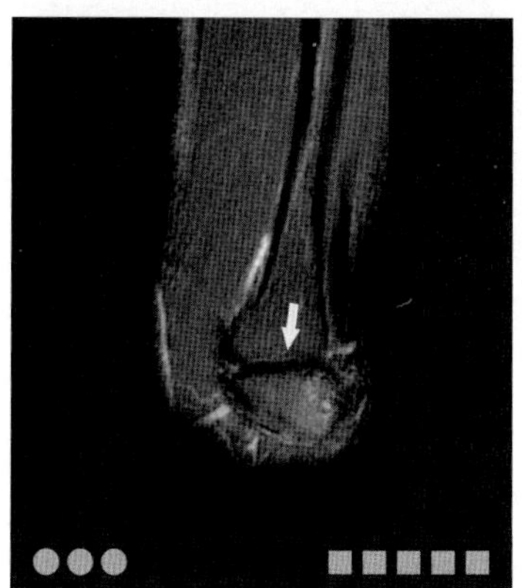

F. Postoperative change: Sagittal T2-weighted fat-saturated image shows linear low signal in the distal fibula (arrow) consistent with a tunnel for ligament repair.

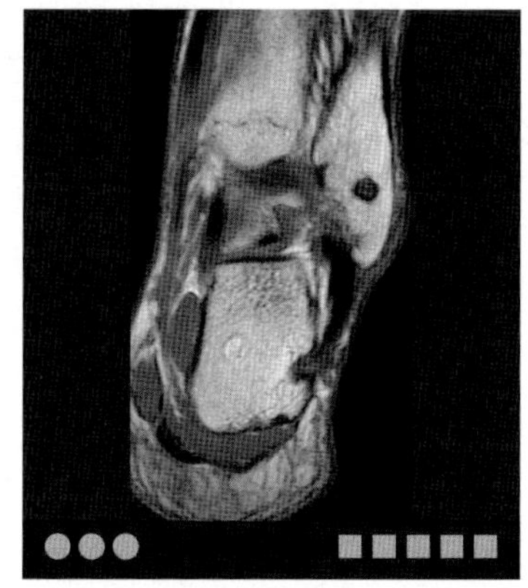

G. Postoperative change: Coronal T1-weighted image shows the circular defect of the tunnel for ligament repair in the distal fibula.

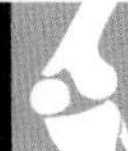

29–25 Juvenile Tillaux Fracture

Tod Abrahams

PRESENTATION

Severe anterior ankle pain and swelling

FINDINGS

Radiograph shows vertical fracture lucent line through the lateral aspect of the distal tibial epiphysis.

DIFFERENTIAL DIAGNOSES

- *Transitional fracture:* Coronally oriented metaphyseal fracture present on lateral view.
- *Osteochondral talar dome fracture:* The lucent defect disrupts the subchondral bone of the talus.

COMMENTS

The patient presented with anterior ankle swelling after sliding into second base. The term Tillaux fracture is an eponym used to describe a fracture of the distal anterolateral tibial epiphysis in adolescents. The common age of incidence is 14 in boys and 12 in girls. It is more common in girls. The fracture results from forced external rotation of the foot or medial rotation of the leg on a fixed foot. Skateboarding and baseball (sliding) are common activities associated with it. The fracture is the result of several factors: distal epiphyseal closure starts posteriorly and progresses anteriorly and occurs first in the middle third, next the medial third, and finally the lateral third. The anterolateral epiphysis is therefore at risk. Additionally, in children, ligaments are stronger than the physis and avulsions are more common than ligamentous injury. The posterior tibiofibular ligament is much stronger than the anterior counterpart and thus, the anterior structures are more susceptible to injury. Radiographs of the ankle show a vertically oriented fracture lateral to the midline within the distal tibial epiphysis on the AP or mortise projection. The lateral view may show a displaced fragment anteriorly with soft tissue swelling and an effusion. CT or MR imaging shows more definitive fracture morphology as the vertical fracture begins anterolaterally within the epiphysis and exits laterally on the lateral tibial cortex. The fragment frequently rotates anterolaterally and displacement typically is minimal but can be marked. The more skeletally mature the patient, the more lateral the fracture.

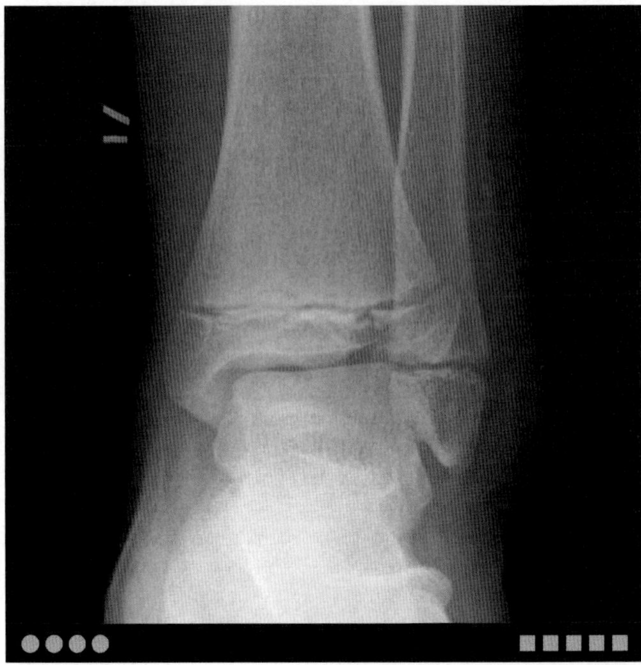

A. Juvenile Tillaux fracture: AP radiograph shows the typical vertically oriented fracture through the lateral aspect of the distal tibial epiphysis.

PEARLS

- **Tillaux fracture occurs in the adolescent age group as the distal tibial epiphysis is undergoing closure.**
- **The anterolateral portion of the epiphysis closes last and is therefore susceptible to fracture.**
- **When minimally displaced the fracture may only be seen on the frontal view as a vertical lucent line lateral to the midline.**
- **CT or MR imaging can demonstrate fracture displacement, rotation and articular surface gap.**

ADDITIONAL IMAGES

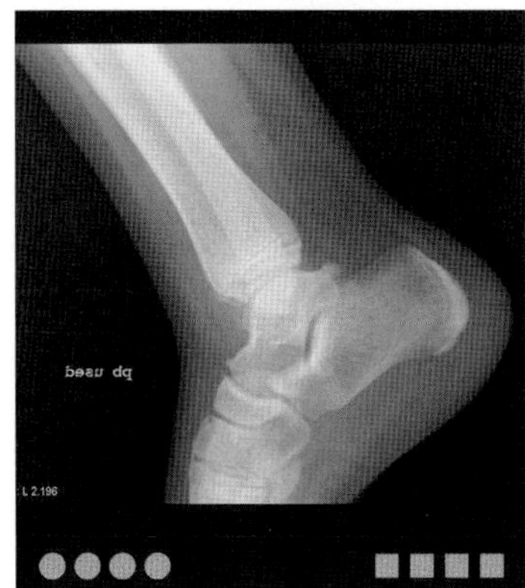

B. Juvenile Tillaux fracture: Lateral radiograph shows the displaced bony fragment anteriorly.

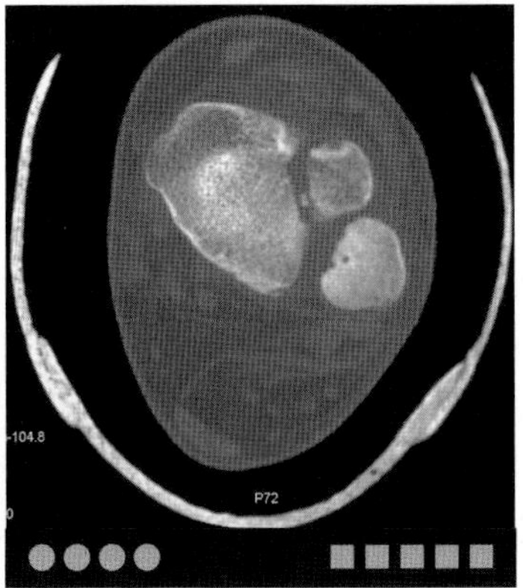

C. Juvenile Tillaux fracture: Axial CT image shows the sagittally oriented fracture through the epiphysis.

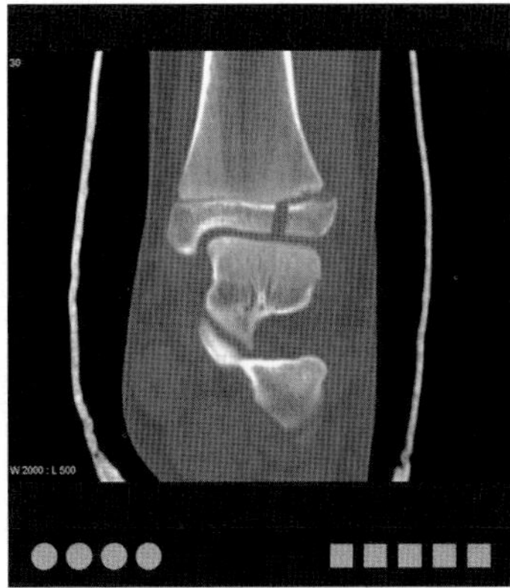

D. Juvenile Tillaux fracture: Coronal CT demonstrates the vertical fracture through the epiphysis with intra-articular extension.

DIFFERENTIAL DIAGNOSES IMAGES

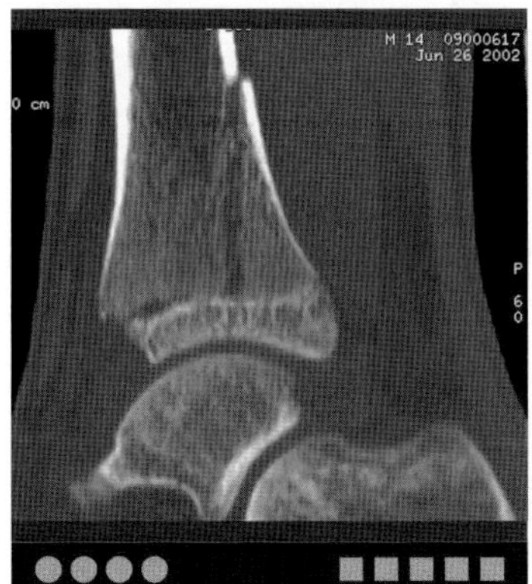

E. Triplane fracture: Sagittal CT image of triplane fracture showing the coronally oriented metaphyseal fracture.

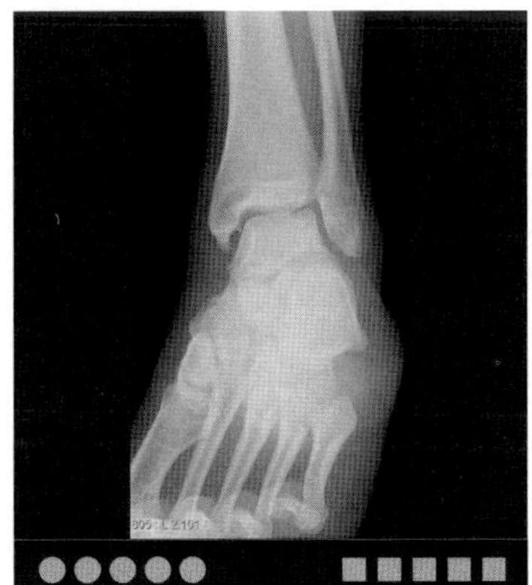

F. Osteochondral fracture (osteochondritis diseccans): AP radiograph demonstrating an osteochondral lesion of the lateral talar dome inferior to the epiphysis.

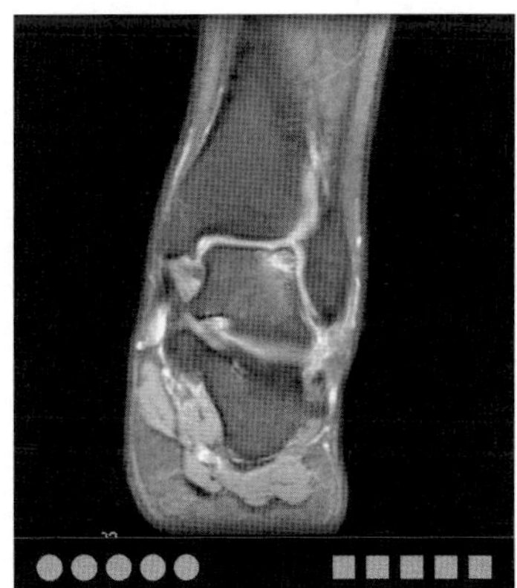

G. Osteochondral fracture (osteochondritis diseccans): Coronal MR image shows the osteochondral lesion with associated edema.

IMAGE KEY

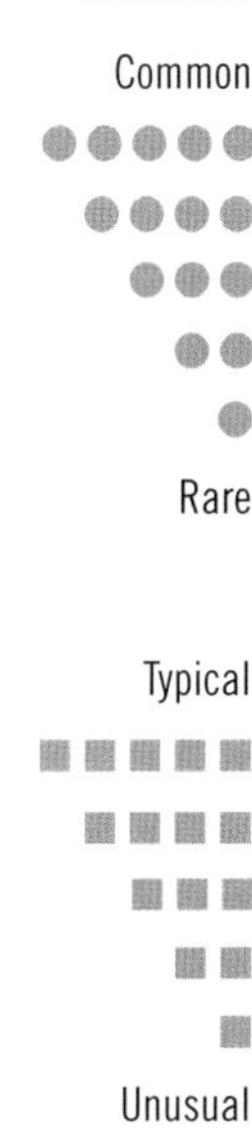

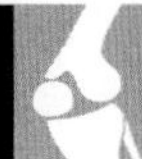

29–26 Talar Body Fractures

Tod Abrahams

PRESENTATION

Diffuse ankle swelling and pain

FINDINGS

Radiograph shows a vertically oriented fracture line through the talar body.

DIFFERENTIAL DIAGNOSES

- *Talar neck fracture:* The fracture line is more anterior in the constricted portion of the talus.
- *Talar head fracture:* An oblique fracture in the articular portion of the talus anteriorly.
- *Lateral talar process fractures:* A horizontal fracture is seen on the lateral view. The mortise view shows a fracture below the level of the lateral malleolus.
- *Posterior talar process fracture:* Fracture line is vertically oriented but posterior to the articular surface of the talus.

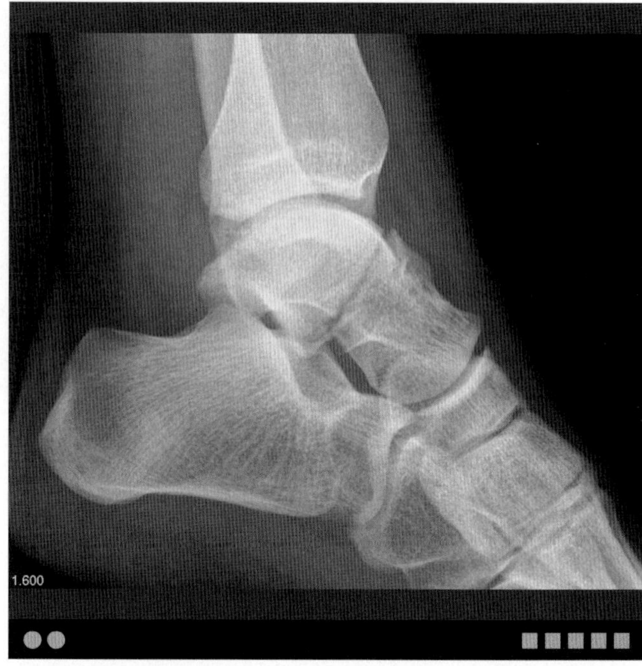

A. Talar body fracture: Lateral radiograph shows a vertical fracture through the talar body with soft tissue swelling and effusion.

COMMENTS

The patient presented with diffuse ankle swelling after a fall from a ladder. Talar fractures can be divided based on three anatomic regions: body, neck, and head. Body fractures can be further subdivided based on involvement of the main portion of the body, lateral process, posterior process, or talar dome. Lateral process fractures are commonly seen with snowboarding injuries as the result of eversion or inversion and dorsiflexion. Posterior process fractures result from three mechanisms: excessive plantar flexion, avulsion of the posterior talofibular ligament, or as stress injuries particularly in ballet dancers. Talar dome fractures (osteochondritis dissecans) result from an inversion injury. Fractures through the main portion of the body are uncommon and typically the result of an axial load or shearing injury secondary to a fall from a height. This is the same mechanism that causes the more frequent calcaneal fracture. The fracture orientation may be coronal or sagittal. The radiologist must consider this type of fracture in the following setting: an axial load injury has occurred; there is diffuse ankle swelling and evidence clinically or radiographically of an ankle effusion; and no other fracture, particularly calcaneal, is identified on initial radiographs. Further imaging may be necessary if the radiographs are not diagnostic and may include CT or MRI. Both modalities will assess fracture plane, degree of comminution, articular surface disruption, and other fractures that may be present. Talar body fractures can be associated with fractures of the tibia and calcaneus. The most common late complication is subtalar arthritis.

PEARLS

- **Talar body fractures can be divided anatomically into three types: main body, process (posterior or lateral), or dome.**
- **Fractures of the main body are uncommon but need to be considered in the setting of an axial load injury with diffuse ankle swelling and a joint effusion.**
- **Radiographs may show a vertical fracture line through the body and an effusion on the lateral projection; however, CT or MRI may be necessary to make the diagnosis.**
- **CT or MR imaging demonstrates the extent of fracture, articular involvement, comminution, and the presence of other fractures.**

ADDITIONAL IMAGES

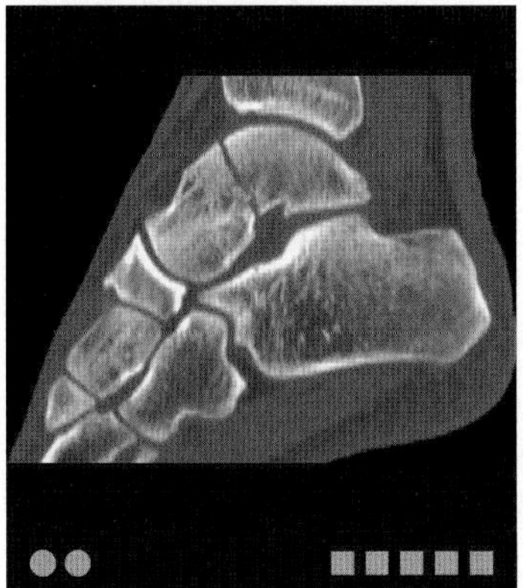

B. Talar body fracture: Sagittal CT shows the fracture extent and intra-articular extension.

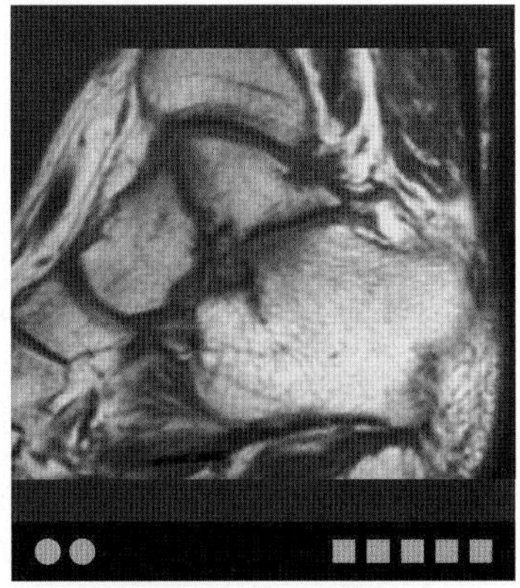

C. Talar body fractures: Sagittal MR T1-weighted image shows the fracture as a region of linear signal void.

DIFFERENTIAL DIAGNOSES IMAGES

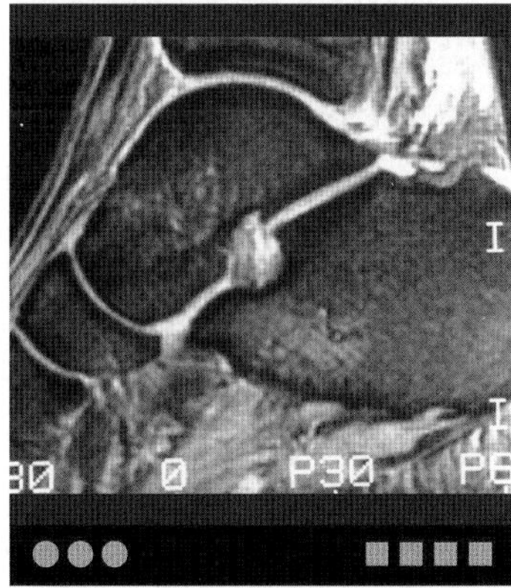

D. Nondisplaced talar neck fracture: Sagittal T2-weighted fat-saturated MR image shows linear bone marrow edema anterior to the talar body.

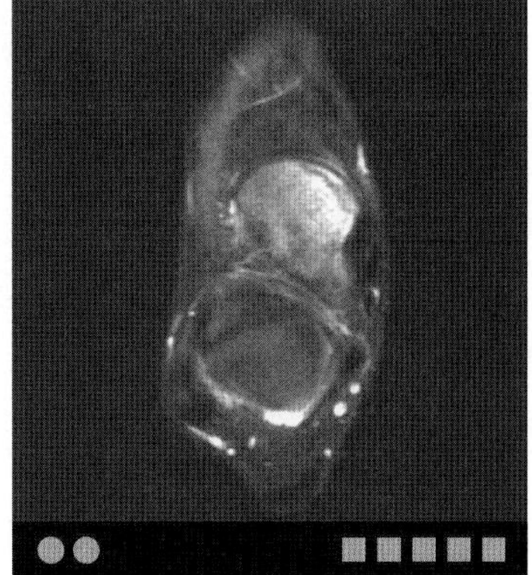

E. Talar head fracture: Axial T2-weighted fat-saturated image shows talar head fracture with oblique linear signal void and associated edema.

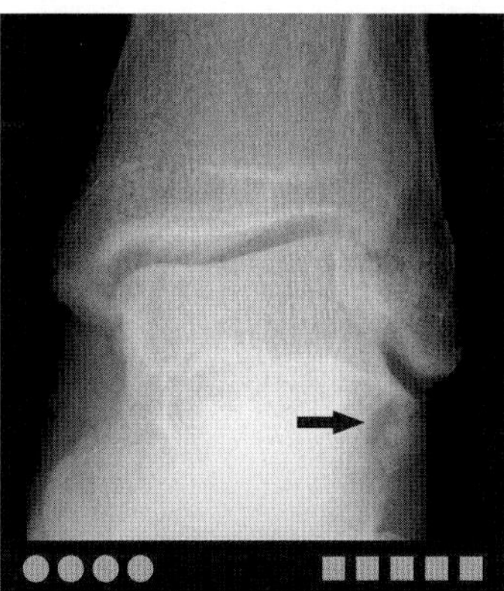

F. Lateral talar process fracture: AP radiograph shows fracture of the lateral talar process (arrow).

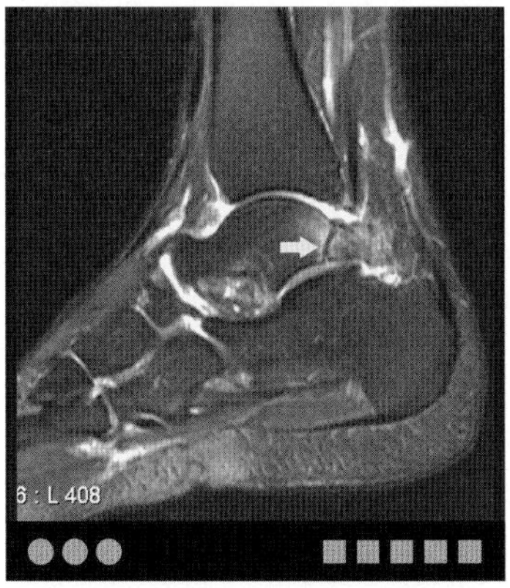

G. Posterior talar process fracture: Axial T2-weighted MR image shows findings of a nondisplaced posterior talar process fracture with adjacent bone marrow edema (arrow).

IMAGE KEY

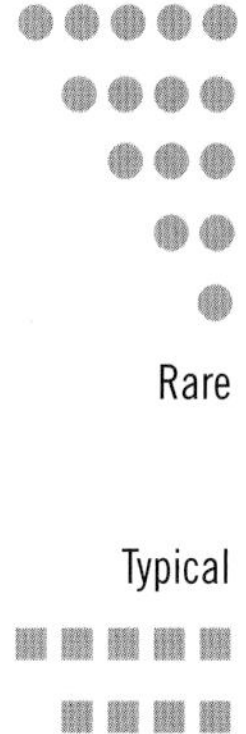

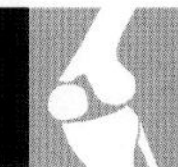

29–27 Calcaneal Insufficiency Avulsion Fracture (CIA)

Oganes Ashikyan and Jamshid Tehranzadeh

PRESENTATION

Pain, erythema, edema of the heel

FINDINGS

Calcaneal avulsion fracture with associated osteomyelitis and cellulitis.

DIFFERENTIAL DIAGNOSES

- *Fatigue fracture of calcaneus:* This fracture occurs in normal individuals such as athletes with normal bones when excessive force is applied to the calcaneus.
- *Insufficiency fracture related to osteoporosis:* Fractures of osteoporotic calcaneus are usually seen in elderly females such as postmenopausal or those with chronic rheumatoid arthritis who present with spontaneous pain in the ankle.
- *Osteomyelitis of the calcaneus without a fracture:* These are often seen in diabetic patients especially adjacent to the skin ulceration.

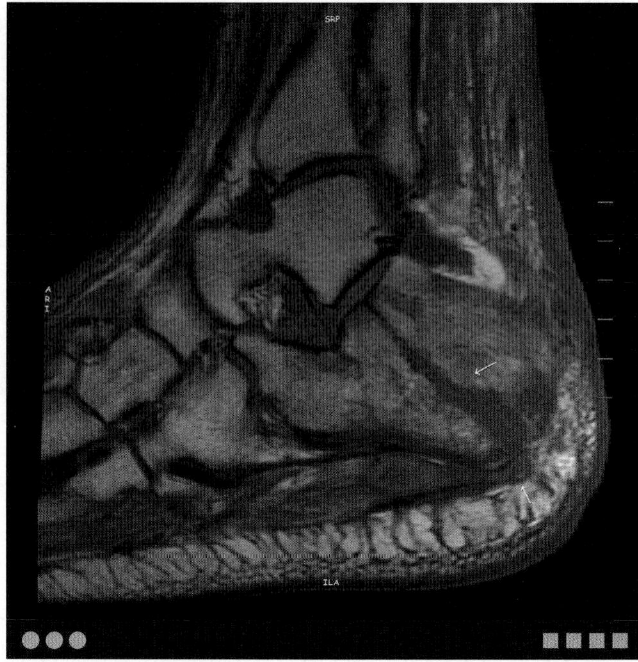

A. Calcaneal insufficiency avulsion fracture: Sagittal T1-weighted image demonstrates fracture of the calcaneus with slight superior angulation of the avulsed fragment.

COMMENTS

The patient is a 47-year-old man with diabetes, who presented with right heel pain. Patient was found to have cellulitis of the right foot and calcaneal fracture extending into the subtalar joint. Calcaneal insufficiency avulsion fractures in diabetic patients were originally described as extra-articular fractures of the posterior calcaneus with fracture line coursing in parallel to the apophysis of the calcaneus. This type of fracture is sometimes referred to as "Iowa" type in reference to the institution of authors who coined the term "Calcaneal Insufficiency Avulsion" fractures. The second type is "mid-body" compression fracture, which is a horizontal fracture oriented in parallel to the talocalcaneal joint again without joint involvement. Wedge or cleavage type of calcaneal fracture in diabetic patients extends from the calcaneal tubercle distal to the insertion site of the Achilles tendon to the talonavicular joint without joint involvement. The majority of the reported cases in the literature describes and classifies extra-articular fractures of the calcaneus in the diabetic patients. However, intra-articular fracture of the calcaneus in diabetic patient has also been described. Calcaneal insufficiency fractures can occur in the absence of any trauma or after normal activities usually not expected to result in fractures such as dancing or running. Calcaneal insufficiency avulsion fractures have been reported to occur in patients who were non-weight bearing at the time of fracture discovery. Associated cellulitis and soft tissue ulceration can be seen. Insufficiency fractures of calcaneus have also been described in patients with neurological impairment related to meningomyeloceles, congenital insensitivity to pain, peripheral nerve damage, and amyloid associated neuropathy. Patients with osteoporosis related to rheumatoid arthritis or aging can also present with insufficiency fractures. Treatment depends on a variety of factors and surgical intervention maybe needed in some cases.

PEARLS

- **Calcaneal insufficiency avulsion fractures occur in diabetic patients with no history of significant trauma.**
- **Both intra-articular and extra-articular calcaneal insufficiency avulsion fractures have been described with extra-articular fractures reported more commonly.**
- **In a nondiabetic patient, calcaneal insufficiency fractures maybe related to osteoporosis or neuropathies.**

ADDITIONAL IMAGES

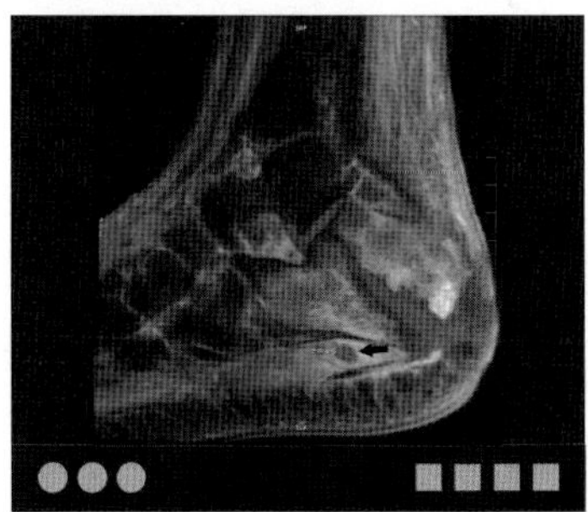

B. Calcaneal insufficiency avulsion fracture: Sagittal T1-weighted image with fat saturation post-contrast demonstrates fracture and osteomyelitis of the calcaneus. There is contrast enhancement of the adjacent soft tissues, which represents cellulitis and plantar fasciitis. Small abscess can be seen in the plantar soft tissues (arrow).

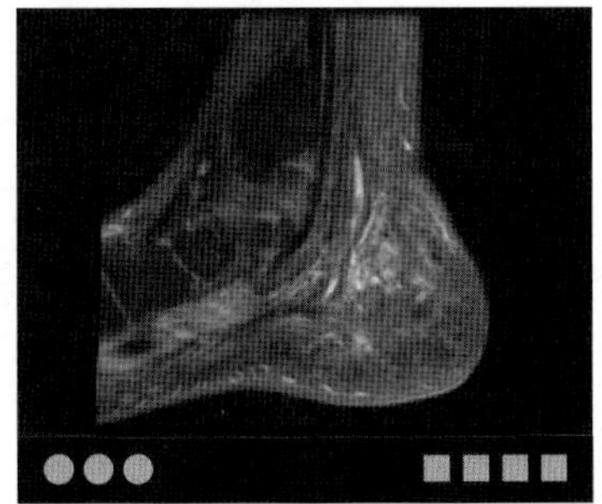

C. Calcaneal insufficiency avulsion fracture showing cellulitis of the foot: Sagittal T1-weighted image with fat saturation obtained after administration of intravenous contrast demonstrates extensive cellulitis of soft tissues with heterogeneous enhancement.

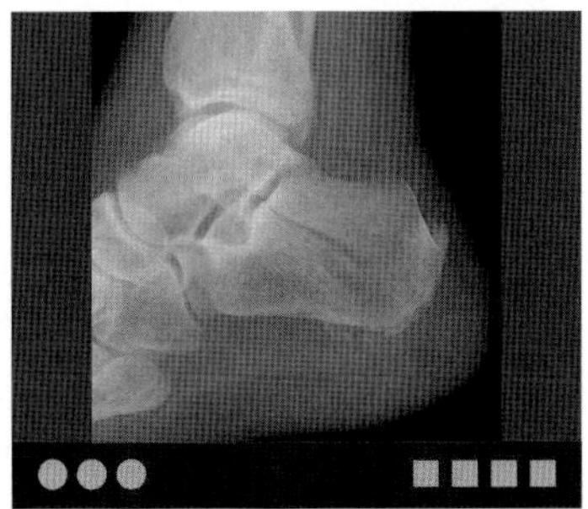

D. Calcaneal insufficiency avulsion fracture: Lateral radiograph of the calcaneus obtained 2 days prior to MRI demonstrates nondisplaced intra-articular fracture of the calcaneus.

E. Calcaneal insufficiency avulsion fracture: Lateral radiograph obtained one month after the radiograph of image D shows cephalic angulation of avulsed fracture fragment. There is also fragmentation and osteopenia of the calcaneus, which represent progression of osteomyelitis.

IMAGE KEY

Common

Rare

Typical

Unusual

DIFFERENTIAL DIAGNOSES IMAGES

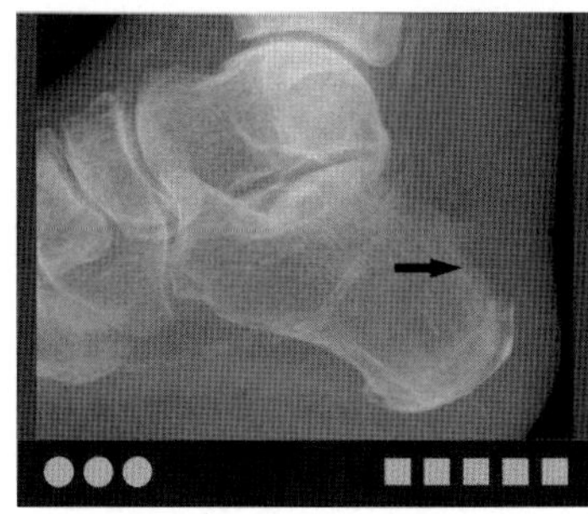

F. Osteomyelitis of the calcaneus: Lateral radiograph of the calcaneus in another patient demonstrates large osseous defect at the posterior aspect of the calcaneus (arrow), which is adjacent to edematous soft tissues. This patient presented with soft tissue ulcer that progressed to osteomyelitis of calcaneus. Note vascular calcifications.

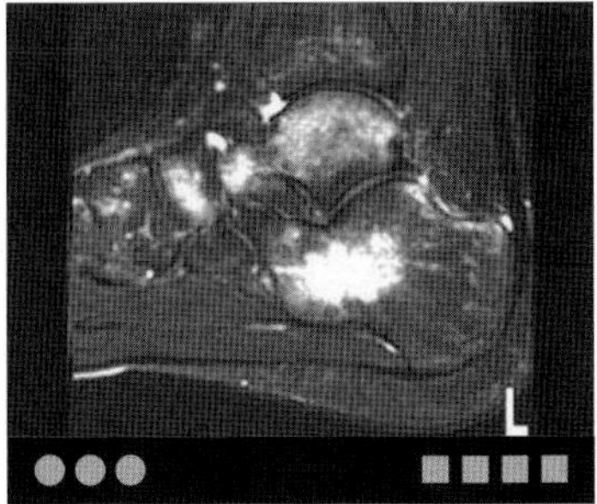

G. Fatigue fractures of ankle: Lateral T2-weighted image with fat saturation demonstrates bone marrow edema caused by fractures and bone contusions in the anterior aspect of calcaneus and also in talus, navicular and medial cuneiform. Note increased signal intensity representing injuries in these bones.

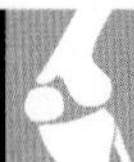

29–28 Triplane Fracture of the Ankle

Wilfred CG Peh

PRESENTATION

Acute pain and swelling following twisting injury

FINDINGS

Radiograph and CT show fractures in three planes, producing a rectangular anteromedial epiphyseal fragment and a large posterior epiphyseal–metaphyseal triangular fragment.

DIFFERENTIAL DIAGNOSES

- *Osteochondral fracture:* Regarded as a subchondral fatigue fracture, it consists of an osteochondral fragment ("mouse") with sclerosed pit in the articular surface ("mouse bed").
- *Stress fractures:* These are recognized in the distal tibia, distal fibula, and calcaneus. Seen on radiographs as a sclerotic linear area in a weight-bearing bone, biopsy should be avoided. Undiagnosed fractures may progress to complete fractures.

COMMENTS

The patient is a 15-year-old boy, who sustained a forced external rotation (eversion) injury to his right ankle. Triplane fracture of the ankle occurs in the distal tibia during adolescence, before complete closure of the distal tibia physis. External rotation (eversion) of the foot on the tibia with resultant shearing through the unfused distal lateral tibial growth plate is the essential force that initiates this type of fracture. Triplane fracture occurs most commonly in patients aged 12 to 15 years, and represents 5% to 10% of pediatric intra-articular ankle injuries. This fracture extends through three anatomical planes, namely: transversely through the growth plate, sagittally through the epiphysis, and coronally through the distal tibial metaphysis, resulting in intra-articular tibial plafond disruption. Triplane fracture may be classified as being two-part or three-part, with two-part fractures being more common and occurring at a younger age. In the three-part triplane fracture, the three fracture lines in each of the three anatomic planes produce three fragments, namely: a rectangular fragment of the anterolateral portion of the epiphysis, the remainder of the epiphysis with an attached posterior spike of the distal tibial metaphysis, and the tibial shaft with the anteromedial epiphysis. There may be an associated fibular fracture. On radiographs, triplane fractures may be missed or incompletely diagnosed initially. CT is useful for full assessment of this complex multiplane fracture of the ankle. CT is able to demonstrate all the fracture lines, intra-articular involvement, and accurately show the orientation and displacement of fragments in anticipation of internal fixation.

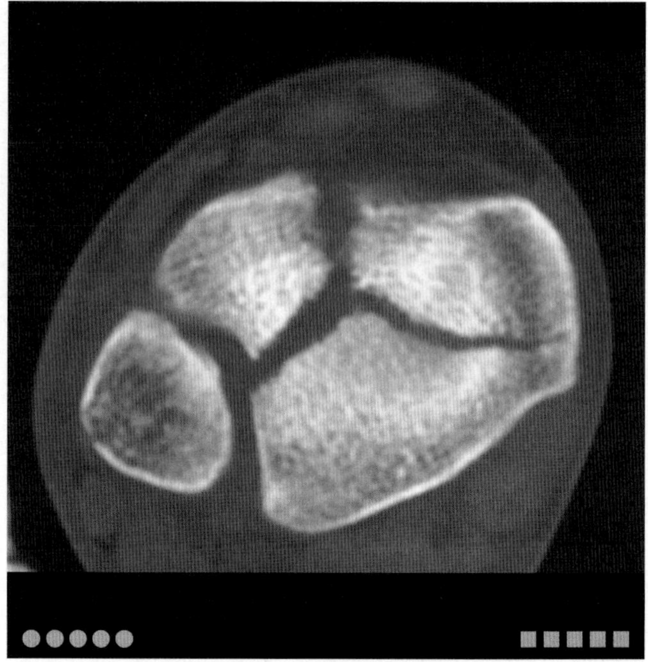

A. Three-part triplane fracture: Axial CT image shows fractures in the coronal and sagittal planes, producing a rectangular anterolateral fragment. The distal tibiofibular joint is involved. An undisplaced distal fibular fracture is also noted.

PEARLS

- **Triplane fractures may be initially missed or incompletely diagnosed on radiographs alone.**
- **CT with 2D reformatting is useful in showing the full extent of fracture planes, fragments, and intra-articular involvement.**
- **CT is useful in excluding other causes of ankle pain such as osteochondral fractures.**

ADDITIONAL IMAGES

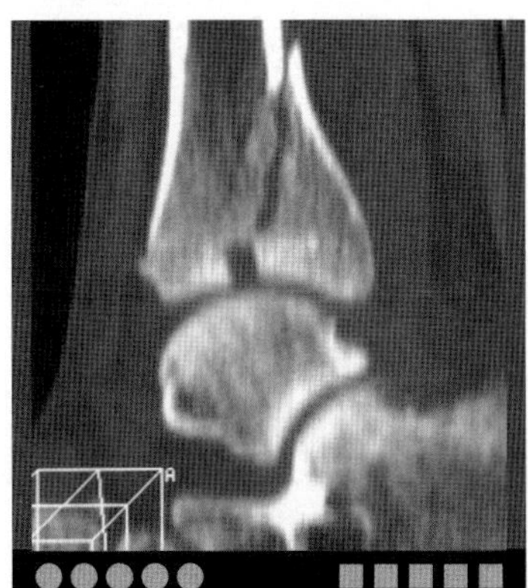

B. Three-part triplane fracture: Reconstructed sagittal CT image shows a coronal fracture extending through the epiphysis and metaphysis, producing a large triangular fragment. A transverse fracture through the growth plate results in a rectangular anterior fragment.

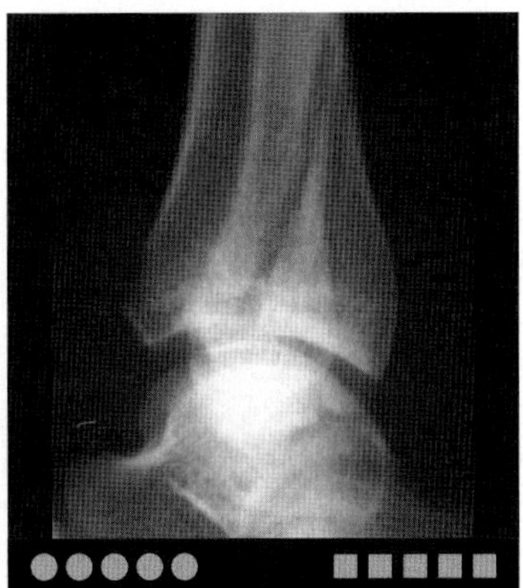

C. Three-part triplane fracture: Lateral radiograph shows the transverse fracture through the growth plate and a coronal fracture through the epiphysis and metaphysis, producing a metaphyseal spike.

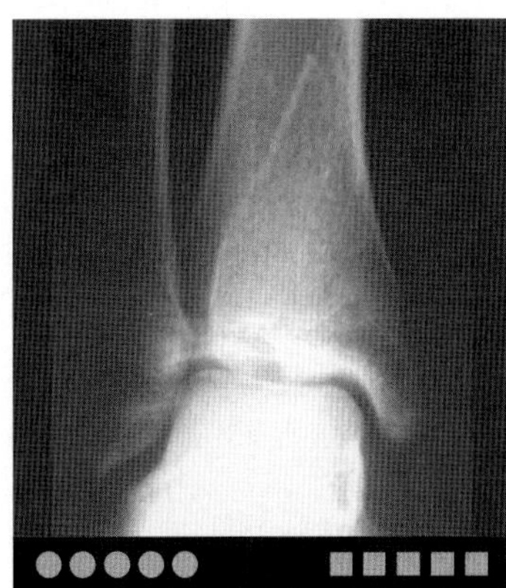

D. Three-part triplane fracture: Frontal radiograph shows the vertical fracture through the epiphysis. The outline of the metaphyseal spike is seen. The horizontal fracture through the growth plate is visible. From analysis of lateral and frontal radiographs, all components of a three-part triplane fracture, including the rectangular anterolateral fragment, can be discerned.

IMAGE KEY

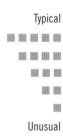

DIFFERENTIAL DIAGNOSES IMAGES

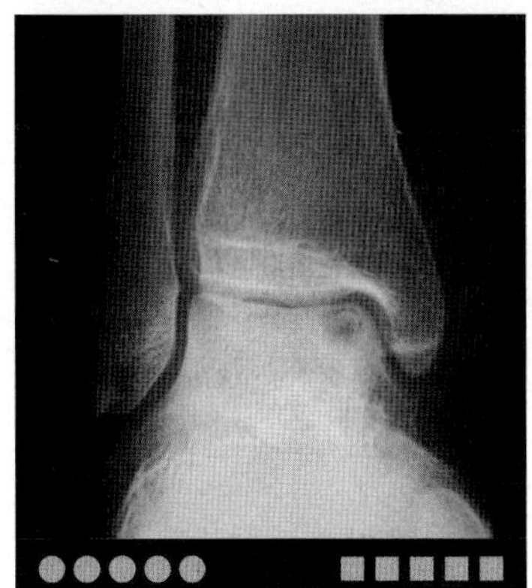

E. Osteochondral fracture of the talus: Frontal radiograph shows a rounded osteolytic area in the medial dome of the talus. It has sclerotic margins and suggestion of a detached fragment within.

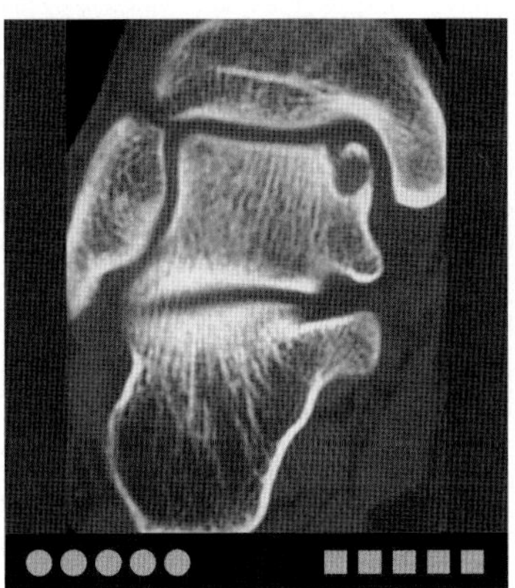

F. Osteochondral fracture of the talus: Axial CT image shows a large rounded defect in the superomedial talar dome, with an osteochondral fragment adjacent to it.

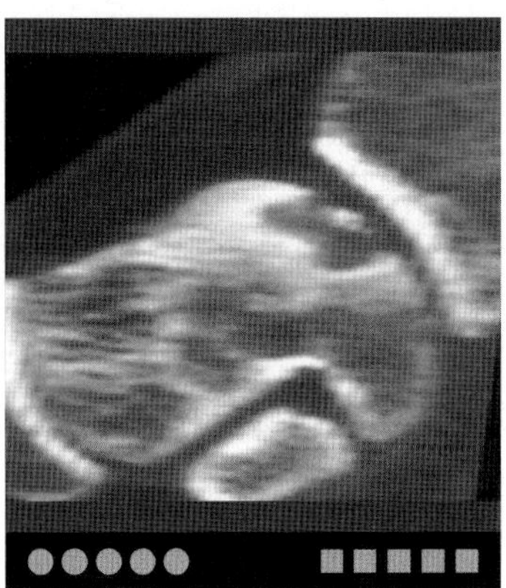

G. Osteochondral fracture of the talus: Reconstructed sagittal CT image shows the osteochondral fragment and the talar pit with a thick sclerotic rim.

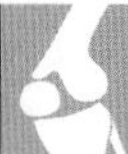

29–29 Posterior Tibial Tendinosis

Ashkan Afshin and Joshua Farber

PRESENTATION

Ankle pain

FINDINGS

MR images demonstrate thickening and enlargement of the posterior tibial tendon.

DIFFERENTIAL DIAGNOSES

- *Split tear of posterior tibial tendon:* MR images in these patients exhibit longitudinal increased signal in posterior tibial tendon as well as enlargement of the tendon.
- *Complete tear of posterior tibial tendon:* MRI shows complete tear or absence of this tendon (empty tendon sheath filled with fluid) with retraction of proximal segment of the tendon.
- *Tenosynovitis and tendinopathy of posterior tibial tendon:* MR images show hyperintense fluid around the tendon in the tendon sheath consistent with tenosynovitis. Tendinopathy is also observed in these patients as thickening and possible intermediate signal in the tendon.

COMMENTS

The patient is a 39-year-old man diagnosed with posterior tibial tendinosis and mild synovitis of peroneal tendon. Posterior tibial tendon provides stability for the plantar arch and medial ankle and performs inversion and plantar flexion of the foot. The anterior component of the tendon inserts to the navicular tuberosity and the middle component continues to insert into the cuneiforms, cuboid and the medial three metatarsal bases. Posterior tibial tendinosis represents degeneration of this tendon which results from chronic problems such as excessive pronation in obese people. Patients with this injury complain of the pain over the tendon especially distal to the medial malleolus. With progression of the pain, they may experience difficulty in normal standing and walking. Physical examination of the patient reveals swelling and tenderness in the region of the medial malleolus. The clinical examination may identify the anatomic locus of the symptoms but often can not precisely distinguish posterior tibial tendinosis from other causes of similar symptoms. Standing on the toes is also painful in these patients. Conventional radiographs can be beneficial in assessing the extent of structural changes; however, it is not of diagnostic value. Injury to the posterior tibial tendon is confirmed by MRI. MR images show enlargement and thickening of the posterior tibial tendon with possible intermediate signal inside the tendon.

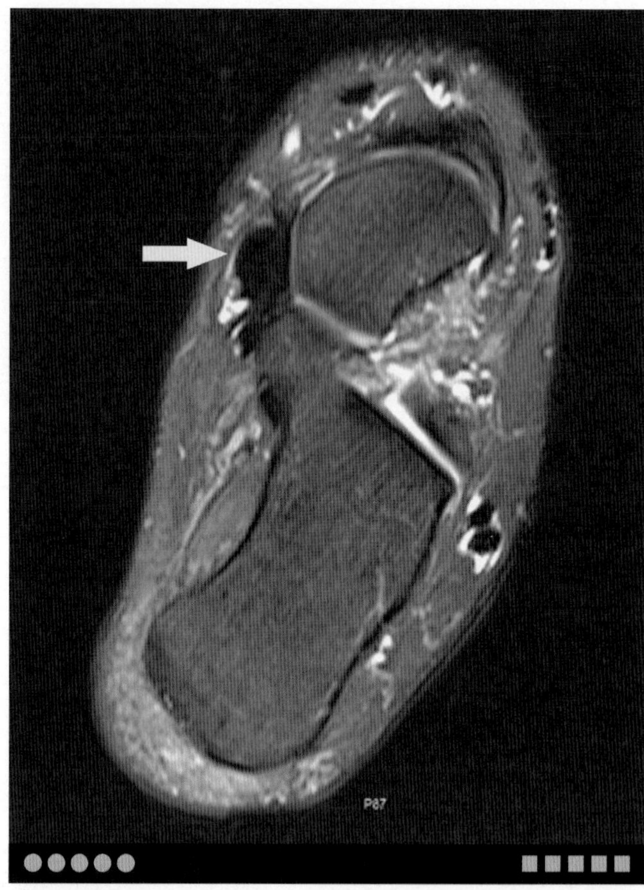

A. Chronic tendinosis of posterior tibial tendon: Axial T2-weighted fat-saturated image shows thickening and enlargement of the posterior tibial tendon (arrow). Mild synovitis of the peroneal tendons is also noted.

PEARLS

- **Degeneration of posterior tibial tendon resulting from long-standing problems.**
- **Pain over the medial malleolus is a common complaint of these patients.**
- **Swelling and tenderness over the medial malleolus and painful standing on the toes are observed in physical exams.**
- **Thickening and enlargement of the tendon with possible intermediate intrasubstance signals are observed on MR images.**

ADDITIONAL IMAGES

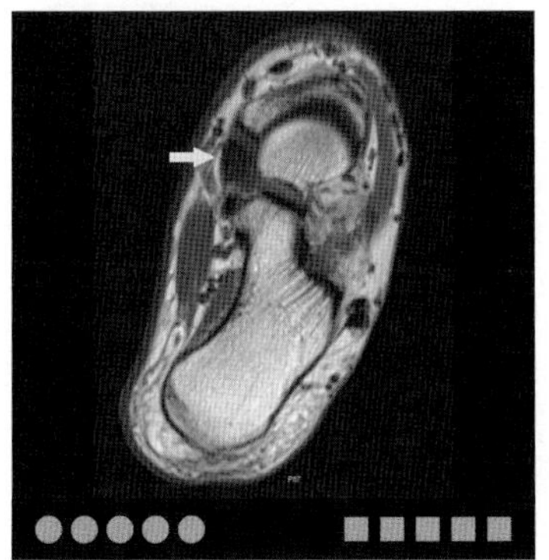

B. Chronic tendinosis of posterior tibial tendon: Axial T1-weighted image shows enlargement of the posterior tibial tendon (arrow).

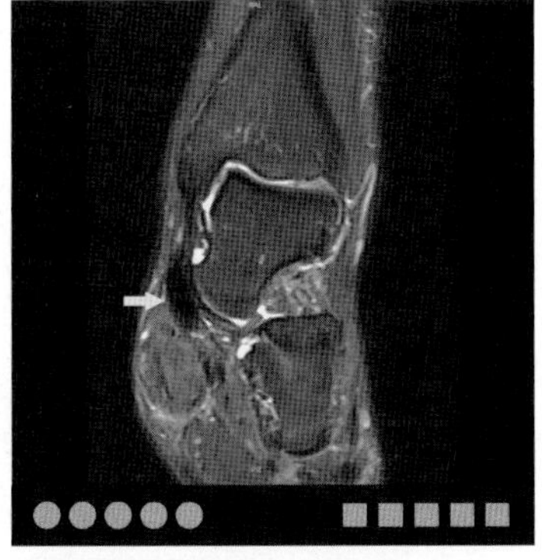

C. Chronic tendinosis of posterior tibial tendon: Coronal T2-weighted fat-saturated image shows marked thickening of the posterior tibial tendon (arrow).

DIFFERENTIAL DIAGNOSES IMAGES

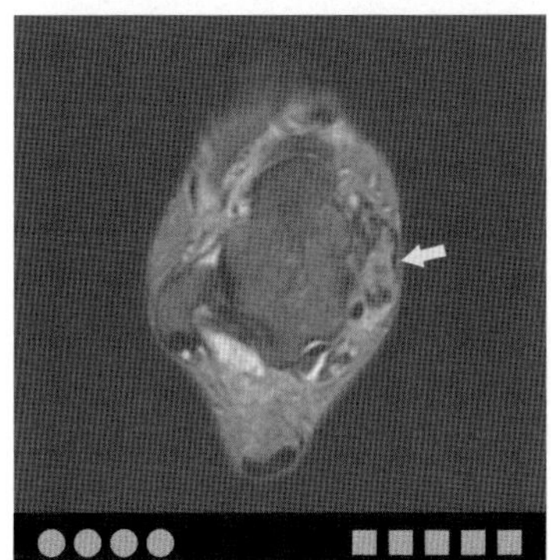

D. Split tear of posterior tibial tendon: Axial fat-saturated T2-weighted image shows increased signal in the posterior tibial tendon (arrow) caused by the split tear of this tendon.

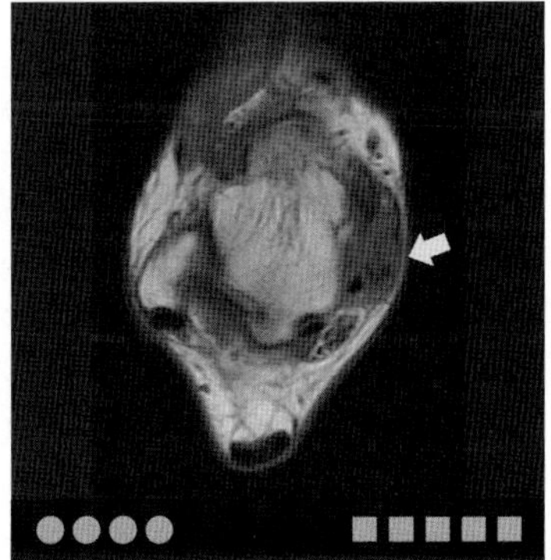

E. Split tear of posterior tibial tendon: Axial T1-weighted image shows enlargement of the posterior tibial tendon (arrow) with intrasubstance intermediate signal.

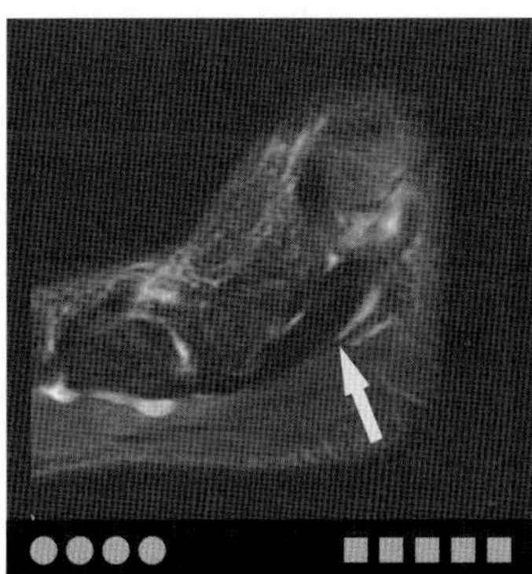

F. Split tear of posterior tibial tendon: Sagittal fat-saturated T2-weighted image shows thickening and enlargement of the posterior tibial tendon with intrasubstance signal caused by split tear.

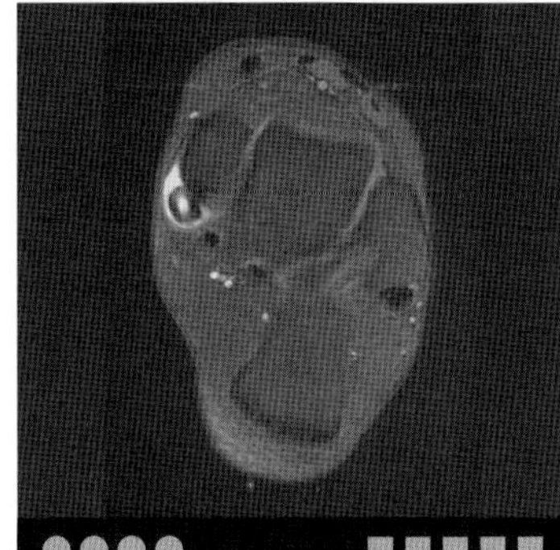

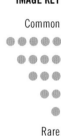

G. Tenosynovitis, tendinopathy, and intrasubstance tear of posterior tibial tendon: Axial MR T2-weighted fat-saturated image exhibits hyperintense fluid in the tendon sheath. Intratendinous focal high signal corresponds to tendinopathy and intrasubstance tear.

IMAGE KEY

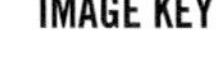

Common

Rare

Typical

Unusual

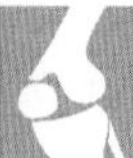

29–30 Lisfranc Fracture/Dislocation

Alipasha Adrangui and Jamshid Tehranzadeh

PRESENTATION

Pain and swelling in the midfoot.

FINDINGS

Coronal CT image of the foot shows comminuted fracture/dislocation of tarsometatarsal joints with divergence of second from the third metatarsal bony fragments seen at the Lisfranc joint level.

DIFFERENTIAL DIAGNOSES

- *Longitudinal stress injuries of mid-tarsal joints:* Usually severe mid-tarsal injury with a high incidence of associated fracture.
- *Cuboid fracture:* Stress fractures have linear low signal appearance on T1-weighted image associated with adjacent marrow edema on T2-weighted or STIR imaging.

COMMENTS

The patient is a 29-year-old man with midfoot trauma diagnosed with Lisfranc fracture. Lisfranc joint fracture/dislocations and sprains can be caused by high-energy forces in motor vehicle crashes, industrial accidents and falls from high places. There are three classifications for Lisfranc fracture: the homo-lateral which all five metatarsals are displaced in the same direction; the isolated which one or two metatarsals are displaced from the others; and the divergent form which metatarsals are displaced in sagittal and coronal planes. Diabetic foot is also a common cause of Lisfranc fracture/dislocation. On the radiographs, dislocation of the tarsometatarsal joint is indicated by the loss of in-line arrangement of the lateral margin of the first metatarsal base with the lateral edge of the medial (first) cuneiform and loss of in-line arrangement of the medial margin of the second metatarsal base with the medial edge of the middle (second) cuneiform in the weight-bearing AP view and the presence of small avulsed fragments (fleck sign), which are further indications of ligamentous injury and probable joint disruption. The lateral radiographic view of the foot may show a diagnostic "step-off," which means that the dorsal surface of the proximal second metatarsal is higher than the dorsal surface of the middle cuneiform. On an oblique view, the medial edge of the fourth metatarsal base should be aligned with the medial edge of the cuboid. The CT scan is useful in formulating the surgical treatment plans. Open reduction and internal fixation is necessary for management; closed reduction would not maintain the alignment and leads to osteoarthritis.

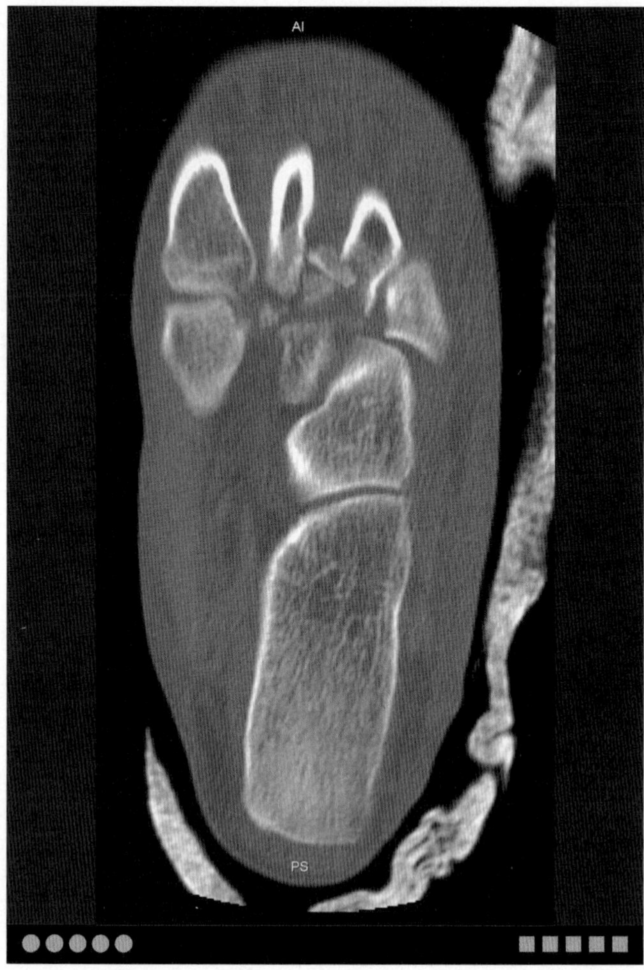

A. Lisfranc fracture/dislocation: Coronal CT image of the foot shows comminuted fracture/dislocation of tarsometatarsal joints. Note divergence of second from the third metatarsal bony fragments seen at the Lisfranc joint level.

PEARLS

- **A weight-bearing radiograph is necessary, because a non-weight-bearing view may not reveal the injury.**
- **Besides trauma, diabetic foot is a common cause of Lisfranc fracture/dislocation.**
- **Routine CT scan through the midfoot is helpful to visualize any bony injury to the plantar bony structures. CT scan allows a three-dimensional assessment of surrounding joint stability.**
- **The three major complications of this injury are nonanatomic reduction or alignment, posttraumatic arthritis and pain with weight bearing.**

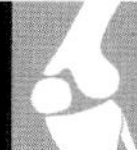

ADDITIONAL IMAGES

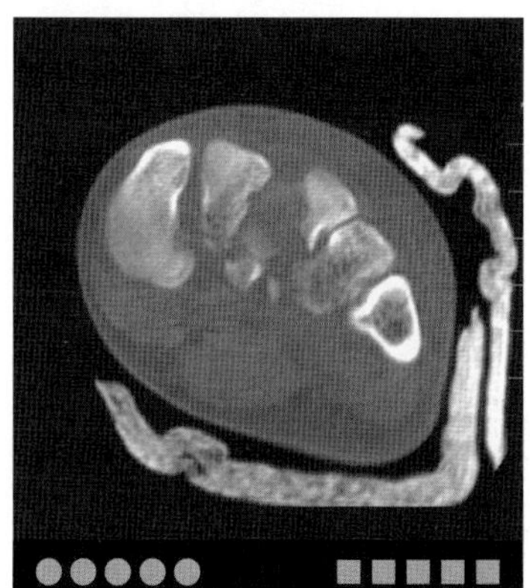

B. Lisfranc fracture/dislocation: Axial CT image shows divergence of the second from the third rays with bony fragments in between.

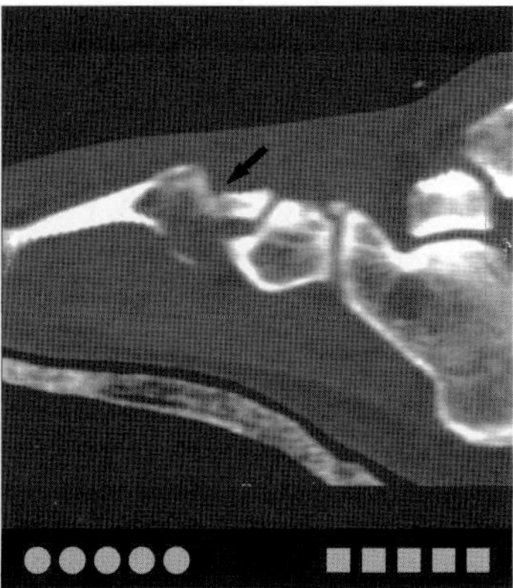

C. Lisfranc fracture/dislocation: Sagittal CT of the ankle shows a big step off at level of the tarsometatarsal joints (arrow).

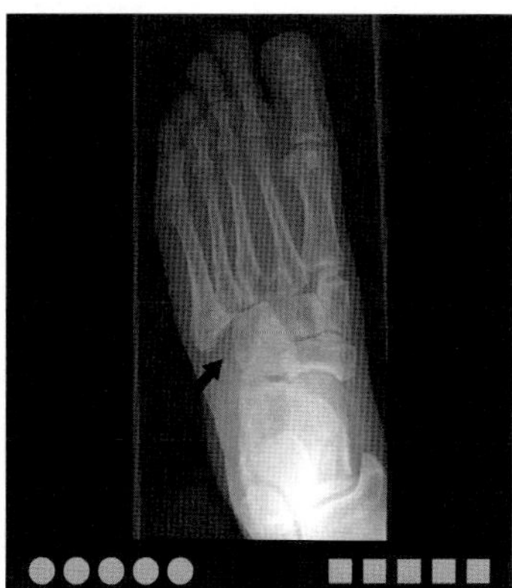

D. Lisfranc fracture/dislocation: AP radiograph of the same patient shows divergence of the second from the third metatarsal. Note bony fracture fragments at the tarsometatarsal joints. Dislocation of the cuboid fifth metatarsal joint is obvious (arrow).

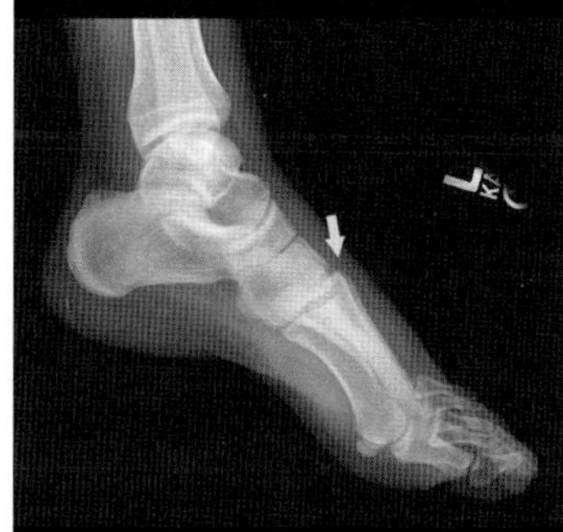

E. Lisfranc fracture/dislocation: Lateral radiograph of the foot shows step off at the tarsometatarsal joints (arrow).

IMAGE KEY

Common

Rare

Typical

Unusual

DIFFERENTIAL DIAGNOSES IMAGES

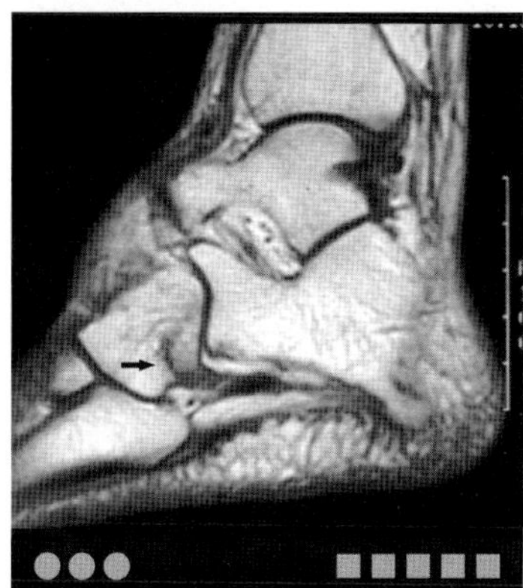

F. Stress fracture of cuboid bone: Sagittal proton density image of the ankle shows stress fracture of cuboid (arrow).

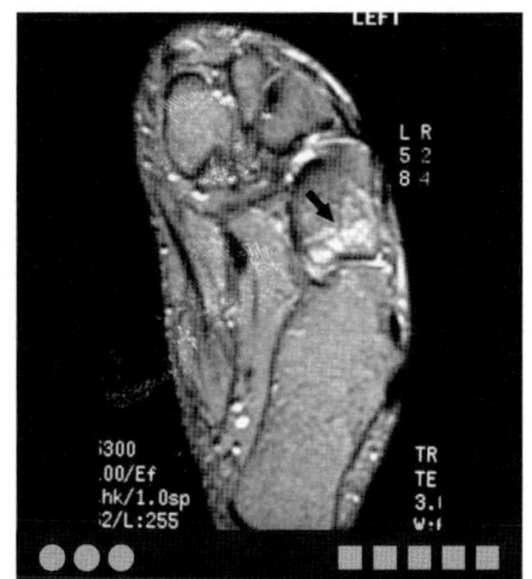

G. Stress fracture of cuboid bone: Coronal T2-weighted image shows increased marrow signal at the site of the stress fracture of cuboid (arrow).

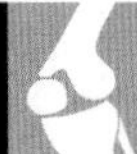

29–31 Stress Fracture of Metatarsal Bone

Rosemary J. Klecker

PRESENTATION

Forefoot pain following training for marathon

FINDINGS

MR images show bone marrow edema in the mid-shaft of the second metatarsal and adjacent soft tissues edema.

DIFFERENTIAL DIAGNOSES

- *Osteomyelitis:* Unlike a stress fracture, a discrete fracture line is not present. Instead there is history of diabetes or penetrating injury.
- *Freiberg's infraction:* Initially restricted to the dorsal subchondral bone. Imaging findings of sclerosis and flattening of the metatarsal head are diagnostic.
- *Tumor:* Unlike stress a fracture there is associated soft tissue mass or bony destruction.

COMMENTS

The patient is a 32-year-old woman with forefoot pain. Patient has been training for upcoming marathon. Stress fractures are fatigue fractures that occur as the result of abnormal stresses placed on normal bone. These differ from insufficiency fractures that occur when normal stresses are placed on abnormal bone. Stress fractures are commonly seen in runners, gymnasts, ballet dancers, and military recruits. When present in the foot, stress fractures most commonly occur in the second and third metatarsals but may be seen in other bones of the foot including the cuneiforms and cuboid bones. Conditions that result in altered weight bearing such as hallux valgus deformity, recent surgery of the foot, or flat foot deformity, increase the risk of developing a stress fracture. On MR imaging a stress fracture is identified by edema signal in the medullary cavity of the bone associated with a nondisplaced fracture line which is a band of low signal intensity contiguous with the cortex on both T1-weighted and on T2-weighted images. Edema may be present in the adjacent soft tissues. A stress reaction or phenomenon is a precursor to the stress fracture and presents on MR imaging as edema signal of the marrow without a fracture line. The imaging characteristics of a stress reaction are nonspecific and correlation with clinical findings is essential for making a correct diagnosis. A stress reaction may progress to a stress fracture or may resolve if recognized early and treatment is initiated.

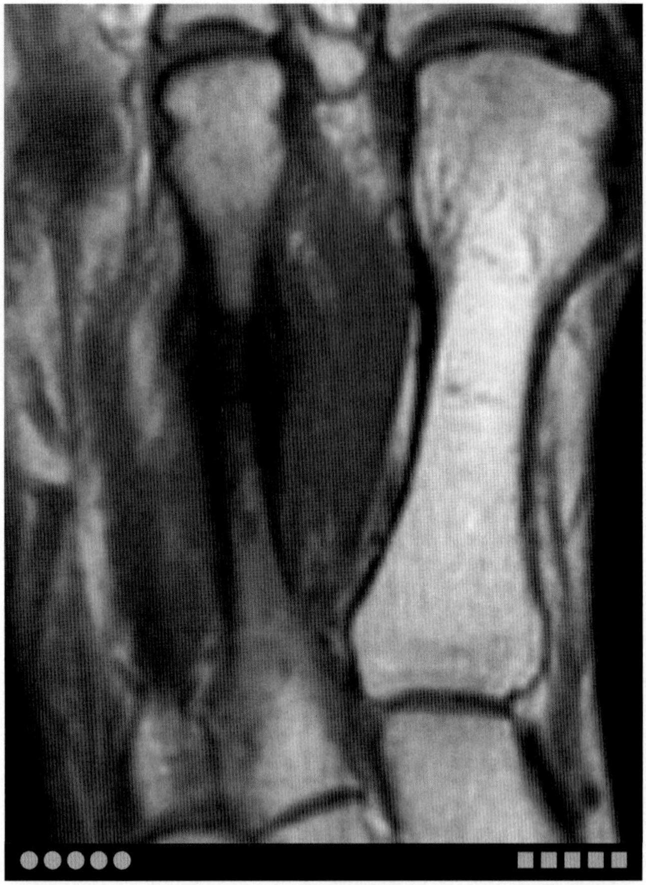

A. Stress fracture: Axial T1-weighted image of a stress fracture in the mid-diaphysis of the second metatarsal with marrow edema and periosteal reaction and thickening.

PEARLS

- **In the foot, stress fractures are most commonly seen in the second through fourth metatarsals and, less commonly, in the cuneiforms and cuboid bones.**
- **Stress fractures occur secondary to abnormal stresses placed on normal bone and anything that alters the weight-bearing mechanics of the bone which predispose the bone to a stress fracture.**
- **The diagnosis of a stress fracture is made on MR imaging by a band of T1 and T2 low signal intensity contiguous with the cortex.**

ADDITIONAL IMAGES

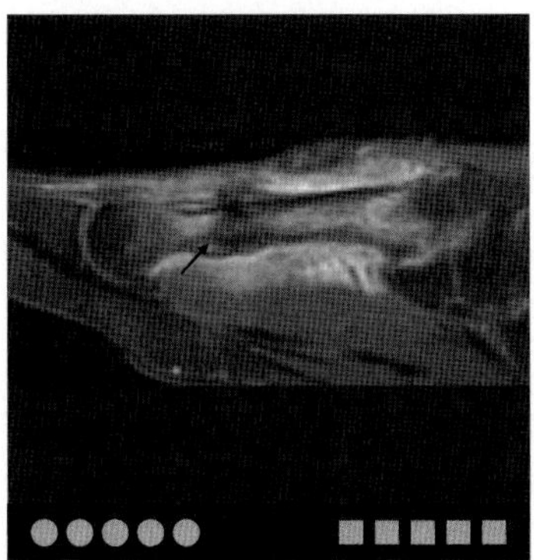

B. Stress fracture: Sagittal STIR-weighted image shows the fracture line (arrow) and associated marrow edema and cortical reaction. There is edema of the surrounding soft tissues.

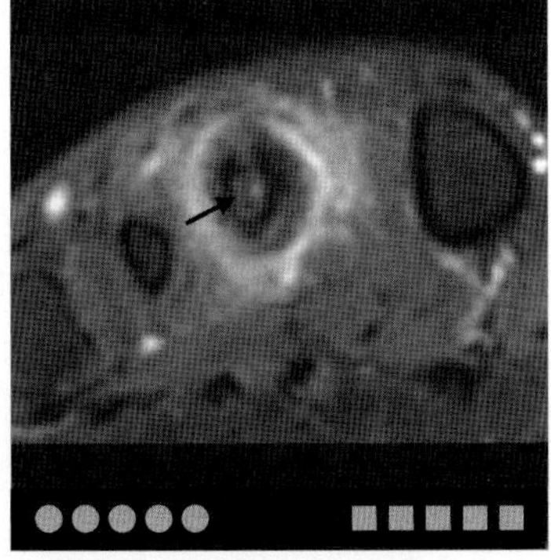

C. Stress fracture: Coronal T2-weighted image of the second metatarsal shows the diffuse cortical thickening and periosteal reaction. The fracture line is seen centrally (arrow).

DIFFERENTIAL DIAGNOSES IMAGES

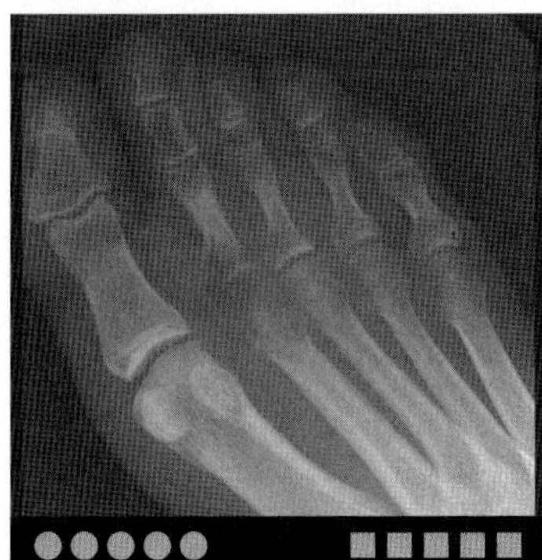

D. Osteomyelitis: Radiograph of the forefoot shows periarticular osteopenia with cortical destruction at the second MTP joint.

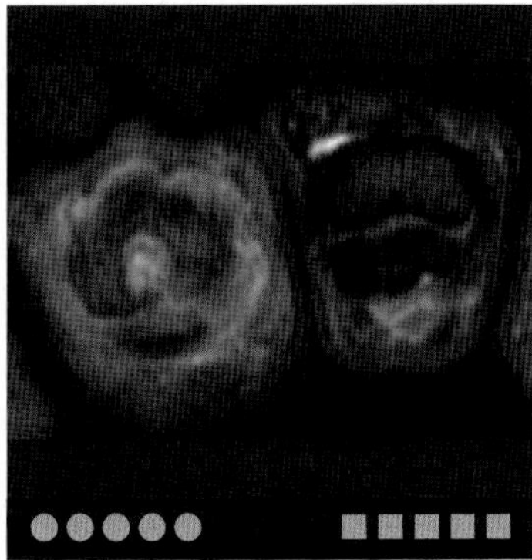

E. Osteomyelitis: Coronal T2-weighted image of the third metatarsal shows an intraosseous abscess with a sinus tract through the plantar cortex.

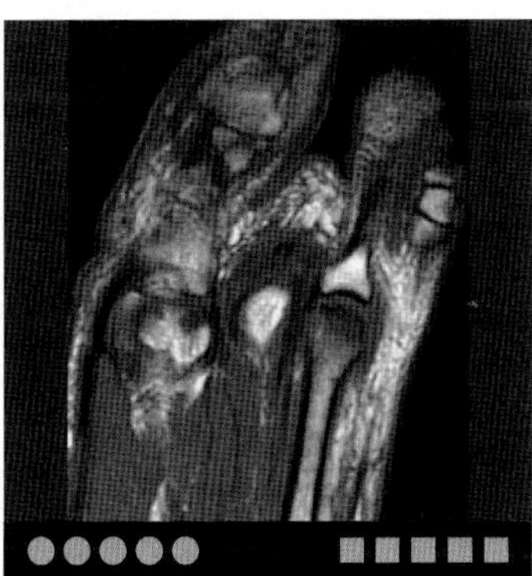

F. Freiberg's infraction: Axial T1-weighted MR image shows focal, well-marginated sclerosis of the second metatarsal head.

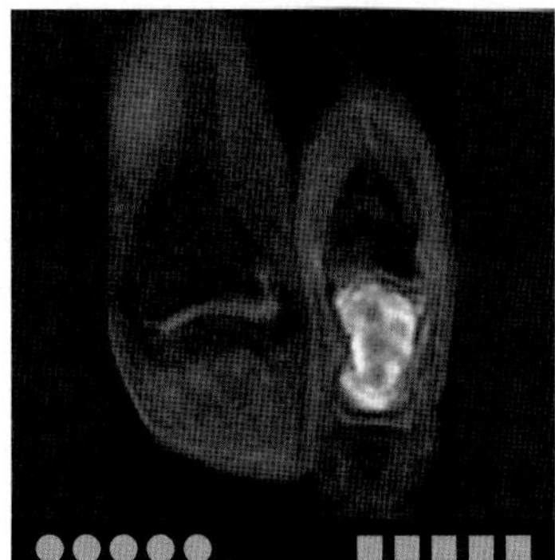

G. Enchondroma: Axial T2-weighted image of the second toe shows an expansile lesion of high and intermediate signal intensity in the proximal phalanx. MR and radiographic findings are compatible with an enchondroma.

IMAGE KEY

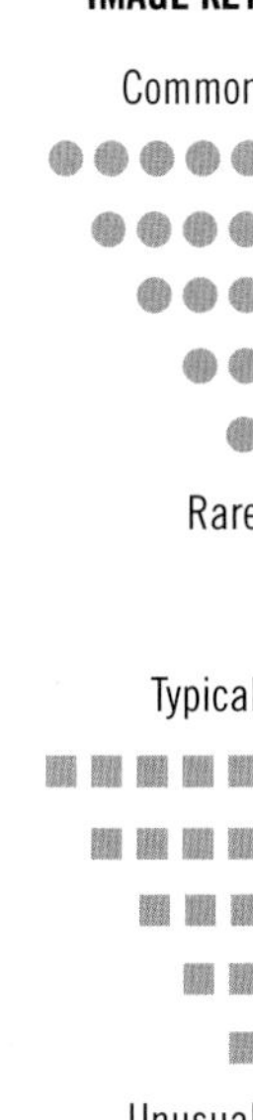

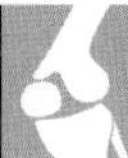

29–32 Avascular Necrosis of Medial Sesamoid Bone of the Great Toe

Mohammad Reza Hayeri and Jamshid Tehranzadeh

PRESENTATION

Pain in the great toe

FINDINGS

On MRI increased signal intensity on T2/STIR images and decreased signal intensity on T1-weighted images are noted. Cortical irregularity, bone collapse, and cysts formation are seen in a later stage of osteonecrosis.

DIFFERENTIAL DIAGNOSES

- *Freiberg disease:* This is osteochondrosis of the head of the second or third metatarsal bone caused by vascular compromise or trauma insult.
- *Stress fracture:* Also known as "fatigue fracture" is the result of overuse injury. The weight-bearing bones are the most common site of these fractures.

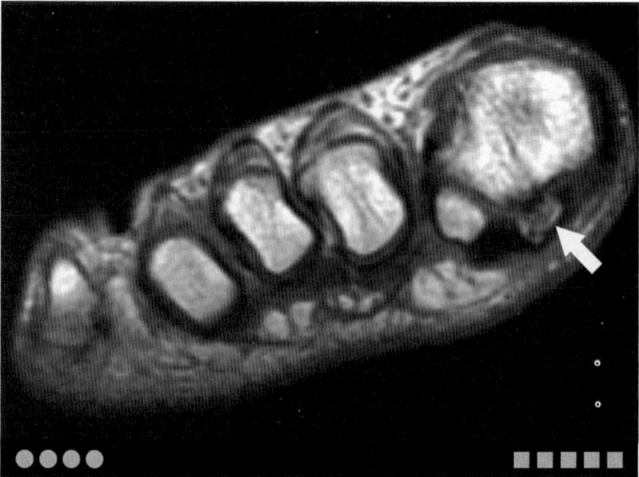

A. AVN of the medial sesamoid of the great toe: Axial T1-weighted image of the forefoot shows low signal intensity and partial collapse of the medial sesamoid indicating AVN caused by stress fracture (arrow).

COMMENTS

Sesamoid bones are normal radiologic finding and are generally asymptomatic; however, occasionally they might become painful as a result of fracture, degenerative changes, avascular necrosis, and irritation or impingement of adjacent soft tissue. Sesamoid bones are partially or totally embedded in the substance of a corresponding tendon. Being adjacent to synovial bursae; they can also get involved in inflammatory conditions such as rheumatoid arthritis. They act as a part of gliding mechanism that protects tendons by reducing friction. The medial and lateral hallux sesamoids are embedded within the medial and lateral slips of the flexor hallucis brevis tendon at the level of the first metatarsal head. They are separated from each other by a small bony ridge, the crista, on the plantar aspect of the metatarsal head. The medial sesamoid is further stabilized by attachments of the abductor hallucis tendon, while the lateral sesamoid receives attachments from the adductor hallucis tendon. Chronic stress may cause painful conditions in the hallux sesamoids, and is most commonly associated with chondromalacia, osteochondritis, osteonecrosis, and stress fracture. All these entities are part of the same pathologic spectrum, share a common etiological factor, and present clinically with a painful syndrome that has been termed sesamoiditis. Unlike stress fracture which affects medial sesamoid more commonly, lateral sesamoid is more prone to osteonecrosis. On MRI increased signal intensity on T2/STIR images and decreased or normal signal intensity on T1-weighted images are noted.

PEARLS

- **The medial and lateral hallux sesamoids are embedded within the medial and lateral slips of the flexor hallucis brevis tendon at the level of the first metatarsal head.**
- **Sesamoid bones might become painful as a result of fracture, degenerative changes, avascular necrosis, and irritation or impingement of adjacent soft tissue.**
- **Osteonecrosis is more common in lateral sesamoid bone while stress fracture is more common in the medial sesamoid bone.**
- **MRI shows high signal intensity on T2/STIR images, with decreased or normal signal intensity on T1-weighted images.**

ADDITIONAL IMAGES

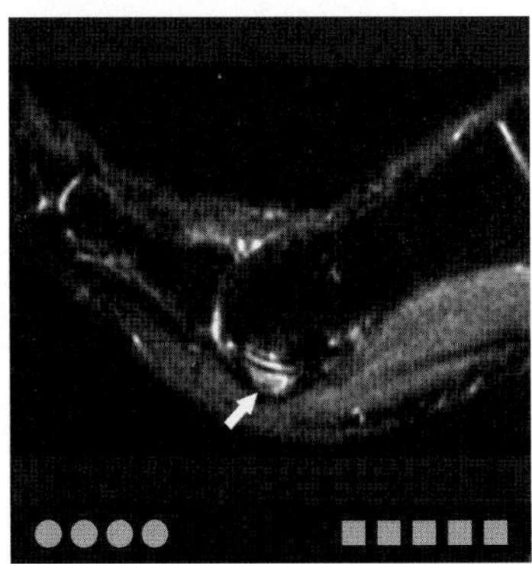

B. AVN of the medial sesamoid of the great toe: Sagittal fat-saturated T2-weighted image shows bright signal of the medial sesamoid of the great toe (arrow) (same patient as image A).

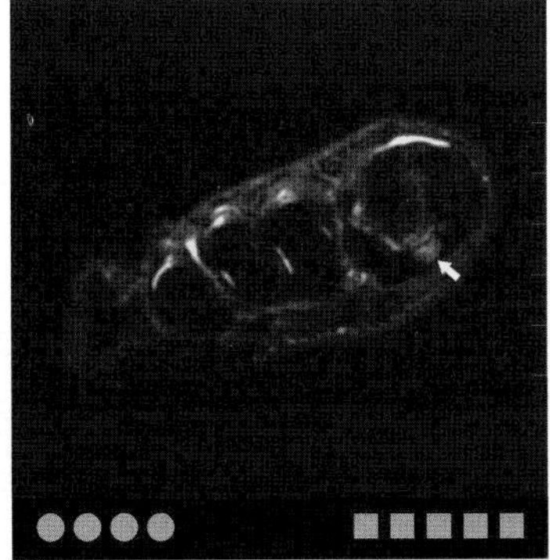

C. AVN of the medial sesamoid of the great toe: Axial fat-saturated T2-weighted image shows increased signal intensity in the medial sesamoid of the great toe (arrow) (same patient as image A).

DIFFERENTIAL DIAGNOSES IMAGES

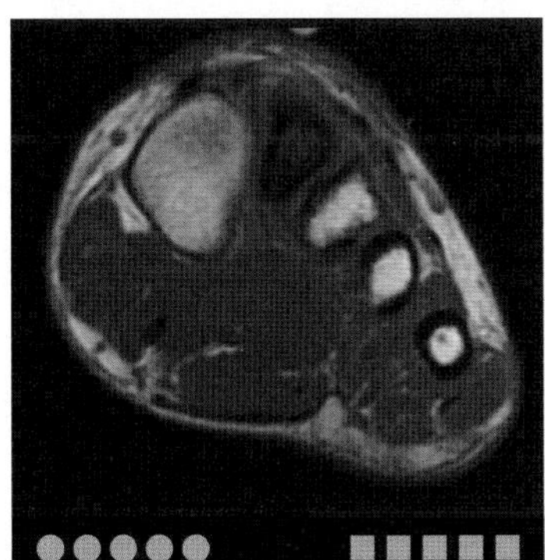

D. Stress fracture of the second metatarsal: Axial T1-weighted image shows low signal intensity of the marrow of the second metatarsal as a result of marrow edema secondary to stress fracture.

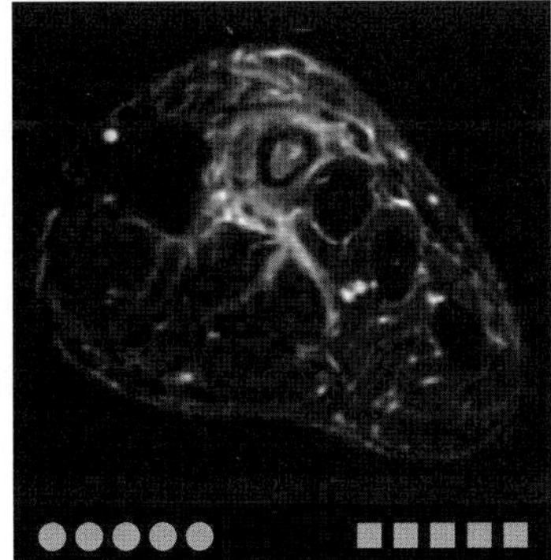

E. Stress fracture of the second metatarsal: Axial fat-saturated T2 image shows marrow edema of the second metatarsal associated with surrounding soft tissue swelling secondary to stress fracture.

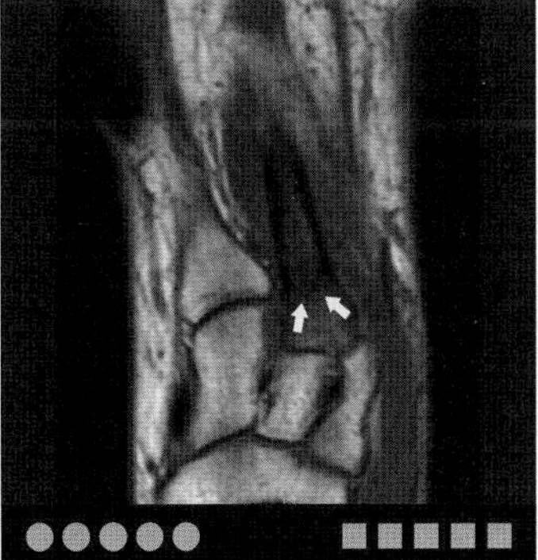

F. Stress fracture of the second metatarsal: Coronal T1-weighted image shows low signal of the second metatarsal as a result of marrow edema with linear darker signal (arrow) indicating stress fracture.

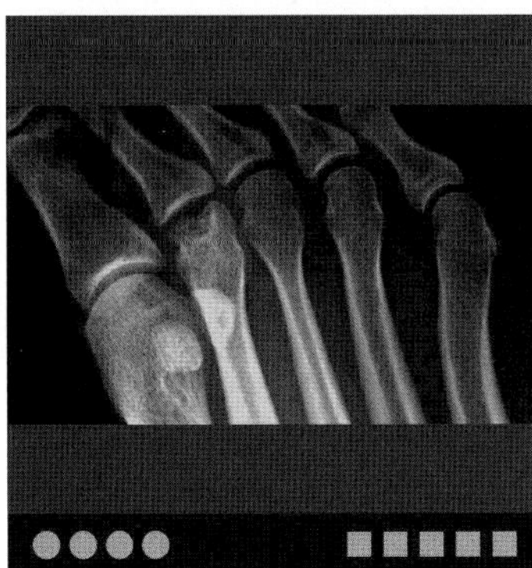

G. Osteochondritis dissecans as a result of Freiberg disease: Oblique radiograph of the forefoot shows osteochondral fracture with bony defect and sclerosis of the second metatarsal head because of osteochondrosis or AVN (Freiberg disease).

IMAGE KEY

Common

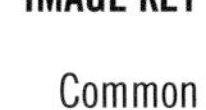

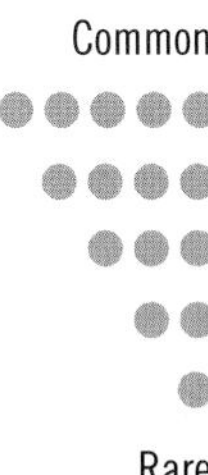

Rare

Typical

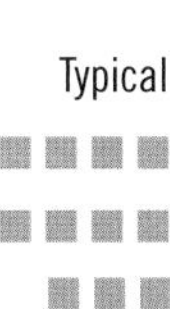

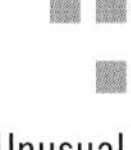

Unusual

Chapter 30

Congenital, Systemic and Metabolic Diseases

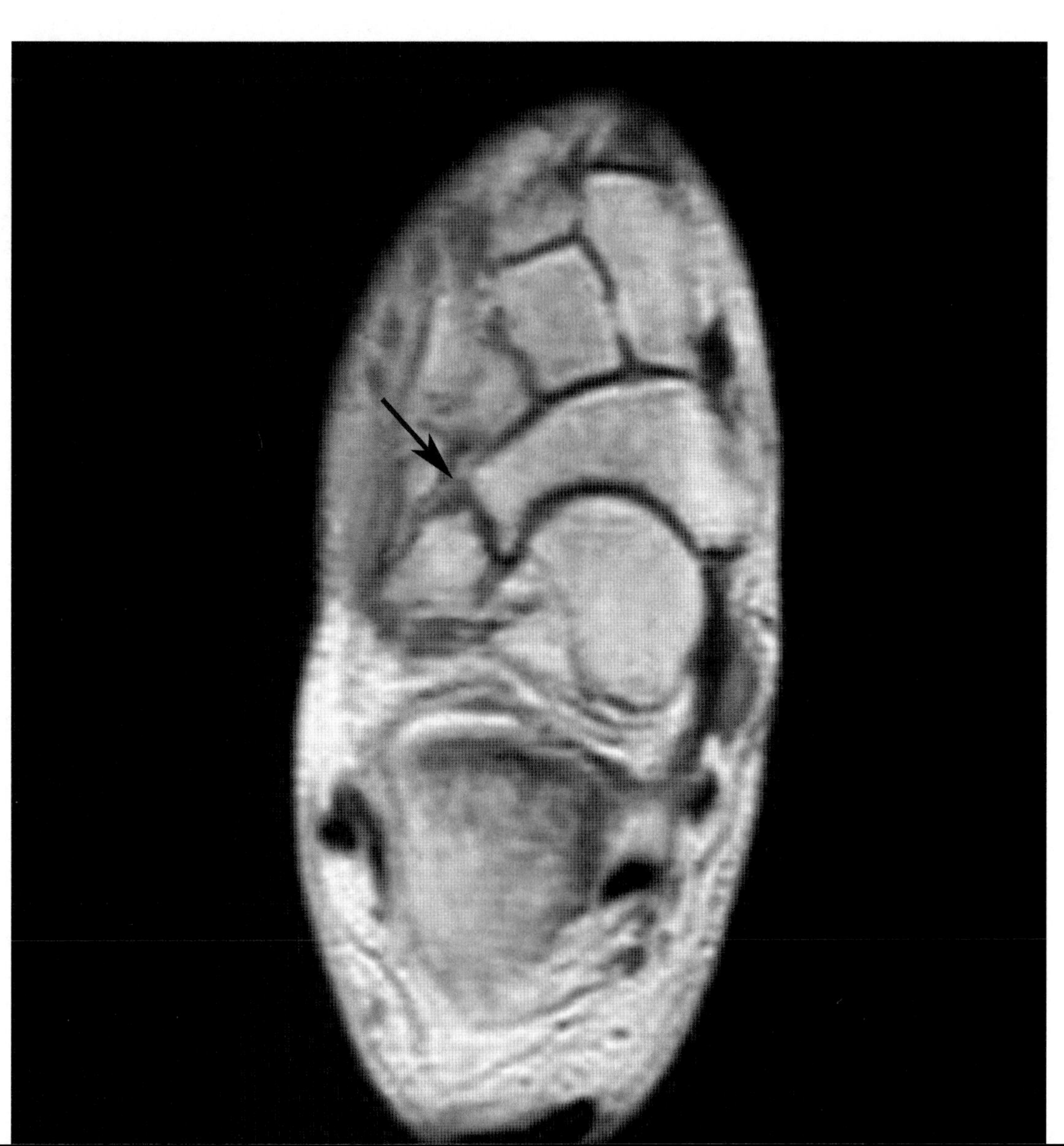

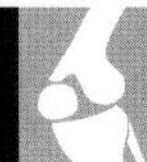

30–1 Fibrous Calcaneonavicular Coalition

Amilcare Gentili

PRESENTATION

Foot pain

FINDINGS

Fibrous calcaneonavicular coalition is noted with marked narrowing of the space between the calcaneus and navicular.

DIFFERENTIAL DIAGNOSES

- *Talonavicular coalition:* This is relatively rare.
- *Pes planus:* This is often present in patients with tarsal coalition, but can be caused by other pathology such as posterior tibial tendon dysfunction.
- *Osteoarthrosis:* Primary osteoarthrosis of the talonavicular and subtalar joint is uncommon; osteoarthrosis of these joints is often caused by pes planus, prior trauma or coalition.
- *Subtalar coalition:* This type and calcaneonavicular coalitions are the most common forms of tarsal coalitions. Subtalar coalition is usually seen at mid-subtalar joint (Sustentaculum tali joint) and may be associated with rigid flat foot.

COMMENTS

The patient is 25-year-old with foot pain. Tarsal coalitions involving the calcaneonavicular or talocalcaneal joints account for more than 90% of tarsal coalitions. Calcaneal navicular coalitions were considered more frequent than subtalar coalition probably because subtalar coalition is more difficult to diagnose on radiographs. With the use of cross sectional imaging, calcaneonavicular coalitions appear to be the second most common type of coalition. Calcaneonavicular coalition may present at ages between 8 and 12 when bony fusion occurs, but may remain asymptomatic and be found as an incidental finding on imaging performed for unrelated reasons. Calcaneonavicular coalition is often bilateral. The symptoms and secondary signs are often less severe than in subtalar coalition. A classic sign is elongation of the anterior process of the calcaneus that has been likened to the elongated nose of an anteater. Calcaneonavicular coalitions are best visualized on sagittal and axial MR images. Tarsal coalitions are subclassified as fibrous, cartilaginous, or osseous on the basis of the tissue of the abnormal bridging. In osseous coalition, there is bone marrow bridging the space between the calcaneus and navicular bones. In nonosseous coalition, the space between the calcaneus and navicular bones is narrowed. In fibrous coalitions, low signal intensity is present in the space between the calcaneus and navicular bones on all sequences. In cartilaginous coalition, signal intensity similar to fluid is present in the coalition. On fluid sensitive sequences, high signal intensity may be present in the bone adjacent to the fused joint secondary to stress reaction.

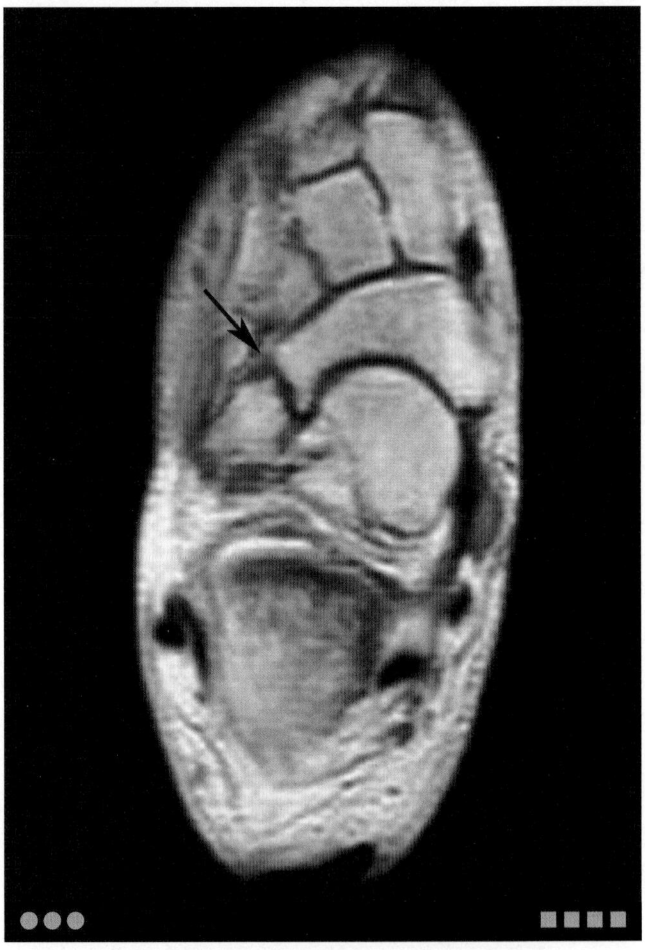

A. Fibrous calcaneonavicular coalition: Axial proton density image shows marked narrowing between the calcaneus and navicular (arrow).

PEARLS

- **The second most common type of tarsal coalition after subtalar coalition.**
- **Abnormal bone marrow signal is often present in the bone adjacent to the coalition.**
- **Best seen on sagittal and axial images.**

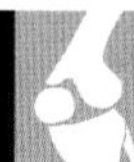

ADDITIONAL IMAGES

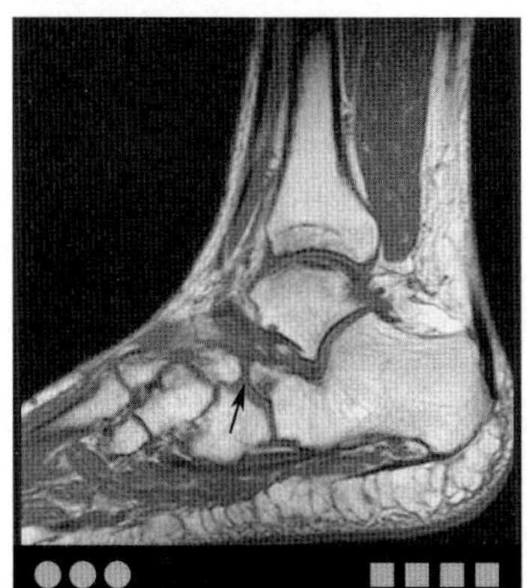

B. Fibrous calcaneonavicular coalition: Sagittal T1-weighted image shows marked narrowing between the calcaneus and navicular (arrow) with reactive changes in the underlying bone.

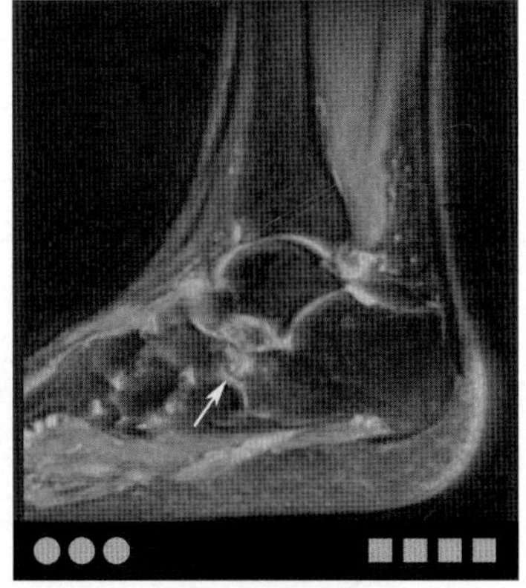

C. Fibrous calcaneonavicular coalition: Sagittal T2-weighted fat-suppressed image shows marked narrowing between the calcaneus and navicular with reactive changes in the underlying bone (arrow).

DIFFERENTIAL DIAGNOSES IMAGES

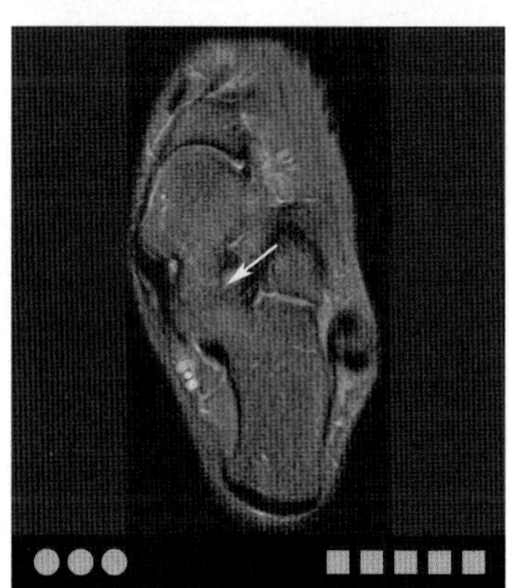

D. Osseous talocalcaneal coalition: Axial T2-weighted fat-suppressed image shows bony fusion (arrow) of the sustentaculum tali with the talus. No bone marrow edema is present.

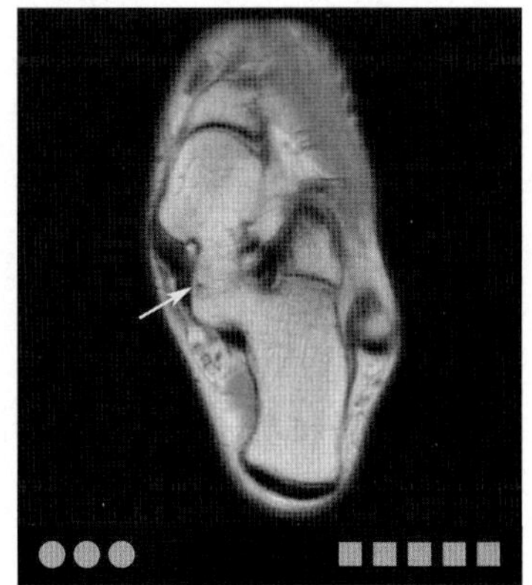

E. Osseous talocalcaneal coalition: Axial T1-weighted image shows bony fusion (arrow) of the sustentaculum tali with the talus.

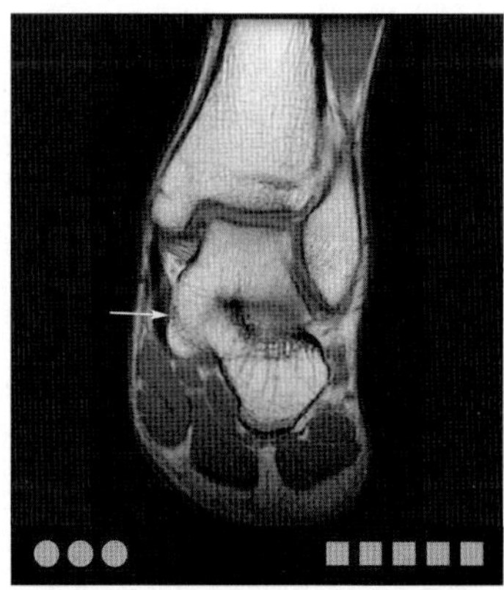

F. Osseous talocalcaneal coalition: Coronal T1-weighted image shows bony fusion (arrow) of the sustentaculum tali with the talus.

IMAGE KEY

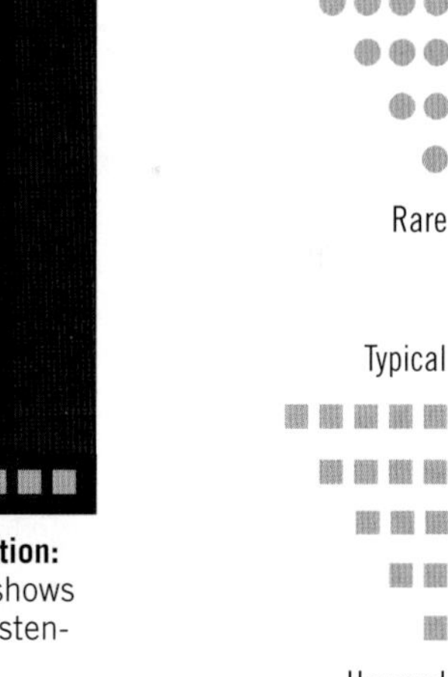

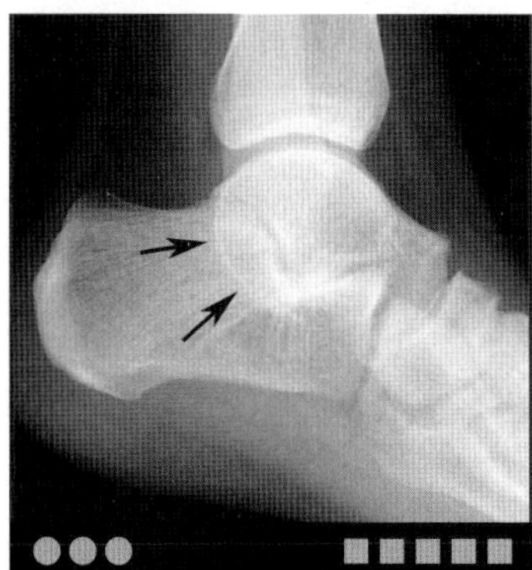

G. Osseous talocalcaneal coalition: Lateral radiograph of the ankle shows a "C" sign (black arrows).

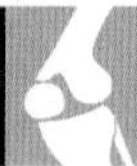

30–2 Symptomatic Accessory Navicular

Tod G. Abrahams

PRESENTATION

Medial foot pain

FINDINGS

Bone marrow edema in the bones adjacent to the synchondrosis associated with the accessory navicular.

DIFFERENTIAL DIAGNOSES

- Cornuate navicular bone: Elongated navicular bone
- Os tibiale externum: Normal sesamoid.
- Medial tuberosity fracture: Best seen on CT.

COMMENTS

The patient is a 40-year-old female with medial foot pain. Normal variants in skeletal development may be the cause of patient symptoms. There are three variants involving the medial aspect of the navicular. Type 1 or os tibiale externum is a sesamoid in the posterior tibialis tendon and has no cartilaginous connection to the navicular tuberosity. It accounts for approximately 30% of accessory navicular bones and are generally asymptomatic. Type 2 is a secondary ossification center and is united with the tuberosity by a cartilaginous or fibrocartilaginous bar. This type accounts for approximately 70% of accessory navicular bones and is the dominant type in symptomatic patients. Type 3 represents a fused type 2 accessory navicular and as such produces a cornuate process (cornuate naviculare). The prevalence of accessory navicular bones is in the range of 4% to14% and when symptomatic occurs more often in females. The most frequent complaint is medial foot pain and tenderness associated with soft tissue swelling. The cause of pain is likely the result of repetitive tension and/or shearing stress secondary to the functional pull of the posterior tibialis tendon across the synchondrosis. Radiograph or CT will show the accessory bone with an irregular and generally broad based connection to the tuberosity. MR imaging in symptomatic patients shows bone marrow edema, which is most prominent in the bone adjacent to the synchondrosis and may be seen in the synchondrosis itself. Adjacent soft tissue swelling as well as posterior tibialis tendon pathology may be present.

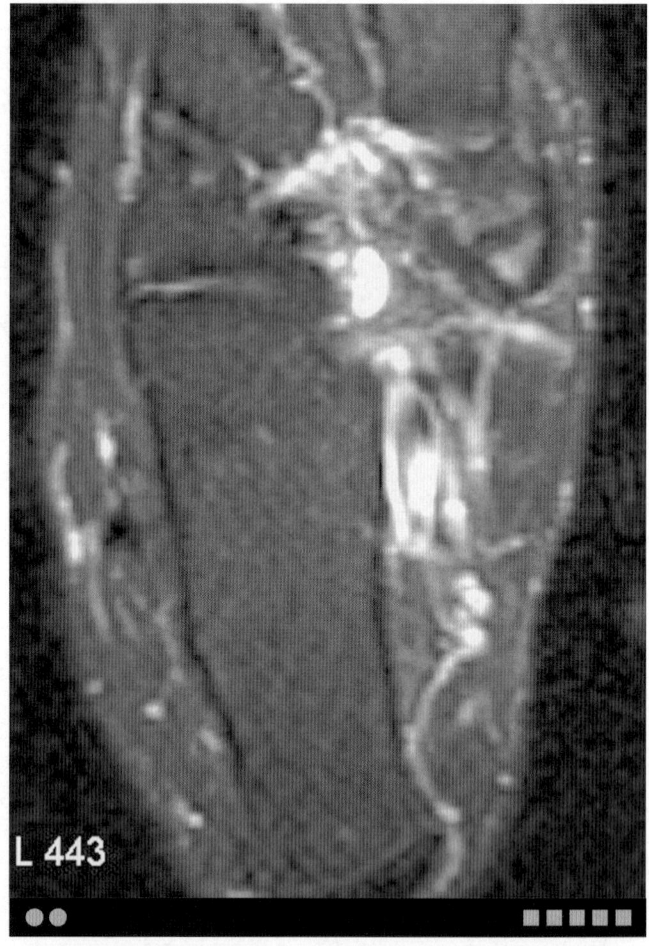

A. Symptomatic accessory navicular: Axial T2-weighted fat-saturated image shows bone marrow edema in the accessory navicular bone and medial tuberosity.

PEARLS

- **Normal variants may be symptomatic.**
- **The synchondrosis associated with an accessory navicular is predisposed to tension and/or shearing stress and can lead to medial foot pain.**
- **MR imaging is the modality of choice and shows bone marrow edema in the bones and soft tissues adjacent to the synchondrosis.**

ADDITIONAL IMAGES

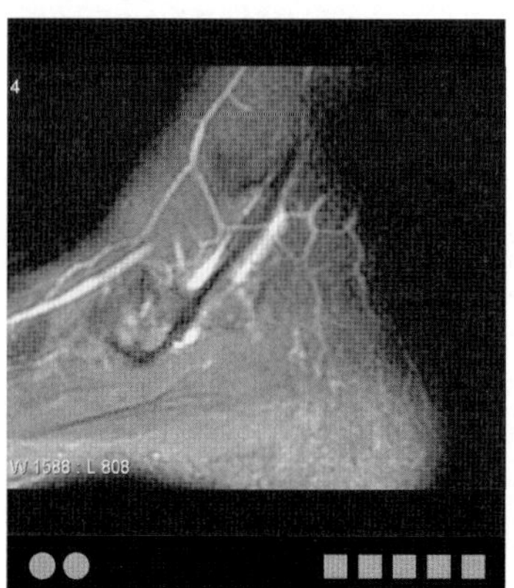

B. Symptomatic accessory navicular: Sagittal T2-weighted fat-saturated image shows insertion of the posterior tibialis tendon and bone marrow edema in the accessory navicular and adjacent tuberosity.

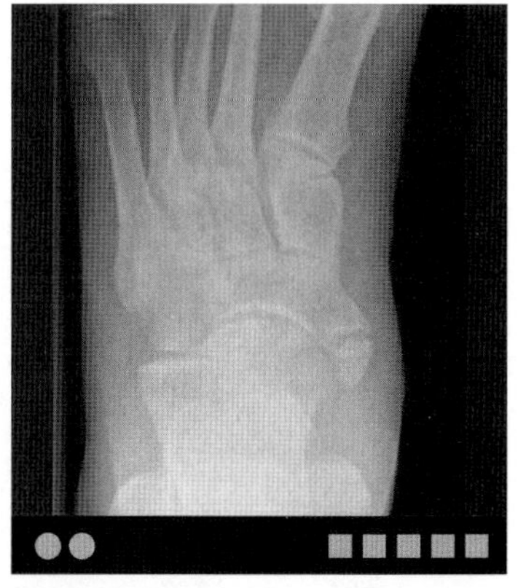

C. Symptomatic accessory navicular: Radiograph shows the anomalous articulation of the accessory bone.

DIFFERENTIAL DIAGNOSES IMAGES

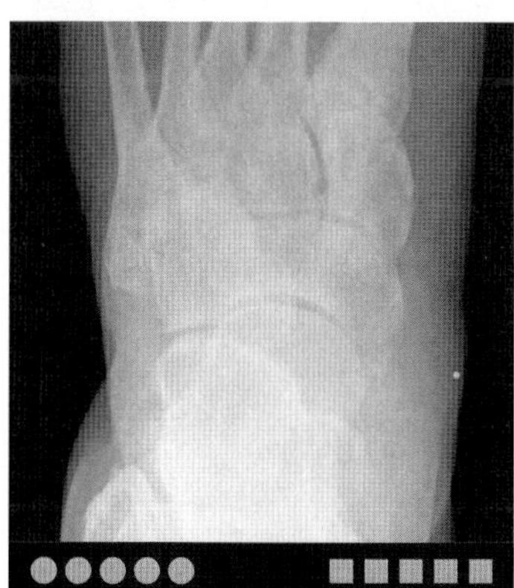

D. Os tibiale externum: Radiograph shows an os tibiale externum as a rounded ossicle with no connection to the medial navicular tuberosity.

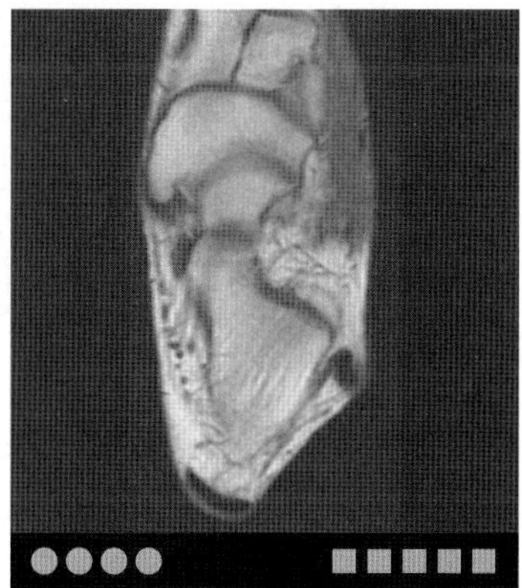

E. Cornuate naviculare bone: MR image shows a cornuate navicular bone with prominence of the posteromedial margin of the tuberosity.

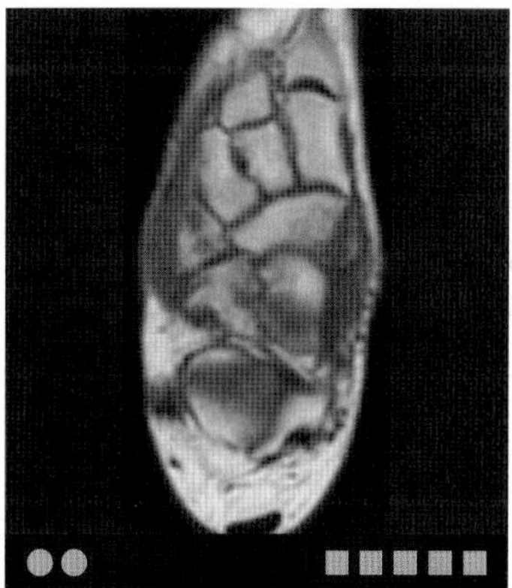

F. Fracture of navicular bone: Axial T1-weighted image shows fracture of the medial navicular tuberosity. The fracture plane is sagittally oriented and the medial aspect of the navicular is not prominent.

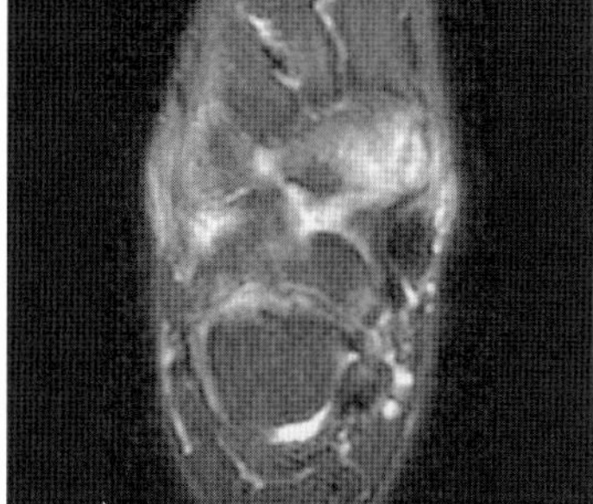

G. Fracture of navicular bone: Axial T2-weighted MR image shows the medial tuberosity fracture with surrounding edema.

IMAGE KEY

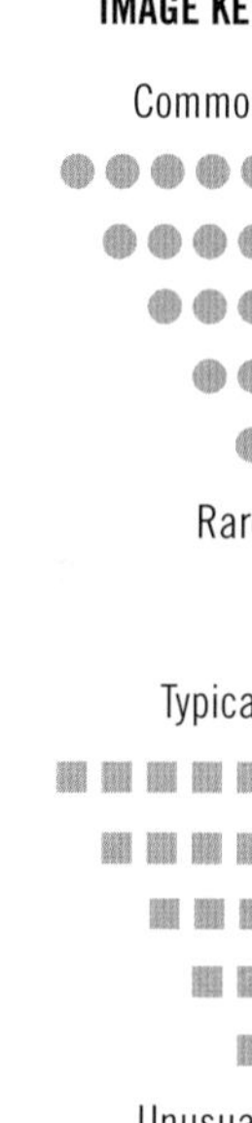

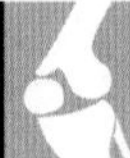

30–3 Subtalar (Talocalcaneal) Coalition

Amilcare Gentili

PRESENTATION

Hindfoot pain

FINDINGS

MR images show bony bridge between the sustentaculum tali and the middle facet of the talus.

DIFFERENTIAL DIAGNOSES

- *Talonavicular coalition:* Best seen on lateral view.
- *Pes Planus:* It is often present in patients with tarsal coalition, but can be caused by other pathology such as posterior tibial tendon dysfunction.
- *Osteoarthrosis:* Primary osteoarthrosis of the talonavicular and subtalar joint is uncommon. Osteoarthrosis of these joints is often caused by pes planus, prior trauma, or coalition.

COMMENTS

Coalitions involving the calcaneonavicular or talocalcaneal joints account for more than 90% of tarsal coalitions. Subtalar coalitions were considered less frequent than calcaneonavicular coalitions. Cross-sectional imaging has revealed that the subtalar coalition appears to be the most common type of coalition, is more frequent in males, and usually presents during the second decade of life. It is bilateral in 50% of cases, and classic presentation is stiffness of the foot accentuated by standing and walking, pes planus deformity, peroneal spasm, and limitation of inversion and eversion. The pain is not caused by the fusion itself, but is related to alteration in the motion of the talocalcaneonavicular complex. Subtalar coalition usually involves the middle facet of the subtalar joint. The anterior and posterior facets are rarely involved. Limitation of motion of the subtalar joint can cause adaptive changes of the ankle joint; the talar dome becomes hemispherical in both the anterior-posterior and medio-lateral dimensions, and the tibial plafond becomes concave giving the ankle joint a "ball-and-socket" appearance. Tarsal coalitions are subclassified as fibrous, cartilaginous, or osseous on the basis of the tissue of the abnormal bridging. In osseous coalition, there is bone marrow bridging the fused joint. In nonosseous coalition, the joint space is narrowed and more oblique than normal. In fibrous coalitions, low signal intensity is present in the joint space on all sequences. In cartilaginous coalitions, signal intensity similar to fluid is present in the joint space. On fluid sensitive sequences, high signal intensity may be present in the bone adjacent to the fused joint.

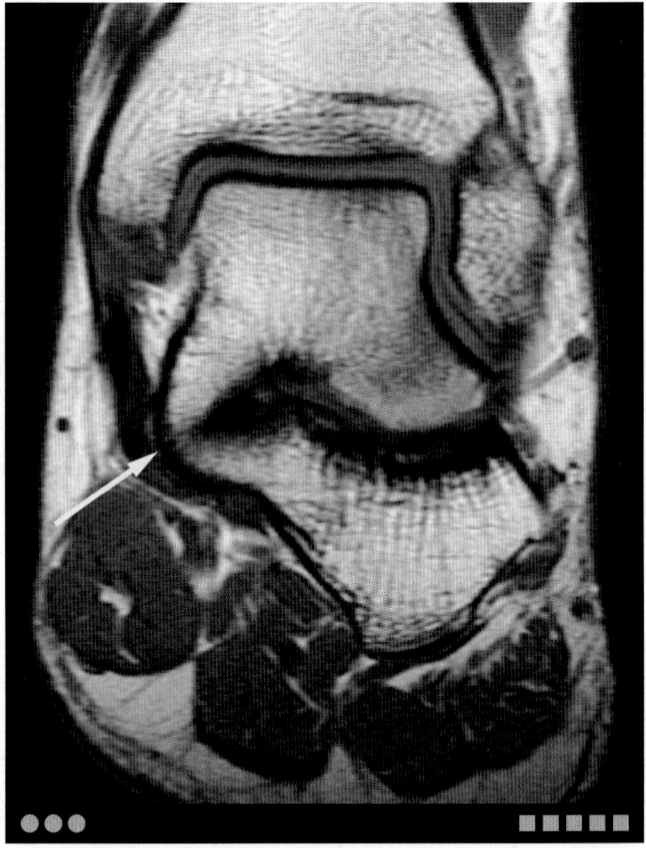

A. Osseous talocalcaneal coalition: Coronal T1-weighted image shows bony fusion (arrow) of the sustentaculum tali with the talus.

PEARLS

- **The most common type of tarsal coalition.**
- **It may be associated with rigid flat foot.**
- **Abnormal bone marrow signal is often present in the bone adjacent to the coalition.**
- **Best seen on coronal images.**

ADDITIONAL IMAGES

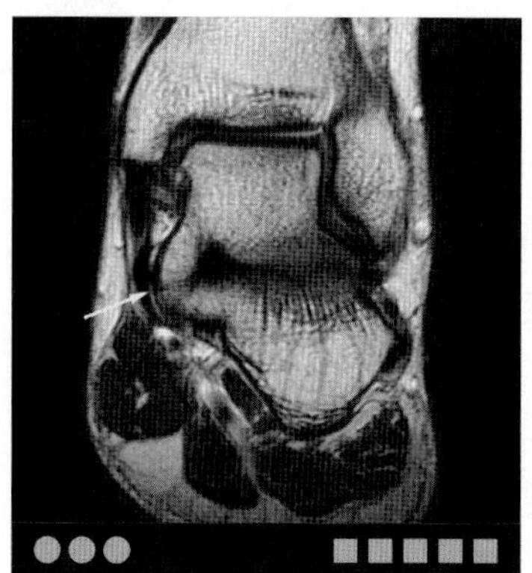

B. Osseous talocalcaneal coalition: Coronal T2-weighted image shows bony fusion (arrow) of the sustentaculum tali with the talus.

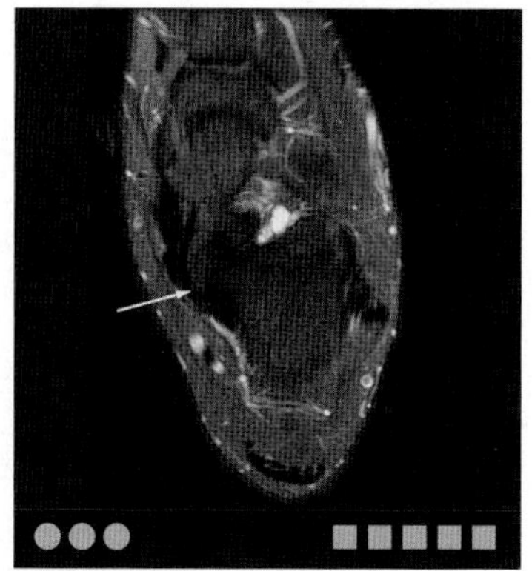

C. Osseous talocalcaneal coalition: Axial T2-weighted fat-suppressed image shows bony fusion (arrow) of the sustentaculum tali with the talus. No bone marrow edema is present.

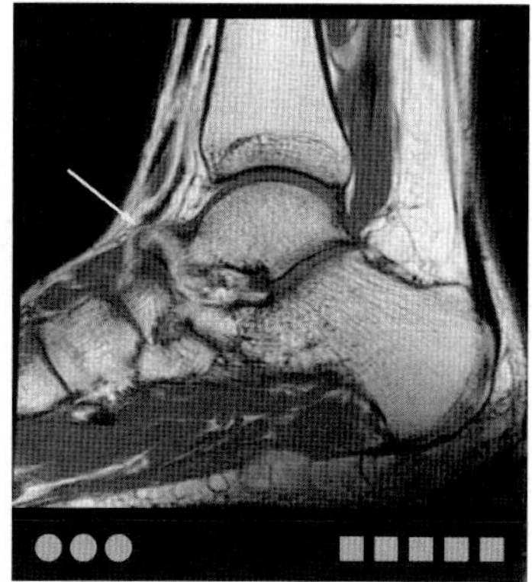

D. Osseous talocalcaneal coalition: Sagittal T1-weighted image shows a large talar beak (arrow).

DIFFERENTIAL DIAGNOSES IMAGES

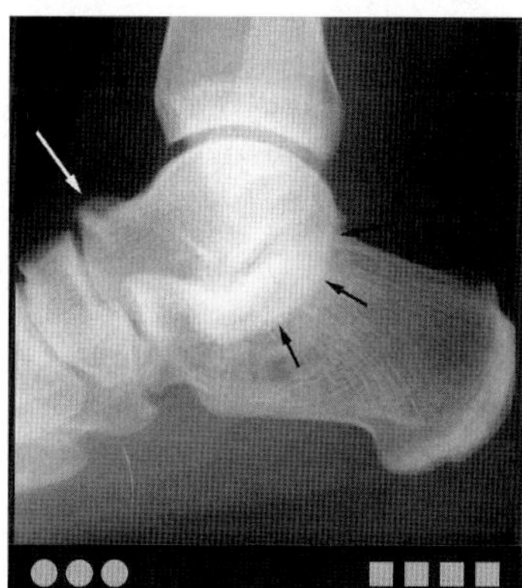

E. Fibrous talocalcaneal coalition: Lateral radiograph of the ankle shows a talar beak (white arrow) and a "C" sign (black arrows)

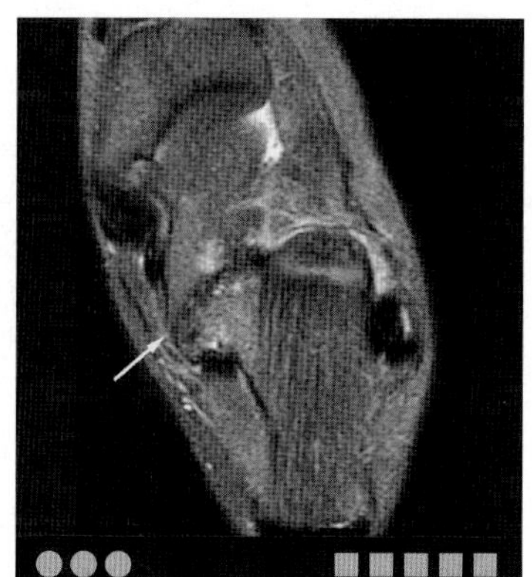

F. Fibrous talocalcaneal coalition: Axial T2-weighted fat-suppressed image shows fibrous coalition (arrow) of the sustentaculum tali with the talus. Note bone marrow edema adjacent to the subtalar joint.

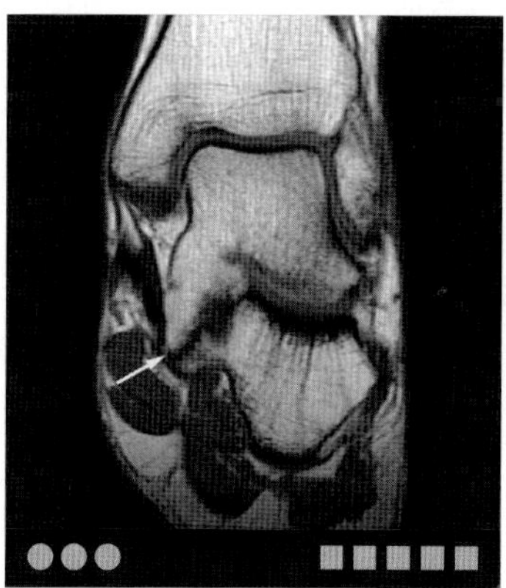

G. Fibrous talocalcaneal coalition: Coronal T1-weighted MR image shows fibrous coalition (arrow) of the subtalar joint. Note oblique orientation of the sustentaculum tali.

IMAGE KEY

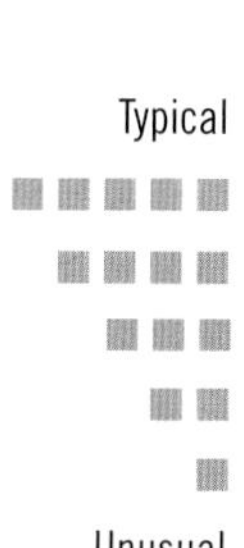

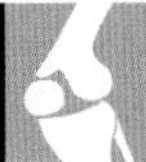

30–4 Familial Hyperlipidemia Syndrome (Xanthoma)

Sulabha Masih

PRESENTATION

Bilateral lower extremity nonhealing ulcers

FINDINGS

MR images demonstrate diffuse enlargement of Achilles, peroneus longus, posterior tibialis tendons and plantar fascia. Radiograph shows nodular, subcutaneous soft tissue mass lesions in the hands.

DIFFERENTIAL DIAGNOSES

- *Gout affecting tendons:* Shows as intermediate signal lobulated tophi on MRI surrounding the tendon, with associated intraosseous gouty deposits.
- *Partial Achilles tendon tear:* In hypertrophic partial tears, the tendon is thickened with variable signal intensity on MR imaging depending on duration.
- *Calcific tendinosis:* Easily diagnosed on radiographs.
- *Haglund deformity and tendinosis:* Bony protuberance of posterior calcaneus leading to tendinosis.
- *Giant cell tumor of tendon sheath:* Painless soft tissue mass in the hands or feet.

Lobulated low-intermediate signal mass on MR imaging adjacent to the tendon.

COMMENTS

This is the case of a 45-year-old male with a history of hypercholesterolemia and bilateral lower extremity nonhealing ulcers. Familial hyperlipidemia syndrome (xanthoma) can occur in all five types of hyperlipoproteinemias. Type 2 is the most common. Types 2 and 3 have affinity for the Achilles' tendon as well as extensor tendons of the hands. Plasma cholesterol levels are normal or slightly elevated. Plasma triglyceride levels are elevated. Some of these tumors are associated with endocrine and metabolic disorders such as hypothyroidism, multiple myeloma, macroglobulinemia, diabetes, and hepatitis. Calcification is noted in approximately 25% of cases. Xhanthomas are classified in four groups:

1. *Eruptive xanthomas:* Yellow triglyceride papules with surrounding erythema in shoulders, knees, buttocks, and back.
2. *Tendinous xanthomas:* Lipid deposits in Achilles, peroneal, posterior tibialis, and patellar tendons. These may erode into adjacent bone.

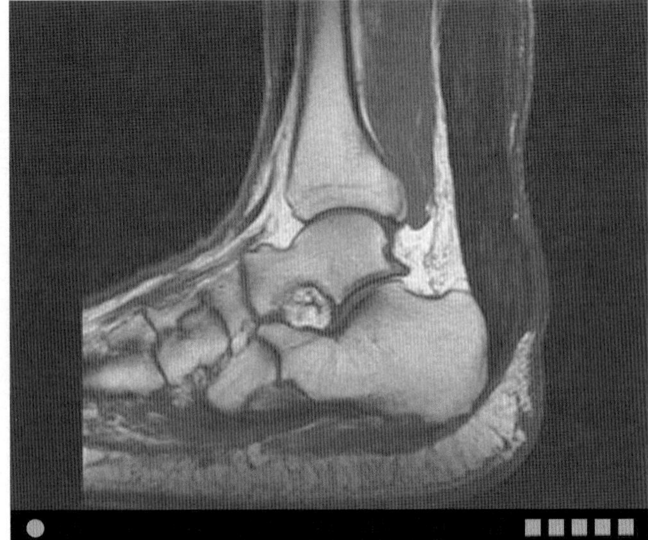

A. Xanthoma: Sagittal PD image shows diffuse enlargement of Achilles tendon with stippled appearance.

3. *Tuberous xanthomas:* Subcutaneous masses in the hands.
4. *Subperiosteal and osseous xanthomas:* Lipid deposits under the periosteum, causing scalloping and osteolytic lesions in the cortex and osteonecrosis.

MR is diagnostic and T1- and T2-weighted images demonstrate low signal intensity of Achilles tendon fibers infiltrated by intermediate signal intensity lipid-laden foamy histiocytes, with resultant stippled appearance and focal or diffuse markedly enlarged tendon size. Usually bilateral Achilles tendons are involved and it is hard to distinguish them from partial tendon tears on MR imaging. Radiography can show nodular soft tissue masses over the extensor surfaces of hands. Ultrasound may be helpful to visualize enlarged tendons.

PEARLS

- **Plasma cholesterol levels are normal or slightly elevated. Plasma triglyceride levels are elevated.**
- **Tendinous xanthomas may cause diffuse enlargement of Achilles, tibialis posterior, peroneus longus, patellar tendons and plantar fascia.**
- **Tuberous xanthomas present as subcutaneous soft tissue masses over the extensor surfaces of hands.**
- **MR shows low signal intensity enlarged tendons infiltrated by intermediate signal intensity lipid-laden foamy histiocytes resulting into stippled appearance.**

ADDITIONAL IMAGES

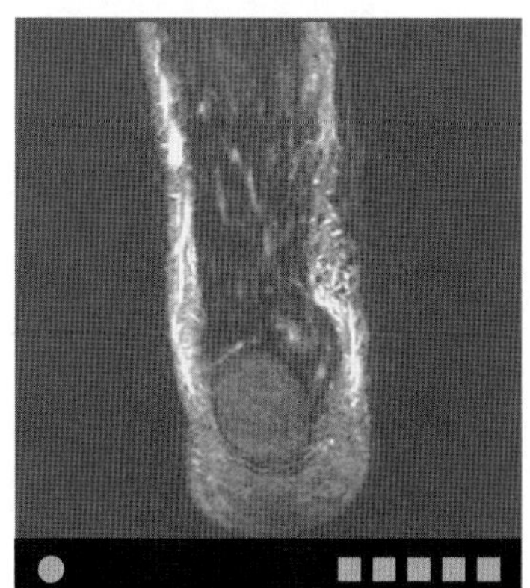

B. Xanthoma: Coronal T2 image also shows diffuse enlargement of Achilles tendon with stippled appearance.

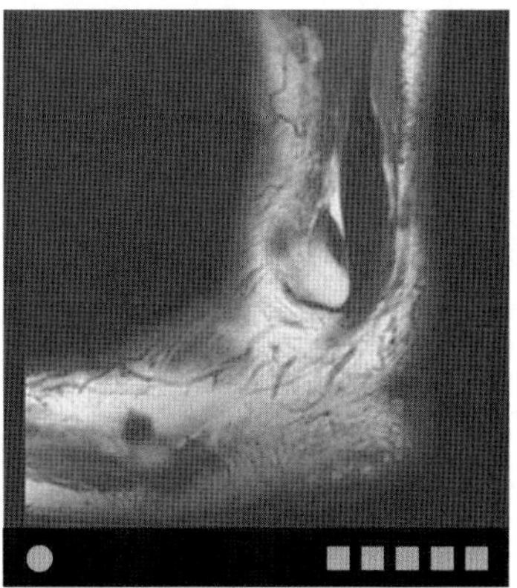

C. Xanthoma: Sagittal PD image shows enlarged peroneus longus tendon.

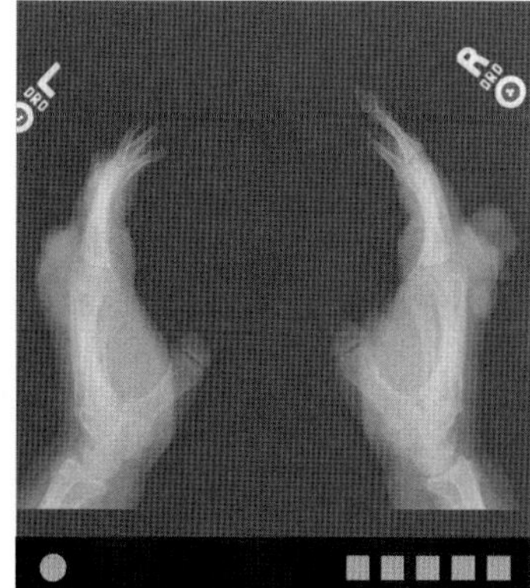

D. Xanthoma: Hand radiographs demonstrating soft tissue masses.

DIFFERENTIAL DIAGNOSES IMAGES

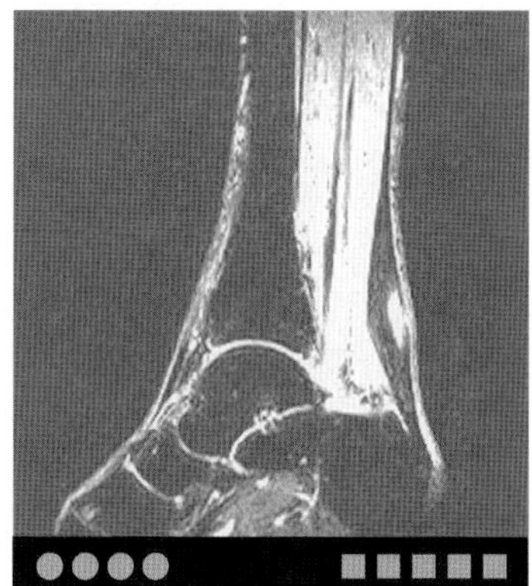

E. Partial Achilles tendon tear: Sagittal PD fat-saturated image demonstrates partial Achilles tendon tear.

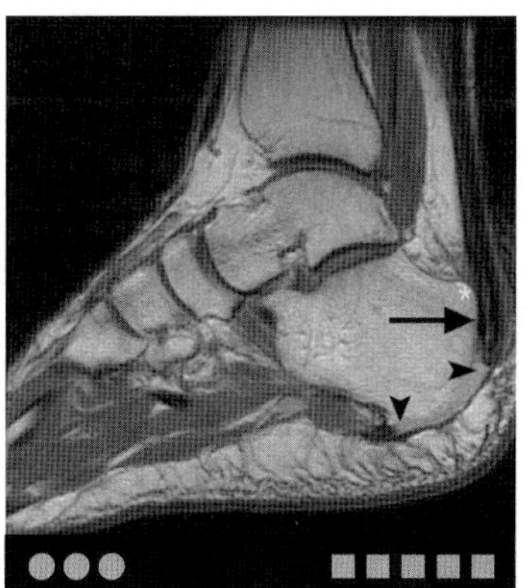

F. Haglund deformity and Achilles tendinosis: Sagittal T2-weighted image shows bony protuberance of posterior calcaneus (*) leading to chronic tendinosis (large arrow). Note plantar and posterior calcaneal spurs (arrowheads).

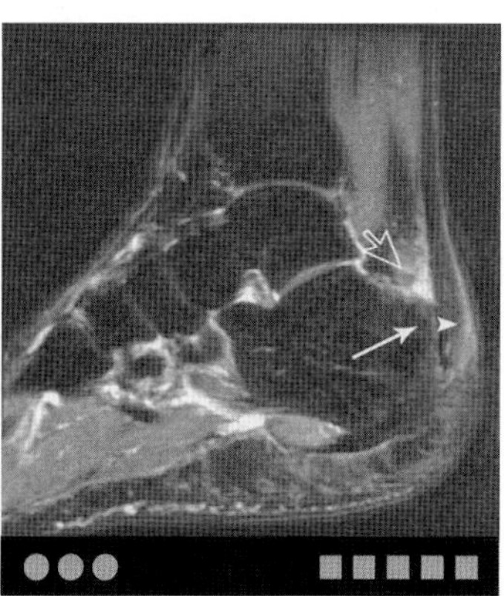

G. Haglund deformity and Achilles tendinosis: Sagittal STIR image shows chronic tendinosis and thickening of Achilles tendon and pre- (black arrow) and post-Achilles tendon fluid and edema (arrowhead).

IMAGE KEY

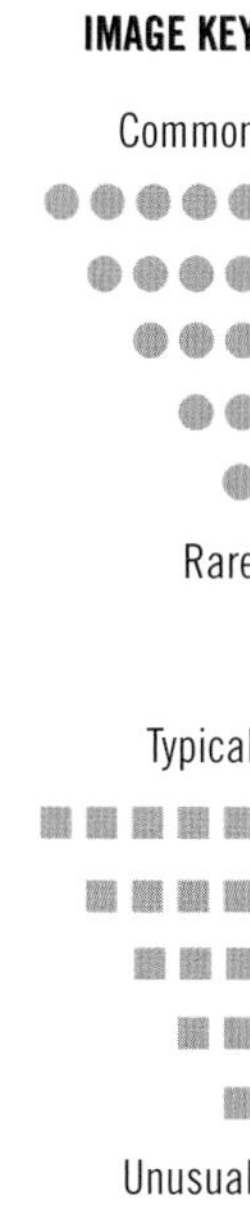

Chapter 31

Arthritis, Connective Tissue and Crystal Deposition Disorders

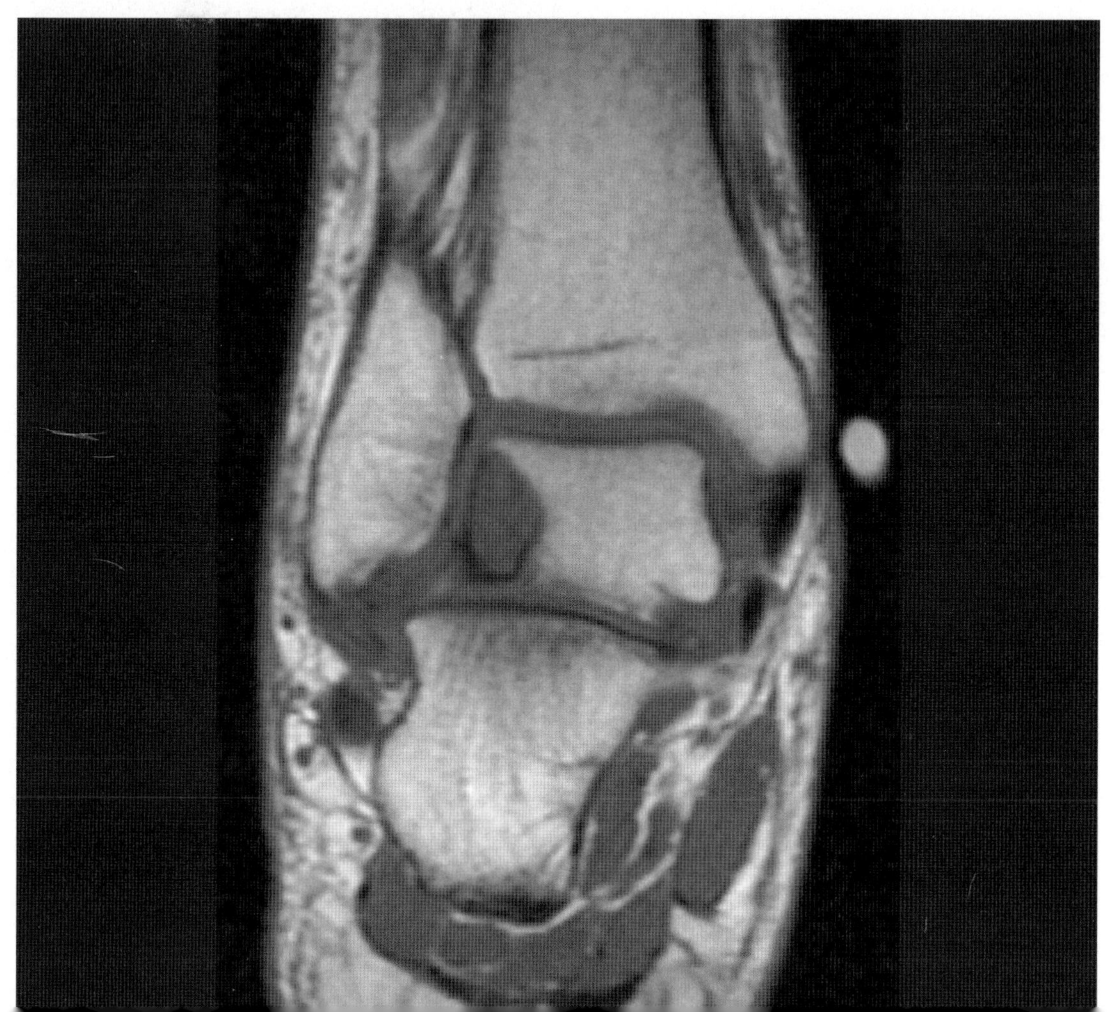

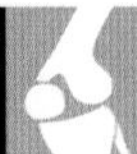

31–1 Gout of the Ankle

Melitus Maryam Golshan and Jamshid Tehranzadeh

PRESENTATION

Foot pain

FINDINGS

MR images show erosion of talus with low signal intensity on T1-weighted image which enhances after intravenous administration of contrast.

DIFFERENTIAL DIAGNOSES

- *PVNS (localized form):* Owing to hemosiderin content, this aggressive but benign villonodular synovial lesion often presents with dark signal on most MR sequences.
- Amyloidosis often presents with similar MR signal appearance with more homogenous enhancement.
- Synovial chondromatosis may be associated with joint effusion.
- Indolent infections such as TB or Coccidiomycosis have joint fluid and additional adjacent soft tissue findings.

COMMENTS

This case is of a 60-year-old man who presented with a 2-year history of foot pain. Gout is the most common inflammatory arthritis in men over the age of 30. Women are infrequently affected. Acute gouty arthritis commonly presents as monoarticular arthritis, occurring in the metatarsophalangeal (MTP) joints, predominantly the first MTP joint. Involvement of the dorsum of the foot, heel, and ankle are less frequent. In the acute stage of gout MR imaging findings of the joint effusion and synovial thickening are nonspecific.

If the acute attack of gout is not treated or if treated ineffectively, after an undetermined period, the clinical syndrome of tophaceous gout may appear. Tophaceous deposits account for the bone erosions seen in gouty arthritis. These large erosions with "overhanging edge" may be para-articular, intra-articular, or located at a considerable distance from the joint. Gouty tophi may produce bony erosions and cystic changes of the adjacent bone resulting in chronic deforming arthritis. Large deposits of urate crystals are also seen in adjacent bursae, tendon, ligaments, and subcutaneous layers of the skin. Gouty tophi are mostly of low or intermediate signal intensity on T1-weighted images and reveal an increase in signal intensity after intravenous administration of gadolinium. The imaging findings of tophi on T2-weighted images are variable but usually contain low signal regions.

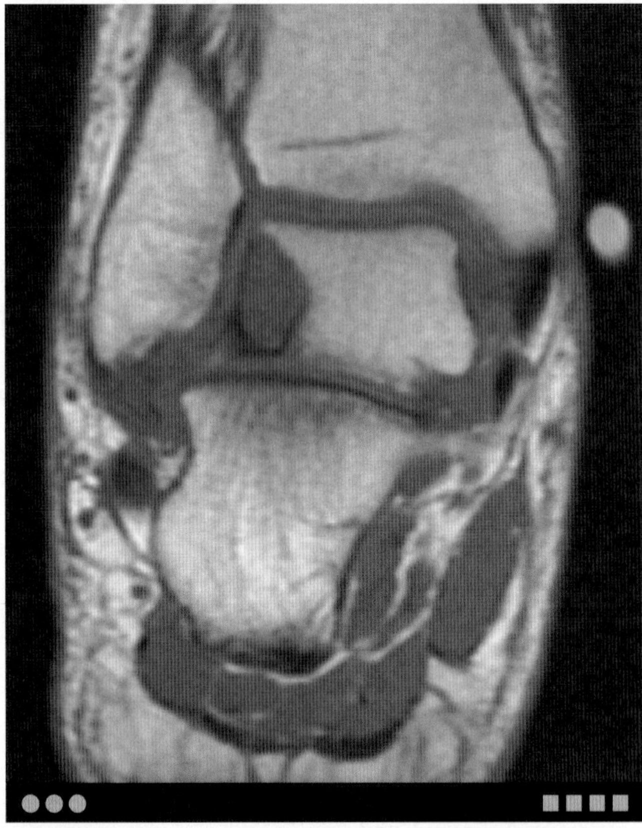

A. Gout: Coronal T1-weighted image shows an almost elliptical, intermediate signal intensity lesion in the lateral aspect of talus. Note synovial thickening of the ankle mortis joint and small erosions at the tip of fibula.

PEARLS

- **Gout is an important cause of foot pain in middle-age men.**
- **First metatarsophalangeal joint is considered the main target.**
- **MRI shows tophi as a low to intermediate signal intensity mass on T1-weighted image, which enhances with contrast agent. T2-weighted images are more variable, and it may have mixed high or low signal intensity.**

ADDITIONAL IMAGES

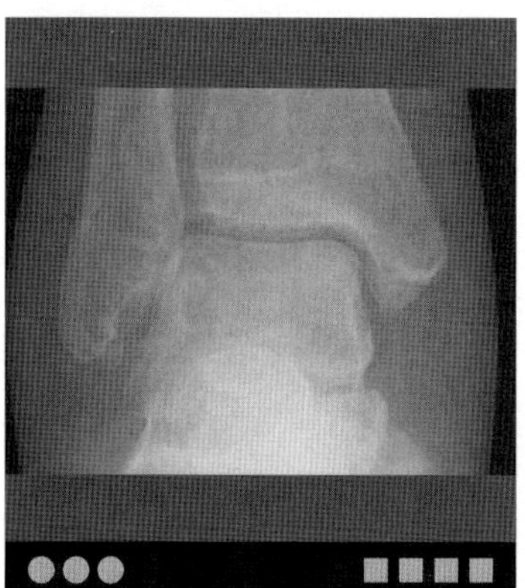

B. Gout: AP radiograph of ankle shows osteolytic lesion in lateral talus with sclerotic margin. Note cystic changes in the tip of fibula.

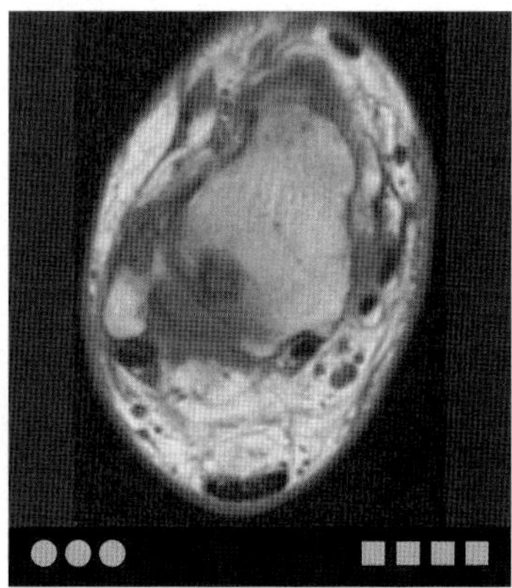

C. Gout: Axial T1-weighted image shows large erosion in the lateral aspect of the talus with small erosions of fibula.

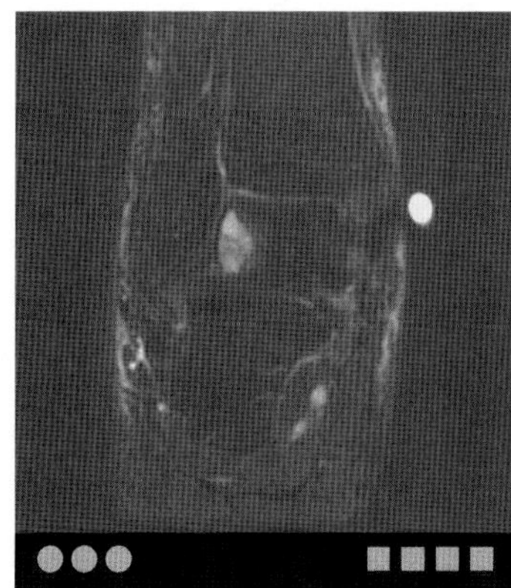

D. Gout: Coronal T2-weighted image with fat saturation shows bright and intermediate signal in lesion in the lateral aspect of the talus.

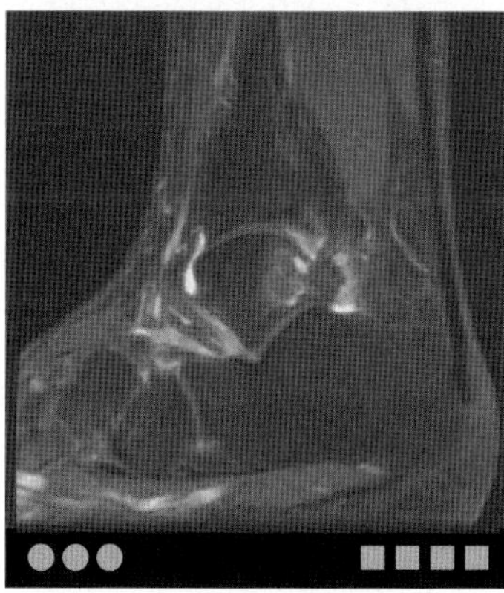

E. Gout: Sagittal postcontrast fat-saturated T1-weighted image shows synovial enhancement in the joint and peripheral enhancement of the lesion in the talus.

IMAGE KEY

Common

Rare

Typical

Unusual

DIFFERENTIAL DIAGNOSES IMAGES

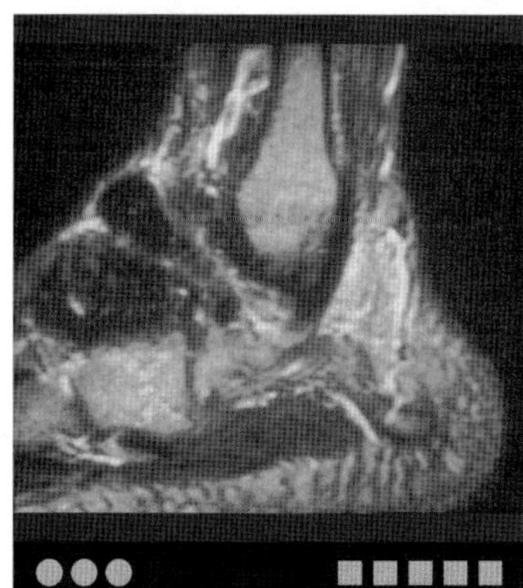

F. PVNS: Sagittal T2-weighted spin echo MR image shows low signal intensity mass infiltrating the subtalar joint and extending to the anterior and posterior ankle mortis joint in a patient with PVNS.

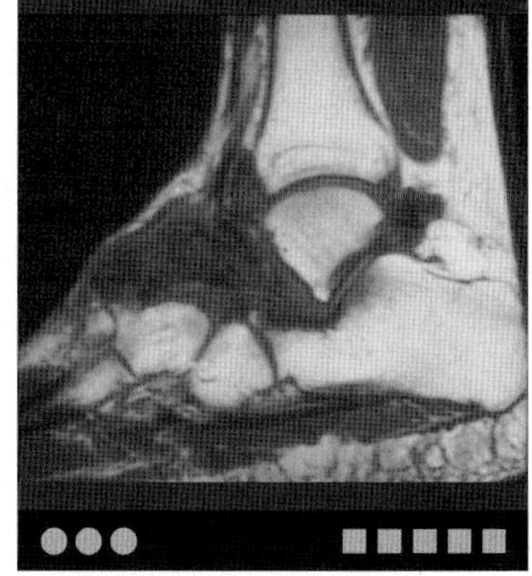

G. PVNS: Sagittal T1-weighted spin echo MR image shows low signal intensity mass infiltrating the subtalar joint and extending to the anterior and posterior ankle mortis joint.

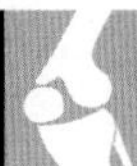

31–2 Pseudogout

Mélanie Morel, Nathalie Boutry, and Anne Cotten

PRESENTATION

Pain of the forefoot for 3 weeks

FINDINGS

Imaging shows fragmentation and prominent subchondral cysts of the talonavicular and cuneonavicular joints.

DIFFERENTIAL DIAGNOSES

- *Gouty arthropathy:* Periarticular nonmarginal erosions with overhanging margins and bony proliferations are located next to calcified soft tissue masses. Intraosseous tophi may be present.
- *Neuropathic osteoarthropathy:* No chondrocalcinosis is found. Joint destruction, bone fragmentation, and sclerosis are prominent. Often, a history of long-standing diabetes is present.
- *Osteoarthritis:* Weight-bearing surfaces are involved, with marked osteophytes, and rare fragmentation.
- *Hemochromatosis:* Foot involvement is rare. The fourth and fifth metacarpophalangeal joints are frequently involved, in addition to the second and third ones. Drooping osteophytes along the radial sides of the metacarpal heads and subchondral cysts are distinctive features. Osteopenia may be present.
- *Rheumatoid arthritis and septic arthritis:* These are accompanied by osteopenia and marginal erosions.

COMMENTS

This is an image of a 62-year-old woman complaining of subacute pain of the forefoot associated with dorsal soft tissue swelling. Pseudogout is a goutlike clinical syndrome produced by calcium pyrophosphate dihydrate (CPPD) crystal deposition disease that is characterized by intermittent acute attacks of arthritis. It may be sporadic, hereditary, or secondary (hyperparathyroidism, hemochromatosis). The pseudogout pattern represents 10% to 20% of the clinical presentations, which is caused by shedding of pyrophosphate crystals into the joint fluid. It occurs most frequently in the knee, but may also affect the hip, shoulder, elbow, ankle, wrist, acromioclavicular, talocalcaneal, and metatarsophalangeal joints. Fever and elevated erythrocyte sedimentation rate are encountered. Chondrocalcinosis, defined by hyaline and fibrocartilage calcification may be present; linear calcifications parallel to the subchondral plate of the articular surfaces are commonly found in the knee, wrist, elbow, and hip joints. Thick, granular, or stratified calcifications may outline the menisci of the knee, triangular fibrocartilage of the wrist, labra of the acetabulum or glenoid, symphysis pubis, annulus fibrosus of the intervertebral disk, or even the sternoclavicular, and acromioclavicular joints. Synovial membranes, articular capsules, tendons, ligaments, and vessels may also be calcified. Pyrophosphate arthropathy affects non–weight-bearing surfaces and is usually bilateral but asymmetric. The knee, wrist (radioscaphoid and trapezioscaphoid joints), and metacarpophalangeal joints (second and third mostly) are most frequently involved. At radiography, femoropatellar joint is characteristically involved. Scapholunate dissociation is often seen in the wrist with scapholunate advanced collapse (SLAC). The spine may also be affected, with crystal deposition involving spinal ligaments and the annulus fibrosus.

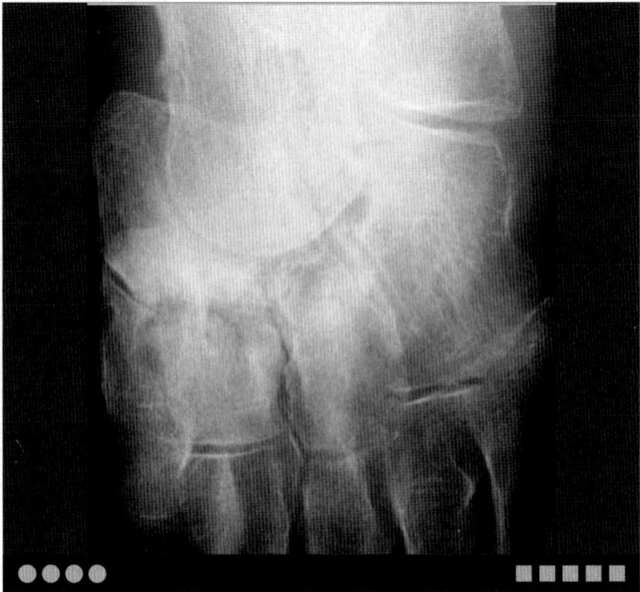

A. CPPD: Radiograph of the forefoot exhibits joint space narrowing of the cuneonavicular joint with prominent subchondral cysts. Note the absence of osteophytes.

PEARLS

- **Pseudogout is a clinical syndrome produced by calcium pyrophosphate dihydrate (CPPD) crystal deposition.**
- **Chondrocalcinosis with hyaline and fibrocartilage calcification is helpful for diagnosis. It may be absent at the joint involved by the arthropathy, but should be looked for in other joints (wrist, knee, and pelvis).**
- **Pyrophosphate arthropathy affects non–weight-bearing surfaces with joint space narrowing, marked subchondral sclerosis, and prominent subchondral cysts. Fragmentation of the affected joints is commonly encountered.**

ADDITIONAL IMAGES

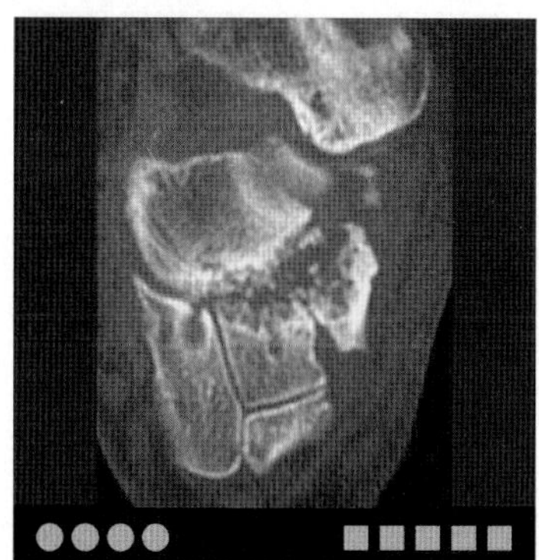

B. CPPD: Axial CT scan image exhibits fragmentation of the cuneonavicular joint with subchondral sclerosis, erosions, and cysts.

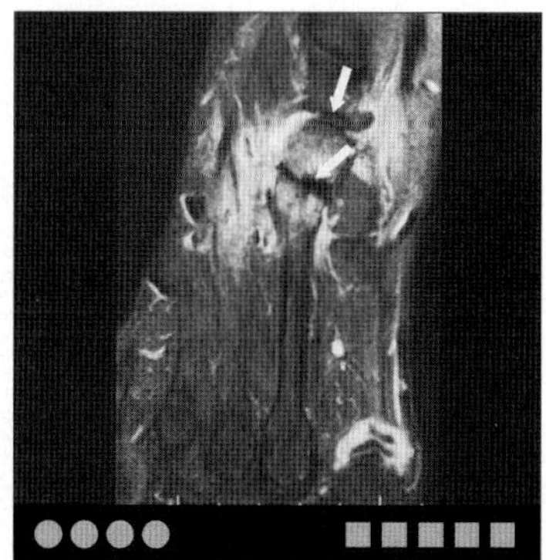

C. CPPD disease: Axial T2-weighted fat-saturated image shows low signal intensity subchondral bands along the cuneonavicular and cuneometatarsal joints (arrows) and bone edema.

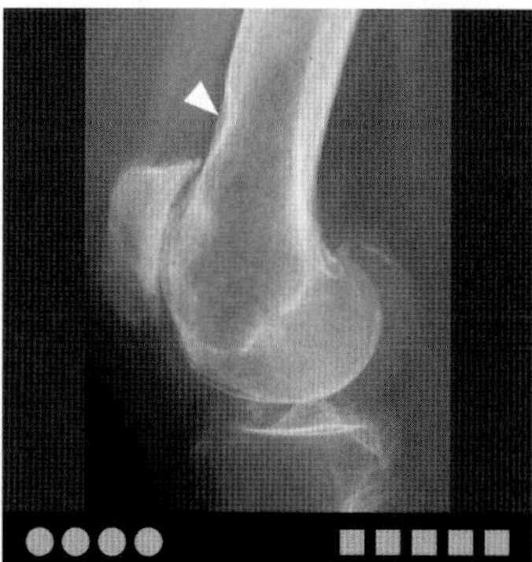

D. CPPD disease: Lateral knee radiograph exhibits narrowing of the patellofemoral joint with a suprapatellar femoral erosion (arrowhead). Chondrocalcinosis (calcification of the menisci, hyaline cartilage, and tendon of the gastrocnemius muscle) is also found. Subchondral sclerosis (arrowheads) of the lateral tibiofemoral compartment.

E. CPPD disease: Frontal knee radiograph shows linear calcification within the medial meniscus (chondrocalcinosis) and joint space narrowing with marked and well-defined subchondral sclerosis (arrowheads) of the lateral tibiofemoral compartment.

DIFFERENTIAL DIAGNOSES IMAGES

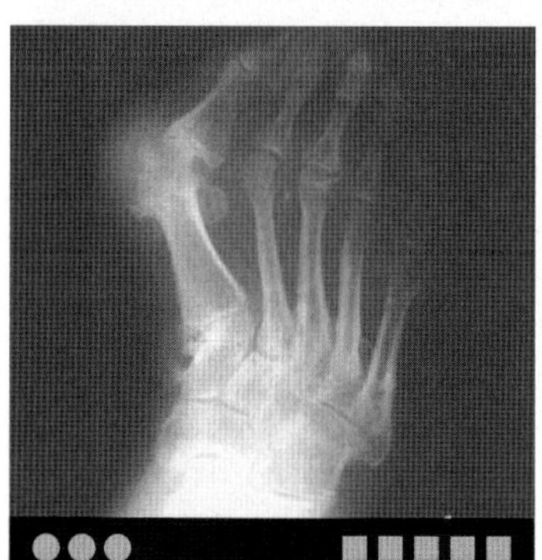

F. Gouty arthropathy: Soft tissue tophus is typically located along the first MTP joint with adjacent paraarticular erosion and overhanging margins. Note bone proliferations along the first metatarsal and the medial cuneiform bones.

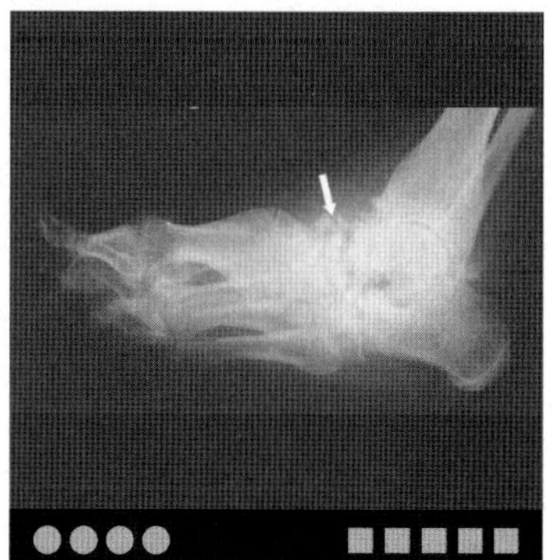

G. Neuropathic (Charcot) osteoarthropathy: Lateral radiograph of the foot exhibits fragmentation of the navicular bone (arrow) and destruction of the talonavicular, calcaneocuboidal, and cuneonavicular joints. Note associated bone sclerosis.

IMAGE KEY

Common

Rare

Typical

Unusual

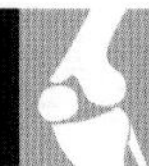

31–3 Amyloidosis of the Ankle

Melitus Maryam Golshan and Jamshid Tehranzadeh

PRESENTATION

Bilateral ankle pain and swelling

IMAGING FINDINGS

MRI shows extensive thickening of the tendons of the ankle.

DIFFERENTIAL DIAGNOSES

- *Chronic tendinosis:* It shows thickening of tendons associated with intermediate to dark signal in most MR sequences. The findings are often localized.
- *Xanthoma:* This is an infiltrating lesion of the tendon, which results in intermediate signal change in proton density images. T2-weighted images may show mixed bright signal. The condition leads to degenerative shredding of the tendon.
- *Gout:* Tophaceous material have low signal in T1 and proton density images and dark to mixed dark and bright signal on T2-weighted sequences. Gout finally leads to erosions mostly at first metatarsophalangeal joint and intertarsal joints.

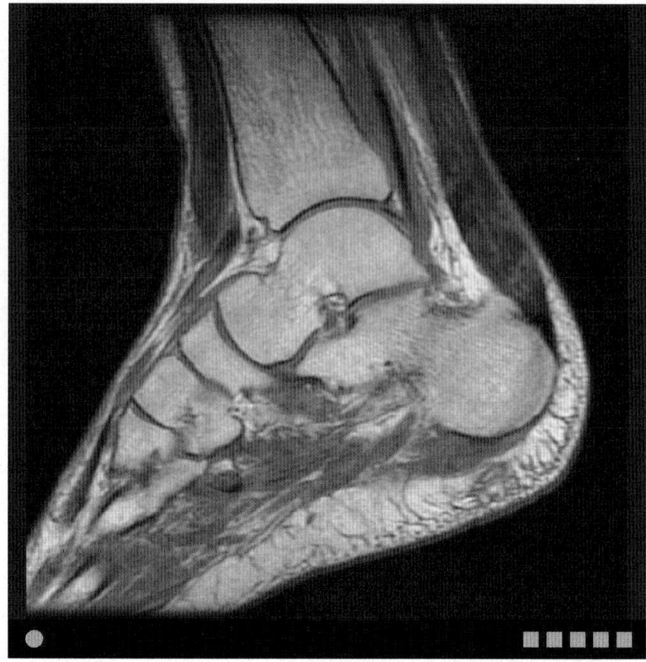

A. Amyloidosis: Sagittal T1-weighted image of the ankle shows marked thickening and low signal intensity of the anterior tibialis and Achilles tendons with intermediate signal intensity within.

COMMENTS

This is an image of a 29-year-old man who presented with end-stage renal disease for 19 years complaining of bilateral ankle pain for weeks. Amyloidosis is defined as the extracellular deposition of the fibrous protein (β_2-microglobulin) in one or more sites in the body. This low molecular weight serum protein is not filtered by standard dialysis membranes and tends to accumulate within the musculoskeletal system. In large joints, amyloid arthropathy resembles inflammatory arthritis with juxtaarticular soft tissue swelling, mild periarticular osteoporosis, and subchondral cystic lesions, usually with well-defined sclerotic margins. The joint space is often normal in width until late in the course of the disease. Two types of lesions are noted: (1) Capsular and tendon lesions show thickened hypointense areas, which enhance by gadolinium (Gd) on T1-weighted image and have intermediate signal on T2-weighted image. (2) Periarticular and osseous lesions appear to be tumor forming and hypointense on both T1-weighted image and T2-weighted image; they are not enhanced by Gd. The MR imaging appearance of amyloid infiltration within or around the joint consists of extensive deposition of an abnormal soft tissue that has low or intermediate signal intensity on both T1- and T2-weighted image. This abnormal material covers the synovial membrane, tendons which may fills subchondral defects, and extends to periarticular soft tissues. Joint effusion is usually present.

PEARLS

- **Amyloidosis is defined as the extracellular deposition of the fibrous protein (β_2–microglobulin).**
- **Two types of lesions are noted which include capsular and tendon lesions, and the second category is periarticular and osseous lesions.**
- **Amyloid deposition is low to intermediate signal intensity on T1- and T2-weighted image. This abnormal material covers the synovial membrane, tendon sheets, and may fills subchondral defects.**

ADDITIONAL IMAGES

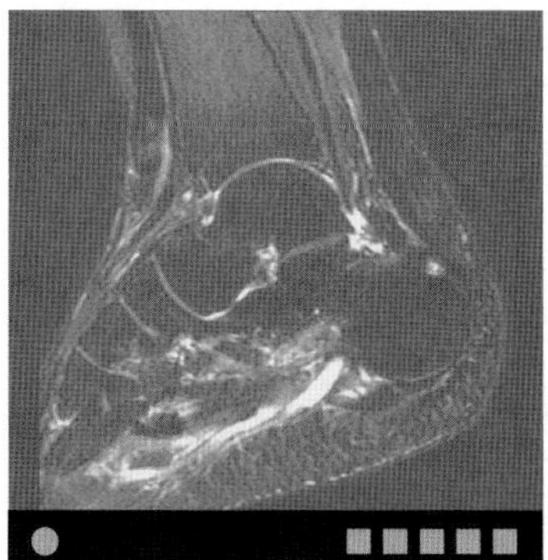

B. Amyloidosis: Sagittal fat-saturated fast spin echo (FSE) T2-weighted image shows thickening and low signal intensity of anterior tibialis and Achilles tendon with intermediate signal intensity within.

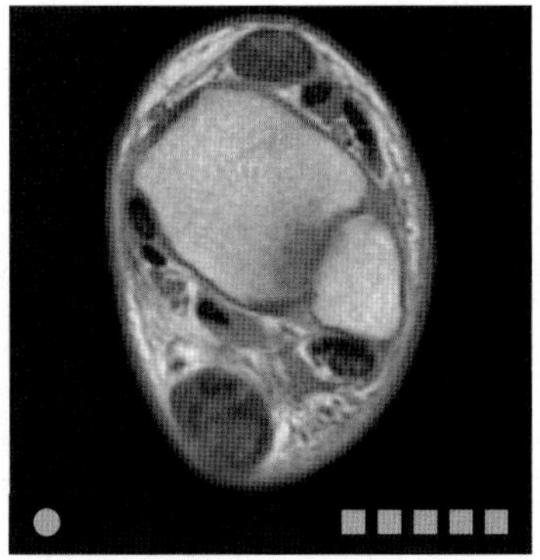

C. Amyloidosis: Axial T1-weighted image shows intermediate signal intensity within thickened Achilles, anterior tibialis, peroneus longus, and brevis tendons.

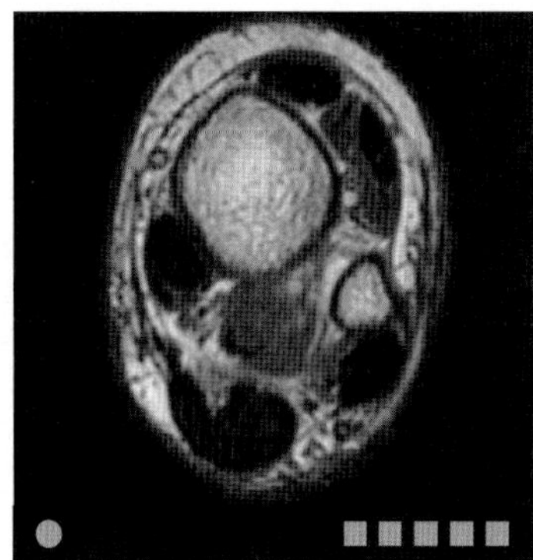

D. Amyloidosis: Axial FSE T2-weighted image shows thickened Achilles, peroneal tendons, and anterior and posterior tibialis tendons.

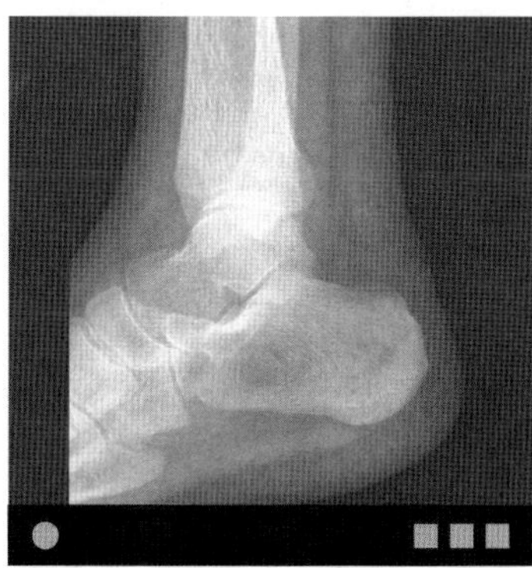

E. Amyloidosis: Lateral radiograph of the ankle shows soft tissue swelling caused by thickening of anterior tibialis and Achilles tendons.

DIFFERENTIAL DIAGNOSES IMAGES

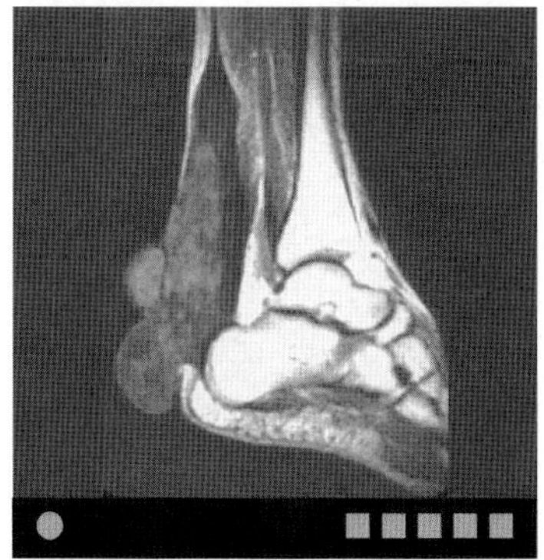

F. Xanthoma of Achilles tendon: Sagittal SE T1-weighted image shows large infiltrating and lobulated intermediate signal soft tissue mass within the thickened Achilles tendon.

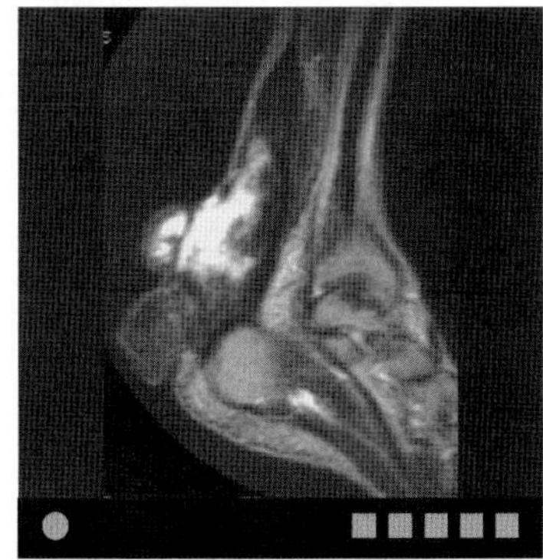

G. Xanthoma of Achilles tendon: Sagittal SE T2-weighted image shows low signal intensity with internal bright signals in the Achilles tendon.

IMAGE KEY

Common

●●●●●
●●●●
●●●
●●
●

Rare

Typical

■■■■■
■■■■
■■■
■■
■

Unusual

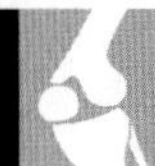

31–4 Dermatomyositis

John C. Hunter

PRESENTATION

Progressive muscle weakness of lower extremities

FINDINGS

Axial inversion recovery images of both lower extremities demonstrate diffuse muscle hyperintensity in the thighs and scattered muscle groups in the lower legs.

DIFFERENTIAL DIAGNOSES

- *Autoimmune myopathies:* Besides dermatomyositis and polymyositis, other autoimmune myopathies (Sjogren's syndrome, mixed connective disease), lymphoma, sarcoidosis, denervation, diabetic muscle necrosis, infectious fasciitis/myositis (necrotizing fasciitis, HIV myositis, etc.), trauma, rhabdomyolysis, and muscular dystrophy exist.
- *Denervation muscle atrophy:* High SI early with eventual fatty atrophy can be seen in the distribution of the affected nerve(s)
- *Sarcoidosis:* This is associated with hilar adenopathy and other systemic manifestations.
- *Lymphoma:* Muscle involvement may mimic myositis. Other systemic manifestations are present.
- Infectious fasciitis/myositis including necrotizing fasciitis, HIV myositis, and other deep infection is considered.

COMMENTS

This is an image of a 14-year-old female who presents with progressive muscle weakness of lower extremities. Dermatomyositis/polymyositis is a progressive disease of muscle which typically starts in proximal muscles of the thigh and upper extremity. These entities are distinguished by the presence of a skin rash in dermatomyositis. Weakness and tenderness in early stages progress to atrophy and contractures in the later phase of the disease. This is generally a disease of the third to fifth decades of life with female predominance; it may also be seen in the pediatric population. One form of the disease has a significant association with visceral malignancy. Imaging early with MR shows muscle edema on fluid sensitive sequences such as STIR or T2-weighted images with fat saturation. With treatment, the symptoms and edema may revert to normal, but flares of the disease may show recurrent muscle edema accompanied by clinical weakness. As the disease progresses, atrophy dominates with fatty infiltration of muscles, and is best seen on T1-weighted images. Steroid related myopathy may be difficult to distinguish on imaging. Differential diagnosis includes other autoimmune myopathies (Sjogren's syndrome, mixed connective disease), lymphoma, sarcoidosis, denervation, diabetic muscle necrosis, infectious fasciitis/myositis (necrotizing fasciitis, HIV myositis, etc.), trauma, rhabdomyolysis, and muscular dystrophy. Clinical presentation, physical findings, and history help to distinguish these entities. With recurrent symptoms in dermatomyositis/polymyositis, flare of disease and steroid induced myopathy can be implicated. MR imaging helps to establish the diagnosis, provide a site for confirmatory biopsy, and evaluate for the presence of atrophy.

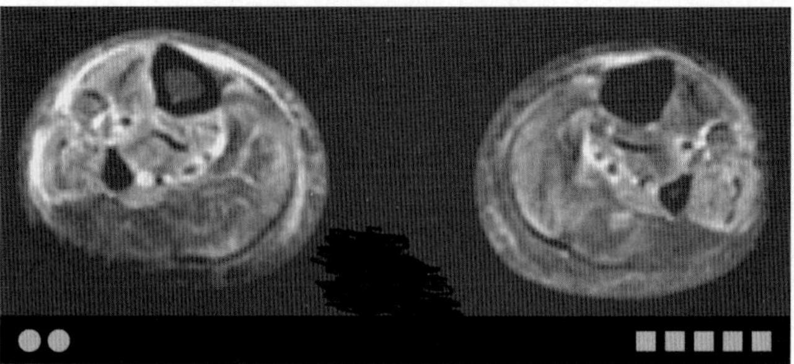

A. Dermatomyositis: Axial T2 images with fat saturation through the lower leg shows increased signal in the anterior muscles with relative sparing of the posterior calf muscles. Subcutaneous edema is seen.

PEARLS

- **While dermatomyositis is most commonly seen in the third to fifth decades, childhood disease can occur and is often quite severe.**
- **The muscle, fascial, and subcutaneous edema is nonspecific on imaging, and may be secondary to a variety of etiologies and clinical correlation is essential.**
- **Autoimmune myositis is characterized clinically by insidious onset of muscle weakness, where as infectious myositis/fasciitis has a far different clinical course.**
- **The main indication for MR imaging is to find areas of active disease for biopsy and to follow recurrence and progression of disease.**

ADDITIONAL IMAGE

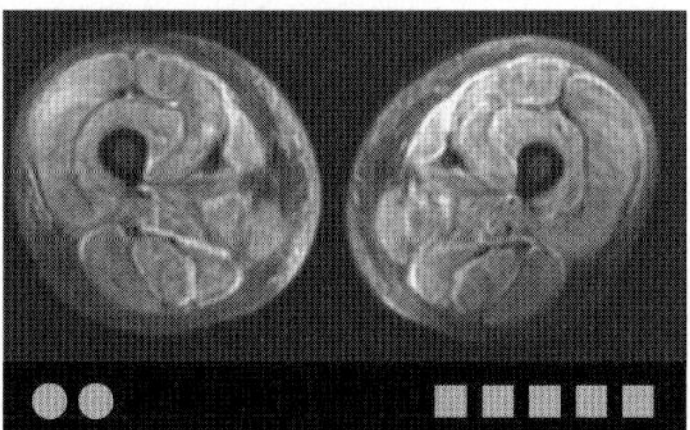

B. Dermatomyositis: Axial T2 images with fat saturation through the thighs shows diffused, increased in signal intensity in all muscle groups.

DIFFERENTIAL DIAGNOSES IMAGES

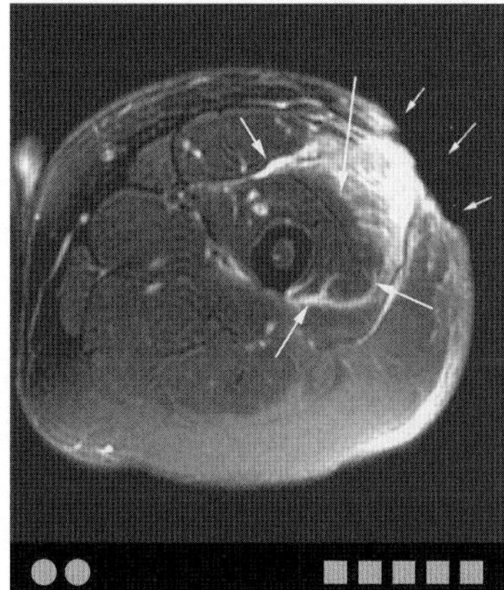

C. Bacterial myositis and fasciitis: Axial T2-weighted image with fat saturation in this 26-year-old male with an ulcer on the lateral thigh (arrow) shows increased SI in the underlying muscle (arrow) and fascial planes (arrow). Infected open wound with underlying inflammation is seen.

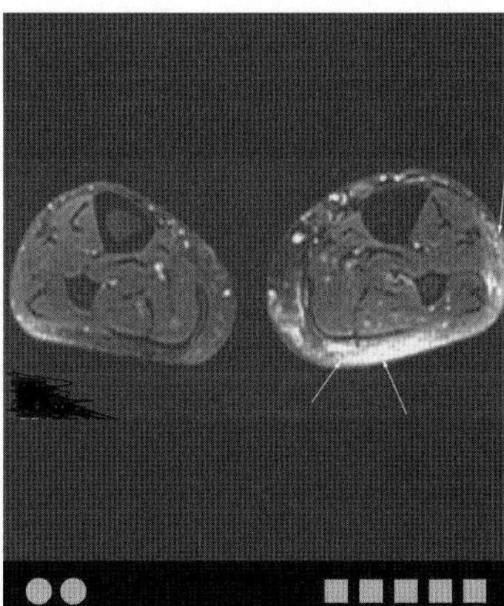

D. Cellulitis: Axial T2-weighted image with fat saturation in left lower leg of this 47-year-old diabetic man shows extensive subcutaneous edema with sparing of the subfascial structures.

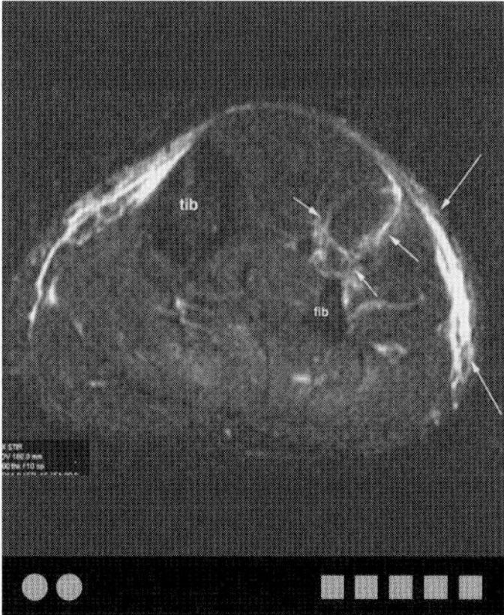

E. Early necrotizing fasciitis: Axial inversion recovery image through the lower leg shows subcutaneous edema (arrow) as well as increased SI in the anterior-lateral intermuscular fascial planes (arrows), particularly those surrounding the extensor digitorum longus (arrows). The muscles are spared.

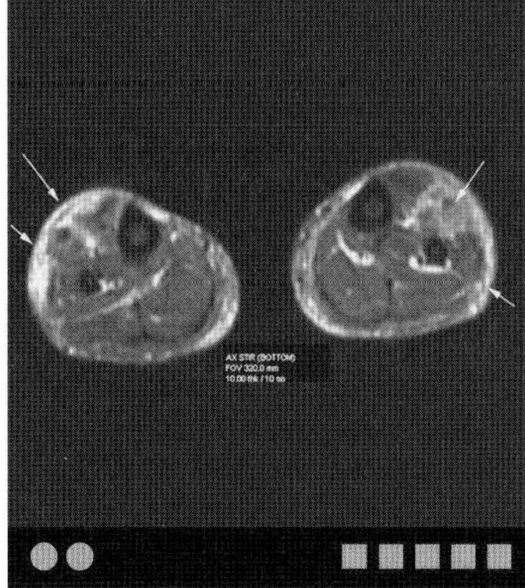

F. Sjogren's syndrome (autoimmune myositis): Axial image through the lower legs in this 39-year-old female shows bilateral subcutaneous edema (arrows) as well as focal myositis in the anterior-lateral muscles (arrow).

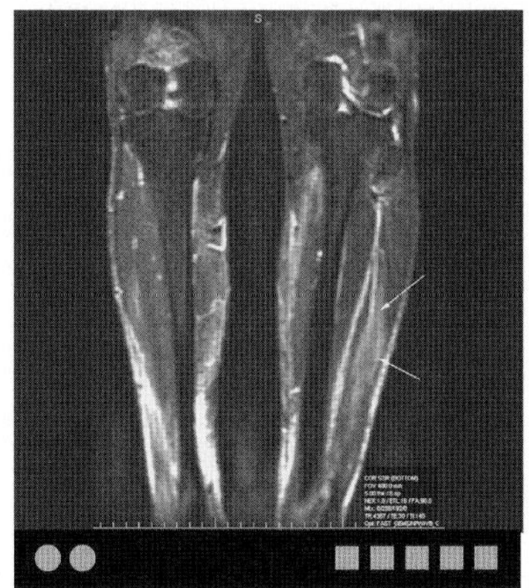

G. Sjogren's syndrome (Autoimmune myositis): Coronal IR images through the lower legs in this 39-year-old female shows bilateral subcutaneous edema (arrows) as well as focal myositis in the anterior lateral muscles (arrow).

IMAGE KEY

Common

Rare

Typical

Unusual

Chapter 32

Infections

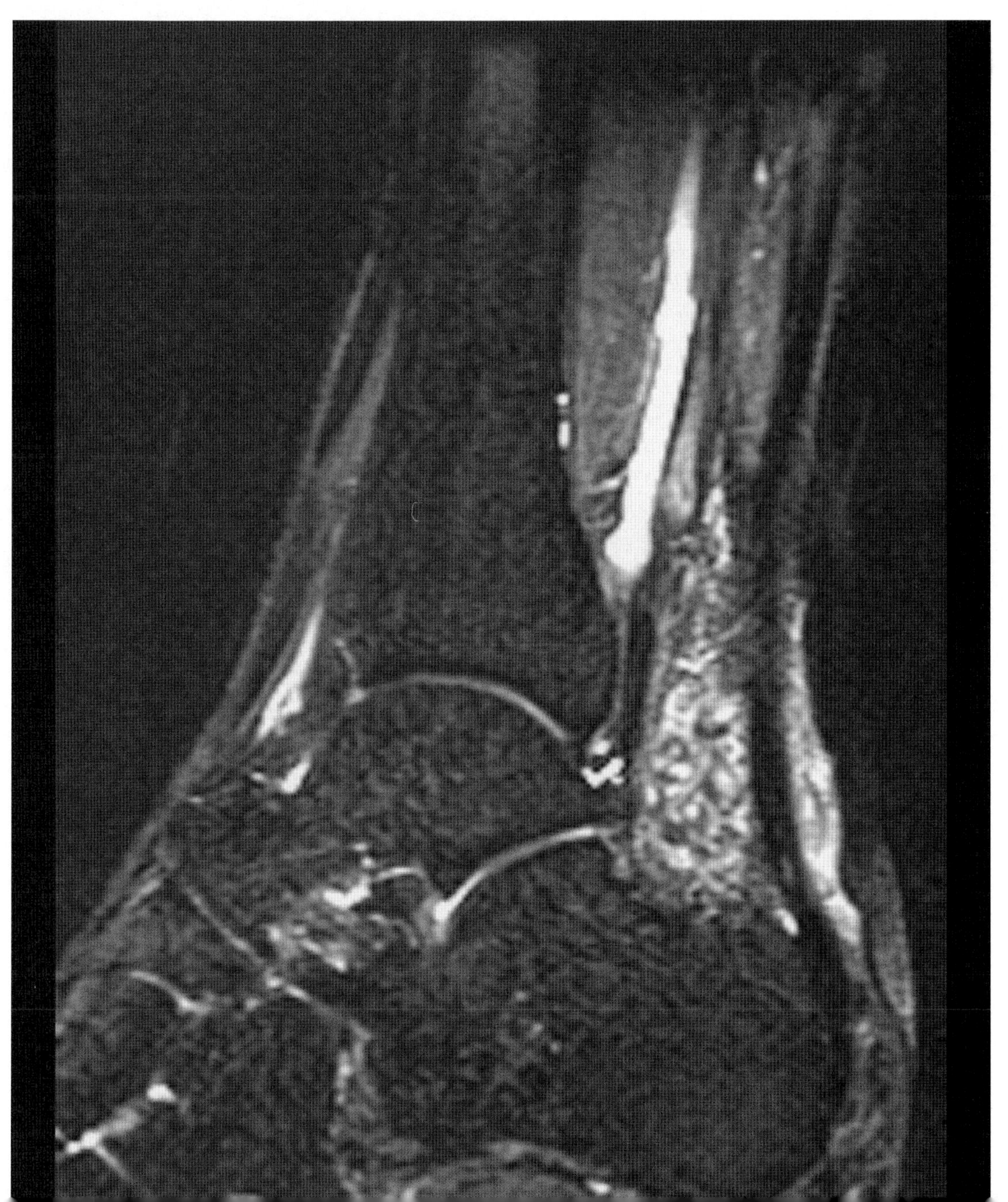

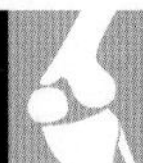

32–1 Eumycetoma of the Ankle

Timothy Auran and Rajeev K. Varma

PRESENTATION

Enlarging ankle mass with occasional purulent discharge

FINDINGS

MR images show an ill-defined, heterogeneous mass posterior to the talus with low signal intensity on T1-weighted image, which enhances after contrast administration.

DIFFERENTIAL DIAGNOSES

- *Nonfungal mycetoma:* Most cases of nonfungal mycetoma are of actinomycetes.
- Other indolent cutaneous infections such as coccidioidomycosis, onychomycosis, or tuberculosis.
- Soft tissue malignancy may mimic fungal infection.

COMMENTS

This is the case of a 27-year-old Hispanic male field worker, who suffered a cut over his left ankle while working in the fields. After initial treatment with oral antibiotics failed to resolve his ankle pain and swelling, an anti-fungal regimen was started based on culture results. Failure of further outpatient treatment leads to MRI to evaluate the extent of disease and eventually surgical debridement. The earliest reports of eumycetoma occurred in Chennai (previously Madras), India, where a characteristic indolent fungal infection of the sole of the foot was termed "Madura foot." Eumycetoma is most frequently seen in the tropical and subtropical zones between the latitudes of 15 degrees south and 30 degrees north. As such, eumycetoma is a rare condition in the United States, although it is somewhat common in Mexico and cases infrequently present in the Southwest United States. The foot is the most frequent site of infection, however, almost any tissue may be involved. The disease is usually limited to the cutaneous and subcutaneous tissues, but extension through fascial planes may occur. A history of trauma to the area is often found as well as direct exposure to the soil such as during frequently walking barefoot outdoors or agricultural work. Treatment of eumycetoma is frequently difficult. Outpatient therapy with oral azole antifungal agents is occasionally effective; however amphotericin B is not effective in treatment.

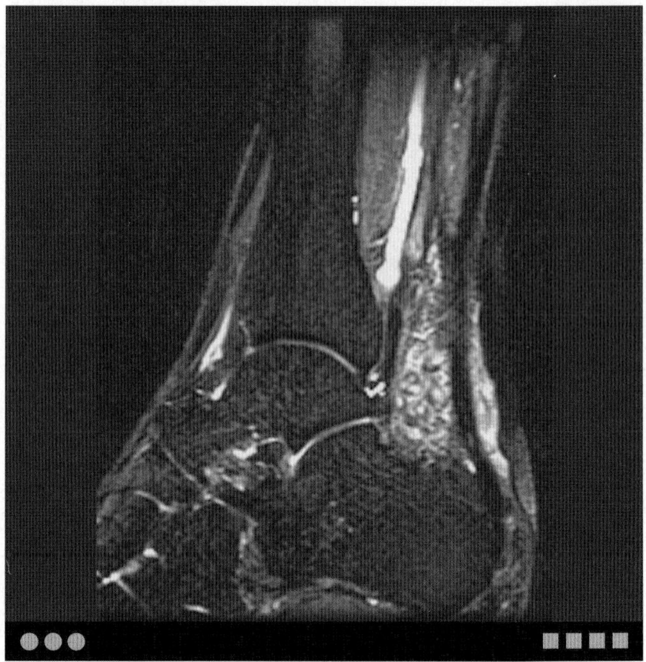

A. Eumycetoma: Sagittal STIR image of the ankle shows heterogeneous high and low signal intensity in the pre-Achilles' fat pad and cutaneous tissues.

Following failure of medical therapy, wide surgical debridement is usually necessary, and postsurgical recurrence rates are high.

PEARLS

- **Eumycetoma is a true fungal infection of the cutaneous and subcutaneous tissues.**
- **Eumycetoma is usually seen in the tropical and subtropical regions of the world.**
- **The foot is the most common site of infection.**
- **MRI shows low signal intensity mass on T1-weighted image, which enhances with contrast administration. T2-weighted images are more variable and may have heterogeneous signal.**

ADDITIONAL IMAGES

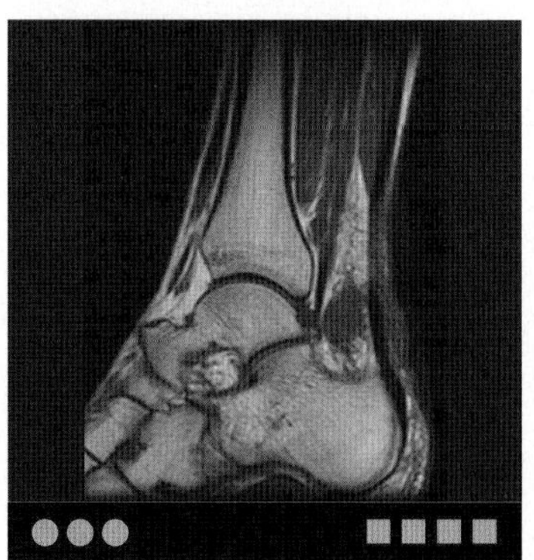

B. Eumycetoma: Sagittal T1-weighted image of the ankle shows ill-defined, low signal intensity mass in the pre-Achilles' fat pad, as well as low signal within the cutaneous fat posterior to the Achilles' tendon.

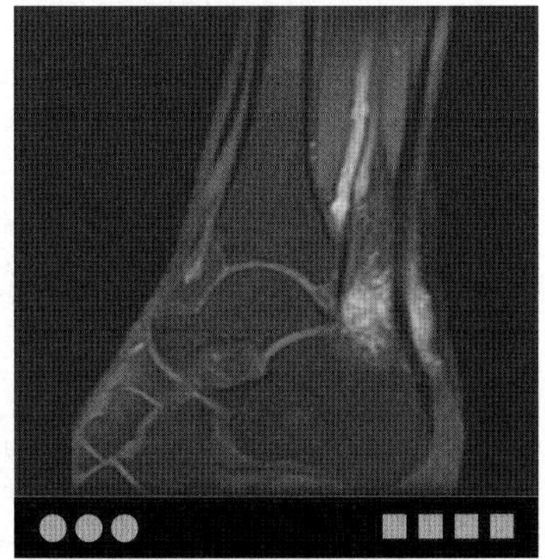

C. Eumycetoma: Sagittal fat-saturated, postcontrast T1-weighted images show avid enhancement through the corresponding low-signal regions seen in images A and B.

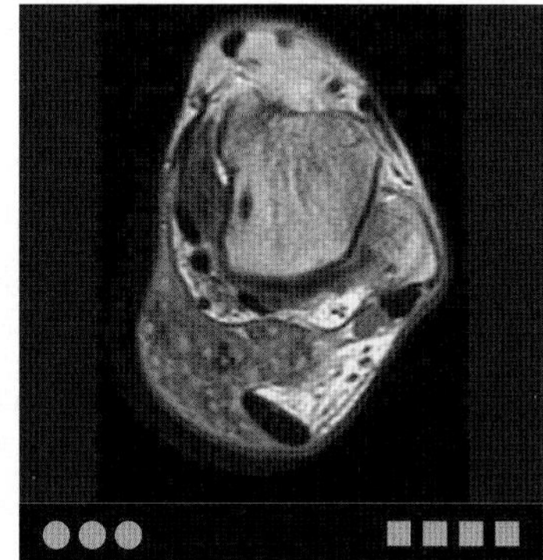

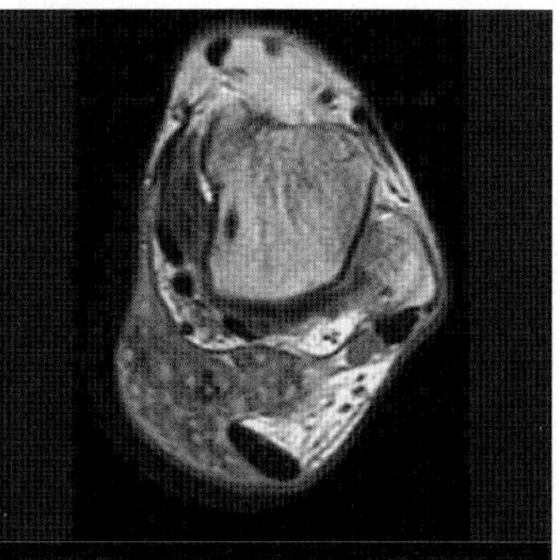

D. Eumycetoma: Axial PDW image shows an isointense, heterogeneous mass in the posteromedial ankle. Note the extension through facial planes, without frank involvement of the Achilles' tendon.

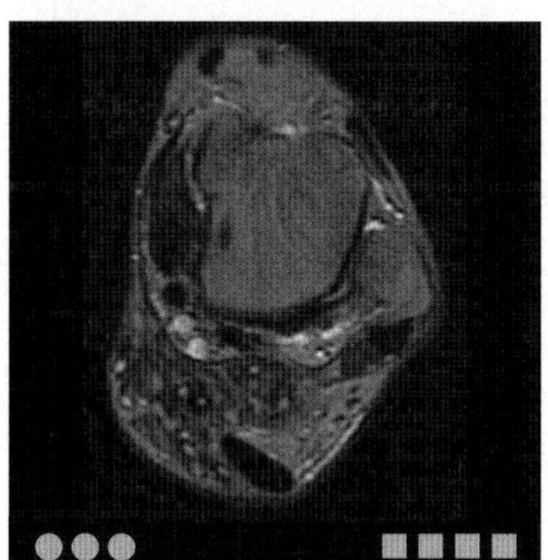

E. Eumycetoma: Axial T2-weighted image through the same level as image D shows the mass with mixed internal high and low signal.

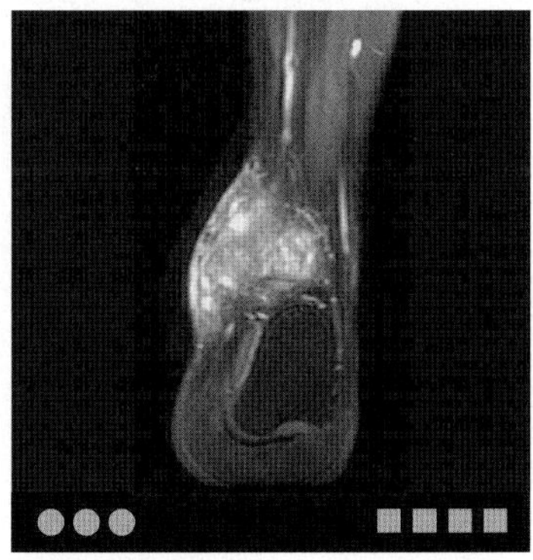

F. Eumycetoma: Coronal fat-saturated, postcontrast T1-weighted images show avid enhancement through the corresponding low-signal regions seen in images A and B.

DIFFERENTIAL DIAGNOSIS IMAGE

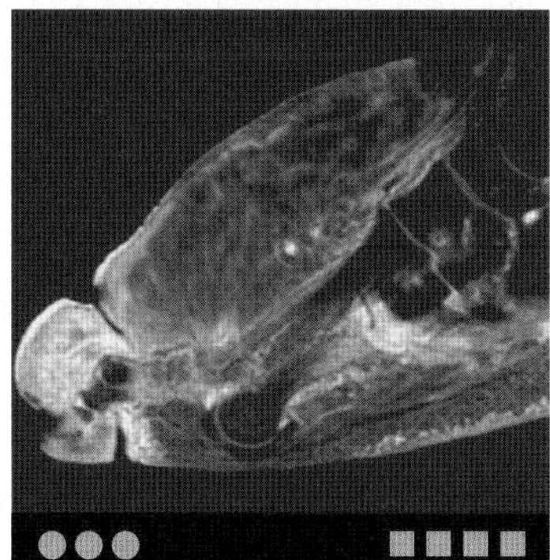

G. Onychomycosis: Sagittal T1-weighted FS postcontrast image shows large soft tissue mass of the foot with heterogeneous enhancement.

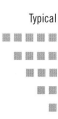

IMAGE KEY

Common

Rare

Typical

Unusual

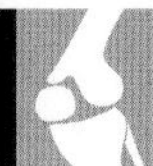

32–2 Pyomyositis, Fasciitis, and Myonecrosis of the Leg

Melitus Maryam Golshan and Jamshid Tehranzadeh

PRESENTATION

Fever, calf pain, and swelling

FINDINGS

MRI shows abscess formation in posterior and middle compartment of leg and partial myonecrosis of the gastrocnemius muscle.

DIFFERENTIAL DIAGNOSES

- *Polymyositis:* It shows bright muscle signal on T2-weighted and STIR imaging and enhancement of involved muscle after contrast administration.
- *Fasciitis:* It shows enhancement along fascial planes between muscles with contrast injection.
- *Cellulitis:* This shows stranding and edema of skin and the soft tissue, with postcontrast enhancement.
- *Myonecrosis:* There is focal area of lack of contrast enhancement with rim of increased signal inside the muscle.

COMMENTS

The patient is a 52-year-old man with history of chronic liver disease presenting with fever and severe leg pain. Pyomyositis (infection of muscle) can be divided into three clinical stages. Stage one is characterized by localized pain in one muscle group with induration of overlying skin, low-grade fever, and mild elevation of the WBC. Stage two is characterized by escalating pain, fever, and edema of affected muscle. Aspiration of muscle reveals pus. In stage three, a fluctuant abscess may be noted with necrosis of muscle, and patient may become septic. CT shows areas of muscle enlargement with decreased attenuation of edematous muscle. With administration of intravenous contrast material, necrotic tissue will demonstrate lack of enhancement and abscess appears as well-defined fluid collection with enhancing wall. MRI in pyomyositis shows a central area of low signal intensity within muscle on T1-weighted image, in some cases surrounded by a peripheral rim of high signal intensity that probably represents blood products. Pus inside abscess can be either isointense or hyperintense in T1-weighted image depending on the proteinaceous content of fluid collection. On T2-weighted image, abscess collection is hyperintense. Areas of abnormal high signal intensity in adjacent muscles represent unorganized phlegmon collections, edema, or hyperemia. After contrast injection, necrotic tissue manifests as a low signal intensity area surrounded by a hyperintense-enhancing rim on T1-weighted image.

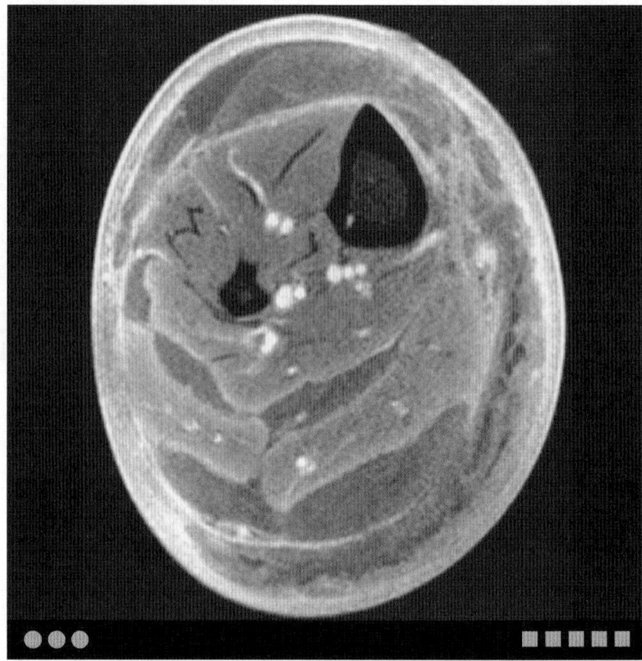

A. Pyomyositis: Axial postcontrast fat-saturated T1-weighted images shows fluid collections anterior to the tibia, between soleus and gastrocnemius muscles and posterior to the gastrocnemius with rim enhancement indicating fasciitis and abscess formation. There is also extensive cellulitis.

PEARLS

- **Pyomyositis has three stages. It starts with pain and indurations and leads to abscess formation and finally myonecrosis occurs.**
- **CT with contrast in pyomyositis shows areas of muscle enlargement with decreased attenuation of edematous muscle with rim enhancement.**
- **Pyomyositis and abscess appear as hypointense areas on T1weighted image and hyperintense on T2-weighted image.**
- **Myonecrosis is characteristically low signal intensity area of muscle, which is nonenhancing in the center but has enhancing rim after contrast injection.**

ADDITIONAL IMAGES

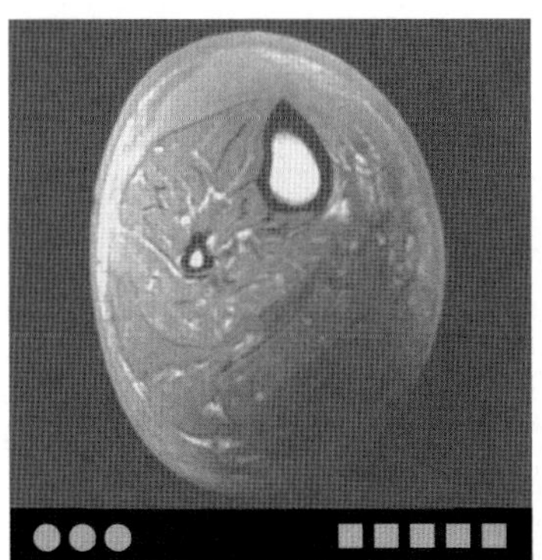

B. Pyomyositis: Axial T1-weighted image shows areas of hypointense signal intensity inside the gastrocnemius muscle as well as low signal intensity in posterior and middle compartments and anteriorly in subcutaneous tissue.

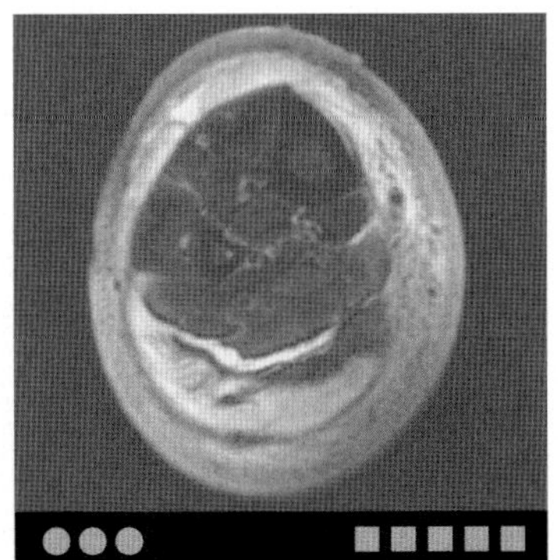

C. Pyomyositis: Axial fat-saturated T2-weighted image shows fluid collections in front of anterior compartment myositis and myonecrosis with fluid collection in the region of gastrocnemius muscle and between soleus and gastrocnemius fascial planes.

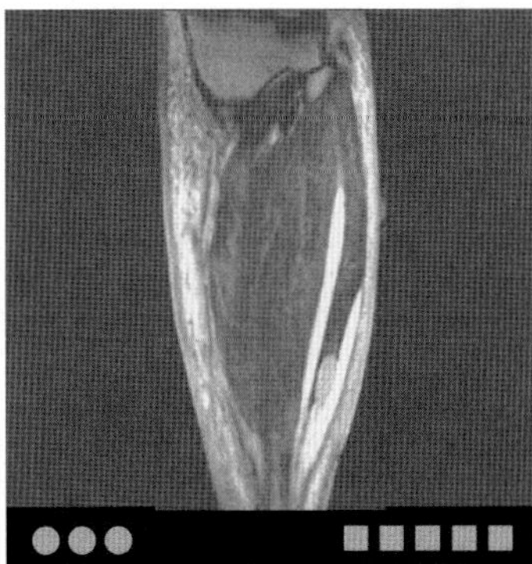

D. Pyomyositis: Coronal T2-weighted image shows bright signal fluid collections along fascial planes and between peroneus longus and soleus muscles.

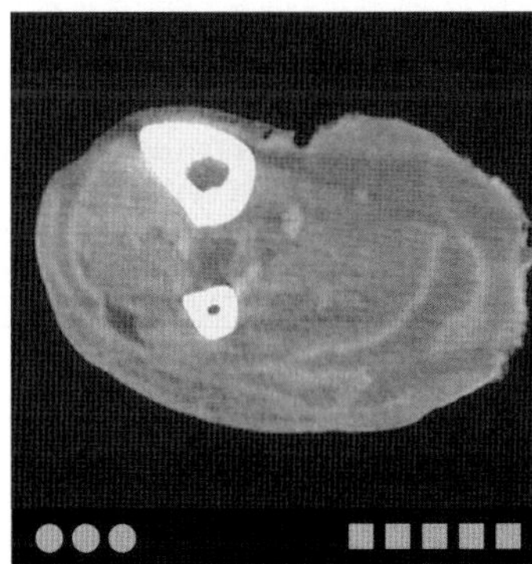

E. Pyomyositis: CT following surgery shows rim enhancing fluid collection anteriorly and posteriorly indicating residual abscesses.

IMAGE KEY

Common

Rare

Typical

Unusual

DIFFERENTIAL DIAGNOSES IMAGES

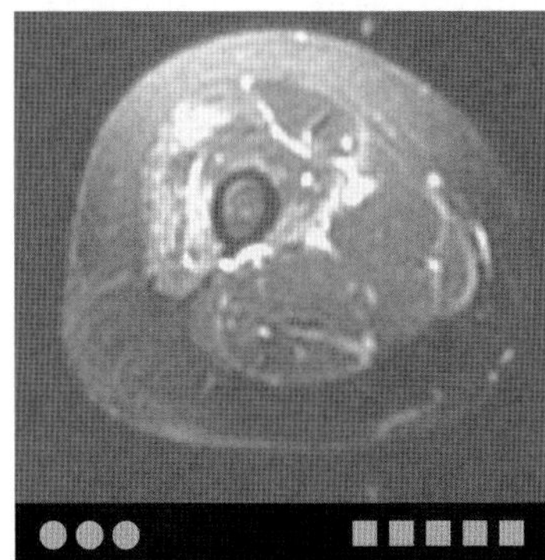

F. Polymyositis: Axial fat-saturated FSE T2-weighted image shows bright signal in vastus lateralis and intermedius muscles suggesting myositis in a 37-year-old female with dermatomyositis.

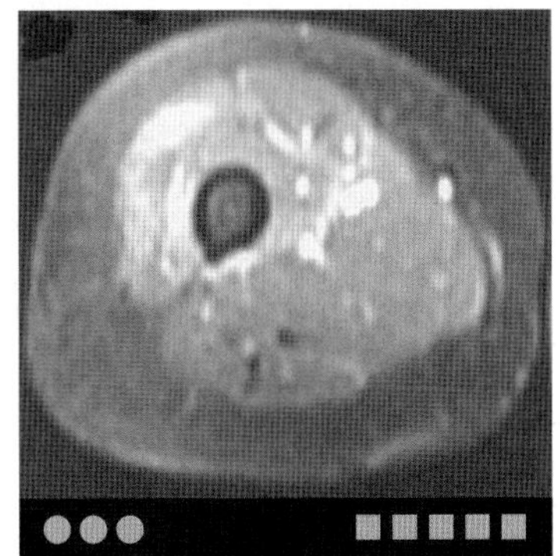

G. Polymyositis: Axial post-contrast fat-saturated T1-weighted image shows enhancement in vastus lateralis and intermedius muscles in the same patient with dermatomyositis.

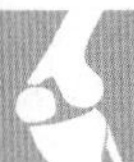

32–3 Osteomyelitis in Diabetes Mellitus

Melitus Maryam Golshan and Jamshid Tehranzadeh

PRESENTATION

Heel ulcer, pain

FINDINGS

MR imaging shows a deep plantar ulcer with adjacent soft tissue swelling and osteomyelitis of calcaneus.

DIFFERENTIAL DIAGNOSES

- *Neuropathic osteoarthropathy:* It is associated with increased density on radiograph, multiple fractures, dislocation, disorganization, and debris. MR shows low signal intensity in T1- and T2-weighted image. Contusion and fractures may lead to high signal on T2-weighted image, which makes differentiation from osteomyelitis difficult, especially in the midfoot.
- *Cellulitis:* It shows soft tissue edema, stranding, and postgadolinium enhancement.
- Tarsal bone contusions or fractures, which show irregular foci of low signal on T1 and high signal intensity on T2-weighted images.

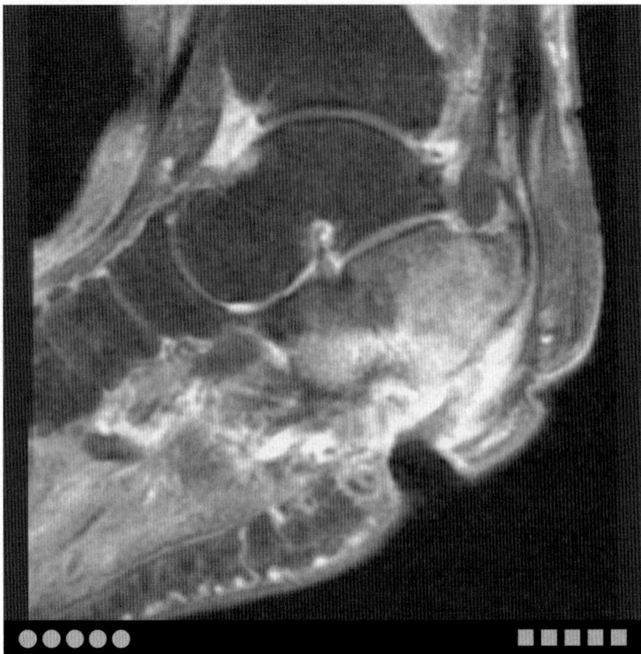

A. Osteomyelitis: Sagittal postcontrast fat-saturated T1-weighted image shows a large ulcer in heel with high signal intensity in soft tissue around it indicating cellulitis. Note erosion in calcaneus with high signal in the bone suggesting osteomyelitis of os calcis, there is also effusion in ankle joint.

COMMENTS

This is the case of a 54-year-old diabetic woman presenting with long-standing heel ulcer, drainage, and pain. Diabetic patients are predisposed to foot infections because of a compromised vascular supply secondary to diabetes. In addition to microvascular disease, local trauma or pressure (often in association with lack of sensation because of neuropathy) may result in a variety of diabetic foot infections. The spectrum of foot infections in diabetes ranges from simple superficial cellulitis to chronic osteomyelitis. Ninety-four percent of cases of diabetic foot osteomyelitis are associated with ulcers. Ulcers are commonly found beneath weight bearing bony prominences, such as metatarsal heads and calcaneal tuberosity. Radiology findings are delayed in acute osteomyelitis for 1 to 3 weeks. It includes localized osteoporosis, bone destruction, and periosteal reaction. MR imaging shows subtle soft tissue changes, which are best evaluated by unenhanced and enhanced MRI. In general, MRI permits differentiation of cellulitis from osteomyelitis. MR imaging demonstrates low signal intensity on T1-weighted image and high signal intensity on T2-weighted image and particularly STIR images in osteomyelitis. Foci of osteomyelitis greatly enhance with contrast. Homogenous fat suppression and STIR imaging are essential for the evaluation of osteomyelitis in the diabetic foot. Proximity to the typical ulcer site and presence of adjacent abnormal soft tissue favors osteomyelitis as a cause of abnormal marrow signal.

PEARLS

- **Foot infection is a common problem in diabetic patients; it ranges from cellulitis to chronic osteomyelitis. In most cases the lesion is adjacent to a pressure point ulcer.**
- **Radiographic findings are late in osteomyelitis, which include localized osteoporosis, soft tissue swelling, bone destruction, and periosteal reaction. The latter finding is not common in toes and hindfoot.**
- **MR imaging demonstrates low signal intensity on T1-weighted image and high signal intensity on T2-weighted image and particularly STIR images in osteomyelitis. It shows marked postcontrast enhancement in foci with osteomyelitis.**

ADDITIONAL IMAGES

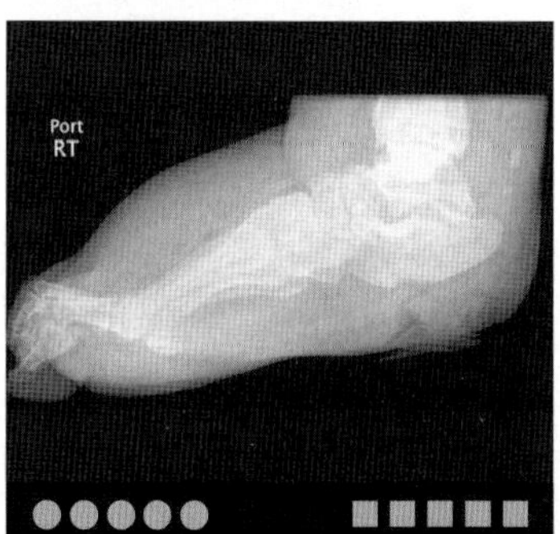

B. Osteomyelitis: Lateral radiograph of the ankle shows vascular calcification and soft tissue swelling with air containing ulcer in soft tissue of the heel. Note erosion of plantar cortex of calcaneus indicating osteomyelitis. There is also calcification in the Achilles tendon.

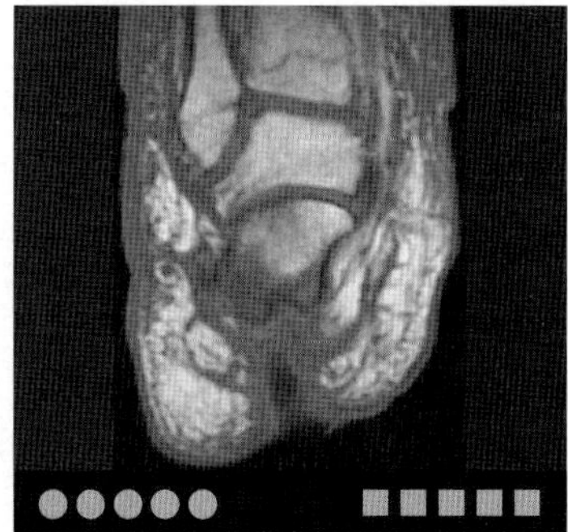

C. Osteomyelitis: Coronal T1-weighted image shows large ulcer in the heel and erosion of calcaneus with low signal marrow changes indicating osteomyelitis.

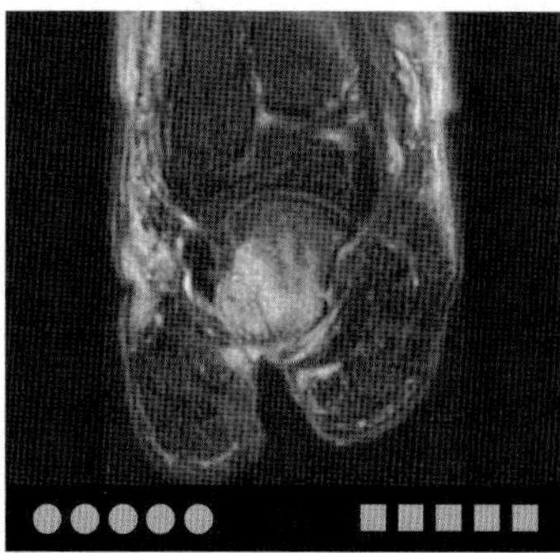

D. Osteomyelitis: Coronal fat-saturated T2-weighted image shows heel ulcer and high signal in the calcaneus indicating osteomyelitis.

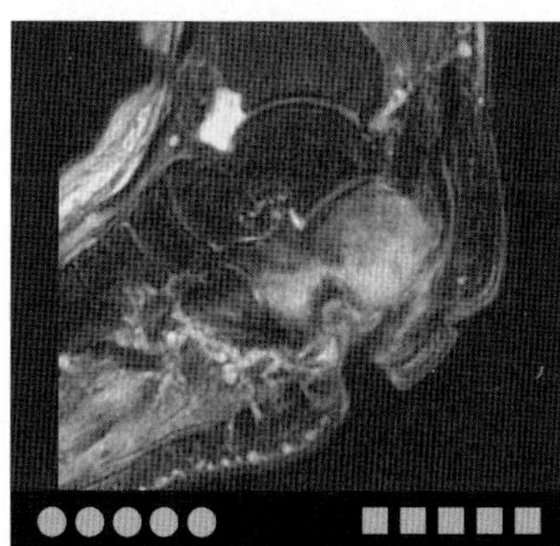

E. Osteomyelitis: Sagittal fat-saturated T2-weighted image shows a large ulcer in heel with bright signal in surrounding soft tissues with edema indicating cellulitis. There is calcaneus erosion adjacent to the ulcer with high signal in the marrow consistent with osteomyelitis. Note fluid in the ankle joint.

IMAGE KEY

Common

Rare

Typical

Unusual

DIFFERENTIAL DIAGNOSES IMAGES

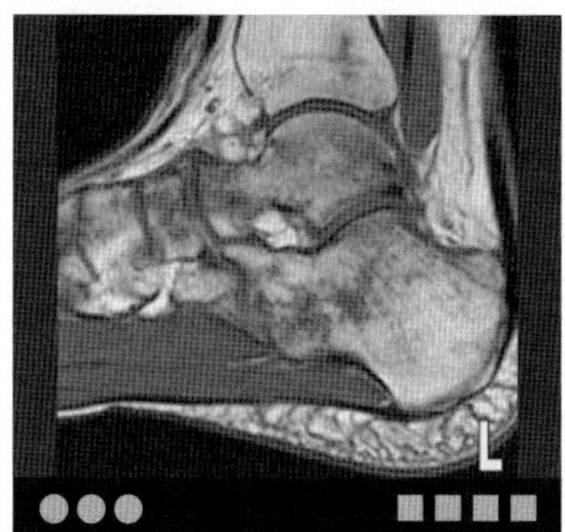

F. Multiple bone contusion: Sagittal T1-weighted image shows low signal intensity foci in distal tibia, calcaneus, talus, navicular, and cuneiform in a 19-year-old kick boxer with ankle and foot pain indicating tarsal bones contusion.

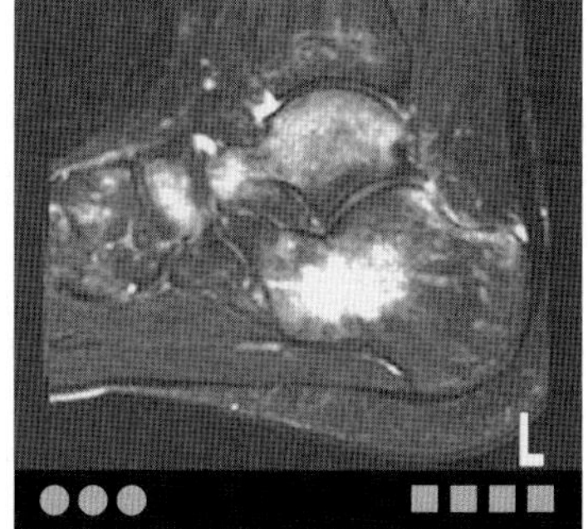

G. Multiple bone contusion: Sagittal SPIR image of the ankle shows foci of high signal intensity in tarsal bones indicating multiple bone contusion in the same patient shown in image F.

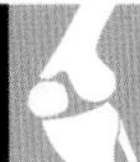

32–4 Tuberculosis of Ankle

Melitus Maryam Golshan and Jamshid Tehranzadeh

PRESENTATION

Chronic pain, swelling, and discharge

FINDINGS

MR images show extensive bone edema with postcontrast enhancement in distal tibia, fibula, and tarsal bones consistent with osteomyelitis.

DIFFERENTIAL DIAGNOSES

- *Septic arthritis:* The changes are more acute and rapidly progressive. Neglected cases lead to severe and early joint destruction.
- Fungal arthritis shows a high signal intensity rim on unenhanced T1-weighted image. A sinus tract formation, seen as linear high signals on T2-weighted image with marginal "tram track enhancement," might also be seen, which may differentiate it from tuberculosis (TB) arthritis.
- Rheumatoid arthritis shows earlier loss of articular space and usually affects more than one joint.
- Pigmented villonodular synovitis shows intra-articular nodules, low signal hemosiderin deposits on all MR sequences.
- Gouty tophi are mostly of low or intermediate signal intensity of T1-weighted image and reveal a characteristic increase in signal intensity after contrast.

COMMENTS

The patient is a 59-year-old man with ankle pain and swelling. Ankle tuberculosis occurs in less than 1% of all cases of osteoarticular TB. The talus being the most commonly involved bone in ankle. The pain is slowly growing with mild fever, inflamed joint, and high ESR. Tenosynovitis and bone marrow changes are the most common abnormalities.

Osteoporosis reflects chronicity of the disease process. Joint narrowing and bony erosions are often late findings in TB arthritis. MRI shows earliest findings, which are ankle and subtalar joint effusions that are hypointense on T1-weighted image and hyperintense on T2-weighted image. Further sequel of the disease is in the form of bone marrow signal alterations of varying grades. The altered signal intensities are in the form of fat replacement on T1-weighted image and bone marrow edema on T2-weighted image. Capsular thickening and synovial thickening with granulation tissue formation are revealed with further progression of the disease. Caseation of granulation tissue leads to abscess formation. Cellulitis, tenosynovitis, and myositis in the form of inflammation of the Achilles, peroneal and tibialis muscle groups, and invasion and displacement of anterior, medial, and lateral neurovascular bundles may be seen in TB arthritis. Use of MRI contrast reveals synovial, soft tissue and marrow enhancements, which surround low-signal foci of joint fluid and abscess formation.

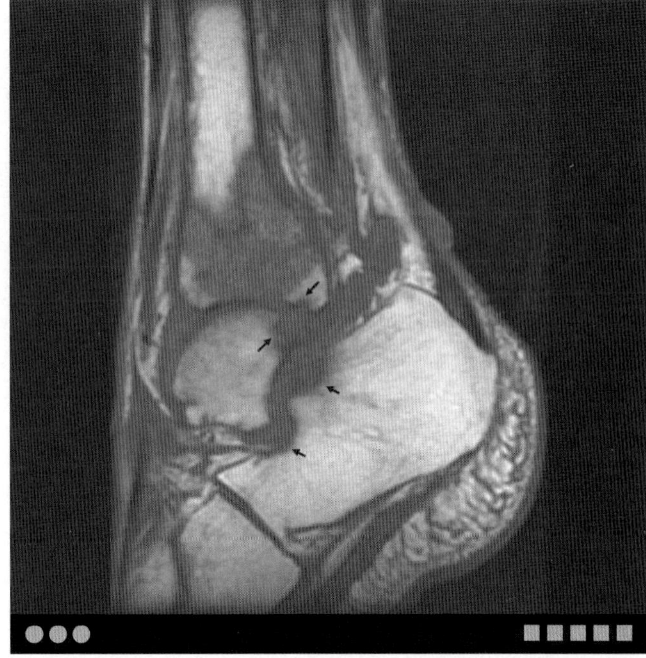

A. Tuberculosis: Sagittal T1-weighted image shows low signal bone marrow changes in tibia with synovial proliferation in ankle and subtalar joint. Note erosion in tibia plafond, talus, and calcaneus (black arrows). Anterior tibialis tendon, plantaris fascia, and flexor hallucis longus tendon are thickened. Intermediate signal sinus tract in posterior ankle is noted.

PEARLS

- **Ankle tuberculosis is an uncommon entity; however, when it occurs, talus is the most commonly involved bone.**
- **Tenosynovitis and bone marrow changes are the most common abnormalities in TB osteoarthritis.**
- **The earliest findings were ankle and subtalar joint effusions that were hypointense on T1-weighted image and hyperintense on T2weighted image.**
- **Cellulitis, tenosynovitis, and myositis in the form of inflammation of the Achilles, peroneal and tibialis muscle groups may be seen in TB arthritis.**
- **Use of MRI contrast reveals synovial, soft tissue, and marrow enhancements surrounding low-signal foci of joint fluid and abscess formation.**

ADDITIONAL IMAGES

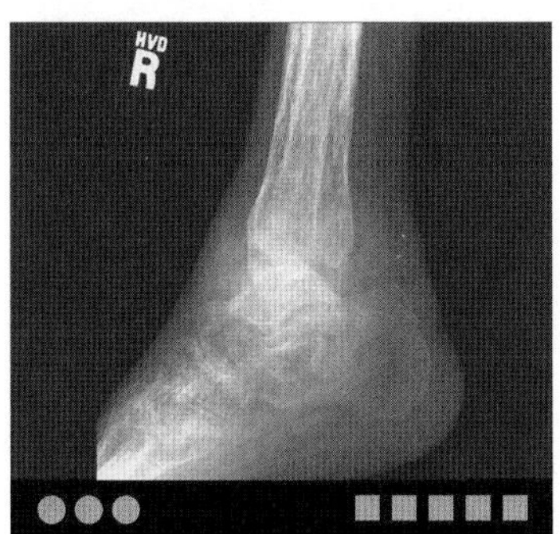

B. Tuberculosis: Lateral radiograph of ankle shows severe osteopenia with synovial proliferation in anterior ankle joint with erosion of anterior tibia. Note soft tissue swelling in posterior part of ankle and fullness of Kager's fat pad.

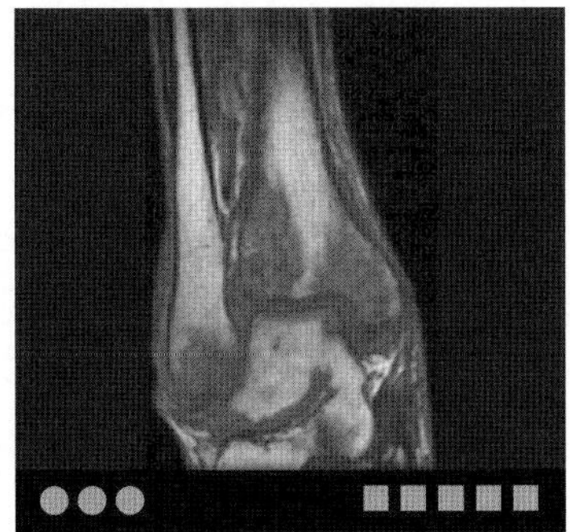

C. Tuberculosis: Coronal T1-weighted image shows low signal bone marrow foci in tibia and calcaneus. Note erosions in tibia, fibula, and talus.

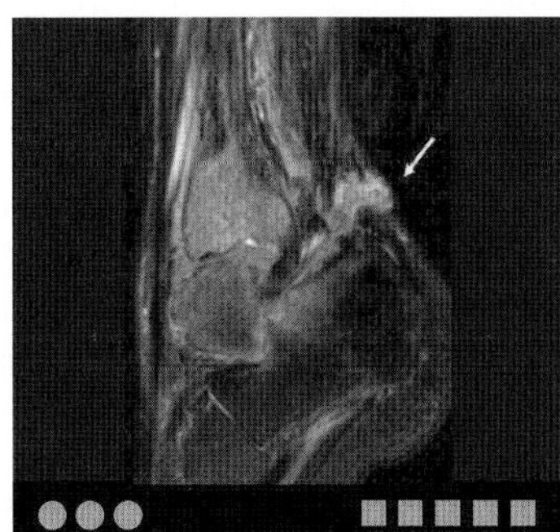

D. Tuberculosis: Sagittal fat-saturated fast spin echo T2-weighted image shows bright signal in tibia, talus, and calcaneus. Note bright signal sinus tract in posterior ankle (arrow).

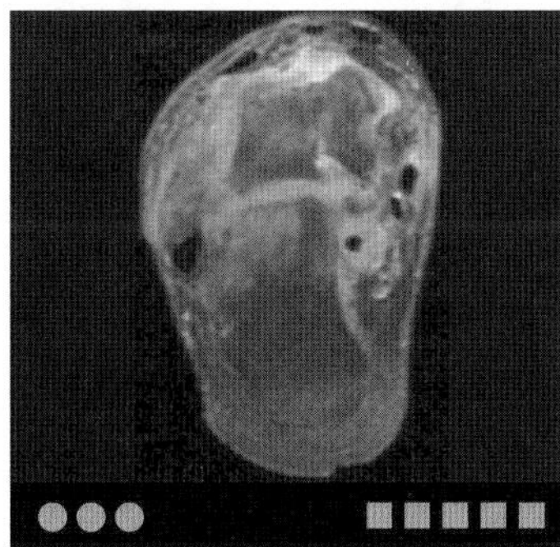

E. Tuberculosis: Axial fat-saturated postcontrast T1-weighted image shows extensive soft tissue enhancement around ankle with tenosynovitis of peroneal, posterior tibialis, flexor digitorum longus, and hallucis longus tendons. Note talus and calcaneus enhancement with erosions.

IMAGE KEY

Common

Rare

Typical

Unusual

DIFFERENTIAL DIAGNOSES IMAGES

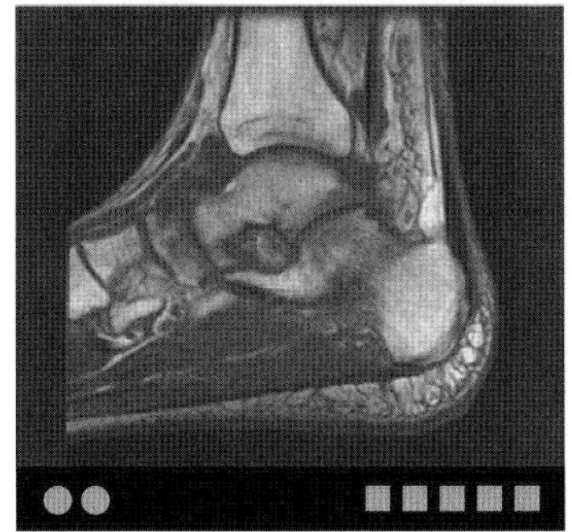

F. HIV arthritis: Sagittal T1-weighted image shows low signal bone marrow changes in calcaneus, talus, navicular, and medial cuneiform bones and soft tissue swelling. Note fluid in the ankle joint and around flexor tendons in a 36-year-old HIV positive man with acute ankle pain.

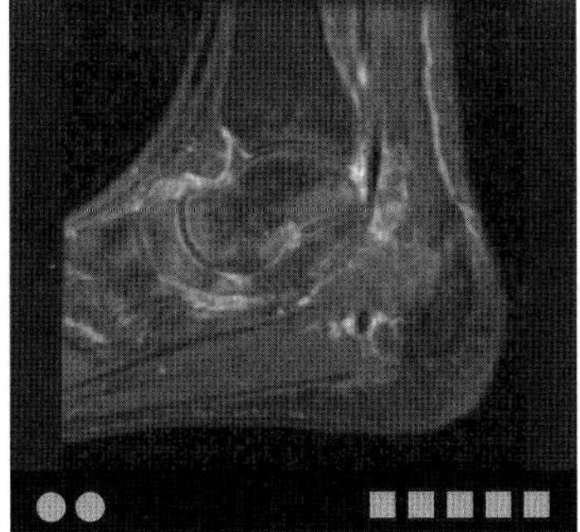

G. HIV arthritis: Sagittal fat-saturated postcontrast T1-weighted image shows bright signal in calcaneus, talus, navicular, and medial cuneiform bones with enhanced synovium and soft tissue swelling.

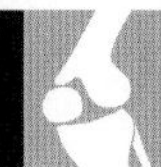

32–5 Onychomycosis and Fungal Infection of the Foot

Shahla Modarresi and Daria Motamedi

PRESENTATION

Swelling of the foot, ulceration of toes

FINDINGS

MR imaging shows diffuse soft tissue edema and low T1 signal mass in dorsal aspect of second digit.

DIFFERENTIAL DIAGNOSES

- *Squamous cell carcinoma:* Most nail bed malignancies are squamous cell carcinoma. MR imaging of squamous cell carcinoma shows superficial cutaneous mass with low to intermediate PD and high T2-weighted signal showing contrast enhancement.
- *Hematoma:* The signal intensity of hematoma varies depending on its age duration. MR shows intermediate to low signal mass in case of acute and chronic hematoma.
- *PVNS, Giant cell tumor of tendon sheet:* MRI shows a mass with intermediate to low signal on T1-weighted and heterogeneous signal intensity on T2-weighted images, with areas of decreased signal related to hemosiderin.
- *Synovial soft tissue sarcoma:* MR signal intensity is usually nonspecific showing low to intermediate T1, high T2 signal and contrast enhancement. Histologic analysis of tissue is usually required for definitive diagnosis.
- *Elephantiasis:* Chronic, extreme enlargement and hardening of cutaneous and subcutaneous tissue, especially the legs from lymphatic obstruction, usually caused by infestation of the lymph glands and vessels with a filarial worm.

COMMENTS

The patient is a 65-year-old man, with sever lymphedema and ulceration on the dorsum of the second and third toes. Onychomycosis is a chronic, highly resistant fungal infection of the nail, accounting for 30% of all cutaneous fungal infections. Onychomycosis is mostly caused by a dermatophyte, but nondermatophyte fungi (yeast or mold) may also be causative agents. The term tinea unguium is used specifically to describe invasive dermatophytic onychomycosis. The infection can be acquired by walking barefoot in public places or most commonly as part of an infection called athlete's foot. The disease is twice as frequent among men as women and increases with age, likely secondary to decreased peripheral circulation, inactivity, poor nail hygiene and diabetes.

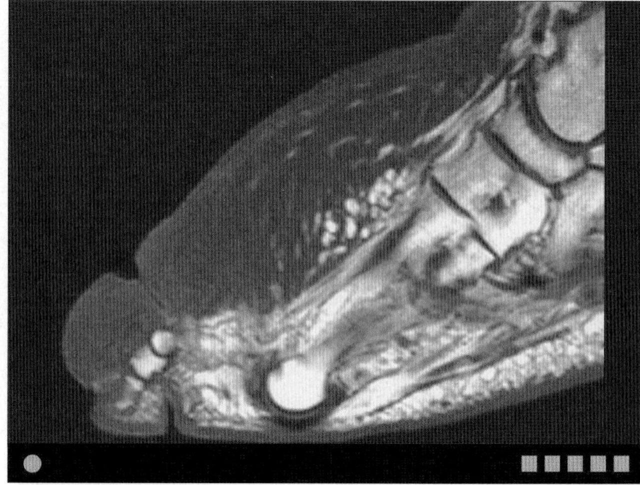

A. Onychomycosis: Sagittal T1-weighted image showing diffuse edema and exophytic mass dorsal to the second toe.

The prevalence of onychomycosis in patient with diabetes is about 26% with three times increase risk of infection than nondiabetic individuals. Immunosuppressed individuals, HIV, and non-HIV, are more prone to this infection. Other risk factors include nail trauma, hyperhydrosis, and tinea pedis. Fungal nail infections may precipitate secondary bacterial infections, diffuse cellulitis, and chronic urticaria. Infected toenails may act as reservoirs for fungi, causing transmission to other areas of the body and perhaps to other people. Diagnosis of the disease is purely clinical, and is made by microscopy and culture of the nail specimen. In the presence of adjacent soft tissue involvement and secondary infection, MR imaging may be valuable to see the extent of the disease, underlying bone, and to rule out other etiologies.

PEARLS

- **Onychomycosis is a chronic, highly resistant fungal infection of the nail accounting for 30% of all cutaneous fungal infections.**
- **The infection can be acquired by walking barefoot in public places or most commonly as part of an infection called athlete's foot.**
- **The disease likely results from the decreased peripheral circulation, seen with poor nail hygiene, old age, diabetes, and immunosuppressed individuals.**
- **Secondary bacterial infections, diffuse cellulitis, chronic urticaria; and transmission to other areas of the body and to other individuals are complications of the disease.**
- **Diagnosis is purely clinical with specimen culture. With soft tissue involvement and secondary infection, MRI is valuable to see the extent of the disease and underlying bone.**

ADDITIONAL IMAGES

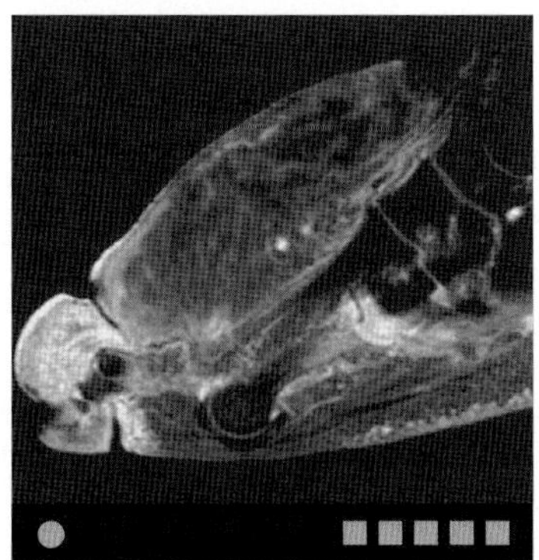

B. Onychomycosis: Sagittal T1-weighted postcontrast image shows enhancement of the exophytic mass on the dorsum of the second toe.

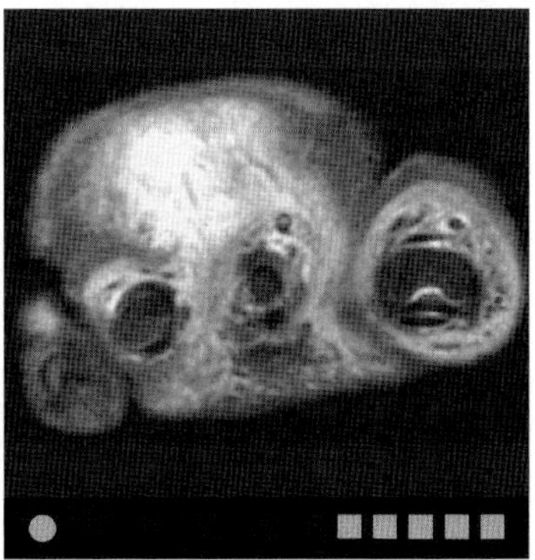

C. Onychomycosis: Axial STIR image shows exophytic hyperintense mass dorsal to second and third digits.

DIFFERENTIAL DIAGNOSES IMAGES

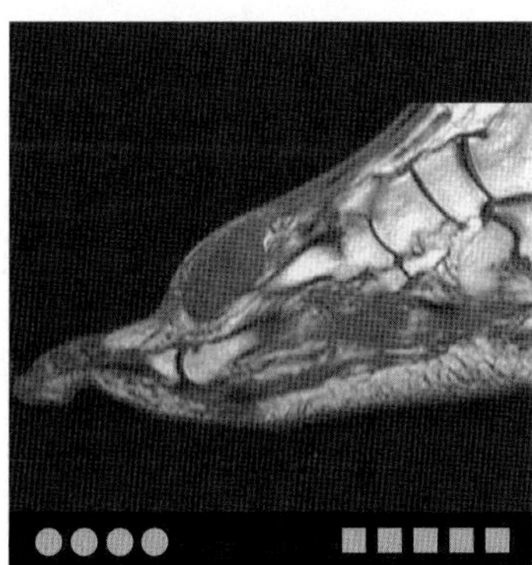

D. Hematoma: Sagittal T1-weighted image shows a well defined low signal mass on the dorsum of the foot consistent with hematoma.

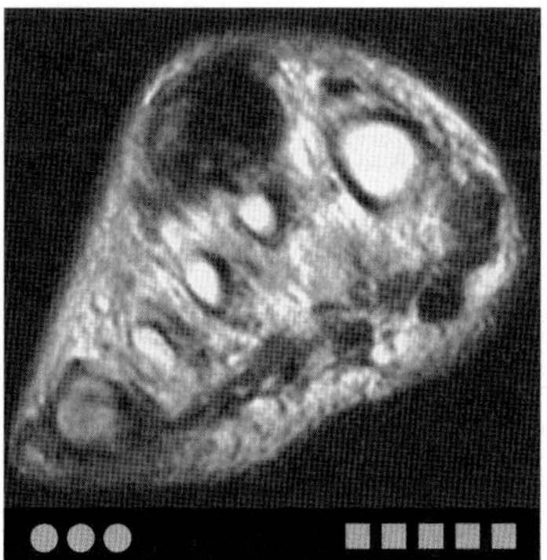

E. Giant cell tumor: Axial T1-weighted image shows rounded low signal mass dorsal to second and third digit consistent with giant cell tumor of the tendon sheet.

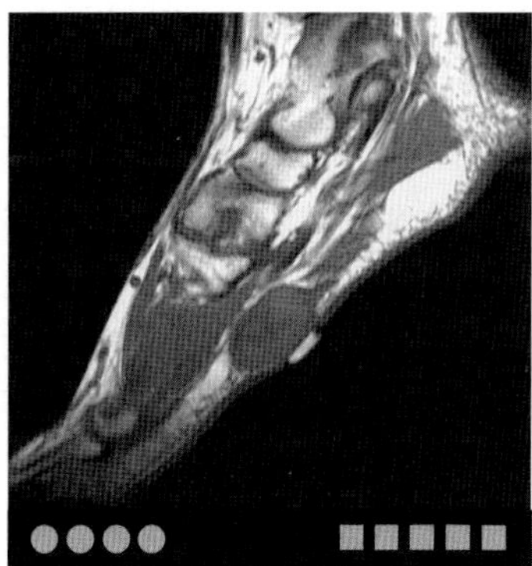

F. Soft tissue sarcoma: Sagittal T1-weighted image shows well-defined low signal mass in the plantar surface of the foot, which showed bright signal on STIR image consistent with soft tissue sarcoma.

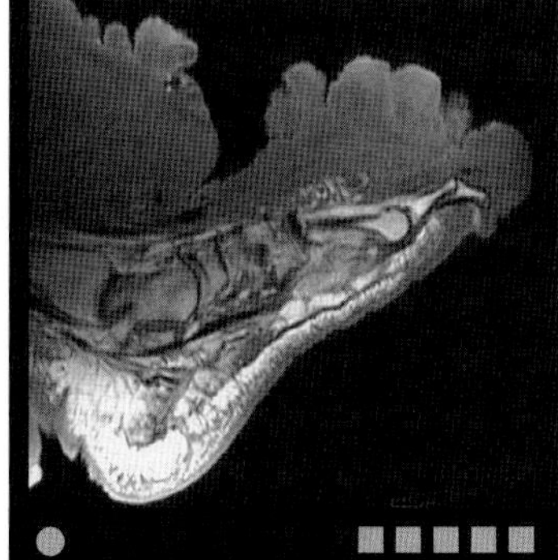

G. Elephantiasis: Sagittal T1-weighted image shows extreme enlargement and villous projections of cutaneous and subcutaneous tissue consistent with edema in this patient with elephantiasis.

IMAGE KEY

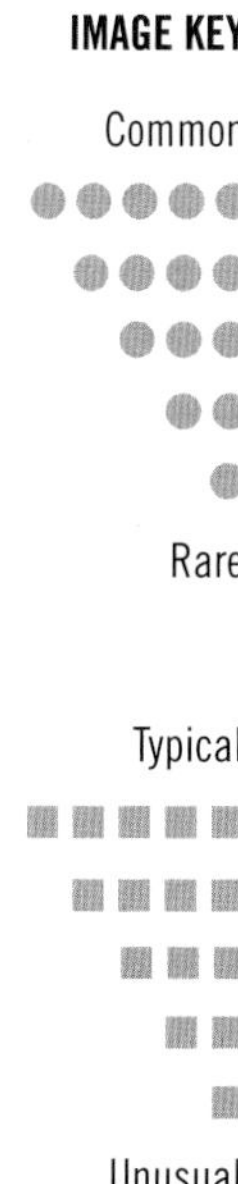

Chapter 33

Tumors and Tumor Like Lesions

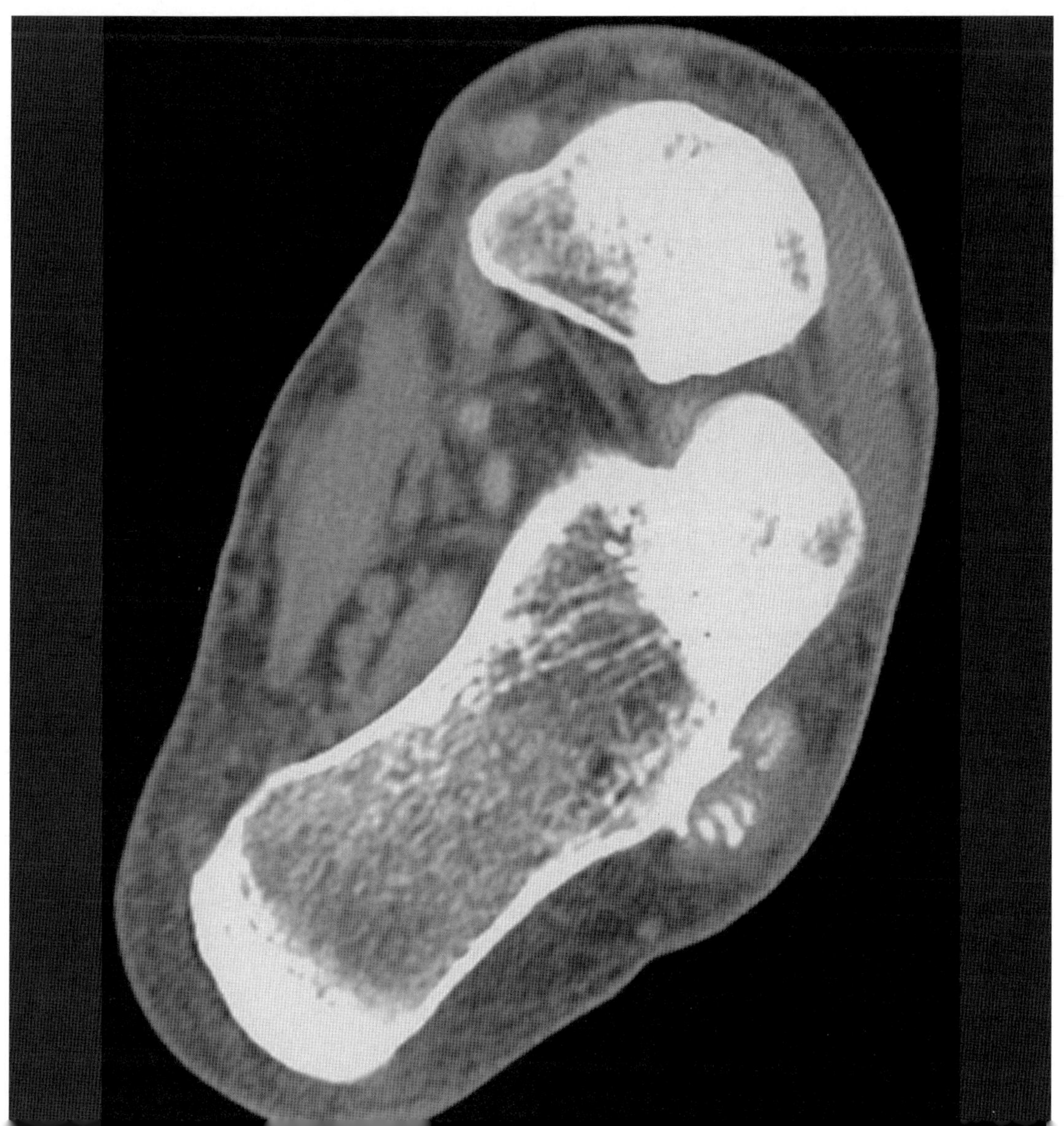

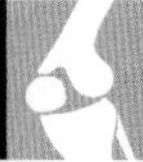

33–1 Synovial Hemangioma of the Peroneal Tendon Sheath

Kambiz Motamedi

PRESENTATION

Palpable mass of the ankle and hind foot

FINDINGS

CT shows a soft tissue mass along the course of the peroneal tendons with round calcifications.

DIFFERENTIAL DIAGNOSES

- *Tenosynovitis of the tendon sheath:* Cross-sectional imaging will show fluid within the tendon sheath. This can be focal nodular indicating stenosing variant.
- *Partial or split tear of the tendon:* On MR or ultrasound an interstitial tear of the tendon becomes evident. There may be small amount of fluid within the tendon sheath.
- *Synovial chondromatosis of the tendon sheath:* MRI shows a mass adjacent to the tendon displaying high signal on fluid sensitive sequences.

COMMENTS

This is a 48-year-old male patient who presented with a painless mass of his lateral aspect of the ankle and hind foot. He denied any previous trauma to this ankle. A hemangioma is an abnormal proliferation of blood vessels that may occur in any vascularized tissue. It is yet not agreed upon as to whether these lesions are neoplasms, hamartomas, or vascular malformations. Hemangiomas occur most often in the skin or subcutaneous tissue, but hemangiomas of the deeper tissues such as intramuscular hemangiomas are not uncommon. Synovial hemangiomas are extremely rare. They can arise from any surface that is lined by synovium, particularly tendon or joint space. They typically occur in young patients. In tendinous synovium, they typically present as a painless mass. In the synovium of a joint, they may present with recurrent effusions, pain, and even mechanical symptoms suggesting intra-articular derangement. A palpable, spongy, compressible mass may be present, and it may decrease in size with elevation of the extremity. The knee is by far the most common joint involved, where the presentation may be confused with meniscal or ligamentous pathology. Both localized and diffuse forms exist. The natural history of many deep tissue hemangiomas is that of gradual fatty replacement, atrophy, and involution over time. This is supported by their greater frequency in individuals younger than 30 years and relative rarity in older adults. Treatment may be considered if pain is substantial.

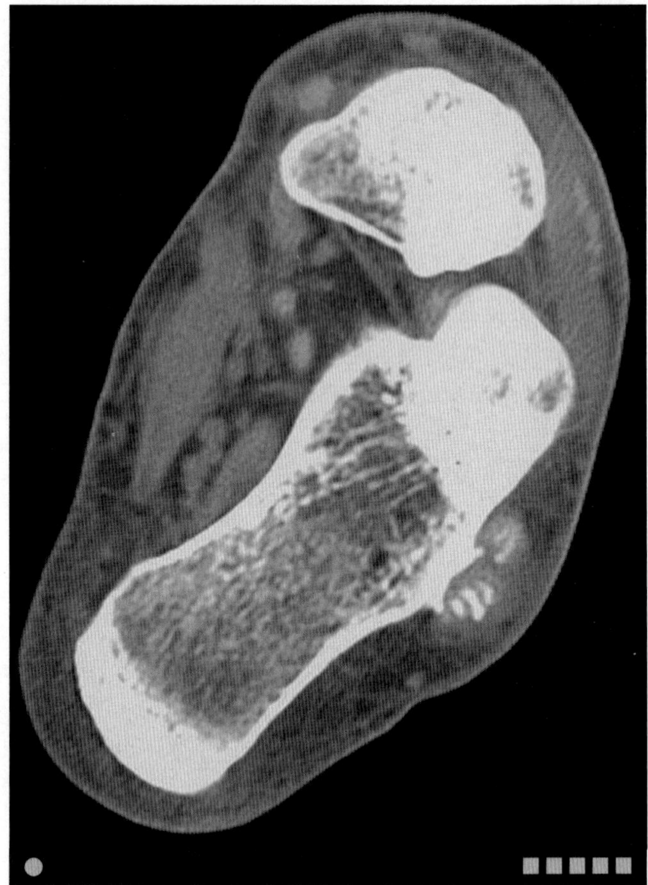

A. Synovial hemangioma: Nonenhanced axial CT scan (soft tissue window) through calcaneus shows a soft tissue mass along the course of the peroneal tendons with calcifications.

PEARLS

- **Radiographs may readily show round calcifications in the course of a tendon.**
- **CT scan may be performed if calcifications are faint.**
- **Both MRI and CT would show tubular structures with interspersed fatty tissue.**

ADDITIONAL IMAGES

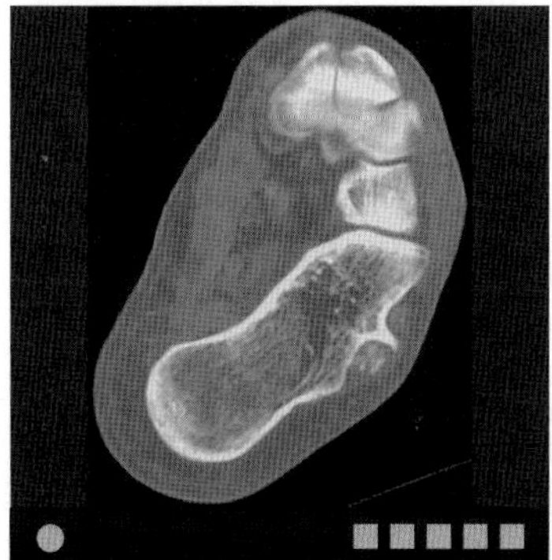

B. Synovial hemangioma: Nonenhanced CT scan (bone window) shows a hypertrophic lateral spur of the calcaneus between the peroneal brevis and longus tendon sheaths with a hemangioma.

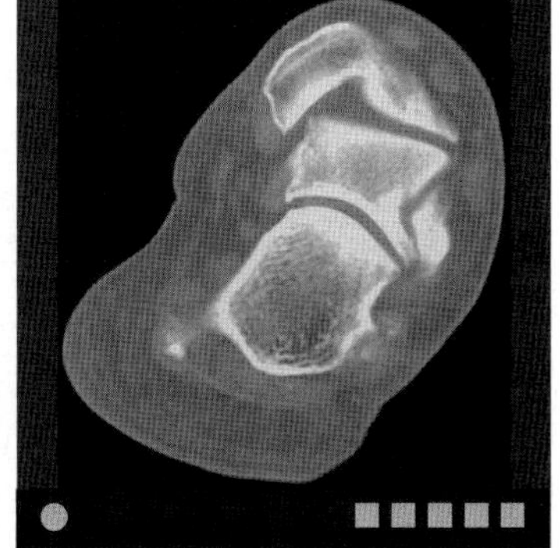

C. Synovial hemangioma: Nonenhanced coronal CT scan (bone window) of the ankle confirms the location of the elongated soft tissue mass within the tendon sheath of the peroneal tendons.

DIFFERENTIAL DIAGNOSES IMAGES

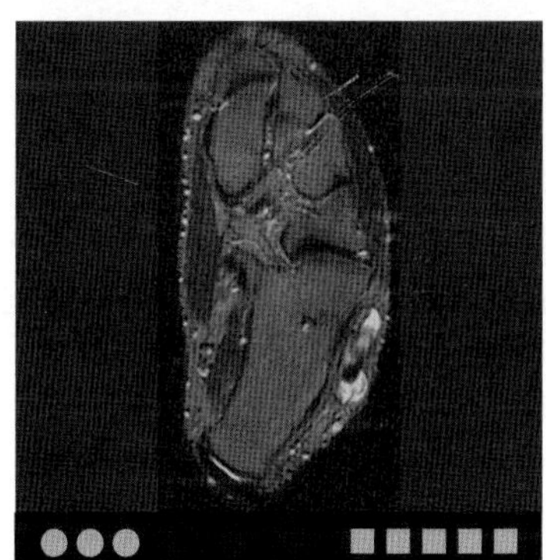

D. Peroneal brevis tendon tear: Axial fat-saturated T2WI of the hind foot shows fluid accumulation within the tendon sheath of the peroneal tendons lateral to the calcaneus.

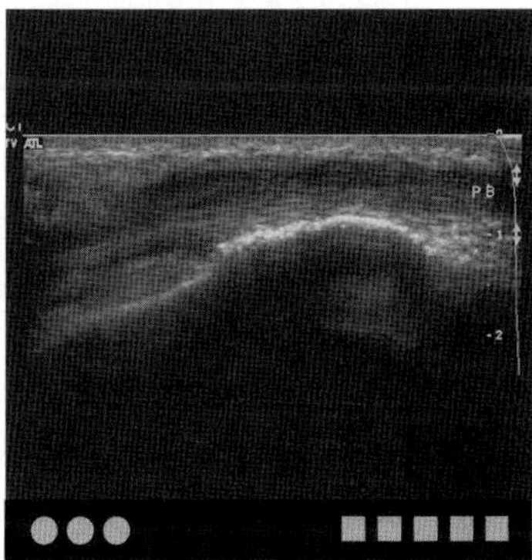

E. Peroneal brevis tenosynovitis: Longitudinal sonographic image of the lateral ankle shows fluid accumulation within the peroneal brevis tendon sheath. Note there is thickening of the tendon sheath as well.

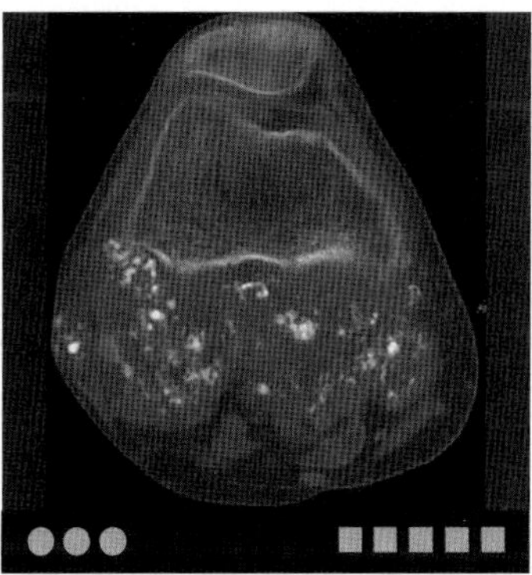

F. Synovial chondromatosis: Nonenhanced axial CT scan (bone window) of the knee reveals a large soft tissue mass with innumerable foci of calcifications. There are several erosions of the posterior femur.

IMAGE KEY

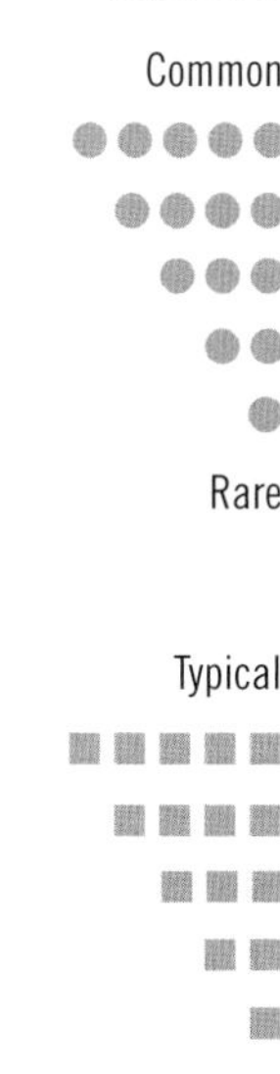

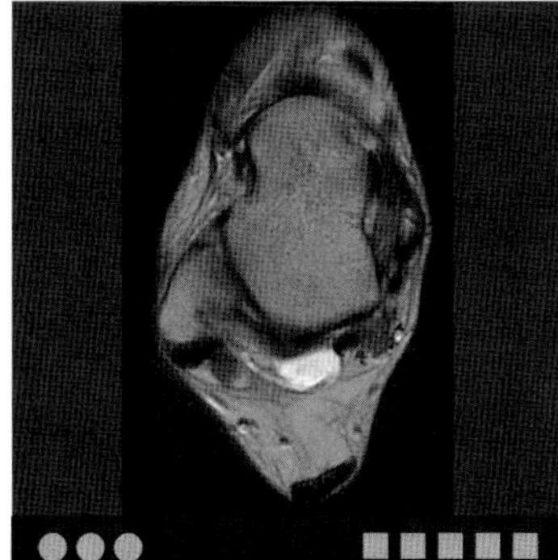

G. Focal nodular synovitis: Axial fat-saturated T2W FSE image of the ankle demonstrates high signal intensity soft tissue mass of the posterior ankle adjacent to the flexor hallucis longus tendon.

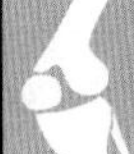

33–2 Pigmented Villonodular Synovitis

Ayodale S. Odulate and Piran Aliabadi

PRESENTATION

Increased swelling, pain, and decreased range of motion

FINDINGS

Joint effusion and mass in the anterior ankle.

DIFFERENTIAL DIAGNOSES

- *Hemophilic arthropathy:* Epiphyseal hypertrophy, linear striation of bones.
- *Synovial chondromatosis:* Multiple small calcified loose bodies in the joint.
- *Tuberculous arthritis:* Monoarticular, involving mainly large and medium joints. Usually diagnosis is made by synovial biopsy and culture.
- *Spondyloarthropathy:* Polyarticular, erosions, cartilage space narrowing, and soft tissue swelling.

COMMENTS

This is a 38-year-old female with chronic intermittent ankle pain. Pigmented villonodular synovitis (PVNS) is a benign tumor of the synovium that can become locally aggressive most common in the knee, shoulder, and ankle. Two types of PVNS are described, diffuse and nodular. The diffuse form is much more common and associated with cystic changes of the joint and periarticular erosions. The nodular form of PVNS usually does not cause local destruction to the joint and diagnosis is difficult as a hemarthrosis may be the only findings. The etiology is unknown with an age range of 20 to 50 years. Patients often present clinically with swelling and pain of the joint. Early MRI findings include a synovial mass with hypointense T1-T2-weighted and proton density signal intensity with a joint effusion. The hypointense signal on T1W imaging results from hemosiderin deposition from multiple bouts of hemarthrosis. Isointense to hyperintense T2W signal intensity can also be seen secondary to the localized synovitis. During the early presentation of the disease, no cartilage space narrowing or destructive changes are present. Later in the course of the disease, cartilage space narrowing and pressure erosions in the bones from the hypertrophied synovium develop. The synovial mass can become locally aggressive and advance into surrounding tendons and ligaments. Imaging plays a crucial role in the diagnosis and direction of surgical management as the treatment is total synovectomy. If the mass is not completely resected, recurrence is likely.

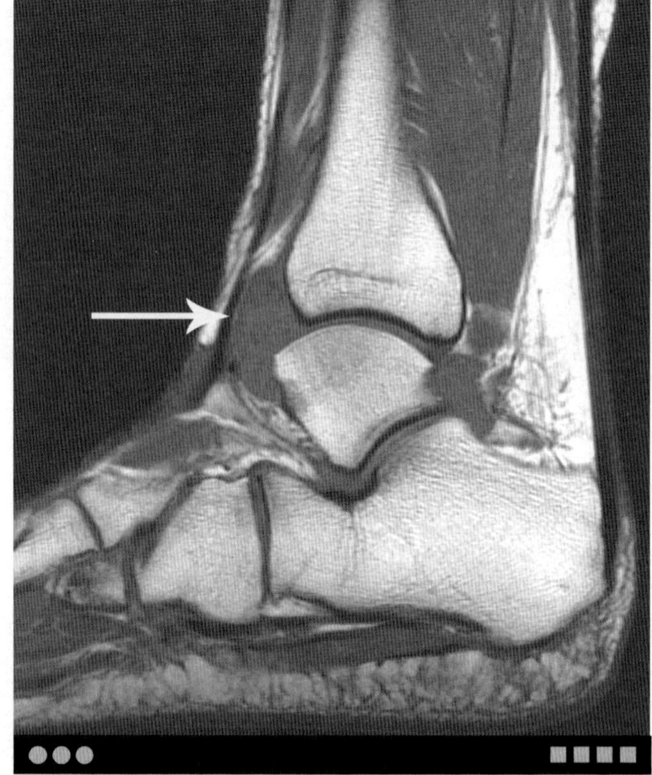

A. PVNS: Sagittal T1WI shows a mass (arrow) in the anterior joint.

PEARLS

- **Episodic monoarticular hemarthrosis and soft tissue swelling with locking or snapping sensation.**
- **Hypointense synovial mass on T1W, T2W, and proton density imaging with blooming artifact seen on gradient echo imaging because of hemosiderin deposition.**
- **Radiographs cannot differentiate pigmented villonodular synovitis from nonossified synovial osteochromatosis.**

ADDITIONAL IMAGES

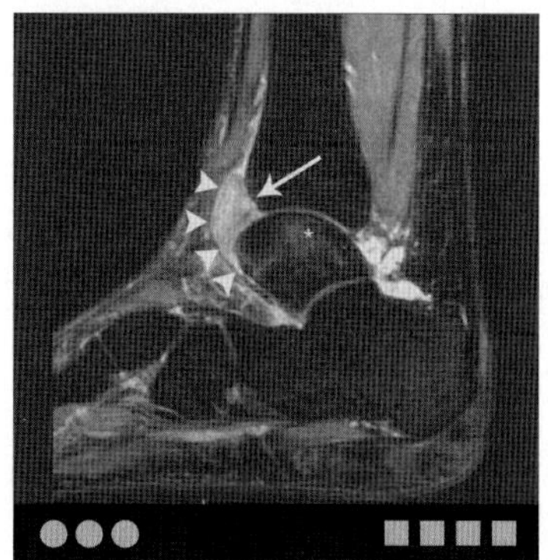

B. PVNS: Sagittal STIR image shows distention of the joint capsule (arrowheads) and heterogeneous signal intensity mass in the anterior joint (arrow). Edema in the talar dome is also seen (asterisk).

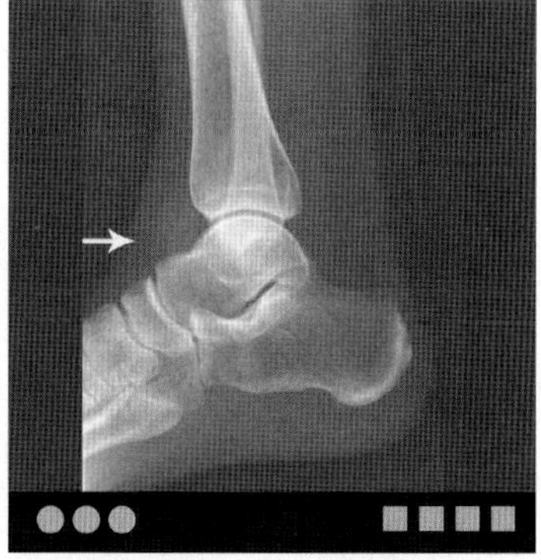

C. PVNS: Lateral radiograph of the left ankle shows a large well-defined dense joint effusion (arrow). The cartilage space and bone density are maintained. No calcifications are seen.

DIFFERENTIAL DIAGNOSES IMAGES

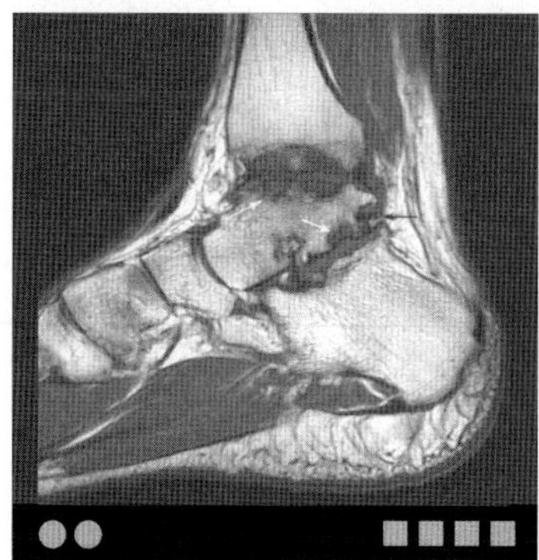

D. Hemophilic arthritis: Sagittal T1WI demonstrates multiple bone erosions of the tibiotalar and subtalar joints (arrows). Flattening of the talar dome is seen.

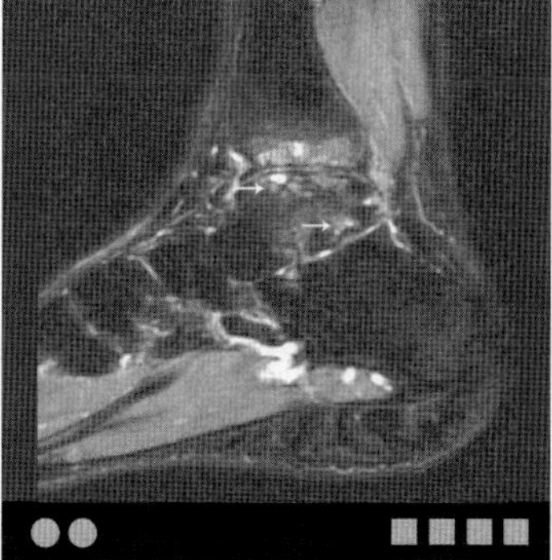

E. Hemophilic arthritis: Sagittal STIR image shows subchondral cysts (arrow) and edema of the talar dome and subtalar joint. Repeated episodes of hemarthrosis have led to secondary degenerative changes in the joint.

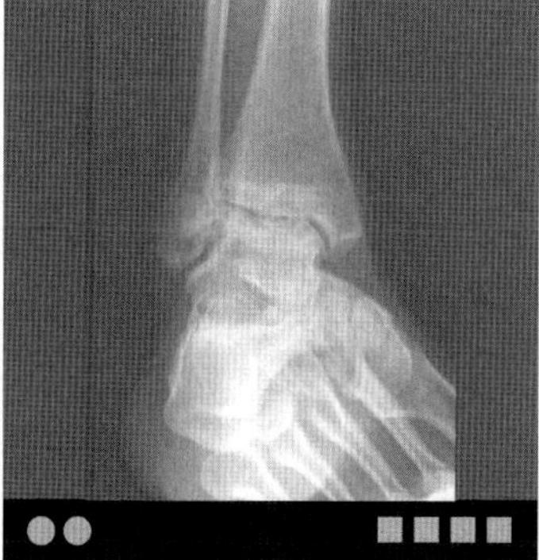

F. Hemophilic arthritis: Mortise radiograph of the same patient again demonstrates secondary degenerative changes of the ankle joints. Note the well-described talar tilt caused by asymmetric growth of the tibial epiphysis.

IMAGE KEY

Common

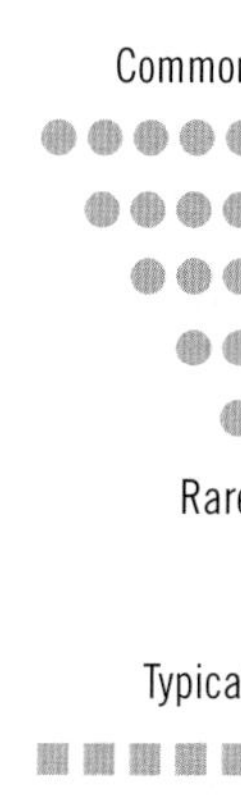

Rare

Typical

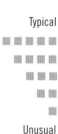

Unusual

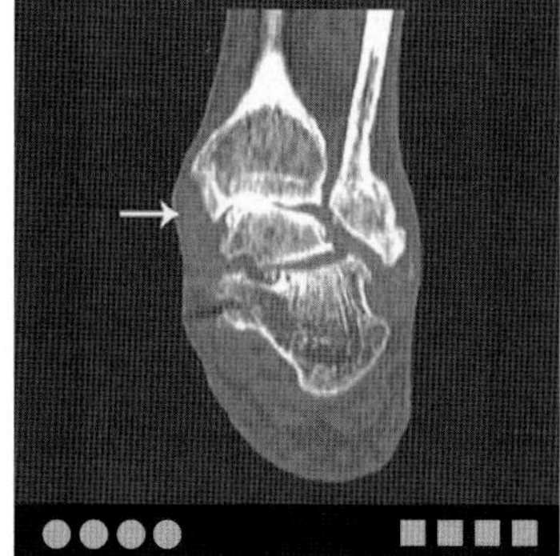

G. Rheumatoid arthritis: Reformatted coronal computed tomography image of the ankle shows diffuse osteopenia, soft tissue swelling, cartilage space narrowing, and bone on bone articulation of the tibiotalar joint.

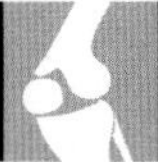

33–3 Osteoblastoma

Mohammad Reza Hayeri and Jamshid Tehranzadeh

PRESENTATION

Pain, redness, and swelling of ankle

FINDINGS

The CT examination showed an oval lucency with surrounding sclerosis and cortical break in diametaphysis of distal fibula. There is central calcification in this osteolytic lesion.

DIFFERENTIAL DIAGNOSES

- *Osteoid osteoma:* This is a benign active osteoblastic lesion of the bone. The hallmark of these tumors is night pains relieved with small doses of salicylates. This has similar histology to osteoblastoma but the lesion is less than 2 cm in size.
- *Brodie's abscess:* This subacute form of osteomyelitis is minimally or totally asymptomatic and is usually localized to the metaphysis.
- *Chondroblastoma:* This is a benign aggressive giant cell and chondroid type tumor and has a predilection for epiphysis or apophysis of bones prior to epiphyseal closure.
- *Giant cell tumor:* This aggressive subchondral lesion account for 15% of symptomatic benign bone tumors and is most commonly found in distal femur and proximal tibia.

COMMENTS

This is a 16-year-old girl with ankle pain and swelling. Osteoblastoma is a benign, rare osseous tumor that develops in the bony spongiosa. These tumors resemble osteoid osteoma histologically and radiologically. They present with long history of pain but they do not usually have the nocturnal worsening commonly associated with osteoid osteoma and are not as readily relieved by salicylates. Osteoblastomas also referred as giant osteoid osteomas and are usually over 2 cm in diameter and the intense bony reaction noted in osteoid osteoma may not be always seen in osteoblastomas. It accounts for less than 1% of primary bone tumors and usually affects adolescents and young adults. There is a 2 to 3:1 male predilection. The common sites are vertebral neural arches, spinous processes, metaphysic or diaphysis of long bones, and rarely in pelvis. In about 25% of patients, an associated soft tissue mass is also noted. These tumors may be accompanied by aneurysmal bone cyst. On gross examination they are fairly well circumscribed, red to tan in colors with hemorrhagic areas. On rare cases the malignant transformation with histologic features to osteosarcoma may be seen. Osteoblastomas present as lytic lesion of bone, with or without matrix mineralization. This mineralization is surrounded by a narrow or broader zone of sclerosis or if expansive, a thin bony shell. On T1W MRI image, low-to-intermediate signal intensity and foci of signal void corresponding to calcification are noted. On T2WI intermediate-to-high signal intensity is seen with foci of signal void representing calcification.

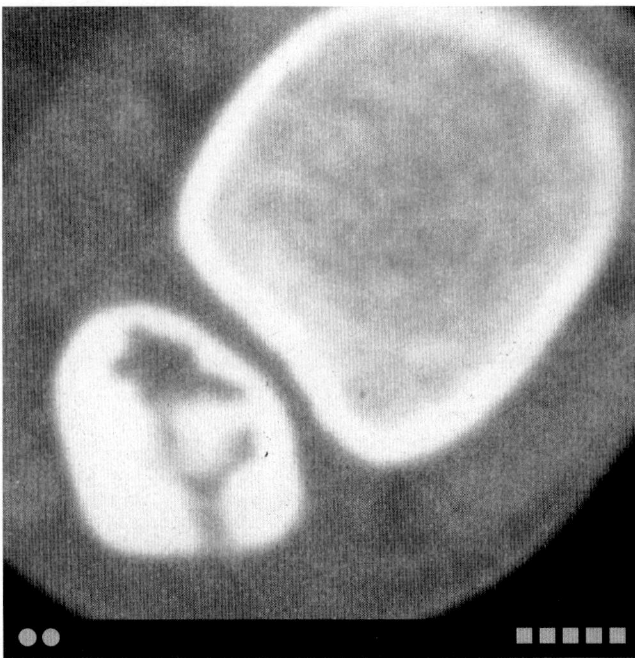

A. Osteoblastoma of distal fibula: Axial CT of ankle shows osteolytic lesions of distal fibular shaft with central calcification and cortical break.

PEARLS

- **Osteoblastoma is a rare, benign tumor involving vertebral neural arches, spinous processes, metaphysis or diaphysis of long bones, and rarely pelvis.**
- **Osteoblastoma histologically resembles osteoid osteoma but is larger (≥2cm), and the intense bony reaction seen in osteoid osteomas may not always be present.**
- **Radiologically osteoblastoma is an expansile, circumscribed lytic lesion of bone, surrounded by a narrow or broader zone of sclerosis or if expansive, a thin bony shell.**
- **T1W MRI image shows low-to-intermediate signal intensity. On T2WI intermediate-to-high signal intensity is seen. Foci of signal void corresponding to calcification may be noted.**

ADDITIONAL IMAGES

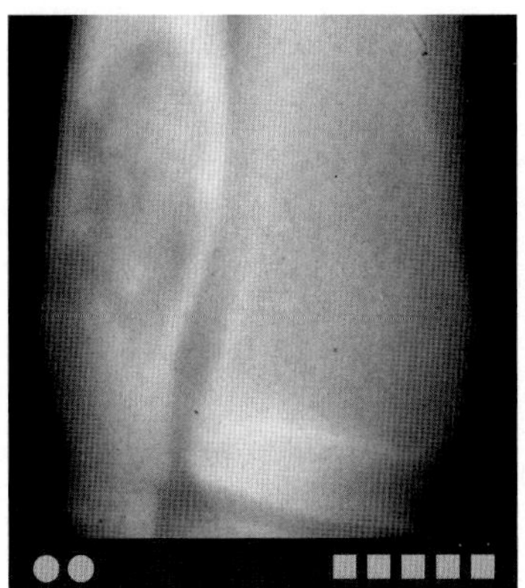

B. Osteoblastoma of distal fibula: AP radiograph of the ankle shows osteolytic lesion of the distal fibular shaft with central calcification.

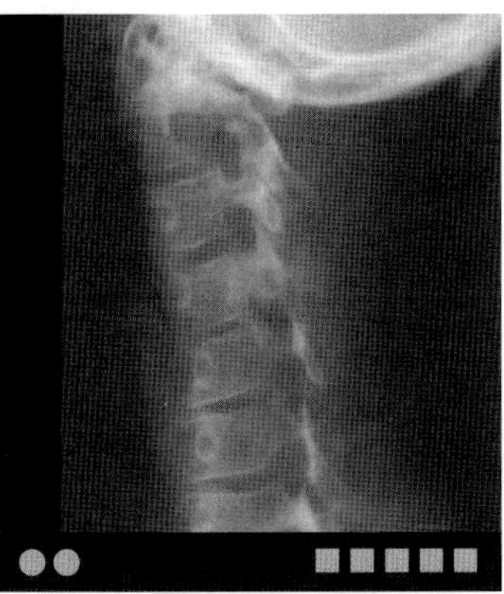

C. Recurrent osteoblastoma: Oblique radiograph of cervical spine shows sclerotic lesion of the pedicle and lamina of C4 vertebra on the right.

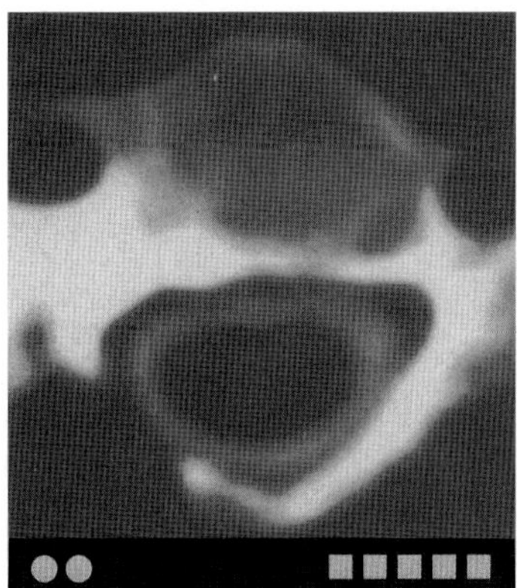

D. Recurrent osteoblastoma: CT myelogram of C4 vertebra shows osteosclerotic changes of the right pedicle and transverse process of this vertebra. Note previous laminectomy for removal of original osteoblastoma.

IMAGE KEY

Common

Rare

Typical

Unusual

DIFFERENTIAL DIAGNOSES IMAGES

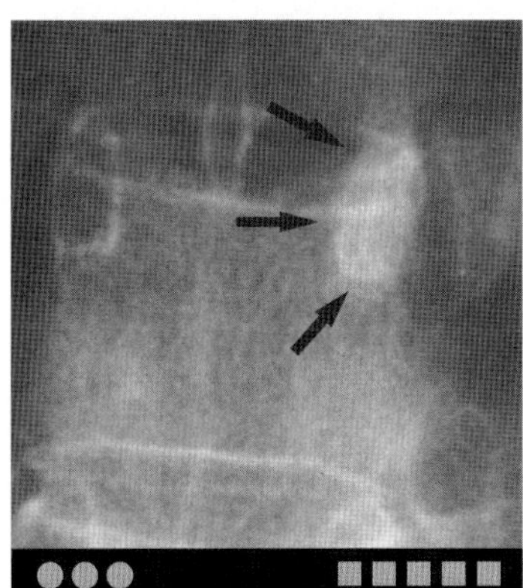

E. Osteoid osteoma of the left pedicle in thoracic spine: AP radiograph of thoracic spine shows sclerotic left pedicle (arrows) representing osteoid osteoma.

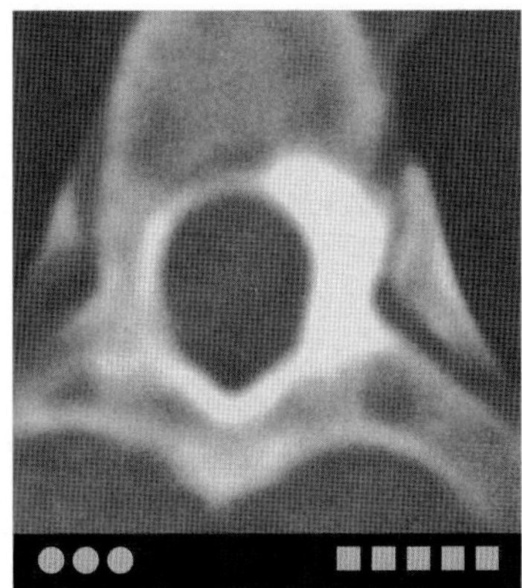

F. Osteoid osteoma of the left pedicle in thoracic spine: Axial CT of thoracic spine shows sclerotic density of the left pedicle of the thoracic vertebra. The nidus is hidden in the sclerosis.

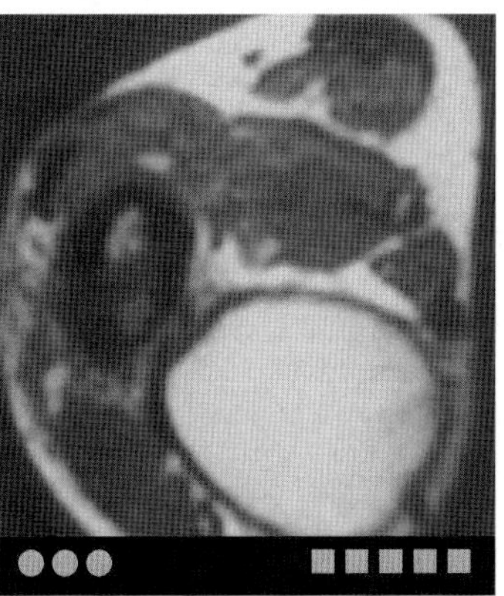

G. Cortical osteoid osteoma of distal fibula: MRI of distal fibula shows a cortical defect with intermediate signal representing cortical osteoid osteoma.

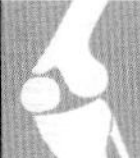

33–4 Sonographic Appearance of Nodular PVNS of the Talonavicular Joint

Stefano Bianchi and Ibrahim F. Abdelwahab

PRESENTATION

Soft tissue mass of the instep

FINDINGS

US demonstrates a solid mass located close to the talus.

DIFFERENTIAL DIAGNOSES

- *Malignant tumor:* Presents as hyperintense mass in T2W MR images.
- *Soft tissue ganglion:* Appears as an anechoic cystic mass in US.
- *Tibialis anterior tendon tear:* Spontaneous tears affect aged patients. The swollen proximal tendon stump mimics a soft tissue mass. US easily demonstrates the torn retracted tendon.

COMMENTS

This 35-year-old woman developed a painless lump of the anterior aspect of the left ankle. Physical examination showed normal skin overlying an ill-defined fusiform mass that was not attached to the skin but was adherent to the underlying tissues. Pigmented villonodular synovitis (PVNS) is an uncommon benign proliferative disease of the synovium that affects joints, bursae, or tendons' sheaths and can present macroscopically as a diffuse or a nodular form. Pathologically, PVNS demonstrates a fibrous stroma covered by hyperplastic lining cells, histiocytes containing fat or hemosiderin and multinucleated giant cells. When the nodular type of PVNS involves the tendon sheath, it is called giant cell tumor of the tendon sheath. Intra-articular PVNS mainly affects the knee and the ankle and presents with nonspecific clinical findings or symptoms often referred to as intra-articular loose bodies or meniscal tears. Radiographs can be normal or show a paraarticular soft tissue dense mass without internal calcifications. In the long-standing disease, pressure erosions on adjacent bones can be evident. CT can show evidence of hemosiderin and fat deposits inside the mass and easily detects bone erosions not evident on the radiographs. MR shows a well-delimited soft tissue mass containing scattered areas, related to hemosiderin deposits that show low signal both in T1 and T2W sequences, which usually enhance with contrast. US shows a hypoechoic well marginated mass that may contain some internal flow signals at color-Doppler. The US appearance is nonspecific.

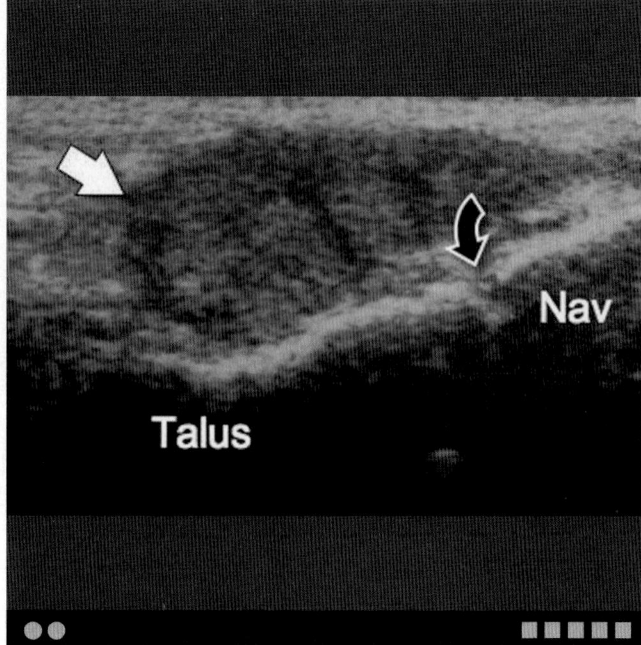

A. Nodular PVNS of the talonavicular joint: Sagittal US image over the anterior aspect of the ankle shows a hypoechoic, well-delimited mass (arrow) located anterior to the talus. The mass presents a homogeneous internal structure. Curved arrow = talonavicular joint, Nav = navicular.

PEARLS

- **Nodular PVNS can affect the peritendinous or para-articular structures and presents mainly as an indolent soft tissue mass.**
- **When located anterior to the ankle joint nodular, PVNS can be easily differentiated from ganglia, lipoma, and tears of the tibialis anterior tendon by US.**
- **A definite diagnosis relies on MRI demonstration of internal hemosiderin deposits appearing as hypointense signal on both T1WI and T2WI.**

ADDITIONAL IMAGES

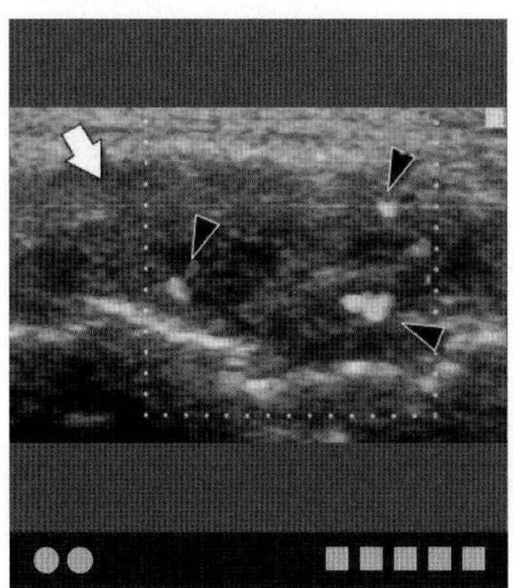

B. Nodular PVNS of the talonavicular joint: Coronal color Doppler US image of the mass (arrow) shows internal flow signals (arrowheads).

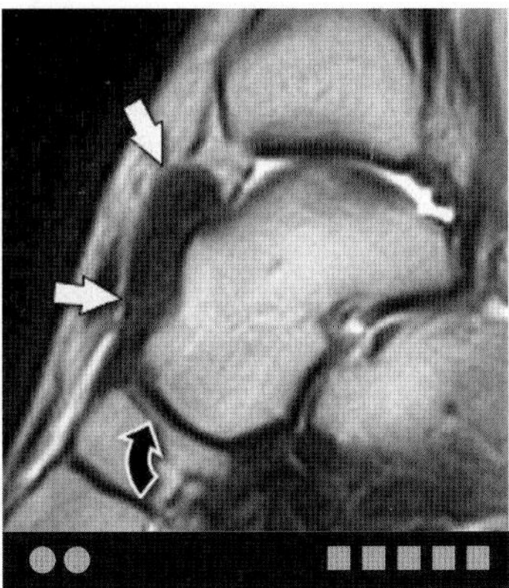

C. Nodular PVNS of the talonavicular joint: Sagittal T2W MRI image shows the well-marginated mass (arrows) presenting a hypointense signal. Note the relation with the talus and the normal appearing talonavicular joint (curved arrow).

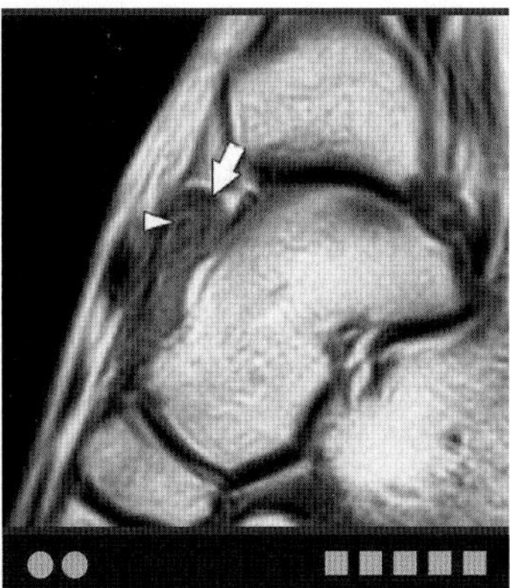

D. Nodular PVNS of the talonavicular joint: Sagittal gadolinium-enhanced T1W MRI image shows contrast enhancement of the mass (arrow). Note persistence of internal hypointense spots (arrowhead) consistent with hemosiderin deposits.

DIFFERENTIAL DIAGNOSES IMAGES

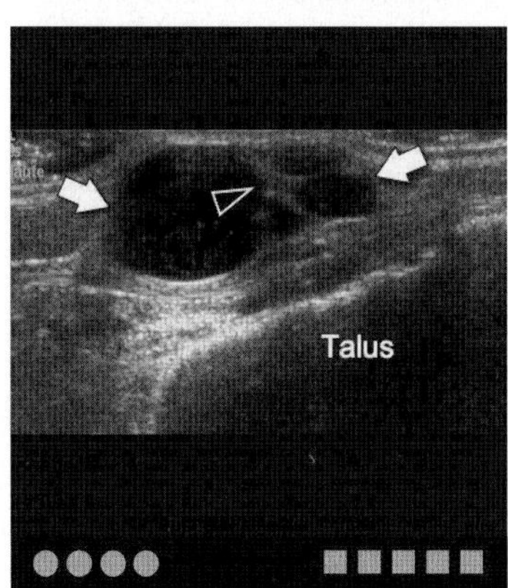

E. Soft tissue ganglion: Axial US image obtained over the anterior aspect of the talus shows a mass (arrows) with well-marginated border. The mass is hypoanechoic with internal echogenic septa (arrowhead).

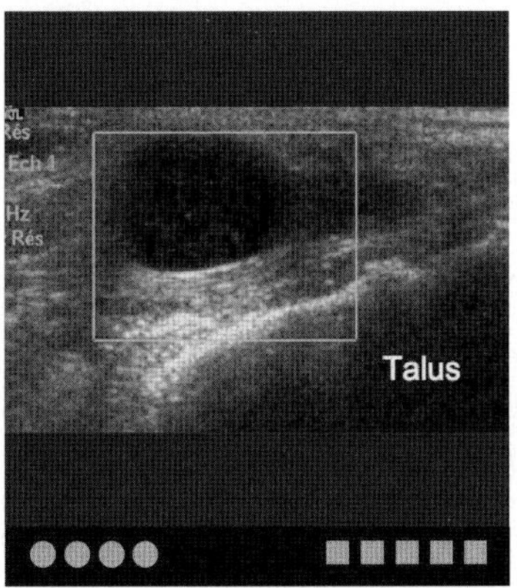

F. Soft tissue ganglion: Axial color Doppler US image, obtained at the same level asimage E, shows absence of internal flow signals.

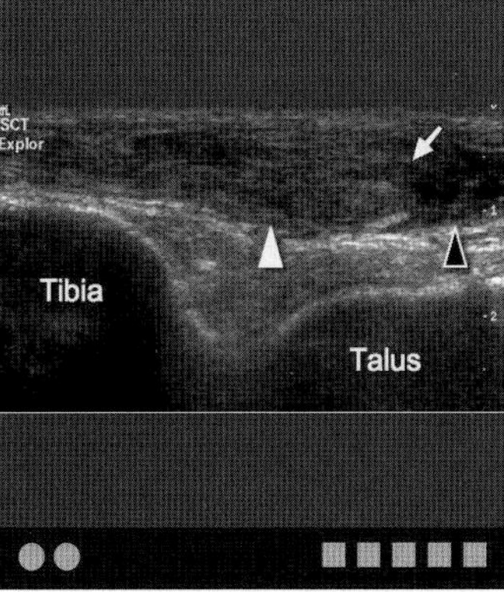

G. Tibialis anterior tendon tear: Sagittal US image obtained over the ankle joint in a patient presenting with a soft tissue mass. Image demonstrates a complete tear of the tibialis anterior tendon (arrow). Note swelling and internal irregularity of the proximal tendon stump (white arrowhead). Distal to the tear the tendon sheath is filled by anechoic synovial fluid (black arrowhead).

IMAGE KEY

Common

Rare

Typical

Unusual

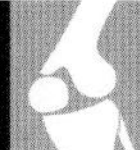

33–5 Kaposi Sarcoma

Ricky Kim and Rajeev K. Varma

PRESENTATION

Recurrent skin lesions

FINDINGS

MR images show numerous small well-circumscribed lesions within the soft tissues of both legs.

DIFFERENTIAL DIAGNOSES

- Bacillary angiomatosis can present with a cutaneous angiomatous lesions that appear similar to those in Kaposi sarcoma. Osseous lesions are more common in bacillary angiomatosis and can predate cutaneous lesions by several months.
- *Lymphoma:* It has been described as resembling vascular lesions; again a biopsy will be needed.
- *Infection:* Cat scratch disease may show osteolytic lesions but clinical history might help.

COMMENTS

This is a 40-year-old HIV+ male who presented with recurrent skin lesions. Kaposi's sarcoma is the most common tumor in HIV+ patients. It is a vascular neoplasm that is generally multifocal and can involve virtually any organ. The most frequent sites of involvement are the skin, mucous membranes, lymph nodes, and gastrointestinal tract. Osseous involvement by Kaposi's sarcoma is rare. When seen, it usually occurs in the endemic form of Kaposi's sarcoma in Africa. Osseous involvement is usually from local extension of an adjacent skin lesion. Primary osseous involvement without adjacent skin lesion is very rare. Osseous lesions appear similar to osseous findings seen in bacillary angiomatosis, tuberculosis, and lymphoma. Findings can range from cortical erosions to osseous destruction with possible periosteal reaction. CT scanning can more precisely characterize the lytic lesion. MR can identify marrow abnormalities that appear similar to changes seen in lymphoma and osteomyelitis. MR can also better detect soft tissue masses. The primary differential diagnosis is bacillary angiomatosis, which can present with cutaneous and osseous lesion that appear similar to those of Kaposi. Osseous lesions are more commonly seen in bacillary angiomatosis than in Kaposi and can predate cutaneous lesions by several months. Skin biopsy is usually necessary for definitive diagnosis. Prompt diagnosis is critical as both entities require different treatment and delay of treatment can quickly lead to fatal complications.

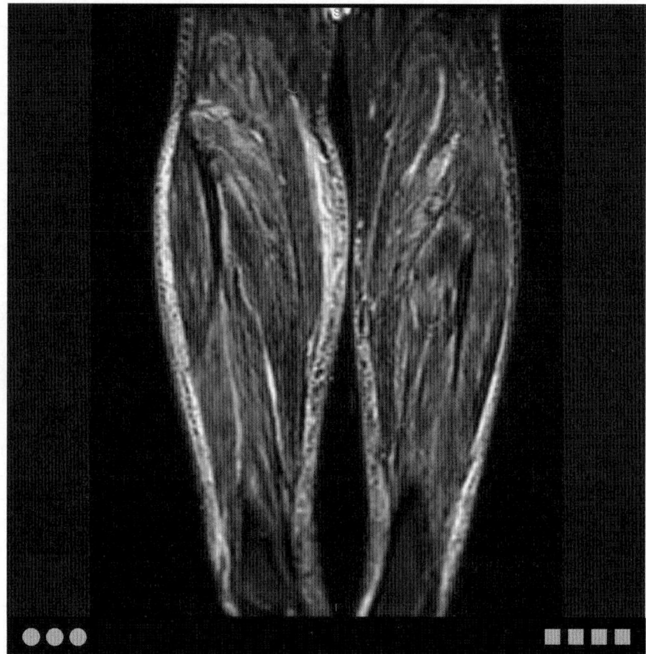

A. Kaposi sarcoma: Coronal T2WI shows diffuse edema of the subcutaneous tissue with numerous tortuous hypointense structures correspond to blood vessels. There is also reactive edema in the underlying muscles. Bones though not fully seen on this figure were unremarkable.

PEARLS

- **Primary differential diagnosis is bacillary angiomatosis, which can present with cutaneous and osseous lesions that appear similar to those seen Kaposi.**
- **Osseous findings range from cortical erosions to destruction with possible periosteal reaction.**
- **Prompt differentiation between bacillary angiomatosis and Kaposi's sarcoma is critical as delay of treatment can quickly lead to fatal complications. The former is treatable with a course of antibiotics.**

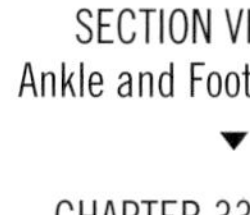

ADDITIONAL IMAGES

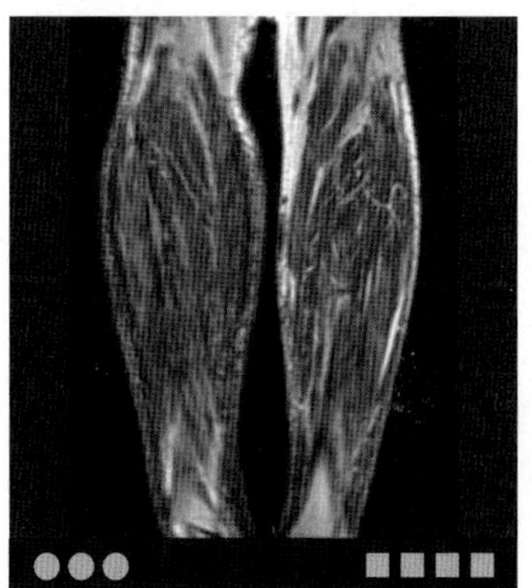

B. Kaposi sarcoma: Coronal T1WI in the same patient shows hypointensity in the subcutaneous fat corresponding to vascular lesions seen on fluid sensitive sequences.

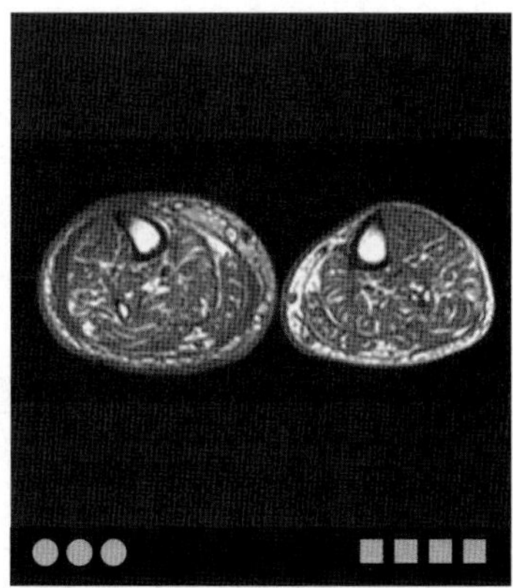

C. Kaposi sarcoma: Axial T1WI shows hypointense subcutaneous tissue and fatty infiltration of the muscles likely related to disuse atrophy.

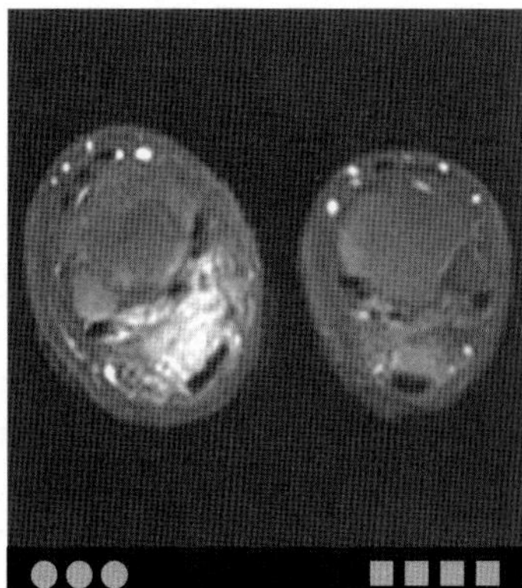

D. Kaposi sarcoma: Axial T1WI with IV contrast and fat saturation shows enhancement at the level of the ankle (same patient as in previous figure).

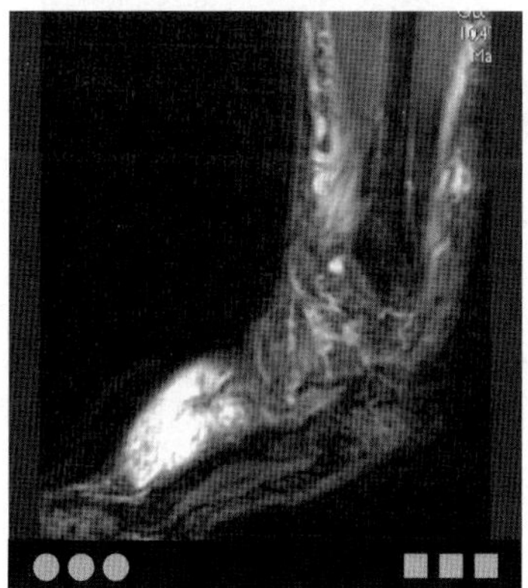

E. Kaposi sarcoma of ankle: Sagittal STIR sequence in a different patient with known Kaposi sarcoma shows increased signal in the subcutaneous tissue over the ankle.

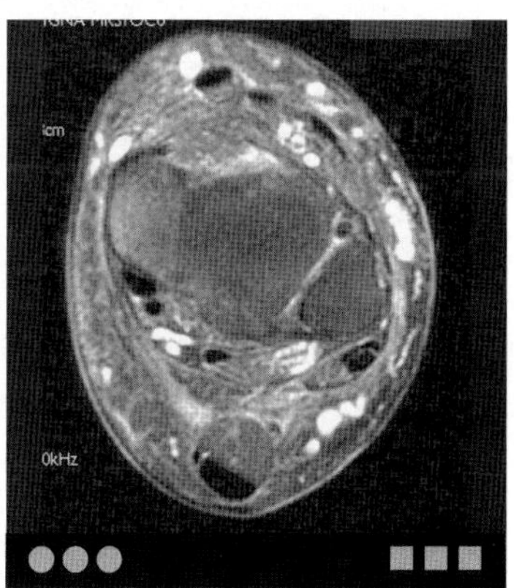

F. Kaposi ankle: Axial contrast enhanced T1WI with Fat suppression demonstrated increased vascularity in the subcutaneous tissue. The bones appear to be normal.

DIFFERENTIAL DIAGNOSIS IMAGE

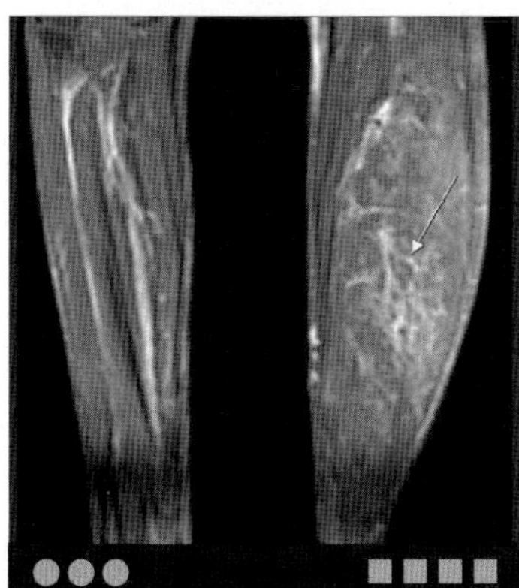

G. Lymphoma versus aggressive vascular lesion: Coronal contrast enhanced T1W image with fat saturation shows an enhancing vascular mass (arrow) in the leg muscles.

IMAGE KEY

Common

Rare

Typical

Unusual

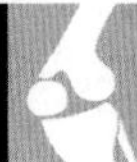

33–6 Soft Tissue Hemangioma of Foot

Sulabha Masih

PRESENTATION

Painful slowly growing mass of foot

FINDINGS

On MRI mass is isointense to muscle on T1W images with variable amount of increase signal related to fat. Mass shows serpiginous high signal intensity on T2W images with foci of decreased signal intensity because of calcified phleboliths.

DIFFERENTIAL DIAGNOSES

- *Hibernoma:* Presents as a heterogeneous signal intensity mass, with increased fat signal and branching, serpentine low signal vascular structures on MR imaging.
- *Lipoma:* Presents as homogeneous, fatty radiolucent mass on radiographs. MR imaging will show homogenous fatty increased signal intensity on T1WI.
- *Angiolipoma:* Radiographs and CT scanning demonstrate inhomogeneous fat and water density mass lesion with phleboliths, and infiltration into adjacent tissue.
- *Hemangiopericytoma:* Commonly presents as a soft tissue vascular tumor arising from pericytes of Zimmerman, which surround the capillary wall. Imaging shows soft tissue mass with occasional calcification, bone erosion, and hypervascularity.
- *Synovial hemangioma:* Commonly associated with cutaneous and deep soft tissue hemangiomas. Arthrography usually shows intraarticular mass with villo-nodular filling defects. On MRI, T2W and STIR images show inhomogeneous intraarticular villonodular high signal intensity lesion.

COMMENTS

This case is a 40-year-old male with painful slowly growing soft tissue mass in plantar aspect of midfoot. Soft tissue hemangiomas are benign lesions and histologically may classify into capillary type involving small caliber vessels, cavernous type comprised of dilated blood filled spaces, arteriovenous type with persistent fetal capillary bed, with abnormal communication of the arteries and veins and venous type comprised of thick walled vessels containing muscle. Soft tissue hemangioma is one of the most common soft tissue tumors and constitute 7% of all benign tumors. They are relatively common in females and typically involve the skeletal muscles of lower extremities. They are associated with several clinical syndromes, such as Maffucci syndrome, which is the combination of multiple enchondromatosis and soft tissue hemangiomas, Klippel-Trenaunay-Weber syndrome, which includes varicose veins, soft tissue and bony hypertrophy, and cutaneous hemangiomas, and Kasabach-Merrit syndrome, which consists of papillary hemangiomas and extensive purpura. On radiographs, there is nonspecific soft tissue mass. It may contain phleboliths or varying amount of fat. On CT, mass is poorly defined with attenuation similar to muscles, interspersed with decreased attenuation, similar to fat and increased attenuation because of phleboliths. On MR, mass is isointense to muscle, with areas of high signal intensity because of fat on T1WI. There is serpiginous high signal intensity on T2WI, with foci of decreased signal intensity caused by calcified phleboliths.

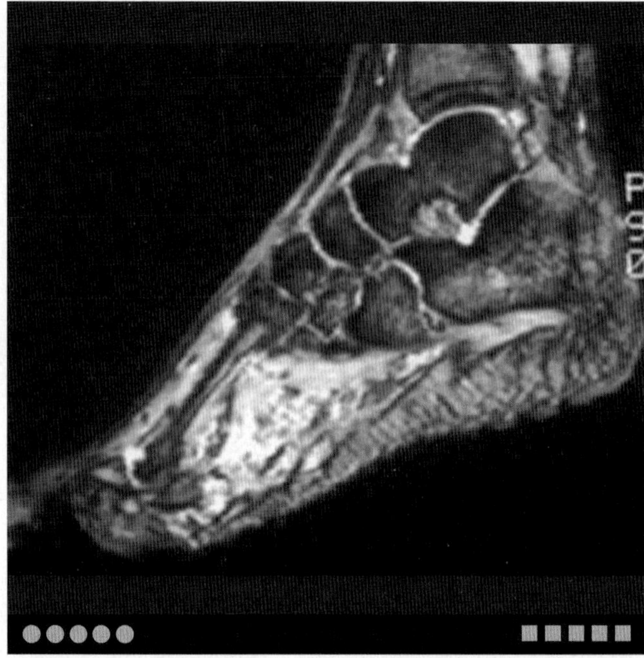

A. Soft tissue hemangioma: Sagittal STIR image demonstrates serpiginous high signal intensity, with few areas of low signal intensity-calcified phleboliths.

PEARLS

- **Typically divided into capillary type involving small caliber vessels and cavernous type comprised of dilated blood filled spaces.**
- **Maffucci syndrome, Klippel-Trenaunay-Weber syndrome, and Kasabach-Merritt syndrome are the associated clinical syndromes.**
- **On MR, the mass is isointense to muscle, with areas of high signal intensity because of fat on T1WI and serpiginous high signal intensity on T2WI, with foci of decreased signal intensity because of calcified phleboliths.**

ADDITIONAL IMAGES

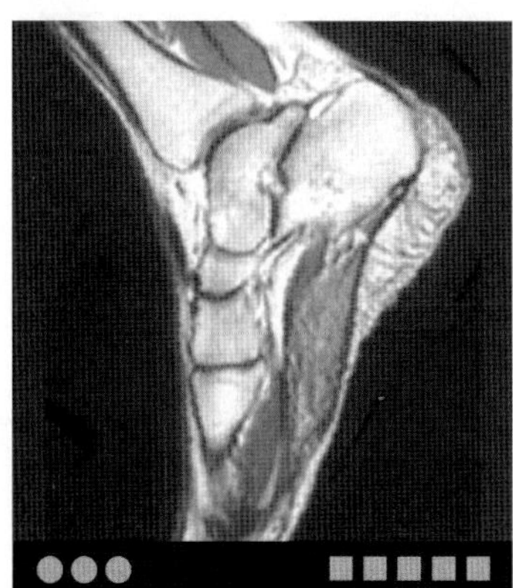

B. Soft tissue hemangioma: Sagittal proton density (PD) weighted image demonstrates mass at the plantar aspect of the foot, isointense to the muscles with foci of high signal intensity fat.

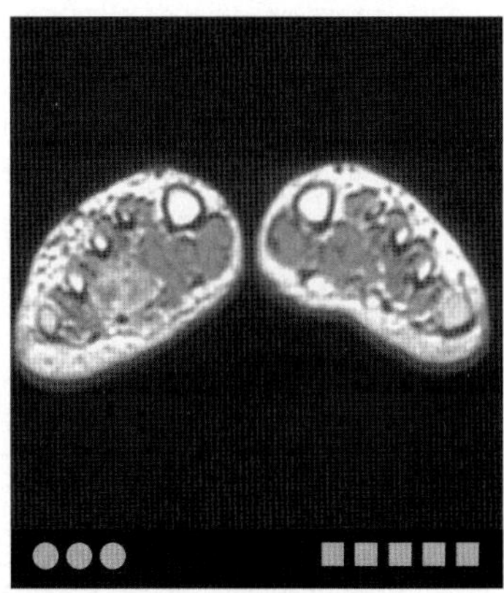

C. Soft tissue hemangioma: Axial PD image demonstrates isointense mass with foci of high signal intensity fat.

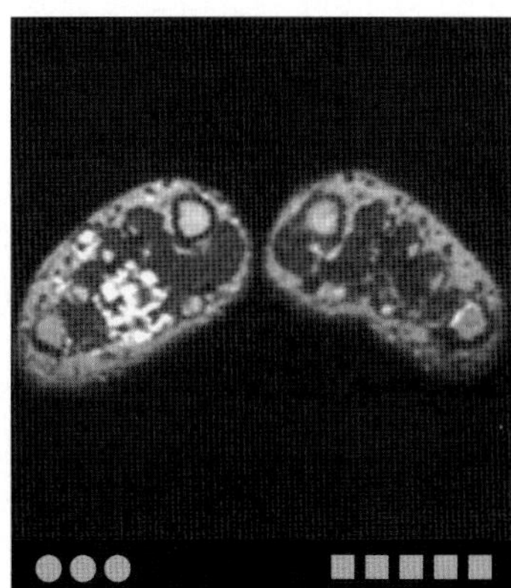

D. Soft tissue hemangioma: Axial T2WI demonstrates serpiginous high signal intensity with few areas of low signal intensity calcified phleboliths.

IMAGE KEY

Common

Rare

Typical

Unusual

DIFFERENTIAL DIAGNOSES IMAGES

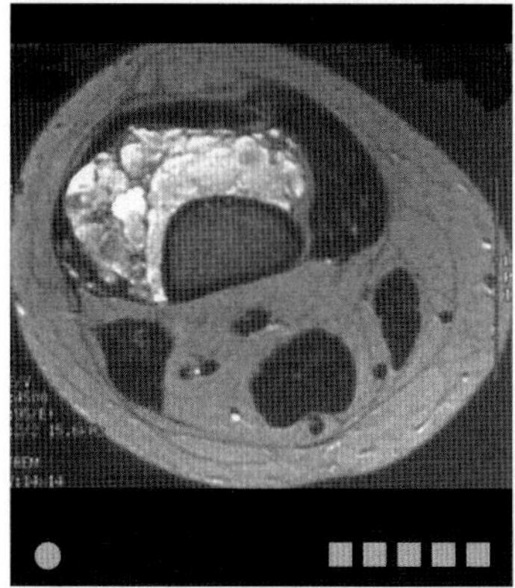

E. Synovial Hemangioma: Axial T2WI shows inhomogeneous intraarticular villonodular high signal intensity lesion.

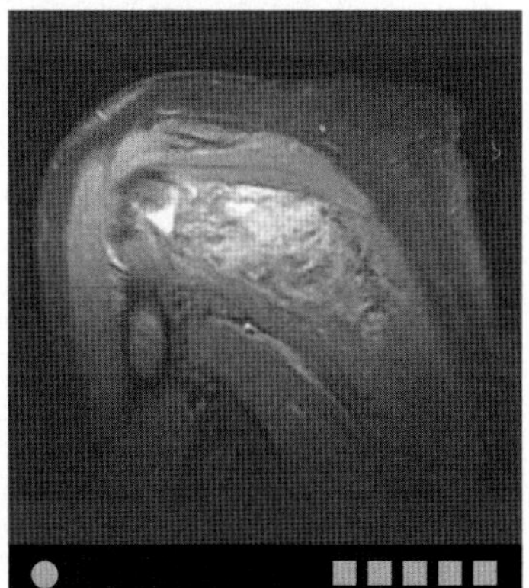

F. Hibernoma: Coronal T2WI shows heterogenous signal intensity mass, with branching, serpentine low signal vascular structures.

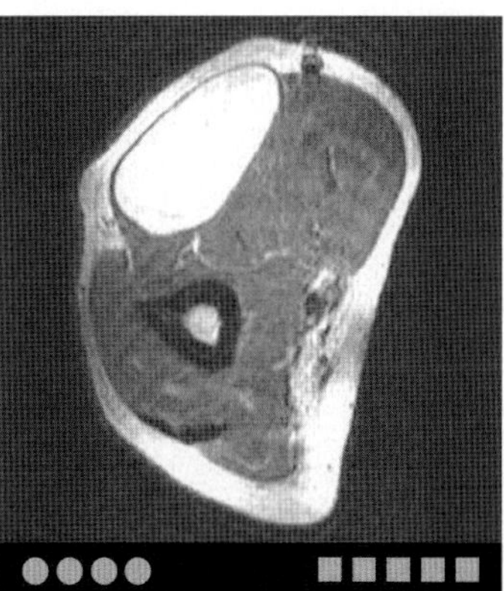

G. Lipoma: Axial T1WI shows homogenous increase signal intensity fatty mass.

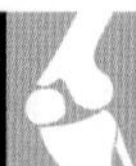

33–7 Fibroma of the Tendon Sheath in the Ankle

Minh-Chau Vu and Rajeev K. Varma

PRESENTATION

Left ankle mass for 1 year, with increasing size

FINDINGS

MRI shows well-circumscribed mass in the lateral ankle that is superficial to the peroneal tendons and contains areas of enhancement and low signal foci.

DIFFERENTIAL DIAGNOSES

- *Giant cell tumor of the tendon sheath:* One of the most common tumors of the hand with a slight female predominance; has avid contrast enhancement
- *Malignant fibrous histiocytoma:* Most common soft tissue sarcoma of late adult life, usually occurring in the lower extremities. Lesions are usually deep intramuscular masses.
- *Synovial sarcoma:* Like most soft tissue sarcomas; these tumors are intermediate-to-low signal on T1 and high signal on T2WI.

COMMENTS

This is a 58-year-old woman with biopsy proven fibroma of the tendon sheath of the ankle. Fibroma of the tendon sheath is a benign fibroblastic proliferation that commonly affects the tendons and tendon sheaths of the distal extremities, particularly the wrists, hands, and fingers. As a result, this tumor can clinically be confused with a giant cell tumor of the tendon sheath. It usually affects adults in the third to fifth decades of life with a slight male predominance of 1.5 to 3:1. Patients present with a firm, slowly enlarging, and painless mass of duration ranging from months to years. Radiographic findings are often negative but may demonstrate a soft tissue mass. Scalloping of the adjacent bone because of pressure erosions has been reported but is very rare. MRI classically shows a superficial focal nodular mass adjacent to a tendon sheath that is hypointense on all pulse sequences with little or no contrast enhancement. These findings, however, may vary depending if there is increased cellularity or myxoid changes within the mass, resulting in increased signal on T2WI and variable contrast enhancement. The main differential is with giant cell tumor of the tendon sheath, which is more common than fibroma of the tendon sheath. Histologically, the two tumors have separate and distinct radiological features. Fibroma of the tendon sheath is hypovascular with slit-like vascular channels within a dense collagen matrix, whereas giant cell tumor of tendon sheath is more cellular and contains multiloculated giant cell from histiocytes and hemosiderin.

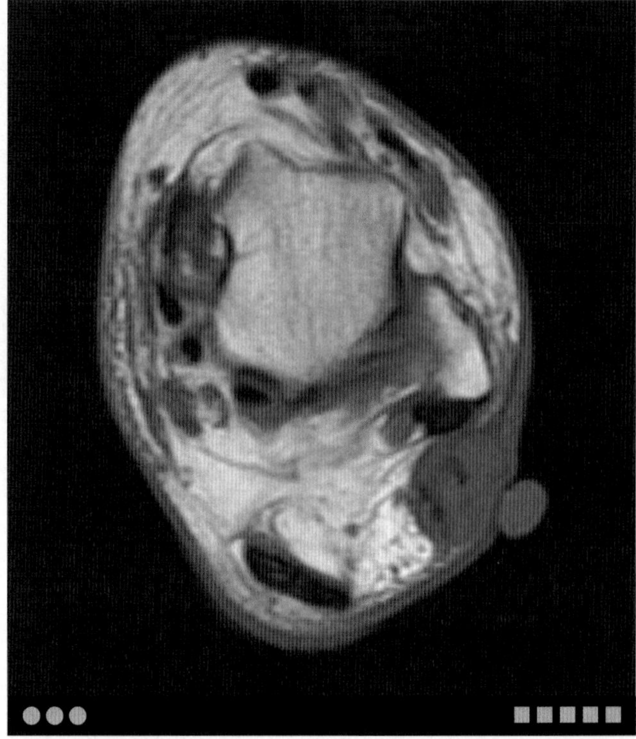

A. Fibroma of the tendon sheath: Axial T1WI shows a hypointense mass seen next to posterolateral tendons.

PEARLS

- **Fibroma of the tendon sheath is a benign fibroblastic proliferation that most commonly affects the tendons or tendon sheaths of the wrists, hands, and fingers.**
- **Affects young to middle-aged adults with a slight male predominance.**
- **Often confused with giant cell tumor of the tendon sheath.**
- **Radiographs can be normal or show soft tissue mass.**
- **MRI classically shows a focal, nodular mass adjacent to a tendon sheath that has decreased signal on all pulse sequences with little or no contrast enhancement.**

ADDITIONAL IMAGES

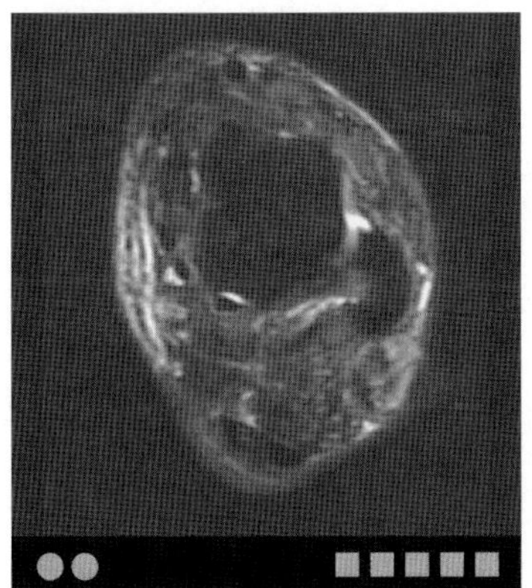

B. Fibroma of the tendon sheath: Axial STIR image shows mixed hyperintensity.

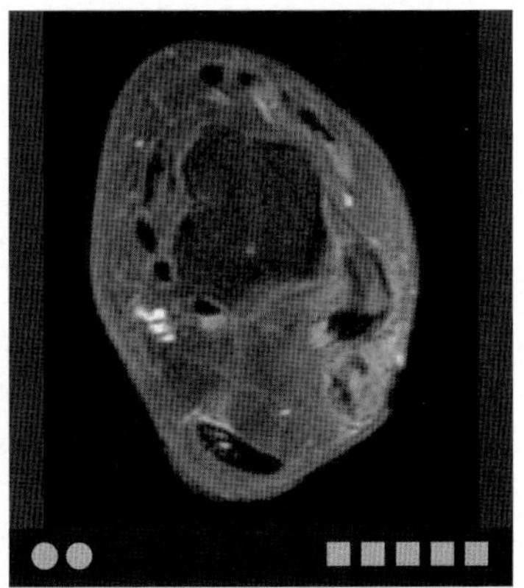

C. Fibroma of the tendon sheath: Axial T1W fat-saturated post Gd image shows mixed enhancement.

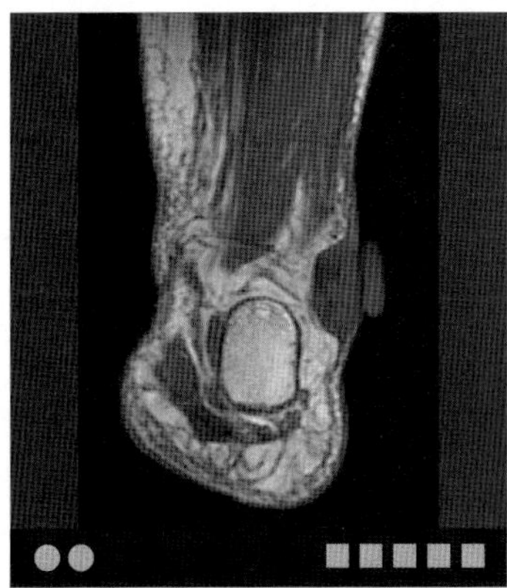

D. Fibroma of the tendon sheath: Coronal T1WI shows the subcutaneous hypointense mass.

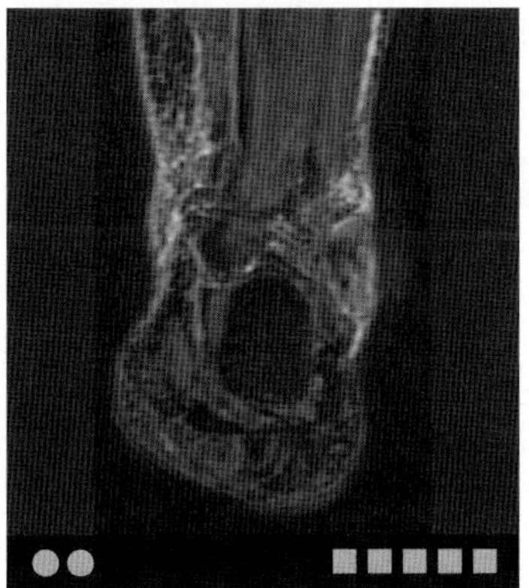

E. Fibroma of the tendon sheath: Coronal STIR sequence showing mixed hyperintensity.

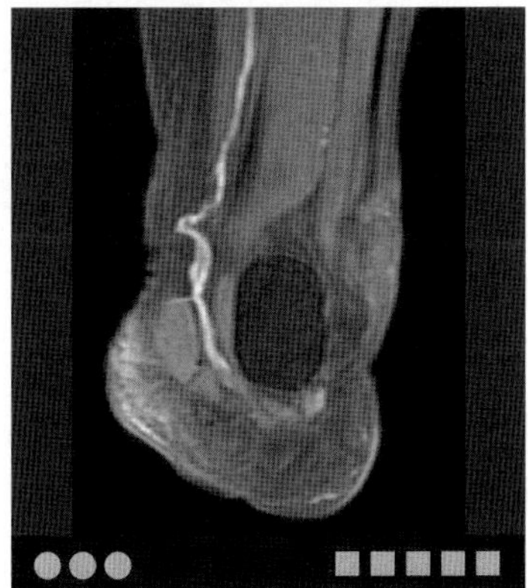

F. Fibroma of the tendon sheath: Coronal T1W fat-saturated, post Gd image showing minimal to mixed enhancement pattern.

DIFFERENTIAL DIAGNOSIS IMAGE

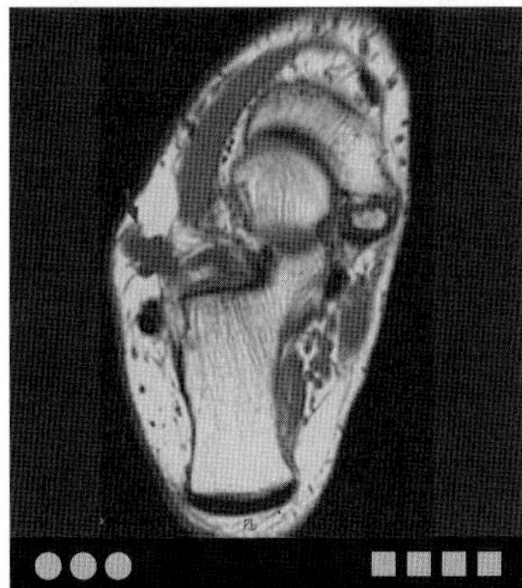

G. Synovial sarcoma: Axial T1WI shows an intermediate signal within an irregular nodule anterior to peroneal tendon in subcutaneous region (arrow).

IMAGE KEY

Common

●●●●●
●●●●
●●●
●●
●

Rare

Typical

■■■■■
■■■■
■■■
■■
■

Unusual

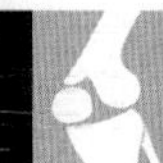

33–8 Morton Neuroma

Ayodale S. Odulate and Piran Aliabadi

PRESENTATION

Chronic forefoot pain

FINDINGS

MRI image shows intermediate signal intensity mass between the second and third metatarsal head interspace.

DIFFERENTIAL DIAGNOSES

- *Metatarsal stress fracture:* Acute onset of pain and swelling with periostitis and/or bone edema.
- *Rheumatoid nodule:* Dumbbell-shaped metatarsal nodule bright on fluid sensitive MRI sequences.
- *Peripheral nerve sheath tumor:* Irregular enhancing heterogeneous mass.
- *Freiburg osteonecrosis:* Uncommon, aseptic osteonecrosis with flattening, and sclerosis of the second metatarsal head.

COMMENTS

This is a 56-year-old female with chronic forefoot pain that is radiating proximally and distally to the toes. A Morton neuroma is a common finding that often presents with radiating sharp pain in the forefoot with or without numbness of the toes originating between the second and third web space or between the second through fourth metatarsal heads. The pain is relieved by ceasing activity. The predominant patient population is females wearing tight-fitting shoes and athletes. The exact pathophysiology of the lesion is unknown; however, it is believed to result from repetitive stress and trauma to the plantar digital nerve with subsequent hyperplasia and perineural fibrosis of the intermetatarsal plantar digital nerve. It is the compression of the nerve that is the cause of pain. The treatment is usually conservative or with surgical excision. On examination, the patient may have a positive Tinel's sign. No imaging findings are present on plain radiography; however, this is an important first-line examination to exclude other causes of foot pain such as metatarsal fracture, tumor, or underlying arthropathy. MRI is considered the imaging modality of choice and the location of the lesion in the third webspace is characteristic of a Morton neuroma. The lesion is hypo to isointense on T1WI and T2WI relating to the fibrous histology of the lesion. Intravenous contrast is not indicated for evaluation of this lesion, but if administered, will be avidly enhancing owing to the inflammatory nature of the disease.

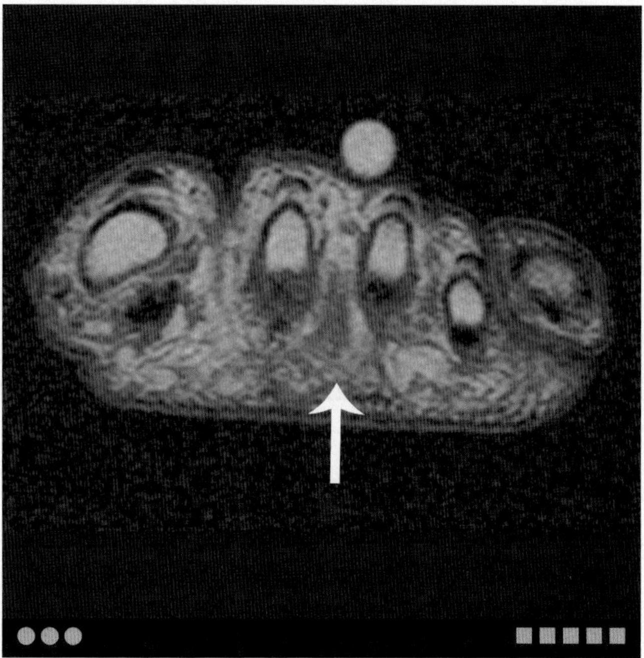

A. Morton Neuroma: Coronal fat-saturated proton density image shows a hypointense ovoid mass (arrow) between the second and third metatarsal heads.

PEARLS

- **Most commonly found in the third plantar metatarsal interspace, between the third and fourth metatarsals and usually solitary.**
- **Hypointense lesion on T1WI and T2WI that may enhance.**
- **Associated with radiating pain in the forefoot relieved by stoppage of activity.**

ADDITIONAL IMAGE

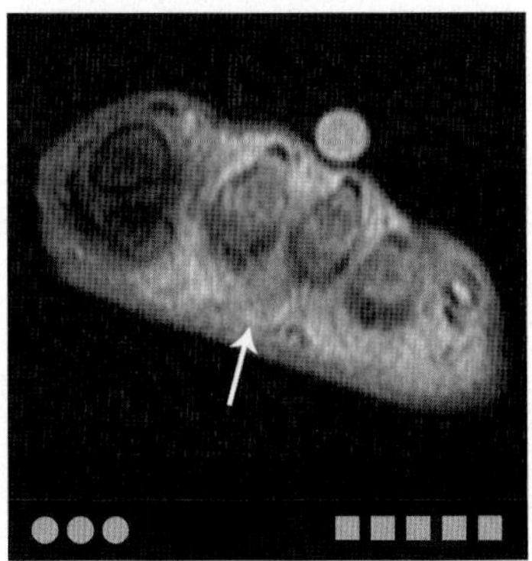

B. Morton neuroma: Coronal T1WI shows an isointense ovoid lesion (arrow) between the second and third metatarsal plantar interspace representing the neuroma.

DIFFERENTIAL DIAGNOSES IMAGES

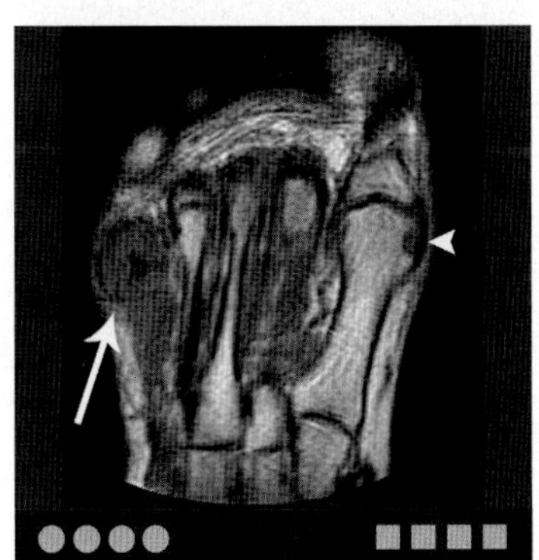

C. Rheumatoid nodule: Axial T1WI shows a hypointense nodule (arrow) adjacent to the fifth metatarsal head. Note the erosion of the medial bare area of the first metatarsal head (arrowhead).

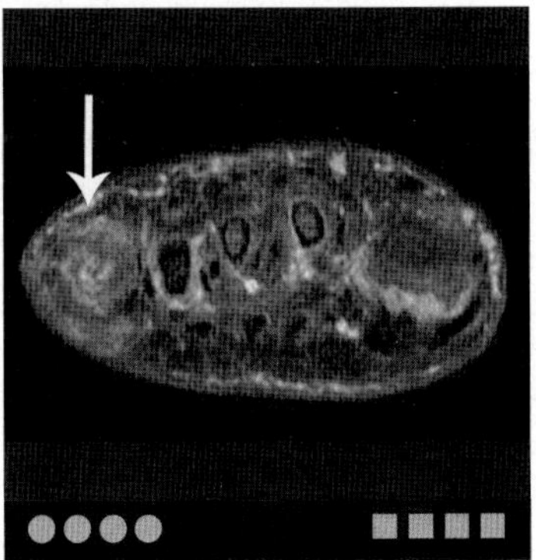

D. Rheumatoid nodule: Coronal post-gadolinium T1WI shows irregular enhancement of the soft tissue nodule (arrow) adjacent to the fifth metatarsal.

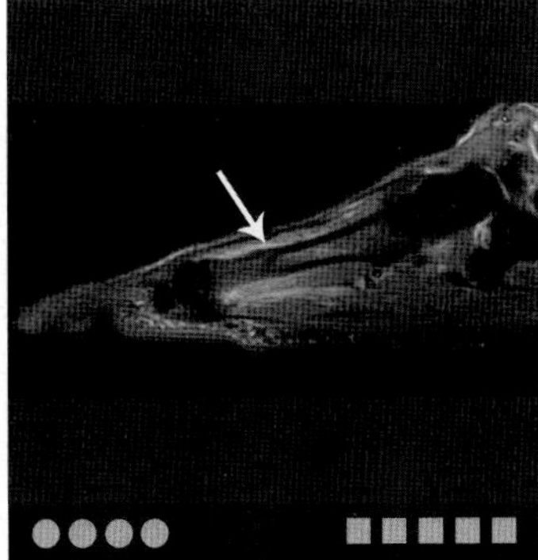

E. Metatarsal stress fracture: Sagittal STIR shows edema of the third metatarsal with a linear stress fracture in the distal metadiaphysis (arrow) characterized by linear hypointensity.

IMAGE KEY

Common

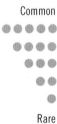

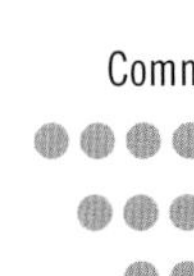

Rare

Typical

Unusual

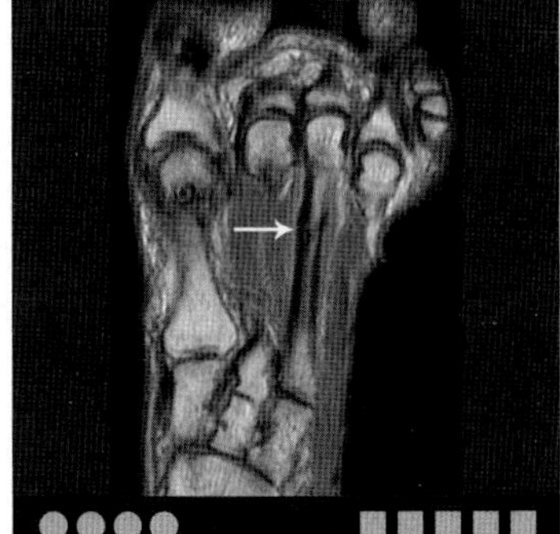

F. Metatarsal stress fracture: Axial T2WI of the same patient shows the oblique linear hypointense line in the distal metadiaphysis representing the stress fracture. Note the hypertrophied cortex representing bone callus (arrow).

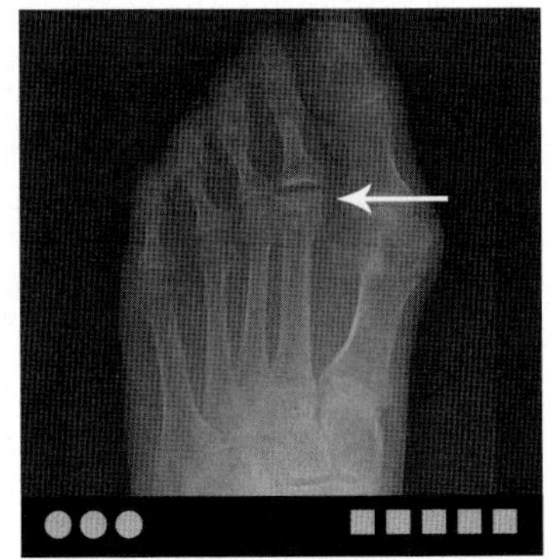

G. Freiburg osteonecrosis: Radiograph of the left foot demonstrates flattening of the head of the second metatarsal (arrow).

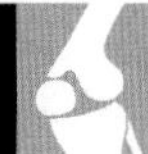

33–9 Plantar Fibromatosis

Arash Anavim

PRESENTATION

Longstanding foot mass

FINDINGS

MRI shows two soft tissue masses at the plantar aspect of the foot, close to the aponeurosis

DIFFERENTIAL DIAGNOSES

- *Soft tissue sarcoma:* In some cases, it might be difficult to differentiate the two. Typically sarcomas are aggressive and demonstrate low signal on T1WI and high signal on T2WI with intense and sometimes heterogeneous contrast enhancement.
- *Plantar Fasciitis:* It shows high signal in fluid-sensitive sequences and does not present as a mass lesion.

COMMENTS

This is a 55-year-old man who was diagnosed with Plantar Fibromatosis 4 years ago. Now the mass has enlarged and a new mass is found. Plantar fibromatosis (also known as Ledderhose disease) represents not a single entity, but rather, a heterogeneous group of conditions with the common characteristics of plantar location and histologic features of mature collagen and fibroblasts with no malignant cytologic features. Like other types of fibromatosis conditions, it is three to four times more common in males. It occurs between the ages of 30 and 50 and is seen bilaterally in 20% to 50% of cases. It is associated with palmar fibromatosis 10% to 65% of the time. The fibromas are most commonly seen on the medial aspect of the plantar aponeurosis. The lesions are often asymptomatic. Biopsy of the masses is not recommended. The act of biopsy may cause the fibroma to enlarge. Surgical excision of the mass requires removal of most of the plantar fascia. Simple excision of mass without removal of the entire ligament generally results in recurrence of the mass. Postsurgical radiation treatment may diminish the chance of recurrence. Typical appearance of plantar fibromatosis on MR is a poorly defined, infiltrative mass in the aponeurosis next to the plantar muscles. They are typically heterogeneously low signal when compared to muscle on both T1 and T2. Lesions with an increased T2 signal have more cellularity and are more likely to recur; therefore, some surgeons may postpone resection until the lesion is more fibrous (i.e., low T2 signal). Enhancement following gadolinium administration is variable.

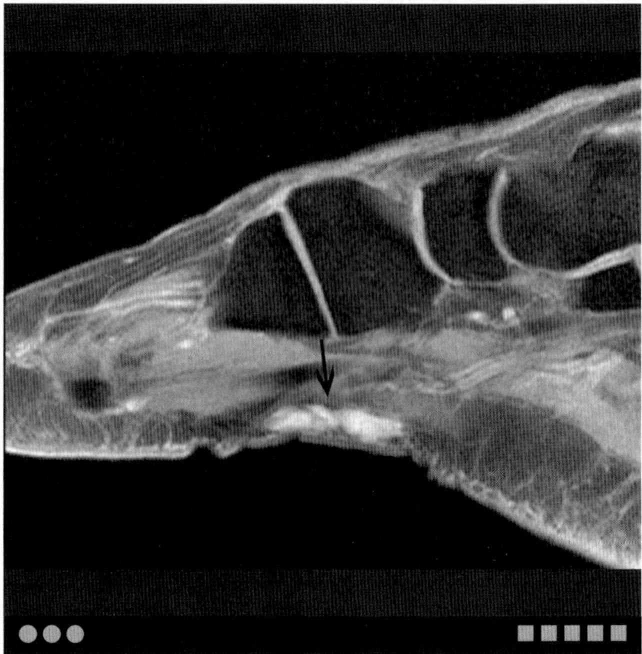

A. Plantar fibromatosis: Sagittal fat-saturated T1 postcontrast demonstrates enhancing subcutaneous mass along the plantar fascia (arrow).

PEARLS

- **Plantar fibromatosis appears as a nodular thickening of the plantar aponeurosis, which has low-to-intermediate signal intensity on both T1WI and T2WI.**
- **Biopsy of the masses is not recommended. The act of biopsy may cause the fibroma to enlarge.**

ADDITIONAL IMAGES

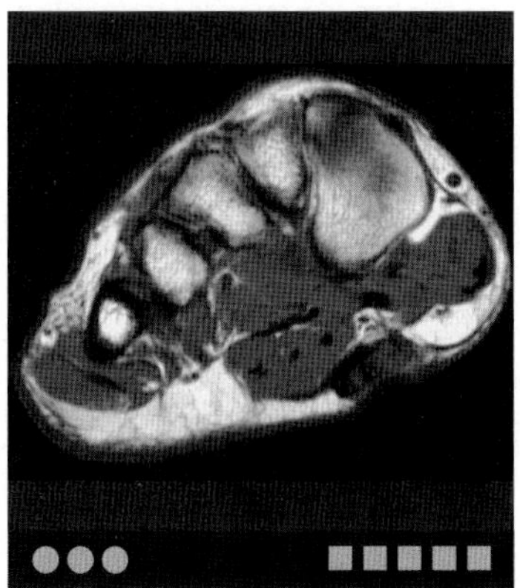

B. Plantar fibromatosis: Coronal T1 shows a low signal mass in the plantar aspect of the foot.

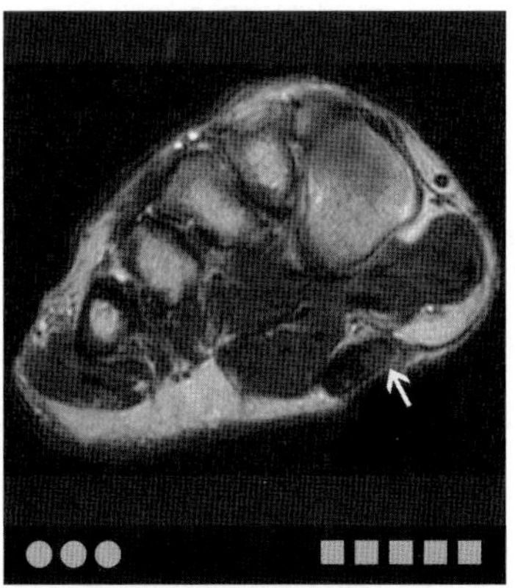

C. Plantar fibromatosis: Coronal T2 demonstrates the plantar mass to be in inhomogeneous with areas of high signal (arrow) indicating high cellularity and areas of low signal, showing fibrous tissue.

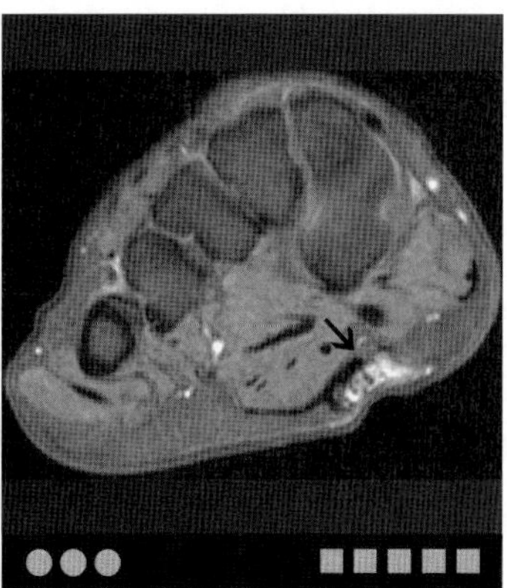

D. Plantar Fibromatosis: Coronal T1 fat-saturated postcontrast shows the mass to be enhancing adjacent to the plantar fascia (arrow).

IMAGE KEY

Common

Rare

Typical

Unusual

DIFFERENTIAL DIAGNOSES IMAGES

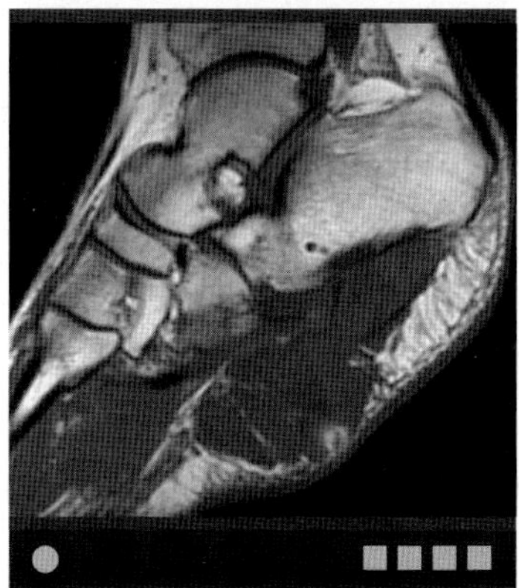

E. Synovial sarcoma of the foot: Sagittal T1 shows a large infiltrating low signal mass invading through the plantar fascia to the deep soft tissues of the foot.

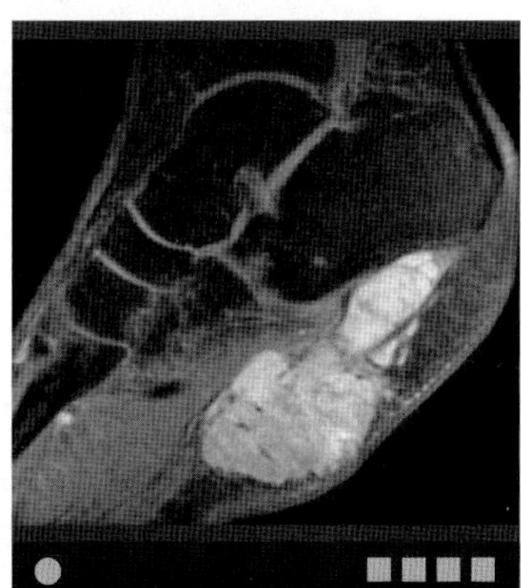

F. Synovial sarcoma of the foot: Sagittal fat-saturated T1 postcontrast shows intense enhancement of the infiltrating plantar mass.

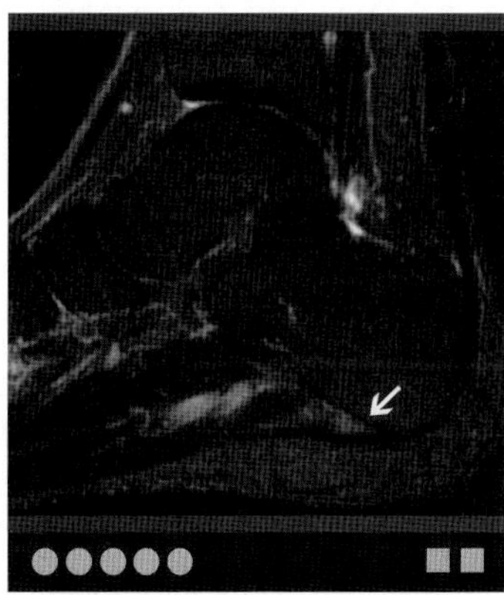

G. Plantar fasciitis: Sagittal fat-saturated T2 demonstrates mild edema at the attachment site of the plantar fascia (arrow).

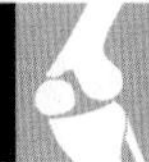

33–10 Extraskeletal Soft Tissue Chondrosarcoma

Sulabha Masih

PRESENTATION

Painless soft tissue mass of right heel

FINDINGS

MR images demonstrate a mass which is isointense to muscle on T1WI and hyperintense on T2WI with central hypointense calcification.

DIFFERENTIAL DIAGNOSES

- *Extraskeletal chondroma:* Rare tumor, predominantly occur in adults, in the hands and feet. Commonly arise in close association with tendon, tendon sheath, or joint capsule.
- *Synovial Sarcoma:* This tumor occurs in the third and fourth decade and has predilection for thigh and lower extremity. Angiography usually shows capillary blush and neovascularity.
- *Synovial osteochondromatosis:* The most common sites are knee, hips, and shoulders. Multiple ossified or calcified bodies of equal size are seen in the joint cavity.
- *Synovial chondrosarcoma:* Extremely rare. It is usually primary or secondary to idiopathic synovial osteochondromatosis.

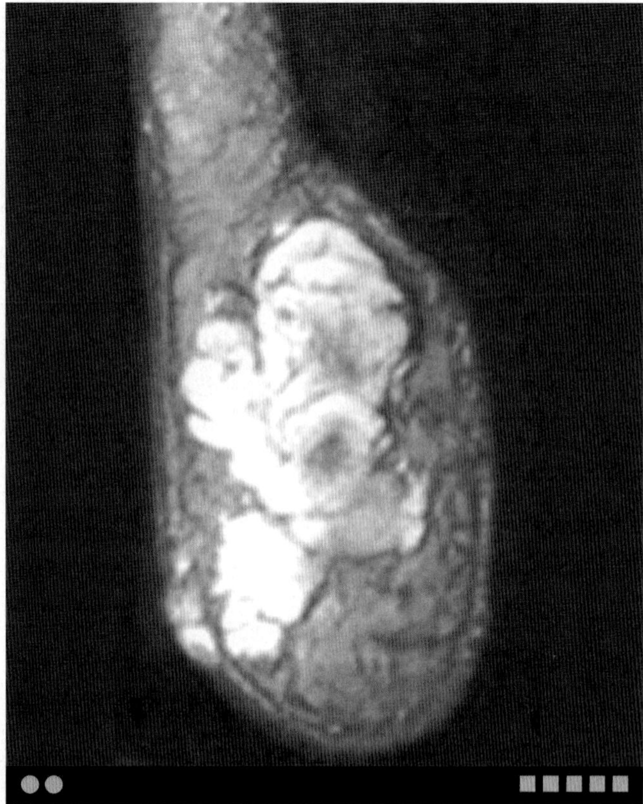

A. Extraskeletal chondrosarcoma: Coronal T2W MR image shows hyperintense mass with scattered foci of low signal intensity calcification.

COMMENTS

This case is of a 64-year-old male with painless soft tissue mass at lateral and plantar side of the heel. Extraskeletal soft tissue chondrosarcoma is a very rare, slow growing, low-grade tumor. It often presents as painful, tender soft tissue mass. At presentation, 40% already have metastasis. Typical locations are soft tissues of head and neck, extremities, shoulders, and buttocks. They typically occur in the fifth decade. On radiographs and CT, radiopaque calcified mass or stippled calcification in the soft tissues may be noted. On MR imaging, the mass is usually isointense to muscle on T1 weighted and inhomogeneously hyperintense on T2WI. Low signal intensity foci of calcification on all the sequences are seen scattered in the mass. Contrast enhancement is typically present. Although there are no definite characteristics on MR imaging to distinguish histologic type or grade of chondrosarcoma, MR imaging is an excellent tool for exact delineation of tumor extent. Radionuclide imaging with dynamic Tc-99m MDP and Tc-99m DTPA scintigraphy shows increased blood flow in the mass. Delayed 3 hour images show moderate Tc-99m DTPA accumulation in the tumor. Histologically the tumor consists of lobules containing tumor cells arranged in strand cords. The tumor is myxoid variant of chondrosarcoma with relatively good prognosis.

PEARLS

- **Extraskeletal chondrosarcoma is a rare, slow growing, painful, low-grade tumor.**
- **Typical locations are head and neck, extremities, shoulders, and buttocks.**
- **Radiographs and CT show calcified soft tissue mass. On MR imaging it is isointense to muscle on T1W and hyperintense on T2WI, with scattered foci of low signal intensity calcification.**

ADDITIONAL IMAGES

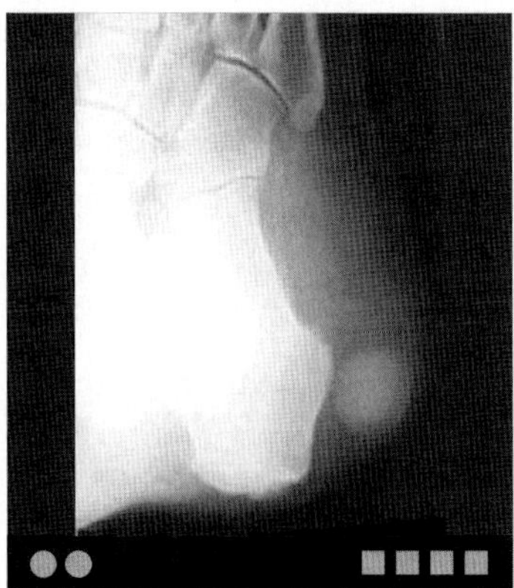

B. Extraskeletal chondrosarcoma: Oblique foot radiograph demonstrates densely calcified mass in the lateral and plantar aspect of right heel.

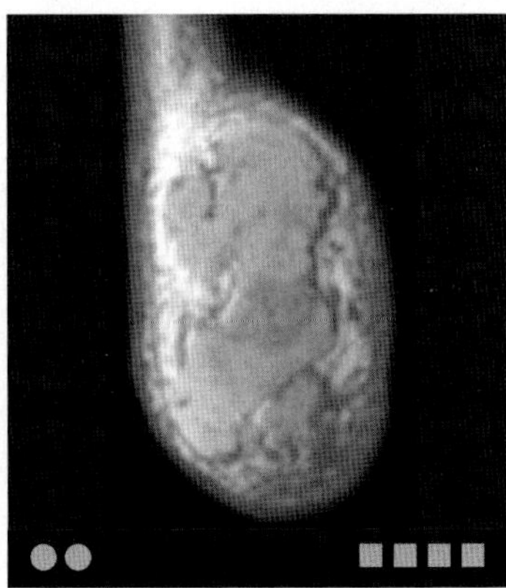

C. Extraskeletal chondrosarcoma: Coronal T1W MR image shows isointense mass with scattered foci of low signal intensity calcification.

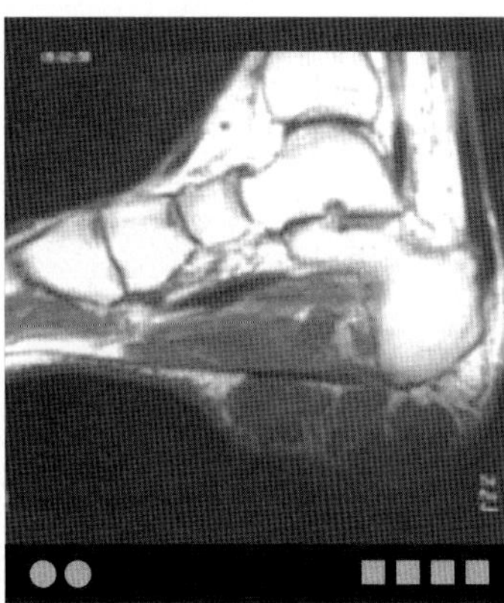

D. Extraskeletal chondrosarcoma: Sagittal T1W MR image shows low signal intensity mass of the heel.

DIFFERENTIAL DIAGNOSES IMAGES

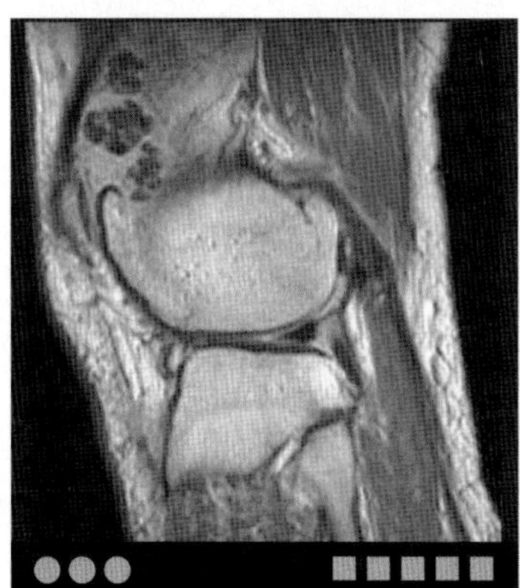

E. Synovial chondromatosis: Sagittal proton density image shows multiple low signal intensity calcified loose bodies.

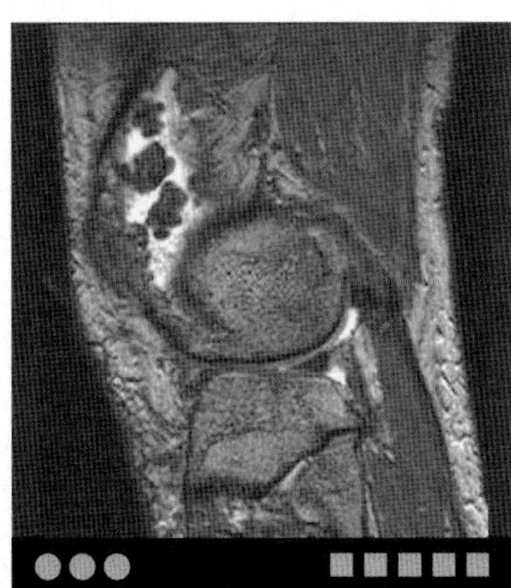

F. Synovial chondromatosis: Sagittal T2 W image shows intraarticular loose bodies.

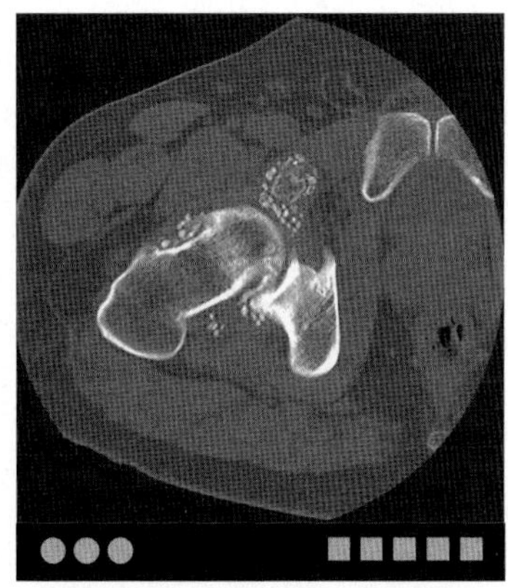

G. Synovial osteochondromatosis: CT exam shows multiple calcified loose bodies in the hip joint.

IMAGE KEY

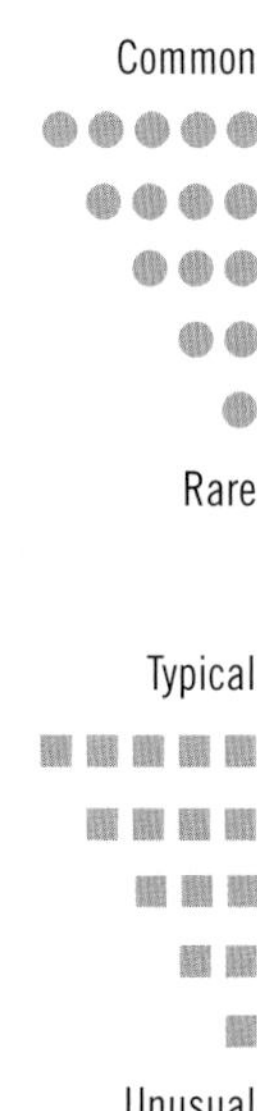

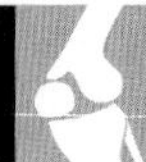

33–11 Malignant Melanoma of Foot

Sulabha Masih

PRESENTATION

Mass in plantar aspect of second and third toes

FINDINGS

MR imaging shows increased signal intensity on T1W and intermediate-to-low signal intensity on STIR and T2WI.

DIFFERENTIAL DIAGNOSES

- *Mortons neuroma:* This is degenerative fibrosis in the plantar digital nerve. Most often arises at the second or third intermetatarsal space at the level of metatarsophalangeal joint. On MRI, lesion is low intermediate signal intensity on T1W and T2WI. It may show mild homogenous contrast enhancement.
- *Gout:* Gouty tophi have homogenous low signal intensity on T1WI and inhomogeneous low-to-intermediate signal intensity on T2WI because of urate crystals and calcium deposition.
- *Giant cell tumor of the tendon sheath:* Local form of pigmented villonodular synovitis. Usually involves tendon sheaths of the hands and feet. On MRI, the lesion has low signal on proton density, T1WI, and T2WI because of deposition of hemosiderin.
- *Chronic hematoma:* Hemosiderin deposition demonstrates decrease signal intensity on both T1WI and T2WI.

COMMENTS

This case is a 64-year-old male with slowly growing mass between the proximal phalanges of second and third toes. Melanoma is a malignant transformation of melanocytes derived from neural crest cells, arising in preexisting benign nevi. They are induced by solar radiation and are more common in whites than blacks and Asians. Melanoma may occur at any age, and up to 75% of patients are younger than 70 years. Melanoma is the most common malignancy in women aged 25 to 29 years. It has two growth phases, radial and vertical. During the radial growth phase, malignant cells grow in radial direction in the epidermis. After a latent period of 2 to 20 years, most melanomas progress to the vertical growth phase, invading the dermis with metastasis to lymph nodes, skin, adrenal glands, bone, lung, liver, spleen, and other viscera. If detected early, melanoma can be cured with surgical excision. Majority of tumors contain melanin, on rare occasion, anaplastic melanocytes do not form pigment and are called amelanotic melanomas. Malignant melanoma demonstrates variable signal characteristics on MR, depending on melanin content. Primary melanomas and nonhemorrhagic melanotic metastasis demonstrates increase signal intensity on T1WI and intermediate-to-low signal intensity on T2WI because of intrinsic paramagnetic effects. However amelanotic melanoma without hemorrhage may present low signal on T1WI and high signal on T2WI.

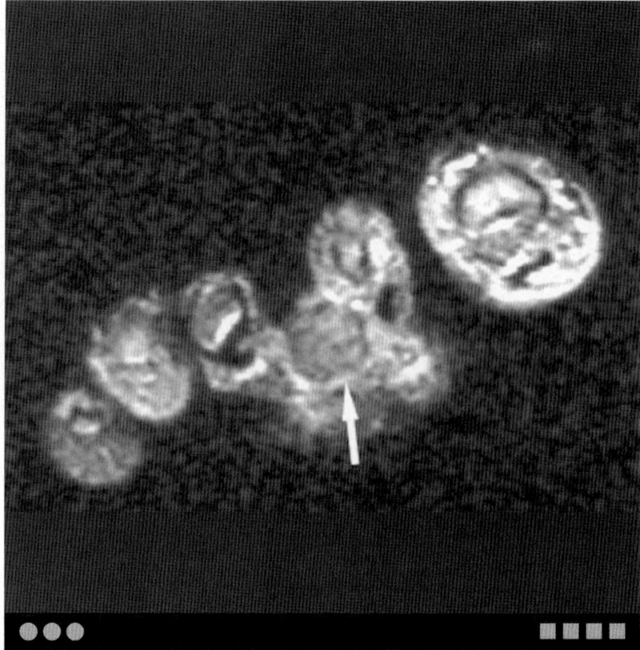

A. Malignant melanoma: Axial T2WI shows well-defined low signal intensity mass (arrow) at plantar aspect between the second and third toes.

PEARLS

- **Melanoma develops from melanocytes derived from neural crest cells.**
- **Primary melanomas and nonhemorrhagic melanotic metastasis demonstrate increase signal intensity on T1W and intermediate-to-low signal intensity on T2WI.**
- **Amelanotic melanomas without hemorrhage, present low signal on T1WI and high signal on T2WI.**

ADDITIONAL IMAGES

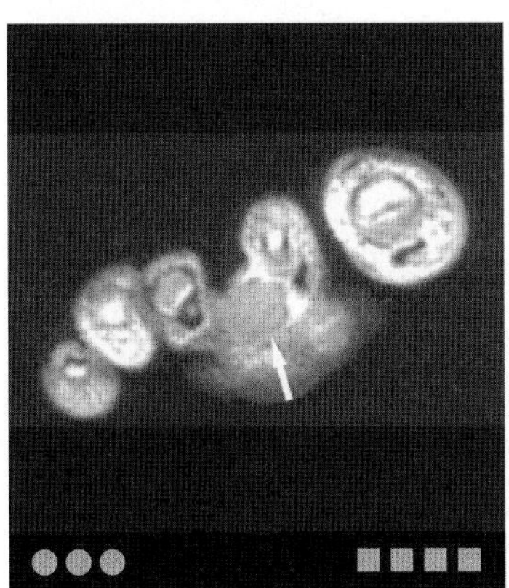

B. Malignant melanoma: Axial proton density image shows low-to-intermediate signal intensity mass (arrow) at plantar aspect between the second and third toes.

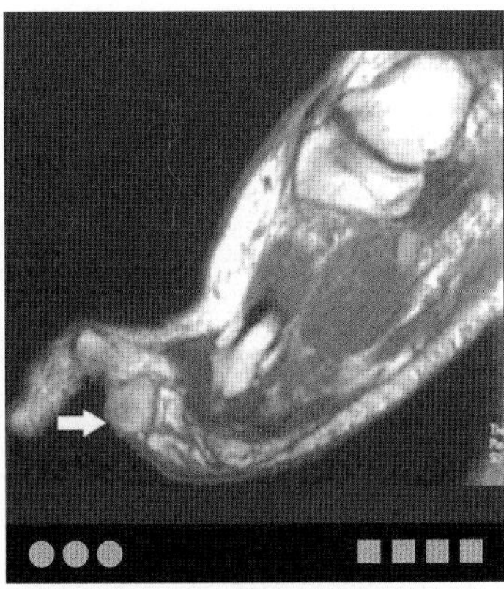

C. Malignant melanoma: Sagittal T1WI shows low-to-intermediate signal intensity mass (arrow) at the plantar aspect of foot.

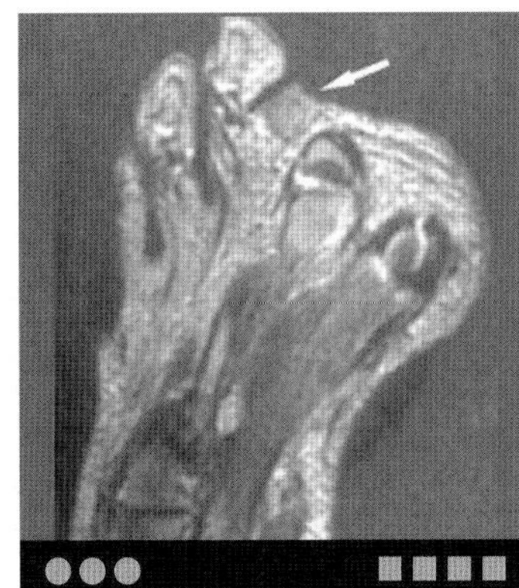

D. Malignant melanoma: Coronal T2WI shows low signal intensity mass (arrow) at plantar aspect between the second and third toes.

IMAGE KEY

Common

Rare

Typical

Unusual

DIFFERENTIAL DIAGNOSES IMAGES

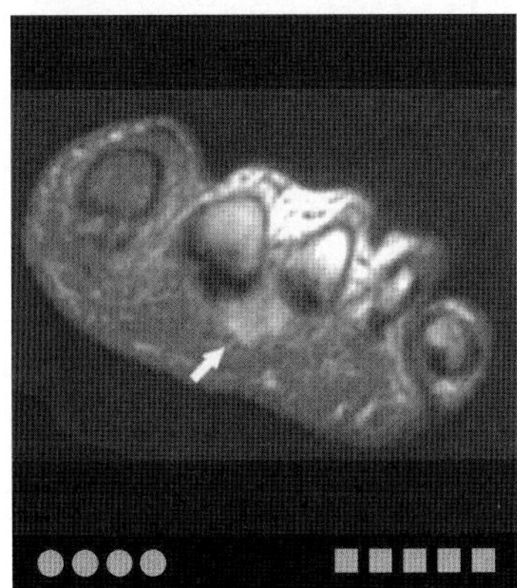

E. Mortons neuroma: Axial T1W fat-saturated postcontrast image shows mild contrast enhancement (arrow).

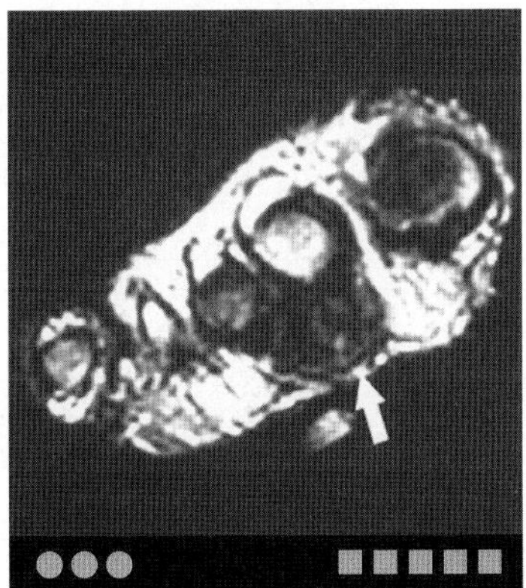

F. Gout: Axial T2WI shows low signal intensity tophus (arrow) between the second and third toes. Note bone marrow edema at the base of proximal phalanx of second toe.

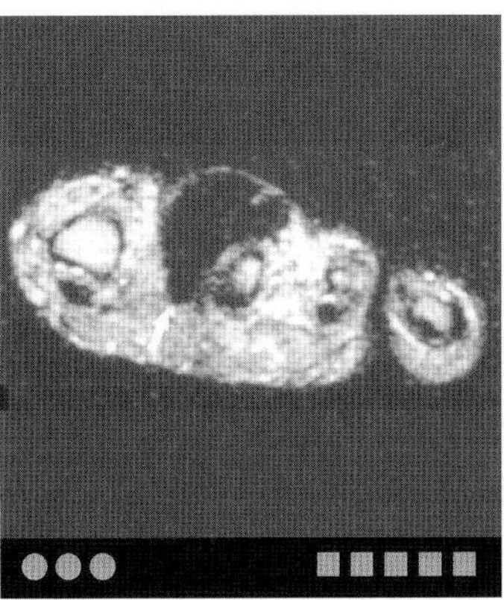

G. Giant cell tumor of tendon sheath: Axial T2WI shows low signal intensity mass (arrow) eroding proximal phalanx of second toe.

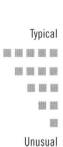

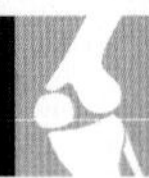

33–12 Malignant Peripheral Nerve Sheath Tumor (MPNST) of

Joon Kim

PRESENTATION

Painful soft tissue forefoot mass

FINDINGS

MR images show a soft tissue mass between the second and third metatarsal shafts.

DIFFERENTIAL DIAGNOSES

- *Morton's Neuroma:* Typically seen as a T1W and T2W hypointense mass arising between the metatarsal heads.
- *Hemangioma:* Usually shows high signal on both T1W and T2W sequences. Presence of fat and serpentine signal voids assist with diagnosis.
- *Desmoid Tumor:* MR signal characteristics vary depending on the abundance of collagen fibers versus fibroblasts, but are generally isointense to hypointense on both T1WI and T2WI.
- *Other soft tissue sarcomas:* Variable MR signal characteristics.

COMMENTS

Malignant peripheral nerve sheath tumors (MPNSTs) are the malignant counterparts to benign peripheral nerve sheath tumors, such as schwannomas and neurofibromas. These tumors are commonly located within the deep soft tissue, usually adjacent to a nerve trunk. MPNSTs account for 10% of all soft tissue sarcomas, and approximately 30% to 50% are associated with neurofibromatosis Type 1 (NF1). Another 10% of MPNST cases are associated with prior radiation. MPNSTs are usually seen in 20 to 50 year olds, but patients with NF1 may develop these tumors at an earlier age as well. These tumors also tend to be more aggressive in patients with NF1. Clinically, the classic presenting symptom is pain. Neurologic deficits as a result of mass effect may also occur. As with most soft tissue tumors, MPNSTs are best evaluated with MR imaging. The MR characteristics are usually nonspecific and vary depending on the degree of necrosis and its histology, but MPNSTs are typically isointense on T1W and hyperintense on T2WI with enhancement seen on the post-gadolinium sequences. Distinguishing MPNSTs from their benign counterparts or other soft tissue sarcomas can be extremely difficult. Therefore, these masses often require tissue diagnosis.

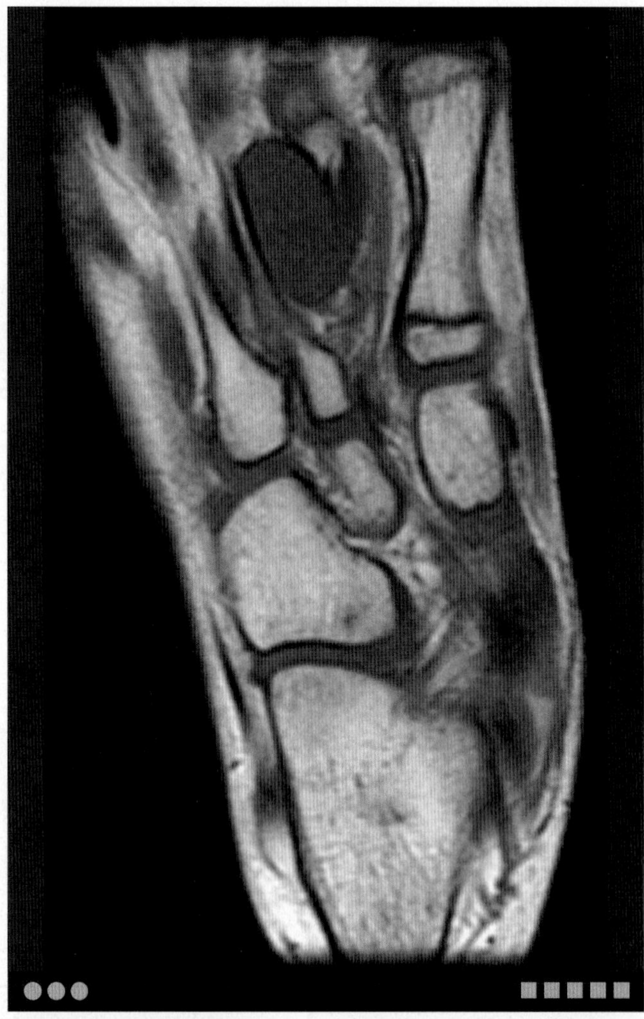

A. MPNST: Axial T1W MR image of the forefoot again demonstrates a mass located between the second and third metatarsal shafts.

PEARLS

- **MPNSTs are the malignant counterparts to benign peripheral nerve sheath tumors.**
- **MPNSTs account for 10% of all soft tissue sarcomas. Approximately 30% to 50% of cases are associated with NF1 with another 10% associated with prior irradiation.**
- **The classic presenting symptom is pain. Neurologic deficits may occur as well.**
- **MR characteristics are typically nonspecific and vary depending on the degree of necrosis and its histology. Therefore, these masses often require tissue diagnosis.**

ADDITIONAL IMAGES

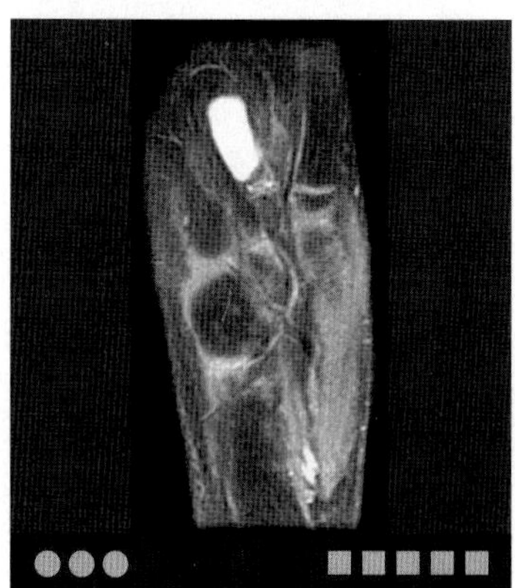

B. MPNST: Axial T1W fat-suppressed post-gadolinium MR image of the forefoot demonstrates intense enhancement of this inter-metatarsal space mass.

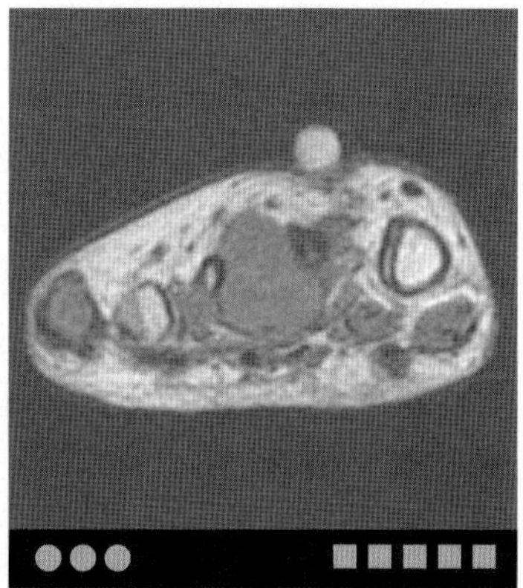

C. MPNST: Coronal T1W MR image of the forefoot demonstrates an isointense mass located between the second and third metatarsal shafts. Note the mass effect, resulting in splaying of the metatarsal shafts.

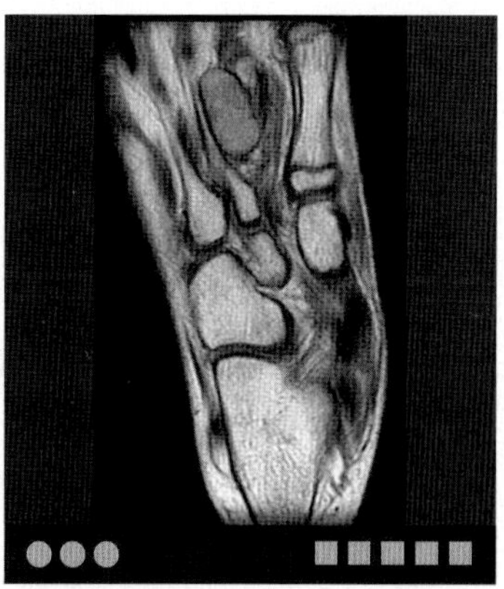

D. MPNST: Axial T2W MR image of the forefoot shows that the mass is mildly hyperintense.

DIFFERENTIAL DIAGNOSES IMAGES

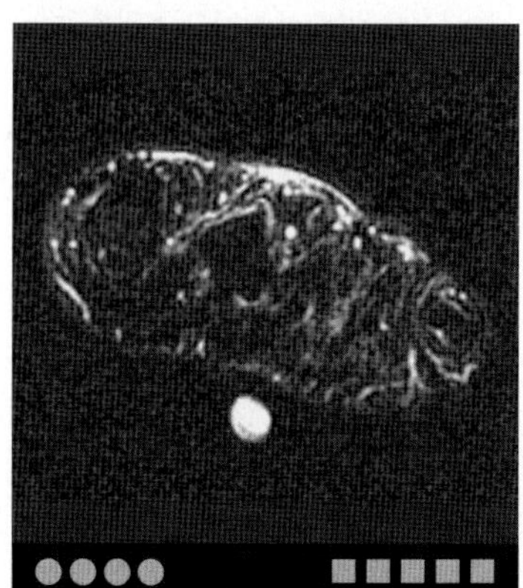

E. Morton's Neuroma: Coronal T2W fat-suppressed MR image of the forefoot demonstrates a small hypointense mass located between the second and third distal metatarsal shafts. This mass was also hypointense on the T1W images (not shown).

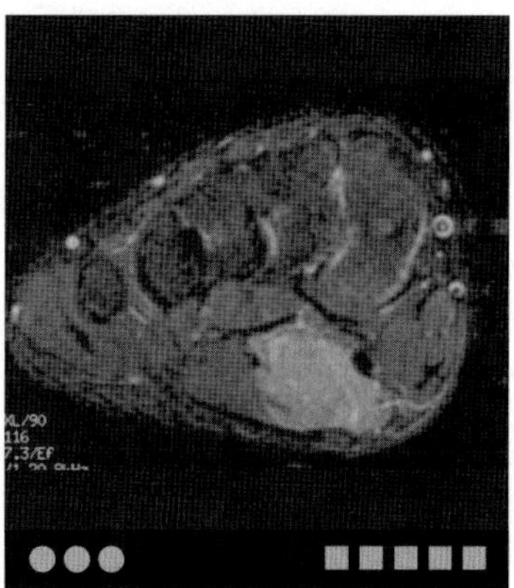

F. Hemangioma: Coronal T2W fat-suppressed MR image of the forefoot demonstrates a hyperintense intramuscular mass within the plantar aspect of the forefoot. Note the lack of significant mass effect, which is often seen with hemangiomas.

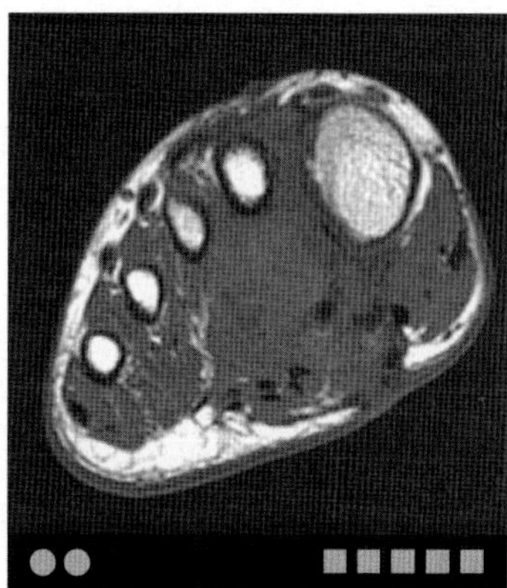

G. Desmoid: Coronal T1W MR image of the forefoot demonstrates a large, isointense, ill-defined, intramuscular mass within the plantar aspect of the forefoot. Note its significant mass effect on the flexor digitorum tendons.

IMAGE KEY

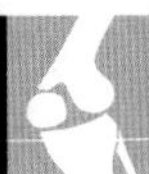

33–13 Intraosseous Lipoma of Calcaneus

Amilcare Gentili

PRESENTATION

Heel pain

FINDINGS

MR images show a lesion in the calcaneus with the same signal as fat on all sequences.

DIFFERENTIAL DIAGNOSES

- *Normal trabecular calcaneal pattern:* Paucity of the trabeculae in the anterior aspect of the calcaneus at area of "neutral triangle" of calcaneus may simulate a lytic lesion in the calcaneus.
- *Unicameral bone cyst:* A homogeneous single, fluid-filled cavity.
- *Giant Cell Tumor:* May contain area of low signal due to hemosiderin deposits.
- *Aneurysmal bone cyst:* There is usually expansion of bone and fluid–fluid levels
- *Chondroblastoma:* In 50% of cases contains calcifications.
- *Bone infarct:* This form of bone infarct is called cystic infarct.

COMMENTS

Lipoma is a benign lesion composed of mature adipose tissue. It is the most frequent benign soft tissue tumor, but is a rare osseous lesion. The etiology of intraosseous lipomas is controversial: hypotheses range from a primary benign neoplasm to a reactive bone lesion following trauma or bone infarct. The intraosseous lipoma can be asymptomatic, and may be found incidentally during radiological investigation following trauma. However, occasionally intraosseous lipomas may cause pain. Rarely, a pathologic fracture occurs. The age peak for lipomas is between 40 and 60 years. Intraosseous lipomas are seen in both males and females with the same frequency. The most common locations are the fibula, femur, calcaneus, and tibia. The majority of intraosseous lipomas present classic radiographic features and cross-sectional imaging is not needed. Based on histology, intraosseous lipoma is divided in three stages. Stage 1 contains only viable fat. Stage 2 lesions typically contain viable fat, fat necrosis, and dystrophic calcifications. In stage 3 there is involution of the lesion with extensive fat necrosis, cyst formation, calcification, and reactive new bone formation. The MR appearance in stage 1 shows the entire lesion having the same signal intensity as fat on all sequences. Areas of fat necrosis with calcification (stage 2 and 3) have low signal intensity on all sequences. Areas of cystic degeneration (stage 3) have high signal intensity on fluid sensitive (T2 and STIR) sequences. The identification of fat in the lesion permits definitive diagnosis of intraosseous lipoma.

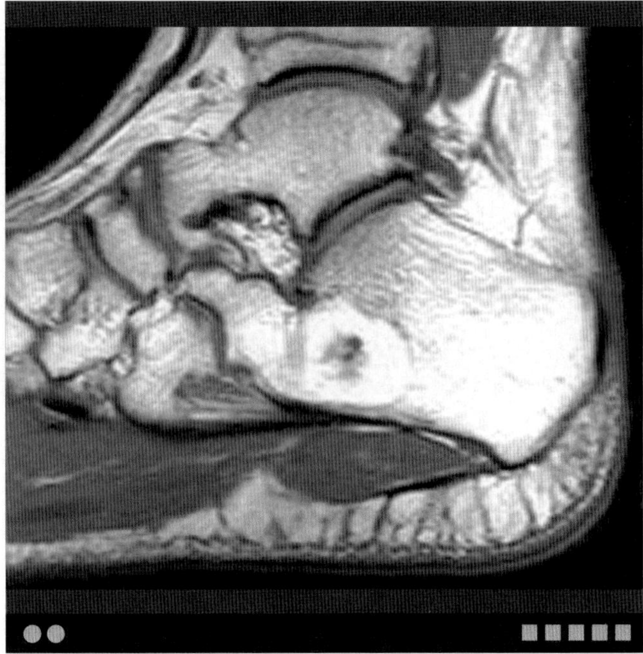

A. Intraosseous Lipoma: Sagittal T1WI shows a high signal intensity lesion with a low signal center in the calcaneus.

PEARLS

- **At least portion of the lesion has same signal as subcutaneous fat on all sequences.**
- **It may contain dystrophic calcifications in the center of the lesion.**
- **Cystic degeneration can be present.**
- **Intraosseous lesions containing fat are benign.**

ADDITIONAL IMAGES

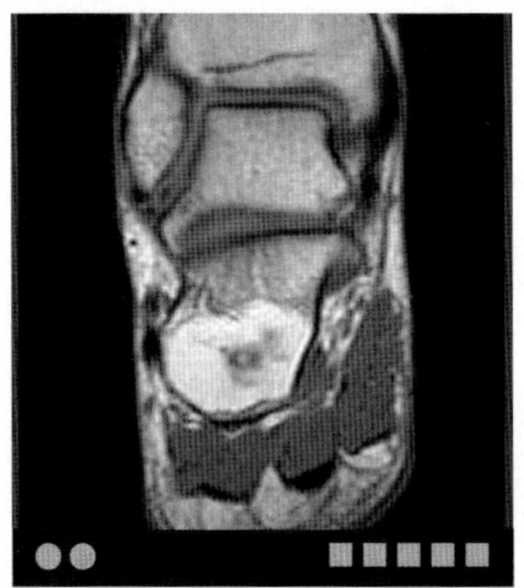

B. Intraosseous Lipoma: Coronal proton density image shows a high signal intensity lesion with a low signal center in the calcaneus.

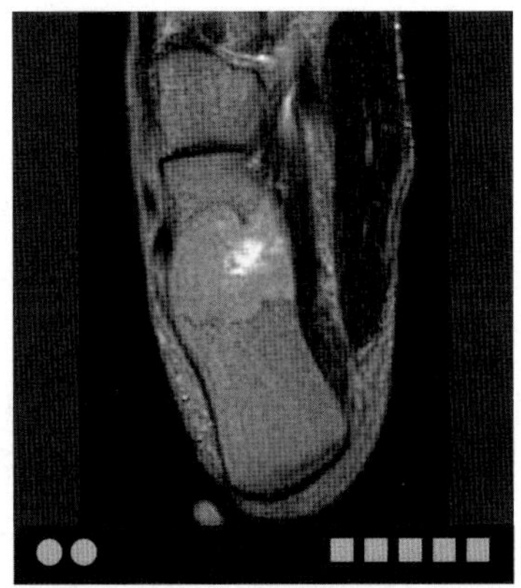

C. Intraosseous Lipoma: Axial T2WI shows reversal of the signal pattern, the periphery of the lesion has intermediate signal as subcutaneous fat, the center is mostly high signal, with the exception of few specks of low signal corresponding to calcifications.

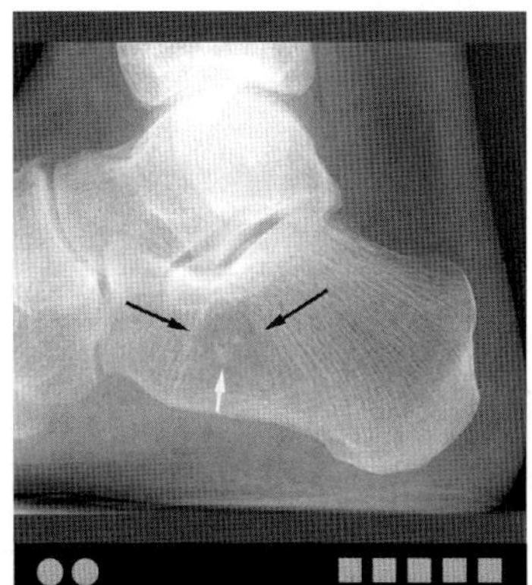

D. Intraosseous Lipoma: Radiograph of the ankle shows a well-defined lytic lesion of the calcaneus (black arrows) with several central calcifications (white arrow).

IMAGE KEY

Common

●●●●●
●●●●
●●●
●●
●

Rare

Typical

■■■■■
■■■■
■■■
■■
■

Unusual

DIFFERENTIAL DIAGNOSES IMAGES

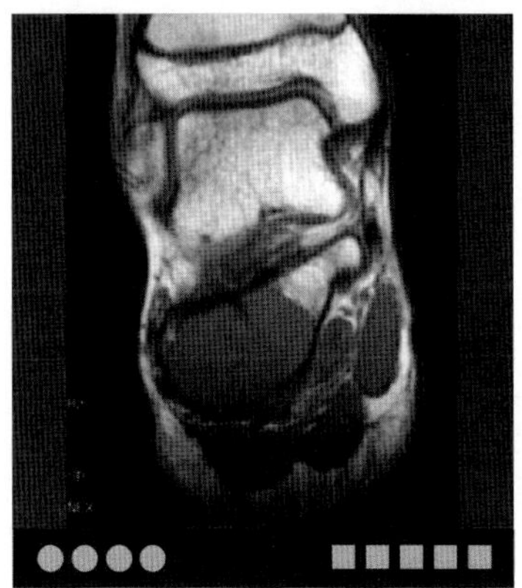

E. Unicameral bone cyst: Coronal T1WI shows a mass with low signal intensity in the calcaneus.

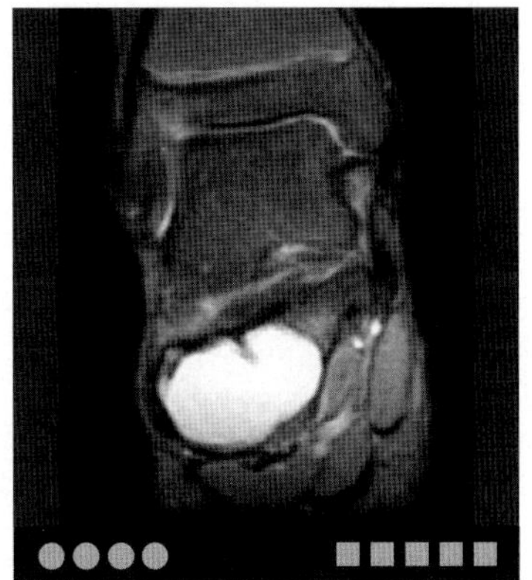

F. Unicameral bone cyst: Coronal T2W fat-saturated fast spin echo MR image shows a high signal intensity mass infiltrating in the calcaneus.

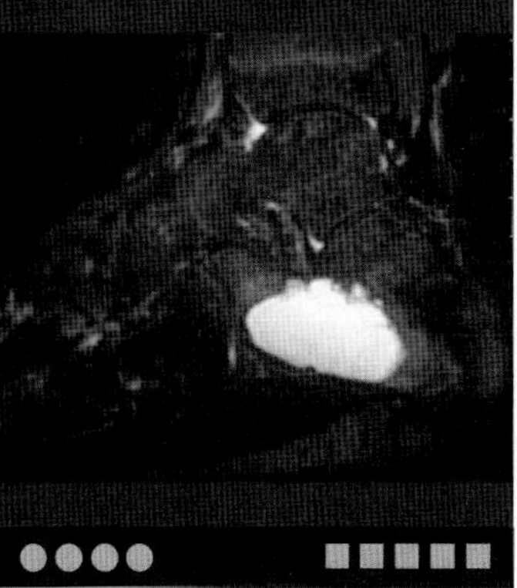

G. Unicameral bone cyst: Sagittal STIR image shows high signal intensity mass in the calcaneus.

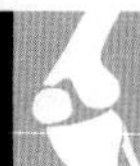

33–14 Giant Cell Tumor of Calcaneus

Robert D. Simon and Rajeev K. Varma

PRESENTATION

Foot pain

FINDINGS

MR images demonstrate a well-defined lesion in the calcaneus with low-to-intermediate signal intensity on T1WI, high signal on STIR and T2WI, and avid enhancement with contrast.

DIFFERENTIAL DIAGNOSES

- *Aneurysmal bone cyst:* Unlikely, usually found in younger population and contains a thin sclerotic rim best seen on CT. Multiple fluid- fluid levels are often noted.
- *Simple bone cyst of calcaneus:* This is a common lesion at the center of calcaneus where paucity of bone trabeculae creates the neutral triangle.
- *Chondroblastoma:* Unlikely here; it is found in skeletally immature patients and typically has a sclerotic margin.
- *Brown Tumor:* Possible, these tumors have a similar appearance. One should correlate with clinical history and other radiographic features of hyperparathyroidism.

COMMENTS

This is a 27-year-old male with foot pain. Giant cell tumor (GCT), consisting of multinucleated giant cells in a fibroid stroma, is a common benign tumor representing 4% to 9% of all primary bone tumors. They almost always occur after epiphyseal fusion appearing as a geographic expansile lesion that originates in the metaphysis and usually extends to the subarticular region. GCTs most commonly occur in between the third and fifth decades of life and are usually found at the knee and wrist in long bones and the sacrum and vertebral body in the spine. The lesion usually appears benign with a narrow zone of transition and without a sclerotic margin. Rarely, do GCTs demonstrate cortical breakthrough and soft tissue mass. The vast majority have a low histologic grade; however, 5% are malignant and can metastasize to the lungs. The typical MR appearance of GCT is that of a solid lesion with nonspecific low signal intensity on T1 imaging. On T2 imaging, 60% of lesions will demonstrate predominately high signal intensity with low signal regions correlating to hemosiderin or collagen content. The remaining 40% will have more homogenous high signal intensity. Moreover, GCTs enhance on gadolinium contrast imaging.

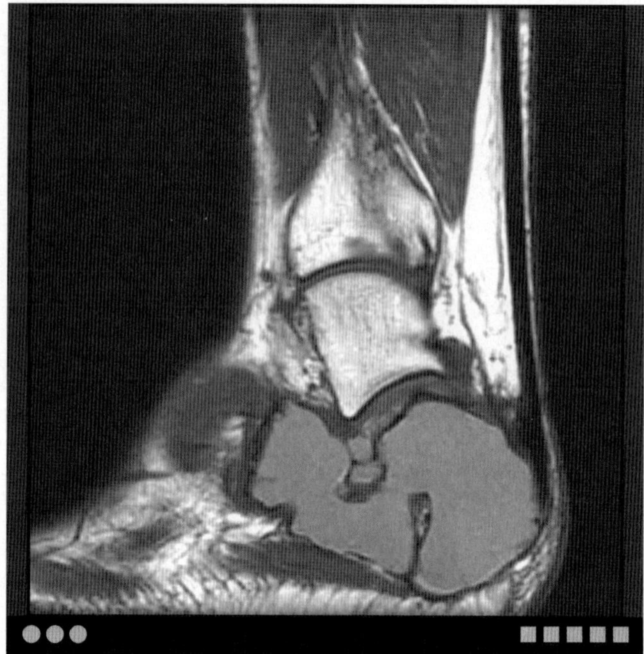

A. GCT: Sagittal T1W image demonstrates a low signal lesion in the calcaneus with septations.

PEARLS

- **Benign appearing expansile lytic lesion originating in the metaphysis extending to the subarticular region.**
- **Commonly occurring between the third and fifth decades of life in the knee, wrist sacrum, and vertebral body.**
- **Low signal on T1, mostly high signal on T2, and enhances with gadolinium.**

ADDITIONAL IMAGES

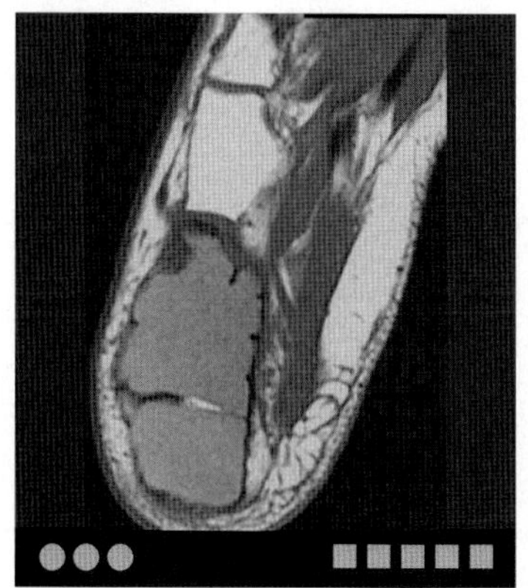

B. GCT: Axial T1WI in axial plane demonstrates a low signal lesion in the calcaneus with septations.

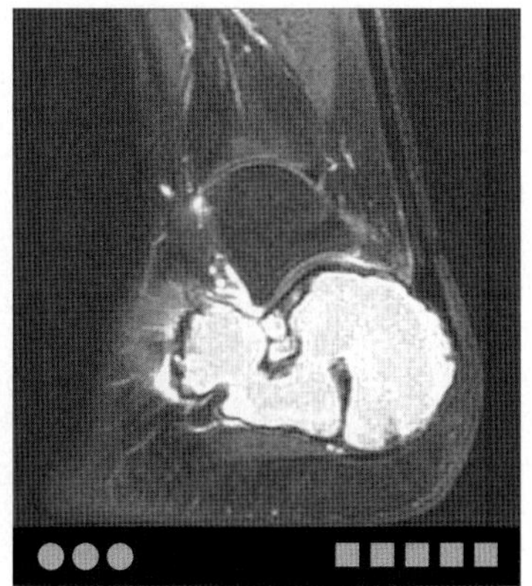

C. GCT: Sagittal T1WI with fat saturation and gadolinium enhanced image shows a markedly enhancing lesion.

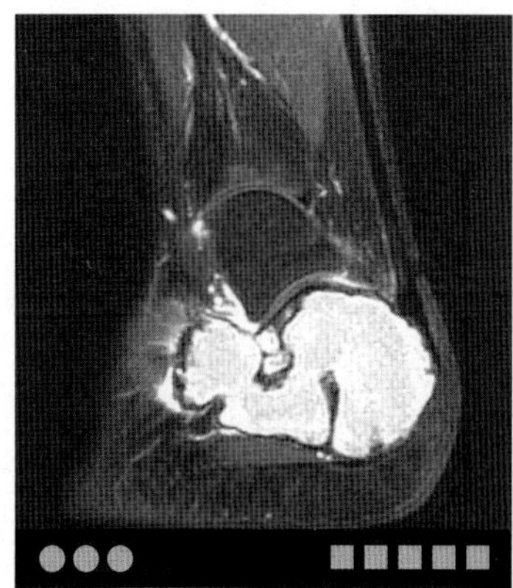

D. GCT: Sagittal STIR image shows high signal intensity lesion encompassing the calcaneus.

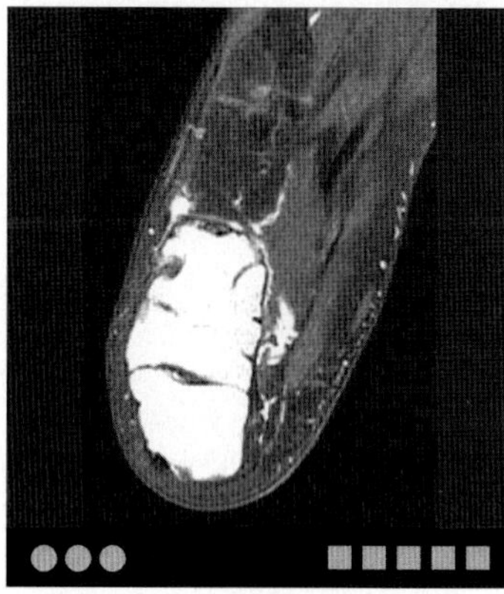

E. GCT: STIR sequence in axial plane showing high intensity lesion in the calcaneus.

IMAGE KEY

Common

Rare

Typical

Unusual

DIFFERENTIAL DIAGNOSES IMAGES

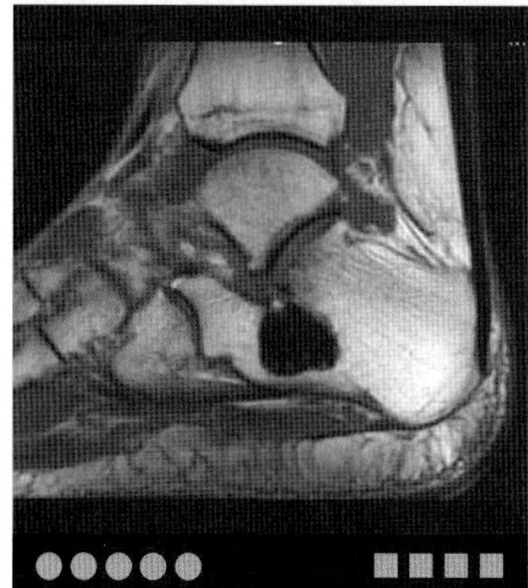

F. Treated calcaneal cyst: Sagittal T1W image shows a calcaneal cyst treated with intralesional cement.

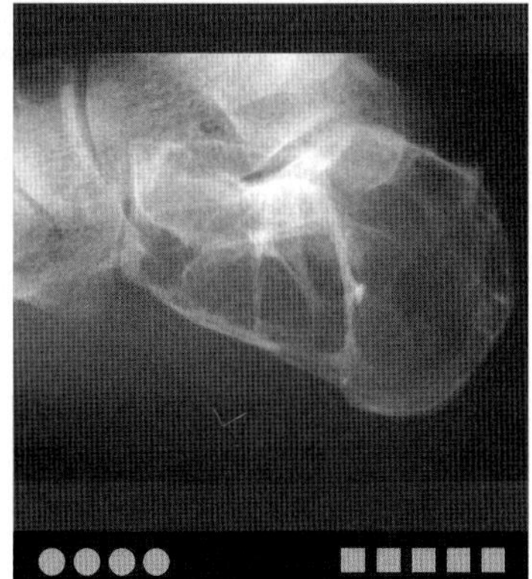

G. Calcaneal cyst: Radiograph of the ankle shows mildly expansile cyst with multiple septations.

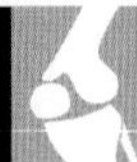

33–15 Unicameral Bone Cyst of Calcaneus

Amilcare Gentili

PRESENTATION

An incidental finding on radiograph

FINDINGS

MR images show a lesion in the calcaneus with low signal intensity on T1WI and homogenous high signal on fluid-sensitive sequences.

DIFFERENTIAL DIAGNOSES

- *Intraosseous lipoma:* This lesion shows dark signal on fat-suppressed images. Central specks of calcification are often observed.
- *Giant Cell Tumor:* Mimics unicameral bone cyst (UBC); may show multiple fluid levels and deposits of dark hemosiderin.
- *Osteoblastoma:* Shows significant reactive sclerosis.
- *Chondroblastoma:* It is an epiphyseal lesion and has matrix calcification in more than 50% of cases

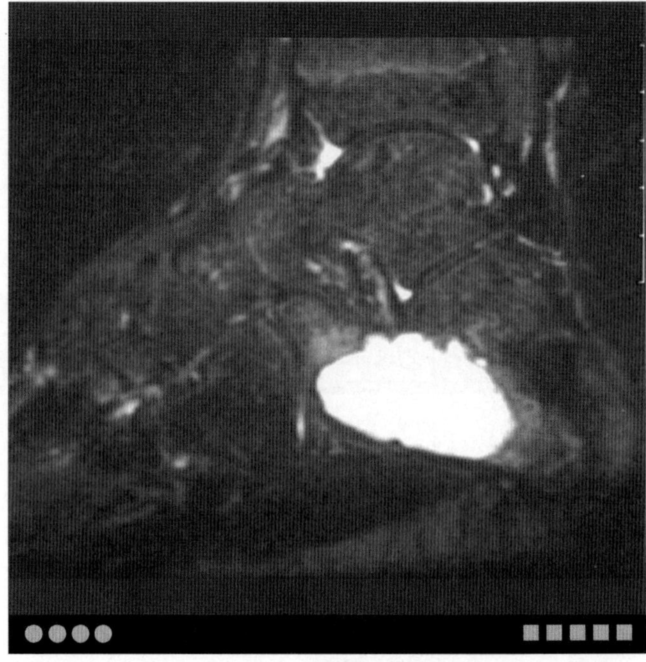

A. Unicameral bone cyst: Sagittal STIR shows an almost elliptical high signal intensity lesion in the calcaneus.

COMMENTS

This is an incidental finding on a radiograph done after an ankle sprain in a 30-year-old male. Simple bone cyst is a benign cystic lesion of bone of unknown etiology. It can be seen in any age group but is very rare before 5 and after 20 years of age. In children simple bone cyst are usually seen in long bones (the proximal humerus followed by the proximal femur), in adults have a predilection for the calcaneus and the iliac bone. It is more common in males with a 2.5 to 1 male-to-female ratio. Simple cysts are central, lytic, expansile lesions. Their radiographic appearance is usually diagnostic and neither MR nor CT is usually necessary. On MRI they are well defined with low signal intensity on T1WI and high signal intensity on T2WI because of the fluid content of the cyst. Typically, they are homogeneous on both T1WI and T2WI, unless hemorrhage has occurred. Peripheral low signal intensity borders represent reactive sclerosis. No edema is present in the surrounding bone marrow or muscle unless a pathological fracture is present. CT is superior to MRI in detecting subtle infractions of the lesion. The "fallen fragment sign" is pathognomonic for this cyst. It is seen with pathological fractures of simple bone cysts, a fragment of cortical bone become dislodged and gravitate to the dependent portion of the unicameral bone cyst.

PEARLS

- **The most common locations of simple bone cysts are the proximal humerus and proximal femur in children and the calcaneus and pelvis in adults.**
- **Usually asymptomatic unless fractured.**
- **"Fallen fragment sign" present in UBC with fracture.**

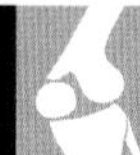

ADDITIONAL IMAGES

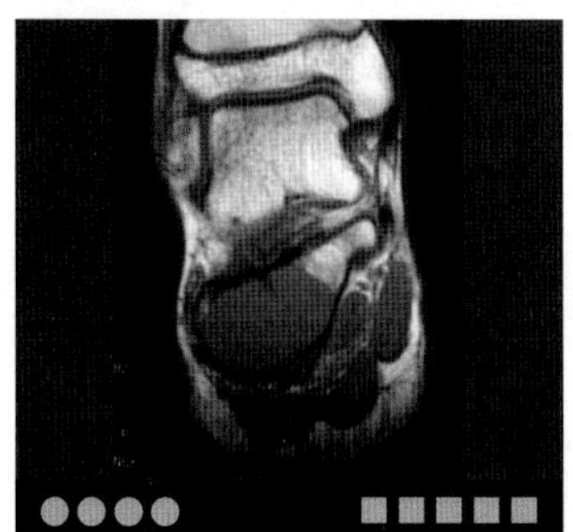

B. Unicameral bone cyst: Coronal T1WI shows the lesion with the same signal intensity as muscle.

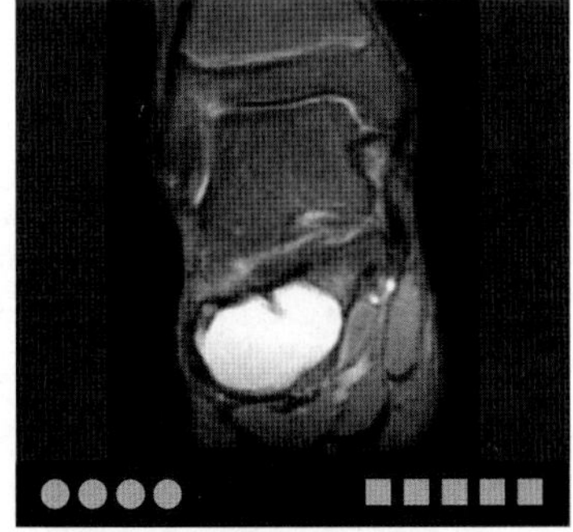

C. Unicameral bone cyst: Coronal T2W fat-saturated image shows the lesion with high signal intensity.

DIFFERENTIAL DIAGNOSES IMAGES

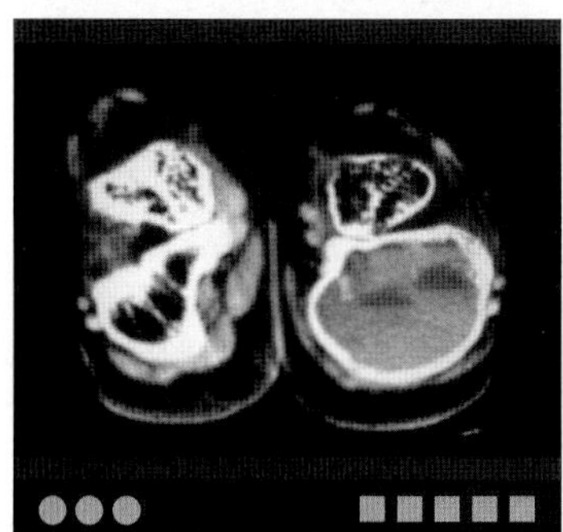

D. Aneurysmal bone cyst: Coronal CT image shows an expansile lesion of the left calcaneus. Note multiple fluid levels typical of an aneurysmal bone cyst although it can be seen in other bone lesions such as giant cell tumors, chondroblastoma, and telangiectatic osteosarcomas.

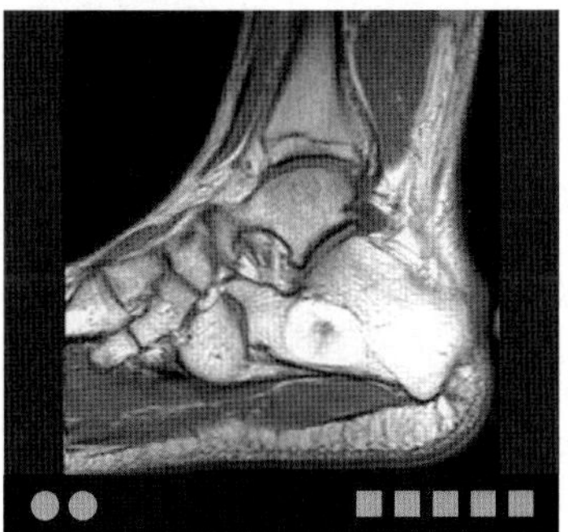

E. Intraosseous lipoma: Sagittal T1WI shows a high signal intensity lesion with a low signal center in the calcaneus.

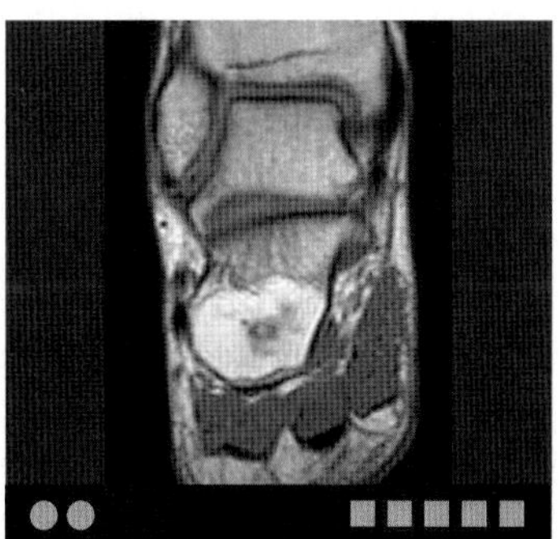

F. Intraosseous lipoma: Coronal proton density image shows a high signal intensity lesion with a low signal center in the calcaneus.

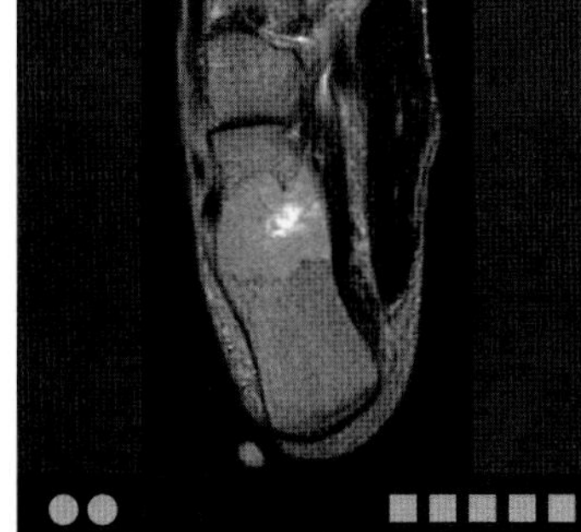

G. Intraosseous lipoma: Axial T2WI shows reversal of the signal pattern, the periphery of the lesion has intermediate signal as subcutaneous fat, and the center is mostly high signal, with the exception of few specks of low signal corresponding to calcifications. The identification of fat in the lesion permits definitive diagnosis of intraosseous lipoma.

IMAGE KEY

Common

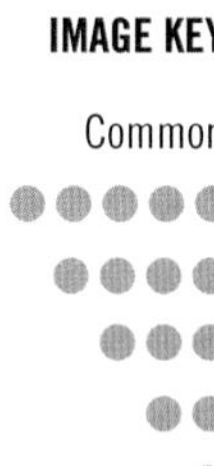

Rare

Typical

Unusual

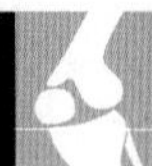

33–16 Osteoid Osteoma of the Talus

Kambiz Motamedi

PRESENTATION

Ankle pain

FINDINGS

CT shows a small lytic lesion of the talar dome with a central nidus calcification.

DIFFERENTIAL DIAGNOSES

- *Osteochondritis dissecans:* Radiographs and cross-sectional imaging show an osteochondral defect of the medial or lateral aspect of the talar dome.
- *Avascular necrosis:* Imaging demonstrates increased sclerosis of the talus. There may be a structural collapse of the talar dome.
- *Giant cell tumor:* CT shows a lytic lesion of the subchondral bone without a mineralized matrix and narrow zone of transition.

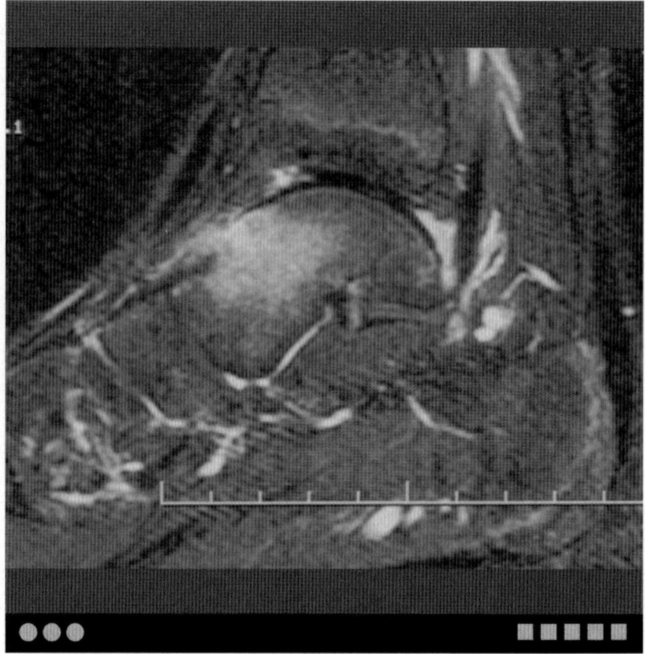

A. Osteoid osteoma: Sagittal inversion recovery image reveals a patchy edema of the anterior and medial aspect of the talus.

COMMENTS

This is a 13-year-old male with a 7-month history of ankle pain. Imaging revealed an osteoid osteoma of the ankle for which he underwent surgical resection. He spent 4 months with pain. Imaging revealed the presence of an osteoid osteoma for which he underwent a radiofrequency ablation. Osteoid osteoma is a benign skeletal neoplasm of unknown etiology that is composed of osteoid and woven bone. The tumor is usually smaller than 1.5 cm in diameter. It can occur in any bone, but in approximately two thirds of patients, the appendicular skeleton is involved. The patients are young. The classic presentation is that of focal bone pain at the site of the tumor. The condition worsens at night and increases with activity, and it is dramatically relieved with small doses of aspirin. The lesion initially appears as a small sclerotic bone island within a circular lucent defect. This central nidus is seldom larger than 1.5 cm in diameter, and it may be associated with considerable overlying cortical and endosteal bone sclerosis. The tumors may regress spontaneously. The mechanism of this involution is not known, but tumor infarction is a possibility. Osteoid osteoma is classified as cortical, cancellous, or subperiosteal. Cortical tumors are the most common. Intra-articular osteoid osteomas are difficult to identify because of the lack of periosteal thickening and may lead to early osteoarthrosis. The hallmark of imaging is the smooth periosteal thickening at the site of the lesion, which is absent with the intra-articular location. MRI readily demonstrates the marrow edema.

PEARLS

- **Smooth periosteal thickening of a tubular bone is the hallmark of the lesion.**
- **The cortical thickening is absent in intra-articular osteoid osteomas because of the lack of periosteum. MRI shows the marrow edema, and CT with reformats may be helpful to detect the nidus.**
- **Clinical history of night pain relieved with aspirin is most helpful to confirm the diagnosis.**

ADDITIONAL IMAGES

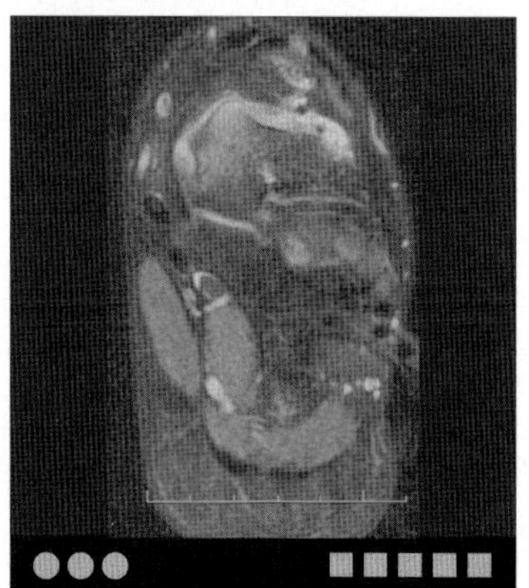

B. Osteoid osteoma: Coronal fat-saturated PD image shows edema of the medial aspect of the talar dome. There is a small joint effusion.

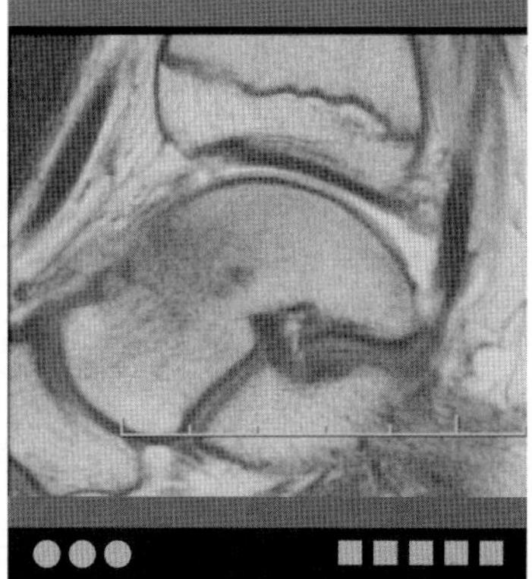

C. Osteoid osteoma: Sagittal T1W image corresponding to image A shows the patchy edema as an ill-defined area of marrow replacement.

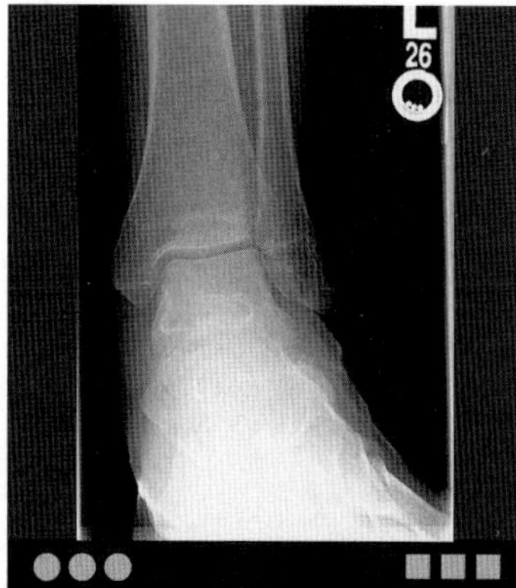

D. Osteoid osteoma: AP radiograph of the ankle shows no abnormalities.

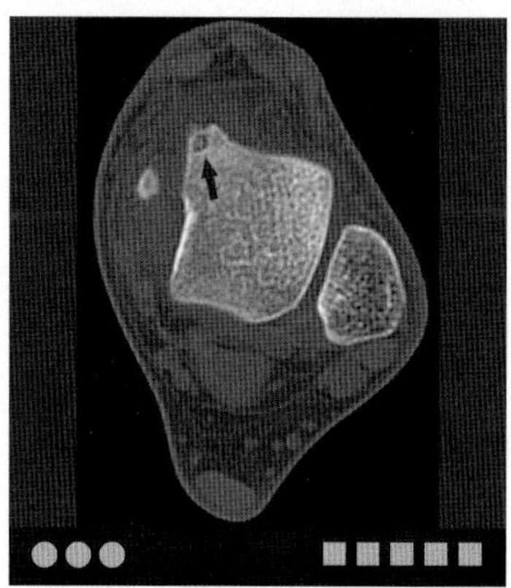

E. Osteoid osteoma: Axial nonenhanced CT scan in bone algorithm demonstrates a subcentimeter lytic lesion of the anterior talus with a sclerotic nidus pathognomonic for osteoid osteoma (arrow).

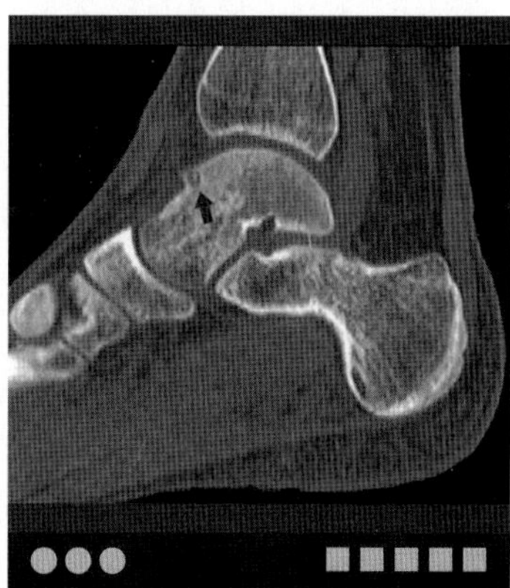

F. Osteoid osteoma: The sagittal reformats reveal the focus of osteoid osteoma (arrow) in the center of the patchy edema seen on the MRI.

DIFFERENTIAL DIAGNOSIS IMAGE

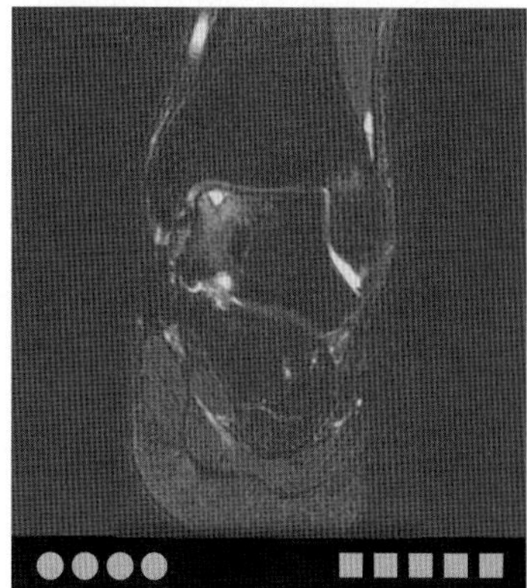

G. Osteochondritis dissecans: Coronal fat-saturated T2W MR image shows a tiny cystic lesion of the subchondral medial talar dome with surrounding edema in this young patient consistent with osteochondritis dissecans.

IMAGE KEY

Common

Rare

Typical

Unusual

Chapter 34

Miscellaneous

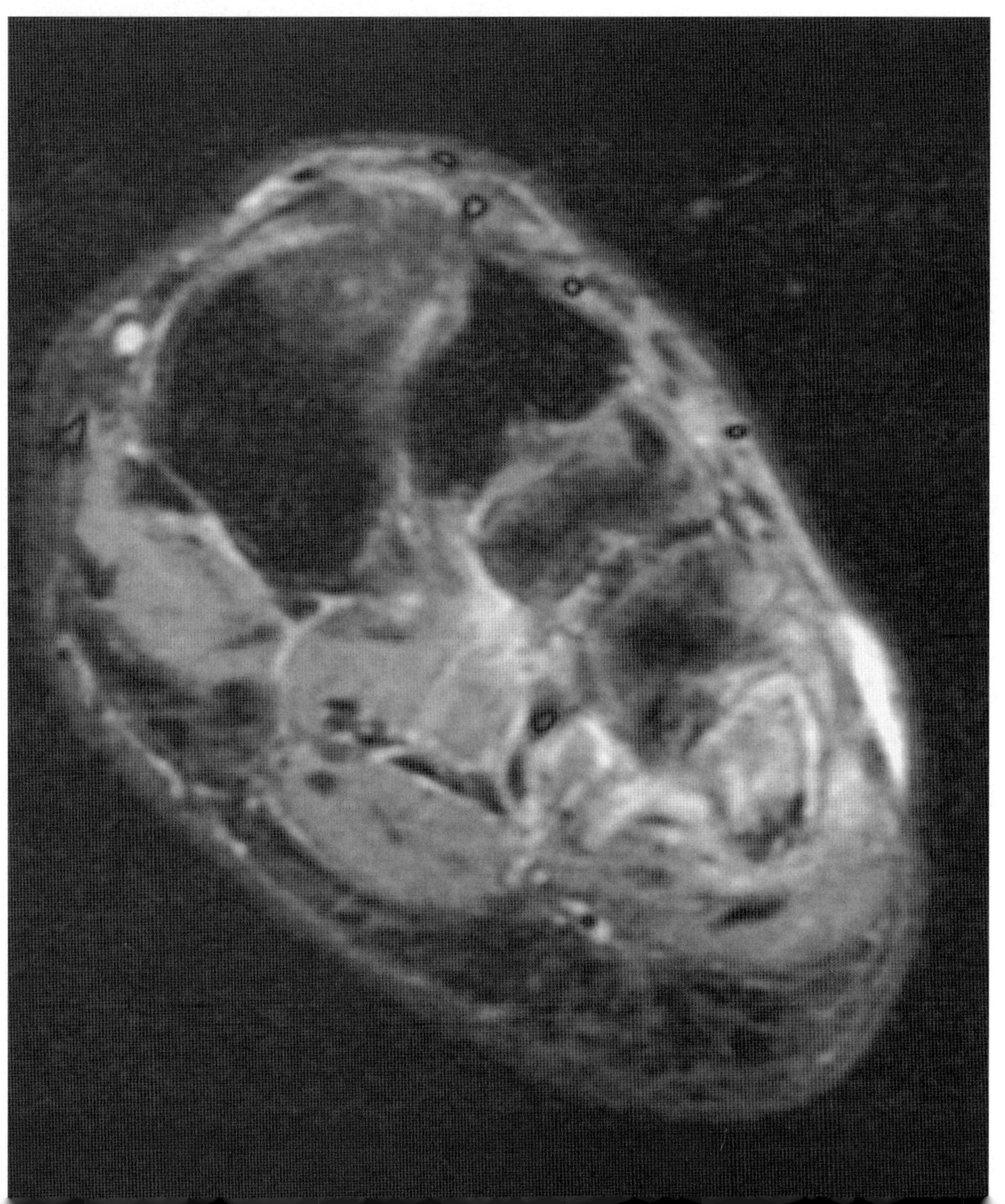

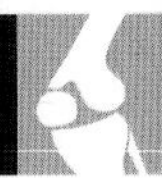

34–1 Reflex Sympathetic Dystrophy (Sudeck's Atrophy)

Rosemary J. Klecker

PRESENTATION

Foot pain and swelling 2 months after injury

FINDINGS

MR image shows soft tissue edema of the midfoot and forefoot.

DIFFERENTIAL DIAGNOSES

- *Disuse osteopenia:* Results from immobilization of a joint and it is not painful. The periarticular osteopenia seen on MR and radiographic imaging is usually more diffused than that of Reflex sympathetic dystrophy (RSD). Clinical history is useful in making this diagnosis
- *Infection:* Early osteomyelitis presents radiographically as periarticular osteopenia associated with soft tissue edema. On MR imaging, marrow edema signal of the affected joint is diffuse.
- *Inflammatory arthropathy:* Although it may demonstrate periarticular osteopenia and soft tissue edema on MR imaging, this process is differentiated from RSD by clinical history, laboratory values, and joint aspiration if needed.

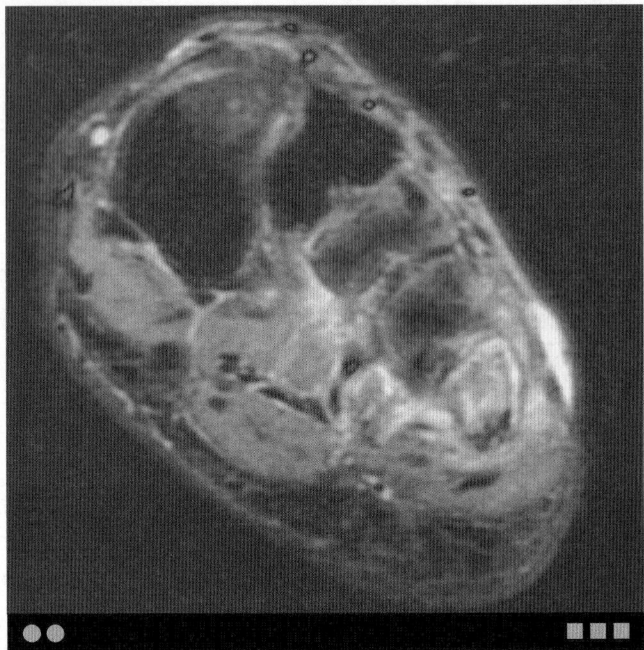

A. Reflex sympathetic dystrophy: Coronal STIR weighted image acquired 2 months after injury shows edema of the superficial and deep soft tissues and periarticular osteopenia at the tarsometatarsal joints.

COMMENTS

This is an image of a 63-year-old female who presented with foot pain and swelling two months after injury. The imaging characteristics of reflex sympathetic dystrophy depend on the stage of the disease. The first stage lasts from 1 to 7 weeks and is characterized by vasomotor instability, burning pain, and edema of the affected joint. The findings of soft tissue edema on MR images and radiographs are nonspecific. If imaging is performed after increased bone resorption and turnover has begun, periarticular osteopenia of the symptomatic joint may be seen radiographically manifesting as periarticular edema on MR images. During this stage, increased blood flow is seen on the radionuclide angiogram and blood pool images. Delayed scintigraphs demonstrate increased radionuclide uptake, which is typically greater in the periarticular regions. A 111-WBC radionuclide, scan is useful to differentiate this disease from infection. The second stage may last from 3 to 24 months and manifests as hypesthesia, osteoporosis, and early skin and muscle atrophy. In this phase, the blood flow and blood pool images return to normal, but the delayed image will remain abnormal. Periarticular osteopenia is more likely to be seen on MR and radiographic imaging during this phase. After the second stage, the disease may go into remission with no clinical sequella or rarely progress to the final, atrophic stage. In this stage, radionuclide scans may be virtually normal although clinically, there is scleroderma like skin changes and aponeurotic or tendinous retractions may occur. MR and radiographic images may demonstrate soft tissue atrophy and muscular wasting.

PEARLS

- **In stage I RSD, three-phase radionuclide bone scan shows increased blood flow on the radionuclide and blood pool images and increased bone uptake on the delayed scintigraphs.**
- **MR images and radiographs demonstrate soft tissue edema during stage I RSD. If bone resorption has begun, periarticular osteopenia may also be seen.**
- **Imaging studies demonstrate periarticular osteopenia and early skin and muscular atrophic changes in stage II RSD.**
- **The three-phase radionuclide bone scan may be virtually normal in the final or atrophic stage of RSD.**

ADDITIONAL IMAGES

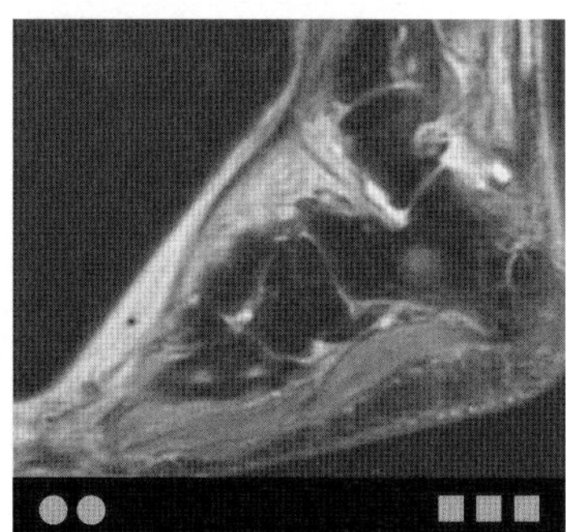

B. Reflex sympathetic dystrophy: Sagittal STIR weighted image acquired 2 months after injury shows edema of the superficial and deep soft tissues and periarticular osteopenia at the tarsometatarsal joints.

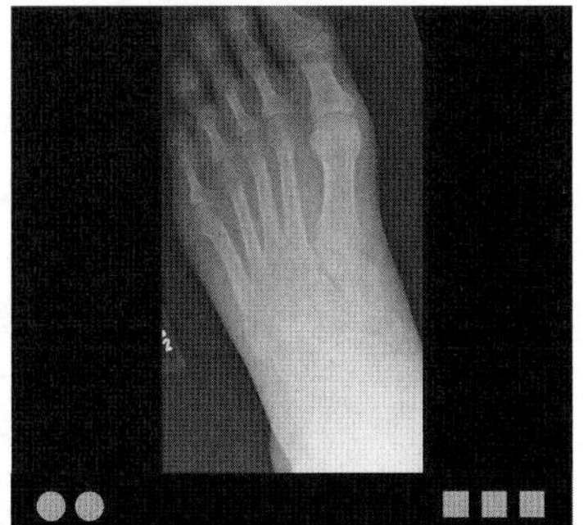

C. Reflex sympathetic dystrophy: Radiograph of the left foot acquired at time of imaging of image **B** shows diffuse, periarticular osteopenia at the tarsometatarsal joints and at the second through fifth metatarsophalangeal joints.

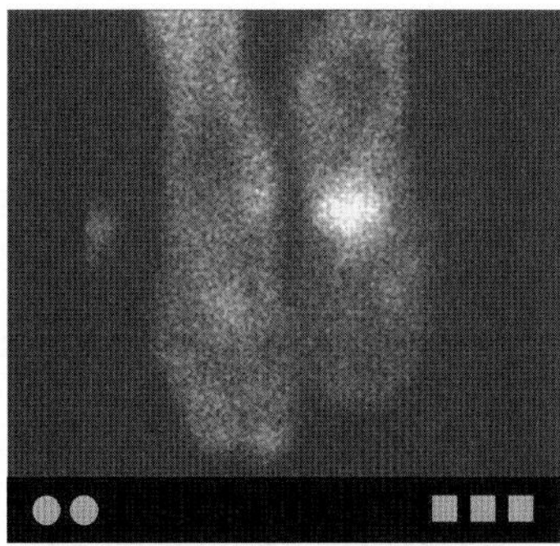

D. Reflex sympathetic dystrophy: Blood flow phase of triple-phase bone scan show increased radionuclide uptake at the TMT and lateral MTP joints.

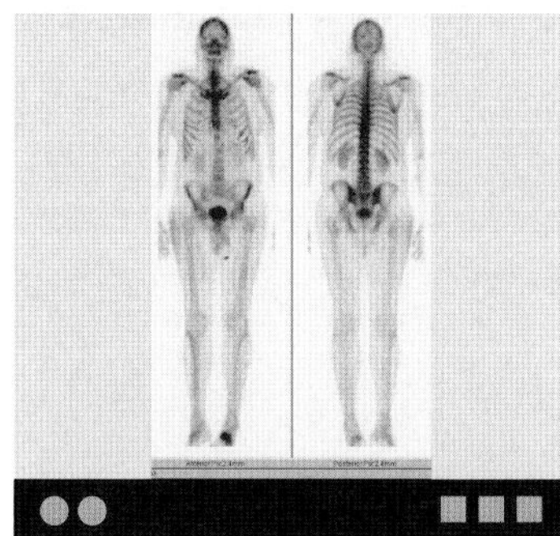

E. Reflex sympathetic dystrophy: Delayed phase of triple-phase bone scan show increased radionuclide uptake at the TMT and lateral MTP joints.

IMAGE KEY

Common

Rare

Typical

Unusual

DIFFERENTIAL DIAGNOSES IMAGES

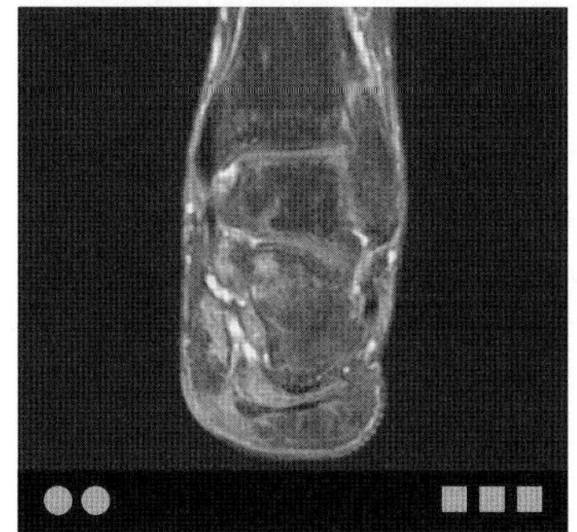

F. Disuse osteopenia: Coronal T1-weighted image with fat saturation after gadolinium shows diffused, periarticular osteopenia of the hindfoot. The patient was immobilized secondary to talar and calcaneal fractures not completely seen on this image.

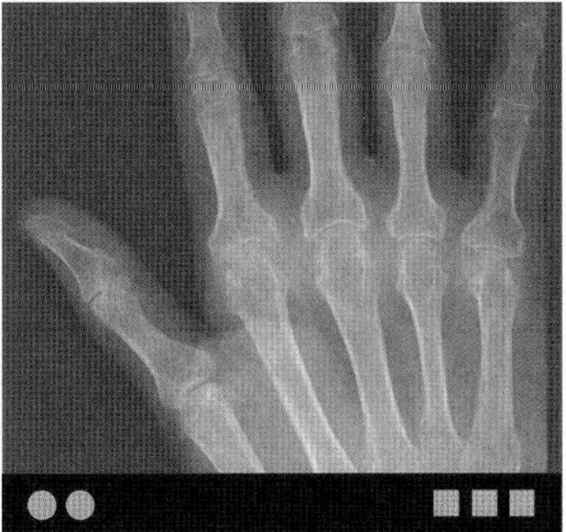

G. Inflammatory arthropathy: There is diffused, periarticular osteopenia and soft tissues swelling at the metacarpophalangeal joints. There are MCP and PIP joint marginal erosions.

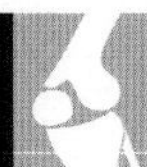

34–2 Baxter's Neuropathy

Rosemary J. Klecker

PRESENTATION

A 55-year-old female with flatfoot and heal pain

FINDINGS

MR image shows selective fatty atrophy of the abductor digiti quinti muscle.

DIFFERENTIAL DIAGNOSES

- *Diabetic neuropathy:* MR imaging findings include fatty replacement of all the intrinsic muscles of the foot.
- *Plantar fibromatosis:* Lesions located plantar to the intrinsic foot muscles. On MR imaging, these lesions classically demonstrate decreased signal intensity on all MR pulse sequences, although it may be hyperintense on T2-weighted image.
- *Fibrolipomatous hamartoma:* MR imaging shows fat signal intensity infiltrating the interfascicular connective tissue of a nerve. Nerve fascicles may be seen as cylindrical areas of signal void.

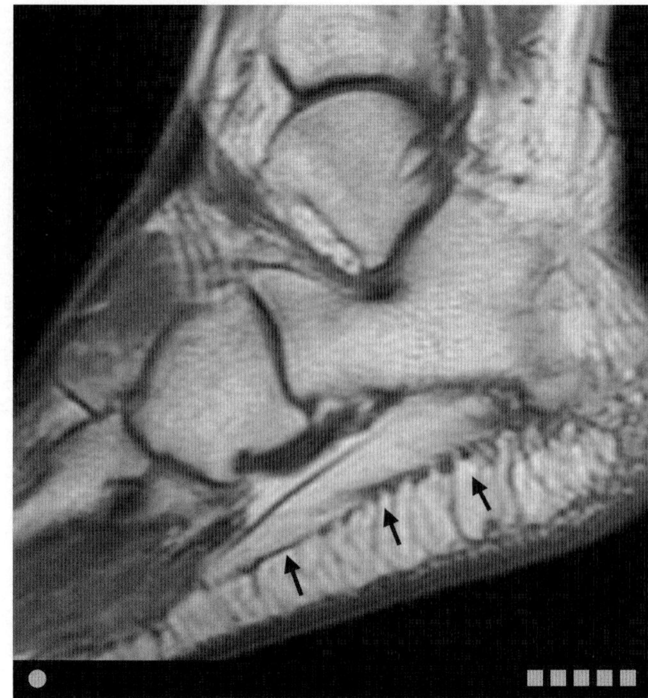

A. Baxter neuropathy: Sagittal T2-weighted image of the hindfoot shows replacement of the abductor digiti quinti muscle replaced by fat signal intensity (arrows).

COMMENTS

Baxter neuropathy is neuropathy or compression of the inferior calcaneal nerve and is diagnosed on MR imaging by isolated fatty atrophy of the abductor digiti quinti muscle (ADQM). The inferior calcaneal nerve originates as a branch from the lateral plantar nerve at the level of the medial malleolus and courses distally between the adbuctor hallucis and the quadratus plantae muscles. At the lower border of the abductor hallucis, it turns and courses laterally, passing just anterior to the medial calcaneal tuberosity and between the quadratus plantae and the flexor digitorum brevis muscle sending branches to the ADQM. Compression of the inferior calcaneal nerve may result from chronic microtrauma secondary to a calcaneal enthesophyte or to internal foot derangement. Plantar fasciitis, particularly if associated with flexor digitorum brevis muscle and soft tissue edema, may also result in inferior calcaneal neuropathy. The inferior calcaneal nerve is a mixed nerve with both motor and sensory branches, nerve entrapment first manifests as medial hindfoot pain, often indistinguishable from the pain of plantar fasciitis. As a result, early MR imaging findings of muscle denervation such as increased T2-weighted signal intensity and muscle enlargement are usually not seen. MR imaging of the hindfoot is usually reserved for those who have failed conservative management and therefore, the late manifestation of muscular denervation, and fatty atrophy of the ADQM is seen on MR imaging.

PEARLS

- **Baxter neuropathy is compression of the inferior calcaneal nerve, a branch of the lateral plantar nerve.**
- **Etiologies of inferior calcaneal nerve entrapment include chronic microtrauma from an enlarged calcaneal enthesophyte or internal derangement and plantar fasciitis.**
- **The symptoms of Baxter neuropathy are identical to those of plantar fasciitis and the two entities may coexist.**
- **MR imaging findings of Baxter neuropathy is isolated fatty atrophy of the Abductor digiti quinti muscle.**

ADDITIONAL IMAGE

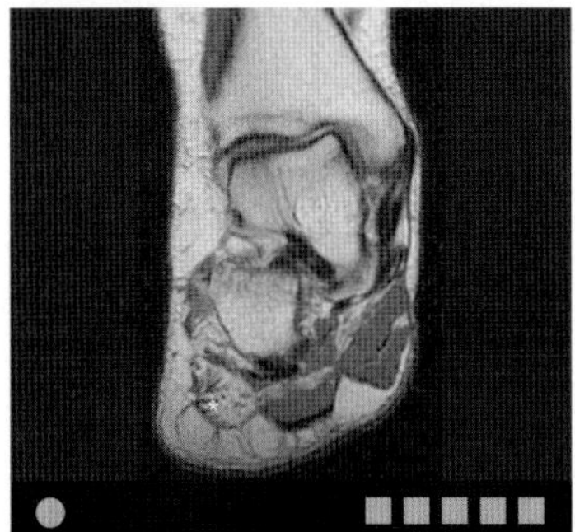

B. Baxter neuropathy: Coronal T2-weighted image shows fat signal intensity of the abductor digiti quinti muscle (asterix). Note the normal low signal intensity of the adjacent intrinsic muscles.

DIFFERENTIAL DIAGNOSES IMAGES

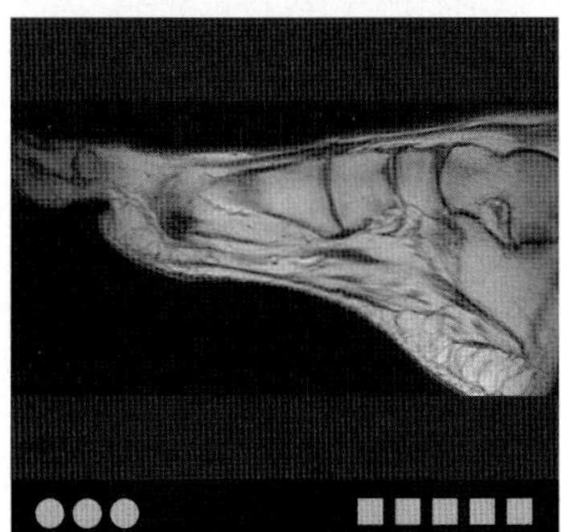

C. Diabetic neuropathy: Sagittal T2-weighted image shows diffused muscle signal intensity of all the intrinsic muscles of the foot secondary to diffused fatty atrophy. The low signal intensity of the tendons is preserved.

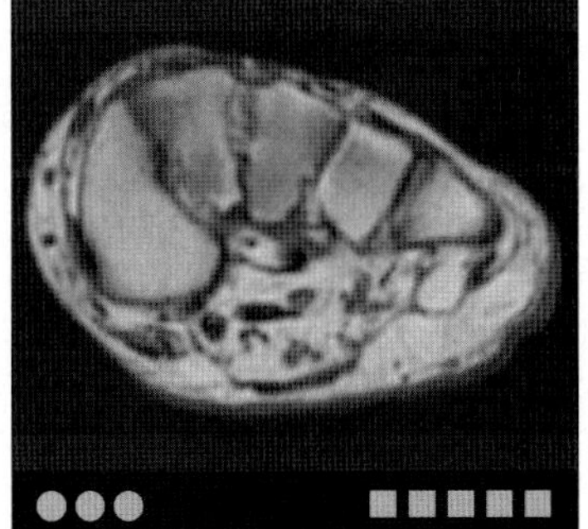

D. Diabetic neuropathy: CoronalT2-weighted image shows diffused muscle signal intensity of all the intrinsic muscles of the foot secondary to diffused fatty atrophy. The low signal intensity of the tendons is preserved.

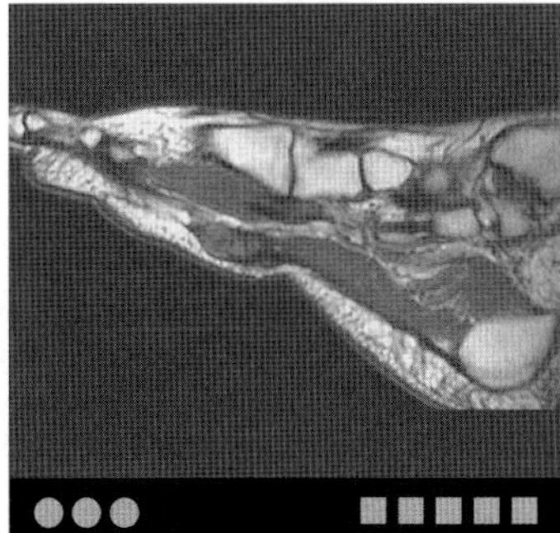

E. Plantar fibromatosis: Sagittal PD weighted image shows a lobulated mass associated with the plantar aponeurosis that is isointense to the muscle.

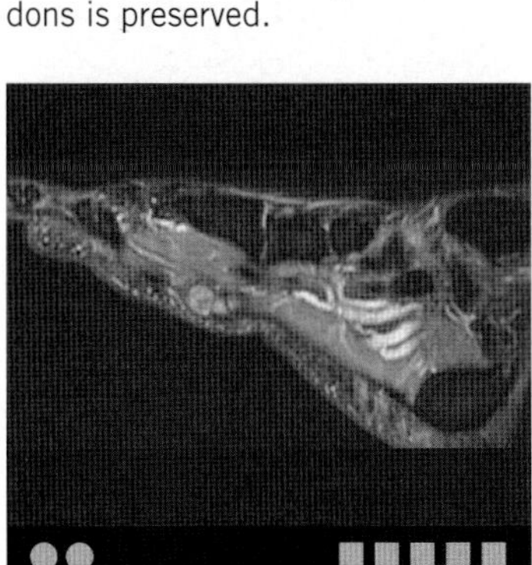

F. Plantar fibromatosis: Sagittal T2-weighted fat saturation image shows a lobulated mass associated with the plantar aponeurosis that is isointense to the muscle. There is mild increased T2 signal in the mass secondary to a higher than normal cell to collagen ratio.

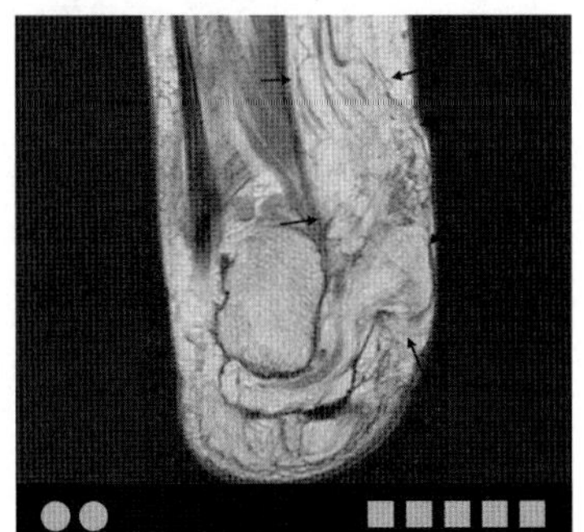

G. Fibrolipomatous hamartoma: Coronal T2-weighted images shows fusiform enlargement of the posterior, tibial nerve infiltrated by a mass of fat signal intensity (arrows). There is fatty atrophy of the plantar muscles of the foot secondary to posterior, tibial nerve compression.

IMAGE KEY

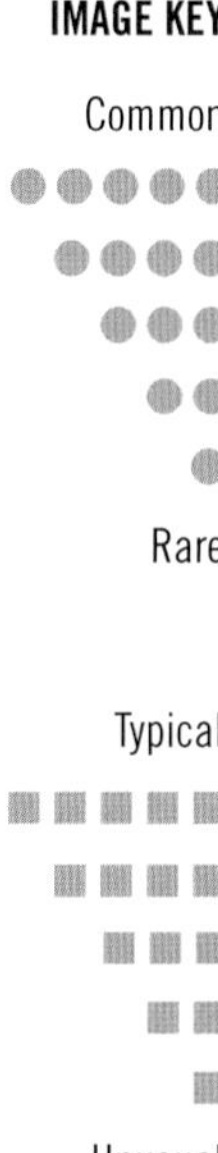

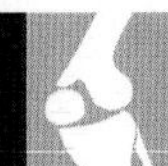

34–3 Freiberg Disease

Mohammad Reza Hayeri and Jamshid Tehranzadeh

PRESENTATION

Pain in the forefoot

FINDINGS

Early MR imaging findings include low-signal-intensity changes in the head of the second or third metatarsal on T1-weighted images, with increased or mixed signal intensity on corresponding T2-weighted or STIR images

DIFFERENTIAL DIAGNOSES

- *Stress fracture:* Occurs as the result of repetitive subthreshold loading on bones and is most common in lower extremity.
- *Avascular necrosis (AVN) of sesamoid bone:* Osteonecrosis of Sesamoid bones occurs because of lack of blood supply or following stress fracture of these bones. The bone signal intensity changes are similar to those caused by a stress response.

COMMENTS

Freiberg infraction also known as osteochondrosis of the metatarsal head is caused by avascular necrosis of the metatarsal head. Unilateral involvement of the second metatarsal is the most common presentation; however, it may occur in the third and more rarely the fourth and fifth metatarsals. In 7% of cases bilateral involvement is noted. Unlike other kinds of osteochondrosis this type is 5 to 11 times more common in females especially adolescent girls with athletic activities and during the skeletal growth .The etiology most likely is multifactorial .The most popular theories are traumatic insult in the form of either acute or repetitive injury or vascular compromise. In many cases patient remain symptom free and do not seek medical attention. Patients may present with localized pain and swelling in forefoot and limitation of motion in metacarpophalangeal joint. The pain is exacerbated with activity and increases over time. Five stage classification based on radiographic changes has been described: Fissuring of the epiphysis (stage I), central depression of articular surface (stage II), central depression which leads to medial and lateral projection at the margins with intact plantar hinge (stage III), loose body formation with fracture of medial and lateral projection (stage IV), and flattening of the metatarsal head with secondary degenerative changes (stage V). MRI image shows low signal intensity in T1-weighted images and high or mixed signal in T2-weighted and STIR images. With disease progression, flattening of the metatarsal head occurs, and low signal intensity changes develop on T2-weighted images as the bone becomes sclerotic.

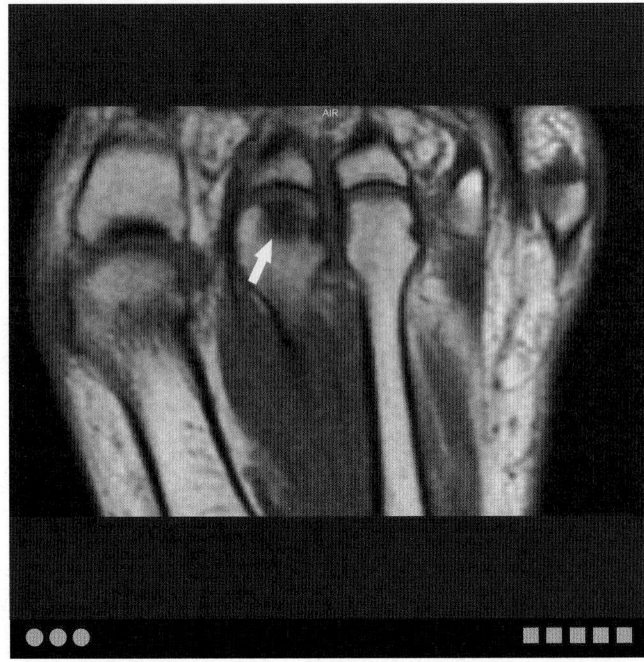

A. Freiberg disease: Coronal T1-weighted image of the forefoot shows a focus of low signal intensity in the head of second metatarsal consistent with osteonecrosis or AVN of the second metatarsal head (arrow).

PEARLS

- **Freiberg infraction is osteochondrosis of the head of the second or less commonly of the third metatarsal heads.**
- **It is seen more commonly in adolescent girls and present with focal pain and tenderness over the second metatarsal bone.**
- **Radiographs show early osteopenia with subchondral fracture. Subchondral sclerosis can develop over time. Flattening of the metatarsal head is a classic sign. Loose bodies can form over time.**
- **MRI image shows low signal intensity in T1-weighted images and high or mixed signal in T2-weighted or STIR images.**

ADDITIONAL IMAGES

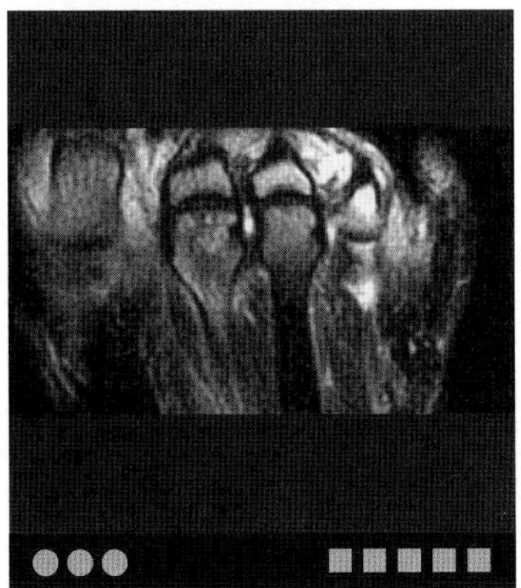

B. Freiberg disease: Coronal T2-weighted image of the forefoot shows a focus of increased and decreased or mixed signal intensity in the head of second metatarsal consistent with osteonecrosis or AVN of the second metatarsal head (same patient as shown in image A).

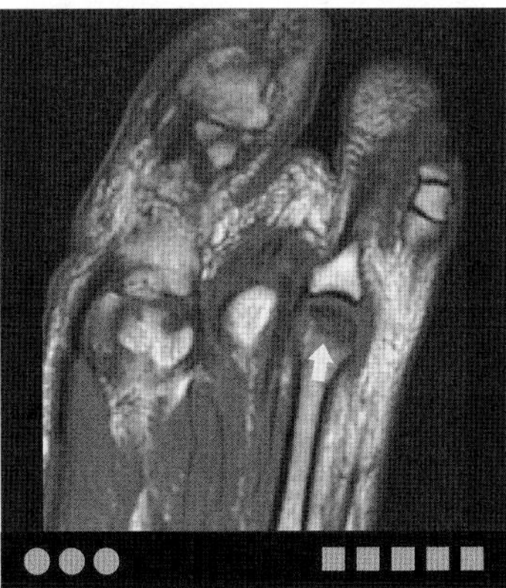

C. Freiberg disease: Coronal T1-weighted image of the forefoot (in another patient) shows a focus of low signal intensity in the head of third metatarsal consistent with AVN of the third metatarsal head (arrow). Subchondral cystic changes of the head of the first metatarsal head are also seen.

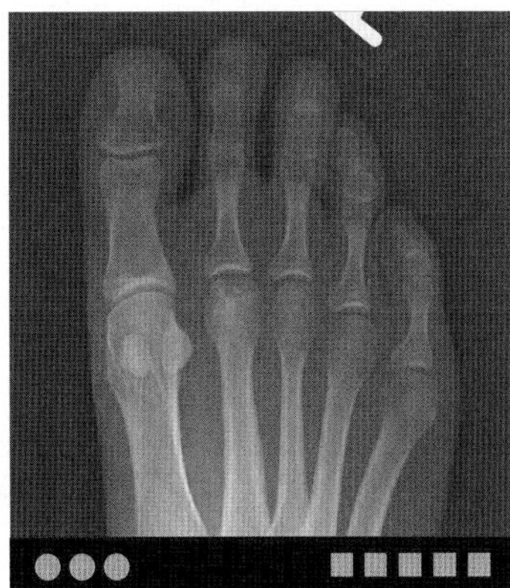

D. Freiberg disease: AP radiograph of forefoot (in another patient) shows osteochondritis dissecans as a result of osteochondrosis of the second metatarsal bone.

IMAGE KEY

Common

Rare

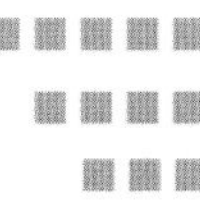

Typical

Unusual

DIFFERENTIAL DIAGNOSES IMAGES

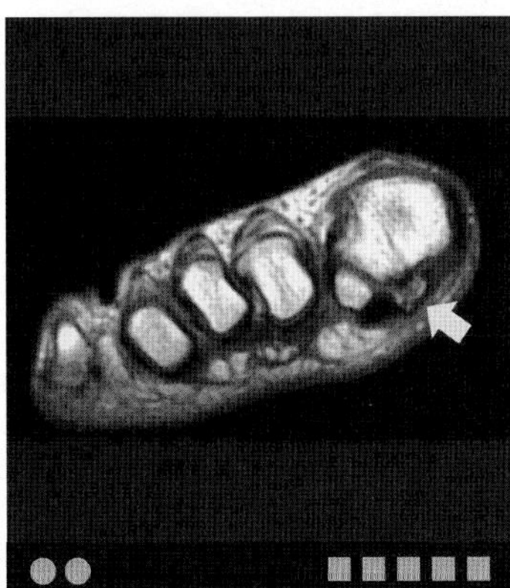

E. AVN of the sesamoid of the great toe: Axial T1-weighted image of the forefoot shows low signal intensity and partial collapse of the medial sesamoid indicating AVN caused by stress fracture (arrow).

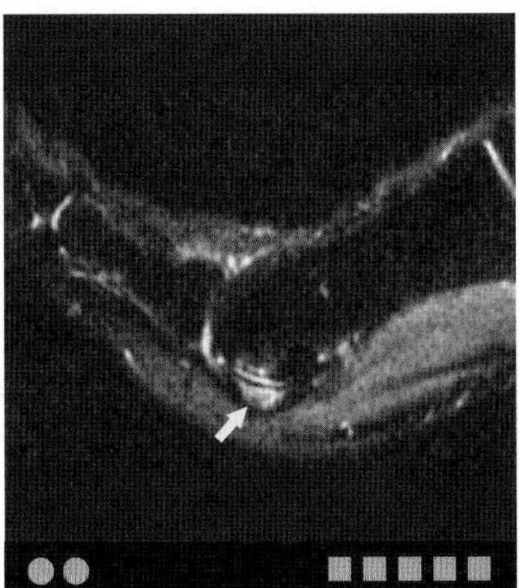

F. AVN of the sesamoid of the great toe: Sagittal fat-saturated T2-weighted image shows bright signal of the medial sesamoid of the great toe (arrow). (Same patient as shown in image E.)

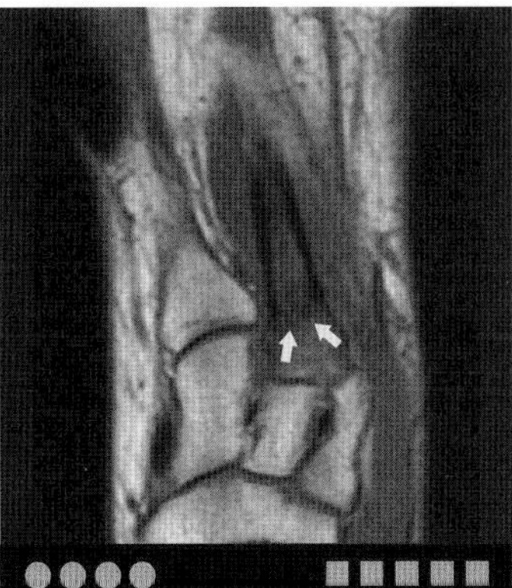

G. Stress fracture: Coronal T1-weighted image of the second metatarsal shows low signal of the second metatarsal caused by marrow edema with linear, darker signal (arrows) indicating stress fracture.

SECTION VII

SPINE

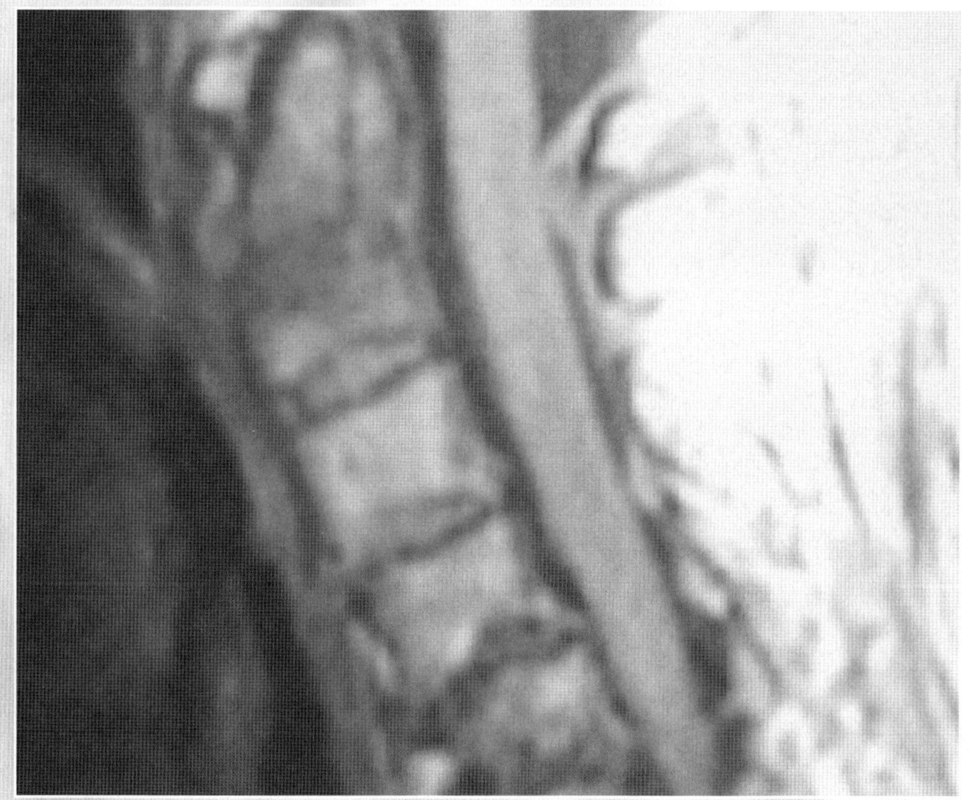

Chapter 35

Sport Medicine and Trauma

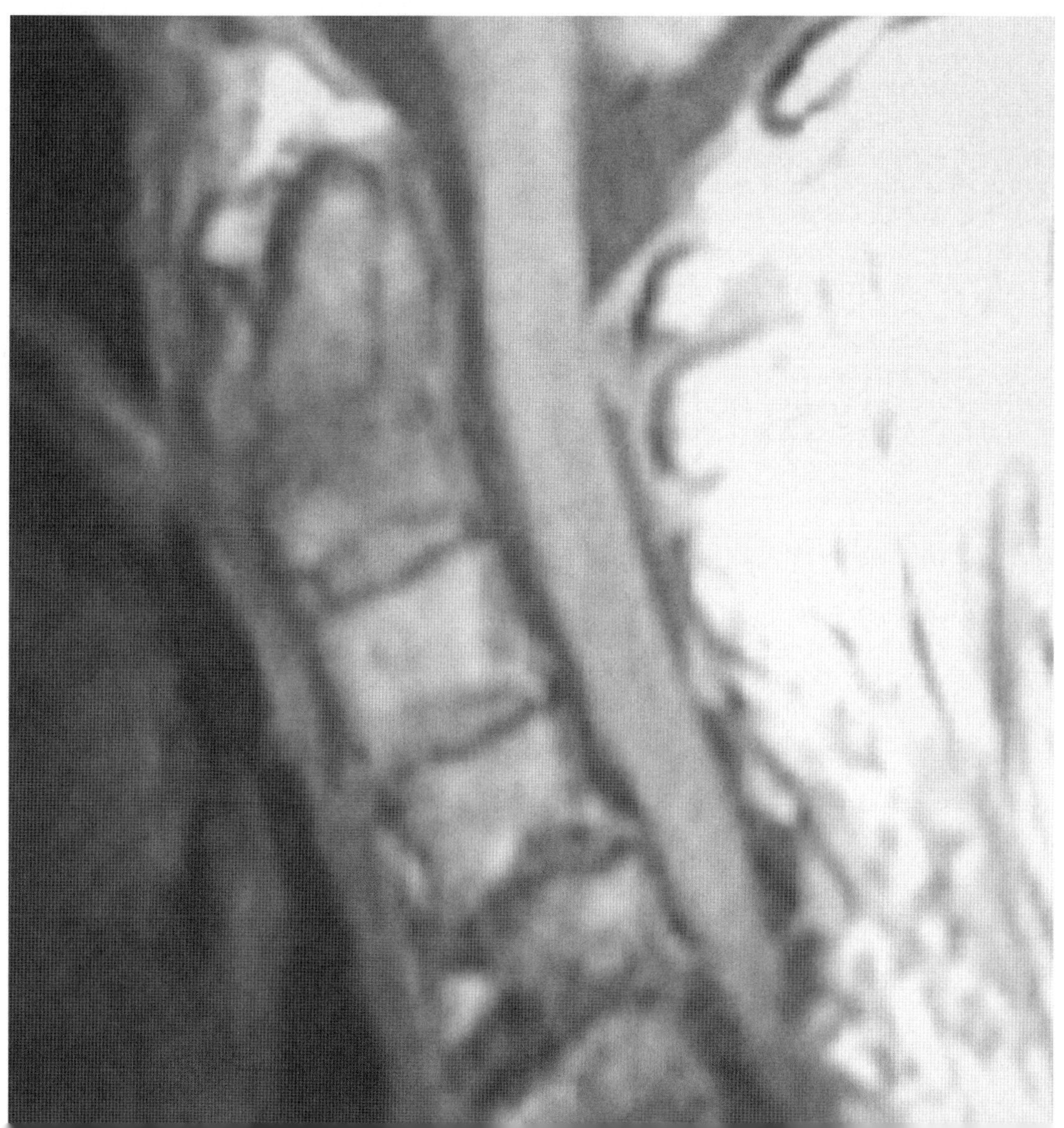

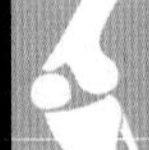

35–1 MR Imaging of Odontoid Fracture

Wilfred CG Peh

PRESENTATION

Neck pain and limitation of neck movement

FINDINGS

MR images show a transverse fracture line extending through the base of the odontoid peg, with adjacent marrow edema. There is fluid within the fracture line.

DIFFERENTIAL DIAGNOSES

- *Os odontoideum:* Normal variant thought by some to be post-traumatic in origin. Unfused dens may move independently of the body of the odontoid peg with associated compensatory hypertrophy of the arch of atlas.
- *Jefferson's fracture:* Owing to axial compression force on the top of the skull that causes the C1 lateral masses to split apart. CT is much better than radiographs for showing the C1 ring fractures.

COMMENTS

The patient is a 77-year-old woman, who complained of neck pain and an occult odontoid fracture was incidentally found on MR imaging. She could not recall the initial traumatic episode. She had limitation of neck movement and sensation of instability. Odontoid fractures account for about 10% of cervical spine injuries, and are usually caused by motor vehicular accidents or falls. These fractures can be classified into three types. Type I fracture occurs at the tip of the odontoid process, and is regarded as an avulsion injury, and is stable. Type II fractures are the commonest type, are located at the base of the odontoid peg, and have the tendency to displace. Type III fractures extend from the base into the body of C2 vertebra and almost always unite. The precise mechanism of odontoid fractures is unknown, but is likely to be caused by a combination of flexion, extension, and rotation. Radiographs are able to show these fracture types, particularly on adequately taken lateral and open mouth views. CT images show better bony detail, with reconstructed 2D images being especially useful in showing transverse fractures and displacement. On radiographs, a pseudofracture may be caused by the "mach band" artifact, seen as a radiolucent line across the base of the odontoid peg. It is important to exclude concomitant cervical spine injuries, such as C1 anterior ring fractures. MR imaging is useful for detection and diagnosis of radiographically occult fractures, and for assessment of cord injury.

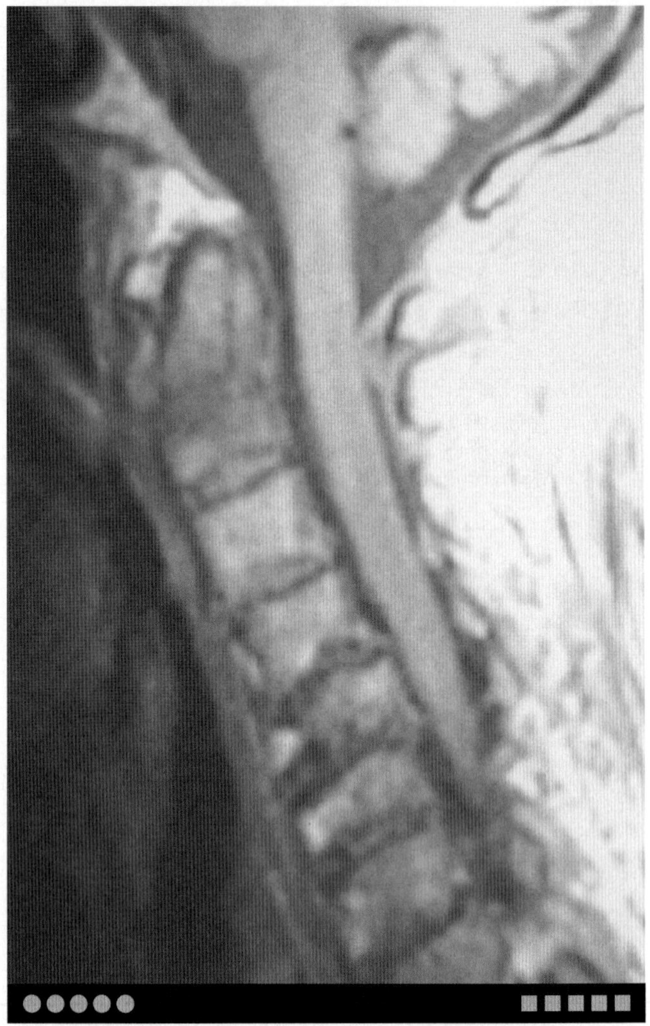

A. Odontoid fracture: Sagittal SE T1-weighted MR image shows an ill-defined area of hypointense signal at the base of the odontoid peg.

PEARLS

- **Type II odontoid fractures are inherently unstable and have the tendency to displace.**
- **MR imaging is useful for detection of occult odontoid fractures.**
- **Injury to the cord and adjacent soft tissues are best demonstrated on MR imaging.**

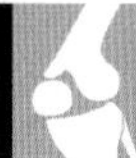

ADDITIONAL IMAGES

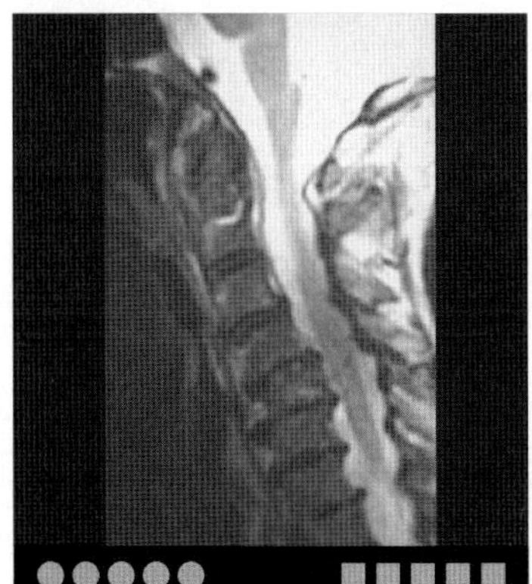

B. Odontoid fracture: Sagittal FSE T2-weighted MR image shows a linear area of hyperintense fluid within the fracture line. There is adjacent patchy moderately hyper-intense marrow edema.

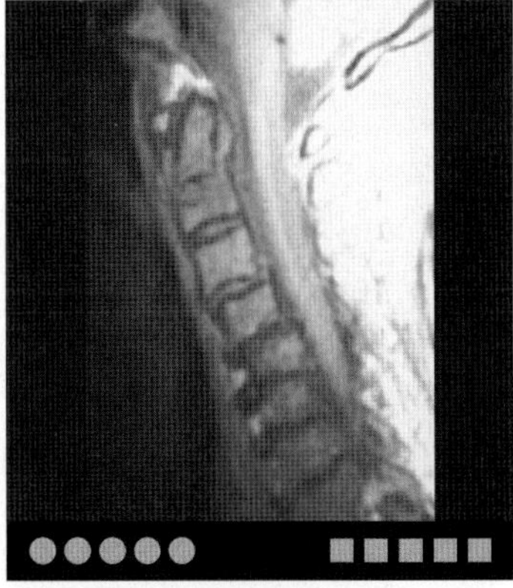

C. Odontoid fracture: Sagittal FSE proton density weighted MR image shows the nondisplaced transverse fracture of the odontoid peg. This is a type II fracture.

DIFFERENTIAL DIAGNOSES IMAGES

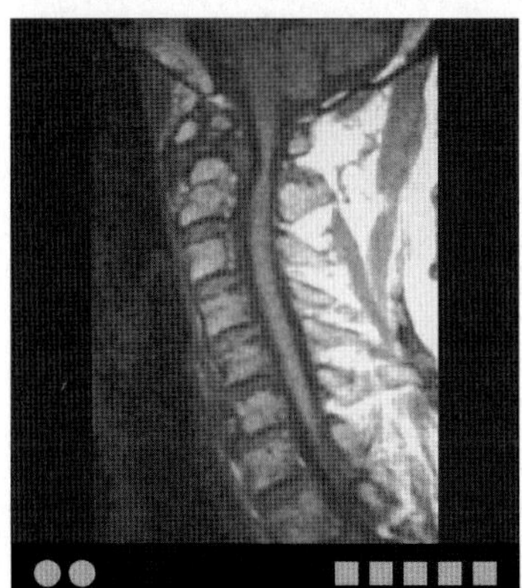

D. Os odontoideum: Sagittal SE T1-weighted MR image shows a rounded well-corticated os that is separated from the rest of the odontoid peg.

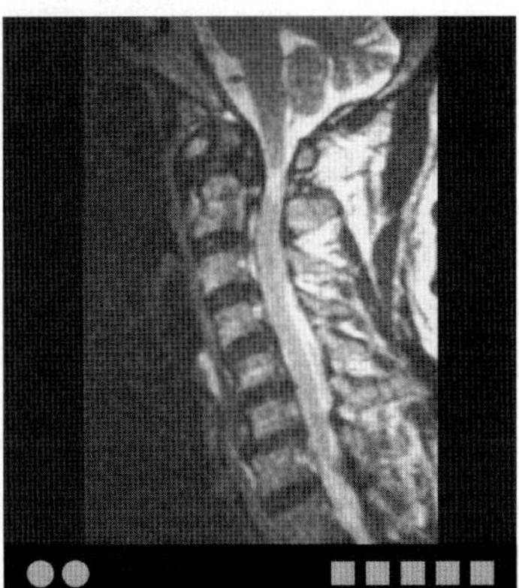

E. Os odontoideum: Sagittal FSE T2-weighted MR image shows an area of hyperintense signal within the narrowed upper cervical spinal cord. If unstable, surgical stabilization may be required.

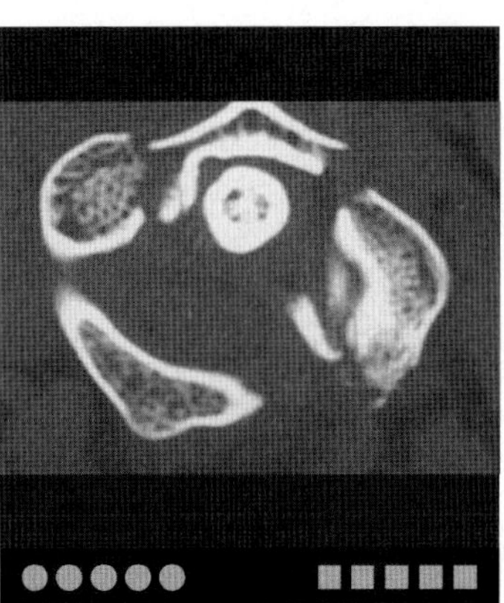

F. Jefferson's fracture of the atlas: Axial CT image shows multiple fractures of the C1 ring.

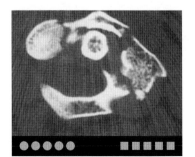

G. Jefferson's fracture of the atlas: Axial CT image shows multiple fractures of the C1 ring.

IMAGE KEY

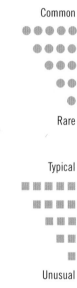

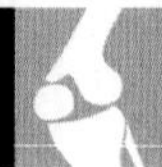

35–2 CT Imaging of Type II Odontoid Fracture

Stephen E. Ling and William R. Reinus

PRESENTATION

Pain, spasm, neurological deficit

FINDINGS

C2 fracture involving the top of the dens, base of the dens, or vertebral body.

DIFFERENTIAL DIAGNOSES

- *Odontoid fracture (Type I): Oblique tip fracture as a result of alar ligament avulsion.*
- *Odontoid fracture (Type III): This fracture extends into the vertebral body with or without involvement of the base of the dens.*

COMMENTS

Patients generally present, not only with pain, but also with a sensation of instability and may actually be holding their heads in their hands to prevent motion. Neurological loss may range from absent to quadriplegia and respiratory center suppression. The exact mechanism that causes an odontoid fracture is unknown, but is most commonly a combination of flexion, extension, and rotation. Anderson and D'Alonzo classified these fractures into three types: Type I: oblique tip fracture (<5%) as a result of alar ligament avulsion, no instability unless cranio-cervical diastasis (Atlanto-occipital dislocation). Type II: the fracture (60%) occurs at the base of the dens at its junction with the vertebral body. Nonunion is frequent (30–50%) and related to the recurrent blood supply. It is associated with transverse ligament rupture (10%) and instability. Type III: This fracture extends into the vertebral body with or without involvement of the base of the dens (~33%), and has a symmetric or oblique fracture line. Instability may occur with this type of fracture although it is less common than with Type II fractures. Methods of treatment include collar, halo orthosis, anterior screw fixation, and posterior atlantoaxial arthrodesis. The poor blood supply and increased instability present in Type II fractures give these the worst prognosis of all three types of odontoid fracture.

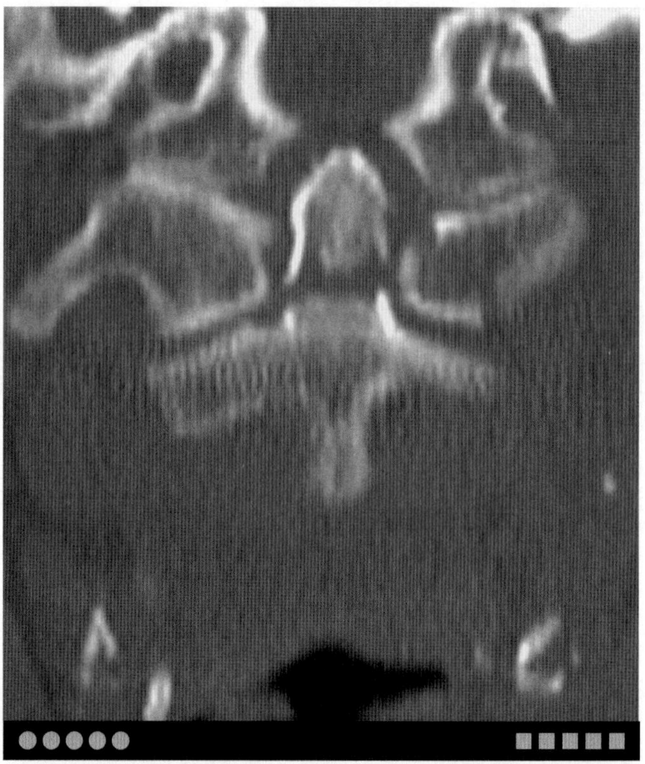

A. Dens fracture (Type II): Coronal CT image demonstrates a fracture at the base of the dens at its junction with the vertebral body.

PEARLS

- **Interruption of the Ring of Harris on the lateral radiograph may tip the radiologist off to a subtle, minimally displaced odontoid fracture.**
- **CT with coronal reconstruction makes classification of odontoid fractures much more accurate.**
- **Watershed blood supply at the base/waist of the dens, displacement (>5 mm)/angulation (>10°), and relative paucity of medullary bone in contact at the fracture site all contribute to a high rate of non-union in Type II fractures.**
- **Many radiologists currently believe that os odontoidium represents an old non-united occult odontoid fracture (Type II), rather than a normal variant resulting from incomplete fusion of the dens to the vertebral body.**

ADDITIONAL IMAGES

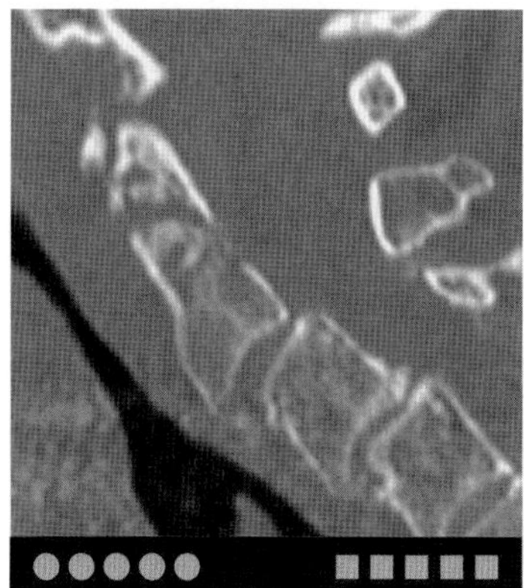

B. Dens fracture (Type II): Sagittal CT image demonstrates a fracture at the base of the dens at its junction with the vertebral body.

DIFFERENTIAL DIAGNOSES IMAGES

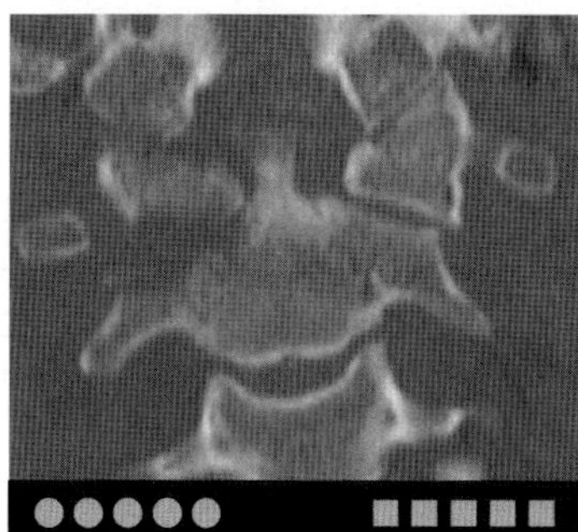

C. Dens fracture (Type I): Coronal CT image shows a fracture of the tip of the dens.

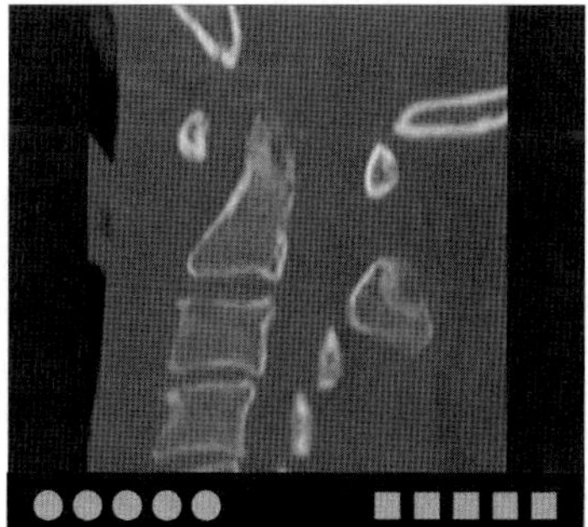

D. Dens fracture (Type I): Sagittal CT image shows a fracture of the tip of the dens. Note the widening of the Atlanto-dens interval, indicating transverse ligament insufficiency.

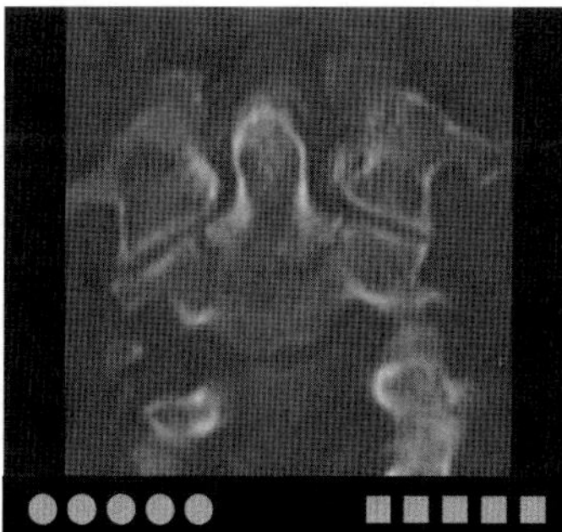

E. Dens fracture (Type III): Coronal CT image demonstrates a fracture of the C2 vertebral body. Note that these fractures may additionally involve the base of the dens, a finding not present in this case.

IMAGE KEY

Common

Rare

Typical

Unusual

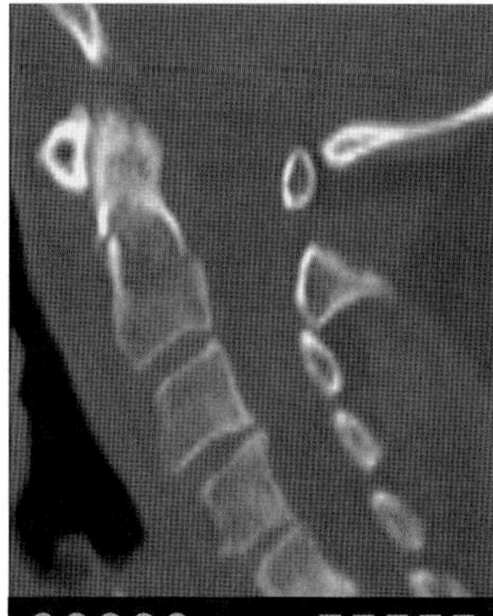

F. Dens fracture (Type III): Sagittal CT image demonstrates a fracture of the C2 vertebral body. Note that these fractures may additionally involve the base of the dens, a finding not present in this case.

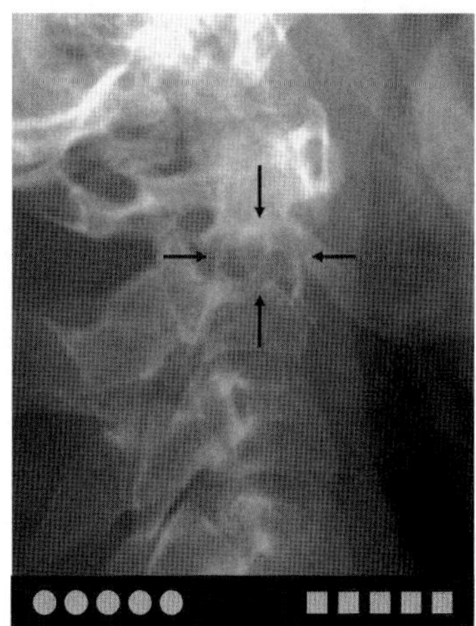

G. Dens fracture: Lateral radiograph demonstrates a dens fracture manifesting as interruption of the Ring of Harris (arrows) formed by the lateral masses of C2 and the base of the dens.

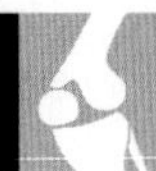

35–3 Traumatic Atlanto-Occipital Subluxation (AOS)

Edward Mossop and Jamshid Tehranzadeh

PRESENTATION

Acute trauma and pain

FINDINGS

Perching of superior facet of atlas with occipital condyle and associated osteochondral defect.

DIFFERENTIAL DIAGNOSES

- *Atlanto-axial subluxation:* This condition may occur in trauma as a result of tear of the transverse ligament or as the result of inflammatory arthritis such as rheumatoid arthritis.
- *Normal for comparison:* Image F is an example of normal anatomy which shows the relationship of atlanto-occipital joint.
- *Atlantoaxial rotatory fixation (subluxation):* A condition in which there is fixed rotation of C1 on C2. CT demonstrates rotational displacement of the atlantoaxial complex with asymmetrical space between odontoid process and lateral masses of atlas.

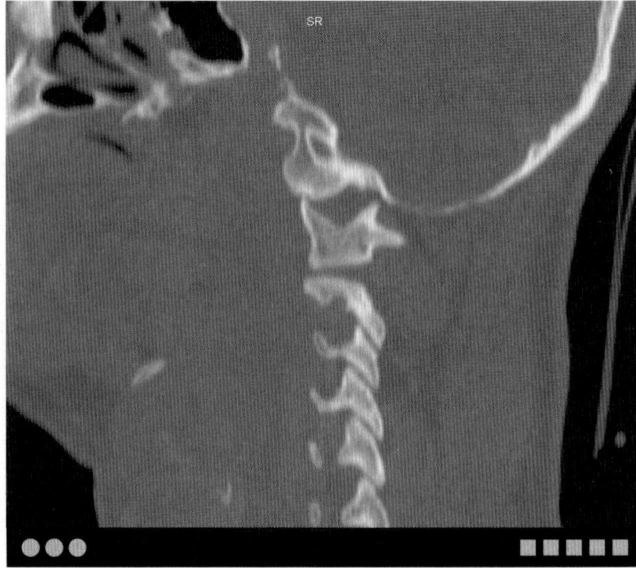

A. AOS: Sagittal reformatted CT of the occipito-cervical junction shows perching of the superior articular process of the atlas with the occipital condyle creating an osteochondral defect on the occipital condyle surface.

COMMENTS

The patient is a 30-year-old man involved in a motor vehicle accident. Traumatic atlanto-occipital dislocation (AOD) is usually a fatal injury. AOD occurs more frequently in children because of the relatively small occipital condyles, ligamentous laxity, and a flat articulation between the occiput and the atlas. These injuries are frequently ligamentous or other soft-tissue disruptions rather than fractures. AOD has been divided into three specific types: Type I involves anterior displacement of the occiput with respect to the atlas; Type II is primarily a longitudinal distraction with separation of the occiput from the atlas; and Type III denotes posterior displacement of the occiput on the atlas. Cervical radiographs often show the subluxation. CT is far more sensitive at demonstrating translatory or distractive lesions. MR imaging of the cervical spine with fat-suppressed gradient-echo T2-weighted or STIR sequences can demonstrate increased signal intensity in the atlanto-axial and atlanto-occipital joints, craniocervical ligaments, prevertebral soft tissues, and spinal cord. Axial gradient-echo MR images may be particularly useful in assessing the integrity of the transverse ligament. Disruption of the apical ligament can often be seen on sagittal and coronal images. A high T2 signal intensity may fill the space created by the bowing of the tectorial membrane and may extend across the apical dens to the anterior atlanto-occipital membrane or anterior longitudinal ligament. Bone injuries can include epiphysiolysis of C-2 and occasional C-2 pedicle fractures.

PEARLS

- **Traumatic AOD is usually a fatal injury.**
- **AOD occurs more frequently in children because of the relatively small occipital condyles, ligamentous laxity, and a flat articulation between the occiput and the atlas.**
- **Injuries are frequently ligamentous or other soft-tissue disruptions rather than fractures.**
- **CT scanning is highly sensitive at demonstrating translatory or distractive lesions.**
- **MRI is excellent for visualizing soft tissues, ligaments, and associated spinal cord injury.**

ADDITIONAL IMAGES

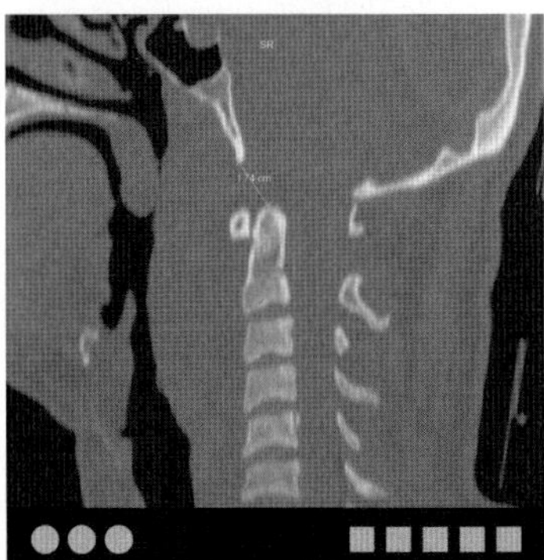

B. AOS: Sagittal reformatted CT of the occipito-cervical junction shows excessive (1.74 cm) distance between the basion and the tip of the odontoid process. The normal distance should be 1.2 cm or less.

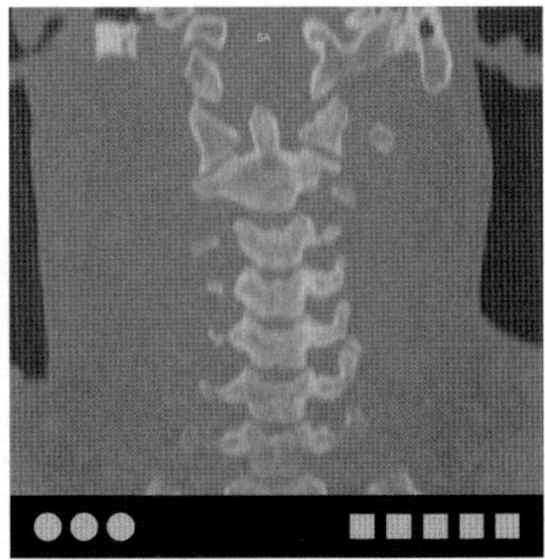

C. AOS: Coronal reformatted CT of the occipito-cervical junction shows the abnormal relation of the occipital condyles with the superior articular processes of the atlas with widening of the facet joints at this level.

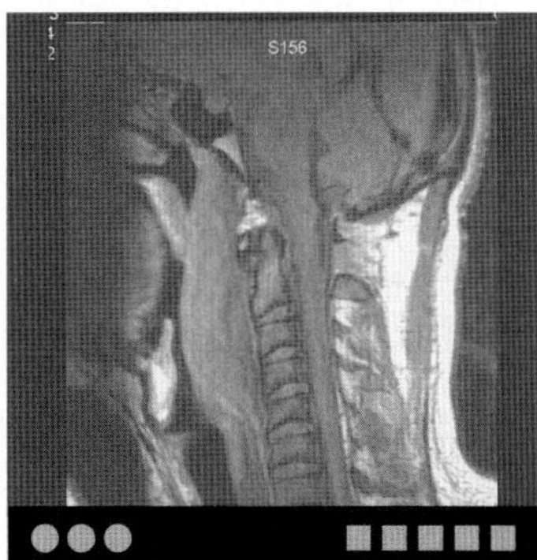

D. AOS: Sagittal T1-weighted MRI shows excessive soft tissue swelling at the preodontoid space with increased distance of basion to the tip of the odontoid.

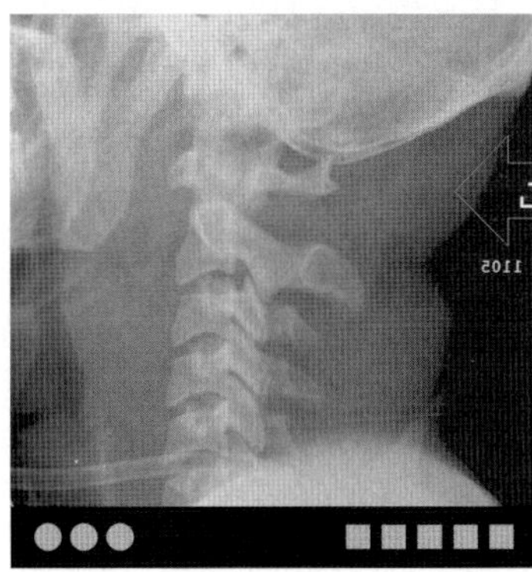

E. AOS: Lateral radiograph of the cervical spine shows a wide space between the occiput and the tip of the odontoid process.

DIFFERENTIAL DIAGNOSES IMAGES

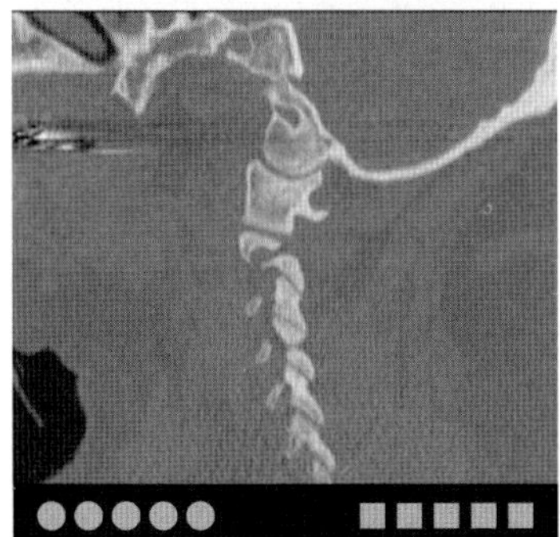

F. Normal: Sagittal reformatted CT of the cervical spine shows the normal relationship of the occipital condyle with superior facet of the atlas.

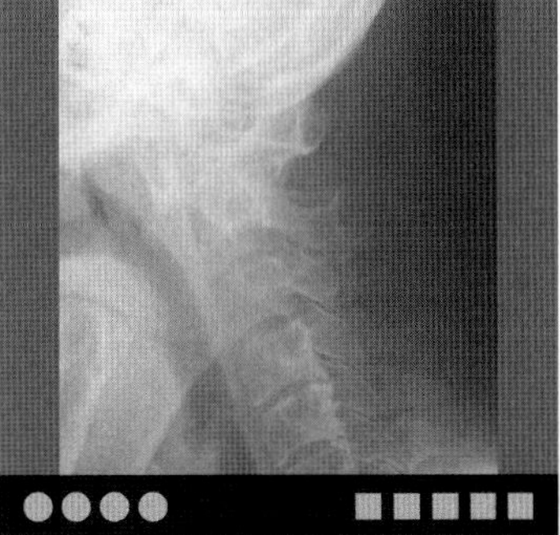

G. Atlanto-axial subluxation: Lateral radiograph of the cervical spine in a patient with rheumatoid arthritis shows bony erosions of the odontoid process with a wide space between the anterior cortex of the odontoid and posterior cortex of the anterior tubercle of the atlas.

IMAGE KEY

Common

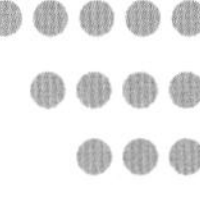

Rare

Typical

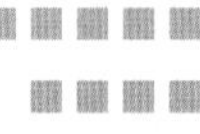

Unusual

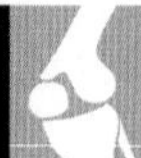

35–4 Atlantoaxial Rotatory Fixation

Nuttya Pattamapasong and Wilfred CG Peh

PRESENTATION

Limited neck mobility, torticollis

FINDINGS

Axial CT images taken with the head turned to the right and left show consistent (fixed) widening of the right atlantoaxial interval.

DIFFERENTIAL DIAGNOSES

- *Pseudosubluxation in children:* Ligamentous laxity in infants and young children allows for movement of the vertebral bodies on each other.
- *Traumatic subluxation:* This is almost always associated with a fracture of the odontoid peg. In hyperflexion injuries, the odontoid peg is displaced anteriorly while in hyperextension injuries, it is displaced posteriorly.
- *Rheumatoid arthritis:* In inflammatory arthritides, laxity of the transverse ligament is caused by synovial inflammation and hyperemia of the adjacent articulation, particularly between the posterior odontoid peg and the anterior transverse ligament.

COMMENTS

The patient is a 41-year-old man with stiffness and limitation of neck movement. The distance between the odontoid peg and the lateral mass of the atlas (C1) is not corrected by changes in head position and remains asymmetrical.

The principal motion at the atlantoaxial articulation is rotation. Stability of this joint mostly relies on transverse ligament that binds the C1 lateral masses and holds the odontoid peg in position. Atlantoaxial subluxation refers to translation of atlas on the axis, and usually results from injury or laxity of the transverse ligament. Common causes include rheumatoid arthritis, seronegative spondyloarthropathies, and congenital anomalies such as Down's syndrome. Atlantoaxial rotatory subluxation may be transient and is especially frequent in children who present with torticollis following minor trauma. When abnormal atlantoaxial subluxation persists, the condition is called rotatory fixation. This fixation may occur as an isolated injury or in combination with transverse ligament rupture or C1/C2 fractures. Atlantoaxial rotatory fixation is diagnosed by recognition of a persistent asymmetry between the odontoid peg and the lateral masses of the atlas during rotation and lateral bending of the neck. In normal subjects, the relative positions of the odontoid peg and atlas will vary with patient movement, i.e. with head rotation to the right, the space on the right widens. Imaging documentation is classically provided by performing open-mouth radiographs in five positions, namely anteroposterior (AP) view in neutral, AP views with head tilted 10 degrees to either side, and AP views with head rotated 10 degrees to either side.

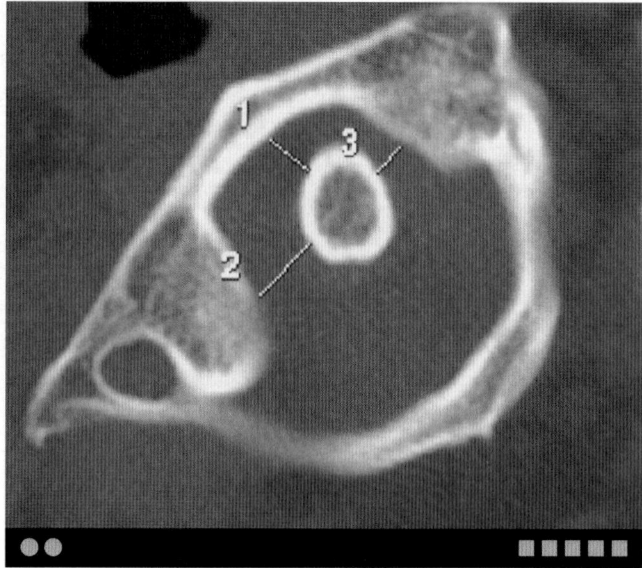

A. Atlantoaxial rotatory fixation: Axial CT image with the patient's head turned to the right shows widening of the right lateral atlantoaxial interval.

PEARLS

- **Atlantoaxial subluxation is related with congenital abnormality, inflammation, or injury of the transverse ligament.**
- **Rotatory subluxation may be transient or fixed. The diagnosis of atlantoaxial rotatory fixation is dependent on understanding that rotation is the principal motion at the atlantoaxial articulation and that in normal subjects, the lateral atlantoaxial interval is variable.**
- **Imaging diagnosis is made on performing either open-mouth radiographs or axial CT with the patient's head turned to the right and left, and looking for persistent asymmetry of the lateral atlantoaxial interval.**

ADDITIONAL IMAGES

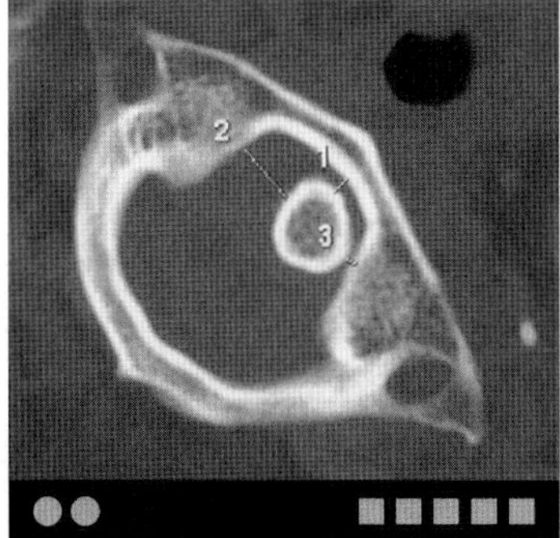

B. Atlantoaxial rotatory fixation: Axial CT image with the patient's head turned to the left shows persistent widening of the right lateral atlantoaxial interval.

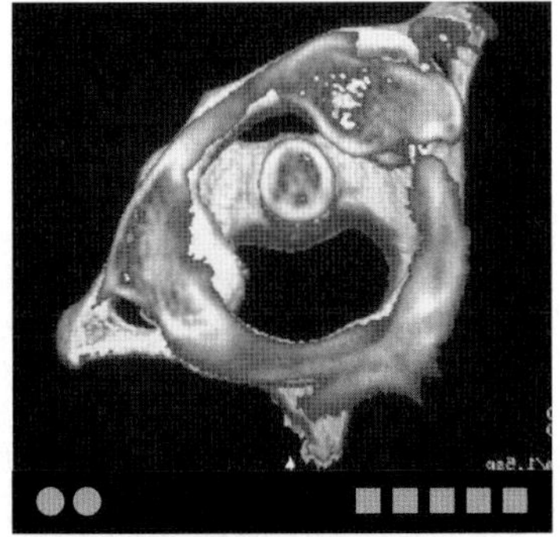

C. Atlantoaxial rotatory fixation: Reconstructed 3D CT image with the patient's head turned to the right shows widening of the right lateral atlantoaxial interval.

DIFFERENTIAL DIAGNOSES IMAGES

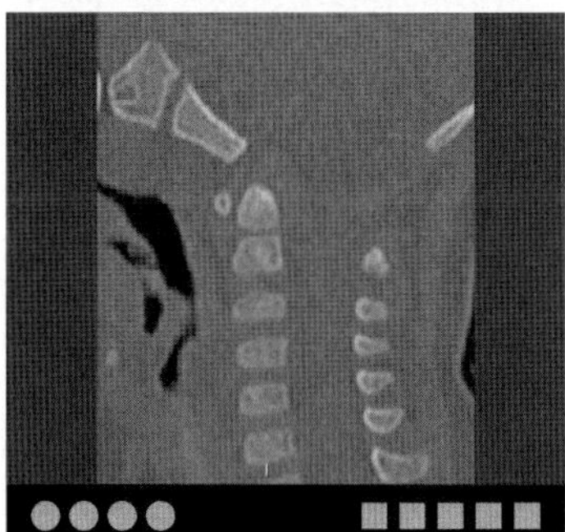

D. Childhood pseudosubluxation: Reconstructed 2D sagittal CT image shows from apparent anterior atlantoaxial widening because of ligament laxity and unossified dens. Further displacement during flexion is less than 1 mm.

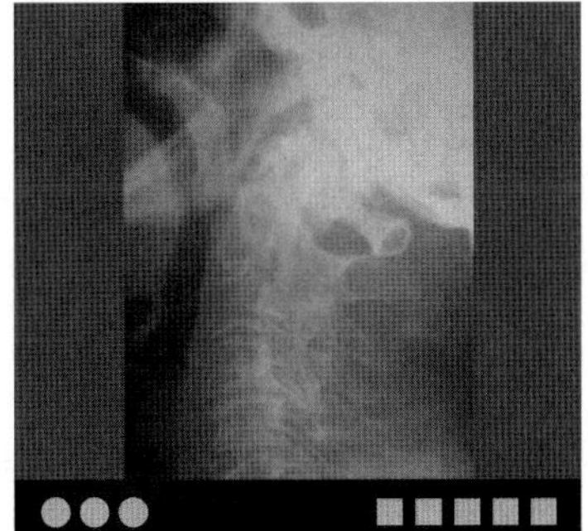

E. Odontoid fracture with associated atlantoaxial subluxation: Lateral radiograph shows a displaced transverse fracture through the base of the odontoid peg which is displaced posteriorly, indicative of a hyperextension injury.

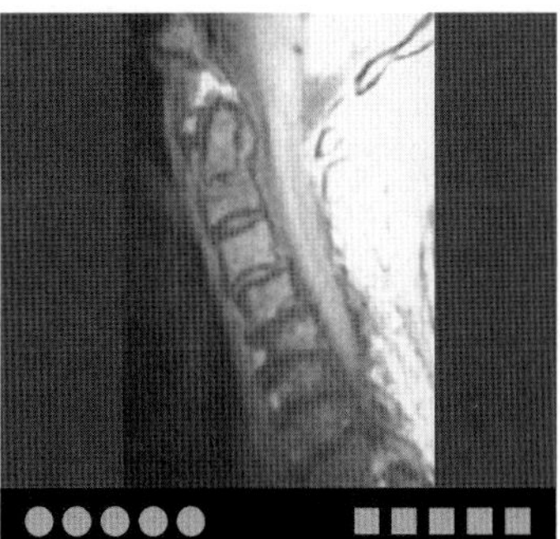

F. Odontoid fracture: Sagittal FSE proton density weighted MR image shows an undisplaced transverse fracture through the base of the odontoid peg. Spinal alignment is still maintained.

IMAGE KEY

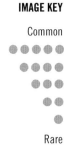

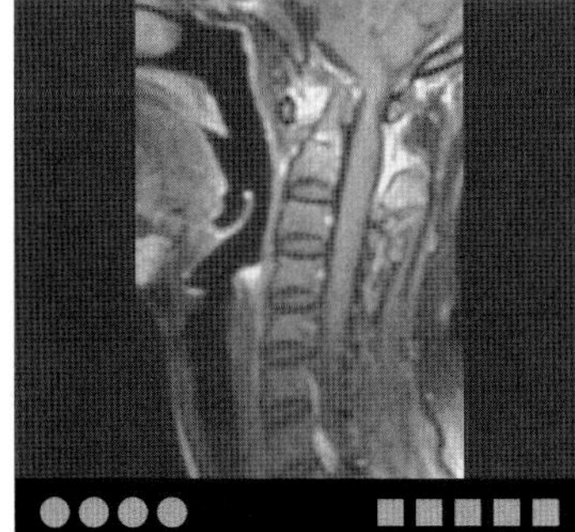

G. Rheumatoid arthritis: Contrast-enhanced sagittal fat-suppressed SE T1-weighted MR image shows an enhancing pannus surrounding and causing erosion of the tip of the odontoid peg, with widening of the anterior atlantoaxial joint. There is slight resultant angulated indentation of the cervicomedullary junction.

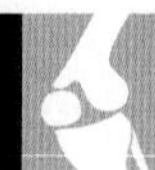

35–5 Hangman Fracture (Type I)

Stephen E. Ling and William R. Reinus

PRESENTATION

Pain, instability, neurological deficit

FINDINGS

Bilateral pars interarticularis fracture at C2 with or without anterolisthesis at C2–C3 so-called type I Hangman fracture.

DIFFERENTIAL DIAGNOSES

- *Hangman fracture type II:* Type II (30%: unstable): >3 mm translation, angulation >10°, disrupted longitudinal ligaments and C2–C3 disc; C3 compression fracture.
- *Hangman fracture type III:* Type III (10%: unstable): >3 mm translation, >10° angulation, disrupted ligaments and C2–C3 disc; unilateral or bilateral facet dislocation.

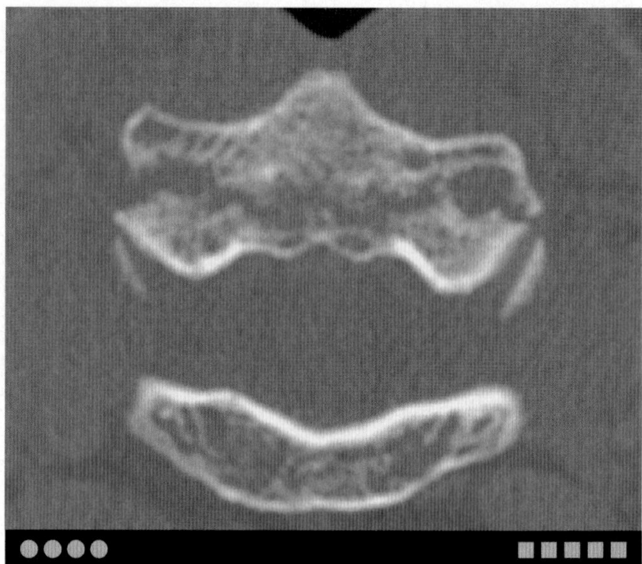

A. Hangman fracture (Type I): Axial CT image shows fracture through the posterior vertebral body of C2.

COMMENTS

The Hangman fracture, accounting for 4% to 7% of traumatic injuries to the cervical spine, is a bilateral fracture of the pedicles or pars interarticularis of C2. They are common in adults, but rare in children. The typical cause of these fractures is sudden severe hyperextension as occurs in a head-on motor vehicle collision. Hyperflexion, however, may be the etiology in some cases. Fractures of the posterior arch of C1 and the odontoid may occur concomitantly. Levine and Edwards classify these fractures into three types: Type I (60%: stable): <3 mm translation, no angulation, intact longitudinal ligaments, and C2–C3 disc. Type II (30%: unstable): >3 mm translation, angulation >10°, disrupted longitudinal ligaments and C2–C3 disc; C3 compression fracture. Type III (10%: unstable): >3 mm translation, >10° angulation, disrupted ligaments and C2–C3 disc; unilateral or bilateral facet dislocation. Neurologic deficits are uncommon with these fractures (~10%) because of the high central canal to cord ratio at the C2 level, and the automatic decompression of the canal by the pars fractures. Deficits are more common with Type II and III fractures and are typically mild and short lived. Dissection or embolization of the vertebral artery injury from extension of the fracture into the transverse foramen is a recognized, serious complication. The importance of evaluating the integrity of the longitudinal ligaments and the C2–C3 disc to determine stability makes CT or MRI essential in this injury. Treatment options range from conservative use of a collar in stable injuries to fusion of the posterior elements in unstable ones. Following treatment, malunion or nonunion is rare.

PEARLS

- **The moniker "Hangman fracture" is somewhat of a misnomer, as most cases do not involve the traction component of the hyperextension distraction mechanism occurring in judicial hangings.**
- **Neurological deficit is unusual in the setting of Hangman fracture as a result of "auto-decompression" of the central canal and the baseline relatively wide canal at the level of C2.**
- **Vertebral artery injury is often life threatening.**

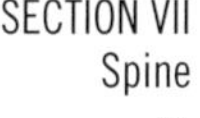

ADDITIONAL IMAGE

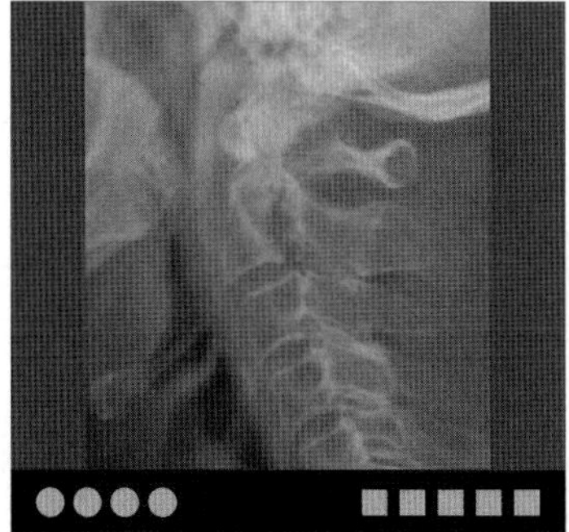

B. Hangman fracture (Type I): Lateral radiograph from the same patient as image A shows displacement of less than 3 mm and minimal angulation. Note the absence of stenosis of the central canal at the C2 level.

DIFFERENTIAL DIAGNOSES IMAGES

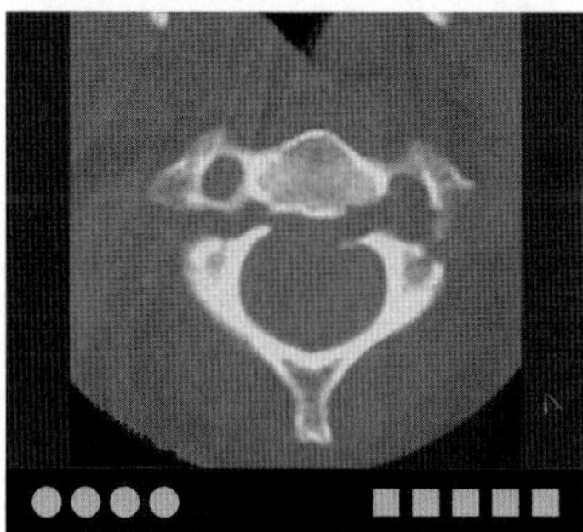

C. Hangman fracture (Type II): Axial CT image shows bilateral pars interarticularis fracture at C2 with displacement of more than 3 mm. Concomitant C3 compression fracture seen in some patients with these fractures is not present in this case.

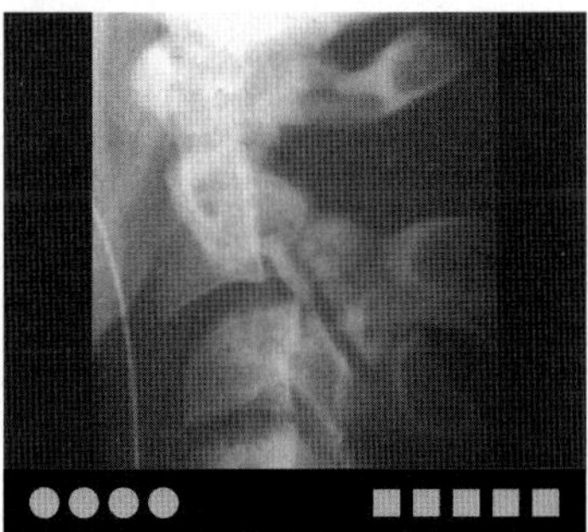

D. Hangman fracture (Type II): Lateral radiograph shows bilateral pars interarticularis fracture at C2 with displacement of more than 3 mm and angulation apex superior greater than 10°. Concomitant C3 compression fracture seen in some patients with these fractures is not present in this case.

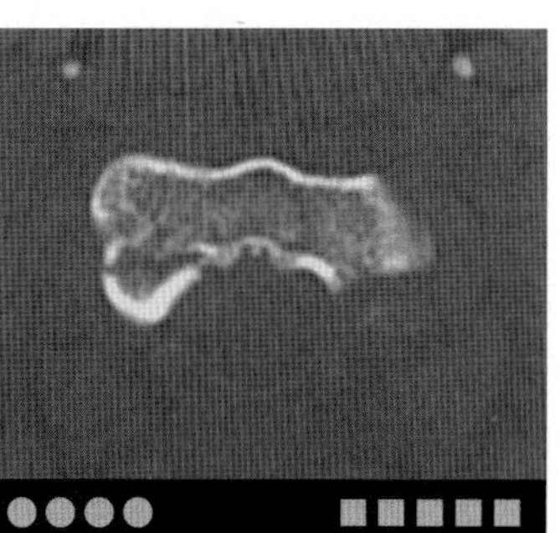

E. Hangman fracture (Type III): Axial CT image in another patient shows findings similar to those seen in images C and D.

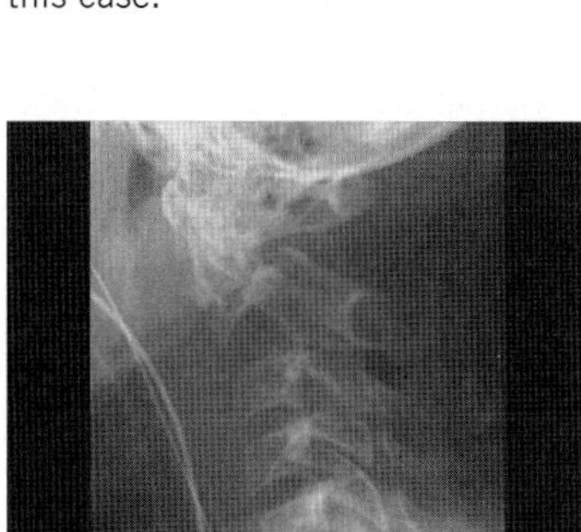

F. Hangman fracture (Type III): Lateral radiograph in another patient shows findings similar to those seen in images C and D. In addition, there is facet dislocation at C2–C3.

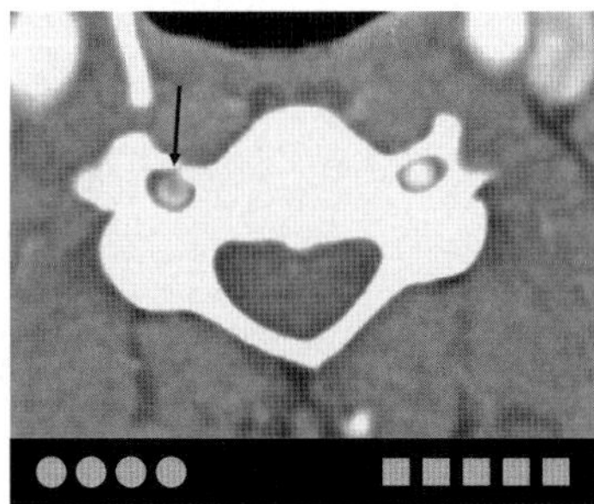

G. Hangman fracture–vertebral artery dissection: Axial CT image shows a filling defect in the right vertebral artery indicating dissection, which in this case was secondary to extension of the fracture (not shown) into the transverse foramen at C2 on the right.

IMAGE KEY

Common

Rare

Typical

Unusual

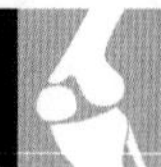

35–6 Flexion Teardrop Fracture of the Cervical Spine

Michael A. Bruno

PRESENTATION

Diving injury

FINDINGS

There is a fracture involving anterior, middle, and posterior columns of C5 with marked kyphosis, a triangular "teardrop" fragment anteriorly, and retropulsion of bony fragments into the cervical canal. The fracture pattern is shown to good advantage on CT reconstruction. On MRI there is noted to be evidence of cervical cord injury.

DIFFERENTIAL DIAGNOSES

- *Fracture-dislocation or "burst" fracture* can have a similar appearance. This devastating injury may result in cord compression and paralysis.
- *Extension tear-drop fracture:* This avulsion fracture occurs as a result of pull of anterior longitudinal ligament during hyperextension and results in a triangular fracture fragment avulsed from anterior inferior end plate of C2 vertebra.
- *Hyperextension dislocation of axis:* Severe hyperextension injury of the neck results in dislocation of C2–C3 vertebra which often results in cord transection and quadriplegia. A sliver of horizontal subtle fracture will be seen at inferior endplate of axis with marked prevertebral soft tissue injury. There is rupture of ACL and avulsion of axis from subjacent disc or horizontal rupture of the disc.
- *Avulsion fracture of posterior cortex of axis:* This is because of pull of posterior longitudinal ligament which occurs during flexion injury.

COMMENTS

The "flexion teardrop" fracture of the cervical spine is considered by many experts to be the worst possible fracture of the cervical spine. The mechanism of injury usually involves significant axial loading and flexion, as commonly occurs when diving headfirst into shallow water. Severe cord injury usually results, with quadriplegia. The fracture is extremely unstable, with disruption of both osseous and ligamentous structures. Retropulson of bony fragments into the spinal canal is a characteristic feature. The name "teardrop" is derived from the shape of the small anterior fragment. This should not be mistaken for the "extension teardrop injury," in which there is no disruption of the middle or posterior columns (in that case, which is related to hyperextension mechanism, a small "teardrop" anterior fragment is avulsed from the lower anterior corner of a vertebral body). The degree of spinal canal compromise is variable; however, as a result of the large forces required to produce this fracture pattern, some degree of spinal cord injury is universally seen. A severe three-column fracture-dislocation injury, which can occur in a wide variety of mechanisms, is a similar lesion mechanically, but without the combined flexion and axial loading vectors in the mechanism, the "teardrop" fragment is not seen.

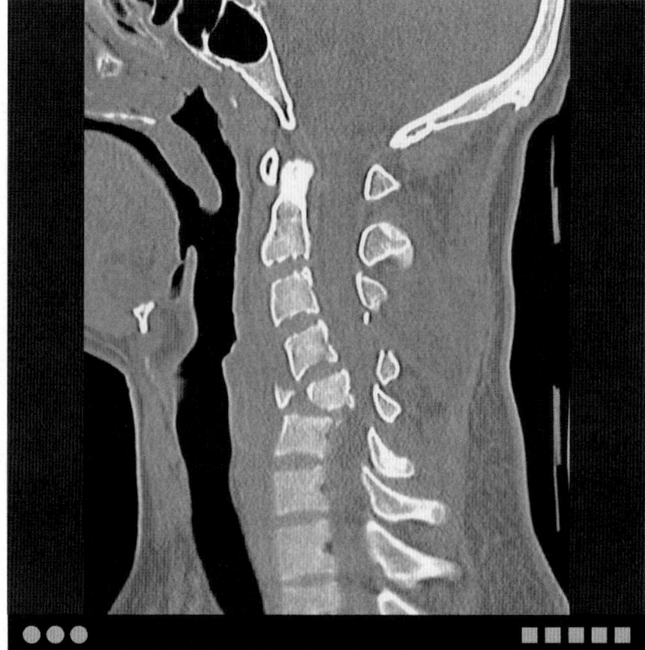

A. Flexion teardrop fracture: Sagittal CT reformatting shows the characteristic injury pattern at C5. Note the retropulsed fragment, the spinal canal compromise, the marked kyphosis, and the "teardrop" fragment.

PEARLS

- **The flexion teardrop fracture of the cervical spine is widely regarded as the most severe type of C-spine fracture.**
- **An extension-avulsion injury can mimic the appearance of the "teardrop" fragment, but is a dissimilar injury.**
- **When the mechanism does not include significant flexion force vectors, a fracture-dislocation or "burst" fracture may be seen, with similar clinical significance, but without the characteristic "teardrop" fragment.**

ADDITIONAL IMAGE

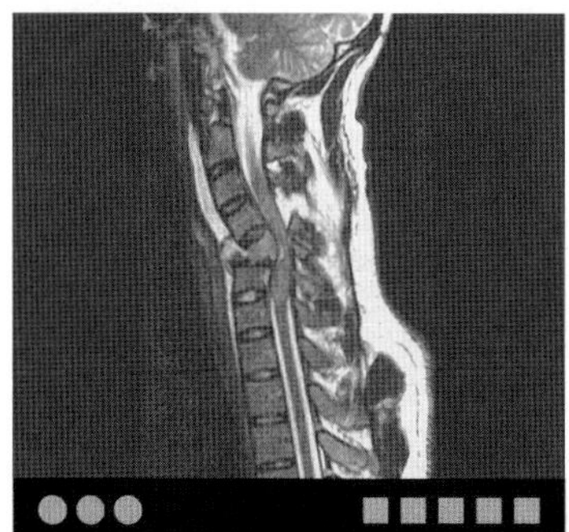

B. Flexion teardrop fracture: T2-weighted spin-echo midsagittal MR image of the cervical spine demonstrates the fracture pattern, the spinal canal compromise, and the cord contusion/compression resulting from this fracture.

DIFFERENTIAL DIAGNOSES IMAGES

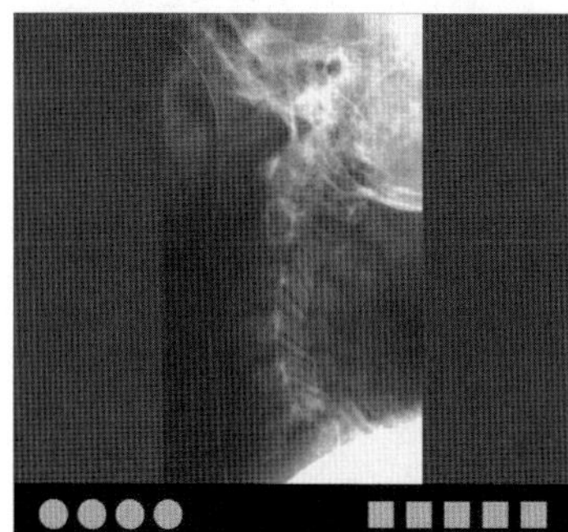

C. Non-teardrop "burst" fracture-dislocation: Lateral radiograph of cervical spine. By comparison, this fracture pattern is similarly unstable, with similar compromise of the spinal canal. Note the absence of the "teardrop" fragment, and kyphosis. Significant flexion force vectors were not part of the mechanism of injury in this case.

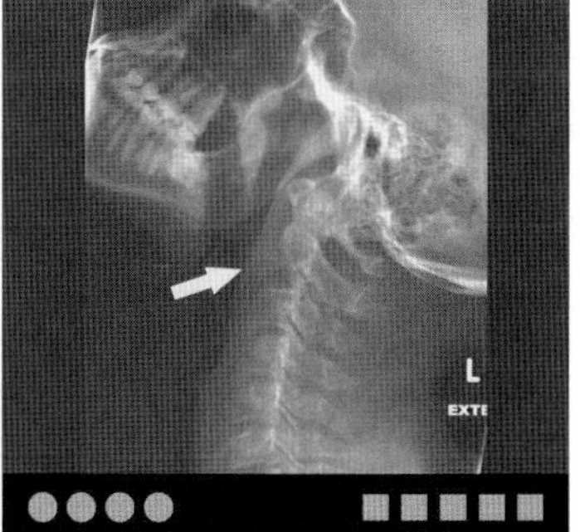

D. Extension tear drop: Lateral radiograph of the cervical spine shows triangular fracture of the anterior inferior endplate of axis (arrow).

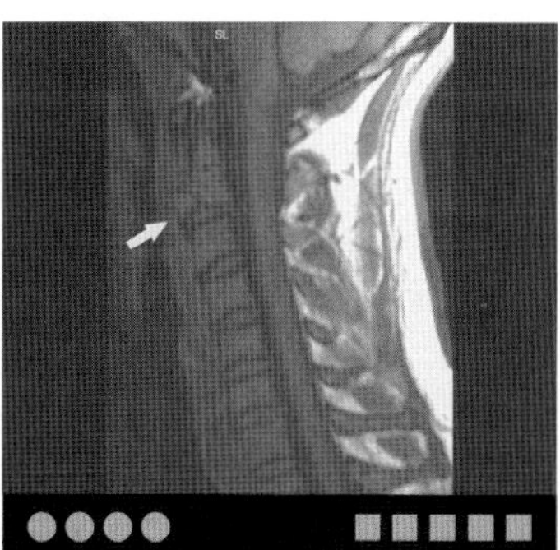

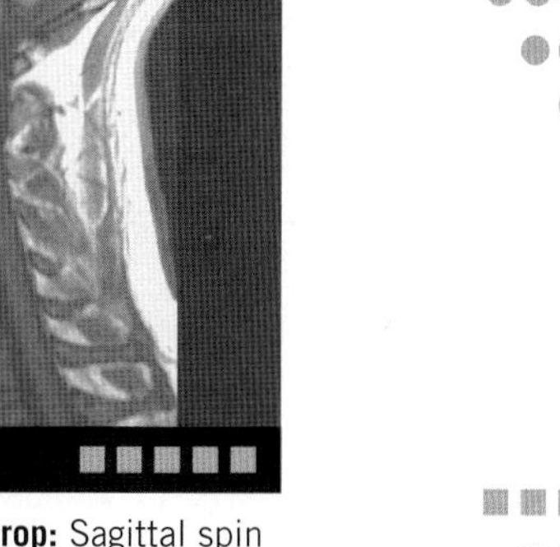

E. Extension tear drop: Sagittal spin echo T1-weighted image shows the same fracture (arrow).

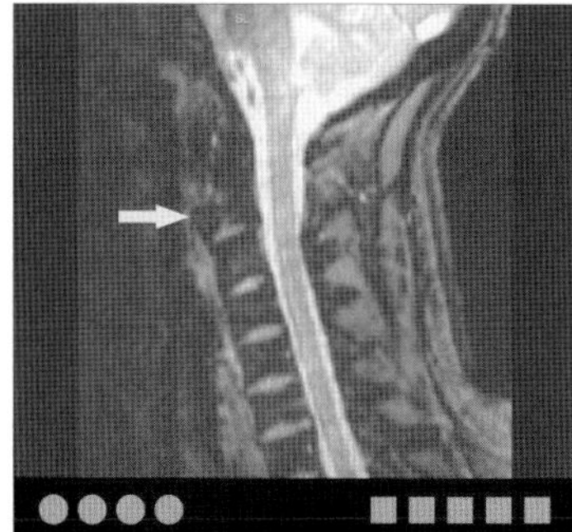

F. Extension tear drop: Sagittal GE T2*-weighted image shows the same fracture (arrow).

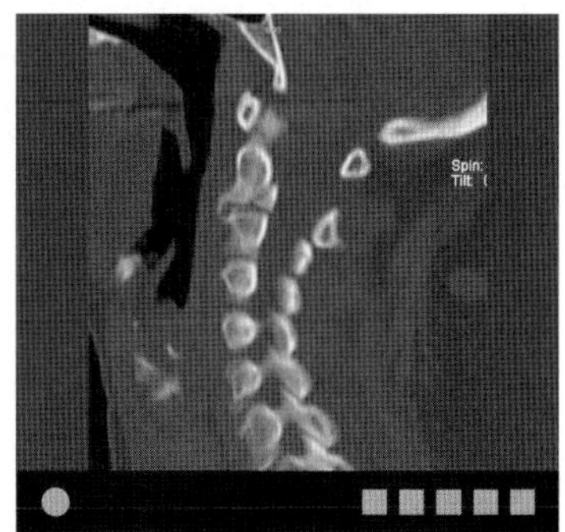

G. Avulsion fracture of posterior inferior cortex of axis: A small bony fragment is avulsed from posterior inferior endplate of axis vertebra.

IMAGE KEY

Common

Rare

Typical

Unusual

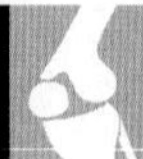

35–7 Hyperextension Injury of Cervical Spine

Mohammad Reza Hayeri and Robert Ward

PRESENTATION

Pain

FINDINGS

Avulsion fracture of cervical spine caused by disruption of anterior longitudinal ligament is associated with widening of disk space and prevertebral soft tissue swelling.

DIFFERENTIAL DIAGNOSIS

- *Flexion tear drop fracture:* The mechanism of injury usually involves significant axial loading and flexion, as commonly occurs when diving headfirst into shallow water. Severe cord injury usually results, with quadriplegia. The fracture is extremely unstable, with disruption of both osseous and ligamentous structures.

COMMENTS

Hyperextension injury is a common injury of cervical spine with significant morbidity. Different injuries to cervical spine have been described as a result of hyperextension such as hyperextension sprains, hyperextension dislocation, burst fracture of atlas (Jefferson fracture), traumatic spondylolisthesis (Hangman's fracture), extension teardrop fracture, and isolated laminar fractures. The two main mechanisms contributing to hyperextension injury of cervical spine are rear-end motor-vehicle collisions resulting in acceleration extension "whiplash injuries" or hyperextension injuries as a result of direct anterior craniofacial trauma. In the whiplash mechanism hyperextension generally centers on the C-5 to C-6 level, and is limited by the occiput striking the back, and may be followed by recoil flexion. The disks and ligaments are susceptible to rupture if a rotational element is also contributed. Pain occurring hours or days after injury is the main symptom of the injury. Associated anterior longitudinal ligament tear, stretch and tear of the lower cervical disk anulus, and traction of sympathetic and cervical plexus nerves or roots cause an immediate and more severe symptoms. Hyperextension dislocation is a serious injury which may be associated with the cord transection, but usually has subtle manifestation in radiographs. Prevertebral soft tissue swelling may be the only sign on the radiograph. Avulsion fracture fragment of endplate in this injury has shorter vertical height compared to cases of hyperextension tear drop. The diagnosis is usually established by the presence of an acute central cervical spinal cord syndrome in a patient, who has sustained facial or craniofacial trauma and in whom the cervical vertebrae are normally aligned in the lateral projection.

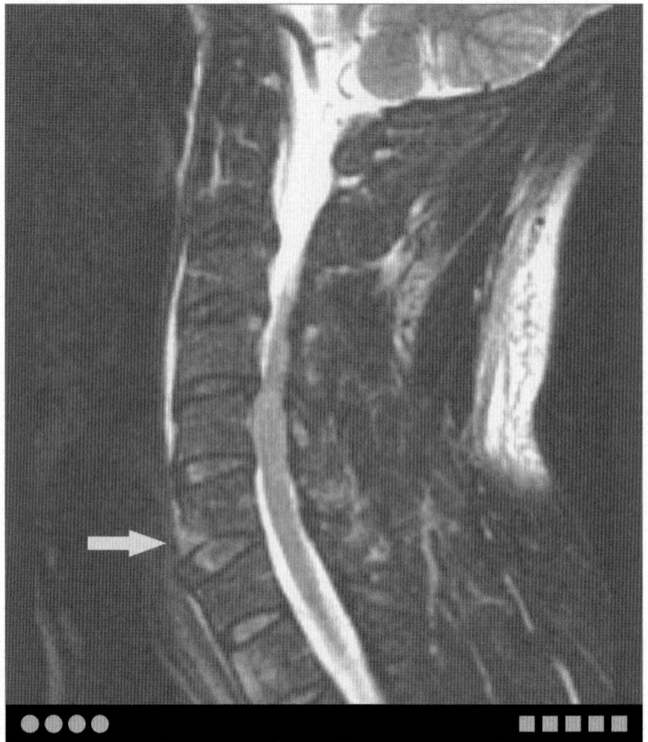

A. Hyperextension teardrop avulsion of C6: Sagittal T2 fat-saturated image shows avulsion fracture of inferior endplate of C6 vertebra (arrow) as a result of hyperextension injury and avulsion fracture of anterior longitudinal ligament. Note widening of the disc space. Narrowing of spinal canal and mild cord edema are also noted. (Courtesy of Adam Zoga.)

PEARLS

- **Hyperextension injuries may manifest in different forms including hyperextension sprains, hyperextension dislocation, burst fracture of atlas (Jefferson fracture), traumatic spondylolisthesis (Hangman's fracture), extension teardrop fracture, and isolated laminar fractures.**
- **Hyperextension tear drop is caused by avulsion of anterior longitudinal ligament, which is associated with triangular endplate fracture fragment that has taller vertical height.**
- **Hyperextension dislocation is a serious injury which may be associated with the cord transection. Prevertebral soft tissue swelling may be the only sign on the radiograph. Avulsion fracture fragment of endplate in this injury has shorter vertical height compared to cases of hyperextension tear drop.**

ADDITIONAL IMAGES

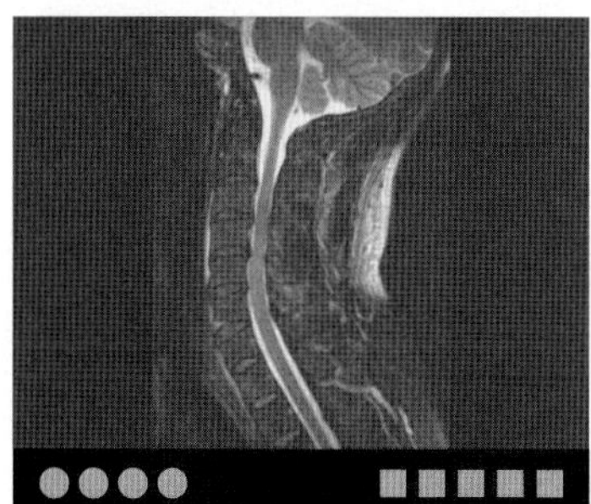

B. Hyperextension teardrop avulsion of C6: Sagittal T2 fat-saturated image shows avulsion fracture of inferior endplate of C6 vertebra as a result of hyperextension injury and avulsion fracture of anterior longitudinal ligament. Note widening of the disc space. Narrowing of spinal canal and mild cord edema are also noted. (Courtesy of Adam Zoga.)

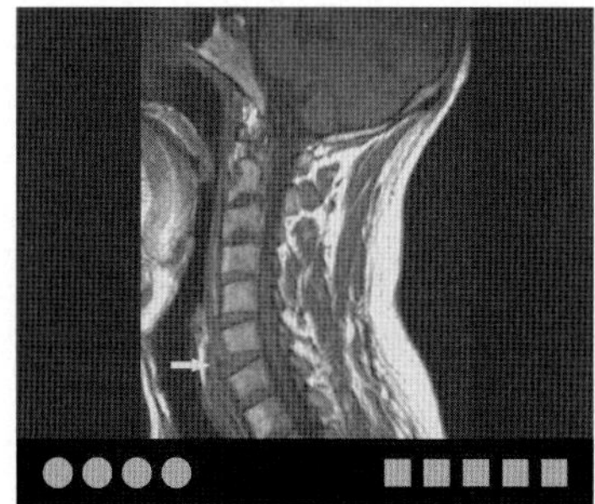

C. Hyperextension teardrop avulsion of C6: Sagittal T1-weighted image shows avulsion fracture of inferior endplate of C6 vertebra as a result of hyperextension injury and avulsion fracture of anterior longitudinal ligament. Note widening of the disc space. Narrowing of spinal canal and mild cord edema are also noted. (Courtesy of Adam Zoga)

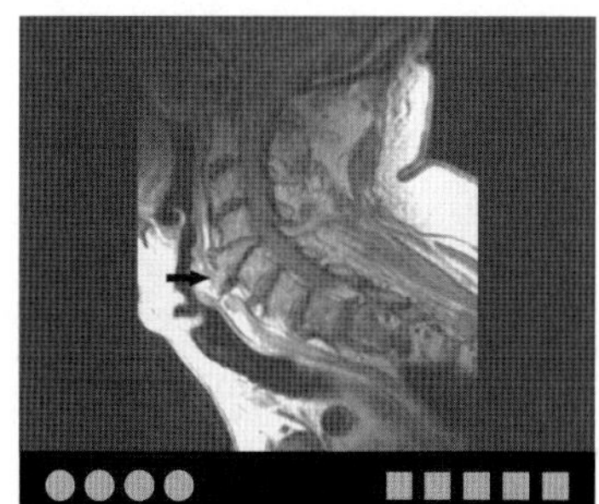

D. Hyperextension injury of C4-C5 vertebra: Sagittal T1-weighted image shows tear of anterior longitudinal ligament and widening of disc space at C4-C5 level. (Courtesy of Adam Zoga.)

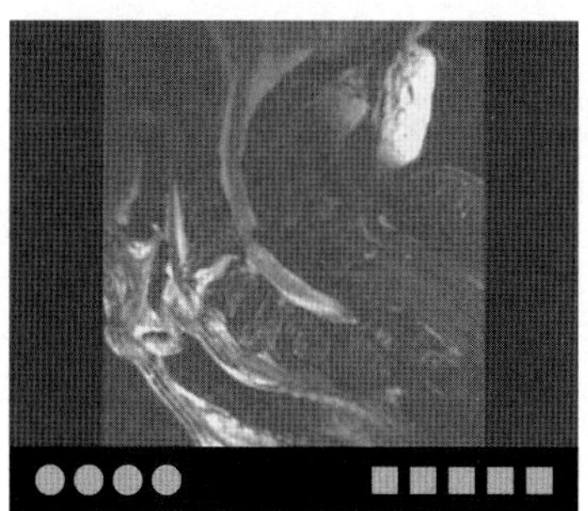

E. Hyperextension injury of C4-C5 vertebra: Sagittal T1-weighted image shows tear of anterior longitudinal ligament and widening of disc space at C4-C5 level. (Courtesy of Adam Zoga.)

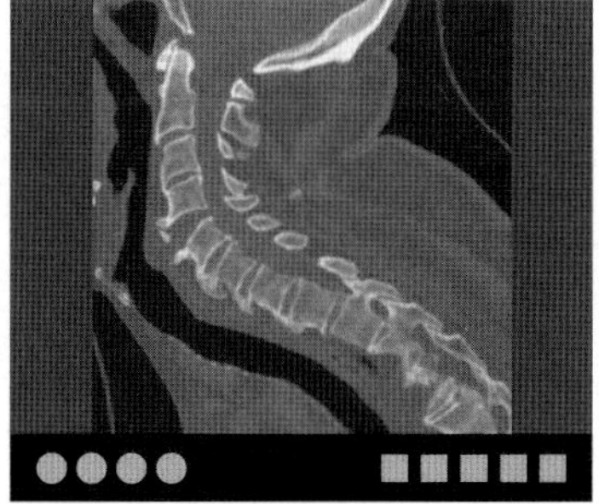

F. Hyperextension injury of C4-C5 vertebra: Sagittal reformatting CT of cervical spine shows tear of anterior longitudinal ligament and widening of disc space at C4-C5 level. Prevertebral soft tissue swelling is also noted. (Courtesy of Adam Zoga.)

IMAGE KEY

Common

Rare

Typical

Unusual

DIFFERENTIAL DIAGNOSES IMAGES

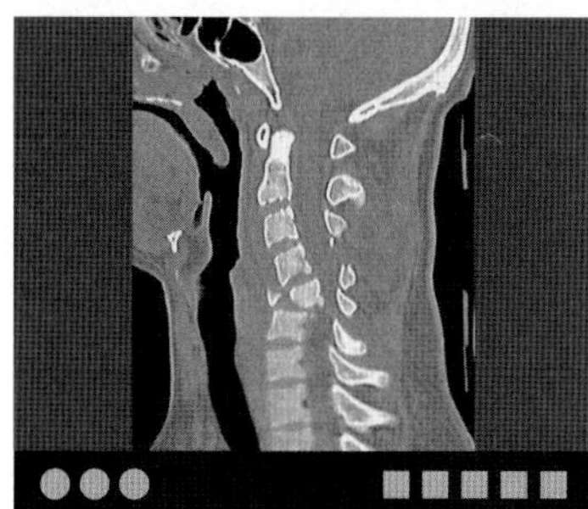

G. Flexion teardrop fracture: Sagittal CT reformatting shows the characteristic injury pattern at C5. Note the retropulsed fragment, the spinal canal compromise, the marked kyphosis, and the "teardrop" fragment.

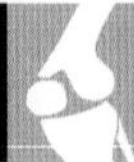

35–8 Extension Teardrop Fracture of C2

Ashkan Afshin and Jamshid Tehranzadeh

PRESENTATION

Neck pain

FINDINGS

Lateral radiograph, CT, and MRI show triangular fracture of the anterior inferior endplate of the body of C2. The height of the avulsed fragment is greater than its width.

DIFFERENTIAL DIAGNOSES

- *Hyperextension dislocation of axis:* Severe hyperextension injury of the neck results in dislocation of C2-C3 vertebra, which often results in cord transection and quadriplegia. A sliver of horizontal subtle fracture will be seen at inferior endplate of axis with marked prevertebral soft tissue injury. Rupture of anterior longitudinal ligament and avulsion of axis from subjacent disc or horizontal rupture of the disc are observed.
- *Flexion teardrop fracture:* This is the worst possible fracture of the cervical spine and manifests with severe cord injury and quadriplegia. Retropulson of bony fragments into the spinal canal is a characteristic feature.
- *Avulsion fracture of posterior cortex of axis:* This is caused by the pull of posterior longitudinal ligament, which occurs during flexion injury.

COMMENTS

Extension teardrop fracture is an avulsion fracture of the anterior inferior endplate of the vertebral body. The name "teardrop" is derived from the shape of the small anterior fragment. As the name implies, this rare type of fracture usually results from severe hyperextension of the neck. Hyperextension force causes the anterior longitudinal ligament to pull a fragment away from its insertion site on the inferior aspect of the vertebra. This condition is most common in elderly patients with osteoporotic bone and is associated with little or no prevertebral hematoma. Extension teardrop fracture usually involves second cervical vertebra. It is usually not associated with neurologic manifestations. Extension teardrop fracture is unstable in extension but stable in flexion. This injury should not be mistaken for the "flexion teardrop injury," which is extremely unstable, with disruption of both osseous and ligamentous structures, and manifests with severe cord injury and quadriplegia. The size of the avulsed fragment in extension teardrop fracture is small and is not greater than one quarter of the sagittal diameter of the vertebral body. Lateral radiograph of the neck shows that the vertical height of the fragment is greater than its horizontal dimension. This finding is the most characteristic radiographic feature of the fracture. Little or no prevertebral soft tissue swelling is also present.

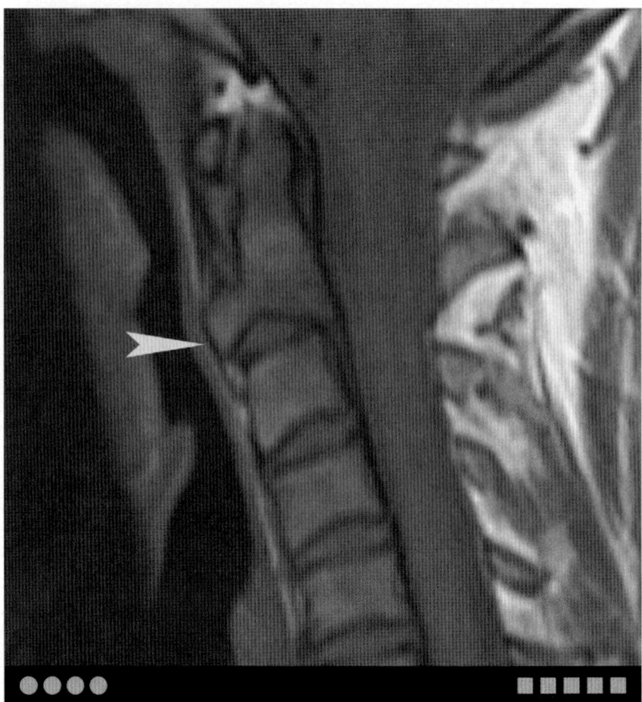

A. Extension teardrop fracture of C2: Sagittal T1-weighted image shows teardrop fracture of the inferior endplate of C2 vertebra with anterior displacement (arrowhead).

PEARLS

- **Extension teardrop fracture is an avulsion fracture of the anterior inferior endplate of the vertebral body**
- **It usually results from severe hyperextension of the neck**
- **It is most common in elderly patients**
- **It is unstable in extension but stable in flexion**
- **The most characteristic radiographic finding is that the vertical height of the fragment is greater than its horizontal dimension**
- **Little or no prevertebral soft tissue swelling is present**

ADDITIONAL IMAGES

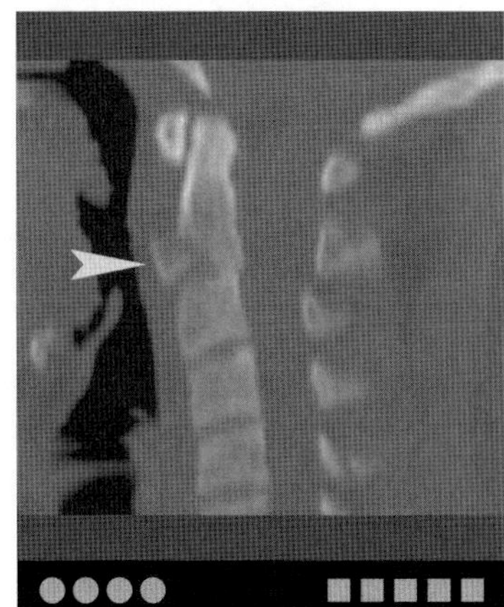

B. Extension teardrop fracture of C2: Sagittal CT reformatting of the cervical spine shows anteriorly displaced teardrop fracture of the inferior endplate of C2 vertebra (arrowhead).

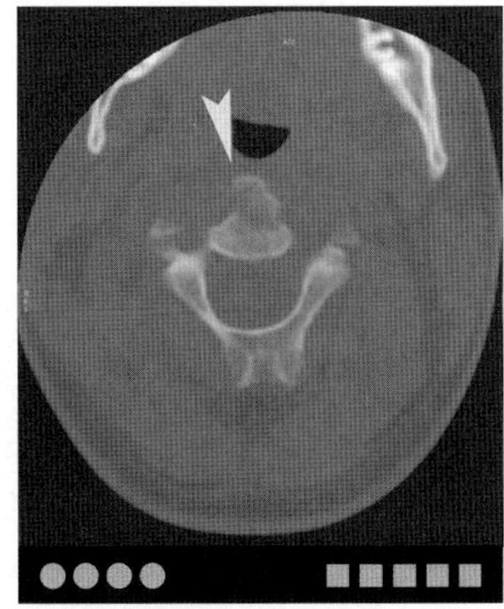

C. Extension teardrop fracture of C2: Axial CT of the cervical spine shows anteriorly displaced teardrop fracture of the inferior endplate of C2 vertebra (arrowhead).

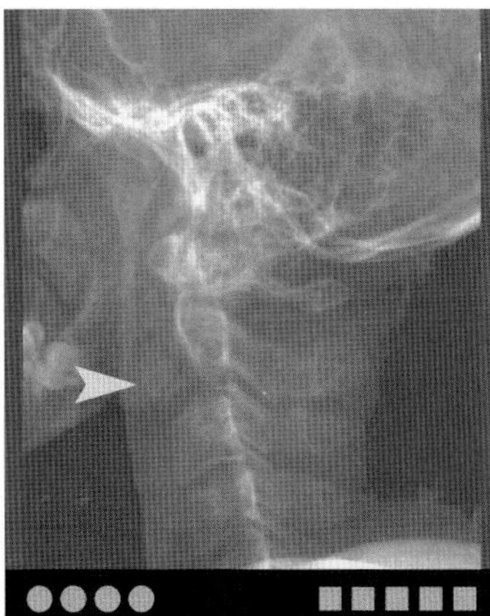

D. Extension teardrop fracture of C2: Lateral radiograph of the upper cervical spine shows anteriorly displaced teardrop fracture of the inferior endplate of C2 vertebra (arrowhead).

DIFFERENTIAL DIAGNOSES IMAGES

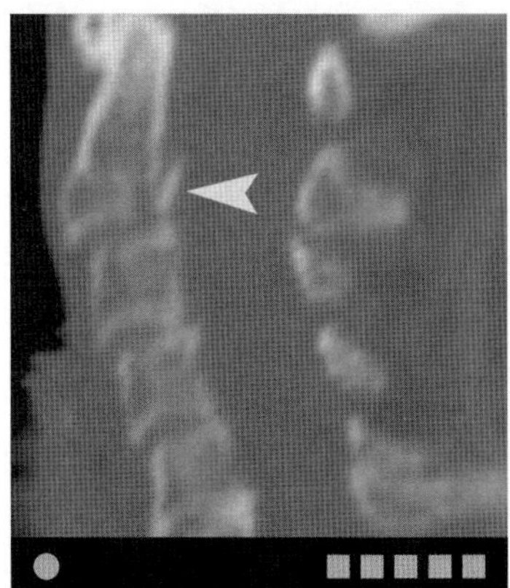

E. Avulsion of the posterior aspect of the inferior endplate of the C2 vertebra: Sagittal CT reconstruction shows a bony fragment avulsed from the posterior aspect of the inferior endplate of the C2 vertebra (arrowhead).

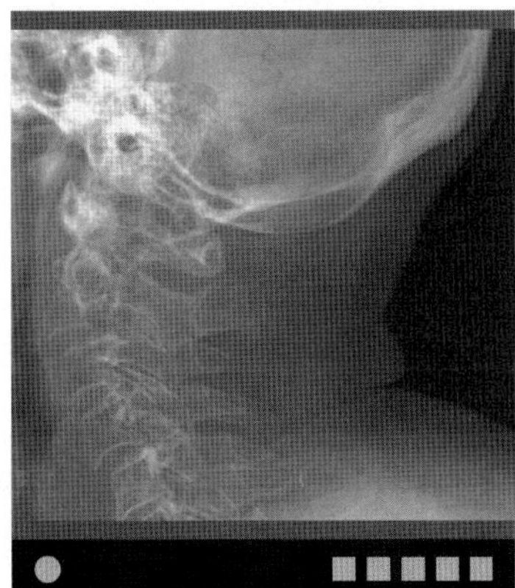

F. Avulsion of the posterior aspect of the inferior endplate of the C2 vertebra: Lateral radiograph of the upper cervical spine shows a bony fragment avulsed from the posterior aspect of the inferior endplate of the C2 vertebra.

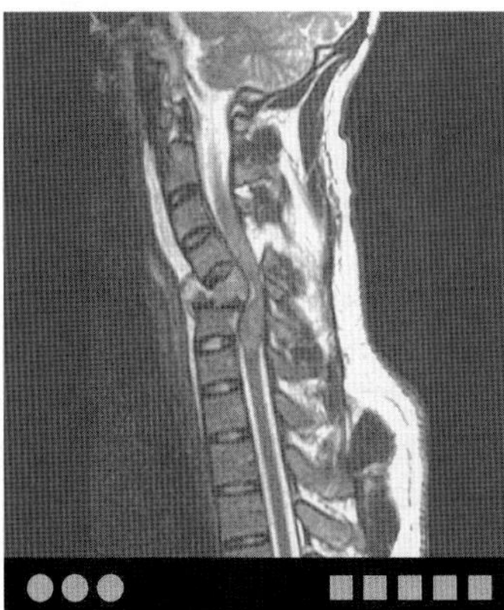

G. Flexion teardrop fracture: T2-weighted spin-echo midsagittal MR image of the cervical spine demonstrates the fracture pattern, the spinal canal compromise, and the cord contusion/compression resulting from this fracture.

IMAGE KEY

Common

●●●●●
●●●●
●●●
●●
●

Rare

Typical

■■■■■
■■■■
■■■
■■
■

Unusual

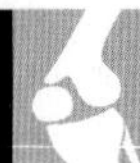

35–9 Unilateral and Bilateral "Jumped" Facets

Michael A. Bruno

PRESENTATION

Motor vehicle trauma

FINDINGS

Radiographs of the cervical spine demonstrate malalignment of the facet joints of the cervical spine, either bilateral (image A) or unilateral (image B).

DIFFERENTIAL DIAGNOSES

- *"Perched" facets:* an unstable configuration in which the tip of the superior facet rests on the tip of the inferior facet. This is not a stable configuration and can spontaneously self-reduce or progress to the full "jumped" or "locked" configuration without the application of traction. See images C to F.
- *Fracture/dislocation:* Fracture, which can co-exist, can usually be excluded by multiple views and CT.

COMMENTS

For a facet joint to be "jumped," or "locked," the superior articulating process, which normally lies anterior to its lower, or inferior "mate," is transposed to lie in a posterior position, where it is in a fairly stable state and is said to be "locked." Significant upward head traction is usually needed to reduce this malalignment. Note that there is a greater degree of AP misalignment and spinal canal compromise with bilateral jumped facets, while rotatory subluxation is a prominent feature in unilateral jumped facets. This type of injury is the result of substantial ligamentous injury and typically results from high-energy trauma, such as a high-speed motor vehicle accident or fall from a significant height. The bilateral jumped facet dislocation case illustrated here occurred when an oblique high-speed freeway collision resulted in the driver's vehicle penetrating the guard rails on an overpass and falling approximately 30 feet. In the case of unilateral jumped facets, the head was turned at the time of impact. Spinal cord injury commonly occurs with bilateral jumped facets caused by significant canal compromise. In contrast, unilateral facet dislocation can occur with a lower-energy mechanism, as was reported in this case involving a young pregnant female who drove her car at a moderate speed into the rear bumper of the stopped car ahead of her while she was distracted, her head turned posteriorly, scolding children in the back seat of her own car. The unstable condition where one articulating facet is "perched" upon another can spontaneously reduce or spontaneously advance to the "locked" configuration, often with abrupt spinal canal compromise.

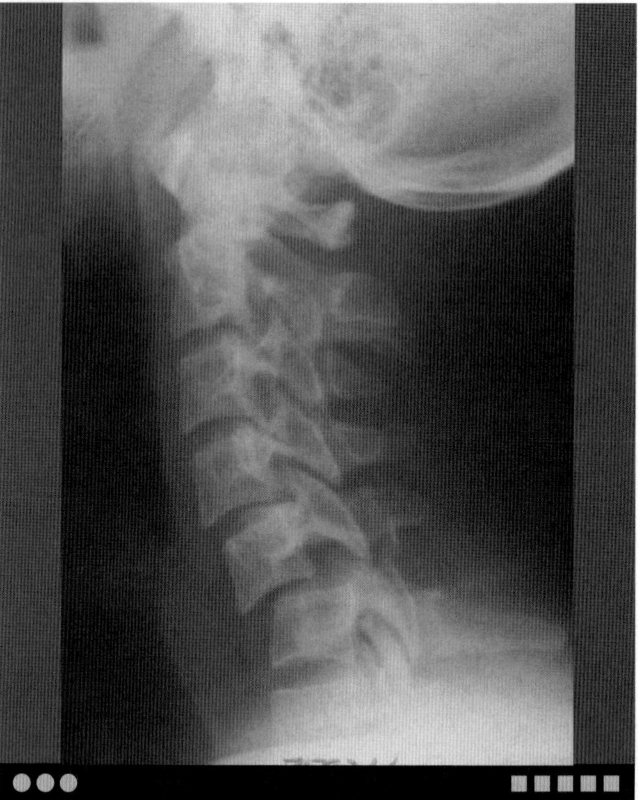

A. Bilateral jumped facets: Lateral planar radiograph of the cervical spine in a case of bilateral jumped facets. Note the degree of anterior displacement and the high degree of spinal canal compromise. Cord injury is common.

PEARLS

- **Bilateral jumped facets are characterized by significant ligamentous instability and spinal canal compromise, usually resulting in severe cord injury. They tend to occur in the setting of high-energy blunt trauma.**
- **Unilateral jumped facets are characterized by rotatory vertebral displacement, have less spinal canal compromise, and are less likely to result in severe spinal cord injury.**
- **"Perched" facets are extremely unstable and can abruptly progress to the "locked" position, with abrupt spinal canal compromise. They can also be radiographically subtle. Prompt, accurate radiological diagnosis can help to avert significant neurological injury.**

ADDITIONAL IMAGES

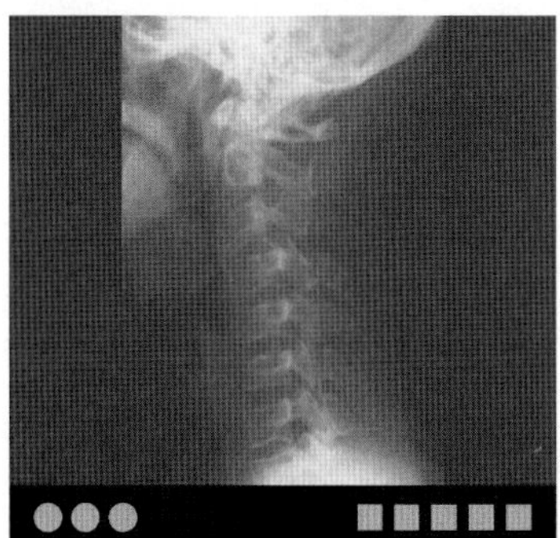

B. Unilateral jumped facets: "Lateral" radiograph in a case of unilateral jumped facets. Note the presence of rotatory subluxation, with the neuoforamina visible above the level of the dislocation, but not below (neuroforamina are normally only seen on oblique views). There is a lesser degree of spinal canal compromise than was seen in the bilaterally dislocated facet case of image A.

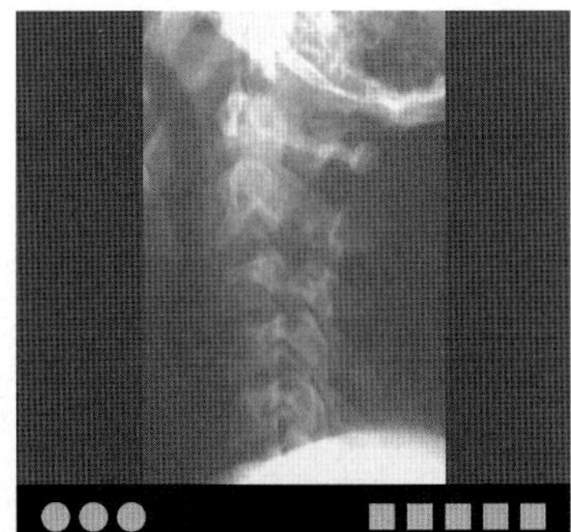

C. Unilateral "perched" facets: This is a somewhat more subtle case than the unilaterally "locked" facets seen in image B. Note that the spinal–laminar alignment is only minimally perturbed relative to anterior alignment. This injury is frequently missed by radiologists in the Emergency setting.

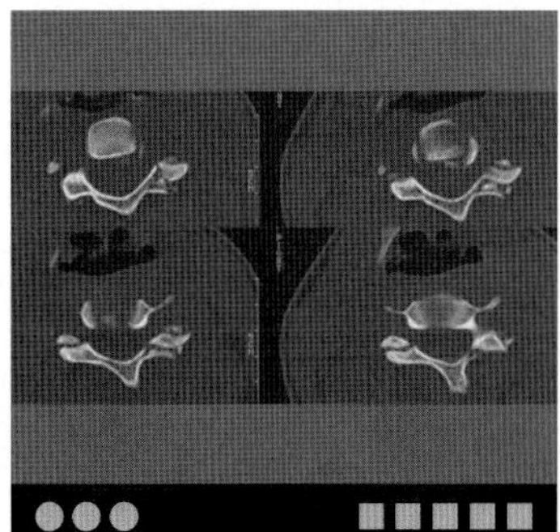

D. Unilateral "perched" facets: CT scan in a case of unilateral "perched" facet—axial plane; note the rotational subluxation of the superior level and the relationship of the articulating facets to each other. This is a very unstable lesion, which in this case was complicated by facet fracture.

E. Unilateral "perched" facets: CT scan, sagittal reconstruction images better delineate the precarious "perched" relationship of the articulating facets.

DIFFERENTIAL DIAGNOSES IMAGES

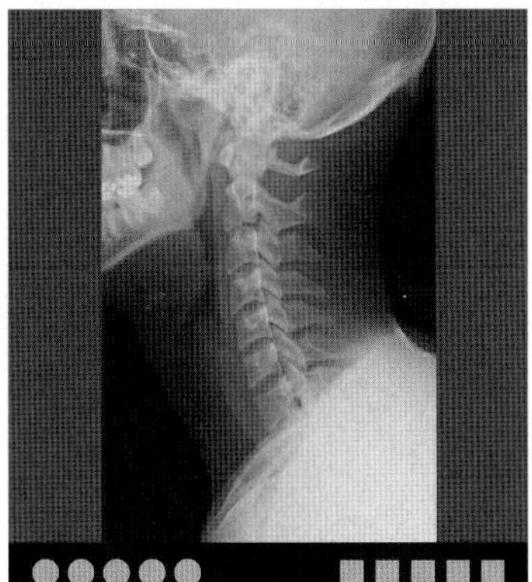

F. A normal lateral C-spine: Lateral radiograph is provided for comparison. Note normal arrangement of the facets.

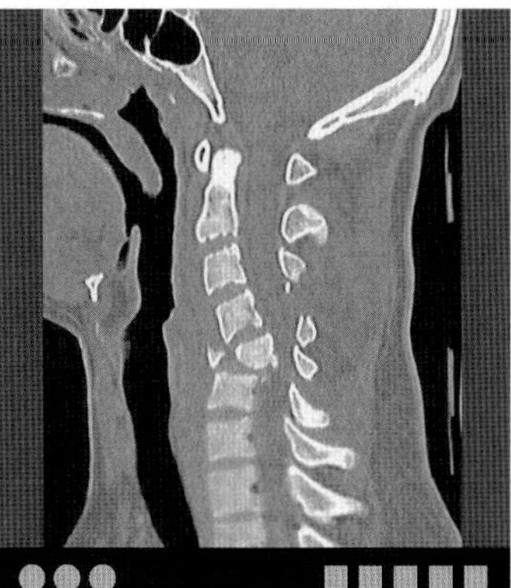

G. Flexion teardrop fracture: Sagittal CT reformatting shows the characteristic injury pattern at C5. Note the retropulsed fragment, the spinal canal compromise, the marked kyphosis and the "teardrop" fragment.

IMAGE KEY

Common

Rare

Typical

Unusual

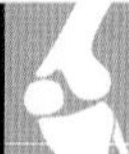

35–10 Burst Compression Fracture

Eric Chen and Jamshid Tehranzadeh

PRESENTATION

Back pain following trauma

FINDINGS

MRI shows burst fracture of T7 vertebra with transverse anterior to posterior disruption and perched articular processes at T7-T8 and stripping of anterior longitudinal ligament.

DIFFERENTIAL DIAGNOSES

- *Osteoporotic compression fracture:* This is a nontraumatic compression commonly seen in postmenopausal women.
- *Malignant compression fracture:* This may be associated with presence of pre-existing primary malignancy. It has the MRI feature of malignant involvement of the spine.
- *Spondylitis:* The disc space and the endplates of two adjacent vertebrae are involved with soft tissue inflammation and possible epidural abscess.

COMMENTS

The patient is a 42-year-old male with a history of head trauma. The concept of burst compression fracture was defined by Denis in 1983 as a combination of a wedge compression of the anterior column and fracture of the middle column with retropulsion of a bone fragment into the spinal canal. Involvement of the posterior column defines an unstable burst fracture. Conventional radiography can detect most cases of burst fractures but misdiagnoses 20% as simple wedge compression fractures. Typical findings on radiography include loss of anterior and posterior vertebral body height, retropulsion of bone into spinal canal, and comminution of the superior and/or inferior end-plates. CT provides additional information regarding the nature of injury such as degree of canal compromise, identification of rotational or translational components, and assessment of the pedicles above and below the fracture. CT also better identifies laminar fractures and fracture-dislocations of the facets. MRI is particularly useful to evaluate ligamentous injury and injury to the spinal cord. Posterior longitudinal ligament (PLL) can be completely ruptured, manifesting as a discontinuous black stripe on sagittal MRI or more commonly, the PLL is stripped from the vertebral body by a hematoma or bone manifesting as a continuous black stripe. Interspinous ligament (ISL) rupture is seen as a high intensity signal on T2-weighted image in the region of the ISL. Acute injury to the spinal cord is manifested as a poorly defined high signal on T2-weighted image.

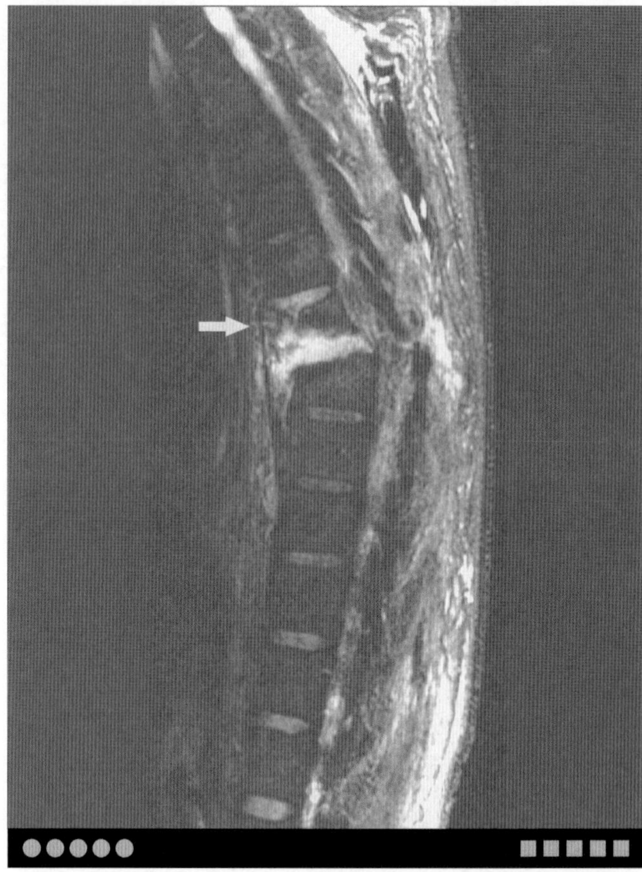

A. Burst fracture: Sagittal fat-saturated T2-weighted MR image shows compression fracture of the T7 vertebrae with fragmentation of the vertebral body and fluid accumulation at the fracture site at the disc space of T7-T8. Note stripping of anterior longitudinal ligament (arrow).

PEARLS

- **Bone retropulsion into spinal canal is classically associated with burst fractures.**
- **Most cases of burst fractures can be diagnosed with radiography as widening of interpediculate distance or widening of the facet joint spaces but CT is recommended to better differentiate between burst and simple wedge compression.**
- **MRI better diagnoses ligamentous and spinal injury.**

ADDITIONAL IMAGES

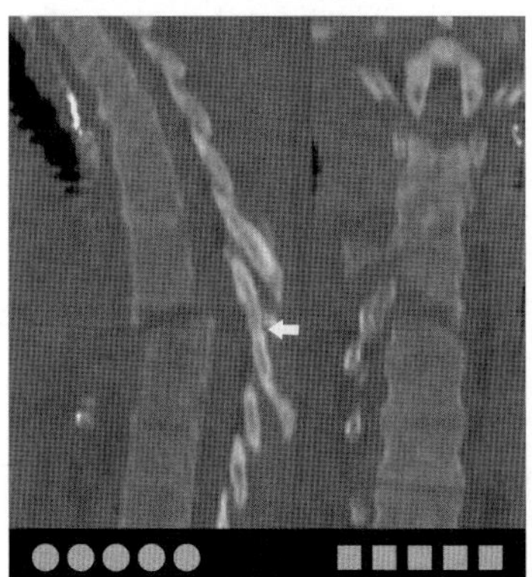

B. Burst fracture: Coronal and sagittal reformatted CT views of the thoracic spine shows burst fracture of T7. There is subluxation of T7 on T8 with perching of the articular processes of the facet joint (arrow).

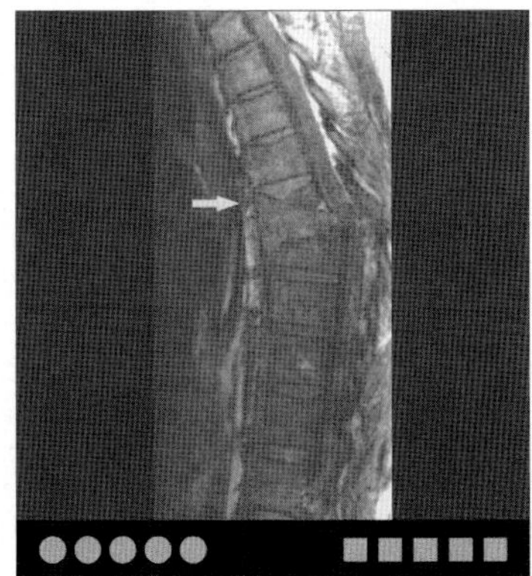

C. Burst fracture: Sagittal fat-saturated T1-weighted image shows compression (burst) fracture of T7 (arrow) with subluxation of T7 on T8. Note kyphotic deformity at the fracture site.

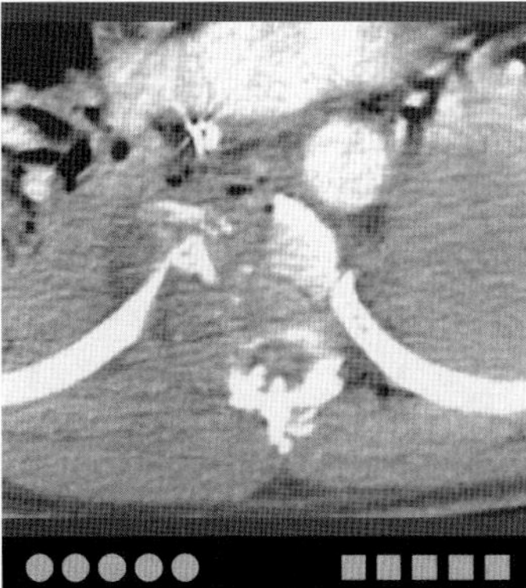

D. Burst fracture: Axial CT soft tissue window at level of T7 shows comminuted fracture of body and posterior elements of T7. Note bony fragments in the spinal canal. Air in soft tissue is because of pneumomediastinum. There is also bilateral pleural effusion, pulmonary contusion, and atelectasis.

E. Burst fracture: Axial fat-saturated T2-weighted image at T7 level shows the comminuted fracture with fluid accumulation at fracture site. Note the paraspinal soft tissue edema especially on the right side.

DIFFERENTIAL DIAGNOSES IMAGES

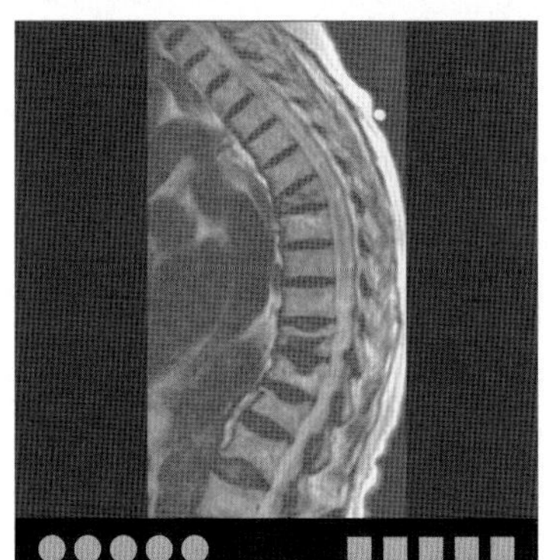

F. Osteoporotic compression fracture: Sagittal T1-weighted image shows multiple wedge compression of the vertebral bodies caused by osteoporosis. Note the preservation of the marrow in the collapsed vertebrae.

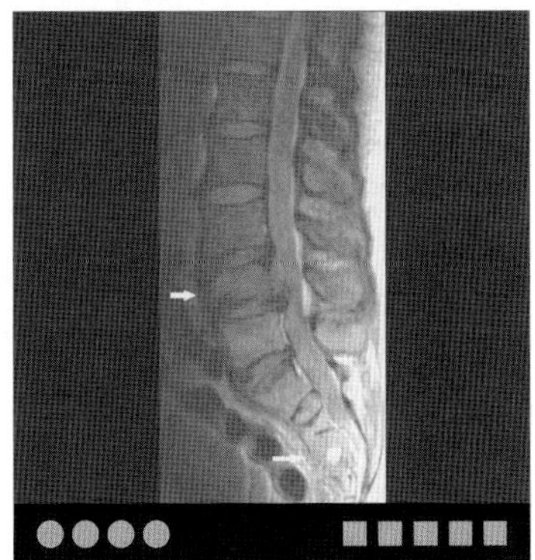

G. Malignant compression fracture: Sagittal fat-saturated T1-weighted post-contrast image shows compression of L4 and S2-S3 vertebrae (arrows). Note posterior cortex of L4 shows convexity toward the spinal canal. There are also abnormal marrow signals in the metastatic vertebrae.

IMAGE KEY

Common

Rare

Typical

Unusual

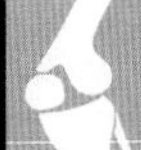

35–11 Chance (Seat Belt) Fracture

Ingrid B. Kjellin

PRESENTATION

Severe back pain after a car accident

FINDINGS

MRI shows a horizontal fracture through the L1 vertebral body and the spinous process.

DIFFERENTIAL DIAGNOSES

- *A compression fracture:* Also known as wedge fracture, only involves the anterior aspect of the vertebral body, and is a stable injury.
- *A burst fracture:* Typically has retropulsion of bone fragments into the spinal canal, which results in decreased diameter of the spinal canal. It may or may not be stable.
- *Fracture-dislocation:* There is anterior translation of the upper vertebral body. The interspinous distance and facet joints are widened. This is an unstable injury with high incidence of neurological injury.
- *Translational injury:* This is unstable, with shear forces causing neurological deficit in most cases.

COMMENTS

Of all the thoracic and lumbar fractures, approximately 60% are at the T12-L2 levels. Three features predispose this region to injury: (1) there is a change from a kyphosis to a lordosis; (2) there is a loss of stability provided by the ribs; and (3) there is a change in facet joint orientation from the coronal plane in the thoracic spine to the sagittal plane in the lumbar spine. Thoracolumbar injuries are stable or unstable. In stable injuries the posterior ligamentous complex is intact, and in unstable injuries the posterior elements are disrupted. Signs of instability on radiographs include a widened interpediculate space, increased distance between the spinous processes, widened facet joints, and lateral displacement of a vertebral body. The basic types of thoracolumbar injuries include compression fracture, burst fracture, seat-belt type (chance fracture) injury, and fracture-dislocation. Seat belt injuries occur when the spine is flexed against a seat belt, which acts a fulcrum. These injuries most commonly are seen at L1 and L2. In approximately 15% of these patients there are abdominal and neurological injuries. The flexion-distraction forces in seat belt injuries may result in bony, ligamentous, or a combination of bony and ligamentous injury. In the classic chance fracture the fracture line passes through the spinous process, laminae, facet joints, pedicles, and vertebral body. To address the surgeon's concern regarding stability at the fracture site, deformity, and neural compression, both CT and MRI are often performed preoperatively.

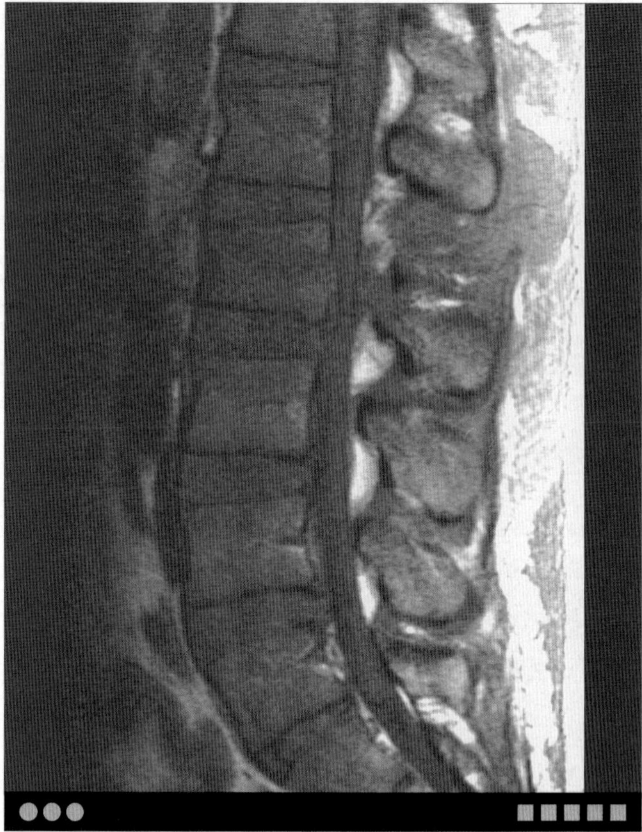

A. Chance fracture: A sagittal T1-weighted image shows a transverse fracture through the L2 vertebral body and the L2 spinous process. There is also a tear of the interspinous ligament between L1 and L2.

PEARLS

- **In seat belt injuries there are flexion-distraction forces, because the seat belt functions as a fulcrum.**
- **In 15% of patients with seat belt injury there are abdominal and neurological injuries.**
- **In the classic chance fracture the fracture line passes through the spinous process, laminae, facet joints, pedicles, and vertebral body.**

ADDITIONAL IMAGES

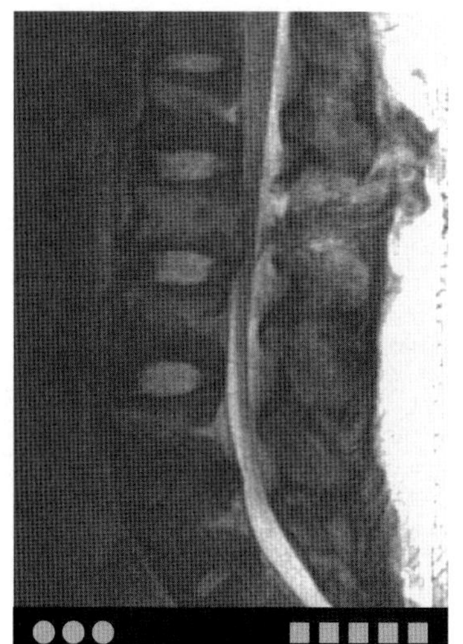

B. Chance fracture: A sagittal T2-weighted image shows the tear of the interspinous ligament between L1 and L2 more clearly than the T1-weighted image. There are also contusive changes in several vertebral bodies and spinous processes.

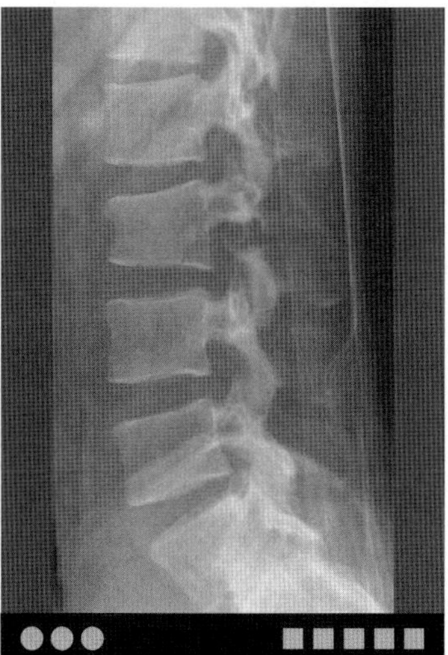

C. Chance fracture: A lateral radiograph shows mild anterior wedging of the L2 vertebral body and a transverse fracture through the posterior elements.

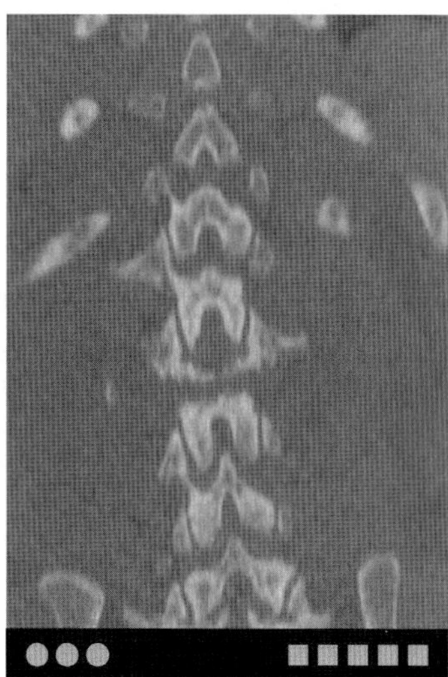

D. Chance fracture: A CT image in the coronal plane depicts the transverse fracture plane through the lamina of L2.

IMAGE KEY

Common

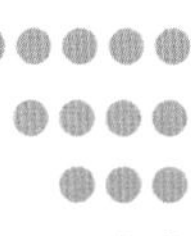

Rare

Typical

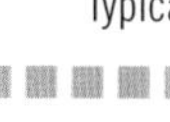

Unusual

DIFFERENTIAL DIAGNOSES IMAGES

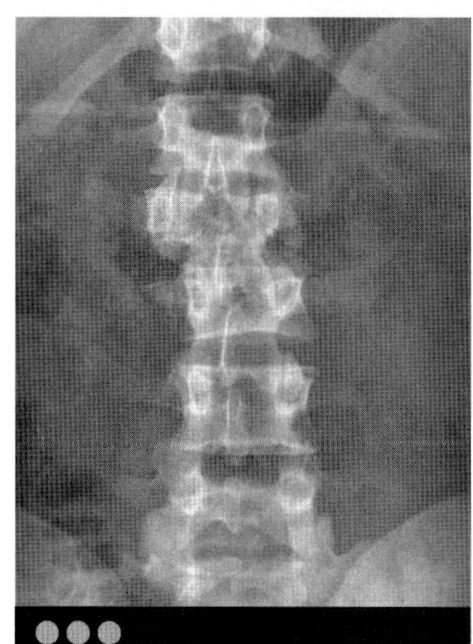

E. Translational injury: A frontal radiograph of the lumbar spine shows subluxation of L2 to the right, with respect to L3. There is also a comminuted fracture of L2 with mildly increased interpediculate distance at L2. The interspinous distance is also mildly increased at L1-2.

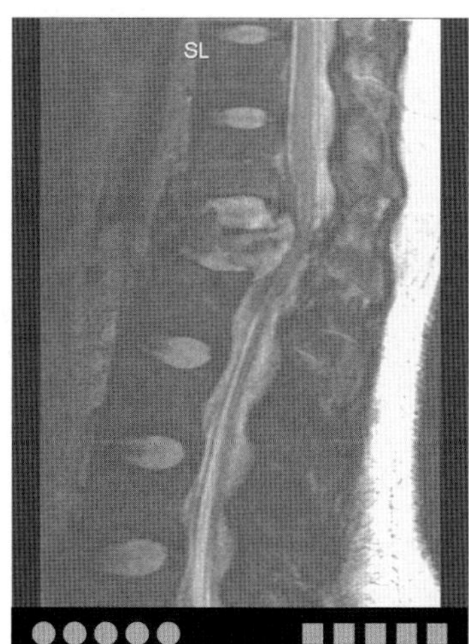

F. Burst fracture: A T2-weighted sagittal image shows a fracture of L1 with severe height loss and retropulsion of bone fragments.

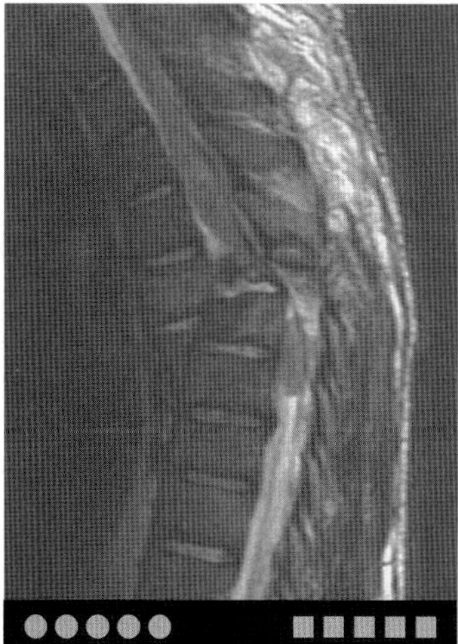

G. Fracture-dislocation: A T2-weighted image shows fracture-dislocation in the lower thoracic spine with severe anterior translation of the vertebral above, and disruption of the facet joints. There is also transection of the spinal cord.

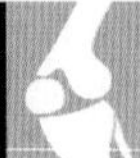

35–12 Avulsion of the Posterior Vertebral Endplate

Mohammad Reza Hayeri and Jamshid Tehranzadeh

PRESENTATION

Low back pain following trauma

FINDINGS

CT examination shows avulsion fracture of posterior inferior endplate of L4 vertebra associated with disc protrusion. There is also bilateral spondylolysis of L5-S1 level caused by pars interarticularis fractures.

DIFFERENTIAL DIAGNOSES

- *Disc calcification:* Intervertebral disc calcification can be seen in conditions such as pseudogout, hyperparathyroidism, ochronosis, hemochromatosis, or chronic disc protrusion and degeneration.
- *Osteophyte formation:* Bone spurs, or osteophytes, are bony projections that form along joints, and are often seen in conditions such as arthritis and disc degeneration.
- *Disc protrusion:* Disc protrusion consists of a tear in the annulus fibrosus that leads to outpouring of gelatinous nucleus pulposus.
- *Ossification posterior longitudinal ligament (OPLL):* OPLL represents a continuum beginning with hypertrophy of the posterior longitudinal ligament followed by progressive coalescence of centers of chondrification and ossification.

COMMENTS

The patient is a 31-year-old man involved in motor vehicle accident. Avulsion of the vertebral ring or endplate also known as epiphyseal dislocation usually presents in adolescence and early adult life. Lower lumbar spine is the most common place of occurrence. Avulsions at the endplate are caused by abrupt acceleration–deceleration movements although there is frequently no history of trauma. The intervertebral disc is attached to the endplate by Sharpey's fibers, which are the outermost fibers of annulus fibrosus. The endplate is separated from the remainder of the vertebral body by a cartilaginous plate that is replaced by bone at 18 to 25 years. Disc herniation through the cartilage plate and fracture or fragmentation of the ring apophysis occurs together in response to shearing or recurrent stress. The presenting symptoms are back and leg pain and restricted leg rising similar to those of disc propose. There are four types based on vertebral rim fracture: Type I is simple, thin avulsion fractures in the posterior cortex of endplate with no obvious defect in the vertebral body except an arcuate fracture fragment. In Type II the fracture also includes medullary bone and there is a defect in vertebral body. Type III is small lateral fractures. Type IV runs the full height of the vertebral body and extends to both vertebral endplates. CT scan shows bony avulsed fragment and associated disc prolapse and bone defect. On MRI the avulsed fragment can be best seen in proton density or gradient echo sequences as an arcuate or angular low signal area lying posteriorly.

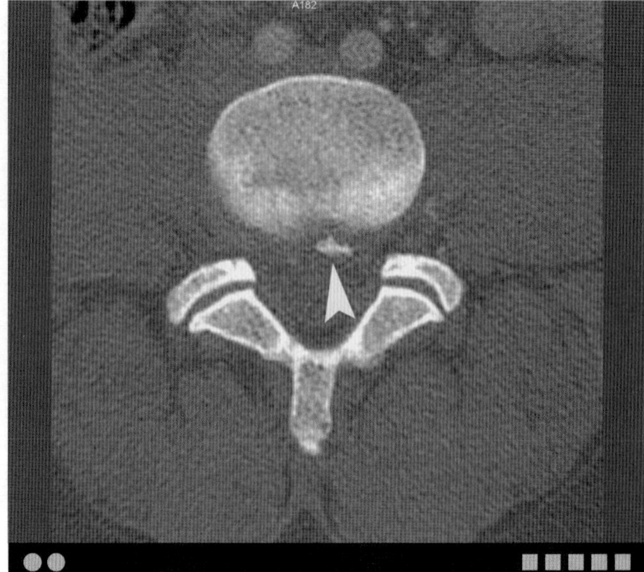

A. Avulsion of posterior vertebral endplate: Axial CT scan of the lumbar spine shows a fracture of the posterior endplate caused by avulsion of the posterior longitudinal ligament and Sharpey's fibers. A piece of fractured bone fragment (arrowhead) is displaced posteriorly.

PEARLS

- **Avulsions at the endplate are caused by abrupt acceleration–deceleration movements although there is frequently no history of trauma.**
- **Disc herniation through the cartilage plate and fracture or fragmentation of the ring apophysis occurs together in response to shearing or recurrent stress.**
- **CT scan shows bony avulsed fragment and associated disc prolapse and bone defect.**
- **On MRI the avulsed fragment can be best seen in proton density or gradient echo sequences as an arcuate or angular low signal area lying posteriorly.**

ADDITIONAL IMAGES

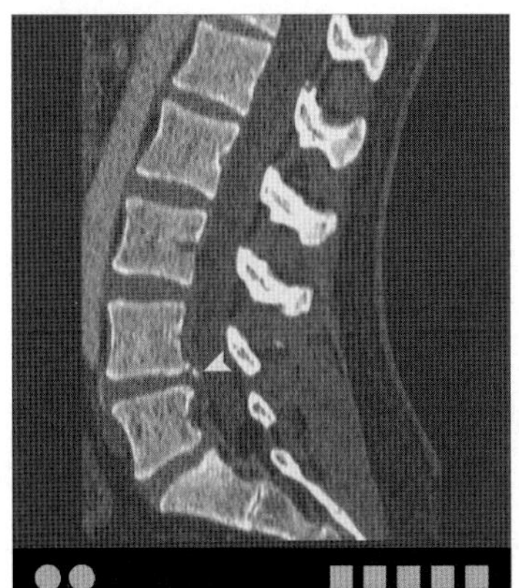

B. Avulsion of posterior vertebral endplate: Sagittal CT reformatting scan of the lumbar spine (same patient as image A) shows a fracture of the posterior endplate caused by avulsion of the posterior longitudinal ligament and Sharpey's fibers. A piece of fractured bone fragment (arrowhead) displaced posteriorly.

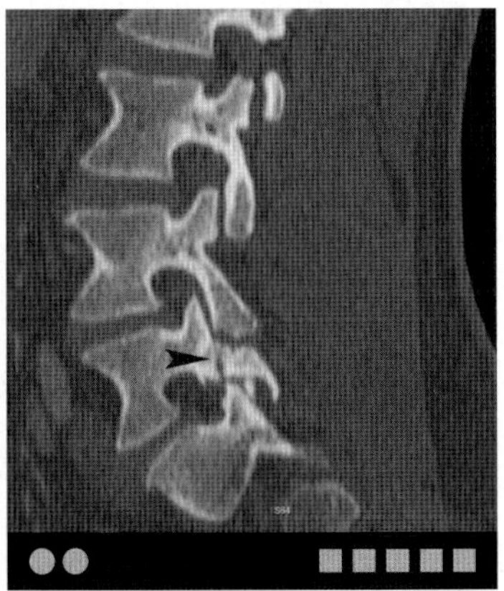

C. Bilateral spondylolysis: Parasagittal CT reformatting scan of the lumbar spine (same patient as A and B) shows pars interarticularis defect (arrowhead) indicating spondylolysis at L5-S1 level.

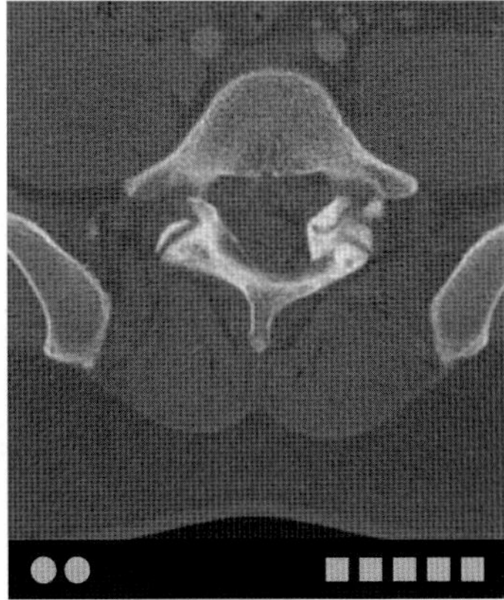

D. Bilateral spondylolysis: Axial CT scan of the lumbosacral spine (same patient as A, B, and C) shows double facet joints on both sides indicating bilateral spondylolysis at L5-S1 level.

IMAGE KEY

Common

●●●●●
●●●●
●●●
●●
●

Rare

Typical

■■■■■
■■■■
■■■
■■
■

Unusual

DIFFERENTIAL DIAGNOSES IMAGES

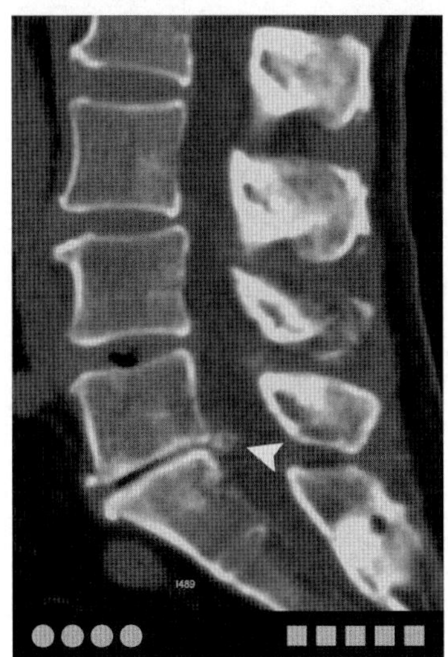

E. Calcified protruded disc: Sagittal CT reformatting scan shows degenerated disc at multiple levels with vaccum phenomenon at L4-L5 and L5-S1 and protruded calcified disc (arrowhead) at the L5-S1 level.

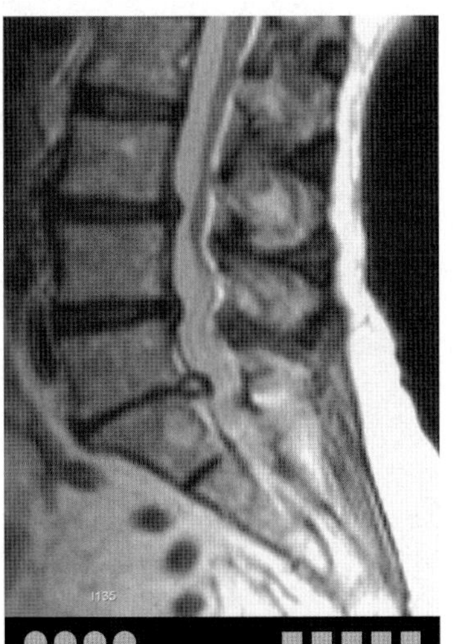

F. Calcified protruded disc: Sagittal T2-weighted MR image shows degenerated low signal discs at multiple levels. Bulging annulus fibrosus at L3-L4 and L4-L5 are noted. There is a calcified protruded disc at L5-S1 level.

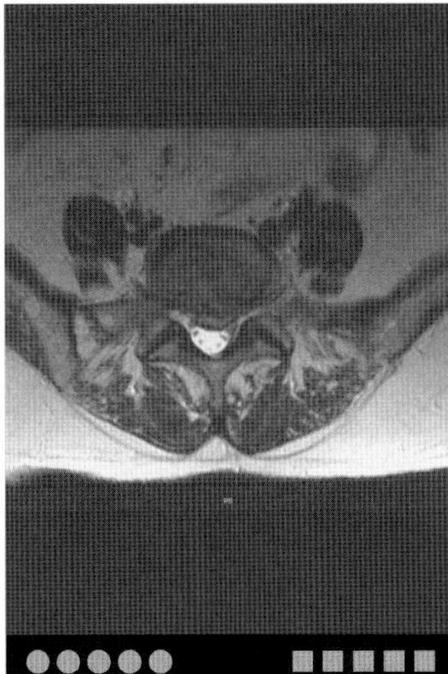

G. Calcified protruded disc: Axial T2-weighted MR image shows central calcified protruded disc at L5-S1 level.

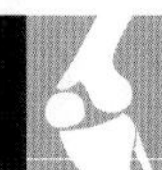

35–13 Spondylolysis Secondary to Fatigue Fracture

Ashkan Afshin and Jamshid Tehranzadeh

PRESENTATION

Low back pain

FINDINGS

There are bilateral subtle fatigue fractures of the pars interarticularis at L4 level with adjacent sclerosis.

DIFFERENTIAL DIAGNOSIS

- *Degenerative spondylolisthesis:* This subluxation is because of facet disease and ligamentous laxity. Unlike spondylolisthesis secondary to pars interarticularis defect, which results in widening of AP diameter of spinal canal, degenerative spondylolisthesis cause narrowing of spinal canal in axial plane.

COMMENTS

The patient is a 17-year-old male baseball player with low back pain. Spondylolysis is a clinical condition characterized by a defect in the pars interarticularis (Isthmus) of the spine. This disorder is relatively common and has prevalence of 3% to 7%.Great majority of cases occur at L5; however, it can be found at L4 and rarely at a higher level (thoracic spine). In bilateral cases, the posterior articulations can no longer provide the posterior stability, and anterior slipping of the vertebra results in a condition called spondylolisthesis. Stress fracture as a result of repeated microtrauma and heredity are two important etiologic factors in occurrence of spondylolysis. Patients are often asymptomatic. For symptomatic patients, back pain with extension or rotation of the lumbar spine is the most common symptom. Athletes who participate in sports, such as baseball and gymnastics, are more likely to have symptomatic spondylolysis at some point. Lateral radiographs of patient with spondylolysis shows a linear lucency in the pars interarticularis. This lucency on oblique radiograph is typically called the "Scottie dog has lost its collar"; the collar being pars interarticularis. Associated sclerosis at the fracture site may be present. CT and MR examinations can confirm doubtful cases on radiographs. "Double facet sign" are best detected on CT examinations. MRI may show the fracture line or bone edema in the pars interarticularis or the lamina. The spinal canal size appears wider in the AP diameter on axial planes in spondylolisthesis secondary to spondylolysis; while degenerative spondylolisthesis will result in narrowing of the spinal canal AP diameter on axial plane.

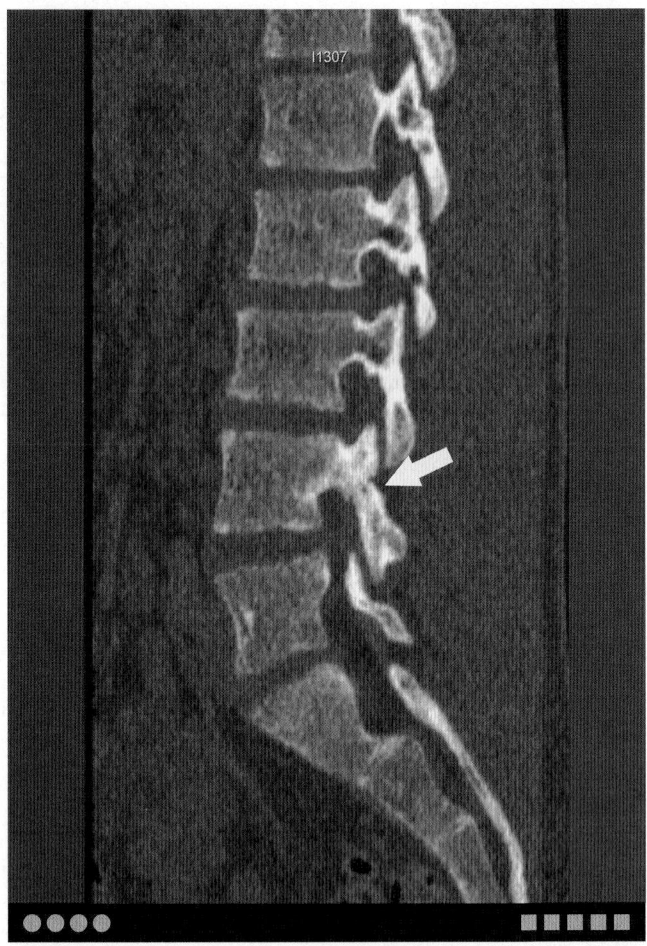

A. Spondylolysis secondary to fatigue fracture: Sagittal reformatted CT from fine 1 mm sections through lumbar spine shows subtle fracture (arrow) of pars interarticularis at L4 level.

PEARLS

- **Defect in pars interarticularis**
- **Most common anatomic location is L5**
- **Bilateral spondylolysis results in spondylolisthesis**
- **Back pain is the most common symptom**
- **On oblique radiograph appears as the collar on the neck of the Scottie dog**
- **Double facet sign is seen on axial imaging**

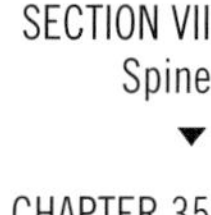

ADDITIONAL IMAGES

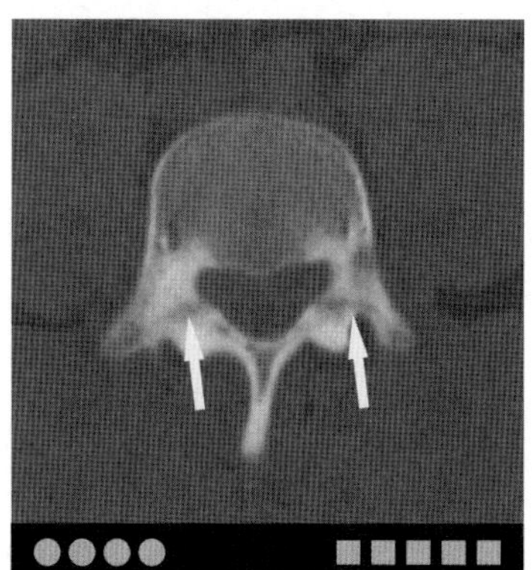

B. Spondylolysis secondary to fatigue fracture: Axial CT scan from fine 1 mm sections through L4 level shows bilateral subtle fatigue fractures (arrows) at the region of lamina of L4 level. Note adjacent sclerosis at fracture sites.

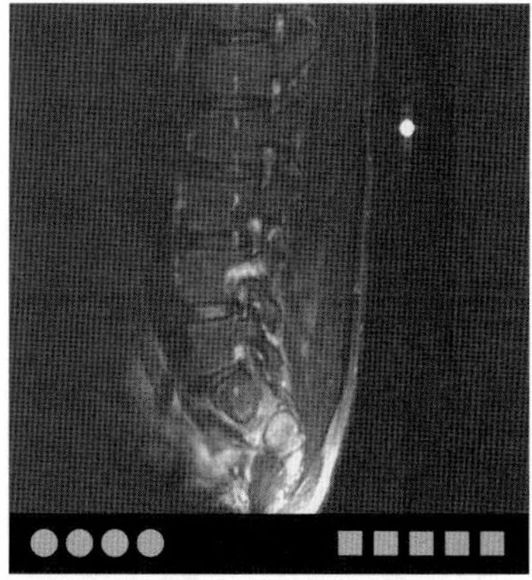

C. Spondylolysis secondary to fatigue fracture: Sagittal fat-saturated T2-weighted image of the lumbar spine shows bone edema at the lamina and pars interarticularis of L4 level.

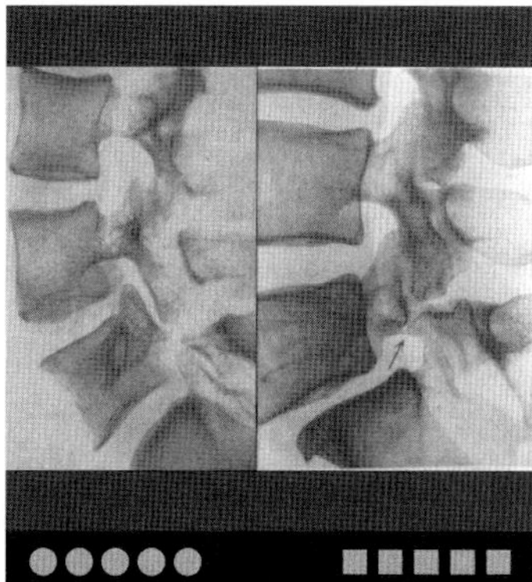

D. Spondylolysis and spondylolisthesis: Radiograph of lumbar spine in another patient shows a defect in the pars interarticularis at L5-S1 level (arrow) with spondylolisthesis at the L5-S1 level.

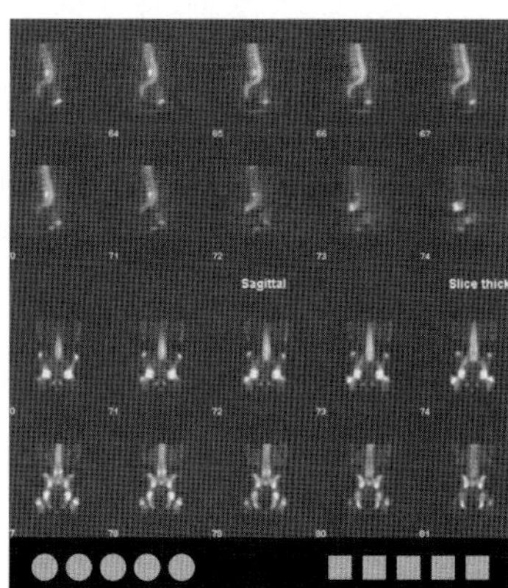

E. Spondylolysis and spondylolisthesis: Single photon emission computed tomography (SPECT) of the lumbar spine in a 14-year-old gymnast girl shows focal increased uptake in the region of spondylolysis.

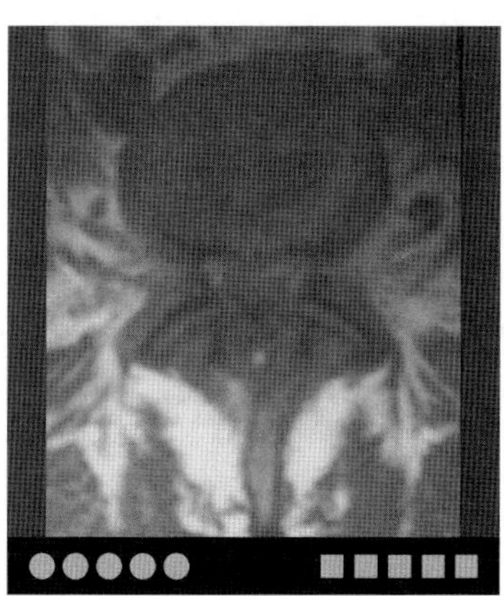

F. Spondylolysis and spondylolisthesis: Axial T1-weighted MRI of the spine in another patient shows increase in the AP diameter of canal associated with spondylolisthesis secondary to spondylolysis.

IMAGE KEY

Common

Rare

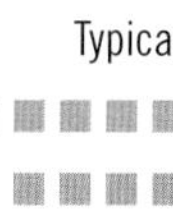

Typical

Unusual

DIFFERENTIAL DIAGNOSES IMAGES

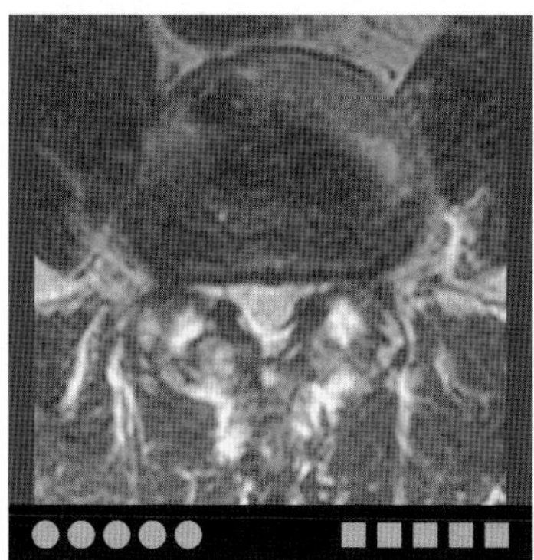

G. Degenerative spondylolisthesis: Axial T2-weighted image shows marked degenerative facet disease. Note the spinal canal is narrowed.

Chapter 36

Congenital, Systemic and Metabolic Diseases

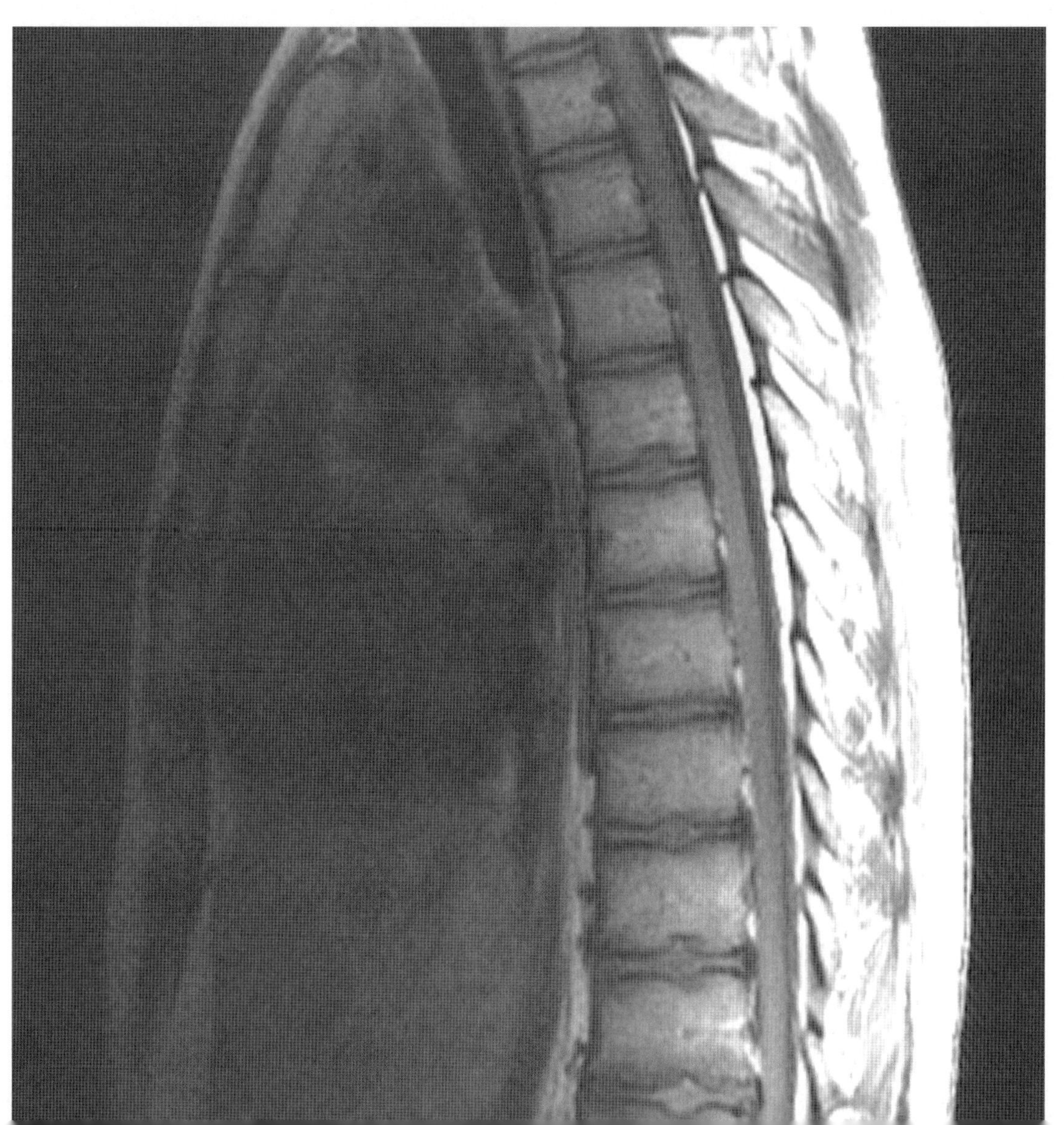

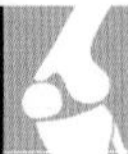

36–1 Scheuermann Disease (Juvenile Kyphosis, Vertebral Osteochondrosis)

Rajendra Kumar

PRESENTATION

Progressive back pain

FINDINGS

Discogenic degenerative changes are seen on sagittal T1-weighted and fat-saturated T2-weighted MR images of the thoracic spine consisting of disk space narrowing, endplate irregularity, and presence of Schmorl nodes without marginal osteophytes. A mild wedge deformity of T12 vertebral body is present with mild kyphosis at T11-T12.

DIFFERENTIAL DIAGNOSES

- *Discitis:* In this condition, there is narrowing of the disk space with bony destruction at the apposing endplates and paraspinal soft tissue edema.
- *Spondylosis deformans:* The findings on radiographs and MR images are similar to those seen with Scheuermann disease; however, marginal osteophytes are invariably present at the affected vertebrae, and the disease affects the elderly.

COMMENTS

The patient is a 15-year-old boy with progressive back pain. Scheuermann disease, an autosomal dominant disorder, is the most common cause of kyphosis in skeletally immature adolescents. The exact etiology is not known; however, chronic physical stress on congenitally weak vertebrae may be responsible for the retarded growth of the anterior cartilage at the vertebral endplates resulting in anteriorly wedged vertebrae and irregular endplates. The condition is seen more often in adolescent boys between the ages of 13 and 17 years. The disease can be asymptomatic, and discovered incidentally on lateral radiographs of the thoracic spine. In other cases, exaggerated thoracic kyphosis or back pain may bring the patient to medical attention. On lateral radiographs of the thoracic spine, irregularity of the superior and inferior endplates of at least three contiguous thoracic vertebrae is seen with disk space narrowing and anterior wedge vertebral body deformity of 5 degrees or more, resulting in kyphosis. The kyphosis of normal thoracic spine varies between 25 to 40 degrees. However, in Scheuermann disease the thoracic kyphosis is >45 degrees. The thoracic spine is most often involved (75%), followed by thoracolumbar (20–25%) and lumbar spine (0–5%). Narrowing of the disk spaces at the affected levels resembles spondylosis deformans; however, no osteophytes are present and the patient is young. Rarely, disk herniation may occur. Anterior disk herniation may lead to a limbus vertebra. MRI not only confirms the radiographic findings, but also demonstrates Schmorl nodes and disk herniation with advantage.

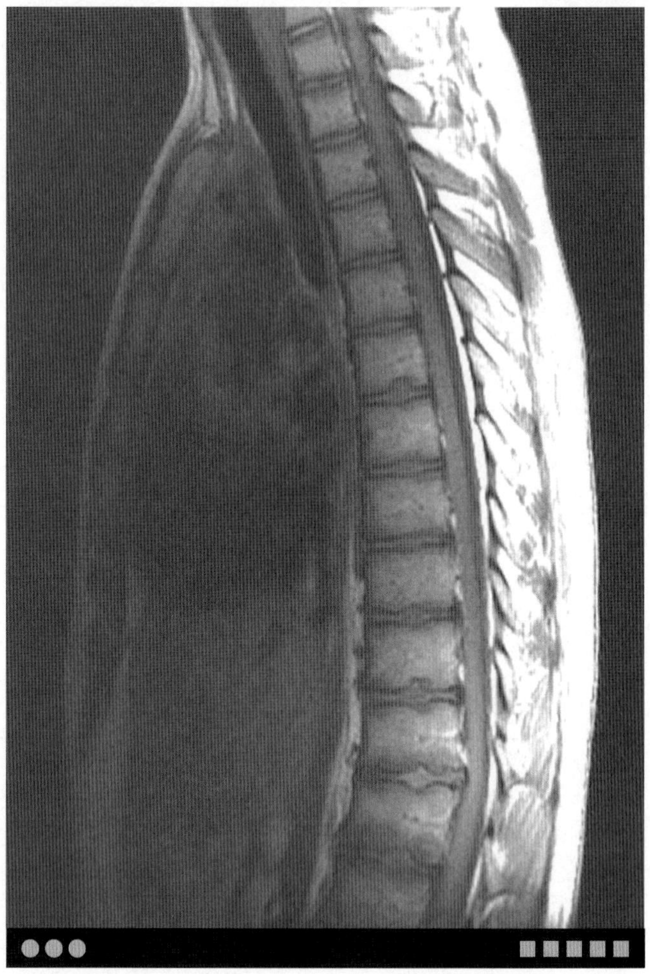

A. Scheuermann disease: Sagittal T1-weighted thoracic spine MR image shows multilevel desiccated disks with disk space narrowing, endplate irregularity, and presence of Schmorl nodes.

PEARLS

- **Adolescent patient with back pain or kyphosis.**
- **Radiographic findings of spondylosis; however, without osteophytosis.**
- **No bony destruction or paraspinal abscess.**

ADDITIONAL IMAGES

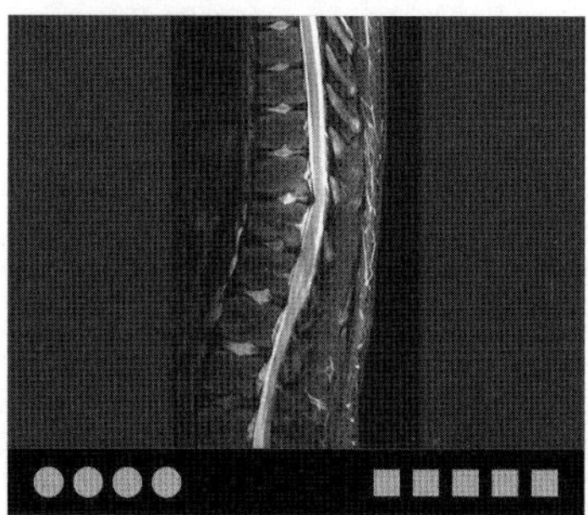

B. Scheuermann disease: Sagittal fat-saturated T2-weighted thoracolumbar spine MR image shows multilevel desiccated disks with disk space narrowing, endplate irregularity, and presence of Schmorl nodes. A posteriorly protruded disk is present at T11-T12 with epidural impression and sharp angle kyphosis.

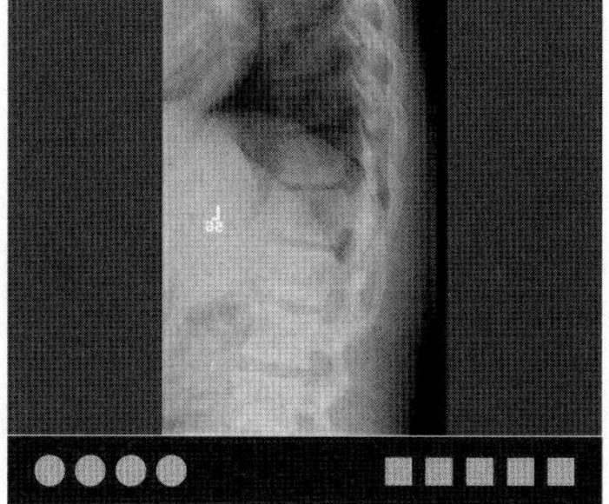

C. Scheuermann disease: A coned-down lateral radiograph of the thoracolumbar junction shows disk space narrowing and endplate irregularity of the lower thoracic vertebrae with anterior wedge compression deformity of T12 and mild kyphosis at T11-T12. Note absence of marginal osteophytes.

IMAGE KEY

Common

Rare

Typical

Unusual

DIFFERENTIAL DIAGNOSES IMAGES

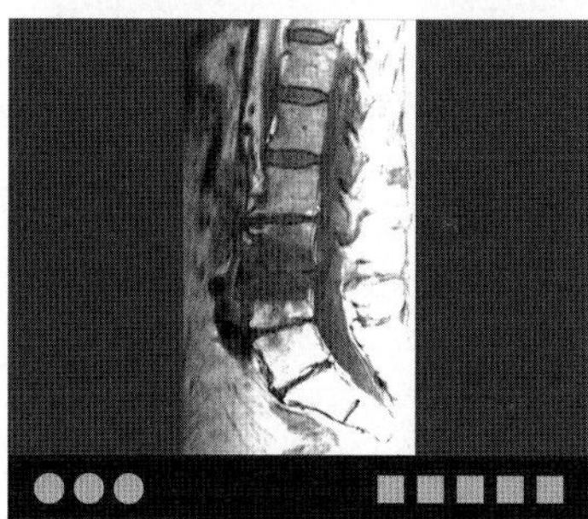

D. Discitis: Sagittal T1-weighted image of the lumbar spine shows marked narrowing of the disk space at L3-L4 with bony destruction at the adjoining endplates.

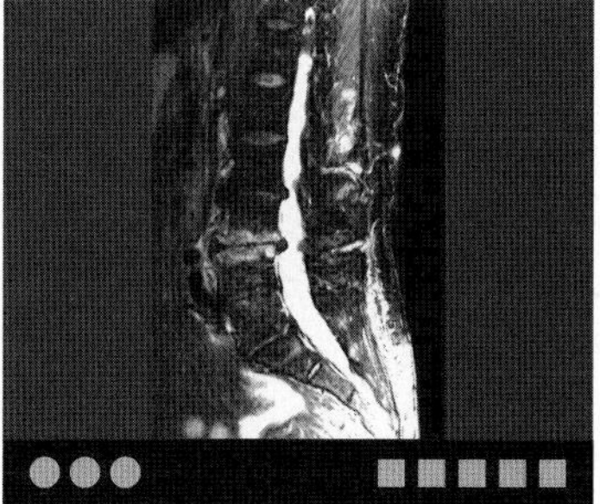

E. Discitis: Sagittal FS T2-weighted image of the lumbar spine shows marked narrowing of the disk space at L3-L4 with bony destruction at the adjoining endplates. Note marrow edema in the involved vertebral bodies and paraspinal soft tissue edema/abscess anteriorly presenting as hyperintense T2-weighted signal.

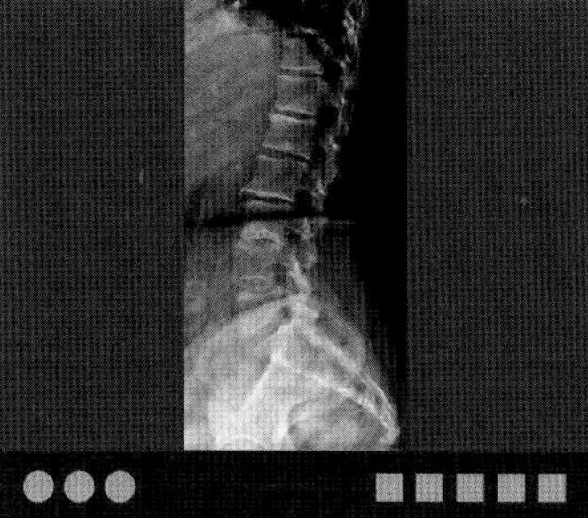

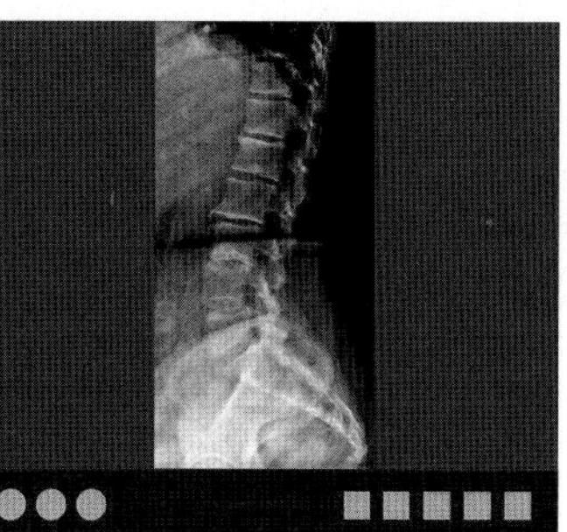

F. Spondylosis deformans: This is a 68-year-old man: A lateral radiograph of lumbar spine shows disk space narrowing and eburnation at T12-L4 with anterior osteophytes at L2-L3. Also note presence of vacuum phenomena at several levels.

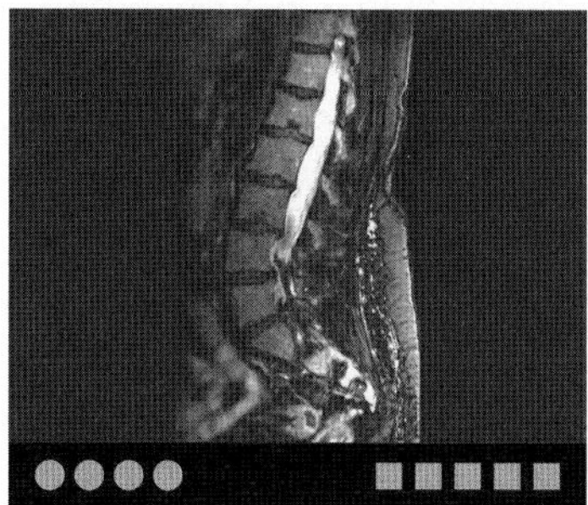

G. Spondylosis deformans: Sagittal fat-saturated T2-weighted MR image shows multilevel degenerative discogenic disease with Schmorl nodes in the lumbar spine. Note presence of osteophytes at several levels.

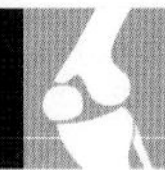

36–2 Os Odontoideum

Ingrid B. Kjellin

PRESENTATION

Neck pain after mild trauma

FINDINGS

MRI shows two separate marrow-containing structures superior to the axis body, and mild hypertrophy of the anterior arch of C1.

DIFFERENTIAL DIAGNOSES

- *Odontoid fractures are three types:* Type I fracture is a fracture through the tip of the odontoid process. Type 2 fracture is a fracture at the junction of the odontoid and the body of C2, and type 3 fracture is seen adjacent to the base of the odontoid with extension into the body of C2.
- *Odontoid erosions:* These are seen in arthritic conditions, such as rheumatoid arthritis, psoriasis, and pyrophosphate arthropathy. An eroded odontoid process can fracture after minor trauma.
- *Os terminale:* This is a normal ossicle located at the superior tip of the odontoid process. The typical round and corticated appearance of an os terminale allows easy differentiation from a Type I odontoid fracture.
- *Odontoid hypoplasia:* This is often associated with various syndromes, such as spondyloepiphyseal dysplasia, achondroplasia, Klippel-Feil syndrome, Morquio's disease, Hurler's disease, metatropic dysplasia, and Down syndrome. Increased rotation of the atlas, caused by incompetence of the transverse ligament, may be present.

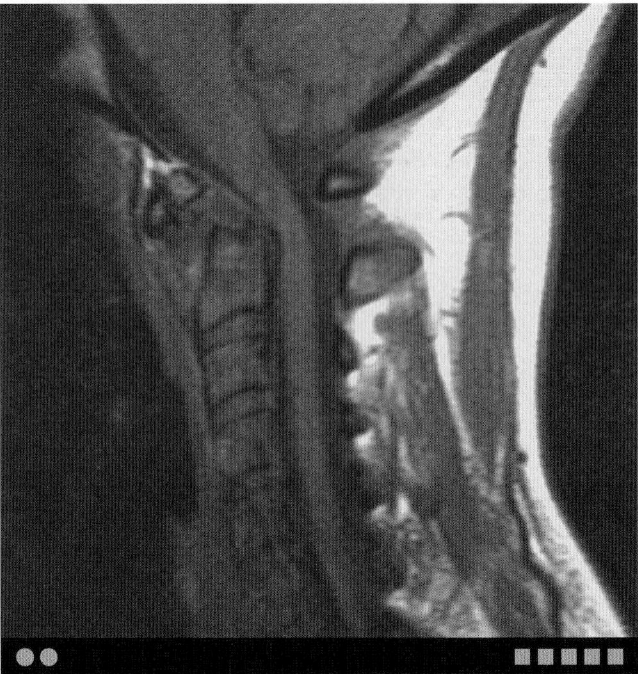

A. Os odontoideum: A sagittal T1-weighted image shows absence of the dens. There is a small ossicle just below the basion (anterior margin of the foramen magnum). The anterior arch of C1 lies too far anterior to the C2 vertebral body.

COMMENTS

The patient is a 40-year-old female, who was assaulted, and was initially thought to have a Type II odontoid fracture. An os odontoideum is an ossicle located superior to the base of the dens and is separated from it by a lucent gap. This gap is wider than that of a fracture. There is controversy over whether the os odontoideum represents a congenital anomaly or a nonunited Type II odontoid fracture. One theory describes an early insult to the odontoid process with overgrowth of the os terminale. There are two types of os odontoideum, an orthotopic variety and a dystopic variety. In the former, the ossicle is in the expected position of the dens. In the latter, the ossicle lies immediately under the anterior foramen magnum, to which it may be fused. The anterior arch of the atlas is often hypertrophied, which could be a useful finding when attempting to differentiate an os odontoideum from a Type II odontoid fracture. The transverse ligament may not be appropriately attached, which could lead to instability. A secondary sign of instability is signal abnormality in the cervical cord. Some congenital conditions, such as Down syndrome, spondyloepiphyseal dysplasia, Morquio's syndrome, and the Klippel-Feil anomaly, have an increased incidence of os odontoideum. The treatment is conservative, unless there is instability (>3 mm translation on flexion–extension radiographs) or neurological symptoms, in which case posterior C1-C2 fusion is performed.

PEARLS

- **Os odontoideum is an osseous structure positioned cephalad to the body of C2.**
- **Hypertrophy of the anterior arch of C1 is a useful finding when attempting to differentiate an os odontoideum from a Type II odontoid fracture.**
- **Signs of instability include abnormal flexion–extension radiographs and signal abnormality in the cervical spinal cord on MRI, and is treated with posterior surgical fusion.**

ADDITIONAL IMAGES

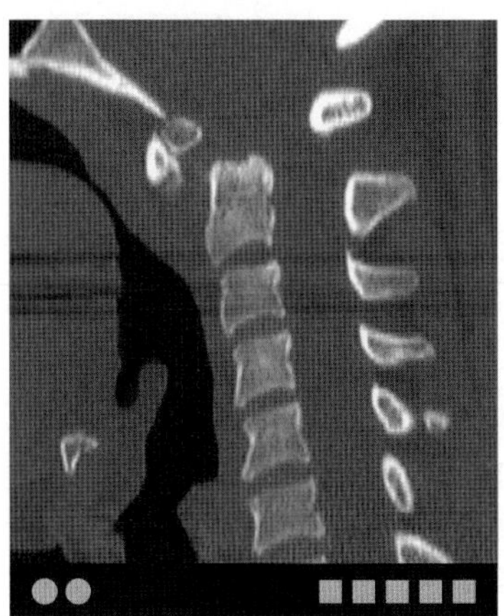

B. Os odontoideum: CT of the cervical spine in the sagittal plane shows the small well-corticated ossicle, consistent with an os odontoideum. There is mild hypertrophy of the anterior arch of C1.

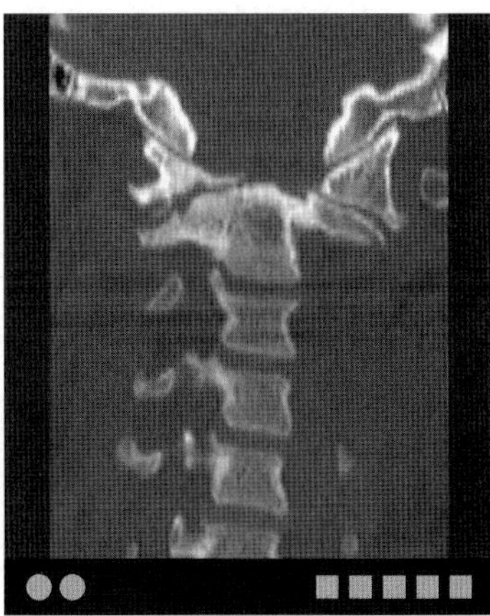

C. Os odontoideum: CT of the cervical spine in the coronal plane shows chronic arthritis between the lateral masses of C1 and C2 on the right, which could be related to chronic instability.

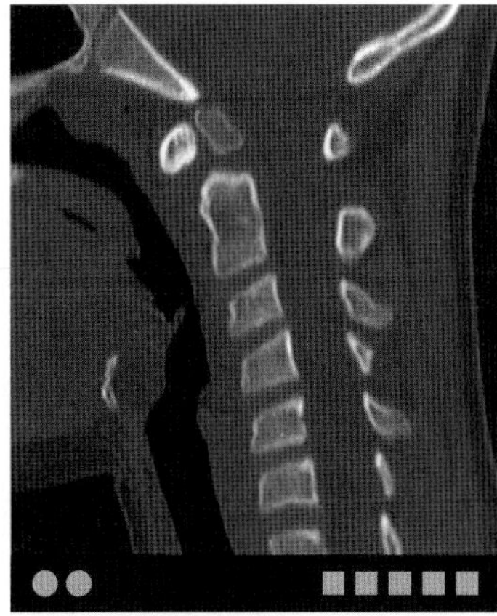

D. Os odontoideum: In a different case CT in the sagittal plane shows a larger os odontoideum with marked hypertrophy of the anterior arch of the atlas.

IMAGE KEY

Common

Rare

Typical

Unusual

DIFFERENTIAL DIAGNOSES IMAGES

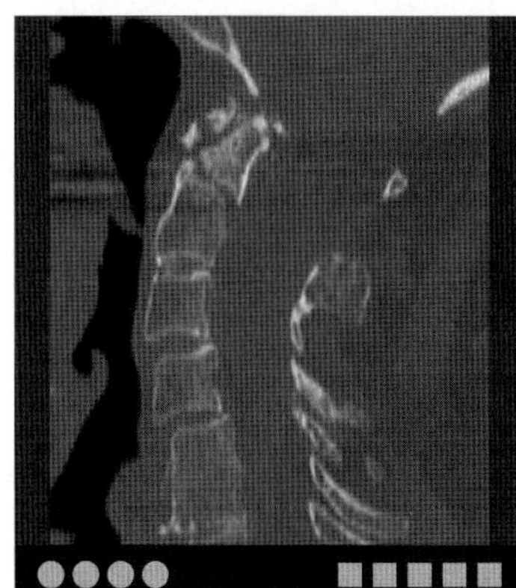

E. Type 2 odontoid fracture: CT of the cervical spine in the sagittal plane shows a nonacute, nondisplaced fracture through the odontoid at the junction with the C2 vertebral body. There is also a transverse fracture through the anterior arch of C1.

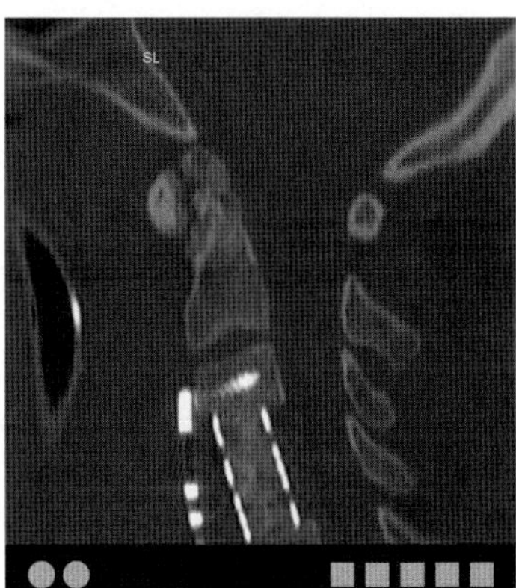

F. Os terminale: A well-corticated ossicle is seen along the superior margin of the odontoid process on a CT with sagittal reformatted images.

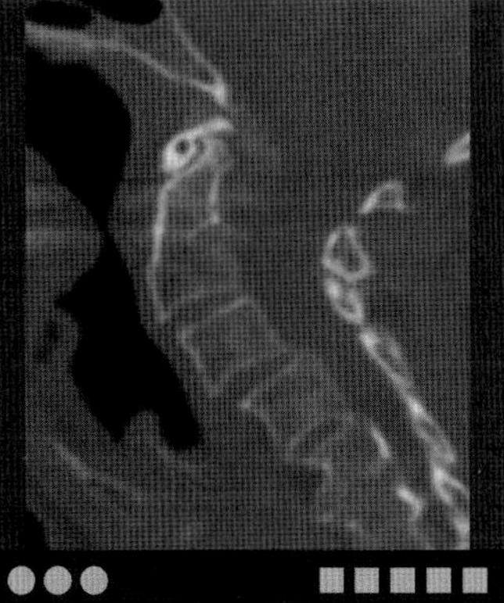

G. Odontoid erosions in pyrophosphate arthropathy: CT of the cervical spine in the sagittal plane shows decreased size of the odontoid and the anterior arch of C1, with a surrounding calcified mass (crystal deposition in a region of synovial thickening).

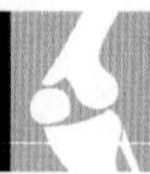

36–3 Spondyloepiphyseal Dysplasia

Ingrid B. Kjellin

PRESENTATION

Dwarfism, hypotonia, and short extremities

FINDINGS

MRI shows pear-shaped vertebral bodies with decreased height, shorter than the intervertebral disks.

DIFFERENTIAL DIAGNOSES

- *Achondroplasia:* Short rectangular vertebral bodies with relatively wide disk spaces and narrowing of the distal lumbar spinal canal are typical findings.
- *Hypothyroidism:* Marked vertebral body flattening with a beak-like projection from the anterior inferior aspect of lumbar vertebrae are present in neonates. There is also a delay in skeletal age.
- Other dysplasias with universal platyspondyly in the neonates and young children are metatropic dysplasia, thanatophoric dysplasia, achondrogenesis, and hypophosphatasia,
- The differential diagnosis for universal platyspondyly detected in older children includes spondyloepiphyseal dysplasia, spondylometaphyseal dysplasia, osteogenesis imperfecta, osteoporosis, mucopolysaccharidosis, Dyggve–Melchior–Clausen dysplasia, pseudoachondroplasia, Kniest syndrome, Stickler syndrome, and dysosteosclerosis.

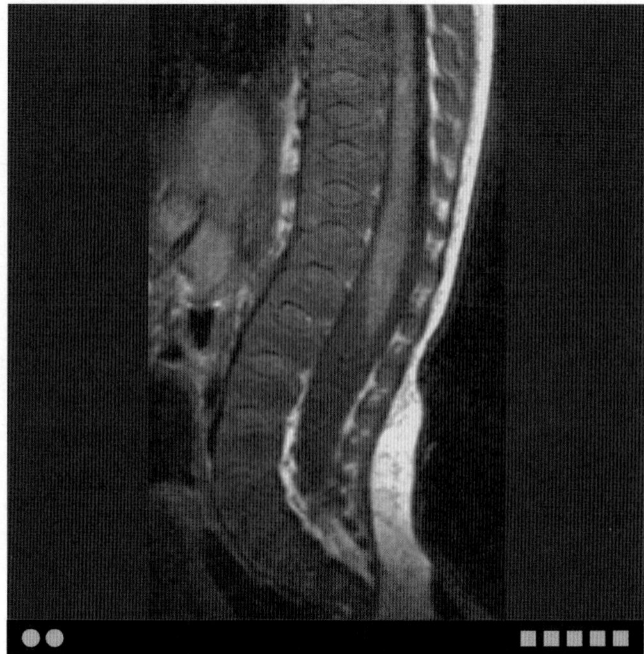

A. Spondyloepiphyseal dysplasia: A sagittal T1-weighted image of the lumbar spine shows small, pear-shaped vertebral bodies. There is also a mild kyphosis at the thoracolumbar junction.

COMMENTS

The patient is an 18-month-old girl with dwarfism, hypotonia, and short extremities. The spondyloepiphyseal dysplasias may occur in the congenita form or the tarda form, with considerable genetic heterogeneity. In the congenita form there are even lethal variants. Spondyloepiphyseal dysplasia congenita is characterized by short-trunk dwarfism, mild shortening of the limbs, flat face, short neck, lumbar lordosis, thoracolumbar kyposis, and joint restriction. Imaging findings include universal platyspondyly, kyphoscoliosis, and delayed epiphyseal ossification. In the infant, the vertebral bodies are pear-shaped, and in the child, the vertebral bodies have anterior wedging and irregularity. Odontoid hypoplasia may occur, and can be associated with atlantoaxial instability. Spondyloepiphyseal dysplasia tarda typically becomes evident between the ages of 5 and 10 years, with complaints of pain in the back and hips. In distinction to the congenita form, the face and extremities are normal. Radiographic findings are most prominent in the lumbar region and consist of diminished height of the anterior portion of the vertebral bodies with a hump-shaped area of bone on the central and posterior regions of the endplates. The disk spaces are narrow posteriorly and wide anteriorly. Abnormal spinal curvatures and odontoid hypoplasia are less frequently seen in spondyloepiphyseal dysplasia tarda than in spondyloepiphyseal dysplasia congenita. There is mild flattening of the epiphyses about large joints. Premature osteoarthritis often develops in both types of spondyloepiphyseal dysplasia.

PEARLS

- **The spondyloepiphyseal dysplasias may occur in the congenital form or the tarda form.**
- **Platyspondyly, kyphoscoliosis, and delayed epiphyseal ossification are important imaging findings.**
- **Odontoid hypoplasia and associated atlantoaxial instability may produce cord compression early in life and require spinal fusion.**
- **Premature osteoarthritis can become disabling.**

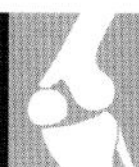

ADDITIONAL IMAGES

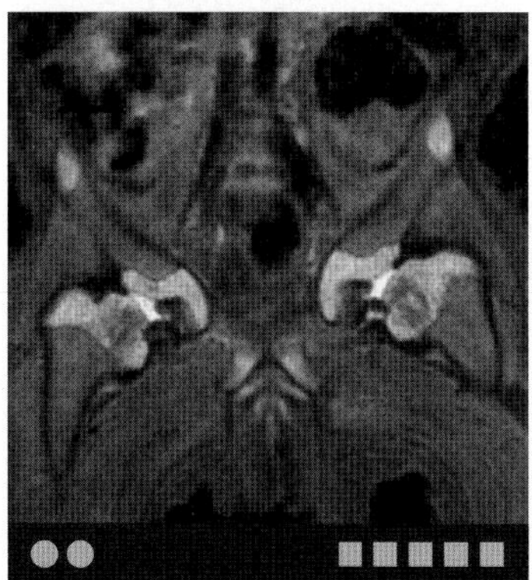

B. Spondyloepiphyseal dysplasia: A coronal STIR image of the pelvis and hips shows delayed ossification of the pelvic bones and proximal femurs, shortening of the femoral necks, decreased size of the femoral heads, and bilateral hip subluxation.

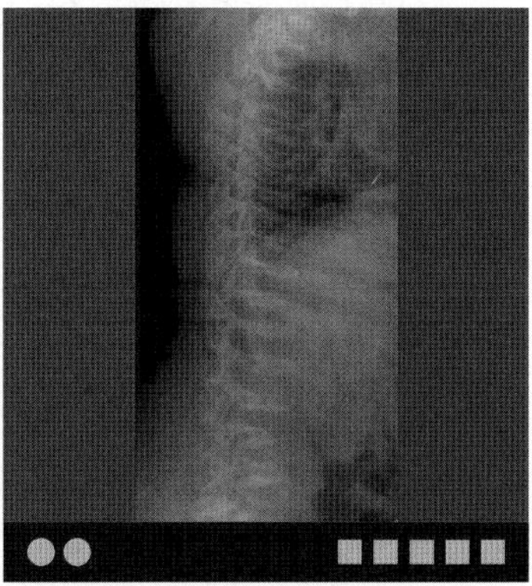

C. Spondyloepiphyseal dysplasia: A lateral radiograph of the spine in a 12-year-old patient shows decreased height of the vertebral bodies with wedging and endplate deformity.

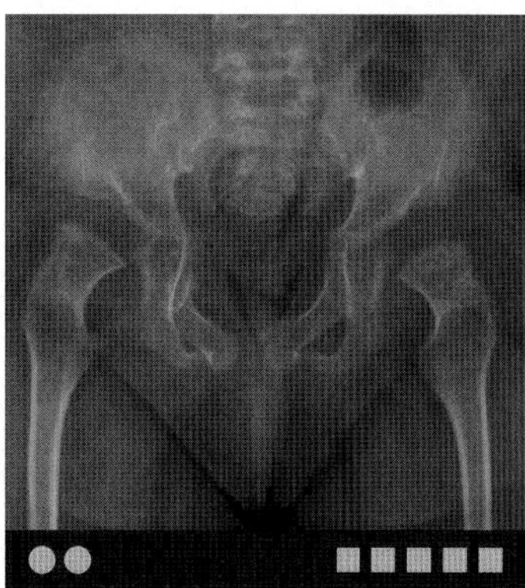

D. Spondyloepiphyseal dysplasia: A frontal radiograph of the pelvis and hips in a 12-year-old patient shows delayed ossification of the femoral heads and bilateral hip subluxation.

IMAGE KEY

Common

Rare

Typical

Unusual

DIFFERENTIAL DIAGNOSES IMAGES

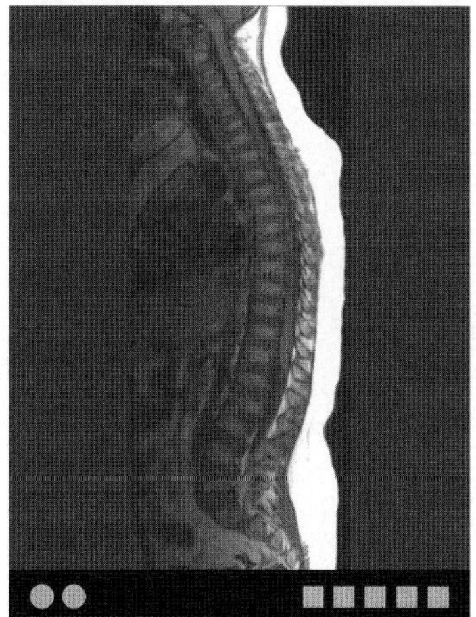

E. Morquio's syndrome: Sagittal T1-weighted, large field-of-view, sagittal MR image of the spine shows platyspondyly, anterior vertebral beaking, and L2 vertebral wedging with an associated focal kyphosis.

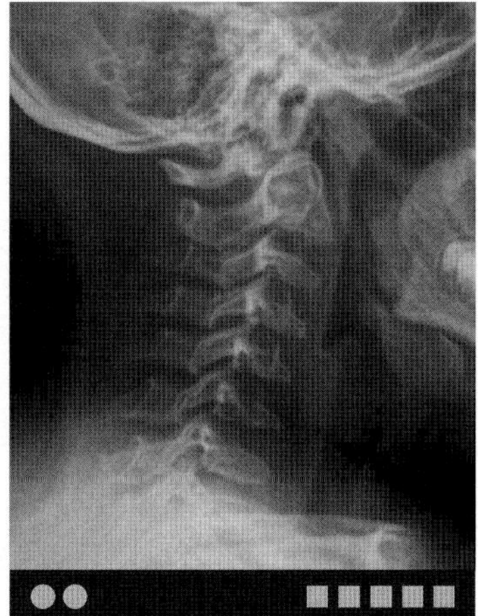

F. Morquio's syndrome: A lateral radiograph of the cervical spine shows platyspondyly and odontoid hypoplasia.

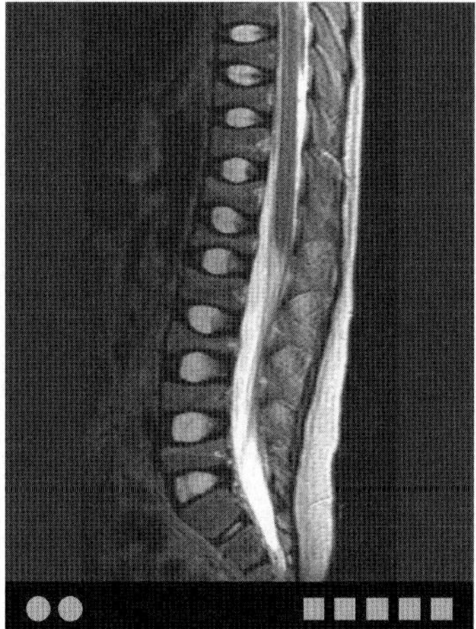

G. Osteogenesis imperfecta: A T2-weighted sagittal image of the lumbar spine shows mildly decreased height of the vertebral bodies, consistent with fractures.

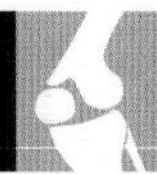

36–4 Diastematomyelia of Thoracic Spine

Ingrid B. Kjellin

PRESENTATION

Severe scoliosis and weakness of the lower extremities

FINDINGS

MRI shows two hemicord, separated by a spur.

DIFFERENTIAL DIAGNOSES

- *Diplomyelia:* This condition is extremely rare
- *Spina bifida:* This condition may be associated with meningomyelocele and lipomyelomeningocele.
- Other congenital vertebral anomalies such as hemivertebra and butterfly vertebra.

COMMENTS

In diastematomyelia, there is splitting of the cord into two parts, which are usually of different sizes. Diastematomyelia is seen in 1% to 5% of patients with scoliosis and in up to 30% of patients with open spinal dysraphism. Over 90% are girls. Clinical features include weakness of the lower extremities, foot deformities, and urinary problems. A cutaneous lesion over the back, such as a patch of hair or a nevus, is seen in 50% to 75% of patients. A mesodermal spur or septum between the two hemicords is not always seen, but when present, it may be fatty, cartilaginous, or osseous. A bony septum frequently extends from the neural arch forward, toward the vertebral body. Spurs can be found in the thoracic and lumbar regions, and can be multiple in 6% of cases. Common radiological findings in diastematomyelia include intersegmental laminar fusion associated with a defect in the neural arch at the same level or at an adjacent level, as well as increased interpediculate distance, scoliosis, kyphosis, and segmentation anomalies (hemivertebra, butterfly vertebra, or block vertebra). MRI is utilized to assess the cord abnormalities. The hemicords are often asymmetric in size and are usually fused above and below the level of splitting. Additional imaging findings include fluid-filled spinal cord cyst, a low-lying conus medullaris, a thickened filum terminale, epidermoids, and dermoids.

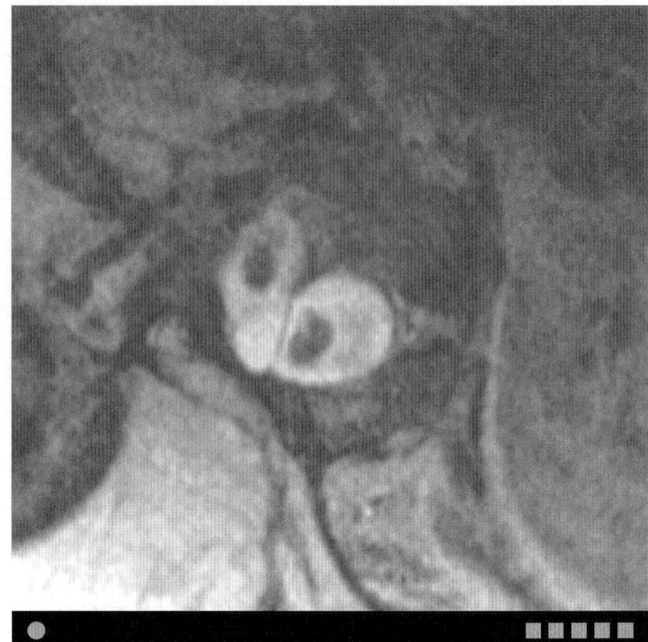

A. Diastematomyelia: An axial T2-weighted image shows a split cord with the two hemicords separated by a sagittally oriented thin, probably fibrous spur. The hemicords are of different sizes, with slightly increased caliber of the left hemicord. A small syrinx is present on the left.

PEARLS

- **Diastematomyelia refers to splitting of the cord into two hemicords by a mesodermal spur.**
- **A spur may be composed of fibrous tissue, fat, cartilage, bone, or a combination of these.**
- **A segmentation anomaly is present in over 95% of patients. Other findings include a low-lying conus medullaris, a thickened filum terminale, epidermoids, and dermoids.**
- **Spurs are multiple in 6% of patients.**

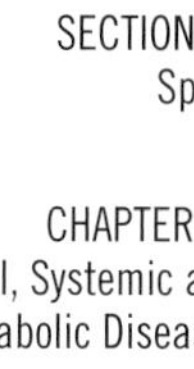

ADDITIONAL IMAGES

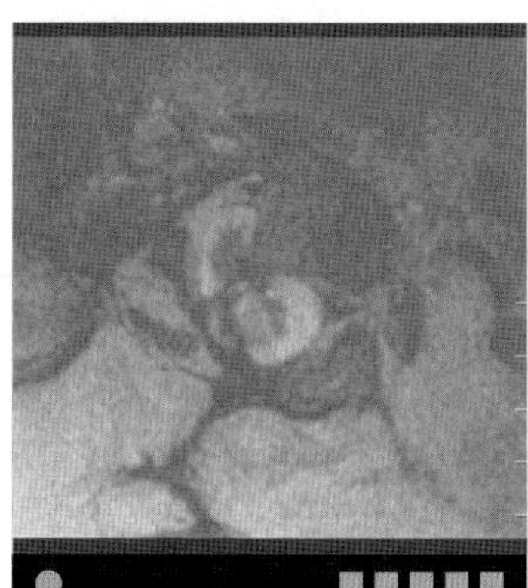

B. Diastematomyelia: An axial T2-weighted image shows the two hemicords with a thicker midline spur at a different level.

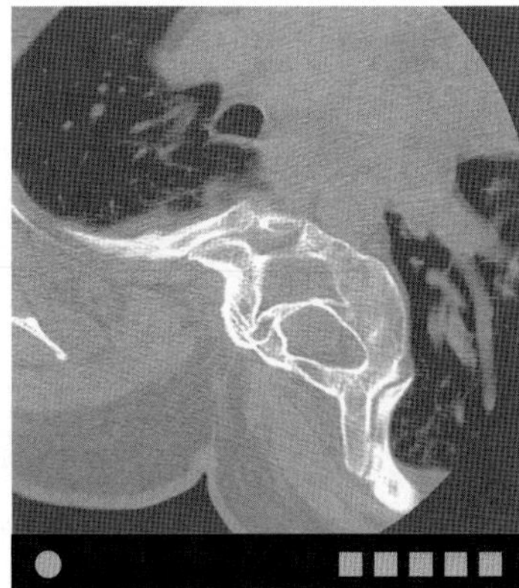

C. Diastematomyelia: An axial CT image of the thoracic spine demonstrates a thick bone spur extending from the lamina to the vertebral body.

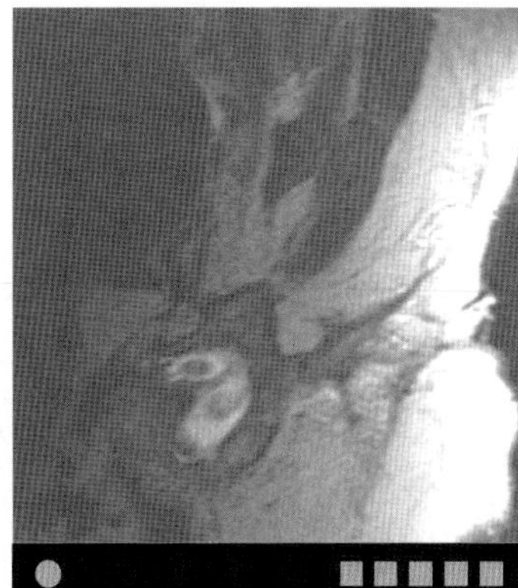

D. Diastematomyelia: Axial T2-weighted image demonstrates again mild asymmetry of the two hemicords. Mild expansion and hyperintense signal of the left hemicord are related to a fluid-filled cyst. Each hemicord has its own pial-arachnoid covering.

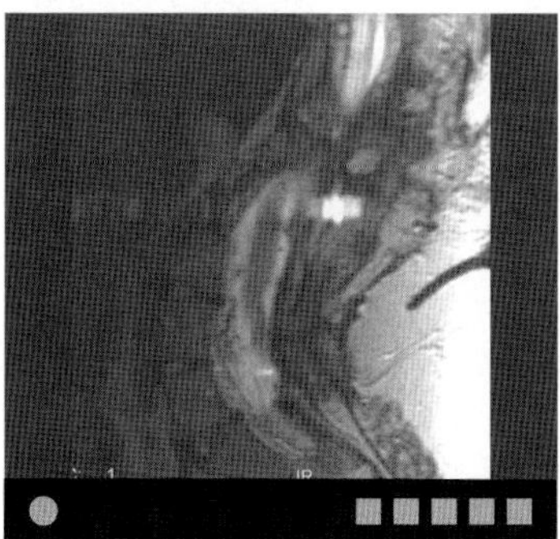

E. Diastematomyelia: A sagittal T2-weighted image shows a low-lying conus medullaris, at L3.

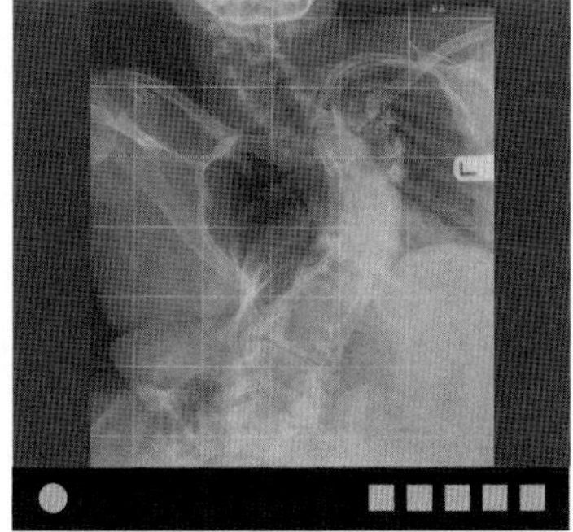

F. Diastematomyelia: A frontal radiograph in the same patient shows marked scoliosis and spinal anomaly with widening of the interpedicular distance at multiple levels.

DIFFERENTIAL DIAGNOSIS IMAGE

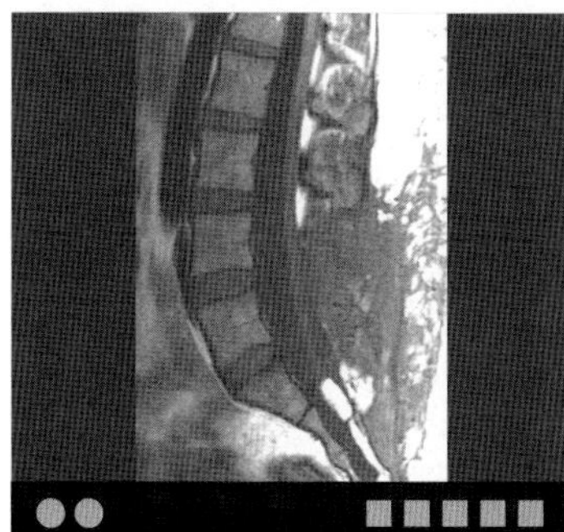

G. Lipomyelomeningocele: A T1-weighted sagittal image shows a low-lying cord in a patient with a history of repair of a myelomeningocele. A lipoma posterior to the neural placode at the level of the sacrum is tethering the cord. The subarachnoid space is expanded posteriorly.

IMAGE KEY

Common

Rare

Typical

Unusual

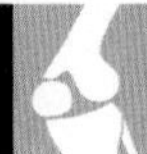

36–5 Diastematomyelia

James Coumas

PRESENTATION

Numbness in left toes with pain in right toes

FINDINGS

MR images show abnormal extension of the spinal cord to the L4 level with a focus of inhomogeneity of the spinal cord at the L3-L4 level. There are associated bony abnormalities of posterior elements of the lumbar spine noted.

DIFFERENTIAL DIAGNOSES

- *Tethered cord:* In this condition, the spinal cord or specifically the conus medullaris extends below the L2 vertebral level and is characterized by a thickened filum terminale. A tethered cord is associated with spina bifida occulta, Chiari malformations, intradural lipoma, myelomeningocele, scoliosis, and hydrosyringomyelia.
- *Spinal dysraphism:* Spinal dysraphism represents a multiplicity of vertebral, spinal cord, and intracranial congenital and acquired abnormalities.
- *Diplomyelia:* With diplomyelia there are two distinct spinal cords (in contrast to hemicords) within two distinct sacs. It is a rare as well as controversial entity, as many authors suggest complementary hemicords rather than true duplication of the spinal cord.

COMMENTS

The patient is an 11-year-old female with a history of prior surgery for a tethered cord. Diastematomyelia is a longitudinal split of the spinal cord with the split most commonly localized to the upper lumbar spine (60%) or lower thoracic spine (25%). Two distinct dural sacs may occur; however, more commonly two hemicords exist in a single dural sac. Associated bony abnormalities are found in 85% of cases. These include spina bifida, hemivertebra, and scoliosis. Diastematomyelia can be seen in conjunction with various congenital and acquired abnormalities including tethered cord, Chiari II malformation, myelomeningocele, and hydrosyringomyelia. There is a strong female predilection for cases presenting in the pediatric age group. Spinal segmentation anomalies with laminar fusion are highly suggestive of diastematomyelia. Diastematomyelia is frequently associated with additional congenital abnormalities requiring extensive diagnostic imaging incorporating CT as well as MR modalities. Because of these associated findings, radiological assessment of the entire spine and skull base and brain is recommended. A cutaneous stigmata such as a hairy patch on the back is not an uncommon clinical finding. The etiology of the "split cord" is a bony (cartilaginous) or fibrous band, which traverses the spinal canal during embryogenesis. It is best shown on CT or CT/myelography.

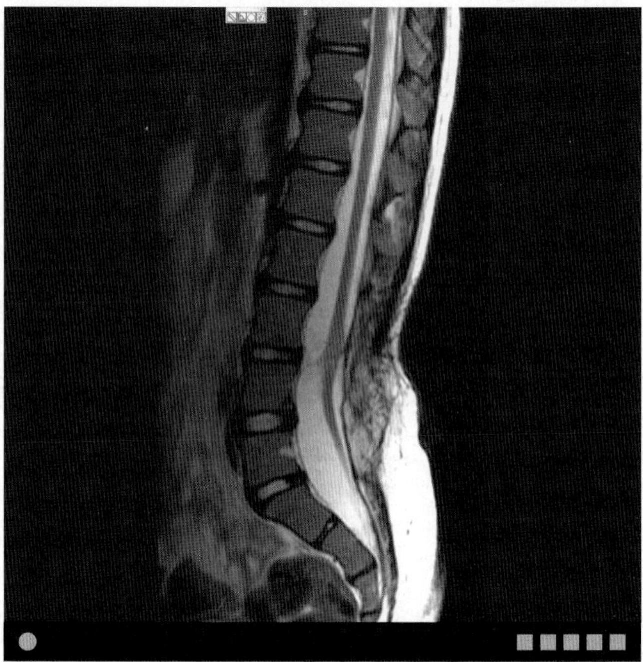

A. Diastematomyelia: Sagittal T2-weighted MR image shows extension of the spinal cord to the L4 level with an oblique horizontal band traversing the cord at the L3-L4 level.

PEARLS

- **Diastematomyelia is frequently associated with additional congenital abnormalities requiring extensive diagnostic imaging incorporating CT as well as MR modalities.**
- **There is a strong female predilection for cases presenting in the pediatric age group.**
- **Spinal segmentation anomalies with laminar fusion are highly suggestive of diastematomyelia.**

ADDITIONAL IMAGES

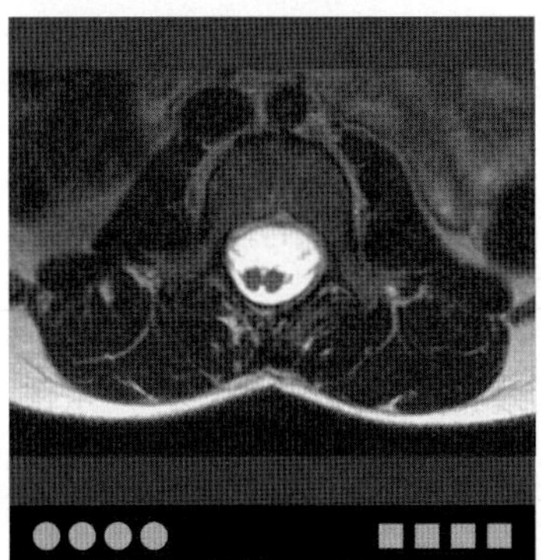

B. Diastematomyelia: Axial T2-weighted MR image shows two hemicords in a single dural sac.

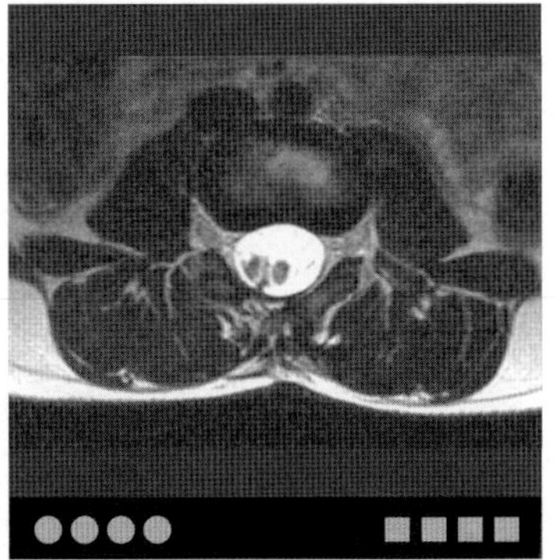

C. Diastematomyelia: Axial T2-weighted MR image shows fibrous band traversing the split in cord.

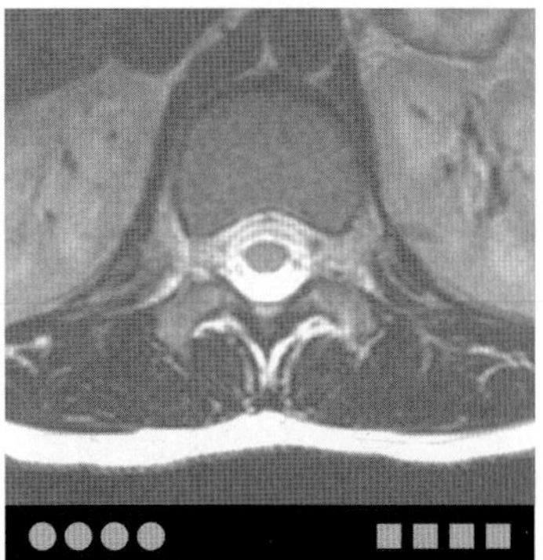

D. Diastematomyelia: Axial T2-weighted MR image shows a normal spinal cord just above the level of the hemicords.

IMAGE KEY

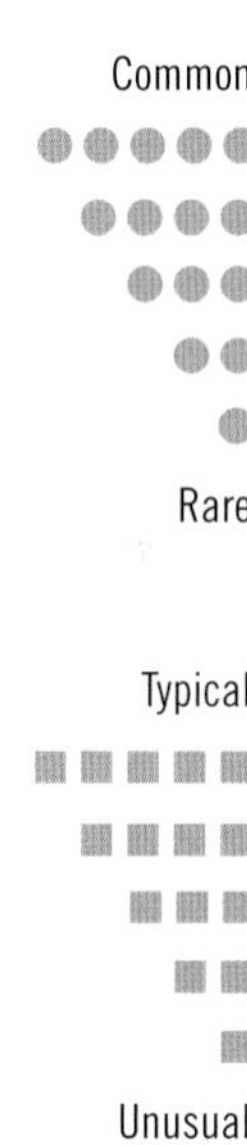

DIFFERENTIAL DIAGNOSES IMAGES

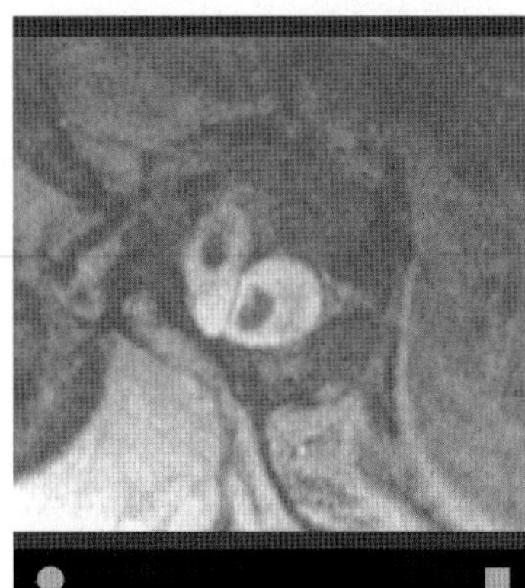

E. Diastematomyelia with separate dural sac: Axial T2-weighted image shows diplomyelia with two distinct dural sacs.

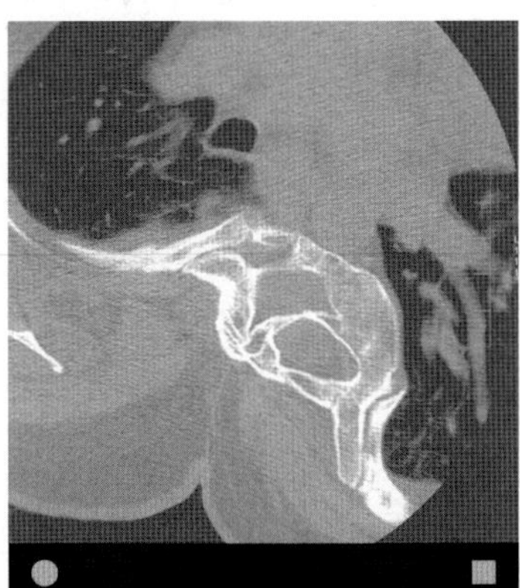

F. Diastematomyelia with separate dural sac: Axial CT scan (same patient as image E).

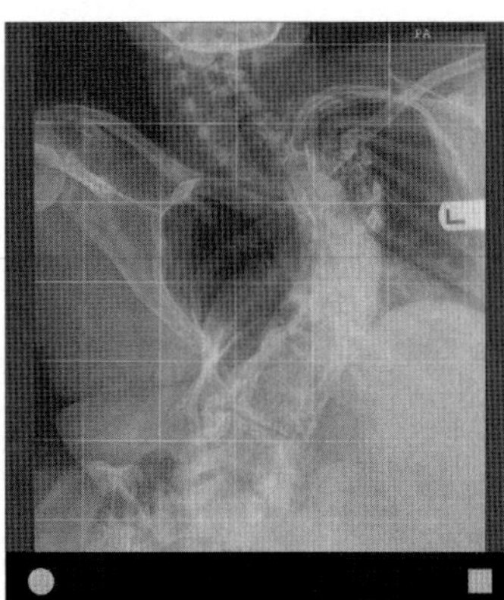

G. Diastematomyelia with separate dural sac: AP radiograph (same patient as images E and F) shows scoliosis with widening of the spinal canal and spinal dysraphism.

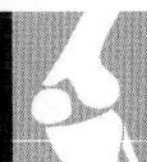

36–6 Achondroplasia

Ingrid B. Kjellin

PRESENTATION

Macrocephaly and mild hypotonia

FINDINGS

MRI shows a constricted skull base with a small foramen magnum. There is also frontal bossing. The ventricles were normal in size.

DIFFERENTIAL DIAGNOSES

- A small foramen magnum may be present in achondrogenesis, thanatophoric dysplasia, metatropic and diastrophic dysplasia, occipitalization of C1, spondyloepiphyseal dysplasia, and Morquio's syndrome.
- Another craniocervical junction disorder is basilar invagination or basilar impression, which is upward displacement of the margins of the foramen magnum and the upper cervical vertebrae into the posterior fossa.
- Odontoid anomalies include aplasia, hypoplasia, and os odontoideum, which commonly produce craniocervical instability. These anomalies may be idiopathic or part of a syndrome, such as Down's syndrome.

COMMENTS

The patient is a 1-year-old girl with craniofacial dysmorphia, consistent with achondroplasia. This is the most common type of dwarfism to involve the spine and craniovertebral junction. It occurs in about 1:25,000 live births, and is autosomal dominant, although approximately 80% of cases are spontaneous mutations. The basic abnormality in achondroplasia is defective enchondral bone formation. The clinical manifestations are short stature, short limbs (rhizomelic micromelia), relative or absolute macrocephaly, prominent forehead, nasal bridge flattening, constricted skull base, thoracolumbar kyphosis in infancy, and increased lumbar lordosis in children and adults. Thoracolumbar scoliosis is common. Foramen magnum stenosis, probably a result of early fusion of basal synchondrosis, occurs in about one-third of cases, and may lead to cervicomedullary compromise below the age of 5 years. Teenagers and adults may be symptomatic from spinal canal stenosis at lower levels, and symptoms often worsen with superimposed degenerative changes. Hydrocephalus occurs in approximately 15% of patients. Imaging findings include a skull that is large as compared to the size of the face, with a narrow skull base.

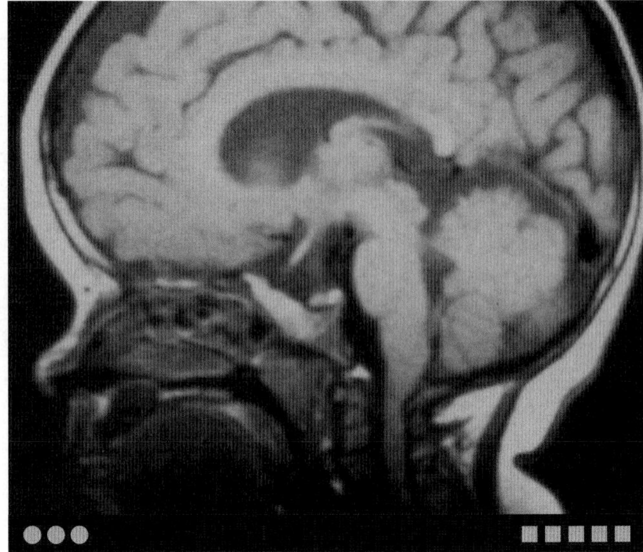

A. Achondroplasia: A sagittal T1-weighted image of the head shows a small foramen magnum with impingement of the upper cervical cord by the posterior lip of the foramen magnum. There is also prominence of the forehead.

The small size of the foramen magnum is best appreciated with CT and MR imaging. The spinal canal is small with short pedicles and decreased interpediculate distances. The vertebral bodies are short and rectangular. There is flaring of the iliac wings with small sacrosciatic notches and horizontal acetabular roofs. Shortening of the tubular bones and ribs are also seen.

PEARLS

- **Achondroplasia is a defect of enchondral bone formation and is autosomal dominant, but most cases are spontaneous mutations.**
- **Clinical manifestations include short stature with short limbs, a large head with a prominent forehead, abnormal kyphosis and lordosis.**
- **Compression of the spinal cord, cauda equina and nerve roots may develop at any age and may lead to neurologic problems.**

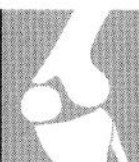

ADDITIONAL IMAGES

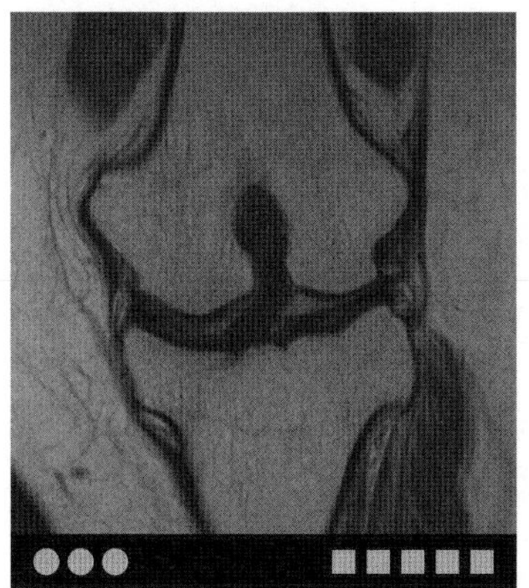

B. Achondroplasia: A coronal proton density image of the knee shows severe deformity of the femoral condyles and tibial plateaus with a narrowed intercondylar notch.

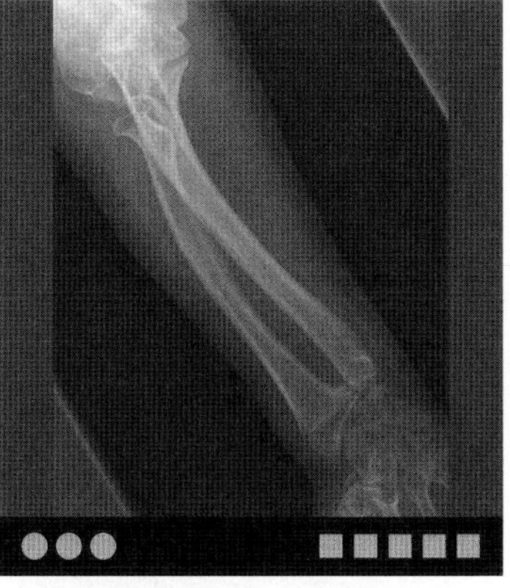

C. Achondroplasia: A frontal radiograph of the forearm shows short tubular bones, mild bowing, and mild metaphyseal flaring.

DIFFERENTIAL DIAGNOSES IMAGES

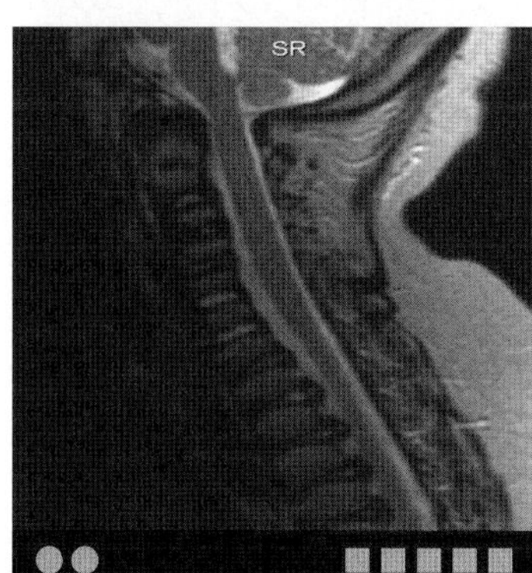

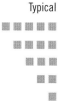

D. Morquio's syndrome: A T2-weighted sagittal MR image shows a mildly narrowed foramen magnum, mild platyspondyly, and vertebral beaking.

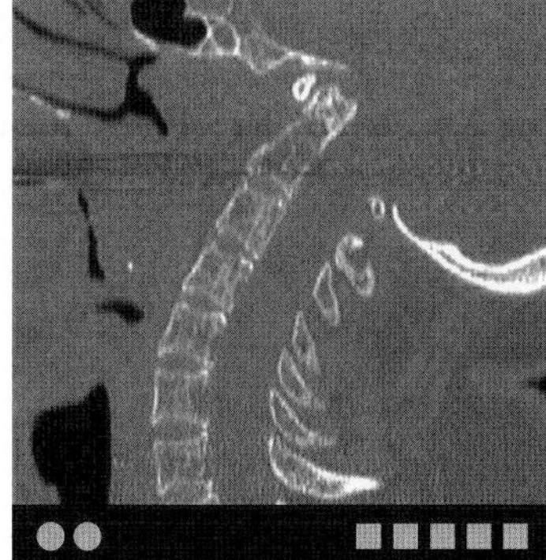

E. Osteogenesis imperfecta: A CT image in the sagittal plane shows basilar impression with high-riding dens. There is upward displacement also of the margins of the foramen magnum.

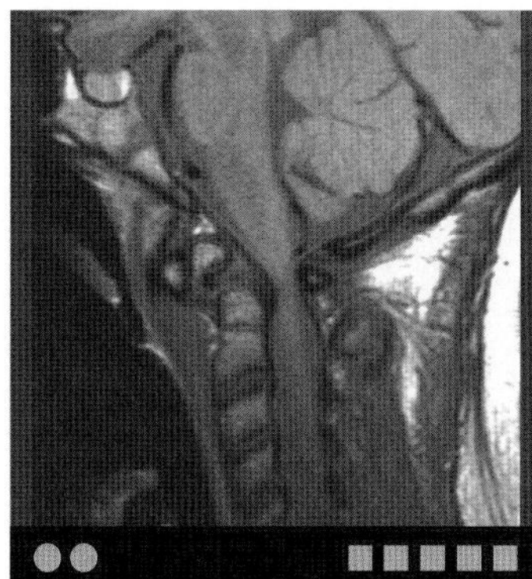

F. Down's syndrome: A sagittal T1-weighted image shows a small ossicle below the anterior margin of the foramen magnum, consistent with an os odontoideum. There is also atlantoaxial instability with associated narrowing of spinal canal.

IMAGE KEY

Common

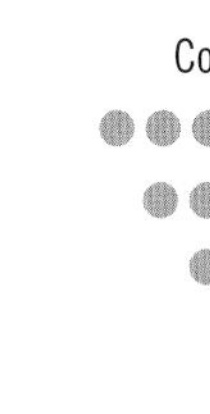
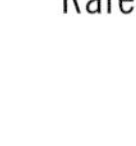

Rare

Typical

Unusual

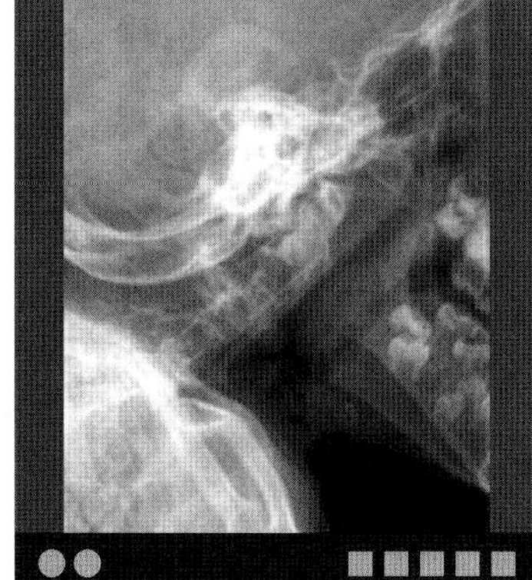

G. Klippel–Feil anomaly: A lateral radiograph of the cervical spine shows fusion of several cervical vertebrae, including C2 and C3. There is also occipitalization of the atlas.

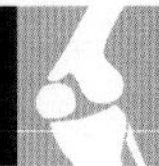

36–7 Osteogenesis Imperfecta

Peyman Borghei and Jamshid Tehranzadeh

PRESENTATION

Low back pain

FINDINGS

MRI shows compression and increased T2 marrow signal in T11 and L4 representing acute fracture. Posterior cortical bulging of T11 and L4 vertebral bodies is also evident. Other findings include increased disk space height and widening of the spinal canal.

DIFFERENTIAL DIAGNOSES

- *Osteoporotic compression fracture:* This is a common finding especially in older postmenopausal females.
- *Battered child syndrome:* This diagnosis often comes in differential with osteogenesis imperfecta (OI) in long bone. Battered child syndrome is associated with metaphyseal corner fracture (bucket handle fracture), posterior rib fracture, and multiple fractures at different stages of healing.

COMMENTS

The patient is a 4-year-old girl with osteogenesis imperfecta complaining of back pain, diagnosed with acute fracture of the vertebrae. OI is a disorder with congenital bone fragility, caused by mutations in the genes that code for Type I procollagen. Patients present with fractures after minor trauma and may bruise easily. Other features include blue sclera, dental problems, soft skull, hyperlaxity of joints, and thin loose skin. There are two related clinical types: (1) Congenital type which is autosomal dominant, manifests at birth and is the lethal variety; (2) Tarda type which is autosomal recessive, manifests after birth and is the nonlethal variety. Radiography shows diffuse osteoporosis, cortical thinning, and defective cortical bone with multiple cystic areas and increased diameter of proximal humerus and femur. Other features include evidence of multiple fractures, pseudoarthrosis, and bowing. The consequences of multiple long bone fractures and bowing are short stature and limb deformity. There is no mental retardation in this disease. Spine radiography may show biconcave vertebral bodies, Schmorl's node, widened canal, and increased height of intervertebral disk space. MRI may show signs of acute fracture as decreased marrow signal intensity on T1-weighted and increased marrow signal intensity on T2-weighted images representing marrow edema and fracture.

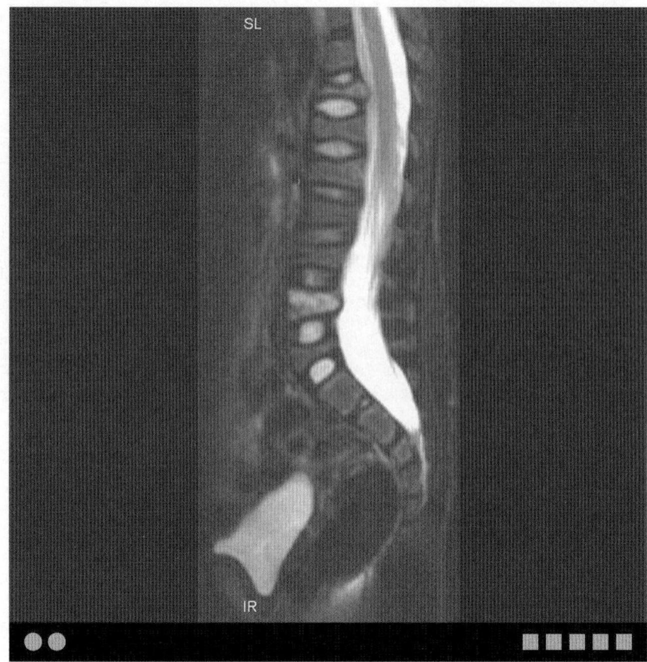

A. Osteogenesis imperfecta: Sagittal T2-weighted fat-saturated image shows partial compression and increased signal intensity in L4 and T11 caused by acute fracture and marrow edema.

PEARLS

- **Osteogenesis imperfecta is a connective tissue disorder characterized by severe osteoporosis, multiple skeletal fractures, soft and brittle bones, blue sclera, and easy bruising of skin.**
- **The congenital type manifests at birth and is lethal; however, the tarda type manifests later and is associated with morbidity.**
- **Radiograph shows diffuse osteoporosis, multiple fractures, widening of spinal canal, flattened vertebrae, and increased disk spaces.**
- **MRI may show evidence of acute fractures and bone marrow edema.**

ADDITIONAL IMAGES

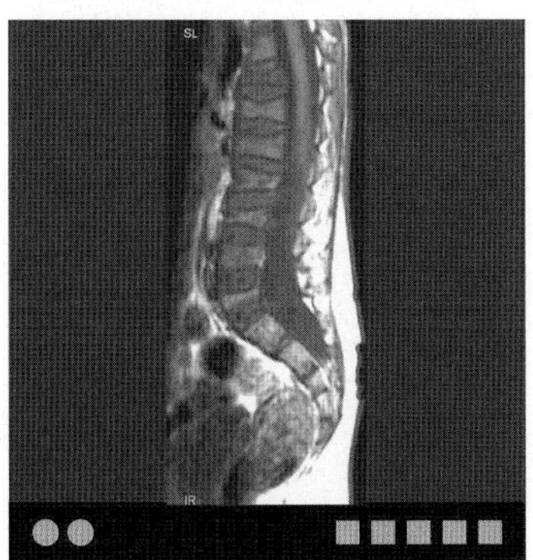

B. Osteogenesis imperfecta: Sagittal T1-weighted image shows flattened vertebrae and increased disk height. Marrow edema caused by acute fractures at L4 and T11 is noted as decreased marrow signal.

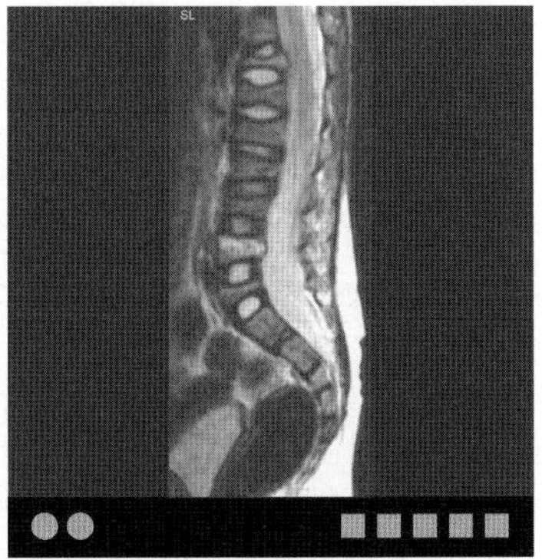

C. Osteogenesis imperfecta: Sagittal T2-weighted image shows increased signal intensity and marrow edema at the level of L4 and T11. Also note well-hydrated disks and widened spinal canal.

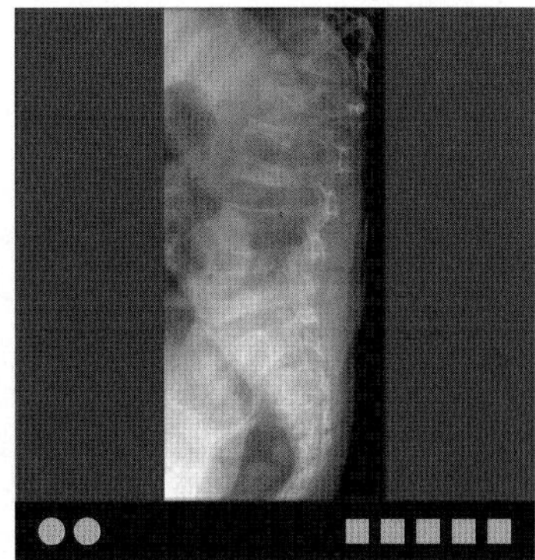

D. Osteogenesis imperfecta: Lateral radiography of lumbar spine shows flattened vertebrae and increased intervertebral disk spaces. There is good vertebral alignment.

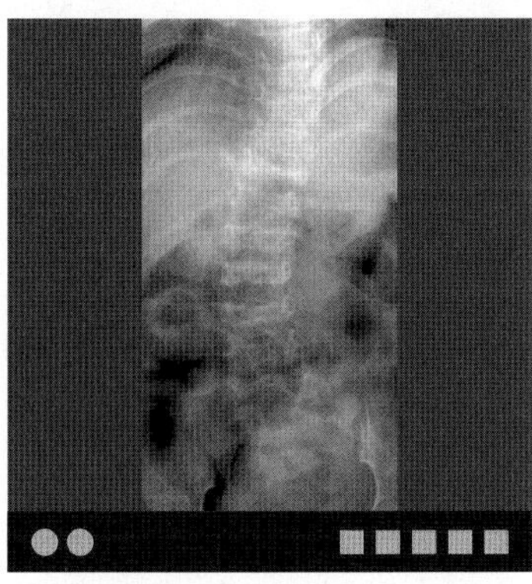

E. Osteogenesis imperfecta: AP radiograph of the lumbar spine shows osteoporosis and flattened vertebrae.

DIFFERENTIAL DIAGNOSES IMAGES

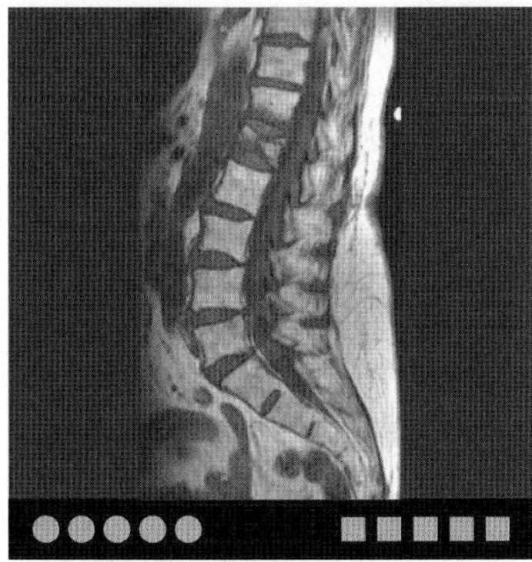

F. Compression fracture: Sagittal T1-weighted image shows decreased marrow signal and compression fracture of L1 vertebrae caused by osteoporosis in a 72-year-old woman. Also note decreased signal intensity in the lower end plate of T12 caused by partial compression.

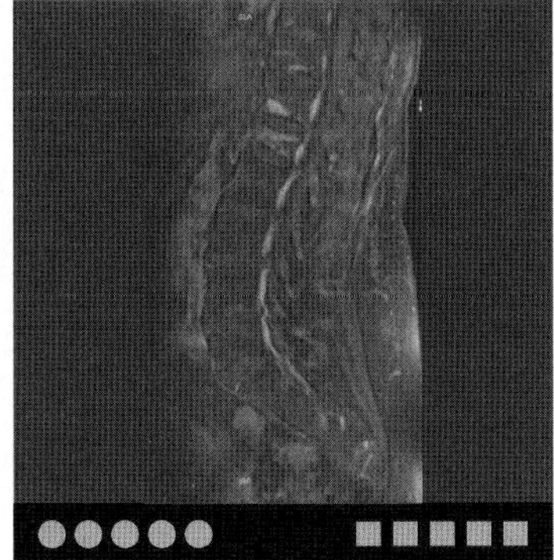

G. Compression fracture: Sagittal T1-weighted fat-saturated post-contrast image shows compression of L1 and T12 demonstrating contrast enhancement caused by acute fracture.

IMAGE KEY

Common

●●●●●
●●●●
●●●
●●
●

Rare

Typical

■■■■■
■■■■
■■■
■■
■

Unusual

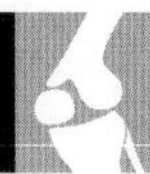

36–8 Ossification of the Posterior Longitudinal Ligament (OPLL)

Tatiana Voci

PRESENTATION

Arm weakness and paresthesias

FINDINGS

Radiograph, CT, and MRI of the cervical spine demonstrates bulky flowing ossifications posterior to the vertebral bodies with a characteristic appearance of "inverted T" shape. MRI shows linear low T1 and T2 signal ossification.

DIFFERENTIAL DIAGNOSES

- *Extruded disk:* Originate from disk level and is centered at a single disk space with upward and downward migration along the adjacent vertebral bodies posteriorly.
- *Osteochondroma:* Similar to OPLL, this also can result from head and neck radiation and may mimic OPLL.
- *Meningioma:* Although low in signal on precontrast T1-weighted image, enhances densely and reveals a dural tail.
- *Epidural abscess or hematoma:* These are associated with adjacent soft tissue inflammation and edema of the bone marrow. There is heterogeneous signal intensity in the epidural hematoma caused by hemorrhagic products and rim enhancement in the epidural abscess.

COMMENTS

Ossification of the posterior longitudinal ligament is most common in the Asian population with an incidence of approximately 2%. The estimated incidence in Caucasians is significantly less (0.2%). Patients can present with symptoms of spinal stenosis or may present acutely secondary to cord contusion with even minimal trauma. Most patients are symptom-free. Ossification most commonly involves the posterior longitudinal ligament of the cervical spine but can also affect the thoracic and lumbar spine. The etiology is unknown but 20% of cases are associated with diffuse idiopathic skeletal hyperostosis (DISH). The ossification can be directly adjacent to the vertebral bodies or separated by connective tissue. OPLL should be distinguished from DISH as well as from ossification of the ligamentum flavum (OLF). DISH also called Forestier's disease is marked by ossification of the anterior longitudinal ligament (ALL) most commonly in the thoracolumbar spine. The ligamentum flavum runs posterior to the spinal canal anterior to the lamina. Ossification occurs most frequently in the lower thoracic spine. Ossification can narrow the spinal canal and/or lateral recesses producing symptoms of spinal stenosis or nerve root compression. OPLL appears as thick, smooth, linear calcification posterior to the vertebral bodies and disks. CT and MR can be helpful for more accurate delineation as well as to assess the degree of narrowing of the spinal canal and to evaluate the spinal cord for contusion.

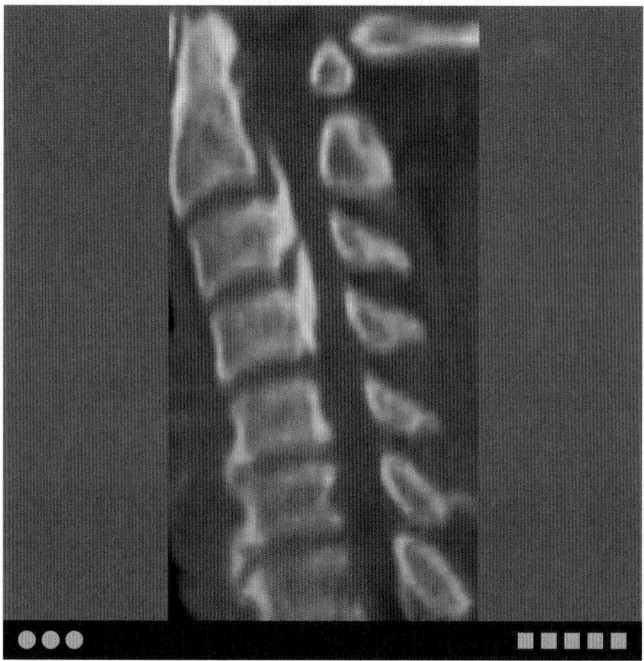

A. Ossification of posterior longitudinal ligament: Sagittal CT of the cervical spine confirms prominent linear ossification of posterior longitudinal ligament extending from C2 to C4.

PEARLS

- **Ossification of the posterior longitudinal ligament primarily affects Asian patients.**
- **OPLL can result in spinal stenosis and put effected individuals at risk for cord contusion with minimal trauma.**
- **OPLL can easily be distinguished from DISH and ossification of the ligamentum flavum by the location of the ossification directly posterior to the vertebral bodies.**
- **20% of cases of DISH will be associated with OPLL.**

ADDITIONAL IMAGES

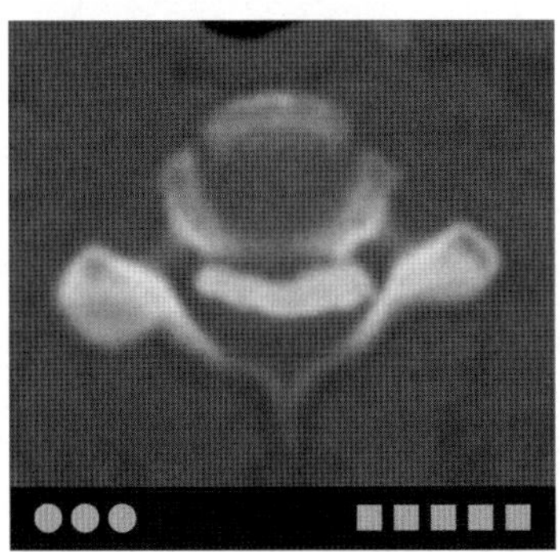

B. Ossification of posterior longitudinal ligament: Axial CT of the cervical spine shows severe narrowing of the spinal canal.

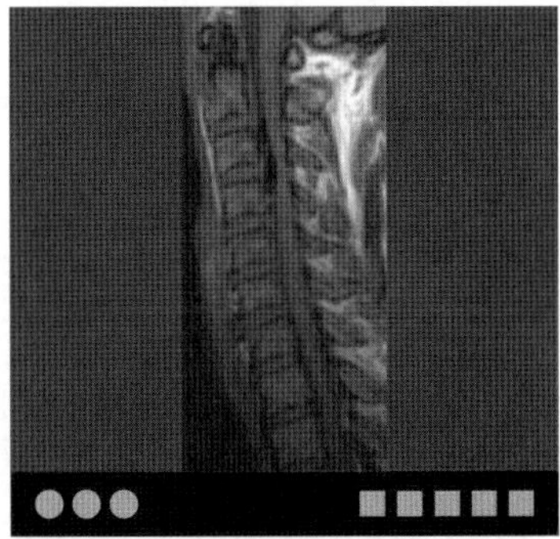

C. Ossification of posterior longitudinal ligament: Sagittal T1-weighted image shows linear signal void posterior to C2-C4 vertebral bodies' correlation with thick calcifications seen on CT.

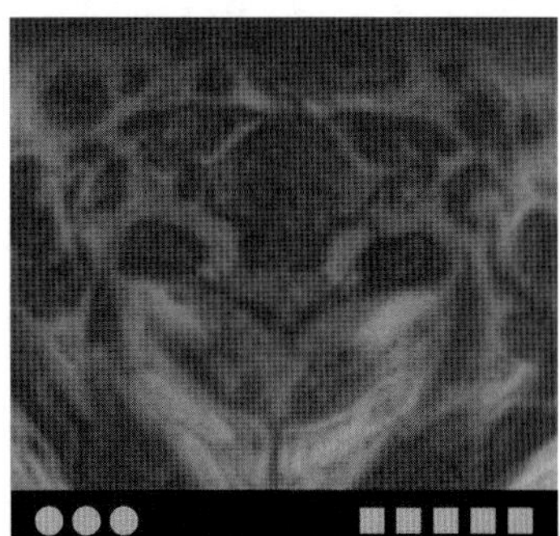

D. Ossification of posterior longitudinal ligament: Axial T2-weighted image shows cord compression with intramedullary high signal. Cord is flattened. There is obliteration of ventral and dorsal cerebrospinal fluid spaces as a result of OPLL superimposed onto congenital canal stenosis.

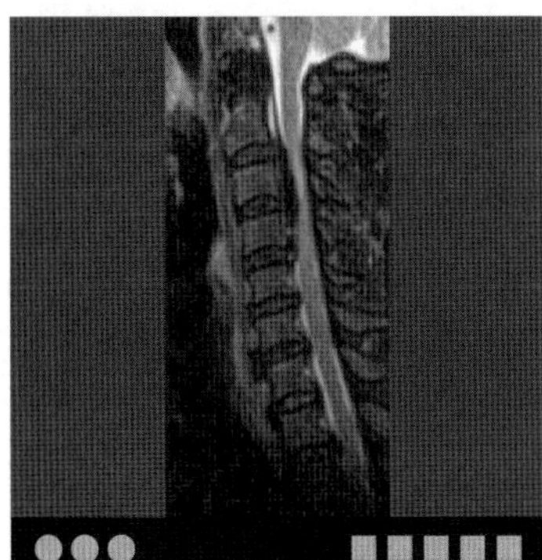

E. Ossification of posterior longitudinal ligament: Sagittal T2-weighted image shows similar signal void as a result of calcium. Note dural and cord compression.

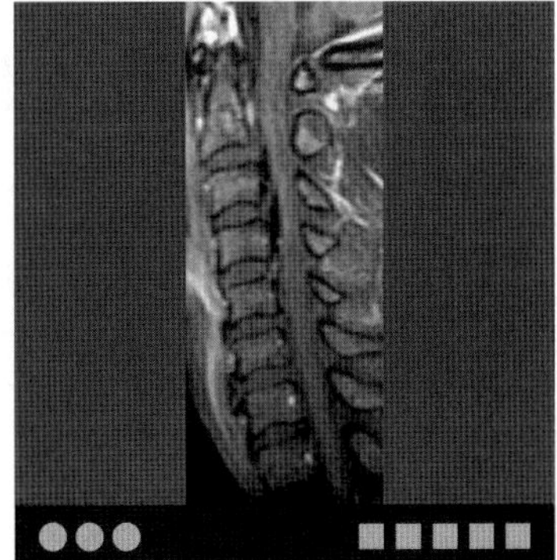

F. Ossification of posterior longitudinal ligament: Sagittal post gadolinium T1-weighted image shows no enhancement of OPLL.

DIFFERENTIAL DIAGNOSES IMAGES

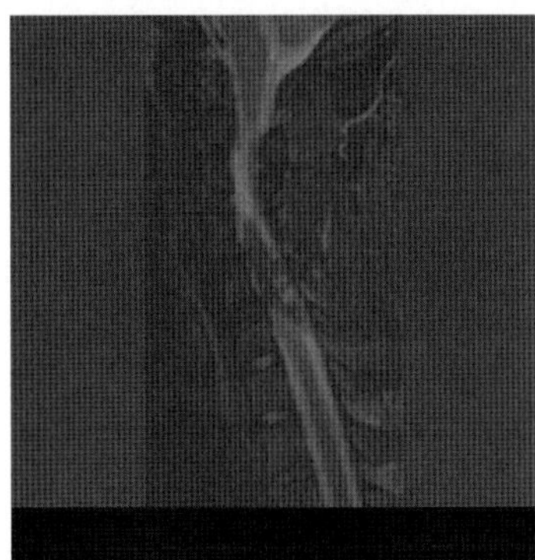

G. Subdural and epidural hematoma: Sagittal T2-weighted image shows amorphous low signal intensity subdural and epidural hematoma secondary to traumatic nerve roots avulsion at C3-C5 level.

IMAGE KEY

Common

Rare

Typical

Unusual

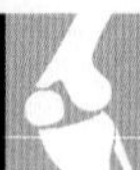

36–9 Ochronotic Arthropathy

Mélanie Morel, Nathalie Boutry, and Anne Cotten

PRESENTATION

Chronic low back pain and stiffness of the hip

FINDINGS

Radiographs show widespread lumbar discal calcifications and disk space narrowing with osteophytosis.

DIFFERENTIAL DIAGNOSES

- *Ankylosing spondylitis:* Ankylosis and ossification of the apophyseal joints and spine ligaments, in addition to syndesmophytes lead to a bamboo column. Central discal calcifications are linked with motion restriction. Osseous erosion and osteitis at the anterior aspects of the vertebral bodies are associated with "squaring". Sacroiliitis and peripheral enthesitis are major findings.
- *Calcium pyrophosphate dehydrate deposition disease:* Spinal involvement may be isolated, with thin linear peripheral disk calcifications, widespread degenerative discopathy, intradiscal vacuum phenomenon, and rare endplate sclerosis. Disk calcifications may be diffuse, but are less radiodense than in ochronosis. Spinal ligament calcification is encountered. Other peripheral joints are often affected.
- *Calcium hydroxyapatite deposition disease:* Discal calcifications are central and radiodense. Calcification within longus colli muscle is characteristic.

COMMENTS

This patient presents with chronic low back pain, stiffness of the hip, and long-standing history of dark urine. Ochronotic arthropathy arises from ochronotic deposition in joints. This rare (1:250,000) hereditary metabolic disorder is because of absence of homogentisic acid oxidase, leading to presence of homogentisic acid in urine, which is called alkaptonuria. Deposits in connective tissues give rise to a brown-black pigmentation of the skin, sclera, and ear cartilage. The abnormality is present at birth, but remains asymptomatic until 30 or 40 years of age. Ochronotic depositions in many organs lead to a great variety of dysfunctions (coronary and valvular calcification, nephrolithiasis). Ochronotic arthropathy initially affects the spine (lumbar, then thoracic and eventually cervical spine) and leads to motion restriction, lumbar hyperlordosis, and thoracic kyphosis. Sacroiliac joints are rarely involved. Acute exacerbations of arthritis, joint effusions, and progressive stiffness are also encountered in large appendicular joints (shoulder, hip, knee) several years after spinal involvement. Radiographs of spine show disk degeneration and central or diffuse disk calcification. Marked diffuse narrowing of intervertebral disk spaces with intradiscal vacuum phenomenon is distinctive. Vertebral body osteoporosis, endplate sclerosis, and mild osteophytosis are also found. Widespread ossification of spinal ligaments and vertebral disks and complete ankylosis can be seen at a late stage. MRI demonstrates high signal intensity intradiscal areas on T1-weighted image because of diffuse calcification and ossification (bone marrow). Intradiscal low signal intensity may be related to vacuum phenomenon. Appendicular joints show accelerated and severe degenerative changes, with diffuse joint space narrowing, sclerosis, moderate osteophytosis, fragmentation, and intra-articular loose bodies.

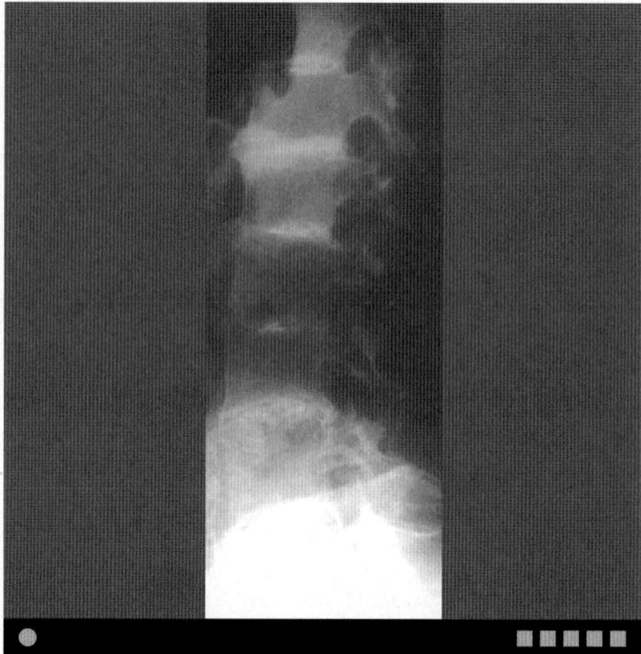

A. Ochronosis: Lateral view of the lumbar column exhibits osteoporosis of vertebral bodies, disk space narrowing and discal calcifications.

PEARLS

- **Alkaptonuria is a rare hereditary metabolic disorder.**
- **Ochronotic arthropathy results from pigmented deposits in the joints of axial and appendicular skeleton.**
- **Spinal abnormalities include discal calcification, characteristic diffused disk space narrowing with vacuum phenomena and osteoporosis.**

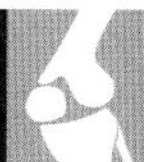

ADDITIONAL IMAGES

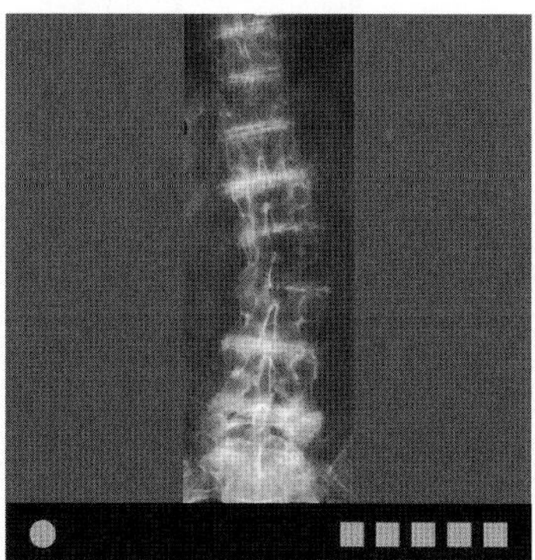

B. Ochronosis: AP view of the lumbar column reveals severe and extensive loss of disk space contrasting with moderate osteophytosis.

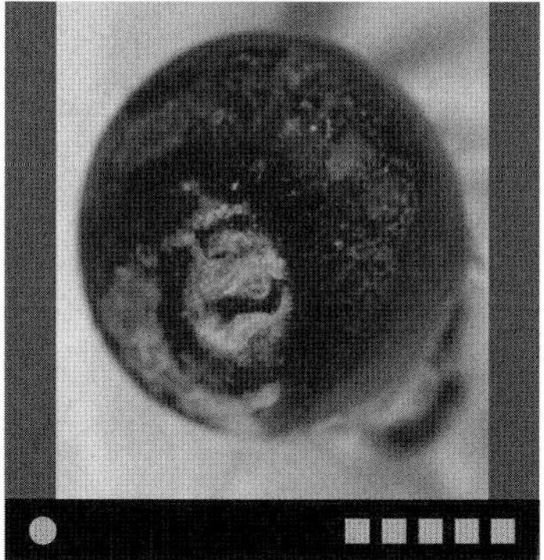

C. Ochronosis: Photograph of a femoral head demonstrates the brown-black pigmentation of the head cartilage.

DIFFERENTIAL DIAGNOSES IMAGES

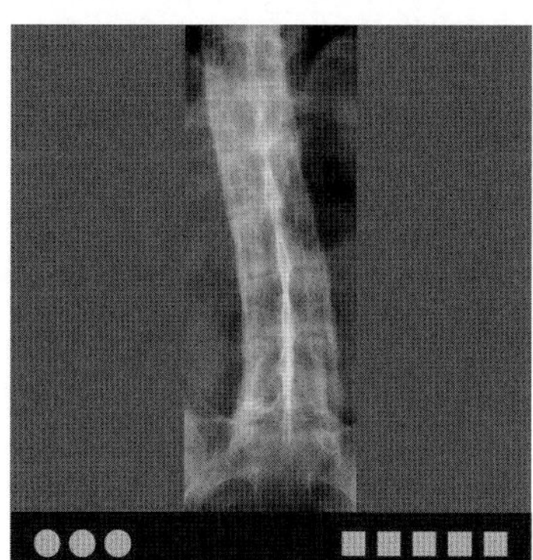

D. Ankylosing spondylitis: Frontal radiograph reveals continuous marginal syndesmophytes (bamboo spine), ossification of the supraspinous and interspinous ligaments, and ankylosis of the apophyseal joints.

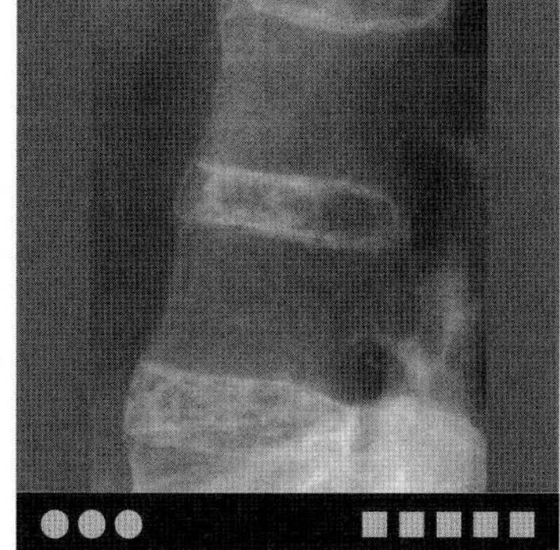

E. Ankylosing spondylitis: Lateral radiograph demonstrates continuous syndesmophytes, ballooning of the disk spaces, and discal calcifications.

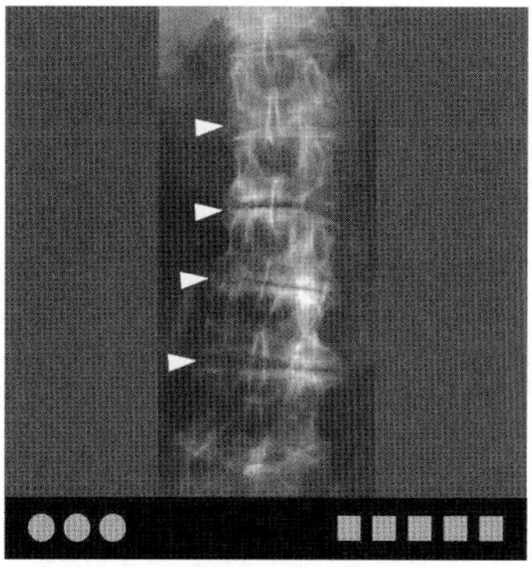

F. Calcium pyrophosphate dehydrate deposition disease: AP radiograph shows peripheral discal calcifications (arrowheads) in addition to disk space narrowing and vacuum phenomenon.

IMAGE KEY

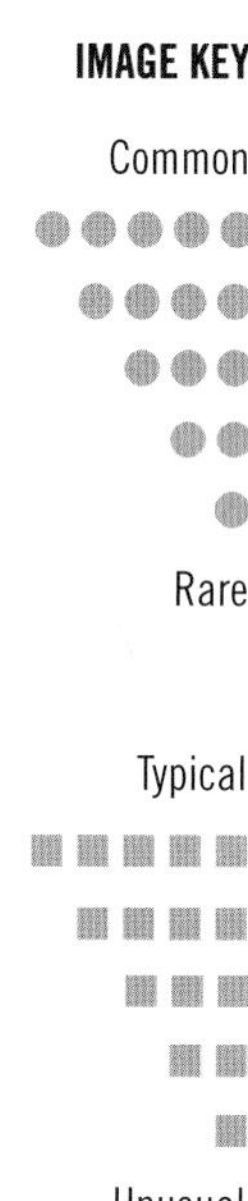

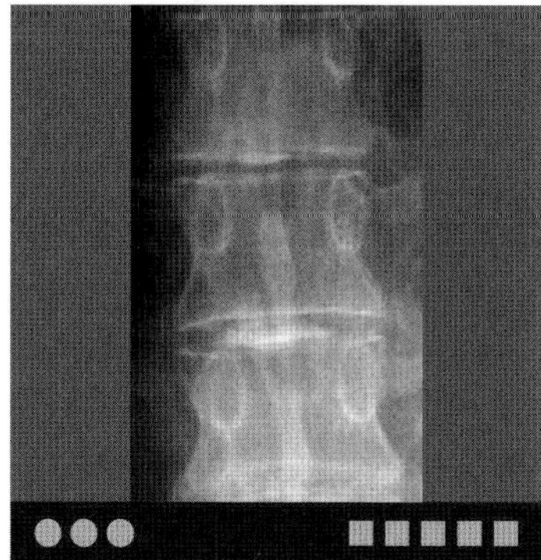

G. Calcium hydroxyapatite deposition disease: Discal calcification is dense, homogeneous, and located in the central part of the disk.

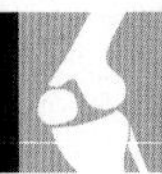

36–10 Tarlov Cyst (Perineural Root Sleeve Cyst)

Tatiana Voci and Melitus Maryam Golshan

PRESENTATION

Low back pain

FINDINGS

MR images show low T1-weighted image and high T2-weighted image signal intensity nonenhancing perineural cysts remodeling the neural foramina and causing posterior vertebral scalloping. S2 and S3 nerve roots are most commonly involved.

DIFFERENTIAL DIAGNOSES

- *Facet synovial cyst:* Are more common at lower lumbar spine, especially L4-5, and are immediately adjacent to the facet joint, often there are fluid and hypertrophic changes in the facet.
- *Spinal masses; e.g. Lipoma:* They usually present with neurologic symptoms and subcutaneous lipoma. Lipoma is bright in both T1 and T2-weighted images.
- *Meningocele:* Often it is not a diagnostic dilemma to distinguish between anterior, lateral, posterior meningocele, and Tarlov cyst. Look for CSF intensity mass filling the sacral canal, and a pedicle connection is present between the meningocele and thecal sac more distally.
- *Spinal nerve root avulsion:* Is more common in lower cervical and upper thoracic spine, usually unilateral or at contiguous levels.
- *Nerve sheath tumor:* Presents with soft tissue rather than CSF density and shows post-contrast enhancement.

COMMENTS

The patient is a 47-year-old female with low back pain. Tarlov cysts affect men and women equally in their 30s and 40s. About 5% to 9% of adults are affected. The majority of patients are asymptomatic (about 80%), those with symptoms complain of low back pain, paresthesia, weakness, and bladder and bowel dysfunction. There is no reliable imaging method to differentiate symptomatic from asymptomatic lesions. Perineurial (Tarlov) cysts are meningeal dilations of the posterior spinal nerve root sheath that most often affect sacral roots. The most common location is S2 and S3 neural foramina. Tarlov cysts are most commonly diagnosed by lumbosacral magnetic resonance imaging and can often be demonstrated by computerized tomography myelography to communicate with the spinal subarachnoid space-thecal sac. These are best seen on T2-weighted image as well-circumscribed high signal intensity lesions, unilaterally or bilaterally, they show no post-contrast enhancement. The cyst can enlarge via a net inflow of cerebrospinal fluid, eventually causing symptoms by distorting, compressing, or stretching adjacent nerve roots. It is generally agreed that asymptomatic Tarlov cysts do not require treatment. The natural history of these lesions is slow progressive growth, they often recur following aspiration. Spontaneous rupture can cause intracranial hypotension and sacral insufficiency fracture. These lesions can be treated conservatively with physical therapy, cyst aspiration, and surgically with laminectomy and cyst/nerve root resection.

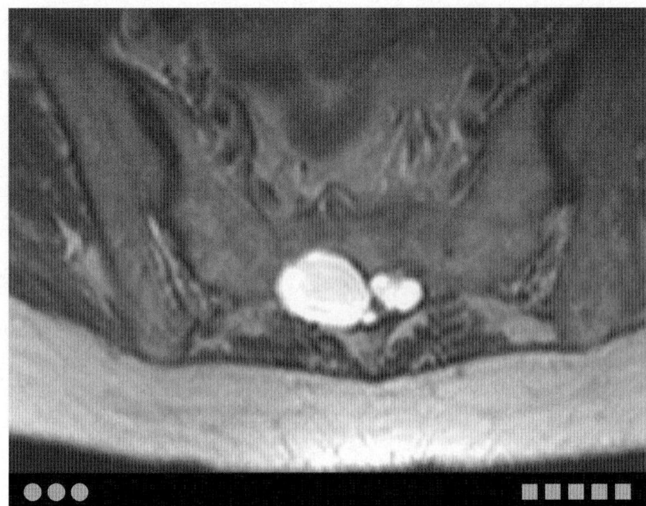

A. Tarlov cyst: Axial T2-weighted image shows bilateral, right greater than left, high signal intensity lesions within S2 neural foramina. Right neural foramen is markedly scalloped.

PEARLS

- **Most Tarlov cysts are incidental finding and are asymptomatic (leave alone lesions)**
- **MR images show low T1-weighted image and high T2-weighted image signal intensity nonenhancing perineural cysts remodeling the neural foramina and causing posterior vertebral scalloping.**
- **S2 and S3 nerve roots are most commonly involved.**

ADDITIONAL IMAGES

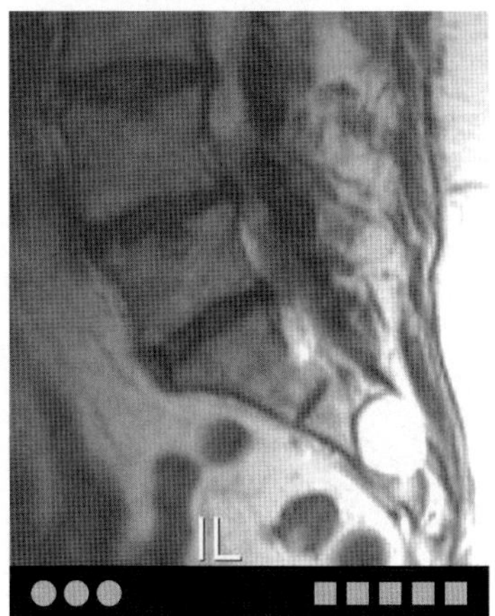

B. Tarlov cyst: Sagittal T2-weighted image shows CSF signal intensity lesion in the right S2 neural foramen.

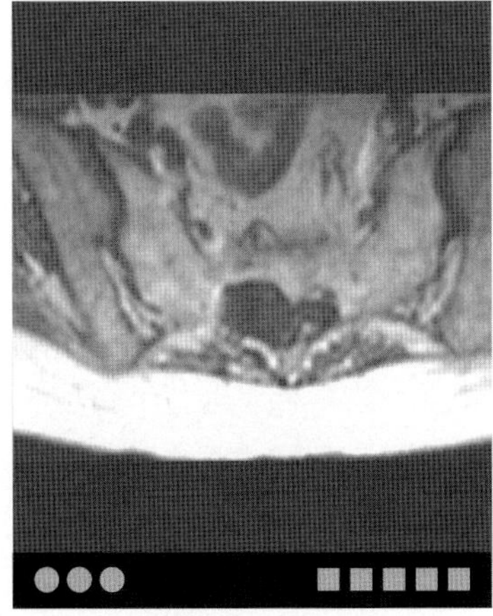

C. Tarlov cyst: Axial T1-weighted image shows two low signal intensity Tarlov cysts within S2 neural foramina.

DIFFERENTIAL DIAGNOSES IMAGES

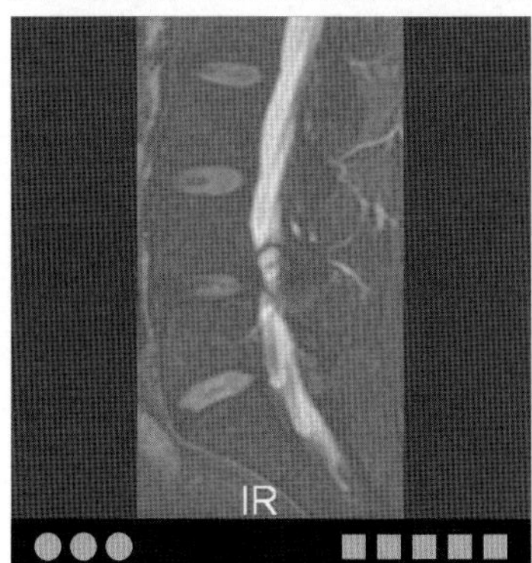

D. Synovial cyst: Sagittal T2-weighted image shows a synovial cyst adjacent to the right L4-5 facet joint, it has low peripheral signal intensity consistent with calcification.

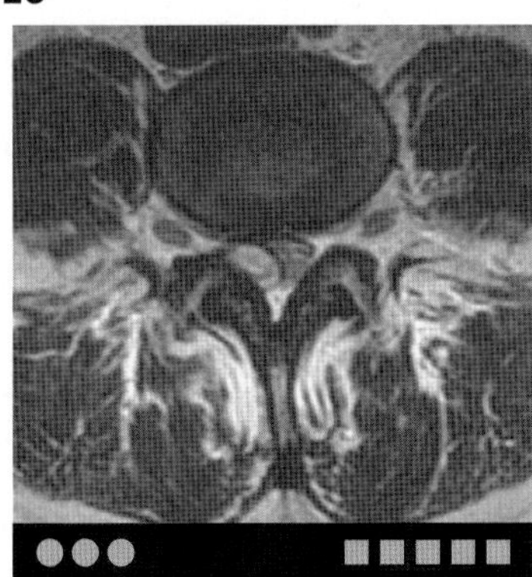

E. Synovial cyst: Axial T2-weighted image shows right L4-5 synovial cyst.

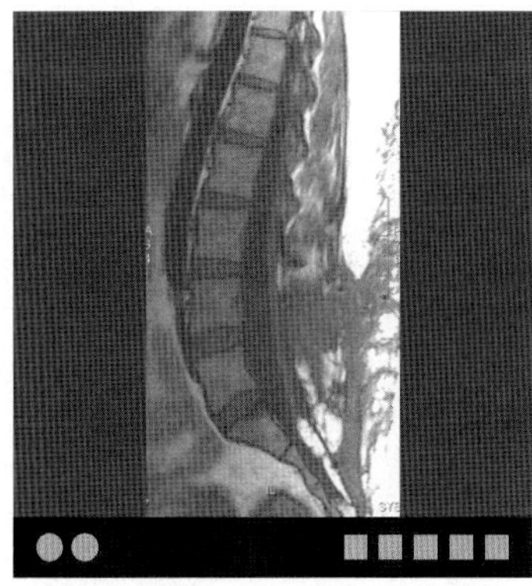

F. Lipoma: Sagittal T1-weighted image shows high signal intensity lipomatose masses in filum terminalis in a 34-year-old woman.

IMAGE KEY

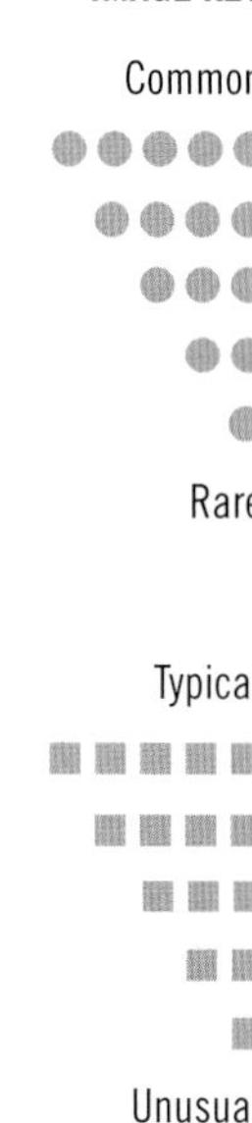

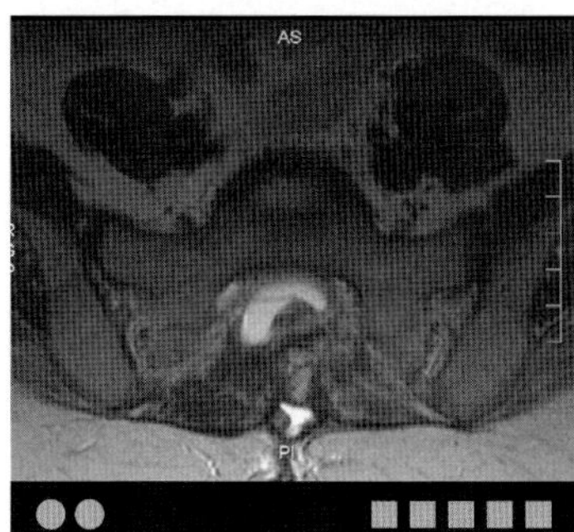

G. Lipoma: Axial T2-weighted image shows areas of high signal intensity in the side of filum terminalis consistent with lipoma.

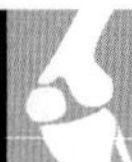

36–11 Extramedullary Hematopoiesis

Stephen E. Ling and William R. Reinus

PRESENTATION

Asymptomatic, space occupying symptoms

FINDINGS

Extra-osseous lobular soft tissue masses

DIFFERENTIAL DIAGNOSES

- *Plasmacytoma, metastases:* More destructive than extramedullary hematopoiesis
- *Lymphoma:* Usually bulkier than EMH and remote from osseous structures
- *Nerve sheath tumors:* Typically seen along the course of nerves and show an elliptical shape with very bright signal on T2-weighted images.

COMMENTS

Extramedullary hematopoiesis (EMH) is a compensatory response to chronic pathologically increased red cell production. This phenomenon most commonly arises in the setting of hemolytic anemia, e.g. β-thalassemia, sickle cell disease, hereditary spherocytosis, or sideroblastic anemia. Myeloproliferative disorders, e.g. myeloid metaplasia and polcythemia vera; bone marrow neoplasm, e.g. leukemia and lymphoma; and other marrow packing disorders, e.g. Gaucher's disease, also may give rise to EMH. Although patients may have symptoms secondary to the underlying systemic disorder, EMH usually is asymptomatic. Paracostal, paravertebral, and mediastinal involvement are frequent, particularly in patients with hemolytic anemia. The hematopoietic masses typically arise adjacent to bones that normally contain red marrow and can exert mass effect on adjacent structures, but are noninvasive and hence benign in appearance. Organs that make up the reticuloendothelial system (RES), including the liver, spleen, and lymph nodes, can also be affected and enlarged but usually only in the setting of destroyed or ineffective bone marrow. In addition, EMH of the thymus, kidneys, adrenals, bowel, uterus, and breast have also been reported. If the EMH results from hemolytic anemia, radiographs show one or more lobulated, well-defined soft tissue masses. These may be bilateral. These masses are often paravertebral and located between T8 and L2. Chronic hemolytic anemia also may lead to osseous medullary space expansion with thinned cortices, and even loss of cortex or cortical transgression. On CT, similar findings are present although the herniation of bone marrow through cortex with subsequent extraosseous formation of erythropoietic soft tissue masses is better shown on CT than radiographs.

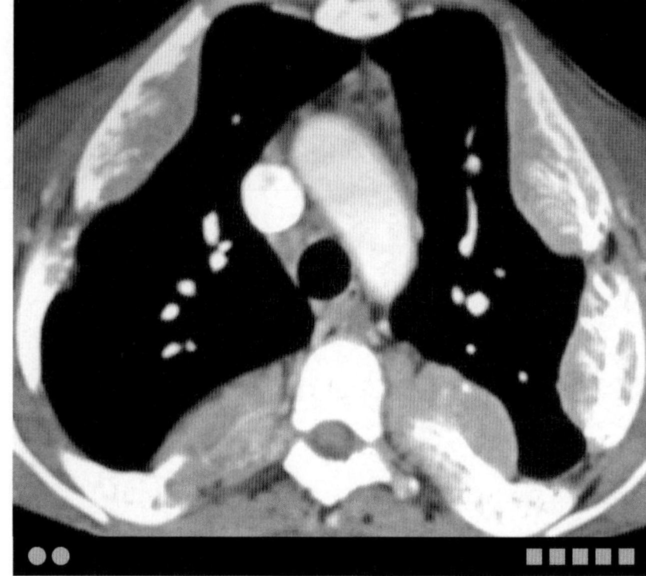

A. Extramedullary hematopoiesis: Axial CT image through the upper thorax in a patient with thalassemia major demonstrates multiple bilateral, extra-pleural lobular soft tissue masses associated with several enlarged ribs.

PEARLS

- **Tc-99m-sulfur colloid scan may be helpful in making the diagnosis of extramedullary hematopoiesis, especially for involvement of the RES.**
- **The hematopoietic tissue of EMH tends to take the path of least resistance, such as through the anterior cortex of the ribs and into the central canal of the spine.**
- **A paravertebral soft tissue mass to the right of the spine between T8 and T12 should suggest EMH, particularly in the presence of diseases that affect the RES.**

ADDITIONAL IMAGES

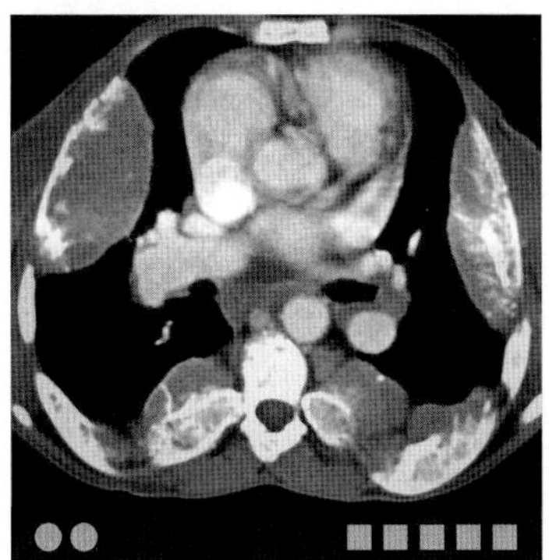

B. Extramedullary hematopoiesis: Axial CT image shows additional bilateral soft tissue masses and ribs with expanded medullary spaces in the mid thorax similar to those seen in Figure A.

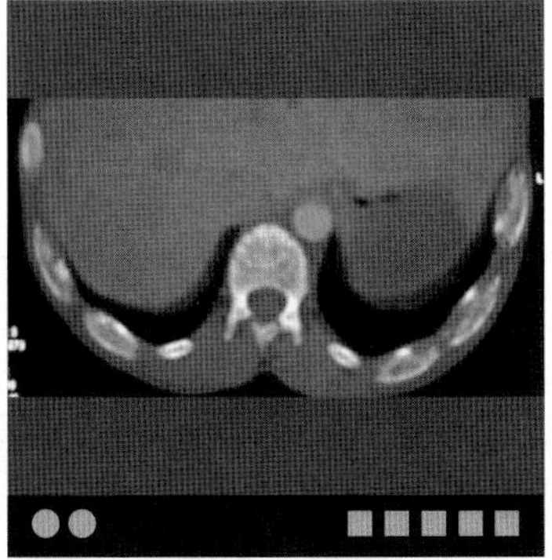

C. Extramedullary hematopoiesis: Axial CT image through the lower thorax and upper abdomen shows widening of the medullary cavity of multiple ribs bilaterally and adjacent early extraosseous hematopoietic soft tissue.

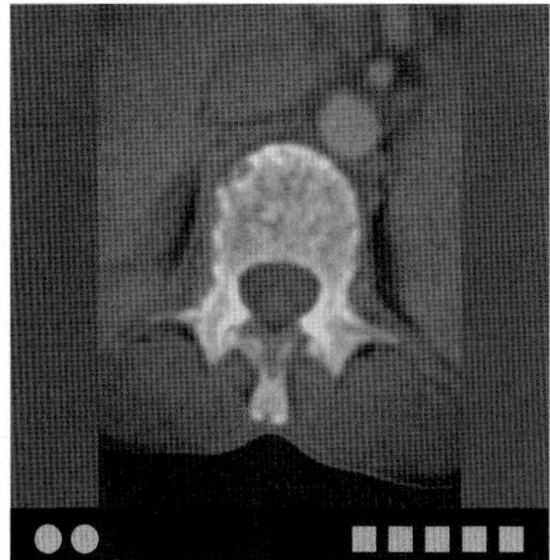

D. Extramedullary hematopoiesis: Axial CT image shows diffuse heterogeneity of the medullary bone and coarsening of trabeculae in the vertebral body at this level as a result of red marrow hyperplasia.

IMAGE KEY

Common

Rare

Typical

Unusual

DIFFERENTIAL DIAGNOSES IMAGES

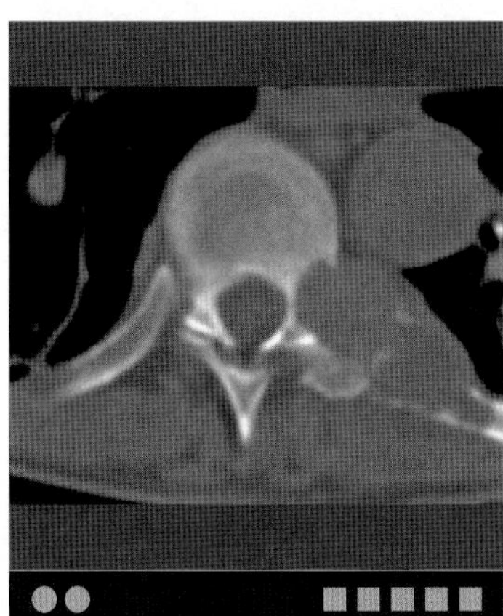

E. Plasmacytoma: Axial CT image demonstrates a very destructive, asymmetric left-sided soft tissue mass involving the pedicle, transverse process, and a posterior rib at this level.

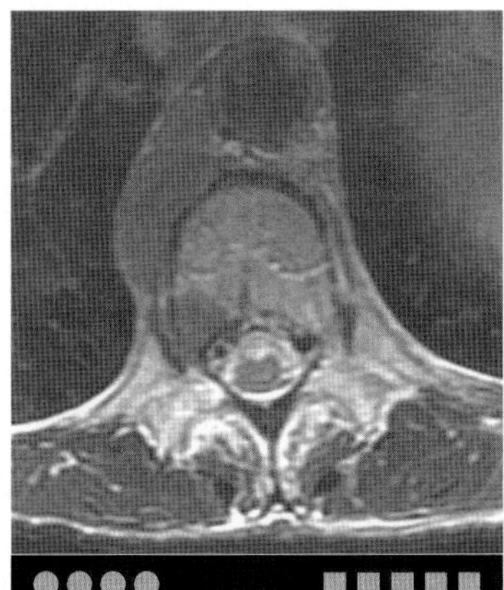

F. Metastases: Axial T2-weighted images in this patient with history of carcinoid primary shows bilateral paraspinal soft tissue masses at adjacent levels in the lower thoracic spine consistent with metastases. Note the involvement of the neighboring posterior vertebral body and pedicle on the right and posterior rib on the left by tumor.

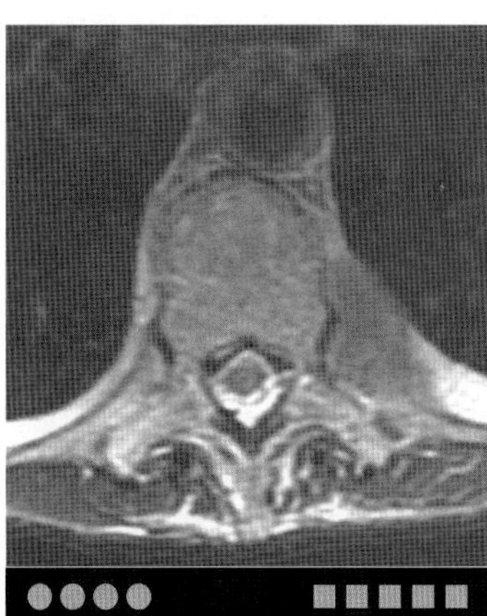

G. Metastases: Axial T2-weighted images in this patient with history of carcinoid primary shows bilateral paraspinal soft tissue masses at adjacent levels in the lower thoracic spine consistent with metastases. Note the involvement of the neighboring posterior vertebral body and pedicle on the right and posterior rib on the left by tumor.

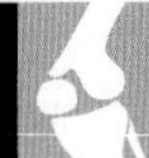

36–12 Brown Tumor

Ingrid B. Kjellin

PRESENTATION

Chronic renal failure and back pain

FINDINGS

MRI shows a focal lytic lesion in the L3 vertebral body.

DIFFERENTIAL DIAGNOSES

- *Metastatic disease to the skeleton:* It is the most common type of malignant bone tumor. Carcinoma of the prostate, breast, kidney, and lung account for more than 75% of the cases of skeletal metastases in adults.
- *Multiple myeloma:* This is the most common primary bone neoplasm in adults. The typical pattern on imaging is focal or diffuse bone destruction with osteolysis. The axial skeleton is the most common site of involvement. Other round cell tumors, such as lymphoma, should also be considered.
- *Intraosseous hemangioma:* This can occasionally be very large and simulate an aggressive lesion.
- *Chordoma:* Spinal chordomas initially show destruction of the vertebral body. Sclerosis and a large soft tissue mass will subsequently develop. Adjacent vertebral bodies and intervertebral disks may also be involved.
- *Osteoblastoma and aneurysmal bone cyst:* These are benign tumors that may involve the spine, typically in the posterior elements, and rarely in the vertebral body.

COMMENTS

The patient is a 33-year-old male with chronic renal failure. Long-standing renal insufficiency will result in osteitis fibrosa cystica, osteomalacia or rickets, osteosclerosis and osteoporosis, as a result of secondary hyperparathyroidism and abnormal vitamin D metabolism. Characteristic biochemical findings are hypercalcemia, hypophosphatemia, and elevated parathormone levels. Bone resorption at various sites, along with regions of bone sclerosis along the vertebral endplates, the so-called rugger-jersey spine, is frequently seen on imaging studies. Periosteal neostosis and soft tissue calcifications are additional findings. Brown tumors are seen in primary, as well as secondary hyperparathyroidism. It has been reported that the frequency of these lesions is higher in primary hyperparathyroidism than in secondary hyperparathyroidism. With the development of more effective treatments, that may no longer be true. Brown tumors are seen at any age, at any location in the skeleton, and can be single or multiple. Reports of spinal involvement are limited

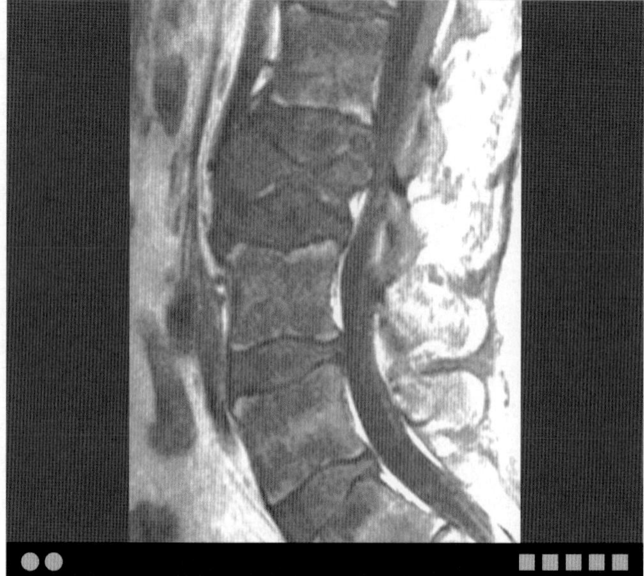

A. Brown tumor: A T1-weighted sagittal image of the lumbar spine shows a destructive lesion of the L3 vertebral body with cortical expansion and fracture. There is diffuse signal abnormality throughout the visualized bone marrow, which may be a result of diffuse osteosclerosis and red marrow hyperplasia.

in number. The vertebral body as well as the posterior elements can be involved. Associated cortical expansion and fracture may be causes of pain and neurological deficit. After treatment of renal failure these lesions may decrease in size or completely resolve, although progression of lesions has also been reported. Histologically, the brown tumors have a fibrous stroma with giant cells and hemosiderin deposits. Imaging findings include an osteolytic lesion with a well-defined, nonsclerotic margin. On CT, there is a uniform soft tissue density, replacing the bone trabeculae. On MR imaging, the signal is intermediate on T1-weighted images and variable on T2-weighted images.

PEARLS

- **Brown tumors are found in hyperparathyroidism, both primary and secondary.**
- **They are seen in any age group and at any location in bone.**
- **Other imaging features of renal osteodystrophy are diffuse bone resorption, rickets or osteomalacia, osteosclerosis, rugger-jersey spine, and soft tissue calcification.**
- **Brown tumors may decrease in size or resolve after adequate treatment of hyperparathyroidism.**

ADDITIONAL IMAGES

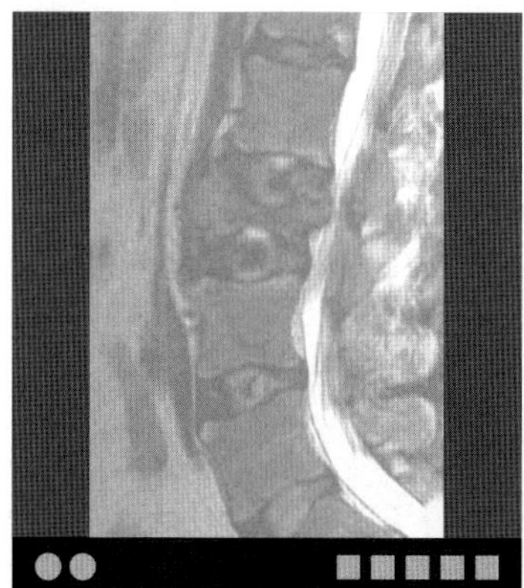

B. Brown tumor: A T2-weighted sagittal image shows low signal of the lesion in the L3 vertebra.

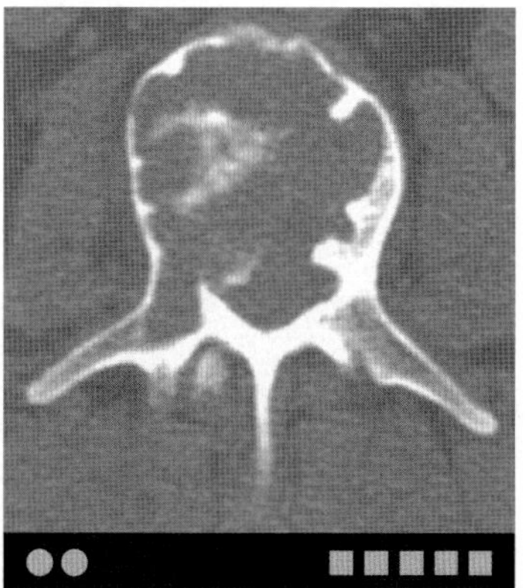

C. Brown tumor: A CT axial image of L3 shows an expansile lytic lesion without calcified tumor matrix.

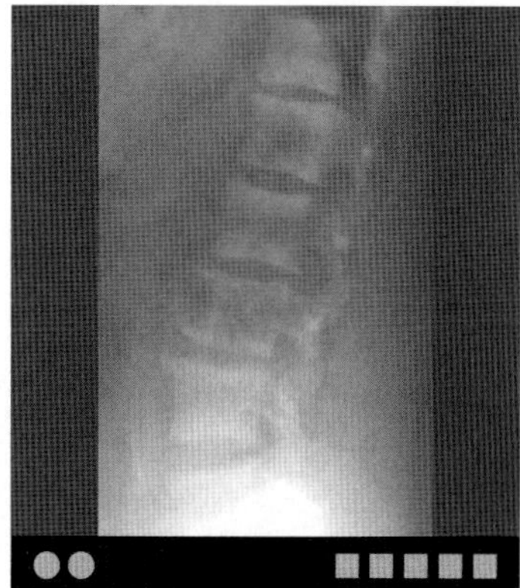

D. Brown tumor: A lateral radiograph of the lumbar spine shows sclerosis along the vertebral endplates (rugger-jersey spine). The lytic lesion of L3 is also demonstrated.

IMAGE KEY

Common

●●●●●
●●●●
●●●
●●
●

Rare

Typical

■■■■■
■■■■
■■■
■■
■

Unusual

DIFFERENTIAL DIAGNOSES IMAGES

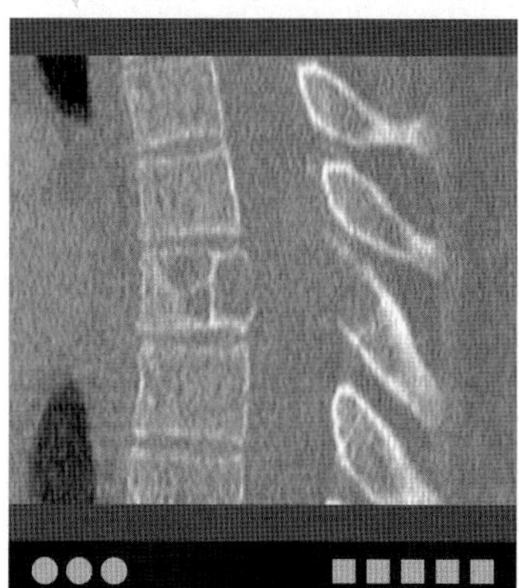

E. Aneurysmal bone cyst: A CT of the thoracic spine, reformatted in the sagittal plane, shows a lytic lesion involving a mid-thoracic vertebra. There is no calcified tumor matrix. Both the body and the posterior elements of the vertebra are involved.

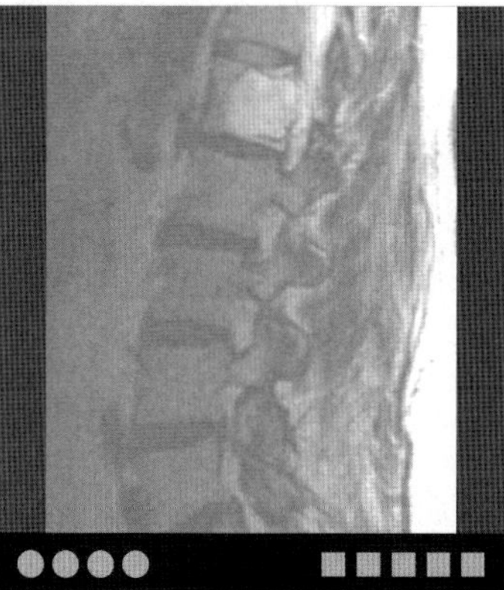

F. Hemangioma with epidural extension: A sagittal post-contrast fat-saturated T1-weighted image of the lumbar spine shows a well-demarcated lesion in the L1 vertebral body with strong enhancement and deformity of the posterior cortex of the vertebral body. The lesion extends into the anterior epidural space.

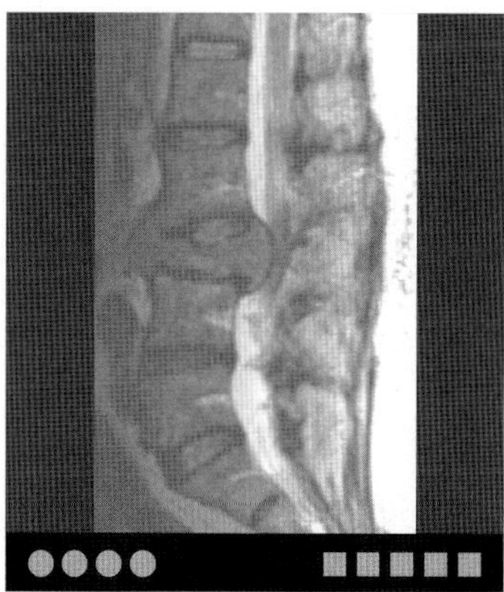

G. Multiple myeloma: A T2-weighted sagittal image of the lumbar spine shows a focal expansile lesion of the L3 vertebral body with associated vertebral collapse. There is low signal within the lesion on T2-weighted, which may be a result of the high nucleus cytoplasm ratio in round cell tumors. A characteristic feature of multiple myeloma is extension of the tumor across the intervertebral disk, in this case anteriorly into the L2 vertebral body.

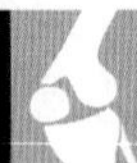

36–13 Diffuse Skeletal Sarcoidosis

Sandra Leigh Moore

PRESENTATION

Vague back and pelvic pain

FINDINGS

MRI shows innumerable round intramedullary lesions throughout the spine, sacrum, and pelvis, resembling osseous metastases. Bone scan and radiographs were interpreted as normal.

DIFFERENTIAL DIAGNOSES

- *Osseous metastases:* The patient may have a known primary malignancy.
- *Bone lymphoma:* Osteolytic, osteosclerotic or often mixed lesions are noted.
- *Multiple myeloma:* Elderly patients are often affected with presence of diffuse osteoporosis or multiple lytic lesions.
- *Disseminated nonmalignant entities:* Such as fibrous dysplasia, fungal, or mycobacterial infection, and serious atrophy.

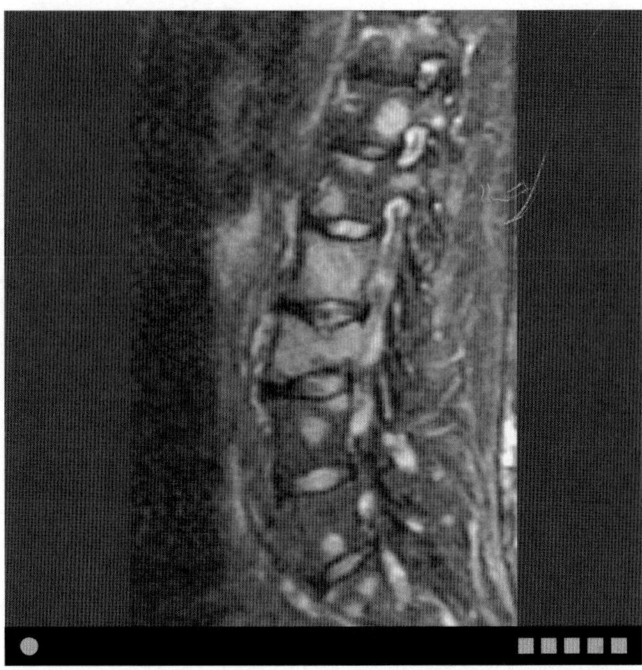

A. Bone sarcoidosis: Middle-aged female with sarcoidosis. Sagittal STIR image shows marrow infiltration and compression fracture. Patient declined biopsy. Follow-up imaging 6 years later showed near-complete resolution of these lesions.

COMMENTS

The patient is a middle-aged woman with sarcoidosis complaining of vague back and pelvic pain. Sarcoidal bone involvement, which occurs in about 5% of sarcoidosis patients, may be symptomatic or asymptomatic, and is considered more common among patients with skin lesions. The clinical diagnosis of sarcoidosis in most cases has already been established prior to the biopsy of a suspicious bone lesion, by clinical presentation, laboratory findings, or biopsy (lymph node, skin, etc). Bone lesions may be biopsied to confirm sarcoidosis, and/or exclude co-existent etiologies such as neoplasm. Sarcoidosis is a common cause of bone marrow granulomas at biopsy (about 3% to 32%, average 10%) with sarcoidal pulmonary involvement in over 90% of patients with marrow lesions. The radiographic appearance of lacy lesions in the small bones of the hands and feet is virtually pathognomonic. Large bone and axial skeletal involvement are uncommon radiographic findings and lesions show variable uptake on bone scan. Large bone and spinal sarcoidal lesions, often occult on radiographs, may be detected on MRI either as an incidental finding, or for work-up of musculoskeletal symptoms. These demonstrate a range of appearances from vague, patchy marrow infiltration to well-defined discrete lesions. The signal characteristics (low on T1-weighted image, increased on water-sensitive images, enhancing with contrast) are nonspecific. Signal intensity drop on in- and out-of-phase images is variable with sarcoidal bone lesions, and therefore may not contribute to the differentiation of sarcoidosis lesions from infiltrative/neoplastic disease.

PEARLS

- **On MR sarcoidal bone lesions resemble disseminated infiltrative disease including osseous metastases.**
- **In the setting of clinical sarcoidosis, sarcoidal bone lesions should be included in the differential diagnosis.**
- **There are no pathognomonic MR imaging findings, but sarcoidal bone lesions may resolve on follow-up imaging, with or without treatment.**

ADDITIONAL IMAGES

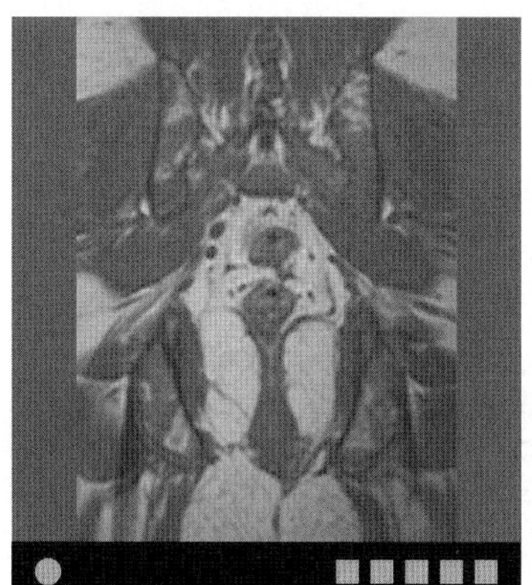

B. Bone sarcoidosis: Middle-aged male with sarcoidosis. Coronal T1-weighted image shows patchy diffuse marrow signal abnormality, revealing non-caseating granulomata at biopsy.

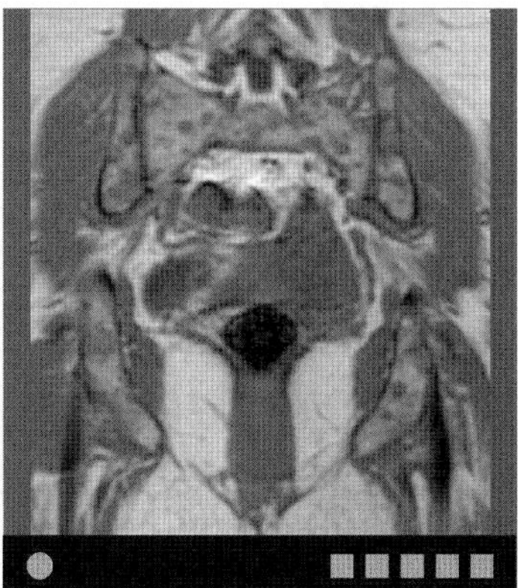

C. Bone sarcoidosis: Middle-aged woman with sarcoidosis. Coronal proton density image shows innumerable round intramedullary lesions resembling osseous metastases. Biopsy revealed non-caseating granulomata.

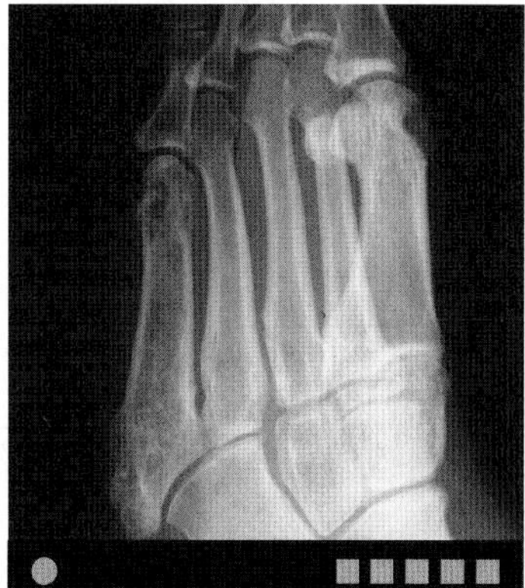

D. Bone sarcoidosis: Oblique radiograph of the foot shows the familiar lacy lytic pattern of small bone sarcoidosis, virtually pathognomonic in the setting of clinical sarcoidosis.

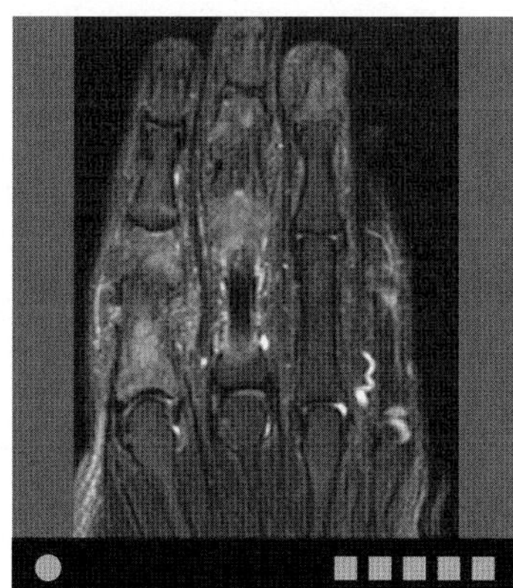

E. Bone sarcoidosis: Coronal T2 fat-saturated image of the hand shows sarcoid granulomas in digits 2 to 4.

IMAGE KEY

Common

Rare

Typical

Unusual

DIFFERENTIAL DIAGNOSES IMAGES

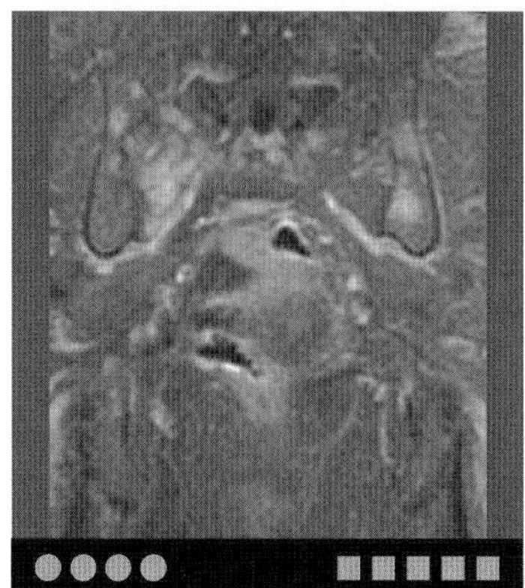

F. Osseous metastases: Coronal proton density image shows multiple round foci of marrow infiltration in this patient with breast cancer and proven osseous metastases.

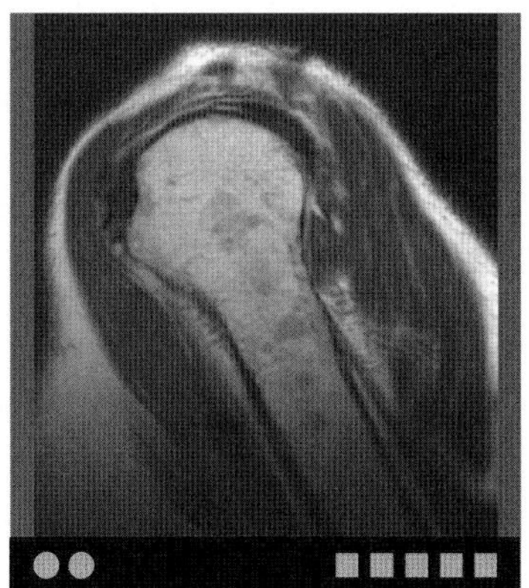

G. Bone lymphoma: Sagittal T1-weighted image shows multiple faint round intramedullary foci. Biopsy revealed osseous lymphoma.

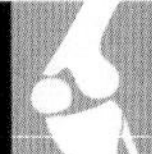

36–14 Tuberous Sclerosis

Mohammad Reza Hayeri and Jamshid Tehranzadeh

PRESENTATION

A 37-year-old female with renal mass and skin lesion

FINDINGS

The CT images show foci of sclerotic densities in spine and pelvis and a renal mass.

DIFFERENTIAL DIAGNOSES

- *Osteoblastic metastases:* Malignancies such as prostate, breast, and lung may present with osteoblastic metastasis.
- *Osteopoikilosis:* Osteopoikilosis is a benign, usually asymptomatic condition characterized by osteosclerotic dysplasia of bones in childhood and persists throughout life. Multiple, small, variably shaped radio densities usually in the periarticular areas especially in pelvis, carpal, and tarsal bones and epiphyseal ends of the long bones.

COMMENTS

The patient is a 37-year-old women presenting with renal mass and history of prior resection of angiofibroma of scalp. Tuberous sclerosis is a rare autosomal dominant trait neurocutaneous multisystem disorder. Neurologic symptoms vary from minimally affected patients with normal intelligence and no seizure to profound mental retardation and frequent seizure. Autism, attention deficit hyperactivity disorder (ADHD), and sleep problems are the most frequent behavioral disorders. Skin abnormalities include "ash leaf spots," which are depigmented or hypopigmented lesions; "Shagreen patches," which are collagen accumulation manifested as raised patches on the lower back in an orange peel texture; and adenoma sebaceums, which are high vascular lumps on the face that resemble irritated acne. Brain is affected by benign tumors such as giant cell astrocytoma, which can block the flow of fluid within the brain; subependymal nodules, which form in the wall of ventricles with calcification; and cortical tubers, which generally form on the brain cortex. The most common renal manifestation is angiomyolipoma, which is a benign tumor, often multiple and bilateral and affect female 3 to 4 times more than male. Rhabdomyomas are benign tumors of heart, which affect two-thirds of newborn infants with tuberous sclerosis. Other manifestations include Hamartomatous polyps in the gastrointestinal tract, lymphangioleiomyomatosis in the lung, pitting in the permanent teeth, retinal hamartomas, and arterial aneurysms. The bones may show areas of cyst formation mainly in phalanges of the hands and feet, periosteal new bone growth, and foci of sclerosis resembling bone islands. Symptomatic bone diseases are rare.

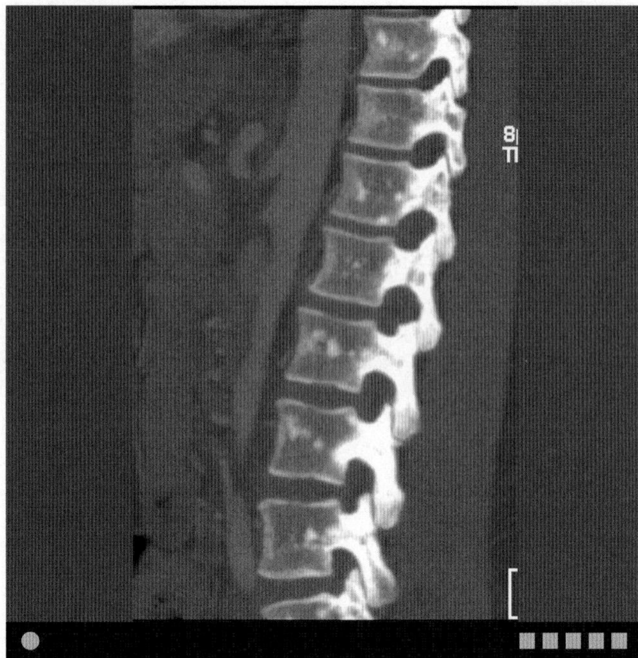

A. Tuberous sclerosis: Sagittal CT reformatting shows multiple foci of sclerotic lesions in vertebral bodies of lumbar spine resembling "bone islands."

PEARLS

- **Tuberous sclerosis is a rare autosomal dominant disease.**
- **The main manifestations include skin lesions, epilepsy, mental retardation, and benign tumors of multiple organs such as kidney, heart, eye, and brain.**
- **Neurologic symptoms vary from minimally affected patients with normal intelligence and no seizure to profound mental retardation and frequent seizure.**
- **Areas of cyst formation mainly in phalanges of the hands and feet, periosteal new bone formation, and foci of sclerosis are the main bone radiographic manifestation of tuberous sclerosis.**

ADDITIONAL IMAGES

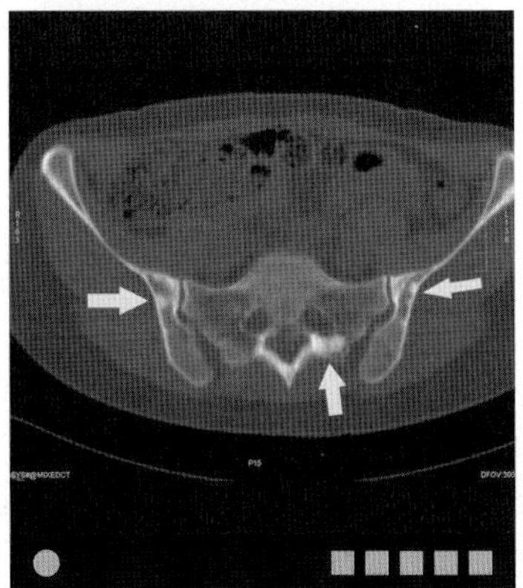

B. Tuberous sclerosis axial: CT of the pelvis shows multiple foci of sclerotic lesions (arrows).

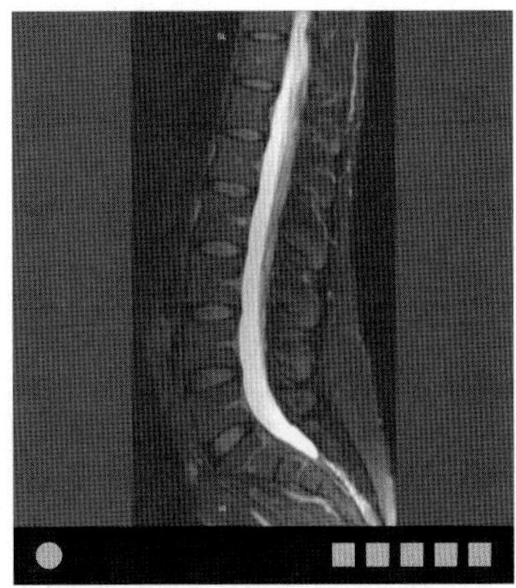

C. Tuberous sclerosis: T2-weighted fat-saturated sagittal MR images of lumbar spine are basically unremarkable.

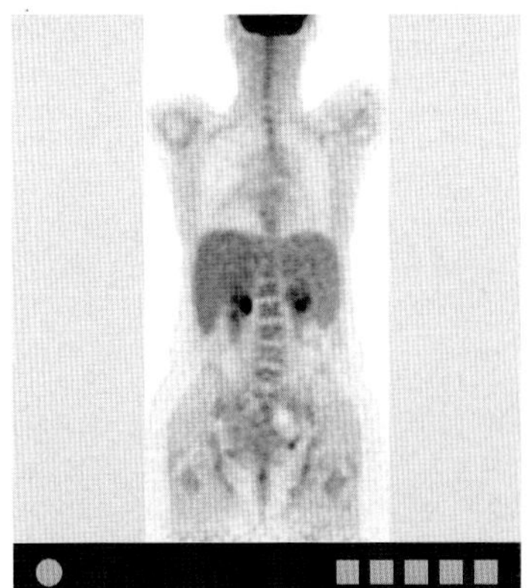

D. Tuberous sclerosis: Coronal image of PET scan shows spinal lesions do not have significant scintigraphic uptake.

IMAGE KEY

Common

Rare

Typical

Unusual

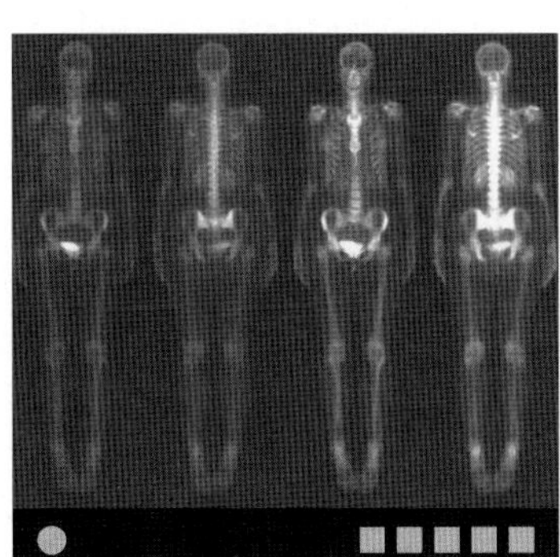

E. Tuberous sclerosis: TC-99m-MDP scan shows spinal lesions do not have significant uptake.

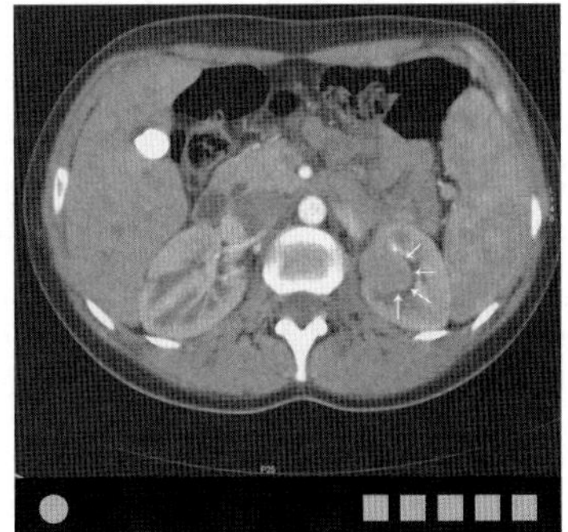

F. Tuberous sclerosis: Axial CT of abdomen with IV contrast shows a mass lesion in the left kidney (arrows) which on biopsy was angiomyolipoma.

DIFFERENTIAL DIAGNOSIS IMAGE

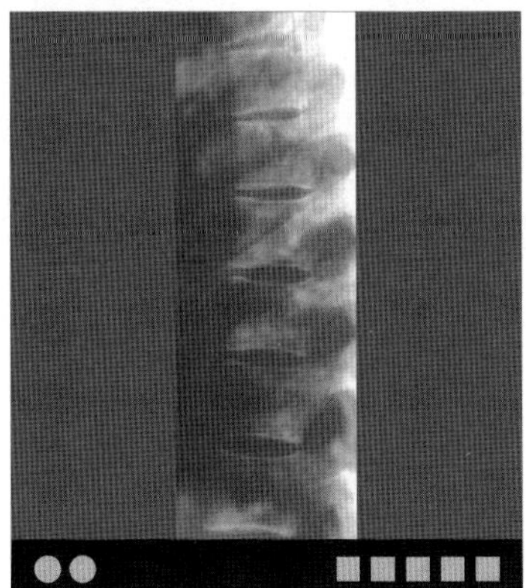

G. Osteopoikilosis: Lateral radiograph of thoracic spine: shows small foci of sclerotic lesions in the vertebrae bodies.

Chapter 37

Arthritis, Connective Tissue and Crystal Deposition Disorders

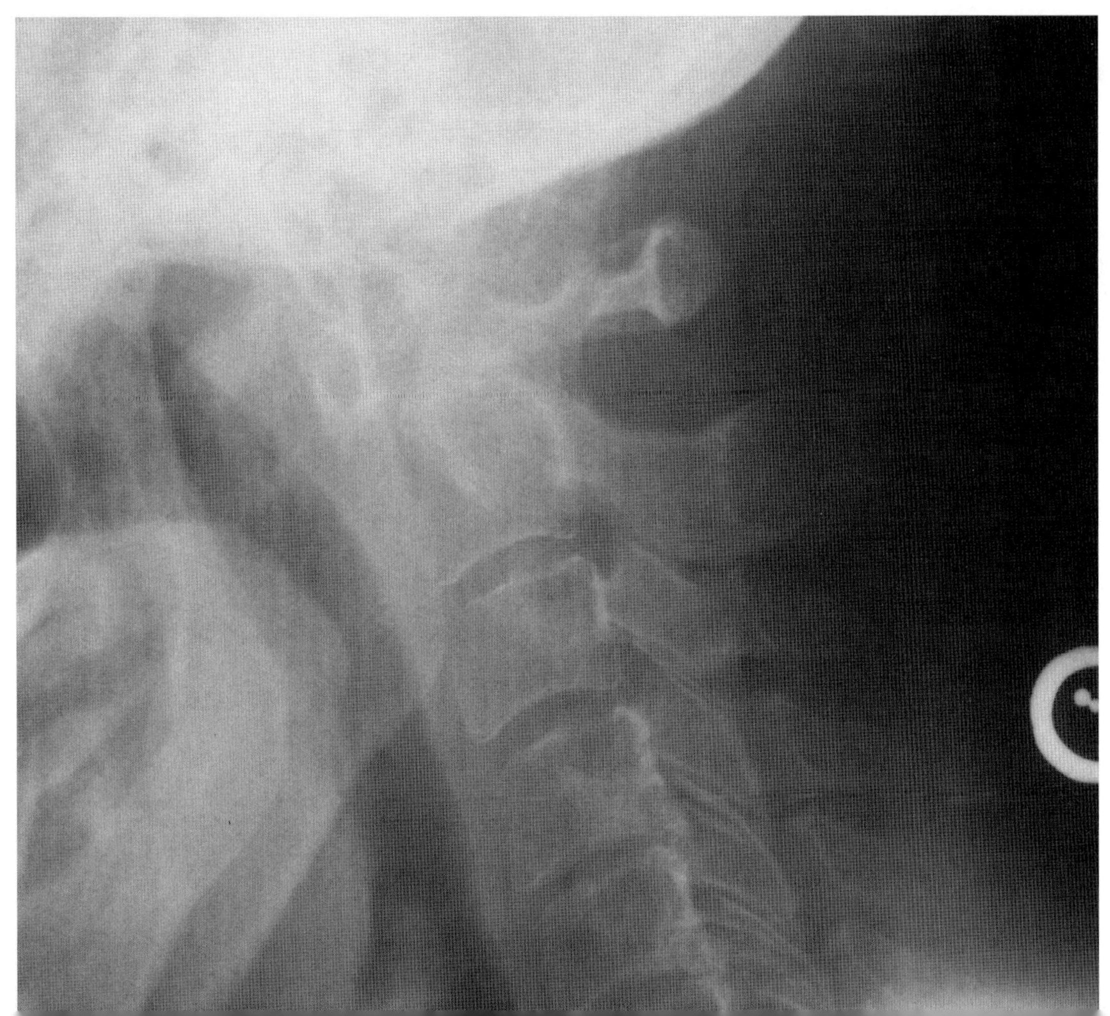

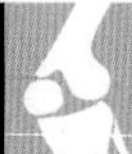

37–1 Atlantoaxial Instability in Rheumatoid Arthritis

Michael A. Bruno

PRESENTATION

History of rheumatoid arthritis

FINDINGS

Flexion/extension radiographs of the cervical spine demonstrate C1–C2 malalignment in flexion that reduces in extension (i.e., C1–C2 instability) because of ligamentous laxity. The preodontoid interval, defined as the space between the posterior cortex of the anterior arch of C1 and the anterior margin of the odontoid process of C2, should never exceed 3 mm in an adult. This space should also not change on flexion or extension.

DIFFERENTIAL DIAGNOSES

- Odontoid fracture, most commonly occurring through the base of the odontoid process (known as a type II odontoid fracture) can alter the normal relationships of the upper cervical spine.
- Atlanto-occipital subluxation is considered a devastating injury with often higher mortality.

COMMENTS

These case examples illustrate the phenomena of C1–C2 instability, which can occur as a result of ligamentous laxity involving the transverse ligament of the cervical spine, which serves to maintain the preodontoid interval. Normally, this space should never exceed 3 mm in an adult and 5 mm in children. Common causes are trauma and rheumatoid arthritis, in which, rheumatoid pannus can cause ligamentous laxity or even bony erosion of the odontoid. The major stabilizer of the atlantoaxial joint is the transverse ligament. This relatively thick ligament is located posterior to odontoid process. Synovial bursae surrounding the odontoid process become severely inflamed in rheumatoid arthritis, psoriatic arthritis, and ankylosing spondylitis. Formation of pannus and granulation tissue by inflamed synovium eventually erodes and tears the transverse ligament, leading to atlanto-axial subluxation. Retropharyngeal abscesses in children, which drain into deep cervical nodes and cause inflammation of lymph nodes in periodontal region, also lead to C1–C2 instability. In Down syndrome, the odontoid process may be dysmorphic, leading to similar instability at C1–C2. Trauma and rupture of transverse ligament also lead to atlantoaxial subluxation. Fractures of the odontoid process can mimic this instability; although in most cases the preodontoid interval is not altered. The most common fracture involving the odontoid process is transversely through the base, known as the "Type II" odontoid fracture, illustrated here.

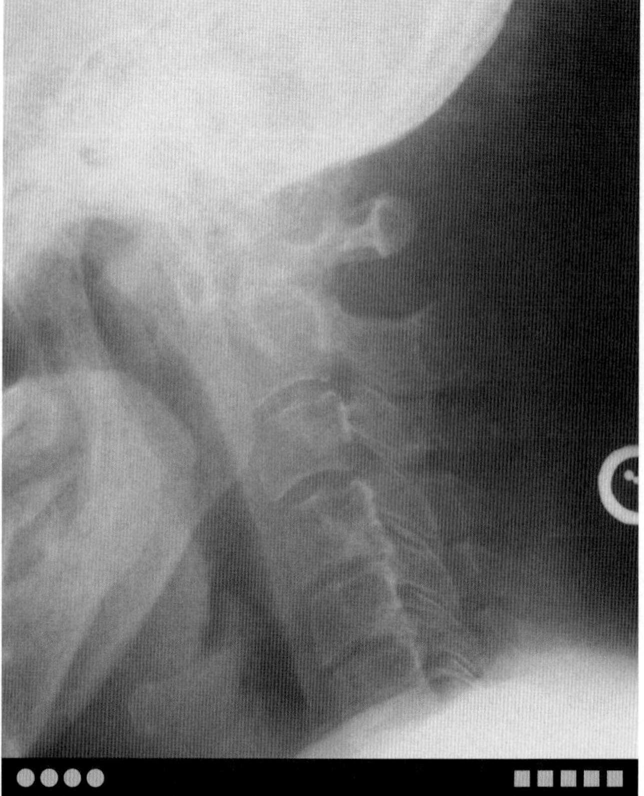

A. Rheumatoid arthritis: Lateral planar radiograph of the cervical spine in neutral position shows normal preodontoid interval. There is some suggestion that the cortex of the odontoid process may be somewhat thinned.

PEARLS

- **The normal C1–C2 relationship precludes the widening of the preodontoid space beyond 3 mm in an adult and 5 mm in children.**
- **Rheumatoid arthritis commonly involves this joint as it is a synovial joint. Laxity at C1–C2 leads to instability with widening of the preodontoid interval on flexion, with reduction on extension.**
- **Similar findings can be seen in other inflammatory processes, acute trauma, and in Down syndrome.**

ADDITIONAL IMAGES

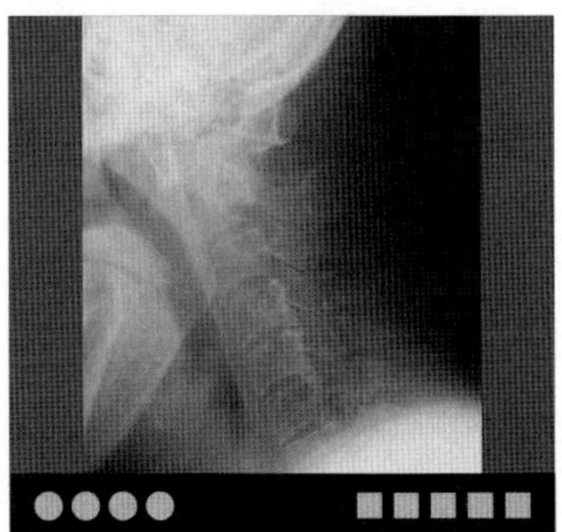

B. Rheumatoid arthritis: Lateral attempted flexion view of the cervical spine in the same patient shows gross instability at C1–C2 with marked widening of the preodontoid interval on flexion as compared to the neutral position.

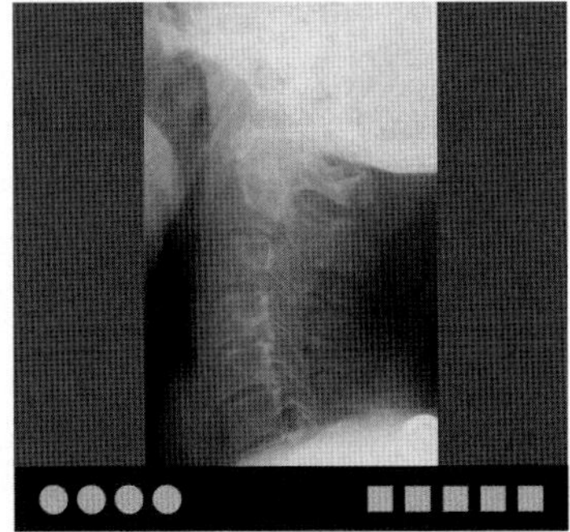

C. Rheumatoid arthritis: Lateral attempted extension view in the same patient shows reduction of the preodontoid interval in extension.

DIFFERENTIAL DIAGNOSES IMAGES

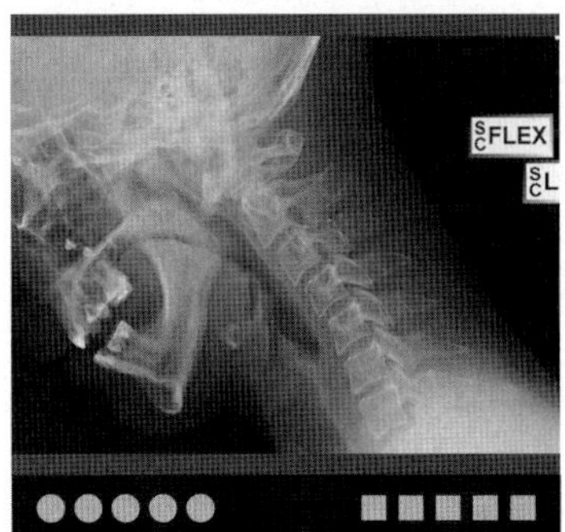

D. Type II odontoid fracture: Lateral flexion view shows abnormal alignment at C1–C2, although the preodontoid interval is maintained. Note the fracture plane at the base of the odontoid process. Note the position of the C1 and C2 lamina and spinous processes. There is some spinal canal compromise in flexion.

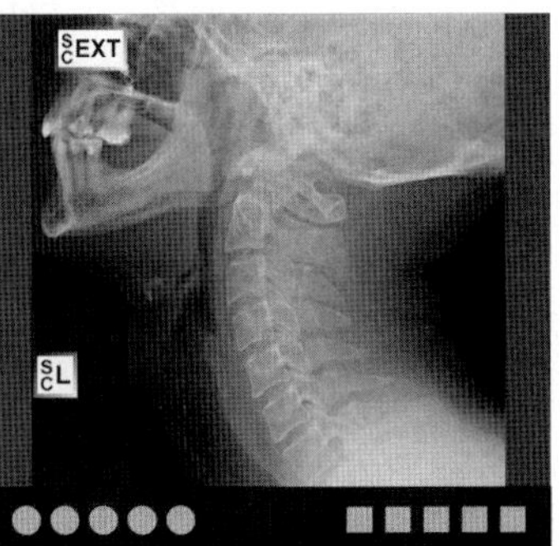

E. Type II odontoid fracture: Lateral extension view of same patient as in image D. Note the change in the fracture plane at the base of the odontoid process, and the alteration in alignment at C1–C2, nearly restoring the spinolaminar alignment and spinal canal diameter. This is a markedly unstable fracture, which must be stabilized to obviate the risk of neurological injury.

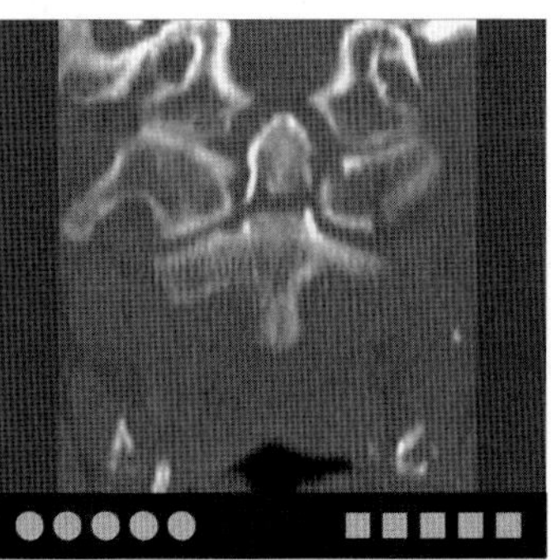

F. Dens fracture (Type II): Coronal CT image in another patient demonstrates a fracture at the base of the dens at its junction with the vertebral body.

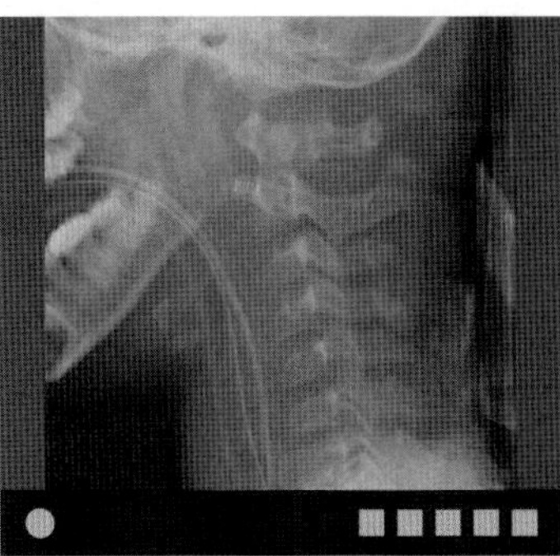

G. Atlanto-occipital dislocation: This lateral image, showing dislocation of the atlanto-occipital joint (e.g., above the level of C1) is provided for comparison to images A to F.

IMAGE KEY

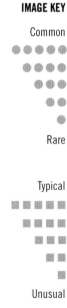

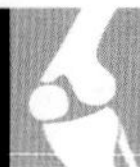

37–2 Spinal Pseudoarthrosis in Ankylosing Spondylitis

Wilfred CG Peh

PRESENTATION

Increasing spinal pain and neurological deficits

FINDINGS

Radiographs and CT images show a destructive discovertebral T12/L1 lesion with a transverse linear osteolytic lesion, extending through the fused posterior elements. There are background changes of established ankylosing spondylitis.

DIFFERENTIAL DIAGNOSES

- *Infective spondylodiscitis:* In subacute infection, there is reduced disc space, height, and endplate erosion. In the chronic period, adjacent vertebral body collapse and sclerosis may occur. The posterior elements are usually normal.
- *Renal osteodystrophy:* Osteosclerosis seen as sclerotic bands along the vertebral body endplates are also known as the rugger-jersey spine. The disc spaces are preserved and the posterior elements are normal.
- *Spinal fracture:* Seat belt fractures occur secondary to hyperflexion at the waist level during a motor vehicular accident. Usually affects L1 or L2 vertebrae, with anterior vertebral body compression and posterior element distraction. Fracture of the spinous process is called a chance fracture.

COMMENTS

The patient is a 32-year-old male known to have longstanding ankylosing spondylitis, who had exacerbation of thoracolumbar junction pain over the recent 1 year. He had increasing onset of spinal pain and neurological deficits. Ankylosing spondylitis is a type of seronegative arthropathy that is characterized by inflammation of multiple articular and paraarticular structures, frequently resulting in bony ankylosis. This entity has a predilection for the axial skeleton, particularly the sacroiliac and spinal facet joints. Young males are typically affected, with the peak age of onset being 15 to 35 years, and a male-to-female ratio of 4–10:1. Sacroiliitis is the hallmark of the disease, and is detected on radiographs as indistinctness of the joint in the early stage. This is followed by subchondral erosions, subchondral sclerosis, bony proliferation, and eventual bony fusion of both sacroiliac joints. In the spine, radiographic changes include corner erosions and sclerosis (Romanus lesions), vertebral body squaring, syndesmophyte formation, paraspinal ligament ossification, and erosion and fusion of the apophyseal and costovertebral joints. In established ankylosing spondylitis, where the spine is usually fused and rigid, complications include fractures and pseudoarthrosis formation. Pseudoarthrosis usually develops secondary to a previously undetected fracture, or an unfused segment. Radiographically, pseudoarthrosis is seen as an area of discovertebral destruction with adjacent endplate sclerosis. This may resemble disc infection. An important distinguishing feature is the involvement of the posterior elements at the level of the pseudoarthrotic lesion, where a linear hypodense area with sclerotic borders is typically seen.

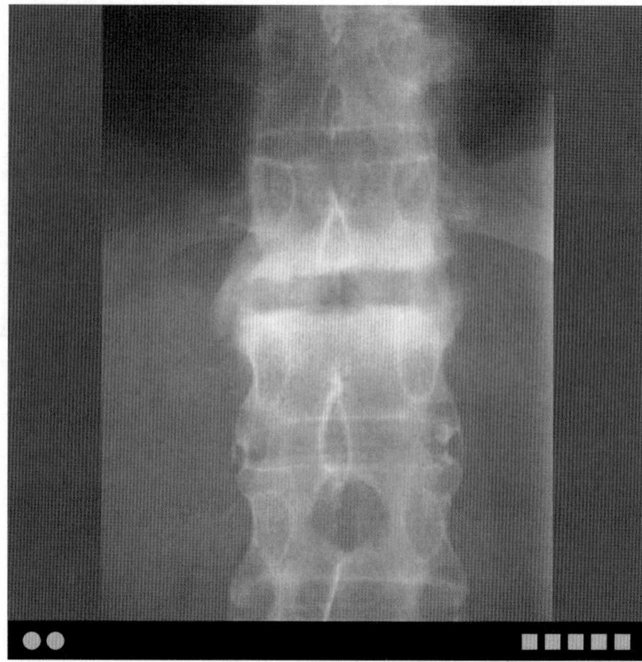

A. Spinal pseudoarthrosis in ankylosing spondylitis: Frontal radiograph shows T11/12 discovertebral destructive changes with adjacent sclerosis. There are syndesmophyte in the rest of the vertebral column, typical of ankylosing spondylitis.

PEARLS

- **Spinal pseudoarthrosis is a well-known complication and should be suspected when a patient with long-standing ankylosing spondylitis develops new onset of spinal pain.**
- **Discovertebral destruction resembling infective spondylodiscitis is seen. Involvement of the posterior element is the key distinguishing feature.**
- **CT with 2D reconstructions is useful for assessing posterior element linear osteolytic lesion.**

ADDITIONAL IMAGES

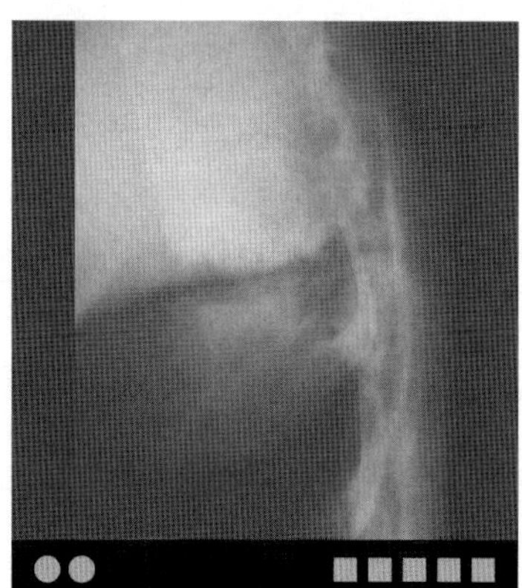

B. Spinal pseudoarthrosis in ankylosing spondylitis: Lateral radiograph shows irregularity of the adjacent lower T12 and upper L1 vertebral endplates, with adjacent subchondral sclerosis. The rest of the spine is ankylosed but there is a transverse linear osteolytic area in the T12/L1 posterior elements.

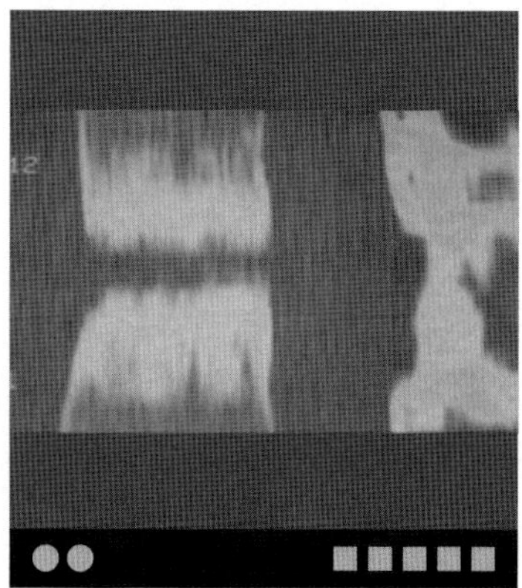

C. Spinal pseudoarthrosis in ankylosing spondylitis: Reconstructed sagittal CT image shows T12/L1 endplate irregularity and prominent sclerosis.

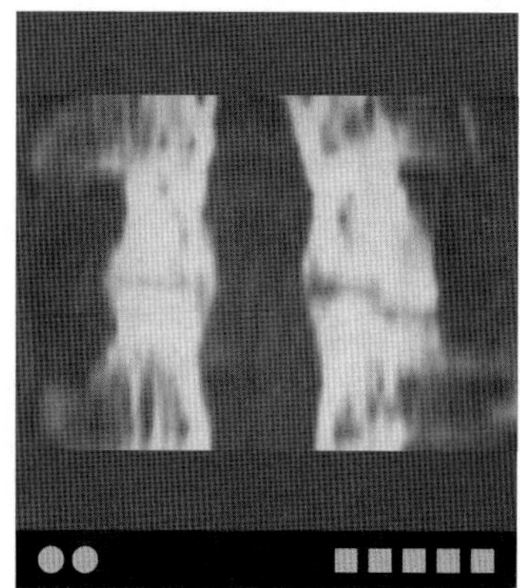

D. Spinal pseudoarthrosis in ankylosing spondylitis: Reconstructed coronal CT image shows bilateral transverse linear breaks through the otherwise fused posterior elements at T12/L1 level.

IMAGE KEY

Common

Rare

Typical

Unusual

DIFFERENTIAL DIAGNOSES IMAGES

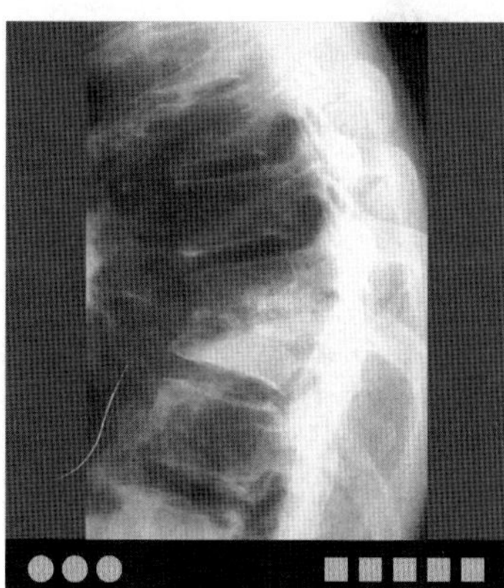

E. Pyogenic spondylodiscitis: This is a 42-year-old man. Lateral radiograph shows anterior wedging of T9 and T10 vertebral bodies, with loss of the adjacent T9/10 disc space.

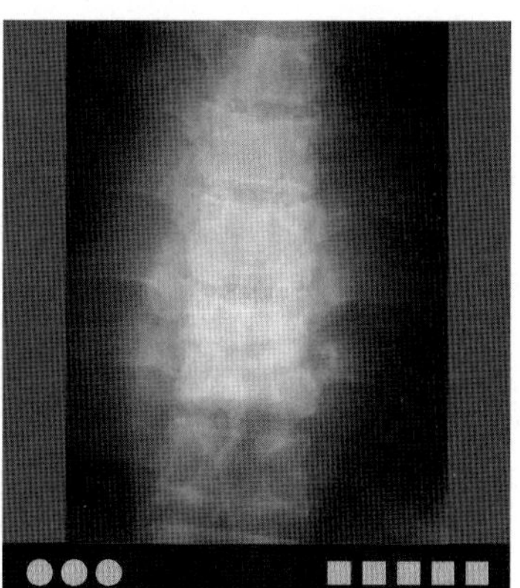

F. Pyogenic spondylodiscitis: This is the same 42-year-old man as shown in image E. Frontal radiograph shows marked narrowing and marginal irregularity of the T9/10 disc with prominent sclerosis of the adjacent vertebral bodies. A large paravertebral soft tissue mass is present.

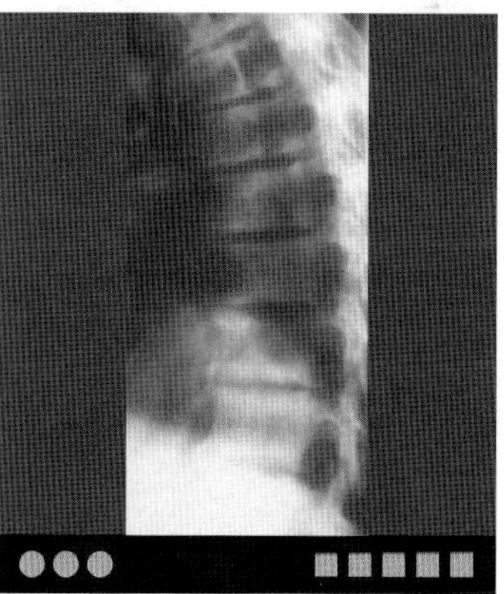

G. Rugger jersey spine: This is a 57-year-old man with renal osteodystrophy. Lateral radiograph shows band-like endplate sclerosis in all the vertebral bodies. The posterior elements are normal.

Chapter 38

Infections

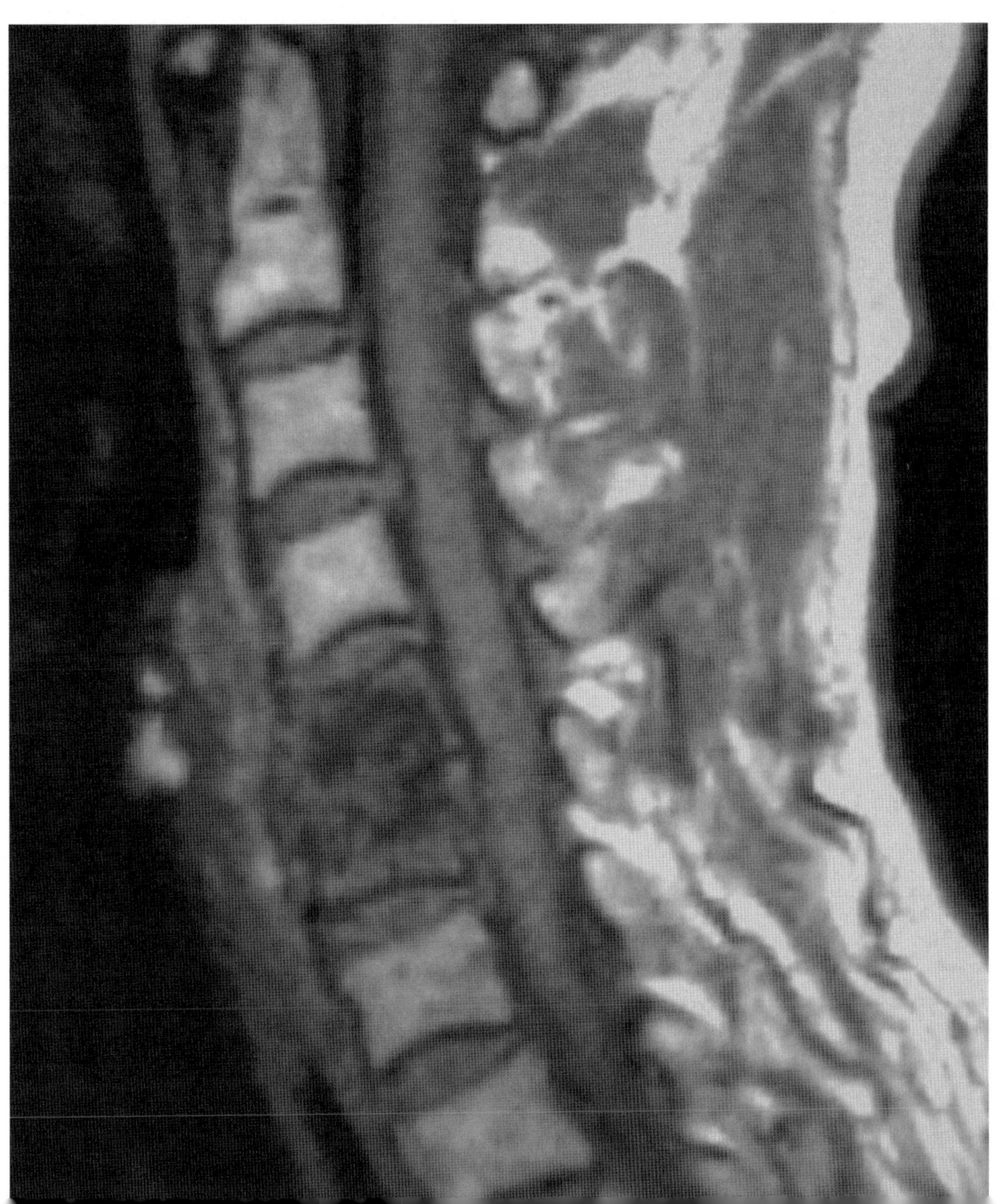

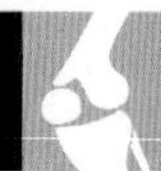

38–1 Spondylodiscitis of Cervical Spine

Wilfred CG Peh

PRESENTATION

Localized neck pain, malaise, and fever

FINDINGS

MR images show signal changes in adjacent C5 and C6 vertebral bodies and disk. Fluid is seen in this disk space, which tracks anteriorly. There is marked enhancement of all these structures as well as of the surrounding soft tissues.

DIFFERENTIAL DIAGNOSES

- *Compression fracture:* History of trauma because of moderate axial loading. Vertebral body compression is most common at C5 level, with central depression of superior endplate.
- *Disk protrusion:* Disk is often degenerated with loss of T2 signal and reduced disk height on MR imaging. Axial images are important for assessment of full extent of disk protrusion.
- *Metastases:* History of known primary tumor. MR imaging shows replacement of fatty marrow by tumor deposits and any soft tissue extension, particularly to epidural space.

COMMENTS

The patient is a 71-year-old woman with stiffness and pain in her neck. Infections of the spine usually present as spinal osteomyelitis, diskitis, or both. The most common organisms are *Staphylococcus aureus* and *Enterobacter* species. *Mycobacterium tuberculosis* causes most nonpyogenic spinal infections. Risk factors include old age, diabetes mellitus, and immunosuppression. The three main routes of spinal infection are hematogenous spread, direct inoculation (usually after a spinal procedure), and contiguous spread. In adults, infection enters the disk by means of contiguous involvement from adjacent vertebral osteomyelitis or by neovascular proliferation. In children, disk infection is usually hematogenous. Residual vascular channels lead directly to the disk. These channels typically regress by 15 years. Pyogenic organisms usually release proteolytic enzymes that dissolve the nucleus pulposus, resulting in the loss of disk height. In contrast, nonpyogenic organisms such as those that cause tuberculosis lack these enzymes and tend to spare the disk. Complications include paraspinal and epidural abscess formation. Radiographs are not sensitive for detecting early infective changes. In the subacute period, reduced disk space height and endplate erosion may be seen while in chronic infection, there may be vertebral body sclerosis and collapse. MR imaging is effective for detecting and precisely delineating the extent of acute infection, and involvement of adjacent soft tissue structures. Typically, there are T2 hyperintense and T1 hypointense signal changes in the disk and adjacent vertebral endplates, with loss of margin between disk and endplate. Paraspinal and epidural abscesses are usually T1 isointense and T2 hyperintense with rim enhancement.

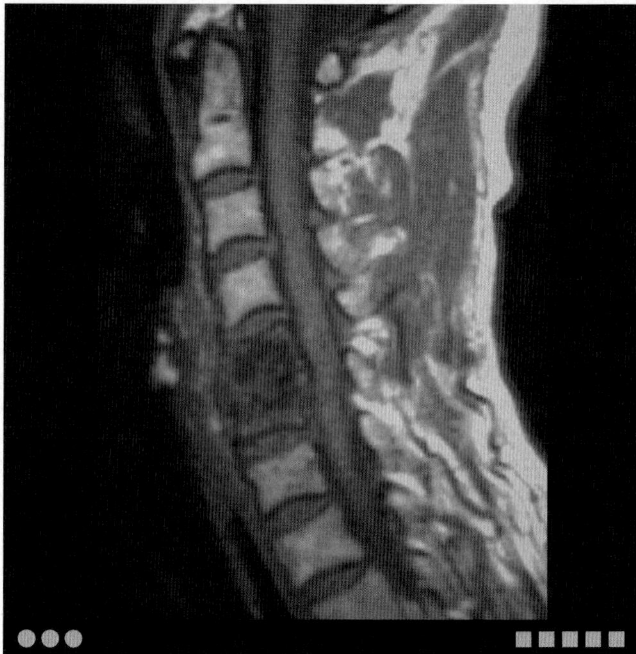

A. Cervical spine infective diskitis: Sagittal SE T1-weighted MR image shows wedging and loss of signal of C5 and C6 vertebral bodies, with loss of definition of the intervening disk.

PEARLS

- **MR imaging is the modality of choice for evaluating the presence and severity of spine infection.**
- **On MR imaging, the presence of hyperintense signal in the disk is highly suggestive of diskitis.**
- **MR imaging is useful for evaluating involvement of neural structures and extradural soft tissues.**

ADDITIONAL IMAGES

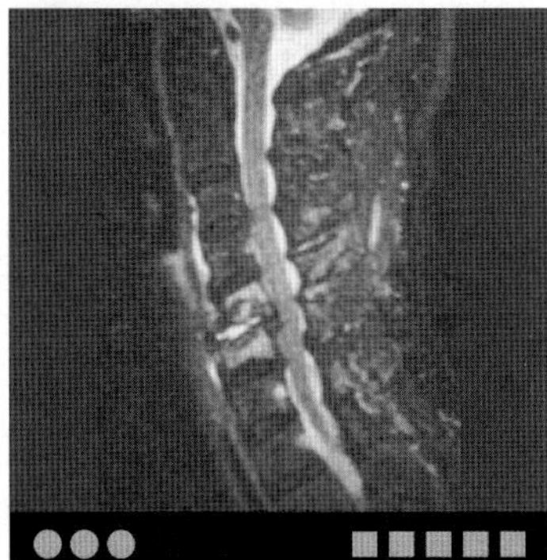

B. Cervical spine infective diskitis: Sagittal STIR MR image shows hyperintense signal within C5 and C6 vertebral bodies. A sliver of fluid is seen within the C5/C6 disk, which is irregularly narrowed. There is also tracking of fluid anterior to C3–C6 vertebral bodies.

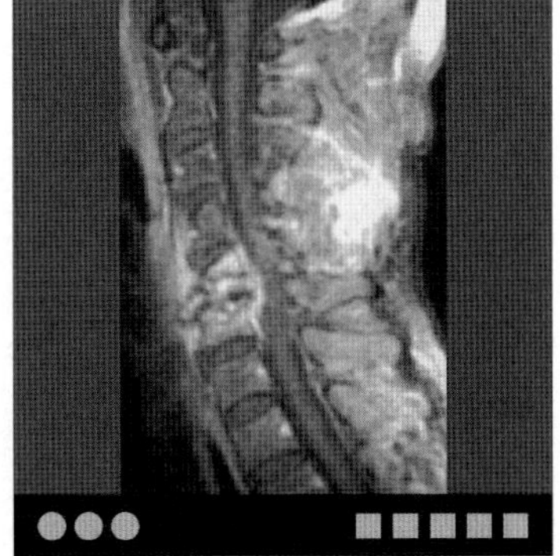

C. Cervical spine infective diskitis: Contrast-enhanced sagittal fat-suppressed SE T1-weighted MR image shows marked enhancement of the C5/C6 disk, adjacent vertebral bodies, and anterior soft tissues. There is also patchy enhancement of the posterior interspinous soft tissues.

DIFFERENTIAL DIAGNOSES IMAGES

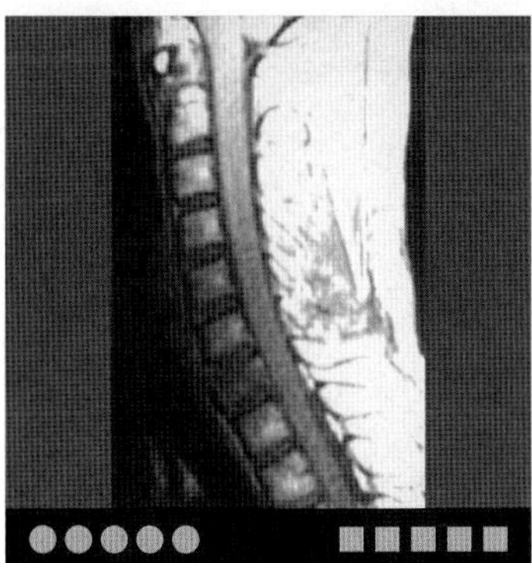

D. Compression fracture of vertebral body: Sagittal SE T1-weighted MR image shows loss in height and slight retropulsion of C7 vertebral body. There is loss of the normal fatty signal in C7 vertebral body.

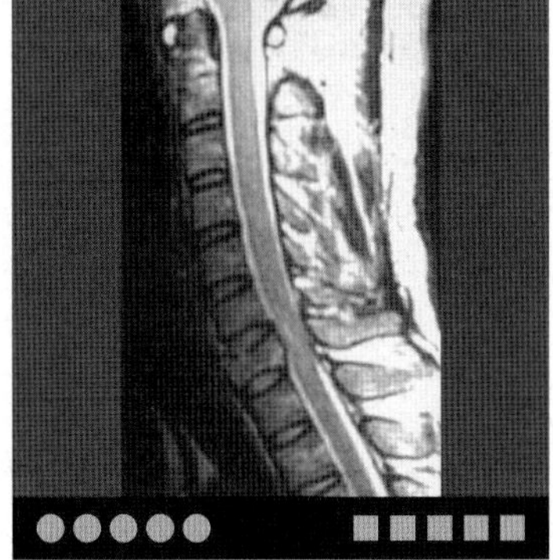

E. Compression fracture of vertebral body: Sagittal FSE T2-weighted MR image shows hyperintense signal within the compressed C7 vertebral body, indicative of marrow edema. Note small herniation of C6/C7 disk through the C7 superior endplate. There is also a small area of hyperintense signal within the adjacent cord, consistent with mild cord edema.

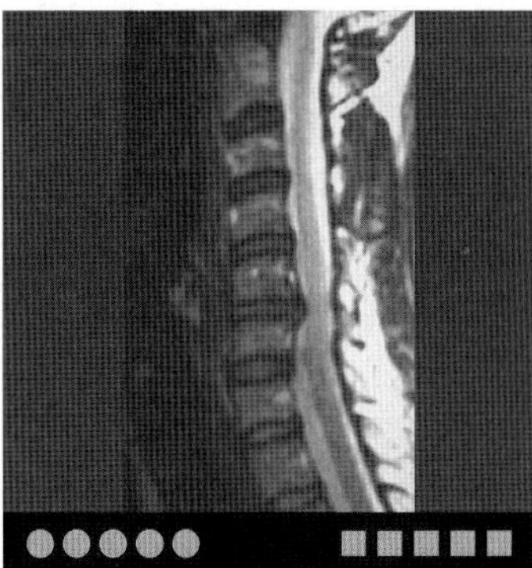

F. Disk protrusion: Sagittal FSE T2-weighted MR image shows posterior protrusion of the C5/C6 disk with indentation of the adjacent thecal sac.

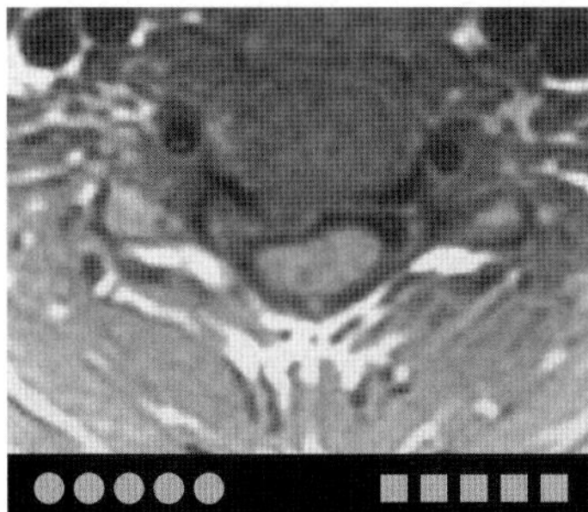

G. Disk protrusion: Axial SE T1-weighted MR image shows right posterolateral protrusion of the C5/C6 disk with slight compression of the cord.

IMAGE KEY

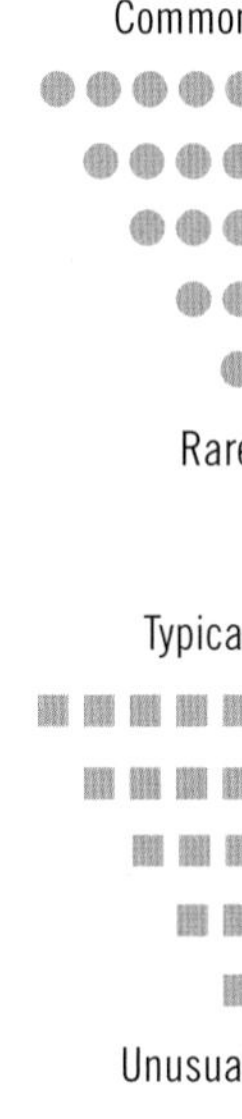

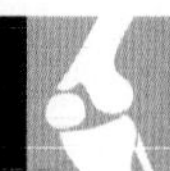

38–2 Diskitis

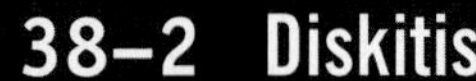

James Coumas

PRESENTATION

Pain in the lower back

FINDINGS

MR images show abnormal marrow signal within adjacent vertebral bodies, with destruction of the endplates and increased fluid within the disk space.

DIFFERENTIAL DIAGNOSES

- *Severe degenerative arthritis:* With this condition, bone production rather than destruction is usually the predominant feature.
- *Metastasis:* Metastatic disease typically neither involves adjacent endplates nor it causes a decrease in disk space height.
- *Spondyloarthropathy:* Bone changes are typically erosive with mineralization of associated ligaments and a high incidence of sacroiliac joint involvement, especially in seronegative spondyloarthropathies.
- *Charcot arthropathy:* Destructive arthropathy seen principally in diabetic patients with ununited fractures, fragmentation/debris, preservation of vacuum disk, and instability.

COMMENTS

The patient is a 67-year-old male with total colectomy for idiopathic inflammatory bowel disease, now with back pain. Diskitis is an inflammation of the disk space often in response to infection. In the adult, the disk space is essentially avascular receiving nutrients by diffusion from the adjacent vertebral endplates. Most infections of the disk space are the result of hematogenous dissemination to the vertebral body and subsequent extension to the disk space. The most common sources of infection include the urinary tract, pneumonia, and soft tissue wound infections. *Staphylococcus aureus* is the most common bacterial pathogen. Less than 0.5% of infections of the disk space are secondary to surgery or attributed to contiguous extension. The incidence of diskitis is twofold greater in males. A bimodal curve exists with childhood involvement peaking at the age of seven years, and adult involvement occurring in the fifth and sixth decades of life. Mortality is variably reported at between 2% and 12%, depending on the age of the patient, the patient's immunologic status, the level of spinal involvement, and predisposing health factors such as diabetes. MR is the imaging modality of choice. Accurate assessment of the vertebra, disk space, epidural space, and paravertebral soft tissues is performed. In cases of neurological compromise, the entire spine should be examined for multifocal involvement and the site of greatest neurological deficit. Appropriate treatment requires percutaneous aspiration and culture to optimize antibiotic selection. Therapy requires 6 to 8 weeks of intravenous antibiotics. Open biopsy/surgery is indicated in patients with progressive neurological deficits despite antibiotic treatment, spinal deformity, or antibiotic toxicity.

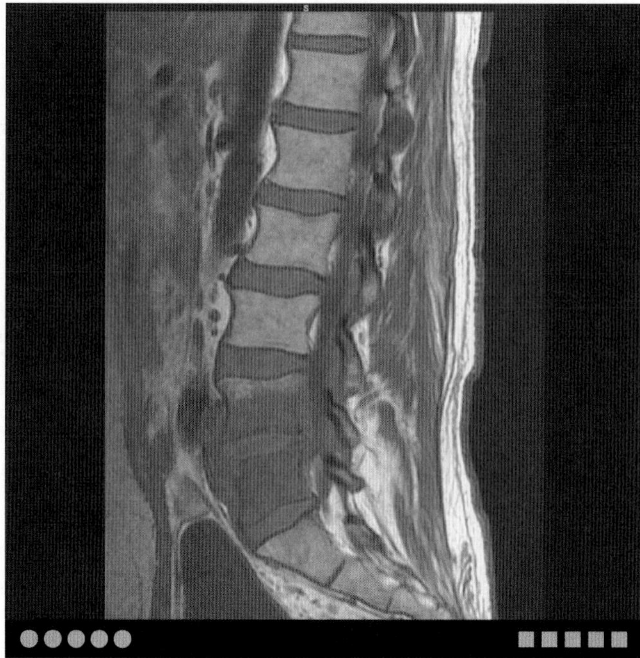

A. Diskitis: Sagittal T1-weighted MR image shows loss of normal marrow signal within adjacent vertebral bodies (L4 and L5), destruction of the endplate (L5), and loss of paravertebral and epidural fat signal.

PEARLS

- **Subtle physiologic changes of diskitis are readily apparent on MR imaging.**
- **Contrast enhancement is helpful in assessing involvement of the paravertebral and epidural soft tissues.**
- **Contrast enhancement is helpful in directing percutaneous CT-guided aspiration of fluid collections.**

ADDITIONAL IMAGES

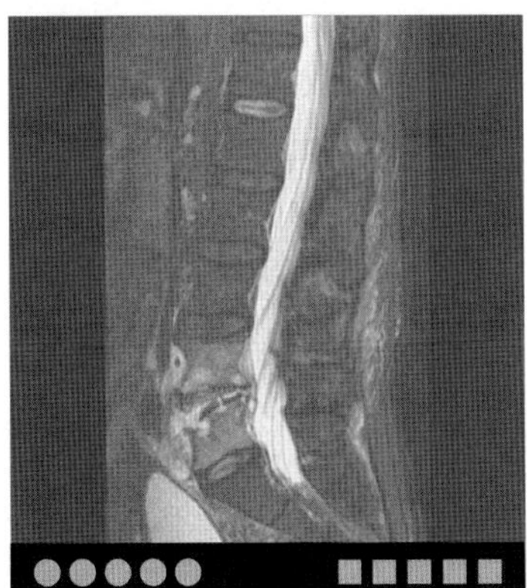

B. Diskitis with osteomyelitis and epidural abscess: Sagittal T2-weighted MR images show the destruction of the endplates as well as the destruction of the vertebral body. Epidural abscess is well shown at levels of the L4 and L5 vertebral bodies.

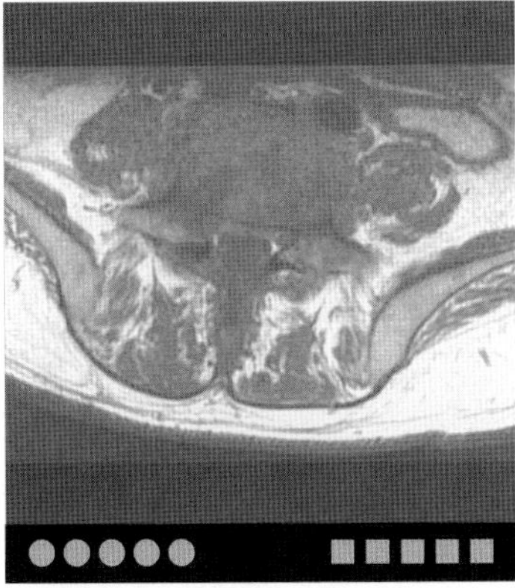

C. Diskitis with paravertebral and epidural extension: Axial T1-weighted MR image shows loss of the paravertebral fat stripe typically interposed between psoas muscle and vertebral body.

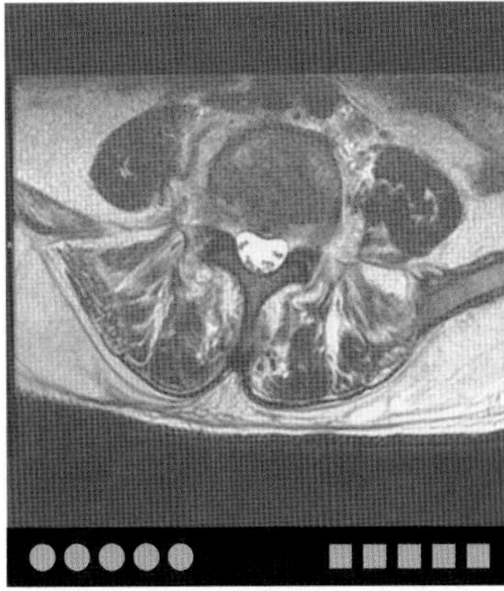

D. Diskitis with epidural abscess: Axial T2-weighted MR image shows an abnormal paravertebral soft tissue mass, which does extend to the epidural soft tissues.

IMAGE KEY

Common
●●●●●
●●●●
●●●
●●
●
Rare

Typical
■■■■■
■■■■
■■■
■■
■
Unusual

DIFFERENTIAL DIAGNOSES IMAGES

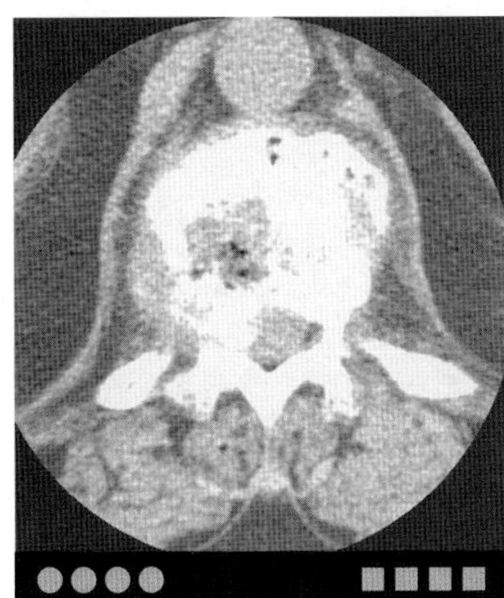

E. Discal spondyloarthropathy: CT axial section shows circumferential bulge with epidural soft tissue mineralization associated with crystal deposition arthropathy. Note the fat planes are preserved and vacuum gas persists.

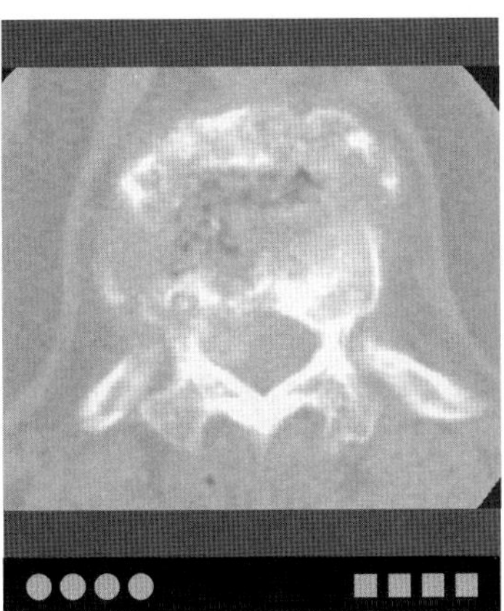

F. Discal spondyloarthropathy: Bone window on CT shows anterior spur formation but no bony destruction.

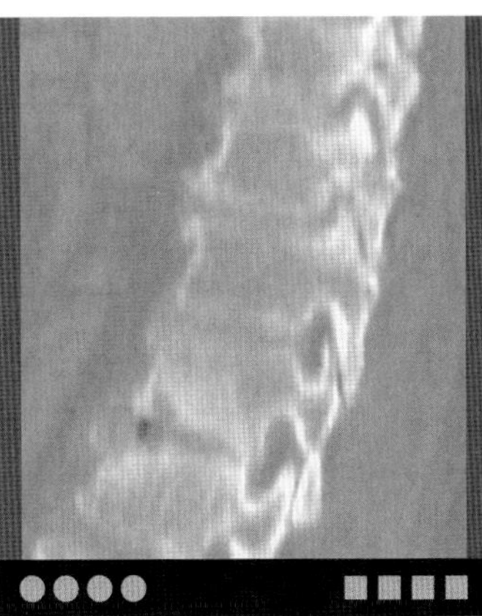

G. Spondyloarthropathy: Sagittal CT reconstruction shows reactive bony sclerosis and vacuum gas.

Chapter 39

Tumors and Tumor Like Lesions

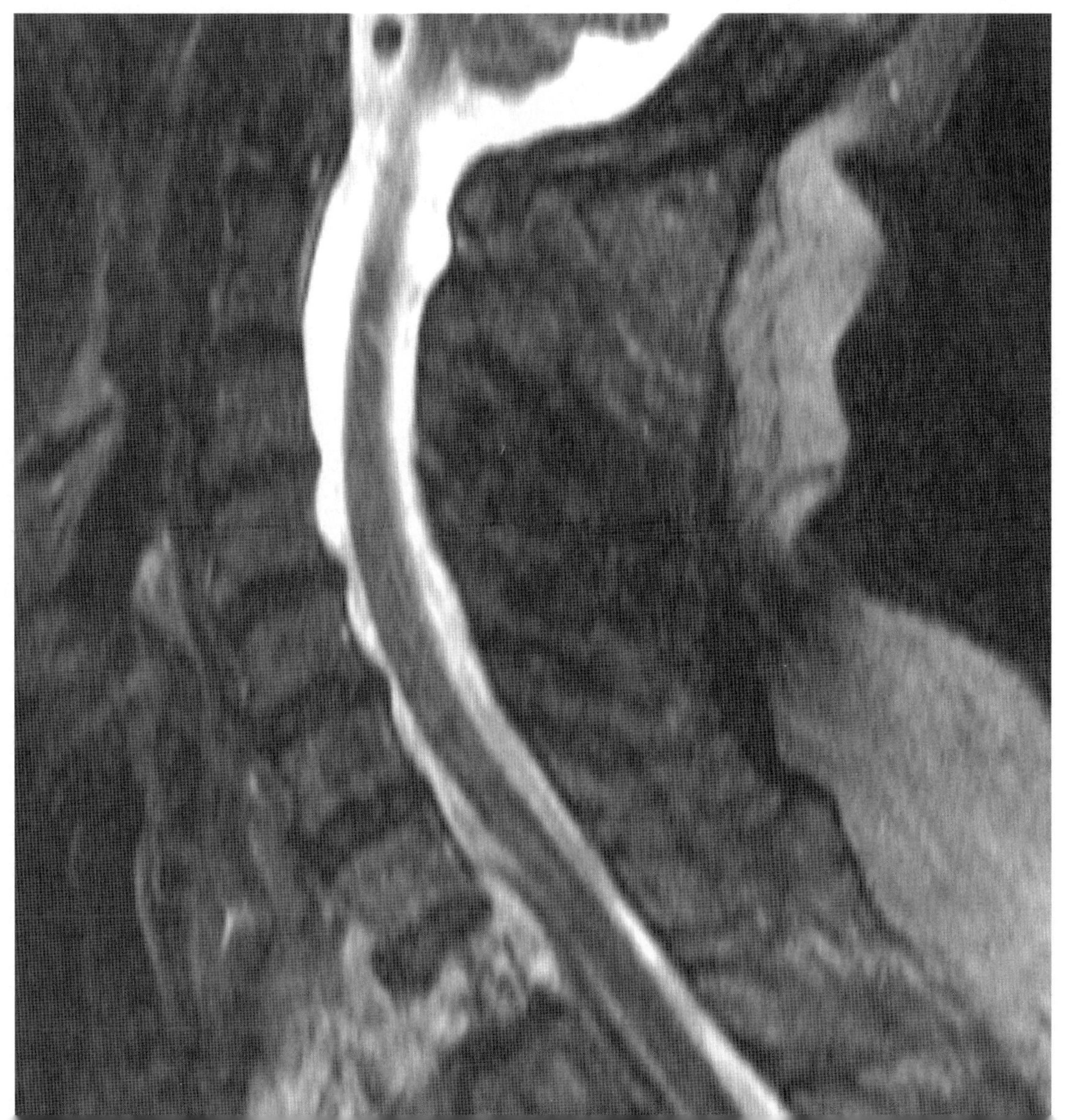

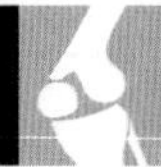

39–1 Chordoma of Cervicothoracic Junction

Melitus Maryam Golshan and Jamshid Tehranzadeh

PRESENTATION

Weakness of extremities

FINDINGS

MR imaging shows a lobulated, heterogeneous midline mass in cervicothoracic junction at T1 vertebra with low signal intensity (SI) on T1-weighted and high SI on T2-weighted images relatively sparing intervertebral discs.

DIFFERENTIAL DIAGNOSES

- *Plasmacytoma:* It has well-circumscribed or diffused low to intermediate SI marrow changes on T1 and intermediate to high SI on T2-weighted image with contrast enhancement. It often involves older age group.
- *Lymphoma:* It shows diffused, homogenous marrow SI change with extension to extra osseous soft tissue without bone destruction (wrap around sign).
- *Metastases:* It usually cause heterogeneous signal in the marrow with bone destruction and epidural soft tissue mass.
- *Giant notochordal hemangioma:* The most important discriminating factor from chordoma in this lesion is the absence of soft tissue mass and the absence of any osteolysis of vertebral trabeculae.
- *Neurogenic tumors:* They usually enlarge neural foramen and are unilateral with dumbbell appearance.

COMMENTS

This is an image of a 60-year-old woman who presented with a history of extremities weakness. Cervical chordomas are rare, slow-growing, but locally aggressive tumors. Chordomas are predominantly found in people 50 to 69 years old and are derived from remnants of primitive notochord. It is most often found in the sacrococcygeal or skull base areas. However, it can occur throughout the spine more commonly in cervical region. Vertebral chordomas tend to occur in somewhat younger populations and are more aggressive. Chordomas are slow-growing tumors as a result, they may reach considerable size before the patient becomes symptomatic. Surgical resection with a wide margin is the only curative procedure. Chordomas may occur without bone and disc involvement. However, malignant chordomas are usually extradural and cause local bone destruction. Local invasion is associated with bone erosion and destruction, which usually involves the dorsal portion of vertebral body with extension toward the spinal canal. Radiography shows osteolytic lesion of vertebra, secondary reactive osteosclerosis because of vertebral collapse, and characteristic amorphous soft tissue calcifications or ossifications. CT scan may demonstrate ivory vertebral body, paravertebral tumor, and intraspinal extension. Contrast enhancement is mild to moderate and heterogeneous. Septate areas of low attenuation within the tumor or multiple zones of hypodensity with correlating areas of cystic degeneration may be present. Chordoma is well-circumscribed, lobulated lesion with low to intermediate signal on T1-weighted and high signal on T2-weighted MR images. Chordomas contain low signal fibrous septa in all sequences, and it has moderate to mark heterogeneous contrast enhancement.

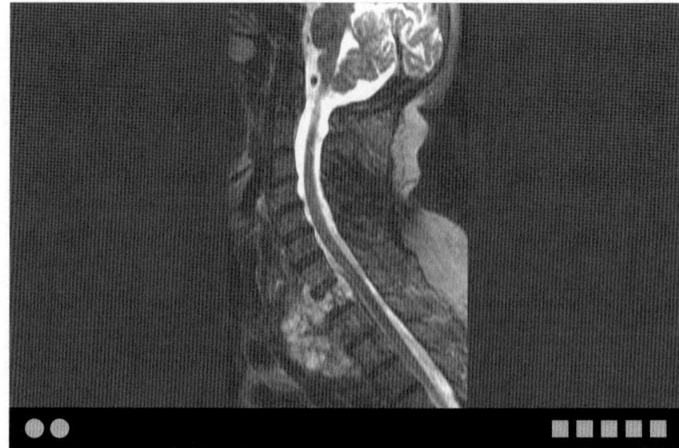

A. Chordoma: Sagittal T2-weighted image shows a nonhomogeneous high SI mass in T1 vertebral body extending to prevertebral soft tissue at C7 proximally and to T3 distally. Tumor involves the body of T1 creating a small mass posteriorly at the anterior epidural space and a large mass anteriorly. Note low SI strands in the mass probably corresponding to fibrous septa.

PEARLS

- **Chordomas are slow growing midline bone tumors spanning several vertebral segments and sparing intervertebral discs.**
- **CT scan may demonstrate ivory vertebral body, paravertebral soft tissue tumor, and intraspinal extension.**
- **Chordoma is a well-circumscribed, lobulated lesion with low to intermediate signal on T1-weighted and high signal on T2-weighted MR images. It demonstrates moderate to mark heterogeneous enhancement after gadolinium administration.**
- **Low signal fibrous septa may be seen in all sequences in chordomas.**

ADDITIONAL IMAGES

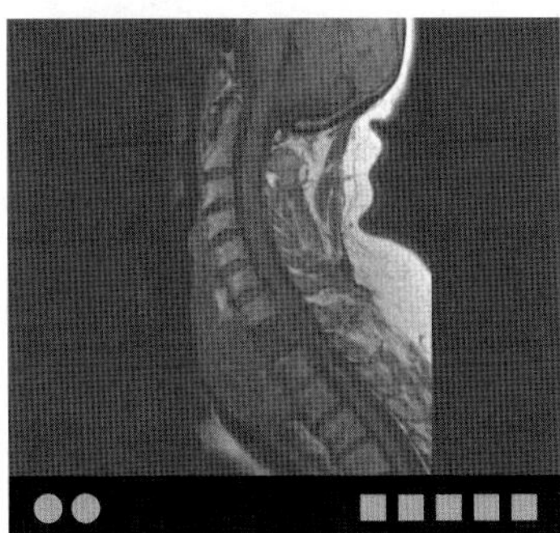

B. Chordoma: Sagittal T1-weighted image shows low to intermediate SI mass involving T1 vertebral body with anterior and posterior extension. Note marrow changes in T2 and T3 vertebral bodies with relatively intact discs.

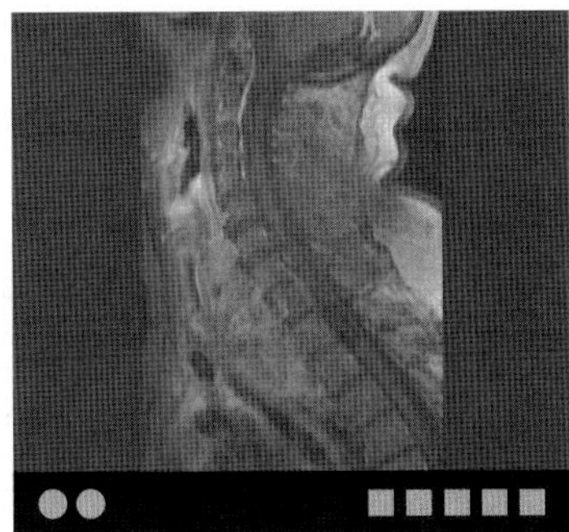

C. Chordoma: Sagittal postcontrast T1-weighted image shows heterogeneous marked enhancement in the mass. Note nonenhancing low SI septa in the mass consistent with fibrous bands.

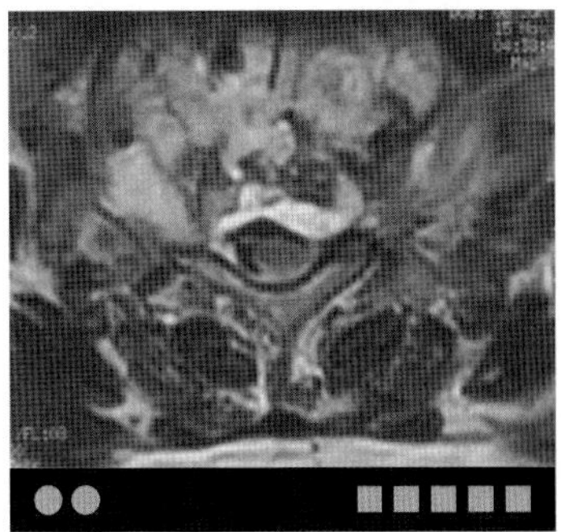

D. Chordoma: Axial T2-weighted image shows large soft tissue mass extending from vertebral body into prevertebral soft tissues anteriorly and with some extension to anterior epidural space posteriorly.

E. Chordoma: Axial CT scan shows mixed, destructive, and lytic lesion of vertebral body. Note large soft tissue mass with displacement of anterior mediastinal structures as well as extension of the mass to spinal canal.

IMAGE KEY

Common

Rare

Typical

Unusual

DIFFERENTIAL DIAGNOSES IMAGES

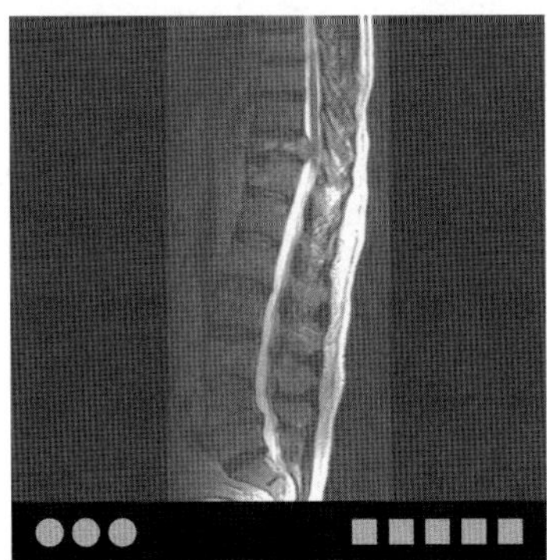

F. Plasmacytoma: Sagittal T2-weighted image shows collapse of T10 and partial collapse of T11 with intermediate signal in the vertebrae. Note convex cortex of T10 extending to spinal canal.

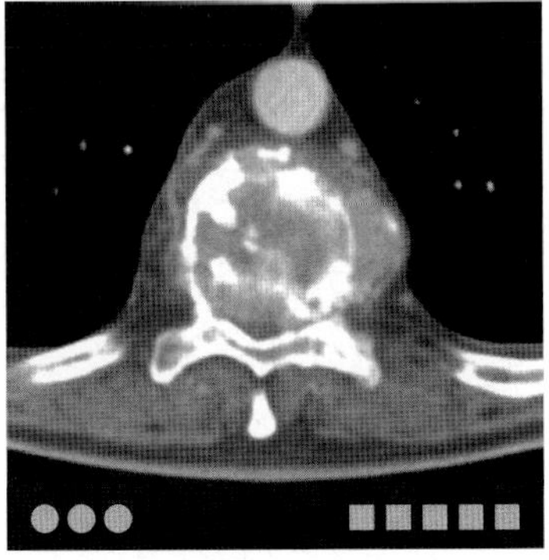

G. Plasmacytoma: Axial CT scan shows lytic, destructive lesion of vertebral body. Note extension of the lesion to paravertebral region and to the spinal canal.

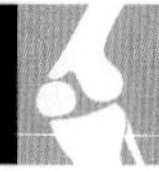

39–2 Giant Osteochondroma of the Cervical Spine

Neerjana Doda and Wilfred CG Peh

PRESENTATION

Soft tissue mass, pain, and paraesthesia

FINDINGS

Lateral radiograph shows a large, lobulated, and calcified mass arising from C3 spinous process. MR images show that the lobulated lesion is markedly T2-hyperintense, has thin septations, with an enhancement pattern that is typical of osteochondroma.

DIFFERENTIAL DIAGNOSES

- *Degenerative changes:* Osteophytes related to degenerate discs are located anteriorly, adjacent to the vertebral bodies, and are usually not a diagnostic problem. Sometimes, those associated with facet degeneration may appear prominent because of bony outgrowths.
- *Osteoblastoma:* Uncommon, usually symptomatic. CT scan often shows a well-defined, scalloped, or lobulated expansile lytic lesion that is predominantly lucent, but may show matrix mineralization. Usually has a thin bony or sclerotic rim.

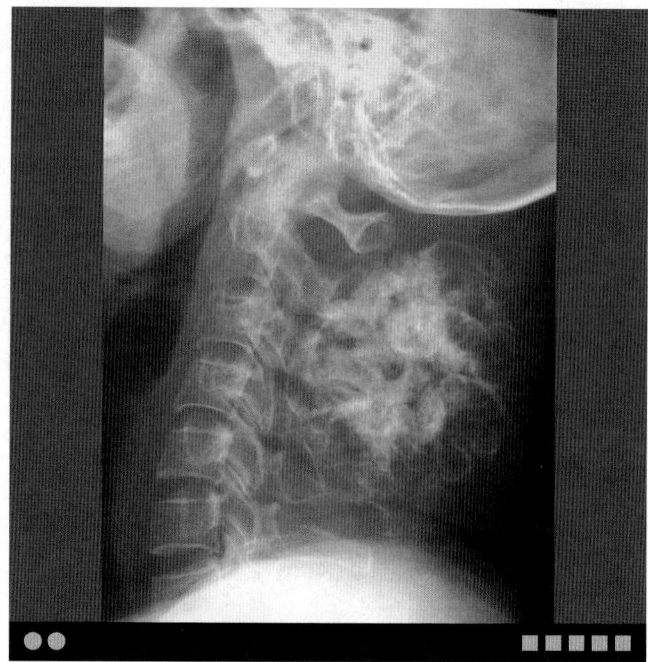

A. Giant osteochondroma of the cervical spine: Lateral radiograph shows a large calcified cauliflowerlike mass arising from C3 spinous process. It is well-defined and contains central areas of dense calcifications.

COMMENTS

This is an image of a 32-year-old man who felt a hard painless mass at the back of his neck. Osteochondromas (or exostoses) are the most common benign bone tumors and constitute 10% to 15% of all bone tumours. This lesion arises from the surface of a bone, and is seen as a bony excrescence with a cartilaginous covered cortex and a medullary cavity that is contiguous with the parent bone. It may be solitary or multiple, with the latter being associated with an autosomal dominant syndrome called hereditary multiple exostoses. Malignant transformation is estimated to occur in 1% of solitary and 1% to 20% of multiple osteochondromas. This lesion usually occurs between the age of 10 to 25 years. The male: female predominance is 1.5 to 2.5: 1. It most commonly affects the long bones, usually around knee, and the proximal humerus. Spinal osteochondromas account for only 1% to 4% of osteochondromas, and most frequently affect the spinous or transverse process. Fifty percent occur in the cervical vertebra, with the C2 vertebra being the most common location. Clinically, the lesions present as asymptomatic, palpable, and bony masses or more unusually, with neurological deficit. Radiographs show a sessile or pedunculated bone-like mass. CT scan shows a cauliflowerlike lobulated mass with ringlike mineralization as well as calcifications. MR imaging demonstrates medullary continuity between the osteochondroma and the parent bone. The cartilaginous portion of the lesion is T1 hypo- to isointense and markedly T2 hyperintense and shows the characteristic "rings and arcs" and septal patterns of contrast enhancement. A cap thicker than 2 cm should raise suspicion of possible sarcomatous transformation.

PEARLS

- **Only 1% to 4% of osteochondromas occur in the spine. It is most common in cervical spine, 50% of which occur in C2 vertebra.**
- **Spinal osteochondromas typically involves the spinous or transverse process. They present as palpable, bony-hard masses that are usually asymptomatic.**
- **Pedunculated or sessile cauliflowerlike mass with ring-like mineralization and calcification. Shows marrow continuity with the parent bone.**
- **Cartilaginous cap, which often contains calcific foci. Best evaluated on MR imaging which shows low signal on T1- and high signal on T2-weighted sequences.**

ADDITIONAL IMAGES

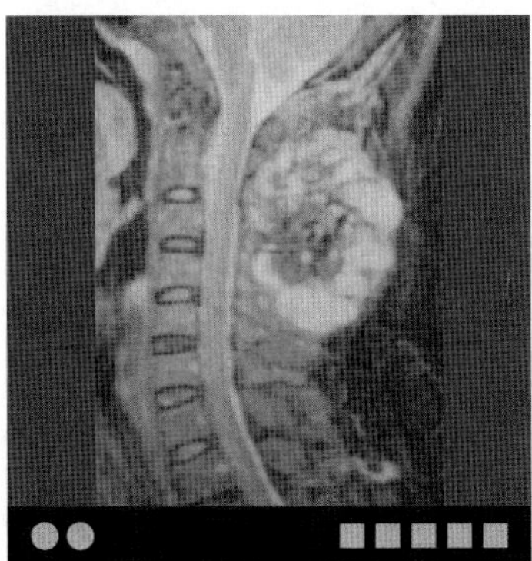

B. Giant osteochondroma of the cervical spine: Sagittal T2-weighted MR image shows a lobulated mass that is mostly hyperintense in signal. There are internal septations and a central cluster of hypointense signal, consistent with calcifications.

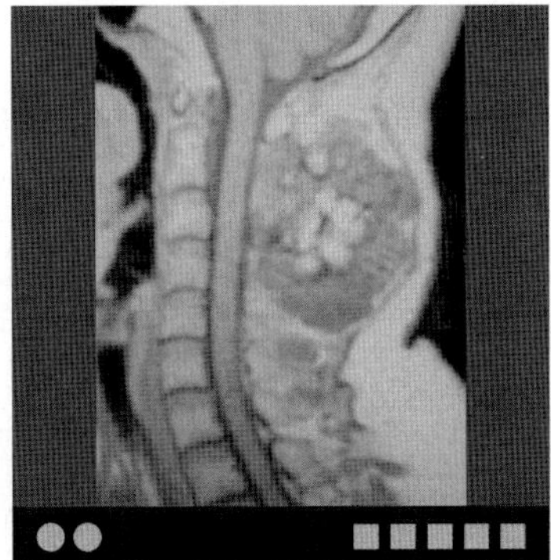

C. Giant osteochondroma of the cervical spine: Sagittal T1-weighted MR image shows a lobulated mass that is largely isointense in signal. Hypertintense areas correspond to fatty marrow, while hypointense areas represent calcifications.

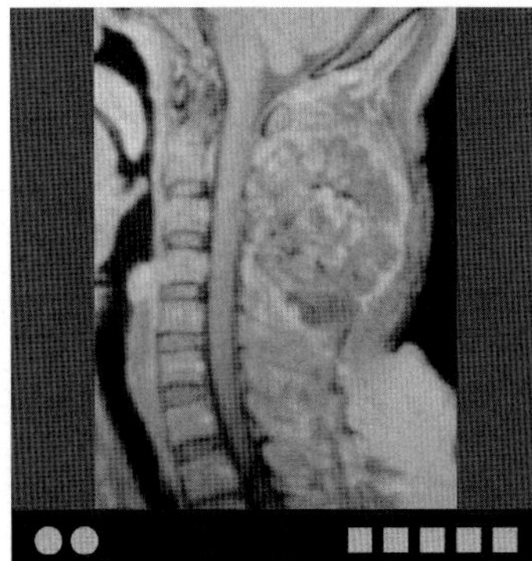

D. Giant osteochondroma of the cervical spine: Sagittal contrast-enhanced T1-weighted MR image shows a pattern of rings and arcs and septal enhancement.

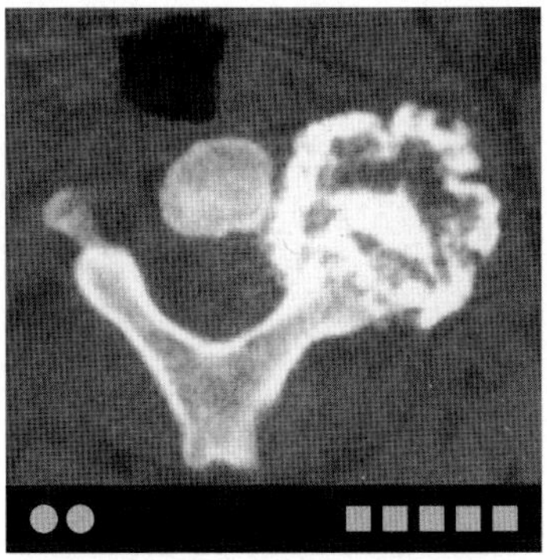

E. Osteochondroma of the facet joint: Axial CT scan image of cervical spine shows a large osteochondroma arising from the articular processes at facet joint on the left side.

DIFFERENTIAL DIAGNOSES IMAGES

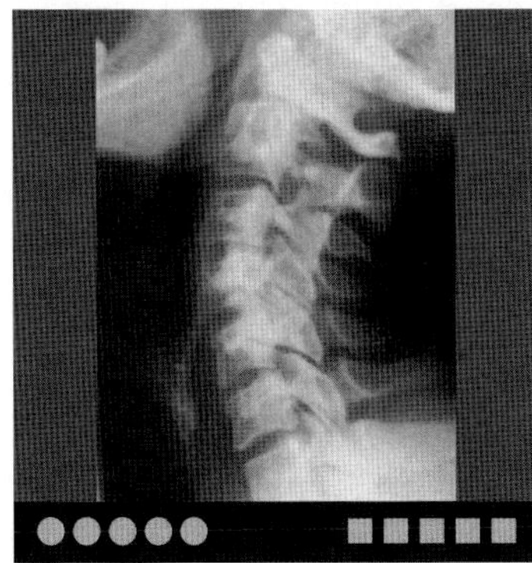

F. Cervical spine facet degeneration: Lateral radiograph of the cervical spine shows a sclerotic and hypertrophic right C4/5 facet joint.

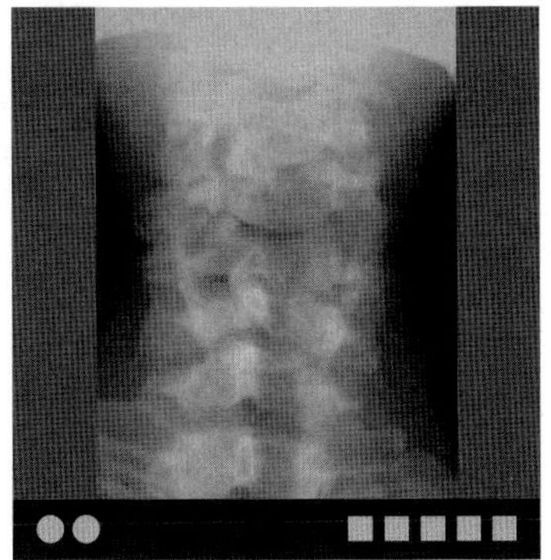

G. Cervical spine facet degeneration: Frontal radiograph of the cervical spine shows a sclerotic and hypertrophic right C4/5 facet joint.

IMAGE KEY

Common

●●●●●
●●●●
●●●
●●
●

Rare

Typical

■■■■■
■■■■
■■■
■■
■

Unusual

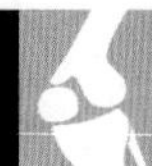

39–3 Cavernous Hemangioma Malformation of the Cervical Spinal Cord

Tatiana Voci and Peyman Borghei

PRESENTATION

Upper extremity weakness

FINDINGS

MRI shows a bright, intramedullary, spinal lesion with an irregular border of low signal intensity on T2-weighted image because of hemosiderin. On T1-weighted image, this peripheral rim is hyperintense because of subacute hemorrhage.

DIFFERENTIAL DIAGNOSES

- *Inflammation and myelitis:* It is caused by inflammation and edema; T2-weighted images show high signal intensity foci within the cord, which enhances with contrast.
- *Cord contusion caused by trauma:* MRI shows poorly defined low signal intensity foci within the cord on T1-weighted image and high signal intensity foci on T2-weighted image.
- *Syringohydromyelia:* MRI shows cystic areas of low signal intensity on T1-weighted image and high signal intensity on T2-weighted image, with a sharp border between these cystic lesions and the cord. No contrast enhancement is seen.
- *Astrocytoma or ependymoma of spine:* They are large, expansile lesions usually extending over several vertebrae with cystic and solid components. Astrocytomas appear ill-defined; however, ependymomas are sharply marginated.
- *Hemorrhagic metastasis:* History of a primary malignancy with tendency to hemorrhage such as thyroid cancer, renal cell carcinoma, and melanoma is essential. MRI shows contrast enhancement with surrounding edema (high signal on T2-weighted image).

COMMENTS

Cavernous hemangioma is a vascular lesion consisting of thin, vascular channels with no interspersed neural tissue. Only 3% to 5% of these lesions are found in the spinal cord, and the remainders are seen in the brain. Patients with spinal, intramedullary, and cavernous hemangioma present with either an acute onset of neurological compromise or a slowly progressive neurological deficit. Acute neurological decline is usually secondary to hemorrhage within the spinal cord. Chronic progressive myelopathy occurs as a result of micro hemorrhages and the resulting gliotic reaction to hemorrhagic products. There is no evidence that cavernous hemangiomas increased in size. The rate of rebleeding is unknown, but spinal cavernous hemangiomas appear to be clinically more aggressive than the cranial one, probably because the spinal cord is less tolerant of mass lesions. CT scan is often normal apart from subtle cord enlargement. MRI is virtually diagnostic for spinal cavernous hemangioma. It confirms the presence of lesions containing heterogeneous blood products of different ages, with typical "popcorn" heterogeneous signal. T2-weighted image shows characteristic hypointense signal rim because of hemosiderin. T1-weighted postcontrast image shows minimal or no enhancement. The size of the cavernous hemangioma may vary from few millimeters to over a centimeter with well-defined borders. These lesions usually are angiographically occult. MRI of the entire neuraxis (brain and spine) is recommended for lesion multiplicity.

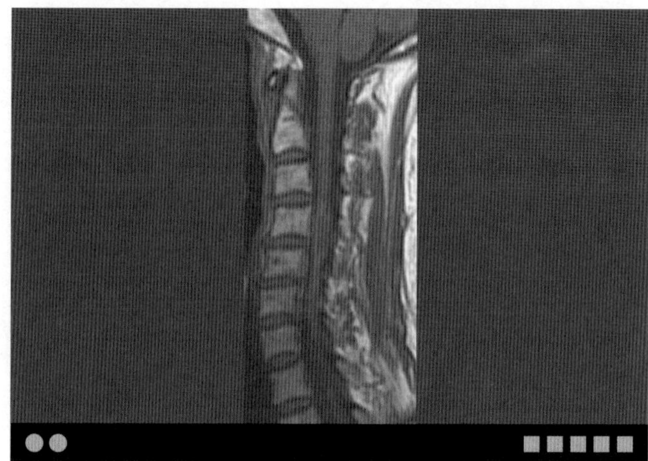

A. Cavernous hemangioma: Sagittal T1-weighted image shows an oval, approximately 2 cm long, intermediate intensity lesion within the cord with subtle, hyperintense periphery representing hemorrhagic products.

PEARLS

- **Clinical patterns seen with cavernous hemangioma are diverse, including slow progressive neurological decline, sudden onset of hemi-or paraplegia, multiple episodes of gradually worsening neurological deterioration with intermittent recovery, and a rare presentation with subarachnoid hemorrhage.**
- **MR imaging characteristics of the cavernous hemangioma is a low signal rim on T2-weighted images caused by hemosiderin.**
- **MRI of the entire neuraxis is recommended for lesion multiplicity.**

ADDITIONAL IMAGES

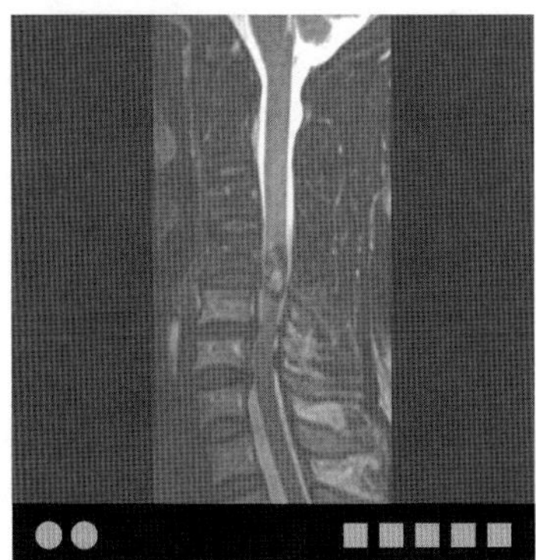

B. Cavernous hemangioma: Sagittal T2-weighted image shows peripheral foci of hypointensity consistent with hemosiderin ring which is surrounding a central area of mixed low and high signal.

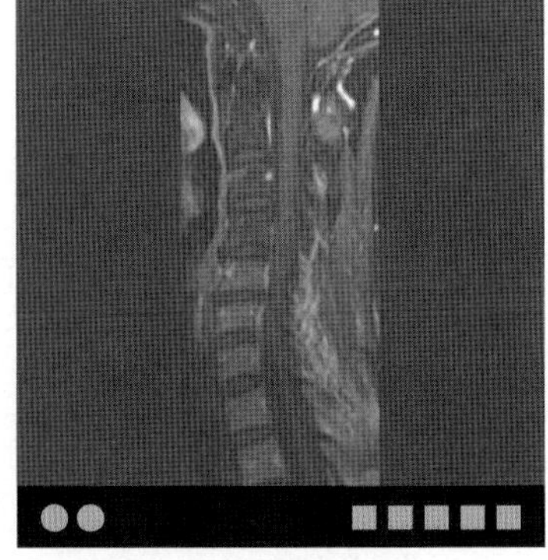

C. Cavernous hemangioma: Sagittal T2-weighted postcontrast image demonstrates no appreciable enhancement.

DIFFERENTIAL DIAGNOSES IMAGES

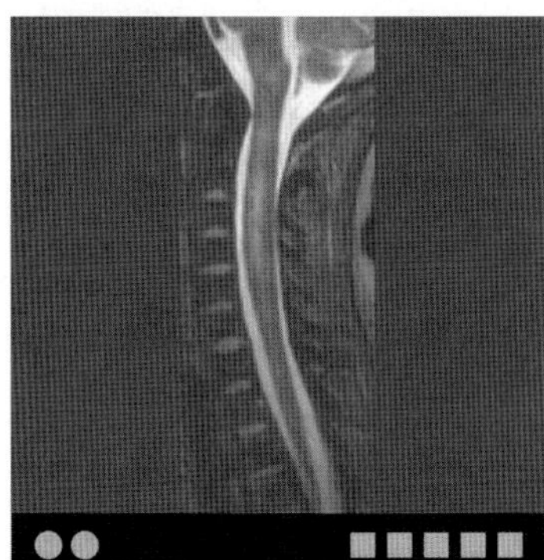

D. Postviral myelitis: Sagittal T2-weighted image shows entire cervical cord expansion and edema secondary to longitudinal postviral myelitis

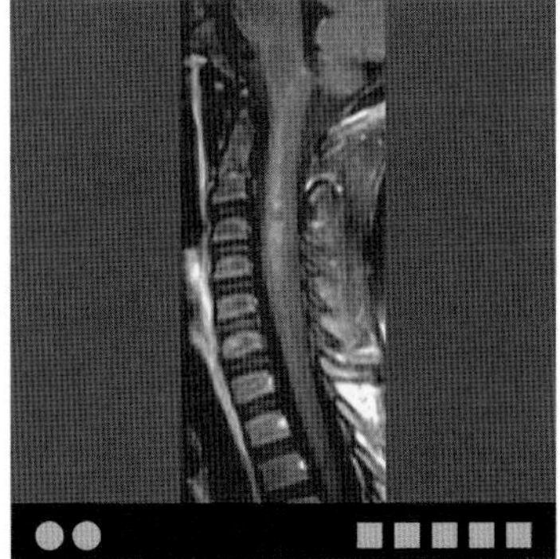

E. Postviral myelitis: Sagittal post-contrast T1-weighted image shows heterogeneous enhancement of the affected cervical cord extending to the medulla.

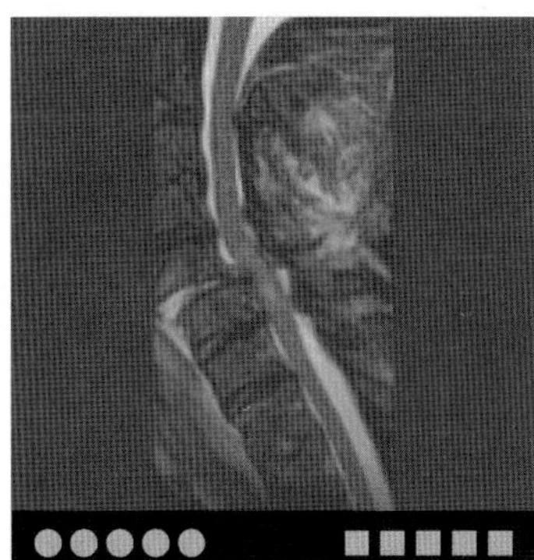

F. Posttraumatic cord contusion: Sagittal T2-weighted image shows cord contusion and low signal intensity hemorrhage posteriorly caused by extensive traumatic injury including tear of anterior longitudinal ligament, posterior longitudinal ligament, ligamentum nuchae, traumatic C5-6 fracture –dislocation, and disk extrusion.

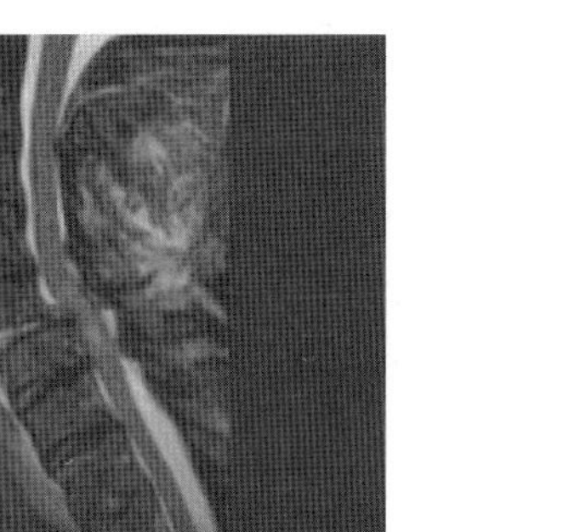

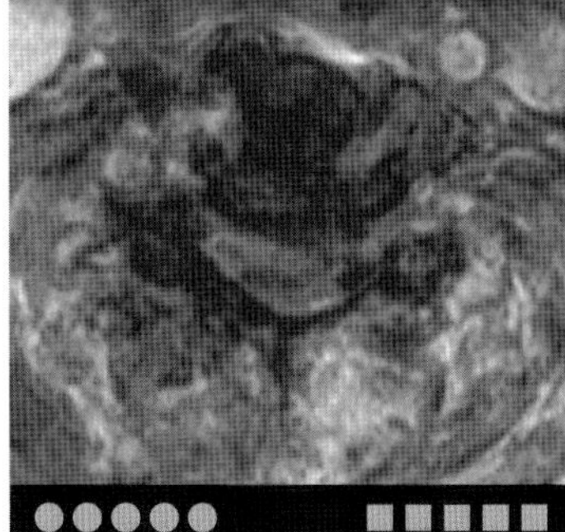

G. Posttraumatic cord contusion: Axial T2-weighted image shows traumatic cord compression and low signal intensity hemorrhage within the cord posteriorly.

IMAGE KEY

Common
●●●●●
●●●●
●●●
●●
●
Rare

Typical
■■■■■
■■■■
■■■
■■
■
Unusual

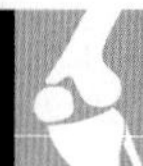

39–4 Spinal Intramedullary Astrocytoma

Edward Mossop and Jamshid Tehranzadeh

PRESENTATION

Back pain and progressive weakness

FINDINGS

MRI shows long, intramedullary, expansile lesion of mid to lower thoracic spine, which enhances with contrast.

DIFFERENTIAL DIAGNOSES

- *Neurofibromatosis: (NF):* These tumors in NF are isointense or slightly hyperintense on T1-weighted image. On T2 images and enhanced T1-weighted images, a target pattern with a peripheral hyperintense rim and central low intensity is seen.
- *Ependymoma:* Heterogeneity and hyperintensity on T1-weighted image may be consistent with a hemorrhagic component to the mass. Ependymomas are homogeneously and intensely enhancing. The tumor often has well-defined borders with contrast enhancement.
- *Hemangioblastoma:* MRI usually shows an enhancing mass clearly delineated from the surrounding spinal cord tissue. The tumor may be hypointense or isointense on precontrast T1-weighted image and hyperintense on T2-weighted image.
- *Schwannoma:* MRI shows a mass, isointense, or slightly hypointense on T1-weighted mage and slightly hypointense to CSF on T2-weighted image. Enhancement is typically homogeneous. Larger schwannomas can show areas of cystic degeneration and heterogeneous signal intensity.

COMMENTS

This is an image of a 3-year-old boy presenting with progressive weakness. Astrocytomas are CNS neoplasms in which the predominant cell type is derived from an immortalized astrocyte. Two classes of astrocytic tumors are recognized—-those with narrow zones of infiltration (e.g., pilocytic astrocytoma, and subependymal giant cell astrocytoma) and those with diffused zones of infiltration (e.g., low-grade astrocytoma, anaplastic astrocytoma, and glioblastoma). Approximately 3% of CNS astrocytomas arise within the spinal cord. Astrocytomas affect the very young and middle-aged people. Patients with astrocytomas of the spinal cord most frequently present with pain, weakness, gait disturbance, and sphincter dysfunction. Paresthesias and loss of sensation occur later in the disease course. On a CT scan, low-grade astrocytomas appear as poorly defined, homogeneous, and low-density masses without contrast enhancement. However, slight enhancement, calcification, and cystic changes may be evident early in the course of the disease. MRI will show widening of the cord. Astrocytomas generally are isointense on T1-weighted image compared to normal spinal tissue. On T2-weighted image, a high signal reflects the tumor and the associated edema. Pilocytic astrocytomas often are associated with a cyst, which may be particularly prominent on T2-weighted sequences. While low-grade astrocytomas uncommonly enhance on MRI, most anaplastic astrocytomas enhance with paramagnetic contrast agents. Angiography may be employed to rule out vascular malformations and to evaluate tumor blood supply. Positron emission tomography (PET) and single-photon emission computed tomography (SPECT) imaging sometimes are used to try to differentiate low-grade gliomas from either high-grade tumors or other types of pathology.

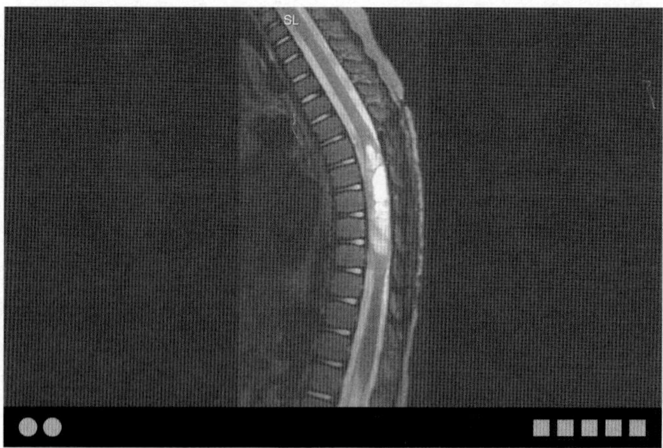

A. Astrocytoma: Sagittal T2-weighted fat-saturated image of the thoracic spine shows a long, expansile lesion with inhomogeneous bright signal inside the spinal cord extending from mid to lower thoracic spine.

PEARLS

- **Approximately 3% of central nervous system astrocytomas arise within the spinal cord.**
- **Patients with astrocytomas of the spinal cord most frequently present with pain, weakness, gait disturbance, and sphincter dysfunction.**
- **Astrocytomas generally are isointense on T1-weighted images compared to normal spinal tissue.**
- **On T2-weighted image, a high signal reflects the tumor and the associated edema.**
- **While low-grade astrocytomas uncommonly enhance on MRI, most anaplastic astrocytomas enhance with paramagnetic contrast agent**

ADDITIONAL IMAGES

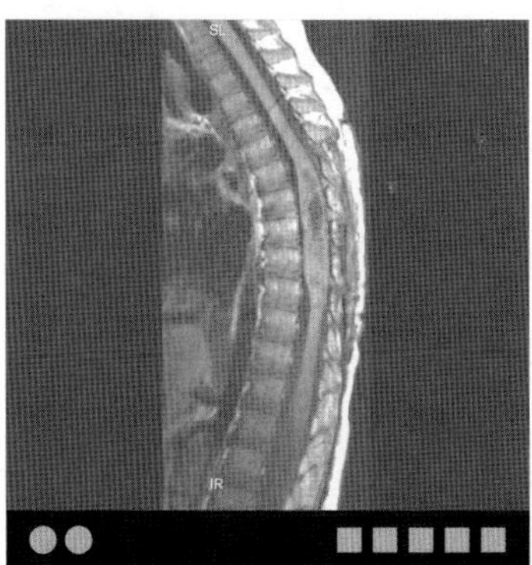

B. Astrocytoma: Sagittal T1-weighted image of the thoracic spine shows an intramedullary, expansile lesion of the mid to lower thoracic region with central low signal intensity, which may represent necrosis or fluid.

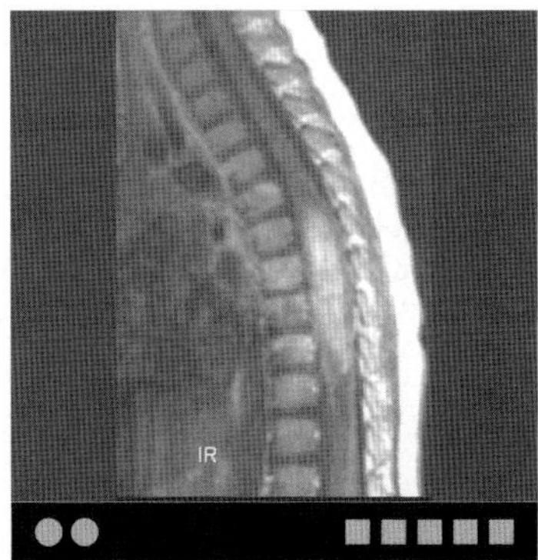

C. Astrocytoma: Sagittal T1-weighted postcontrast image shows enhancement of the expansile, intramedullary lesion of the mid to lower thoracic spine.

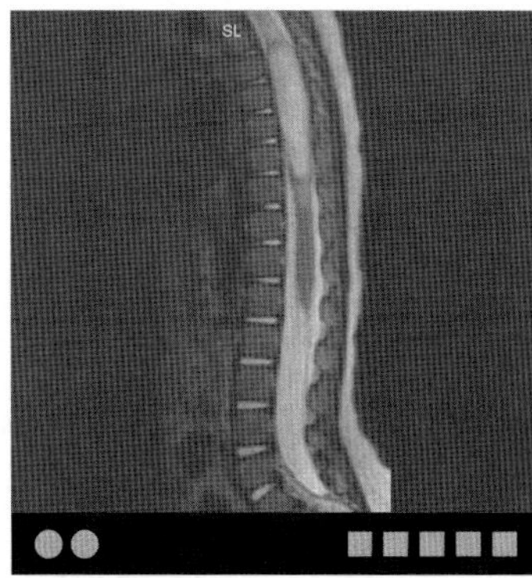

D. Astrocytoma: Sagittal T2-weighted fat-saturated image of the lumbar spine shows the expansile, intramedullary lesion in the lower thoracic region.

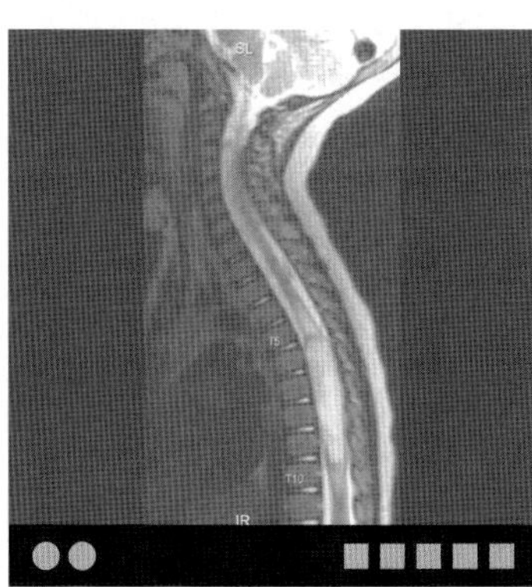

E. Astrocytoma: Sagittal T2-weighted fat-saturated image of the cervical/thoracic spine shows the inhomogeneous, bright, expansile, and intramedullary lesion to be at the level of T5 to T10.

IMAGE KEY

Common

Rare

Typical

Unusual

DIFFERENTIAL DIAGNOSES IMAGES

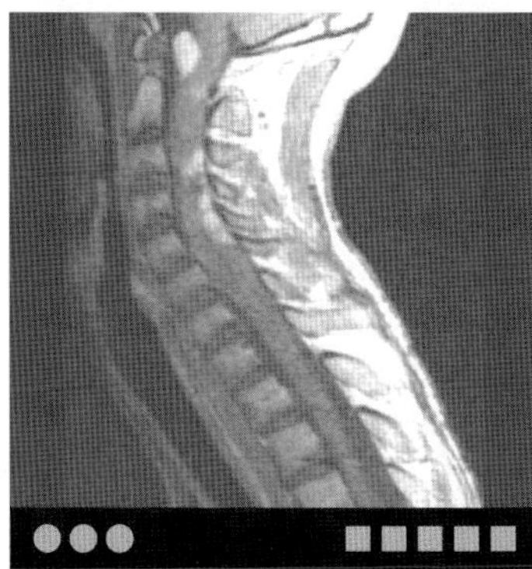

F. Plexiform neurofibroma: T1-weighted image shows a plexiform neurofibroma of the cervical spine.

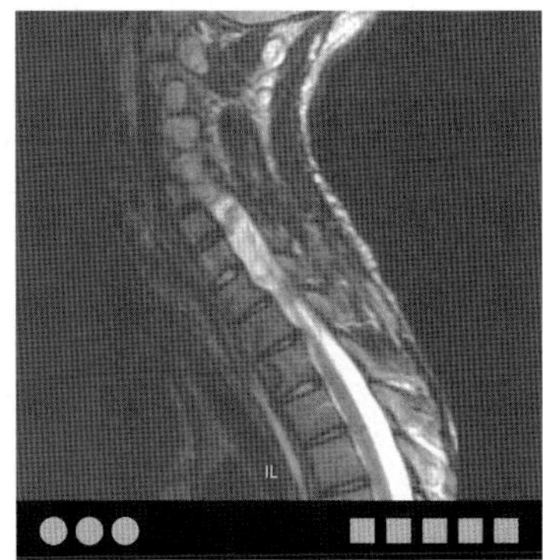

G. Plexiform neurofibroma: T2- weighted image shows a plexiform neurofibroma of the cervical spine.

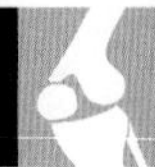

39–5 Malignant Compression Fracture of the Spine

Eric Chen and Jamshid Tehranzadeh

PRESENTATION

Back pain, progressive kyphosis

FINDINGS

MR images show multiple, vertebral compression fractures as a result of metastasis.

DIFFERENTIAL DIAGNOSES

- Osteoporotic vertebral compression occurs in postmenopausal women and MRI shows normal bone marrow signal.
- Multiple myeloma may be difficult to differentiate from metastasis, but it usually does not demonstrate complete marrow replacement.
- Traumatic fractures are often associated with a history of trauma.
- Tuberculous spondylitis is diagnosed by the presence of contiguous spinal involvement.

COMMENTS

This is an image of a 48-year-old man who presented with thyroid carcinoma with skeletal and pulmonary metastasis. The most common cause of malignant compression fracture of the spine is metastatic disease; including most commonly breast, bronchogenic, prostatic, or renal carcinoma. Primary malignancies of the spine such as osteosarcoma or multiple myeloma are less common. Up to one-third of all cases of vertebral collapse are benign in patients with a history of primary malignancy. Patients usually present with back pain and progressive kyphosis. Differential diagnosis between malignant collapse, and osteoporotic collapse is difficult especially when there is no history of significant trauma. Furthermore, malignant compression fractures share some MRI signal characteristics with benign compression fractures caused by osteoporosis such as hypointensity on T1-weighted, hyperintensity on T2-weighted, and enhancement on postcontrast images. However, malignant compression fractures of the spine also show specific MRI signs. Most specific indicators of malignant spinal compression fracture are presence of a nodular, irregular, and paraspinal soft tissue mass and complete involvement of the pedicle. Other characteristic findings include abnormal marrow signal, multifocal involvement, posterior vertebral convexity or bulging, well-defined round foci in other vertebrae, and epidural soft tissue masses. In contrast, the presence of normal marrow, fracture line, intravertebral fluid, posterior-angulated fragment, and fragmentation are signs favoring benign collapse.

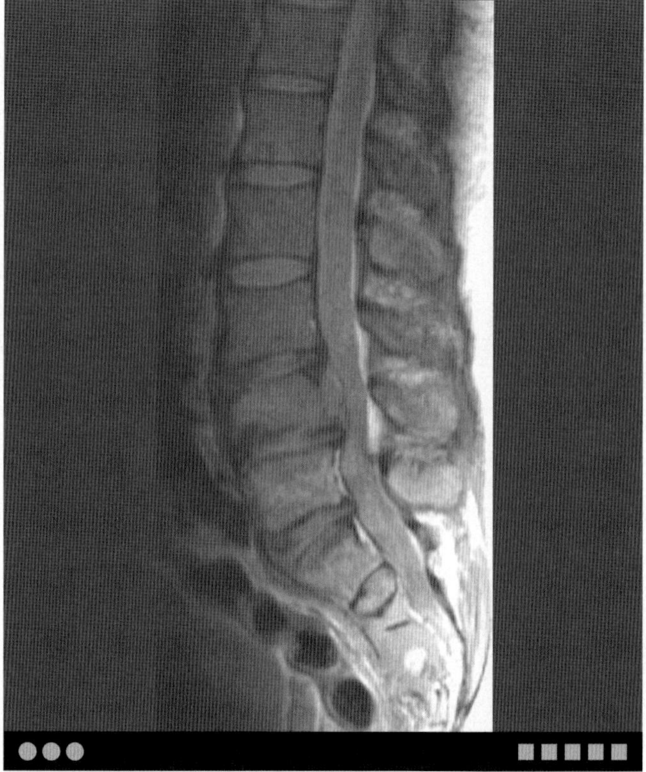

A. Metastatic collapse: Sagittal proton density T2-weighted image of L spine shows partial compression of L4. Note the convex margin of the posterior cortex of L4 vertebra. There is also metastatic involvement at the S2 level.

PEARLS

- **Irregular, paraspinal soft tissue masses and pediculate involvement are highly specific MRI findings indicating malignant collapse.**
- **Abnormal marrow replacement, posterior vertebral convexity, and well-defined round foci in other vertebrae are additional findings for malignant collapse with good specificity.**
- **Epidural soft tissue extension helps to differentiate malignancy from osteoporosis.**
- **Presence of normal marrow, fracture line, intravertebral fluid, posterior-angulated fragment, and fragmentation are signs favoring benign collapse.**

ADDITIONAL IMAGES

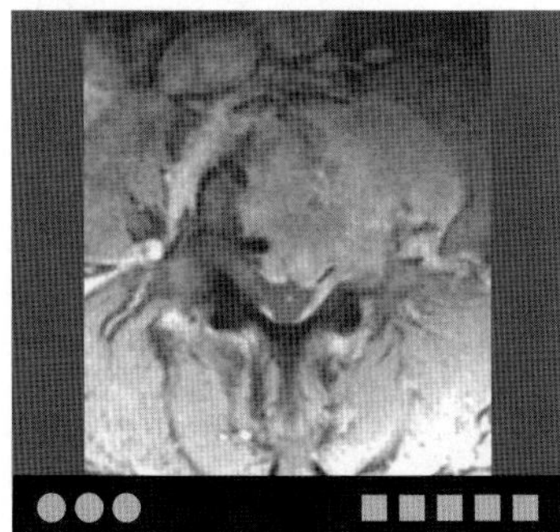

B. Metastatic collapse: Axial postcontrast Fat Sat T1-weighted image shows large soft tissue mass with destruction of the left side of L4 vertebrae with extension into the spinal canal and epidural space and lateral expansion into the left psoas muscle.

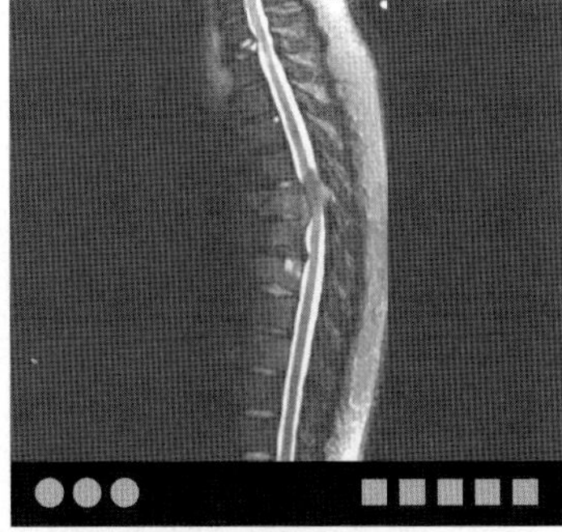

C. Metastatic collapse: Sagittal Fat Sat T2-weighted image shows thoracic spine of same patient with multiple osseous metastases. Notice bulging or convex posterior cortices with cord impingement.

DIFFERENTIAL DIAGNOSES IMAGES

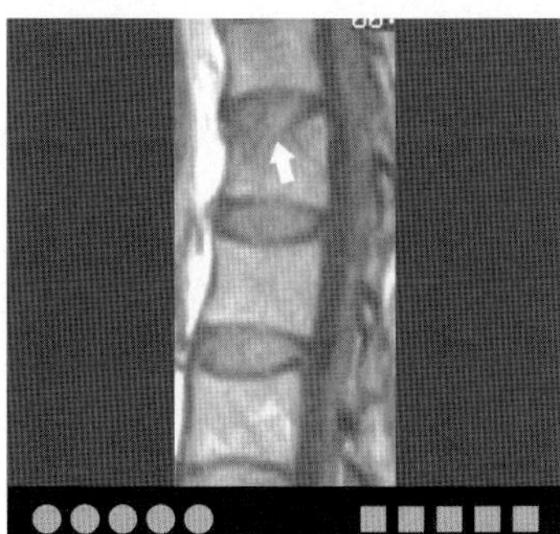

D. Benign compression: Sagittal spin echo T1-weighted image shows partial compression of the superior endplate of the vertebra (arrow).

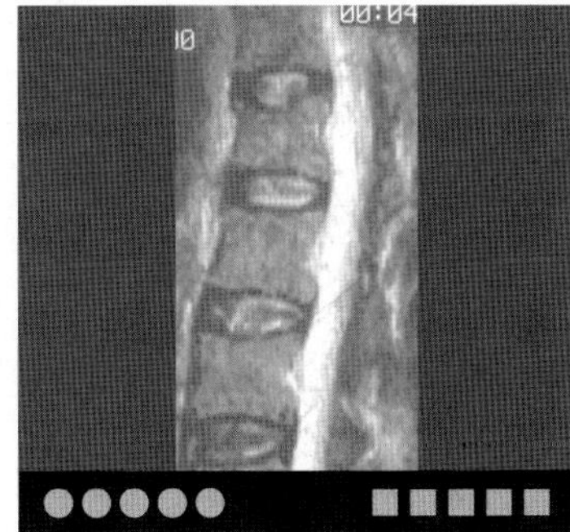

E. Benign compression: Sagittal spin echo T2-weighted image shows partial compression of the superior endplate of the lumbar vertebra. Note normal marrow.

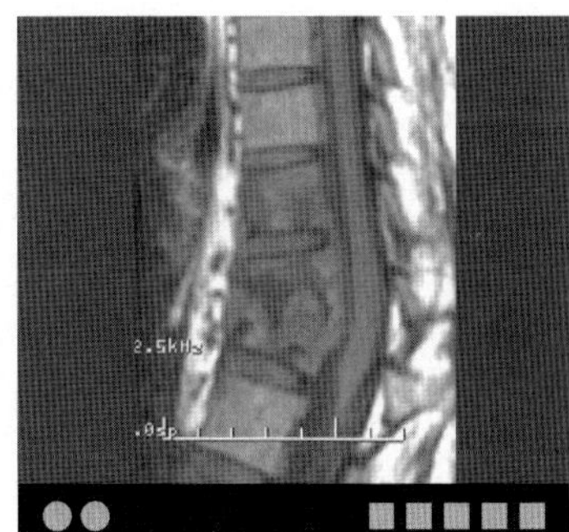

F. Tuberculosis spondylitis: Sagittal T1-weighted image shows collapse of two adjacent vertebral bodies with destruction of the intervertebral discs associated with narrowing of the spinal canal at the same level. (With permission from Tehranzadeh J. Advances in MR imaging of vertebral collapse. *Semin Ultrasound CT MRI* 2004;25:440-460.)

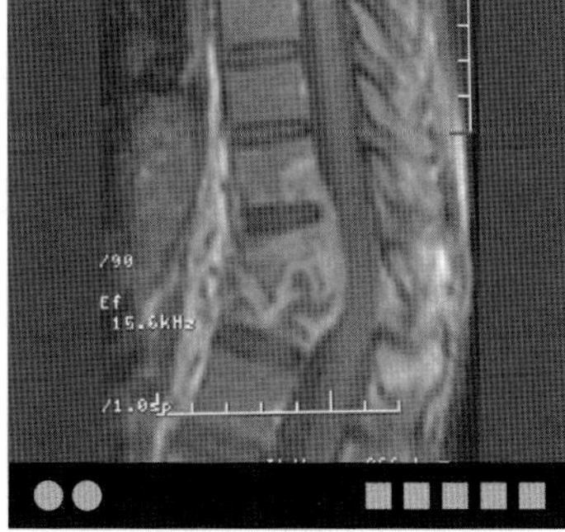

G. Tuberculosis spondylitis: Sagittal T1 postcontrast image shows collapse of two adjacent vertebral bodies with enhancement of the bone marrow, endplate, and destroyed intervertebral disc. Note kyphosis and compression of the spinal cord at this level. (With permission from Tehranzadeh J. Advances in MR imaging of vertebral collapse. *Semin Ultrasound CT MRI* 2004;25:440-460.)

IMAGE KEY

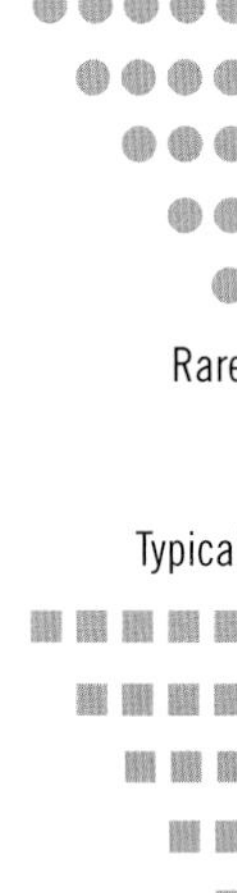

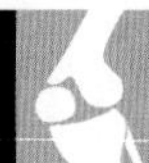

39–6 Multiple Myeloma

Tatiana Voci

PRESENTATION

Back pain

FINDINGS

Skeletal survey and CT scan demonstrate numerous lytic lesions. MR images show bone marrow replacement with multifocal patchy or diffused low T1- and high T2-weighted image signal intensity lesions and variable amount of heterogeneous mottled enhancement. Epidural/paravertebral extension may be present as well as compression fractures resulting in central canal stenosis.

DIFFERENTIAL DIAGNOSES

- *Metastatic disease:* The pedicles involvement is characteristic for metastatic disease and usually appears earlier than in cases of multiple myeloma. Although both multiple myeloma and metastasis show low T1-weighted image and high T2-weighted image signal on MRI, radiographs and CT scan may demonstrate sclerotic or mixed lytic-sclerotic nature of the metastasis, not typical of multiple myeloma. Many metastasis present with increased uptake of tracer of bone scans and will not have monoclonal gammopathy of plasma electrophoresis.
- *Osteoporosis:* Admittedly, it is difficult to distinguish diffused marrow involvement of multiple myeloma from osteopenia.
- *Myeloproliferative disorder:* As a result of polycythemia vera, chronic myelogenous leukemia, primary thrombocytopenia, and myelofibrosis with myeloid hyperplasia. These processes tend to have both low T1-weighted image and T2-weighted image signal intensities and show no discrete lesion and no significant gadolinium enhancement. Tc-99m diphosphonate bone scan and Tc-99m sulfur colloid scans show sites of increased uptake because of marrow expansion in distal appendicular skeleton and calvaria.

COMMENTS

Multiple myeloma is a malignancy of the plasma cells. It is characterized by bone destruction, paraprotein formation, and replacement of bone marrow. Destruction of bone can lead to bone pain, lytic lesions, osteoporosis, and pathological fractures. The median age at presentation is 65 years. Common presenting complaints can include those related to anemia, infection, or bone pain. The back or ribs are the most common places where bone pain is identified. The predominant sites of involvement are the vertebrae, ribs, skull, pelvis, and femora. The classic appearances are multiple, well-circumscribed, and "punched out" lytic lesions. In some cases, structures can appear normal or osteopenic. Lesions may be expansile. 1% of multiple myeloma cases were reported to present with sclerotic lesions. Radiography does rely on approximately one-third of the bone cortex to be removed before lesions are detected, so it can be less sensitive than CT scan or MRI. MRI findings of diffused or focal bone marrow involvement replacement of fatty marrow by abnormal low T1-weighted image signal intensity, which is conspicuously hypointense to signal of intervertebral disks (never a normal finding); it is high signal of T2-weighted image or STIR and shows variable degree of enhancement. Also bone marrow can have a prominently variegated low T1-weighted image intensity with patchy, mottled enhancement. Bone scintigraphy detects only about 10% of the lesions. Whole body PET shows metabolically active lesions with sensitivity of 84% to 92% and specificity of 83% to 100% and is useful in monitoring treatment response.

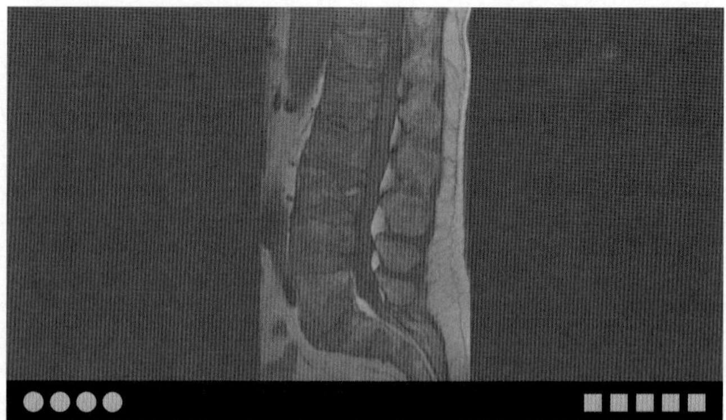

A. Multiple myeloma: Sagittal image T1-weighted image shows mottled low signal intensity lesions throughout the bone marrow. The signal intensity of the majority of the vertebral bodies is abnormally isointense or hypointense compared to the adjacent intervertebral disks. Various degrees of compression fractures and endplates collapse involve T12, L1, L2, L3, L4, and L5.

PEARLS

- **Multiple myeloma involves primarily axial skeleton followed by the long bones, skull, mandible, ribs, and pelvis. Punches out lesions or diffused osteopenia are the most common findings.**
- **MR images show homogeneous or patchy low T1-weighted image and high T2-weighted image signal intensity abnormality replacing fatty bone marrow with associated epidural or paraspinous extension of the tumor mass. Multiple compression fractures are common.**

ADDITIONAL IMAGES

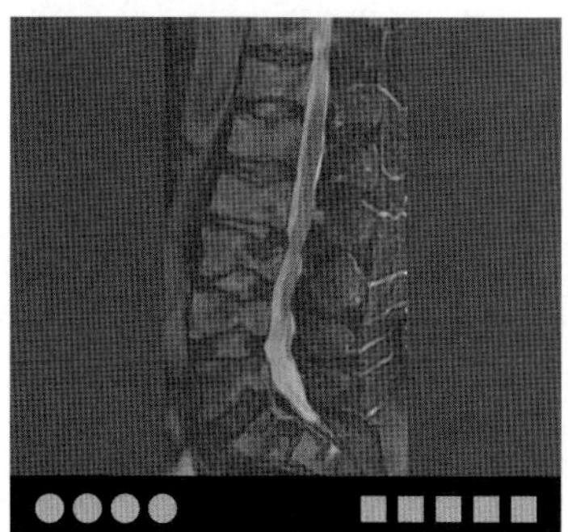

B. Multiple myeloma: Sagittal T2-weighted image show patchy high signal intensity lesions throughout the bone marrow. There is no epidural extension or paraspinous mass.

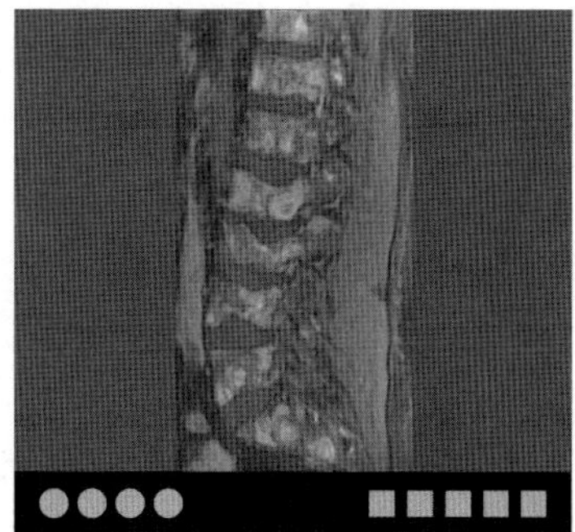

C. Multiple myeloma: Sagittal T1-weighted image postcontrast show innumerable amorphous enhancing vertebral myelomatous lesions. There is "variegated" appearance to T11-L1. There is some involvement of the posterior elements.

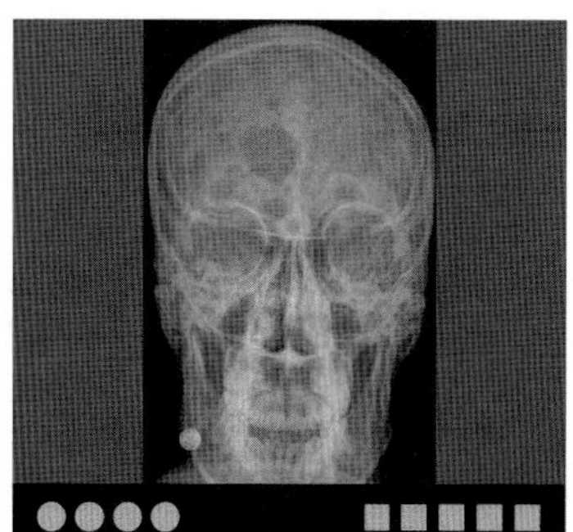

D. Multiple myeloma: Frontal radiograph of the skull shows multiple punched out lesions in the calvaria and the ramus of the right mandible.

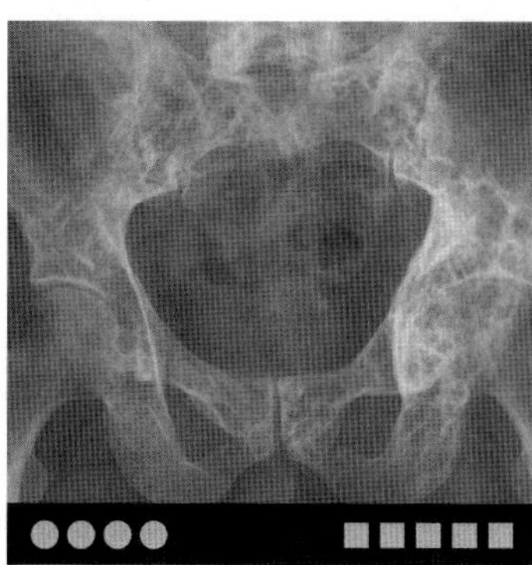

E. Multiple myeloma: Frontal radiograph of the pelvis shows replacement of normal bony architecture by innumerable lytic lesions of different sizes. There is some expansion of the left ischium/inferior pubic ramus.

IMAGE KEY

Common

●●●●●
●●●●
●●●
●●
●

Rare

Typical

■■■■■
■■■■
■■■
■■
■

Unusual

DIFFERENTIAL DIAGNOSES IMAGES

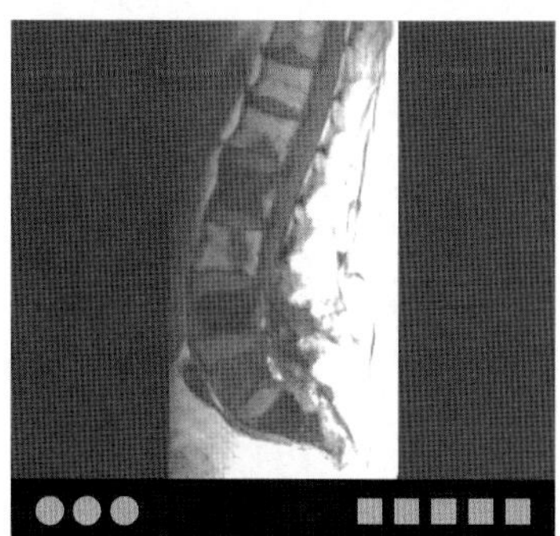

F. Metastatic lesion of prostate carcinoma: Sagittal image T1-weighted image shows marked low signal intensity discrete lesions in all visualized, vertebral bodies with most prominent involvement of L2, L4, and L5. These are metastatic lesions of prostatic carcinoma.

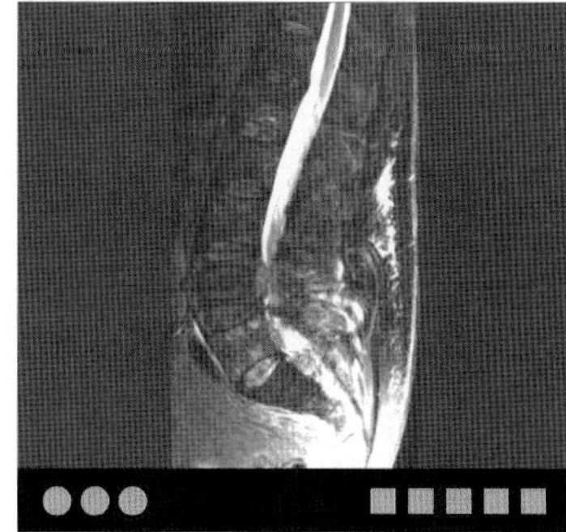

G. Metastatic lesion of prostate carcinoma: Sagittal T2-weighted image fat sat show low signal intensity corresponding to low signal intensity lesions seen on T1-weighted image, typical of sclerotic metastasis—low on T1 and low on T2. The remainder of low signal in the bone marrow is the result of fat saturation.

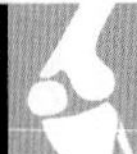

39–7 Sclerosing Myeloma

George Hermann

PRESENTATION

Back pain

FINDINGS

MRI shows signal alteration of the thoracolumbar area.

DIFFERENTIAL DIAGNOSES

- Metastatic carcinoid may present as scattered, osteoblastic lesions in the skeleton.
- Hodgkin's lymphoma occasionally presents as osteoblastic lesions on radiograph. On MRI, it demonstrates decreased SI on T1-weighted and T2-weighted images.
- Metastatic breast carcinoma may be mixed, lytic, and blastic.
- Metastatic prostate carcinoma in most cases presents as osteoblastic lesions. They are discrete, scattered primarily, involving the axial skeleton. On MRI, the lesions show decreased SI on T1-weighted image and T2-weighted images.

COMMENTS

This is an image of a 47-year-old man who complained of general weakness and back pain. He was diagnosed with sclerosing myeloma. Multiple myeloma is the most common primary malignant neoplasm of bone. It is composed of proliferating plasma cells and manifested by multiple lesions in the skeleton with or without osteoporosis. Osteosclerotic myeloma is a rare but well-defined entity. The incidence is only less than 3%. Primary osteosclerosis has been described in association with polyneuropathy, organomegaly, endocrinopathy, monoclonal gammopathy, and skin changes (POEMS syndrome). This type of myeloma and POEMS syndrome are considered to be part of the clinical spectrum of plasma cell dyscrasia with polyneuropathy. Osteosclerotic myeloma differs from multiple myeloma in that the patients are younger; the marrow contains less than 5% plasma cells. Multiple myelomas on the other hand contain more than 10% plasma cells in the marrow. Radiologically, the bone lesion may present as a uniform sclerosis target sign or marginal rim sclerosis. The vertebrae show localized osteosclerotic lesions on CT scan (image A). MRI demonstrates scattered decreased SI lesions both on T1-and T2-weighted images along the vertebrae, which are usually more extensive than seen on CT scan.

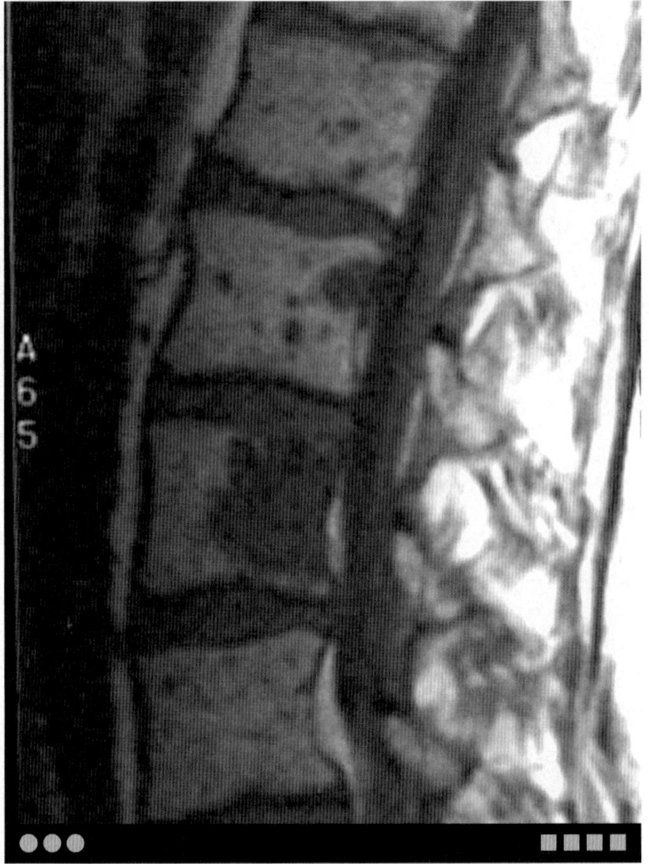

A. Sclerosing myeloma: MRI of spine: sagittal plane T1-weighted image shows focal spots of decreased SI involving the vertebral bodies.

PEARLS

- **Sclerosing myeloma is a rare presentation of myeloma.**
- **It involves predominantly the axial skeleton.**
- **It is difficult to differentiate it from osteoblastic metastasis such as breast, carcinoma of the gastrointestinal tract, and carcinoid metastasis.**

ADDITIONAL IMAGES

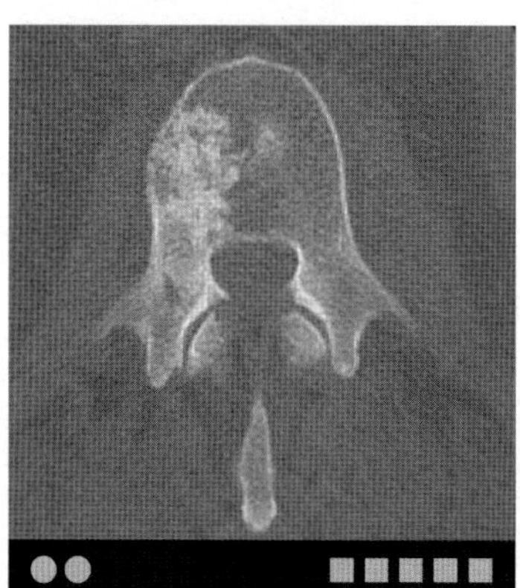

B. Sclerosing myeloma: CT scan of the thoracolumbar area reveals localized, osteoblastic lesions in the body of L3.

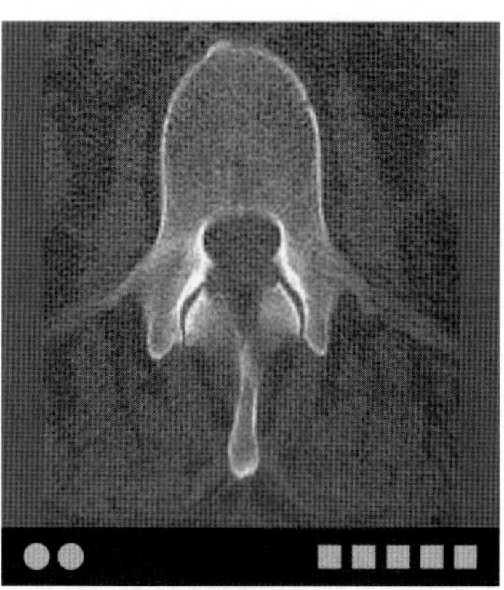

C. Sclerosing myeloma: CT scan of L2 appears uninvolved.

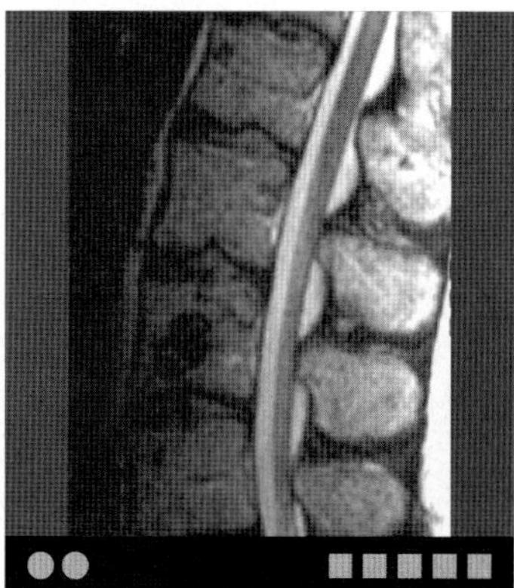

D. Sclerosing myeloma: On sagittal T2-weighted image focal spots of decreased SI are noted at T12-L5. Note the extensive involvement of the spine that is not seen on CT scan.

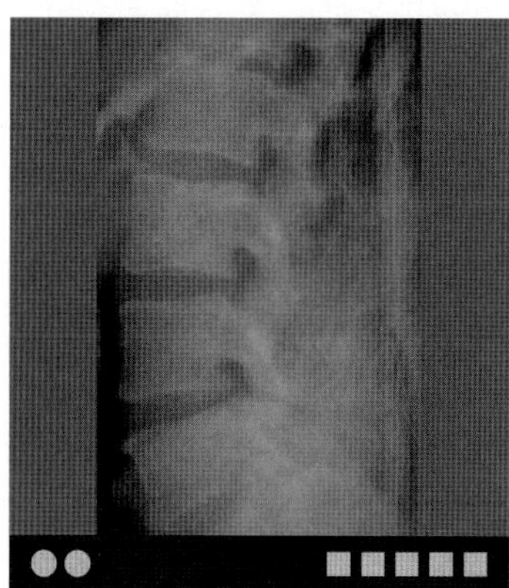

E. Sclerosing myeloma: Lumbar spine, lateral view. There is an osteoblastic lesion on L3.

IMAGE KEY

Common

Rare

Typical

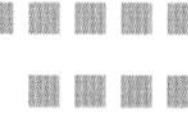

Unusual

DIFFERENTIAL DIAGNOSES IMAGES

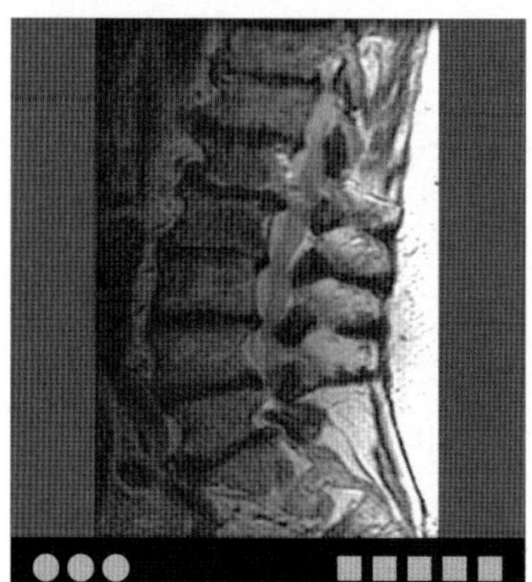

F. Metastatic carcinoma of prostate: Sagittal MR T1-weighted image demonstrates multiple decreased SI spots of the vertebral bodies.

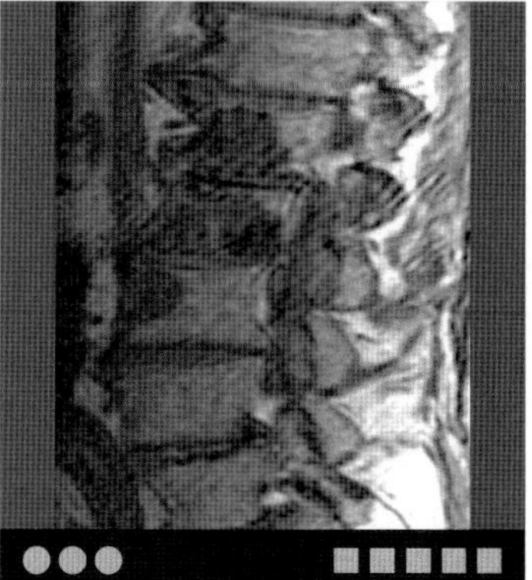

G. Metastatic carcinoma of prostate: On T2-weighted image, the decreased SI of the vertebrae remains unchanged representing osteoblastic metastasis.

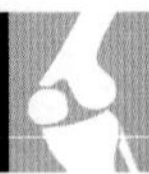

39–8 Intradural Schwannoma of Lumbar Spine

Peyman Borghei and Jamshid Tehranzadeh

PRESENTATION

Low back pain and leg weakness

FINDINGS

MRI shows a well-circumscribed, low signal intensity, and oval mass at the level of L5 on T1-weighted and intermediate to high signal on T2-weighted images, which enhances with the contrast.

DIFFERENTIAL DIAGNOSES

- *Astrocytoma:* Astrocytomas generally are isointense on T1-weighted image compared to normal spinal tissue and high intense on T2-weighted image. While anaplastic astrocytomas enhance with the contrast agent, the low-grade types usually do not.
- *Meningioma:* MRI shows low to intermediate signal intensity lesion on T1-weighted and intermediate to high signal intensity on T2-weighted image with marked contrast enhancement. Calcification may also be present.
- *Ependymoma:* MRI shows low to intermediate heterogeneous signal intensity on T1-weighted image and intermediate to high signal intensity on T2-weighted image. High signal intensity foci on T1-weighted image are caused by mucin or hemorrhage.
- *Neurofibroma:* Tumor of nerve sheaths are composed of Schwann cells and fibroblasts. T2-wighted MR image shows "target sign," which is a low signal-intensity center because of collagen accumulation.
- *Dermoid:* MRI shows intermediate to high signal intensity on T1-weighted and intermediate to high signal lesion on T2-weighted image without contrast enhancement.

COMMENTS

This is an image of a 22-year-old woman with the complaint of low back pain and weakness of the lower extremities, diagnosed with the schwannoma of the spine. Schwannoma is an encapsulated benign tumor arising from the Schwann cells that surround the nerve roots and mostly involves a spinal nerve and has intradural and extramedullary location. Middle-aged adults are commonly affected, with the thoracic spine being involved in 50%, the cervical spine in 30%, and the lumbosacral spine in 20% of the cases. Radicular pain is the initial symptom in the majority of cases, while motor disorders are less common and occur later in the course of the disease. Clinically, the compression of the nerve root within the foramen by the tumor causes lancinating pain from nerve root irritation and perhaps muscle atrophy. The tumor may grow to compress the spinal cord, resulting in pyramidal tract and posterior column signs below the level of compression. On MRI, schwannoma is visible as an oval mass with a vertical long axis, usually located within the dural sheath but outside the spinal cord. On MRI, the lesion generates a signal intensity that is slightly decreased or normal on T1-weighted and increased on T2-weighted image, which homogeneously enhances with the contrast. MRI also provides a highly accurate evaluation of the mass including detection of intraforaminal extensions and assessment of spinal cord compression. Inhomogeneous contrast enhancement may suggest cystic degeneration and hemorrhage.

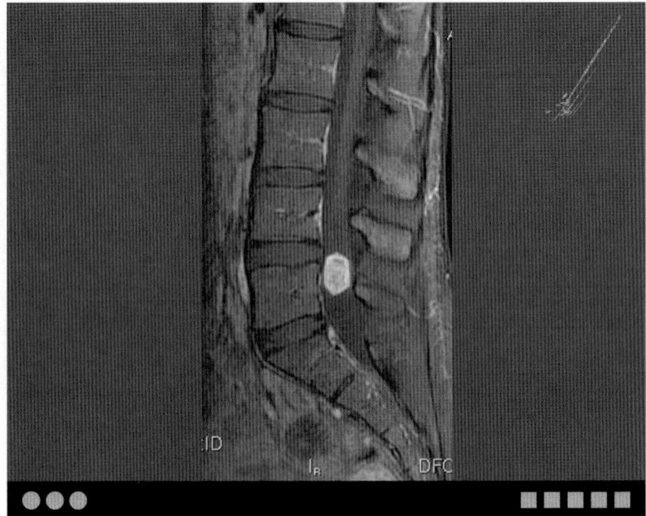

A. Schwannoma: Sagittal FS T1-weighted postcontrast image shows an oval, well-marginated, and intradural mass at the level of L5 at cauda equina, which enhances with contrast with an additional ring enhancement.

PEARLS

- **Schwannoma is the most common intradural extramedullary neoplasm usually presenting with pain, radiculopathy, and weakness.**
- **The presenting radicular pain might be confused with disc protrusion.**
- **MRI shows an oval mass, low signal on T1-weighted and high signal on T2-weighted image, which homogeneously enhances with contrast.**
- **Inhomogeneous contrast enhancement may suggest cystic degeneration and hemorrhage.**

ADDITIONAL IMAGES

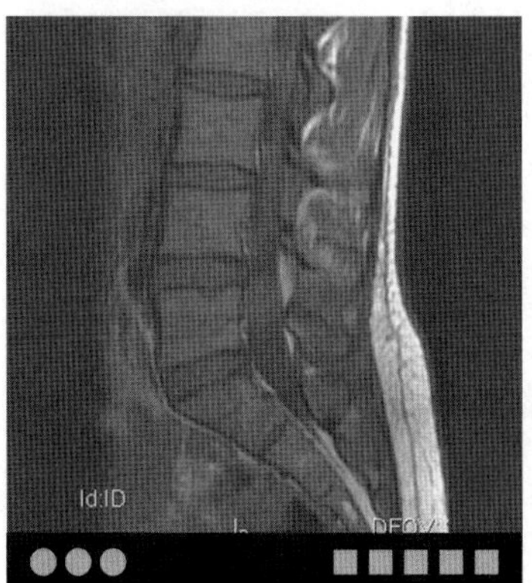

B. Schwannoma: Sagittal T1-weighted image shows a low signal intensity oval-shaped, intradural mass at the level of L5.

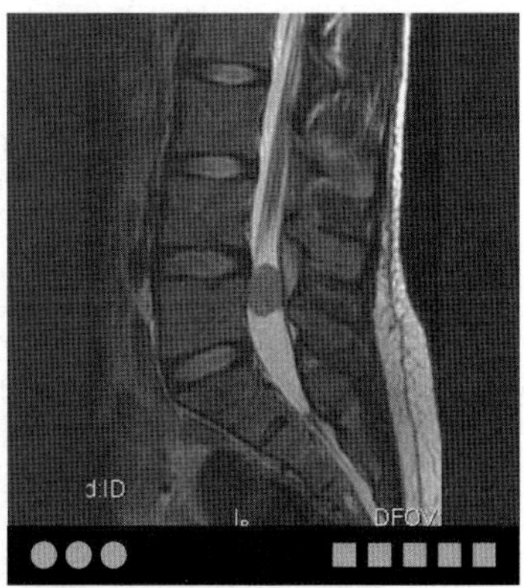

C. Schwannoma: Sagittal T2-weighted image shows an intermediate signal intensity oval-shaped, intradural mass at the level of L5.

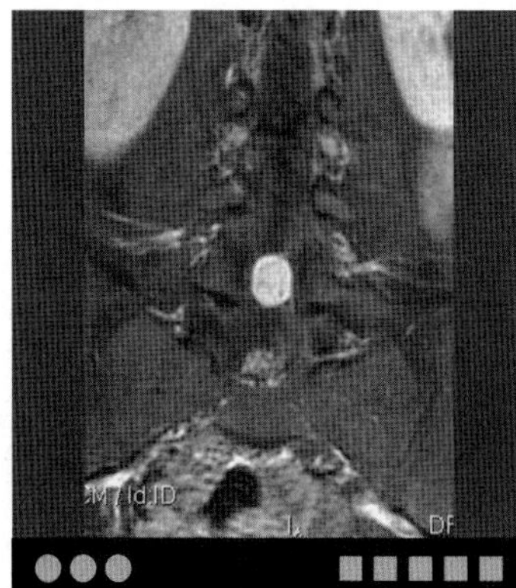

D. Schwannoma: Coronal T1-weighted postcontrast image shows a well-circumscribed, oval-shaped, and intradural mass. Note more prominent enhancement of the rim of the lesion.

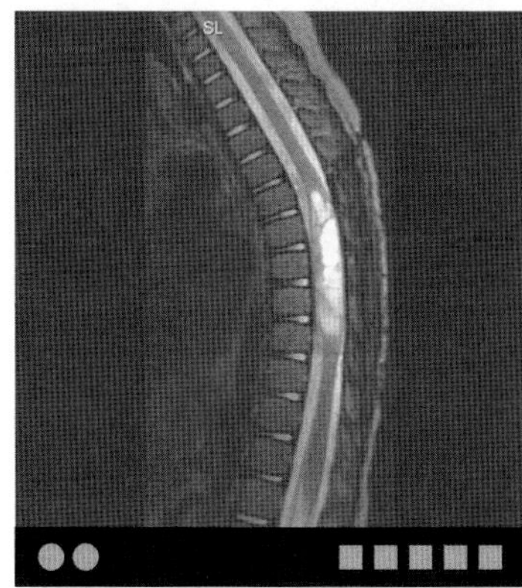

E. Schwannoma: Axial T1-weighted postcontrast image shows slightly in- homogeneous enhancement of this mass.

DIFFERENTIAL DIAGNOSES IMAGES

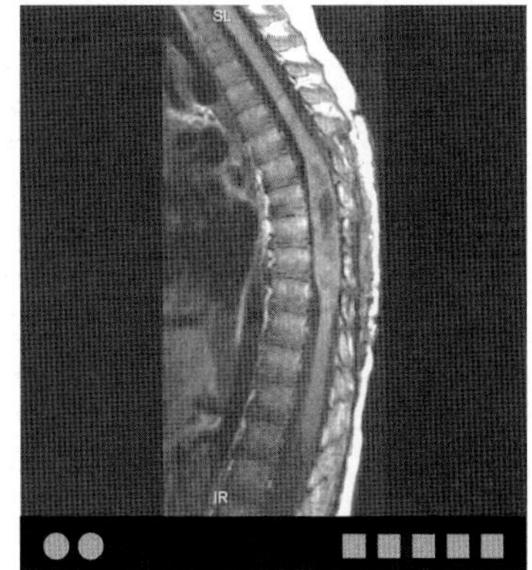

F. Spinal astrocytoma: Sagittal T2-weighted fat-saturated image of the thoracic spine shows a long, expansile lesion with inhomogeneous, bright signal inside the spinal cord extending from mid to lower thoracic spine.

G. Spinal astrocytoma: Sagittal T1-weighted image of the thoracic spine shows an intramedullary, expansile lesion of the mid to lower thoracic region with central low signal intensity, which may represent necrosis or fluid.

IMAGE KEY

Common

Rare

Typical

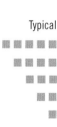

Unusual

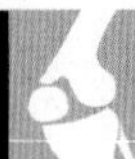

39–9 Mazabraud Syndrome

Ingrid B. Kjellin

PRESENTATION

Chronic back pain and a focal mass in the lower back

FINDINGS

MRI shows multiple focal lesions in the lumbar spine and lower thoracic spine and deformity of vertebral bodies and posterior elements.

DIFFERENTIAL DIAGNOSES

- *Metastatic disease:* Metastasis to the skeleton is the most common type of malignant bone tumor. In adult patients; carcinomas of the prostate, breast, kidney, and lung account for more than 75% of the cases of skeletal metastases.
- *Multiple myeloma:* This is the most common primary bone neoplasm in adults. The typical pattern on imaging is focal or diffused bone destruction with osteolysis. The axial skeleton is the most common site of involvement.
- *Neurofibromatosis:* This is one of the most common genetic diseases with skeletal abnormalities occurring in about 40% of patients. These include kyphoscoliosis, sphenoid dysplasia, pseudarthrosis, nonossifying fibromas, rib deformity, and posterior vertebral scalloping.
- *Enchondromatosis and soft tissue hemangiomas:* These are seen in Maffucci's syndrome, a rare nonhereditary mesodermal dysplasia. The metacarpals and phalanges of the hand are the most frequently affected regions.

COMMENTS

This is an image of a 46-year-old woman who presented with chronic polyostotic bone disease for over 20 years. A small soft tissue mass in her lower back had been present for many years and would vary slightly in size. Fibrous dysplasia is a developmental anomaly of mesenchymal origin and is monostotic (70%–80%) or polyostotic (20%–30%). Rib, femur, tibia, gnathic bone, skull, and humerus are frequently affected. Spine is rarely involved, but when it is involved, there could be neurological consequences because of vertebral expansion and fractures. Endocrine dysfunction and cutaneous pigmentation are sometimes seen with fibrous dysplasia, and is referred to as McCune-Albright syndrome. The rare association of intramuscular myxomas and polyostotic fibrous dysplasia is known as Mazabraud syndrome. The myxomas are found near severely affected bones and may be multiple. The incidence of malignant transformation in fibrous dysplasia is low, only 0.5%. There is a suggestion that patients with Mazabraud syndrome may have a greater risk for malignant transformation than patients having fibrous dysplasia alone. Radiographically, fibrous dysplasia is typically a radiolucent lesion with "ground-glass" appearance and expansion. On MRI, fibrous dysplasia is low in signal on T1-weighted images and variable on T2-weighted and gadolinium-enhanced images. Myxomas are well-defined and appear similar to fluid on MRI. After the administration of contrast, there is usually only peripheral and septal enhancement.

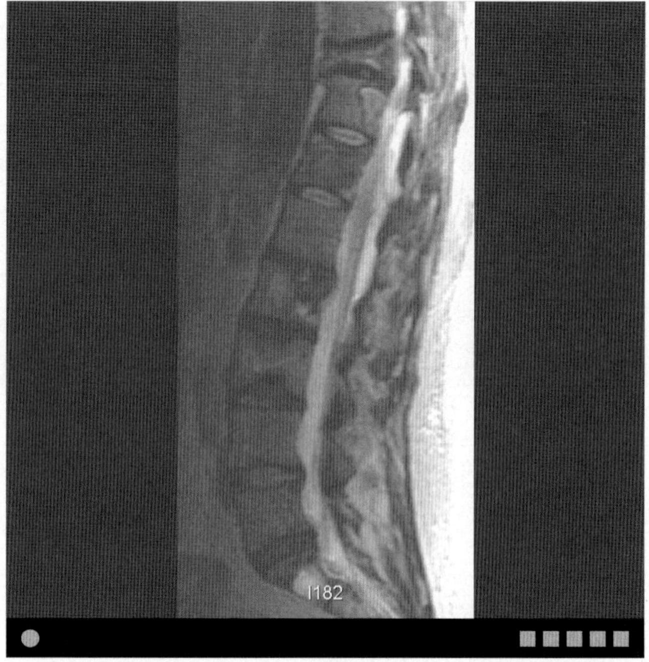

A. Mazabraud syndrome: A T2-weighted sagittal image through the lumbar spine shows multiple well-defined, vertebral lesions of varying signal intensity, and a fracture of T10.

PEARLS

- **Fibrous dysplasia is monostotic or polyostotic.**
- **The typical radiographic features include a radiolucent lesion with ground-glass appearance and expansion.**
- **The signal intensity is low on T1-weighted images and low, intermediate, or high on T2-weighted images.**
- **The rare combination of intramuscular myxomas with polyostotic fibrous dysplasia has been termed Mazabraud syndrome.**

ADDITIONAL IMAGES

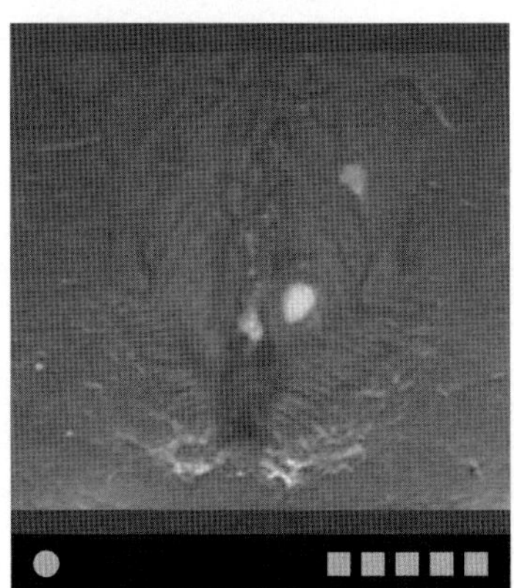

B. Mazabraud syndrome: A T2-weighted axial oblique image shows two small intramuscular, hyperintense masses, consistent with myxomas, posterior to the sacrum.

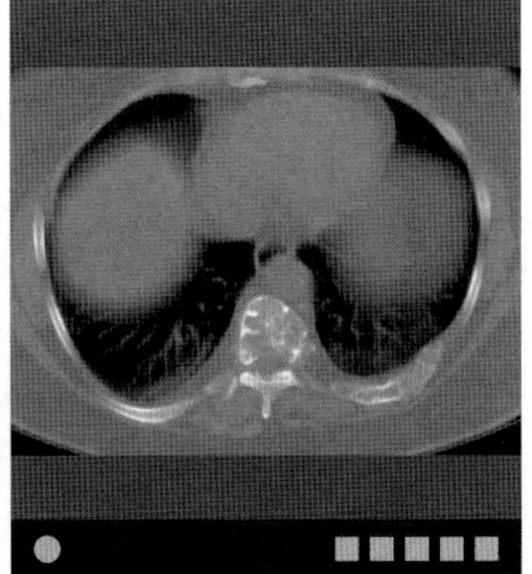

C. Mazabraud syndrome: A CT scan axial image through the lower thorax shows multiple lytic, expansile lesions in the ribs and spine, some of which have a ground-glass appearance.

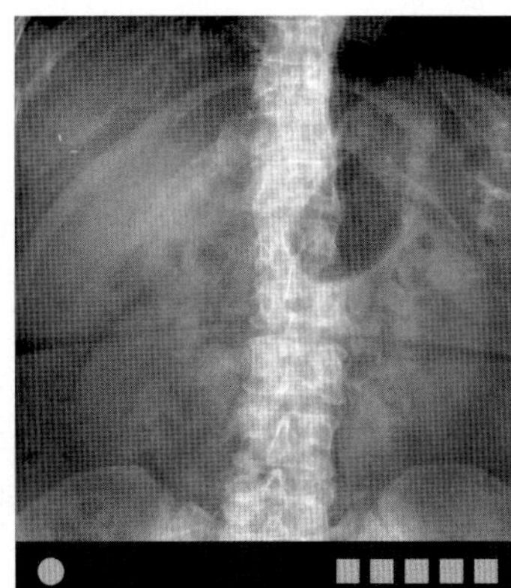

D. Mazabraud syndrome: A frontal radiograph of the lumbar spine shows multifocal vertebral and rib deformity.

IMAGE KEY

Common

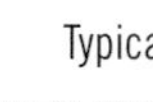

Rare

Typical

Unusual

DIFFERENTIAL DIAGNOSES IMAGES

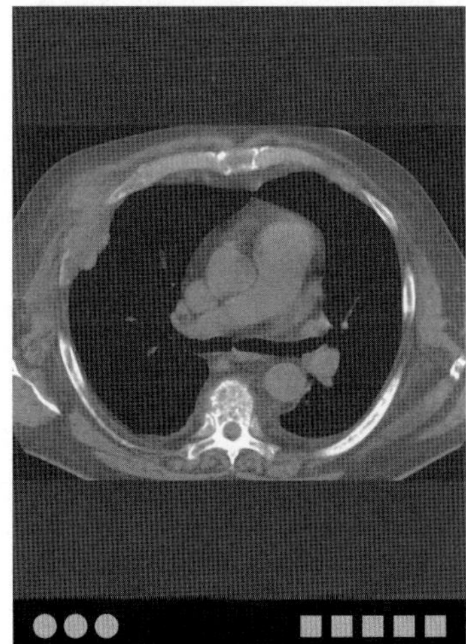

E. Multiple myeloma: An axial CT scan image through the lower thorax shows diffused destruction and expansion of a rib, expansion of the sternum, and focal lytic lesions in a vertebra.

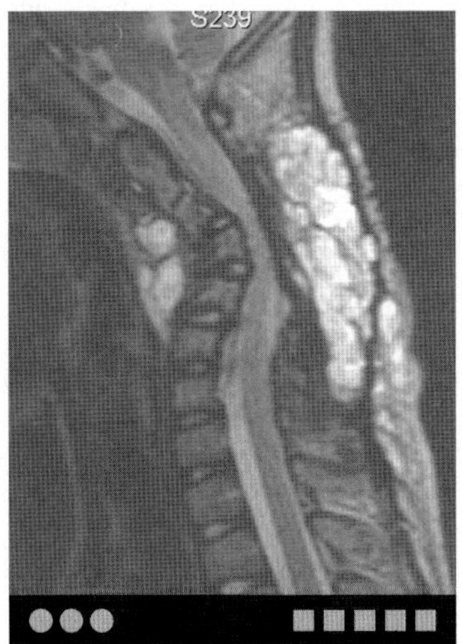

F. Neurofibromatosis: A sagittal T2-weighted image of the cervical spine in a child shows kyphosis with severe deformities of the vertebral bodies and neurofibromas in the surrounding soft tissues.

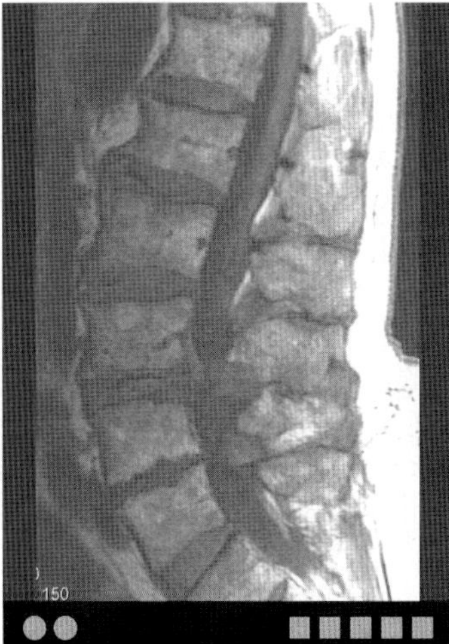

G. Paget's disease: A sagittal T1-weighted image of the lumbar spine shows marked heterogeneity of the bone marrow with enlargement of some bones, especially the spinous processes.

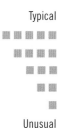

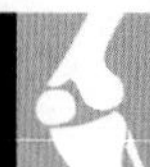

39–10 Langerhans Cell Histiocytosis

Kira Chow

PRESENTATION

Back pain

FINDINGS

Sagittal MR images demonstrate marked loss of vertebral body height in a child.

DIFFERENTIAL DIAGNOSES

- *Osteomyelitis:* May result in compression of vertebra; however, adjacent disk is often involved.
- *Malignancy:* Ewing sarcoma, osteosarcoma, metastatic disease (neuroblastoma), leukemia, and lymphoma show abnormal marrow with possible pedicle involvement, soft tissue mass, and multilevel lesions.
- *Compression fracture:* Post-traumatic history or postmenopausal status.
- *Dysplasias or systemic conditions:* Mucopolysaccharidosis, spondyloepiphyseal dysplasia, and Gaucher disease: Multiple vertebrae involvement are noted. Vertebral beakings are present in cases of dysplasias.

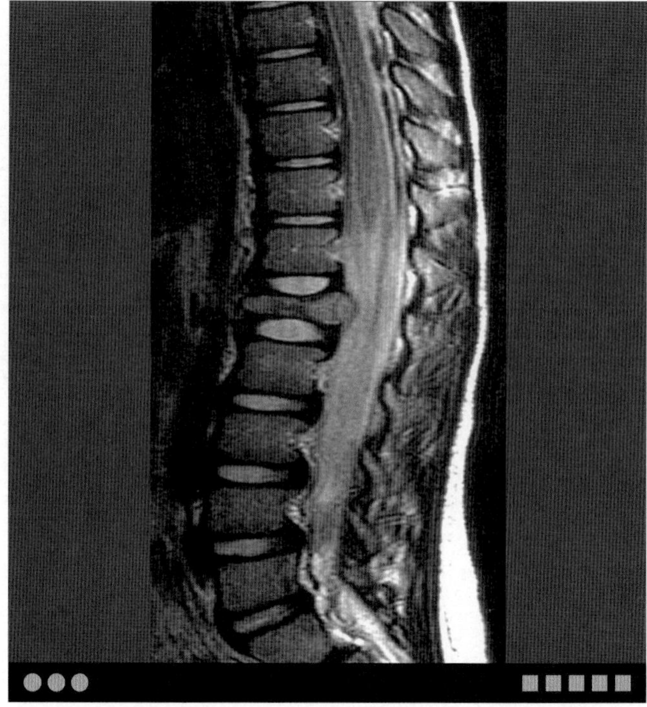

A. Langerhans cell histiocytosis: Sagittal T2-weighted MRI demonstrates marked loss of L1 vertebral body height in a child.

COMMENTS

Langerhans cell histiocytosis (LCH) is a spectrum of diseases with the common link of overproliferation of LCH (antigen presenting cells). Letterer-Siwe disease is a malignant variety with extensive deposits of Langerhans histiocytes in skeletal and extraskeletal locations. Hand-Schuller-Christian disease involves the skull, presenting with osseous lesions, exophthalmos, and diabetes insipidus. Eosinophilic granuloma is the benign form, with histiocytic infiltration of the medullary cavity. Most patients with LCH have at least one skeletal lesion. The most common sites of monostotic involvement are the skull, mandible, ribs, upper extremity long bones, pelvis, and spine. In the spine, as in this case, there can be involvement of one vertebral level or many. Therefore, if LCH in spine is suspected, bone scan or skeletal survey is useful because the presence of multiple lesions affects treatment. Radiographic findings include vertebral collapse, which can range from minimal to severe and can be uniform collapse or anterior/lateral wedging; well-maintained, intervertebral disc space; lack of soft tissue mass. In other skeletal locations, lesions have a variable appearance. Usually they are well-defined lucent lesions with scalloped borders. However, they can have aggressive features with cortical erosion, periosteal reaction, osseous expansion, and cortical breakthrough with associated soft tissue mass. Interestingly, the classically described vertebra plana is not the typical appearance, and when present, it is in children. LCH is the most common cause of vertebra plana. Collapsed vertebrae often regain height on follow up imaging and clinical symptoms typically resolve.

PEARLS

- **If a spine lesion is suspected to be LCH, bone scan or skeletal survey should be obtained to check for other lesions.**
- **The classic vertebra plana appearance of vertebral collapse is not the most common manifestation of LCH in the spine.**
- **Vertebral collapse may resolve on follow-up imaging.**

ADDITIONAL IMAGES

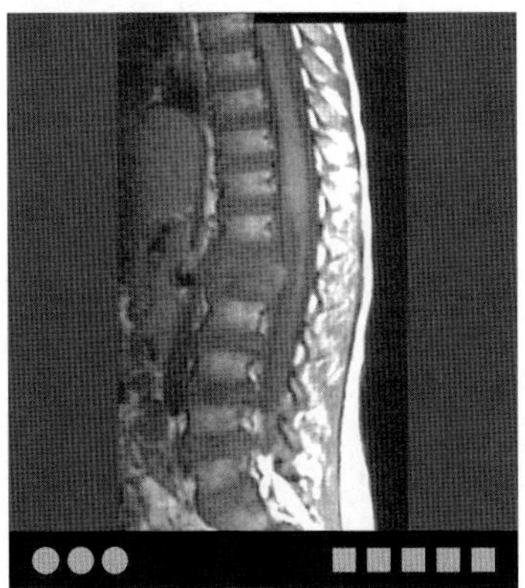

B. Langerhans cell histiocytosis: Sagittal T1-weighted image demonstrates marked loss of L1 vertebral body height in this child.

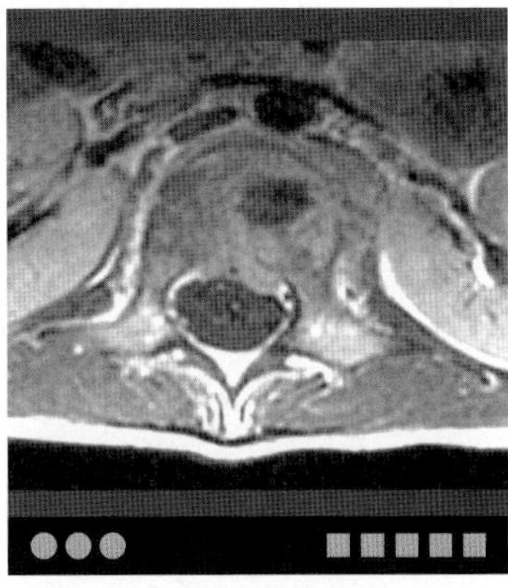

C. Langerhans cell histiocytosis: Axial T1-weighed image demonstrates contour abnormality along the anterior thecal sac secondary to abnormal soft tissue. There is also prevertebral soft tissue along the left anterior vertebral body

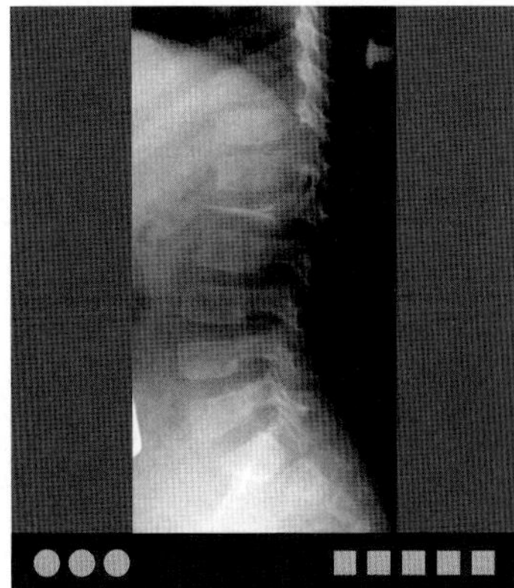

D. Langerhans cell histiocytosis: Lateral lumbar spine radiograph shows the classic radiographic sign vertebra plana with severe symmetric vertebral body collapse.

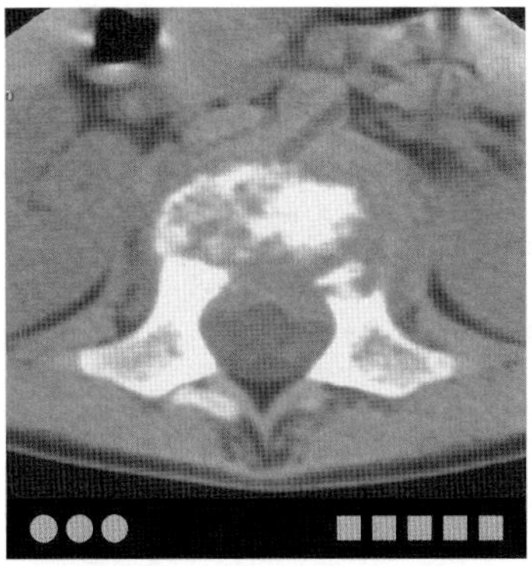

IMAGE KEY

Common

Rare

Typical

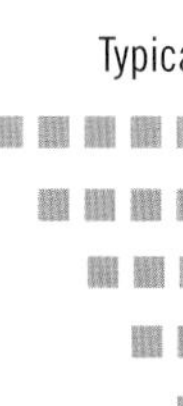

Unusual

E. Langerhans cell histiocytosis: Axial CT scan in soft tissue window demonstrates a circumferential prevertebral soft tissue rind. There is sclerosis and destruction of the vertebral body.

DIFFERENTIAL DIAGNOSES IMAGES

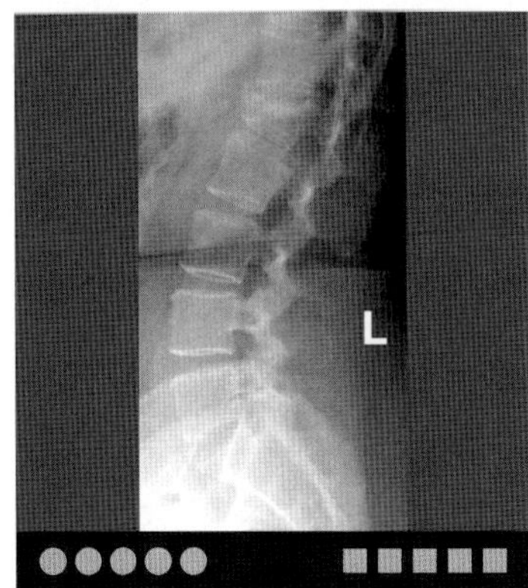

F. Compression fracture: Lateral radiograph of the lumbar spine demonstrates compression fracture with loss of height at L1 vertebra

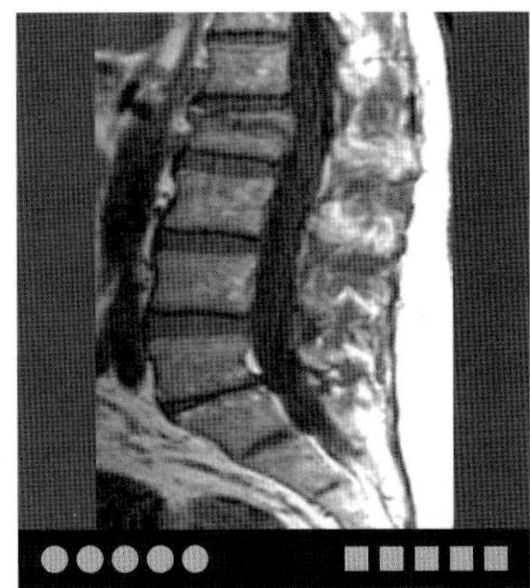

G. Compression fracture: T1-weighted sagittal MRI in another patient shows L2 superior endplate compression fracture with curvilinear T1-weighted hypointense fracture line.

Chapter 40

Miscellaneous

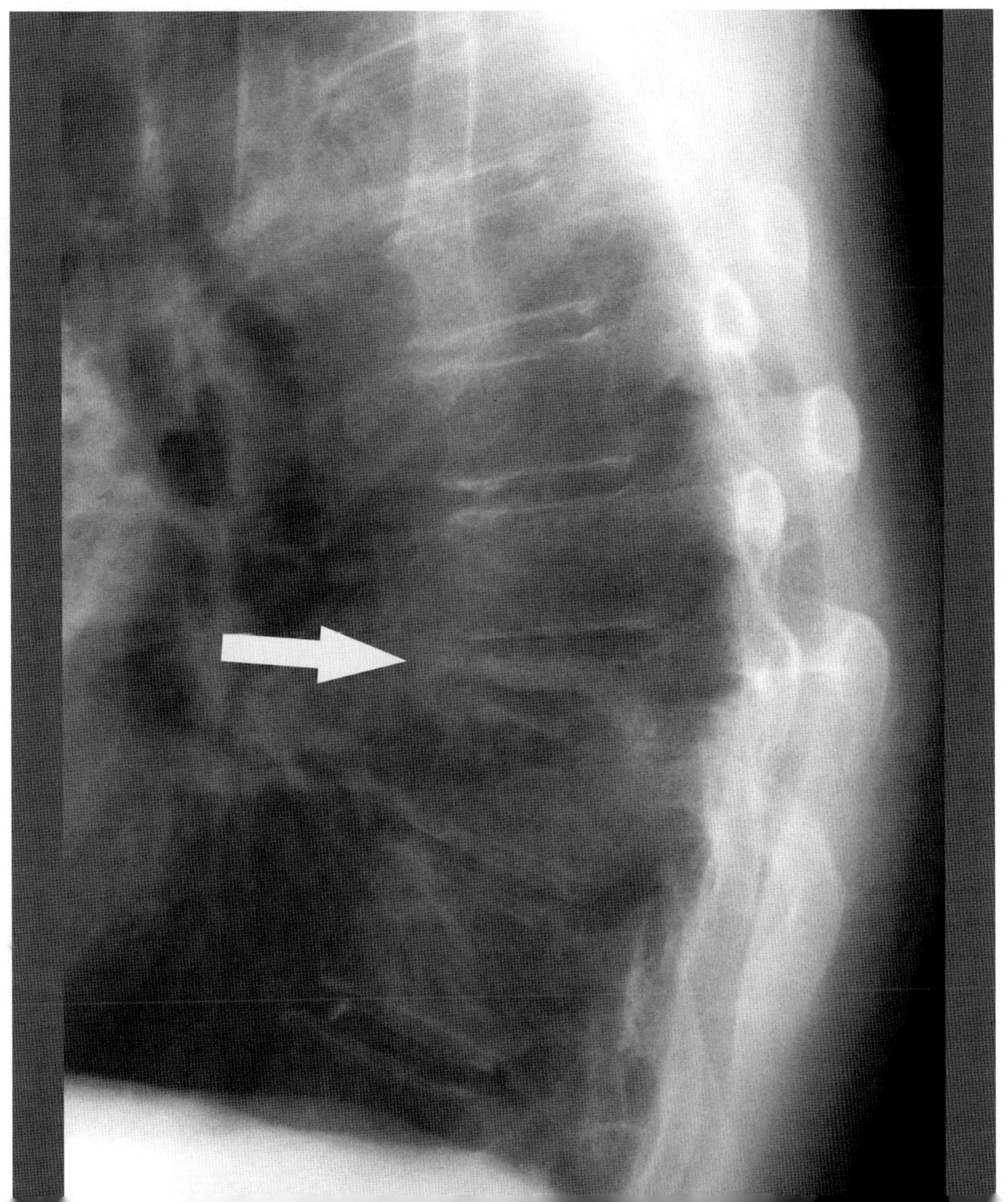

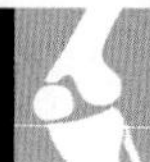

40–1 Vertebral Osteonecrosis (*Kümmell Disease*)

Charles H. Bush

PRESENTATION

Compression fracture of lower thoracic spine

FINDINGS

A lateral radiograph of the thoracic spine shows a wedge compression fracture in the lower thoracic spine, which was not present on radiographs from 3 years earlier. CT scan was obtained to evaluate for underlying lymphomatous involvement.

DIFFERENTIAL DIAGNOSES

- *Lymphoma:* This must be considered in a patient with non-Hodgkin lymphoma. However, involvement of the spine by diffused lymphoma almost always consists of multiple lesions, while primary lymphoma of bone usually occurs in the appendicular skeleton.
- Osteoporotic compression fracture is certainly possible in this elderly male patient, but osteoporotic compression fractures are more common in postmenopausal Caucasian and Asian females.
- *Eosinophilic granuloma:* These vertebral wedge compression fractures are much more common in children, where the appearance is termed *vertebra plana.*

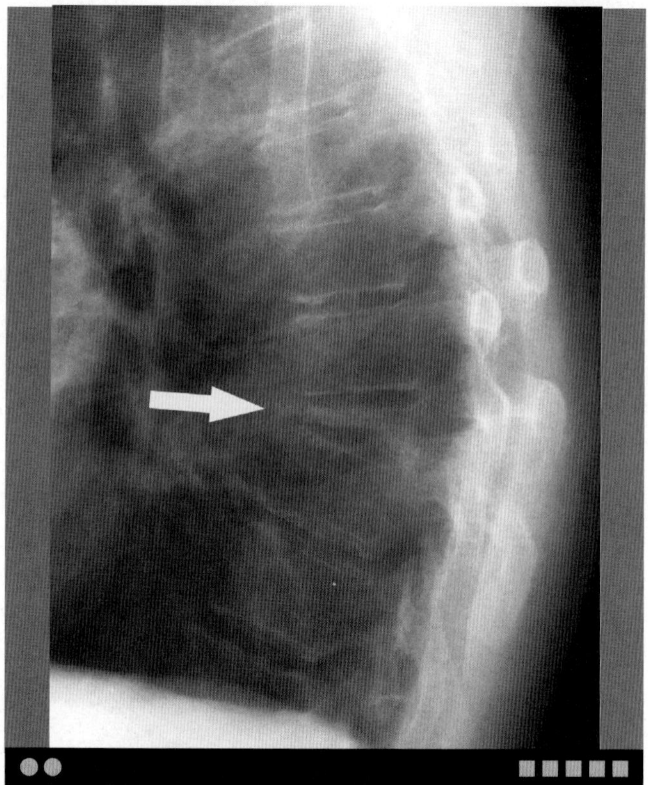

A. Vertebral osteonecrosis: A lateral radiograph of the chest during staging for lymphoma shows a wedge compression fracture (arrow) of a midthoracic vertebral body.

COMMENTS

A 68-year-old male had routine chest radiography for staging of non-Hodgkin lymphoma, when a new lower thoracic compression fracture was discovered. Ischemic necrosis of a vertebral body can occur as a delayed response to trauma, sometimes called by the eponym of *Kümmell disease.* This affliction is typically seen in both men and women past the sixth decade. Vertebral osteonecrosis can also be secondary to the usual causes of ischemic necrosis of bone (hypercorticoidism, Gaucher disease, irradiation, pancreatitis, etc.). What is distinctive about post-traumatic vertebral osteonecrosis is its characteristic appearance as the "vacuum vertebral body" sign of gas bubbles within a fractured, often markedly compressed vertebral body. The gas, which consists of almost pure nitrogen, the least soluble of the blood gases, accumulates because of the very slightly negative pressure in the ischemic vertebral body relative to the cellular interstitial space. This sign is virtually diagnostic, and can be useful in excluding other etiologies, such as neoplasia. Although vertebral osteomyelitis with gas forming organisms is theoretically possible, this is extremely rare, particularly in the absence of systemic signs, and infection is also virtually excluded by this sign. Cross-sectional imaging, particularly CT scan, is quite useful in distinguishing vertebral osteonecrosis from neoplasia, both in confirming the presence of small amounts of gas within a collapsed vertebral segment, as well as excluding the presence of a paraspinous mass, bone destruction, and other occult vertebral lesions at other levels that are frequently associated with the latter.

PEARLS

- **Sometimes a large Schmorl node can accumulate gas within its cavity, and mimic the appearance of gas within the vertebral body.**
- **Another clue to the benign etiology of vertebral collapse in patients with vertebral osteonecrosis is the presence of the "puzzle sign," where all of the fragments of the collapsed body considered together show no net bone destruction.**

ADDITIONAL IMAGES

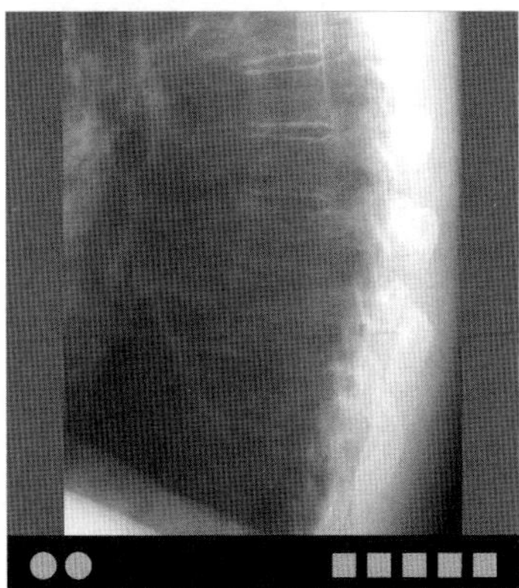

B. Vertebral osteonecrosis: A lateral radiograph of the chest 3 years earlier shows no evidence of thoracic, vertebral abnormality.

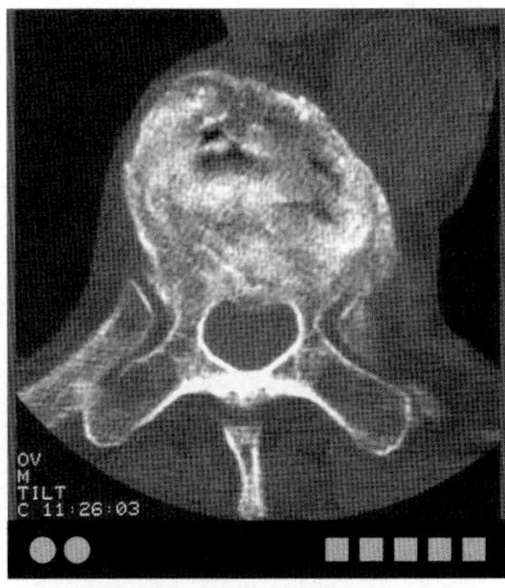

C. Vertebral osteonecrosis: CT scan through the affected level shows radiolucent gas bubbles within the fractured vertebral segment, with absence of a paraspinous soft tissue mass, diagnostic for vertebral osteonecrosis.

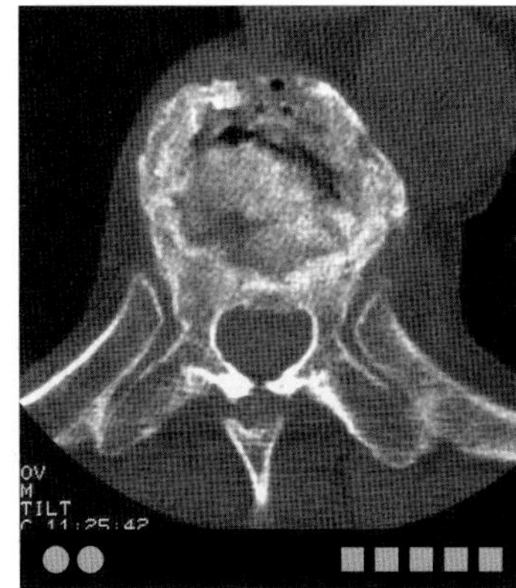

D. Vertebral osteonecrosis: CT scan section through the ischemic vertebral body at a slightly different level. Both sections also show a positive puzzle sign, with the vertebral fragments showing no net bone destruction.

IMAGE KEY

Common

Rare

Typical

Unusual

DIFFERENTIAL DIAGNOSES IMAGES

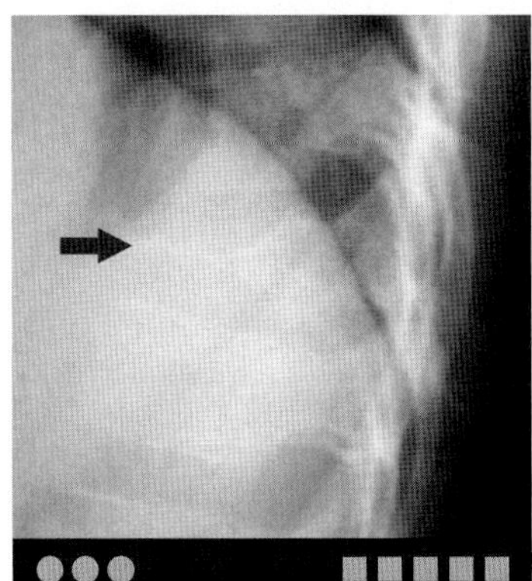

E. Eosinophilic granuloma: Lateral radiograph of a 13-year-old boy with vertebral collapse (arrow) from eosinophilic granuloma.

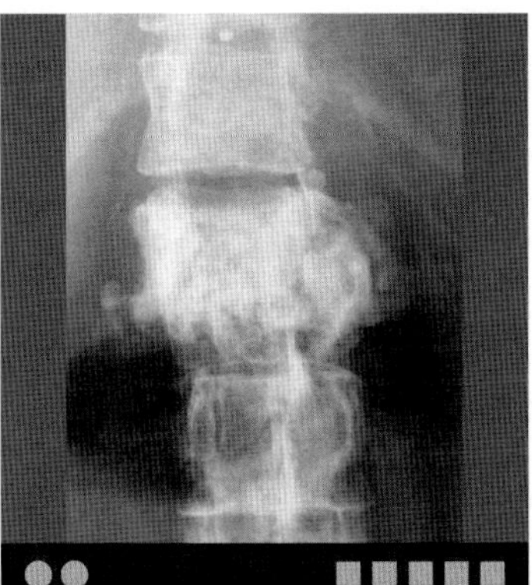

F. Radiation osteonecrosis: AP radiograph of another patient irradiated at the thoracolumbar junction 14 years previously after resection of conus ependymoma, showing collapse of two adjacent segments secondary to osteonecrosis.

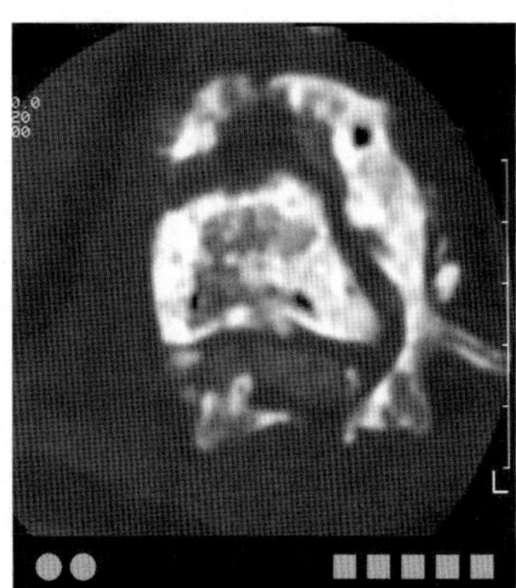

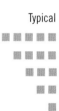

G. Radiation osteonecrosis: Axial section from a CT scan myelogram of the same patient (as in image F), showing small pockets of lucent gas within the collapsed segments, with no paraspinous mass.

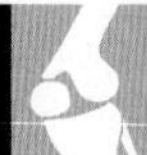

40–2 Kümmell Disease

Ashkan Afshin and Jamshid Tehranzadeh

PRESENTATION

Back pain

FINDINGS

Conventional radiographs show sclerosis of collapsed vertebra with transverse radiolucent line in the center of the vertebral body (intravertebral vacuum cleft sign). Bone scan demonstrates increased uptake in the collapsed vertebra. MR images show decreased signal intensity in both T1-weighted and T2-weighted images in the collapsed vertebra.

DIFFERENTIAL DIAGNOSES

- *Malignancy:* Primary malignancies of the spine such as multiple myeloma or lymphoma and metastasis may lead to vertebral collapse. Collapsed vertebra in children because of leukemia may also be considered.
- *Spinal osteomyelitis:* Lumbar spine is most often affected by spinal osteomyelitis. Disk involvement and vertebral endplate erosions are the clues to the diagnosis.
- *Eosinophilic granuloma of the spine:* Thoracic spine in children is most often affected.
- *Osteochondritis (Calvé's disease) of a vertebral body:* It is a rare condition with flattening of the vertebral body in children. It may be acute or insidious and is most frequent in boys. Eosinophilic granuloma may be the cause.
- *Osteogenesis imperfecta:* Osteoporosis in this disease is the cause of multiple vertebral collapses, which can occur at any age and may lead to symptomatic back deformities.

COMMENTS

Kümmell disease is a rare spinal disorder which is characterized by delayed post-traumatic collapse of the vertebral body. The pathophysiology of this disease is not clear; however, osteonecrosis is the most widely accepted mechanism of injury. Kümmell disease usually affects middle-aged or elderly men or women with the interval between the acute traumatic episode and the vertebral collapse varying from days to years. It usually involves one vertebral body at T8 through L4 level. Acute back pain is the most prominent symptom in early phase of disease. When the pain recurs kyphotic deformity is often found in thoracolumbar region of the back corresponding to affected vertebral body. Neurologic manifestation of the disease may also develop during later stages of the disease. The highly suggestive, but not pathognomic, radiographic finding of Kümmell disease is intravertebral vacuum cleft sign.

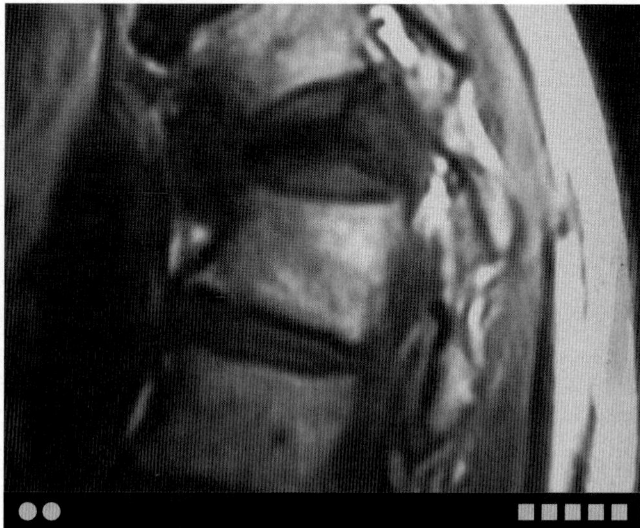

A. Kümmell disease of thoracic spine: Sagittal T1-weighted image of thoracic spine in this 60-year-old man with collapsed thoracic vertebra shows anterior wedging with low signal of the body of this collapsed vertebra.

It results from collection of gas within the collapsed vertebral body and appears as a transverse radiolucent line in the center of the vertebral body or adjacent to one of its endplates. This vacuum cleft is exaggerated with extension views. It is seen on CT scans as low signal intensity on all pulse sequences. Bone scan demonstrates increased uptake in the collapsed vertebra. MRI can differentiate Kümmell disease and spontaneous vertebral osteonecrosis from osteoporotic compression fractures. Osteoporotic fractures shows no signal change on MR images, while osteonecrotic collapse of the vertebral body shows decreased signal intensity in T1-weighted and T2-weighted images.

PEARLS

- **It is a delayed post-traumatic collapse of the vertebral body.**
- **Osteonecrosis is the most widely accepted mechanism of injury.**
- **Usually, it affects one vertebral body at T8 through L4 levels.**
- **Back pain, kyphotic deformity in thoracolumbar region of the back, and neurologic manifestations are common clinical findings.**
- **Intravertebral vacuum cleft sign is the highly suggestive radiographic finding.**
- **MR images show collapse of the vertebral body with decreased signal intensity in T1-weighted and T2-weighted images.**

ADDITIONAL IMAGES

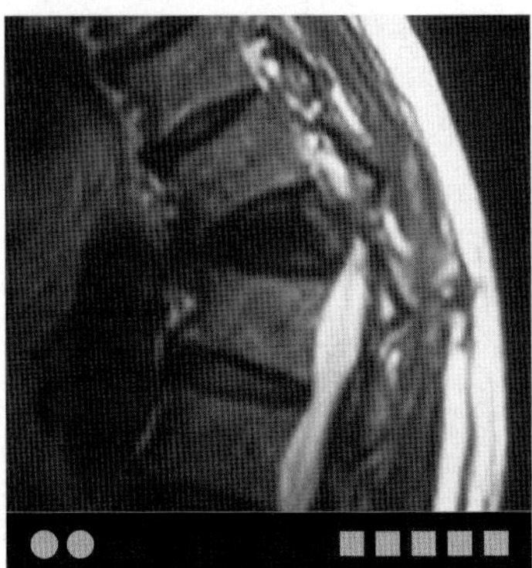

B. Kümmell disease of thoracic spine: Sagittal T2-weighted image of thoracic spine (same patient as in image A) shows anterior wedging with low signal of the body of this collapsed vertebra. Note acute angle kyphosis at the fracture site.

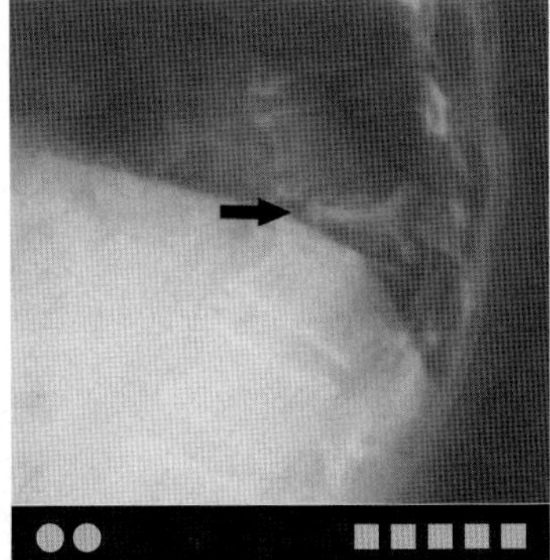

C. Kümmell disease of thoracic spine: Lateral radiograph of thoracic spine (same patient as in image A and B) shows collapse, sclerosis, and intraosseous air (vacuum phenomenon) (arrow).

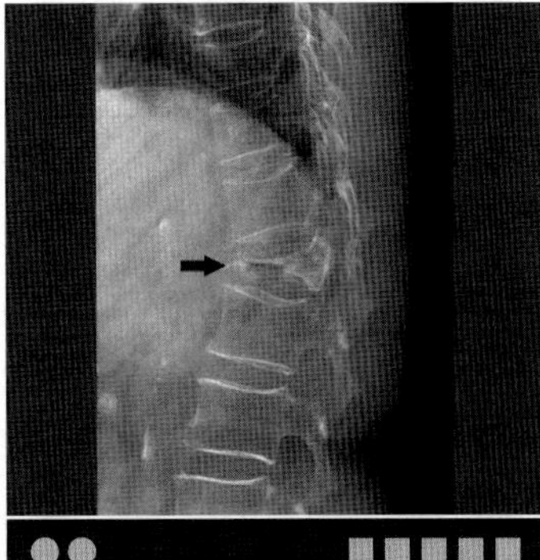

D. Kümmell disease of lumbar spine: Lateral radiograph of lumbar spine in another patient shows collapse of the L1 vertebra with intraosseous air (vacuum phenomenon).

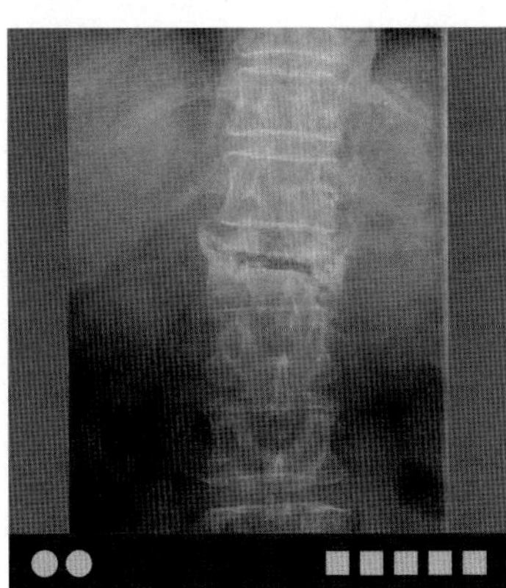

E. Kümmell disease of lumbar spine: AP radiograph of thoracic spine (same patient as in image D) shows collapse of the L1 vertebra with intraosseous air (vacuum phenomenon).

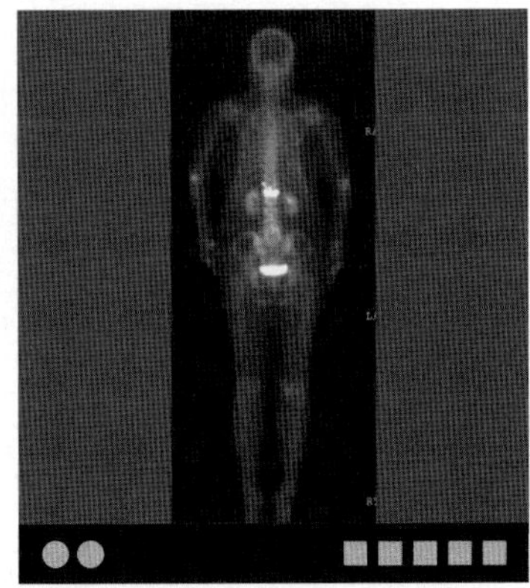

F. Kümmell disease of lumbar spine: Posterior view of the bone scan (same patient as image D and E) shows increased uptake in the collapsed vertebra.

DIFFERENTIAL DIAGNOSIS IMAGE

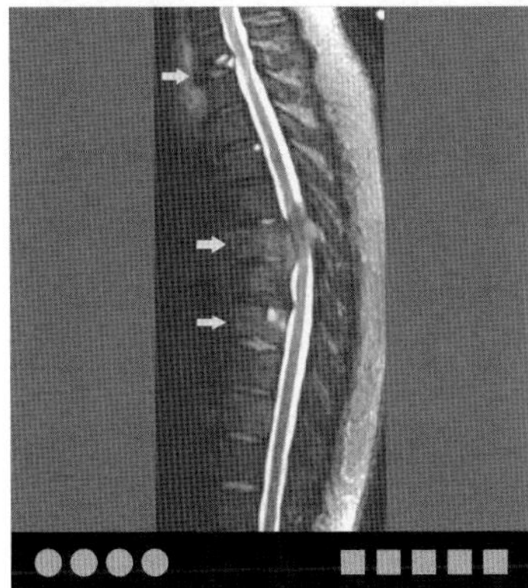

G. Multiple collapsed vertebrae caused by metastasis: Sagittal T2-weighted image shows multiple collapsed vertebral bodies (arrows) caused by metastasis to spine.

IMAGE KEY

Common

Rare

Typical

Unusual

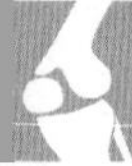

40–3 Degenerative Spondylolisthesis

Cliff Tao

PRESENTATION

Chronic low back pain

FINDINGS

MRI shows anterior translation of L4 on L5 with marked facet arthrosis and degenerative disc disease. The pars interarticularis is intact.

DIFFERENTIAL DIAGNOSES

- *Spondylolytic spondylolisthesis:* May occur at any level but usually at L5. There is a unilateral or bilateral defect at the pars interarticularis (spondylolysis). Unlike degenerative type; in this type the size of spinal canal is normal or even enlarged.
- *Traumatic spondylolisthesis*: This is a spondylolisthesis with a posterior arch fracture in an area other than the pars interarticularis. Classically seen at C2–hangman's (or hangee's) fracture.
- *Facet dislocation:* There is spondylolisthesis secondary to unilateral or bilateral facet dislocation ("jumped" or "perched" facet). The disc space is usually anterior wedged-shaped.
- *Normal variant:* At C6, the pars region may be elongated, resulting in 1 mm to 2 mm of anterolisthesis. At C2, there may be slight (1–2 mm) anterolisthesis, particularly in the pediatric spine.

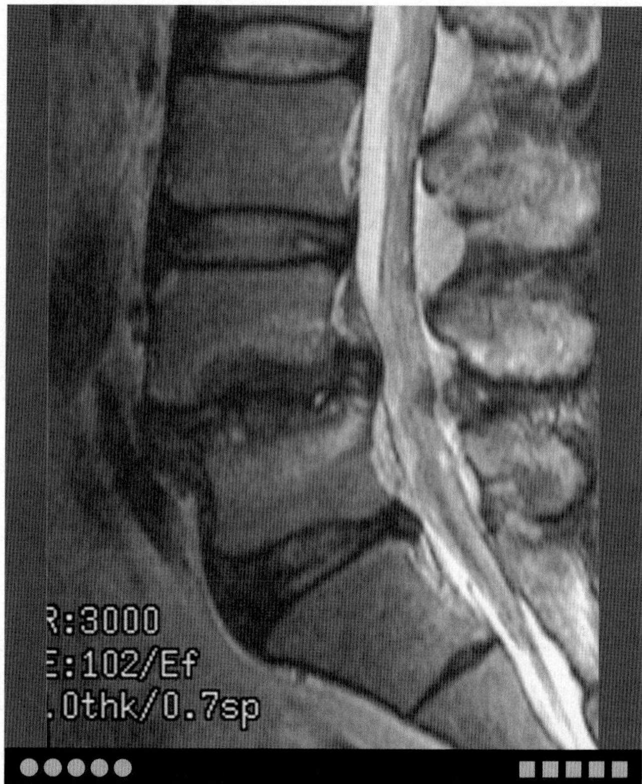

A. Degenerative spondylolisthesis: Sagittal T2-weighted image shows anterolisthesis of L4 on L5. Note the severe degenerative disc disease.

COMMENTS

This is an image of a 53-year-old male who presented with chronic low back pain and a degenerative spondylolisthesis at L4 with severe degenerative disc and facet disease. All findings contribute to bilateral foraminal stenosis, and any, all, or none of these findings may account for the clinical presentation. There are at least five types of spondylolisthesis: dysplastic, isthmic, degenerative, traumatic, and pathologic. The isthmic or pars variety is broken into subtypes of fatigue fracture (spondylolytic), elongated pars, and acute fracture. This case is the most common type at L4 because of degenerative disc and facet disease. Women are affected more than men, especially black women, and the patient is usually older than 40 years. There is narrowing of the central spinal canal and intervertebral foramina, which may result in sciatica-like symptoms or even neurogenic claudication. Although most of these are stable, there is a possibility of instability and surgical stabilization may be considered. Weight-bearing radiographs may accentuate the anterolisthesis. If the pars interarticularis cannot be directly visualized, secondary findings specific to degenerative spondylolisthesis include: anterior position of the spinous process; normal or narrowed AP diameter of the spinal canal; marked degenerative facet arthrosis; and normal AP diameter of the posterior epidural fat.

PEARLS

- **The most common type of spondylolisthesis at L4 is degenerative, caused by disc and facet disease.**
- **Check the pars interarticularis region on sagittal and axial images for spondylolysis.**
- **Use secondary signs (spinous process, spinal canal, and posterior epidural fat diameter) if the pars interarticularis is not directly visualized.**
- **Follow-up to assess for instability may be necessary.**
- **The spinal canal is narrowed at subluxation level.**

ADDITIONAL IMAGES

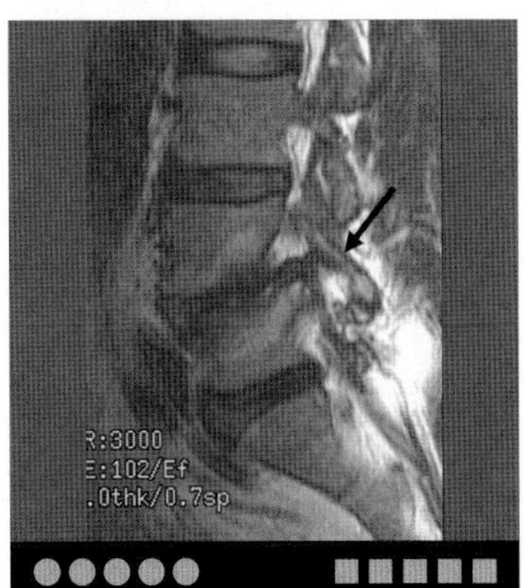

B. Degenerative spondylolisthesis: Sagittal T2-weighted image shows intact pars interarticularis (arrow).

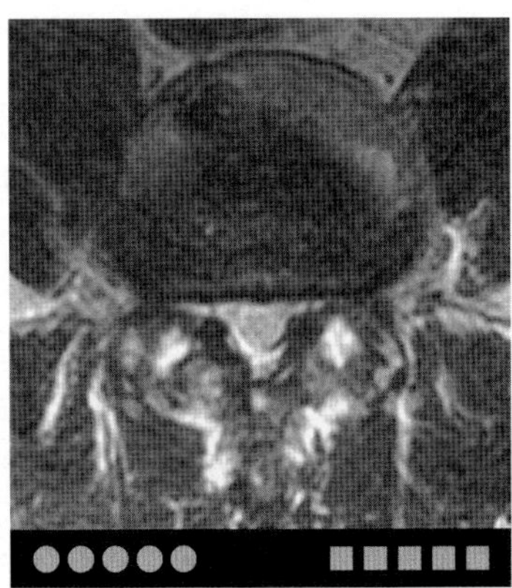

C. Degenerative spondylolisthesis: Axial T2-weighted image shows marked degenerative facet arthrosis. Note the spinal canal is narrowed.

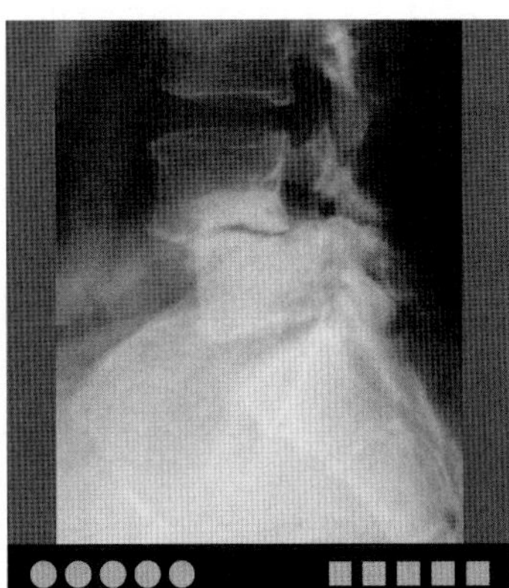

D. Degenerative spondylolisthesis: Lateral weight-bearing radiograph increases the anterior translation. There is marked degenerative disc and facet disease. Superimposed, iliac crest has created a mach effect on posterior elements.

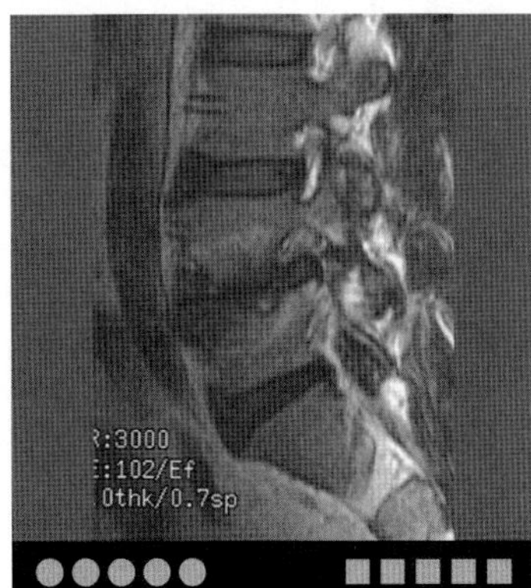

E. Degenerative spondylolisthesis: Sagittal T2-weighted image shows intervertebral foraminal narrowing.

IMAGE KEY

Common

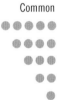

Rare

Typical

Unusual

DIFFERENTIAL DIAGNOSES IMAGES

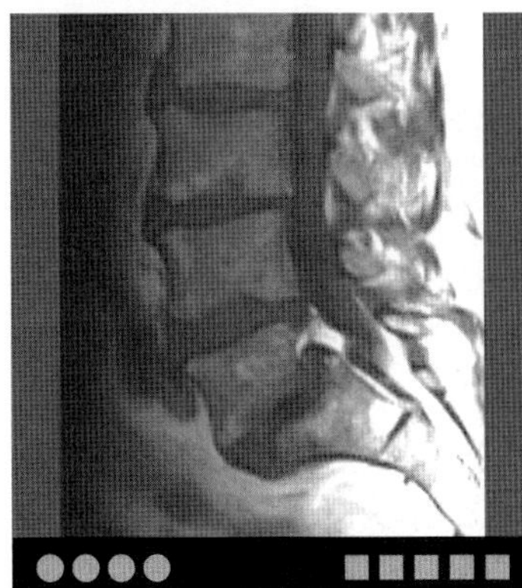

F. Spondylolytic spondylolisthesis: Note the increase in canal diameter and normal position of spinous process.

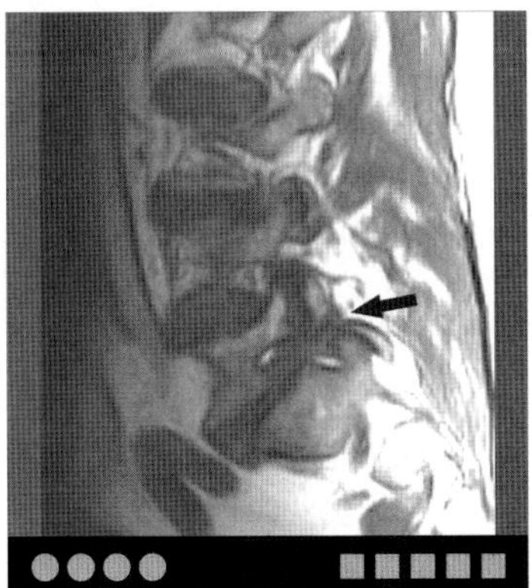

G. Spondylolytic spondylolisthesis: Same patient as in image F. There is a spondylolysis (arrow) and narrowing of the intervertebral foramen.

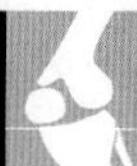

40–4 Diffuse Idiopathic Skeletal Hyperostosis (DISH)

Oganes Ashikyan and Jamshid Tehranzadeh

PRESENTATION

Trauma

FINDINGS

Exuberant flowing ossifications along anterior spine with relatively preserved disk spaces.

DIFFERENTIAL DIAGNOSES

- *Ankylosing spondylitis:* Fusion of sacroiliac and facet joints can help differentiate ankylosing spondylitis from DISH.
- *Intervertebral osteochondrosis:* Narrowed disk spaces in this condition differentiate intervertebral osteochondrosis from DISH.
- *Spondylosis deformans:* In some cases, this condition can be differentiated from DISH by the degree of disk prolapse and size of osteophytes. However, findings of one of the pathologic subtypes of DISH (type II) may be identical to spondylosis deformans.
- *Acromegaly:* Periosteal new bone formation and osseous outgrowth may be present in patients with acromegaly. Peripheral manifestation of acromegaly such as excessive height and distal bone enlargement are absent in patients with DISH.

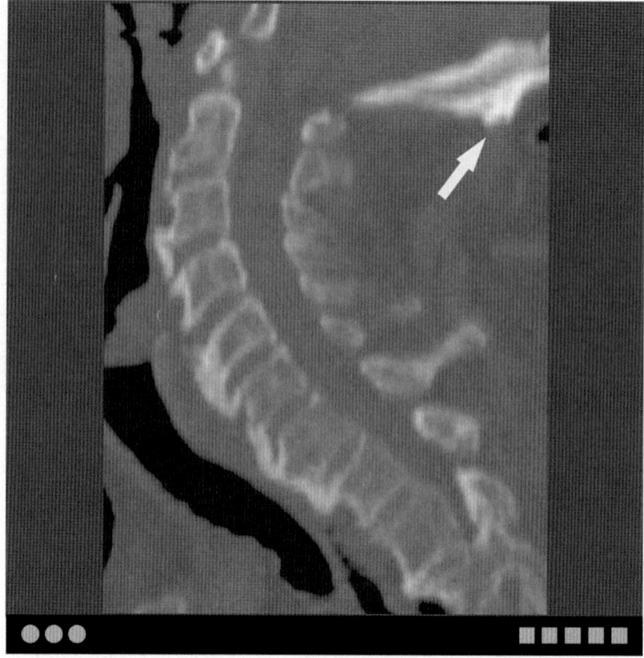

A. Diffuse idiopathic skeletal hyperostosis: Reformatted sagittal CT scan image of the cervical spine demonstrates exuberant ossification and bridging osteophytes along the anterior aspect of the spine. The disk spaces appear relatively well preserved. Note prominence of origin of the nuchal ligament at the occiput (arrow).

COMMENTS

This is an image of a 69-year-old male who sustained multiple fractures after falling onto cement surface. Findings related to DISH were discovered incidentally on the CT scan obtained for evaluation of trauma. The etiology of DISH is unknown. This disorder also called Forestier disease, and it usually presents in the elderly patients with and without a remote history of trauma. DISH may first present with spinal stiffness and back pain. Dysphagia in patients with large cervical osteophytes may also be the presenting symptom. This disorder may be discovered incidentally during work-up of other abnormalities. Characteristic radiographic finding in patients with DISH is that of exuberant flowing ossification along the anterior aspect of the spine. The abnormalities are usually seen in the thoracic spine, but lower cervical and upper lumbar levels may also be involved. Posterior osteophytosis is rare, but may occur. Disk space narrowing is usually mild. The bones may appear radiodense for patient's age. Bony ankylosis may be present in the thoracic spine and less frequently in the cervical and lumbar spine. Ankylosing spondylitis can be differentiated from DISH by the presence of fusion of the sacroiliac and/or facet joints. In addition to spinal involvement, DISH may manifest in a variety of other sites including pelvis and heel; and at the sites of other ligament and tendon attachments in the upper and lower extremities. Proliferative bony changes at the sites of ligament and tendon attachment (enthesis) have been reported to occur more frequently in patients with DISH compared to other patients. Even hyperostosis frontalis interna of the skull has been reported in the context of DISH.

PEARLS

- **DISH usually presents as an exuberant flowing ossification along the anterior aspect of the spine.**
- **Thoracic spine, lower cervical spine, and upper lumbar spine are usual sites of this disease.**
- **Large ossifications at the sites of tendon and ligament attachments may be related to DISH, though these are not specific findings.**
- **Continuous flowing ankylosing ossification in the thoracic spine will require evaluation of other sites to differentiate DISH from ankylosing spondylitis.**

ADDITIONAL IMAGES

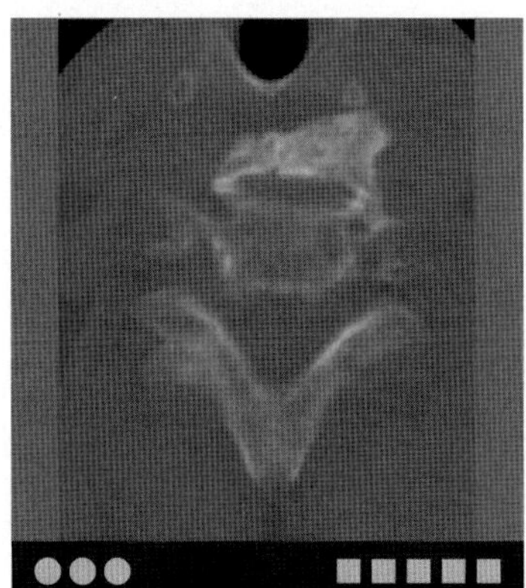

B. Diffuse idiopathic skeletal hyperostosis: Axial CT scan image of the cervical spine at C5 level demonstrates extensive ossification anterior to the vertebral body.

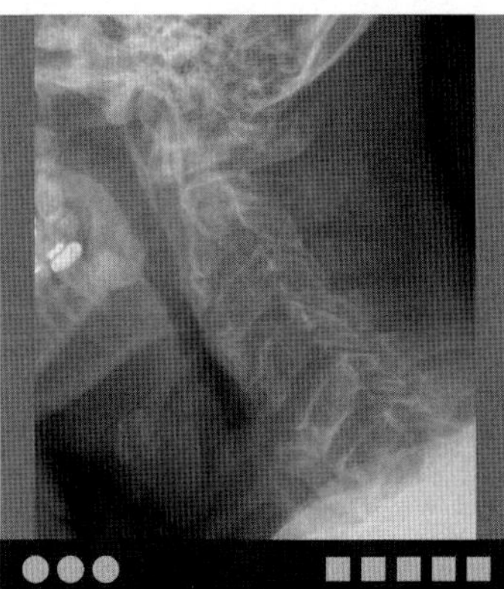

C. Diffuse idiopathic skeletal hyperostosis: Lateral radiograph of the cervical spine again shows extensive ossification of the anterior longitudinal ligament. Note that the facet joints are relatively spared.

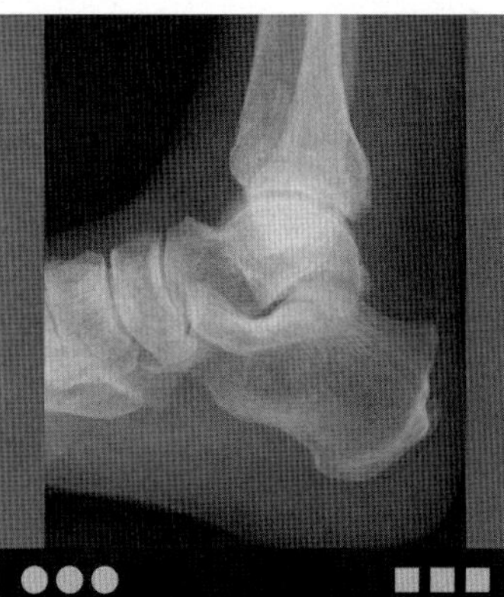

D. Diffuse idiopathic skeletal hyperostosis: Lateral view of the ankle demonstrates large calcification at the Achilles tendon insertion site onto calcaneus.

IMAGE KEY

Common

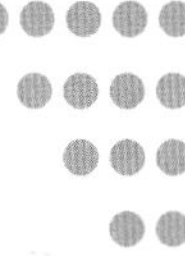

Rare

Typical

Unusual

DIFFERENTIAL DIAGNOSES IMAGES

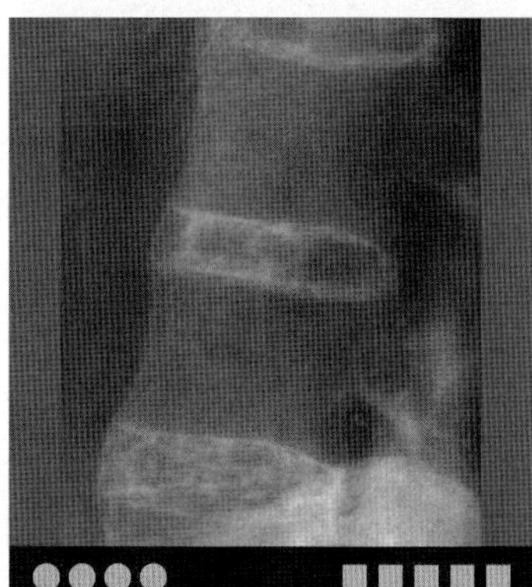

E. Ankylosing spondylitis: Lateral radiograph of the spine shows fine syndesmophytes in the margin of the spine with intervertebral calcifications and facets and spine fusion.

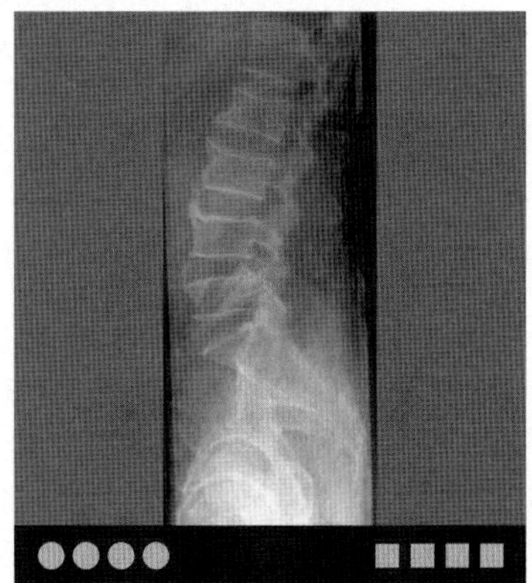

F. Ankylosing spondylitis in a 79-year-old man: Lateral view of the lumbar spine demonstrates flowing anterior ossification with preservation of disk spaces.

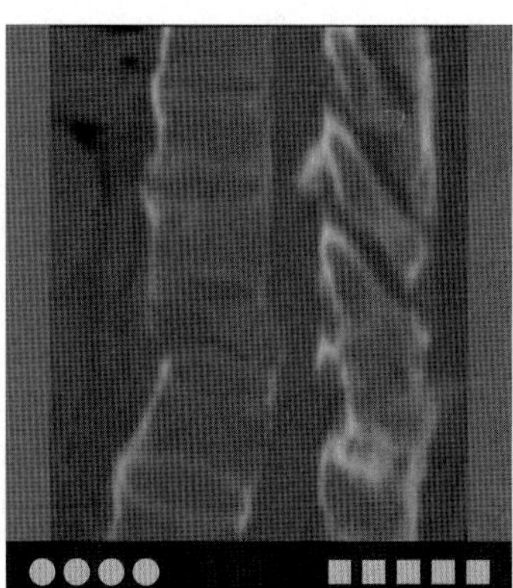

G. Ankylosing spondylitis in a 79-year-old man and vertebral body fracture: Reformatted sagittal CT scan image of the thoracolumbar junction in the same patient as in image F shows ankylosing ossification along the thoracolumbar spine above and below T11 vertebral body fracture.

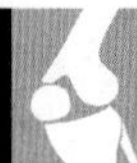

40–5 Primary Hyperparathyroidism

Michael A. Bruno

PRESENTATION

Hypercalcemia; asymptomatic

FINDINGS

The bone scan is characteristic of a "superscan" with intense, generalized skeletal uptake and nonvisualization of the kidneys. The mandible is visualized on this bone scan. Radiograph of the skull shows the classic "salt and pepper" pattern. Radiographs reveal subperiosteal bone resorption, cortical tunneling, osteoporosis, and distal tuft erosions so called acro-osteolysis.

DIFFERENTIAL DIAGNOSES

- Paget disease is the primary differential diagnosis. Paget disease generally results in higher density of the affected bones, and a greater degree of bony expansion. On bone scan (not shown) the mandible is generally spared.
- Secondary hyperparathyroidism, e.g., renal osteodystrophy may have identical manifestations.

COMMENTS

This case illustrates radiographic and imaging manifestations of primary hyperparathyroidism, with characteristic radiographic and nuclear medicine bone scan findings. The imaging hallmark of the disease is subperiosteal bone resorption. Other signs include endocortical and intracortical bone resorption, also known as cortical tunneling. Acro-osteolysis is bone resorption at the distal phalangeal tufts, which may be the earliest finding and is a sensitive sign to monitor healing following treatment. Osteoporosis is a common finding and is the result of osteoclastic activity and bone resorption. Chondrocalcinosis and tendon and ligament erosions may be seen. Focal bone resorption or osteitis fibrosa cystica may occur which is called Brown tumor. This classic finding (Brown tumor) or (osteoclastoma) which is absent in this case can occur in both primary and secondary hyperparathyroidism, but is not seen in all cases. It can be readily distinguished from its main differential diagnosis which is Paget disease of bone, by conventional radiograph and bone scan. Secondary hyperparathyroidism, caused by renal disease or other factors, can have a similar appearance on all modalities of imaging. In approximately 80% of cases of primary hyperparathyroidism, one or more discrete parathyroid adenomas can be identified as the cause; resection is curative. Diffused hyperplasia of all four parathyroid glands accounts for the bulk of the remainder of the cases. Hyperfunctioning carcinoma of the parathyroid is a very rare cause of hyperparathyroidism. Rare in children, the incidence of disease peaks around the age of 50.

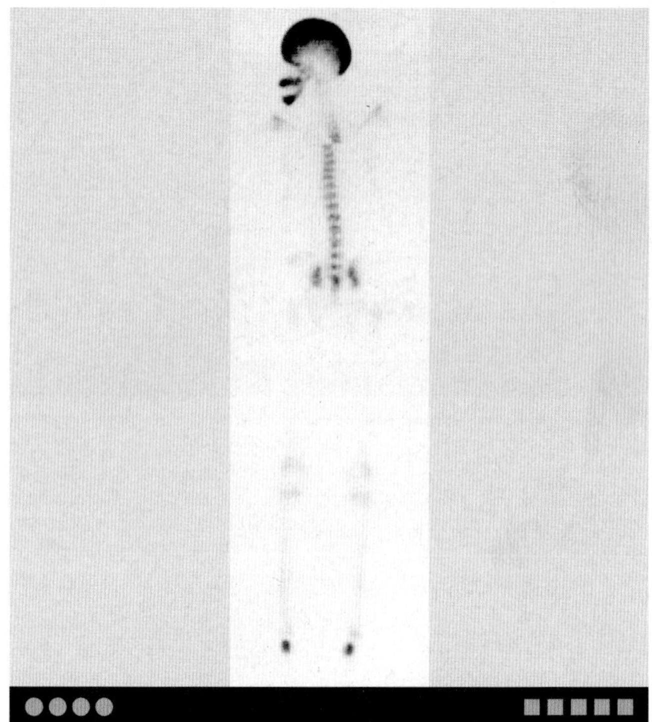

A. Primary hyperparathyroidism: Whole body image of the bone scan in this patient shows a superscan, with intense uptake in the skeleton and essentially no renal excretion of tracer (nonvisualization of the kidneys). Note that the mandible is visualized.

PEARLS

- **Usually patients are asymptomatic, and the diagnosis is made on the basis of laboratory results (abnormal serum calcium) and the finding of osteopenia on radiographs obtained for other reasons.**
- **Subperiosteal bone resorption is considered the hallmark of imaging signs.**
- **Most commonly secondary to discrete parathyroid adenomas.**
- **Peak age of incidence is around 50 years; rare in children.**
- **Radiographic and/or nuclear imaging may not distinguish primary from secondary hyperparathyroidism, such as renal osteodystrophy.**

ADDITIONAL IMAGES

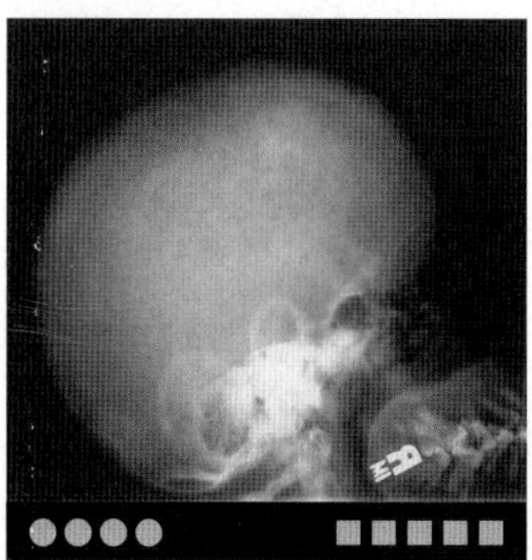

B. Primary hyperparathyroidism: Lateral skull radiograph shows classic salt and pepper appearance of bony resorption in the skull.

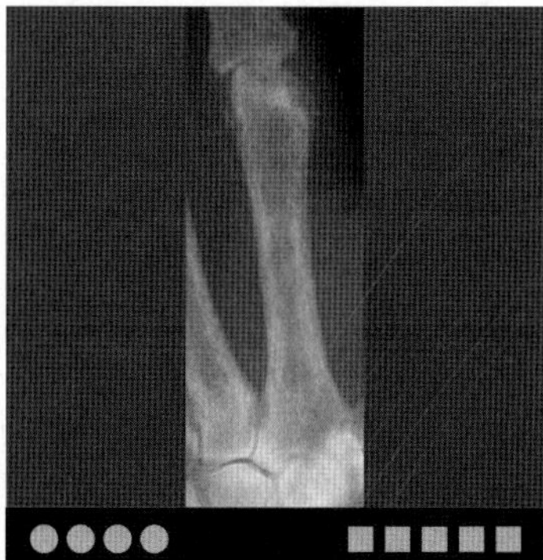

C. Primary hyperparathyroidism: PA radiograph of the finger in the same patient shows subperiosteal and endosteal resorption and osteopenia.

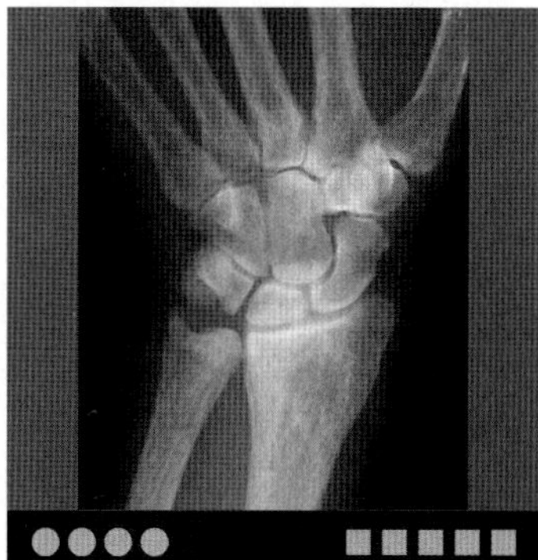

D. Primary hyperparathyroidism: PA radiograph of the wrist in the same patient, just proximal to image C, shows osteopenia and chondrocalcinosis of triangular fibrocartilage.

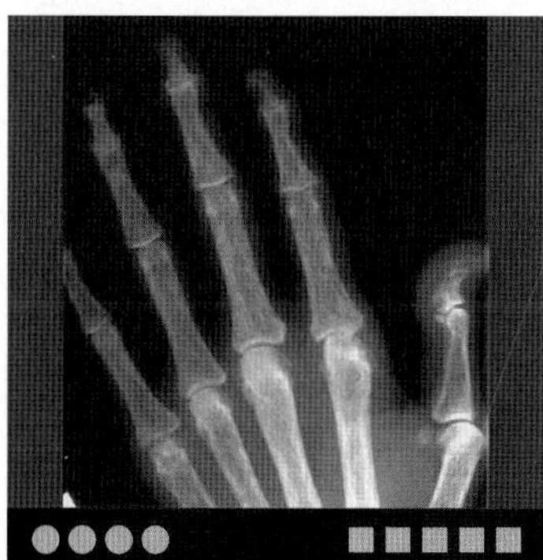

E. Primary hyperparathyroidism: Detail view radiograph of the fingers of the same patient reveals distal tuft resorption in the fingertips and thumb.

IMAGE KEY

Common

Rare

Typical

Unusual

DIFFERENTIAL DIAGNOSES IMAGES

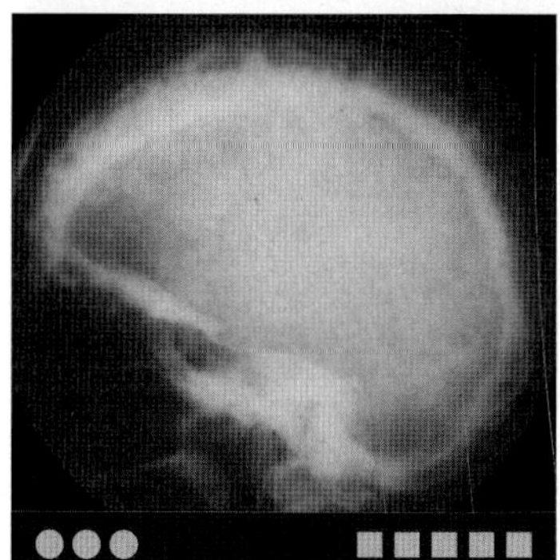

F. Paget disease of bone: Lateral radiograph of the skull in Paget disease (compare to image B) shows cortical thickening and increased density of the bony calvaria. After secondary hyperparathyroidism, Paget disease of bone would be the principal differential diagnosis. Note that the mandible is spared.

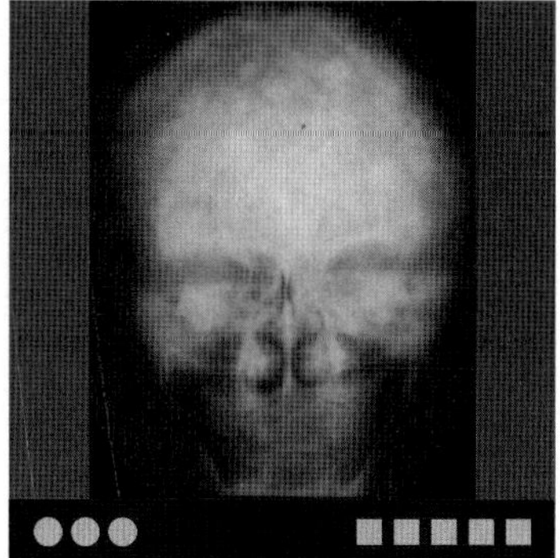

G. Paget disease of bone: AP skull radiograph in the same patient shows the mandible is spared.

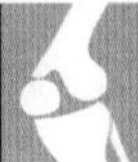

40–6 Gorham-Stout Disease/Lymphangiomatosis Cranium

Michelle Chandler

PRESENTATION

Pain, swelling, and breathlessness

FINDINGS

Radiograph of the skull shows innumerable lytic defects without sclerotic borders.

DIFFERENTIAL DIAGNOSES

- *Metastatic disease:* This would be difficult to distinguish from metastatic disease by imaging and clinical history would help to differentiate.
- *Histiocytosis X:* The patient may have constitutional symptoms and the osseous defects characteristically have a beveled edge in the cranium.

COMMENTS

This patient is a pediatric male who presented with lymphangiomatosis of multiple bones and soft tissue involvement of the mediastinum. The generalized term for this condition is angiomatosis, which is a benign process without a genetic mode of transmission and is characterized by abnormal vessels that contain lymph or blood within a fibrous background. Isolated skeletal involvement referred to as "Gorham-Stout disease," "vanishing bone disease," or "idiopathic massive osteolysis" is now better understood as part of a continuum or spectrum of disease that involves lymphangiomatosis predominating in the soft tissues or viscera to predominately bony involvement. The disease is of unknown etiology, but can follow major trauma and results in progressive osseous destruction by vascular and lymph malformations, and/or soft tissue involvement. The course of the disease is unpredictable and an osseous reparative response is notably absent. Treatment is palliative. Craniocervical involvement may be associated with neural compression or craniocervical instability leading to death. More characteristic in the pediatric or younger patient pulmonary visceral involvement or presence of a chylous effusion portends a poor prognosis often leading to death. Radiograph evaluation may initially demonstrate osteopenia with eventual development of ill-defined areas of lysis without an associated sclerotic border or periosteal reaction. Bone scan findings are complimentary to radiograph as not all lesions are demonstrated by either modality and lesions may be "hot" or "cold." Lymphoscintigraphy may show pooling of tracer in the lesions. MR imaging will demonstrate low signal on T1 and high signal on T2 with enhancement. Lesions appear cystic in the viscera.

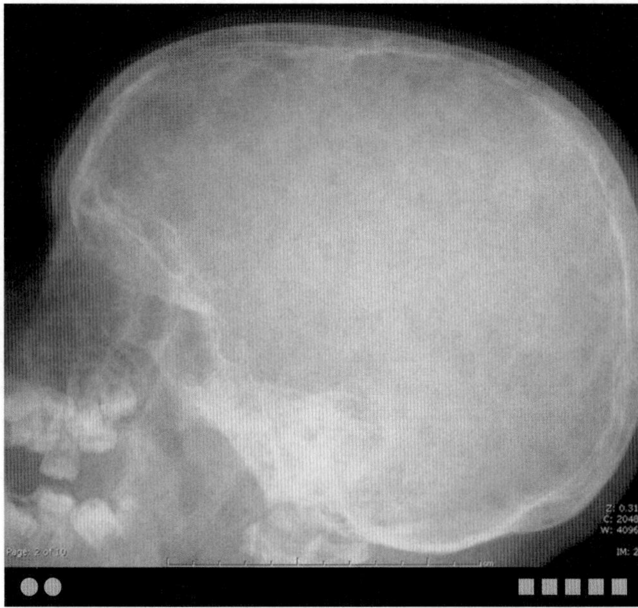

A. Gorham stout/lymphangiomatosis: Lateral radiograph evaluation of the skull shows numerous lytic defects without borders centered in the diploic space.

PEARLS

- **Multiple, lytic, and osseous lesions without associated periosteal reaction or sclerosis particularly in the region of the pelvis or shoulder should lead one to consider lymphangiomatous involvement.**
- **This condition is better described as part of a spectrum of lymphangiomatous involvement that may predominate in the skeleton, viscera, and soft tissues or both.**
- **Craniocervical lysis, pulmonary parenchymal involvement, and chylous effusion tend to be associated with the most serious complications including death.**

ADDITIONAL IMAGES

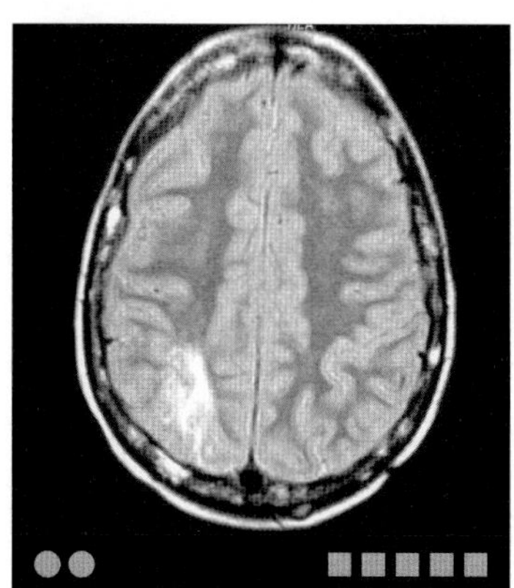

B. Gorham stout/lymphangiomatosis: Axial T2 MR image of the brain demonstrates homogeneous high signal in the cranium corresponding to the lytic defects demonstrated by radiography.

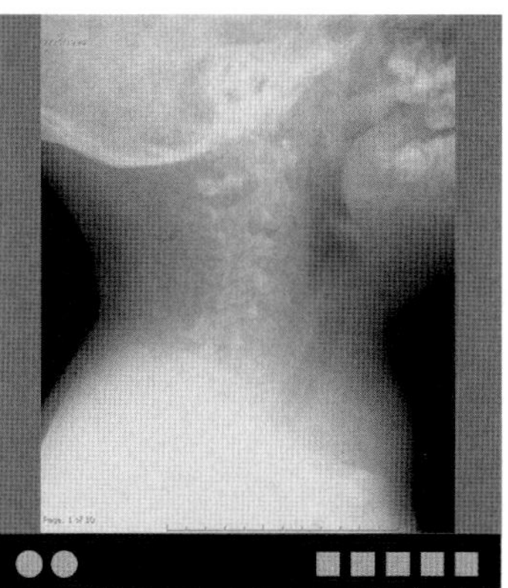

C. Gorham stout/lymphangiomatosis: Radiograph of the cervical spine demonstrates subtle diffused lysis of the cervical spine and an accompanying soft tissue lesion in the inferior anterior neck.

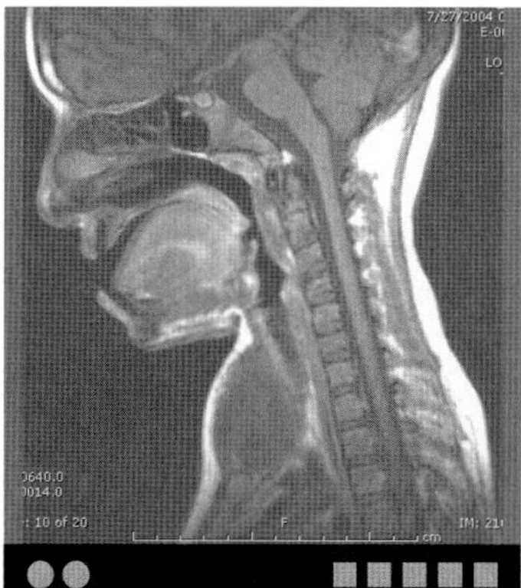

D. Gorham stout/lymphangiomatosis: Sagittal T1 MR image of the cervical spine demonstrates a heterogenous pattern of the bone marrow and a soft tissue mass in the anterior neck both representing lymphangiomatous involvement.

IMAGE KEY

Common

Rare

Typical

Unusual

DIFFERENTIAL DIAGNOSES IMAGES

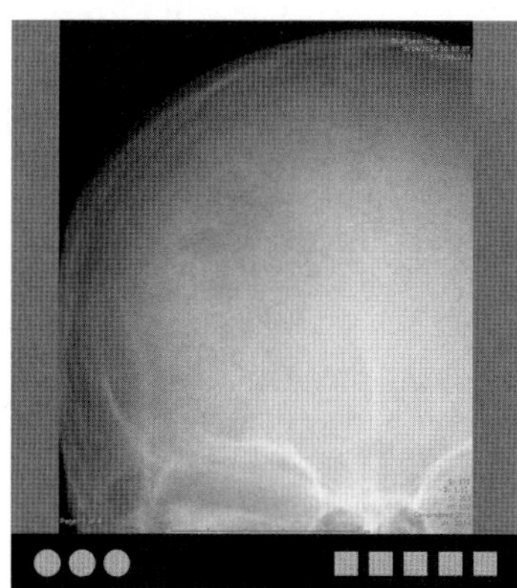

E. Histiocytosis X: Radiograph of the skull demonstrates a solitary, lytic lesion without defined borders in the right frontal region. This was associated with a palpable soft tissue mass and diagnosed as histiocytosis X the leading differential consideration.

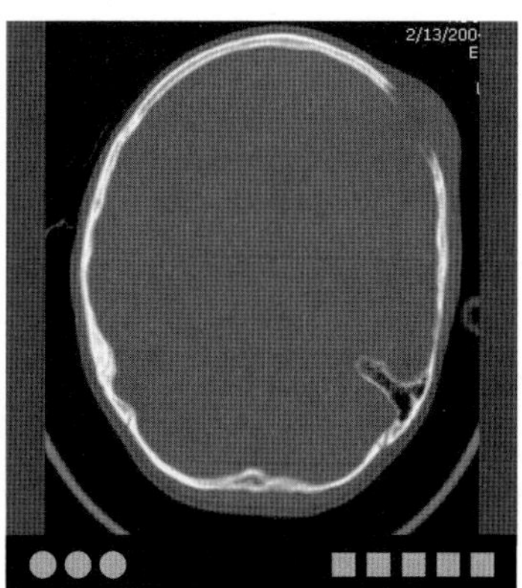

F. Histiocytosis X: Axial CT scan of the head in bone windows demonstrates the classic beveled edge commonly associated with histiocytosis X involvement of the cranium.

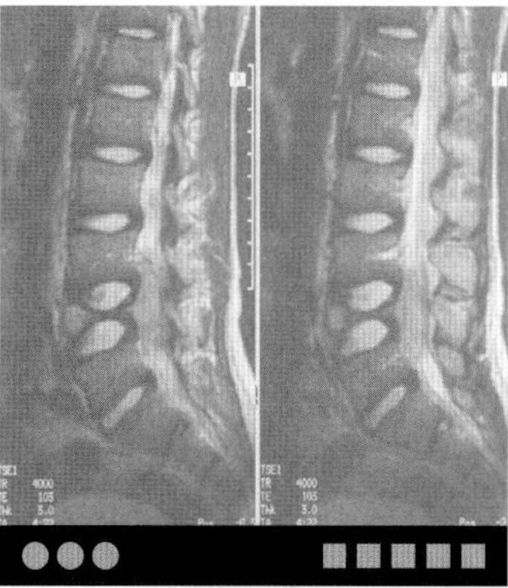

G. Histiocytosis: Sagittal T2 MR image of the lumbar spine in a patient with histiocytosis X demonstrates classic vertebra plana of L4.

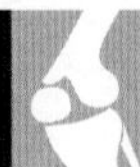

40–7 Hyperostosis Frontalis Interna

Ayodale S. Odulate and Piran Aliabadi

PRESENTATION

Headache

FINDINGS

Symmetrical thickening of the internal table of the frontal bones.

DIFFERENTIAL DIAGNOSES

- *Interosseous meningoma:* Sclerotic changes to the surrounding bones can be seen with meningiomata.
- *Sclerosing osteomyelitis:* Can present as sequelae of prior infection. This is likely to be asymmetric and originate from sinus disease.
- *Osteosclerotic metastases:* Discrete sclerotic foci scattered in a random pattern.
- *Paget's disease:* Thickening of the cortex, trabeculae, and bone enlargement. Bone scan uptake is variable depending on the stage of the disease; in the active stage there is uptake of radiotracer.

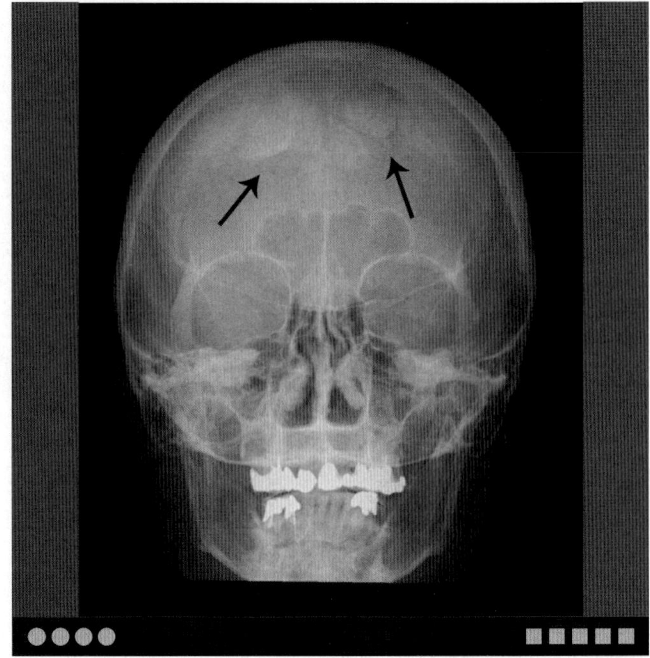

A. Hyperostosis frontalis interna: Frontal radiograph of the skull demonstrates nodular sclerosis in the calvarium (arrows).

COMMENTS

This is an image of a 58-year-old woman who presented with chronic headaches. Hyperostosis frontalis interna is a benign condition of the skull bones, primarily the frontal bones, and rarely involves the parietal bones. This benign entity is mostly seen in the postmenopausal patient population. Hyperostosis frontalis interna is often an incidental finding in asymptomatic patients. This entity has been described as part of a triad of findings that have been reported in patients with Morgagni-Stewart-Morel syndrome (*adipositas*, virilism and hirsutism are the other symptoms). An association of obesity and headache symptoms has been reported; however, no direct correlation has been proved. This finding should be differentiated from a neoplastic process. Metastases will often appear as random discrete foci of sclerosis or lytic lesions depending on the primary tumor. Paget's disease will have characteristic cortical thickening, trabecular thickening, and enlargement of the bone. Intraosseous meningioma can appear as diffuse sclerosis in the surrounding bone. Histologically, thickening of cancellous bone in the inner table is often symmetric; however, a nodular asymmetric appearance has been reported in case reports. Radiographs demonstrate symmetric thickening of the inner table of the frontal bones with preservation of the cortex. Imaging characteristics are similar by computed tomography, where one often finds lens-shaped thickening of the frontal bones. Radiopharmaceutical uptake on bone scintigraphy can be variable. A variant of hyperostosis frontalis is hyperostosis calvariae diffusa; distinguished by both inner and outer table thickening.

PEARLS

- **Symmetric lobulated thickening of the inner table of the frontal bones.**
- **Asymptomatic benign finding commonly seen in postmenopausal women.**
- **Found in patients with Morgagni-Stewart-Morel syndrome.**

ADDITIONAL IMAGES

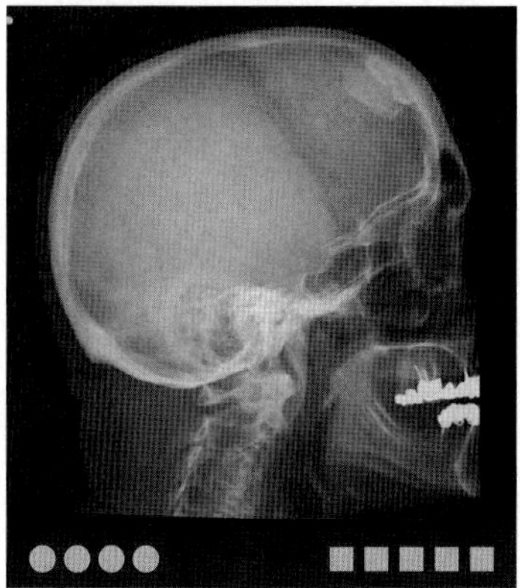

B. Hyperostosis frontalis interna: Lateral radiograph of the skull from the same patient shows a butterfly appearance of thickening of the frontal bones.

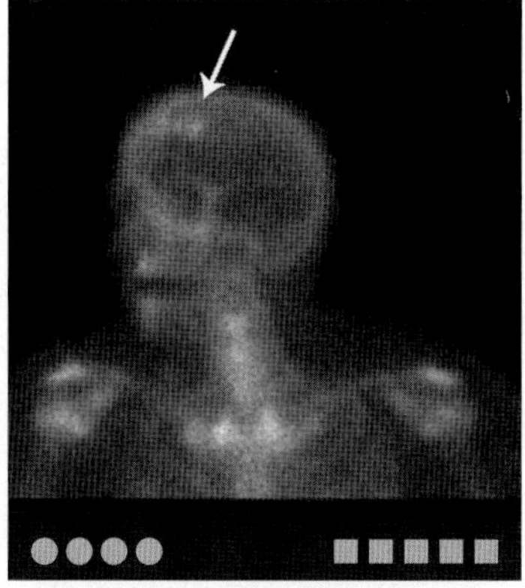

C. Hyperostosis frontalis interna: Bone scan from the same patient shows discrete foci of increased uptake in the region of the frontal bones that correspond to the plain film imaging.

DIFFERENTIAL DIAGNOSES IMAGES

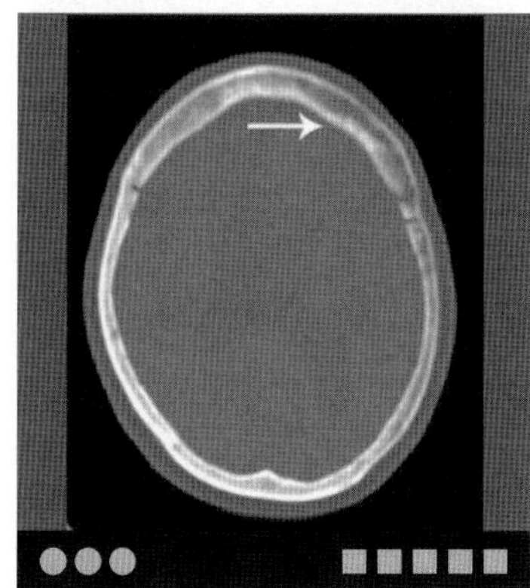

D. Paget's disease: Axial computed tomography image of the skull at the level of the frontal lobes demonstrates thickening of the cortex and trabeculae (arrow).

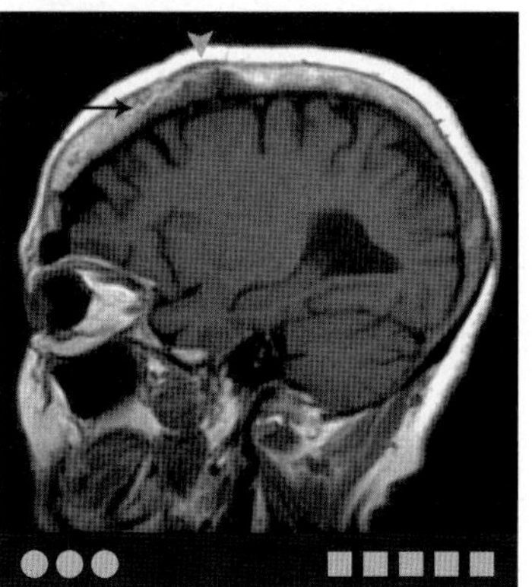

E. Paget's disease: Sagittal T1-weighted image from the same patient demonstrates enlargement of the frontal bone, cortical thickening (arrowhead), and coarsened trabeculae represented by hypointense foci (arrow).

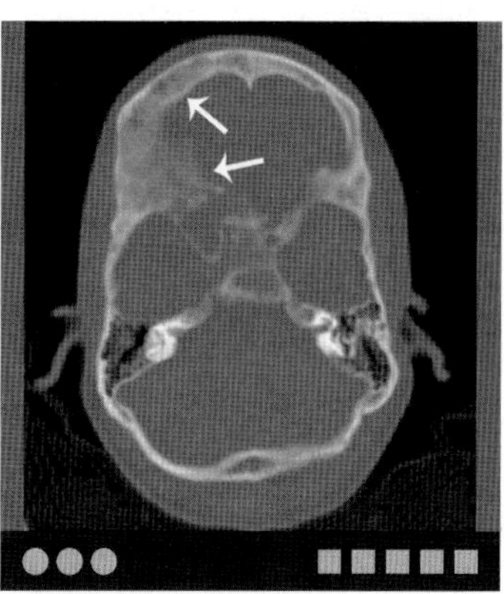

F. Fibrous dysplasia: Axial computed tomography shows the right frontal bone and greater wing of the sphenoid are expanded with a ground-glass matrix (arrow).

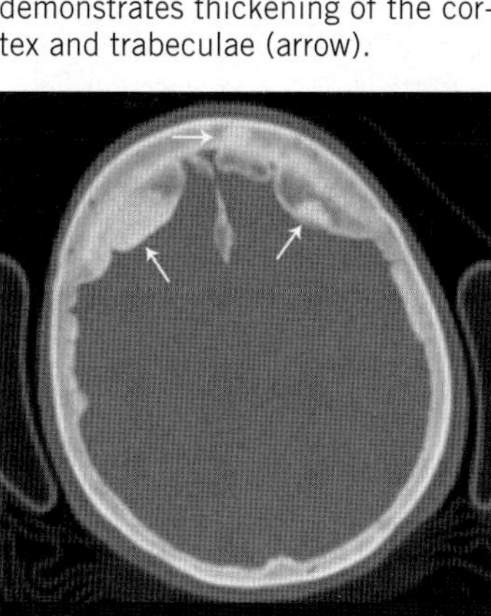

G. Osteoblastic metastases: Axial computed tomography shows discrete round foci of sclerosis (arrow) represent breast metastases in this patient with hyperostosis frontalis interna. Note the expansion of the inner table only.

IMAGE KEY

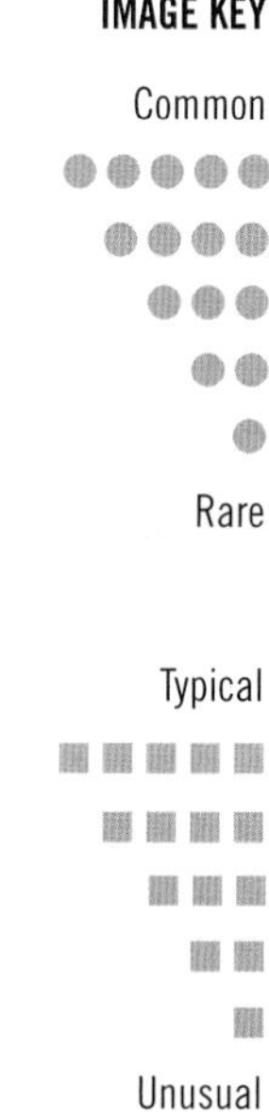

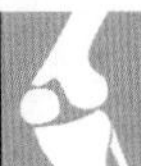

40–8 Costochondral Gout

Kambiz Motamedi

PRESENTATION

Anterior chest wall mass

FINDINGS

CT scan shows a mineralized mass arising from the first costochondral junction.

DIFFERENTIAL DIAGNOSES

- *Chondrosarcoma:* CT scan of chondrosarcoma may be very similar with a destructive mineralized mass.
- *Metastatic disease:* CT scan may reveal rib destruction and a soft tissue mass. The mass may be sclerotic or lytic depending on the primary disease.
- *Pancoast tumor:* Apical bronchogenic carcinoma may breakthrough the chest wall and cause rib destruction. A lung mass would be evident.
- *Healing rib fracture:* CT scan may reveal callus surrounding a rib fracture.

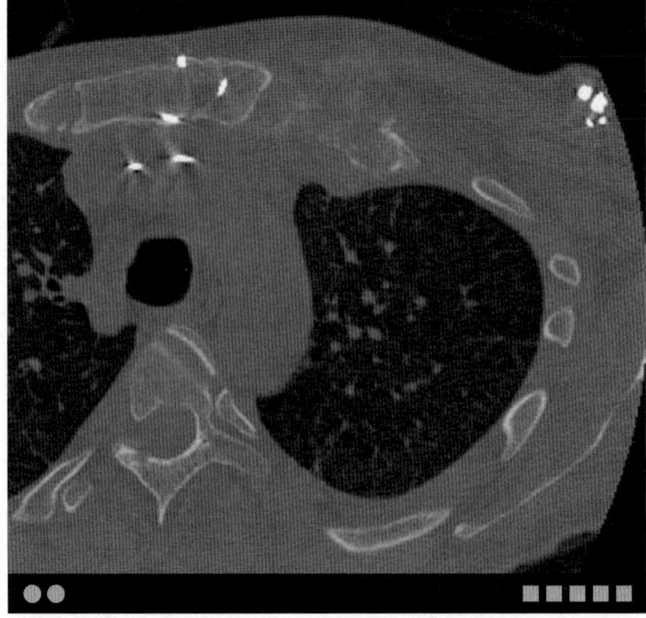

A. Gout: Axial CT scan (bone window) through the upper thorax reveals an ill-defined, large mass arising from the first costochondral junction. This mass has a mineralized matrix.

COMMENTS

This is an image of a 49-year-old male heart transplant recipient with a 10-year history of gout, who presented with a painful left first costochondral junction mass. CT scan shows a mineralized mass arising from the first costochondral junction. A CT-guided biopsy of the mass revealed foreign body giant cell reaction and crystalline deposition consistent with tophaceous gout. Gout is a common inflammatory disorder caused by hyperuricemia and deposition of urate crystals in and around joints and soft tissues. Gout primarily affects the peripheral skeleton and has two major stages of disease. Gouty arthritis results from acute inflammation secondary to urate crystal deposition within the joint. First metatarsophalangeal joint and intertarsal joints are mainly involved. Other common locations include the extensor surfaces such Achilles insertion site, olecranon, and quadriceps insertion on patella. Chronic tophaceous gout develops from established disease and is secondary to urate, protein matrix, and inflammatory cell deposition in cartilage, bone, tendon, and other soft tissues. Recent studies have demonstrated an increased incidence of gout in transplant recipients, especially in those patients who have undergone heart transplants. Noncontrast chest CT scan may demonstrate an irregular mass arising from the costochondral junction. It shows soft tissue density and adjacent rib destruction. There is no finding of pulmonary airspace disease. Chest radiography may reveal lung zone opacity, simulating pneumonia.

PEARLS

- **Gout is a common disease and with some chemotherapeutic, specifically cyclosporine, there is an increasing incidence.**
- **Tophaceous gout usually presents with a mineralized mass along with bone or cartilage destruction.**
- **Tophaceous gout may show a soft tissue mass and crystal deposition in any tissue, including cartilage, bone, tendon, and other soft tissues. This may not be in a joint.**

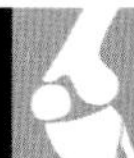

ADDITIONAL IMAGES

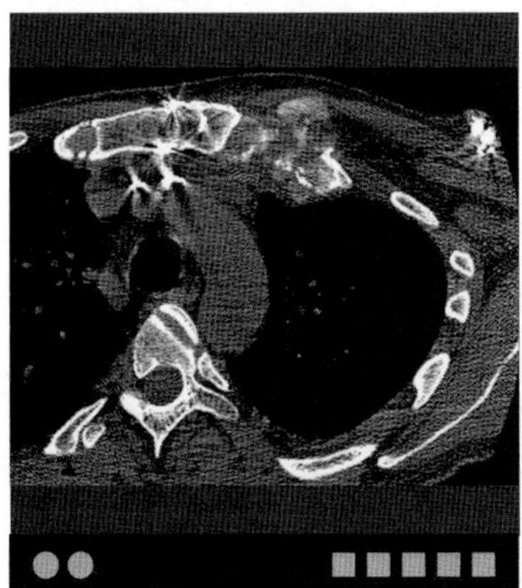

B. Gout: Axial CT scan (soft tissue window) readily demonstrates the mineralized matrix.

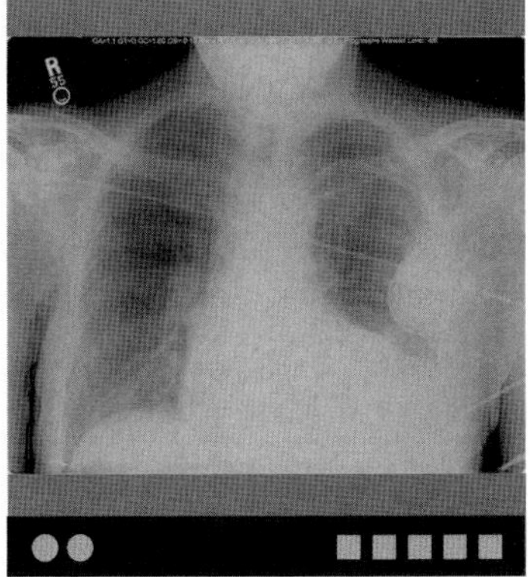

C. Gout: The AP chest radiograph shows an upper left lung opacity suggesting pneumonia.

DIFFERENTIAL DIAGNOSES IMAGES

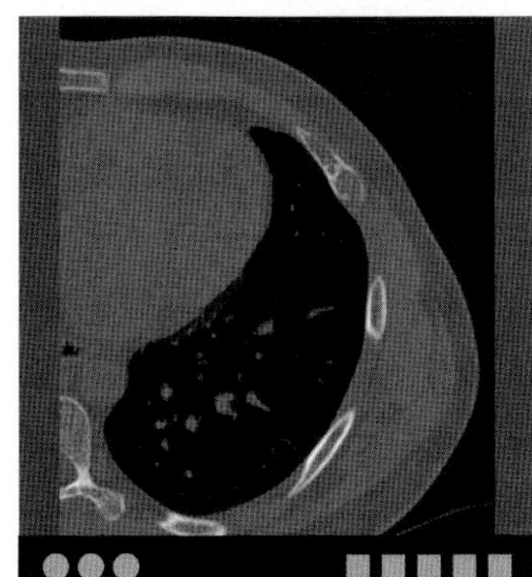

D. Chondroid lesion of the rib: CT scan shows a mineralized, expansile lesion of the rib.

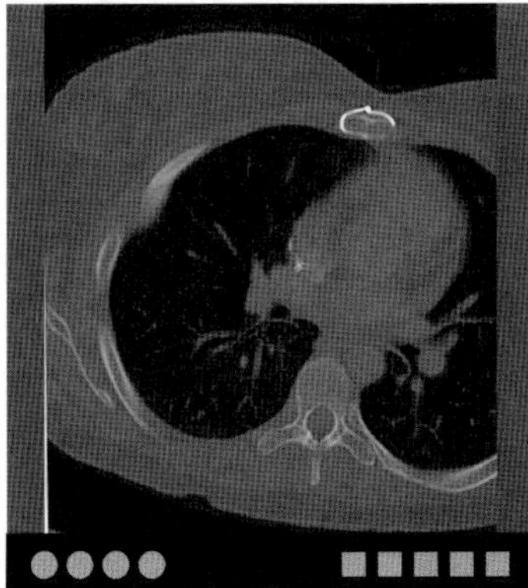

E. Metastatic rib lesion: The nonenhanced CT scan in bone window shows a sclerotic, mildly expansile of lateral aspect of a mid left rib known to be a metastatic focus of an adrenal primary.

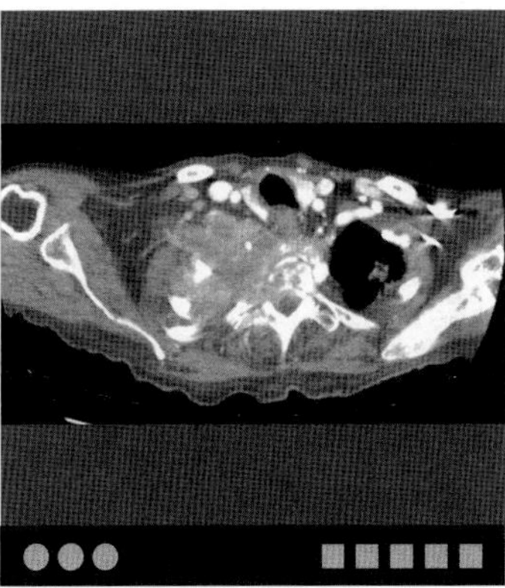

F. Pancoast tumor: CT scan shows a destructive lung mass extending to the apical chest wall.

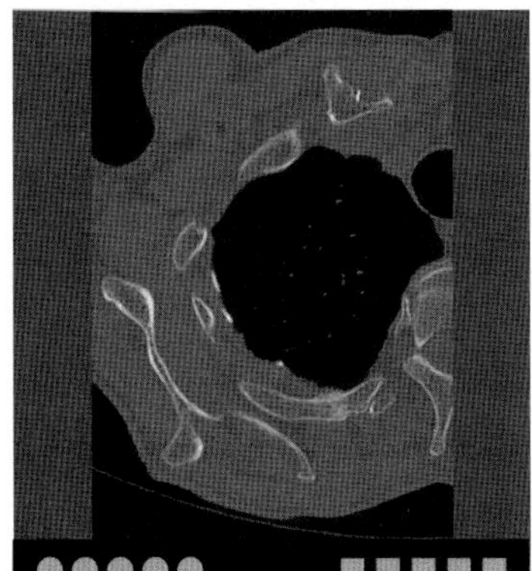

G. Rib fracture: CT scan reveals periosteal thickening and subtle callus formation of the posterior aspect of a lower left rib.

IMAGE KEY

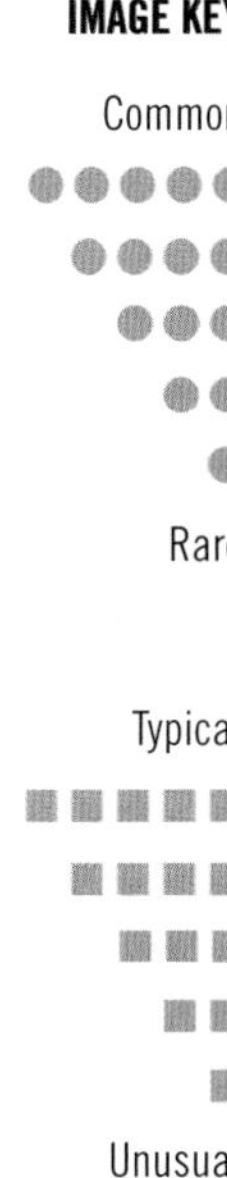

INDEX

Page number with *f* indicates figure

E

F

G

H

O

T

U

V

W

X

Y

Z